HUMAN BRAIN FUNCTION

SECOND EDITION

HUMAN BRAIN FUNCTION

SECOND EDITION

Editors

Richard S.J. Frackowiak, Karl J. Friston Christopher D. Frith, Raymond J. Dolan, Cathy J. Price, Semir Zeki, John Ashburner, William Penny

Functional Imaging Laboratory
Wellcome Department of Imaging Neuroscience
University College London
London, United Kingdom

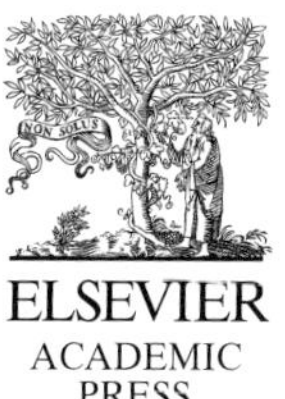

ELSEVIER
ACADEMIC
PRESS

Amsterdam Boston Heidelberg London New York Oxford
Paris San Diego San Francisco Singapore Sydney Tokyo

This book is printed on acid-free paper. ∞

Academic Press
An imprint of Elsevier Science
525 B Street, Suite 1900, San Diego, California 92101-4495, USA
http://www.academicpress.com

Academic Press
84 Theobald's Road, London WC1X 8RR, UK
http://www.academicpress.com

Library of Congress Catalog Card Number: 2003113436

International Standard Book Number: 0-12-264841-2

PRINTED IN CHILE
04 05 06 07 08 9 8 7 6 5 4 3 2 1

To our families and loved ones;
To our students, fellows, teachers, and collaborators;
And to the memory of Sir Henry Wellcome, philanthropist

Contents

PART ONE

IMAGING NEUROSCIENCE—BRAIN SYSTEMS

SECTION ONE

SENSORY, MOTOR AND PLASTICITY

SECTION TWO

VISION AND VISUAL PERCEPTION

SECTION THREE

HIGHER COGNITIVE FUNCTIONS

SECTION FOUR

EMOTION AND MEMORY

SECTION FIVE

LANGUAGE AND SEMANTICS

PART TWO

IMAGING NEUROSCIENCE—THEORY AND ANALYSIS

SECTION ONE
COMPUTATIONAL NEUROANATOMY

SECTION TWO
MODELLING

SECTION THREE
INFERENCE

SECTION FOUR
FUNCTIONAL INTEGRATION

Authors

INTRODUCTION R. S. J. Frackowiak

PART I

IMAGING NEUROSCIENCE—BRAIN SYSTEMS

SECTION ONE

SENSORY, MOTOR AND PLASTICITY
R. S. J. Frackowiak

1. R. E. Passingham, N. Ramnani, and J. B. Rowe
2. D. Corfield
3. A. Kleinschmidt
4. T. Griffiths and A. L. Giraud
5. D. McGonigle
6. N. Ward and R. S. J. Frackowiak
7. T. Good and R. S. J. Frackowiak
8. A. L. Giraud

SECTION TWO

VISION AND VISUAL PERCEPTION
S. Zeki

9. S. Zeki
10. S. Zeki
11. S. Zeki and K. Moutoussis
12. K. Moutoussis and S. Zeki
13. A. Bartels and S. Zeki
14. R. Perry

SECTION THREE

HIGHER COGNITIVE FUNCTIONS
C. Frith

15. C. Frith, G. Rees, E. Macaluso, and S. Blakemore
16. C. Portas, P. Maquet, G. Rees, S. Blakemore, and C. Frith
17. J. Coull and C. Thiele
18. C. Frith, H. Gallagher, and E. Maguire

SECTION FOUR

EMOTION AND MEMORY
R. Dolan

19. J. Morris and R. Dolan
20. H. Critchley and R. Dolan
21. P. Vuilleumier, J. L. Armony, and R. J. Dolan
22. R. Elliott
23. R. N. A. Henson
24. R. N. A. Henson
25. P. Fletcher and R. N. A. Henson

SECTION FIVE

LANGUAGE AND SEMANTICS
C. Price

26. C. Price
27. U. Noppeney
28. C. Price
29. E. McCrory
30. A. Mechelli

PART TWO

IMAGING NEUROSCIENCE—THEORY AND ANALYSIS

31. K. Friston

SECTION ONE

COMPUTATIONAL NEUROANATOMY

J. Ashburner

32. J. Ashburner and K. Friston
33. J. Ashburner and K. Friston
34. J. Ashburner and K. Friston
35. J. Ashburner and K. Friston
36. J. Ashburner and K. Friston

SECTION TWO

MODELLING

W. Penny

37. S. Kiebel and A. Holmes
38. J. B. Poline, F. Kherif, and W. Penny
39. D. Glaser and K. Friston
40. R. Henson
41. D. Glaser, K. Friston, A. Mechelli, R. Turner, and C. Price
42. W. Penny and A. Holmes
43. W. Penny and K. Friston

SECTION THREE

INFERENCE

W. Penny

44. M. Brett, W. Penny, and S. Kiebel
45. K. Worsley
46. T. Nichols and A. Holmes
47. K. Friston and W. Penny

SECTION FOUR

FUNCTIONAL INTEGRATION

K. Friston

48. K. Friston
49. K. Friston and C. Büchel
50. L. Harrison and K. Friston

51. K. Friston
52. K. Friston
53. K. Friston

POSTSCRIPT A. Roepstorff

INTRODUCTION

It is almost a decade since the first edition of *Human Brain Function* was conceived and planned. It was a unique book in that it tried to set out the thoughts and achievements of a school, or more accurately a laboratory working in the field of functional and structural human neuroanatomy. Historically, it marked the border between the application of tracer-based methods to brain imaging, exemplified by the PET technique of local blood flow mapping, and the blood oxygen level dependent (BOLD) technique based on magnetic resonance imaging (fMRI). The concept of a 'group' book was comparatively unusual in the biosciences where the tradition of the solitary scientist (often assisted by 'juniors') was still the dominant ethos. The evolution of human brain mapping depended on much diverse expertise from mathematics and statistics, through physics and biology to neurology, neuropsychiatry, and neuropsychology. The realisation of this dependence on the expertise of many individuals from many disciplines motivated the principal investigators to create a laboratory environment that was collegiate, interactive, collaborative, and also amicable. That laboratory emerged from the Medical Research Council's Cyclotron Unit and was incarnated in the then nascent Wellcome Trust funded Functional Imaging Laboratory, known as The FIL. The first edition marked the emigration of that group from the MRC CU to the FIL and represented the beginning of a new enterprise focussed on understanding the functional and structural architecture of the human brain and methodological developments that supported the achievement of that mission. The beginnings of statistical parametric mapping (SPM) were already described, but the advances made possible by fMRI did not make it into the first edition.

This second edition, like the previous one, is written exclusively by members of the FIL, past and present and long-term collaborators. The chapters are knit together like a book rather than a series of reviews. In that sense the book remains a 'personal' reflection on the state of our knowledge of how human thinking, feeling, and action are instantiated in the brain. However, the methodological advances of the last 6 years that include event-related fMRI, massive improvements in image acquisition and pre-processing and an escape from the relative constraints of classical inference are huge. These combined with a courageous, sometimes foolhardy wish to attack interesting problems that include consciousness, free will, and feelings make it possible that the book is becoming perhaps too big for its boots. We think this may be the last time we can put together theory and application in a single volume, even though they would be focussed by a common mission.

The book is now organised in sections, edited by each of The FIL's Principal Investigators who have promoted their component of the common programme. The theory and analysis section edited by Karl Friston, abetted by John Ashburner and Will Penny, is entirely up to date and gives readers an approachable and yet professional overview of all that is possible with modern imaging of brain structure and function. The adoption of a common analytic approach internationally, though sometimes in different guises, means that this section contains contributions from 'honorary' FIL members who have worked with Karl in the context of developing and supporting SPM. Chris Frith tackles the roles of the frontal lobes including mechanisms for attention and control of action and the relevance of these mechanisms to understanding the neural correlates of consciousness. Cathy Price continues her revision of the psychological theories of the organisation of human language by marshalling more and more experimental evidence that challenges older theories based purely on behavioural observation. Ray Dolan explores the difficult areas of feeling, emotion, and their interaction with memory and cognition and provides many new insights that complement the explosion in knowledge in this area that has occurred in animal and basic biology. Semir Zeki explores the visual world that has become his unique domain and extends our understanding of why it constitutes such a paradigmatic sensation in the history of neuroscience. He approaches the problems with his usual panache and delight in intellectual exploration through controversy. I deal with action and sensation with an ever-vigilant eye on implications for recovery of function and mechanisms underlying this phenomenon. I am abetted in this work by Dick Passingham whose contributions have been massive.

What of the future, for which this volume will act as our springboard? The integration of temporally resolved methods such as EEG and MEG, spontaneous or evoked, is a big challenge. It is a challenge that has received a major boost from experiments by others that have elucidated the physiological correlates of the BOLD signal and the relationship between changes in each. Mapping one type of signal onto the anatomy of the other is trivial compared to relating the biological basis of each into a common framework. A common framework should result in inferences that lead to new predictions and experiments which focus on distributions of brain activity and their correlation in time. The second area where we foresee great advances is in the application of the knowledge obtained in over a decade of experimentation in normal humans to the diseased condition. An understanding of the principles of normal functional organisation and an elaboration of experimental approaches and principled, reproducible methods of data now make this task feasible. The questions to be asked are unlikely to be primarily diagnostic but will generate ideas and facts about disease mechanisms as well as information about how these can be altered by therapy. The possibility of assessing drug effects on small well-defined groups of patients instead of by costly large population studies that last years will have to be explored. The idea that the genetic understanding of brain disease will be aided by a description of correlated changes in the working of brain systems and associated with the identification of abnormal proteins or their absence might be dismissed as a flight of fantasy except for the fact that preliminary data suggest otherwise. In brain diseases of ageing or neurodegenerations it is entirely possible that proteomic data will most readily be interpreted by a mixture of physiological data obtained via human imaging neuroscience and behavioural correlation.

We hope that the reader will forgive the hubris that underlies the decision to produce this volume. This scientific field has excited us so much that we see no reason to hide our enthusiasm to communicate it. However, it should not be thought that we do not recognise the enormous contribution of many others worldwide to this science. Without that, much that is recorded in this book would not have been possible. The field is now so huge that one volume cannot hope to cover it completely. There is much missing in these pages that will be found elsewhere; some of it in the first edition. There is much that in the time required for printing and publication will already be out of date. However, when a field is expanding fast, a book should try to convey the process of acquisition of knowledge as much as content. In the internet-based information age, it is perhaps that function which a book can fulfill in a way that papers themselves, read individually cannot. So, we hope the reader will share our excitement when reading this volume; that the reader will be stimulated at times and at others perplexed. We will even consider it a success if the book irritates the reader or causes reflection that leads to new experiments that refute (or support) the claims and speculations based on our work recorded within.

It remains for me to thank, on behalf of all my colleagues, the Wellcome Trust for its munificence. Without the decision to fund the FIL in 1994 and to renew funding in 1999 very little of the work contained in this volume would have been possible.

Richard S. J. Frackowiak
London
September 2003

PART ONE

IMAGING NEUROSCIENCE—BRAIN SYSTEMS

SECTION ONE

SENSORY, MOTOR AND PLASTICITY

CHAPTER

1

The Motor System

MOTOR AREAS

Just as there are a host of *visual areas*—defined loosely as areas with visual inputs (Felleman and van Essen, 1990)—so are there many *motor areas* — defined loosely as regions with projections to the premotor and motor areas. Thus. the term *motor system* will be used in this chapter to include parietal and prefrontal cortex, as well as the premotor and motor areas. All are involved in the selection, guidance or execution of action.

One advantage of studying the motor system is that, as for the visual system (see Section 2, Vision and Visual Perception), the anatomy and physiology are well worked out in non-human primates. We can identify the different motor and premotor areas in the macaque monkey using cytoarchitectonics (Brodmann, 1909; von Bonin and Bailey, 1947) and receptor architectonics (Zilles *et al.*, 1996). The anatomical connections between the different areas are well described, and an exhaustive database of these, CoCoMac, is available (Stephan *et al.*, 2001; http://www.cocomac.org). There are also many studies in which single units have been recorded, and comparisons are available between recordings taken in different areas (*e.g.*, Crutcher and Alexander, 1990; Muskiake *et al.*, 1991; Matsuzaka and Tanji, 1996; Nakamura *et al.*, 1998; Shima and Tanji, 2000). Thus, the motor system provides an excellent case study of how the findings of imaging experiments can be grounded in anatomy and physiology.

ANATOMY

The anatomical basis of functional localisation is the unique set of inputs and outputs for each cytoarchitectonic area. Passingham *et al.* (2002) have suggested the term *connectional fingerprint* for this set. Young (1993) has shown that each area has a unique set of inputs and outputs. The most stringent test is to compare the set of connections for regions within a single functional area. Passingham *et al.* (2002) have formally done this for the subregions of prefrontal cortex. The connections are plotted as *fingerprints*. This term was used by Zilles and colleagues (Geyer *et al.*, 1998) to describe the particular pattern of receptor–architecture for each cortical region as demonstrated by the degree of binding for the different receptor types. They plotted the binding in a radial plot. Figure 1.1 shows connectional fingerprints in the form of radial plots for the inputs and outputs of two prefrontal areas, 9 and 14. The data are taken from CoCoMac (Stephan *et al.*, 2001). Figure 1.2 uses multidimensional scaling to plot the data for all prefrontal regions in two dimensions. If any pair of areas shared the same set of connections, they would also share the identical location, but it can be seen from Fig. 1.2 that this is not true for any of these areas.

We have very little direct information, other than from silver studies (Di Virgilio and Clarke, 1997), about the connections of the human brain (Crick and Jones, 1993). It is not yet clear to what extent diffusion-weighted imaging (Conturo *et al.*, 1999; Poupon *et al.*, 2000; Parker *et al.*,

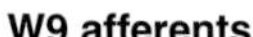

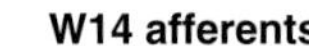

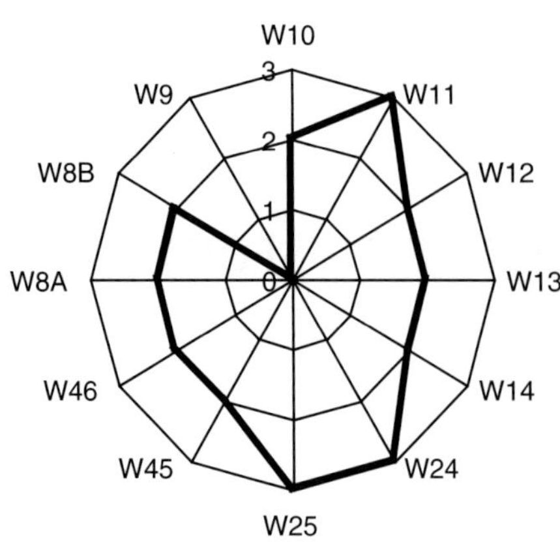

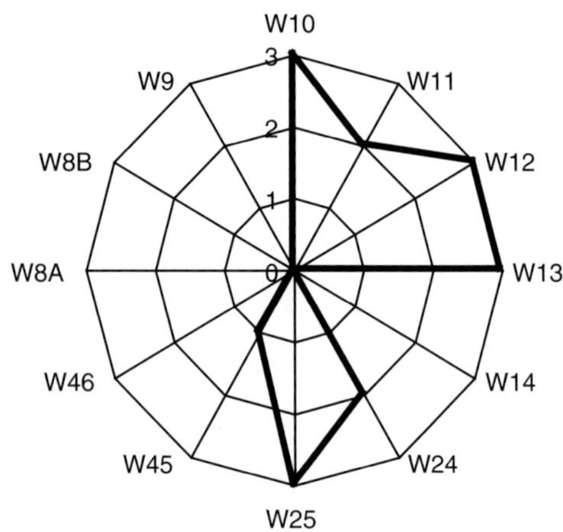

W9 efferents

W14 efferents

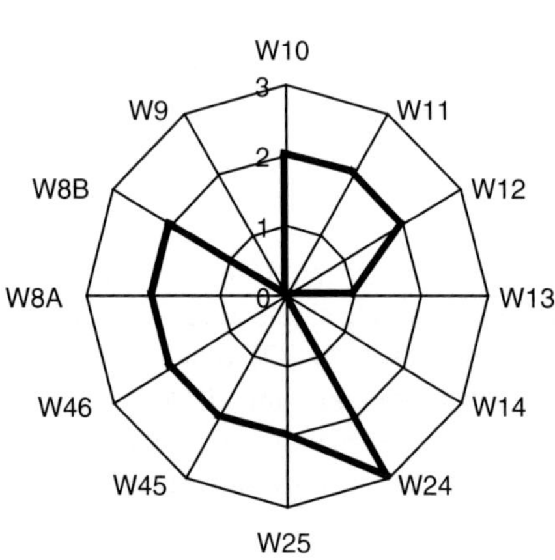

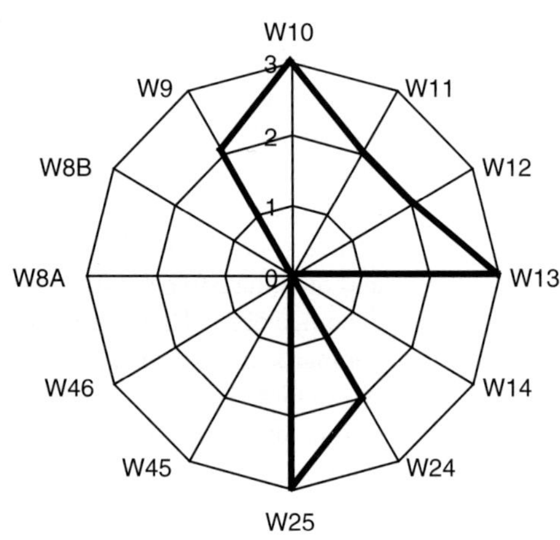

FIGURE 1.1
Diagram of anatomical fingerprints for two prefrontal areas, Walker's areas 9 and 14. The upper row shows the afferent and the lower row the efferent connections of the two areas, with 12 other prefrontal areas identified by their cytoarchitectonic numbers as designated by Walker (1940). The strength of any connection (rated as weak = 1, medium = 2, strong = 3) is shown by the radial distance. (From Passingham *et al.*, (2002). Nature Publishing Group. With permission.)

2002) will be able to discriminate among the fine details of anatomical connections as shown by transport methods. Though it has been used to chart the course of the pyramidal tract in the macaque and human brain (Parker *et al.*, 2002), the technique has yet to be tried for other connections in the motor system. For the moment, the information on connections comes from studies on non-human primates.

The only way to access this information for human imaging studies is the mapping of activations to specific cytoarchitectonic areas. The connections between areas in the macaque brain are identified by infusing tracers into discrete cytoarchitectonic areas (Young *et al.*, 1993; Stephan *et al.*, 2001), and homologies are assumed between areas in the macaque and human brain that have the same cytoarchitectonic characteristics. Since the last edition of the book, advances have been made in producing probability maps for some of the areas within the motor system. This has been done for the primary somatosensory cortex (Geyer *et al.*, 2000), area 6 (Geyer *et al.*, 2001), area 44 (Tomaiulo *et al.*, 1999), and the lateral prefrontal cortex (Rajkowska

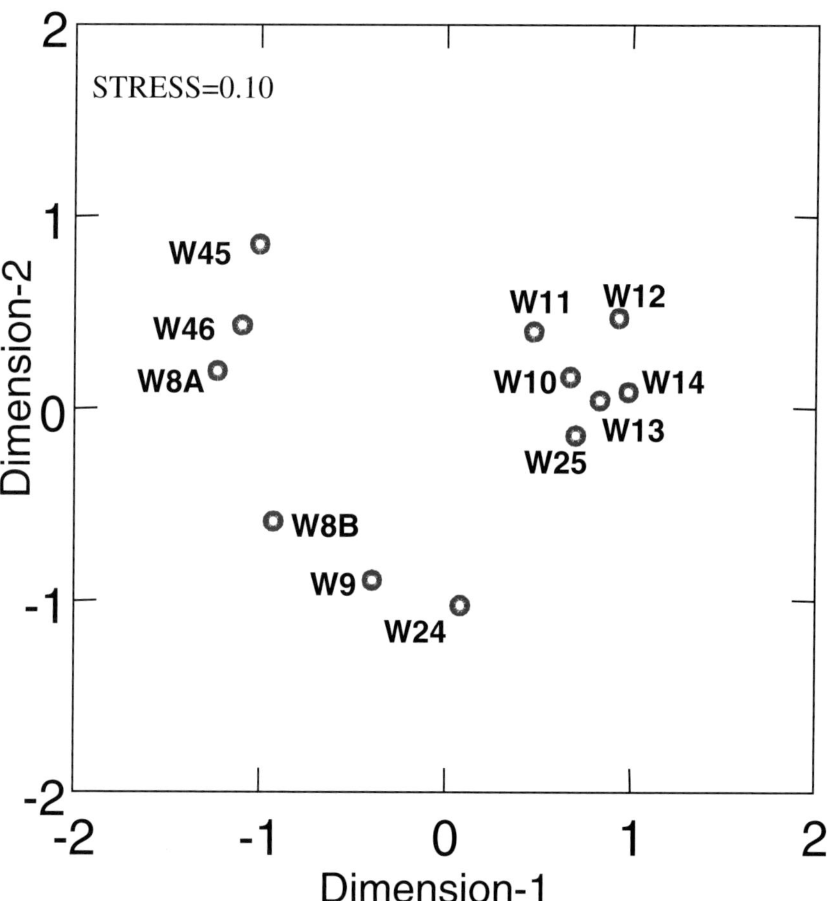

FIGURE 1.2
Multidimensional scaling (MDS) showing two-dimensional space in which prefrontal areas are plotted according to their anatomical connections. MDS gives a high-dimensional metric representation in which distances between elements optimally reflect the overall similarity between their properties—in this case, the connections between the areas. (From Passingham *et al.*, (2002). Nature Publishing Group. With permission.)

and Goldman-Rakic, 1995). Probability maps are also available for sulci within the motor system cortex (Paus *et al.*, 1996; Le Goualher *et al.*, 1999; Chiavaras and Petrides, 2000). The variation in cytoarchitectural boundaries has also been demonstrated for the motor cortex (Roland and Zilles, 1994) and Broca's area (Amunts *et al.*, 1999).

PHYSIOLOGY

Functional specialisation can be studied by comparing the proportions of cells that fire in association with a particular task or component of a task. For example, Mushiake *et al.* (1991) trained monkeys on two sequence tasks: in one task, visual cues specified the sequence, and in the other the animals performed from memory and without visual cues. Figure 1.3 shows that cells in motor cortex fired equally on both tasks (category 4). Many cells in the supplementary motor area (SMA) and premotor cortex also fired equally on both tasks (category 4). However, in the SMA, there was an overall tendency for cells to fire only (category 7) or preferentially (categories 5 and 6) in association with movements performed from memory. By contrast, in the premotor cortex there was an overall tendency for cells to fire only (category 1) or preferentially (categories 2 and 3) in association with movements specified by external cues. Thus, these two areas differ in the activity of the populations of cells as a whole. The difference can be explained in part by the fact that there are projections to the premotor cortex from visually receiving areas of the parietal cortex such as the medial intraparietal cortex (MIP) and anterior intraparietal cortex (AIP) (Rizzolatti *et al.*, 1998).

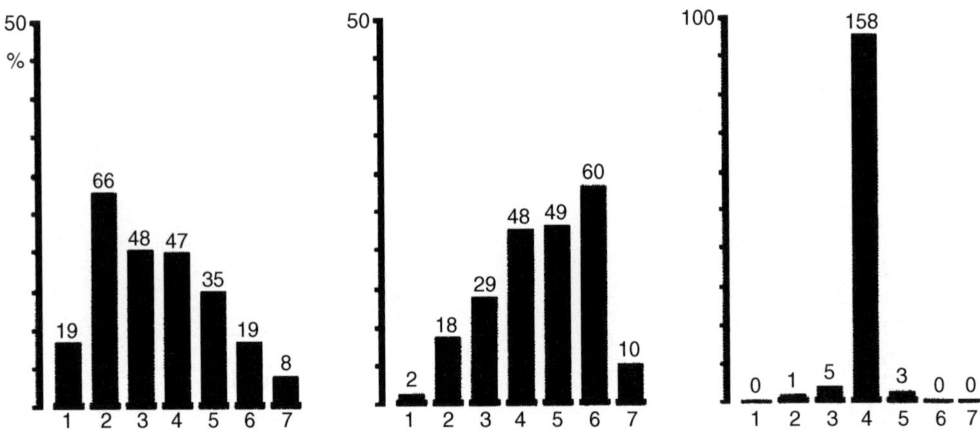

FIGURE 1.3
Distribution of cells in lateral premotor cortex (PMv), SMA, and motor cortex (MI) classified according to the degree to which they were active in association with the visually guided sequence (VS) or the sequence performed from memory (MS). 1 = exclusively related to VS, 2 = predominantly related to VS, 3 = more related to VS than MS, 4 = equally related to VS and MS, 5 = more related to MS, 6 = predominantly related to MS, and 7 = exclusively related to MS. The ordinate shows the percentage of cells and the numbers above the histograms show the number of cells. (Data from Mushiake *et al.*, (1991). American Physiology Society. With permission.)

It is the proportional differences in cell activity within the population that allow imaging studies to reveal differences between areas. For example, more cells in the SMA than in the motor cortex fire in advance of movement (Okano and Tanji, 1987; Tanji and Shima, 1994), and it has been shown using functional magnetic resonance imaging (fMRI) that there is more activity in the SMA than in motor cortex during preparation for movement (Richter *et al.*, 1997). More cells in the pre-SMA than in the SMA increase their firing rate during the learning of new motor sequences (Nakamura *et al.*, 1998) or change between movements (Matsuzaka and Tanji, 1996), and imaging studies have shown that there is more activity in the pre-SMA than in the SMA when subjects learn new sequences (Hikosaka *et al.*,1996) or vary the time at which they respond (Deiber *et al.*, 1999). Finally, more cells in the premotor cortex than in the SMA fire when movements are externally specified, whereas more cells in the SMA fire when sequences are performed from memory (Muskiake *et al.*, 1991; Halsband *et al.*, 1994). Correspondingly, imaging studies have shown more activity in the premotor cortex than in the SMA early in sequence learning when the subjects are dependent on feedback cues, but more activity in the SMA than in premotor cortex when the task is automated and performed from memory (Jenkins *et al.*, 1994; Toni *et al.*, 1998).

The high temporal resolution of single unit recording means that one can also study cell firing at different times during a task. For example, Weinrich *et al.* (1984) have recorded single units in the dorsal premotor cortex while monkeys perform a delayed visuomotor task. The authors report that 47% of the cells fired at the time of presentation of the cue, 34% during the delay period, and 65% at the time of response. Event-related fMRI have also made it possible to associate activations with particular event *within* a trial. Thus, Toni *et al.*, (Passingham and Toni, 2001) were able to demonstrate that in the human brain there are activations in premotor cortex at the time of the instruction cue and at the time of the response, and that there is set activity during the delay (Toni *et al.*, 1999, submitted) (Fig. 1.4).

Functional MRI has also been used to distinguish prefrontal activity related to the maintenance of information in memory from the activity at the time of retrieval (D'Esposito *et al.*, 1999; Rowe *et al.*, 2000; Rowe and Passingham, 2001). Again, the results can be related to single-unit experiments on monkeys. For example, several studies have reported activity in prefrontal area 8 while subjects remember spatial locations (Belger *et al.*, 1998; Courtney *et al.*, 1998; Rowe *et al.*, 2000; Rowe and Passingham, in press). Correspondingly, activity has been recorded in area 8A during the delay period in monkeys performing a spatial memory task (Chafee and Goldman-Rakic, 1999; Sawaguchi *et al.*, 1999).

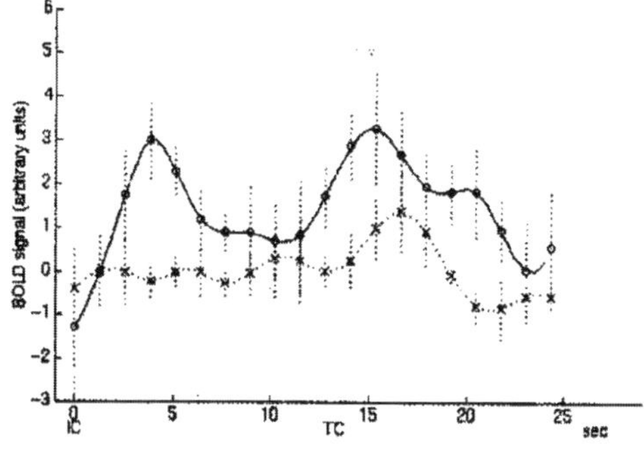

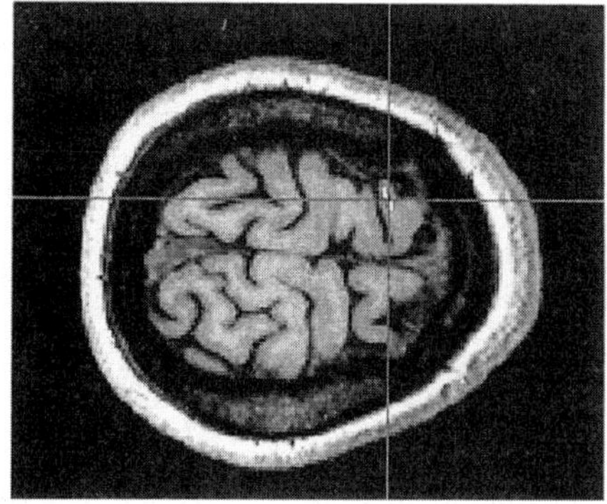

FIGURE 1.4
Activation in dorsal premotor cortex (see MRI) during a visuomotor association task. In this area, the BOLD signal shows a response associated with the presentation of the instruction cue (IC) and another with presentation of the trigger cue (TC). There is also set activity during the delay period. For comparison, the dotted line shows the signal for motor cortex where there is only a response associated with the trigger cue. (Data from Toni *et al.*, (1999). Oxford University Press. With permssion.)

The *mechanisms* by which single areas operate, however, are only accessible to single-unit and multi-unit physiology. For example, in a human imaging study, it was found that the population signal from the premotor cortex is the same whether the subject is preparing to move a lever to the left or right. It is necessary to record cells at once to show that there are cells in this area that fire differentially according to the spatial target of the action (Weinrich and Wise, 1984; Shen *et al.*, 1997). Furthermore, with unit recording one can show a shift in the *vector* of the population response as learning proceeds (Chen and Wise, 1997; Wise and Murray, 2000); this vector represents the net directional signal of the population of cells where the cells have *votes* (Georgopoulos *et al.*, 1988). The BOLD (blood-oxygen-level-dependent) signal also reflects the population response; however, it has an amplitude but no direction. Understanding the motor system, as with other systems, requires a combination of methods available to neuroscience. The following sections show that imaging makes a major contribution to this enterprise.

This section is not an exhaustive review of imaging studies on the motor system Instead, it considers three topics that we believe to be of fundamental importance. The first is how visual information can influence action, the second is how actions are selected when there are no external cues at the time of selection, and the last is how novel actions are learned until they become automatic with practice.

VISUAL GUIDANCE OF ACTION

Visual Guidance of Movement

The brain converts light and sound into muscle activity. In the case of vision, we think that we know the pathways by which it does this. The first stage involves projections from striate cortex to the inferior parietal cortex via prestriate areas (Ungerleider and Desimone, 1986; Young, 1992). There are then connections from the anterior intraparietal cortex (AIP) to the ventral premotor cortex (PMv) (Matelli *et al.*, 1986; Tanne *et al.*, 1995; Johnson *et al.*, 1996) and from the intraparietal area MIP to the dorsal premotor cortex (PMd) (Matelli *et al.*, 1998; Marconi *et al.*, 2001). The final link is from these premotor areas to the motor cortex (Strick, 1985).

These dorsal paths can be distinguished from the ventral visual paths running to the temporal lobe (Ungerleider and Desimone, 1986; Young, 1992, 1993). Ungerleider and Mishkin (1982) proposed that information about form was processed exclusively in the ventral stream, but there is now evidence that cells in the parietal area LIP (dorsal system) are sensitive to information about form (Sereno and Maunsell, 1998; Toth and Asaad, 1999; Murata *et al.*, 2000). Milner and Goodale (1997) have therefore proposed that the dorsal system differs from the ventral system in the use to which this information is put, suggesting that the dorsal system uses information about shape to guide action. Both recording and lesion studies implicate these pathways in the pre-shaping of the hand and wrist in preparation for grasping (Jeannerod *et al.*, 1995; Murata *et al.*, 1997, 2000; Sakata *et al.*, 1997; Fogassi *et al.*, 2001).

When human subjects reach for and grasp objects, there is activation in an anterior parietal area in the region in which the intraparietal sulcus touches the postcentral sulcus (Faillenot *et al.*, 1997; Passingham *et al.*, 1998). This area is also activated when subjects manipulate objects (Binkofski *et al.*, 1999), and it is a candidate for the human homologue of the macaque AIP. When subjects reach for and grasp objects, activation is also observed in the ventral premotor cortex (Passingham *et al.*, 1998).

Activity is also detected in the parietal cortex when subjects reach for targets (Grafton *et al.*, 1992). If subjects are scanned when they learn to adapt their reaching movements while wearing laterally distorting prisms, the activity lies deep in the intraparietal sulcus in an area that has been identified as PEG (Clower *et al.*, 1996). Reaching is also associated with activation in the dorsal premotor cortex (Grafton *et al.*, 1998). The greater the precision of aiming required, the greater the activation (Winstein *et al.*, 1997).

In macaque monkeys, there are also cells that fire when the animal observes a person grasping an object. These "mirror neurons" (Gallese and Goldman, 1998) have been found in the anterior inferior parietal cortex (area 7b) (Fogassi *et al.*, 1998) and the inferior premotor area F5 (Gallese *et al.*, 1996). Several groups have imaged subjects while they watch videos of people performing simple actions: in some studies the subjects are simply required to observe (Decety *et al.*, 1997; Decety and Grezes, 1999; Grezes *et al.*, 1999; Buccino *et al.*, 2001) and in others to imitate the actions (Decety *et al.*, 1997; Grezes *et al.*, 1999; Iacaboni *et al.*, 1999). The aim of these studies has been to identify the location of mirror neurons in the human brain. Activation has been reported for observation of movements in the inferior parietal cortex (Buccino *et al.*, 2001; Grezes and Decety, 2001) and dorsal premotor cortex (Buccino *et al.*, 2001). It could be argued that these activations might simply represent the perception of movements, but Buccino *et al.* (2001) have shown that the parietal and premotor activations are somatotopically mapped; that is, the peaks differ according to whether the subject observes hand, mouth, or leg movements. This shows that they are associated with the perception of actions.

Activation has also been reported in the inferior frontal gyrus (area 44) when subjects imitate finger movements (Iacaboni *et al.*, 1999), prepare finger movements (Rushworth *et al.*, 2001), or imagine that they are watching their own actions (Binofski *et al.*, 2000). This region is the classical Broca's area. It could be argued that this area is activated because the subjects code the movements verbally. However, in the study by Iacaboni *et al.* (1999), the area was more active in the imitation condition than in other conditions, yet all involved the same finger movements and if the subjects verbalised the responses they would have done so in all cases. Rizzolatti and Arbib (1998) have argued that area 44 in the human brain may be the homologue of the ventral premotor area F5 in the brain of the macaque monkey. They further suggest that the human speech system might have evolved from a system for recognising hand and facial gestures.

Arbitrary Visuomotor Associations

The system for reaching and grasping can function without the subject paying attention to the movements. The movements area performed on line and with a short time constant (Milner, 1997). It has also been shown that the parietal/premotor system for grasping can operate without the subject being able to identify the shapes. Patient DF, with a large lesion in the ventral visual system, is unable to identify shapes and yet can accurately grasp them (Carey *et al.*, 1996). The parietal/premotor system can be contrasted with the ventral visual system, which is specialised for the use of colour and form so as to identify objects (Ungerleider and Mishkin, 1982). This involves the formation of an explicit representation (Frith *et al.*, 1999). For example, for a visual choice reaction time task, the subject must first identify the stimulus and then select the appropriate finger. Here, the subject does not respond to the object itself but performs an action that is linked with the stimulus by an arbitrary rule (Passingham, 1993; Wise and Murray, 2000). The action that is appropriate depends on the visual context.

The two tasks have been contrasted by Farrer *et al.* (2002). A visual stimulus was moved to the left or right; in one condition ("follow"), the subjects tracked the stimulus itself with their finger, and in the other ("report") they touched the screen to the left or right to indicate the direction of movement. When they had to identify the direction of movement and report it, there was activation in the middle and inferior temporal gyrus and in the ventral prefrontal cortex to which the temporal lobe projects (Webster *et al.*, 1994; Bullier *et al.*, 1996; Pandya and Yeterian, 1998). Activation has also been reported in the ventral prefrontal cortex in a related study that contrasted making arbitrary gestures to objects compared with grasping them (Passingham *et al.*, 1998; Toni *et al.*, 2001). This area has also been shown to be activated when subjects evaluated whether a particular action was appropriate given the stimulus (Deiber *et al.*, 1997).

If the appropriate response is arbitrary, it must be learned. Learning-related increases occur in the temporal lobe and ventral prefrontal cortex when subjects learn the responses that are appropriate given specific visual stimuli (Passingham and Toni, 2001; Toni *et al.*, 2001) (Fig. 1.5). It could be argued that the activity simply reflects the fact that the subjects became familiar with the nonsense figures during learning; however, Toni *et al.* (1999) introduced a novel event-related method for identifying whether activity is associated with the visual cue, the response, or both. By introducing a variable delay between the visual stimulus and the response, it is possible to decorrelate activity related in time with the presentation of the visual stimulus and activity related in time with the response. Using this method, it can be shown that activation in the temporal lobe is associated with the presentation of the visual stimulus, whereas activation in the ventral prefrontal cortex is associated both with presentation of the stimulus and with the response (Toni *et al.*, 1999; Passingham and Toni, 2001). This suggests that the prefrontal activation may reflect the association between the context and response. This suggestion is supported by the finding that there is more activity in this region when pianists sight read music and play the notes than when they sight read alone and another person plays the notes (Sergent, 1992).

It could be argued that there might be subpopulations, one for visual activity and another for motor activity. This can be tested by single-unit studies in animals. Asaad and Miller (1998) taught monkeys to make a saccade to the left given visual stimulus A and to the right given B; they then trained the monkeys on the reverse associations; that is, if A then look right, and if B then look left. This enabled the authors to identify whether cell activity in the lateral prefrontal cortex reflected the cue (*e.g.*, A, irrespective of response), the response (*e.g.*, left, irrespective of the cue), or the association between a specific cue and a specific response. The activity of 44% of the cells reflected the association of a specific stimulus and specific response. Furthermore, it was shown that cells modified their activity with learning.

The prefrontal cortex lies at the top of the processing hierarchy, receiving inputs from both the parietal and premotor cortex and the temporal lobe (Passingham, 1993; Rushworth, 2000). This means that it is in a position to integrate the dorsal and ventral systems (Rao *et al.*, 1997), as there are interconnections between the dorsal and ventral prefrontal cortex (Barbas, 1988; Petrides and Pandya, 1999). There are prefrontal cells that code both for objects (ventral) and locations (dorsal) (Rao *et al.*, 1997; Rainer *et al.*, 1998), and it has been shown using fMRI that there is activation in the dorsal prefrontal cortex of the human brain both when subjects remember objects and when they remember locations (Postle and D'Esposito, 1999).

The same mechanism could integrate information about the identity of visual stimuli and the targets of action. For example, there are cells in the macaque prefrontal cortex that fire when the animal is remembering a specific pattern and waiting to make a saccade to a specific location (Asaad *et al.*, 1998). When a human subject is learning to press key 1 given pattern A or key 2 given pattern B, the association is either between a pattern and specific finger or between a pattern and the spatial position of the appropriate key. Ramnani and Miall (2003) have also shown that prepatory activity in the human frontal polar cortex is modulated by expectation of reward.

The correct choice depends on the subject's goals. In the case of an animal, these are the rewards that are contingent on performance. In the case of a human subject, the goals are provided by the instructions given and the feedback received. We know that there are cells in the ventral and orbital prefrontal cortex of non-human primates that code for the association between visual cues and rewards of particular value (Watanabe, 1996; Tremblay and Schultz, 1999; Shultz *et al.*, 2000). Correspondingly, there is activation in the orbital frontal cortex of the human brain when subjects receive visual feedback concerning monetary rewards (Elliott *et al.*, 1997; Thut *et al.*, 1997; O'Doherty *et al.*, 2001).

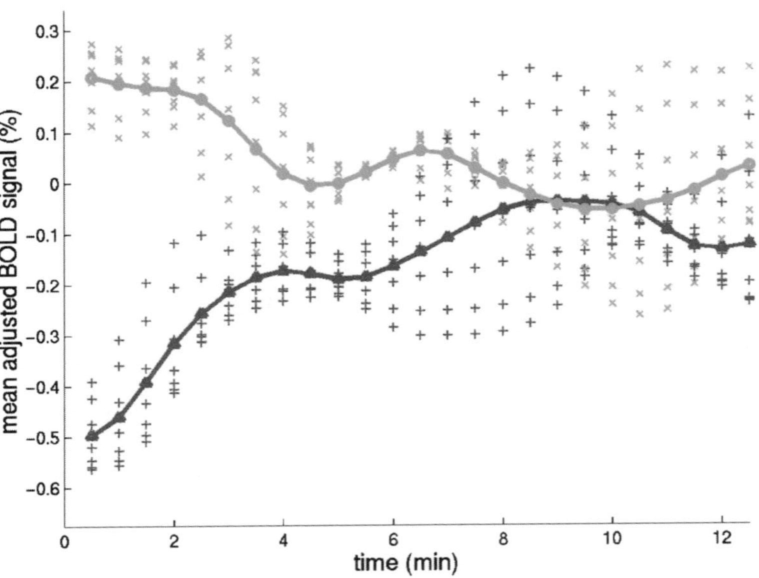

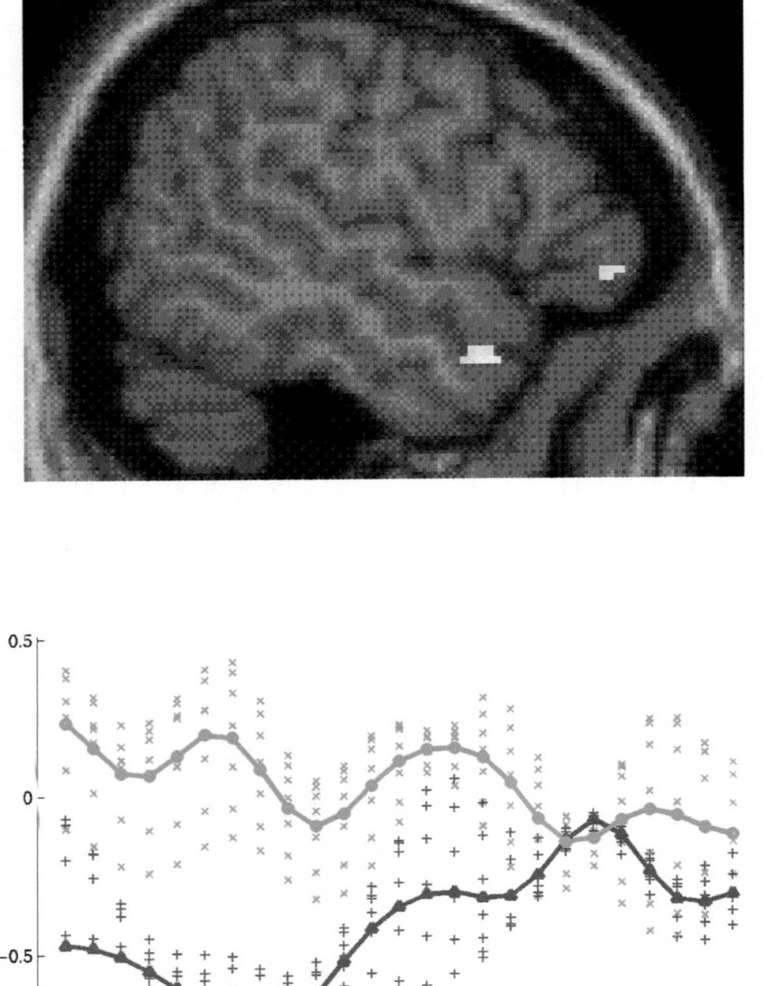

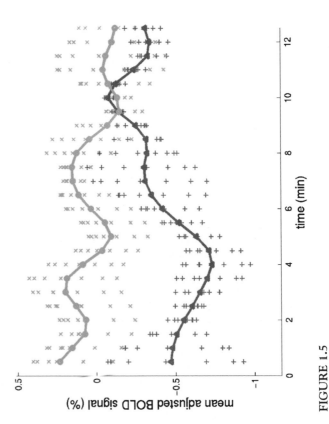

FIGURE 1.5
The MRI shows peaks voxels at which there were learning-related increases on a visuomotor association task. The increases are shown by the curves—lower curves for inferotemporal cortex and curves at the top right for the ventral prefrontal cortex. Red curves for learning task, green curves for control task. (Data from Toni *et al.* (2001). Elseveier. With permission.)

Thus, the prefrontal cortex is in a position to integrate information concerning the context and the response that is appropriate given the subject's goals (Passingham *et al.*, 2000; Miller and Cohen, 2001). On a visuomotor association task, response 1 is associated with positive feedback given cue A and with negative feedback given cue B. Thus, there is a need for a mechanism to learn the association between the cue and response as the result of success or failure. The prefrontal cortex receives high-level information from all the senses (Barbas, 2000; Miller and Asaad, in press), including taste and smell (Rolls, 2000). Furthermore, different modalities can be integrated at the single cell level (*e.g.*, Rolls and Baylis, 1994). Thus, the prefrontal cortex is in a position to specify the current context as well as the current goals. Cohen *et al.* (1996) have used a computational model in which the context as specified by the prefrontal cortex influences linkages between visual cues and motor responses that are stored elsewhere in the system. However, this model was devised to account for performance on the Stroop task. The imaging (Toni and Passingham, in press) and single unit data (Asaad *et al.*, 1998) suggest that the prefrontal cortex is involved in the *learning* of arbitrary linkages, even if with further training they are stored elsewhere. Wallis *et al.* (2001) have shown that cells in the lateral and orbital prefrontal cortex can encode abstract rules linking visual cues and responses, and that different cells can encode different rules. The learning of visuomotor tasks is further discussed in the section below on motor learning.

THE SELECTION OF ACTION

Free Selection

The term *voluntary action* can be used for actions that are not prompted by others. Voluntary actions have been tested in the scanner on the free selection task (Deiber *et al.*, 1991), where subjects are given a free choice on each trial as to which of several actions to perform. Many imaging studies have reported activation in the dorsal prefrontal cortex when subjects freely select between actions such as movements of a joystick (Deiber *et al.*, 1991; Spence *et al.*, 1998) or finger movements (Frith *et al.*, 1991; Jueptner, 1997; Hyder *et al.*, 1999; Weeks *et al.*, 2001). The same area is activated when subjects freely select between mouth movements (Spence *et al.*, 1998) or randomly generate numbers (Jahanshahi *et al.*, 2000).

Subjects can also be required to select the time at which they act; thus, Jahanshahi *et al.* (1995) used positron emission tomography (PET) to scan subjects while they initiated finger movements at times that they decided. The only constraint was that they should achieve a mean interval of 3 seconds. The only difference between this condition and a condition in which tones specified the time to move was activation in the dorsal prefrontal cortex, area 46. This finding depends critically on the fact that the intervals were matched in the two conditions, and the standard deviation of the intervals in the self-initiated condition was relatively small. Thus, in the externally triggered condition, the subjects knew roughly when the tones would occur and could prepare their response. In a later study by Jenkins *et al.* (2000) the subjects were required to vary the intervals through a greater range. The self-initiated and externally triggered conditions therefore differed in two respects—free selection and preparation—and there were now additional activations in the pre-SMA, premotor cortex, and parietal cortex. Deiber *et al.* (1999) also found activation in the pre-SMA for self-initiated versus externally triggered movements where the intervals were not predictable. The conclusion is that these additional activations may relate to response preparation rather than to the free selection of time intervals and that it is the activation in the dorsal prefrontal cortex that is associated specifically with selecting the time intervals.

It could, however, be argued that the prefrontal activation on free selection tasks reflects working memory' that is, the subjects decide which action to perform on the basis of their memory of their most recent actions. There are two reasons for thinking that this may not be so. First, Hadland *et al.* (2001) gave subjects the task of moving each of their eight fingers once on any one trial, but no memory was required because, when the subject moved a finger, a light came on to indicate for the rest of the trial that that finger had been moved. Repetitive transcranial magnetic stimulation over the dorsal prefrontal cortex delayed movements that were freely selected but had no effect on movements that were made in response to external cues. This shows that prefrontal area 46 plays a role in the selection of responses.

Second, it can also be shown that activation occurs in this area when there is selection on a task with no working memory load. Desmond *et al.* (1998) used a stem completion task in which subjects supplied one work for each stem, and each stem was only presented once. Thus, no memory was required for previous words that were generated. There was more activation in the dorsal prefrontal cortex when selection was taxed because the stem fitted many words compared with stems that fitted only two words in English.

Selection from Working Memory

When subjects freely select between actions, there are no external cues at the time to specify the appropriate response. This is also the case where subjects are required to select between items in memory. Rowe *et al.* (2000; Rowe and Passingham, 2001) used event-related fMRI to scan subjects on working memory tasks on which they were required to remember three locations for a delay period and then to select one of the locations and respond to that location. By varying the delay period, it was possible to decorrelate activity occurring during the delay from activity occurring at selection.

In the first experiment, three dots were presented simultaneously and at selection a line indicated the correct location (Rowe *et al.*, 2000). In the second experiment, the dots were presented in sequence and a number indicated the correct dot; for example, the number 2 specified the second dot in the sequence (Rowe and Passingham, 2001). In both cases, the subjects selected the location of the remembered dot by moving a cursor to that location with a joystick.

Activity that persisted throughout the delay was found in prefrontal area 8 as well as in parietal cortex; however, no significant activity was observed during the delay in prefrontal area 46. The activity in this area was associated with the selection period (Rowe *et al.*, 2000) (Fig. 1.6). This figure plots the data for the different delay lengths. It could, of course, be argued that the method for detecting activity during the delay was not sufficiently sensitive or that activity during the maintenance period might have been found had the memory load been increased by using more items. Indeed Leung *et al.*, (2003) have reported that with very long delays activity can be recorded in area 46 if the subjects have to remember five rather than three items. Nevertheless it remains that in the studies by Rowe and collegues (Rowe *et al.*, 2000,

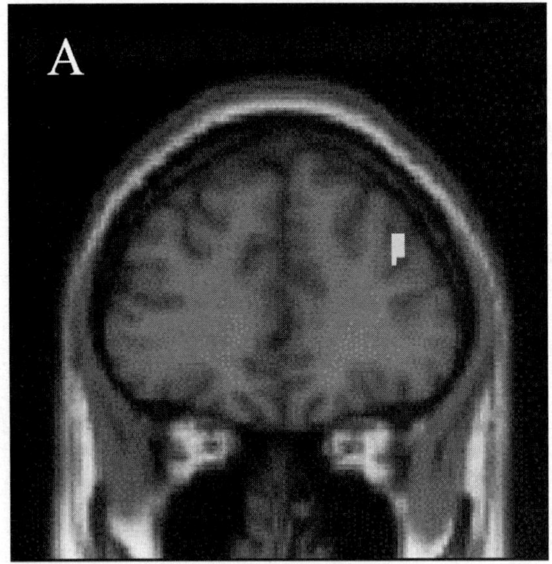

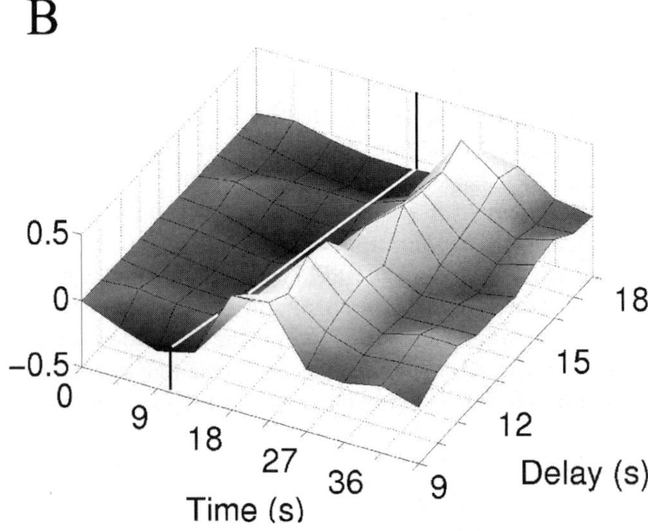

FIGURE 1.6
The MRI shows voxels in prefrontal area 46 (48, 32, 30) which were significantly more active when selection was from memory rather than being externally specified. The BOLD data from the peak voxel have been temporally realigned to the onset of working memory trials and are shown as changes in BOLD signal (z-axis) over time (x-axis) for each delay length of working memory (y-axis). The grey scale indicates the relative change in BOLD signal from the start of each trial. (From Passingham and Rowe (2002). Oxford University Press. With permssion.)

Rowe and Passingham, 2001) with three items and shorter delays it was the activity at selection that was predominant.

Others have also argued that the activation in prefrontal area 46 reflects executive processes. Thus, Petrides (1998) has suggested that it reflects the monitoring of items in memory. He argues that activation of prefrontal area 46 on the "self-ordered task" (Petrides *et al.*, 1993) or the "*n*-back" task (Owen *et al.*, 1999) is associated with the requirement to pick out the one that is currently relevant. Similarly, D'Esposito and colleagues (1999) have argued that activation of this area is associated with the requirement to manipulate items in memory. For example, they report that activation of area 46 occurs when subjects must reorder a list of items but not when they simply report them in the order given (Postle *et al.*, 1999).

Rowe *et al.* (2000) have proposed that activation of area 46 reflects attentional selection—that is, the process by which the representation of one item in memory is enhanced in competition with other items. The term *attentional selection* has two advantages. The first is that it can be applied both to the selection between items in memory and the free selection of responses; in both cases, the subject must select a representation without guidance from any external cue that is present at the time of selection. The second advantage is that it is associated with the *biased competition* model of visual attention by which voluntary shifts in attention lead to top–down signals that enhance the representation of one stimulus at the expense of the representations of other stimuli (Desimone and Duncan, 1995). Frith (2000) has suggested the prefrontal cortex may select between actions by modulating activity in other brain regions where the relevant responses are represented. Rowe *et al.* (2002a) have used fMRI to compare two conditions. In one, the subjects performed a simple manual sequence (1, 2, 3, 4, 1, 2, 3, 4, ...); in the other, they performed the same sequence but were instructed to attend to the next move. Only activity in the dorsal prefrontal area 46 was observed in the attention condition. There was also enhanced activity in the premotor, supplementary motor, and parietal cortex when the subjects attended to their actions (Fig. 1.7).

One way to study the relation between activity in prefrontal cortex and other areas is to measure *effective connectivity* (Friston *et al.*, 1993). For example, Buchel and Friston (1997) used structural equation modelling to study the effect of attention on visual motion processing. They showed that there was a difference in the connectivity of area V5 and the parietal cortex depending on whether activity in the prefrontal cortex was low or high. Rowe *et al.* (2002b)

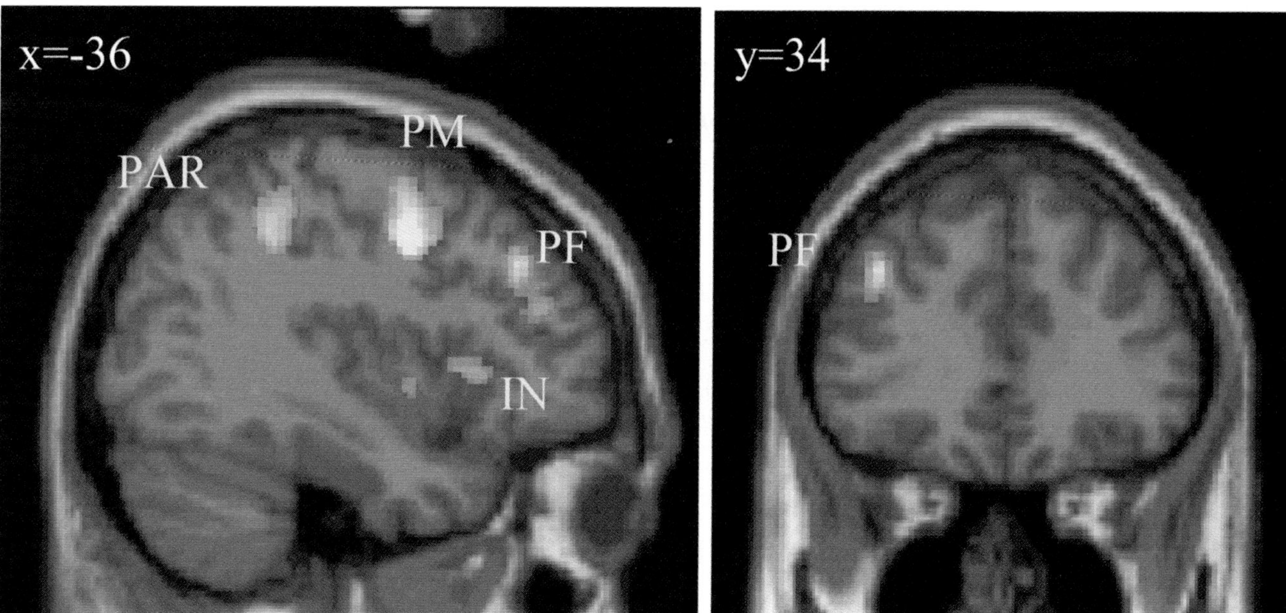

FIGURE 1.7
The prefrontal area 46, dorsal premotor cortex, and intraparietal cortex were more activated when the subjects specifically attended to action than when the subjects performed the simple motor sequence alone. The activations are shown on a parassagital MRI and also for the prefrontal cortex on a coronal section. (From Rowe *et al.*, (2002a). Elsevier. With permission.)

therefore used structural equation modelling to study the attentional modulation of the path coefficients. Figure 1.8 shows four paths linking prefrontal cortex, premotor cortex, the SMA, and motor cortex. The histograms show the extent of the modulatory effect of attention on the strength of the coupling for these paths. It can be seen that there was a significant increase in the strength of the paths linking prefrontal cortex with the premotor cortex and SMA, but no significant change in the strength of the paths linking the latter areas with the motor cortex. In a related study, it was shown that attention to action did not modulate the path strength between parietal and premotor cortex (Rowe *et al.*, 2002a).

To test the claim that the top–down signal comes from the dorsal prefrontal cortex, one would need to interfere with activity in the prefrontal cortex. Fuster *et al.* (1985), for example, cooled the prefrontal cortex and recorded from cells in the inferotemporal cortex while the monkeys performed a delayed colour-matching task. They found that the cooling abolished activity in the inferotemporal cortex that discriminated between the stimuli during the delay period. Similarly, Tomita *et al.* (1999) showed that prefrontal cortex can influence memory retrieval in the inferotemporal cortex. They presented visual stimuli to one inferotemporal cortex, having

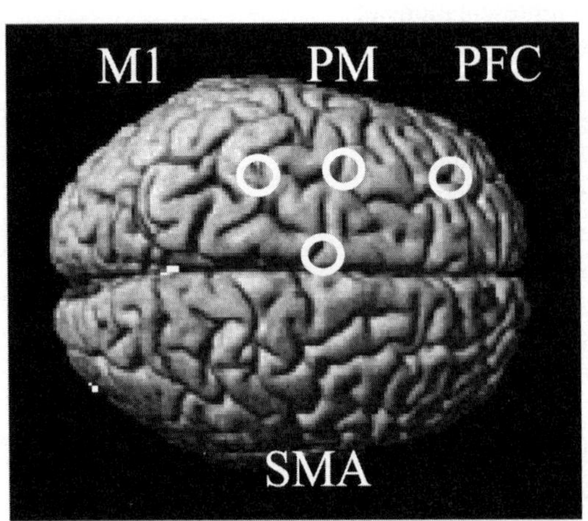

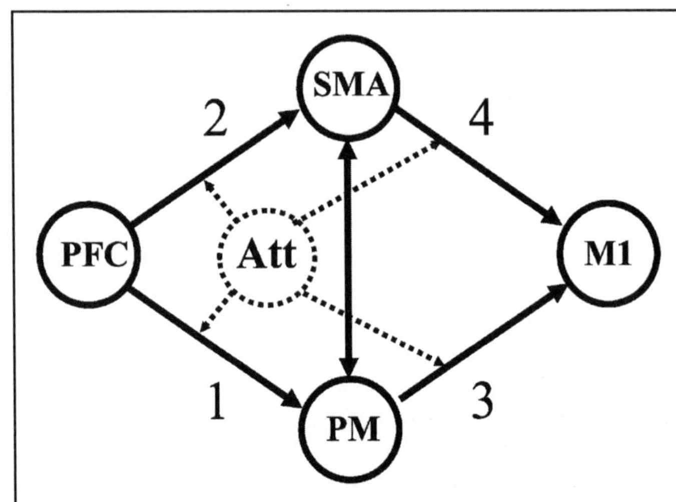

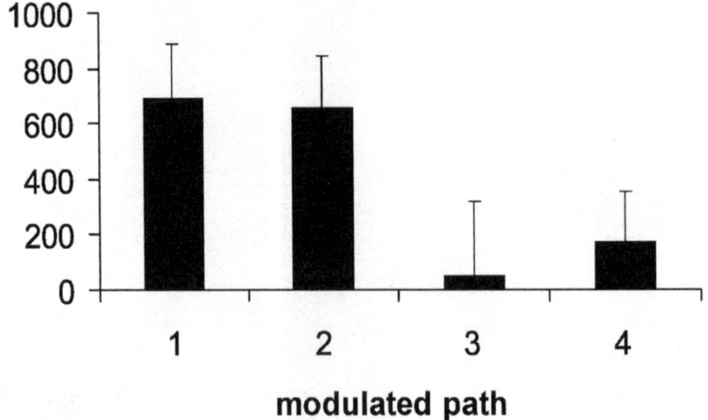

FIGURE 1.8
The model used for structural equation modelling includes the prefrontal cortex (PFC), premotor cortex (PM), supplementary motor cortex (SMA), and primary motor cortex (MI) (top left) with their interconnections (top right). The strength of these connections may be modulated by attention to action (Att) as shown by the dotted lines (top right). The histograms (lower) show the mean (±SE) coefficients for each of the four modulatory pathways numbered in the model (top right). There was a significant increase in the path coefficient for the connections between PFC and SMA and between the PFC and PM. (Data from Rowe *et al.*, (2002b). Oxford University Press. With permission.)

disconnected it from the inferotemporal cortex in the other hemisphere. During an associative task, they could still record activity related to memory retrieval in the other inferotemporal cortex, but this was abolished when the pathway from the prefrontal cortex was disrupted. Barcelo *et al.* (2000) studied patients with unilateral infarcts localised to the dorsal prefrontal cortex and recorded event-related potentials (ERPs) from extrastriate areas. The task was to detect target in a sequence of stimuli presented to one or other hemifield. The lesion abolished the N2 to targets presented in the hemifield contralateral to the lesion but had less effect on the N2 for targets presented in the hemifield ipsilateral to the lesion.

The Planning of Actions

Human subjects can select actions in advance of performing them. Jeannerod (1994, 1997) has suggested that motor imagery and motor preparation share a common mechanism. Planning involves the selection and representation of potential actions and preparation of those actions. Brain imaging can be used to scan subjects while they are required to imagine actions, to prepare for actions, or to solve tasks that require planning. Deiber *et al.* (1998) used PET to scan subjects while they imagined either adducting or abducting a finger. Compared with a resting condition, there were activations in the dorsal prefrontal cortex, the pre-SMA and premotor cortex, and the cortex in the intraparietal sulcus. Gerardin *et al.* (2000) directly compared the imagination of hand movements with the execution of the movements and reported that many of the same areas were activated.

Motor preparation is also associated with activations in the premotor cortex (Richter *et al.*, 1997; Toni *et al.*, 2001; Rushworth *et al.*, 2001), medial frontal cortex (Richter *et al.*, 1997; Lee, 1999), and parietal cortex (Deiber *et al.*, 1996; Rushworth *et al.*, 2001; Toni *et al.*, 2001). There is also activation in the dorsal prefrontal cortex if subjects are required to prepare for action over a long period. Pochon *et al.* (2001) used event-related fMRI to compare a condition in which subjects could prepare a sequence of movements with a condition in which they were not required to do so. In both conditions, they were given a sequence of five locations to remember for six seconds: In the preparation condition they pointed to the locations in turn, and in the other condition they simply reported whether a comparison sequence was the same as the first sequence presented. There was activation in the dorsal prefrontal area 46 during the delay period only in the condition in which the subjects prepared to point to the locations. Single-unit studies in monkeys have also demonstrated activity during motor preparation in prefrontal cortex (Fuster, 1997), the supplementary motor cortex (Romo and Schultz,1987), the premotor cortex (Weinrich *et al.*, 1984), and parietal cortex (Crammond and Kalaska, 1989). Taken together, these findings for motor preparation confirm the suggested association with motor imagery as measured in imaging studies of humans.

Planning has been assessed by scanning subjects while they perform variants of the Tower of Hanoi. Shallice (1982) introduced the Tower of London, and Owen *et al.* (1990) utilised a computerised version of the same task. The dorsal prefrontal cortex is activated whether subjects are required to plan and perform the moves (Owen *et al.*, 1996; Dagher *et al.*, 2001; Rowe *et al.*, 2001) or just evaluate how many moves are required to solve the problem (Baker *et al.*, 1996; Elliott *et al.*, 1997). Other areas, such as the premotor cortex and parietal cortex, are also activated when subjects perform the Tower task (Baker *et al.*, 1996; Owen *et al.*, 1996; Dagher *et al.*, 1999; Rowe *et al.*, 2001). It is therefore necessary to find a means of distinguishing between the role of the prefrontal cortex and these other areas. Dagher *et al.* (1999) have done this by performing a correlational analysis to detect activations that are greater as the number of moves required to solve the problem increases. Whereas the activations in the dorsal prefrontal cortex, anterior cingulate, and lateral premotor cortex correlated with task difficulty, the activations in the pre-SMA and intraparietal cortex did not. The authors concluded that it is the anterior areas, the prefrontal cortex and cingulate and premotor cortex, that are part of a circuit for planning.

Planning involves several components, however, including selecting moves, holding them in working memory, and evaluating the moves as appropriate to the goal. It is clear that the activation in the dorsal prefrontal cortex reflects several of these components. The activation is eliminated if planning is compared with monitoring moves in working memory (Owen *et al.*,

1996), with free selection and memory (Rowe *et al.*, 2001), or with free selection alone (Elliott *et al.*, 1997). Prefrontal cortex is involved both in the selection of moves on a planning task and in representing these moves during the preparation period.

Pathways for the Selection of Action

The evidence that the dorsal prefrontal cortex is involved in the selection and representation of action raises the question as to how it influences performance. The dorsal prefrontal cortex lies at the top of the motor hierarchy (Rushworth, 2000). It can influence the manual action indirectly by projections to the premotor areas. Thus, there are projections from prefrontal area 46 to the pre-SMA and rostral cingulate motor area (rCMA) (Luppino *et al.*, 1993; Lu *et al.*, 1994) and in turn from the pre-SMA to the SMA (Luppino *et al.*, 1993); both the CMAr and SMA project to motor cortex (Dum and Strick, 1993). There are also projections from area 46 to the dorsal and ventral premotor cortex (Dum and Strick, 1997; Matelli *et al.*, 1986) and from these areas to the motor cortex (Muakkasa and Strick, 1979). The dorsal, but not ventral, prefrontal cortex projects to the cerebellum via the pons (Schmahmann and Pandya, 1997), and there are corresponding projections from the cerebellum back to the dorsal prefrontal cortex via the ventral thalamus (Middleton and Strick, 2001).

It is possible to measure the order of events when subjects select actions. Using MEG, Pedersen *et al.* (1998) were able to show that, when subjects move a finger at will, the first activity is in the dorsal prefrontal cortex. This is followed by activity in the SMA and then in the motor cortex (Pedersen *et al.*, 1998; Erdler *et al.*, 2000). Lee (1999) has also claimed on the basis of an fMRI that there is a tendency for activation of the pre-SMA early in a preparatory period and the SMA later in that period; however, the data are only suggestive because one cannot assume that the vascular bed is similar in different areas (Menon *et al.*, 1998). The problem has been overcome in a recent study using single-shot fMRI (Weilke *et al.*, 2001). For self-initiated movements, the activation in the SMA preceded that in the motor cortex. No time difference was found for externally triggered movements. This shows that the difference for self-initiated movements cannot be attributed to differences in the vascular bed.

Richter *et al.* (1997) have also used fMRI at 4 Tesla to demonstrate that, when subjects must wait before performing movements, preparatory activity is more evident in the SMA and premotor cortex than in the motor cortex itself. This is an accord with the finding that, well in advance of movement, there is activity in the SMA and premotor cortex (Romo and Schultz, 1987; Tanji and Shima, 1994; Shima and Tanji, 2000) but not the motor cortex (Tanji and Shima, 1994; Halsband *et al.*, 1994). Taken together, the imaging studies are consistent with the view that when a subject performs a voluntary action, the prefrontal cortex influences action via connections with the medial and lateral premotor areas.

MOTOR LEARNING

Motor learning has been studied in animals by recording changes in cell firing in particular areas as the animal learns. Such changes have, for example, been demonstrated in the premotor cortex (Mitz *et al.*, 1991), the supplementary eye field (Chen and Wise, 1995a,b), and the prefrontal cortex (Asaad *et al.*, 1998); however, such recordings in animals can only be taken from one area at a time. The advantage of brain imaging is that it is a whole brain method. In the previous edition, the motor learning section reported PET studies. Such studies have the disadvantage that it is only possible to plot changes over four or six learning sessions, and only linear changes can be established. fMRI has the advantage that it is possible to scan continuously for up to 45 minutes and to plot changes that are nonlinear (Toni *et al.*, 1998).

Motor learning can be subdivided into associative learning and the learning of skills. Associative learning involves the learning of associations between antecedent and consequent events. The antecedent can be a visual context, as in visuomotor associative (Wise and Murray, 2000), or a previous action, as in motor sequence learning. Here, the subject learns *what* to do. By contrast, the learning of skills involves learning *how* to perform the movement—for example, learning the appropriate control parameters such as timing, muscle synergy, and force.

Eyeblink Conditioning

Eyeblink conditioning has been used as a simple model of motor learning; however, although the task appears simple, there are two aspects to eyeblink conditioning. First, a tone (conditioned stimulus, CS) is associated with an air puff (unconditioned stimulus, US). In well-trained subjects, eyeblinks (conditioned responses, CRs) are given only to tones that are reinforced by a US; tones at other frequencies are far less effective at evoking CRs. Second, the CRs are well timed. The CRs peak at the time at which the US is expected. Thus, eyeblink conditioning involves both the learning of association and the learning of appropriate control parameters.

We know from animal studies that the US information is carried from the trigeminal system directly to the facial nucleus, where motoneurons are activated to produce a reflexive UR (Van Ham and Yeo, 1996). Lesion and anatomical studies have revealed that the CR pathway starts and ends at these places, but its path includes in addition, the precerebellar nuclei, the cerebellum, and facial cortical motor areas (Yeo, 1991). Lesions to these areas do not abolish the UR, but eyeblink conditioning is either impaired or abolished by lesions in the face regions of the cerebellar cortex (lobule HVI and Crus I of Larsell) (Yeo and Hardiman, 1992; Gruart and Yeo, 1995), anterior parts of the cerebellar interpositus to which the cerebellar cortical areas project (Yeo *et al.*, 1985), and in the face areas of the motor cortex that are reciprocally interconnected with these corticonuclear modules in the cerebellum (Hoover and Strick, 1999).

It remains to be demonstrated that learning-related changes occur in these areas during eyeblink conditioning. Single-unit recordings taken from Purkinje cells in the rabbit (Berthier and Moore, 1990) and cat (Aou *et al.*, 1992) have shown activity that is specific to CRs; however, no study has demonstrated the evolution of activity in the cerebellar cortex as animals acquired CRs. Ramnani *et al.* (2000) used event-related fMRI to reveal areas of the human brain in which activity progressively increases as subjects learn during classical eyeblink conditioning. The subjects were presented pseudorandomly with CS tones that were partially reinforced, with both paired and unpaired CS^+ trials. On unpaired CS^+ trials, the CS^+ was presented but no US was given. In order to ensure that conditioned responses and brain activity were specific to the CS^+, CS^- trials were also presented in which the CS was an auditory tone of a different frequency, and these were never reinforced. By simultaneously sampling all trial types, it was possible to remove nonspecific changes over time. The data were analysed for time-by-condition interactions to find differential, trial-by-trial changes in haemodynamic response amplitude to unpaired CS^+ and CS^- trials. There were learning-related changes in activity in the cerebellum (on the border between Crus I and lobule HVI) and in a ventral motor or neighbouring premotor face area. The activity in these areas increased with training on unpaired CS^+ trials relative to CS^- trials; this is shown for the cerebellum in Fig. 1.9. Other imaging studies have also reported learning-related changes in the cerebellum (Logan and Grafton, 1995; Blaxton *et al.*, 1996; Schreurs *et al.*, 1997), but these have not controlled for nonspecific time effects, which confound learning-related signal.

As mentioned above, CRs have very precise temporal characteristics. The peak of the CR occurs at the time that the US is expected. This is governed by the CS–US interval. If the CS–US interval is altered during conditioning, then subjects readapt the temporal characteristics of the CR to the new interval. It is therefore possible that the cerebellum is important for learning the timing of responses (Ivry, 1997). Ramnani and Passingham (2000) therefore conducted a further study in which subjects were only required to readapt the timings of the CRs. The subjects were overtrained to produce CRs to the CS^+ before scanning and were not required to learn associations between the CS^+ and the CR during scanning. These CRs peaked at 400 ms. In phase 1, they continued conditioning with an ISI of 400 ms during scanning, but in phase 2 the CS–US interval was altered to a longer latency (700 ms). All other variables, including the CS^+/US contingency, remained exactly the same. The subjects initially produced CRs that peaked at 400 ms (inappropriate for this phase), and then the CR peak latency gradually adapted to the appropriate time (700 ms). In this study, therefore, *only* the timing of the CR was learned.

In phase 1, the peak of the CRs matched the CS–US interval (low temporal error); however, at the start of phase 2, the mismatch between the actual CR latency and the CS–US interval was large. This declined as training progressed. The subjects were not aware of the temporal mismatch or of the switch between phase 1 and phase 2, even though their responses had

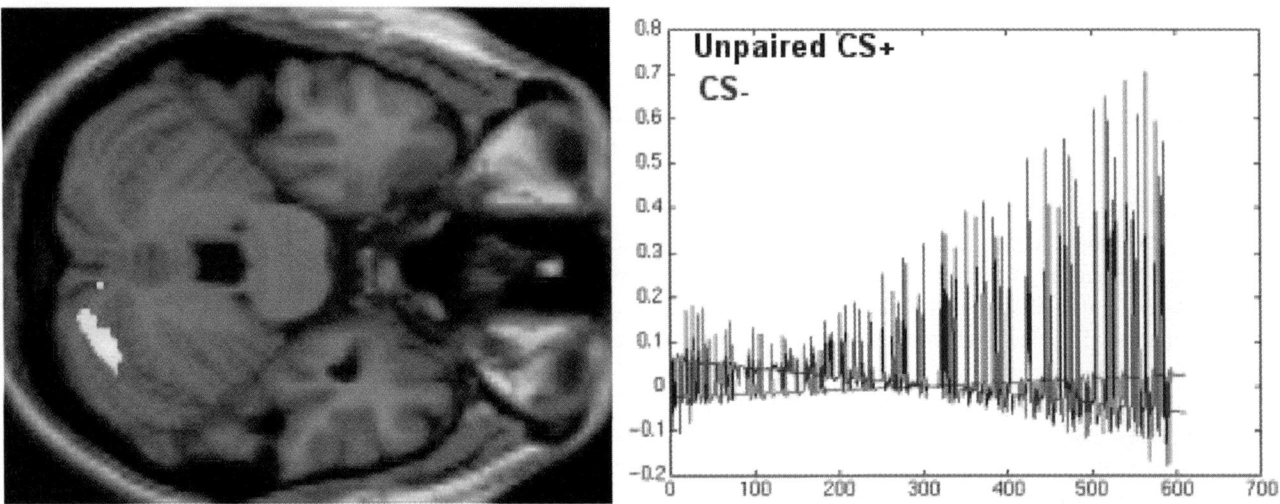

FIGURE 1.9
The MRI shows the peak voxels in the cerebellum (Crus I/lobule HV1) for learning-related increases during eye-blink conditioning. The plot to the right shows the best fitting event-related functions for the BOLD response. Blue = unpaired CS^+, red = CS^-. During unpaired CS^+ trials, the CS^+ was presented but no US. (Data from Ramnani *et al.*, (2000). American Physiology Society. With permission.)

adapted. The analysis looked for trial-by-trial activity that followed the same time course as this error signal. Such activity was found in two regions of the brain. The first was the cerebellar cortex, on the borders of lobules HV and HVI (Fig. 1.10). This confirms a cerebellar role in learning the timing of responses. The second area was the hippocampus and adjacent parahippocampal gyrus which is consistent with a role for the hippocampus in monitoring sensory inputs and responding to mismatches between expectation and outcome.

Visuomotor Learning

Lesions in specific brain regions are known to severely impair visuomotor learning in nonhuman primates. Lesions in the ventral and orbital prefrontal cortex severely impair the learning of visuomotor associations (Murray *et al.*, 2000). It was shown in Fig. 1.5 that there are learning-related increases in the ventral prefrontal cortex when human subjects learn visuomotor associations; however, impairments are also found after lesions of the dorsal premotor (Halsband and Passingham, 1985; Petrides, 1985), the basal ganglia territory of the ventral thalamus (Canavan *et al.*, 1989), and the hippocampus (Murray and Wise, 1996).

Lesion studies show that these areas are essential for visuomotor learning, but physiological studies are needed to demonstrate the changes in activity that occur with learning. Learning-related changes have been shown in macaques in the dorsal premotor cortex (Mitz *et al.*, 1991), basal ganglia (Tremblay *et al.*, 1998), and hippocampus (Cahusac *et al.*, 1993). Chen and Wise (1995a,b) have also demonstrated learning-related changes in the supplementary eye field when monkeys learn arbitrary mappings between visual cues and saccades.

Both PET (Toni and Passingham, 1999) and fMRI (Toni *et al.*, 2001) studies have shown changes in activity during visuomotor learning in the basal ganglia and hippocampus. The learning-related changes in the hippocampus occur early in learning (Toni *et al.*, 2001), and this may relate to the fact the hippocampal lesions prevent new learning but leave intact retention of stimulus–response mapping learned before surgery (Wise and Murrary, 1999). No learning-related changes were found in the dorsal premotor cortex. It is not clear why this was so, because such changes have been reported from single-unit studies in monkeys (Mitz *et al.*, 1991). However, Toni *et al.* (2002a) have been able to demonstrate an increase in effective connectivity between the caudate and dorsal premotor cortex as learning progresses.

No learning-related changes were found in the cerebellum. This is consistent with the finding that lesions in the output nuclei of the cerebellum do not impair retention of visuomotor associations in monkeys (Nixon and Passingham, 2000), though some patients with cerebellar

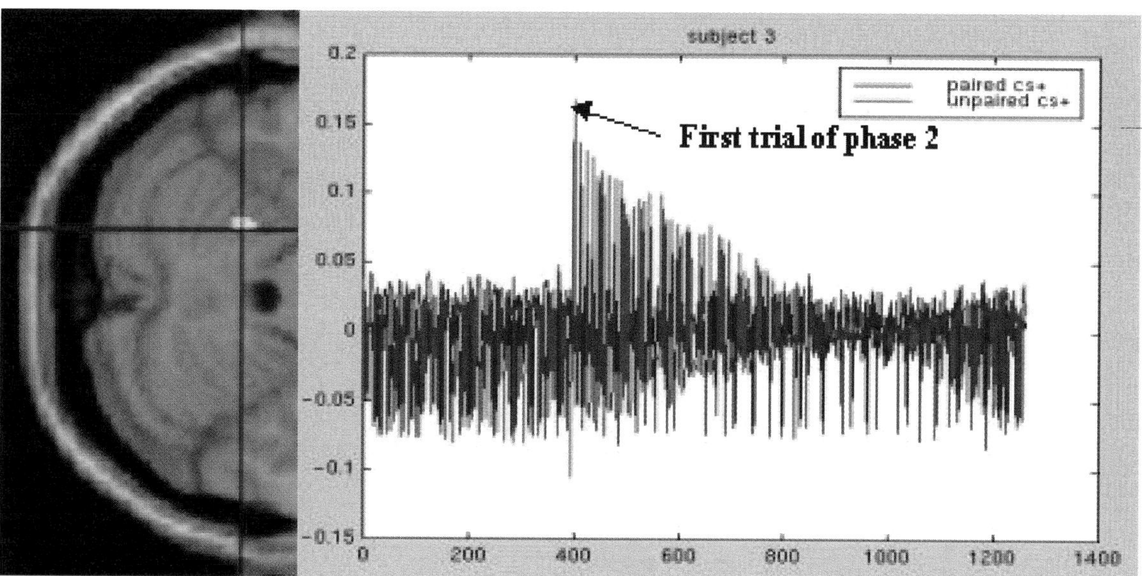

FIGURE 1.10
The MRI shows the peak voxels in the cerebellum (lobule HV/HVI) where there was activation associated with the time at which the CS–US interval was altered from 400 to 700 ms (phase 2). The plot to the right shows the best-fitting, event-related functions for the BOLD response. Red = paired CS, blue = unpaired CS$^+$. During unpaired CS$^+$ trials, the CS$^+$ was presented but no US. (Data from Ramnani and Passingham, 2001.)

pathology have been reported to be impaired at learning such tasks (Tucker *et al.*, 1997). The ventral system plays a role in the identification of the visual cues, and there no projections to the cerebellum via the pons from the ventral visual system (Schmahmann and Pandya, 1997). On the other hand, there are projections from the temporal lobe to the striatum (van Hoesen *et al.*, 1981), and Toni and Passingham (2002a) have demonstrated increases in effective connectivity between the inferotemporal cortex and caudate with learning.

Motor Sequence Learning

Sequence learning has been tested in three ways. First, Hikosaka *et al.* (1995) have taught monkeys sequences by trial and error. Sixteen buttons are arranged in a 4 × 4 matrix. In the task, two of the buttons in the matrix illuminate simultaneously, and the task is to press them in the correct order. If correct, the next set of two buttons then illuminate. There are typically five sets in a fixed order (known as a hyperset). The same task has been used in fMRI studies (Hikosaka *et al.*, 1996). Second, human subjects have been explicitly taught finger sequences eight long by trial and error (Jenkins *et al.*, 1994; Jueptner *et al.*, 1997a,b; Toni *et al.*, 1998). Third, the serial reaction time task has been used for human subjects. Here, the sequence is prompted by visual cues. Learning can take place either implicitly (Doyon *et al.*, 1996; Hazeltine *et al.*, 1997) or explicitly (Honda *et al.*, 1998).

Nakamura *et al.* (1998) have recorded in the medial frontal cortex in monkeys. They have shown that in the pre-SMA neurons fired on presentation of a new hyperset and typically decreased in activity over the course of learning. Activity remained at a low rate if the animal was presented with a hyperset that had been prelearned. Temporary inactivation using muscimol infusions into the pre-SMA significantly impaired learning if applied before new hypersets but did not affect performance if applied before learned hypersets (Miyashita *et al.*, 1996). This supports the view that the pre-SMA is required for learning motor sequences but is not required for retrieval of motor sequences from memory.

In a related fMRI study, Sakai *et al.* (1998) scanned human subjects during the learning of task in which they had to press 10 pairs of buttons in the correct order, a variant of the task used for monkeys. The authors report that activity was present in the pre-SMA early in learning. Activation in the dorsal prefrontal cortex also occurs early in explicit learning of a motor sequence (Jenkins *et al.*, 1994; Jueptner *et al.*, 1997a,b; Toni *et al.*, 1998). The dorsal prefrontal cortex and the pre-SMA are interconnected (Lu *et al.*, 1998); however, in the study by Toni *et al.* (1998), this activity reduced with learning until it reached baseline as the task became automatic (Fig. 1.11A). The dorsal prefrontal cortex also projects to the caudate nucleus (Selemon and Goldman-Rakic, 1985). In the study by Jueptner *et al.* (1997), there was more activity in the caudate early than late in learning. Miyachi *et al.* (1997) infused muscimol into the head of the caudate and anterior putamen and showed that it impaired the learning of new hypersets.

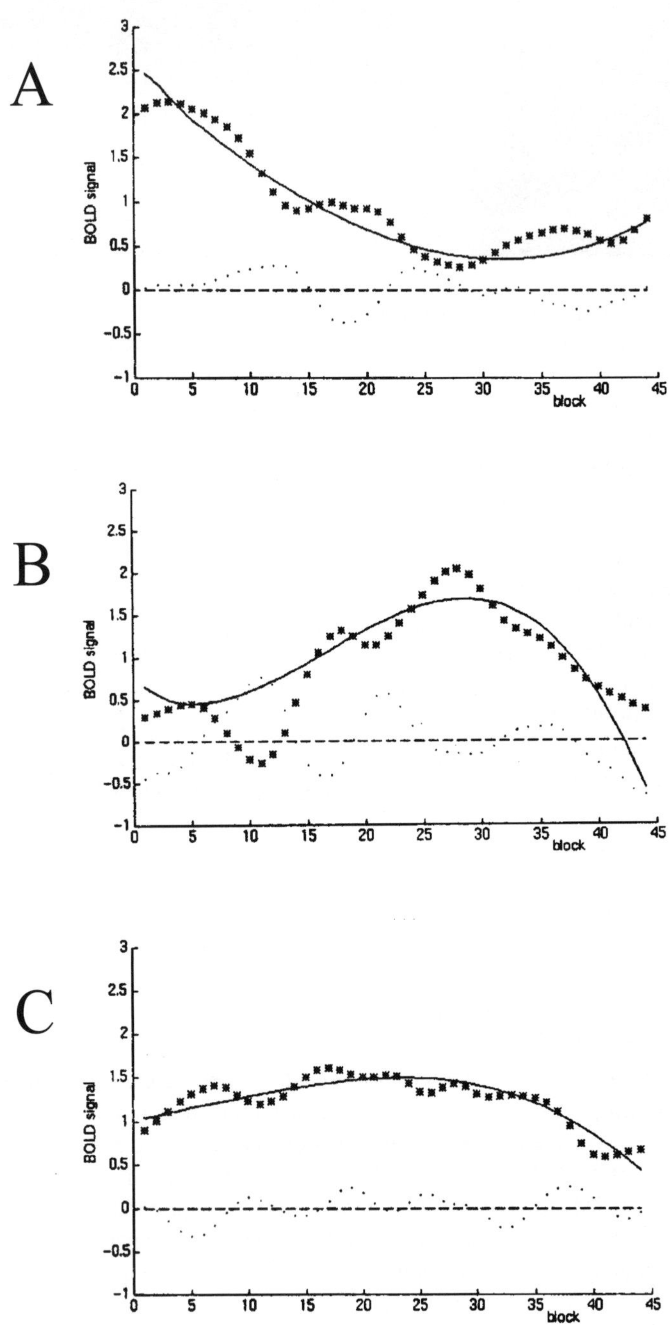

FIGURE 1.11
Learning-related changes in BOLD signal on a sequence learning task, averaged over three subjects. The adjusted data from the activation and baseline blocks are shown by the stars and dots, respectively; the fitted response is shown by the solid line (activation) and the dashed line (baseline). A = right dorsolateral prefrontal cortex (42, 32, 24), B = SMA (–6, –2, 70), C = right anterior cerebellar lobe (26, –44, 30). (From Toni *et al.* (1998). Elsevier. With permission.)

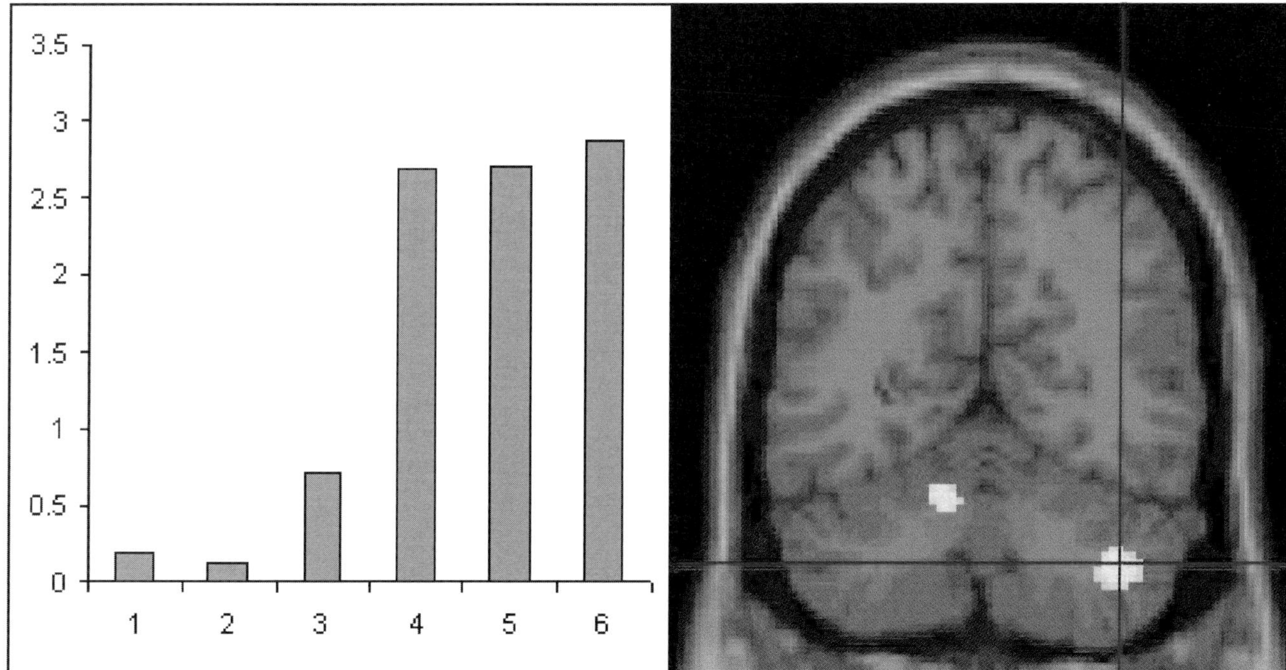

FIGURE 1.12
The MRI shows the peak voxels in the cerebellum (vermis and lateral cortex) at which there were learning-related changes when subjects learned a manual rhythm compared with performing a task on which the timings were random. The histograms on the left show the data for Crus I/Crus II (lobule HVI-A). The abscissa shows the changes during six learning sessions (1–6), and the ordinate shows the relative rCBF. (Data from Ramnani and Passingham, in press.)

Hikosaka *et al.* (1999) have proposed that two systems are involved in motor sequence learning. The sequence is first coded spatially. They suggest that this abstract representation of the sequence depends on a corticobasal ganglia system. As learning progresses, the sequence is recoded motorically. They suggest that this motor representation depends on cortico-cerebellar circuitry. The model suggests that in the early stages of sequence learning, sequences are learned as associations between sensory elements, but that as learning progresses, they are coded as associations between motor elements.

Evidence for a change in coding comes from a study by Ramnani *et al.* (2001) on the learning of a manual rhythm. The rhythm was cued by visual stimuli, but as the task became automatic it could be performed as a motor sequence without reference to the pacing cues. There were decreases with learning in a series of interconnected visual areas; these included the prestriate cortex, the inferior temporal cortex, and the ventral prefrontal cortex to which it projects (Webster *et al.*, 1994). There were also decreases in the dorsal cortex. These results suggest that sequences were first learned as a series of sensory events. There were corresponding increases in the cerebellum (Fig. 1.12) and premotor cortex consistent with the view that the task was then coded in motor coordinates.

Skilled Performance

Lu *et al.* (1998) have shown that temporary inactivation of the cerebellar nuclei impairs automated performance of sequences. Infusion of muscimol into the dorsal parts of the dentate nucleus caused an increase in the number of errors and the reaction time for learned hypersets, but not for new hypersets. This effect was specific to the limb ipsilateral to the inactivation, suggesting that the sequence was coded in motoric terms. Nixon and Passingham (2000) have also demonstrated that monkeys with bilateral lesions in the dentate and interpositus are able to learn motor sequences, but they never achieve the same level of automation as unoperated monkeys. The monkeys were tested on the serial reaction time task. Patients with cerebellar lesions also improve on this task over days, but their curve flattens off (Doyon, 1997), and the patients showed impaired retention one year later (Doyon *et al.*, 1998).

In imaging studies, learning-related changes have also been reported in the cerebellum. An increase in cerebellar activity with learning has been reported (Toni *et al.*, 1998), but this is then followed by a decrease at the end of overlearning (Fig. 1.11C). This may account for the inconsistency in reports of changes in activity in the cerebellum. Comparing new learning with performance of an overlearned task, Jenkins *et al.* (1994) and Jueptner *et al.* (1997a) reported greater activation in the cerebellum for new learning. On the other hand, Doyon *et al.* (1996) compared performance of a highly learned sequence with a random control using the serial reaction time task and reported activation in the dentate nucleus. Ramnani *et al.* (2001) taught manual rhythms but scanned for a shorter time than Toni *et al.* (1998). Relative to a random control, learning related increases were observed in three regions of the cerebellar cortex (Fig. 12), but no changes in the basal ganglia.

The cerebellar cortex projects to the ventral thalamus, and there are projections from the cerebellar territory of the thalamus to motor cortex, premotor cortex, and SMA (Matelli and Luppino, 1996; Middleton and Strick, 1997). In PET studies, learning-related increases have been found for the serial reaction time task in the SMA (Hazeltine *et al.*, 1997). Van Mier *et al.* (1998) also trained subjects on a maze task with their eyes closed, and skilled performance was associated with activity in the SMA. Using fMRI, Toni *et al.* (1998) also found a striking learning-related increase in activity in the SMA as an explicit sequence task became automated (Fig. 1.11B); however, it was suggested that at the end of overtraining there was a subsequent decrease in activity. This may relate to the finding by Aizawa *et al.* (1991) that, when macaques had been overtrained on a motor task for one year, it was no longer possible to find task-related neurons in the SMA. Task-related neurons returned, however, if motor cortex was then lesioned. Changes have also been reported in motor cortex as motor tasks become automatic. Karni *et al.* (1995) trained subjects on finger sequences every day for three weeks and found large gains in performance that were limited to the use of the practiced hand. The authors compared performance of the overtrained sequence with performance of a novel sequence and found more voxels activated in motor cortex for the overtrained sequence. Monkeys have also been trained on a task requiring the skilled use of their digits, and electrophysiological recording showed an expansion of the digit representations in motor cortex with a corresponding contraction of the representation of the wrist and forearm (Nudo *et al.*, 1996).

In the study of Karni *et al.* (1995), the subjects were trained *across* days. Most imaging studies of motor learning had been restricted to changes in learning within a day when practice was either continuous (*e.g.*, Toni *et al.*, 1998) or the runs were only separated by 10 minutes (Hazeltine *et al.*, 1997). Karni *et al.* (1998) also found complex changes within the first session when comparing performance of two sequences. At first, more voxels were activated for the sequence performed first rather than second, suggesting a habituation effect, but after 30 minutes this effect reversed.

Training across days allows consolidation, that is the stabilisation of labile memory traces. Consolidation occurs as a function of intervening time. It has been demonstrated in two ways. First, the performance of subjects on a motor task can be better at the beginning of the second day than the end of the first (Brashers-Krug *et al.*, 1996; Karni *et al.*, 1998). Second, if subjects are trained on a motor task A and then trained on the opposite task B just 10 minutes later, there is considerable interference, but this interference is less if more time is allowed to elapse before task B is trained (Brashers-Krug *et al.*, 1996; Shadmehr and Holcomb, 1997). Shadmeyr and Holcomb (1997) used PET to scan subjects while they learned to move a cursor with a joystick against a force field; the same subjects were then rescanned 5 hours later. The authors report that after the interval there was an increase in activation in the cerebellum, parietal cortex, and premotor cortex.

CONCLUSIONS

A distinction can be drawn for human subjects between declarative and procedural learning. Declarative learning is necessarily explicit. Explicit learning has the advantage of being faster than implicit learning–for example, on the serial reaction time task (Honda *et al.*, 1998). The declarative learning of associations, whether between visual cues and movements (Toni *et al.*,

2002a,b) or between elements in a sequence (Jueptner *et al.*, 1997a; Toni *et al.*, 1998) involves a prefrontal–basal ganglia system. It is this fast learning that is impaired by prefrontal lesions in monkeys: Monkeys with ventral prefrontal lesions are unable to learn visuomotor associations within a day but can learn them slowly across days (Murray and Bussey, 2001). The prefrontal cortex projects to the anterior cingulate and pre-SMA (Lu *et al.*, 1994), and both the anterior cingulate (Toni *et al.*, 1998) and pre-SMA (Hikosaka *et al.*, 1996) are active early in the learning of associations between the movements in a sequence.

This system can represent cues, responses, and the associations between them (Asaad *et al.*, 1998a; Toni and Passingham, 1999; Toni *et al.*, 2002b). These are explicit representations: human subjects attend to them (Passingham, 1996) and are aware of them (Frith *et al.*, 2000). They concern actions rather than movements, where an action is defined by its target rather than by the muscle activity that brings the effector to that target. Neither the prefrontal cortex nor pre-SMA have direct projections to the motor cortex (Lu *et al.*, 1994) or spinal cord (Dum Richard and Strick Peter, 1996). This system makes explicit decisions as to *what* action to perform (Frith *et al.*, 1991, 2001; Jueptner *et al.*, 1997b).

This system can be contrasted with a system for determining *how* movements are performed. Such a system involves the parietal cortex and its projections to the premotor cortex, as well as the cerebellum and its projections to motor cortex and the premotor areas. As motor sequences are learned, there are learning-related increases in the parietal cortex (Toni *et al.*, 1998; Ramnani and Sakai *et al.*, 2000; Passingham, 2001), as well as in the cerebellum and SMA. If learning sessions are separated by hours to allow consolidation, there are increases with the passage of time alone in the cerebellum, parietal, and premotor cortex (Shadmehr and Holcomb, 1997). This system is involved in determining the kinematics and timing of movements. There are learning-related increases in parietal and cerebellar cortex when subjects learn a new set of timings (Ramnani and Passingham, 2001). Imaging studies have also shown that the parietal–cerebellar system is involved in motor coordination, whether it be coordination of eye and hand movements (Miall *et al.*, 2001), finger and arm coordination (Ramnani *et al.*, 2001), or changes in visuomotor coordination with prisms (Clower *et al.*, 1996).

When a sequences has been overlearned, subjects can perform the task without attention, as shown by the relative lack of interference by the simultaneous performance of a secondary task (Passingham, 1996). The system can learn implicitly—that is, without the subject being aware that there is a task to be learned. In studies of eyeblink conditioning, the subjects are not aware of the explicit linkage between a CS^+ and an air puff (Ramnani *et al.*, 2000) or that the timing of the air puff has changed (Ramnani *et al.*, 2001). When a complex motor task has become automatic, it can be performed as a series of coordinated movements. The advantage of automation is that the subject can then attend to other more pressing tasks.

References

Aizawa, H., Inase, M., Mushiake, H., Shima, K., and Tanji, J. (1991). Reorganisation of activity in the supplementary motor area associated with motor learning and functional recovery. *Exp. Brain Res.*, **84**, 668–671.

Amunts, K., Schleicher, A., Burgel, U., Mohlberg, H., Uylings, H. B. M., and Zilles, K. (1999). Broca's region revisited: cytoarchitecture and intersubject variability. *J. Comp. Neurol.*, **412**, 319–341.

Aou, S., Woody, C. D., and Birt, D. (1992). Changes in the activity of units of the cat motor cortex with rapid conditioning and extinction of a compound eye blink movement. *J. Neurosci.,* **12**, 549–559.

Asaad, W. F., Rainer, G., and Miller, E. K. (1998). Neural activity in the primate prefrontal cortex during associative learning. *Neuron*, **21**, 1399–1407.

Baker, S. C., Rogers, R. D., Owen, A. M., Frith, C. D., Dolan, R. J., Frackowiak, R. S. J., and Robbins, T. W. (1996). Neural systems engaged by planning: a PET study of the Tower of London task. *Neuropsychology*, **34**, 515–526.

Barbas, H. (1988). Anatomical organisation of basoventral and mediodorsal visual recipient prefrontal region in the rhesus monkey. *J. Comp. Neurol.*,**76**, 313–342.

Barbas, H. (2000). Connections underlying the synthesis of cognition, memory, and emotion in primate prefrontal cortices. *Brain Res. Bull.*, **52**, 319–330.

Barcelo, F., Suwazono, S., and Knight, R. T. (2000). Prefrontal modulation of visual processing in humans. *Nat. Neurosci.*, **3**, 399–403.

Belger, A., Puce, A., Krystal, J. H., Gore, J. C., Goldman-Rakic, P., and McCarthy, G. (1998). Dissociation of mnemonic and perceptual processes during spatial and nonspatial working memory using fMRI. *Hum. Brain Mapping.*, **6**, 14–32.

Berthier, N. E. and Moore, J. W. (1990). Activity of deep cerebellar nuclear cells during classical conditioning of nictitating membrane extension in rabbits. *Exp. Brain Res.*, **83**,44–54.

Binkofski, F., Buccioino, G., Stephan, K. M., Rizzolatti, G., Seitz, R. J., and Freund, H.-J. (1999). A parieto-premotor network for object manipulation: evidence from neuroimaging. *Exp. Brain Res.*, **128**, 210–213.

Binkofski, F., Amunts, K., Stephan, K. M., Posse, S., Schormann, T., Freund, H. J., Zilles, K., and Seitz, R. J. (2000). Broca's region subserves imagery of motion: a combined cytoarchitectonic and fMRI study. *Hum. Brain Mapping*, **11**, 273–285.

Blaxton, T. A., Zeffiro, T. A., Gabrieli, J. D. E., Bookheime, S. Y., Carrillo, M. C., Theodore, W. H., and Disterhoft, J. F. (1996). Functional mapping of human learning: a positron emission tomography activation study of eyeblink conditioning. *J. Neurosci.*, **16**, 4032–4040.

Brashers-Krug, T., Shadmehr, R., and Bizzi, E. (1996). Consolidation in human motor memory. *Nature*, **382**,252–255.

Brodmann, K. (1909). *Vergleichende Lokalisationlehre der Grosshirnrinde*. Barth, Leipzig.

Buccino, G., Binkofski, F., Fink, G. R., Fadiga, L., Fogassi, L., Gallese, V., Seitz, R. J., Zilles, K., Rizzolatti, G., and Freund, H.-J. (2001). Action observation activates premotor and parietal areas in a somatotopic manner: an fMRI study. *Eur. J. Neurosci.*, **13**, 400–404.

Buchel, C. and Friston, K. J. (1997). Modulation of connectivity in visual pathways by attention: cortical interactions evaluated with structural equation modelling and fMRI. *Cereb. Cortex*, **7**, 768–778.

Bullier, J., Schall, J. D., and Morel, A. (1996). Functional streams in occipito-frontal connections in the monkey. *Behav. Brain Res.*, **76**, 89–97.

Cahusac, P. M., Rolls, E. T., Miyashita, Y., and Niki, H. (1993). Modification of the responses of hippocampal neurons in the monkey during the learning of a conditional spatial response task. *Hippocampus*, **3**, 29–42.

Canavan, A. G., Nixon, P. D., and Passingham, R. E. (1989). Motor learning in monkeys (*Macaca fascicularis*) with lesions in motor thalamus. *Exp. Brain Res.*, **77**,113–126.

Carey, D. P., Harvey, M., and Milner, A. D. (1996). Visuomotor sensitivity for shape and orientation in a patient with visual form agnosia. *Neuropsychology*, **34**, 329–337.

Chafee, M. V. and Goldman-Rakic, P. S. (1998). Matching patterns of activity in primate prefrontal area 8a and parietal area 7ip during a spatial working memory task. *J. Neurophysiol.*, 79, 2919–2940.

Chen, L. L. and Wise, S. P. (1995a). Neuronal activity in the supplementary eye field during acquisition of conditional oculomotor associations. *J. Neurophysiol.*, **73**, 1101–1121.

Chen, L. L. and Wise, S. P. (1995b). Supplementary eye field contrasted with the frontal eye field during acquisition of conditional oculomotor associations. *J.Neurophysiol.*, **73**, 1122–1134.

Chen, L. L. and Wise, S. P. (1997). Conditional oculomotor learning in the supplementary eye field during acquisition of oculomotor associations. *J. Neurophysiol.*, **78**, 1166–1169.

Chiavaras, M. M. and Petrides, M. (2000). Orbitofrontal sulci of the human and macaque monkey brain. *J. Comp. Neurol.*, **422**, 35–54.

Clower, D. M., Hoffmann, J. M., Votaw, J. R., Faber, T. L., Woods, R. P., and Alexander, G. E. (1996). Role of posterior parietal cortex in the recalibration of visually guided reaching. *Nature*, **383**, 618–621.

Cohen, J. D., Dunbar, K., and McClelland, J. L. (1996). On the control of automatic processes: a parallel distributed model of the Stroop effect. *Psychol. Rev.*, **97**, 332–361.

Conturo, T. E., Lori, N. F., Cull, T. S., Akbudak, E., Snyder, A. Z., Shimony, J. S., McKinstry, R. C., Burton, H., and Raichle, M. E. (1999). Tracking neuronal fiber pathways in the living human brain. *Proc. Nat. Acad. Sci. USA*, **96**, 10422–10427.

Courtney, S. M., Petit, L., Maisog, J. M., Ungerleider, L. G., and Haxby, J. V. (1998). An area specialised for spatial working memory in human frontal cortex. *Science*, **279**, 1347–1351.

Crammond, D. J. and Kalaska, J. F. (1989). Neuronal activity in primate parietal cortex area 5 varies with intended movement direction during an instructed-delay period. *Exp. Brain Res.*, **76**, 458–462.

Crick, F. and Jones, E. (1993). Backwardness of human neuroanatomy. *Nature*, **361**, 109–110.

Crutcher, M. D. and Alexander, G. E. (1990). Movement-related neuronal activity selectively coding either direction or muscle pattern in three motor areas of the monkey. *J. Neurophysiol.*, **64**, 151–163.

Dagher, A., Owen, A. M., Boecker, H., and Brooks, D. J. (1999). Mapping the network for planning: a correlational PET activation study with the Tower of London. *Brain*, **122**, 1973–1987.

Decety, J. and Grezes, J. (1999). Neural mechanisms subserving the perception of human actions. *TICS*, **3**, 172–178.

Decety, J., Grezes, J., Costes, N., Perani, D., Jeannerod, M., Procyk, E., Grassi, F., and Fazio, F. (1997). Brain activity during observation of actions: influence of action content and subject's strategy. *Brain*, **120**, 1763–1777.

Deiber, M.-P., Passingham, R. E., Colebatch, J. G., Friston, K. J., Nixon, P. D., and Frackowiak, R. S. J. (1991). Cortical areas and the selection of movement: a study with positron emission tomography. *Exp. Brain Res.*, **84**, 393–402.

Deiber, M.-P., Ibanez, V., Sadato, N., and Hallett, M. (1996). Cerebral structures participating in motor preparation in humans: a positron emission tomography study. *J. Neurophysiol.*, **75**, 233–247.

Deiber, M.-P., Wise, S. P., Honda, M., Catalan, M. J., Grafman, J., and Hallett, M. (1997). Frontal and parietal networks for conditional motor learning; a positron emission tomography study. *J. Neurophysiol.*, **78**, 977–991.

Deiber, M.-P., Ibanez, V., Honda, M., Sadato, N., Raman, R., and Hallett, M. (1998). Cerebral processes related to visuomotor imagery and generation of simple finger movements studied with positron emission tomography. *NeuroImage*, **7**, 73–85.

Desimone, R. and Duncan, J. (1995). Neural mechanisms of selective visual attention. *Ann. Rev. Neurosci.*, **18**, 193–222.

Desmond, J. E., Gabrieli, J. D. E., and Glover, G. H. (1998). Dissociation of frontal and cerebellar activity in a cognitive task: evidence for a distinction between selection and search. *NeuroImage*, **7**, 368–376.

D'Esposito, M., Postle, B. R., Ballard, D., and Lease, J. (1999). Maintenance versus manipulation of information held in working memory: an event-related fMRI study. *Brain Cognition*, **41**, 66–86.

D'Esposito, M., Postle, B. R., Jonides, J., and Smith, E. E. (1999). The neural substrate and temporal dynamics of interference effects in working memory as revealed by event-related functional MRI. *Proc. Nat. Acad. Sci.*, **96**, 7514–7519.

Di Virgilio, G. and Clarke, S. (1997). Direct interhemispheric visual inputs to human speech areas. *Hum. Brain Mapping*, **5**, 347–354.

Doyon, J. (1997). Skill learning. *Int. Rev. Neurobiol.*, 41273–41294.

Doyon, J., Owen, A. M., Petrides, M., Sziklas, V., and Evans, A. C. (1996). Functional anatomy of visuomotor skill learning in human subjects examined with positron emission tomography. *Eur. J. Neurosci.*, **8**, 637–648.

Doyon, J., Laforce, R., Bouchard, G., Gaudreau, D., Roy, J., Poirier, M., Bedard, P. J., Bedard, F., and Bouchard, J. P. (1998). Role of the striatum, cerebellum and frontal lobes in the automatisation of a repeated visuomotor sequence of movements. *Neuropsychology*, **36**, 625–641.

Dum, R. P. and Strick, P. L. (1996). Spinal cord terminations of the medial wall motor areas in macaque monkeys. *J. Neurosci.*, **16**, 6513–6525.

Dum, R. P. and Strick, P. L. (1997). Cortical inputs to the digit representations in the primary motor cortex and the dorsal premotor area of the cebus monkey. *Soc. Neurosci. Abs.*, **23**, 502–512.

Elliott, R., Frith, C. D., and Dolan, R. J. (1997). Differential neural responses to positive and negative feedback in planning and guessing tasks. *Neuropsychology*, **35**, 1395–1404.

Faillenot, I., Toni, I., Decety, J., Greoire, M.-C., and Jeannerod, M. (1997). Visual pathways for object-oriented action and object recognition: functional anatomy with PET. *Cereb. Cortex*, **7**, 77–85.

Farrer, C, Passingham, R. E., Frith, C. D. (2002). A role for the ventral visual stream in reporting movements. *NeuroImage*, **15**, 587–595.

Felleman, D. J. and van Essen, D. C. (1991). Distributed hierarchical processing in primate cerebral cortex. *Cereb. Cortex*, **1**, 1–47.

Fogassi, L., Gallese, V., Fadiga, L., and Rizzolatti, G. (1998). Neurons responding to the sight of goal-directed hand/arm actions in the parietal area PF (7b*). Soc. Neurosci. Abs.*, **257**, 654.

Fogassi, L., Gallese, V., Buccino, G., Craighero, L., Fadiga, L., and Rizzolatti, G. (2001). Cortical mechanism for the visual guidance of hand grasping movements in the monkey: a reversible inactivation study. *Brain*, **124**, 571–586.

Friston, K. J., Frith, C. D., and Frackowiak, R. S. J. (1993). Time-dependent changes in effective connectivity measured with PET. *Hum. Brain Mapping*, **1**, 69–79.

Frith, C. D. (2000). The role of dorsolateral prefrontal cortex in the selection of action, in *Control of Cognitive Processes: Attention and Performance*, Vol. XVIII, Monsell, S. and Driver, J., Eds., pp. 549–565. MIT Press, Cambridge, MA.

Frith, C. D., Friston, K., Liddle, P. F., and Frackowiak, R. S. J. (1991). Willed action and the prefrontal cortex in man: a study with PET. *Proc. Roy. Soc. London Ser. B*, **244**, 241–246.

Frith, C. D., Perry, R., and Lumer, E. (1999). The neural correlates of conscious experience: an experimental framework. *Trends Cogn. Sci.*, **3**, 105–114.

Frith, C. D., Blakemore, S. J., and Wolpert, D. M. (2000). Abnormalities in the awareness and control of action. *Phil. Trans. Roy. Soc. London Ser. B*, **355**, 1771–1788.

Fuster, J. (1997). *The Prefrontal Cortex*. Lippincott-Raven, Philadelphia.

Fuster, J., Bauer, R. H., and Jervey, J. P. (1985). Functional interactions between inferotemporal and prefrontal cortex in a cognitive task. *Brain Res.*, **330**, 299–307.

Gallese, G. and Goldman, A. (1998). Mirror neurons and the simulation theory of mind reading. *Trends Cognit. Sci.*, **2**, 493–500.

Gallese, V., Fadiga, L., Fogassi, L., and Rizzolatti, G. (1996). Action recognition in the premotor cortex. *Brain*, **119**, 593–610.

Georgopoulos, A. P., Caminiti, R., Kalaska, J. F., and Massey, J. T. (1983). Spatial coding of movements: a hypothesis concerning the coding of movement directions by motor cortical populations. *Exp. Brain Res.*, **7**, 327–336.

Gerardin, A., Sirigu, A., Lehericy, S., Poline, J.-B., Gaymard, B., Marsault, C., Agid, Y., and Le Bihan, D. (2000). Partially overlapping neural networks for real and imagined hand movements. *Cereb. Cortex*, **10**, 1093–1104.

Geyer, S., Matelli, M., Luppino, G., Schleicher, A., Jansen, Y., Palomero-Gallagher, N., Zilles, K. (1998). Receptor autoradiographic mapping of the mesial and premotor cortex of the macaque monkey. *J. Comp. Neurol.*, **397**, 231–250.

Geyer, S., Schormann, T., Mohlberg, H., and Zilles, K. (2000). Areas 3a, 3b, and 1 of human primary somatosensory cortex. II. Spatial normalisation to standard anatomical space. *NeuroImage*, **11**, 684–696.

Geyer, S., Grefkes, C., Schormann, T., Mohlberg, H., and Zilles, K. (2001). The microstructural border between the agranular frontal (Brodmann's area 6) and the granular prefrontal cortex: a population map in standard anatomical space. *NeuroImage*, **13**, S1171.

Grafton, S. T., Mazziotta, J. C., Woods, R. P., and Phelps, M. E. (1992). Human functional anatomy of visually guided finger movements. *Brain*, **115**, 565–587.

Grafton, S. T., Fagg, A. H., and Arbib, M. A. (1998). Dorsal premotor cortex and conditional movement selection: a PET functional mapping study. *J. Neurophysiol.*, **79**, 1092–1097.

Grezes, J. and Decety, J. (2001). Functional anatomy of execution, mental simulation, observation, and verbal generation of actions: a meta-analysis. *Hum. Brain Mapping*, **12**, 1–19.

Grezes, J., Costes, N., and Decety, J. (1999). The effect of learning and intention on the neural network involved in the perception of meaningless actions. *Brain*, **122**, 1875–1887.

Gruart, A. and Yeo, C. H. (1995). Cerebellar cortex and eyeblink conditioning: bilateral regulation of conditioned responses. *Exp. Brain Res.*, **104**, 431–448.

Hadland, K. A., Rushworth, M. F. S., Passingham, R. E., Jahanshahi, M., and Rothwell, J. (2001). Interference with performance of a response selection task that has no working memory component: an rTMS comparison of the dorsolateral prefrontal and medial frontal cortex. *J. Cog. Neurosci.*, **13**, 1097–1108.

Halsband, U. and Passingham, R. E. (1985). Premotor cortex and the conditions for movement in monkeys (*Macaca fascicularis*). *Behav. Brain Res.*, **18**, 269–277.

Halsband, U., Matsuzaka, Y., and Tanji, J. (1994). Neuronal activity in the primate supplementary, pre-supplementary and premotor cortex during externally and internally instructed sequential movements. *Neurosci. Res.*, **20**, 149–155.

Hazeltine, E., Grafton, S. T., and Ivry, R. (1997). Attention and stimulus characteristic determine the locus of motor-sequence encoding. A PET study. *Brain*, **120**, 123–140.

Hikosaka, O., Rand, M. K., Miyachi, S., and Miyashita, K. (1995). Learning of sequential movements in the monkey: process of learning and retention of memory. *J. Neurophysiol.*, **74**, 1652–1661.

Hikosaka, O., Sakai, K., Miyauchi, S., Takino, R., Sasaki, Y., and Putz, B. (1996). Activation of human presupplementary motor area in learning of sequential procedures: a functional MRI study. *J. Neurophysiol.*, **76**, 617–621.

Hikosaka, O., Nakahara, H., Rand, M. K., Sakai, K., Lu, X., Nakamura, K., Miyachi, S., and Doya, K. (1999). Parallel neural networks for learning sequential procedures. *Trends Neurosci.*, **22**, 464–471.

Honda, M., Wise, S. P., Weeks, R. A., Deiber, M. P., and Hallett, M. (1998). Cortical areas with enhanced activation during object-centred spatial information processing. A PET study. *Brain,* **121**, 2145–2158.

Hoover, J. E. and Strick, P. L. (1999). The organisation of cerebellar and basal ganglia outputs to primary motor cortex as revealed by retrograde transneuronal transport of herpes simplex virus type 1. *J. Neurosci* ., **19**, 1446–1463.

Hyder, F., Phelps, E. A., Wiggins, C. J., Labar, K. S., Blamire, A. M., and Shulman, R. G. (1997). Willed action: a functional MRI study of the human prefrontal cortex during a sensorimotor task. *Proc. Nat. Acad. Sci. USA*, **94**, 6989–6994.

Iacaboni, M., Woods, R. P., Brass, M., Bekkering, H., Mazziotta, J. C., and Rizzolatti, G. (1999). Cortical mechanisms of human imitation. *Science*, **286**, 2526–2528.

Ivry, R. (1997). Cerebellar timing systems. *Int. Rev. Neurobiol.*, 41555–41573.

Jahanshahi, M., Jenkins, I. H., Brown, R. G., Marsden, C. D., Passingham, R. E., and Brooks, D. J. (1995). Self-initiated versus externally triggered movements. I. An investigation using regional cerebral blood flow and movement-related potentials in normals and Parkinson's disease. *Brain*, **118**, 913–934.

Jahanshahi, M., Dinberger, G., Fuller, R., and Frith, C. D. (2000). The role of the dorsolateral prefrontal cortex in random number generation: a study with positron emission tomography. *NeuroImage*, **12**, 713–725.

Jeannerod, M. (1994). The representing brain: neural correlates of motor intention and imagery. *Beh. Brain Sci.*, **17**, 187–245.

Jeannerod, M. (1997). *The Cognitive Neuroscience of Action*. Blackwell's, Oxford.

Jeannerod, M., Arbib, M. A., Rizolatti, G., and Sakata, H. (1995). Grasping objects: the cortical mechanisms of visuomotor transformation. *TINS*, **18**, 314–320.

Jenkins, I. H., Brooks, D. J., Nixon, P. D., Frackowiak, R. S. J., and Passingham, R. E. (1994). Motor sequence learning: a study with positron emission tomography. *J. Neurosci.*, **14**, 3775–3790.

Jenkins, I. H., Jahanshahi, M., Brown, R. G., Jueptner, M., Marsden, C. D., Passingham, R. E., and Brooks, D. J. (2000). Self-initiated versus externally triggered movements. II. The effect of response predictability and movement-related potentials. *Brain*, **123**, 1142–1154.

Johnson, P. B., Ferraina, S., Bianchi, L., and Caminiti, R. (1996). Cortical networks for visual reaching: physiological and anatomical organisation of frontal and parietal lobe arm regions. *Cereb. Cortex*, **6**, 102–119.

Jueptner, M., Frith, C. D., Brooks, D. J., Frackowiak, R. S., and Passingham, R. E. (1997a). Anatomy of motor learning. II. Subcortical structures and learning by trial and error. *J. Neurophysiol.*, **77**, 1325–1337.

Jueptner, M., Stephan, K. M., Frith, C. D., Brooks, D. J., Frackowiak, R. S. J., and Passingham, R. E. (1997b). Anatomy of motor learning. I. Frontal cortex and attention to action. *J. Neurophysiol.*,**77**, 1313–1324.

Karni, A., Meyer, G., Jezzard, P., Adams, M. M., Turner, R., and Ungerleider, L. G. (1995). Functional MRI evidence for adult motor cortex plasticity during motor skill learning. *Nature*, **377**, 155–158.

Karni, A., Meyer, G., Rey Hipolito, C., Jezzard, P., Adams, M. M., Turner, R., and Ungerleider, L. G. (1998). The acquisition of skilled motor performance: fast and slow experience-driven changes in primary motor cortex. *Proc. Nat. Acad. Sci. USA*, **95**, 861–868.

Le Goualher, G., Procyk, E., Collins, D. L., Venugopal, R., Barillot, C., and Evans, A. (1999). Automated extraction and variability analysis of sulcal neuroanatomy. *Trans. Med. Imaging*, **18**, 206–217.

Lee, K.-M., Change, K. H., and Roh, J.-K. (1999). Subregions within the supplementary motor area activated at different stages of movement preparation and execution. *NeuroImage*, **9**, 117–123.

Leung, H. C., Gore, J. C., Goldman–Rakic, P. S. (2002). Sustained mnemonic response in the human middle frontal gyrus during on-line storage of spacial memoranda. *J. Cogn. Neurosci.*, **14**, 659–671.

Logan, C. G. and Grafton, S. T. (1995). Functional anatomy of human eyeblink conditioning determined with regional cerebral glucose metabolism and positron-emission tomography. *Proc. Nat. Acad.Sci. USA.*, **92**, 7500–7504.

Lu, T., Preston, J. B., and Strick P. L. (1994). Interconnections between the prefrontal cortex and the premotor areas in the frontal lobe. *J. Comp. Neurol.*, **341**, 375–392.

Lu, X., Hikosaka, O., and Miyachi, S. (1998). Role of monkey cerebellar nuclei in skill for sequential movement. *J. Neurophysiol.*, **79**, 2245–2254.

Luppino, G., Matelli, M., Camarda, R., and Rizzolatti, G. (1993). Corticocortical connections of area F3 (SMA-proper) and area F6 (Pre-SMA) in the macaque monkey. *J. Comp. Neurol.*, **338**, 114–140.

Marconi, B., Genovesio, A., Battaglia-Mayer, A., Ferraina, S., Squatrito, S., Molinari, M., Lacquaniti, F., and Caminiti, R. (2001). Eye-hand coordination during reaching. 1. Anatomical relationships between parietal and frontal cortex. *Cereb. Cortex*, **11**, 513–528.

Matelli, M. and Luppino, G. (1996). Thalamic input to mesial and superior area 6 in the macaque monkey. *J. Comp. Neurol.*, **372**, 59–87.

Matelli, M., Camarda, M., Glickstein, M., and Rizzolatti, G. (1986). Afferent and efferent projections of the inferior area 6 in the macaque monkey. *J. Comp. Neurol*, **251**, 281–298.

Matelli, M., Govoni, P., Galletti, C., Kutz, D. F., and Luppino, G. (1998). Superior area 6 afferents from the superior parietal lobule in the macaque monkey. *J. Comp. Neurol.*, **402**, 327–352.

Matsuzaka, Y. and Tanji, J. (1996). Changing directions of forthcoming arm movements: neuronal activity in the presupplementary and supplementary motor area of monkey cerebral cortex. *J. Neurophysiol.*, **76**, 2327–2342.

Menon, R. S., Luknowsky, D. C., and Gati, J. S. (1998). Mental chronometry using latency-resolved functional MRI. *Proc. Nat. Acad. Sci.USA*, **95**, 10902–10907.

Miall, R. C., Reckess, G. Z., and Imamizu, H. (2001). The cerebellum coordinates eye and hand tracking movements. *Nat. Neurosci.*, **4**, 638–644.

Middleton, F. A. and Strick, P. L. (1997). Dentate output channels: motor and cognitive components. *Prog. Brain Res.*, **114**, 553–566.

Middleton, F. A. and Strick, P. L. (2001). Cerebellar projections to the prefrontal cortex of the primate. *J. Neurosci.*, **21**, 700–712.

Miller, E. K. and Asaad, W. F. (in press). The prefrontal cortex: conjunction and cognition, in *Handbook of Neuropsychology*, Grafman, J., Ed.

Miller, E. K. and Cohen, J. D. (2001). An integrative theory of prefrontal cortex function. *Ann. Rev. Neurosci.*, **24**, 167–202.

Milner, A. D. (1997). Vision without knowledge. *Philos. Trans. Roy. Soc. London B*, **352**, 1249–1256.

Milner, A. D. and Goodale, M. A. (1997). *The Visual Brain in Action*, Oxford University Press, London.

Mitz, A. R., Godschalk, M., and Wise, S. P. (1991). Learning-dependent neuronal activity in the premotor cortex: activity during the acquisition of conditional motor associations. *J. Neurosci.*, **11**, 1855–1872.

Miyachi, S., Hikosaka, O., Miyashita, K., Karadi, Z., and Rand, M. K. (1997). Differential roles of monkey striatum in learning of sequential hand movement. *Exp. Brain Res.*, **115**, 1–5.

Miyashita, K., Rand, M. K., Miyachi, S., and Hikosaka, O. (1996). Anticipatory saccades in sequential procedural learning in monkeys. *J. Neurophysiol.*, **76**, 1361–1366.

Muakkassa, K. F. and Strick, P. L. (1979). Frontal lobe inputs to primate motor cortex: evidence for four somatotopically organised "premotor areas". *Brain Res.*, **177**, 176–182.

Murata, A., Fadiga, L., Foigassi, L., Gallese, V., Raos, V., and Rizzolatti, G. (1997). Object representation in the ventral premotor cortex (area F5) of the monkey. *J. Neurophysiol.*, **78**, 2226–2230.

Murata, A., Gallese, V., Luppino, G., Kaseda, M., and Sakata, H. (2000). Selectivity for the shape, sise and orientation of objects for grasping in neurones of monkey parietal AIP. *J. Neurophysiol.*, **83**, 2580–2601.

Murray, E. A. and Bussey, T. J. (2001). Consolidation and the medial temporal lobe revisited: methodological considerations. *Hippocampus*, **11**, 1–7.

Murray, E. A. and Wise, S. P. (1996). Role of the hippocampus plus subjacent cortex but not amygdala in visuomotor conditional learning in rhesus monkeys. *Behav. Neurosci.*, **110**, 1261–1270.

Murray, E. A., Bussey, T. J., and Wise, S. P. (2000). Role of prefrontal cortex in a network for arbitrary visuomotor mapping. *Exp. Brain Res.*, **133**, 114–129.

Mushiake, H., Inase, M., and Tanji, J. (1991). Neuronal activity in the primate premotor, supplementary, and precentral motor cortex during visually guided and internally determined sequential movements. *J. Neurophysiol.*, **66**, 705–718.

Nakamura, K., Sakai, K., and Hikosaka, O. (1998). Neuronal activity in medial frontal cortex during learning of sequential procedures. *J. Neurophysiol.*, **80**, 2688–2698.

Nixon, P. D. and Passingham, R. E. (2000). The cerebellum and cognition: cerebellar lesions impair sequence learning but not conditional visuomotor learning in monkeys. *Neuropsychology*, **38**, 1054–1072.

Nudo, R. J., Milliken, G. W., Jenkins, W. M., and Merzenich, M. M. (1996). Use-dependent alterations of movement representations in primary motor cortex of adult squirrel monkeys. *J. Neurosci.*, **16**, 785–807.

O'Doherty, J., Kringelbach, M. L., Rolls, E. T., Hornak, J., and Andrews, C. (2001). Abstract reward and punishment representations in human orbitofrontal cortex. *Nat. Neurosci.*, **4**, 95–102.

Okano, K. and Tanji, J. (1987). Neuronal activity in the primate motor fields of the agranular frontal cortex preceding visually triggered and self-paced movements. *Exp. Brain Res.*, **66**, 155–166.

Owen, A. M., Downes, J. J., Sahakian, B. J., Polkey, C. E., and Robbins, T. W. (1990). Planning and spatial working memory following frontal lobe lesions in man. *Neuropsychology*, **28**, 1021–1034.

Owen, A. M., Doyon, J., Petrides, M., and Evans, A. C. (1996). Planning and spatial working memory: a positron emission tomography study in humans. *Eur. J. Neurosci.*, **8**, 353–364.

Owen, A., Herrod, N. J., Menon, D. K., Clark, J. C., Downey, S. P. M. J., Carpenter, A., Minhas, P. S., Turkhemier, F. E., Williams, E. J., Robbins, T. W., Sahakian, B. J., Petrides, M., and Pichard, J. D. (1999). Redefining the functional organisation of working memory processes within human lateral prefrontal cortex. *Eur. J. Neurosci.*, **11**, 567–574.

Pandya, D. N. and Yeterian, E. H. (1998). Comparison of prefrontal architecture and connections, in *The Prefrontal Cortex*, Roberts, A. C., Robbins, T. W., and Weiskrantz, L., Eds., pp. 51–66. Oxford University Press, London.

Parker, G. J. M., Stephan, K. E., Barker, G. J., Rowe, J. B, MacManus, D. G., Wheeler-Kingshott, A. M., Ciccarrelli, Passingham, R. E., Spinks, R. L., Lemon, R. N., and Turner, R. (2002). Initial demonstration of *in vivo* tracing of axonal projections in the macaque brain and comparison with the human brain using diffusion tensor imaging and fast marching tractography. *Neuroimage*, **15**, 797–809.

Passingham, R. E. (1993). *The Frontal Lobes and Voluntary Action*, Oxford University Press, London.

Passingham, R. E. (1996). Attention to action, *Philos. Trans. Roy. Soc. London B: Biol. Sci.*, **351**, 1473–1479.

Passingham, R. E. and Rowe, J. B. (2002). Dorsal prefrontal cortex: maintenance in memory or attentional selection. In *Principles of Frontal Lobe Function*, Stuss, D. T. and Knight, R. T. Eds., pp. 221–232, Oxford University Press, Oxford.

Passingham, R. E. and Toni, I. (2001). Contrasting the dorsal and ventral visual systems: guidance of movement versus decision making. *NeuroImage*, **14**, S125–S131.

Passingham, R. E., Toni, I., Schluter, N., and Rushworth, M. F. S. (1998). How do visual instructions influence the motor system?, in *Sensory Guidance of Movement*, Bock, C. R. and Goode, J., Eds., pp. 129–141. Wiley, Chichester.

Passingham, R. E., Toni, I., and Rushworth, M. F. S. (2000). Specialisation within the prefrontal cortex: the ventral prefrontal cortex and associative learning. *Exp. Brain Res.*, **113**, 103–113.

Passingham, R. E., Stephan, K., and Kotter, R. (2002). The anatomical basis of functional localisation in the cortex. *Nat. Rev. Neurosci.*, **3**, 606–616.

Paus, T., Tomaiuolo, F., Otaky, N., MacDonald, D., Petrides, M., Atlas, J., Morris, R., and Evans, A. C. (1996). Human cingulate and paracingulate sulci: pattern, variability, asymmetry, and probabilistic map. *Cereb. Cortex*, **6**, 207–214.

Pedersen, J. R., Johansoen, P., Bak, C. K., Kofoed, B., Saermark, K., and Gjedde, A. (1998). Origin of human readiness field linked to left middle frontal gyrus by MEG and PET. *NeuroImage*, **8**, 214–220.

Petrides, M. (1985). Deficits in non-spatial conditional associative learning after periarcuate lesions in the monkey. *Behav. Brain Res.*, **16**, 95–101.

Petrides, M. (1998). Specialised systems for the processing of mnemonic information within the primate frontal cortex, in *The Prefrontal Cortex*, Roberts, A. C., Robbins, T. W., and Weiskrantz, L., Eds., pp. 103–116. Oxford University Press, London.

Petrides, M., Alivisatos, B., Evans, A. C., and Meyer, E. (1993). Dissociation of human mid-dorsolateral from posterior dorsolateral frontal cortex in memory processing. *Proc. Nat. Acad. Sci. USA*, **90**, 873–877.

Petrides, M. and Pandya, D. N. (1999). Dorsolateral prefrontal cortex: comparative cytoarchitectonic analysis in the human and the macaque brain and corticocortical connection patterns. *Eur. J. Neurosci.*, **11**, 1011–1036.

Pochon, J.-B., Levy, R., Poline, J.-B., Crozier, S., Lehericy, S., Pillon, B., Deweer, B., Bihan, D. L., and Dubois, B. (2001). The role of dorsolateral prefrontal cortex in the preparation of forthcoming actions: an fMRI study. *Cereb. Cortex*, **11**, 260–266.

Postle, B. R. and D'Esposito, M. (1999). "What–then–where" in visual working memory: an event-related fMRI study. *J. Cog. Neurosci.*, **11**, 585–597.

Poupon, C., Clark, C. A., Frouin, V., Regis, J., Bloch, I., Le Bihan, D., and Mangin, J.-F. (2000). Regularisation of diffused-based direction maps for the tracking of brain white matter fascicles. *NeuroImage*, **12**, 184–195.

Rainer, G., Asaad, W. F., and Miller, E. K. (1998). Memory fields of neurons in the primate prefrontal cortex. *Proc. Nat. Acad. of Sci. USA*, **95**, 15008–15013.

Ramnani, N. and Miall, R. C. (2003). Instructed delay activity in the human prefrontal cortex is modulated by monetary reward expectation. *Cer. Cortex*, **13**, 318–327.

Ramnani, N. and Passingham, R. E. (2000). Timing error in the human brain during classical eyeblink conditioning: an event-related fMRI study. *Soc. NeuroSci. Abstr.*, **26**, 1851.

Ramnani, N. and Passingham, R. E. (2001). Changes in the human brain during rhythm learning. *J. Cog. Neurosci.*, **13**, 1–15.

Ramnani, N., Toni, I., Josephs, O., Ashburner, J., and Passingham, R. E. (2000). Learning- and expectation-related changes in the human brain during motor learning. *J. Neurophysiol.*, **84**, 3026–3035.

Ramnani, N., Toni, I., Passingham, R. E., and Haggard, P. (2001). The cerebellum and parietal cortex play a specific role in coordination: a PET study. *Neuroimage*, **14**, 885–911.

Rao, S. C., Rainer, G., and Miller, E. K. (1997). Integration of what and where in the primate prefrontal cortex. *Science*, **276**, 821–824.

Rajkowska, G. and Goldman-Rakic, P. S. (1995). Cytoarchitectonic definition of prefrontal areas in the normal human cortex. II. Variability in locations of areas 9 and 46 and relationship to Talairach coordinate system. *Cer. Cortex*, **5**, 323–337.

Richter, W., Andersen, P. M., Georgopoulos, A. P., and Kim, S.-G. (1997). Sequential activity in human motor areas during a delayed cued finger movement task studied by time-resolved fMRI. *Neuroreport*, **8**, 1257–1261.

Rizzolatti, G. and Arbib, M. A. (1998). Language within our grasp. *TINS*, **21**, 188–194.

Rizzolatti, G., Luppino, G., and Matelli, M. (1998). The organisation of the cortical motor system: new concepts. *EEG Clin. Neurophysiol.*, **106**, 283–296.

Romo, R. and Schultz, W. (1987). Neuronal activity preceding self-initiated or externally timed arm movements in area 6 of monkey cortex. *Exp. Brain Res.*, **67**, 656–662.

Roland, P. E. and Zilles, K. (1994). Brain atlases: a new research tool? *Trends Neurosci.*, **17**, 458–467.

Rolls, E. T. (2000). The orbitofrontal cortex and reward. *Cer. Cortex*, **10**, 284–294.

Rolls, E. T. and Baylis, L.L. (1994). Gustatory, olfactory and visual convergence within the primate orbitofrontal cortex. *J. Neurosci.*, **14**, 5432–5452.

Rowe, J. and Passingham, R. E. (2001). Working memory for location and time: activity in prefrontal area 46 relates to selection rather than to maintenance in memory. *NeuroImage*, **14**, 77–86.

Rowe, J. B., Toni, I., Josephs, O., Frackowiak, R. S. J., and Passingham, R. E. (2000). Prefrontal cortex: response selection or maintenance within working memory. *Science*, **288**, 1656–1660

Rowe, J., Johnstrude, I., Owen, A. M., and Passingham, R. E. (2001). Imaging the mental components of a planning task. *Neuropsychology*, **39**, 315–327.

Rowe, J., Frackowiak, R. S. J., Friston, K., and Passingham, R. E. (2002a). Attention to action: specific modulation of corticocortical interactions in humans. *NeuroImage*, **17**, 988–998.

Rowe, J., Stephan, K. E., Friston, K., Frackowiak, R. S. J., Lees, A., and Passingham, R. E. (2002b). Attention to action in Parkinson's disease: impaired effective connectivity among frontal cortical regions. *Brain*, **125**, 276–239.

Rushworth, M. (2000). Anatomical and functional subdivision within the primate lateral frontal cortex. *Psychobiology*, **28**, 187–196.

Rushworth, M., Krams, M., and Passingham, R. E. (2001). The attentional role of the left parietal cortex: the distinct lateralisation and localisation of motor attention in the human brain. *J. Cog. Neurosci.*, **13**, 698–710.

Sakai, K., Hikosaka, O., Miyauchi, S., Takino, R., Sasaki, Y., and Putz, B. (1998). Transition of brain activation from frontal to parietal areas in visuomotor sequence learning. *J. Neurosci.*, **18**, 1827–1840.

Sakai, K., Hikosaka, O., Takino, R., Miyauchi, S., Nielsen, M., and Tamada, T. (2000). What and when: parallel and convergent processing in motor control. *J. Neurosci.*, **20**, 2691–2700.

Sakata, H., Taira, M., Kusonoki, M., Murata, A., and Tanaka, V. (1997). The parietal association cortex in depth perception and visual control of hand action. *Trends Neurosci.*, **20**, 350–356.

Sawaguchi, T. and Yamane, I. (1999). Properties of delay-period activity in the monkey dorsolateral prefrontal cortex during a spatial delayed matching to sample task. *J. Neurophysiol.*, **82**, 2070–2080.

Schmahmann, J. D. and Pandya, D. N. (1997). The cerebrocerellar system, in *The Cerebellum and Cognition*, Schmahmann, J. E., Ed., pp. 31–60. Academic Press, San Diego.

Schreurs, B. G., McIntosh, A. R., Bahro, M., Herscovich, P., Sunderland, T., and Molchan, S. E. (1997). Lateralisation and behavioural correlation of changes in regional cerebral blood flow with classical conditioning of the human eyeblink response. *J. Neurophysiol. Bethesda*, **77**, 2153–2163.

Schultz, W., Tremblay, L., and Hollerman, J. R. (2000). Reward processing in primate orbitofrontal cortex and basal ganglia. *Cereb. Cortex*, **10**, 272–283.

Selemon, L. D. and Goldman-Rakic, P. S. (1985). Longitudinal topography and interdigitation of corticostriatal projections in the rhesus monkey. *J. Neurosci.*, **5**, 776–794.

Sereno, A. B. and Maunsell, J. H. R. (1998). Shape selectivity in primate lateral intraparietal cortex. *Nature*, **395**, 500–503.

Sergent, J., Zuck, E., Terriah, S., and MacDonald, B. (1992). Distributed neural network underlying musical sight-reading and keyboard performance. *Science*, **257**, 106–109.

Shadmehr, R. and Holcomb, H. H. (1997). Neural correlates of motor memory consolidation. *Science*, **277**, 821–825.

Shallice, T. (1982). Specific impairments of planning. *Philos. Trans. Roy. Soc. London B*, **298**, 199–209.

Shen, L. and Alexander, G. E. (1997). Preferential representation of instructed target location versus limb trajectory in dorsal premotor cortex. *J. Neurophysiol.*, **77**, 1195–1212.

Shima, K. and Tanji, J. (2000). Neuronal activity in the supplementary and presupplementary motor areas for temporal organisation of multiple movements. *J. Neurophysiol.*, **84**, 2148–2160.

Spence, S. A., Hirsch, S. R., Brooks, D. J., and Grasby, P. M. (1998). Prefrontal cortex activity in people with schizophrenia and control subjects. *J. Psychiatry*, **172**, 1–8.

Stephan, K. E., Kamper, L., Bozkurt, A., Burns, G. A., Young, M. P., and Kötter, R. Advanced database methodology for the collation of connectivity data on the Macoque brain (CoCoMac). *Philos. Trans. R. Soc. Lond. B Biol. Sci.*, **356**, 1159–1186.

Tanji, J. and Shima, K. (1994). Role for supplementary motor area cells in planning several moves ahead. *Nature*, **371**, 413–416.

Tanne, J., Boussaoud, D., Boyer-Zeller, N., and Roullier, E. (1995). Parietal inputs to physiologically defined regions of dorsal premotor cortex in macaque monkey. *NeuroReport*, **7**, 267–272.

Thut, G., Schultz, W., Nienhusmeier, M., Missimer, J., Maguire, R. P., and Leenders, K. L. (1997). Activation of the human brain by monetary reward. *NeuroReport*, **8**, 1225–1228.

Tomaiulo, F., MacDonald, J. D., Caramanos, Z., Posner, G., Chiavaras, M., Evans, A. C., and Petrides, M. (1999). Morphology, morphometry and probability mapping of the pars opercularis of the inferior frontal gyrus: an *in vivo* MRI analysis. *Eur. J. Neurosci.*, **11**, 3033–3046.

Tomita, H., Ohbayashi, M., Namahara, K., Hasaegawa, I., and Miyashita, M. (1999). Top–down signal from prefrontal cortex in executive control of memory retrieval. *Nature*, **401**, 699–703.

Toni, I. and Passingham, R. E. (1999). Prefrontal-basal ganglia pathways are involved in the learning of arbitrary visuomotor associations: a PET study. *Exp. Brain Res.*, **127**, 19–32.

Toni, I., Ramnani, N., Josephs, O., Asburner, J., and Passingham, R. E. (2001). Learning arbitrary visuomotor associations: temporal dynamic of brain activity. *NeuroImage*, **14**, 1048–1057.

Toni, I., Krams, M., Turner, R., and Passingham, R. E. (1998). The time course of changes during motor sequence learning: a whole brain fMRI study. *NeuroImage*, **8**, 50–61.

Toni, I., Schluter, N. D., Josephs, O., Friston, K., and Passingham, R. E. (1999). Signal-, set- and movement-related activity in the human brain: an event-related fMRI study. *Cer. Cortex*, **9**, 35–49.

Toni, I., Rowe, J., and Passingham, R. E. (2002a). Changes of cortico-striatal effective connectivity during visuo-motor learning. *Cereb. Cortex*, **12**, 1040–1047.

Toni, I., Rushworth, M. F. S., and Passingham, R. E. (2001). Neural correlates of visuomotor associations: spatial vs arbitrary rules. *Exp. Brain Res.*, **141**, 359–369.

Toni, I., Shah, N. J., Fink, G. R., Thoenissen, D., Passingham, R. E., and Zilles, K. (2002b). Multiple movement representations in the human brain: an event-related fMRI study. *J. Cogn. Neurosci.*, **14**, 769–784.

Toth, L. J. and Asaad, J. A. (1999). Visual stimulus selectivity during an association task in LIP. *Soc. Neurosci. Abs.*, **25**, 1546.

Tremblay, L., Hollerman, J. R., and Schultz, W. (1998). Modifications of reward expectation-related neuronal activity during learning in primate striatum. *J. Neurophysiol.*, **80**, 964–977.

Tremblay, L. and Schultz, W. (1999). Relative reward preference in primate orbitofrontal cortex. *Nature*, **398**, 704–708.

Tucker, J., Harding, A., Jananshahi, M., Nixon, P. E., Rushworth, M., Quinn, N., Thompson, P., Passingham, R. E. (1997). Associative learning in patients with cerebellar ataxia. *Beh. Neurosci.* **110**, 1229–1234.

Ungerleider, L. G. and Desimone, R. (1986). Cortical connections of visual area MT in the macaque. *J. Comp. Neurol.*, **248**, 190–222.

Ungerleider, L. G. and Mishkin, M. (1982). Two cortical visual systems, in *Advances in the Analysis of Visual_Behavior*, Ingle, D. J., Mansfield, J. W., and Goodale, M. A., Eds., pp. 549–586. MIT Press, Cambridge, MA.

Van Ham, J. J. and Yeo, C. H. (1996). Trigeminal inputs to eyeblink motoneurons in the rabbit. *Exp. Neurol.*, **142**, 244–257.

van Hoesen, G., Yeterian, E. H., and Lavizzo-Mourey, R. (1981). Widespread corticostriate projection from temporal cortex of the rhesus monkey. *J. Comp. Neurol.*, **199**, 205–219.

Van Mier, H., Tempel, L. W., Perlmutter, J. S., Raichle, M. E., and Petersen, S. E. (1998). Changes in brain activity during motor learning measured with PET: effects of hand of performance and practice. *J. Neurophysiol.*, **80**, 2177–2199.

von Bonin, G. and Bailey, P. (1947). *The Neocortex of Macaca Mulatta*. University of Illinois Press, Urbana.

Wallis, J. D., Anderson, K. C., and Miller, E. K. (2001). Single neurons in prefrontal cortex encode abstract rules. *Nature*, **411**, 953–956.

Watanabe, M. (1996). Reward expectancy in primate prefrontal neurones. *Nature*, **382**, 629–632.

Webster, M. J., Bachevalier, J., and Ungerleider, L. G. (1994). Connections of inferior temporal areas TEO and TE with parietal and frontal cortex in macaque monkeys. *Cer. Cortex*, **4**, 471–483.

Weeks, R. A., Honda, H., Gatalan, M.-J., and Hallett, M. (2001). Comparison of auditory, somatosensory, and visually instructed and internally generated finger movements: a PET study. *NeuroImage*, **14**, 219–230.

Weilke, F., Spiegel, S., Boecker, H., von Einsiedel, H. G., Conrad, B., Schwaiger, M., and Erhard, P. (2001). Time-resolved fMRI of activation patterns in MI and SMA during complex voluntary movement. *J. Neurophysiol.*, **85**, 1858–1863.

Weinrich, M., Wise, S. P., and Mauritz, K.-H. (1984). A neurophysiological study of the premotor cortex in the rhesus monkey. *Brain*, **107**, 385–414.

Winstein, C. J., Grafton, S. T., and Pohl, P. S. (1997). Motor task difficulty and brain activity: an investigation of reciprocal aiming using positron emission tomography. *J. Neurophysiol.*, **77**, 1581–1594.

Wise, S. P. and Murray, E. A. (1999). Role of the hippocampal system in conditional motor learning: mapping antecedents to action. *Hippocampus*, **9**, 101–117.

Wise, S. P. and Murray, E. A. (2000). Arbitrary associations between antecedents and actions. *Trends Neurosci.*, **23**, 271–276.

Yeo, C. H. (1991). Cerebellum and classical conditioning of motor responses. *Ann. N.Y. Acad. Sci.*, 627292–627304.

Yeo, C. H. and Hardiman, M. J. (1992). Cerebellar cortex and eyeblink conditioning: a reexamination. *Exp. Brain Res.*, **88**, 623–638.

Yeo, C. H., Hardiman, M. J., and Glickstein, M. (1985). Classical conditioning of the nictitating membrane response of the rabbit. I. Lesions of the cerebellar nuclei. *Exp. Brain Res.*, **60**, 87–98.

Young, M. P. (1992). Objective analysis of the topological organisation of the primate cortical visual system. *Nature*, **358**, 152–154.

Young, M. P. (1993). The organisation of neural systems in the primate cerebral cortex. *Proc. Roy. Soc. London B*, **252**, 13–18.

Zilles, K., Schlaug, G., Geyer, S., Luppino, G., Matelli, M., Qu, M., Schleicher, A., and Schormann, T. (1996). Anatomy and transmitter receptors of the supplementary motor area in the human and nonhuman primate brain. *Adv. Neurol.*, **70**, 29–44.

CHAPTER

2

Motor Control of Breathing

INTRODUCTION

Breathing is an unusual motor act. Rhythmic breathing is essential for gas exchange, each inspiration bringing oxygen-rich air into the lungs, and each expiration removing carbon dioxide. However, in addition to automatic rhythm generation for gas exchange at rest, breathing must be controlled for other acts such as coughing, sneezing, and swallowing and for complex behaviours such as vocalisation and exercise. In humans, breathing can also be controlled voluntarily; breaths can be taken or held at will. Breathing is further modulated by arousal and by emotion.

A wealth of evidence from non-human species indicates that specialised structures within the brain stem are essential for the generation of the rhythmic motor activity (Feldman, 1986; Rekling and Feldman, 1998). It is understandable that relatively little has been learned about the behavioural control of breathing from studies on non-humans; however, with the advent of methodologies to study human brain function—$H_2{}^{15}O$ positron emission tomography (PET) and functional magnetic resonance imaging (fMRI), in particular—we have begun to gain significant new information about the control of breathing in humans. The purpose of this chapter is to summarise what we have learned from a series of related functional imaging studies of breathing in humans and, from these, to compare the control of breathing with the control of other motor acts.

BACKGROUND

To most neuroscientists, and to the likely readership of this book, the control of breathing is a small and unfamiliar niche. So, as background to the subsequent discussion of the neuroimaging studies, it is useful to summarise a few essential elements of breathing physiology and breathing behaviour.

An Outline of Breathing Physiology

At rest, contraction of the diaphragm and of the inspiratory intercostals muscles expands the chest wall; this stretches the lungs. As a result, pressure within the lungs falls and an inspiratory flow of air occurs. On expiration, the inspiratory muscles relax and the elastic recoil of the stretched tissues compresses the lungs, leading to expiration; thus, expiration at rest is passive and requires no active muscle contraction. When breathing is sufficiently fast or deep or performed against a resistance, inspiration will be augmented by the recruitment of further muscle groups acting on the chest wall, most notably by the sternocleidomastoid, scalene, and pectoral muscles. Expiration can be augmented by contraction of the expiratory intercostal muscles and by the abdominal muscles; this active process is essential for expirations that require more force than that achieved by elastic recoil or to expel air out of the lungs below a normal end-expiratory lung volume. For breathing to occur, contraction of the "pump" muscles must be accompanied by the appropriate control of upper airways calibre; this is achieved by the coordinated control of the muscles of the larynx and pharynx.

In animals, specialised areas within the pons and medulla, the *respiratory centres*, generate a rhythmic motor output to the muscles of the pump and upper airways (Feldman, 1986; Rekling and Feldman, 1998). The respiratory centres contain a group of pace-making neurons that generate a regular rhythm (Smith *et al.*, 1991; Gray *et al.*, 2001); this rhythm is converted into a patterned motor output. Respiratory activity is modulated by afferent feedback, most importantly from stretch receptors in the lungs and from chemoreceptors in the carotid bodies and within the brainstem. Increasing the level of arterial CO_2 or decreasing arterial O_2 stimulates breathing as part of a homeostatic negative feedback loop. Classically, in lower mammals, stretching the lungs inhibits inspiration and prolongs expiration; the importance of this mechanism in humans is not clear. The respiratory centres in the brainstem are closely related to, but independent of, areas responsible for cardiovascular control (Taylor *et al.*, 1999). It is worth remembering that, although rhythmic breathing is controlled automatically, it is not under the control of the autonomic nervous system; the pump and upper airways muscles are all striated and innervated by either spinal or cranial nerves.

CO_2 and the Control of Breathing in Humans

In humans, during sleep and under anaesthesia, rhythmic breathing is critically dependent on the level of arterial PCO_2; even a slight reduction in arterial PCO_2 leads to a cessation of breathing rhythm (Datta *et al.*, 1991). Although there is no direct evidence, the neural control of such rhythmic breathing in humans is presumably similar to that in other mammals; however, during wakefulness, human breathing is far less dependent on CO_2. Ventilation may be stimulated when the level of CO_2 is artificially increased, but, in direct contrast to sleep, breathing will continue despite marked reductions in PCO_2 (Fink, 1961; Corfield *et al.*, 1995b). Fink (1961) used the term *wakefulness stimulus* to describe this non-reflex phenomenon that maintains breathing during wakefulness. The importance of the wakefulness drive is demonstrated by many abnormalities of respiratory control that are most evident during sleep. For example, patients with lesions in the rostrolateral medulla breathe normally during wakefulness but suffer from sleep-disordered breathing (Morrell *et al.*, 1999). Additionally, patients with congenital central hypoventilation syndrome (who lack any respiratory sensitivity to CO_2) maintain adequate ventilation during wakefulness but markedly hypoventilate or cease breathing during non-rapid eye movement (NREM) sleep (Shea, 1997). The neural basis for this CO_2-independent wakefulness drive is uncertain, but it is likely to include supra-brainstem structures.

Any complete description of the neural control of breathing in humans must be able to explain the full range of human breathing activities including such state-related differences in control. The subsequent sections describe what we have learned of this control up to the present from respiratory neuroimaging studies.

VOLUNTARY CONTROL OF BREATHING

The first neurophysiological evidence that breathing muscles are represented within the human primary motor cortex was obtained by Foerster (1936) in his neurosurgical studies to map sensory and motor representations on the human cortex. He reported that direct electrical stimulation of the exposed cortical surface could result in a "hiccup" caused by diaphragm contraction. The focus for this response was a site slightly anterior to the representation of the thorax on the dorsal portion of the motor homunculus (see figure reproduced in Maskill *et al.*, 1991). More recently, percutaneous electrical stimulation in humans has demonstrated that the excitatory pathway from the motor cortex to the diaphragm is fast conducting and oligosynaptic (Gandevia and Rothwell, 1987). Observations using transcranial magnetic stimulation (TMS) have confirmed these findings (Murphy *et al.*, 1990). Focal TMS of the motor cortex has demonstrated that the activation of the diaphragm is predominantly contralateral (Maskill *et al.*, 1991), with its anatomical focus on the scalp slightly lateral to and behind the vertex—a site

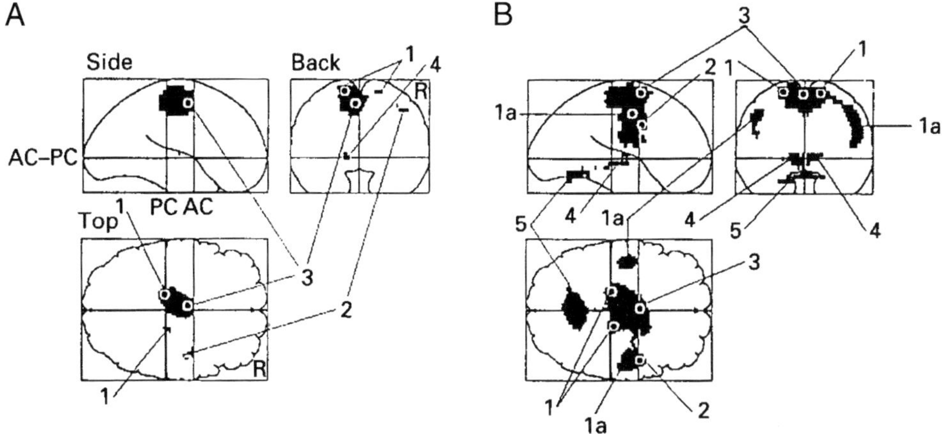

FIGURE 2.1
Voluntary breathing: PET. Glass brain projection identifying sites of significantly increased regional cerebral blood flow ($H_2{}^{15}O$ PET) associated with (A) volitional inspiration and (B) volitional expiration, each compared with passive ventilation as the control. 1, Superolateral left and right primary motor cortex; 2, right premotor area; 3, supplementary motor area; 4, thalamus; 5, cerebellum. $N = 5$; $p < 0.05$ corrected. (From Ramsay, S. C. *et al.*, *J. Physiol.*, 461, 85–101, 1993. With permission.)

consistent with Foerster's original observation. It is noteworthy that, despite the representation of each hemidiaphragm in each contralateral motor cortex, we cannot control the two halves independently; the site of this integration is unknown.

Colebatch *et al.* (1991) performed the first PET study of voluntary breathing. Regional cerebral blood flow was determined during voluntary, self-paced overbreathing, with active inspiration and relaxed (passive) expiration. As a control, breathing was performed at the same increased level using positive pressure mechanical ventilation (passive inspiration/passive expiration). To maintain a normal and unchanged global cerebral blood flow, each condition was performed at a constant arterial PCO_2, close to a resting level. Voluntary inspiration was associated with increased activity bilaterally within the primary motor cortex at a dorsolateral position compatible with the findings of both Foerster (1936) and Maskill *et al.* (1991). Additionally, activity was identified in the premotor cortex, the supplementary motor area (SMA), and the cerebellum. With an extended protocol, Ramsay *et al.* (1993a) confirmed these findings (Fig. 2.1A) and demonstrated that voluntary active expiration was also associated with increased activity bilaterally within the dorsolateral primary motor cortex (Fig. 2.1B). This area overlapped that associated with voluntary inspiration and presumably reflects the close representation of inspiratory (diaphragm and intercostals) and expiratory (intercostals and abdominal) muscles in the primary motor cortex. More surprisingly, active expiration was associated with extensive activity in more ventrolateral motor cortical areas (Fig. 2.1B). Neither the cortical map of Foerster (1936) nor that of Penfield and Boldrey (1938) shows representations of the chest and abdomen at these sites and so does not readily explain the observed activity. However, active expiration may also be associated with increased activity in the muscles of the larynx, pharynx, and mouth; these do have representations in this area. The lower half of the precentral gyrus is also associated with the representation of vocalisation (Penfield and Boldrey, 1938). Precise control of expiratory airflow is an important component of vocalisation, and the ventrolateral activity reported by Ramsay *et al.* (1993a) may reflect the needs of this task. The control of breathing for speech is discussed further below.

A PET study designed principally to investigate the pattern of neural activity associated with increasing inspiratory force (self-paced breathing against increasing inspiratory loads) highlights both the extent of the corticomotor representation of breathing-related muscles and also the importance of the baseline/control condition in determining the pattern of observed activity (Fink *et al.*, 1996). When compared with passive, positive-pressure breathing, inspiratory force generation was associated with increased activity principally within the superolateral primary motor cortex, the premotor cortex, the SMA, cingulate cortex, and medial and lateral areas of the

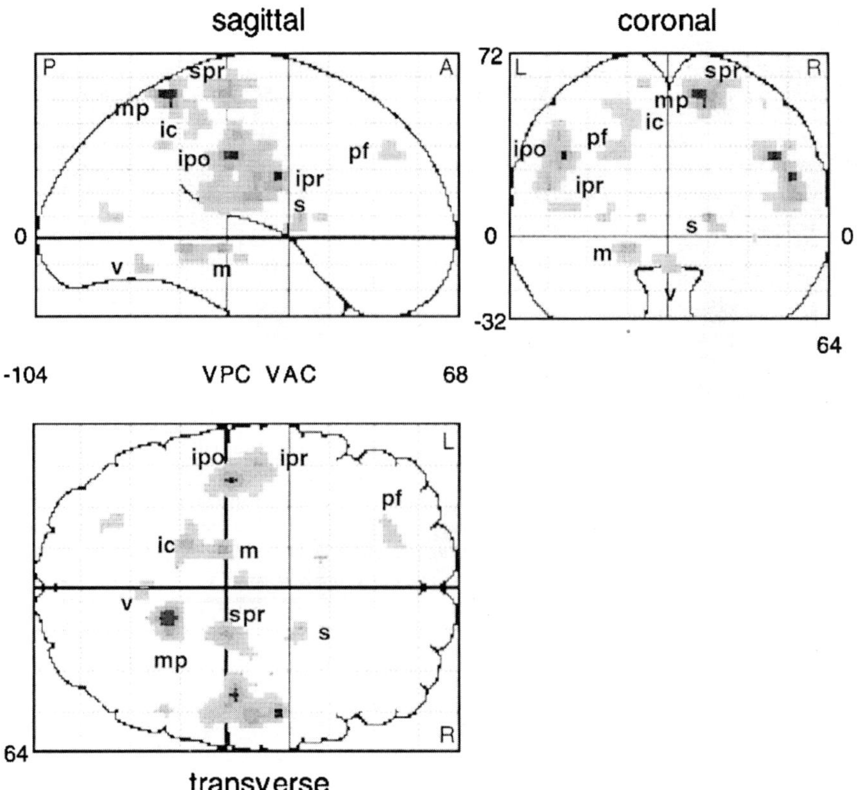

FIGURE 2.2
Forced inspiration. Glass brain projection identifying significant increases in relative regional cerebral blood flow ($H_2{}^{15}O$ PET) associated with forced inspiration, when compared with unloaded volitional breathing as a control. spr, Superolateral precentral gyrus; ipr, inferolateral precentral gyrus; ipo, inferolateral postcentral gyrus; mp, medial parietal cortex; m, midbrain; pf, prefrontal cortex (*); ic, intermediate cingulate cortex (*); s, striatum (*); v, vermis (*). $N = 6$; $p < 0.001$; $*0.001 < p < 0.01$ uncorrected. (From Fink, G. R. *et al.*, *J. Appl. Physiol.*, 81, 1295–1305, 1996. With permission.)

parietal cortex. When unloaded paced breathing was used as a control (Fig. 2.2), the SMA signal change failed to reach significance, and the superolateral motor cortical signal was weaker, indicating a significant role for these structures in the generation of unloaded paced breathing. With this latter condition as control, strong and extensive activity was revealed in inferolateral primary sensory and motor areas during both loaded breathing and passive, positive-pressure breathing. Activity within these regions of the cortex suggest that active control of muscles in the upper airways and mouth are important in stabilising these structures during both respiratory manoeuvres. Passive ventilation may therefore be an appropriate control condition for the breathing pump muscles but not for other respiratory-related muscle actions.

The most complete pattern of activity associated with voluntary breathing has been obtained more recently utilising the greater sensitivity of fMRI (McKay *et al.*, 2003). When voluntary hyperventilation is compared with spontaneous breathing (*i.e.*, passive ventilation is not the control), clear focal activity is seen bilaterally within the same superolateral primary motor cortical areas identified using PET and in the immediately adjacent primary sensory cortex. With the enhanced spatial resolution of fMRI, the activity within the superolateral areas can be resolved into two distinct foci, one with a more anterior location (Fig. 2.3). With reference to the cortical map of Foerster, it is most likely that the more anterior focus represents, specifically, the diaphragm, and the focus closer to the sulcus represents the intercostals muscles. Additionally, voluntary breathing is associated with focal activity within the SMA; the parietal, temporal, and anterior cingulate cortices; and subcortical structures, including the anterior thalamic nuclei, the basal ganglia (globus pallidus and caudate nucleus), the medulla, and a number of foci within the cerebellum.

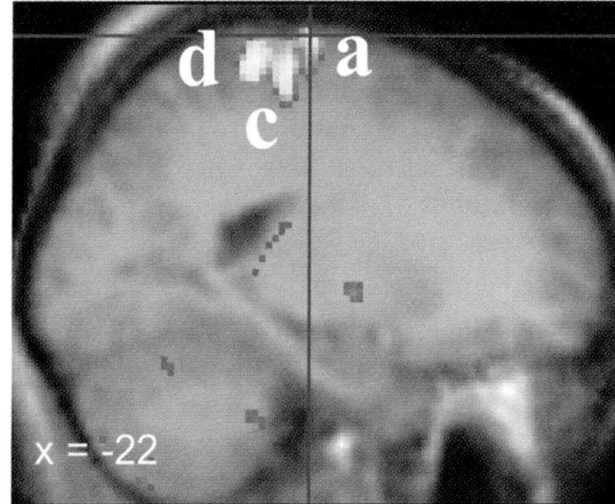

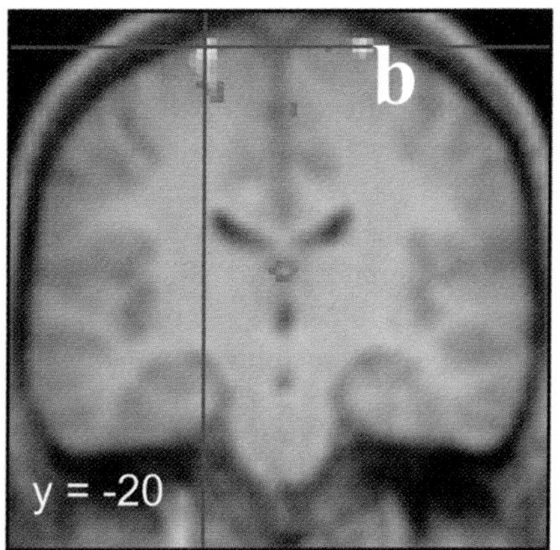

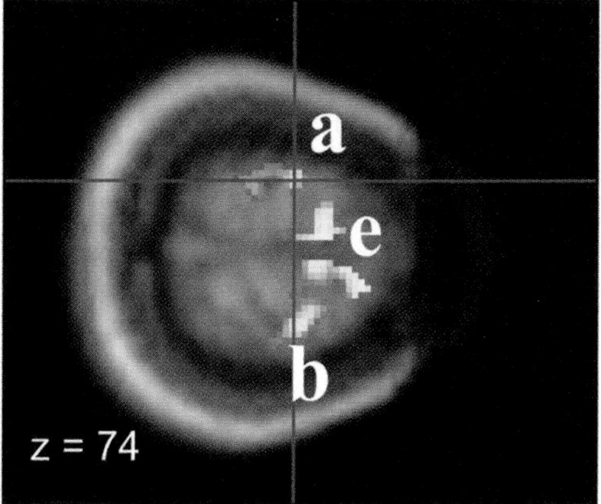

FIGURE 2.3
Voluntary breathing: fMRI. Significant activity associated with voluntary hyperventilation determined using BOLD (blood-oxygen-level-dependent) fMRI with spontaneous breathing as a control. Foci can be identified bilaterally in the anterior, superolateral primary motor cortex (a, b; cross hair at maximum a). Additional sites of activity can be seen, with the foci maxima out of plane: posterior primary motor cortex (c), primary sensory cortex (d), supplementary motor cortex (e). With reference to Foerster (1936), foci at a and b may represent the diaphragm. $N = 6$; $p < 0.05$ corrected. (Data from Mckay *et al.*, 2003.)

In summary, these PET and fMRI studies clearly indicate that the control of voluntary breathing, taking deliberate breaths in or out, is mediated in a similar way as other voluntary motor tasks (Fink *et al.*, 1997; Passingham, 1997).

CONTROL FOR OTHER BREATHING BEHAVIOURS

It might be argued that voluntary breathing is not a typical breathing act and that the neural basis for its control is not relevant to the control of other breathing behaviours; however, an underlying hypothesis drove the voluntary breathing studies described above: The restricted structures defined in animals that generate reflex rhythmic breathing could not alone control most human breathing behaviours. Further, the neural basis for much behavioural breathing in humans might be mediated by the voluntary motor system. The purpose of this section is to summarise the finding of some neuroimaging studies that have tested these hypotheses.

Breathing for Exercise

Physical exercise increases ventilation in proportion to the workload by mechanisms that are generally assumed to be reflex in nature, acting via brainstem respiratory neurons. These reflex stimuli may include signals from the peripheral chemoreceptors in the carotid bodies, exercising muscles, lungs and heart. However, studies in patients following carotid body resection

(Wasserman *et al.*, 1975), heart–lung transplantation (Banner *et al.*, 1989), and spinal cord transection (Adams *et al.*, 1984) show a virtually normal ventilatory response to steady-state exercise. Alternatively, ventilation may be driven by "central command" as part of a feed-forward motor program for exercise. This concept was first proposed by Krogh and Lindhart (1913) but has remained largely untested (and untestable) until the advent of human neuro-imaging. In the first of two complementary experiments (Fink *et al.*, 1995), volunteers performed right-leg exercise during PET scanning; the exercise was adequate to increase oxygen consumption 2.5-fold. As a control, scanning was performed during passive right-leg movement and passive positive-pressure ventilation. Both group and single subject analyses revealed that exercise was associated with increased activity within superomedial primary motor cortex (the motor "leg" area); this activity was present on the left side in those individuals who performed the task satisfactorily and present bilaterally in those who co-contracted the left leg. Activity was also present bilaterally in the superolateral primary motor cortex (Fig. 2.4A) at a location consistent with the voluntary breathing motor cortical foci (discussed above). To address concerns that: (1) the volunteers were not naïve to the outcome (all six were co-authors of the paper) and (2) the superolateral motor cortical activity might reflect involuntary contraction of trunk muscles, a second study was performed in naïve subjects. These subjects were scanned immediately following bicycle exercise, when breathing was still increased but when all exercising muscles were relaxed (Fink *et al.*, 1995). When compared to the passive positive ventilation control, this study again revealed activity bilaterally within the superolateral primary motor cortex in the areas activated during exercise (Fig. 4B). Taken together, these two studies provide direct evidence for motor cortical involvement in the control of breathing during exercise in humans.

Breathing for Speech

The act of speaking demands simultaneous control of muscles of the respiratory pump, the larynx, the palate, and the face, this motor control being in addition to the cognitive processes required for language. Breathing for speech itself requires coordinated activity of inspiratory- and expiratory-related muscles. Each utterance is preceded by a controlled and rapid intake of

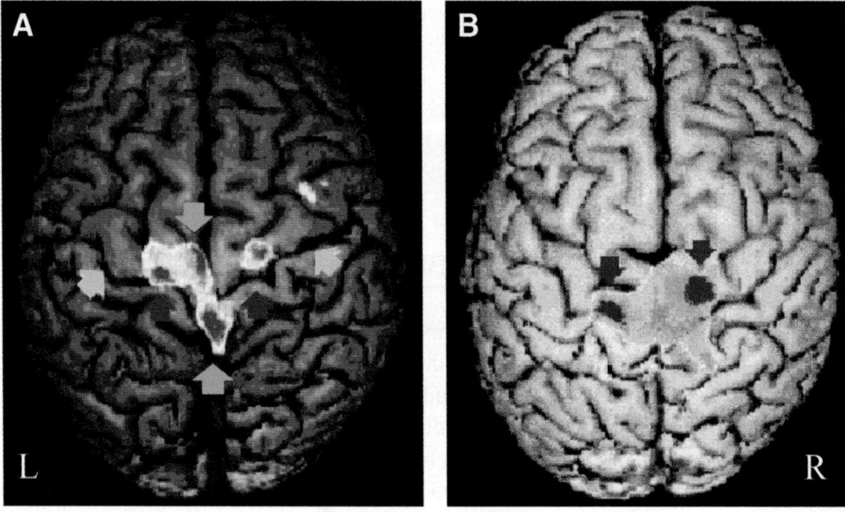

FIGURE 2.4
Breathing during exercise/post exercise. Significant relative regional cerebral blood flow increases ($H_2{}^{15}O$ PET) can be observed (A) during right leg exercise and (B) immediately following exercise; passive ventilation was the control. Ventilation is increased in both A and B, but exercising leg is only active in A. The activation maps, from two different individuals, are superimposed upon surface renderings of each individual's MRI. Yellow arrows indicate the central sulcus. Red arrows indicate significant activations bilaterally in the superolateral primary motor cortex both during and after exercise; these foci presumably represent the ventilatory motor activity. In A, green arrows indicate activity in superomedial sensory and motor corticies. Individual analyses: $p < 0.001$ not corrected. (From Fink, G. R. *et al.*, *J. Physiol.*, 489, 663–675, 1995. With permission.)

air appropriate for the volume and duration of the passage of speech. Vocalisation is performed during expiration when subglottic pressure must be regulated for the control of loudness as the thoracic volume reduces; this function uses a combination of both inspiratory and expiratory muscles (Draper *et al.*, 1959). Similar coordination is required for singing and for wind-instrument playing.

Given the complexity of the control of breathing for speech, it is a reasonable hypothesis that breathing for speech would involve cortical networks similar to those used for voluntary breathing. In principle, we would wish to determine the neural correlates of each component of speech production separately; in practice, this is not possible. In particular, the control of breathing cannot be separated from the control of laryngeal function, as airflow will depend on laryngeal resistance, which in turn will depend on the laryngeal tone required for sound production. Given this constraint, Murphy *et al.* (1997) determined neural activity for four conditions, during each of which subjects continuously repeated a simple phrase: (A) spoken aloud, (B) mouthed silently, (C) vocalised aloud without articulation, and (D) thought silently. Articulation alone ([A-C] + [B-D]) revealed activity bilaterally within the inferolateral sensorimotor cortex, thalamus, caudate nucleus, and cerebellum. Control of breathing for speech and vocalisation (in the presence of hearing but in the absence of articulation, [A-B]+[C-D]) was associated with activity in the sensorimotor cortex, close to, but distinct from, the articulatory focus, together with activity in the SMA, thalamus, and cerebellum. The sensorimotor foci for breathing and vocalisation were not identical to, but did overlap with, the inferolateral foci previously associated with expiration (Ramsay *et al.*, 1993a). No activity was detected at the superolateral motor cortical sites associated with inspiratory and expiratory control (Colebatch *et al.*, 1991; Ramsay *et al.*, 1993a; Fink *et al.*, 1996; McKay *et al.*, 2003). It is understandable that no representation of inspiration was identified; given the pattern of breathing for speech, neural activity for inspiration will form a very small fraction of the scanning period, and the signal may be too weak to detect. More surprising is the absence of any activity in the superolateral motor cortex that might be associated with expiratory control for speech. This raises two possibilities. First, breathing for speech is not mediated via the primary motor cortex. Second, the inferolateral motor representation identified by both Ramsay *et al.* (1993a) and Murphy *et al.* (1997) represents not only control of the upper airway during expiration but also control of expiratory flow by pump muscles. This functional representation of expiratory airflow in the inferolateral region of the primary motor cortex would be consistent with Penfield and Boldrew's (1938) localisation of vocalisation in this region (vocalisation requiring expiratory airflow for sound production), if not the somatotopic representation of the thorax and abdomen more superiorly. The second explanation is more attractive but the question requires further experimentation.

C. CO_2-Stimulated Breathing

Carbon dioxide is a classic respiratory stimulus. The increase in ventilation associated with inhaling carbon dioxide is mediated by the increased partial pressure of CO_2 (PCO_2) in the blood, stimulating chemoreceptors in the carotid body and in the brainstem; this leads to increased efferent output from the respiratory centres in the medulla to the respiratory muscles. Increasing ventilation will minimise the increased PCO_2 that results from the CO_2 loading. This reflex mechanism forms an essential part of the normal homeostatic control of the blood gasses; however, the ventilatory response to inhaled CO_2 is highly variable in awake humans. The ventilatory response to CO_2 is also associated with the unpleasant sensation of dyspnea, particularly of breathlessness; indeed, the sensory and motor components of the response to dyspnea are probably not separable. Such observations suggest that supra-brainstem structures might modulate the ventilatory response to CO_2 in humans. To test this, PET scans were performed in a group of individuals during CO_2-stimulated breathing (Corfield *et al.*, 1995a). The CO_2 stimulation was sufficient to increase the arterial PCO_2 to 50 mmHg and to stimulate breathing by about fourfold when compared to rest. As a control, passive mechanical ventilation was performed at a comparable level, but at a normal PCO_2 of 38 mmHg. To account for the increase in global cerebral blood flow during CO_2 stimulation, when compared to the control condition, a voxel by voxel analysis of covariance was performed using global blood flow as the covariate. With this approach, CO_2-stimulated breathing was not associated with activity within the primary motor cortex (and in particular within the superiolateral motor cortex), despite an increase in ventilation that was comparable to the previous studies of voluntary breathing and of breathing during exercise.

CO_2 stimulation was, however, associated with increased activity in the upper brainstem; midbrain; hypothalamus; hippocampus and parahippocampus; fusiform gyrus; anterior, intermediate, and posterior cingulate cortex; insula; frontal cortex; temporo-occipital cortex; parietal cortex; and cerebellar vermis (Fig. 2.5). These results indicated that CO_2 stimulation was associated with widespread activation of the limbic system as well as other attentional areas of the cortex; this pattern of stimulation would be consistent with the subjects' awareness of the unpleasant nature of the CO_2 stimulation and the symptoms of dyspnea. A caveat on this interpretation relates to the global effect of CO_2 on cerebral blood flow. The statistical model relies on the local neural effects on blood flow being independent of and additive with the global pharmacological effects of CO_2 on blood flow; this is supported by other data (Ramsay *et al.*, 1993b; Corfield *et al.*, 2001). In addition, it is possible that the blood-flow changes result from an inhomogeneity in the cerebrovascular response to CO_2. It is difficult to test this question, as in conscious humans CO_2 administration will always produce global (pharmacological) effects together with local (neural) effects associated with CO_2 stimulation. However, more recently, a number of neuroimaging studies have investigated the neural basis for dyspnea by inducing this

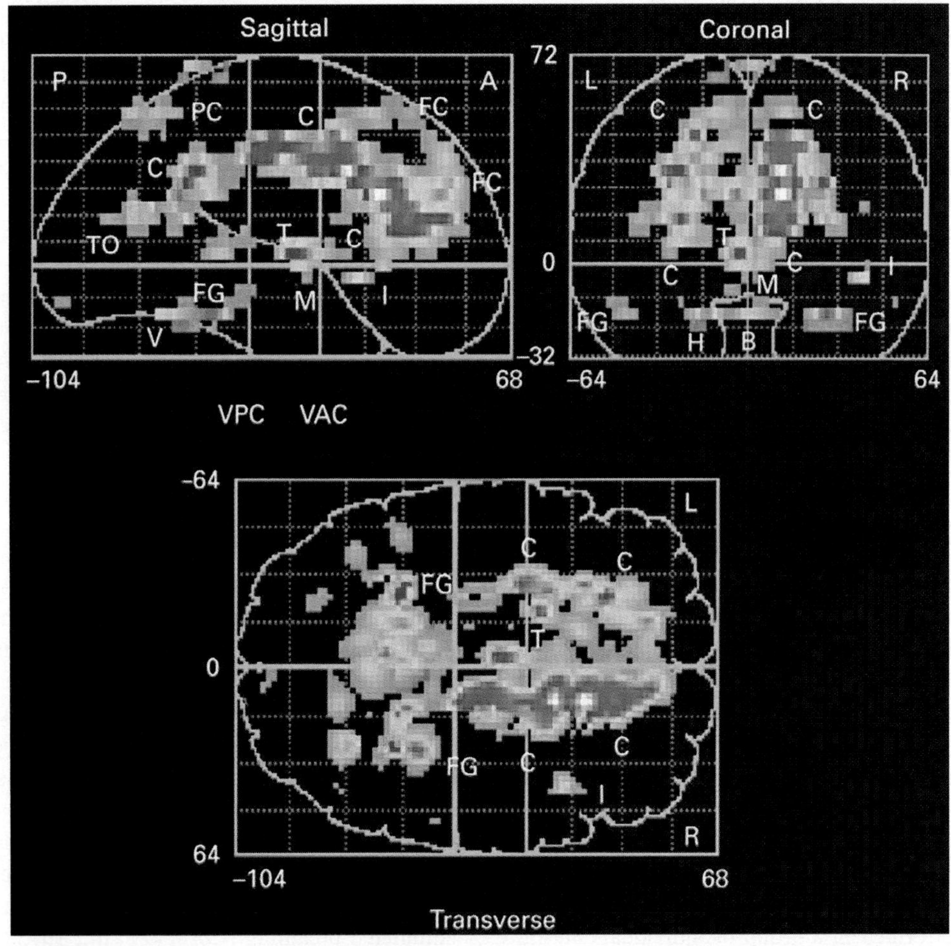

FIGURE 2.5
CO_2-stimulated breathing. Glass brain projection identifying significant increases in relative regional cerebral blood flow ($H_2{}^{15}O$ PET) associated with CO_2-stimulated breathing, with passive ventilation as a control. B, Upper brainstem; M, midbrain/hypothalamus; T, thalamus; H, hippocampus/parahippocampus; FG, fusiform gyrus; C, cingulate cortex; I, insula; FC, frontal cortex; TO, temporo-occipital cortex; PC, parietal cortex; V, cerebellar vermis. $N = 5$; $p < 0.05$ corrected. (From Corfield, D. R. *et al.*, *J. Physiol.*, 488, 77–84, 1995. With permission.)

symptom in ways that were largely independent of CO_2 related global effects (Banzett *et al.*, 2000; Brannan *et al.*, 2001; Liotti *et al.*, 2001; Peiffer *et al.*, 2001; Evans *et al.*, 2002). Despite the diversity of experimental approaches, and in support of the findings of the earlier study (Corfield *et al.*, 1995a), limbic-related areas, in general, and the anterior insula, in particular, are consistently associated with the perception and response to dyspnea (Fig. 2.6).

Ventilatory Load Compensation

The spontaneous ventilatory response to an external load has been much studied by respiratory physiologists. It is a model of how the system may respond to physiological changes in load during health. For example, it models the intrinsic change in load that occurs with the change from nose to mouth breathing and the increased effort of breathing that is present during exercise. Importantly, increases in intrinsic load will be present during disease, when airway resistance increases; some causes of respiratory failure can be considered a failure to respond adequately to the imposed load. There is broad agreement that spontaneous ventilatory response to a moderate inspiratory load in an awake human consists of an almost immediate prolongation of inspiratory time and the maintenance of tidal volume; arterial PCO_2 remains essentially unchanged. This response is severely blunted in sleep. There is no agreement on the mechanisms underlying this ventilatory response (Von Euler, 1974), but the dependence of this response on wakefulness strongly suggests that it may be behaviourally mediated.

A first study of the spontaneous ventilatory response to loaded breathing was performed by Gozal *et al.* (1995) using fMRI; single slice data, acquired through regions of interest, revealed increased activity in the ventral and dorsal pons, the basal forebrain, the putamen, and multiple cerebellar regions; motor cortical areas were not studied. Subsequently Isaev *et al.* (2002) used PET to determine activity across the whole brain. The spontaneous ventilatory response to loaded breathing in naïve subjects was associated with significant activations in inferior parietal cortex, prefrontal cortex, midbrain (red nucleus), basal ganglia, and multiple cerebellar sites

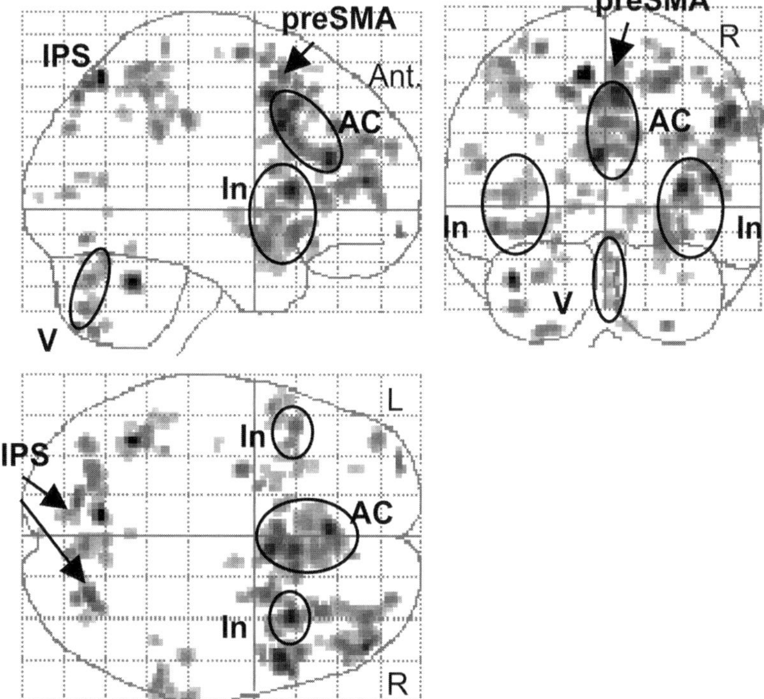

FIGURE 2.6
Air hunger. Glass brain projection identifying significant increases in BOLD fMRI signal associated with periods of air hunger. AC, Anterior cingulate; In, insula; IPS, intraparietal sulcus; SMA, supplementary motor area, V, cerebellar vermis. N = 6; p @ 0.05 corrected; T : 5.1. (From Evans, K. C. *et al.*, *J. Neurophysiol.*, **88**, 1500–1511, 2002. With permission.)

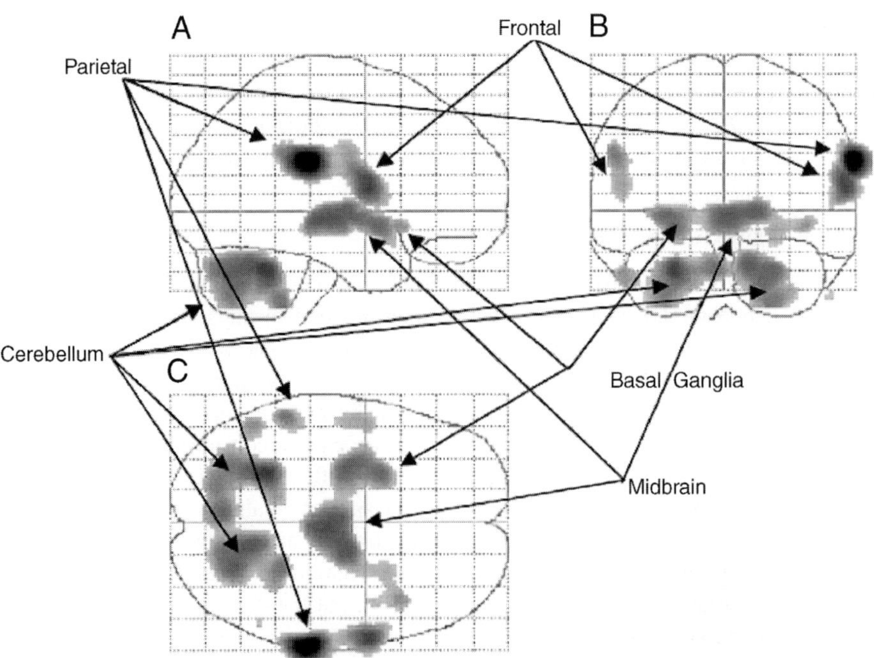

FIGURE 2.7
Ventilatory load compensation. Glass brain projection identifying significant increases in relative regional cerebral blood flow ($H_2{}^{15}O$ PET) associated with ventilatory load compensation. $N = 6$; $p < 0.0001$ uncorrected. (From Isaev, G. *et al.*, *J. Physiol.*, 539, 935–945, 2002. With permission.)

(Fig. 2.7). The authors suggested that this pattern of activity reflects a behavioural motor response to the uncomfortable sensation that inspiration is impeded. This response results in a prolongation of inspiratory time, the maintenance of tidal volume, and a reduction in the degree of discomfort, presumably because of the reduction of mean negative pressure in the airways. Assuming that this pattern of activity reflects a motor-related response to the loading, it is surprising that no activity was detected either in the thalamus or in the primary motor cortex. The authors concluded that the physiological changes in response to the load were associated with motor cortical activation too small to be detected by the scanning methodology. Indeed, loaded breathing induces changes in respiratory timing and not in tidal volume; it was increases in the latter that produced activation in the superolateral motor cortex (Colebatch *et al.*, 1991; Ramsay *et al.*, 1993a; Fink *et al.*, 1996; McKay *et al.*, 2003).

INTEGRATION OF BEHAVIOURAL AND REFLEX BREATHING

Behavioural breathing acts can clearly override reflex breathing, for example during voluntary paced breathing (see above); however such behavioural breathing cannot be performed wholly independently of the demands of gas exchange and of reflex breathing. This is most clearly illustrated by breath holding: The voluntary ability to inhibit reflex breathing is subsequently overcome by an overwhelming reflex drive and urge to breathe. This competition is also seen in other behaviours; breathing for speech is clearly impaired with the increased breathing demands of exercise and is commonly impaired during lung disease when breathlessness is present. Even small increases in the prevailing level of arterial CO_2 impair the ability to control breathing voluntarily (Corfield *et al.*, 1999b). Further, emotional changes, such as laughter, crying, or anxiety, can overwhelm other aspects of respiratory control. The neural basis for such integration, or competition, is not known. Evidence from animals indicates that integration of reflex and behavioural breathing occurs within the respiratory centres of the brainstem (Orem and Netick, 1986; Orem, 1988); however, indirect evidence from humans suggests greater functional separation of reflex and voluntary control (Corfield *et al.*, 1998). In addition, the neural basis for the control of breathing for laughter appears distinct from that for voluntary breathing (Heywood *et al.*, 1996).

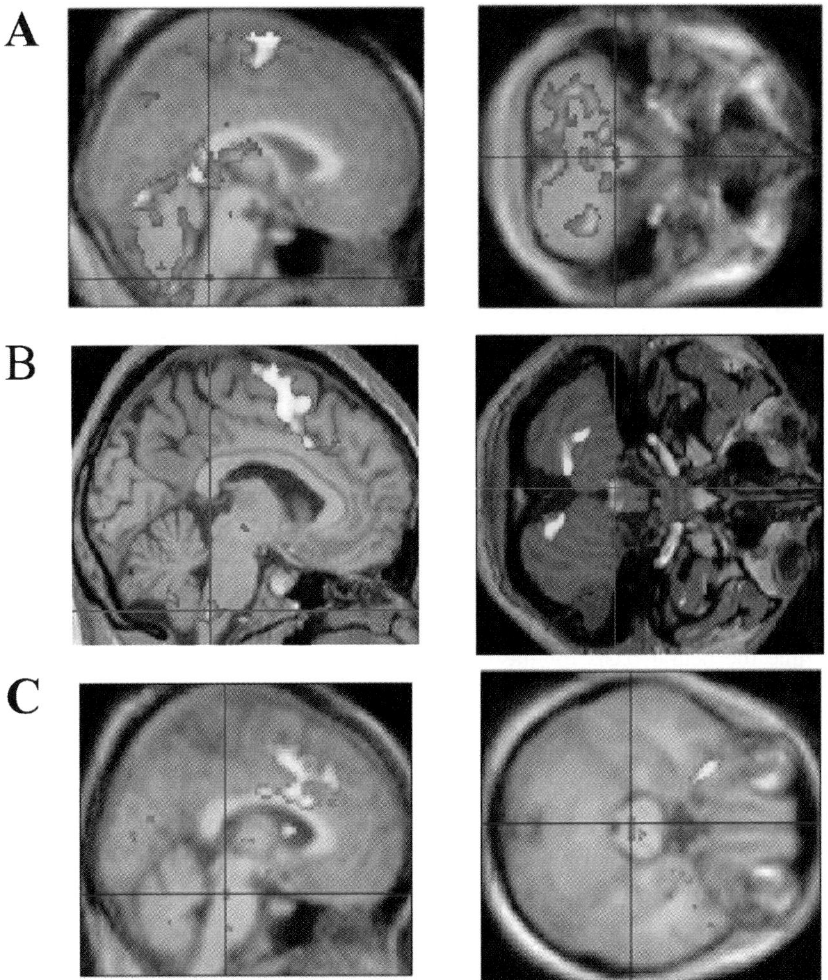

FIGURE 2.8
Breathing-related brain stem activity: fMRI. (A) Voluntary breathing. Cross hair indicates maximum of medullary activation associated with voluntary breathing (same data as Figure 2.3). $N = 6$; maximum at $x = 0$, $y = -38$, $z = -52$; $p = 0.012$; $T = 3.2$ (small volume correction, 10-mm radius from centre of medulla). The cluster is located in the superior dorsal medulla extending bilaterally from the midline. (Data from Mckay *et al.*, 2003.) (B) Voluntary tongue contraction. Separate bilateral maxima, reflecting medullary activation in the hypoglossal nucleus, were associated with voluntary tongue contraction. Cross hair indicates maximum at $x = -4$, $y = -38$, $z = -48$; $p < 0.001$ (uncorrected, Z = 6.2). (From Corfield, D. R. *et al.*, *J. Appl. Physiol.*, 86, 1468–1477, 1999. With permission.) (C) Voluntary breathholding. Suppression of reflex breathing (breath holding at end expiration) was associated with significant activation in the mid-superior dorsal pons, extending bilaterally from the mid line. $N = 6$; $p < 0.05$ corrected; maximum at $x = -2$, $y = -30$, $z = -24$; $T = 6.86$. (Data from Mckay *et al.*, 2000.)

Functional neuroimaging should help address these questions; however, technically it is challenging to image activity within the human brainstem: The neural structures are small, and the brainstem is subject to more cardiorespiratory-related motion than the cortex. Nevertheless, fMRI has now reliably identified respiratory-related activity in this region. Voluntary paced breathing, in addition to its cortical components, is associated with activity in the superior dorsal medulla (McKay *et al.*, 2000) (Fig. 2.8a). This signal presumably reflects increased activity of respiratory neurons in the region of the nucleus of the solitary tract or the nucleus ambiguous. However, the functional significance of the activity associated with voluntary breathing is unclear as, with this paradigm, it could represent changes in either sensory or motor activity. This medullary focus is distinct from that produced in the hypoglossal nucleus by voluntary tongue movement (Corfield *et al.*, 1999a) (Fig. 2.8b). The ability of fMRI to usefully separate functionally distinct regions of the medulla should allow further progress with this question.

In contrast with voluntary breathing, the voluntary suppression of reflex breathing (*i.e.*, breath holding) is associated with increased activity within the dorsal pons close to the parabrachial nucleus (McKay *et al.*, 2000) (Fig. 2.8c). In animals, this region (the pontine respiratory group or the parabrachial complex) is known to exert strong influences on reflex breathing activity (Feldman, 1986). Stimulation of these regions can result in both hyperpnea and apnea (Dick *et al.*, 1994; Fung and St. John, 1994a,b). It is an attractive hypothesis that, in humans, this region mediates the corticomotor inhibition of reflex breathing.

CONCLUSIONS

The reported studies have defined the neural substrates for a broad range of breathing acts. Taken together, they emphasise the importance of supra-brainstem structures for the control of many breathing behaviours in awake humans. In particular, these studies identify an extensive representation of breathing-related muscles within the primary motor cortex. The neural structures that mediate the deliberate taking of a breath have much in common with those that control other voluntary motor acts. It is clear that the motor network controlling voluntary breathing is also important for mediating other spontaneous breathing behaviours, including exercise, speech, and the response to loaded breathing.

Currently, much remains unknown in regard to breathing. In particular, we do not know what controls breathing during emotional changes such as laughter or stress or what underlies the state-dependent differences in breathing control associated with waking and sleep. We must further define the neural basis for the integration of brainstem and supra-brainstem control. Behaviours and states that change breathing frequently produce changes in the cardiovascular system; important elements of autonomic cardiovascular control reside in the forebrain (Critchley *et al.*, 2000, 2001), and the basis for the integration of respiratory and cardiovascular control must be identified. Importantly, the motor control of the breathing muscles is intimately linked to sensory aspects of respiration, and a fuller characterisation of the neural basis of respiratory sensation is essential for a complete understanding of respiratory control.

References

Adams, L., Frankel, H., Garlick, J., Guz, A., Murphy, K., and Semple, S. J. G. (1984). The role of spinal cord transmission in the ventilatory response to exercise in man. *J. Physiol.*, **355,** 85–97.

Banner, N. R., LLoyd, M. H., Hamilton, R. D., Innes, J. A., Guz, A., and Yacoub, M. H. (1989). Cardiopulmonary response to dynamic exercise after heart and combined heart–lung transplantation. *Br. Heart J.*, **61,** 215–223.

Banzett, R. B., Mulnier, H. E., Murphy, K., Rosen, S. D., Wise, R. J. S., and Adams, L. (2000). Breathlessness in humans activates insular cortex. *NeuroReport*, **11,** 2117–2120.

Brannan, S., Liotti, M., Egan, G., Shade, R., Madden, L., Robillard, R., Abplanalp, B., Stofer, K., Denton, D., and Fox, P. T. (2001). Neuroimaging of cerebral activations and deactivations associated with hypercapnia and hunger for air. *Proc. Natl. Acad. Sci. USA*, **98,** 2029–2034.

Colebatch, J. G., Murphy, K., Martin, A. J., Lammertsma, A. A., Tochon-Danguy Clark, H., Friston, K. J., Guz, A., and Adams, L. (1991). Regional cerebral blood flow during volitional breathing in man. *J. Physiol.*, **443,** 91–103.

Corfield, D. R., Fink, G. R., Ramsay, S. C., Murphy, K., Harty, H. R., Watson, J. D. G., Adams, L., Frackowiak, R. S. J., and Guz, A. (1995a). Evidence for limbic system activation during CO_2-stimulated breathing in man. *J. of Physiol.*, **488,** 77–84.

Corfield, D. R., Morrell, M. J., and Guz, A. (1995b). The nature of breathing during hypocapnia in awake man. *Respir. Physiol.*, **101,** 145–159.

Corfield, D. R., Murphy, K., and Guz, A. (1998). Does the motor cortical control of the diaphragm 'bypass' the brain stem respiratory centres in man? *Respir. Physiol.*, **114,** 109–117.

Corfield, D. R., Murphy, K., Josephs, O., Fink, G. R., Frackowiak, R. S. J., Guz, A., Adams, L., and Turner, R. (1999a). Cortical and subcortical control of tongue movement in humans: a functional neuroimaging study using fMRI. *J. Appl. Physiol.*, **86,** 1468–1477.

Corfield, D. R., Roberts, C. A., Guz, A., Murphy, K., and Adams, L. (1999b). Modulation of the corticospinal control of ventilation by changes in reflex respiratory drive. *J. Appl. Physiol.*, 1923–1930.

Corfield, D. R., Murphy, K., Josephs, O., Adams, L., and Turner, R. (2001). Does hypercapnia-induced cerebral vasodilation modulate the hemodynamic response to neural activation? *NeuroImage*, **13,** 1207–1211.

Critchley, H. D., Corfield, D. R., Chandler, M. P., Mathias, C. J., and Dolan, R. J. (2000). Cerebral correlates of autonomic cardiovascular arousal: a functional neuroimaging investigation in humans. *J. Physiol.*, **523,** 259–270.

Critchley, H. D., Mathias, C. J., and Dolan, R. J. (2001). Neural activity in the human brain relating to uncertainty and arousal during anticipation. *Neuron*, **29,** 537–545.

Datta, A. K., Shea, S. A., Horner, R. L., and Guz, A. (1991). The influence of induced hypocapnia and sleep on the endogenous respiratory rhythm in humans. *J. Physiol.*, **440,** 17–33.

Dick, T. E., Bellingham, M. C., and Richter, D. W. (1994). Pontine respiratory neurons in anesthetised cats. *Brain Res.*, **636,** 259–269.

Draper, M. H., Ladefoged, P., and Whitteridge, D. (1959). Respiratory muscles in speech. *J. Speech Hearing Res.*, **2,** 16–27.

Evans, K. C., Banzett, R. B., Adams, L., Makay, L. C., Frackowiak, R. S. J., and Corfield, D. R. (2002). BOLD fMRI identifies limbic, para-limbic and cerebellar activation during air hunger. *J. Neurophysiol.*, **88,** 1500–1511.

Feldman, J. L. (1986). Neurophysiology of breathing in mammals, in *Handbook of Physiology: The Nervous System. Intrinsic Regulatory System in the Brain*, Bloom, F. E., Ed., Vol. IV, pp. 463–524. American Physiology Society, Washington, D.C.

Fink, B. R. (1961). Influence of cerebral activity in wakefulness on regulation of breathing. *J. Appl. Physiol.*, **16,** 15–20.

Fink, G. R., Adams, L., Watson, J. D. G., Innes, J. A., Wuyam, B., Kobayashi, I., Corfield, D. R., Murphy, K., Jones, T., Frackowiak, R. S. J., and Guz, A. (1995). Hyperpnoea during and immediately after exercise in man: evidence of motor cortical involvement. *J. Physiol.*, **489,** 663–675.

Fink, G. R., Corfield, D. R., Murphy, K., Kobayashi, I., Dettmers, C., Adams, L., Frackowiak, R. S. J., and Guz, A. (1996). Human cerebral activity with increasing inspiratory force: a study using positron emission tomography. *J. Appl. Physiol.*, **81,** 1295–1305.

Fink, G. R., Frackowiak, R. S. J., Pietrzyk, U., and Passingham, R. E. (1997). Multiple nonprimary motor areas in the human cortex. *J. Neurophysiol.*, **77,** 2164–2174.

Foerster, O. (1936). Motorische Felder und Bahnen, in *Handbuch der Neurologie*, Bumke, O. and Foerster, O., Eds., pp. 50–51. Springer, Berlin.

Fung, M. L. and St. John, W. M. (1994a). Neuronal activities underlying inspiratory termination by pneumotaxic mechanisms. *Respir. Physiol.*, **98,** 267–281.

Fung, M. L. and St. John, W. M. (1994b). Separation of multiple functions in the ventilatory control of pneumotaxic mechanisms. *Respir. Physiol.*, **96,** 83–98.

Gandevia, S. C. and Rothwell, J. C. (1987). Activation of the human diaphragm from the motor cortex. *J. Physiol. (London)*, **384,** 109–118.

Gozal, D., Omidvar, O., Kirlew, K. A., Hathout, G. M., Hamilton, R., Lufkin, R. B., and Harper, R. M. (1995). Identification of human brain regions underlying responses to resistive inspiratory loading with functional magnetic resonance imaging. *Proc. Natl. Acad. Sci. USA*, **92,** 6607–6611.

Gray, P. A., Janczewski, W. A., Mellen, N., McCrimmon, D. R., and Feldman, J. L. (2001). Normal breathing requires preBotzinger complex neurokinin-1 receptor-expressing neurons. *Nat. Neurosci.*, **4,** 927–930.

Heywood, P., Murphy, K., Corfield, D. R., Morrell, M. J., Howard, R. S., and Guz, A. (1996). Control of breathing in man; insights from the 'locked-in' syndrome. *Respir. Physiol.*, **106,** 13–20.

Isaev, G., Murphy, K., Guz, A., and Adams, L. (2002). Areas of the brain concerned with ventilatory load compensation in awake man. *J. Physiol.*, **539,** 935–945.

Krogh, A. and Lindhard, J. (1913). The regulation of respiration and circulation during the initial stages of muscular work. *J. Physiol.*, **47,** 112–136.

Liotti, M., Brannan, S., Egan, G., Shade, R., Madden, L., Abplanalp, B., Robillard, R., Lancaster, J., Zamarripa, F. E., Fox, P. T., and Denton, D. (2001). Brain responses associated with consciousness of breathlessness (air hunger). *Proc. Natl. Acad. Sci. USA*, **98,** 2035–2040.

Maskill, D., Murphy, K., Mier, A., Owen, M., and Guz, A. (1991). Motor cortical representation of the diaphragm in man. *J. Physiol.*, **443,** 105–121.

McKay, L. C., Adams, L., Frackowiak, R. S. J., and Corfield, D. R. (2000). The neural basis of breath holding in humans determined by functional magnetic resonance imaging. *J. Physiol.*, **525,** 29P–30P.

McKay, L. C., Evans, K. C., Frackowiak, R. S. J., and Corfield, D. R. (2003). Neural correlates of voluntary breathing in humans. *J. Appl. Physiol.*, **95,** 1170–1178.

Morrell, M. J., Heywood, P., Moosavi, S. H., Guz, A., and Stevens, J. (1999). Unilateral focal lesions in the rostrolateral medulla influence chemosensitivity and breathing measured during wakefulness, sleep, and exercise. *J. Neurol. Neurosurg. Psychiatry*, **67,** 637–645.

Murphy, K., Mier, A., Adams, L., and Guz, A. (1990). Putative cerebral cortical involvement in the ventilatory response to inhaled CO_2 in conscious man. *J. Physiol.*, **420,** 1–18.

Murphy, K., Corfield, D. R., Guz, A., Fink, G. R., Wise, R. J., Harrison, J., and Adams, L. (1997). Cerebral areas associated with motor control of speech in humans. *J. Appl. Physiol.*, **83,** 1438–1447.

Orem, J. (1988). Neural basis of behavioural and state-dependant control of breathing, in *Clinical Physiology of Sleep*, Lydic, R. and Biebuyck, J. F., Eds., pp. 79–95. American Physiological Society, Bethesda, MD.

Orem, J. and Netick, A. (1986). Behavioural control of breathing in the cat. *Brain Res.*, **366,** 238–253.

Passingham, R. E. (1997). Functional organisation of the motor system, in *Human Brain Function*, Frackowiak, R. S. J., Friston, K. J., Frith, C. D., Dolan, R. J., and Mazziotta, J. C., Eds., pp. 243–274. Academic Press, San Diego.

Peiffer, C., Poline, J. B., Thivard, L., Aubier, M., and Samson, Y. (2001). Neural substrates for the perception of acutely induced dyspnea. *Am. J. Respir. Crit. Care Med.*, **163,** 951–957.

Penfield, W. and Boldrey, E. (1938). Somatic motor and sensory representation in the cerebral cortex as studied by electrical stimulation. *Brain*, **15,** 389–443.

Ramsay, S. C., Adams, L., Murphy, K., Corfield, D. R., Grootoonk, S., Bailey, D. L., Frackowiak, R. S. J., and Guz, A. (1993a). Regional cerebral blood flow during volitional expiration in man: a comparison with volitional inspiration. *J. Physiol.*, **461,** 85–101.

Ramsay, S. C., Murphy, K., Shea, S. A., Friston, K. J., Lammertsma, A. A., Clark, J. C., Adams, L., Guz, A., and

Frackowiak, R. S. J. (1993b). Changes in global cerebral blood flow in humans: effect on regional cerebral blood flow during a neural activation task. *J. Physiol.*, **471,** 521–534.

Rekling, J. C. and Feldman, J. L. (1998). PreBotzinger complex and pacemaker neurons: hypothesised site and kernel for respiratory rhythm generation. *Annu. Rev. Physiol.*, **60,** 385–405.

Shea, S. A. (1997). Life without ventilatory chemosensitivity. *Respir. Physiol.,* **110,** 199–210.

Smith, J. C., Ellenberger, H. H., Ballanyi, K., Richter, D. W., and Feldman, J. L. (1991). Pre-Botzinger complex: a brainstem region that may generate respiratory rhythm in mammals. *Science*, **254,** 726–729.

Taylor, E. W., Jordan, D., and Coote, J. H. (1999). Central control of the cardiovascular and respiratory systems and their interactions in vertebrates. *Physiol. Rev.*, **79,** 855–916.

Von Euler, C. (1974). On the role of proprioceptors in perception and execution of motor acts with special reference to breathing, in *Loaded Breathing*., Pengelly, L. D., Rebuck, A. S., and Cambell, E. J. M., Eds., pp. 139–149. Longman, Canada.

Wasserman, K., Whipp, B. J., Koyal, S. N., and Cleary, M. G. (1975). Effect of carotid body resection on ventilatory and acid-base control during exercise. *J. Appl. Physiol.*, **39,** 354–358.

CHAPTER

3

Perceptual Construction

INTRODUCTION

What one perceives visually is not a passive and veridical translation of the stimulation received at the retina. Sensory input provides abundant information about certain physical properties in the surrounding world, and the reception, processing, and transmission of such information are often framed as a neural bottom-up process. This view of the associated neural processes refers to the visually responsive brain structures as a distributed hierarchical system — that is, a system in which functional specialisation and segregation can be demonstrated by differences in the stimulus–response functions recorded at different sites. Yet, in neurophysiological experiments with awake behaving subjects it can be shown that stimulus-induced neural activity is modulated by additional extraretinal influences such as attention. Such modulations are the likely substrate of, for instance, improved task performance, and their sources are commonly addressed as top-down processes, again reflecting a hierarchical view of the visual system. The neural correlates of each of these aspects—bottom-up and top-down—can be studied in their own right by suitable experimental paradigms, and functional magnetic resonance imaging (fMRI) has proven very valuable for such studies in humans and, more recently, non-human primates (see, for instance, Tootell *et al.*, 1998).

Within this framework, visual perception may be conceptualised as resulting from an interaction of bottom-up and top-down processes. If we postulate such an interaction as the neural basis for visual percepts, we would hypothesise that detectable neural activity correlates of perception are accounted for by neither of the two factors by themselves (i.e., bottom-up or top-down). In experimental studies of the visual system, these two factors correspond explicitly to sensory input and task instruction. In other words, we would seek to demonstrate this interaction by studying paradigms where brain activity changes occur in correlation with subjective visual perceptual experience but not in correlation with changes in sensory input or compliance with task instructions. Appropriate visual stimulus paradigms that elicit such a behaviour have been employed by perceptual psychologists for a long time (see, for instance, Gregory, 1998; Kruse and Stadler, 1995), and this chapter reviews some more recent functional imaging experiments that have exploited these perceptual phenomena so as to define neural correlates of visual perception and, in a broader sense, of phenomenal visual awareness.

HYSTERESIS IN VISUAL PERCEPTION

Think of the starting point of visual object perception (*e.g.*, the detection of a figure in a noisy ground). The functional challenge for the visual system in this situation is to determine which parts of the picture belong together and constitute an object and which parts belong to the rest of the scene. This problem is generally referred to as the *binding problem*, and from the perspective of pure visual scene analysis it is believed to be solved by detecting the coherence

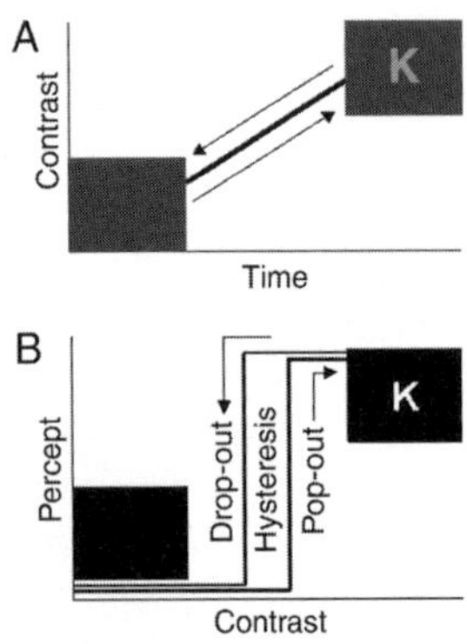

FIGURE 3.1
Gradual contrast changes of a visual letter initially hidden in a dot pattern providing a noisy background (A) yields categorical changes in perception that occur when an identification threshold is passed. The contrast level at which this perceptual transition occurs depends on the direction of contrast change, and systematic differences between contrast values at pop-out and at drop-out yield a hysteresis effect when plotting a stimulus–response function. (Adapted from Kleinschmidt *et al.*, 2002a.)

in low-level visual cues or attributes such as luminance, colour, or motion displayed by object parts but not by the background.

An object can easily be hidden in a noisy visual background, and gradually increasing its contrast relative to the background will eventually lead to perceptual pop-out. While the actual degree of stimulus change required to induce pop-out may be minor, the perceptual significance of transition across this threshold is high. Related neural activity can therefore be expected to display highly nonlinear behaviour in the contrast range that covers this threshold; however, the absolute value of this threshold contrast is not a fixed variable determined purely on the grounds of the physical properties that contrast the stimulus against the background. Once a percept has been evoked, the structures that process the visual input can rely on a powerful hypothesis of what this input means. In a psychophysical experiment, this is demonstrated by reversing the direction of contrast change. Setting out at supra-threshold levels, perception during progressive deterioration of physical stimulus contrast may be preserved down to much lower threshold values than those required for pop-out. At some level of contrast, however, a critical boundary will be reached, and passing it will engender perceptual drop-out (*i.e.*, loss of the percept) (Fig. 3.1).

If in a neurophysiological experiment one increases and decreases contrast of a stimulus in this way and expresses the resulting activity time series as a function of contrast, the phenomenon of direction-dependent perceptual threshold shift should manifest as a so-called hysteresis effect in the stimulus–response function of this neural structure, provided it is sensitive to the perceptual consequence and not merely to the physical characteristics of a visual stimulus. There are many ways of framing the hysteresis effect conceptually, but to the neurophysiological experimentalist it offers the opportunity of comparing brain states during which the same stimuli either induce a meaningful percept or not. In other words, the perceptual effect accounting for hysteresis is orthogonal to the sensory stimulus as the other determinant of the stimulus–response function.

From the perspective of functional neuroimaging, this experimental design is interesting because the actual stimulation undergoes continuous slow parameter changes instead of following a structure of epochs or events; however, in the perceptual domain, this stimulation induces changes and states that can be analysed as events (pop-out) and epochs (percepts), respectively. Especially the event-related changes rely on the all-or-none character of the stimulus chosen. For example, somebody approaching you in a forest will produce a series of recognition levels: realising something is moving toward you, identifying the figure as a human being, identifying the human's gender, and so on and so forth until you maybe even recognise somebody you know. Presumably, the neural signatures of these levels of recognition are different, but at this stage it would still present a considerable challenge to enter the study of such a multilayered process with sufficiently refined starting hypotheses.

For this reason, for our study (Kleinschmidt *et al.*, 2002a) we chose visual letters as a stimulus category and density of random dots within their form as the sensory contrast source. This paradigm minimises component-related processing and results in a rather categorical transition from preconscious processing of shaped elements to a meaningful percept. Performing a functional magnetic resonance imaging experiment this way, we obtained time-series data for subjects who indicated by key presses pop-out and drop-out of the visual letter percepts. In a first step, these behavioural reports allowed us to contrast those images during which visual stimulation evoked a categorically meaningful percept to those when it did not. This comparison showed significantly greater activity in brain structures ranging from the fusiform gyrus to the so-called lateral occipital complex (LOC) bilaterally (Malach *et al.*, 1995) and predominantly right-hemispheric in inferior parietal, premotor, and inferior frontal cortex (Fig. 3.2, left).

This analysis served only as a mapping procedure to identify candidate areas and is compromised by the fact that meaningful percepts occurred during higher contrast levels than those when only noise was perceived. The analysis of interest was performed on time-course data that were plotted as a stimulus–response function, splitting the data into the ascending and descending direction of contrast change. Haemodynamic response latencies already generate a temporal order effect; therefore, it was important to compare these data to those from trials during which no perceptual hysteresis occurred. When performed this way, the analysis revealed that the areas mapped in a nonspecific way displayed hysteresis in their activity time courses and

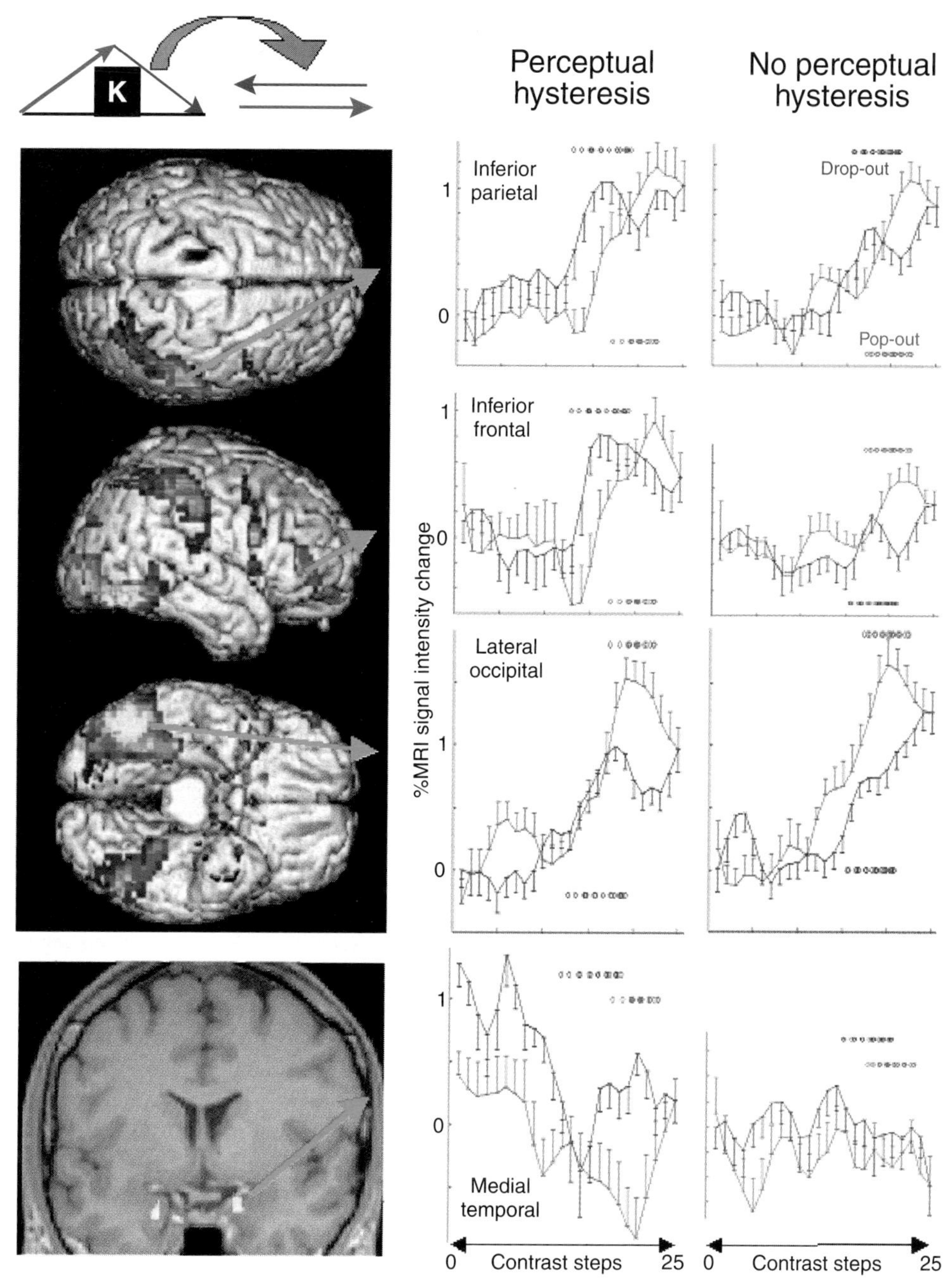

FIGURE 3.2
Perceptual and mnemonic functional behaviour in a visual letter identification task. (Adapted from Kleinschmidt *et al.*, 2002a.)

did so only in those trials when perceptual hysteresis occurred (Fig. 3.2, right). This underscores the fact that their activity was indeed related to the perceptual consequence of visual stimulation rather than to its physical properties. The result was confirmed by a mapping procedure that was based trial-by-trial only on those images that covered the contrast range over which perceptual hysteresis occurred.

The only exception was the lateral occipital cortex because its activity expressed another time-dependent effect that can be termed adaptation or repetition suppression. It has been established recently that this LOC response property occurs not only with identical stimuli but also with trains of stimuli that, despite constant perceptual meaning (invariance), differ in physical properties such as size and position (Grill-Spector *et al.*, 1998, 1999; Kourtzi and Kanwisher, 2000). Response adaptation in LOC also occurred in the experiment described here when stimuli changed progressively but activity after pop-out nonetheless underwent profound adaptation as long as a stable percept was maintained. Only in trials with perceptual hysteresis, however, was there an additional relative response increase in LOC that counteracted and cancelled adaptation. In addition to the aforementioned parietal and frontal areas, then, LOC also proved sensitive to visual perceptual awareness.

This is in line with findings from other studies that analysed LOC activity during blocks of brief masked presentations (20–500 ms) and found it to display the highest correlation with visual recognition performance. Also, if recognition at given presentation durations was improved by training, this was accompanied by an enhanced fMRI signal in LOC (Grill-Spector *et al.*, 2000). A more recent fMRI study in a similar vein used event-related analyses to address explicit recognition of briefly presented and masked visual objects and found a gradual increase of event-related responses in LOC as well as in an anterior region of the fusiform gyrus (Bar *et al.*, 2001). The authors also showed an anterior progression of activation along ventral temporal cortex as a function of the level of recognition success.

These studies differ from our experiment in several important ways: (1) They used rich composite stimuli that could be recognised in a gradual way, reflecting multiple successful recognitions at the component level. We attempted to minimise the importance of these subprocesses by using visual letters (*i.e.*, stimuli that are not composed of meaningful percepts at the component level). (2) They also used brief and masked presentations, thereby focusing on the recognition (*i.e.*, onset) of a percept. In the study presented here visual stimulation underwent continuous but only subtle changes. Therefore, pop-out and the presence of a percept could be addressed separately, and related activity was identified by transient and sustained regressor shapes, respectively. Hysteresis lasted for only relatively short time spans in relation to haemodynamic latencies, so it is important to realise that the related sustained activity was not only modelled differently but also occurred with different timing. The epochs over which hysteresis could be observed precede the transient activations related to the perceptual transitions of pop-out and drop-out (see Fig. 3.1).

These various neuroimaging findings thus converge in identifying brain structures in which activity correlates with the appearance and presence of meaningful visual percepts. The more fundamental question is whether local computations performed in these structures fully account for perceptual synthesis. Theoretical models suggest that perceptually successful processing of sensory input in visual association areas could depend on backward signals (Carpenter and Grossberg, 1993; Ullman, 1995), and studies in non-human primates suggest that such a signal could originate from the medial temporal lobe system (Miyashita *et al.*, 1996; Tanaka, 1997; Naya *et al.*, 2001). In our experimental setting, a backward signal should be detectable over the hysteresis range if one considers that it might account for the fact that identical stimulation either does or does not evoke a meaningful percept. In line with this assumption and in addition to the aforementioned areas, the hysteresis contrast also showed significantly higher activity in the medial temporal lobe. This region did not change activity as a function of whether visual stimulation elicited a percept or not and consequently did not show up in the related mapping contrast. Instead, it loaded with activity once pop-out had occurred and maintained this activity level up to the point at which drop-out occurred.

Event-related analyses further confirmed a different functional behaviour for the percept-sensitive areas, where we found activations during pop-out and drop-out, and the medial temporal lobe, where deactivations occurred at these time points. One interpretation is that medial temporal activity reflects the matching of perceptual or mnemonic representations against the incoming sensory input with the aim of minimising error registered in lower visual processing areas by providing them with progressively refined predictions. This activity should transiently collapse once the pop-out is achieved by supra-threshold sensory input and thus a particular representation is selected. Such a collapse should also occur when percept stabilisation by a backward signal finally fails and subjects experience the drop-out.

Apart from these transient decreases related to perceptual transitions, however, a mnemonic response component in this area could provide a sustained backward signal. This signal should rise once a specific representation has been evoked by supra-threshold sensory input and persist despite subsequent gradual deterioration of the sensory input. Again, this behaviour corresponds precisely to the activity time courses we observed in medial temporal cortex. If perception relies on the interaction of this backward signal with sensory input in visual associative areas, the backward signal could delay but not infinitely prevent drop-out, thus yielding hysteresis in the stimulus–response functions. The medial temporal system thus appears to be a candidate structure for mediating the prolonged activity increase in visual associative areas and may thereby account for perceptual hysteresis.

Conversely, a persisting mnemonic trace could carry over into a second run of percept build-up and account for priming of perceptual pop-out. This is what we found when repeating the same trial a second time (data not shown). The interpretation of a combined perceptual and mnemonic functional role of medial temporal cortex is compatible not only with theoretical models (Gluck and Myers, 1993) but also with recent neuroimaging findings of enduring activation in medial temporal and dorsolateral inferior frontal structures during maintenance of a percept (Portas *et al.*, 2000) and of sustained medial temporal activation during maintenance of information that is no longer supported by sensory input (Ranganath and d'Esposito, 2001). It is also compatible with longstanding human and non-human primate studies relating visual recognition memory to basal medial temporal cortex (Scoville and Milner, 1957; Zola-Morgan et al., 1994; Buckley and Gaffan, 1998; Murray and Bussey, 1999; Brown and Aggleton, 2001).

Regarding activations, the event-related analyses showed transient responses to perceptual transitions in areas largely overlapping with those that responded to perceptual awareness in a sustained way. In the setting of this experiment, an initial transient component of a sustained response to a percept cannot be distinguished from a purely transient response related to the instant of pop-out or recognition. This is because we used a paradigm where one single percept appears and disappears in an all-or-none fashion. The isolation of transient responses related to perceptual transitions from the initial responses related to the onset of a percept would require a stimulation where the same type of perceptual transitions (pop-out and drop-out) occur but each transition leads into a meaningful and ideally equivalent percept. These requirements are fulfilled by ambiguous visual stimuli that engender perceptual rivalry.

BISTABLE VISUAL PERCEPTION

Ambiguity of Object Perception

Over the last couple of years, several neuroimaging studies have been performed with constant visual stimuli that produce bistable percepts. Focusing on ventral temporal areas with high-level categorical response preferences (faces or places), Tong *et al.* (1998) used the technique of binocular rivalry with dichoptically different stimuli (*e.g.*, faces shown to one eye and places to the other eye). They showed that activity levels in ventral temporal visual areas reflected which percept dominated. In other words, while the subjects perceived a face, activity was elevated in the fusiform face area; while they perceived a place, activity was elevated in the parahippocampal place area. This study hence addressed sustained, percept-related activity levels during bistable perception.

Another study using binocular rivalry investigated the transient activations associated with switches between two percepts, a face and a moving grating, and found widely distributed responses in occipital, parietal, and frontal areas (Lumer *et al.*, 1998). More specifically, however, these activations were compared to those from a non-rivalrous monocular alternation of the two different stimuli that mimicked the previously experienced sequence of fluctuating dominance between the two stimuli presented to either eye. Greater activity in the rivalry as opposed to this replay condition was observed in a right-sided frontoparietal network. These findings were related to neural processes subserving attentional selection, assuming that the subjects experienced no attentional set shift between the two conditions. Conversely, responses from that experiment could not be conclusively related to changes in perception for two reasons: (1) In either of the two single conditions, the brain activity changes recorded pooled the perceptual shift and the congruent behavioural report, as confirmed by prominent activations in several motor areas; and (2) when attempting to control for the motor response component by comparing rivalrous and non-rivalrous conditions, the resulting comparison eliminated those signal changes related to perceptual alternation, instead focusing on those related to the difference between the rivalrous and non-rivalrous conditions (*i.e.*, to the processes of attentional selection).

In another study, we elicited perceptual rivalry using classical ambiguous pictures such as the "vase/face" stimulus by Rubin and the "my-wife-and-my-mother-in-law" stimulus by Boring (Kleinschmidt *et al.*, 1998). We also addressed event (transition)-related brain activity changes and disambiguated them from state (percept)-related activity modulations. For that purpose and in contrast to the aforementioned studies, we not only chose stimuli with little categorical change between the two percepts (1 face–object, 2 face–body, 1 face–face reversals) but also set up the stimuli so as to yield temporally well-spaced reversals that were interleaved with periods of perceptual stability of comparable duration. These experimental and behavioural characteristics were necessary because with the sluggishness of haemodynamic responses an imbalance between the mean duration of the two percepts could confound event-related responses to transitions with state-related responses during the briefer percept. This confound could be an important bias in the case when one percept was more powerful than the other (*e.g.*, an object or face compared to a mere texture).

During scanning, we obtained behavioural reports that tagged the alternation of perceptual flips and stable percepts (*i.e.*, that were interspersed in real-time). This was achieved by instructing subjects to press one key at perceptual transitions and another during the ensuing stable percept. This experimental design is different from the aforementioned experiment, which compared similar perceptual alternations resulting from two different stimulus types (rivalrous and non-rivalrous) because we used only one stimulus (ambiguous picture). For analysis of our experiment, we computed differential event-related responses, matching for percept-related brain activity as well as motor reports, thus isolating switch-related activations. This analysis was robust against category-related activity shifts because perceptual reversals in *both* directions were contrasted with time points locked to *both* percepts. The findings therefore could not be explained by differences in activity associated with differential categorical (or spatial) features of the two percepts. We found no differential activity when comparing one direction of perceptual reversal with the other or by comparing the two stable percepts. Hence, the dominant source of variance in our data was the fact that a perceptual change occurred and not which percept was available for awareness. In other words, these findings reflected the spontaneous appearance (and disappearance) rather than the specific presence of a percept. Confirming our expectations, we found this cognitive event to transiently engage multiple segregated visual areas that process different attributes of visual stimuli.

Transient bilateral activations associated with perceptual reversals occurred in regions of ventral occipital and intraparietal cortex (Fig. 3.3a). Previous studies emphasised functional segregation between separate visual pathways rather than their integrative cooperation in the context of natural visual perception. Our findings using ambiguous figures provide an experimental demonstration of how these areas dynamically activate together when processing meaningful and relatively natural stimuli instead of experimentally isolated visual attributes. Functionally, this conjoint activation in ventral occipital and parietal areas can be understood to show that the reversal-related reinterpretation of an ambiguous figure (like the novel perception of any object in a visual scene) inevitably induces a perceived change in both categorical and spatial aspects.

A different view on these findings is that, in each of these areas, activity can be modulated by selectively directing attention to specific visual attributes. Attention in our paradigm, however, was not continuously directed to any type of attribute but flexibly recruited by the fluctuations between the two percepts, each of which is composed of a set of attributes. In other words, the perceptual ambiguity of our stimuli meant that we were able to study endogenously emergent, as opposed to externally instructed attentional modulation of brain activity. Salience from percept appearance (and disappearance) is inevitably transient and bridges perceptual and attentional domains. With ambiguous figures, it is exclusively related to the subjects' visual awareness, in which stable, figure/ground distinctions are only briefly disrupted during change from one percept to another. These reversals generate repetitive pop-out (and drop-out) equivalents even though the stimulus remains unchanged. The transient activations during perceptual flips may therefore form a substrate of perceived salience.

In line with this interpretation, we also observed switch-related activations in the frontal eye fields. The link between attention and gaze orientation, although dissociated by many experimental paradigms, including ours, is manifest in behaviour (Bowman *et al.*, 1993; Sheliga

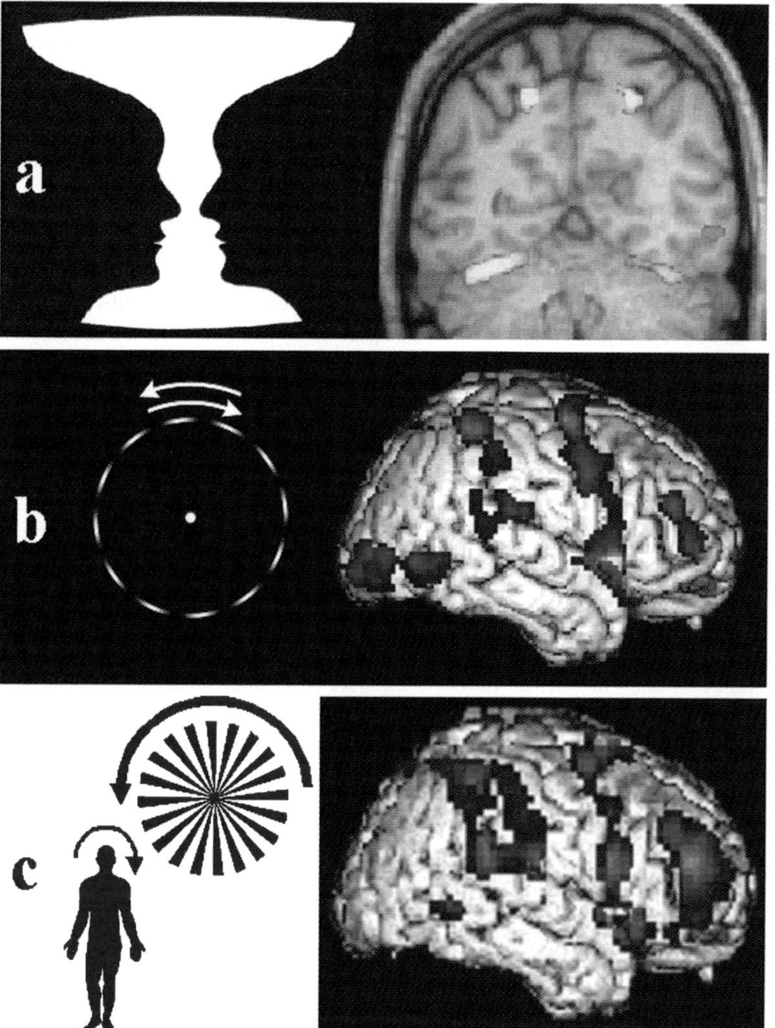

FIGURE 3.3
Stimuli (left) and neuroimaging findings (right) for transitions during bistable perception of objects (a), direction of apparent motion (c), and source of visual motion (*i.e.*, object or self motion) (c). (Adapted from Kleinschmidt *et al.*, 1998 and 2002b, and Sterzer *et al.*, 2002.)

et al., 1995) and implemented by a co-localised or even shared functional anatomy (Nobre *et al.*, 1997; Corbetta, 1998). The frontal eye fields integrate visual and attentional with coulometer processes. Indeed, visual and attentional components have been shown to activate this area in the absence of eye movements (Mohler *et al.*, 1973; Burman and Segraves, 1994; Bichot *et al.*, 1996; Paus, 1996; Kodaka *et al.*, 1997; Law *et al.*, 1997; Nobre *et al.*, 1997).

Even if due to sensitivity limitations the significant foci represent only the tip of the iceberg of transient activations in the visual system during perceptual reversals, it is noteworthy that these activations occur across areas with considerably differing responsiveness to visual stimulus properties. When construing a hierarchical functional specialisation in the primate visual system (Zeki, 1978; Ungerleider and Mishkin, 1982; Felleman and Van Essen, 1991), these areas are not only very distinct from each other but also represent quite advanced processing levels in the two separate pathways that preferentially process either categorical or spatial stimulus attributes. We concluded from this that the perceptual transitions (*i.e.*, changes of meaning assigned to a [constant] stimulus) engage cortical activity most prominently in visual areas remote from multidimensional and elemental early processing but dedicated to specialised higher order attributes of the scene viewed (Milner, 1995; Logothetis, 1998; Treisman and Kanwisher 1998).

Conversely, because the actual visual input remained constant in our experiment, we expected no pronounced signal increase in early visual processing stages where activity is more rigidly locked to the afferent input. In a hierarchical view of the visual system, primary visual cortex is at the trunk end of the tree compared to the branches leading into ventral and parietal areas. It is by far the most prominent target of retinogeniculate afferents and, as the dominant "early" visual area, forms the shared cortical origin for processing multiple visual stimulus features and relaying them into divergent, functionally more specialised visual areas (Felleman and Van Essen 1991). We thus expected to find no activity increases in primary visual cortex during perceptual reversals but were surprised to find that activity there actually displayed transient decreases during flips as it did in the pulvinar. The latter deactivation in particular underscores the fact that the activations in bilateral ventral occipital and parietal cortex are not merely a nonspecific activity gain that occurs across all visual structures modulated by attention. Instead, the activity modulation during perceptual flips differed regionally in sign and therefore presumably in functional significance. In such a more differentiated picture, the deactivations in early structures as primary visual cortex and the pulvinar might reflect an activity breakdown during transitions (i.e., the un- and rebinding of percepts).

Ambiguity of Motion Perception

Ambiguity of Motion Direction

One remaining question after this study was whether the spatial pattern of the activations in extrastriate visual areas is meaningful in relation to the perceptual content that changes during transitions. The classical ambiguous figures we used are perceptually rich in the sense that at flips there is a change in category of the perceived object *(e.g.*, face or vase) or at least in exemplar within a category (*e.g.*, old and young woman). Along with this, there is a change in the spatial configuration and consequently the distribution of interest within the scene that presumably engenders spatial attention shifts. To address whether the cerebral pattern of activations during perceptual switches with ambiguous visual stimuli is related to the perceptual content that changes with these switches, we chose to study with functional neuroimaging a perceptually sparse visual ambiguity, the so-called spinning-wheel illusion (Sterzer *et al.*, 2002). The spinning-wheel illusion is generated by presenting in alternation two frames showing wheels that are offset to each other by half the interspoke angular distance, resulting in a bistable apparent motion stimulus (Fig. 3.3, middle) (see Wertheimer, 1912; Purves *et al.*, 1996). Both possible percepts correspond to the same object and share the same spatial extent and centre. They are perceived as identically patterned stimuli moving at the same speed and changing only in direction.

As opposed to the ambiguities described before, the cognitive difference between the two percepts is minimised in the case of the spinning wheel; therefore, we could study whether the activations in extrastriate cortices during perceptual switches of a single attribute occur selectively in those visual areas that are sensitive to this attribute within a sensory stimulus. According to the perceptual content (motion direction) of switches with the spinning wheel, we expected and confirmed such activations in the area commonly referred to as the human motion complex (hMT+/V5) (Tootell *et al.*, 1995; Watson *et al.*, 1993). This brain region has been shown to be activated by continuous motion perception and direction changes of visual motion stimuli (Cornette *et al.*, 1998; Morrone *et al.*, 2000), as well as during apparent motion perception and motion imagery (Goebel *et al.*, 1998; Zeki *et al.*, 1993). Another site of activation, about 15 mm posterior to, and obviously distinct from, area hMT+/V5 (Fig. 3.3), was found in the lateral occipital sulcus of both hemispheres, putatively corresponding to a region that has been previously described as kinetic occipital (KO) area (Dupont *et al.*, 1997; Van Oostende *et al.*, 1997). This response pattern was hence different from the fusiform activations observed in previous studies on bistable perception, the latter presumably being related to categorical changes in perception. At the same time, we confirmed that even with a perceptually sparse ambiguity, such as the spinning wheel, switch-related responses also occurred in a similar frontoparietal network as in the aforementioned studies on perceptual rivalry (Kleinschmidt *et al.*, 1998; Lumer *et al.*, 1998).

Ambiguity of Self vs. Object Motion

The findings with ambiguous visual stimuli showed activations in areas that seem to be necessary for perceiving specific visual attributes or categories. Akinetopsia presumably results from (bilateral) damage to the occipitotemporal junction in the area of the motion complex (Zihl *et al.*, 1983), and selective agnosias as prosopagnosia can be related to lesions in the fusiform gyrus (see Farah, 1990). These areas are also the structures where the endpoint of specialised sensory processing overlaps with the specific responses associated with bistable percepts. Of course, sensory processing of visual input also involves earlier visual structures and requires their integrity, and the activations observed with bistable percepts during constant visual input also include frontoparietal structures that presumably subserve more general functions as attentional selection. Yet, the overlap of activations in certain extrastriate visual areas both in purely sensory and in purely perceptual experiments suggests that studies with bistable percepts may be used to identify those areas of the brain with the highest perceptual specificity for a certain aspect of the visual scene.

The study with the spinning wheel addressed an ambiguity of motion direction that can be elicited by an apparent motion stimulus. The use of an illusion in that experiment was driven by the need to create a bistable motion percept from a single stimulus. Yet, the far more fundamental ambiguity that the brain has to resolve when receiving visual-motion stimulation at the retina is whether it originates from motion of an object in the world or the observer. Visual motion reflects only relative motion information between object and observer. Within the visual sense, wide visual field coverage by the object and/or impoverished information from the stationary background can suggest that retinal shifting of an object is caused by observer motion (Mach, 1875; Helmholtz, 1896; Gibson, 1954; Warren, 1995; Lappe *et al.*, 1999). Yet, additional cues from other spatial senses usually help to disambiguate object from self motion. Vestibular and proprioceptive sensory feedback and efference copies of body, head, and eye movements can prevent us from mistaking the origin of visual motion (Wertheim, 1994; Wexler *et al.*, 2001). However, when visual motion is the sole informative cue for reconstructing self-motion, a perceptual ambiguity may arise and induce *vection*, an illusion of self motion (Dichgans and Brandt, 1978). This illusion is, for instance, commonly experienced when a sensation of self motion is evoked by a train slowly moving on a neighbouring track as we watch from a stationary position.

We hypothesised that this illusion could be used to address the neural correlates of self-motion perception and that, similar to the aforementioned studies, a neuroimaging experiment could identify the specific brain structures underlying this percept (Kleinschmidt *et al.*, 2002b). Using an illusion in this case is inevitable because the requirements of functional neuroimaging currently preclude studies with true observer motion; however, this experimental approach provides a valid model to study visual processing of one type of self-motion. A not actively moving, but steadily displaced, observer (zero acceleration) will lack congruent proprioceptive and vestibular input (i.e., afferent input during circular vection imitates that from constant velocity self-motion). That this illusion cannot be considered a failure of the brain's perceptual mechanisms is illustrated by contemporary real-life situations that depend exclusively on visual-motion input (e.g., while driving a car at constant velocity and fixating on the end of a straight road). Correspondingly, an appropriate visual-motion stimulus can evoke the sensation of self motion in a stationary observer. We used a windmill pattern rotating around its centre and adjusted the stimulus properties that support circular vection such that while being scanned the subjects perceived the two perceptual states of object and self motion for roughly equivalent lengths of time. This allowed us to compare brain activity while stimulation was constant but perception fluctuated between two different states (i.e., object vs. self motion). In that sense, this experiment was similar to the one reported by Tong *et al.* (1998).

In a first step, we determined brain areas sensitive to the type of visual-motion stimulus we used (coherent, wide-field stimulation) by contrasting brain activity between the whole period of rotation and a preceding stationary phase. We found multiple brain regions activated, and our findings largely conform with reports from previous neuroimaging studies mapping the responses to visual-motion (Watson *et al.*, 1993; Dupont *et al.*, 1994; de Jong *et al.*, 1994; Cheng *et al.*, 1995; McCarthy *et al.*, 1995; Tootell *et al.*, 1995; McKeefry *et al.*, 1997, Dieterich *et al.*, 1998; Greenlee, 2000; Previc *et al.*, 2000).

In a second step, we analysed brain activity levels as a function of the percept (i.e, object vs. self motion). We expected that areas where lesions result in disturbed self-motion perception would display enhanced activity during self-motion; yet, this was not the case. While all of the candidate areas were strongly responsive to our rotatory flow stimulus, their activity remained unchanged across the two different perceptual interpretations of this sensory input. These regions included (1) dorsomedial cortex (DM), comprising cuneus and parieto-occipital cortex (Heide *et al.*, 1990; also see Richer *et al.*, 1991, for electrostimulation), and (2) the anterior portion of the human visual-motion complex (V5/MT complex) at the occipitotemporal junction (hypothetical V5a/MST), i.e., the hypothetical homologue of monkey medial superior temporal cortex (V5a/MST) (Duffy and Wurtz, 1991; Orban, 1997; Tanaka, 1998; Vaina, 1998; Wurtz, 1998).

This finding became more plausible when we contrasted the areas that did show activity differences related to the percept. Apart from a cerebellar region that presumably corresponds to the nodulus and therefore might be related to a slight gain increase of the torsional nystagmus occurring during vection (Angelaki and Hess, 1994; Thilo *et al.*, 1999), no activations were observed during vection. Conversely, virtually the entire visual system was more active during perceived object motion as opposed to self motion. The aforementioned candidate areas were thus the only structures that stood out in that they resisted what can also be considered a general suppressive influence on the visual system that arises during vection. Likewise, the parieto-insular cortex, a putative human homologue of a vestibular cortex (Bottini *et al.*, 1994; see also Guldin and Grüsser, 1998) that was not responsive to the motion stimulus per se, showed significant deactivation during vection in line with previous findings by Brandt *et al.* (1998).

Together, these observations suggested that during vection there are suppressive visuo-visual and visuo-vestibular interactions (Brandt, 1999). This could be taken as indirect evidence that the areas not showing this suppression are of crucial importance for perceiving visual self motion. More direct evidence was obtained when investigating transition- instead of percept-related brain activity. One would postulate that, if an area is sensitive to the perceptual consequence of a visual stimulus, then it should also display transient signal changes whenever the perceptual interpretation changes. The sustained response levels we found, for example, in the presumptive human homologue of the dorsal medial superior temporal area (MSTd) indicated that it was responsive to our stimulus but that its response level was identical across the two percepts. Such a behaviour could correspond to one continuous sustained response unaffected by perceptual switches, but it could also be that every perceptual change was accompanied by a transient response and that the activity level between such switches remained constant. Our event-related analyses showed that the latter was the case (Fig. 3.3, bottom). In other words, the continuous response of several brain areas, including putative MSTd, to our visual-motion stimulus was modulated by transient activations each time the perceptual interpretation changed from one possible percept to the other, and the strength of these activations was identical for both directions of perceptual change, as were the sustained activity levels for both percepts. Interestingly, in the aforementioned study by Morrone *et al.* (2000), the best temporo-occipital responses were elicited by changes in optic flow direction rather than constant flow, which is in line with electrophysiological findings in MST (Paolini *et al.*, 2000, see also Duffy and Wurtz, 1997) but also with our finding of transient activations occurring at each perceptual switch (*i.e.*, each perceived change of optic flow). Together, these findings provide support for the idea that MSTd is of crucial importance for visually perceiving self motion but also participates in analysing complex visual-motion stimuli arising from sources other than observer motion (Geesaman and Andersen, 1996; Zemel and Sejnowski, 1998). If these different functional contexts are processed using the same specialised neural architecture, it is not surprising that they may interfere behaviourally (Probst *et al.*, 1984).

Our event-related analyses showed the same functional behaviour during perceptual transitions in other brain areas such as dorsomedial cortex, whereas areas related to object perception such as the fusiform gyrus only activated with the onset of perceived object motion. We also reproduced the event-related response pattern in frontoparietal brain areas that seem related to more general aspects of perceptual synthesis and selection.

This experiment, then, addressed the neural correlates of two spontaneously rivalling and profoundly different perceptual interpretations of one constant visual-motion stimulus. The intermittently generated illusion of self-motion provides a model of how the brain deals with retinal stimulation that results from our own actions. While we found a general suppression of activity in visual and vestibular cortex during vection, the activity levels in advanced visual processing stages remain unaffected and thus presumably allow for continued reconstruction of self motion. These effects can be functionally framed as mechanisms that allow us to stabilise our perception of the visual environment and to use our visual sense to guide our locomotion. The findings also underscore the fact that findings on neural processes (*e.g.*, related to object perception) cannot simply be extrapolated from a fixating stationary observer to the more realistic and relevant setting of a human in motion.

SUMMARY

This chapter has illustrated some recent functional neuroimaging experiments on the constructive side of visual perception. These experiments addressed very different neurobiological questions ranging from object to motion perception but share in common the methodological approach of relating brain activity levels and changes to perceptual states and transitions instead of to the physical characteristics of the stimuli employed. This approach was introduced by referring to bottom-up and top-down perspectives on brain function, a view that may be of some practical usefulness but that turns vulnerable once one asks what is at the top. In that sense, it is relevant to point out that phenomena such as hysteresis and bistability are readily generated by theories of brain function that model the emergence of higher layers of meaning, (*e.g.*, perception in relation to sensation) purely from the intrinsic properties of a sophisticated network (Kelso, 1995). Whether or not this is an appropriate model of brain function cannot be said at this stage, but many of the pertinent hypotheses have become experimentally testable by the novel tools available to human brain research.

References

Angelaki, D. E. and Hess, B. J. M. (1994). The cerebellar nodulus and ventral uvula control the torsional vestibuloocular reflex. *J. Neurophysiol.*, **72**, 1443–1447.

Bar, M., Tootell, R. B. H., Schacter, D. L., Greve, D. N., Fischl, B., Mendola, J. D., Rosen, B. R., and Dale, A. M. (2001). Cortical mechanisms specific to explicit object recognition. *Neuron*, **29**, 529–535.

Bichot, N. P., Schall, J. D., and Thompson, K. G. (1996). Visual feature selectivity in frontal eye fields induced by experience in mature macaques. *Nature (London)*, **381**, 697–699.

Bottini, G., Sterzi, R., Paulesu, E., Vallar, G., Cappa, S. F., Erminio, F., Passingham, R. E., Frith, C. D., and Frackowiak, R. S. F. (1994). Identification of the central vestibular projections in man: a positron emission tomography activation study. *Exp. Brain Res.*, **99**, 164–169.

Bowman, E. M., Brown, V. J., Kertzman, C., Schwarz, U., and Robinson, D. L. (1993). Covert orienting of attention in macaques. 1. Effects of behavioural context. *J. Neurophysiol.*, **70**, 431–443.

Brandt, T. (1999). Cortical visual-vestibular interaction for spatial orientation and self-motion perception. *Curr. Opin. Neurol.*, **12**, 1–4.

Brandt, T., Bartenstein, P., Janek, A., and Dieterich, M. (1998). Reciprocal inhibitory visual-vestibular interaction: visual motion stimulation deactivates the parieto-insular vestibular cortex. *Brain*, **121**, 1749–1758.

Brown, M. W. and Aggleton, J. P. (2001). Recognition memory: what are the roles of the perirhinal cortex and hippocampus? *Nat. Rev. Neurosci.*, **2**, 51–61.

Buckley, M. J. and Gaffan, D. (1998). Perirhinal cortex ablation impairs visual object identification. *J. Neurosci.*, **18**, 2268–2275.

Buckner, R. L., Goodman, J., Burock, M., Rotte, M., Koutstaal, W., Schacter, D., Rosen, B., and Dale, A. M. (1998). Functional-anatomic correlates of object priming in humans revealed by rapid presentation event-related fMRI. *Neuron*, **20**, 285–296.

Burman, D. D. and Segraves, M. A. (1994). Primate frontal eye field activity during natural scanning eye movements. *J. Neurophysiol.*, **71**, 1266–1271.

Carpenter, G. A. and Grossberg, S. (1993). Normal and amnesic learning, recognition and memory by a neural model of cortico-hippocampal interactions. *Trends Neurosci.*, **16**, 131–137.

Cheng, K., Fujita, H., Kanno, I., Miura, S., and Tanaka, K. (1995). Human cortical regions activated by wide-field visual motion: an $H_2{}^{15}O$ PET study. *J. Neurophysiol.*, **74**, 413–427.

Corbetta, M. (1998). Frontoparietal cortical networks for directing attention and the eye to visual locations: identical, independent, or overlapping neural systems? *Proc. Natl. Acad. Sci. USA*, **95**, 831–838.

Cornette, L., Dupont, P., Rosier, A., Sunaert, S., Hecke, P. V., Michiels, J., Mortelmans, L., and Orban, G. A. (1998. Human brain regions involved in direction discrimination. *J Neurophysiol.*, **79**, 2749–2765.

de Jong, B. M., Shipp, S., Skidmore, B., Frackowiak, R. S. J., and Zeki, S. (1994). The cerebral activity related to the visual perception of forward motion in depth. *Brain*, **117**, 1039–1054.

Dichgans, J. and Brandt, T. (1978). Visual-vestibular interaction: effects on self-motion perception and postural control, in *Handbook of Sensory Physiology*, Vol. 8, Held, R., Leibowitz, H. W., Teuber, H. L., Eds., pp., 755–804. Springer, Heidelberg.

Dieterich, M., Bucher, S. F., Seelos, K. C., and Brandt, T. (1998). Horizontal or vertical optokinetic stimulation activates visual motion-sensitive, ocular motor and vestibular cortex areas with right hemispheric dominance. *Brain*, **121**, 1479–1495.

Driver, J. and Mattingley, J. B. (1998). Parietal neglect and visual awareness. *Nat. Neurosci.*, **1**, 17–22.

Duffy, C. J. and Wurtz, R. H. (1991). Sensitivity of MST neurons to optic flow stimuli. 1. A continuum of response selectivity to large-field stimuli. *J. Neurophysiol.*, **65**, 1329–1345.

Duffy C. J. and Wurtz R. H. (1997). Multiple temporal components of optic flow responses in MST neurons. *Exp. Brain Res.*, **114**, 472–482.

Dupont, P., DeBruyn, B., Vandenberghe, R., Rosier, A. M., Michiels, J., Marchal, G., Mortelmans, L., and Orban G. A. (1997). The kinetic occipital region in human visual cortex. *Cereb. Cortex*, **7**, 283–292.

Dupont, P., Orban, G. A., de Bruyn, B., Verbruggen, A., and Mortelmans, L. (1994). Many areas in the human brain respond to visual motion. *J. Neurophysiol.*, **72**, 1420–1424.

Farah, M. J. (1990). *Visual Agnosia*. MIT Press, Cambridge, MA.

Felleman, D. J. and Van Essen, D. C. (1991). Distributed hierarchical processing in the primate cerebral cortex. *Cereb. Cortex*, **1**, 1–81.

Geesaman, B. J. and Andersen, R. A. (1996). The analysis of complex motion patterns by form/cue invariant MSTd neurons. *J. Neurosci.*, **16**, 4716–4732.

Gibson, J. J. (1954). The visual perception of objective motion and subjective movement. *Psychol. Rev.*, **61**, 304–314.

Gluck, M. A. and Myers, C. E. (1993). Hippocampal mediation of stimulus representation: a computational theory. *Hippocampus*, **3**, 491–516.

Goebel, R., Khorram-Sefat, D., Muckli, L., Hacker, H., and Singer, W. (1998). The constructive nature of vision: direct evidence from functional magnetic resonance imaging studies of apparent motion and motion imagery. *Eur. J. Neurosci.*, **10**, 1563–1573.

Greenlee, M. W. (2000). Human cortical areas underlying the perception of optic flow: brain imaging studies. *Int. Rev. Neurobiol.*, **44**, 269–292.

Gregory, R. L. (1969/1998). *Eye and Brain: The Psychology of Seeing*, 5th ed., pp. 194–243. Oxford University Press, London.

Grill-Spector, K., Kushnir, T., Edelman, S., Itzchak, Y., and Malach, R. (1998). Cue-invariant activation in object-related areas of the human occipital lobe. *Neuron*, **21**, 191–202.

Grill-Spector, K., Kushnir, T., Edelman, S., Avidan, G., Itzchak, Y., and Malach, R. (1999). Differential processing of objects under various viewing conditions in the human lateral occipital complex. *Neuron*, **24**, 187–203.

Grill-Spector, K., Kushnir, T., Hendler, T., and Malach, R. (2000). The dynamics of object-selective activation correlate with recognition performance in humans. *Nat. Neurosci.*, **3**, 837–843.

Guldin, W. O. and Grüsser, O. J. (1998). Is there a vestibular cortex? *Trends Neurosci.*, **21**, 254–259.

Heide, W., Koenig, E., and Dichgans, J. (1990). Optokinetic nystagmus, self-motion sensation and their aftereffects in patients with occipito-parietal lesions. *Clin. Vis. Sci.*, **5**, 145–156.

Helmholtz, H. (1896). *Handbuch der Physiologischen Optik*. Voss, Leipzig.

Kelso, J. A. S. (1995). *Dynamic Patterns*, MIT Press, Cambridge, MA.

Kleinschmidt, A., Büchel, C., Hutton, C., Friston, K. J., and Frackowiak, R. S. J. (2002a). The neural structures expressing perceptual hysteresis in visual letter recognitition. *Neuron*, **34**, 659–666.

Kleinschmidt, A., Thilo, K. V., Büchel, C., Gresty, M. A., Bronstein, A. M., and Frackowiak, R. S. J. (2002b). Neural correlates in the human brain of visual-motion perception as object- or self-motion. *NeuroImage*, **16**, 873–882.

Kodaka, Y., Mikami, A., and Kubota, K. (1997). Neuronal activity in the frontal eye field of the monkey is modulated while attention is focused on to a stimulus in the peripheral visual field, irrespective of eye movement. *Neurosci. Res.*, **28**, 291–298.

Kourtzi, Z. and Kanwisher N. (2000). Cortical regions involved in perceiving object shape. *J. Neurosci.*, **20**, 3310–3318.

Kruse, P. and Stadler, M., Eds. (1995). *Ambiguity in Mind and Nature*. Springer, Berlin.

Lappe, M., Bremmer, F., and van den Berg, A. V. (1999). Perception of self-motion from visual flow. *Trends Cogn. Sci.*, **3**, 329–336.

Law, I., Svarer, C., Holm, S., and Paulson, O.B. (1997). The activation pattern in normal humans during suppression, imagination and performance of saccadic eye movements. *Acta Physiol. Scand.*, **161**, 419–434.

Logothetis, N. (1998). Object vision and visual awareness. *Curr. Opin. Neurobiol.*, **8**, 536–544.

Lumer, E. D., Friston, K. J., and Rees, G. (1998). Neural correlates of perceptual rivalry in the human brain. *Science*, **280**, 1930–1934.

Mach, E. (1875). *Grundlinie der Lehre von den Bewegungsempfindungen*. Engelmann, Leipzig.

Malach, R., Reppas, J. B., Benson, R. R., Kwong, K. K., Jiang, H., Kennedy, W. A., Ledden, P. J., Brady, T. J., Rosen, B. R., and Tootell, R. B. H. (1995). Object-related activity revealed by functional magnetic resonance imaging in human occipital cortex. *Proc. Natl. Acad. Sci. USA*, **92**, 8135–8139.

McCarthy, G., Spicer, M., Adrignolo, A., Luby, M., Gore, J., and Allison, T. (1995). Brain activation associated with visual motion studied by functional magnetic resonance imaging in humans. *Hum. Brain Mapping*, **2**, 234–243.

McKeefry, D. J., Watson, J. D. G., Frackowiak, R. S. J., and Zeki, S. (1997). The activity in human areas V1/V2, V3, and V5 during the perception of coherent and incoherent motion. *NeuroImage*, **5**, 1–12.

Milner, A. D. (1995). Cerebral correlates of visual awareness. *Neuropsychology*, **33**, 1117–1130.

Miyashita, Y., Okuno, H., Tokuyama, W., Ihara, T., and Nakajima, K. (1996). Feedback signal from medial temporal lobe mediates visual associative mnemonic codes of inferotemporal neurons. *Cogn. Brain Res.*, **5**, 81–86.

Mohler, C. W., Goldberg, M. E., and Wurtz R. H. (1973). Visual receptive fields of frontal eye field neurons. *Brain Res.*, **61**, 385–389.

Morrone, M. C., Tosetti, M., Montanaro, D., Fiorentini, A., Cioni, G., and Burr, D. C. (2000). A cortical area that responds specifically to optic flow, revealed by fMRI. *Nat Neurosci.*, **3**, 1322–1328.

Murray, E. A. and Bussey, T. J. (1999). Perceptual-mnemonic functions of the perirhinal cortex. *Trends Cogn. Sci.*, **3**, 142–151.

Naya, Y., Yoshida, M., and Miyashita, Y. (2001). Backward spreading of memory-retrieval signal in the primate temporal cortex. *Science*, **291**, 661–664.

Nobre, A. C., Sebestyen, G. N., Gitelman, D. R., Mesulam, M. M., Frackowiak, R. S. J., and Frith, C. D. (1997). Functional localisation of the system for visuospatial attention using positron emission tomography. *Brain*, **120,** 515–533.

Orban, G. A. (1997). Visual processing in macaque area MT/V5 and its satellites (MSTd and MSTv), in *Cerebral Cortex*. Vol. 12. *Extrastriate Cortex*, Rockland, K. S., Kaas, J. H., and Peters, A., Eds., pp. 359–434. Plenum, New York.

Paolini, M., Distler, C., Bremmer, F., Lappe, M., and Hoffmann, K. P. (2000). Responses to continuously changing optic flow in area MST. *J Neurophysiol.*, **84**, 730–743.

Paus, T. (1996). Location and function of the human frontal eye-field: a selective review. *Neuropsychologia*, **34**, 475–483.

Portas, C. M., Strange, B. A., Friston, K. J., Dolan, R. J., and Frith, C. D. (2000). How does the brain sustain a visual percept? *Proc. Roy. Soc. London Ser. B*, **267**, 845–850.

Previc, F. H., Liotti, M., Blakemore, C., Beer, J., and Fox, P. (2000). Functional imaging of brain areas involved in the processing of coherent and incoherent wide field-of-view visual motion. *Exp. Brain Res.*, **131**, 393–405.

Probst, T., Krafczyk, S., Brandt, T., and Wist, E. R. (1984). Interaction between perceived self-motion and object-motion impairs vehicle guidance. *Science*, **225**, 536–538.

Purves, D., Paydarfar, J. A., and Andrews, T. J. (1996). The wagon wheel illusion in movies and reality. *Proc. Natl. Acad. Sci. USA*, **93**, 3693–3697.

Ranganath, C. and d'Esposito, M. (2001). Medial temporal lobe activity associated with active maintenance of novel information. *Neuron*, **31**, 865–873.

Rao, R. P. and Ballard, D. H. (1999). Predictive coding in the visual cortex: a functional interpretation of some extra-classical receptive-field effects. *Nat. Neurosci.*, **2**, 79–87.

Richer, F., Martinez, M., Cohen, H., and Saint-Hilaire, J. M. (1991). Visual-motion perception from stimulation of the human medial parietooccipital cortex. *Exp. Brain Res.*, **87**, 649–652.

Scoville, W. B. and Milner, B. (1957). Loss of recent memory after bilateral hippocampal lesions. *J. Neurol. Neurosurg. Psych.*, **20**, 11–21.

Sekuler, R. (1996). Motion perception: a modern view of Wertheimer's 1912 monograph. *Perception*, **25**, 1243–1258.

Sheliga, B. M., Riggio, L., and Rizzolatti, G. (1995). Spatial attention and eye movements. *Exp. Brain Res.*, **105**, 261–275.

Solomon, J. A. and Pelli, D. G. (1994). The visual filter mediating letter identification. *Nature*, **369**, 395–397.

Sterzer, P., Russ, M. O., Preibisch, C., and Kleinschmidt, A. (2002). Neural correlates of spontaneous direction reversals in ambiguous apparent visual-motion. *NeuroImage*, **15**, 908–916.

Suzuki, W. A., Zola-Morgan, S., Squire, L. R., and Amaral, D. G. (1993). Lesions of the perirhinal and parahippocampal cortices in the monkey produce long-lasting memory impairment in the visual and tactual modalities. *J. Neurosci.*, **13**, 2430–2451.

Tanaka, K. (1997). Mechanisms of visual object recognition: monkey and human studies. *Curr. Opin. Neurobiol.*, **7**, 523–529.

Tanaka, K. (1998). Representation of visual motion in the extrastriate visual cortex, in *High-Level Motion Processing*, Watanabe, T., Ed., pp., 295–313. MIT Press, Cambridge, MA.

Thilo, K. V., Probst, T., Bronstein, A. M., Ito, Y., and Gresty, M. A. (1999). Torsional eye movements are facilitated during perception of self-motion. *Exp. Brain Res.*, **126**, 495–500.

Tong F., Nakayama K., Vaughan J. T., and Kanwisher N. (1998). Binocular rivalry and visual awareness in human extrastriate cortex. *Neuron*, **21**, 753–759.

Tootell, R. B. H., Hadjikhani, N. K., Mendola, J. D., Marrett, S., and Dale, A. M. (1998). From retinotopy to recognition: fMRI in human visual cortex. *Trends Cog. Sci.*, **2**, 174–183.

Tootell, R. B. H., Reppas, J. B., Kwong, K. K., Malach, R., Born, R. T., Brady, T. J., Rosen, B. R., and Belliveau, J. W. (1995). Functional analysis of human MT and related visual cortical areas using magnetic resonance imaging. *J. Neurosci.*, **15**, 3215–3230.

Treisman, A. M. and Kanwisher, N. G. (1998). Perceiving visually presented objects: recognition, awareness, and modularity. *Curr. Opin. Neurobiol.*, **8**, 218–226.

Ullman, S. (1995). Sequence seeking and counter streams: a computational model for bi-directional information flow in the visual cortex. *Cereb. Cortex*, **5**, 1–11.

Ungerleider, L.G. and Mishkin, M. (1982). Two cortical visual systems, in *Analysis of Visual Behaviour*, Ingle, D. J., Goodale, M. A., and Mansfield, R. J. W., Eds., pp. 549–586. MIT Press, Cambridge, MA.

Vaina, L. M. (1998). Complex motion perception and its deficits. *Curr. Opin. Neurobiol.*, **8**, 494–502.

Van Oostende, S., Sunaert, S., VanHecke, P., Marchal, G., and Orban, G. A. (1997). The kinetic occipital (KO) region in man: an fMRI study. *Cereb Cortex*, **7**, 690–701.

Warren, W. H. (1995). *Self-Motion: Visual Perception and Visual Control*. Academic Press, San Diego.

Watson J. D., Myers R., Frackowiak R. S., Hajnal J. V., Woods R. P., Mazziotta J. C., Ship S., and Zeki S. (1993). Area V5 of the human brain: evidence from a combined study using positron emission tomography and magnetic resonance imaging. *Cereb. Cortex*, **3**, 79–94.

Wertheim, A. (1994). Motion perception during self-motion — the direct versus inferential controversy revisited. *Behav. Brain Sci.*, **17**, 293–311.

Wertheimer, M. (1912). Experimentelle Studien über das Sehen von Bewegung. *Zeitschrift für Psychologie*, 61.

Wexler, M., Panerai, F., Lamouret, I., and Droulez, J. (2001). Self-motion and the perception of stationary objects. *Nature*, **409**, 85–88.

Wurtz, R. H. (1978). Optic flow: a brain region devoted to optic flow analysis. *Curr. Biol.*, **8**, R554–R556.

Zeki, S. M. (1978). Functional specialisation in the visual cortex of the monkey. *Nature*, **274**, 423–428.

Zeki, S., Watson, J. D., and Frackowiak, R. S. (1993). Going beyond the information given: the relation of illusory visual motion to brain activity. *Proc. Roy. Soc. London Ser. B, Biol Sci.*, **252**, 215–222.

Zemel, R. S. and Sejnowski, T. J. (1998). A model for encoding multiple object motions and self-motion in area MST of primate visual cortex. *J. Neurosci.*, **18**, 531–547.

Zihl, J., von Cramon, D., and Mai, N. (1983). Selective disturbance of movement vision after bilateral brain damage. *Brain*, **106**, 313–340.

Zola-Morgan, S., Squire, L. R., and Ramus, S. J. (1994). Severity of memory impairment in monkeys as a function of locus and extent of damage within the medial temporal lobe memory system. *Hippocampus*, **4**, 483–495.

CHAPTER

4

Auditory Function

INTRODUCTION

This chapter considers the processing of sound at the level of patterns in sound that are used to establish sound-object properties. This synthesis is therefore based on a type of sound processing rather than the processing of a particular type of sound and is equally relevant to the processing of speech, music, and environmental sounds. *Pattern* is used here in a broad sense to mean a variety of spectrotemporal features, as discussed later. The anatomy of the human auditory system is considered before functional imaging studies as a precondition for understanding the functional studies. The aim is to assess how the anatomical and functional studies have added to our understanding of the human auditory brain.

ANATOMICAL SUBSTRATES

Ascending Pathway

The ascending pathway in humans between the cochlea and primary cortex contains a number of processing centres with multiple interconnections, as shown in a simplified schematic form in Fig. 4.1. Spectrotemporal processing of sound can occur as early as the cochlear nucleus, while interaural cues for spatial analysis are first processed in the superior olive. Extensive processing of sound pattern is therefore possible before sound signals reach the cortex. In addition to the ascending pathway, there is an extensive corticofugal mechanism (not shown in Fig. 4.1) that has been shown in animals (Yan and Suga, 1998) and humans (Giraud et al., 1997) to have an important modifying influence on the processing of behaviourally relevant sound. Much information about the anatomy of the ascending pathway is derived from animal work (see Irvine, 1986), but there are differences between the structure of the ascending pathway in humans and other species (Moore, 1994). For example, the nucleus of the trapezoid body and lateral superior olive, implicated in interaural intensity analysis in animals, is diminished or absent in humans.

Cortex

Homology between animals and humans is less straightforward in the auditory cortex than in the ascending auditory pathway. The human primary auditory cortex is located in the region of the transverse gyrus of Heschl (HG) in the superior temporal plane (Fig. 4.2). It is possible to have more than one HG on one or both sides in approximately 20% of hemispheres and when the primary auditory cortex is located in the region of the most anterior gyrus. Variability of the gross anatomy of HG is demonstrated by probabilistic mapping of HG (Penhune *et al.*, 1996). Primary auditory cortex is located within the cytoarchitectonic area designated by Brodmann (1909) as area 41, although subsequent studies suggest that this area is subdivided (discussed in Morosan

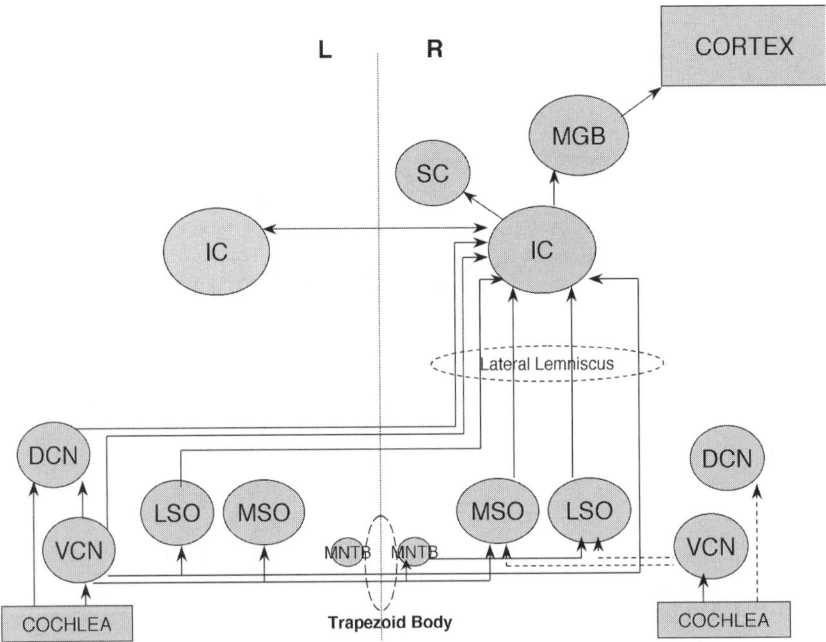

FIGURE 4.1
Simplified schematic showing the ascending auditory areas and their connections. VCN, Ventral cochlear nucleus; DCN, dorsal cochlear nucleus; IC, inferior colliculus; SC, superior colliculus; MGB, medial geniculate body; MNTB, nucleus of the trapezoid body; MSO, medial superior olive; LSO, lateral superior olive.

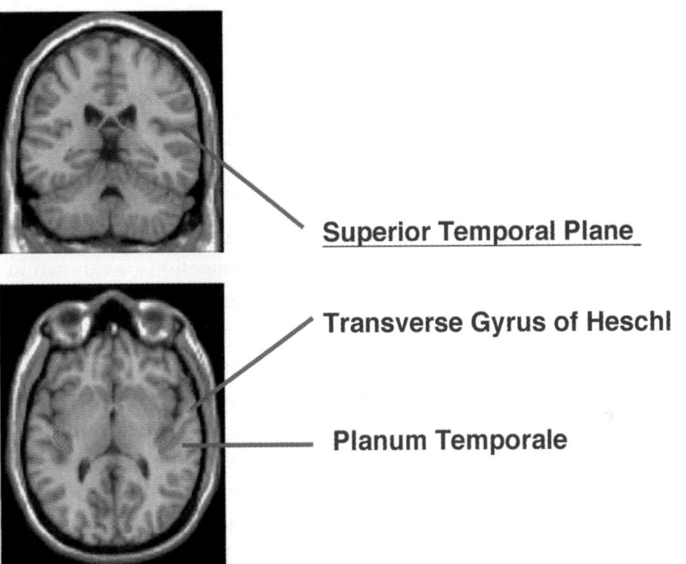

FIGURE 4.2
Location of the primary auditory area (shown in red) rendered onto the canonical brain structural template used in SPM99. A tilted axial slice has been used to show the superior temporal plane containing the transverse gyrus of Heschl and the planum temporale behind it. The primary auditory cortex is situated in the medial part of HG. The relationship between cytoarchitectonically defined primary auditory cortex and HG is not rigid; see Figure 2 in Rademacher *et al.* (2001).

et al., 2001). Recent detailed mapping of auditory cortex using cytoarchitectonic and neurochemical criteria (Hackett *et al.*, 2001; Morosan *et al.*, 2001; Rademacher *et al.*, 2001; Rivier and Clarke, 1997) has not been based on consistent nomenclature, but the studies broadly agree that primary cortex is located in the medial part of HG. The primary cortex is designated A1, core, and Te 1.0 in the studies of Rivier and Clarke, Hackett *et al.*, and Morosan *et al.*, respectively. This area is shown in red in Fig. 4.2, but the figure should only be taken as a guide;

recent studies demonstrate that primary auditory cortex is not consistently defined by the gross pattern of sulci and gyri; specifically, the proportion of HG that is occupied by cytoarchitectonically defined primary cortex can vary between 20 and 80%.

This anatomical information is important in terms of the interpretation of human functional data. The variability of the gross landmarks between subjects means that group functional studies cannot be rigidly interpreted in terms of the involvement of HG, although Penhune's probabilistic map allows the degree of certainty to be attributed. The variability of the cytoarchitectonic areas with respect to gross landmarks means that even when workers relate individual functional data to individual macroscopic anatomy the activations cannot be interpreted rigidly in terms of the involvement of the primary auditory area. Unfortunately, the different cytoarchitectonic areas cannot be distinguished *in vivo* using conventional structural magnetic resonance imaging (MRI) sequences.

The cortex adjacent to the human primary area contains multiple distinct auditory areas on microscopic grounds (Galaburda and Sanides, 1980; Rivier and Clarke, 1997). The lateral part of HG contains secondary auditory cortex, while the planum temporale (Westbury *et al.*, 1999) might be better described as auditory association cortex on the basis of its involvement in visual processes as well as a number of different auditory processes (see below). Few data are related to the anatomical interconnections of the human auditory cortices, but human depth-electrode and magnetoencephalography (MEG) studies of click responses at different latencies allow indirect inference. In the future, MRI diffusion tensor imaging may allow further insight. The earliest electrical responses to click stimuli occur at a latency of less than 30 ms in the region corresponding to primary cortex in medial HG (Liegeois-Chauvel *et al.*, 1991; Yvert *et al.*, 2001). Serial processing in primary cortex followed by non-primary areas can be inferred from measurement of the latency of click responses recorded from the superior temporal plane or directly demonstrated by recording from non-primary areas during electrical stimulation of primary cortex (Howard *et al.*, 2000). Data are scarce, however, as the superior temporal plane is an unusual site for depth-electrode placement in clinical epilepsy studies.

Further studies of the connectivity of human auditory areas are needed to establish whether human auditory cortex affords mechanisms for both serial processing and parallel processing. A basis for parallel processing in addition to serial processing in the macaque has been demonstrated by tracer studies (Rauschecker *et al.*, 1997) that show direct thalamic projections to both primary and non-primary areas.

FUNCTIONAL PROCESSING

Technical Considerations

Activation of structures in the ascending auditory pathway has been shown using positron emission tomography (PET) (Lockwood *et al.*, 1999), but systematic study of the ascending pathway using the greater spatial resolution of functional MRI (fMRI) has only been achieved recently (Griffiths *et al.*, 2001; Guimares *et al.*, 1998). Degradation of brainstem functional images due to the pulsation of the basilar artery represents a major problem in fMRI studies of the ascending auditory pathway. Guimares *et al.* were able to overcome this by triggering the acquisition of a single slice by the electrocardiogram so that images were always acquired at the same point in the cardiac cycle. Our group has developed a cardiac triggering technique for whole brain acquisition based on the use of an ascending axial sequence so that the benefit from the cardiac triggering is maximal in the brainstem where it makes most difference (Griffiths *et al.*, 2001). Using this technique, activation due to sound can be demonstrated in the cochlear nucleus, lateral lemniscus, inferior colliculus, and medial geniculate body (Fig. 4.3).

A problem in fMRI studies of both the ascending pathway and cortex is the noise made by a typical echo planar sequence (Ravicz *et al.*, 1999). Peak sound pressure levels in excess of 100 dB occur in a typical 1.5-Tesla machine, with the greatest source of noise being direct transmission from the gradient coils to the subject's head. This will have two effects. First, there will be a decrease in the difference in fMRI BOLD (blood-oxygen-level-dependent) signals between conditions where sound is presented and those where it is not. Second, the background noise may alter the biological process under investigation in a way that is not constant for

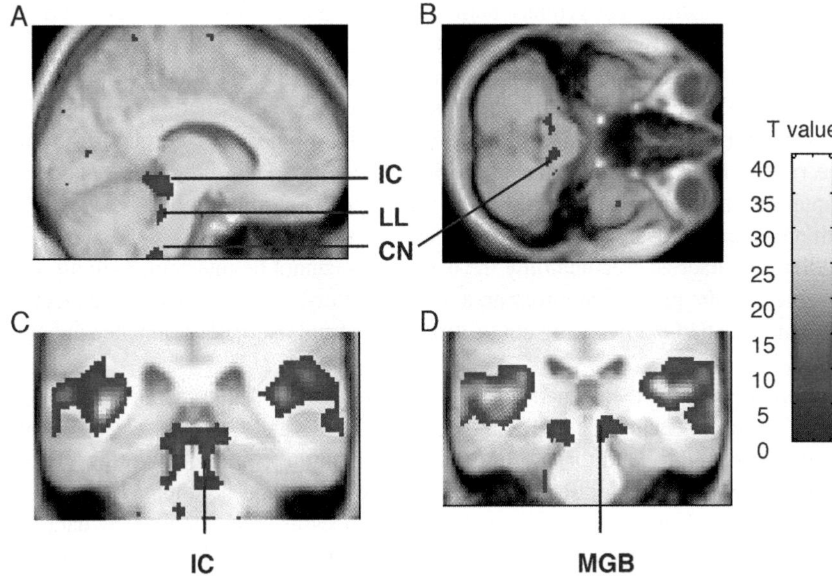

FIGURE 4.3
Demonstration of brain activity in the ascending auditory system using fMRI with cardiac triggering and sparse acquisition (see Griffiths *et al.*, 2001). Group data for eight subjects for a sound-minus-rest-contrast after conventional pre-processing using SPM99. The functional data are rendered onto the mean structural MRI for the group, and the colour map refers to the *t* value for the contrast. CN, cochlear nucleus; LL, lateral lemniscus; IC, inferior colliculus; MGB, medial geniculate body. The data are smoothed using a spatial filter with a full width at half maximum of 5 mm; it is not possible to distinguish the dorsal and ventral CN with this (conventional) level of smoothing.

different sound conditions. The scanner noise renders any auditory task an auditory foreground/background or "streaming" task (Bregman, 1990), thus requiring additional processing. It cannot be assumed that such additional processing will be the same whatever the sound stimulus. In some instances, it is conceivable that the auditory background noise might even make tasks easier—for example, auditory spatial tasks where the scanner noise might act as a fixed positional reference with which to compare the spatial stimulus. There is evidence that auditory cortical areas are not uniformly activated by tasks requiring foreground/background decomposition (Scheich *et al.*, 1998).

The problem of MRI scanner noise has been addressed by the use of *sparse imaging*, developed by a number of groups (Hall *et al.*, 1999; Yang *et al.*, 2000). This turns the sluggishness of the haemodynamic response function (typically ~10 s in auditory cortex) into an advantage (Fig. 4.4). Sound stimuli are presented over a period that is similar to the haemodynamic response function during which time there is no noise from the gradient coils. Single-image volumes are acquired after presentation of the stimulus. The signal measured at this time corresponds to the brain activity during presentation of the stimulus of interest only before the brain response to scanner noise. It takes longer using sparse imaging to acquire sufficient images for statistical analyses compared to standard continuous imaging, but comparable signal changes can be demonstrated in a similar period of time using fewer images (Hall *et al.*, 1999).

Processing of Spectral Information

Spectral mapping corresponding to the spectral analysis occurring in the cochlea is a recurring organisational principle of the auditory system. Although animal neurophysiology has demonstrated mapping of frequency in the auditory centres from the cochlear nucleus (CN) upward (Ehret and Romand, 1997), human functional imaging has only succeeded to date in mapping frequency representation in the cortex. Differential activation of medial and lateral areas in the superior temporal plane according to frequency was one of the first PET findings (Lauter *et al.*, 1985). The initial observation has been refined by studies suggesting more than one tonotopic auditory map along HG (Talavage *et al.*, 2000; Wessinger *et al.*, 1997) and

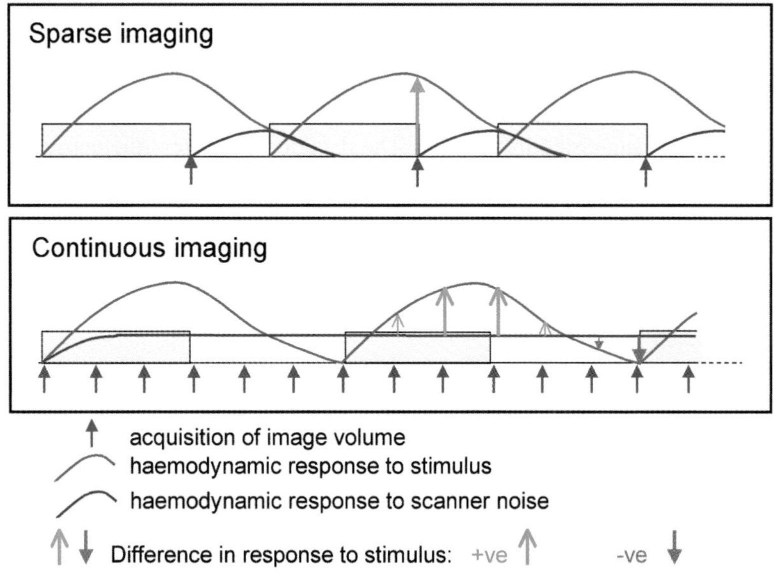

FIGURE 4.4
"Sparse" imaging paradigm for fMRI compared to continuous acquisition (see text). (Modified from an unpublished figure by R. D. Patterson.)

preferred processing of stimuli with greater bandwidth in lateral HG (Wessinger *et al.*, 2001). The study of Talavage *et al.* (2000) suggests at least four tonotopic mappings in the superior temporal plane. This is consistent with the idea that the different microscopically defined areas are associated with distinct tonotopic maps, although the study of Rivier and Clarke (1997) suggests that there are more than four anatomical areas.

Processing of Temporal Information: Sound Regularity or Periodicity

Any sound stimulus in the air can be considered in terms of either its spectral or temporal structure, and at this level the two types of mathematical description are interchangeable (Hartmann, 1997). This begs the question of any mapping of the temporal structure of sound in the human auditory system in addition to the established frequency maps. A model of temporal processing based on animal work (Langner, 1992) postulates orthogonal mapping of spectral and temporal sound features in the ascending pathway, and one human MEG study has been interpreted as showing mapping of sound temporal features in the human auditory cortex (Langner *et al.*, 1997). That study used the missing fundamental stimulus as the periodic stimulus; the envelope of this stimulus has a periodicity that corresponds to the reciprocal of the "missing" fundamental. Other work has used noise stimuli where the degree of temporal regularity that is represented in the auditory nerve can be varied without changing the auditory spectrum (Griffiths *et al.*, 1998, 2001). The fMRI study demonstrated a relationship between the regional local synaptic activity in the centres of the ascending auditory pathway and cortex (as measured indirectly by the BOLD response) and the degree of temporal regularity of the sound. This relationship was demonstrated as early as the CN and was more marked in the inferior colliculus (IC).

How can the data about regularity processing be interpreted? There are two possible interpretations of the data in CN: (1) a subpopulation of cells may become more active when they detect a particular temporal interval, perhaps onset chopper cells (Wiegrebe and Winter, 2001), or (2) the mean activity level of a broader population of cells in the CN may increase due to the synchronising effect of the sound regularity. Modelling work based on excitatory and inhibitory networks of neurons with conventional Hodgkin–Huxley neural dynamics (that could plausibly be applied to brainstem centres) suggests a tight coupling between synchronisation and mean firing rate that is not sensitive to the model parameters (Chawla *et al.*, 1999). At the level of IC, if conversion of regularity into an activity code occurs in a subpopulation of cells in CN, then the data suggest that such conversion is not completed in CN. This would be consistent with the two-stage mechanism suggested by Langner involving *measurement* of time intervals (regularity detection) early in the system and *representation* of those time intervals at a higher level. Alternatively, if the effect of regularity on BOLD response in the CN is due to an effect of synchronisation, this suggests that both measurement and detection of regularity must occur in IC. In either case, a two-stage brainstem mechanism for converting regularity into a more robust population rate code is suggested by the data. The data do not address the question of whether the representation of regularity in the brainstem is in the form of a map.

In the cortex, both PET and fMRI studies have shown a relationship between regularity and local activity in the region of HG. Given the constraints above regarding interpretation of the macroscopic boundaries in terms of functional areas, representation of temporal regularity at the millisecond level is associated with activity along the whole of HG and is likely to involve both primary and secondary auditory cortex.

Processing of Temporal Information: Modulation Processing

Amplitude modulation is an important feature of a number of sounds in the acoustic world, including speech (Saberi and Perrott, 1999; Shannon *et al.*, 1995). Studies of the detection of modulation can extend the study of temporal processing from the millisecond level (considered in the section above as *regularity*) to levels of tens of milliseconds or hundreds of milliseconds. The level of tens of milliseconds and above includes modulation rates below 50 Hz that are likely to be particularly important for speech perception. Psychophysical studies of amplitude modulation detection suggest that this may be centrally processed by a low-pass filtering mechanism in the modulation domain (Viemeister, 1979) or by a bank of parallel filters broadly tuned to different modulation rates (Dau *et al.*, 1997). Further support for the modulation filterbank concept comes from adaptation experiments where the change in detectability of modulation is measured after listening to similar modulation (Kay, 1982; Wojczak and Viemeister, 1999); the essential premise of these studies is that adaptation can occur if two modulations pass through the same modulation filter. Animal neurophysiology suggests tuned responses to amplitude modulation in neurons in CN, IC, and auditory cortex, with the best modulation rates decreasing at higher levels in the pathway (Moller, 1974; Rees and Moller, 1983; Schreiner and Urbas, 1988).

Human fMRI studies show that the amplitude modulation rates producing the largest BOLD responses in the ascending pathway are similar to the best modulation rates shown by single-unit recordings from these centres in animals (Giraud *et al.*, 2000; Harms *et al.*, 1998; Melcher *et al.*, 1999). This suggests that the best following responses of individual units are reflected by the sustained population rate of firing in the centres in which they are situated. Giraud *et al.* (2000) defined both sustained and transient responses to modulation, but it should be noted that these are descriptions of the haemodynamic response, and the transient response is still much slower than the neural following response in an individual neuron. The best modulation rates of hundreds of Hertz occur in the lower brainstem compared to responses of less than 10 Hz in HG, with a range of intermediate best responses for intermediate structures. In the auditory cortex, Giraud *et al.* (2000) found that small clusters responded better to low or high modulation rates, but they were unable to show any systematic mapping of amplitude modulation rate.

Frequency modulation is another form of modulation present in speech. Formant transitions, for example, can be regarded as either amplitude modulation of the harmonic components of voiced sound or as equivalent sweeps of frequency centred on formants (Remez *et al.*, 1981). Studies of frequency modulation by a number of groups also interested in speech perception (Binder *et al.*, 2000; Thivard *et al.*, 2000) suggest preferential responses in the planum temporale.

Work by Hall *et al.* (2000) emphasises the importance of attention in the interpretation of modulation studies. Distinct cortical responses to a mixture of amplitude- and frequency-modulated sounds compared to unmodulated control stimuli were not shown. In contrast, attention to modulation showed activation in the planum temporale.

Processing of Temporal Information: Sound-Sequence Processing

Approaches to auditory temporal processing based on the systematic use of different modulation rates may not allow the complete examination of processes necessary for the analysis of natural patterned sounds. Unlike continuous modulations, speech, music, and environmental sounds are *segmented*, raising the question of how sound sequences are processed. One of the simplest forms of sound sequence is an oddball sequence where infrequent deviants in frequency or duration occur in a stream of similar tones. An extensive body of evidence based on MEG and EEG responses to oddballs (Näätänen *et al.*, 2001) suggests the existence of preattentive auditory feature traces arising from non-primary auditory areas and attentional switching in frontal areas. Oddball responses in auditory cortex have also been demonstrated by PET (Tervaniemi *et al.*, 2000), but haemodynamic techniques such as PET and fMRI do not allow disambiguation of the early preattentive responses and later attentional switches to oddballs.

Processing of sequences that are more complex than oddball trains also involves non-primary auditory cortex. In a study based on sequences of discrete sounds associated with pitch (Griffiths *et al.*, 2001; Patterson *et al.*, 2002), "lively" sequences containing pitch variation between adjacent elements of the sequence produced more activation in secondary cortex in lateral HG than control sequences with a fixed repetitive pitch. This level of temporal structure corresponds to what musicologists refer to as *local structure* (Liegeois-Chauvel *et al.*, 1998; Peretz, 1990). As in lesion studies, a bilateral representation of local structure was suggested, though the imaging study showed greater effect of local structure on the right. This experiment included no task; however, in a PET experiment based on atonal sequences that did include a task, much more distributed bilateral activation was demonstrated, including the planum temporale, frontal operculum, and cerebellum (Griffiths *et al.*, 1999). The cortical activation was similar to that in another PET study of the processing of tonal melodies (Zatorre *et al.*, 1994), where frontal mechanisms were also implicated for the active task. Processing in the previous study was, however, much more lateralised to the right. This may reflect differences in the stimuli (tonal versus atonal) or task (degree of global or contour processing). Other functional imaging studies have examined the processing of sound rhythm (Penhune *et al.*, 1998; Sakai *et al.*, 1999) and implicated the basal ganglia and cerebellum. It is often difficult in these studies requiring motor reproduction of a rhythm to disambiguate the perception of rhythm and motor response preparation and execution.

Identification of Auditory Objects

Spectrotemporal analysis of sound using the processing mechanisms described above allows the identification of objects. This involves the association of the object features with previously learned meanings or schema (Bregman, 1990). The synthesis above demonstrates that complex spectrotemporal analysis occurs in the superior temporal plane in non-primary auditory areas. Further processing to allow object identification has been shown to occur bilaterally in more inferior areas on the temporal convexity. Mechanisms for both voice and environmental sound identification have been demonstrated at this site (Belin *et al.*, 2000; Maeder *et al.*, 2001).

Spatial Processing

There has been considerable recent interest in the hypothesis that distinct "streams" may exist in the human auditory cortex for the localisation of objects in space as opposed to the recognition of auditory objects (Rauschecker and Tian, 2000). This would parallel the concept of dorsal (spatial) and ventral (object) streams in the visual system discussed elsewhere in this book, although there are important differences between the two modalities. First, in the auditory system, the representation of space is not a simple mapping of the distribution of receptor responses. No animal study to date has demonstrated any clear mapping of auditory space in cortex that is similar to a retinotopic map, although this has been done in the superior colliculus (King and Palmer, 1982). Studies of cortex suggest that hundreds of auditory units may be needed to code a point in space (Middlebrooks *et al.*, 1994), making any spatial mapping a population property rather than unit property. Second, considerable sound processing relevant to either spatial or object processing occurs before sound even reaches the cortex.

Table 4.1 lists functional imaging studies of auditory spatial processing using PET and fMRI. These studies fall into two categories: studies of fixed localisation and studies of the processing of sound movement. The studies have used a variety of stimuli, based on either interaural intensity and timing cues or virtual acoustic space techniques, that create over headphones the percept of a sound object in space (Wightman and Kistler, 1989a,b). The term *processing*

TABLE 4.1 Functional Imaging Studies of Sound Spatial Processing

Study	Type	Stimulus	Task	Key Contrast	HG	PT	IPL	Ins	SPL	Premotor	
										Dorsal	Ventral
Fixed Auditory Stimuli											
Weeks *et al.* (1999)	PET	Noise in virtual acoustic space	1. Passive listening 2. Spatial discrimination 3. Spatial discrimination with motor output task	(2 – 1)	No	No	R/L	No	No	R/L	No
Bushara *et al.* (1999)	PET	Noise in virtual acoustic space	1. Passive listening 2. Spatial discrimination 3. Spatial discrimination with motor output task	Conjunction (2 – 1) and (3 – 1)	No	No	R/L	No	R/L	R/L	No
Maeder *et al.* (2001)	fMRI	1. Noise bursts lateralised by interaural time difference 2. Environmental sounds	1. Discrimination of position in hemifield 2. Recognition 3. No task	1. Spatial discrimination minus object recognition 2. Spatial minus environmental stimuli without task	No	R	R/L	L	No	R/L	R/L
Moving Auditory Stimuli											
Griffiths *et al.* (1994)	PET	Binaural beat	None	Movement minus stationary	No	No	No	R	No	No	No
Griffiths *et al.* (1998)	PET	Single object from narrow-band sound with interaural phase/intensity variation	None	Movement minus stationary	No	No	No	No	R	No	No
	fMRI	Single object from narrow-band sound with interaural phase/intensity variation	None	Movement minus stationary	No	No	R/L	R	R > L	R/L	R/L
Griffiths and Green (1999)	PET	Rotation within a virtual sound field	None	Movement minus stationary	No	No	No	No	R	No	R/L
Baumgart *et al.* (1999)	fMRI	Single object from interaural intensity variation of FM sound	None	Movement minus stationary	No	R	Not imaged (limited number of slices)	No	Not imaged	Not imaged	Not imaged
Griffiths *et al.* (2000)	fMRI	Single object from narrow-band sound with interaural phase/intensity variation	None	Movement minus stationary	No	No	R/L	No	R>L	R/L	R/L
Lewis *et al.* (2000)	fMRI	Single object from narrow-band sound with interaural AM	Speed discrimination	Movement minus silence	R/L	R/L	R/L	R/L	R/L	R/L	R/L
Warren *et al.* (2002)	PET	Single object in virtual space with fixed or variable angular velocity	No	Movement minus stationary	No	R/L	R/L	No	No	No	R/L
	fMRI		No	Movement minus stationary	No	R/L	R/L	No	No	No	No

Abbreviations: PET, positron emission tomography; fMRI, functional magnetic resonance imaging; AM, amplitude modulation; FM, frequency modulation, HG, Heschl's gyrus, PT, planum temporale; IPL, inferior parietal lobule; Ins, insula; SPL, superior parietal lobule.

includes obligatory perceptual mechanisms as well as attentional mechanisms and response preparation. The variable presence of a task in these studies will influence the relative involvement of attention and response in addition to perception. Despite these differences, the studies do allow certain generalisations. First and most striking is the absence of any activation in the region of the primary auditory cortex in HG in any single experiment where a condition involving spatial processing is contrasted with a control sound stimulus. This argues against a *specific* involvement of primary auditory cortex in spatial sound processing. In the (plausible) event that the human primary auditory cortex contains neurons sensitive to spatial stimuli as shown in animal auditory cortex (Ahissar *et al.*, 1992; Stumpf *et al.*, 1991), this conclusion is not invalidated, as these neurons could still provide the input to areas for spatial sound processing. The second generalisation is that the majority of the functional imaging studies (indeed, all of the fMRI studies) show specific bilateral involvement of the inferior parietal cortex in auditory spatial processing. Two recent studies of movement processing (Baumgart *et al.*, 1999; Warren *et al.*, 2002) suggest the involvement of the planum temporale as an intermediate stage in processing between the primary cortex and inferior parietal lobule. This would be consistent with a posterior spatial "stream" although the haemodynamic techniques used here do not allow inference about sequential activation.

Much more variation in the spatial studies is seen in the activation of superior parietal and the dorsal and ventral premotor areas, suggesting that this activation is due to processes other than obligatory perception. Such processes include spatial attention and eye- and limb-movement response. The activation often overlaps with the frontoparietal network of activation involved in visiospatial attention (Coull and Nobre, 1998; Nobre *et al.*, 1997). However, the studies of Bushara *et al.* (1999) and Lewis *et al.* (2000) suggest auditory- or visual-specific mechanisms for spatial processing in superior parts of the posterior parietal cortex. Dorsal premotor activation is often seen in the region of the frontal eye fields (Paus, 1996), even when actual eye movements are controlled by fixation. Ventral premotor activation often occurs in an area that might represent a human homologue of the primate ventral premotor areas thought important in limb-movement preparation; units in these areas have both visual and auditory receptive fields (Graziano *et al.*, 1999). Direct support for this interpretation of the importance of attention and task on activation comes from the study of Maeder *et al.* (2001) who demonstrated bilateral activation in the posterior superior temporal lobe and inferior part of the inferior parietal lobule associated with presentation of a spatial stimulus regardless of whether a task was carried out. When a spatial task was carried out, additional activation occurred in more superior parietal cortex and dorsal and ventral premotor areas (Fig. 4.5).

Abnormal Auditory Processing

Tinnitus is a common problem in subjects with and without hearing impairment and represents a form of hallucination: the percept of noise in the absence of any corresponding sensory stimulus. Common forms of tinnitus are difficult to study using functional imaging in the absence of variation of the percept, but unusual forms of tinnitus exist that can be switched on or off by the subject in the scanner. These include tinnitus evoked by orofacial or eye movements (Giraud *et al.*, 1999; Lockwood *et al.*, 1998, 2001). PET studies have demonstrated activation of the auditory cortex during the experience of tinnitus (Lockwood *et al.*, 1998, 2001); however, this has not been a consistent finding (Giraud *et al.*, 1999), and when it does occur the auditory cortex activation has taken a form that would not be produced by actual auditory stimulation. Tinnitus studies have shown strikingly unilateral activation while normal stimulation of the cochlea on one side would always produce some activation of cortex on both sides due to the incomplete decussation of the ascending pathway. Lockwood has suggested that unilateral cortical activation corresponds to a form of central tinnitus that is similar to the "phantom limb" phenomenon in amputees. One fMRI study of subjects with unilateral tinnitus and normal hearing has demonstrated abnormal sound processing in the brainstem in this condition (Melcher *et al.*, 2000). Decreased activation of the IC by noise occurred contralateral to the side on which tinnitus was experienced. This is indirect evidence for abnormal central activity in this form of tinnitus, and the technique allows characterisation of abnormal auditory processing in common forms of tinnitus.

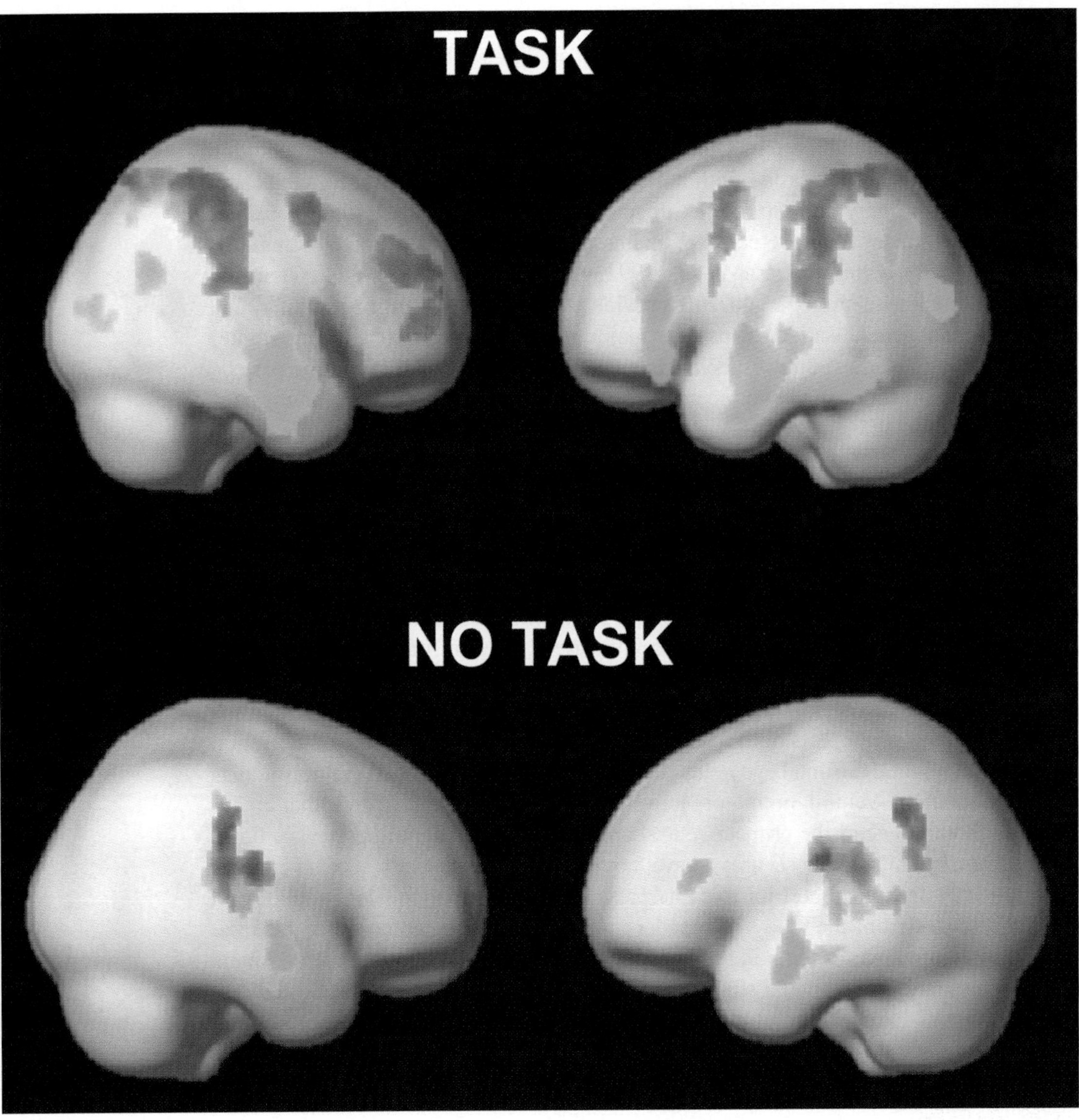

FIGURE 4.5
Areas involved in cortical processing of sound lateralisation and sound object identification. Group data for 18 subjects are rendered onto smoothed normalised brain. Areas more activated in lateralisation shown in red and areas more involved in identification shown in green. (Adapted from Figures 5 and 7 in Maeder *et al.*, 2001. With permission.)

In subjects with hearing impairment, it is also possible to have more complex abnormal perceptions than tinnitus. Musical hallucinations can occur in subjects with acquired deafness, for whom the experience is similar to the normal experience of subjects before they became deaf (Griffiths, 2000). Functional imaging of subjects with this condition demonstrates a network of areas distinct from the primary auditory area that is similar to the network of areas activated in normal subjects when they listen to actual sound sequences. Activation of primary auditory cortex during hallucinations of noise and more distributed temporal lobe areas during musical hallucinations bring to mind the early human stimulation studies of Penfield and colleagues (Penfield and Perot, 1963). In those studies, stimulation of HG could produce the percept of a tone or noise, while stimulation in other areas of the superior temporal lobe could produce more complex percepts, including music. Those studies should be interpreted with caution, however. The studies used rather high current densities that may have led to the activation of mesial temporal lobe structures remote from the stimulation site. More recent stimulation work has not replicated the findings (Howard *et al.*, 2000).

Functional imaging can also allow demonstration of the plasticity of the auditory system. Abnormal activation of the visual cortex by auditory stimuli has been demonstrated in subjects after cochlear implantation (Giraud *et al.*, 2001) and abnormal activation of the auditory cortex by visual stimuli (Calvert *et al.*, 1997). These studies concur to some extent with animal studies suggesting the existence of general processing mechanisms in the sensory cortices (Sharma *et al.*, 2000; von Melchner *et al.*, 2000). Plastic mechanisms have also been demonstrated following lesions of the auditory cortices (Engelien *et al.*, 1995, 2000). Engelien *et al.* (2000) investigated auditory activation in a subject with bilateral destruction of the auditory cortices who could still hear the onset and offset of sounds with attentional effort. Functional imaging demonstrated activation due to sound in the middle temporal gyri and cerebellum outside the normal area of activation due to sound stimuli.

CONCLUSION

Human anatomical and functional imaging studies are beginning to allow a synthesis of human auditory brain function. Studies of auditory processing in the ascending auditory pathway suggest the existence of spectrotemporal processing mechanisms similar to those previously demonstrated in animals. In the human cortex, evidence is accruing that processing occurs lateral to the primary auditory area for the analysis of sounds with complex spectrotemporal structure. Evidence also suggests that processing occurs posterior to the primary auditory area for the analysis of the spectrotemporal features of sounds in space. It will be important to establish further the anatomical connections of the lateral and posterior human areas to determine if they represent serial processing mechanisms for further analysis after the primary area or if they act in parallel with the primary cortex. It will also be important in the future to further disambiguate the contribution of perception, attention, and response preparation to the networks of activation shown in auditory functional imaging studies. If the normal human auditory system is shown to have a structural and functional organisation similar to that of other primates, such a finding would be tremendously helpful in establishing the relevance of animal studies using techniques such as intracellular recording and destructive lesioning that cannot be used in humans. Additionally, clinical functional imaging studies allow inference about human auditory perception and plasticity that cannot be extrapolated from animal models.

References

Ahissar, M., Ahissar, E., Bergman, H., andVaadia E. (1992). Encoding of sound source location and movement: activity of single neurons and interactions between adjacent neurons in the monkey auditory cortex. *J. Neurophysiol.*, **67**, 203–215.

Baumgart, F., Gaschler-Markefski, B., Woldorff, M. G., Heinze, H.-J., and Scheich, H. (1999). A movement-sensitive area in auditory cortex. *Nature*, **400**, 724–726.

Binder, J. R., Frost, J. A., Hammeke, T. A., Bellgowan, P. S. F., Springer, J. A., Kaufman, J. N. *et al.* (2000). Human temporal lobe activation by speech and nonpeech sounds. *Cerebral Cortex*, **10**, 512–528.

Belin, P., Zatorre, R. J., Lafaille, P., Ahad, P., and Pike, B. (2000). Voice-selective areas in human auditory cortex. *Nature*, **403**, 309–312.

Bregman, A. S. (1990). *Auditory Scene Analysis*. MIT Press, Cambridge, MA.

Brodmann, K. (1909).*Vergleichende lokalisationslehre der grosshirnrinde*. Leipzig, Barth.

Bushara, K. O., Weeks, R. A., Ishii, K., Catalan, M. J., Tian, B., Rauschecker, J. P. *et al.* (1999). Modality-specific frontal and parietal areas for auditory and visual spatial localisation in humans. *Nat. Neurosci.*, **2**, 759–766.

Calvert, G. A., Bullmore, E. T., Brammer, M. J., Campbell, R., Williams, S. C. R., McGuire, P. K. *et al.* (1997). Activation of auditory cortex during silent lipreading. *Science*, **276**, 593–596.

Chawla, D., Lumer, E. D., and Friston, K. J. (1999). The relationship between synchronisation among neuronal populations and their mean activity levels. *Neural Comput.*, **11**, 1389–1411.

Coull, J. T. and Nobre, A. C. (1998). Where and when to pay attention: the neural systems for directing attention to spatial locations and to time intervals as revealed by both PET and fMRI. *J. Neurosci.*, **18**, 7426–7435.

Dau, T., Kollmeier, B., and Kohlrausch, A. (1997). Modeling auditory processing of amplitude modulation. I. Modulation detection and masking with narrow-band carriers. *J. Acoust. Soc. Am.*, **102**, 2892–2905.

Ehret, G. and Romand, R., Eds. (1997). *The Central Auditory System*. Oxford University Press, London.

Engelien, A., Silbersweig, D., Stern, E., Huber, W., Doring, W., Frith, C. *et al.* (1995). The functional anatomy of recovery from auditory agnosia: a PET study of sound categorisation in a neurological patient and normal controls. *Brain*, **118**, 1395–1409.

Engelien, A., Huber, W., Silbersweig, D., Stern, E., Frith, C. D., Doring, W. *et al.* (2000). The neural corrlelates of 'deaf-hearing' in man: conscious sensory awareness enabled by attentional modulation. *Brain*, **123**, 532–545.

Galaburda, A. and Sanides F. (1980). Cytoarchitectonic organisation of the human auditory cortex. *J. Comp. Neurol.*, **190**, 597–610.

Giraud, A. L., Garnier, S., Micheyl, C., Lina, G., Chays, A., and Chery-Croze S. (1997). Auditory efferents involved in speech-in-noise intelligability. *NeuroReport*, **8**, 1779–1783.

Giraud, A. L., Chery-Croze, S., Fischer, G., Fischer, C., Vighetto, A., Gregoire M-C. *et al.* (1999). A selective imaging of tinnitus. *NeuroReport*, **10**, 1–5.

Giraud, A. L., Lorenzi, C., Ashburner, J., Wable, J., Johnsrude, I., Frackowiak, R. *et al.* (2000). Representation of the temporal envelope of sounds in the human brain. *J. Neurophysiol.*, **84**, 1588–1598.

Giraud, A. L., Price, C. J., Graham, J. M., Truy, E., and Frackowiak, R. S. (2001). Cross-modal plasticity underpins language recovery after cochlear implantation. *Neuron*, **30**, 657–663.

Graziano, M. S. A., Reiss, L. A., and Gross, C. G. (1999). A neuronal representation of the location of nearby sounds. *Nature*, **397**, 428–430.

Griffiths, T. D. (2000). Musical hallucinosis in acquired deafness: phenomenology and brain substrate. *Brain*, **123**, 2065–2076.

Griffiths, T. D. and Green, G. G. R. (1999). Cortical activation during perception of a rotating wide-field acoustic stimulus. *NeuroImage*, **10**, 84–90.

Griffiths, T. D., Bench, C. J., and Frackowiak, R. S. J. (1994). Cortical areas in man selectively activated by apparent sound movement. *Curr. Biol.*, **4**, 892–895.

Griffiths, T. D., Buechel, C., Frackowiak, R. S. J., Patterson, R. H. (1998). Analysis of temporal structure in sound by the human brain. *Nat. Neurosci.*, **1**, 421–427.

Griffiths, T. D., Johnsrude, I., Dean, J. L., and Green, G. G. R. (1999). A common neural substrate for the analysis of pitch and duration pattern in segmented sound? *NeuroReport*, **18**, 3825–3830.

Griffiths, T. D., Green, G. G. R., Rees, A., and Rees, G. (2000). Human brain areas involved in the perception of auditory movement. *Hum. Brain Mapping*, **9**, 72–80.

Griffiths, T. D., Uppenkamp, S., Johnsrude, I., Josephs, O., and Patterson, R. D. (2001). Encoding of the temporal regularity of sound in the human brainstem. *Nat. Neurosci.*, **4**, 633–637.

Guimares, A. R., Melcher, J. R., Talavage, T. M., Baker, J. R., Ledden, P., Rosen B. R. *et al.* (1998). Imaging subcortical activity in humans. *Hum. Brain Mapping*, **6**, 33–41.

Hackett, T. A., Preuss, T. M., and Kaas, J. H. (2001). Architectonic identification of the core region in auditory cortex of macaques, chimpanzees, and humans. *J. Comp. Neurol.*, **441**, 197–222.

Hall, D. A., Haggard, M. P., Akeroyd, M. A., Palmer, A. R., Summerfield, A. Q., Elliott, M. R. *et al.* (1999). 'Sparse' temporal sampling in auditory fMRI. *Hum. Brain Mapping*, **7**, 213–223.

Hall, D. A., Haggard, M. P., Akeroyd, M. A., Summerfield, A. Q., Palmer, A. R., Elliott, M. R. *et al.* (2000). Modulation and task effects in auditory processing measured using fMRI. *Hum. Brain Mapping*, **10**, 107–119.

Harms, M. P., Melcher, J. R., and Weisskoff, R. (1998). Time courses of fMRI signals in the inferior colliculus, medial geniculate body, and auditory cortex show different dependencies on noise burst rate. *NeuroImage*, **7**, S365.

Hartmann, W. M. (1997). *Signals, Sound, and Sensation.* AIP Press, New York.

Howard, M. A., Volkov, I. O., Mirsky, R., Garell, P. C., Noh, M. D., Granner, M. *et al.* (2000). Auditory cortex on the human posterior superior temporal gyrus. *J. Comp. Neurol.*, **416**, 79–92.

Irvine, D. R. F. (1986).*The Auditory Brainstem: A Review of the Structure and Function of the Auditory Brainstem Processing Mechanisms*, Vol 7. Springer-Verlag, Berlin.

Kay, R. (1982). Hearing of modulation in sounds. *Physiol. Rev.*, **62**, 894–975.

King, A. J. and Palmer, A. R. (1982). The representation of auditory space in the mammalian superior colliculus. *Nature*, **299**, 248.

Langner, G. (1992). Periodicity encoding in the auditory system. *Hear. Res.*, **60**, 115–142.

Langner, G., Sams, M., Heil, P., and Schulze H. (1997). Frequency and periodicity are represented in orthogonal maps in the human auditory cortex: evidence from magnetoencephalography. *J. Comp. Physiol.*, **181**, 665–676.

Lauter, J. L., Herscovitch, P., Formby, C., and Raichle, M.E. (1985). Tonotopic organisation in the human auditory cortex revealed by positron emission tomography. *Hear. Res.*, **20**, 199–205.

Lewis, J. W., Beauchamp, M. S., and DeYoe, E. A. (2000). A comparison of visual and auditory motion processing in human cerebral cortex. *Cerebral Cortex*, **10**, 873–888.

Liegeois-Chauvel, C., Musolino, A., and Chauvel, P. (1991). Localisation ot the primary auditory area in man. *Brain*, **114**, 139–153.

Liegeois-Chauvel, C., Peretz, I., Babai, M., Laguittin, V., and Chauvel, P. (1998). Contribution of different cortical areas in the temporal lobes to music processing. *Brain*, **121**, 1853–1867.

Lockwood, A. H., Salvi, R. J., Coad, M. L., Towsley, M. L., Wack, D. S., and Murphy, B. W. (1998). The functional neuroanatomy of tinnitus, evidence for limbic system links and neural plasticity. *Neurology*, **50**, 114–120.

Lockwood, A. H., Salvi, R. J., Coad, M. L., Arnold, S. A., Wack, D. S., Murphy, B. W. *et al.* (1999). The functional anatomy of the normal human auditory system: responses to 0.5 and 4.0kHz tones at varied intensities. *Cerebral Cortex*, **9**, 65–76.

Lockwood, A. H., Wack, D. S., Burkard, R. F., Coad, M. L., Reyes, S. A., Arnold. S. A. *et al.* (2001). The functional anatomy of gaze-evoked tinnitus and sustained lateral gaze. *Neurology*, **56**, 472–480.

Maeder, P. P., Meuli, R. A., Adriani, M., Bellmann, A., Fornari, E., Thiran J.-P. *et al.* (2001). Distinct pathways involved in sound recognition and localisation, a human fMRI study. *NeuroImage*, **14**, 802–816.

Melcher, J. R., Talavage, T. M., and Harms, M. P. (1999). Functional MRI of the auditory system, in *Medical Radiology Diagnostic Imaging and Radiation Oncology: Functional MRI*, Moonen, C. and Bandettini, P., Eds., pp. 393–406.

Melcher, J. R., Sigalovsky, I. S., and Guinan, J. J. J., and Levine, R. A. (2000). Lateralised tinnitus studied with functional magnetic resonance imaging: abnormal inferior colliculus activation. *J. Neurophysiol.*, **83**, 1058–1072.

Middlebrooks, J. C., Clock, A. E., Xu, L., and Green, D. M. (1994). A panoramic code for sound location by cortical neurons. *Science*, **264**, 842–844.

Moller, A. R. (1974). Response of units in the cochlear nucleus to sinusoidally amplitude modulated tones. *Exp. Neurol.*, **45**, 104–117.

Moore, J. K. (1994). The human brainstem auditory pathway, in *Neurotology*, Jackier, R. K. and Brackmann, D. E., Eds., Mosby, St. Louis, MO, pp. 1–17.

Morosan, P., Rademacher, J., Schleicher, A., Amunts, K., Schormann, T., and Zilles K. (2001). Human primary auditory cortex: cytoarchitectonic subdivisions and mapping into a spatial reference system. *NeuroImage*, **13**, 684–701.

Näätänen, R., Tervaniemi, M., Sussmann, E., Paavilainen, P., and Winkler, I. (2001). 'Primitive intelligence' in the auditory cortex. *Trends Neurosci.*, **24**, 283–288.

Nobre, A. C., Sebetyen, G. N., Gitelman, D. R., Mesulam, M. M., Frackowiak, R. S. J., and Frith, C. D. (1997). Functional localisation of the system for visiospatial attention using positron emission tomography. *Brain*, **120**, 515–533.

Patterson, R. D., Uppenkamp, S., Johnsrude, I., and Griffiths, T. D. (2002). The processing of temporal pitch and melody information in auditory cortex. *Neuron*, **36**, 767–776.

Paus, T. (1996). Location and function of the human frontal eye fields, a selective review. *Neuropsychologia*, **34**, 475–483.

Penfield, W. and Perot P. (1963). The brain's record of auditory and visual experience. *Brain*, **86**, 595–696.

Penhune, V. B., Zatorre, R. J., MacDonald, J. D., and Evans, A. C. (1996). Interhemispheric anatomical differences in human primary auditory cortex, probabalistic mapping and volume measurement from magnetic resonance scans. *Cerebral Cortex*, **6**, 661–672.

Penhune, V. B., Zatorre, R. J., and Evans, A. C. (1998). Cerebellar contributions to motor timing, a PET study of auditory and visual rhythm reproduction. *J. Cogn. Neurosci.*, **10**, 752–765.

Peretz, I. (1990). Processing of local and global musical information by unilateral brain-damaged patients. *Brain*, **113**, 1185–1205.

Rademacher, J., Morosan, P., Schormann, T., Schleicher, A., Werner, C., Freund, H.-J. *et al.* (2001). Probabalistic mapping and volume measurement of human primary auditory cortex. *NeuroImage*, **13**, 669–683.

Rauschecker, J. P. and Tian, B. (2000). Mechanisms and streams for processing of 'what' and 'where' in auditory cortex. *Proc. Natl. Acad. Sci. USA*, **97**, 11800–11806.

Rauschecker, J. P., Tian, B., Pons, T., and Mishkin, M. (1997). Serial and parallel processing in rhesus monkey auditory cortex. *J. Comp. Neurol.*, **382**, 89–103.

Ravicz, M. E., Melcher, J., and Wald, L. L. (1999). Reducing acoustic noise transmission from gradient coils to subgect during fMRI; an approach and preliminary results. *NeuroImage*, **9**, S1.

Rees, A. and Moller, A. R. (1983). Responses of neurons in the inferior colliculus of the rat to AM and FM tones. *Hear. Res.*, **10**, 301–330.

Remez, R. E., Rubin, P. E., Pisoni, D. B., and Carrell, T. D. (1981). Speech perception without traditional speech cues. *Science*, **212**, 947–949.

Rivier, F. and Clarke S. (1997). Cytochrome oxidase, acetylcholinesterase, and NADPH-diaphorase staining in human supratemporal and insular cortex, evidence for multiple audiotry areas. *NeuroImage*, **6**, 288–304.

Saberi, K. and Perrott, D. R. (1999). Cognitive restoration of reversed speech. *Nature*, **398**, 760.

Sakai, K., Hikosaka, O., Miyauchi, S., Takino, R., Tamada, T., Iwata, N. K. *et al.* (1999). Neural representation of a rhythm depends on its interval ratio. *J. Neurosci.*, **19**, 10074–10081.

Scheich, H., Baumgart, F., Gaschler-Markefski, B., Tegeler, C., Tempelmann, C., Heinze, H. J. *et al.* (1998). Functional magnetic resonance imaging of a human auditory cortex area involved in foreground–background decomposition. *Eur. J. Neurosci.*, **10**, 803–809.

Schreiner, C. E. and Urbas, J. V. (1988). Representation of amplitude modulation in the auditory cortex of the cat. II. Comparison between cortical fields. *Hear. Res.*, **32**, 49–64.

Shannon, R. V., Zeng, F.-G., Kamath, V., Wygonski, J., and Ekelid, M. (1995). Speech recognition with primarily temporal cues. *Science*, **270**, 303–304.

Sharma, J., Angelucci, A., and Sur, M. (2000). Induction of visual orientation modules in auditory cortex. *Nature*, **404**, 841–847.

Stumpf, E., Toronchuk, J. M., and Cynader, M. S. (1991). Neurons in cat primary auditory cortex sensitive to correlates of auditory motion in three-dimensional space. *Exp. Brain Res.*, **88**, 158–168.

Talavage, T. M., Ledden, P. J., Benson, R. R., Rosen, B. R., and Melcher, J. R. (2000). Frequency-dependent responses exhibited by multiple regions in human auditory cortex. *Hear. Res.*, **150**, 225–244.

Tervaniemi, M., Medvedev, S., Alho, K., Pakhomov, S., Roudas, M., van Zuijen, T. L. *et al.* (2000). Lateralised pre-attentive processing of phonetic and musical information: a PET study. *Hum. Brain Mapping*, **10**, 74–79.

Thivard, L., Belin, P., Zilbovicius, M., Poline, J.-B., and Samson, Y. S. (2000). A cortical region sensitive to auditory spectral motion. *NeuroReport*,**11**, 2969–2972.

Viemeister, N. F. (1979). Temporal modulation transfer functions based upon modulation thresholds. *J. Acoust. Soc. Am.*, **66**, 1364–1380.

von Melchner, L., Pallas, S. L., and Sur, M. (2000). Visual behaviour mediated by retinal projections directed to the auditory pathway. *Nature*, **404**, 871–876.

Warren, J. D., Zielinski, B. A., Green, G. G. R., Rauschecker, J. P., and Griffiths, T. D. (2002). *PET and fMRI Studies of the Analysis of Sound-Source Motion by the Human Brain*. Association for Research in Otolaryngology. St Petersburg, FL.

Weeks, R. A., Aziz-Sultan, A., Bushara, K. O., Tian, B., Wessinger, C. M., Dang, N. *et al.* (1999). A PET study of human auditory spatial processing. *Neurosci. Lett.*, **262**, 155–158.

Wessinger, C. M., Buonocore, M. H., Kussmaul, C. L., and Mangun, G. R. (1997). Tonotopy in human auditory cortex examined with functional magnetic resonance imaging. *Hum. Brain Mapping*, **5**, 18–25.

Wessinger, C. M., Van Meter, J., Tian, B., Van Lare, J., Peckar, J., and Rauschecker, J. P. (2001). Hierarchical organisation of the human auditory cortex revealed by functional magnetic resonance imaging. *J. Cogn. Neurosci.*, **13**, 1–7.

Westbury, C. F., Zatorre, R. J., and Evans, A. C. (1999). Quantifying variability in the planum temporale: a probability map. *Cerebral Cortex*, **9**, 392–405.

Wiegrebe, L. and Winter, I. M. (2001). Temporal representation of iterated rippled noise as a function of delay and sound level in the ventral cochlear nucleus. *J. Neurophysiol.*, **85**, 1206–1219.

Wightman, F. L. and Kistler, D. J. (1989a). Headphone simulation of free-field listening. I. Stimulus synthesis. *J. Acoust. Soc. Am.*, **85**, 858–867.

Wightman, F. L. and Kistler, D. J. (1989b). Headphone simulation of free-field listening. II. Psychophysical validation. *J. Acoust. Soc. Am.*, **85**, 868–878.

Wojczak, M. and Viemeister, N. F. (1999). *Adaptation Produced by Amplitude Modulation*. Association for Research in Otolaryngology, St Petersburg, FL, p. 59.

Yan, W. and Suga N. (1998). Corticofugal modulation of the midbrain frequency map in the bat auditory system. *Nat, Neurosci.*, **1**, 54–85.

Yang, Y., Engelien, A., Engelien, W., Xu, S., Stern, E., and Silbersweig, D. A. (2000). A silent event-related functional MRI technique for brain activation studies without interference of scanner noise. *Magn. Reson. Med.*, **43**, 185–190.

Yvert, B., Crouzeix, A., Bertrand, O., Seither-Preisler, A., and Pantev, C. (2001). Multiple supratemporal sources of magnetic and electric auditory evoked middle latency components in humans. *Cerebral Cortex*, **11**, 411–423.

Zatorre, R. J., Evans, A. C., and Meyer, E. (1994). Neural mechanisms underlying melodic perception and memory for pitch. *J. Neurosci.*, **14**, 1908–1919.

CHAPTER

5

Somesthetic Function

INTRODUCTION

To perform meaningful, goal-directed motor behaviour, all organisms must obtain sensory information about their environment. The mechanisms underlying this process vary widely between species (see, for example, Hughes, 1998), but there are a number of underlying similarities. One process common to the majority of sensory systems is *transduction*, by which physical energy (such as different wavelengths of light or different intensities of pressure on the skin) is converted into cell-specific biophysical changes via the action of specialised sense organs or receptors. In humans, this information promulgates from the periphery of the body to the central nervous system (CNS) as patterns of electrochemical events between neurons. In this fashion, all sensory information, independent of modality, is decomposed into a neuronal code of spikes.

The ability to study how nervous systems encode the sensory world has advanced tremendously since the first relationships between stimulus intensity and primary afferent firing rates were suggested by Adrian and Zotterman in Cambridge in the 1920s (Adrian and Zotterman, 1926). New advances in noninvasive human imaging techniques, such as functional magnetic resonance imaging (fMRI), positron emission tomography (PET), and magnetoencephalography (MEG) allow investigators to routinely examine how sensory stimuli are encoded centrally. This chapter is intended as a summary of recent advances in the study of information processing in the somatosensory system of humans that have been furnished, primarily, through the use of such neuroimaging techniques. After a brief summary of the basic physiology and anatomy of somatosensory cortex, the chapter concentrates on three topics and uses their discussion to elucidate wider themes:

1. Neuroimaging studies of topographical organisation within anterior parietal cortex
2. Hierarchical organisation of the somatosensory system
3. Functional specialisation of somatosensory cortical areas

BASIC ORGANISATION: STRUCTURE AND FUNCTION IN THE SOMATOSENSORY SYSTEM

Periphery

The somatosensory system has by far the most receptor types of any of the primate sensory systems, including mechanoreceptors, chemoreceptors, nociceptors, and thermoreceptors. The sensation of touch is primarily mediated by mechanoreceptors, but there are a number of other processing channels within the somatosensory system: pain, proprioception, and temperature or thermal sense. This chapter focuses primarily on studies examining the processing of touch information by mechanoreceptors.

The peripheral afferent fibres that innervate the glabrous skin of the human hand are commonly differentiated into four broad subclasses. Most studies use the definitions first introduced by Talbot and colleagues (1968) in macaques or a similar system introduced by Johansson and Valbo and their colleagues in humans (Johansson, 1976; Valbo and Johansson, 1978; Johansson and Valbo, 1979). Valbo and colleagues classified fibres using physiological criteria and defined four functional types (Fig. 5.1) that vary along two dimensions: skin innervation density and the response of fibres to tonic levels of stimulation (their adaptation properties). These are superficially similar to Talbot's classifications. Valbo's FAI, FAII, and SAI afferents are classified as RA, PC, and SA, respectively, by Talbot, and the macaque does not appear to have any SAII afferents (Talbot *et al.*, 1968). For the rest of this chapter, the definitions of Valbo will be adopted.

It is currently believed that the four classes of afferent fibre are each associated with a specific receptor type in the periphery: fast-adapting type I fibres (FAIs) with Meissner's corpuscles, fast-adapting type II fibres (FAIIs) with Pacinian corpuscles, slow-adapting type I fibres (SAIs) with Merkel complexes, and slow-adapting type II fibres (SAIIs) with Ruffini endings. The number of receptors per afferent fibre varies; while as many as 12 Merkel complexes or 20 Meissner's corpuscles can connect to a single afferent fibre, there is usually a one-to-one correspondence between Pacinian and Ruffini endings and afferents.

The different response properties of the four classes of afferent fibre have led some to suggest that each carries out a specific computational task. For example, SAI afferents are thought to be specialised for the representation of spatial information due to their sensitivity to edges, roughness, and curvature (reviewed in Johnson, 2001). A single SAI afferent fibre connects to several Merkel receptors, spread over an area of roughly 10 mm^2 in humans (Vega-Bermudez and Johnson, 1999). It is believed that this highly specialised peripheral morphology is responsible for the ability of SA1 afferents to shrink their receptive fields. When presented with patterns of tactile form that have a higher spatial frequency than the distribution of SAI receptive fields, the afferents become driven primarily by a subset of the Merkel receptors they contact (Phillips and Johnson, 1981), effectively reducing the receptive field size and producing hyperacute resolution.

In contrast to SAI afferents, FAI afferents display fairly homogenous responses to stimuli delivered within their receptive field. These afferents appear to function as specialised monitors of tactile motion and play a vital role in signalling slip between the skin and held objects, allowing grip-force strength to be adjusted accordingly (Srinivasan *et al.*, 1990; Macefield *et al.*, 1996). The remaining two primary afferent classes (SAII and FAII) are thought to process skin stretch and patterns of vibration transduced through held objects, respectively.

The existence of separate processing channels in touch (conceptually similar to the parvo- and magnocellular channels of the human visual system) is supported by the studies of Bolanowski and colleagues (for a review, see Bolanowski *et al.*, 1988) and Johnson and colleagues (Johnson and Hsiao, 1992). With this level of specialisation already apparent in the periphery, it is tempting to conclude that the hard work of somesthesis is performed before information reaches the central nervous system, and central structures need only possess the ability to preserve the features extracted by the processing of primary afferents. However, as noted by Johnson in a recent review (2001), suprathreshold tactile stimuli have a tendency to activate all four classes of peripheral afferent. Thus, the vital computations involved in separately processing and transforming the information within primary afferents must be carried out by more central structures.

Central Organisation: Spinal Cord, Brainstem Nuclei, and Thalamus

The four different somatic primary afferent fibre types enter the spinal cord via the dorsal horn. In the spinal cord, the termination patterns of the primary afferents are complex but stereotypical, and it is possible to differentiate the different afferent fibre types by the pattern of their axonal collaterals (Brown, 1981). The cell bodies of different spinal tracts lie in separate spinal laminae in the grey matter of the dorsal horn, classified according to the scheme of Rexed (1952, 1954). The processes from these neurons cluster together and form dense columns that project superiorly towards the brain. The two major ascending fibre systems in the somatosensory

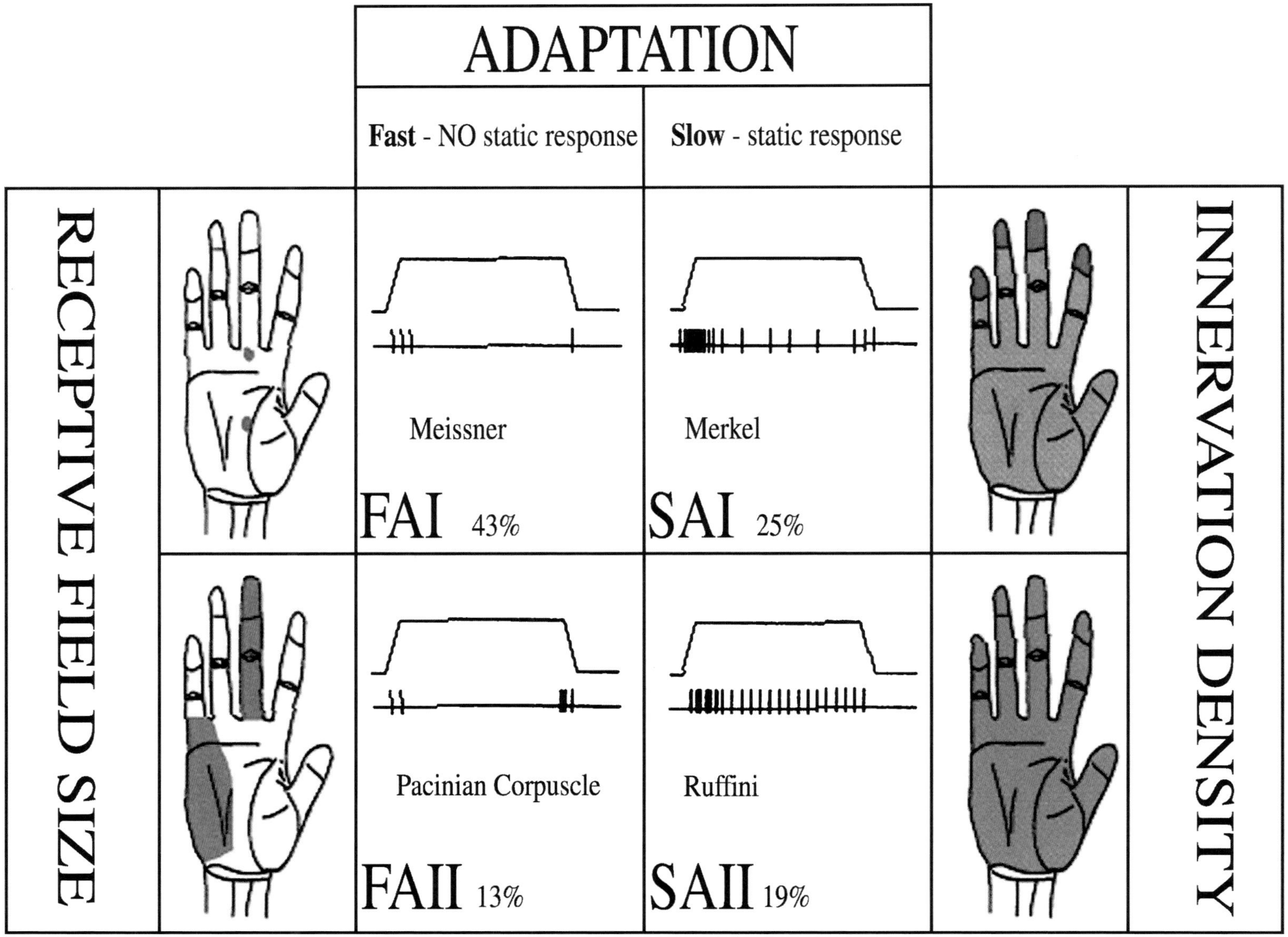

FIGURE 5.1
Depictions of the defining features of the four types of mechanoreceptor afferents innervating human glabrous skin. The centre figures are representative of canonical responses of the afferents to the ramp-and-hold stimulus depicted as the upper trace. The hands to the left show typical receptive field sizes between type I and type II afferents, while the hands on the right indicate the relative densities of the afferents (darker colours represent greater density). (Adapted from Westling, 1986.)

system are the dorsal column and anterolateral projection systems. For the purposes of this chapter, the dorsal column system will be outlined in detail, as it is composed of fibres processing discriminative touch (Fig. 5.2). While ascending information is grossly segregated, cross-talk between ascending fibre systems is possible (Burke *et al.*, 1982).

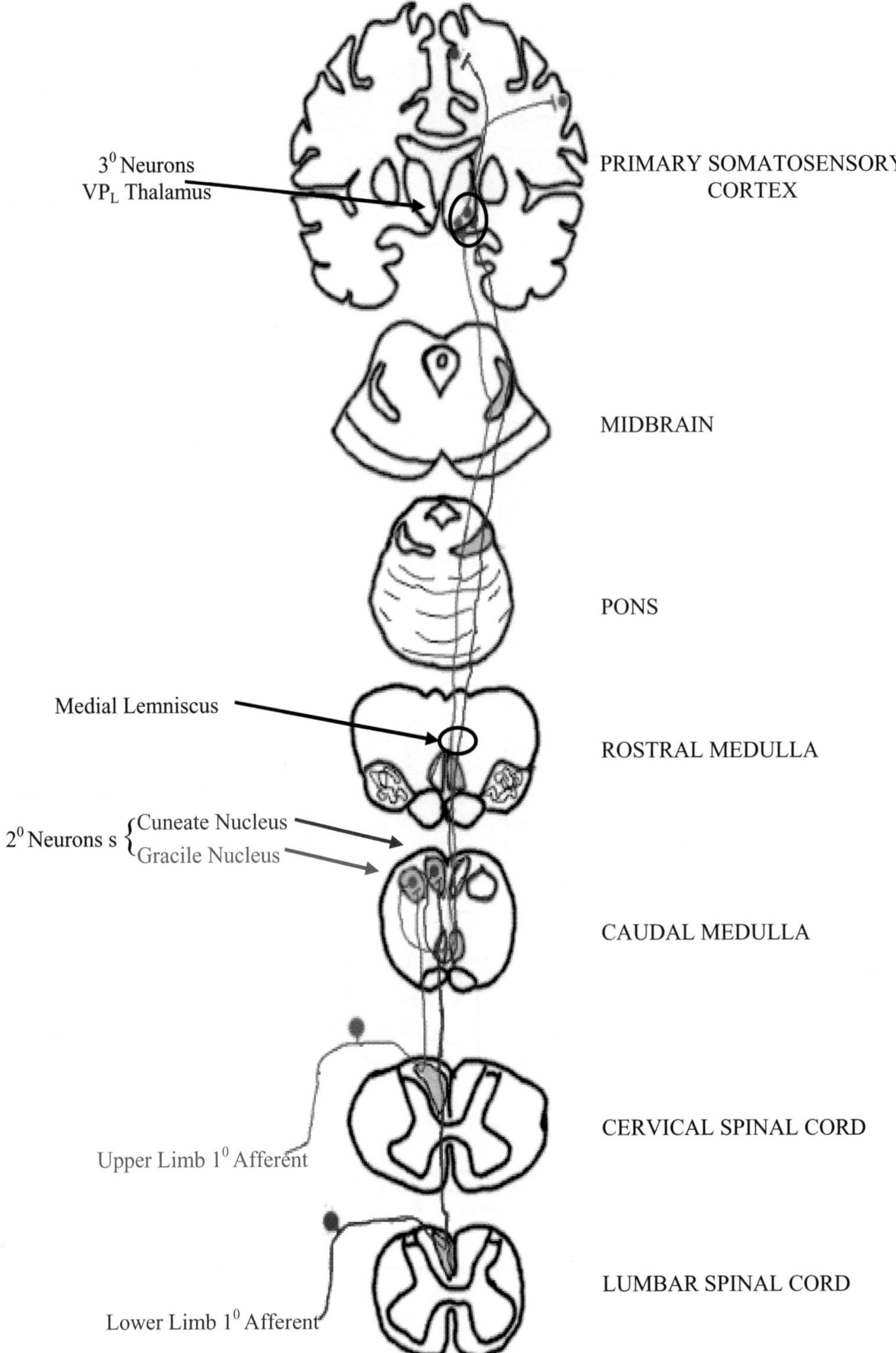

FIGURE 5.2
Ascending pathway for discriminative tactile sensations and the medial lemniscal pathway. Note the decussation of fibres at the level of the caudal medulla; afferent information from the left side of the body is processed by the right hemisphere and vice versa. Axial slices are shown at each level except for cortex (coronal). (Redrawn from Barr and Kiernan, 1993.)

It is possible to delineate separate spinal *tracts* within ascending fibre systems. The dorsal column system forms two principal spinal tracts: the gracile fasiculus, which consists of fibres entering below the midthoracic level, and the cuneate fasiculus, which contains fibres from the upper thoracic and cervical levels. These tracts synapse with second-order neurons in the gracile and cuneate nuclei, respectively, at the level of the lower medulla. The projections from second-order neurons then *decussate* (cross the midline) and ascend as the medial lemniscus system.

A rough level of topography can be seen in the spatial order of ascending fibres of the dorsal columns, and this topography is also observed in the medial lemniscus. Fibres originating from superior spinal segments have a more medial location than those from inferior segments. For example, second-order cervical fibres will be more medial than lumbosacral fibres. The preservation of relative spatial relationships between receptor positions in the periphery and the central neurons to which they project is responsible for the maps of the body that are a ubiquitous feature of early somatosensory cortical areas. These maps are described in more detail later.

Thalamic projections to areas of somatosensory cortex also preserve patterns of peripheral topography, as a mediolateral organisation within the thalamus reflects the terminations of the medial lemniscus. At each synapse from the periphery to the brain, information from adjacent ascending fibres may be combined; however, while there may be local convergence of information at a given level of somatosensory processing, in general this pattern of cross-talk causes extensive *divergence* of ascending somatosensory projections. This becomes most pronounced in the thalamus. For example, the terminal arborisation of a single lemniscal fibre can branch in close proximity with up to 200 thalamic neurons in monkeys (Jones, 1983). Thus, while gross somatotopy is preserved between the periphery and centre, there is ample opportunity for each synaptic relay point to act as a station for the integration of information from spatially separate skin surfaces.

As the medial lemniscal fibres ascend toward the cortex, they synapse with third-order projection neurons in the thalamus. The majority of medial lemniscal fibres terminate in the thalamic venterior posterior lateral (VPL) nucleus. Although the topographic order of the medial lemniscal pathway is, to some extent, preserved, the location of the projection neurons in the thalamus determines the area of cortex to which they project. For example, the central region of VPL sends the majority of its projections to Brodmann's area BA3b. BA1 receives projections from a band of fibres located throughout the entire extent of the VPL, while BA2 primarily receives input from the dorsal and rostral extents of VPL (reviewed in Burton and Sinclair, 1996). BA3a also receives input from VPL, though its primary source of thalamic input appears to be from motor thalamic nuclei, such as the ventral lateral (VL) and mediodorsal (MD) thalamic nuclei (Huffman and Krubitzer, 2001a).

The thalamus also projects to other regions of somatosensory cortex; for example, regions of posterior parietal cortex receive sparse thalamic projections (Burton, 1986). In addition, the somatosensory cortex of the lateral sulcus (including secondary somatosensory cortex, SII) receives direct projections from the VP thalamic nucleus in simian primates (Burton, 1986; Friedman and Murray, 1986) and other mammalian species (cat: Burton and Robinson, 1987; rabbit: Murray *et al.*, 1992; possum: Coleman, 1999). Thalamic neurons projecting to SII appear to be distributed across VP with a density equal to that of the SI-projecting cells (Zhang *et al.*, 2001a), although other groups have found the two groups to be spatially segregated (Krubitzer and Kaas, 1992). The functional significance of these direct thalamic projections to the lateral sulcus is discussed in a later section.

Cortex

Early electrophysiological mapping studies of cortex identified two cortical areas responsive to peripheral tactile stimulation: a primary somatosensory area (SI) and a second somatosensory area (SII) buried in the lateral sulcus (Woolsey and Fairman, 1946). However, most mammals appear to possess at least five somatosensory areas, defined as SI, SII, a parietal ventral area rostral to SII (PV), and bands of cortex flanking the SI field (Kaas and Collins, 2001). Modern connectivity and cytoarchitectonic analysis has defined at least ten separate areas in primates; for example, Burton and Sinclair (1996) divide primate parietal (somatosensory) cortex into four anterior areas (3a, 3b, 1, and 2), two posterior areas (5 and 7b), and four lateral regions (SII rostral, SII posterior, retroinsular, and granular insula). Our discussion begins by focusing on data collected from studies of somatosensory cortex in non-human primates before concentrating on data from noninvasive imaging in humans in later sections.

Anterior Somatosensory Cortex (BA1, 2, 3a, and 3b)

Anterior parietal cortex has been classified both as a single area (SI; for an early example, see Marshall *et al.*, 1937) and as a combination of several subareas delineated by cytoarchitectonic criteria (Brodmann, 1909; Vogt and Vogt, 1919; von Economo and Koskinas, 1925). Although Brodmann's human cytoarchitectonic map (1909) is commonly used to identify active regions in neuroimaging, his study and classification of anterior parietal cortex is not as well documented as those of other studies from the same period. For example, Brodmann defined only three regions in the vicinity of the postcentral gyrus (BA1, 2, and 3), with the first structural definition of a human area 3a being made by the Vogts in 1919. This was followed by the first thorough attempt to use cytoarchitectonic criteria to classify anterior parietal cortex (von Economo and Koskinas, 1925). von Economo and Koskinas defined four areas (PA, PB, PC, and PD) that appear to correspond roughly to areas 3a, 3b, 1, and 2 respectively. Recent work (Geyer *et al.*, 1997, 1999, 2000) has extended the work of these early studies using a more objective method of studying cytoarchitectonics. Some investigators have suggested that, of these regions, only BA3b should be considered as true primary somatosensory cortex, or SI proper (Merzenich *et al.*, 1978; Kaas, 1983). For cross-species comparisons, this is an essential distinction, as the anterior parietal cortex of different species has varying numbers of subdivisions (Krubitzer *et al.*, 1995; Huffman *et al.*, 1999); however, for our purposes, this text will refer to Brodmann areas (BAs) whenever possible, thus avoiding using the term SI.

The topography of the anterior parietal areas and the properties of individual neurons within them have been extensively investigated in monkeys (Kaas, 1983; Iwamura, 1998). Early multiunit electrophysiological mapping studies identified that neurons within areas BA1 and BA3b were primarily responsive to cutaneous inputs, while neurons within BA3a and BA2 were more responsive to deeper stimulation, such as muscle receptors. These investigations established that BA3b and BA1 each contain a complete map of the body's cutaneous receptors, and that the two maps are organised as mirror images of each other, reflected in the BA3b/BA1 border (Merzenich *et al.*, 1978). At least some of BA2 is organised in a similar way, as mapping studies of the hand representation have identified it as a cruder, lower resolution mirror image of the BA1 hand representation (Nelson *et al.*, 1980). Recent work on the topographical organisation of 3a has demonstrated that it has a topographic organisation paralleling that of BA3b (Huffman and Krubitzer, 2001).

Each area within anterior parietal cortex contains neurons with different response properties. Single-unit studies of these regions have determined that, broadly speaking, an anteroposterior gradient of complexity exists (Duffy and Birchfield, 1971; Sakata *et al.*, 1973; Iwamura, 1998). Receptive fields are smallest in BA3b (Sur *et al.*, 1980) and enlarge as one records from progressively posterior areas (in the order 3b, 1, 2), with multidigit receptive fields (rfs) being present in BA2. Between the four areas, BA3b contains the largest representations of the digits (Sur *et al.*, 1980) and the greatest proportion of neurons responsive to simple cutaneous stimuli (Powell and Mountcastle, 1959). Thus, the map of the surface of the body within area 3b is perhaps the least elaborated of the anterior cortical areas; with its small, simple rfs, BA3b contains a fine-grain isomorph of the body surface.

BA1 neurons have more multifaceted receptive field properties than those in BA3b; while the area is still dominated by cutaneous responses, recording studies have identified BA1 neurons that are sensitive to the direction of movement across the skin (Hyvarinen and Poranen, 1978a), that have receptive fields with inhibitory surrounds (Sur, 1980; Sur *et al.*, 1985), and that possess discontinuous receptive fields spanning adjacent digits (Hyvarinen and Poranen, 1978b). This trend in receptive field properties is continued as one moves in a posterior direction from BA1 to 2. Studies by Iwamura and colleagues (1980) demonstrated that the somatotopic map of the digits within BA2 had lower resolution than BA3b or BA1, with overlapping digit representations. Other studies have examined discharges from this area during movement. Burbaud and colleagues (1991) showed a correlation between movement duration and firing duration in area 2 units. A study by Tremblay and colleagues demonstrated that, while some neurons in area 2 had no detectable peripheral receptive fields, they were responsive to changes in surface texture passively applied to the hand (Tremblay *et al.*, 1996). Lesion studies support the general idea of an elaboration of receptive field properties in a posterior direction; lesions of area 1 produce deficits in two-dimensional texture discrimination, while area 2 lesions disrupt three-dimensional discrimination (Randolph and Semmes, 1974). It is worth noting, however, that lesions to region 3b also disrupt these abilities.

In summary, anterior parietal cortex in humans is comprised of four architectonically defined areas: BA3a, BA3b, BA1, and BA2. Electrophysiological investigations of these areas in species of monkeys that possess all four subdivisions show that the distribution of response properties in anterior parietal cortex follows the underlying anatomical structure, such that neurons across the four regions have quite different receptive fields, with the most complex being found in BA2. Most contemporary accounts of these regions consider them as playing an essential role in preprocessing or filtering the representations of tactile stimuli before they are further analysed in more posterior regions.

Areas 5 and 7b: Posterior Parietal Cortex

In the macaque, *posterior parietal cortex* is usually defined as a region encompassing the anterior parietal lobule, the full extent of the intraparietal sulcus (IPS), and the posterior parietal lobule (Cavada, 2001). Defined in this way, posterior parietal cortex occupies the entire cortex of the parietal lobe caudal to area 2 and superior to the lateral sulcus (Kaas, 1990). There have been many attempts to segregate this area of cortex into functionally or structurally defined subunits, as it contains a mosaic of functionally heterogeneous regions. A number of different schemes have been proposed (Pandya and Seltzer, 1982; Colby *et al.*, 1988; Andersen *et al.*, 1990; Felleman and Van Essen, 1991; Lewis and Van Essen, 2000), but a canonical scheme has yet to be agreed upon. This brief review treats posterior parietal cortex simply as the combination of areas defined by Brodmann and the Vogts (5, 7a, and 7b), and refers to further subdivisions only when necessary.

In monkeys, area 5 lies in the superior parietal lobule and on the anterior bank of the intraparietal sulcus, and area 7 lies in the inferior parietal lobule and on the posterior bank. Area 7a lies superior to area 7b, which extends downward to the superior bank of the lateral sulcus. Most electrophysiological recording studies of posterior parietal cortex have stressed the relative complexity of single- and multiunit responses in these areas when compared to responses from neurons in anterior parietal cortex. A number of different explanations for this increase have been proposed. Focusing on area 5, an early hypothesis suggested that the rise in the number of nonclassical receptive fields was due to the pattern of afferent projections to posterior parietal areas. Recording from single neurons in area 5, Duffy and Birchfiel (1971) demonstrated that some units responded to stimulus *conjunctions*, such as simultaneous skin and joint stimulation, or the stimulation of nonadjacent areas of the skin. This scheme explains the emergence of progressively more complex receptive fields downstream from early sensory regions by a process of feedforward integration. Single-cell complexity may therefore be a simple result of a number of simple cells (from anterior parietal cortex, for example) projecting to a single cell in later, higher cortical areas (such as area 5 or 7).

Since these early electrophysiological investigations in monkeys, a number of different roles have been proposed for area 5 and are summarised by Kalaska (1996): The area has been identified as a higher order somatosensory association region (Hyvarinen, 1982), as a region involved in planning movements that require visual guidance (Mountcastle *et al.*, 1975), or as a "command area" required to match appropriate motor responses to sensory inputs (Seal, 1989). In support of the last hypothesis, a number of studies have shown that the firing rates of area 5 neurons can be modulated by certain forms of arm movement and object manipulation (Kalaska *et al.*, 1983; Chapman *et al.*, 1984; Iwamura *et al.*, 1995; Jiang *et al.*, 1997), perhaps suggesting a role for this area in the processing of global shape during the active exploration of objects grasped by the hand. Further evidence for this hypothesis comes from what is currently known about the connectivity of area 5: The area is reciprocally connected to both the primary motor area (M1) and several accessory motor structures, including premotor areas, the supplementary motor area, and the cingulate motor areas (Nelson, 1996).

While neurons within area 5 still possess some clearly somatic (albeit selective) response properties, the responses of area 7 units are more abstract. Hyvarinen and Poranen (1974) found that cells within area 7 were responsive when monkeys looked at a given location in space and also when they reached toward it with their hands. Lesions of cortex in and around the intraparietal sulcus, including areas 5 and 7, result in deficits in reaching and a misalignment of digits, with or without visual guidance (Semmes and Turner, 1977). Yet, some studies have shown that the firing of 7b neurons can be modulated by simple tactile stimulation; recordings from the cynomologus monkey show that in the lateral region of 7b a subset of neurons responds to passive tactile stimulation (Robinson and Burton 1980a,b). This area may also be where a process of selection or competition between different target regions in space may take place; Burton and colleagues (1997b) found evidence for top-down modulation of cell firing rates in this area during an attentional cueing task.

The hypothesis that both areas 7a and 7b code the locations of external objects or body parts in space is one that has received much attention in the last 50 years. Evidence from lesion studies in monkeys and observations on brain-damaged human subjects (Vallar *et al.*, 1994) have provided compelling evidence for the link between the integrity of posterior parietal regions and the ability to respond, attend, or perceive stimuli in space contralateral to the lesion (when this ability is lost due to pathology, the condition is known as *neglect*). Andersen and colleagues (1997) have presented evidence supporting the existence of multiple maps of space within different networks of parietal neurons. They suggest that this area may encode the locations of external objects in either head- or torso-centred space. A different view is advanced by Goldberg *et al.* (Duhamel *et al.*, 1992), who suggest that areas within posterior parietal cortex instead encode the external world in *eye*-centred coordinates. A further viewpoint is that a generic map of space within posterior parietal cortex is used by other areas to construct effector-centred maps (Graziano and Gross, 1998); recordings from monkey ventral premotor cortex (PMv) and its connectivity with parietal areas support this view (Pouget and Sejnowski, 1997). In summary, while few would argue the role of area 7b as an area where afferent information from vision, touch, and proprioception, its exact role is still a matter of debate. Much of this debate may be resolved when a standard anatomical framework for the parcellation of this region is agreed upon.

The posterior parietal regions are densely connected to other regions of somatosensory cortex; for example, there is evidence for connections between areas 7a and 7b and extrastriate visual areas and temporal lobe regions (for a more detailed review of cortical connections, see Darian-Smith *et al.*, 1996). Surprisingly, given that the majority of theories of parietal cortex function identify it as occupying a crucial point in the link between perception and action, the connections of posterior parietal regions to more caudal cortical regions are less certain. Early neuroanatomical tracing studies of posterior parietal regions (Cavada and Goldman-Rakic, 1989a,b; Andersen *et al.*, 1990) pooled data from injection sites and target areas in different animals, making unambiguous conclusions difficult. Only recently have studies focused on delineating the exact projections of the parietal regions to frontal cortex (Rizzolatti *et al.*, 1998). These investigations have identified a number of segregated frontoparietal networks in the macaque, linking regions of posterior parietal cortex to frontal motor areas. While each parietal region (the classification scheme used by Rizzolatti and colleagues is that of von Economo) projects to a number of frontal regions (for example, PE connects to the frontal regions F1 and F3), the authors identify predominant connections between single parietal and frontal areas. These individual circuits are then thought to be used as a blueprint by which structure and function in the parietal cortex are linked (Rizzolatti *et al.*, 1998).

From the evidence presented above, it is clear that, while a number of different hypotheses have been advanced about the function of posterior parietal cortex, a recurring theme is that these areas act to represent space around the body. However, while this region seems specialised in the construction of common spaces in which information from different sensory modalities can be integrated to guide action, it does not seem to be specialised for aspects of action that are germane to the somatosensory system—for example, bilateral coordination of the hands. A potential candidate for these kinds of functions is the cortex lying on the superior bank of the lateral sulcus, or Sylvian fissure, where the second somatosensory area and related areas are located.

The Somatosensory Areas of the Lateral Sulcus

The existence of a second region of cortex responsive to tactile stimuli was first described in the cat by Adrian (1940, 1941). Subsequent to these investigations, Woolsey and colleagues demonstrated that it could be found in a variety of other mammals, including the monkey (Woolsey 1943, 1944; Woolsey and Fairman, 1946). Woolsey defined this region (SII) as located within the parietal operculum, on the upper bank of the lateral sulcus. The existence of a similar region in humans was confirmed after studies showed that stimulation of the parietal operculum in patients undergoing surgery for epilepsy produced paresthetic sensations (Penfield and Jasper, 1954).

Since these early studies, a series of progressively more detailed recording and connectivity studies in monkeys have revealed hitherto-unappreciated aspects of the organisation of the lateral sulcus. Studies by Woolsey in animals demonstrated that the SII area contained a rough somatotopic map of peripheral receptors, although the map appeared less fine-grained than those found in anterior parietal cortex. It is now widely accepted, based on anatomical (Burton *et al.*, 1995) and electrophysiological (Krubitzer *et al.*, 1995) criteria, that the lateral sulcus contains more than one region responsive to somatosensory stimulation. At least two separate representations are present: somatic area II (SII) (SIIp of Burton *et al.*, 1995) and the parietal ventral area (PV) (Krubitzer *et al.*, 1995; SIIa of Burton *et al.*, 1995; SIIr of Whitsel *et al.*, 1969). There is also evidence for a third area, the ventral somatosensory area (VS). This region has been identified in owl monkeys (Cusick *et al.*, 1989), and a partial map of VS has been described in macaque monkeys (Krubitzer *et al.*, 1995). This chapter focuses on areas SII and PV.

Although definitive neuroanatomical delineation of the location of areas SII and PV in the monkey has been achieved only relatively recently (Burton *et al.*, 1995; Krubitzer *et al.*, 1995), the responsiveness of neurons within the lateral sulcus has been studied in detail by a number of researchers. The studies by Krubitzer (1995) and Burton (1995) confirmed and extended the results of Woolsey by demonstrating that both regions contain a complete map of the body surface, though surfaces were represented at a coarser grain than in anterior parietal regions. This may be explained by single-unit studies that show that lateral sulcal neurons have larger receptive fields than those in anterior parietal cortex (Burton, 1986); however, one of the more striking characteristics of neurons within the lateral sulcus is their responsiveness to bilateral stimulation of skin sites. Estimates of the exact number of neurons with bilateral receptive fields in the lateral sulcus vary among investigators; Whitsel and colleagues (1969) reported that 80% of neurons contain bilateral fields, while Robinson and Burton (1980a) found that roughly one-third of neurons were responsive to bilateral stimulation. The presence of these neurons has spurred much speculation regarding the possible functions of lateral sulcal areas; for example, it may be that such bilateral responsiveness facilitates the integration of information between the hands for tasks requiring bimanual coordination (Krubitzer, 1996). Primates rarely use a single hand to explore objects, so the existence of bilateral connections within this area may signal its role in behaviour of this kind.

As the lateral sulcus is traditionally viewed as higher somatosensory cortex, it is not surprising that studies have found that the responses of neurons in this area are modulated by the attentional state of the animal. Early studies by Hyvarinen (Poranen and Hyvarinen, 1982) used a task in which monkeys had to detect the end of a 4-s vibrotactile pulse applied to a single skin location (the *relevant* period). The task also included a phase in which the same stimuli were delivered but the animal was trained to disregard them (the *irrelevant* period). Comparing their results between anterior parietal regions, SII, and the VPL nucleus of the thalamus (Poranen and Hyvarinen used multiunit recording), the authors found little difference between relevant and irrelevant periods in either anterior parietal cortex or the thalamus. Only in SII were recording sites found where there were clear disparities between the relevant and irrelevant periods. In this area, the authors found evidence for two different forms of response. The responses from recording sites with punctate, contralateral receptive fields showed a slight effect of attention when comparing the relevant to irrelevant periods, while the largest differences were found in sites with larger, bilateral receptive fields. The authors concluded that the modulation of activity in SII may reflect its involvement in the analysis of the signals being attended to and the motor response that results. However, any difference in responsiveness between the two periods that could be attributed to attentional modulation is confounded by the fact that the animal has to make a behavioural response (a button press) *only* in the relevant period.

The existence of two separate populations of neurons within the lateral sulcus that are differentially modulated by attention was also found by Hsiao and colleagues (1993). They examined changes in firing rate when comparing mean activity over two different tasks: one in which the monkey had to match visual and tactile stimuli, and one where, although tactile and visual stimuli were delivered as before, the task itself was entirely visual. They found that the majority of single units recorded from (80% of their sample) were modulated by attention, but the effects of attention were different across units: 58% of units in the lateral sulcus increased their firing rate, while 22% showed a decrease. Using a different metric, analysis of a similar task (Steinmetz *et al.*, 2000) suggested that other coding strategies (such as the coherence between firing patterns of single neurons) may be used by somatosensory areas to process information, rather than mean increases of firing rates *per se*. The authors found that roughly 80% of lateral sulcal neurons changed their firing rate when the monkeys had to attend to the tactile stimuli (as in the study of Hsiao and colleagues); however, they also found that synchrony between pairs of neurons within the lateral sulcus increased. Yet, as only 9% of SII neurons showed this effect, its functional significance is currently unknown.

One of the paradigms most frequently employed in the study of spatial attention is the Posner task, which has been used extensively in the study of visual attention (Posner, 1986). This task has also been used to study of tactile spatial attention. Burton and colleagues (1997b) focused on changes in the firing rates of lateral sulcus neurons during a selective attention task (a variant of the Posner cueing paradigm). Monkeys had to detect cued transient increases in the amplitude of vibrotactile stimuli in the cued location, which could be either contralateral or ipsilateral. Because the same stimuli were delivered across all trials, the main effects of cueing could be examined. The authors found enhanced firing rates in lateral sulcal neurons during trials where the contralateral hand was cued compared to trials cued to the ipsilateral location. There was also some evidence for suppression of responses just before the stimuli for discrimination were delivered, which the authors suggest may reflect a decrease in intrinsic neuronal noise that may facilitate the detection of the transient stimuli (Burton *et al.*, 1997). Tactile attention may therefore act to direct processing resources away from irrelevant stimuli (McAdams and Maunsell, 1999a) and increase the signal-to-noise ratio of salient stimuli (McAdams and Maunsell, 1999b).

Fewer studies of the lateral sulcus have attempted to define the receptive fields or stimulus-responses properties of these neurons in detail. Most of these have focused on the differential firing rates of lateral sulcal neurons during the processing of tactile roughness. The interpretation of these results varies depending on whether the authors use active touch (where the animal moves its hand over the stimuli) or passive touch (where the animal's hand is fixed and the stimuli move). Jiang and colleagues (1997) used an active touch paradigm and found that lateral sulcal neurons seemed to code the *transition* between different grades of roughness, rather than representing the actual spatial frequency of each pattern (neurons that displayed graded responses to the different spatial frequencies of roughness were found in anterior parietal cortex). On the other hand, using a passive-touch paradigm, Pruett and colleagues (2001) found that the firing rates of a subset of lateral sulcal neurons correlated with the roughness of the stimuli used.

To tie together these disparate observations on the lateral sulcal regions, some authors have attempted to assign a single function to these areas. In general, these theories have relied in the past on data collected from lesion studies. The removal of cortex around the Sylvian fissure (including SII and adjacent regions) causes impairments of tactile learning and interhemispheric transfer of learned material (Ridley and Ettlinger, 1976; Garcha and Ettlinger, 1978), vibrotactile discrimination (LaMotte and Mountcastle, 1979), and texture and shape discrimination (Murray and Mishkin, 1984). Impairments in tactile discrimination have been found after lateral sulcus lesions by a number of investigators (Ridley and Ettlinger, 1976; Murray and Mishkin, 1984). These observations led to the suggestion that this region may act to link anterior parietal regions subserving short-term information processing with limbic and temporal regions required for long-term storage of tactile memories (Mishkin, 1979). However, while neuroanatomical studies have confirmed the existence of projections from the lateral sulcus to regions of the insula that are connected to the perirhinal cortex, few studies have examined the functional significance of these projections. A single neuroimaging study (Bonda *et al.*, 1996) suggests that such a pathway (lateral sulcus to insula to perirhinal cortex) may be involved in tactile memory. As more researchers begin to probe the role of SII role in tactile discrimination and memory tasks (Romo *et al.*, 2002), our currently incomplete knowledge of the function of this area should begin to change.

NEUROIMAGING STUDIES OF TOPOGRAPHICAL ORGANISATION WITHIN ANTERIOR PARIETAL CORTEX

This section of the chapter concentrates on the use of fMRI to image and interpret somatotopic maps in anterior parietal cortex. The responsiveness of neurons within primary and associated sensory cortices is invariably organised as a mapping, such that neurons with similar response properties are found grouped together. By this process, values along a sensory dimension (*e.g.*, position in the visual field, auditory tone frequency, or position on the body surface) are mapped to corresponding spatial positions within a cortical field. The existence of these maps is a near-invariant feature in mammalian species (Kaas, 2000).

The use of noninvasive neuroimaging technologies allows data from humans to be compared with similar measures from other species. fMRI, PET, electroencephalography (EEG), and MEG represent a first step away from the "backwardness" of much of human neuroscience (*i.e.*, an over-reliance on the use of data from other species to draw conclusions about the human brain; Crick and Jones, 1993) and facilitate the direct study of the human brain, as well as studies in comparative neuroscience. Nevertheless, a major inconvenience facing interspecies work is that different recording techniques are typically used (electrophysiology in non-human species compared with electrical, magnetic, and haemodynamic sensing methods in humans). Any differences detected may be caused by true functional differences or specious differences caused by the use of different imaging methods being used in the different species. This problem is currently being addressed by a number of laboratories using fMRI to study non-human primates (Dubowitz *et al.*, 1998, 2001; Stefanacci *et al.*, 1998; Disbrow *et al.*, 1999, 2000; Logothetis *et al.*, 1999, 2001); however, these methods are still in their infancy. To gain an appreciation of the ability of fMRI to acquire meaningful data from the human somatosensory system, a number of studies have focused on studying the simple topographical structure of the fields within anterior parietal cortex as a benchmark measure.

Early Mapping Studies of Anterior Parietal Cortex

Before focusing on recent developments in mapping anterior parietal areas, it is useful to briefly revisit previous work. Initial attempts at mapping the spatial organisation of somatosensory cortex were far cruder than current noninvasive methods. Penfield and Boldrey (1937) were the first to describe the somatosensory map (*homunculus*, or "little man") in human subjects using direct stimulation of the exposed cortical surface. Their study was one of the first examples of cartographic electrophysiology in the somatosensory system, in which the primary aim was to examine the spatial layout of receptive fields, or how the body's surface was represented in the brain. While other studies from the same period also recorded potentials directly from the brain during surgery (Marshall and Walker, 1948; see also the work summarised in Woolsey *et al.*, 1979), Penfield's homuncular figure became the standard by which all other investigations of localisation in the postcentral gyrus were compared. The majority of subsequent research extending Penfield's work was done in non-human primates and included the initial single-cell somatosensory studies carried out by Mountcastle (1957), the work of Werner and Whitsel on transforming the three-dimensional representation of the body onto a two-dimensional plane (reviewed in Dykes and Ruest, 1986), and, finally, the first demonstrations that each cytoarchitectonic area of primary somatosensory cortex in monkeys contains a complete map of the body surface (Merzenich *et al.*, 1978; Kaas *et al.*, 1979). Later electrophysiological work in non-human primates studied anterior parietal cortex in more detail, as discussed earlier in the chapter.

Early noninvasive neuroelectric and neuromagnetic studies of anterior parietal cortex concentrated on evaluating the ability of these new methods to reproduce the gross patterns of somatotopy found by Penfield and contemporaries. Okada and colleagues (1984) measured the evoked magnetic field resulting from electric stimulation of the ankle and the first, second, and fifth digits (D1, D2, and D5). They found a somatotopic pattern (ankle most medial, thumb most lateral) in the one subject who was stimulated at all four skin sites. As the spatial resolution of PET scanners increased, it became feasible to use this technique to study anterior parietal cortex. The first use of PET to examine somatotopy was published by Fox and colleagues (1987). Using vibrotactile stimulation applied to the lips, fingers, or toes they were able to distinguish separate foci within the postcentral gyrus when stimulating each skin region. This early example showed that it was indeed possible to use haemodynamic measures to obtain an overall picture of the gross pattern of somatotopy within subjects. With the advent of fMRI and its higher spatial resolution, researchers began to investigate the possibility of mapping individual digit foci within anterior parietal regions.

fMRI Investigations of Anterior Parietal Cortex

Early fMRI studies of the anterior parietal cortex used simple stimulation methods such as rubbing the subject's hand with the investigator's hand (Hammeke *et al.*, 1994; Yetkin *et al.*, 1995) or using a brush controlled by one of the investigators (Sakai *et al.*, 1995). More sophisticated stimuli were subsequently used, such as median nerve stimulation (Puce *et al.*, 1995), textured surfaces (Lin *et al.*, 1996), and peripheral electrical stimulation (Kurth *et al.*, 1998), but few systematic studies of the responsiveness of SI to different tactile stimuli were carried out. One notable example was the comparison of two manual stimulation paradigms (air blowing over the palm and brushing the digits) to median nerve stimulation by Puce and colleagues in 1995. The authors found that median nerve simulation was found to be less reliable than other methods of stimulation, but their sample size was small.

Similar to PET and MEG before it, several early fMRI investigations concentrated on evaluating whether it was possible to reproduce the gross pattern of topography in anterior parietal cortex expected from invasive human data and monkey electrophysiology. Investigators thus concentrated on stimulating areas that were maximally separated in the anterior parietal map, such as the foot (superior) and the face (inferior). Sakai and colleagues (1995) were able to reproduce the expected mediolateral pattern of toes, fingers, and lips using a 3-Hz brushing stimulus. A more elaborate method of stimulation was attempted by Servos *et al.* (1998), who used an array of computer-controlled pneumatic valves to map parietal areas responsive to arm stimulation. By using a paradigm that stimulated different regions of the ventral surface of subject's arms in a predetermined sequence, the authors were able to map responsive cortex. The pattern of cortical representation agreed with the classical homunculus and monkey electrophysiology, with distal arm regions (*i.e.*, nearer the palm) being found in inferior regions of cortex and more proximal sites represented more superiorly.

While these demonstrations showed that fMRI possessed sufficient resolution to resolve activation from large areas of skin (*e.g.*, the surface of the palm) and to separate the activation resulting from stimulation of nonadjacent peripheral regions, its ability to resolve activation foci resulting from the stimulation of individual digits was more contentious. As the digits are, in essence, the fovea of touch, it is often desirable to researchers to examine the evoked responses from each digit in isolation. One of the first studies to examine digit somatotopy in fMRI was carried out by Kurth and colleagues (1998). They used nonpainful electrical stimulation to the right D2 and D5 in 20 subjects. Somewhat surprisingly, only eight subjects of this group showed statistically significant responses to stimulation of each finger. Of these eight, only four displayed the expected pattern of somatotopy, with the activation focus for D2 lying inferior and lateral to the focus for D5. A study by Gelnar and colleagues (1998) reported broadly similar results. Using a vibrotactile stimulus, the authors did not find the expected mediolateral pattern of digit representations. Activation foci around the anterior parietal cortex were only observed for all three digits stimulated in 6 out of 8 subjects (these authors suggest that, as the foci lie caudally to the central sulcus, they may lie in area 2).

fMRI as a Tool To Probe Topographic Organisation: Mapping Issues

The studies quoted above demonstrated that, while early fMRI studies of digit somatotopy showed promise, results were not as unambiguous as might have been expected from a knowledge of the neurophysiological literature. The mapping of cortex with topographically oriented stimuli facilitates the study of fundamental questions in sensory neuroscience—for example, how changes in map organisation, secondary to pathology or experimental manipulation, relate to changes in behaviour. If the spatial organisation of activity in topographically mapped areas is thought to be a useful metric of information processing (and there is ample evidence to suggest that map structure in anterior parietal regions is not merely an epiphenomenon of cortical development; see, for example, Kaas, 1997), the stimuli used in mapping experiments must be chosen so that they are able to adequately reveal such a relationship. However, different imaging modalities use different criteria to define receptive fields. While threshold-level stimuli are often used in anaesthetised animals, studies that have mapped anterior parietal cortex in awake monkeys have used suprathreshold stimuli and found overlapping cortical representations of adjacent skin regions (Iwamura *et al.*, 1983; Favorov and Whitsel, 1988a,b). It is accepted that using stimuli of greater intensity will blur representations across cortex, making the delineation of foci specific to stimulation of a particular digit more problematic (Favorov and Diamond, 1990). This may be caused by cells outside the classical receptive fields being excited by the stimulus; as digit representations are organised along a strip of cortex, recruitment/lateral inhibition of surrounding neurons can occur. Different imaging modalities will be differentially responsive to these effects, depending on how reactive they are to inhibitory transmission/subthreshold fluctuations in the postsynaptic membrane caused by excitatory and inhibitory postsynaptic potentials (EPSPs and IPSPs).

Even if the stimuli for mapping experiments are chosen with care, there is evidence that even simple tactile stimuli may cause activation in neurons outside the classical receptive field. Under physiologically normal conditions, approximately 20% of racoon SI cells in which EPSPs can be elicited by stimulation of a single digit *also* display EPSPs to the stimulation of adjacent digits (Smits *et al.*, 1991). Thus the classical receptive fields of cortical neurons in primary sensory areas as mapped under anaesthesia are merely one possible configuration of a dynamic, context-specific map; similar themes have been explored by Sheth and colleagues (1998) using optical imaging in rat barrel cortex. The region of cortex activated by stimulation of a single vibrissa at 1 Hz is *more* diffuse than that activated by greater stimulation rates (up to 10 Hz; see Sheth *et al.*, 1998). The authors concluded that "...the spread of activation in rat barrel cortex is modulated in a dynamic fashion by the frequency of vibrissa stimulation." If the intensities or frequencies of mapping stimuli are not chosen carefully, threshold surround regions may be recruited, making the delineation of classic receptive fields more difficult (Moore *et al.*, 1999). To date, only one systematic investigation of the frequency dependence of the BOLD (blood-oxygen-level-dependent) signal measured with fMRI (Kampe *et al.*, 2000) has been published. The results of this study bear out the concerns voiced above; when stimulating the median nerve, the authors found that increasing stimulus frequency resulted in a linear increase in BOLD signal but with an accompanying increase in the number of activated voxels. Another study of the frequency dependence of anterior parietal cortex (McGonigle and Frackowiak, unpublished observations) found some evidence for a relationship between increasing signal change with increasing rate of stimulation. Therefore, increasing the rate of application of stimuli may act to obscure patterns of somatotopy in SI, as with increasing the intensity of applied stimuli.

The issues discussed above are particularly germane in BOLD fMRI studies. fMRI is handicapped by a low signal-to-noise ratio, which can produce false negatives. This makes mapping studies especially difficult, because if stimulation parameters are optimised to prevent representational overlap, signal changes may be too small to permit reliable detection. Thus, for mapping purposes, the best stimulus is one that causes detectable changes in anterior parietal cortex yet also produces minimal lateral spread to neighbouring representations. Krause and colleagues (Krause *et al.*, 2001) examined the overlap of digit representations in anterior parietal cortex using two different electrical stimulation intensities. They found that higher intensity stimuli produced more overlap between activation foci in foci within the postcentral sulcus (area 3b) and on the crown of the postcentral gyrus (area 1/2). As might be expected from the presence of multiple-digit receptive fields within BA1/2, the overlap between foci in this region was more pronounced; however, as the authors stimulated only two fingers (D2 and D3) with two intensity levels, it is difficult to generalise. Backes and colleagues (2000) examined the relationship between anterior parietal fMRI activation and median nerve stimulation intensity. The authors found, consistent with Krause and colleagues (2001), that higher stimulation intensity was associated with higher levels of signal change in this region. Interestingly, the authors found that activation in lateral sulcal regions did not scale with stimulus intensity, staying relatively constant.

Differentiation of Brodmann Areas in Postcentral Gyrus Using fMRI

Just as different rates of intensity and frequency stimulation may blur representations within subdivisions of cortex, activations may be blurred *across* regions, acting to obscure activation of adjacent areas. This issue is equally important: As each of the four subdivisions of anterior parietal cortex contain neurons with different receptive field properties in monkeys, it is essential that activation in each can be unambiguously ascertained.

Burton and colleagues (1997a) were one of the first groups to report two separate activation foci on the postcentral gyrus. They used a rotating drum to deliver roughness stimuli of different grades in PET; however, as essentially the same stimuli were used across the experiment, they were unable to show differential activation of the two foci. As discussed earlier, while there is no easy relationship between microarchitecture and macroanatomy, the construction of probability maps of anterior parietal cortex by Geyer and colleagues (2000) allows tentative conclusions to be made based on the location of activation foci within the PoG. As noted by the above authors when examining their structural probability maps, constructed from postmortem tissue: "Despite considerable interindividual variability, a clear focus is obvious for each area ... the focus of area 3b [lies] in the rostral bank of the PoG (or posterior bank of the central sulcus), and the focus of area 1 on the crown of the PoG" (Geyer *et al.*, 2000). In fMRI, one of the few studies to directly examine if different activation tasks could be used to distinguish between areas within anterior parietal cortex used punctate tactile stimuli and a squeezing task designed to provide motoric, proprioceptive, and cutaneous mechanoreceptor activation (Moore *et al.*, 2000). In the five subjects studied, dissociation between the areas activated by the two tasks was found: the tactile task activated areas identified by the authors as areas 3b and 1, while the motor/kinaesthetic task also activated regions deep in the postcentral gyrus consistent with the putative location of area 3a.

Other groups have attempted to dissociate anterior parietal regions using PET, by varying the complexity of the tactile stimuli used and by varying task demands (*e.g.*, by using both active and passive touch; see Bodegard *et al.*, 2001). To overcome the low spatial resolution of PET, the authors combined their results with probability maps of the distribution of cytoarchitectonic areas within anterior parietal cortex, allowing them to identify which Brodmann area they were most likely to have activated. They found that areas 3b and 1 did not show any statistically different responses to any of the classes of stimuli that they employed (ellipsoids, a rotating brush, cylinders, etc.), but area 2 showed a preference when subjects had to discriminate shapes when contrasted with rCBF changes to discriminating speeds of a brush that stimulated the hand, although it was also active in all stimulus conditions when contrasted against rest.

While carefully chosen stimuli may allow the segregation of some functionally distinct areas with anterior parietal cortex, the ability to dissociate separate foci in area 3b and area 1 has been less frequently reported. Francis and colleagues (2000) were able to produce Penfieldian somatotopic patterns at 3T using a piezoelectric simulator applied to digits of the right hand. Kurth *et al.* (2000) illustrate particularly impressive activation patterns in multiple regions along the course of the PoG, including BA3b (see Fig. 5.3). Yet, some of these authors found that their highest signal changes lay not within the anterior bank of the PoG (area 3b), but on the crown of the gyrus. In addition, even when taking into account the greater sensitivity afforded them by a 3T magnet and a separate headcoil, Francis and colleagues (2000) found that the most consistently activated area was *not* area 3b, but area 1, lying on the crown of the gyrus (see Fig. 5.4 for another example of this). The more consistent activation of lateral PoG when compared to the anterior bank region is somewhat puzzling. If we accept that this region is BA1, it is likely that BA3b would also be activated when considering the different stimulation methods employed in the studies above. The two areas have some similarities in their cutaneous sensitivity at the single neuron level: BA3b is primarily driven by both slow-adapting (SA) and fast-adapting (FA) cutaneous mechanoreceptors (Sur *et al.*, 1981), and BA1 can be driven by SA afferents also (Kaas, 1983; Iwamura, 1998). Other evidence suggests (Iwamura *et al.*, 1993) that on average both areas have similar *absolute* numbers of cells tuned to cutaneous stimulation, ruling out any differences that might be caused by partial volume effects in voxels.

Population-level responsiveness, however, can be quite different from the rfs of single neurons within an area. Multiple simultaneous recording from sites within the somatosensory

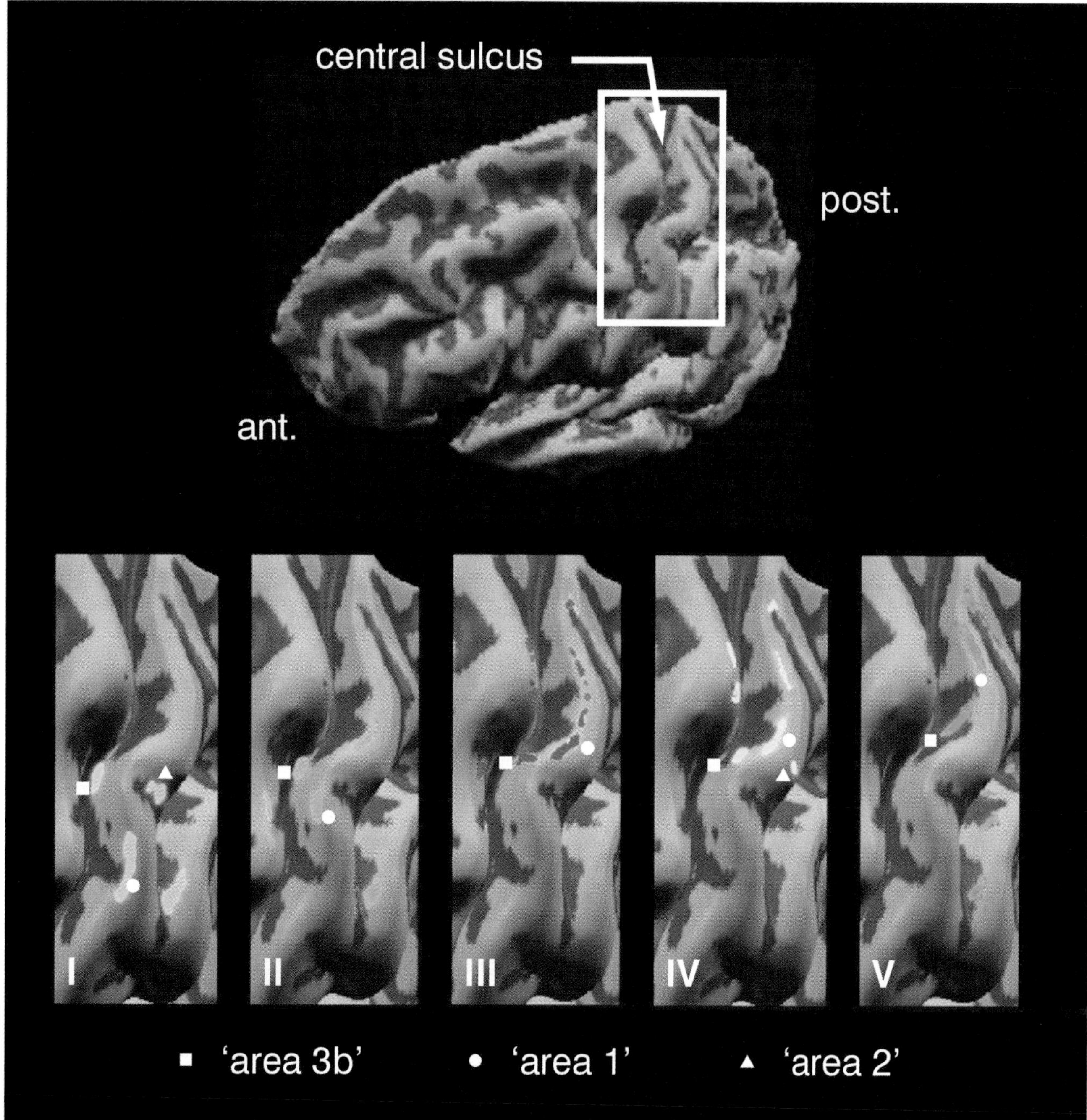

FIGURE 5.3
Somatotopy of digit tip representation in primary somatosensory cortex in humans. Electrical finger stimulation (right digits I to V, block design, group analysis) was consistently associated with significant activation in the regions shown, classified as BA1 and BA3b using the Talairach coordinate system. While the authors found the expected Penfieldian homunculus in BA3b, the spatial ordering of activations in other regions are more equivocal. (Figure courtesy of Dr. Birol Taskin and colleagues, Humboldt University, Berlin, Germany.)

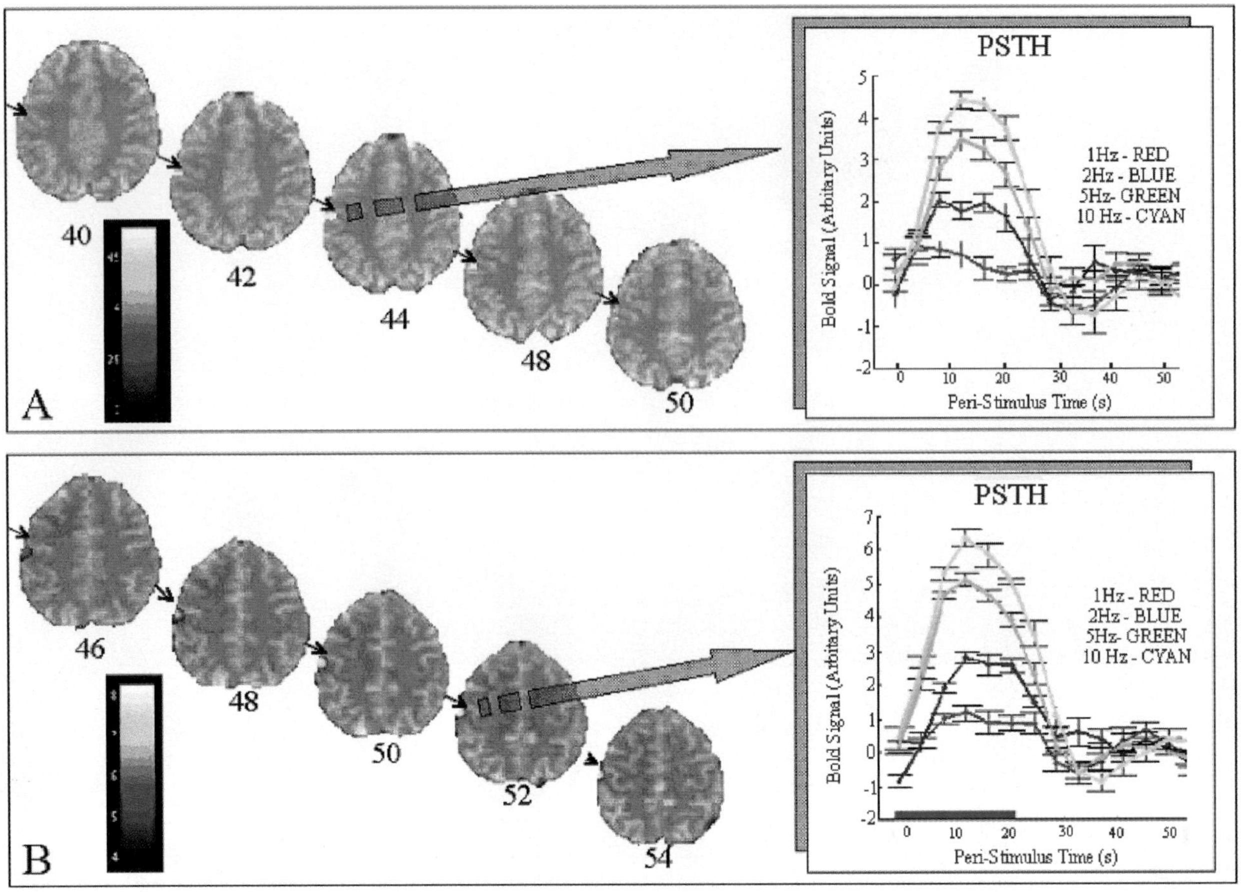

FIGURE 5.4
Effects of stimulation rate on BOLD signal in contralateral SI. (A) 10-Hz thumb stimulation, subject 2; (B) 10-Hz thumb stimulation, subject 5. Activated voxels are shown rendered onto 2-mm axial slices of the subject's mean EPI image. The black arrow points to the central sulcus. The plots to the right of each series of slices represent activity in the peak voxel of the SI cluster, plotted as a function of peri-stimulus time (±SEM). Each rate is plotted in a different colour: 1 Hz, red; 2 Hz, blue; 5 Hz, green; 10 Hz, cyan. The blue bar in B represents stimulus duration. (McGonigle and Frackowiak, unpublished observations.)

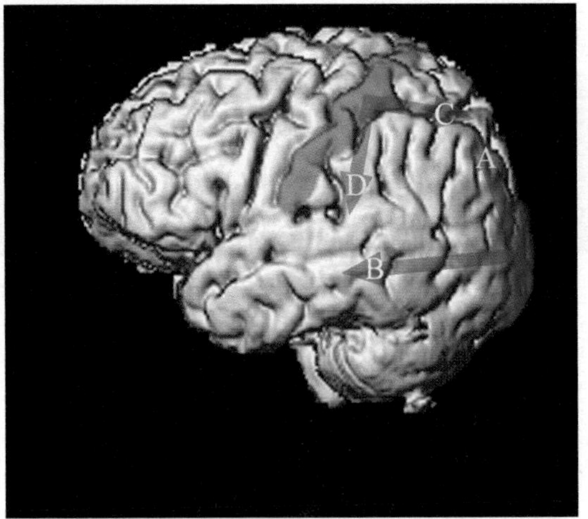

FIGURE 5.5
Illustration of the dorsal and ventral pathway hypotheses in vision and somesthesis. In vision (blue pathways), information flow from VI (solid blue area) is hypothesised to be segregated into dorsal (arrow A) and ventral (B) processing pathways (Ungerleider and Mishkin, 1982). It is not currently clear if a similar distinction exists in somesthesis (SI is shown in red), although a ventrally directed pathway from SI (arrow D) has been proposed by Mishkin (1979) and confirmed by tract-tracing studies (Friedman *et al.*, 1986). In addition, SI sends dense afferent projections to the posterior parietal cortex (C) (Vogt and Pandya, 1978; Jones *et al.*, 1978; Jones and Powell, 1970).

cortex (Nicolelis *et al.*, 1995) suggests that within-area neuronal dynamics code for stimulus properties in a complex fashion that is not apparent from individual rfs or single-cell responses. In other words, while it is useful to know something about the differential response properties of cells across different cortical areas, it is important to note that these results may say as much about the recording method initially used to sample these responses (*i.e.*, using multiunit recording techniques in anaesthetised non-human primates) as the actual *in vivo* dynamics of the network.

Other Investigations of Digit Somatotopy

The discussion in this section assumes that the ability to detect ordered somatotopic maps within the anterior parietal cortex of humans is a good measure of the ability of a noninvasive imaging technique to image patterns of neuronal activity. This assumes that the somatotopic map structure, while subject to some variability and moment–moment fluctuations in order caused by patterns of sensory experience (see Dinse *et al.*, 1997, for some examples), is a robust construct that has been easily imaged previously using other far-field imaging techniques such as EEG and MEG. While group studies using these methods have been able to map out the topography of the body in detail (Hari *et al.*, 1993; Nakamura *et al.*, 1998), single-subject results have been more equivocal (Baumgartner *et al.*, 1991; Hari *et al.*, 1993). In a study of digit somatotopy in four individuals, Baumgartner *et al.* (1991) found that one subject's pattern of digit foci within anterior parietal cortex deviated from the expected homuncular pattern. In the study of Hari and colleagues (1993), "in general, the first finger (thumb) is represented more laterally and the fifth finger most medially," but there was significant individual variability in the patterning of individual digit foci. These studies show that, while it is difficult to directly compare results from different imaging modalities, the variability seen in fMRI investigations of digit somatotopy is mirrored to some extent in MEG and EEG.

Functional MRI is an ideal technique for serial investigations on single subjects. Before embarking on such investigations, it will be useful to optimise the technique to ensure that it possesses the required spatiotemporal resolution to successfully capture ongoing patterns of plastic change. Most non-human primate studies of plasticity or recovery of function have used changes in the representation of the digit pads as their measure of central plasticity (summarised in Buanacomo and Merzenich, 1998). It will be advantageous, therefore, for human studies of reorganisation phenomena to be able to investigate systems similar to those used in monkey neurophysiology.

HIERARCHICAL ORGANISATION OF THE SOMATOSENSORY SYSTEM

Processing Hierarchies in Cortex

The previous section examined issues arising from recent attempts to use fMRI and other non-invasive techniques to study topographic coding within the somatosensory system. Even at the level of anterior parietal cortex, it is apparent that the responses of neurons within each of its four subdivisions are highly selective. As it is possible to define a hierarchy of complexity exclusively within anterior parietal cortex as one progresses from anterior to posterior (Iwamura, 1998), a similar relationship can be mapped between the different, spatially separate areas of somatosensory cortex.

The concept of processing hierarchies, where the patterns of connectivity of cortical areas determine if they primarily send or receive connections from a separate area, was first proposed for the visual system. In general, feedforward connections originate from cortical layers II and III and terminate on cells in layer IV, while feedback connections originate in deeper layers (V/VI) and are usually found to terminate on neurons outside of layer IV (Felleman and Van Essen, 1991). Although feedback connections tend to be more numerous, they are generally regarded as playing a modulatory role in information processing, acting to shape the form of subsequent feedforward volleys. Defined using this criterion, a "higher" visual area is one that receives feedforward connections from a "lower" area, to which it may in turn send feedback projections. In this fashion, visual areas can actively alter the flow of information that they receive from regions lower in the hierarchy (*predictive coding*; see Mehta, 2001).

The basic organisation of the somatosensory system is ostensibly similar to that of vision, the implication being that information should flow from early sensory cortex (anterior parietal cortex), which receives direct thalamocortical projections, to later cortical areas that are specialised for distinct aspects of somesthetic processing (such as posterior parietal areas). This has been confirmed by a number of studies in non-human primates; receptive field complexity and size increase as one proceeds from anterior parietal cortex (SI) to parietal (BA5/7) and temporal (insula) association areas (reviewed in Iwamura, 1998). Thus, at a gross level at least, the somatosensory system can be considered to have an organisation similar to that of the visual system. This segregation of functions and receptive field properties can be advantageous for investigators. In a recent series of studies focusing on tactile perceptual learning (Sathian *et al.*, 1997; Harris *et al.*, 2001), different groups used known receptive field properties to pinpoint the likely cortical regions underlying their behavioural observations, in a fashion similar to that of Karni and Sagi (1991) in the visual system.

While the organisation of the visual system has been the subject of many structural and functional investigations, the current picture of connectivity within the somatosensory system is primarily supported by lesion studies. To investigate connectivity, it is typical for investigators to attempt to disrupt feedforward drive to an area by making targeted lesions in an area downstream and examining the effects this has on the target region. If the lesioned area is the main source of input, there should be an effective silencing of neuronal responses in the target region. In somatosensory cortex, this technique has been used to greatest effect to examine the relationship between anterior parietal cortex and neurons within the lateral sulcus. This relationship is particularly interesting, as both regions receive direct thalamocortical projections in most mammals, yet the lateral sulcus is usually seen as a higher, or *association*, somatosensory region.

Controversies: Parallel and Serial Processing in Somesthesis

The above-mentioned ablation technique has been used across a number of species to examine the direction of connectivity between anterior parietal cortex and the lateral sulcus: in cats (Burton and Robinson, 1987), rabbits (Murray, 1992), marsupials (Coleman *et al.*, 1999), and prosimians (Garraghty *et al.*, 1991). In general, these studies found that removal of a region of anterior parietal cortex failed to affect the responsiveness of lateral sulcal neurons to which this region projected. These studies led to a consensus among investigators that, in these species, the primary somatosensory region and the secondary somatosensory region are organised in parallel (reviewed in Kaas and Garraghty, 1991). This does not necessarily mean that both occupy a similar level in a processing hierarchy; the lateral sulcus receives feedforward projections from anterior parietal cortex in tree shrews and prosimians (Garraghty *et al.*, 1991). However, in the mammalian species outlined above, the parallel projections from thalamus to both anterior parietal cortex and the lateral sulcus suggest a parallel, rather than serial, processing scheme for somesthesis.

Similar techniques used in higher primates have produced more debate. In contrast to the results from lower mammals, ablation of anterior fields in marmoset and macaque monkeys was found to deactivate lateral sulcal neurons that shared receptive fields with the excised region (Garraghty and Sur, 1990; Pons *et al.*, 1987, 1992). Thus, the excision of anterior parietal regions had removed the primary drive to lateral sulcus neurons. These experiments were taken as evidence for the existence of a serial processing scheme for somesthesis in both Old World (Garraghty and Sur, 1990) and New World (Pons *et al.*, 1987) monkeys. The thalamocortical projections to the lateral sulcal region were still present in these species, but the authors of the original reports suggested that these were functionally insignificant (Garraghty and Sur, 1990; Garraghty *et al.*, 1990). These findings supported the existence of a break from a parallel scheme of somesthetic processing in lower mammals to the serial scheme found in the monkey species studied. The functional significance of such an evolutionary divergence was unclear, but the existence of a serial scheme meant that it appeared that, in higher primates at least, the anterior parietal and lateral sulcal regions could be placed in a hierarchical framework, with the earlier anterior parietal regions projecting to the later lateral sulcal regions.

Not all groups found the serial processing scheme suggested by the ablation studies, however. Zhang, Rowe, and colleagues (Zhang *et al.*, 1996; Rowe *et al.*, 1996) used a cooling technique that allowed them to deactivate anterior parietal neurons and then reactivate them again by reversing the cooling effect. During this procedure, the responsiveness of lateral sulcal neurons was studied. The authors did not find compelling evidence for the widespread deactivation of the lateral sulcus found by Pons and colleagues (1987, 1992). In the sample of neurons that they studied, over 90% remained responsive to tactile stimulation during cooling of the anterior parietal region. Their evidence suggested that the parallel processing scheme seen in lower animals persisted to higher primates; thus, the thalamic connections to the lateral sulcus could be thought of as a parallel projection, accompanying the textbook thalamus-to-anterior-parietal projection.

While it is currently unclear which of the two hierarchical frameworks is correct, it is interesting to consider the results of Rowe and colleagues in light of work recording from multiple regions of somatosensory cortex simultaneously. For example, Nicolelis and colleagues (1998) studied the behaviour of groups of neurons across the anterior parietal cortex and lateral sulcus using chronically implanted arrays of microelectrodes in owl monkeys. The authors found that, although anterior parietal cortex and lateral sulcal areas used different coding strategies to encode the location of tactile stimuli, neurons within both areas displayed similar minimal response latencies (anterior parietal neurons, 9.0 ± 2.2 ms; lateral sulcal neurons, 12.5 ± 3.52 ms). Although, by itself, this is not sufficient evidence to prove that both areas were independently activated by their respective thalamic inputs, it does show that neurons within both areas were active concurrently, suggesting parallel inputs.

In humans, it is generally accepted that the latencies of neuronal activity in somatosensory cortical regions detected using far-field measures such as EEG and MEG support a serial processing scheme, with anterior parietal activity present as early as 20 ms after the delivery of tactile stimuli and lateral sulcal sources peaking in the 100- to 180-ms range (Hari *et al.*, 1984, 1993). There is some evidence from MEG, however, that under certain conditions anterior parietal neurons and lateral sulcal neurons contralateral to a tactile stimulus may be active concurrently around 20 to 30 ms after the stimulus (Karhu and Tesche, 1999), considerably earlier than the typical reported latencies. It is currently unclear why these responses were not observed in previous MEG studies of tactile function (see, for example, Mauguiere *et al.*, 1997a,b), although the authors of one study (Karhu and Tesche, 1999) suggested that, as the early responses are typically of low amplitude, their use of a higher than usual number of stimuli may have enhanced their signal-to-noise ratio sufficiently to assist detection. The finding that a direct thalamocortical pathway may drive lateral sulcal neurons as efficiently as their inputs from anterior parietal cortex is supported by lesion studies. Zainos and colleagues (1997) showed that, even when the anterior parietal cortex is excised, animals can still detect the presence of stimuli, although they can no longer perform a trained discrimination task. This ability may be supported by the direct thalamocortical inputs to the lateral sulcus.

FUNCTIONAL SPECIALISATION OF THE SOMATOSENSORY SYSTEM

Task-Related Somatosensory Processing

In the visual system, a number of dominant theories link patterns of connectivity to functional theories on how areas interact to produce complex behavioural and perceptual phenomena (*e.g.*, Ungerleider and Mishkin, 1982; Milner and Goodale, 1996; Zeki and Shipp, 1988). The dissociation between the dorsal and ventral processing of visual information has proven to be an influential classification scheme. Similar schemes have been proposed in other modalities. In the auditory system, recent studies have proposed organisational principles analogous to those for the visual dorsal and ventral regions (Rauschecker, 1998; Romanski *et al.*, 1999). Is there evidence to support a similar organisation in the somatosensory system?

One of the first attempts to subdivide the somatosensory system into functional streams subserving different tasks was made by Mishkin (1979). Arguing from lesion data in non-human primates, he proposed that a pathway between anterior parietal and medial temporal lobe areas may mediate tactile learning and memory. Although subsequent neuroanatomical work (Friedmann *et al.*, 1986) illustrated that such a ventral complex of somatosensory regions does indeed exist in the macaque, its functional significance is still unclear. To date, only a single PET study has reported activation of ventral somatosensory and temporal areas in response to tactile memory paradigms (Bonda *et al.*, 1996); however, preliminary data from a recent study by Reed and colleagues (2000) suggests that under some conditions it may be possible to differentiate between two streams of tactile processing in cortex. They used MEG to compare subjects discriminating either tactile patterns (objects, the "what" task) or different tactile locations (the "where" task). The field pattern for the location task involved mainly bilateral posterior parietal cortex. By contrast, their object discrimination task showed activation of temporal cortical regions. This is broadly similar to the results of Bonda and colleagues (1996), although they found that activation of ventral and temporal cortical areas was observed when comparing activation in passive stimulation epochs *minus* activation during active tactile discrimination (*i.e.*, deactivation of these areas during the active task). Whether this difference is driven by the different imaging modalities is unclear, although it is worth noting that neurophysiological studies examining activity in the inferior temporal region have found that neuronal firing is suppressed in monkeys during match-to-sample tasks similar to those used in the imaging experiments here (Miller *et al.*, 1991, 1993). Further studies combining different modalities should help to clarify these results.

While few neuroimaging studies have attempted to distinguish between different anatomical pathways for different functional tasks in the somatosensory system, a number of patient studies do exist. A series of examinations of the behavioural characterisations of patients with focal cortical lesions carried out by Caselli, Reed, and colleagues (Caselli, 1993; Reed and Caselli, 1994; Reed *et al.*, 1994) and Saetii *et al.* (1999) demonstrated that lesions to different somatosensory cortices could produce different patterns of behavioural deficits. Lesions to dorsomedial cortex (including the supplementary motor area [SMA] and the medial aspects of BA5 and BA7) resulted in the disruption of somesthetic processing *per se*, whereas ventrolateral lesions (around the lateral sulcus) were more likely to disrupt tactile object recognition (Caselli, 1993). These researchers explained their findings as a result of lesions targeting dorsal and ventral somatosensory pathways, thus causing a specific loss of function; however, focal lesions that disrupt only somatosensory cortical areas are rare. Thus, however compelling these results may be, lesion studies considered in isolation are not sufficient evidence for the segregation of cortical areas physiologically.

The two studies above aside, physiological evidence for segregation of function in the somatosensory system has been sparse, although haptic processing and discrimination have been examined in some detail using PET. Roland (1987) was among the first to suggest that, in a fashion similar to that of the parvocellular and magnocellular pathways of the primate visual system, ascending somatosensory information may stay segregated at the level of the cortex, where separate areas may in turn process it. If this assertion is correct, probing the somatosensory system by presenting or requiring subjects to attend to different stimulus dimensions could reveal the functions of different cortical areas. Similarly, reducing more complex tactile objects to their constituent parts may allow one to examine the relative sensitivity of different areas to tasks of this sort. The lack of published studies of this kind in somesthesis is perhaps testament to the practical difficulties in carrying them out; while it is easy to deconstruct a visual stimulus into its component parts, it is more difficult for real three-dimensional objects. Nevertheless, a series of PET studies carried out by Bodegard and colleagues have attempted to address this question (Bodegård *et al.*, 2000a,b, 2001). Earlier work by the same group (Roland, 1987) focused on classifying stimuli according to either surface (*microgeometry*, or roughness) or object features (*macrogeometry*, or length). These features are thought to be combined during active touch (haptic exploration) to build up a three-dimensional percept of an object. By comparing differences in rCBF over a number of different tasks where subjects had to make forced choice discriminations of the speed of moving tactile stimuli (Bodegård *et al.*, 2000a), ellipsoids with differing surface curvatures (Bodegård *et al.*, 2000b), and the length of edges of parallelepipeds (Bodegård *et al.*, 2001), the authors attempted to classify somatosensory cortical regions by their selective involvement in each task. As well as differentiating different regions of anterior parietal cortex by comparing activity between their different tasks, the authors found that more posterior parietal regions along the intraparietal sulcus and supramarginal gyrus were activated during both their active and passive shape discrimination tasks (where subjects had to distinguish the oblongness of different parallelepipeds; Bodegard *et al.*, 2001). Taken together, the results from their three studies suggest parallels between the increasing complexity and specificity of parietal neurons at a single unit level and at the level of population activity imaged using PET, with BA3b and BA1 active indiscriminately to all forms of tactile stimuli, BA2 showing differential responses when subjects had to distinguish surface curvatures, and the posterior parietal regions being specifically active during the active and passive shape discrimination tasks, which the authors interpret as being selectively involved in the processing of global object shape.

One potential problem with interpretation of the results of Bodegard as reflecting activity specific to sensory processing and feature extraction during their tasks is that these studies typically contrasted the activity during each task with a simple rest condition, in which no stimuli were presented to the subjects. The PET subtraction images will therefore contain multiple cognitive components associated: for example, attentional orienting to the location of the tactile stimuli, holding the representation of stimuli online in working memory to compare with a second stimulus, comparing the two stimuli and then planning a concomitant motor response or not, etc. This is a common problem in the analysis of haptic discrimination tasks, where subjects must actively explore objects; the tasks must therefore involve both sensory *and* motoric processes. The analysis of individual haptic features through active touch contributes not just to the identification of a given three-dimensional object but also to the selection of future movements that will optimise a subject's sampling of an object.

This interaction between sensory and motoric processing during haptic discrimination makes it difficult to claim conclusively that one can control for the motoric component of haptic touch by comparing/subtracting movement conditions from active touch conditions, even when using sophisticated measures to characterise movement such as kinaesthetic analysis. Studies by Romo and colleagues (Romo and Salinas, 2001) have shown that each subcomponent of a tactile decision paradigm can be shown to be processed by separate areas, thus care must be taken to control these extraneous variables. For example, O'Sullivan and colleagues (1994) found that, while they could control for finger contact time, number of downward movements, and peak finger velocity when using PET to compare roughness discrimination and length discrimination, subjects used different sampling strategies between the two tasks. During length discrimination, subjects spent far longer exploring the upper edge of the stimulus than during roughness discrimination. However, when comparing active and passive touch tasks, another study (Bodegard *et al.*, 2001) found that qualitatively similar regions were active across both, suggesting that, at least on the time scale of activation measurable with PET, motor confounds during haptic exploration may not be as damaging as first thought. This series of PET studies usefully defines areas where future research using neuroimaging techniques with higher temporal resolution, such as fMRI or EEG/MEG, should be able to separate out the different subprocesses involved in tactile discrimination, in a manner similar to recent electrophysiological studies (Romo and Salinas, 2001).

Vision and Touch

The above discussion demonstrates that neuroimaging can provide detailed *in vivo* investigations of the relative responsiveness of somatosensory cortical areas to qualitatively different tactile stimuli. Furthermore, these results can be used to attempt to construct models of how the inner tactile world is elaborated. As with many other questions in contemporary neuroscience, our current knowledge of how patterns of nerve cell discharges shape perception and cognition is best in the visual system. Much of the human brain has been classified as having a primarily visual function, with other sensory systems occupying relatively smaller volumes of cortex. For example, cortical areas that were traditionally viewed as association cortex in early brain mapping studies are now often labelled as visual areas; however, some of these regions may merely carry out similar kinds of computations that are independent of sensory modality. Their activation may therefore be dependent on the demands of a given experimental task. This section briefly reviews some recent evidence that higher visual areas may also play a role in some aspects of tactile processing in the human brain.

A number of neuroimaging studies have shown that, in blind subjects, tactile stimulation will activate visual regions (Sadato *et al.*, 1996, 1998) and, using transcranial magnetic stimulation (TMS), it has been shown that these visual areas play a functional role in Brail reading in the blind (Cohen *et al.*, 1997). However, there is also evidence from neuroimaging to suggest that some visual or occipital areas may also play a role in tactile processing in normal subjects. One of the first examples of the activation of occipital cortical areas by tactile stimulation using PET was by Sathian and colleagues (1997). They imaged subjects while they performed two different tasks using the same set of stimuli—gratings of variable widths that were presented to subjects' digits in a two-alternate forced choice (2AFC) paradigm. Subjects had to discriminate whether a particular grating had wider or narrower dimensions or was oriented along or across the finger. The authors found that a single focus near the parieto-occipital fissure was more activated when subjects performed the orientation task than when subjects performed the grating width task on the same stimuli.

The authors concluded that visual cortical areas might be useful when tactile discrimination tasks involve the processing of macrogeometric features such as orientation and object shape, as many of their subjects had reported using imagery to perform the task. In a follow-up study, they demonstrated the specificity of activation in the parieto-occipital area for their orientation task (Zangaladze *et al.*, 1999). By giving subjects short pulses of transcranial magnetic stimulation over a region near their PET, focus from the 1997 study while subjects performed a similar tactile orientation discrimination task, they found that they could specifically disrupt task performance; however, TMS over this area did *not* interfere with performance on a tactile grating width discrimination task. Thus, activity in this area appears to be specific to a particular form of tactile processing, and the specificity of the effect argued against the TMS effect disrupting tactile processing in general (Zangaladze *et al.*, 1999).

Other recent neuroimaging studies have suggested the existence of regions of cortex that are not classically somatosensory yet may perform similar tasks between different modalities (Downar *et al.*, 2000). In addition, some higher visual areas have recently been shown to contain neurons with haptic or tactile receptive fields. Area TE lies in the ventral visual pathway and is the final area before the pathway accesses limbic areas. This area is thought to be crucial for primate visual object recognition (Murray and Mishkin, 1984), and neurons within it have large receptive fields that respond to objects independently of how the objects are formed (*e.g*, from motion or contrast differences; see Sary *et al.*, 1993). Mishkin suggested that, on the basis of the proposed tactile ventral stream from anterior parietal regions to lateral sulcus and onward, that regions of the anterior insula may occupy a similar place in the hierarchy of tactile object recognition as area TE occupies in visual object recognition (Mishkin, 1979). However, it may be possible that area TE or regions close to it also play a role in the analysis of haptic form.

An fMRI study by Amedi and colleagues (2001) demonstrated that an occipitotemporal region (across subjects, this varied from posterior fusiform gyrus to the posterior inferior temporal sulcus) responded equally well to visually presented objects and haptically explored objects. The authors had previously found that this region displayed activation specifically to object form rather than similar scrambled images or textures (Malach *et al.*, 1995; Tootell *et al.*, 1996; Kourtzi and Kanwisher, 2000). Analogously, their occipitotemporal region was more activated by tactile objects than tactile textures (Amedi *et al.*, 2001). While optimal haptic sampling of objects and textures will be necessarily different, the authors thought that it was unlikely that differences in motor behaviour could explain their pattern of differences. A more likely confound may be that subjects employed visual imagery in the haptic object recognition task, similarly to subjects in the study of Sathian and colleagues above (1997). However, Amedi and colleagues (2001) included a visual imagery condition in their fMRI paradigm and found a significantly lower effect than when subjects performed the haptic object recognition task.

Does the activation of visual areas in tactile tasks reflect tactile processing or visual processing? It is difficult to answer this question unequivocally. The visual system is very good at representing simple orientation patterns of the sort found used by Sathian and colleagues (1997). As this study did not contain an explicit visual imagery condition, it is difficult to separate out activation associated with tactile orientation discrimination from pure ideation of the stimuli used. In the study by Amedi *et al.* (2001), subjects had to perform object recognition using haptic exploration. Again, the representations constructed by subjects may have been primarily visual, but the authors' use of a visual imagery condition allowed them to say that, while the activity they saw may have included a contribution from subjects forming visual representations of the objects they were exploring, it was not the only process active nor was it likely to be the most significant; thus, there are two possible explanations. First, the areas activated by tactile tasks may truly only process visual information, and their activation may merely reflect subjects relying on visual representations to solve the tactile tasks, perhaps due to their inexperience in employing the somatosensory system in discriminative efforts of this sort. Or, second, the functional identities of the occipital areas where effects were seen by Sathian *et al.* (1997) and Amedi (2001) may have been inadequately explored by previous studies. It is possible to draw parallels with a recent debate in neuroimaging regarding the functional identity of region of visual cortex known as the *fusiform face area*. While some authors have claimed that this area is specialised for the recognition of faces (Kanwisher *et al.*, 1997, 1999), other investigators have suggested that factors other than the simple properties or features of the stimulus are the main determinants of fusiform activity (such as expertise in discriminating objects of a particular category; see Tarr and Gauthier 2000; Gauthier *et al.*, 2000). Thus, it has been argued that the true function of the area or the generality of the computations that it carries out was masked by focusing on differences in visual stimuli, instead of the tasks that the area may perform. It is interesting to speculate whether further investigations of the somatosensory system with neuroimaging will shed light on debates of this sort.

Acknowledgments

The author would like to thank Elizabeth Disbrow, David Blake, and Krish Sathian for comments on this chapter.

References

Adrian, E. D. (1940). Double representation of the feet in the sensory cortex of the cat. *J. Physiol.*, **98**, 16–18.

Adrian, E. D. (1941). Afferent discharges to the cerebral cortex from peripheral sense organs. *J. Physiol.*, **100**, 159–191.

Adrian, E. D. and Zotterman, Y. (1926). The impulses produced by sensory nerve-endings. Part 2. The response of a single end-organ. *J. Physiol.*, **61**, 151–171.

Amedi, A., Malach, R., Hendler,T., Peled, S., and Zohary, E. (2001). Visuo-haptic object-related activation in the ventral visual pathway. *Nat. Neurosci.*, **4**, 324–330.

Andersen, R. A., Asanuma, C., Essick, G., and Siegel, R. M. (1990). Corticocortical connections of anatomically and physiologically defined subdivisions within the inferior parietal lobule. *J. Comp. Neurol.*, **296**, 65–113.

Andersen, R. A., Snyder, L. H., Bradley, D. C., and Xing, J. (1997). Multimodal representation of space in the posterior parietal cortex and its use in planning movements. *Ann. Rev. Neurosci.*, **20**, 303–330.

Backes, W. H., Mess, W. H., van Kranen Mastenbroek, V., and Reulen, J. P. (2000). Somatosensory cortex responses to median nerve stimulation: fMRI effects of current amplitude and selective attention., *Clin. Neurophysiol.*, **111**, 1738–1744.

Barr, M. L., Keirnan, J. A. (1993). *The Human Nervous System: An Anatomical Viewpoint*, pp. 78, J. B. Lippincott, Philadelphia, PA.

Baumgartner, C., Doppelbauer, A., Deecke, L., Barth, D. S., Zeithofer, J., Lindinger, G., and Sutherling, W. W. (1991). Neuromagnetic investigation of somatotopy of human hand somatosensory cortex. *Exp. Brain Res.*, **87**, 641–648.

Bodegard, A., Geyer, S., Naito, E., Zilles, K., and Roland, P. E. (2000a). Somatosensory areas in man activated by moving stimuli: cytoarchitectonic mapping and PET. *NeuroReport*, **11**, 187–191.

Bodegard, A., Ledberg, A., Geyer, S., Naito, E., Zilles, K., and Roland, P. E. (2000b). Object shape differences reflected by somatosensory cortical activation., *J. Neurosci.*, **20**, RC51.

Bodegard, A., Geyer, S., Grefkes, C., Zilles, K., and Roland, P. E. (2001). Hierarchical processing of tactile shape in the human brain. *Neuron*, **31**, 317–328.

Bolanowski, S. J., Jr., Gescheider, G. A., Verrillo, R. T., and Checkosky, C. M. (1988). Four channels mediate the mechanical aspects of touch. *J. Acoust. Soc. Am.*, **84**, 1680–1694.

Bonda, E., Petrides, M., and Evans, A. (1996). Neural systems for tactual memories. *J. Neurophysiol.*, **75**, 1730–7.

Brodmann, K. (1909). *Vergleichende Lokalisationslehre der Grosshirnrinde in ihren Prinzipien dargestellt auf Grund des Zellenbaues*. Barth, Leipzig.

Brown, A. G. (1981). *Organisation in the Spinal Cord: The Anatomy and Physiology of Identified Neurones*. Springer, New York.

Buonomano, D. V. and Merzenich, M. M. (1998). Cortical plasticity: from synapses to maps. *Annu. Rev. Neurosci.*, **21**, 149–186.

Burbaud, P., Doegle, C., Gross, C., and Bioulac, B. (1991). A quantitative study of neuronal discharge in areas 5, 2, and 4 of the monkey during fast arm movements. *J. Neurophysiol.*, **66**, 429–443.

Burke, D., Gandevia, S. C., McKeon, B., and Skuse, N. F. (1982). Interactions between cutaneous and muscle afferent projections to cerebral cortex in man. *Electroencephalogr. Clin. Neurophysiol.*, **53,** 349–360.

Burton, H. (1986). Second somatosensory cortex and related areas, in *Cerebral Cortex*, Jones, E. G. and Peters, A., Eds., pp. 31–98. Plenum, New York.

Burton, H. and Robinson, C. J. (1987). Responses in the first or second somatosensory cortical area in cats during transient inactivation of the other ipsilateral area with lidocaine hydrochloride. *Somatosens. Res.*, **4**(3), 215–236.

Burton, H. and Sinclair, R. J. (1996). Somatosensory cortex, in *Pain and Touch*, Kruger, L., Ed., Academic Press, San Diego.

Burton, H., Sathian, K., and Dian-Hua, S. (1990). Altered responses to cutaneous stimuli in the second somatosensory cortex following lesions of the postcentral gyrus in infant and juvenile macaques. *J. Comp. Neurol.*, **291**, 395–414.

Burton, H., Videen, T. O., and Raichle, M. E. (1993). Tactile-vibration-activated foci in insular and parietal opercular cortex with positron emission tomography: mapping the second somatosensory area in humans. *Somato. Mot. Res.*, **10**, 297–308.

Burton, H., Fabri, M., and Alloway, K. (1995). Cortical areas within the lateral sulcus connected to cutaneous representations in areas 3b and 1: a revised interpretation of the second somatosensory area in macaque monkeys. *J. Comp. Neurol.*, **355**, 539–562.

Burton, H., MacLeod, A. M., Videen, T. O., and Raichle, M. E. (1997a). Multiple foci in parietal and frontal cortex activated by rubbing embossed grating patterns across fingerpads, a positron emission tomography study in humans, *Cereb. Cortex*, **7**, 3–17.

Burton, H., Sinclair, R. J., Hong, S.-Y., Pruett, J. R., and Whang, K. C. (1997b). Tactile-spatial and cross-modal attention effects in the second somatosensory and 7b cortical areas of rhesus monkeys. *Somatosens. Mot. Res.*, **14**, 237–267.

Burton, H., Abend, N. S., MacLeod, A. M., Sinclair, R. J., Snyder, A. Z., and Raichle, M. E. (1999). Tactile attention tasks enhance activation in somatosensory regions of parietal cortex: a positron emission tomography study. *Cereb. Cortex*, **9**, 662–674.

Caselli, R. J. (1993). Ventrolateral and dorsomedial somatosensory association cortex damage produces distinct somesthetic syndromes in humans. *Neurology*, **43**, 762–771.

Cavada, C. (2001). The visual parietal areas in the macaque monkey: current structural knowledge and ignorance. *NeuroImage*, **14**, S21–S26.

Cavada, C. and Goldman-Rakic, P. S. (1989a). Posterior parietal cortex in rhesus monkey. I. Parcellation of areas based on distinctive limbic and sensory corticocortical connections. *J. Comp. Neurol.*, **287**, 393–421.

Cavada, C. and Goldman-Rakic, P. S. (1989b). Posterior parietal cortex in rhesus monkey. II. Evidence for segregated corticocortical networks linking sensory and limbic areas with the frontal lobe. *J. Comp. Neurol.*, **287**, 422–445.

Chapman, C. E., Spidalieri, G., and Lamarre, Y. (1984). Discharge properties of area 5 neurones during arm movements triggered by sensory stimuli in the monkey. *Brain Res.*, **309**, 163–177

Cohen, L. G., Celnik, P., Pascual-Leone, A., Corwell, B., Falz, L., Dambrosia, J., Honda, M., Sadato, N., Gerloff, C., Catala, M. D., and Hallett, M. (1997). Functional relevance of cross-modal plasticity in blind humans. *Nature*, **389**, 180–183.

Colby, C. L., Gattass, R., Olson, C. R., and Gross, C. G. (1988). Topographical organisation of cortical afferents to extrastriate visual area PO in the macaque: a dual tracer study. *J. Comp. Neurol.*, **269**, 392–413.

Coleman, G. T., Zhang, H. Q., Murray, G. M., Zachariah, M. K., and Rowe, M. J. (1999). Organisation of somatosensory areas I and II in marsupial cerebral cortex: parallel processing in the possum sensory cortex. *J. Neurophysiol.*, **81**, 2316–2324.

Crick, E. and Jones, E. (1993). Backwardness of human neuroanatomy. *Nature*, **361,** 109–110.

Cusick, C. G., Wall, J. T., Felleman, D. J., and Kaas, J. H. (1989). Somatotopic organisation of the lateral sulcus of owl monkeys: area 3b, S-II, and a ventral somatosensory area. *J. Comp. Neurol.*, **282**, 169–190.

Darian-Smith, I., Galea, M., Darian, P., Smith, C., Sugitani, M., Tan, A., and Burman, K. (1996). The anatomy of manual dexterity: the new connectivity of the primate sensorimotor thalamus and cerebral cortex. *Adv. Anat. Embryol. Cell Biol.*, **133**, 1–140.

Dinse, H. R., Godde, B., Hilger, T., Haupt, S. S., Spengler, F., and Zepka, R. (1997). Short-term functional plasticity of cortical and thalamic sensory representations and its implication for information processing. *Adv. Neurol.*, **73**, 159–178.

Disbrow, E. A., Roberts, T. P., Slutsky, D., and Krubitzer, L. (1999). The use of fMRI for determining the topographic organisation of cortical fields in human and nonhuman primates. *Brain Res.*, **829**, 167–173.

Disbrow, E. A., Slutsky, D. A., Roberts,T. P., and Krubitzer, L. (2000). Functional MRI at 1.5 Tesla: a comparison of the blood-oxygenation-level-dependent signal and electrophysiology. *PNAS*, **97**, 18–23.

Downar, J., Crawley, A. P., Mikulis, D. J., and Davis, K. D. (2000). A multimodal cortical network for the detection of changes in the sensory environment. *Nat. Neurosci.*, **3**, 277–283.

Dubowitz, D. J, Chen, D. Y., Atkinson, D. J., Grieve, K. L., Gillikin, B., Bradley, W. G., and Andersen, R. A. (1998). Functional magnetic resonance imaging in macaque cortex. *NeuroReport*, **9**, 2213–2218.

Dubowitz, D. J., Chen, D. Y, Atkinson, D. J., Scadeng, M., Martinez, A., Andersen, M. B., Andersen, R. A., and Bradley, W. G. (2001). *J. Neurosci. Methods*, **107**, 71–80.

Duffy, F. H. and Burchfiel, J. L. (1971). Somatosensory system: organisational hierarchy from single units in monkey area 5. *Science*, **172**, 273–275.

Duhamel, J. R., Colby, C. L., and Goldberg, M. E. (1992). The updating of the representation of visual space in parietal cortex by intended eye movements. *Science*, **255,** 90–92.

Dykes, R. W. and Ruest, A. (1986). What makes a map in somatosensory cortex?, in *Cerebral Cortex*, Vol. 5, Sensory-Motor Areas and Aspects of Cortical Connectivity, Jones, E. G. and Peters, A., Eds. Plenum, New York.

Favorov, O. V. and Diamond, M. E. (1990). Demonstration of discrete place-defined columns—segregates—in the cat, *Comp. Neurol.*, **298,** 97–112.

Favorov, O. and Whitsel, B. L. (1988a). Spatial organisation of the peripheral input to area 1 cell columns. I. The detection of 'segregates'. *Brain Res.*, **472,** 25–42.

Favorov, O. and Whitsel, B. L. (1988b). Spatial organisation of the peripheral input to area 1 cell columns. II. The forelimb representation achieved by a mosaic of segregates. *Brain Res.*, **472**, 43–56.

Fellman, D. J. and Van Essen, D. C. (1991). Distributed hierarchical processing in the primate cerebral cortex. *Cerebral Cortex*, **1**, 1–47.

Fox, P. T., Burton, H., and Raichle, M. E. (1987). Mapping human somatosensory cortex with positron emission tomography. *J. Neurosurg.*, **67**, 34–43.

Francis, S. T., Kelly, E. F., Bowtell, R., Dunseath, W. J., Folger, S. E., and McGlone, F. (2000). *Neuroimage*, **11,** 188–202.

Friedman, D. P., Murray, E. A., O'Neill, J. B., and Mishkin, M. (1986). Cortical connections of the somatosensory fields of the lateral sulcus of macaques: evidence for a corticolimbic pathway for touch. *J. Comp. Neurol.*, **252,** 23–47.

Garcha, H. S. and Ettlinger, G. (1978). The effects of unilateral or bilateral removals of the second somatosensory cortex (area SII): a profound tactile disorder in monkeys. *Cortex*, **14**, 319–326.

Garraghty, P. E. and Sur, M. (1990). Morphology of single intracellularly stained axons terminating in area 3b of macaque monkeys. *J. Comp. Neurol.*, **294**, 583–593.

Garraghty, P. E., Pons, T. P., and Kaas, J. H. (1990). Ablations of areas 3b (SI proper) and 3a of somatosensory cortex in marmosets deactivate the second and parietal ventral somatosensory areas. *Somatosens. Mot. Res.*, **7**, 125–135.

Garraghty, P. E., Florence, S. L., Tenhula, W. N., and Kaas, J. H. (1991). Parallel thalamic activation of the first and second somatosensory areas in prosimian primates and tree shrews. *J. Comp. Neurol.*, **311**, 289–299.

Gauthier, I., Tarr, M. J., Moylan, J., Skudlarski, P., Gore, J. C., and Anderson, A. W. (2000). The fusiform 'face area' is part of a network that processes faces at the individual level. *J. Cogn. Neurosci.*, **12**, 495–504.

Gelnar, P. A., Krauss, B. R., Szeverenyi, N. M., and Apkarian, A. V. (1998). Fingertip representation in the human somatosensory cortex: an fMRI study. NeuroImage, **7**, 261–283.

Geyer, S., Schleicher, A., and Zilles, K. (1997). The somatosensory cortex of human, cytoarchitecture and regional distributions of receptor-binding sites. *NeuroImage*, **6**, 27–45.

Geyer, S., Schleicher, A., and Zilles, K. (1999). Areas 3a, 3b and 1 of human primary somatosensory cortex. 1. Microstructural organisation and interindividual variability. *NeuroImage*, **10**, 63–83.

Geyer, S., Schormann, T., Mohlberg, H., and Zilles, K. (2000). Areas 3a, 3b and 1 of human primary somatosensory cortex. 2. Spatial normalisation to standard anatomical space. *NeuroImage*, **11**, 684–696.

Graziano, M. S. and Gross, C. G. (1998). Spatial maps for the control of movement. Curr. Opin. Neurobiol., **8**, 195–201.

Hammeke, T. A., Yetkin, F. Z., Mueller, W. M., Morris, G. L., Haughton, V. M., Rao, S. M., and Binder, J. R. (1994). Functional magnetic resonance imaging of somatosensory stimulation. *Neurosurgery*, **35,** 677–681.

Hari, R., Reinikainen, K., Kaukoranta, E., Hamalainen, M., Ilmoniemi, R., Penttinen, A., Salminen, J., and Teszner, D. (1984). Somatosensory evoked cerebral magnetic fields from, SI and SII in man. *Electroencephalogr. Clin. Neurophysiol.*, **57**, 254–263.

Hari, R., Karhu, J., Hamalainen, M., Knuutila, J., Salonen, O., Sams, M., and Vilkman, V. (1993). Functional organisation of the human first and second somatosensory cortices: a neuromagnetic study. *Eur. J. Neurosci.*, **5**, 724–734.

Harris, J. A., Harris, I. M., and Diamond, M. E. (2001). The topography of tactile working memory. *J. Neurosci.*, **21,** 8262–8269.

Hsiao, S. S., O'Shaughnessy, D. M., and Johnson, K. O. (1993). Effects of selective attention on spatial form processing in monkey primary and secondary somatosensory cortex. *J. Neurophysiol.*, **70**, 444–447.

Huffman, K. J. and Krubitzer, L. (2001a). Area 3a, topographic organisation and cortical connections in marmoset monkeys. *Cereb. Cortex*, **11,** 849–867.

Huffman, K. J, Nelson, J., Clarey, J., and Krubitzer, L. (1999). Organisation of somatosensory cortex in three species of marsupials, *Dasyurus hallucatus*, *Dactylopsila trivirgata*, and, *Monodelphis domestica*, neural correlates of morphological specialisations. *J. Comp. Neurol.*, **403,** 5–32.

Hughes, H. C. (1999). *Sensory Exotica: A World Beyond Human Experience*. MIT Press, Cambridge, MA.

Hughes, H. C. (1998). *Sensory Exotica: A World Beyond Human Experience*, pp. 75, MIT Press, Boston, MA.

Hyvärinen, J. (1982). *The Parietal Cortex of Monkey and Man*. Springer-Verlag, Berlin.

Hyvarinen, J. and Poranen, A. (1974). Function of the parietal associative area 7 as revealed from cellular discharges in alert monkeys. *Brain*, **97**, 673–692.

Hyvarinen, J. and Poranen, A. (1978a). Receptive field integration and submodality convergence in the hand area of the post-central gyrus of the alert monkey. *J. Physiol.*, **283,** 539–556.

Hyvarinen, J. and Poranen, A. (1978b). Movement-sensitive and direction- and orientation-selective cutaneous receptive fields in the hand area of the post-central gyrus in monkeys. *J. Physiol.*, **283,** 523–537.

Iwamura, Y. (1998). Hierarchical somatosensory processing. *Curr. Opin. Neurobiol.*, **8,** 522–528.

Iwamura, Y., Tanaka, M., and Hikosaka, O. (1980). Overlapping representation of fingers in the somatosensory cortex (area 2) of the conscious monkey. *Brain Res.*, **197,** 516–520.

Iwamura, Y. M., Tanaka, M., Sakamoto, M., and Hikosaka, O. (1983). Functional subdivisions representing different finger regions in area 3 of the first somatosensory cortex of the conscious monkey. *Exp. Brain Res.*, **51**, 315–326.

Iwamura, Y., Tanaka, M., Hikosaka, O., and Sakamoto, M. (1995). Postcentral neurons of alert monkeys activated by the contact of the hand with objects other than the monkey's own body. *Neurosci. Lett.*, **186**, 127–130.

Jiang, W., Tremblay, F., and Chapman, C. E. (1997). Neuronal encoding of texture changes in the primary and the secondary somatosensory cortical areas of monkeys during passive texture discrimination. *J. Neurophysiol.*, **77**, 1656–1662.

Johansson, R. S. (1976). Receptive field sensitivity profile of mechanosensitive units innervating the glabrous skin of the human hand. *Brain Res.*, **104**, 330–334.

Johansson, R. S. and Vallbo, A. B. (1979). Tactile sensibility in the human hand, relative and absolute densities of four types of mechanoreceptive units in glabrous skin. *J. Physiol.*, **286**, 283–300.

Johansson, R. S., and Westling, G. (1990). Tactile afferent signals in the control of precision grip. *In Attention and Performance, Vol. XIII,* Jeannerod, M., Ed., pp. 677–713, Erlbaum, Hilldale, NJ.

Johnson, K. O. (2001). The roles and functions of cutaneous mechanoreceptors. *Curr. Opin. Neurobiol.*, **11**(4), 455–461.

Johnson, K. O. and Hsiao, S. S. (1992). Neural mechanisms of tactual form and texture perception. *Annu. Rev. Neurosci.*, **15**, 227–250.

Jones, E. G. (1983). Distribution patterns of individual medial lemniscal axons in thalamic ventrobasal complex of monkeys. *J. Comp. Neurol.*, **215**, 1–16.

Jones, E. G., Coulter, J. D., and Hendry, S. H. C. (1978). Intracortical connectivity of architectonic fields in the somatosensory, motor and parietal cortex of monkeys. *J. Comp. Neurol.,* **181**, 291–348.

Jones, E. G., and Powell, T. P. S. (1970). An anatomical study of converging sensory pathways within the cerebral cortex of the monkey. *Brain,* **93**, 793–820.

Kaas, J. H. (1983). What, if anything, is, SI?: organisation of first somatosensory area of cortex. *Physiol. Rev.*, **63**, 206–230.

Kaas, J. H. (2000). Organising principles of sensory representations. *Novartis Found. Symp.* **228**, 188–198.

Kaas, J. H. (1997). Topographic maps are fundamental to sensory processing. *Brain Res. Bull.*, **44**, 107–112.

Kaas, J. H. and Collins, C. E. (2001). The organisation of sensory cortex. *Curr. Opin. Neurobiol.*, **11,** 498–504.

Kaas, J. H. and Garraghty, P. E. (1991). Hierarchical, parallel, and serial arrangements of sensory cortical areas, connection patterns and functional aspects. *Curr. Opin. Neurobiol.*, **1,** 248–251.

Kaas, J. H., Nelson, R. J., Sur, M., Lin, C. S., and Merzenich, M. M. (1979). Multiple representations of the body within the primary somatosensory cortex of primates. *Science,* **204**, 521–523.

Kalaska, J. F. (1996). Parietal cortex area 5 and visuomotor behaviour. *Can. J. Physiol. Pharmacol.*, **74,** 483–498.

Kalaska, J. F., Caminiti, R., and Georgopoulos, A. P. (1983). Cortical mechanisms related to the direction of two-dimensional arm movements, relations in parietal area 5 and comparison with motor cortex. *Exp. Brain Res.*, **51,** 247–260.

Kampe, K. K., Jones, R. A., and Auer, D. P. (2000). Frequency dependence of the functional MRI response after electrical median nerve stimulation., *Hum. Brain Mapping*, **9,** 106–114.

Kanwisher, N., McDermott, J., and Chun, M. M. (1997). The fusiform face area: a module in human extrastriate cortex specialised for face perception., *J. Neurosci.*, **17**, 4302–4311.

Kanwisher, N., Stanley, D., and Harris, A. (1999). The fusiform face area is selective for faces not animals. *NeuroReport*, **10,** 183–187.

Karhu, J. and Tesche, C. D. (1999). Simultaneous early processing of sensory input in human primary (SI) and secondary (SII) somatosensory cortices. *J. Neurophysiol.*, **81**, 2017–2025.

Karni, A. and Sagi, D. (1991). Where practice makes perfect in texture discrimination: evidence for primary visual cortex plasticity. *Proc. Natl. Acad. Sci. USA*, **88**, 4966–4970.

Kourtzi, Z. and Kanwisher, N. (2000). Cortical regions involved in perceiving object shape. *J. Neurosci.*, **20**, 3310–3318.

Krause, T., Kurth, R., Ruben, J., Schwiemann, J., Villringer, K., Deuchert, M., Moosmann, M., Brandt, S., Wolf, K., Curio, G., and Villringer, A. (2001). Representational overlap of adjacent fingers in multiple areas of human primary somatosensory cortex depends on electrical stimulus intensity: an fMRI study. *Brain Res.*, **899,** 36–46.

Krubitzer, L. A. and Kaas, J. H. (1992). The somatosensory thalamus of monkeys: cortical connections and a redefinition of nuclei in marmosets. *J. Comp. Neurol.*, **319**, 123–140.

Krubitzer, L. A. (1996), *The Organisation of Lateral Somatosensory Areas in Primates and Other Mammals, in* Somesthesis and the Neurobiology of the Somatosensory Cortex, Int. Symp. Series, Franzen, O., Johanson, R., and Terenius, L., Eds., pp. 73–185. Birkhaeuser, Boston.

Krubitzer, L. A., Clarey, J., Tweedale, R., Elston, G., and Calford, M. (1995). A redefinition of somatosensory areas in the lateral sulcus of macaque monkeys. *J. Neurosci.*, **15**, 3821–3839.

Kurth, R., Villringer, K., Mackert, B.-M., Schwiemann, J., Braun, J., Curio, G., Villringer, A., and Wolf, K.-J. (1998). fMRI assessment of somatotopy in human Brodmann area 3b by electrical finger stimulation. *NeuroReport*, **9**, 207–212.

LaMotta, R. H., and Mountcastle, V. B., (1979). Disorders in somesthesis following lesions of parietal lobe. *J. Neurophysiol.,* **42,** 400–419.

Lewis, J. W. and Van Essen, D. C., Mapping of architectonic subdivisions in the macaque monkey, with emphasis on parieto-occipital cortex. *J. Comp. Neurol.*, **428**, 79–111.

Lin, W., Kuppusamy, K., Haacke, E. M., and Burton, H. (1996). Functional MRI in human somatosensory cortex activated by touching textured surfaces. *J.* Magn. Reson. Imaging, **6**, 565–572.

Logothetis, N. K., Guggenberger, H., Peled, S., and Pauls, J. (1999). Functional imaging of the monkey brain. *Nat. Neurosci.*, **2,** 555–562.

Logothetis, N. K., Pauls, J., Augath, M., Trinath, T., and Oeltermann, A. (2001). Neurophysiological investigation of the basis of the fMRI signal. *Nature*, **412,** 150–157.

Macefield, V. G., Hager-Ross, C., and Johansson, R. S. (1996). Control of grip force during restraint of an object held between finger and thumb: responses of cutaneous afferents from the digits. *Exp. Brain Res.*, **108,** 155–171.

Malach, R., Reppas, J. B., Benson, R. R., Kwong, K. K., Jiang, H., Kennedy, W. A., Ledden, P. J., Brady, T. J., Rosen, B. R., and Tootell, R. B. (1995). Object-related activity revealed by functional magnetic resonance imaging in human occipital cortex. *Proc. Natl. Acad. Sci.,* **92,** 8135–8139.

Marshall, C., and Walker, A. E. (1949). Electrocorticography. *Bull. John Hopkins Hosp.,* **85**, 344–359.

Marshall, W. H., Woolsey, C. N., Bard, P. (1937). Cortical representation of tactile sensibility as indicated by cortical potentials. *Science*, **85**, 388–390.

Mauguiere, F., Merlet, I., Forss, N., Vanni, S., Jousmaki, V., Adeleine, P., and Hari, R. (1997). Activation of a distributed somatosensory cortical network in the human brain: a dipole modelling study of magnetic fields evoked by median nerve stimulation. Part I. Location and activation timing of SEF sources. *Electroencephalogr. Clin. Neurophysiol.*, **104**, 281–289.

McAdams, C. J. and Maunsell, J. H. (1999a). Effects of attention on orientation-tuning functions of single neurons in macaque cortical area V4. *J. Neurosci.*, **19**, 431–441.

McAdams, C. J. and Maunsell, J. H. (1999b). Effects of attention on the reliability of individual neurons in monkey visual cortex. *Neuron*, **23**, 765–773.

Mehta, M. R. (2001). Neuronal dynamics of predictive coding. *Neuroscientist*, **7**, 490–495.

Merzenich, M. M., Kaas, J. H., Sur, M., and Lin, C. S. (1978). Double representation of the body surface within cytoarchitectonic areas 3b and 1 in 'SI' in the owl monkey (*Aotus trivirgatus*). *J. Comp. Neurol.*, **181**, 41–73.

Miller, E. K., Li, L., and Desimone, R. (1993). Activity of neurons in anterior inferior temporal cortex during a short-term memory task. *J. Neurosci.,* **13**, 1460–1478.

Miller, E. K., Li, L., and Desimone, R. (1991). A neural mechanism for working and recognition memory in inferior temporal cortex. *Science,* **254**, 1377–1379.

Milner, A. D. and Goodale, M. A. (1996). The Visual Brain in Action. Oxford University Press, London.

Mishkin, M. (1979). Analogous neural models for tactual and visual learning. *Neuropsychologia*, **17,** 139–151.

Moore, C. I., Nelson, S. B., and Sur, M. (1999). Dynamics of neuronal processing in rat somatosensory cortex. *TINS*, **22**, 513–520.

Moore, C. I., Stern, C. E., Corkin, S., Fischl, B., Grey, A. C., Rosen, B. R., and Dale, A. M. (2000). Segregation of somatosensory activation in the human rolandic cortex using fMRI. *J. Neurophysiol.*, **84**, 558–569.

Mountcastle, V. B. (1957). Modality and topographic properties of single neurons of cat's somatosensory cortex. *J.* Neurophysiol., **20**, 408–434.

Mountcastle, V. B., Lynch, J. C., Georgopoulos, A., Sakata, H., and Acuna, C. (1975). Posterior parietal association cortex of the monkey, command functions for operations within extrapersonal space. *J. Neurophysiol.*, **38,** 871–908.

Murray, E. A. and Mishkin, M. (1984). Relative contributions of SII and area 5 to tactile discrimination in monkeys. *Behav. Brain Res.*, **11**, 67–83.

Murray, G. M., Zhang, H. Q., Kaye, A. N., Sinnadurai, T., Campbell, D. H., and Rowe, M. J. (1992). Parallel processing in rabbit first (SI) and second (SII) somatosensory cortical areas: effects of reversible inactivation by cooling of SI on responses in SII. *J. Neurophysiol.*, **68**, 703–710.

Nakamura, A., Yamada, T., Goto, A., Kato, T., Ito, K., Abe, Y., Kachi, T., and Kakigi, R. (1998). Somatosensory homunculus as drawn by MEG. *NeuroImage*, **7**, 377–386.

Nelson, R. J. (1996). Interactions between motor commands and somatic perception in sensorimotor cortex. C*urr. Opin. Neurobiol.*, **6**, 801–810.

Nelson, R. J., Sur, M., Felleman, D. J., and Kaas, J. H. (1980). Representations of the body surface in postcentral parietal cortex of *Macaca fascicularis*. *J. Comp. Neurol.*, **192**, 611–643.

Nicolelis, M. A., Baccala, L. A., Lin, R. C., and Chapin, J. K. (1995). Sensorimotor encoding by synchronous neural ensemble activity at multiple levels of the somatosensory system. *Science*, **268**, 1353–1358.

Nicolelis, M. A., Ghazanfar, A. A., Stambaugh, C. R., Oliveira, L. M., Laubach, M., Chapin, J. K., Nelson, R. J., and Kaas, J. H. (1998). Simultaneous encoding of tactile information by three primate cortical areas. *Nat. Neurosci.*, **1**, 621–630.

Okada, Y. C., Tanenbaum, R., Williamson, S. J., and Kaufman, L. (1984). Somatotopic organisation of the human somatosensory cortex revealed by neuromagnetic measurements. *Exp. Brain Res.*, **56,** 197–205.

O'Sullivan, B. T., Roland, P. E., and Kawashima, R. (1994). A PET study of somatosensory discrimination in man: microgeometry versus macrogeometry. *Eur. J. Neurosci.*, **6**, 137–148.

Pandya, D. N. and Seltzer, B. (1982). Intrinsic connections and architectonics of posterior parietal cortex in the rhesus monkey. *J. Comp. Neurol.*, **204**, 196–210.

Penfield, W. and Boldrey, E. (1937). Somatic and sensory representation in the cerebral cortex of man as studied by electrical stimulation. *Brain*, **60**, 389–443.

Penfield, W. and Jasper, H. (1954). Epilepsy and the Functional Anatomy of the Human Brain. Little, Brown, Boston.

Phillips, J. R. and Johnson, K. O. (1981). Tactile spatial resolution. III. A continuum mechanics model of skin predicting mechanoreceptor responses to bars, edges, and gratings. *J. Neurophysiol.*, **46**, 1204–1225.

Pons, T. P., Garraghty, P. E., Friedman, D. P., and Mishkin, M. (1987). Physiological evidence for serial processing in somatosensory cortex. *Science*, **237**, 417–420.

Pons,T. P., Garraghty, P. E., and Mishkin, M. (1992). Serial and parallel processing of tactual information in somatosensory cortex of rhesus monkeys. *J. Neurophysiol.*, **68,** 518–527.

Poranen, A. and Hyvarinen, J. (1982). Effects of attention on multidigit responses to vibration in the somatosensory regions of the monkey brain. *Electroenceph. Clin. Neurophysiol.*, **53**, 525–537.

Posner, M. I. (1986). A. framework for relating cognitive to neural systems. *Electroencephalogr. Clin. Neurophysiol.*, **38**(suppl.), 155–166.

Pouget, A. and Sejnowski, T. J. (1997). A new view of hemineglect based on the response properties of parietal neurones. *Philos. Trans. Roy. Soc. London B, Biol. Sci.*, **352**, 1449–1459.

Powell, T. P. S., and Mountcastle, V. B. (1959). Some aspects of the functional organisation of the cortex of the post-central gyrus of the monkey: a correlation of findings obtained in a single unit analysis with cytoarchitecture. *Bull. Johns Hopkins Hospital*, **105**, 133–162.

Pruett, J. R., Sinclair, R. J., and Burton, H. (2001). Neural correlates for roughness choice in monkey second somatosensory cortex (SII). *J. Neurophysiol.*, **86,** 2069–2080.

Puce, A. (1995). Comparative assessment of sensorimotor function using functional magnetic resonance imaging and electrophysiological methods., *J. Clin. Neurophysiol.*, **12**, 450–459.

Randolph, M. and Semmes, J. (1974). Behavioural consequences of selective subtotal ablations in the postcentral gyrus of *Macaca mulatta*. *Brain Res.*, **70**, 55–70.

Rauschecker, J. P. (1998). Parallel processing in the auditory cortex of primates. *Audiol. Neuro-Otol.*, **3**, 86–103.

Reed, C. L. and Caselli, R. J. (1994). The nature of tactile agnosia, a case study. *Neuropsychologia*, **32**, 527–539.

Reed, C. L., Caselli, R. J., and Farah, M. J. (1994). Underlying impairment and implications for normal tactile object recognition. *Brain* **119**, 875–888.

Reed, C. L., Dale, A. M., Dhond, R. P., Post, D., Paulson, K., and Halgren, E. (2000). Tactile pattern and location discrimination using MEG. *Soc. Neurosci. Abstr.*, **26**.

Rexed, B. (1952). The cytoarchitectonic organisation of the spinal cord of cat. *J. Comp. Neurol.*, **96**, 415–495.

Rexed, B. (1954). A cytoarchitectonic atlas of the spinal cord of cat. *J. Comp. Neurol.*, **100**, 297–379.

Ridley, R. M. and Ettlinger, G. (1976). Impaired tactile learning and retention after removals of the second somatic sensory projection cortex (SII) in the monkey. *Brain Res.*, **109,** 656–660.

Rizzolatti, G., Luppino, G., and Matelli, M. (1998). The organisation of the cortical motor system, new concepts. *EEG J.*, **106**, 283–296.

Robinson, C. J. and Burton, H. (1980a). Organisation of somatosensory receptive fields in cortical areas 7b, retroinsula, postauditory and granular insula of M. fascicularis. *J. Comp. Neurol.*, **192,** 69–92.

Robinson, C. J. and Burton, H. (1980b). Somatic submodality distribution within the second somatosensory (SII), 7b, retroinsular, postauditory, and granular insular cortical areas of M. fascicularis. *J. Comp. Neurol.*, **192,** 93–108.

Roland, P. E. (1987). Somatosensory detection in patients with circumscribed lesions of the brain. *Exp. Brain Res.*, **66,** 303–331.

Romanski, L. M.,Tian, B., Fritz, J., Mishkin, M., Goldman-Rakic, P. S., and Rauschecker, J. P. (1999). Dual streams of auditory afferents target multiple domains in the primate prefrontal cortex. *Nat. Neurosci.*, **2**, 1131–1136.

Romo, R. and Salinas, E. (2001). Touch and go: decision-making mechanisms in somatosensation, *Annu. Rev. Neurosci.*, **24,** 107–137.

Romo, R., Hernandez, A., Zainos, A., Lemus, L., and Brody, C. D. (2002). Neuronal correlates of decision-making in secondary somatosensory cortex., *Nat. Neurosci.*, **5**, 1217–1225.

Rowe, M. J., Turman, A. B., Murray, G. M., and Zhang, H. Q. (1996). Parallel organisation of somatosensory cortical areas I and II for tactile processing. *Clin. Exp. Pharmacol. Physiol.*, **23,** 931–938.

Sadato, N., Pascual-Leone, A., Grafman, J., Ibanez, V., Deiber, M. P., Dold, G., and Hallett, M. (1996). Activation of the primary visual cortex by Braille reading in blind subjects. *Nature*, **380**, 526–528.

Sadato, N., Pascual-Leone, A., Grafman, J., Deiber, M. P., Ibanez, V., and Hallett, M. (1998). Neural networks for Braille reading by the blind. *Brain*, **121,** 1213–1229

Saetti, M. C. de, Renzi, E., and Comper, M. (1999). Tactile morphagnosia secondary to spatial deficits., *Neuropsychologia*, **37**, 1087–1100.

Sakai, K., Watanabe, E., Onodera, Y., Itagaki, H., Yamamoto, E., Koizumi, H., and Miyashita, Y. (1995). Functional mapping of the human somatosensory cortex with echo-planar MRI. *Magn. Reson. Med.*, **33**, 736–743.

Sakata, H., Takaoka, Y., Kawarasaki, A., and Shibutani, H. (1973). Somatosensory properties of neurons in the superior parietal cortex (area 5) of the rhesus monkey. *Brain Res.*, **64**, 85–102.

Sary, G., Vogels, R., and Orban, G. A. (1993). Cue-invariant shape selectivity of macaque inferior temporal neurons. *Science*, **260**, 995–997.

Sathian, K. and Zangaladze, A. (1997). Tactile learning is task specific but transfers between fingers. *Percept. Psychophys.*, **59,** 119–128.

Sathian, K., Zangaladze, A., Hoffman, J. M., and Grafton, S. T. (1997). Feeling with the mind's eye. *NeuroReport*, **8**, 3877–3881.

Seal, J. (1989). Sensory and motor functions of the superior parietal cortex of the monkey as revealed by single-neuron recordings. *Brain Behav. Evol.*, **33,** 113–117.

Semmes, J. and Turner, B. (1977). Effects of cortical lesions on somatosensory tasks. *J. Invest. Dermatol.*, **69,** 181–189.

Servos, P., Zacks, J., Rumelhart, D. E., and Glover, G. H. (1998). Somatotopy of the human arm using fMRI. *NeuroReport*, **9**, 605–609.

Sheth, B. R., Moore, C. I., and Sur, M. (1998). Temporal modulation of spatial borders in rat barrel cortex. *J. Neurophysiol.*, **79**, 464–470.

Smits, E., Gordon, D. C., Witte, S., Rasmusson, D. D., and Zarecki, P. (1991). Synaptic potential evoked by convergent somatosensory and corticocortical inputs in raccoon somatosensory cortex: substrates for plasticity. *J. Neurophysiol.*, **66**, 688–695.

Srinivasan, M. A., Whitehouse, J. M., and LaMotte, R. H. (1990). Tactile detection of slip, surface microgeometry and peripheral neural codes. *J. Neurophysiol.*, **63,** 1323–1332.

Stefanacci, L., Reber, P., Costanza, J., Wong, E., Buxton, R., Zola, S., Squire, L., and Albright, T. (1998). fMRI of monkey visual cortex. *Neuron*, **20,** 1051–1057.

Steinmetz, P. N., Roy, A., Fitzgerald, P. J., Hsiao, S. S., Johnson, K. O., and Niebur, E. (2000). Attention modulates synchronised neuronal firing in primate somatosensory cortex. *Nature*, **404**, 187–190.

Sur, M. (1980). Receptive fields of neurons in areas 3b and 1 of somatosensory cortex in monkeys. *Brain Res.*, **198,** 465–471.

Sur, M., Merzenich, M. M., and Kaas, J. H. (1980). Magnification, receptive-field area, and 'hypercolumn' size in areas 3b and 1 of somatosensory cortex in owl monkeys. *J. Neurophysiol.*, **44,** 295–311.

Sur, M., Garraghty, P. E., and Bruce, C. J. (1985). Somatosensory cortex in macaque monkeys: laminar differences in receptive field size in areas 3b and 1. *Brain Res.*, **342,** 391–395.

Talbot, W. H., Darian-Smith, I., Kornhuber, H. H., and Mountcastle, V. B. (1968). The sense of flutter-vibration: comparison of the human capacity with response patterns of mechanoreceptive afferents from the monkey hand. *J. Neurophysiol.*, **31**, 301–334.

Tarr, M. J. and Gauthier, I. (2000). FFA, a flexible fusiform area for subordinate-level visual processing automatised by expertise. *Nat. Neurosci.*, **3**, 764–769.

Tootell, R. B., Dale, A. M, Sereno, M. I., and Malach, R. (1996). New images from human visual cortex. *Trends Neurosci.*, **19**, 481–489.

Tremblay, F., Ageranioti-Belanger, S. A., and Chapman, C. E. (1996). Cortical mechanisms underlying tactile discrimination in the monkey. I. Role of primary somatosensory cortex in passive texture discrimination. *J. Neurophysiol.*, **76,** 3382–3403.

Ungerleider, L. G. and Mishkin, M. (1982). Two cortical visual systems, in *Analysis of Visual Behaviour*, Ingle, D. J., Goodale, M. A., and Mansfield R. J. W., Eds., pp. 549–586. MIT Press, Cambridge, MA.

Vallar, G., Rusconi, M. L., Bignamini, L., Geminiani, G., and Perani, D. (1994). Anatomical correlates of visual and tactile extinction in humans, a clinical CT scan study. *J. Neurol. Neurosurg. Psychiatry*, **57,** 464–470.

Vallbo, A. B. and Johansson, R. S. (1978). The tactile sensory innervation of the glabrous skin of the human hand, in *Active Touch: The Mechanism of Recognition of Objects by Manipulation A Multidisciplinary Approach*, Gordon, G., Ed., pp. 29–54. Pergamon Press, London.

Vega-Bermudez, F. and Johnson, K. O. (1999). SA1 and RA receptive fields, response variability, and population responses mapped with a probe array. *J. Neurophysiol.*, **81**, 2701–210.

Vogt, B. A., and Pandya, D. N. (1978). Cortico-cortical connections of somatic sensory cortex (areas 3,1 and 2) in the rhesus monkey. *J. Comp. Neurol.,* **177,** 179–192.

Vogt, C. and Vogt, O. (1919). Allgemeine Ergebnisse unserer Hirnforschung. *Journal für Psychologie und Neurologie Leipzig*, **25**, 273–462.

von Economo, C., and Koskinas, G. N. (1925). *Die Cytoarchitektonik de Hirnrinde des erwachsenen Menschen*, p. 80, Springer, Wein/Berlin.

Whitsel, B. L., Pertrucelli, L. M., and Werner, M. (1969). Symmetry and connectivity in the map of the body surface in somatosensory area II of primates. *J. Neurophysiol.*, **32**, 170–183.

Woolsey, C. N. (1943). 'Second' somatic receiving areas in the cerebral cortex of cat, dog, and monkey. *Fed. Proc.*, **2**, 55.

Woolsey, C. N. (1944). Additional observations on a 'second' somatic receiving area in the cerebral cortex of the monkey. *Fed. Proc.*, **3**, 53.

Woolsey, C. N. and Fairman, D. (1946). Contralateral, ipsilateral, and bilateral representation of cutaneous receptors in somatic areas I and II of the cerebral cortex of pig, sheep, and other mammals. *Surgery*, **19**, 684–702.

Woolsey, C. N., Erickson, T. C., and Gilson, W. E. (1979). Localisation in somatic sensory and motor areas of human cerebral cortex as determined by direct recording of evoked potentials and electrical stimulation. *J. Neurosurg.*, **51,** 476–506.

Yetkin, F. Z., Papke, R. A., Mark, L. P., Daniels, D. L., Mueller, W. M., and Haughton, V. M. (1995). Location of the sensorimotor cortex, functional and conventional MR compared. *AJNR*, **16**, 2109–2113.

Zainos, A., Merchant, H., Hernández, A., Salinas, E., and Romo, R. (1997). Role of primary somatic sensory cortex in the categorisation of tactile stimuli, effects of lesions. *Exp. Brain Res.*, **115**, 357–360.

Zangaladze, A., Epstein, C. M., Grafton, S. T., and Sathian, K. (1999). Involvement of visual cortex in tactile discrimination of orientation. *Nature*, **401**, 587–590.

Zeki, S. M. and Shipp, S. (1988). The functional logic of cortical connections. *Nature*, **355**, 311–317.

Zhang, H. Q., Murray, G. M., Turman, A. B., Mackie, P. D., Coleman, G. T., and Rowe, M. J. (1996). Parallel processing in cerebral cortex of the marmoset monkey: effect of reversible SI inactivation on tactile responses in SII. *J. Neurophysiol.*, **76**, 3633–3655.

Zhang, H. Q., Murray, G. M., Coleman, G. T., Turman, A. B., Zhang, S. P., and Rowe, M. J. (2001). Functional characteristics of the parallel SI- and SII-projecting neurons of the thalamic ventral posterior nucleus in the marmoset. *J. Neurophysiol.*, **85**, 1805–1822.

C H A P T E R

6

The Cerebral Basis of Functional Recovery

BRAIN INJURY AND MOTOR RECOVERY: INTRODUCTION

This chapter begins with a definition of human cerebral plasticity that is predicated on the concept of long-term alterations of patterns of behaviour related activity in distributed brain systems. The theme is developed to show how such a concept and the mechanisms it implies can be investigated using non-invasive functional imaging. A discussion of functional reorganisation following brain injury, which is associated with spontaneous recovery from motor, cognitive and perceptual deficits, is presented from a perspective of activity in large-scale neuronal populations.

In the literature plasticity means different things to different workers, although the central elements remain a change in structure over time resulting in a change in function. It is likely that these changes occur at the level of the synapse, and are consequently reflected at the level of neuronal circuits (Kolb, 1995). From the perspective of functional imaging techniques, we can therefore define plasticity in this chapter as reorganisation of distributed patterns of normal task-associated brain activity that accompany action, perception, and cognition and that compensate impaired function resulting from disease or brain injury. Our results allow for very few conjectures about the molecular or cellular mechanisms responsible for such reorganisation, but non-invasive functional brain monitoring techniques present an experimental opportunity for measuring changes in connectivity and functional segregation that accompany and underpin behavioural change or functional improvement after brain injury. The experimental questions such methods address relate to neural interactions and activity at the level of large scale neuronal populations.

It is a clinical fact that loss of function following acute brain injury, for whatever reason, is often followed by some degree of functional improvement (Twitchell, 1951). Recovery during the acute stage may be related to a number of factors including resolution of oedema and survival of the ischaemic penumbra (Baron *et al.*, 1983). What is remarkable, but is often taken for granted, is that recovery may continue for several months after the acute event. Explanations based on alternative pathways, novel cognitive strategies, or takeover of function by contralateral homologous cortex are common, heuristically valuable, but not explanatory in the absence of empirical evidence (Wall, 1977; Waxman, 1988). At a more basic level, axonal sprouting, alterations of synaptic strengths, and synaptic reorganisation are proposed, largely by analogy with experimental observations *in vitro* and in rodent models of brain damage (Kolb, 1995; Merrill and Wall, 1978; Chambers *et al.*, 1978). The relevance of such mechanisms to human brains remains to be determined. It has been reliably established that both non-human and human brains show considerable plastic change during development (Chugani *et al.*, 1987; Huttenlocher, 1979), and that in animal models at least, this same propensity for plastic change returns in injured adult brains (Cramer and Chopp, 2000). As yet, coherent, system-level, anatomical descriptions of brain mechanisms associated with normal and compensatory change are difficult to formulate. An empirical science of adaptive functional change in normal and lesioned human brain is urgently required. Non-invasive functional imaging provides a means of collecting data with which to generate system-level descriptions, theories, and hypotheses.

EFFECTS OF CIRCUMSCRIBED LESIONS ON RESTING ACTIVITY

A central tenet of brain activation methodology is that typical brain activation patterns can be associated with clearly defined cerebral processes and mental states. This aim is achieved by a combination of judiciously chosen tasks and experimental designs (Frackowiak and Friston, 1994) (categorical, parametric, factorial—see Chapter 39). A rest task is rarely informative even as a control, except when it serves as a reference state for determining whether relative changes found in comparisons of more specified and hence informative tasks are due to differential activations, deactivations, or a mixture of both. Nevertheless, between-group comparisons at rest can be informative especially when patient populations are compared to normal subjects (Weiller *et al.*, 1992). The disturbance of normal patterns of resting brain activity caused by small, restricted cerebral lesions can be large and in some instances unsuspected.

The idea that intact areas of the brain become functionally disconnected from the sites of focal lesions, and that this might have an impact not only on the clinical presentation but also on recovery, was first discussed at the beginning of the last century by Von Monakow (1914) and termed diaschisis. Studies using PET and SPECT have lead to several patterns of diaschisis being recognised, each depending on the site of the lesion (Baron, 1989). These include depressed metabolism and regional cerebral blood flow (rCBF) in the cerebellar hemisphere contralateral to a supratentorial lesion; in the entire cortex ipsilateral to a thalamic infarct; and cortical hypometabolism contralateral to cortical or subcortical middle cerebral territory artery infarcts. Resolution of ipsilateral thalamocortical diaschisis seems to correlate with improvements in cognition and neglect (Baron *et al.*, 1992), but none seems clearly related to motor outcome.

A comparison of resting state brain activity in a group of patients who had recovered from contralateral paralysis due to internal capsule lesions and that of an age matched normal control group showed extensive differences in both the lesioned and unlesioned hemispheres (Weiller *et al.*, 1992). In the lesioned hemisphere relative deactivation occurs in presumed component areas of the cerebral motor system. In addition to very low activity centred on the internal capsule (the site of the lesion) there was deactivation of dorsolateral prefrontal cortex (DLPFC), premotor and parietal cortex, including insular and opercular regions, contralateral cerebellum, and nuclei in the midbrain and pons ipsilateral to the lesioned hemisphere (Fig. 1). These results suggest that, although the various areas subserving motor function are segregated and autonomous, alterations of activity in and between components of the motor system may have far reaching effects on other components of that system. The causes for these disturbances of functionally interdependent regions are presumably anatomical disconnections due to white matter tract lesions. Such lesions can themselves be visualised and identified by appropriate MR scanning. For example, degeneration of human pyramidal tract following capsular infarction has been identified in life (Danek *et al.*, 1990; Fries *et al.*, 1991).

In unlesioned, contralateral cerebral hemispheres in such patients relative hyperactivity was documented in posterior cingulate, ventral premotor cortex, and in the caudate nucleus. The significance of such unexpected changes in hemispheres contralateral to those harbouring internal capsule lesions is as yet poorly understood.

In order to address the question of whether the observed changes have any prognostic implications, Di Piero *et al.* (1992) used serial PET to study regional differences in cerebral metabolic rate of oxygen (CMRO2) in the first week following stroke and again three months later. They found that the degree of recovery in motor function was related to the increase in CMRO2 in intact cortical areas functionally connected to the site of the infarct. Recovery was least pronounced in those with no increase in the relative cortical CMRO2, intermediate in those with increases in cortical areas of the contralesional hemisphere only, and greatest in those with increases in both hemispheres.

Adopting a cross-sectional approach, Pantano *et al.* (1996) measured rCBF in a number of patients 3 months after stroke and found that subsequent functional improvement was predicted

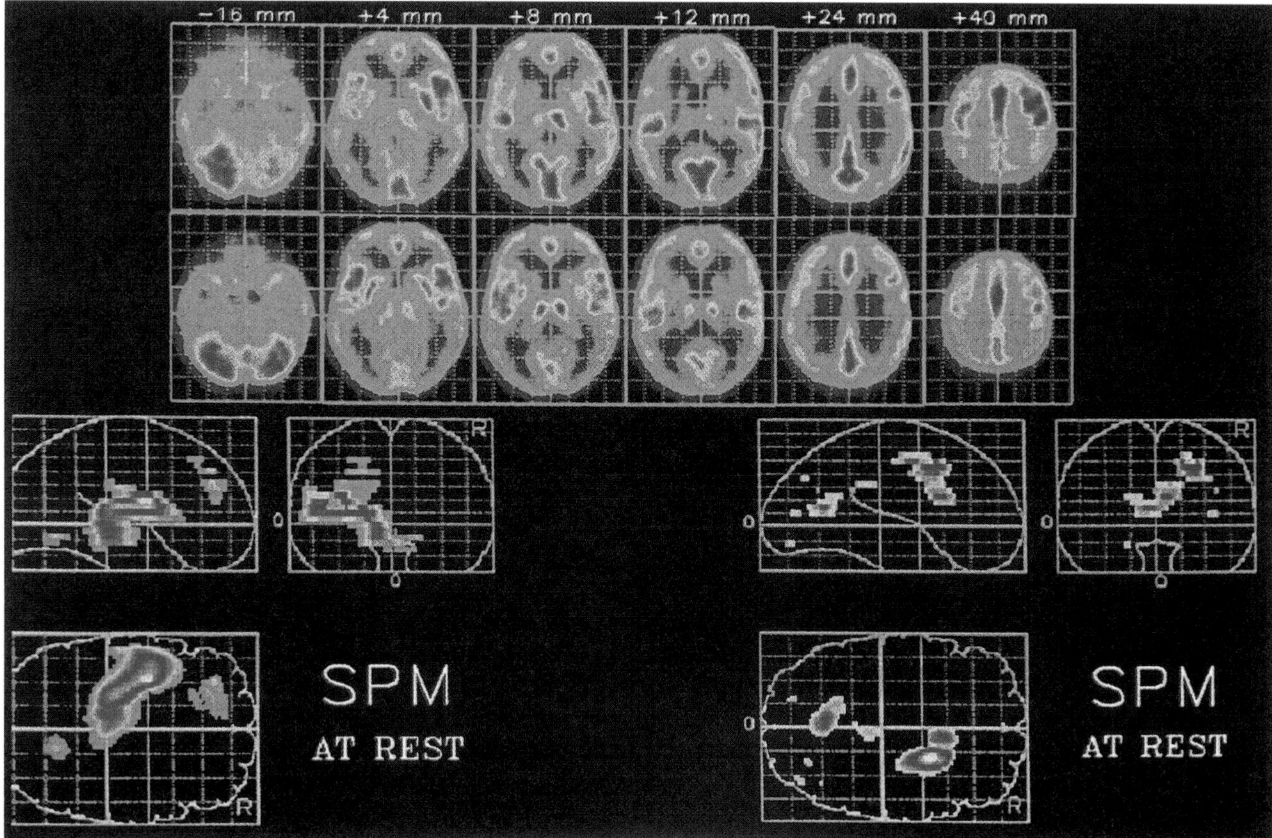

FIGURE 6.1
This figure shows transaxial maps of perfusion in the upper two rows. The first row represents the mean cerebral perfusion in a group of patients all suffering from a lesion in the internal capsule that had led to paralysis of the contralateral limbs with subsequent very substantial recovery. In the second row is the group mean perfusion in an age matched normal control population. The statistical parametric maps show the sagittal, coronal and transaxial views of the results of a comparison of the patient and normal populations at rest. The areas in colour show significant deactivations in patients compared to normal subjects. The right set of SPMs indicate in colour those areas of the brain where there is relative activation in the patient population compared to that seen in the normal group. It is clear that there is substantial reorganisation of resting activity following a relatively small lesion in white matter.

by higher resting levels of rCBF in contralesional thalamus, basal ganglia and premotor cortex. Binkowski *et al.* (1996) found that poorer outcome 4 weeks after stroke was associated with reduced cerebral metabolic rate of glucose (rCMRGlu) in the ipsilesional thalamus measured 2–4 weeks post stroke. It has been suggested that these patterns of diaschisis may reflect other parameters more closely related to prognosis, such as the size of the infarct, but this thalamic hypometabolism was related to the motor evoked potential amplitude (evoked by transcranial magnetic stimulation) recorded from the first dorsal interosseus, as a measure of the integrity of the corticospinal tract, and not to the spatial extent of the infarct. Further analysis of these data suggested that motor recovery (at 4 weeks) was best predicted by a covariance between the resting rCMRGlu in contralesional cerebellum and ipsilesional thalamus, a relationship not seen in patients with poor recovery (Azari *et al.*, 1996). Chollet *et al.* (1991) also reported a functional covariation between the ipsilesional thalamus and contralesional cerebellum during an active motor task (as opposed to rest), when measuring rCBF using PET.

In summary, there is a profound redistribution of resting state activity in both hemispheres associated with recovered motor function, despite the discrete, unilateral location of the lesion in white matter that is responsible for initial motor paralysis. By our working definition these findings suggest plastic change of the cerebral organisation of function that is demonstrable at considerable distances from the site of the original lesion. Furthermore, the plastic changes apparently occur exclusively in brain areas that constitute components of the cerebral motor system.

STUDIES PERFORMED DURING ACTIVE MOVEMENT

Are task related brain activations different in stroke patients?

Chollet *et al.* (1991), and Weiller *et al.* (1992) studied patients using PET whilst performing a finger opposition task some months after full recovery from first ischaemic subcortical stroke. In the first study the patients' unaffected hand was used as the control, whereas the second used normal volunteers. The findings were firstly, that the normal lateralised pattern of cortical and subcortical activity associated with the task became bilateral. The cerebellum was also bilaterally activated. Second, there were additional activations when a recovered limb was moved that were restricted to known (or putative) motor-associated areas. Third, among regions activated there were areas that normally participate in freely selected, complex sequential movement tasks involving the whole limb, but not in simple repetitive tasks performed distally, such as the one used in these experiments (Figs. 2 and 3).

In the above two studies, results of several patients were analysed together, but subsequent methodological advances enabled individual patients to be studied and compared to a group of normal subjects. Weiller *et al.* (1993) studied several patients after recovery from subcortical stroke using the same finger opposition task. Variations in activation patterns were to be expected given the differences in site of lesion (five had lesions involving the posterior limb of the internal capsule, one the genu and three the anterior limb). Overall, these patients were more likely to activate combinations of medial and frontal motor areas bilaterally compared to normal subjects, which was similar to previous studies. However, contralesional primary sensorimotor areas were activated in only four out of eight patients, each of whom displayed mirror movements, and so this finding in particular could not be attributed to reorganisation of the motor system.

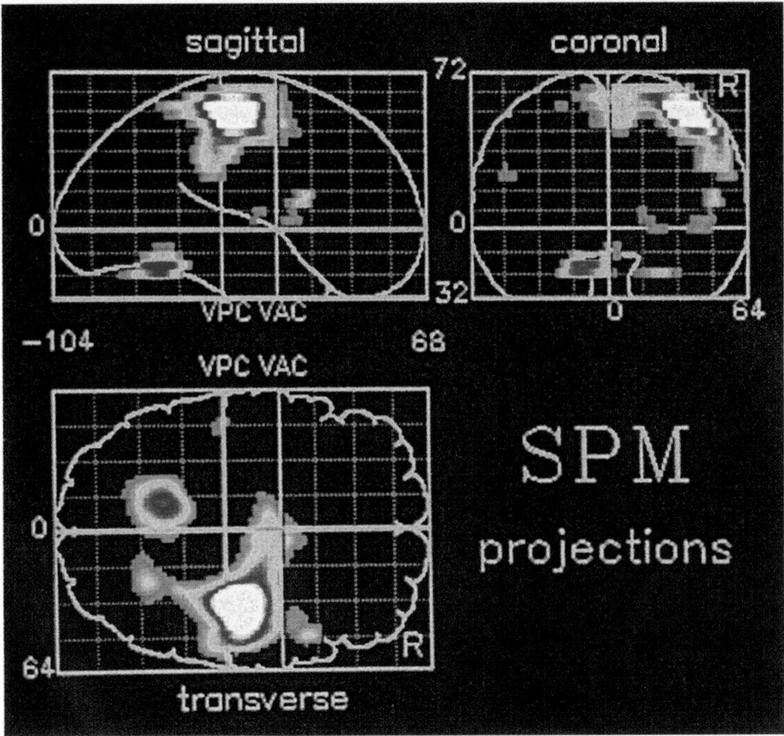

FIGURE 6.2
Statistical parametric maps (SPM) of brain areas normally activated (in comparison with rest) by a paced, sequential, left handed, finger-to-thumb opposition task. Activation is centred on motor, premotor, immediately adjacent parietal and supplementary motor cortices on the right, and in the contralateral cerebellum on the left. The SPMs are presented as projections through the brain seen from side (sagittal), back (coronal), and top (transverse) views. The right side of the figure represents the right side of the brain and the frontal pole is on the right of the transverse section. Highly significant changes of activity between active and resting states are shown in color, coded to represent levels of significance (white, greatest significance).

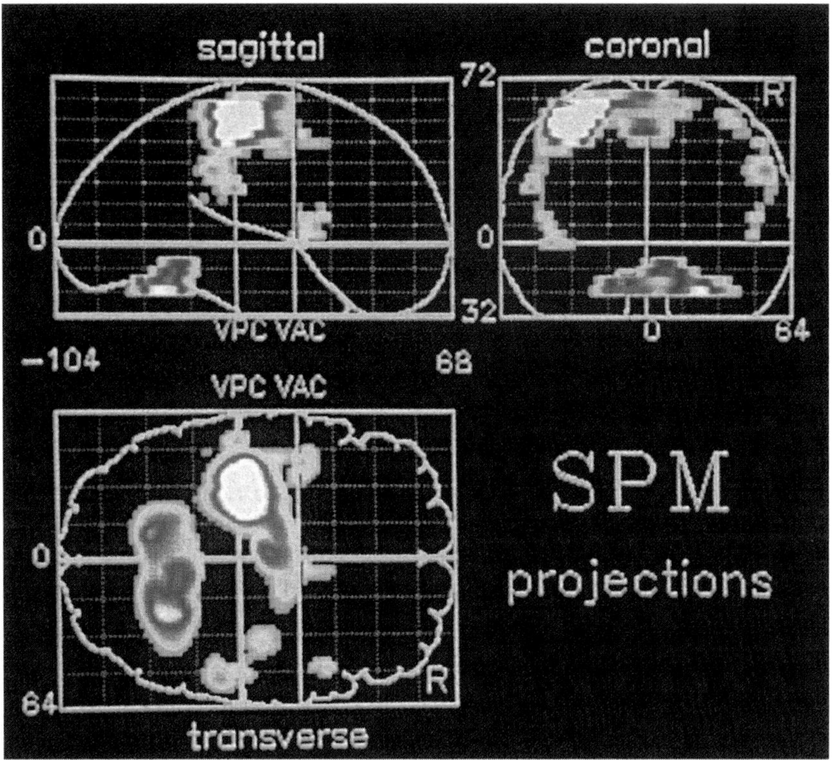

FIGURE 6.3
The pattern of activation found in patients with lesions of the left internal capsule who recover from any resultant paralysis of the right arm. The pattern is obtained by comparing activity during a paced, sequential, right sided, finger-to-thumb opposition task with rest. Activation is bilateral. The prominent activation seen in left (contralateral) motor cortex reflects local and afferent activity onto pyramidal cells of area Ml. The lesion is in motor output fibres of the internal capsule. Both cerebellar hemispheres are activated and there is also some activation in ipsilateral motor cortex. There are also activations in insular areas, both premotor and parietal cortices and in the supplementary motor area and anterior cingulate cortices. This pattern should be compared with Fig. 2 and was obtained from the same patients; the viewing conventions are similar.

Similar experiments using fMRI have been conducted, and throw some light on the question of whether contralesional sensorimotor activations are related to mirror movements of the unaffected hand. Cramer *et al.* (1997) asked patients who had suffered from cortical or subcortical stroke to perform a finger tapping task with their recovered hand during an fMRI study, and demonstrated a greater degree of activation compared to controls in contralesional sensorimotor and premotor cortex, ipsilesional cerebellum, and bilateral supplementary motor areas. Unlike the study by Weiller *et al.* (1993), only one out of ten patients demonstrated mirror movements. Cao *et al.* (1998) also demonstrated contralesional sensorimotor cortex activations during a self paced finger opposition task in six out of eight patients with partly recovered hand function following (mainly) cortical strokes. This contralesional activation was not felt to be a consequence of mirror movements, as these were present in only two out of six patients with contralesional sensorimotor cortex activation. Furthermore, in one patient with mirror movements, there was exclusively contralesional activation during recovered hand movement, suggesting that the contralesional hemisphere was mediating movement in both left and right hands, further evidence against contralesional activations being the result of mirror movements.

The patients employed in the studies described above were largely previously hemiparetic patients described as recovered, in as much as they were able to perform the experimental motor task (often finger to thumb opposition). In general, task related brain activations in a number of non-primary motor regions (particularly lateral premotor cortex, supplementary motor area, cingulate motor areas, parietal cortex, and insula cortex) have been reported in patients described as recovered, over and above control subjects (Weiller *et al.*, 1992; Chollet *et al.*, 1991; Weiller *et al.*, 1993; Cramer *et al.*, 1997; Seitz *et al.*, 1998). Such findings have contributed to the notion that recruitment of these brain regions in the generation of a motor act, particularly those in the unaffected hemisphere, has mediated the recovery process. Longitudinal studies attempting to investigate the dynamic nature of recovery have however not provided clarification. Two studies demonstrated an overall reduction of much of this task related activation over time in patients said to recover fully (Calautti *et al.*, 2001; Marshall *et al.*, 2000) suggesting the recovery process was accompanied by reductions in task related activation, not increases, as had initially been hypothesised. Feydy and co-workers (2002) described differential evolution of motor related activation in stroke patients with different lesion sites, but found no relationship with recovery scores, and another study found no correlates of functional improvement outside of the ipsilateral cerebellum, in which increases in task related activation were seen with recovery (Small *et al.*, 2002).

A number of studies are now emerging which use functional imaging techniques to examine the neural correlates of a motor task before and after a therapeutic intervention such as constraint induced therapy (Johansen-Berg *et al.*, 2002a; Wittenberg *et al.*, 2003; Schaechter *et al.*, 2002) and even pharmacological intervention (Pariente *et al.*, 2000). However, if the relationship between patterns of task related brain activation and outcome, or recovery, is unclear, then it will be very difficult to interpret such studies.

Are Task-Related Brain Activations Related To Outcome In Chronic Stroke Patients?

From the data presented in this chapter so far, the question of whether differences in motor-related brain activations between stroke patients and normal subjects is in any way related to the recovery process remains unanswered. If no such relationship exists, and changes in cerebral reorganisation are purely a function of lesion location then any role for functional imaging in promoting an understanding of the recovery process in humans will be extremely limited.

We performed an experiment designed to answer two questions, (1) is the task-related activation pattern in an individual patient different to the normal population, and (2) if so, is there a correlation between the degree of task-related brain activation and outcome in some brain regions. There are a number of methodological issues which deserve consideration.

Previous studies used finger tapping as their motor task, immediately excluding patients who had not recovered fractionated finger movements. Another choice would be isometric dynamic hand grip, which is well suited to studying not only previously paretic patients, but also those in whom recovery is less than complete, as the ability to perform hand grip returns relatively early compared to fractionated finger movements (Heller *et al.*, 1987) and compares well with other measures of upper limb function (Heller *et al.*, 1987; Sunderland *et al.*, 1989). The neural correlates of handgrip (with 'online' visual feedback of the force exerted) have been studied in detail using fMRI (Ward and Frackowiak, 2003). Because the task involves not only the generation of a motor output, but also significant visuomotor control, it was hypothesised that by employing this task, a large number of motor-related regions would be activated, within which it would be possible to examine for differential effects of recovery. Thus by using hand grip, patients with poor outcome are able to perform the task, and one is not reliant on selecting only patients who can perform fractionated finger movements.

In addition the degree of effort required to perform the task must be taken into consideration. The network subserving motor performance will be differentially engaged depending not only on the task used, but also on the level of difficulty of that task. Any differences in functional imaging results detected in patients compared to normals, or indeed across patients with different degrees of recovery, could be attributed to differences in either neuronal or cognitive reorganisation (Price and Friston, 1999). In studies where patients (with impaired motor performance) are asked to perform a motor task with the same absolute parameters (e.g., rate of finger tapping) as normal controls, patients with less than full recovery will find the task more effortful or cognitively demanding. Relative increases in task-related activation in the patient group may then be attributable to neuronal reorganisation (often termed plasticity) or increasing effort, and complex motor tasks are known to recruit a wider network of motor regions than simple ones (Catalan *et al.*, 1998). In order to control as much as possible for the degree of effort involved in performing a hand grip task, performance levels in our studies, as measured by peak forces exerted, were maintained across all subjects (controls and patients) by asking them to perform at a fixed percentage of their own maximum hand grip (as measured at each session). By performing a motor task (hand grip) that is more reflective of intrinsic motor recovery than adaptation (Sunderland *et al.*, 1989) and controlling for motor effort as much as possible, the results within known motor-related regions are more likely to reflect neuronal reorganisation.

The last point to consider is how to quantify outcome or recovery? There are many scores that one could choose which reflect various aspects of recovery, but it is not clear how they relate to one to another. If one wants to build an overall picture of the degree of recovery, the consensus view is that a range of measures should be used (Duncan *et al.*, 2000). These scores can be combined either by averaging or performing a principal component analysis (Ward *et al.*, 2003a)

Do stroke patients recruit different brain areas compared to normal subjects?

We studied both chronic stroke patients and normal volunteers whilst performing isometric dynamic hand grips. The target grip force was set according to each subject's maximum voluntary contraction (MVC) on the day of scanning (10%, 20%, 40%, and 60%, in equal proportion for each subject). Thus we attempted to control for effort required across subjects. That we were successful was supported by the finding that perceived effort as judged by visual analogue scales was similar across controls and patients. Although the cohort included patients with cortical infarcts, none extended into the hand region of primary motor cortex.

Hand grip with visual feedback activated a network of cortical and subcortical regions known to be involved in the generation of simple motor acts. In addition, activation was seen in a putative human 'grasping circuit' involving rostral ventral premotor cortex (BA 44) and intraparietal sulcus (Ward and Frackowiak, 2003). The most lateralised activations were in contralateral sensorimotor cortex and ipsilateral superior cerebellum. Other activations were bilaterally distributed, including dorsolateral (PMd) and ventrolateral premotor cortex (PMv), supplementary motor area (SMA and pre-SMA), cingulate motor areas (CMA), inferior parietal cortex and intraparietal sulcus, insula cortex, cerebellar vermis, and both inferior and superior cerebellar hemispheres.

Having established the normal pattern of brain activation for this hand grip task, we were able to determine that several patients with poorer recovery were seen to activate a number of brain regions over and above those seen in the control group. These relative overactivations were often bilateral, involving sensorimotor, premotor, posterior parietal, prefrontal and insular cortices, SMA, CMA, and cerebellum (Ward *et al.*, 2003). However, perhaps just as significantly, the task related activation patterns of six patients with near complete recovery were indistinguishable from the control group. Table 1 illustrates that these overactivations compared to the control group, were more often seen in patients with poorer outcome.

Are task-related brain activations correlated with outcome in chronic stroke patients?

When this relationship was formally explored, there was a significant negative linear correlation between the size of brain activation and outcome across chronic stroke patients in a number of brain regions (Fig. 6.4). Thus, the regions that are increasingly likely to be activated by patients with poorer outcome include bilateral PMd, CMA, and prefrontal cortex, ipsilesional SMA, pre-SMA, insular cortex, and bilateral (but more extensively contralesional) cerebellar hemispheres and vermis, together with a number of regions in close proximity to sensorimotor cortex bilaterally (Fig. 6.5). In the ipsilesional hemisphere the regions showing this negative correlation were in central sulcus, but in the contralesional hemisphere they included not only central sulcus but also postcentral gyrus and postcentral sulcus.

Thus, some chronic stroke patients do indeed activate primary and non-primary motor regions over and above normal subjects, but these tend to be patients with poorer outcome, which does not seem to support the notion that recruitment of activity in these regions facilitates recovery. Correlation, however strong, does not prove causality, but neither does the result suggest that this recruitment impedes recovery. In explaining these results, it is useful to consider recent advances in the understanding of the functional neuroanatomy of the premotor (both lateral and medial wall) regions (Dum and Strick, 1991; Strick, 1988). The motor system has long been considered a hierarchical system, with premotor regions at the top and primary motor cortex acting as the common final pathway for the central control of movement. This notion was challenged by

TABLE 6.1 Task related activity for stroke patients compared to control group[a]

	Patients ranked by outcomes score																			
	(poorer outcome)												(better outcome)							
Region	**1**	**2**	**3**	**4**	**5**	**6**	**7**	**8**	**9**	**10**	**11**	**12**	**13**	**14**	**15**	**16**	**17**	**18**	**19**	**20**
SMC - IL	+	+	+		+		+													
SMC - CL	+	+	+	+	+		+													
PMd - IL	+				+		+	+									+			
PMd - CL	+	+	+	+	+	+	+	+												
PMv - IL						+	+													
PMv – CL	+	+		+			+	+	+											
CMA – IL		+	+	+	+	+	+													
CMA – CL		+	+				+													
SMA – IL	+	+	+	+			+													
SMA – CL	+	+	+	+				+												
PPC – IL	+	+		+		+	+		+											
PPC – CL	+	+	+	+	+	+	+		+								+			
PFC – IL	+	+	+		+	+	+													
PFC – CL	+	+		+	+	+	+	+									+			
Insula Cortex – IL			+	+	+	+														
Insula Cortex – CL		+		+			+													
Cerebellum – IL	+	+	+	+	+		+	+			+		+							
Cerebellum – CL	+	+	+	+	+		+	+						+			+			
Cerebellar vermis		+	+		+	+	+						+	+						
Putamen – IL		+			+	+														+
Putamen – CL		+					+													
Thalamus – IL		+																		
Thalamus - CL		+															+			

[a]This table illustrates the finding that patients with poorer outcome activated more brain regions than patients with better outcome. Each column shows the areas of increased task related activation for an individual patient compared to controls. Patients have been ranked by outcome. + = Increased activation present in patient compared to control group (voxels significant at $p < 0.05$, corrected for multiple comparisons across whole brain volume). IL = ipsilesional, CL = contralesional, SMC = sensorimotor cortex, PMd = dorsolateral premotor cortex, PMv = ventrolateral premotor cortex, CMA = cingulate motor area, SMA = supplementary motor area, PPC = posterior parietal cortex, PFC = prefrontal cortex.

observations made supporting the existence of separate parallel motor networks involving cerebellar and basal ganglia afferents and their projections to cortical motor regions *via* ventrolateral thalamus (Strick, 1988). Outputs from deep caudal cerebellar nuclei influence the arcuate premotor area, those from deep rostral cerebellar nuclei influence the primary motor cortex, and those from globus pallidus influence the SMA (Strick, 1988). Furthermore each of these cortical motor regions receives input from different parietal regions. Thus, Strick proposed that these circuits are parallel and independent, with interactions between them occurring at the level of the cortex, the site with the greatest potential for plastic change. Subsequent experiments have indicated that there is a high degree of similarity between the corticospinal projections from the hand regions of primary motor cortex (M1), SMA and CMA (Dum and Strick, 1991; Rouiller *et al.*, 1996), thus providing the substrate whereby a number of motor networks acting in parallel could generate an output to the spinal cord necessary for movement. The implication is that damage in one of these networks could be compensated for by activity in another, thus explaining the recruitment of these regions seen in recovered stroke patients.

However, bilateral recruitment of such regions occured in stroke patients with poor outcome, not in those with good outcome. Recent work has demonstrated that the projections from M1 to the motorneurons in the spinal cord are more numerous and exert a greater excitatory effect than those from SMA (Maier *et al.*, 2002), suggesting that in the situation where SMA projection to spinal cord motor neurons augment or substitute for those from M1, the functional consequences may fall short of fractionated finger movements. Thus in our patient group, in those with

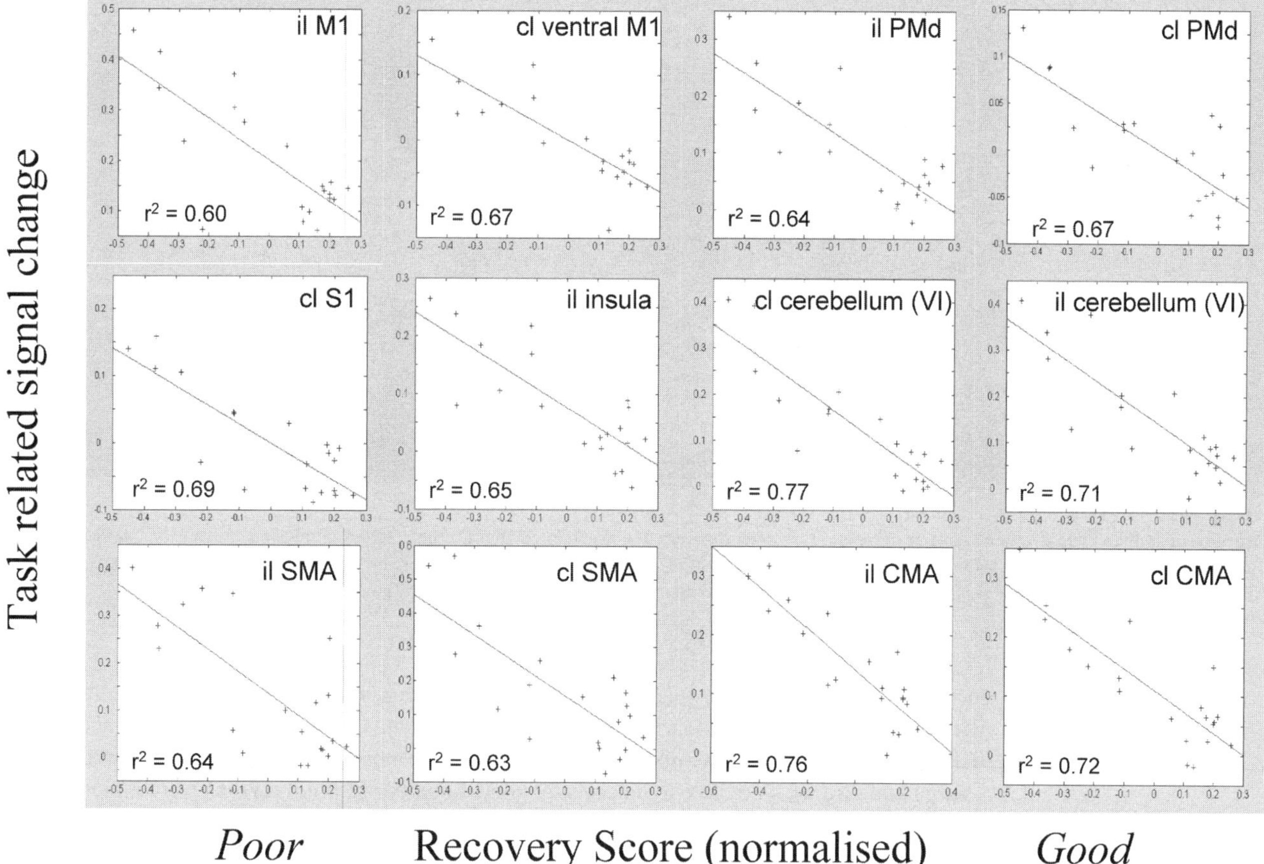

FIGURE 6.4
Plots of task related signal change against relative recovery score (normalised) for all chronic stroke patients in different areas of the brain. The correlation coefficient is also shown. Higher recovery scores represent better outcomes.
M1 = primary motor cortex, PMd = dorsolateral premotor cortex, S1= primary somatosensory cortex, SMA = supplementary motor area, CMA = cingulate motor area, il = ipsilesional, cl = contralesional.

return of fractionated finger movements, cortico-motorneuronal input from M1 is presumably preserved, hence a 'normal' activation pattern, as input from other motor circuits is less important or suppressed. But in those in whom the M1 cortico-motorneuronal input is lost or impaired, there is greater reliance on other parallel motor circuits to generate an alternative output to the spinal motorneurons, resulting in increased task related activation. However, because of the nature of these projections (Maier *et al.*, 2002), functional recovery is incomplete. The observation that preserved transcranial magnetic stimulation induced motor evoked potentials in the hand is associated with good recovery of hand function post stroke supports the importance of M1 cortico-motorneuronal projections for full recovery (Cruz *et al.*, 1999, Heald *et al.*, 1993, Pennisi *et al.*, 1999).

In attempting to reconcile these results with those from previous studies one must first examine how recovery was assessed. It seems likely that patients in many previous studies were not fully recovered, as would be judged by a larger number of outcome measures such as those used in these recent studies. Indeed, three out of six patients in one study (Chollet *et al.*, 1991) described residual slowness of finger movements, and results in these patients were similar to those of ours with residual motor deficit. The importance of *detailed* outcome measurements is clearly crucial.

Patient Studies—force activity correlations

Dettmers and colleagues (1997) described an altered relationship between force exerted in a finger press task and regional cerebral blood flow (rCBF) in several stroke patients with

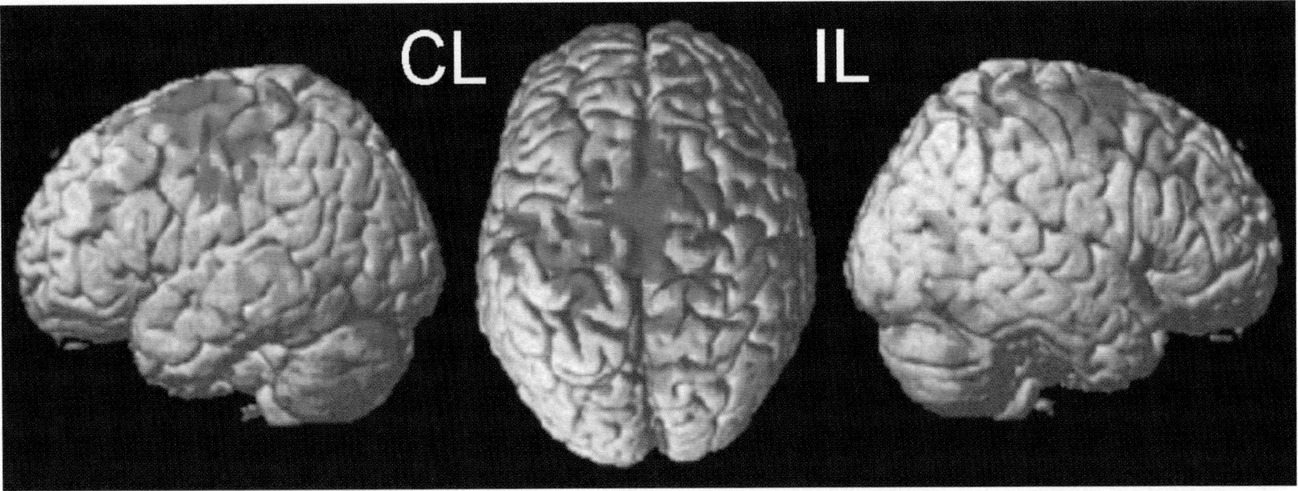

FIGURE 6.5
Brain regions in which there is a linear inverse correlation between recovery and task related BOLD signal across all patients. Results are surface rendered onto a canonical brain. The brain is shown (from left to right) from the left side, from above (left hemisphere on the left), and from the right. All clusters are significant at $p < 0.05$, corrected for multiple comparisons across whole brain. IL = ipsilesional, CL = contralesional.

incomplete recovery. Ipsilesional sensorimotor cortex activity showed a binomial relationship with force compared to a logarithmic relationship in controls. Furthermore, linear increases in rCBF with increasing force, not seen in controls, were observed in SMA and parietal cortex. Using hand grip we were able to demonstrate that a number of brain regions were more likely to exhibit a linear increase in activity in response to increasing grip force in patients with poorer outcome, particularly contralateral central sulcus (deep), postcentral gyrus, dorsolateral premotor cortex, middle temporal gyrus, ipsilateral cerebellum, and bilateral intraparietal sulcus (Ward *et al.*, 2003).

Although it is difficult to interpret these results in terms of their relationship to the recovery process, it is clear that after focal damage the motor system adapts not only in terms of what structures are engaged but also in how those structures respond.

How Are Task-Related Brain Activations Related To Recovery In Individual Patients?

Longitudinal changes in task related activation after stroke

The question of whether task related brain activations are related to the recovery process can also be answered by performing longitudinal studies in individual patients, and examining for correlations with changing outcome scores across a number of sessions. Because of the possibility of session effects in such an experiment, it is advisable to perform as many studies as possible in an individual patient. We performed a longitudinal study, in which eight patients were scanned on an average of eight sessions each (Ward *et al.*, 2003a). The first was performed 10–14 days post stroke, and then approximately weekly for the next 5–6 weeks. Additional studies were performed at approximately 3 months, 6 months, and in some cases 12 months post stroke. It is important to reiterate that at each session, patients performed a repetitive grip task with the target force being 20% of their maximum grip strength (with the affected hand) on the day of scanning, in an attempt to control for effort across sessions as discussed earlier in the chapter.

A negative correlation between task-related increases in brain activation and recovery across sessions was seen in a number of brain regions in all 8 patients. There were clearly differences in the 'recovery maps' of individual patients (Fig. 6), but when examining for consistencies across the group, recovery-related decreases in task-related activation across sessions were identified throughout ipsilesional M1, and in inferior contralesional M1, as well as in anterior and posterior dorsolateral premotor cortex bilaterally (BA 6 and BA 8), contralesional ventrolateral premotor cortex, and ipsilesional SMA, pre-SMA, prefrontal cortex (superior frontal

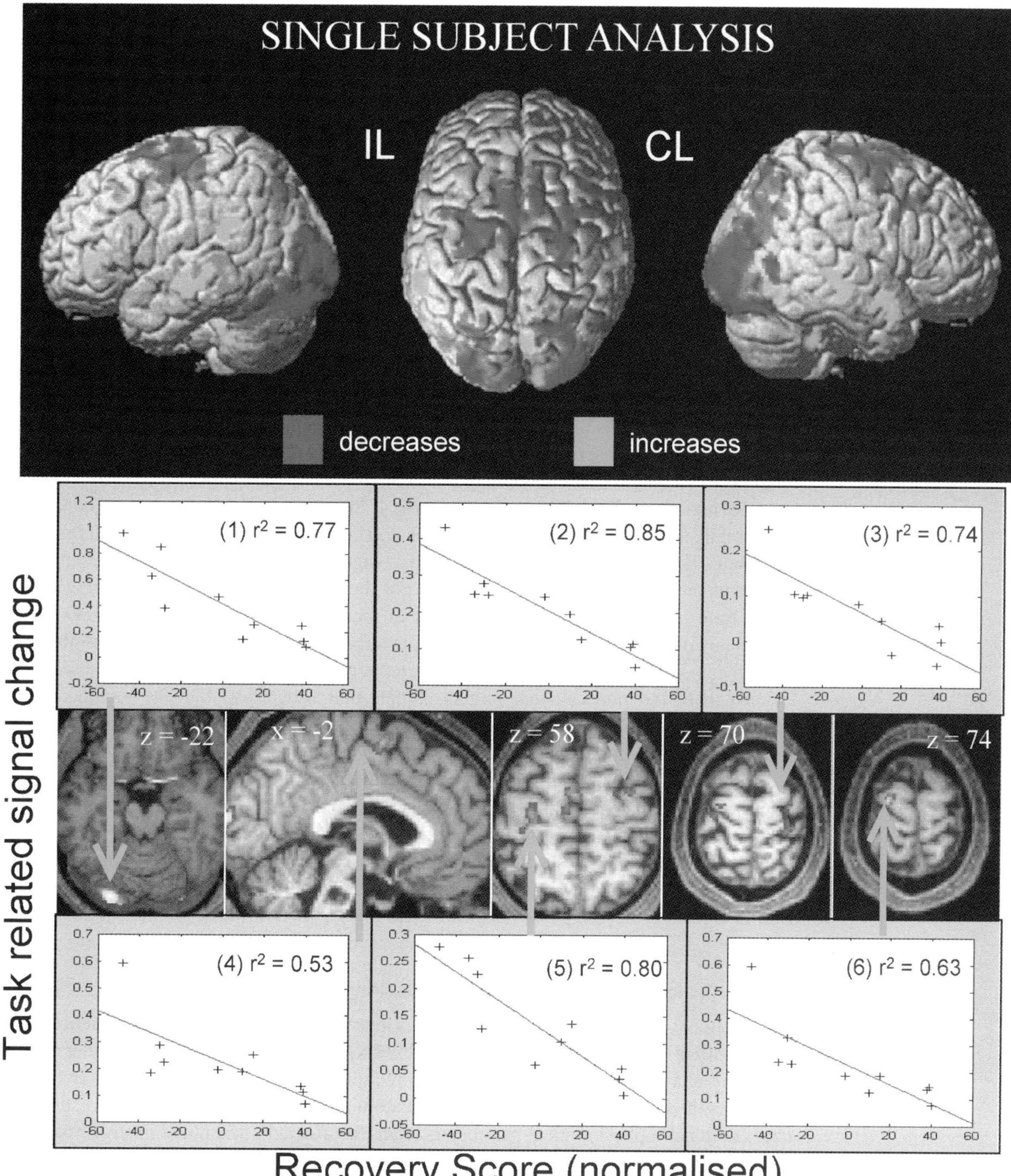

FIGURE 6.6

Results of single subject longitudinal analysis examining for linear changes in task-related brain activations over sessions as a function of recovery. The patient suffered from a left sided pontine infarct resulting in right hemiparesis. Results are surface rendered onto a canonical brain; red areas represent recovery-related decreases in task-related activation across sessions, and green areas represent the equivalent recovery related increases. All voxels are significant at $p < 0.001$ (uncorrected for multiple comparisons) for display purposes. The brain is shown (from left to right) from the left (ipsilesional) side, from above (left hemisphere on the left), and from the right (contralesional). IL = ipsilesional, CL = contralesional.

Results are then displayed on patient's own normalised T_1-weighted anatomical images (voxels significant at $p < 0.05$, corrected for multiple comparisons across the whole brain), with corresponding plots of task–related signal change against overall recovery score (normalised), for selected brain regions. Coordinates of peak voxel in each region are followed by the correlation coefficient and the associated p-value: (1) ipsilesional cerebellum (x=-26, y=-84, z=-22) (r^2=0.77, p<0.01), (2) contralesional dorsolateral premotor cortex (x=38, y=0, z=58) (r^2=0.85, p<0.01), (3) contralesional M1 (x=28, y=-14, z=70) (r^2=0.74, p<0.01), (4) ipsilesional supplementary motor area (x=-2, y=-2, z=60) (r^2=0.53, p=0.02), (5) ipsilesional M1 (x=-30, y=-14, z=58) (r^2=0.80, p<0.01), (6) contralesional dorsolateral premotor cortex (x=-18, y=-10, z=74) (r^2=0.63, p=0.01). Higher recovery scores represent improved recovery.

sulcus) and caudal cingulate sulcus. In addition, these decreases were also seen in parietal, temporal and occipital lobes, as well as thalamus and globus pallidus.

A positive correlation between task-related activation and recovery across sessions was seen in some brain regions in 4 patients (including ipsilesional M1 in 1 patient), but there were no consistent increases in the group analysis (Ward *et al.*, 2003).

Early post-acute changes: the immediate response to injury

When comparing post-acute and chronic phase task-related brain activations, our data and those of others clearly demonstrate greater and more widespread brain activation in early compared to late stages (Calautti, 2001; Marshall *et al.*, 2000; Feydy *et al.*, 2002). Findings in animal models of focal cerebral infarction are helpful in attempting to interpret these results. A number of investigators have observed an increase in both dendritic branching (Jones and Schallert, 1992) and synaptic number (Jones *et al.*, 1996; Stroemer *et al.*, 1995) in both the damaged and undamaged hemispheres days after a lesion. This branching may overshoot and be followed by pruning back, as seen during normal development (Kolb, 1995) which might explain some of the time-related reductions in activation size.

Furthermore, widespread areas of cortical hyperexcitability appear days after cerebral infarction, receding over subsequent months (Buchkremer-Ratzmann *et al.*, 1996). These changes occur in regions structurally connected to the lesion in both hemispheres as a consequence of down-regulation of the α1-GABA receptor subunit and a decrease in GABAergic inhibition (Neumann-Haefelin *et al.*, 1998). The BOLD signal measured by fMRI represents primarily input and processing within a region and not the output signal (Logothetis *et al.*, 2001), so that a state of hyperexcitability will result in increased and more diffuse BOLD signal. The functional consequence of hyperexcitability is a facilitation of activity dependent plastic change (Hagemann *et al.*, 1998). Although these phenomena have been reported in animals with cortical lesions, there is evidence from human studies that subcortical damage to the corticospinal pathway has a similar effect. Enlargement of the motor output zone was observed in patients with pure degeneration of the corticospinal tract (Kew *et al.*, 1994) possibly as a result of loss of recurrent inhibition onto surrounding pyramidal cells (Ghosh and Porter, 1988). There is also evidence for hyperexcitability in the contralesional motor cortex after both cortical and subcortical stroke in humans with at least moderate recovery (Butefisch *et al.*, 2003). Such hyperexcitability decreases with time after infarction, in keeping with the data from animals (Shimizu *et al.*, 2002). Whether these changes result in increased and more diffuse task-related BOLD signal in the early human post-stroke phase, as one would predict, and whether they subserve the recovery process requires further investigation.

How do the longitudinal changes help understand the recovery process?

If recruitment of independent parallel non-primary motor loops is the consequence of impairment to direct M1 cortico-motoneuronal pathways as has been suggested, then the most parsimonious explanation for the reduction of such recruitment is that recovery of motor function is a direct result of restitution of this direct anatomical link. Several studies have demonstrated changes in neurophysiological parameters from the affected hemisphere in stroke patients using transcranial magnetic stimulation suggestive of improving corticospinal function (in particular motor threshold, motor evoked potential amplitude in a hand muscle, and central motor conduction time) that correlate with recovery of hand function (Heald *et al.*, 1993; Pennisi *et al,* 1999; Traversa *et al.*, 1997; Turton *et al.*, 1996). However, it is clear that abnormalities in neurophysiological parameters can persist in patients with complete recovery (Pennisi *et al.*, 1999), suggesting that preservation of fast direct cortico-motoneuronal pathways is not the only means of achieving full recovery, and that cerebral reorganisation may play an important role in generating motor output. A number of mechanisms may be involved in driving this reorganisation.

Changes in cortical motor representation may provide alternative motor output Shifts in the peak ipsilesional (contralateral) sensorimotor task related activations in post stroke patients have been observed in previous studies (Weiller *et al.*, 1993; Pineiro *et al.*, 2001). All our chronic patients activated ipsilesional M1, but only four (with poorer outcome) activated ipsilesional M1 hand region over and above the control group. Across the chronic stroke group, we observed a negative correlation between outcome and task related activity in two parts of ipsilesional M1. The first was situated medial to the hand region, deep in central, and the second was more ventral. In the longitudinal analysis, consistent recovery-related reductions in activation were observed in ipsilesional M1 ventral to the hand area and deep in central sulcus corresponding to area 4p (Geyer *et al.*, 1996). The shifts in ipsilesional M1 representation demonstrated in the cross-sectional and longitudinal studies mirror one another to a remarkable degree.

Changes in cortical maps as a consequence of lesions to the corticospinal pathway have been observed previously (Kew *et al.*, 1994) and may result in early hyperexcitability as discussed. Such changes may enable the lesioned brain to take advantage of considerable redundancy within the somatotopy of M1 (in that a number of combinations of pyramidal cells may produce the same movement (Sanes and Donoghue, 2000) to generate an output to the spinal cord via an intact portion of the pyramidal tract.

Thus early changes such as hyperexcitability may increase the amount of M1 that is activated, facilitating subsequent refocusing towards a shifted sensorimotor representation, with access to undamaged fast cortico-motoneuronal pathways in those with better recovery. In those with poorer recovery, recruitment of additional M1 regions persists (Ward *et al.*, 2003).

One might also speculate that plastic changes in somatotopic representations occur not only in M1, but also in SMA, CMA, and premotor regions (as a consequence of the lesion, or driven by a therapeutic intervention), resulting in (i) stronger connections with different regions of M1 (i.e. with alternative representations of the hand region) in order to generate an output to the spinal cord, and (ii) recruitment of more ischaemia-resistant surviving small diameter myelinated corticospinal fibres, such as those from premotor cortex, which may compensate for the loss of large diameter fibres.

It is worth noting that such a mechanism could not occur with damage to the entire M1 cortical region. In this respect, patients such as ours with preserved M1 are clearly different to those with substantial M1 damage. Clinical improvement in patients with (near) complete M1 damage does occur, but is more limited, and 'reorganised' motor output is likely to come from the undamaged hemisphere.

Does recruitment of contralesional M1 contribute to alternative motor output? The role of contralesional (ipsilateral to the affected hand) M1 in the generation of hand movements remains controversial, but its potential role in recovery of motor function after stroke has always generated much interest. Anatomical studies suggest that both direct (corticospinal) and indirect (corticoreticulospinal) pathways from ipsilateral M1 end in projections to axial and proximal stabilising muscles rather than hand muscles (Carr *et al.*, 1994; Brinkman and Kuypers, 1973). However, repetitive TMS to M1 results in errors in both complex and simple motor tasks using the ipsilateral hand (Chen *et al.*, 1997) suggesting that contralesional M1 may play a role in planning and organisation of hand movement. In our chronic patient group, activation in contralesional M1 was observed in five less well-recovered patients. We did not observe mirror movements of the unaffected arm or hand to explain these activations. These results are similar to those in which TMS to ipsilateral M1 elicited motor evoked potentials in the affected arm only in stroke patients with poor outcome (Turton *et al.*, 1996; Netz *et al.*, 1997), findings which called into question the functional role of contralesional M1. Furthermore, in a group of stroke patients shown to activate contralesional M1 during movement of the affected hand, single pulse TMS to PMd, but not to M1 impaired performance of simple reaction time finger movements, suggesting that contralesional PMd, but not M1, is contributing significantly to motor recovery in those patients (Johansen-Berg *et al.*, 2002b). Interestingly however, in both cross-sectional and longitudinal studies, a negative correlation between task related activity and recovery was observed not in the hand region of contralesional M1, but deep in central sulcus corresponding to area 4p (Geyer *et al.*, 1996). TMS to the motor *hot spot* for hand muscles is unlikely to affect these parts of the motor cortex. Thus it remains plausible that parts of contralesional M1 do generate a motor output to the affected hand in patients with a significant deficit, in whom a dependency on alternative motor projections has developed. There is no evidence however that it is more important than recruitment of non-primary parallel motor networks.

Does attention to motor performance contribute to cerebral reorganisation? Increases in task-related brain activation as a result of increased attention to a simple motor task have been observed in a number of motor regions, including SMA, cingulate cortex, insula, post-central sulcus and deep central sulcus (putative area 4p) (Binkofski *et al.*, 2002; Johansen-Berg and Matthews, 2002). It could be argued therefore, that our results are largely due to the fact that early after stroke, when deficit is greatest; patients need to pay more attention to a task. We attempted to control for attention within a scanning session by incorporating visual feedback to which all subjects were asked to attend. However, a negative correlation was observed between activation and recovery in a number of visual areas as well as posterior parietal cortex, in several patients. Thus attention to the visuomotor task may be greater in those with greater deficit. It is possible that increased attention to a task is a key strategy early after stroke when deficit is greatest. This attentional mechanism will contribute to increased activation in non-primary motor regions, thereby providing a substrate for activity dependent plastic changes in somatotopic representations within the motor system, and consequently increasing access to alternative motor pathways. This is very similar to the notion of accessing latent motor engrams described by Luria and others (Luria, 1963; Meyer, 1972). Evidence that attention can modulate motor performance can be seen in the effect that attending to a neglected limb has in patients with unilateral neglect (Robertson *et al.*, 1997) and may also explain the beneficial effect that d-amphetamine seems to have on motor function (in the context of motor practice) in both animals and stroke patients (Feeney, 1997).

Do stroke patients re-learn motor performance? Current models of motor learning suggest that during early motor learning movements are encoded in terms of spatial coordinates, a process requiring high levels of attention. This encoding is done within a network involving a frontoparietal cortex, and parts of the basal ganglia and cerebellum. Learned or automatic movement is encoded in terms of a kinematic system of joints, muscles, limb trajectories, etc., by a network involving primary motor cortex, and independent parts of the basal ganglia and cerebellum (Hikosaka, 2002)[Hikosaka *et al.* 2002]. Interactions between these parallel systems occur not only in cerebellum and basal ganglia, but also *via* intracortical connections involving particularly premotor cortex and pre-SMA (Hikosaka *et al.*, 2002). A number of empirical findings support such a model. Decreases in brain activation as a function of motor learning have been reported in lateral premotor cortex, prefrontal cortex, pre-SMA, superior parietal cortex, anterior cingulate, cerebellum, cerebellar vermis, and caudate (Jenkins *et al.*, 1994; Nakamura *et al.*, 1998; Toni *et al.*, 1998). The cerebellum is involved in detecting error between internal models of movement and the sensory consequences of actual movement (Blakemore *et al.*, 2001; Imamizu *et al.*, 2000); activation in pre-SMA has been explicitly associated with new motor sequence learning (Hikosaka *et al.*, 1999; Nakamura *et al.*, 1998; Sakai *et al.*, 1999); and a variety of changes in M1, predominantly increases in recruitment, have been observed (Toni *et al.*, 1998; Grafton *et al.*, 1995; Honda *et al.*, 1998; Karni *et al.*, 1995; Muellbacher *et al.*, 2002). The generation of an error signal is key to this model, and it can be seen that attempted movements by hemiparetic patients will result in significant discrepancies between predicted and actual performance, thus generating significant error signals that in normal subjects are used by the cerebellum to optimise subsequent sensorimotor accuracy (Blakemore *et al.*, 2001). We have described decreases in activation with recovery in similar networks consistent with the notion of a transfer of reliance from the frontoparietal to the primary motor system. Increased activation in M1 during motor learning is predicted by such a model as has been observed in normal subjects when learning occurs over several weeks (Karni *et al.*, 1995) but we have observed such an increase in only one patient. However, damage to direct connections between M1 and spinal cord motor neurons may prevent normal responses and result in shifts of peak M1 activation by re-mapping instead. The need to re-learn simple motor tasks after stroke is likely to engage such a mechanism, but the degree to which this can occur will depend on the degree of overall damage to the motor network. An issue such as the role of error signals generated in the damaged motor system is important and unexplored though it may have significant implications for rehabilitative interventions.

STUDIES PERFORMED DURING PASSIVE MOVEMENT

Experiments in which either the elbow or the wrist is passively flexed and extended in normal volunteers have demonstrated activations in ipsilesional sensorimotor cortex, rostral supplementary motor area, and bilateral inferior parietal cortex, when compared to rest (Weiller *et al.*, 1996; Carel *et al.*, 2000). This task may be performed at any stage of recovery, without performance confounds, and Nelles *et al.* (1999) took advantage of this by studying passive movement of the elbow compared to rest in six patients with first pure motor subcortical stroke, using PET. Before hand or forearm recovery had occurred, passive movements lead to activations predominantly in the contralesional hemisphere (inferior parietal, dorsolateral prefrontal, cingulate, and premotor cortices). A second scan was carried out three weeks later when four of the patients had recovered control of forearm movements, but two had little recovery. Bilateral increases in rCBF were again seen in inferior parietal cortex, although now more so on the ipsilesional side, and strong activation was now apparent in ipsilesional sensorimotor cortex. Unfortunately, single subject analysis could not be performed and so correlation with degree of recovery could not be made. In animal models, although there is an increase in the potential for plasticity in post lesioned brains, it is only an increase in activity across synapses, which may come from sensory input that takes advantage of this and leads to an increase in efficacy of that synapse, leading ultimately to improvement in function (Schallert *et al.*, 2000). The studies of the central effects of passive movement are a tantalising link with this work.

CONCLUSIONS

We have observed correlations between changes in motor-related brain activation and recovery of function in stroke patients for the first time, and we postulate that these changes, and thus differential recovery between patients, are likely to be a result of differences in (i) anatomical damage, and (ii) cognitive parameters such as motivation, concentration and attention. In stroke patients with infarcts not involving primary motor cortex, there is a clear negative linear relationship between recovery scores and task-related brain activation in many parts of the motor system.

These results reflect a number of processes occurring after focal brain damage at both cellular and systems levels which contribute to cerebral reorganisation and functional recovery. Early on following cerebral infarction, any voluntary movement is associated with massive recruitment of areas in the motor system, possibly because of alterations in the tonic reciprocal influence of anatomically connected motor-related regions upon each other. In addition a number of mechanisms described in animal models of focal cerebral damage, such as local and distant cortical hyperexcitability, may play a role. Thereafter, it is likely that surviving elements of highly preserved neural systems subserving motor learning are employed to facilitate the transition from attention-dependent movement to a more automated performance. This is accompanied by recovery-dependent decreases in the initial pattern of activation. The degree to which any of these elements are successfully employed in the recovery process will depend on a number of other variables, not least the precise amount and site of anatomical damage caused by the infarct.

One final caveat should be mentioned. After injury-induced reorganisation of the brain, the capacity for subsequent adaptive change is reduced (Kolb *et al.*, 1998). Adaptive changes have been observed in older brains (Ward and Frackowiak, 2003) and these may in turn limit the capacity for further reorganisation after injury. This clearly has implications for what we can expect from therapeutic techniques designed to promote cerebral reorganisation after stroke in older subjects.

Cerebral reorganisation undoubtedly contributes to functional recovery after stroke, but it is clear that a more detailed understanding of the natural history of these processes is required, together with the factors that influence them, before we can utilise such information to rationalise therapeutic strategies in individual patient groups. However, the foundation for such studies is beginning to be laid.

References

Azari, N. P., Binkofski, F., Pettigrew, K. D., Freund, H-J.,and Seitz, R. J. (1996). Enhanced regional cerebral metabolic interactions in thalamic circuitry predicts motor recovery in hemiparetic stroke. *Human Brain Mapping*. **4**, 240–253.

Baron, J. C. (1989). Depression of energy metabolism in distant brain structures: studies with positron emission tomography in stroke patients. *Semin Neurol.* **9**, 281–285.

Baron, J. C., Levasseur, M., and Mazoyer, B. *et al.*, (1992). Thalamocortical diaschisis: positron emission tomography in humans. *J Neurol Neurosurg Psychiatry.* **55**, 935–942.

Baron, J. C., Rougemont, D., Bousser, M. G., Lebrun-Grandie, P., Iba-Zizen, M. T., and Chiras, J. (1983). Local CBF, oxygen extraction fraction (OEF) and CMRO2: prognostic value in recent supratentorial infarction in humans. *J Cereb Blood Flow Metab.* **3** (Suppl 1), S1–S8.

Binkofski, F., Fink, G. R., Geyer, S., Buccino, G., Gruber, O., Shah, N. J., Taylor, J. G., Seitz, R. J., Zilles, K., and Freund, H. J. (2002) Neural activity in human primary motor cortex areas 4a and 4p is modulated differentially by attention to action. *J Neurophysiol* **88,** 514–519.

Binkofski, F., Seitz, R. J., Arnold, S., Classen, J., Benecke, R., and Freund, H-J. (1996). Thalamic metabolism and corticospinal tract integrity determine motor recovery in stroke. *Ann Neurol.* **39**, 460–470.

Blakemore, S. J., Frith, C. D., and Wolpert, D. M. (2001) The cerebellum is involved in predicting the sensory consequences of action. *Neuroreport* **12,** 1879–1884.

Brinkman, J. and Kuypers, H. G. (1973) Cerebral control of contralateral and ipsilateral arm, hand and finger movements in the split-brain rhesus monkey. *Brain* **96,** 653–674.

Buchkremer-Ratzmann, I., August, M., Hagemann, G., and Witte, O. W. (1996) Electrophysiological transcortical diaschisis after cortical photothrombosis in rat brain. *Stroke* **27,** 1105–1109.

Butefisch, C. M., Netz, J., Wessling, M., Seitz, R. J., and Homberg, V. (2003) Remote changes in cortical excitability after stroke. *Brain* **126,** 470–481.

Calautti, C., Leroy, F., Guincestre, J. Y., and Baron, J. C. (2001). Dynamics of motor network overactivation after striatocapsular stroke: a longitudinal PET study using a fixed-performance paradigm. *Stroke* **32,** 2534–2542.

Cao, Y., D'Olhaberriague, L., Vikingstad, E. M., Levne, S. R., and Welch, K. M. A. (1998). Pilot study of functional MRI to assess cerebral activation of motor function after poststroke hemiparesis. *Stroke.* **29,** 112–122.

Carel, C., Loubinoux, I., Boulanouar, K., Manelfe, C., Rascol, O., Celsis, P., and Chollet, F. (2000). Neural substrate for the effects of passive training on sensorimotor cortical representation: a study with functional magnetic resonance imaging in healthy subjects. *J Cereb Blood Flow Metab.* **20**, 478–84.

Carr, L. J., Harrison, L. M., and Stephens, J. A. (1994). Evidence for bilateral innervation of certain homologous motoneurone pools in man. *J Physiol* **475,** 217–227.

Catalan, M. J., Honda, M., Weeks, R. A., Cohen, L. G., and Hallet, M. (1998). The functional neuroanatomy of simple and complex sequential finger movements: a PET study. *Brain.* **121**, 253–264.

Chambers, W. W., Liu, C. N., and McCouch, G. P. (1978). Anatomical and physiological correlates of plasticity in the central nervous system. *Brain Behav Evol.* **8,** 5–26.

Chen, R., Gerloff, C., Hallett, M., and Cohen, L. G. (1997). Involvement of the ipsilateral motor cortex in finger movements of different complexities. *Ann Neurol* **41,** 247–254.

Chollet, F., DiPiero, V., Wise, R. J. S., Brooks, D. J., Dolan, R. J., and Frackowiak, R. S. J. (1991). The functional anatomy of motor recovery after ischaemic stroke in man. *Ann Neurol.* **29**, 63–71.

Chugani, H. T., Phelps, M. E., and Mazziotta, J. C. (1987) Positron emission tomography study of human brain functional development. *Ann Neurol.* **22,** 487–497.

Cramer, S. C. and Chopp, M. (2000). Recovery recapitulates ontogeny. *Trends Neurosci.* **23**, 265–271.

Cramer, S. C., Nelles, G., Benson, R. R., Kaplan, J. D., Parker, R. A., Kwong, K. K., Kennedy, D. N., Finklestein, S. P., and Rosen, B. R. (1997). A functional MRI study of subjects recovered from hemiparetic stroke. *Stroke.* **28**, 2518–2527.

Cruz, M. A., Tejada, J., and Diez, T. E. (1999). Motor hand recovery after stroke. Prognostic yield of early transcranial magnetic stimulation. *Electromyogr Clin Neurophysiol* **39,** 405–410.

Danek, A. , Bauer, M. , and Fries, W. (1990). Tracing of neural connections in the human brain by magnetic resonance imaging in vivo. *Eur J Neurosci.* **2**, 112–115.

Dettmers, C., Stephan, K. M., Lemon, R. N., and Frackowiak, R. S. J. (1997). Reorganization of the executive motor system after stroke. *Cereb. Dis.*, **7**, 187–200.

Di Pierro, V., Chollet, F. M., MacCarthy, P., Lenzi, G. L., and Frackowiak, R. S. J. (1992). Motor recovery after acute ischaemic stroke: a metabolic study. *J Neurol Neurosurg Psychiatry*. **55**, 990–996.

Dum, R. P., and Strick, P. L. (1991). The origin of corticospinal projections from the premotor areas in the frontal lobe. *J Neurosci* **11,** 667–689.

Duncan, P. W., Jorgensen, H. S., and Wade, D. T. (2000). Outcome measures in acute stroke trials: a systematic review and some recommendations to improve practice. *Stroke* **31**, 1429–1438.

Feeney, D. M. (1997). From laboratory to clinic: noradrenergic enhancement of physical therapy for stroke or trauma patients. *Adv Neurol* **73,** 383–394.

Feydy, A., Carlier, R., Roby-Brami, A., Bussel, B., Cazalis, F., Pierot, L., Burnod, Y., and Maier, M. A. (2002). Longitudinal study of motor recovery after stroke: recruitment and focusing of brain activation. *Stroke* **33,** 1610–1617.

Frackowiak, R. S. J., and Friston, K. J. (1994). Functional neuroanatomy of the human brain: positron emission tomography-a new neuroanatomical technique. *J Anat.* **184,** 211–225.

Fries, W., Danek, A., and Witt, T. N. (1991). Motor responses after transcranial electrical stimulation of cerebral hemispheres with a degenerated pyramidal tract. *Ann Neurol.* **29**, 646–650.

Geyer, S., Ledberg, A., Schleicher, A., Kinomura, S., Schormann, T., Burgel, U., Klingberg, T., Larsson, J., Zilles, K., and Roland, P. E. (1996). Two different areas within the primary motor cortex of man. *Nature* **382,** 805–807.

Ghosh, S., and Porter, R. (1988). Corticocortical synaptic influences on morphologically identified pyramidal neurones in the motor cortex of the monkey. *J Physiol.* **400**, 617–629.

Grafton, S. T., Hazeltine, E., and Ivry, R. (1995). Functional mapping of sequence learning in normal humans. *J Cogn Neurosci* **7,** 497–510.

Hagemann, G., Redecker, C., Neumann-Haefelin, T., Freund, H. J., and Witte, O. W. (1998). Increased long-term potentiation in the surround of experimentally induced focal cortical infarction. *Ann Neurol* **44,** 255–258.

Heald, A., Bates, D., Cartlidge, N. E., French, J. M., and Miller, S. (1993). Longitudinal study of central motor conduction time following stroke. 2. Central motor conduction measured within 72 h after stroke as a predictor of functional outcome at 12 months. *Brain* **116 (Pt 6),** 1371–1385.

Heller, A., Wade, D. T., Wood, V. A., Sunderland, A., Hewer, R. L., and Ward, E. (1987). Arm function after stroke: measurement and recovery over the first three months. *J Neurol Neurosurg Psychiatry* **50,** 714–719.

Hikosaka, O., Nakahara, H., Rand, M. K., Sakai, K., Lu, X., Nakamura, K., Miyachi, S., and Doya, K. (1999). Parallel neural networks for learning sequential procedures. *Trends Neurosci* **22,** 464–471.

Hikosaka, O., Nakamura, K., Sakai, K., and Nakahara, H. (2002). Central mechanisms of motor skill learning. *Curr Opin Neurobiol* **12,** 217–222.

Honda, M., Deiber, M. P., Ibanez, V., Pascual-Leone, A., Zhuang, P., and Hallett, M. (1998). Dynamic cortical involvement in implicit and explicit motor sequence learning. A PET study. *Brain* **121 (Pt 11),** 2159–2173.

Huttenlocher, P. R. (1979). Synaptic density in human frontal cortex—developmental changes and effects of aging. *Brain Res.* **163**, 195–205.

Imamizu, H., Miyauchi, S., Tamada, T., Sasaki, Y., Takino, R., Putz, B., Yoshioka, T., and Kawato, M. (2000). Human cerebellar activity reflecting an acquired internal model of a new tool. *Nature* **403,** 192–195.

Jenkins, I. H., Brooks, D. J., Nixon, P. D., Frackowiak, R. S., and Passingham, R. E. (1994). Motor sequence learning: a study with positron emission tomography. *J Neurosci* **14,** 3775–3790.

Johansen-Berg, H., and Matthews, P. M. (2002). Attention to movement modulates activity in sensori-motor areas, including primary motor cortex. *Exp Brain Res* **142,** 13–24.

Johansen-Berg, H., Dawes, H., Guy, C., Smith, S. M., Wade, D. T., and Matthews, P. M. (2002a). Correlation between motor improvements and altered fMRI activity after rehabilitative therapy. *Brain* **125**, 2731–2742.

Johansen-Berg, H., Rushworth, M. F., Bogdanovic, M. D., Kischka, U., Wimalaratna, S., and Matthews, P. M. (2002b). The role of ipsilateral premotor cortex in hand movement after stroke. *Proc Natl Acad Sci USA* **99,** 14518–14523.

Jones, T. A., and Schallert, T. (1992). Overgrowth and pruning of dendrites in adult rats recovering from neocortical damage. *Brain Res* **581,** 156–160.

Jones, T. A., Kleim, J. A., and Greenough, W. T. (1996). Synaptogenesis and dendritic growth in the cortex opposite unilateral sensorimotor cortex damage in adult rats: a quantitative electron microscopic examination. *Brain Res* **733,** 142–148.

Karni, A., Meyer, G., Jezzard, P., Adams, M. M., Turner, R., and Ungerleider, L. G. (1995). Functional MRI evidence for adult motor cortex plasticity during motor skill learning. *Nature* **377,** 155–158.

Kew, J. J., Brooks, D. J., Passingham, R. E., Rothwell, J. C., Frackowiak, R. S. J., and Leigh, P. N. (1994). Cortical function in progressive lower motor neuron disorders and amyotrophic lateral sclerosis: a comparative PET study. *Neurology.* **44**, 1101–1110.

Kolb, B. (1995). "Brain Plasticity and Behaviour", pp.1–194. Lawrence Erlbaum, Mahwah, NJ.

Kolb, B., Forgie, M., Gibb, R., Gorny, G., and Rowntree, S. (1998). Age, experience and the changing brain. *Neurosci. Biobehav. Rev.* **22**, 143–159.

Logothetis, N. K., Pauls, J., Augath, M., Trinath, T., and Oeltermann, A. (2001). Neurophysiological investigation of the basis of the fMRI signal. *Nature* **412,** 150–157.

Luria, A. R. (1963). *Restoration of function after brain injury.* Pergammon Press: Oxford.

Maier, M. A., Armand, J., Kirkwood, P. A., Yang, H. W., Davis, J. N., and Lemon, R. N. (2002). Differences in the corticospinal projection from primary motor cortex and supplementary motor area to macaque upper limb motoneurons: an anatomical and electrophysiological study. *Cereb Cortex* **12,** 281–296.

Marshall, R. S., Perera, G. M., Lazar, R. M., Krakauer, J. W., Constantine, R. C., and DeLaPaz, R. L. (2000). Evolution of cortical activation during recovery from corticospinal tract infarction. *Stroke* **31,** 656–661.

Merrill E. G., and Wall P. D. (1978). Plasticity of connections in the adult nervous system. *In* "Neuronal Plasticity" (C.W. Cottman, Ed.), pp. 97–111. Raven Press, New York.

Meyer, D. R. (1972). Access to engrams. *American Psychologist* **27,** 124–133.

Muellbacher, W., Ziemann, U., Wissel, J., Dang, N., Kofler, M., Facchini, S., Boroojerdi, B., Poewe, W., and Hallett, M. (2002). Early consolidation in human primary motor cortex. *Nature* **415,** 640–644.

Nakamura, K., Sakai, K., and Hikosaka, O. (1998). Neuronal activity in medial frontal cortex during learning of sequential procedures. *J Neurophysiol* **80,** 2671–2687.

Nelles, G., Spiekramann, G., Jueptner, M., Leonhardt, G., Muller, S., Gerhard, H., and Diener, H. C. (1999). Evolution of functional reorganisation in hemiplegic stroke: a serial positron emission tomographic activation study. *Ann Neurol.* **46**, 901–909.

Netz, J., Lammers, T., and Homberg, V. (1997). Reorganisation of motor output in the non-affected hemisphere after stroke. *Brain* **120 (Pt 9),** 1579–1586.

Neumann-Haefelin, T., Staiger, J. F., Redecker, C., Zilles, K., Fritschy, J. M., Mohler, H., and Witte, O. W. (1998). Immunohistochemical evidence for dysregulation of the GABAergic system ipsilateral to photochemically induced cortical infarcts in rats. *Neuroscience* **87,** 871–879.

Pantano, P., Formisano, R., Ricci, M., Di Piero, V., Sabatini, U., Di Pofi, B., Rossi, R., Bozzao, L., and Lenzi, G.L. (1996). Motor recovery after stroke: morphological and functional brain alterations. *Brain.* **119**, 1849–1857.

Pariente, J., Loubinoux, I., Carel, C., Albucher, J. F., Leger, A., Manelfe, C., Rascol, O., and Chollet, F. (2000). Fluoxetine modulates motor performance and cerebral activation of patients recovering from stroke. *Ann Neurol* **50**, 718–729.

Pennisi, G., Rapisarda, G., Bella, R., Calabrese, V., Maertens, D. N., and Delwaide, P. J. (1999). Absence of response to early transcranial magnetic stimulation in ischemic stroke patients: prognostic value for hand motor recovery. *Stroke* **30,** 2666–2670.

Pineiro, R., Pendlebury, S., Johansen-Berg, H., and Matthews, P. M. (2001). Functional MRI detects posterior shifts in primary sensorimotor cortex activation after stroke: evidence of local adaptive reorganisation? *Stroke* **32,** 1134–1139.

Price, C. J., and Friston, K. J. (1999). Scanning patients with tasks they can perform. *Hum Brain Mapp* **8,** 102–108.

Robertson, I. H., Ridgeway, V., Greenfield, E., and Parr, A. (1997). Motor recovery after stroke depends on intact sustained attention: a 2-year follow-up study. *Neuropsychology* **11,** 290–295.

Rouiller, E. M., Moret, V., Tanne, J., and Boussaoud, D. (1996). Evidence for direct connections between the hand region of the supplementary motor area and cervical motoneurons in the macaque monkey. *Eur J Neurosci* **8,** 1055–1059.

Sakai, K., Hikosaka, O., Miyauchi, S., Sasaki, Y., Fujimaki, N., and Putz, B. (1999). Presupplementary motor area activation during sequence learning reflects visuo-motor association. *J Neurosci* **19,** RC1.

Sanes, J. N., and Donoghue, J. P. (2000). Plasticity and primary motor cortex. *Annu Rev Neurosci* **23,** 393–415.

Schaechter, J. D., Kraft, E., Hilliard, T. S., Dijkhuizen, R. M., Benner, T., Finklestein, S. P., Rosen, B. R., and Cramer, S. C. (2002). Motor recovery and cortical reorganisation after constraint-induced movement therapy in stroke patients: a preliminary study. *Neurorehabil Neural Repair* **16**, 326–338.

Schallert, T., Leasure, J. L., and Kolb, B. (2000). Experience-associated structural events, subependymal cellular proliferative activity, and functional recovery after injury to the central nervous system. *J Cereb Blood Flow Metab.* **20**, 1513–1528.

Seitz, R. J., Hoflich, P., Binkofski, F., Tellmann, L., Herzog, H., and Freund, H. J. (1998). Role of the premotor cortex in recovery from middle cerebral artery infarction. *Arch Neurol* **55,** 1081–1088.

Shimizu, T., Hosaki, A., Hino, T., Sato, M., Komori, T., Hirai, S., and Rossini, P. M. (2002). Motor cortical disinhibition in the unaffected hemisphere after unilateral cortical stroke. *Brain* **125,** 1896–1907.

Small, S. L., Hlustik, P., Noll, D. C., Genovese, C., and Solodkin, A. (2002). Cerebellar hemispheric activation ipsilateral to the paretic hand correlates with functional recovery after stroke. *Brain* **125,** 1544–1557.

Strick, P. L. (1988). Anatomical organisation of multiple motor areas in the frontal lobe: implications for recovery of function. *Adv Neurol* **47,** 293–312.

Stroemer, R. P., Kent, T. A., and Hulsebosch, C. E. (1995). Neocortical neural sprouting, synaptogenesis, and behavioural recovery after neocortical infarction in rats. *Stroke* **26,** 2135–2144.

Sunderland, A., Tinson, D., Bradley, L., and Hewer, R. L. (1989). Arm function after stroke. An evaluation of grip strength as a measure of recovery and a prognostic indicator. *J Neurol Neurosurg Psychiatry* **52,** 1267–1272.

Toni, I., Krams, M., Turner, R., and Passingham, R. E. (1998). The time course of changes during motor sequence learning: a whole-brain fMRI study. *Neuroimage* **8,** 50–61.

Traversa, R., Cicinelli, P., Bassi, A., Rossini, P. M., and Bernardi, G. (1997). Mapping of motor cortical reorganisation after stroke. A brain stimulation study with focal magnetic pulses. *Stroke* **28,** 110–117.

Turton, A., Wroe, S., Trepte, N., Fraser, C., and Lemon, R. N. (1996). Contralateral and ipsilateral EMG responses to transcranial magnetic stimulation during recovery of arm and hand function after stroke. *Electroencephalogr Clin Neurophysiol* **101,** 316–328.

Twitchell, T. E. (1951). The restoration of motor function following hemiplegia in man. *Brain.* **74**, 443–480.

Von Monakow, C. (1914). Diaschisis [1914 article translated by G Harris], *In* "Brain and Behaviour I: Moods, states and mind" (K.H. Pribram, Ed) pp. 27-62. Penguin, Baltimore, 1969.

Wall P. D (1977). The presence of ineffective synapses and the circumstances that unmask them. *Philos Trans R Soc London B.* 361–372.

Ward, N. S., and Frackowiak, R. S. J. (2003). Age related changes in the neural correlates of motor performance. *Brain* **126,** 873–888.

Ward, N. S., Brown, M. M., Thompson, A. J., and Frackowiak, R. S. J. (2003a). Neural correlates of outcome after stroke: a cross-sectional fMRI study. *Brain* 126: 1430–1448.

Ward, N. S., Brown, M. M., Thompson, A. J., and Frackowiak, R. S. J. (2003b). Neural correlates of motor recovery after stroke: a longitudinal fMRI study. *Brain* (in press).

Waxman, S. G. (1988). Functional recovery in disease of the nervous system. *In* "Advances in Neurology" (S. G. Waxman, Ed.), Vol. 47, pp 1–7. Raven Press, New York.

Weiller, C., Chollet, F., Friston, K. J., Wise, R. J. S., and Frackowiak, R. S. J. (1992). Functional reorganisation of the brain in recovery from striatocapsular infarction in man. *Ann Neurol.* **31,** 463–472.

Weiller, C., Ramsay, S. C., Wise, R. J. S., Friston, K. J., and Frackowiak, R. S. J. (1993). Individual patterns of functional reorganisation in the human cerebral cortex after capsular infarction. *Ann Neurol.* **33**, 181–189.

Weiller, C., Juptner, M., Fellows, S., Rijntjes, M., Leonhardt, G., Kiebel, S., Muller, S., Diener, H. C., and Thilmann, A. F. (1996). Brain representations of active and passive movements. *Neuroimage.* **4**, 105–110.

Witte, O. W. (1998) Lesion-induced plasticity as a potential mechanism for recovery and rehabilitative training. *Curr Opin Neurol* **11,** 655–662.

Wittenberg, G. F., Chen, R., Ishii, K., Bushara, K. O., Taub, E., Gerber, L. H., Hallett. M., and Cohen, L. G. (2003) Constraint-induced therapy in stroke: magnetic-stimulation motor maps and cerebral activation. *Neurorehabil Neural Repair* **17**, 48–57.

CHAPTER

7

Applied Computational Neuroanatomy in Disease

INTRODUCTION

Recently, there has been renewed interest in brain structural imaging in light of substantial advances in computational power and analytical expertise that permit objective analyses of high-resolution three-dimensional magnetic resonance imaging (MRI) scans. The complementary role of qualitative and quantitative neuroimaging provides greater insight than was previously possible into the structure and function of the human brain in normal and diseased states. Structural differences in brain morphology can be expressed at a macroscopic scale (*e.g.*, global or regional atrophy, regional asymmetries), at a mesoscopic scale (*e.g.*, cortical dysplasia), or at a microscopic scale (*e.g.*, differences in cytoarchitectronics). Computational neuroanatomy is emerging as an exciting new automated methodology to characterise shape and neuroanatomical configuration of structural MRI brain scans on a macroscopic and mesoscopic scale. It encompasses a triad of techniques: voxel-based morphometry (VBM), which interrogates structural MRI brain scans on a voxel-by-voxel basis; deformation-based morphometry (DBM), which provides information about global differences in brain shape; and tensor-based morphometry (TBM), which characterises local shape differences. This chapter describes these techniques and their applications in neurological disease. Comprehensive details of the theory and methodology underpinning computational neuroanatomy can be found in Part II, Section 1.

EVOLUTION OF MORPHOMETRY TECHNIQUES

Although the quest for understanding the structure and function of the human brain started centuries ago, most of the earlier descriptions were qualitative. Qualitative assessments of anatomy and function are preferable but are associated with a number of problems. The human cerebral cortex has a highly complex organisation and architecture with marked interindividual variation in gyral and sulcal anatomy. In addition, brain function is likely to be more closely related to cytoarchitecture, neurotransmitter receptor and enzyme densities, and myeloarchitecture than macroscopic structure. Thus, crude anatomical descriptions on a macroscopic level are generally of limited value, and more sophisticated morphometric methods are required. Quantitative differences in macroscopic brain structure have been assessed by a variety of techniques over the last 3 decades. As early as 1905, changes in brain volume were assessed indirectly postmortem by instilling water into the cranial cavity and measuring the brain/intracranial cavity volume ratio (Reichardt, 1905). Direct postmortem analyses of brain structure, while sensitive to microscopic and macroscopic structural differences, are subject to a number of practical shortcomings. First, postmortem material is not readily available, and, second, these studies are time consuming, as much of the tissue preparation is performed manually. Further confounding effects such as the interval between death and fixation of brain tissue, the timing of measurements (Last, 1953; Messert *et al.*, 1972), and the inclusion or exclusion of brainstem structures and meninges (which can be difficult to control) can vary across studies, making comparisons difficult.

The introduction of modern imaging techniques, including computed tomography (CT) and more recently MRI, have provided the opportunity for noninvasive *in vivo* measurements of intracranial structure. Morphometry methods can be broadly classified as region of interest (ROI)-based or whole brain techniques. To date, a variety of ROI-based volumetric methods have evolved from simple two-dimensional or three-dimensional measurements of specified brain structures on relatively thick-slice, two-dimensional CT or MRI scans to more sophisticated volumetric measurements of chosen regions on high-resolution, three-dimensional MRI scans that have been coregistered and segmented into tissue compartments (Caviness *et al.*, 1996; Cook, 1994; DeLeo *et al.*, 1985; Duncan, 1997; Evans et al., 1993; Filipek *et al.*, 1994; Jack *et al.*, 1990; Jackson *et al.*, 1994; Lee *et al.*, 1998; Murthy *et al.*, 1998; Schulz *et al.*, 1999; Schwartz *et al.*, 1985). Three-dimensional fractal analysis of the grey/white interface (Free *et al.*, 1996) has offered additional information about the structure of the cerebral cortex. These techniques have all been interactive and operator dependent to a greater or lesser extent and subject to bias. The bias is introduced by the small number of regions and metrics used in classical morphometrics that are insensitive to changes elsewhere in the brain. In addition, ROI measurement errors are likely to be greater for smaller structures with complex architectures, particularly if anatomical borders are defined by arbitrary criteria. Furthermore, a number of morphometric features (*e.g.*, thinning of the cortical ribbon) may be difficult to quantify by inspection and thus could be missed by ROI-based techniques.

A number of unbiased whole brain techniques are emerging due to the development of sophisticated image processing tools. The simplest methods apply rigid body registration within a single subject over time; for example, Fox *et al.* (1996) compared age-related changes over one year in patients with Alzheimer's disease. Nonlinear registrations can also be used within a subject (Freeborough and Fox, 1998).

To make meaningful regional comparisons between brains from groups of subjects, confounding factors such as extrinsic differences (*e.g.*, head position and orientation) and intrinsic differences (*e.g.*, brain size and shape) need to be removed. To achieve this, more complex models are required to register multiple images into a common stereotactic space using linear or nonlinear forms of spatial normalisation enabling region-by-region comparisons in cross-sectional or longitudinal studies. For example, voxel-based morphometry allows a voxel-wise comparison of spatially normalised images; deformation-based morphometry and tensor-based morphometry use the deformation fields derived from spatial normalisation to make comparisons. Of these last two techniques, the former is used to identify differences in relative positions of brain structures and the latter to detect local shape differences. There is a developing literature on various forms of such methods (Ashburner *et al.*, 1999; Ashburner *et al.*, 1998; Christensen *et al.*, 1997; Davatzikos and Resnick, 1998) and related techniques using analogous probabilistic methods (Guimond *et al.*, 2000; Thompson and Toga, 1997; Thompson *et al.*, 1996–1998).

Voxel-wise analysis of functional imaging data with statistical parametric mapping (SPM) is well established, and this technique is ideally suited to the interrogation of structural data. An additional advantage is that the same general analytical framework encompasses both structural and functional data, facilitating comparisons between them.

Voxel-Based Morphometry

At its simplest, voxel-based morphometry (VBM) involves the voxel-wise comparison of regional concentrations of grey (or white) matter between groups of subjects. The software is freely available, and the procedure is fully automated and relatively straightforward. High resolution, three-dimensional structural MR images are normalised into the same stereotactic space, segmented into grey and white matter and cerebrospinal fluid (CSF) compartments, and smoothed with an isotropic Gaussian kernel. Voxel-wise parametric statistical tests are then performed on the smoothed grey matter segments employing the framework of the general linear model (Fig. 7.1). We have optimised VBM since its original implementation, and the current method incorporates the following steps

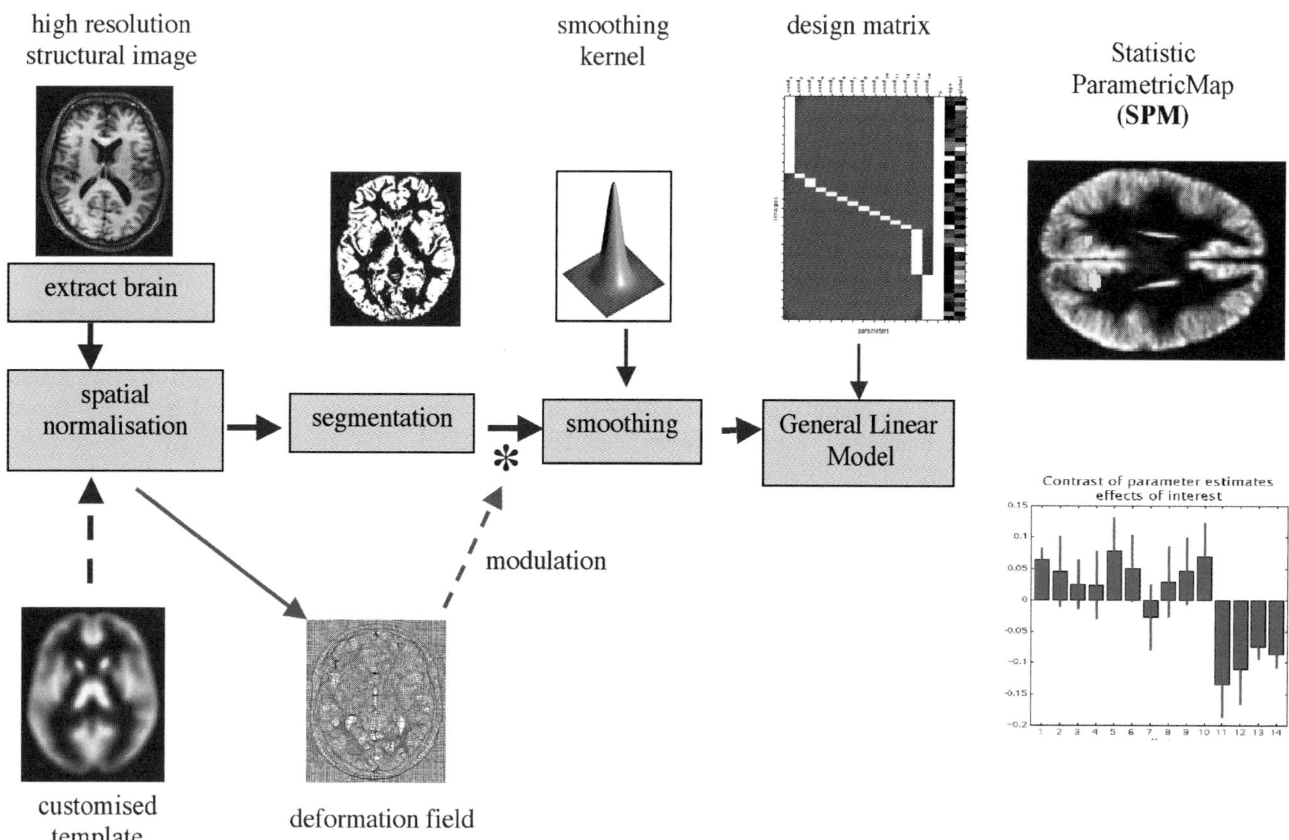

FIGURE 7.1
Schematic representation of the steps involved in voxel-based morphometry (VBM).

Creation of customised templates. An ideal template should consist of the average of a large number of MRI scans that have been registered to within the accuracy of the spatial normalisation technique. The choice of template should not bias the final solution, so we advocate the use of templates matched to the study group. This becomes important when studying disease groups, because diseased brains may differ substantially from a template based on young normal subjects (the default SPM template). In our experience, the best templates are created from the study group itself (all patient and control scans); in this way, the template is customised to the local scanner and disease population, and the spatial normalisation for the diseased brains is balanced to the control brains, so systematic group difference in spatial normalisation is avoided. Practically, we spatially normalise all the study MRI scans to the SPM template, segment into grey and white matter and CSF compartments, and smooth with an 8-mm isotropic Gaussian kernel. Averaging the smoothed segments provides separate grey and white matter templates

Extraction of a brain image. This step is included to remove non-brain voxels. This procedure involves an initial segmentation of the original structural MR images followed by a series of fully automated morphological operations for removing unconnected non-brain voxels from the segmented images (erosion followed by conditional dilation).

Spatial normalisation. The spatial normalisation aims to map each structural MRI to the template in standard stereotactic space and consists of a combination of linear and nonlinear transformations (see Chapters 33–35). The goal of the nonlinear warps is to discount global brain shape differences (*i.e.*, displacement of grey matter from its normal location), but not to match each gyrus and sulcus exactly. VBM thus aims to characterise regional differences in grey and white matter at a local scale, having discounted global shape differences. If the spatial normalisation were perfect, then there would be no structural differences between the normalised images, and all the differences would be encoded in the deformation fields. In such a case, TBM would then be used to characterise the differences. Although this idea is appealing, the high-dimensional warps are computer intensive and time consuming and thus not currently practical.

Segmentation. The segmentation procedure partitions the normalised images into grey and white matter (and CSF) segments based upon *a priori* knowledge from prior probability images. We use the grey and white matter and CSF templates as our prior probability maps, so that they are customised to the study group. Theoretically, prior probability maps from young normal subjects (the default SPM priors) are not optimal for diseased brains. In practice, customised priors allow more precise classification and registration of voxels within healthy and diseased subjects, particularly within the pons and cingulated gyrus (Good *et al.*, 2002).

Modulation. As a result of nonlinear spatial normalisation, the volumes of certain brain regions may grow, whereas others may shrink. In order to preserve the absolute amount of a particular tissue (grey or white matter) within a voxel, a further processing step is incorporated. This involves modulating voxel values by the Jacobian determinants derived from the spatial normalisation step (Ashburner and Friston, 2000). This augmented VBM can thus be considered a combination of VBM and TBM, where TBM employs the testing of the Jacobian determinants themselves. In order to simplify this concept, it is helpful to compare VBM with an analysis using regions of interest. Each voxel in a smoothed grey matter image is the count of the grey matter voxels within the limits of a region defined by the smoothing kernel. After spatial normalisation, the voxels within the region defined by the smoothing kernel can be thought of as being projected onto the original anatomy, but in doing so, their shapes and sizes will be distorted. Without modulating, the proportion of grey matter within each region of interest would be measured. Modulation effectively converts the segments of grey and white matter concentration into grey matter mass (*i.e.*, rendering the inferences about the absolute amounts [volume] of grey matter in a voxel as opposed to the relative amounts) (Ashburner and Friston, 2000). We generally analyse modulated and unmodulated data. A practical illustration of the differences between the two can be seen in male/female comparisons. It is well known that males have larger brains than females, but more interesting is the detection of regionally specific differences (over and above global differences). VBM detects regions of increased grey matter volume in the anteromesial temporal lobes but no regions of significantly increased concentration in males. In females, VBM detects diffusely increased grey matter concentration throughout the cortical mantle as well as regions of increased grey matter volume in the poster lateral temporal lobes (Good *et al.*, 2001) (Fig. 7.2).

Smoothing. The normalised, modulated/unmodulated grey and white matter segments are smoothed using a 12-mm full width half maximum (FWHM) isotropic Gaussian kernel. Smoothing conditions the data to conform more closely to the Gaussian field model underlying the statistical procedures used for making inferences about regionally specific effects. It also helps to compensate for the inexact nature of the spatial normalisation, and has the effect of rendering the data more normally distributed (by the central limit theorem). The intensity in each voxel of smoothed data is a locally weighted average of grey matter volume from a region of surrounding voxels, the size of the region being defined by the size of the smoothing kernel (Ashburner and Friston, 2000). The size of the smoothing kernel should be comparable to the size of the expected regional differences between the groups. In practice, we use smoothing kernels 10 to 12 mm in size as the best balance between rendering more normally distributed data and enhancing the spatial resolution of the inferences.

Statistical analysis. The smoothed data are then analysed using MATLAB 5 (MathWorks; Natick, MA) and SPM99 (Wellcome Department of Cognitive Neurology, ION, London) employing the framework of the general linear model. Global and regionally specific differences in grey (or white) matter or CSF between groups can be assessed statistically using two contrasts: increases or decreases in grey (or white) matter or CSF (two-tailed test). Normalisation for global differences in voxel intensity across scans is done by inclusion of the global mean grey (or white) voxel value as a confounding covariate in an analysis of covariance (ANCOVA) while preserving regional differences in grey (or white) matter. This provides information about regionally specific changes within a tissue compartment, over and above global changes within that compartment. This is important if, for example, we want to detect regionally specific differences between males and females, given the marked global differences in brain volumes. In certain instances, such as in analyses of patients with

Males–females

Females–males

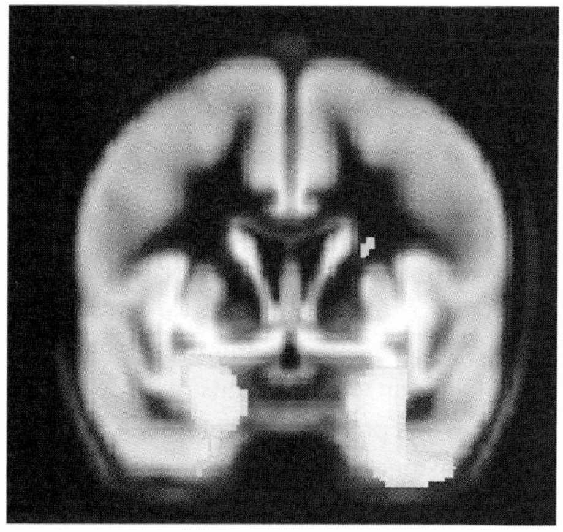

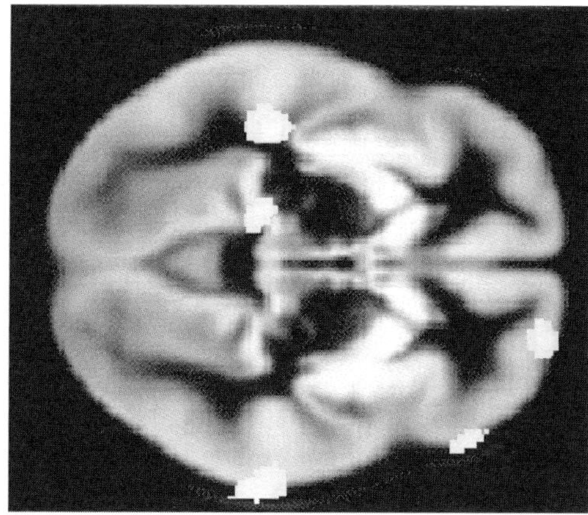

Grey matter volume

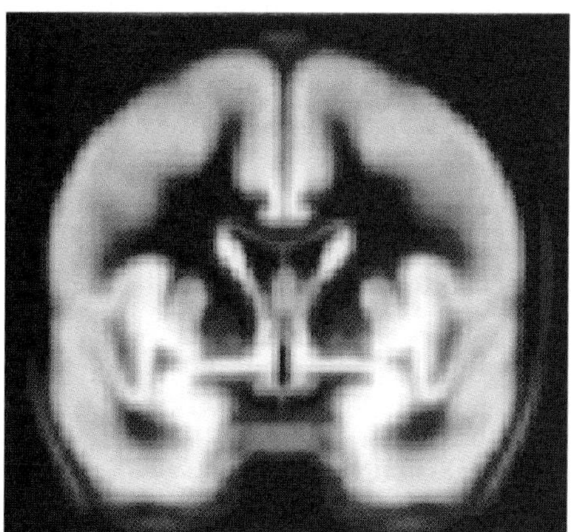

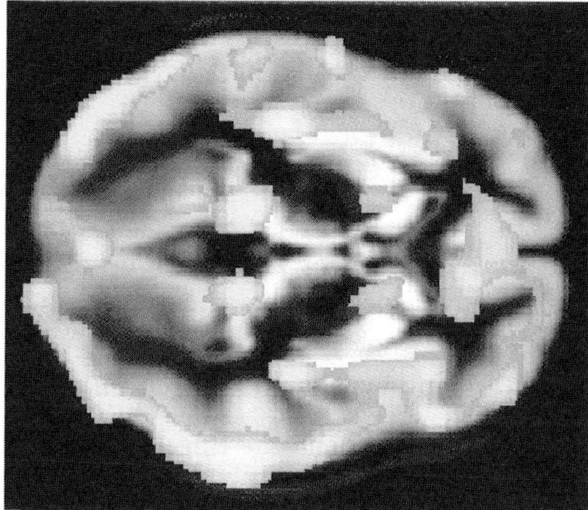

Grey matter concentration

FIGURE 7.2
Regions of increased grey matter volume (modulated data) are superimposed on the normalised symmetrical mean grey matter image. Significant voxels are seen symmetrically in the mesial temporal lobes, in amygdaloid hippocampal complexes, and entorhinal and perirhinal cortex. No regions of increased grey matter concentration (unmodulated data) were observed in males. In females, regions of increased grey matter volume (modulated data) are seen in the right middle temporal gyrus, in the left parahippocampal gyrus, in the right lateral orbital and front marginal gyri, and within the banks of the left superior temporal sulcus. Regions of increased grey matter concentration (unmodulated data) are seen diffusely in the cortical mantle and parahippocampal gyri.

dementia, it may be more appropriate to model total intracranial volume as a confounding covariate, so that differences in head size are removed, while global grey matter changes are preserved (which is generally what ROI approaches measure). This only applies for modulated analyses, which have incorporated a correction for volume changes during spatial normalisation; for unmodulated analyses, total intracranial volume (TIV) would not need to be included, as the global differences have already been removed. In most cases, global and regional inferences are complementary. Corrections for the size of the search volume (multiple comparison correction) are made to the p values using techniques based on Gaussian field theory (Friston *et al.*, 1996; Worsley *et al.*, 1996).

Deformation-Based Morphometry

Whereas VBM analyses the spatially normalised brain segments on a voxel-wise basis, deformation-based morphometry (DBM) analyses differences in the deformation fields themselves. The deformation fields are defined by the affine and nonlinear components of the spatial normalisation. The affine components relate to head position and size, which are not themselves interesting, whereas the nonlinear components relate to head shape. Inferences about these global shape differences can be effected using multivariate statistics (see Chapter 37).

Tensor-Based Morphometry

Tensor-based morphometry (TBM) characterises regional shape differences by interrogating the Jacobian matrices of the deformation fields. The Jacobian matrices encode information about local shearing, stretching, and rotation of voxels when an image is spatially normalised to a template. Inferences about local shape differences can be effected using multivariate statistics (see Chapter 37).

A simpler form of TBM involves analysis of the Jacobian determinants with univariate statistics to provide information about local volume changes. As previously mentioned, the more accurate the spatial normalisation is, the more information is encoded in the deformation fields and the more appropriate TBM is for testing the differences. One can imagine a continuum with simple VBM being performed on images with relatively low-resolution spatial normalisation at one end of the spectrum and TBM being performed on the Jacobian determinants of high-resolution deformation fields at the other end of the spectrum. The augmented VBM (*i.e.*, incorporating the modulation step) could be regarded as a combination or VBM and TBM, becoming more important with faster and more precise spatial normalisation techniques.

CLINICAL APPLICATIONS

An understanding of normal brain structure is fundamental to the appreciation of patterns of pathologically induced structural change.

Characterisation of Normal Anatomy

Cerebral Asymmetry and the Effects of Sex and Handedness on Brain Structure

Morphological asymmetry is common in biological systems (Geschwind and Galaburda, 1985a,b,c), and greater organisational complexity may be reflected in greater functional specialisation and thus in more elaborate asymmetry of function and structure. Humans exhibit structural asymmetry of their hands and feet, sex organs, viscera, facial features, and brains (Beaton, 1997; Geschwind and Galaburda, 1985a; Kimura, 1973; Levy, 1978; Purves *et al.*, 1994) and show lateralised behaviour as early as 10 weeks gestation (Hepper *et al.*, 1997). Hormones may play a role in mediating bodily asymmetry, and it is therefore not surprising to find that phenotypic sex is related in systematic ways to cerebral asymmetry (de Courten-Myers, 1999; Frederikse *et al.*, 1999; Kulynych *et al.*, 1994; Moffat *et al.*, 1998). Likewise, functional asymmetries such as lateralised hand and foot preferences might be expected to correlate with brain structure (Amunts *et al.*, 2000; Beaton, 1997; Moffat *et al.*, 1998).

The optimised VBM method has been used to examine human brain asymmetry and the effects of sex and handedness on brain structure in 465 normal adults (Good *et al.*, 2001). VBM demonstrated significant asymmetry of cerebral grey and white matter in the occipital, frontal, and temporal lobes (petalia), corroborating previous postmortem reports (Geschwind and Galaburda, 1985a) (Fig. 7.3). VBM also detected asymmetric enlargement of grey matter within the anterior transverse temporal (Heschl's) gyrus and adjacent planum temporale on the left, corroborating recent studies using accurate cortical mapping techniques (Thompson *et al.*, 1998, 2001) and postmortem data (Geschwind and Galaburda, 1985a; Geschwind and Levitsky, 1968). Males demonstrated increased leftward asymmetry within Heschl's gyrus and planum temporale (PT) compared to females (Fig. 7.4). There was no significant interaction between asymmetry and handedness and no main effect of handedness, contrary to reported handedness effects on sulcal topography (Amunts *et al.*, 2000; White *et al.*, 1997). There was a significant main effect of sex on brain morphology, even after accounting for the larger global volumes of grey and white matter in males. Females had increased grey matter volume adjacent to the depths of both central sulci and the left superior temporal sulcus, in right Heschl's gyrus and PT, in right inferior

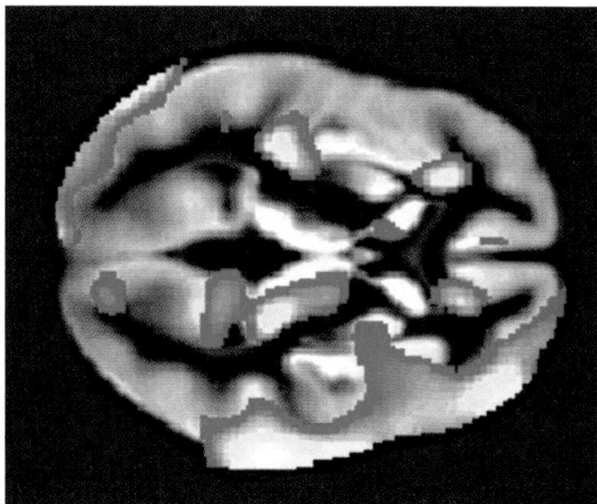

FIGURE 7.3
Regional areas of grey matter volume (modulated data) asymmetry common to males and females superimposed on the normalised symmetrical mean grey matter image. Significant voxels represent ipsilateral side > contralateral side asymmetry (thus also contralateral < ipsilateral asymmetry). The colour bar represents the T score. Significant voxels are seen peripherally in the right frontal and temporal and left occipital lobes (the so-called petalia). More focal leftward (left : right) asymmetry is seen in the frontal operculum and posterior insula (extending into Heschl's gyrus and planum temporale [PT], not shown) and in the depths of the superior and inferior frontal sulci, mesial temporal lobe (including amygdala and hippocampus), anterior cingulate sulcus, and caudate head. Focal rightward (right > left) asymmetry is seen in the lateral thalamus, around the calcarine sulcus and anterior cingulate.

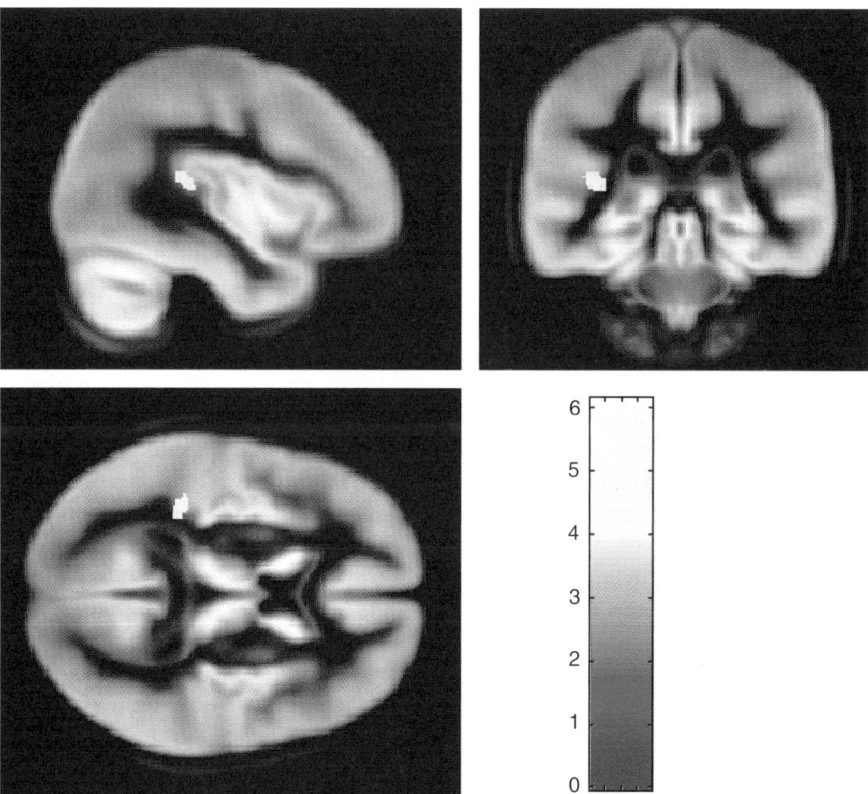

FIGURE 7.4
Regions corresponding to an interaction of asymmetry with sex are superimposed on the normalised symmetrical mean grey matter image. The colour bar represents the T score. Significant voxels are seen at the medial end of left Heschl's sulcus, at the junction with PT, with males having increased leftward asymmetry.

frontal and fronto marginal gyri, and in the cingulate gyrus. Females also demonstrated significantly increased grey matter concentration extensively and relatively symmetrically in the cortical mantle, parahippocampal gyri, and in the banks of the cingulate and calcarine sulci. Males had increased grey matter volume bilaterally in the amygdala and hippocampal heads and entorhinal and perirhinal cortex, corroborating recent work by (Goldstein *et al.*, 2001). Increased grey matter volume was also seen in the anterior lobes of the cerebellum, although no regions of increased grey matter concentration were detected. (Good *et al.*, 2001) (see Fig. 7.2).

In 61 young healthy subjects (20 females and 41 males between 20 and 37 years old), deformation-based morphometry also showed a significant main effect of sex on brain shape, with a more protruding occipital lobe in males and more prominent frontal poles in females. Handedness significantly affected the symmetry of the right frontal lobe (Ashburner *et al.*, 1998).

Age

There is compelling evidence from postmortem and *in vivo* imaging studies that the brain shrinks with age, but accurate quantification of the specific patterns of age-related atrophy has proved more difficult. It is unclear whether there are predictable common patterns of aging or whether individual human brains respond to the aging process idiosyncratically. Many neuropathological studies show that normal aging is characterised by a substantial and extensive loss of neurons in the cerebral cortex, although this is controversial, with recent stereological investigations indicating little neuronal loss with normal aging (Gomez-Isla *et al.*, 1996; Peters *et al.*, 1998) and some reports suggesting that alterations in cerebral white matter and subcortical neuronal loss may be the predominant effect of age (Guttmann *et al.*, 1998). Postmortem analysis of mammalian brains suggest that there may be a gradient of aging from the association areas to the primary sensory regions, with the former showing the most prominent correlations between age and atrophy (Flood and Coleman, 1988).

A number of *in vivo* imaging studies have attempted to quantify age-related change in the brain using CT, two-dimensional MRI, and more recently high-resolution MRI morphometry. Apart from the more obvious limitations of small cohort studies and earlier imaging techniques (Schwartz *et al.*, 1985), as well as variability in reporting absolute or fractional volumes, the majority of these studies have been based on manual or semi-automated region of interest guided measurements (Filipek *et al.*, 1994; Luft *et al.*, 1999; Pfefferbaum *et al.*, 1994; Raz *et al.*, 1997; Xu *et al.*, 2000) which may be inherently biased. Furthermore, if brain weight is related to body height, the progressive increase in height over the past century may limit the applicability of conclusions from many studies that were conducted in the last century (Miller and Corsellis, 1977). More recently, Fox *et al.* (1996), compared age-related changes over one year in a small group of patients with Alzheimer's disease and controls using a semiautomated, rigid-body, co-registration technique; they subsequently showed little change over a year in nine elderly controls using a fluid registration technique (Freeborough and Fox, 1998). Guttmann *et al.* (1998) used a fully automated segmentation technique to evaluate the effects of age on tissue compartments, but provided no information with regional specificity within these compartments. More recently, in a cross-sectional study of 465 normal subjects, VBM detected a linear decrease in global grey matter volume with age, with a significantly steeper decline in males, corroborating previous CT and MRI morphometry studies (Pfefferbaum *et al.*, 1994; Lim *et al.*, 1992; Jernigan *et al.*, 1991; Schwartz, 1985). Although others have suggested accelerated aging in the later decades of life,

Local areas of accelerated loss were observed bilaterally in the insula, superior parietal gyri, central sulci, and cingulate sulci. Little or no age effects (relative preservation) were noted in the amygdala, hippocampi, and entorhinal cortex. Global white matter did not decline with age (Fig. 7.3), but local areas of relative accelerated loss and preservation were seen (Good *et al.*, 2001) (Fig. 7.5). CSF increased linearly with age (Fig. 7.3), with accelerated CSF enlargement in the Sylvian and interhemispheric fissures and little or no CSF enlargement in the pontine cistern (Fig. 7.6).

Characterisation of Plasticity in the Human Hippocampus

Navigation-related structural change has been demonstrated with VBM in the hippocampi of healthy taxi drivers (Maguire *et al.*, 2000). The posterior hippocampi of taxi drivers were

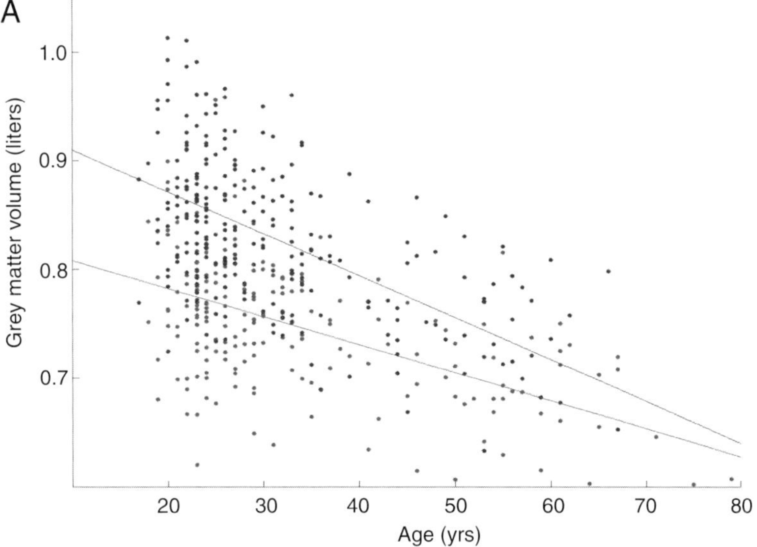

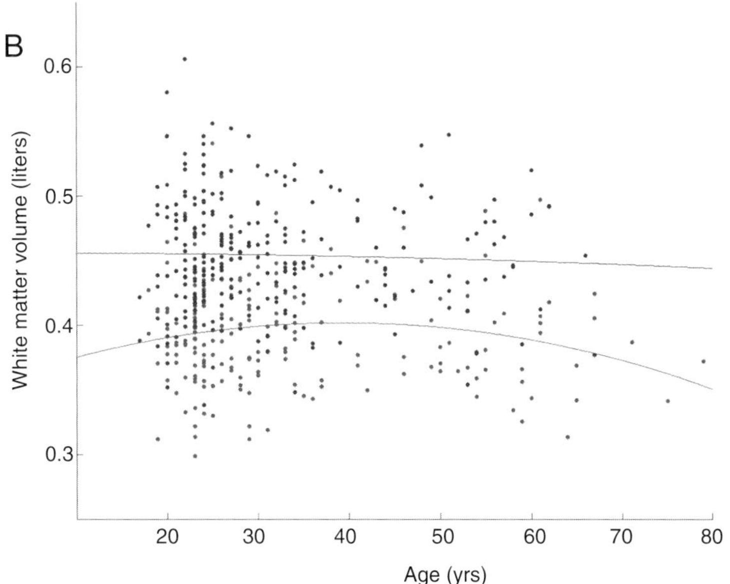

FIGURE 7.5
(a) Scatterplot of total grey matter volume (litres) against age (years) for 465 normal subjects (females in red, males in blue); the best-fitting linear regression curves for females and males are superimposed. (b) Scatterplot of total white matter volume (litres) against age (years) for 465 normal subjects (females in red, males in blue); the best-fitting quadratic regression curves for females and males are superimposed. *(Continued)*

relatively larger than in control subjects (Fig. 7.7), whereas the anterior hippocampi were relatively smaller. The volume changes in the right posterior hippocampus correlated positively with time spent as a taxi driver, suggesting a capacity for local plastic change in healthy adult brains in response to environmental demands. These findings were also confirmed by independent region of interest measurements and correspond well with functional activations observed during navigation tasks in both taxi drivers and control subjects (Maguire *et al.*, 1997, 1998). Another recent VBM study examined a group of non-taxi drivers with navigation abilities ranging from excellent to the very poor (Maguire *et al.*, 2003). VBM detected no correlation of *de novo* navigational skills with brain structure, thus providing further evidence that the structural changes observed in the taxi drivers were acquired and not merely due to innately good navigation skills.

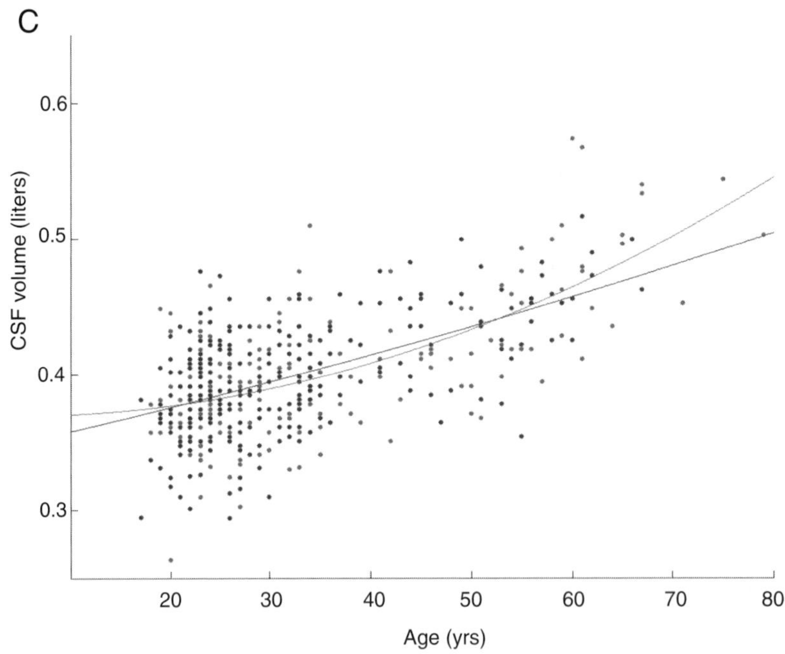

FIGURE 7.5, cont'd.
(c) Scatterplot of total CSF volume (litres) against age (years) for 465 normal subjects (females in red, males in blue); the best-fitting quadratic regression curves for females and males are superimposed.

Neurological and Psychiatric Diseases

The simple method of VBM has already been applied to a number of patient groups, helping to establish the face and construct validity of this technique in disease.

Dementia

The classification of dementias is becoming increasingly complex with advancements in neuropathological, genetic, and neuroimaging techniques, but no true gold standard exists. In practical terms, neuroimaging is commonly used in the diagnostic workup and monitoring of disease progression in patients with dementias, as well as acting as a surrogate marker for assessing disease modifying agents. Region-of-interest-based morphometry can differentiate between various subtypes (Chan *et al.*, 2001), but these techniques are laborious, limited to subregions of the brain, and highly operator dependent; unsurprisingly, results often vary between laboratories. Unbiased automated techniques offer more scope to evaluate the structural correlates of dementias both cross-sectionally and longitudinally, but they need to be validated with the best available gold standard.

In six patients with semantic dementia, VBM delineated regional atrophy correlating with functional data in both temporal lobes (particularly the left), left fusiform gyrus, right temporal pole, bilateral ventromedial frontal cortex, and amygdaloid complex. No significant atrophy was detected in the hippocampus, entorhinal, or caudal perirhinal cortex (Mummery *et al.*, 2000). Several groups are currently applying the simple method of VBM to determine patterns of atrophy in degenerative brain diseases such as Alzheimer's disease. A brief report describes symmetric atrophy in the hippocampus, caudate nucleus, and insula in seven patients with mild to moderate Alzheimer's disease (Rombouts *et al.*, 2000), and a recent report documents symmetric anteromesial temporal, bilateral parietal, and posterior cingulate atrophy in Alzheimer's disease (Baron *et al.*, 2001). Exciting and innovative work using a new computational strategy to map gyral pattern variations across subjects reports the first detailed population-based maps of cortical grey matter loss in Alzheimer's disease (Thompson *et al.*, 2001). This work is an important contribution to the literature, as it models the profiles of early grey matter volume loss having allowed for interindividual gyral variations and mismatch.

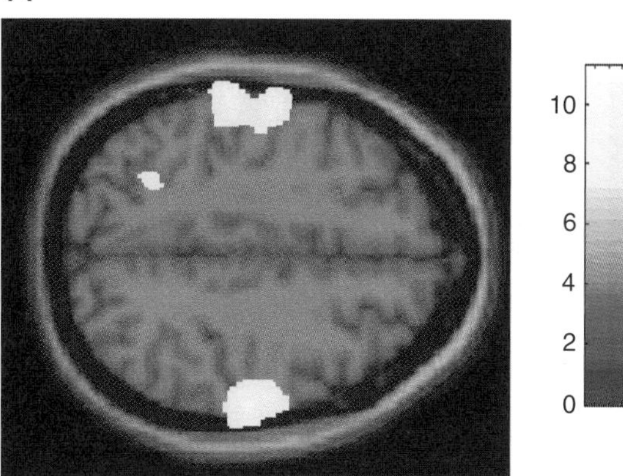

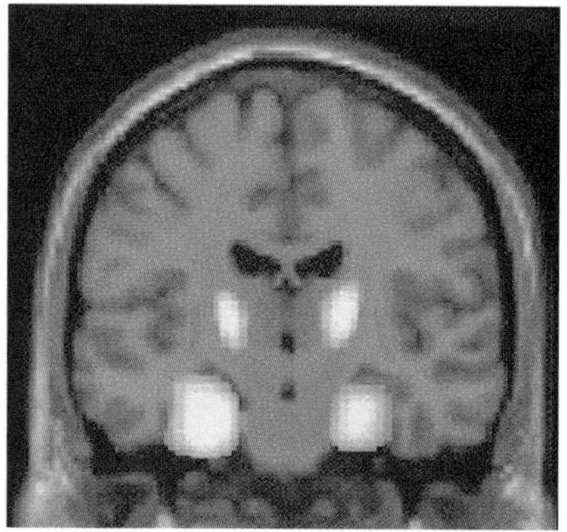

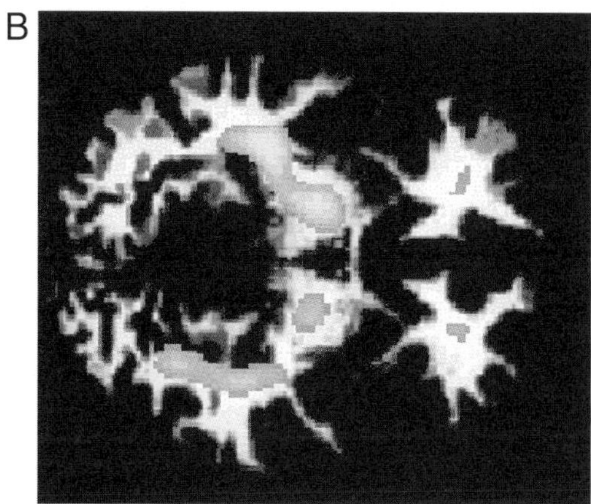

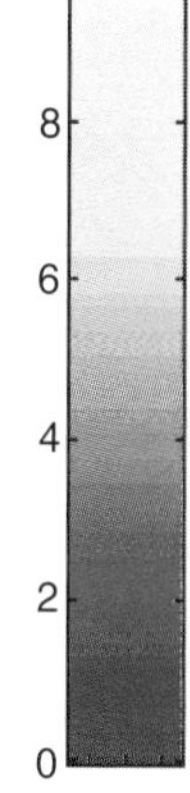

FIGURE 7.6

(A) *Grey matter volume, (modulated) negative correlation with age*: Regions of relative accelerated loss of grey matter volume from 465 normal subjects are superimposed on a normalised structural image in the axial plane. The colour bar represents the T score. Significant voxels ($p < 0.025$, corrected) are seen bilaterally in the pre- and post-central gyri and left angular gyrus (right not shown). The significant cerebellar and anterior insula voxels are not shown. ***Grey matter volume, (modulated) positive correlation with age*:** Regional areas of relative preservation of grey matter are noted bilaterally in amygdala/hippocampal complexes, entorhinal cortex, and lateral thalami. (B) White matter volume, (modulated) negative correlation with age: Regions of accelerated loss of white matter volume from 465 normal subjects are superimposed on a normalised white matter axial image from one of the subjects. The colour bar represents the T score. Significant voxels are seen bilaterally in the corona radiata, bordering on ventral thalamus (voxels classified as white matter) and frontal white matter. *(Continued)*

The optimised method of VBM has recently been compared with independent ROI measurements of temporal lobe structures in patients with Alzheimer's disease (AD) and semantic dementia (SD) (Chan *et al.*, 2001; Good *et al.*, 2002) in order to establish the construct validity of VBM. In AD, VBM detected diffuse and relatively symmetric atrophy of cerebral grey matter, most marked in the parietal lobes and posterior cingulate (Fig. 7.8), matching the distribution of oxygen and glucose hypometabolism on PET studies (Foster *et al.*, 1983; Frackowiak *et al.*, 1981). In the temporal lobe, the right middle temporal gyrus, both hippocampi, and the right fusiform gyrus were most severely atrophied. ROI-based analyses showed a similar pattern of volume loss but differed slightly in the ranking of severity. In SD, VBM showed asymmetric temporal lobe atrophy, more pronounced on the left side (Fig. 9). The most striking grey matter loss was observed in anterior temporal lobe structures, with most severe atrophy observed in the left amygdala, anterior hippocampus, and entorhinal cortex, a finding that closely matches the

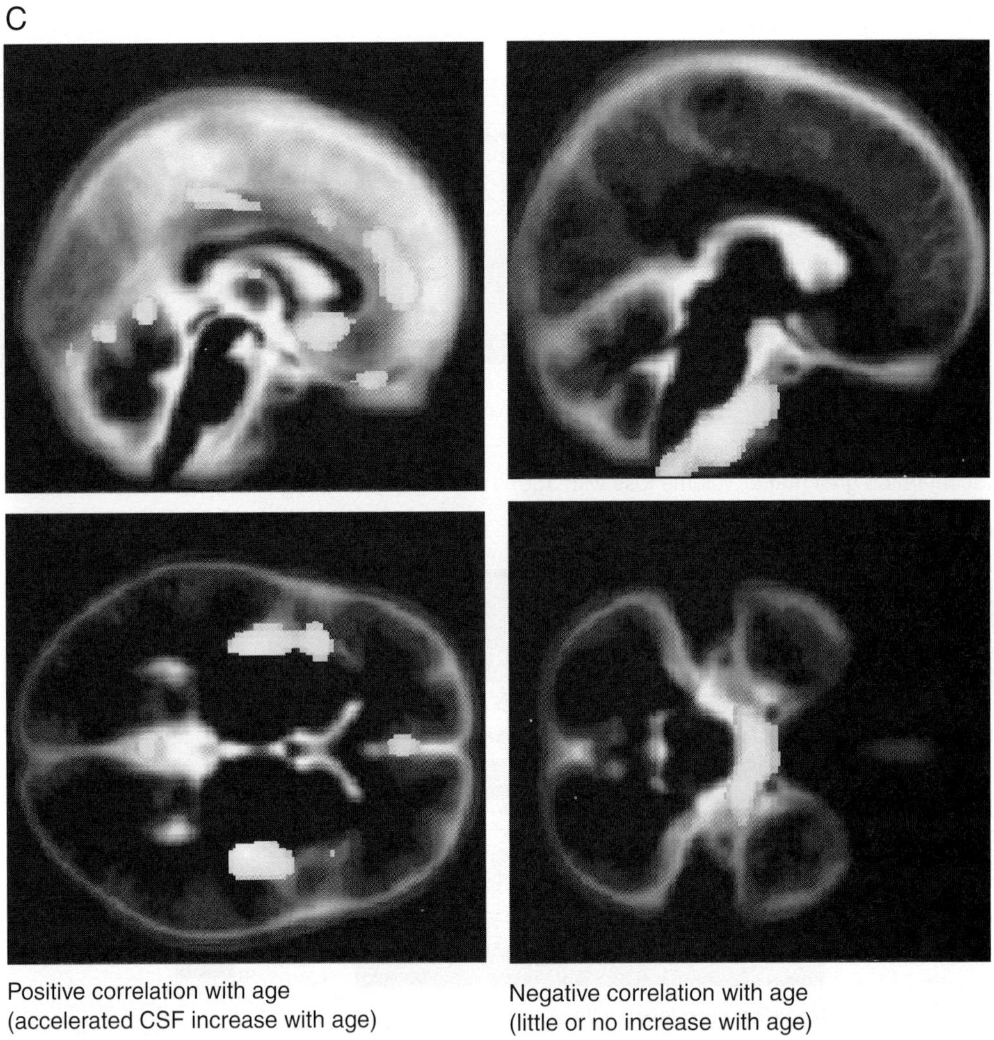

C

Positive correlation with age
(accelerated CSF increase with age)

Negative correlation with age
(little or no increase with age)

FIGURE 7.6, cont'd.
(C) CSF volume, (modulated) positive correlation with age: Accelerated CSF enlargements with age from 465 normal subjects superimposed on a mean normalised CSF image are seen in the Sylvian and interhemispheric fissures. The colour bar represents the T score. *CSF volume, (modulated) negative correlation with age*: Regions of relatively little enlargement of the CSF space are seen in the pontine cistern.

ROI-based analyses. In AD, ROI measurement appear more sensitive for the volume loss in the amygdala, whereas VBM measurements appear more sensitive for volume loss in both superior and right middle temporal gyri, both fusiform gyri and regional hippocampal volumes (right mid and posterior hippocampus, left anterior hippocampus). In SD ROI measurements appear more sensitive for volume loss in the left MITG whereas VBM appears more sensitive to regional hippocampal atrophy. VBM detected more grey matter atrophy in all temporal lobe structures apart from the right middle temporal gyrus in SD than AD (Good *et al.*, 2002). In conclusion, there was a remarkable consistency between VBM and classical ROI-based approaches. This is despite the fact that VBM detects changes in tissue composition (*e.g.*, grey matter atrophy) at a spatial scale defined by the smoothing kernel. The resolution of ROI-based metrics varies according to the size and shape of the ROI and simply reflects volume change across all tissue compartments.

Autistic Disorder

Autism is a developmental disorder marked by impairments in socialisation, communication, and perseverative behaviour and is associated with cognitive impairment and deficits in adaptive functioning. Despite the impressive number of imaging studies attempting to isolate brain regions implicated in autism, the literature remains inconclusive. The most consistent findings

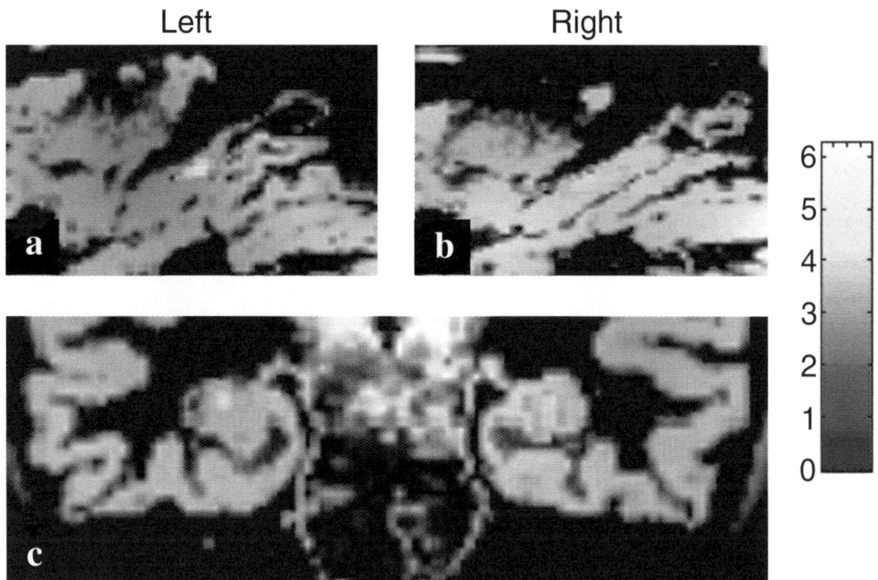

FIGURE 7.7
Focal increase in grey matter in the posterior hippocampi of taxi drivers relative to controls. VBM results are superimposed on grey matter segmented images through the hippocampi, in the sagittal plane (a) and (b) and coronal plane (c). The bar to the right indicates the *Z* score level. (From Maguire, E. A. *et al.*, *Proc. Natl. Acad. Sci. USA*, 97, 4398–4403, 2000.With permission from Dr. E. Maguire.)

include bilateral amygdala enlargement (Howard *et al.*, 2000) and cerebellar abnormalities. In 15 high-functioning patients with autistic disorder, VBM detected regional structural changes in an amygdala-centred system, correlating with PET activations (Abell *et al.*, 1999). Decreases in grey matter were found in the efferent parts of the system (right anterior cingulate, left orbitotemporal junction, left inferior frontal sulcus), and increases in grey matter were found in afferent parts (peri-amygdaloid cortex, superior temporal sulcus, inferior temporal regions) and regions of the cerebellum.

Schizophrenia

Magnetic resonance imaging is an important tool for investigating the brain structural correlates of schizophrenia, but the literature on schizophrenia is large and conflicting. Study sample sizes are often small, and most reports are based upon ROI morphometrics, which vary widely across laboratories. Meta-analyses are being increasingly employed to assist interpretation of the large literature. The most consistent imaging findings in schizophrenia include a reduction in global brain volume and increased CSF volume and regional reductions in the amygdala/hippocampal formations (Wright *et al.*, 2000). In 15 schizophrenic patients, VBM showed a negative correlation between the score for reality distortion syndrome and regional grey matter density in the left superior temporal lobe and regional white matter density in the corpus callosum, correlating with previous functional data (Wright *et al.*, 1995).

Magnetisation transfer imaging (MTI) is a MR technique that provides quantitative assessment of macromolecular structural integrity represented by the magnetisation transfer ratio (MTR). A recent study that used a VBM approach to analyse MTR images showed widespread reductions in MTR in the cortex of 25 patients with schizophrenia, unrelated to volume reduction. Furthermore, bilateral MTR reductions in the parieto-occipital cortex and genu of the corpus callosum correlated with negative symptoms (Foong *et al.*, 2001)

Herpes Simplex Encephalitis

Herpes simplex encephalitis (HSE) is the most common viral encephalitis in humans and is associated with significant morbidity and mortality. Pathologically, HSE has an anatomic predilection for the limbic and paralimbic regions of the brain, including the mesial temporal lobes, orbitofrontal cortex, insula, and cingulate gyri (Damasio and Van Hoesen, 1985). In five

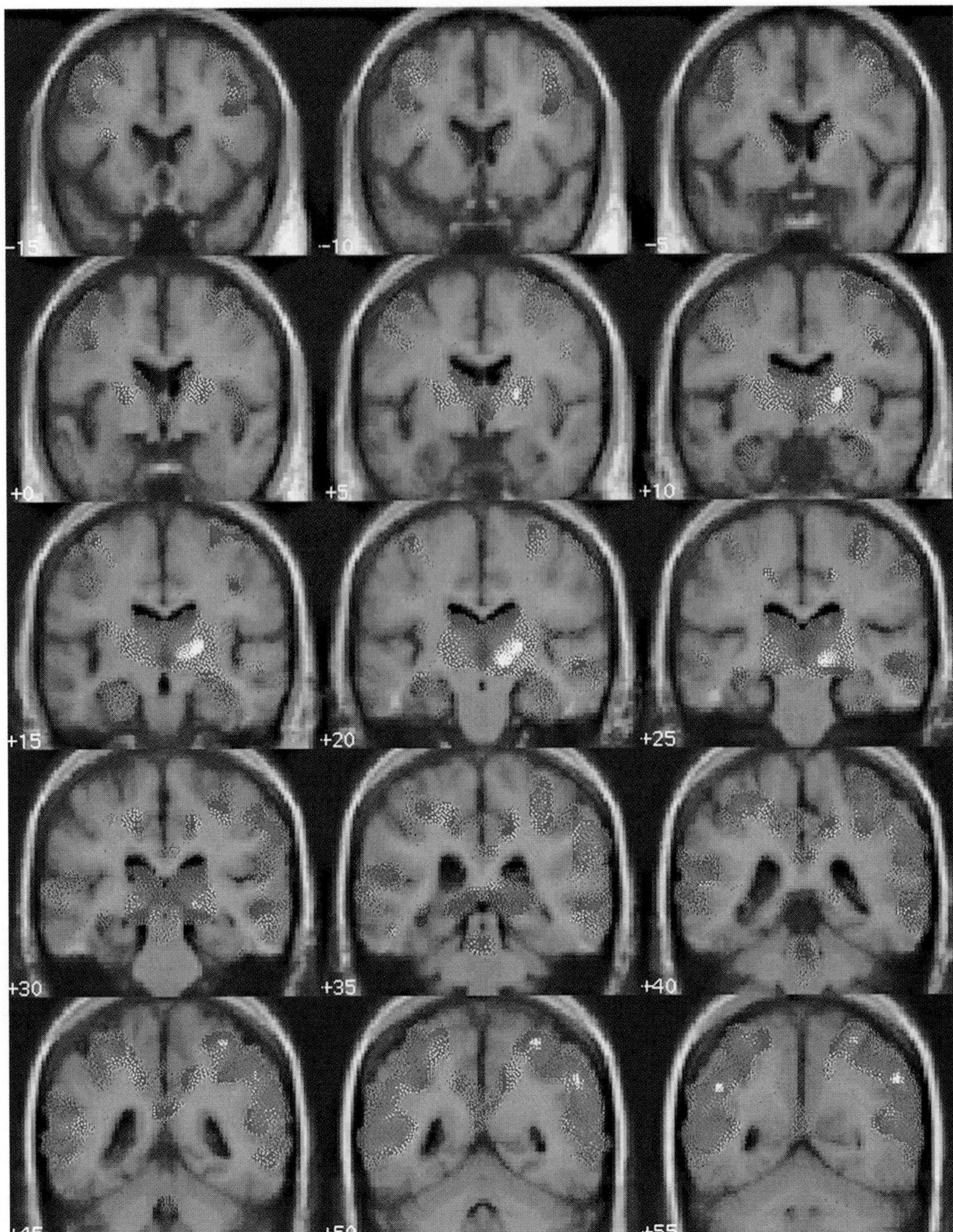

FIGURE 7.8
VBM-detected grey matter atrophy in Alzheimer's disease. Significant voxels (threshold $T > 2.5$, for illustrative purposes only) are projected over coronal slices of the group mean normalised image. Total intracranial volume was included as a confounding covariate. There is a relatively symmetrical and diffuse pattern of atrophy. The most significant voxels are in the parietal cortex, posterior cingulate, and thalami. Within the temporal lobes, atrophy is seen predominantly in the hippocampi and middle and superior temporal gyri.

patients with HSE, VBM detected grey matter abnormalities in limbic and paralimbic areas of cortex, consistent with previous pathological descriptions of the disease (Gitelman *et al.*, 2001).

Primary Autonomic Failure (PAF)

Pure autonomic failure (PAF) is an acquired condition characterised by selective peripheral denervation of the autonomic nervous system. Function neuroimaging studies have demonstrated abnormalities in the cingulate, insula, and pontine regions, suggesting that these regions are involved in autonomic control. Optimised VBM showed associated insula and somatosensory

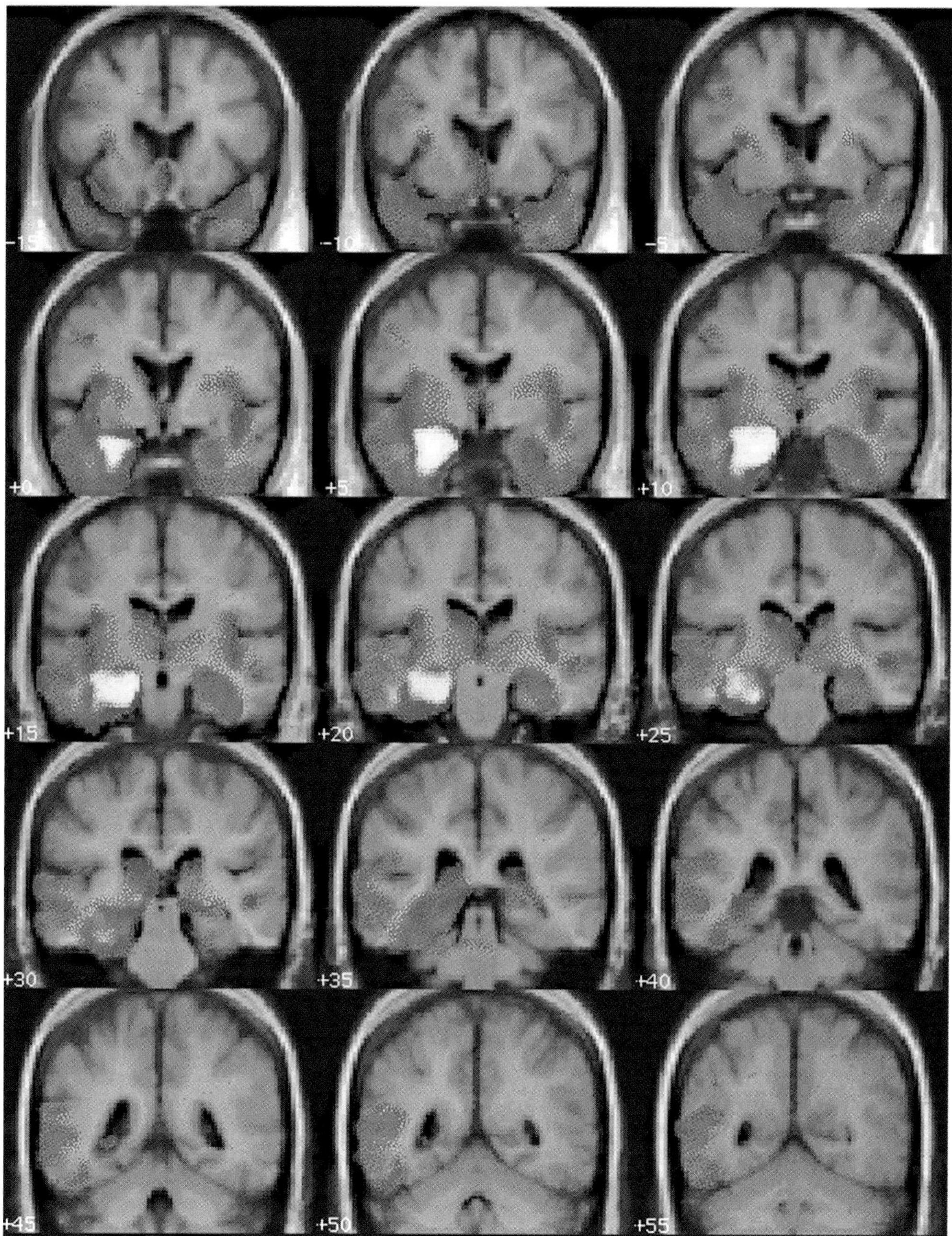

FIGURE 7.9
VBM-detected grey matter atrophy in semantic dementia. Significant voxels (threshold T > 2.5, for illustrative purposes only) are projected over coronal slices of the group mean normalised image. Total intracranial volume was included as a confounding covariate. There is an asymmetric pattern of temporal lobe atrophy, most marked on the left side, particularly in the anteromesial structures.

cortices, associated with homeostatic regulation of body states and changes in cingulate activity attributable to second-order remapping of bodily states (Matharu *et al.*, 2003).

Headache

Focal hypothalamic structural change has been reported in patients with periodic, unilateral diurnal cluster headache, matching PET activations (May *et al.*, 1999). Optimised VBM detected no structural differences within the brains of 22 patients with migraine (11 patients with a history of aura and 11 patients without aura) (unpublished data). This finding may reflect the heterogeneity of the disease, and we are currently studying a pedigree with familial hemiplegic migraine and chromosome 19 P/Q Ca channel mutation in order to identify a more homogeneous phenotype of migraine.

Epilepsy

Regional structural changes correlating with benzodiazepine receptor density have been detected in patients with malformations of cortical development. VBM detected anatomical abnormalities that correlated with functional changes. The anatomical changes were invisible on high-resolution MRI and missed by independent blinded ROI measurements (Richardson *et al.*, 1997). This paper implemented voxel-wise comparisons of structural and functional data for the first time, which may have great potential for future studies if the methodological challenges can be met. In 20 patients with juvenile myoclonic epilepsy and normal diagnostic MRI, VBM detected increased grey matter in the mesial frontal lobes (Woermann *et al.*, 1999b), but interestingly, in another study by the same group, VBM did not identify clearly visible hippocampal atrophy in 10 patients with mesial temporal sclerosis (MTS) (Woermann *et al.*, 1999a). We have recently applied the optimised VBM technique to a group of 62 patients with MTS and 32 age and sex matched controls. VBM clearly identified hippocampal atrophy in these patients and showed more extensive atrophy in left-sided MTS than right-sided MTS (Fig.7.10).

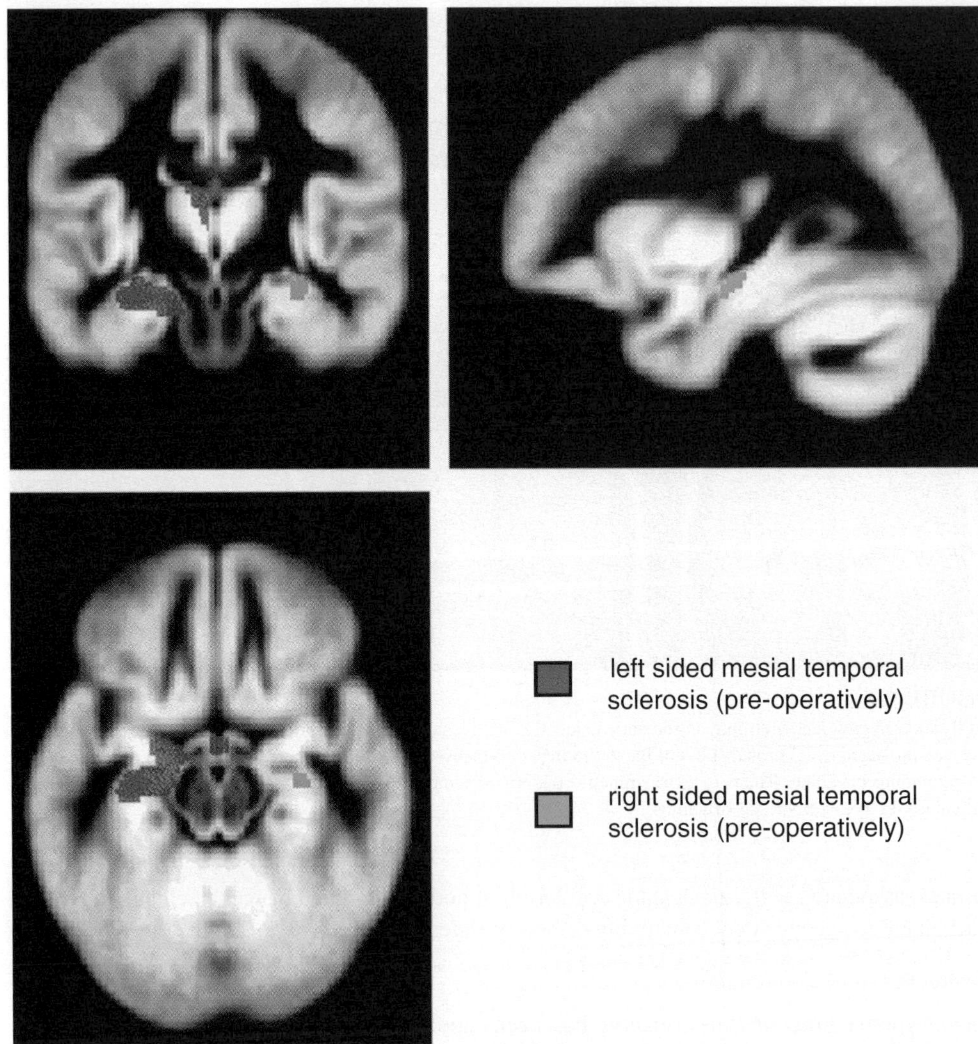

FIGURE 7.10
VBM-detected grey matter atrophy in left mesial temporal sclerosis (MTS) (in red) and right MTS (in green) projected over the group mean normalised image. Atrophy is asymmetric, with more extensive grey matter loss being observed in left MTS.

Furthermore, VBM showed more extensive grey and white matter atrophy in patients who continued to have seizures after temporal lobe surgery, compared with those who remained seizure free post operatively (Fig. 7.11) (manuscript in preparation).

Genotype–Phenotype Mapping

Having cross-validated VBM with independent postmortem data, ROI-based neuroimaging techniques, and functional imaging for a number of pathologies, it is now tempting to investigate whether this technique can bridge the gap between genetics and neurodevelopment. With advancements in molecular techniques and the framework of the Human Genome Project, most genes can now be mapped with a high degree of accuracy. This opens the way for genotype–phenotype correlation and identification of candidate genes coding for specific brain structural and functional phenotypes, with the ultimate aim of further understanding brain development and function.

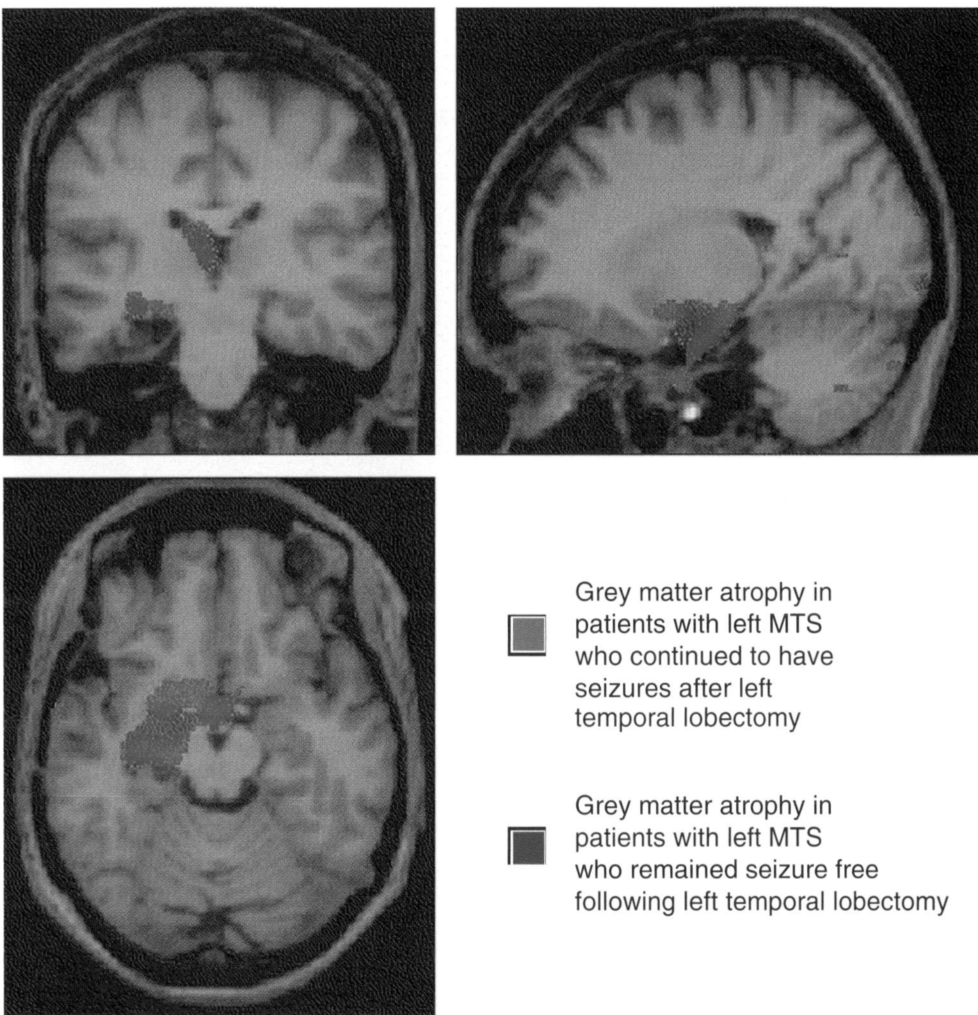

FIGURE 7.11
VBM-detected grey matter atrophy in patients with left MTS projected over a normalised postoperative image from one of the patients. The group that continued to have seizures postoperatively are displayed in red, and those that remained seizure free are displayed in blue. The seizure group shows more extensive mesial temporal atrophy, extending more posteriorly and superiorly than the seizure-free group. In addition, the seizure group shows posterior orbitofrontal atrophy and lateral temporal atrophy, not seen in the seizure-free group.

Gene Mapping of the X Chromosome

The fundamental role of the X chromosome in neurodevelopment has been suggested by a number of reports of altered neurocognitive profiles in sex chromosome aneuploidies. Turner syndrome (TS), a genetic disorder of human females with complete or partial absence of a single X chromosome, offers a convenient natural experiment to study genotype–phenotype correlations of the X chromosome. First, we can characterise the structural and functional phenotype of TS with complete absence of a single X chromosome (the 45X0 karyoptype), compared with normal females with two X chromosomes (46XX). Second, because TS may be associated with partial deletions on one X chromosome, these deletions can be mapped on a molecular level, opening the door for a gene-deletion mapping strategy. The ultimate aim would be to identify regions on the X chromosome containing a candidate gene (or genes) coding for the specific phenotype. TS females have a characteristic cognitive-behavioural phenotype that includes normal verbal skills, impaired visuospatial and constructive skills, and mildly impaired motor function. Behaviourally, they have social adjustment problems, some autistic features, and emotional recognition difficulties, particularly in the fear and anger categories. We used VBM to characterise the structural phenotype of TS and to employ a gene-deletion mapping strategy. VBM detected regions of increased grey matter in the amygdala/hippocampal formations and orbitofrontal cortex bilaterally (Fig. 7.12), regions that have been implicated in face and

TS – normal females

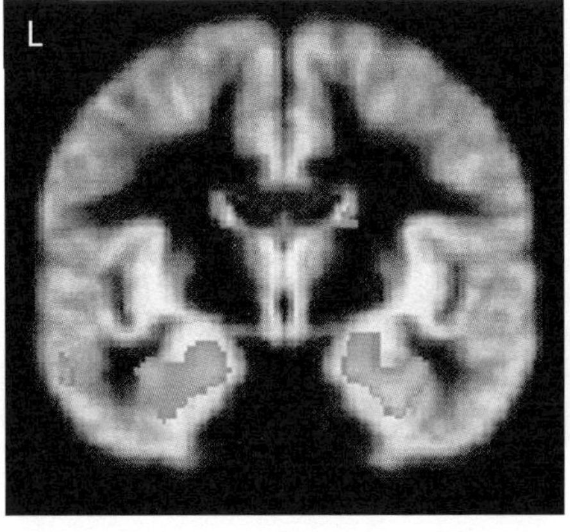

Normal males-normal females
(Good et al)

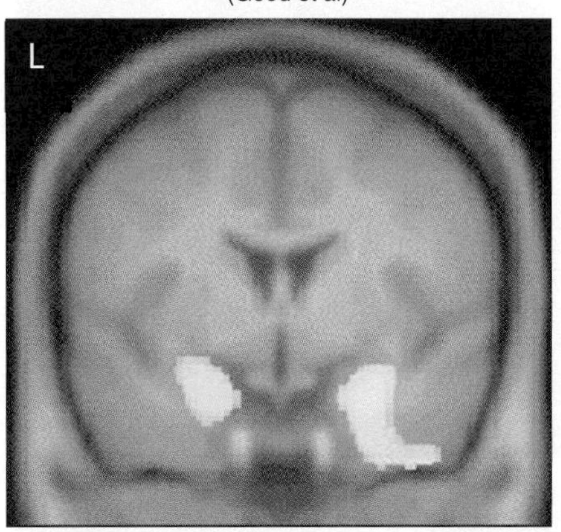

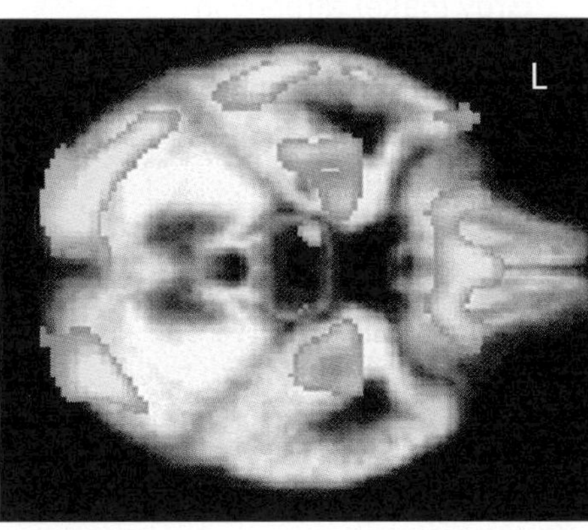

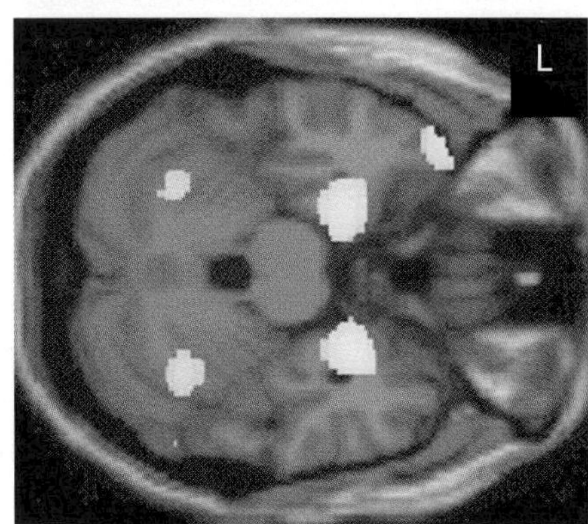

p<0.05 corrected

FIGURE 7.12
VBM-detected increases in grey matter in females with Turner syndrome (45X) compared with normal females (46XX). Regional grey matter increases are noted in the amygdala/hippocampi and cerebellum bilaterally and within the left anterior temporal pole and middle temporal gyrus. Note the striking similarity to the VBM-detected grey matter increases in normal males(46XY) compared with normal females (46XX). (From Good, C. D. *et al.*, *NeuroImage*, 14, 21–36, 2001. With permission.)

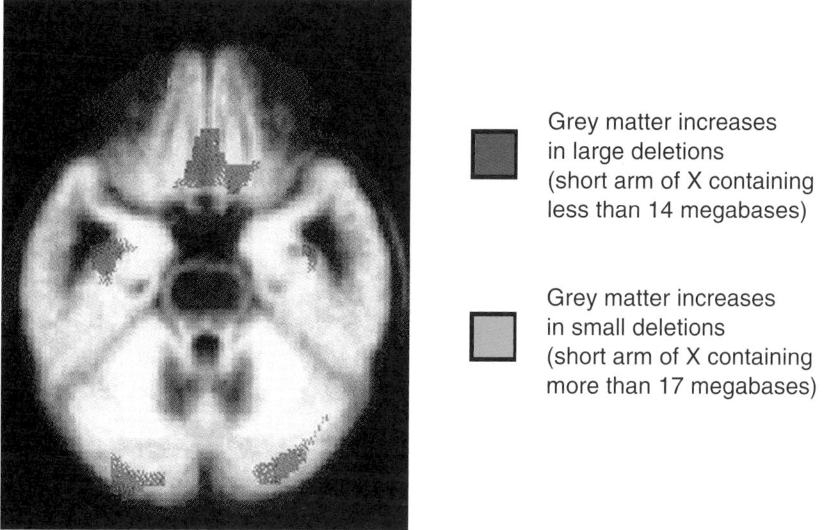

FIGURE 7.13
Grey matter increases in partial deletions of the short arm of the X chromosome projected over the group mean normalised grey matter image. Large deletions (less than 14 megabases present on the short arm) are shown in red; small deletions (more than 17 megabases present on the short arm of X) are shown in green. Large deletions have the Turner syndrome (45X) structural phenotype, whereas small deletions have the structural phenotype of normal females (46XX).

emotional recognition tasks. Interestingly, the VBM-detected structural phenotype of TS (45X0) closely matches the differences between normal males (46XY) and normal females (46XX) (Fig. 7.12). VBM also detected regions of decreased grey matter in the right parieto-occipital region, a region that has been implicated in visuospatial function (Barcelo *et al.*, 1997). Gene-deletion mapping with VBM showed that females with large deletions on the short arm of the X chromosome demonstrated the TS structural and functional phenotype, whereas those with small deletions had normal brain structure (Fig. 7.13). VBM identified two regions on the short arm of the X chromosome that are likely to contain candidate genes (Fig. 7.14) (Good *et al.*, 2003, *Brain*, in press).

Kallmann's Syndrome

Kallmann's syndrome is defined by the association of anosmia with idiopathic hypogonadotropic hypogonadism. The X-linked form of the disease (xKS) is characterised by a high prevalence of mirror movements. Electrophysiological studies suggest abnormality of the ipsilateral corticospinal tract projection in patients exhibiting mirror movements. VBM detected regional white matter changes that correlate with EEG data and independent ROI measurements in Kallmann's syndrome (Krams *et al.*, 1999). In this study, hypertrophy of the corpus callosum was observed in nine patients with xKS with mirror movements and in nine patients with autosomal Kallmann's syndrome (aKS) without mirror movements, but not in normal subjects. Bilateral hypertrophy of the corticospinal tracts was seen only in the group with mirror movements.

Inherited Speech and Language Disorder

Investigation of three generations of a family with an autosomal dominant inherited speech and language disorder resulting from the deletion or disruption of a single gene at 7q31 revealed functional abnormalities in both cortical and subcortical motor-related areas of the frontal lobe. VBM detected structural changes in several of these areas, particularly in the caudate nucleus, corroborating independent ROI-based measurements (Vargha-Khadem *et al.*, 1998).

Narcolepsy

Recent research has implicated the hypothalamic neuropeptides hypocretin 1 and 2 and their receptors in the pathophysiology of narcolepsy. Narcolepsy can be caused by mutations in the

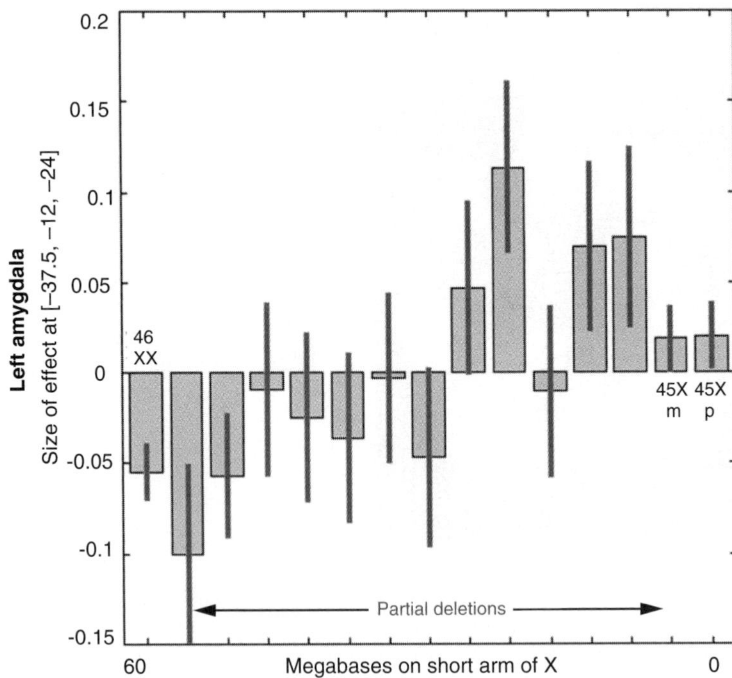

FIGURE 7.14
Fitted and adjusted responses from a local **maximum** in the left amygdala. The columns representing the patient groups are arranged from left to right according to the number of megabases from the centromere on the short arm of the X chromosome. Column 1 represent normal females 46,XX (60 megabases), column 2–3 represent partial deletions arranged in order of increasing size of deletion and decreasing number of megabases, column 14 represents TS, 46X0 (0 megabases) (maternal origin) and column 15 represents TS 46,X0 (0 megabases) (paternal origin). There appears to be a shift from the normal female structural phenotype to the TS phenotype (enlarged amygdala) between 17 and 14 megabases from the centromere. This correlates exactly with the cognitive behavioural findings, suggesting that this locus may contain candidate genes coding for amygdala development.

hypocretin receptor 2 gene in dogs and with preprohypocretin knock-in mice (Chemelli *et al.*, 1999; Lin *et al.*, 1999). In humans, most narcoleptic patients lack hypocretin-1 in the cerebrospinal fluid (Nishino *et al.*, 2000). Furthermore, in a small number of narcoleptic patients, hypocretin mRNA was undetectable, and immunoreactive hypocretin-1 and -2 were greatly diminished in the hypothalamus (Peyron *et al.*, 2000; Thannickal *et al.*, 2000). Based on these findings and the tight association between narcolepsy and the human leukocyte antigen (HLA) subtype DQB1*0602, it has been hypothesised that autoimmune-mediated degeneration of hypocretin neurons is responsible for the disease, although postmortem studies could not formally prove cell loss or gliosis. There have been two VBM studies of narcoleptic patients with conflicting results. One group demonstrated hypothalamic grey matter changes in narcoleptics (Draganski *et al.*, 2002). The other group using the optimised technique detected no significant macroscopic structure between 15 patients with established hypocretin-1 deficiency and narcolepsy compared with controls, even with reduced thresholds (Overeem *et al.*, 2003).

CONCLUSIONS

Voxel-based morphometry (VBM) has been cross-correlated with classical ROI metrics and functional data in a number of studies, establishing the validity of this technique. Importantly, VBM is a fully automated whole brain technique that avoids the subjectivity of ROI approaches and can be practically applied to large study groups. The software is freely available, and the technique can now be applied not only in research units but also within the clinical domain. With further improvements in computational power, more accurate mapping of cortical gyri and sulci will facilitate the detection of more subtle structural differences in health and disease using tensor-based morphometry techniques.

References

Abell, F., Krams, M., Ashburner, J., Passingham, R., Friston, K., and Frackowiak, R. *et al.* (1999). The neuroanatomy of autism: a voxel-based whole brain analysis of structural scans. *NeuroReport*, **10**, 1647–1651.

Amunts, K., Jancke, L., Mohlberg, H., Steinmetz, H., and Zilles, K. (2000). Interhemispheric asymmetry of the human motor cortex related to handedness and gender. *Neuropsychologia*, **38**, 304–312.

Ashburner, J. and Friston, K. J. (2000). Voxel-based morphometry: the methods. *NeuroImage*, **11**, 805–821.

Ashburner, J., Hutton, C., Frackowiak, R., Johnsrude, I., Price, C., and Friston, K. (1998). Identifying global anatomical differences: deformation-based morphometry. *Hum. Brain Mapping*, **6**, 348–357.

Ashburner, J., Andersson, J. L., and Friston, K. J. (1999). High-dimensional image registration using symmetric priors. *Neuroimage.*, **9**, 619–628.

Barcelo, F., Martin-Loeches, M., and Rubia, F. J. (1997). Event-related potentials during memorisation of spatial locations in the auditory and visual modalities. *Electroencephalogr. Clin. Neurophysiol.*, **103**, 257–267.

Baron, J. C., Chetelat, G., Desgranges, B., *et al.* (2001). In vivo mapping of gray matter loss with voxel-based morphometry in mild Alzheimer's disease. *NeuroImage*, **14**, 298–309.

Beaton, A. A. (1997). The relation of planum temporale asymmetry and morphology of the corpus callosum to handedness, gender, and dyslexia: a review of the evidence. *Brain Lang.*, **60**, 255–322.

Caviness, V. S., Kennedy, D. N., Richelme, C., Rademacher, J., and Filipek, P. A. (1996). The human brain age 7–11 years: a volumetric analysis based on magnetic resonance images. *Cereb. Cortex*, **6**, 726–736.

Chan, D., Fox, N. C., Scahill, R. I., Crum, W. R., Whitwell, J. L., Leschziner, G. *et al.* (2001). Patterns of temporal lobe atrophy in semantic dementia and Alzheimer's disease. *Ann Neurol.*, **49**, 433–442.

Chemelli, R. M., Willie, J. T., Sinton, C. M., Elmquist, J. K., Scammell, T., Lee, C. *et al.* (1999). Narcolepsy in orexin knockout mice: molecular genetics of sleep regulation. *Cell.*, **98**, 437–451.

Christensen, G. E., Joshi, S. C., and Miller, M. I. (1997). Volumetric transformation of brain anatomy. *IEEE Trans. Med. Imaging*, **16**, 864–877.

Cook, M. J. (1994). Mesial temporal sclerosis and volumetric investigations. *Acta Neurol. Scand. Suppl.*, **152**, 109–114 (discussion, 115).

Damasio, A. R. and Van Hoesen, G. W. (1985). The limbic system and the localisation of herpes simplex encephalitis. *J. Neurol. Neurosurg. Psychiatry*, **48**, 297–301.

Davatzikos, C. and Resnick, S. M. (1998). Sex differences in anatomic measures of interhemispheric connectivity: correlations with cognition in women but not men. *Cereb. Cortex*, **8**, 635–640.

de Courten-Myers, G. M. (1999). The human cerebral cortex, gender differences in structure and function. *J. Neuropathol. Exp. Neurol.*, **58**, 217–226.

DeLeo, J. M., Schwartz, M., Creasey, H., Cutler, N., and Rapoport, S. I. (1985). Computer-assisted categorisation of brain computerised tomography pixels into cerebrospinal fluid, white matter, and gray matter. *Comput. Biomed. Res.*, **18**, 79–88.

Draganski, B., Geisler, P., Hajak, G., *et al.* (2002, Nov). Hypothalamic gray matter changes in narcoleptic patients. *Nat. Med.*, **8**(11), 1186–1188.

Duncan, J. S. (1997). Imaging and epilepsy. *Brain*, **120**, 339–377.

Evans, A., Collins, D., Mills, S., Brown, E., Kelly, R., and Peters, T. (1993). Three-dimensional statistical neuroanatomical models from 305 MRI volumes, in *Trans. IEEE Nuclear Science Symp. and Medical Imaging Conf.*, 1813–1817.

Filipek, P. A., Richelme, C., Kennedy, D. N., and Caviness, V. S., Jr. (1994). The young adult human brain: an MRI-based morphometric analysis. *Cereb. Cortex*, **4**, 344–360.

Flood, D. and Coleman, P. (1988). Neuron numbers and size in aging brain: comparison of human, monkey and rodent data. *Neurobiol. Aging*, **9**, 453–463.

Foong, J., Symms, M. R., Barker, G. J., Maier, M., Woermann, F. G., Miller, D. H. *et al.* (2001). Neuropathological abnormalities in schizophrenia, evidence from magnetisation transfer imaging. *Brain*, **124**, 882–892.

Foster, N. L., Chase, T. N., Fedio, P., Patronas, N. J., Brooks, R. A., and Di Chiro, G. (1983). Alzheimer's disease: focal cortical changes shown by positron emission tomography. *Neurology*, **33**, 961–965.

Fox, N. C., Freeborough, P. A., and Rossor, M. N. (1996). Visualisation and quantification of rates of atrophy in Alzheimer's disease. *Lancet*, **348**, 94–97.

Frackowiak, R. S., Pozzilli, C., Legg, N. J., Du Boulay, G. H., Marshall, J., Lenzi, G. L. *et al.* (1981). Regional cerebral oxygen supply and utilisation in dementia: a clinical and physiological study with oxygen-15 and positron tomography. *Brain*, **104**, 753–778.

Frederikse, M. E., Lu, A., Aylward, E., Barta, P., and Pearlson, G. (1999). Sex differences in the inferior parietal lobule. *Cereb. Cortex*, **9**, 896–901.

Free, S. L., Sisodiya, S. M., Cook, M. J., Fish, D. R., and Shorvon, S. D. (1996). Three-dimensional fractal analysis of the white matter surface from magnetic resonance images of the human brain. *Cereb. Cortex*, **6**, 830–836.

Freeborough, P. A. and Fox, N. C. (1998). Modeling brain deformations in Alzheimer's disease by fluid registration of serial three-dimensional MR images. *J. Comput. Assist. Tomogr.*, **22**, 838–843.

Friston, K. J., Holmes, A., Poline, J. B., Price, C. J., and Frith, C. D. (1996). Detecting activations in PET and fMRI: levels of inference and power. *NeuroImage*, **4**, 223–235.

Geschwind, N. and Galaburda, A. M. (1985a). Cerebral lateralisation: biological mechanisms, associations, and pathology. I. A hypothesis and a program for research. *Arch Neurol.*, **42**, 428–459.

Geschwind, N. and Galaburda, A. M. (1985b). Cerebral lateralisation: biological mechanisms, associations, and pathology. II. A hypothesis and a program for research. *Arch Neurol.*, **42**, 521–552.

Geschwind, N. and Galaburda, A. M. (1985c).Cerebral lateralisation: biological mechanisms, associations, and pathology, III. A hypothesis and a program for research. *Arch Neurol.*, **42**, 634–654.

Geschwind, N. and Levitsky, W. (1968). Human brain: left-right asymmetries in temporal speech region. *Science*, **161**, 186–187.

Gitelman, D. R., Ashburner, J., Friston, K. J., Tyler, L. K., and Price, C. J. (2001). Voxel-based morphometry of herpes simplex encephalitis. *NeuroImage*, **13**, 623–631.

Goldstein, J. M., Seidman, L. J., Horton, N. J., Makris, N., Kennedy, D. N., and Caviness, V. S., Jr. *et al.* (2001). Normal sexual dimorphism of the adult human brain assessed by *in vivo* magnetic resonance imaging. *Cereb. Cortex*, **11**, 490–497.

Gomez-Isla, T., Price, J. L., McKeel, D. W., Jr., Morris, J. C., Growdon, J. H., and Hyman, B. T. (1996). Profound loss of layer II entorhinal cortex neurons occurs in very mild Alzheimer's disease. *J. Neurosci.*, **16**, 4491–4500.

Good, C. D., Johnsrude, I. S., Ashburner, J. R. N. A. H., Friston, K. J., and Frackowiak, R. S. J. (2001). A voxel-based morphometric study of ageing in 465 normal adult human brains. *NeuroImage*, **14**, 21–36.

Good, C. D., Scahill, R. I., Fox, N. C., Asburner, J., Friston, K. J., Chan, D., Crum, W. R., Rossor, M. N., and Frackowiak, R. S. J. (2002). Automatic differentiation of anatomical patterns in the human brain: validation with studies of degenerative dementias. *NeuroImage*, **17**, 29–46.

Guimond, A., Meunier, J., and Thirion, J. P. (2000). Average barin models: a convergence study. *Comp. Vision Image Understanding*, **77**, 192–210.

Guttmann, C. R., Jolesz, F. A., Kikinis, R., Killiany, R. J., Moss, M. B., Sandor, T. *et al.* (1998). White matter changes with normal aging. *Neurology*, **50**, 972–978.

Hepper, P. G., Shannon, E. A., and Dornan, J. C. (1997). Sex differences in fetal mouth movements [letter]. *Lancet*, **350**, 1820.

Howard, M. A., Cowell, P. E., Boucher, J., Broks, P., Mayes, A., Farrant, A. *et al.* (2000). Convergent neuroanatomical and behavioural evidence of an amygdala hypothesis of autism. *NeuroReport*, **11**, 2931–2935.

Jack, C. R., Sharbrough, F. W., Twomey, C. K., Cascino, G. D., Hirschorn, K. A., Marsh, W. R. *et al.* (1990). Temporal lobe seizures: lateralisation with MR volume measurements of the hippocampal formation. *Radiology*, **175**, 423–429.

Jackson, G. D., Kuzniecky, R. I., and Cascino, G. D. (1994). Hippocampal sclerosis without detectable hippocampal atrophy. *Neurology.*, **44**, 42–46.

Jernigan, T. L., Archibald, S. L., Berhow, M. T., Sowell, E. R., Foster, D. S., and Hesselink, J. R. (1991a). Cerebral structure on MRI, Part I: Localization of age-related changes. *Biol. Psychiatry*, **29**, 55–67.

Kimura D. (1973). The asymmetry of the human brain. *Sci. Am.*, **228**, 70–78.

Krams, M., Quinton, R., Ashburner, J., Friston, K. J., Frackowiak, R. S., Bouloux, P. M. *et al.* (1999). Kallmann's syndrome: mirror movements associated with bilateral corticospinal tract hypertrophy. *Neurology*, **52**, 816–822.

Kulynych, J. J., Vladar, K., Jones, D. W., and Weinberger, D. R. (1994). Gender differences in the normal lateralisation of the supratemporal cortex: MRI surface-rendering morphometry of Heschl's gyrus and the planum temporale. *Cereb. Cortex.*, **4**, 107–118.

Last, RJaT., D.H. (1953). Casts of cerebral ventricles. *Br. J. Surg.*, **40**, 525–543.

Lee, J. W., Andermann, F., Dubeau, F., Bernasconi, A., MacDonald, D., Evans, A. *et al.* (1998). Morphometric analysis of the temporal lobe in temporal lobe epilepsy. *Epilepsia*, **39**, 727–736.

Levy, J. L. (1978). Human lateralisation from head to foot: sex-related factors. *Science*, **200**, 1291–1292.

Lim, K. O., Zipursky, R. B., Watts, M. C., Pfefferbaum, A. (1992). Decreased gray matter in normal aging: an in vivo magnetic resonance study. *J. Gerontol.*, **47**, 26–30.

Lin, L., Faraco, J., Li, R., Kadotani, H., Rogers, W., Lin X. *et al.* (1999). The sleep disorder canine narcolepsy is caused by a mutation in the hypocretin (orexin) receptor 2 gene. *Cell*, **98**, 365–376.

Luft, A. R., Skalej, M., Schulz, J. B., *et al.* (1999). Patterns of age-related shrinkage in cerebellum and brainstem observed in vivo using three-dimensional MRI volumetry. *Cereb. Cortex*, **9**, 712–721.

Maguire, E. A., Frackowiak, R. S., and Frith CD. (1997). Recalling routes around London: activation of the right hippocampus in taxi drivers. *J Neurosci.*, **17**, 7103–1710.

Maguire, E. A., Frith, C. D., Burgess, N., Donnett, J. G., and O'Keefe, J. (1998). Knowing where things are: parahippocampal involvement in encoding object locations in virtual large-scale space. *J. Cogn. Neurosci.*, **10**, 61–76.

Maguire, E. A., Gadian, D. G., Johnsrude, I. S., Good, C. D., Ashburner, J., Frackowiak, R. S. *et al.* (2000). Navigation-related structural change in the hippocampi of taxi drivers. *Proc. Natl. Acad. Sci. USA*, **97**, 4398–4403.

Maguire, E. A., Spiers, H. J., Good, C. D., Hartley, T., Frackowiak, R. S., and Burgess, N. (2003). Navigation expertise and the human hippocampus: a structure brain imaging analysis. *Hippocampus*, **13**(2), 250–259.

Matharu, M. S., Good, C. D., May, A., Bahra, A., and Goadsby, P. J. (2003). No change in the structure of the brain in migrain: a voxel-based morphometric study. *Eur. J. Neurol.*, **10**, 53–57.

May, A., Ashburner, J., Buchel, C., McGonigle, D. J., Friston, K. J., Frackowiak, R. S. *et al.* (1999). Correlation between structural and functional changes in brain in an idiopathic headache syndrome. *Nat. Med.*, **5**, 836–838.

Messert, B., Wannamaker, B. B., and Dudley, A. W., Jr. (1972). Reevaluation of the size of the lateral ventricles of the brain: postmortem study of an adult population. *Neurology*, **22**, 941–951.

Moffat, S. D., Hampson, E., and Lee, D. H. (1998). Morphology of the planum temporale and corpus callosum in left handers with evidence of left and right hemisphere speech representation. *Brain*, **121**, 2369–2379.

Mummery, C. J., Patterson, K., Price, C. J., Ashburner, J., Frackowiak, R. S., and Hodges, J. R. (2000). A voxel-based morphometry study of semantic dementia: relationship between temporal lobe atrophy and semantic memory. *Ann Neurol.*, **47**, 36–45.

Murthy, J. M., Rao, C. M., and Meena, A. K. (1998). Clinical observations of juvenile myoclonic epilepsy in 131 patients: a study in South India. *Seizure.*, **7**, 43–47.

Nishino, S., Ripley, B., Overeem, S., Lammers, G. J., and Mignot, E. (2000). Hypocretin (orexin) deficiency in human narcolepsy. *Lancet*, **355**, 39–40.

Overeem, S., Steens, S. C., Good, C. D., *et al.* (2003, Feb). Voxel-based morphometry in hypocretin-deficient narcolepsy. *Sleep*, **26**(1), 44–46.

Peters, A., Morrison, J. H., Rosene, D. L., and Hyman, B. T. (1998). Feature article, are neurons lost from the primate cerebral cortex during normal aging? *Cereb. Cortex*, **8**, 295–300.

Peyron, C., Faraco, J., Rogers, W., Ripley, B., Overeem, S., Charnay, Y. *et al.* (2000). A mutation in a case of early onset narcolepsy and a generalised absence of hypocretin peptides in human narcoleptic brains. *Nat. Med.*, **6**, 991–997.

Pfefferbaum, A., Mathalon, D. H., Sullivan, E. V., Rawles, J. M., Zipursky, R. B., and Lim, K. O. (1994). A quantitative magnetic resonance imaging study of changes in brain morphology from infancy to late adulthood. *Arch. Neurol.*, **51**, 874–887.

Purves, D., White, L. E., and Andrews, T. J. (1994). Manual asymmetry and handedness. *Proc. Natl. Acad. Sci. USA*, **91**, 5030–5032.

Reichardt, M. (1905). Uber die bestemmung der schadelkapazikat an der leiche. *Allgemeine zeitschrift fur psychiatrie*, **62**, 787–801.

Richardson, M. P., Friston, K. J., Sisodiya, S. M., Koepp, M. J., Ashburner, J., Free, S. L. *et al.* (1997). Cortical grey matter and benzodiazepine receptors in malformations of cortical development: a voxel-based comparison of structural and functional imaging data. *Brain*, **120**, 1961–1973.

Rombouts, S. A., Barkhof, F., Witter, M. P., and Scheltens P. (2000). Unbiased whole-brain analysis of gray matter loss in Alzheimer's disease. *Neurosci. Lett.*, **285**, 231–233.

Schulz, J. B., Skalej, M., Wedekind, D., Luft, A. R., Abele, M., Voigt, K. *et al.* (1999). Magnetic resonance imaging-based volumetry differentiates idiopathic Parkinson's syndrome from multiple system atrophy and progressive supranuclear palsy. *Ann. Neurol.*, **45**, 65–74.

Schwartz, M., Creasey, H., Grady, C. L., DeLeo, J. M., Frederickson, H. A., Cutler, N. R. *et al.* (1985).Computed tomographic analysis of brain morphometrics in 30 healthy men, aged 21 to 81 years. *Ann. Neurol.*, **17**, 146–157.

Thannickal, T. C., Moore, R. Y., Nienhuis, R., Ramanathan, L., Gulyani, S., Aldrich, M. *et al.* (2000). Reduced number of hypocretin neurons in human narcolepsy. *Neuron*, **27**, 469–474.

Thompson, P. M. and Toga, A. W. (1997). Detection, visualisation and animation of abnormal anatomic structure with a deformable probabilistic brain atlas based on random vector field transformations. *Med. Image Anal.*, **1**, 271–294.

Thompson, P. M., Schwartz, C., Lin, R. T., Khan, A. A., and Toga, A. W. (1996a). Three-dimensional statistical analysis of sulcal variability in the human brain. *J. Neurosci.*, **16**, 4261–4274.

Thompson, P. M., Schwartz, C., and Toga, A. W. (1996b). High-resolution random mesh algorithms for creating a probabilistic three-dimensional surface atlas of the human brain. *NeuroImage*, **3**, 19–34.

Thompson, P. M., MacDonald, D., Mega, M. S., Holmes, C. J., Evans, A. C., and Toga, A. W. (1997). Detection and mapping of abnormal brain structure with a probabilistic atlas of cortical surfaces. *J. Comput. Assist. Tomogr.*, **21**, 567–581.

Thompson, P. M., Moussai, J., Zohoori, S., Goldkorn, A., Khan, A. A., Mega, M. S. *et al.* (1998). Cortical variability and asymmetry in normal aging and Alzheimer's disease. *Cereb. Cortex*, **8**, 492–509.

Thompson, P. M., Mega, M. S., Woods, R. P., Zoumalan, C. I., Lindshield, C. J., Blanton, R. E. *et al.* (2001). Cortical change in Alzheimer's disease detected with a disease-specific population-based brain atlas. *Cereb. Cortex*, **11**, 1–16.

Vargha-Khadem, F., Watkins, K. E., Price, C. J., Ashburner, J., and Alcock, K. J., Connelly, A. *et al.* (1998). Neural basis of an inherited speech and language disorder. *Proc. Natl. Acad. Sci. USA*, **95**, 12695–12700.

White, L. E., Andrews, T. J., Hulette, C., Richards, A., Groelle, M., Paydarfar, J. *et al.* (1997). Structure of the human sensorimotor system. II. Lateral symmetry. *Cereb Cortex*, **7**, 31–47.

Woermann, F. G., Free, S. L., Koepp, M. J., Ashburner, J., and Duncan, J. S. (1999a).Voxel-by-voxel comparison of automatically segmented cerebral gray matter: A rater-independent comparison of structural MRI in patients with epilepsy. *NeuroImage*, **10**, 373–384.

Woermann, F. G., Free, S. L., Koepp, M. J., Sisodiya, S. M., and Duncan, J. S. (1999b). Abnormal cerebral structure in juvenile myoclonic epilepsy demonstrated with voxel-based analysis of MRI. *Brain*, **122**, 2101–2108.

Worsley, K. M., Vandal, A. C., Friston, K. J., and Evans, A. C. (1996). A unified statistical approach for determining significant voxels in images of cerebral activation. *Hum. Brain Mapping*, **4**, 58–73.

Wright, I. C., McGuire, P. K., Poline, J. B., Travere, J. M., Murray, R. M., Frith, C. D. *et al.* (1995). A voxel-based method for the statistical analysis of gray and white matter density applied to schizophrenia. *NeuroImage*, **2**, 244–252.

Wright, I. C., Rabe-Hesketh, S., Woodruff, P. W., David, A. S., Murray, R. M., and Bullmore, E. T. (2000). Meta-analysis of regional brain volumes in schizophrenia. *Am. J. Psychiatry*, **157**, 16–25.

Xu, J., Kobayashi, S., Yamaguchi, S., Iijima, K., Okada, K., and Yamashita, K. (2000a). Gender effects on age-related changes in brain structure. *Am. J. Neuroradiol.*, **21**, 112–118.

C H A P T E R

8

Plasticity in Cochlear Implant Patients

INTRODUCTION

One of the most obvious forms of brain plasticity is cross-modal takeover of deafferented cortices by the intact senses. This occurs readily after early sensory deprivation. When the loss of a sense occurs later in life, however, cerebral organisation changes in a more subtle and reversible way. These changes take place at organisational levels that are inferior to the supra- or polymodal level; hence, they must be investigated from within the modality affected. Auditory reafferentation by cochlear implants (CIs) offers a unique opportunity to study such effects. It allows for investigations of brain plasticity resulting both from deafness and from chronic electrical stimulation. Plastic changes are found at the cortical map level, the speech system level, the multimodal language system level, and on up to the cross-modal level. This chapter reviews the insights that functional brain imaging studies of cochlear implant patients have permitted in the domain of human cortical plasticity.

PLASTICITY ASSOCIATED WITH PRE-LINGUAL DEAFNESS

The absence of auditory input during the development of language is responsible for differences that contrast with normal brain organisation and performance (Bavelier and Neville, 2002). These differences mostly consist of a takeover of the peri-Sylvian region, which is normally dedicated to auditory and language processing, by other sensory modalities. In particular, sign language used by congenitally deaf adults activates not only visual areas but also bilateral supratemporal gyri (Nishimura *et al.*, 1999; Pettito *et al.*, 2000). Unlike further connections to higher order auditory areas, connections from the cochlea to the primary auditory cortex develop irrespective of the presence of auditory input. Thus, cross-modal competition remains confined to secondary auditory and association areas and spares primary auditory regions (Nishimura *et al.*, 2000). The selective sparing of primary regions from takeover by other modalities can be deduced from the observation that the primary auditory cortex responds to noise and speech in pre-lingual CI adults (Herzog *et al.*, 1991; Naito *et al.*, 1997; Truy *et al.*, 1995).

Persisting susceptibility of primary regions to potential auditory inputs allows pre-lingual patients to detect stimulation coming from an implant but is insufficient for speech comprehension. The recruitment of auditory association areas by other cognitive processes, particularly by non-auditory language, is probably accompanied by an irreversible depression of connections from the primary auditory regions. Consistently, a reduction of activation in secondary auditory and association language areas in response to speech was observed in pre-lingual CI patients compared to normal and post-lingual CI patients (Naito *et al.*, 1997).

Auditory deprivation is also responsible for an enhancement of visual performance associated with increased activation of areas related to vision. This is illustrated by experiments showing that congenitally deaf people have shorter reaction times and larger evoked responses and recruit cortical visual areas (e.g., V5/V5a) more than normal-hearing subjects' cortical visual areas (*e.g.*, V5/V5a) (Bavelier *et al.*, 2000; Neville and Lawson, 1987a–c; Rettenbach *et al.*, 1999). Electric stimulation of the auditory nerve during preimplantation tests has permitted direct confirmation of the relative sparing of primary auditory regions against takeover by other sensory modalities. Most studies consistently show an activation of the primary auditory cortex in pre-lingual CI adults; however, patients do not systematically experience such stimulation as an "auditory" sensation. Auditory nerve stimulation can be associated with additional manifestations such as eye movements or somatosensory sensations (Ponton *et al.*, 1993) probably due to excitation of other nerves located in the vicinity of the electrodes or perhaps due to the development of cross-modal connections. More surprisingly, some patients report no sensation at all despite significant cortical responses (Truy *et al.*, 1995).

PLASTICITY ASSOCIATED WITH POST-LINGUAL DEAFNESS

Studies in humans and animals illustrate critical periods for both language and hearing development. If implantation is performed later, its usefulness for oral communication is generally compromised. In contrast to pre-lingual CI patients, those patients who lose hearing after the critical stages of language development show sound-induced responses after implantation that extend to secondary auditory and association cortices, often very soon after implantation (*i.e.*, before significant language rehabilitation) (Naito *et al.*, 1997; Okazawa *et al.*, 1996).

We observed in a recent study that post-lingual CI patients scanned in the first week after implant switch-on recruited primary and nonprimary auditory cortices contralateral to the implant. The activation of nonprimary auditory areas, however, was not specific and occurred in response to any sound (Fig. 8.1). This observation correlated with the inability of patients to distinguish speech from noises at that stage.

Nonspecific cortical responses contralateral to auditory nerve stimulation are not very informative about deafness-induced plasticity, as similar responses persist after implantation in both pre- and post-lingual CI patients (Naito *et al.*, 1995). Responses specifically associated with speech stimuli very early after implantation reveal more about the impact of deafness on the organisation of the language system. Although secondary auditory and association areas can be recruited by sounds, even after a long period of deafness, their specificity is profoundly altered. The response patterns resulting from deafness undergo major reorganisation in the months following implantation.

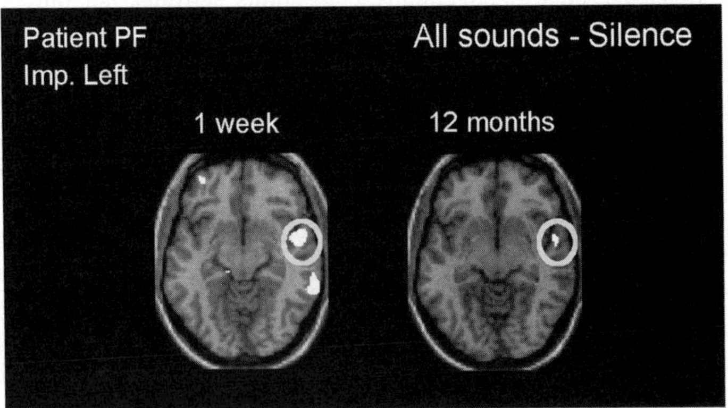

FIGURE 8.1
In a post-lingually deaf patient implanted on the left side, auditory cortex activation in response to speech and noise was contrasted with silent baseline (implant switched on). The patient was scanned with PET one week after the implant was first switched on and one year later. Activation of primary and nonprimary auditory cortices is observed one week after the implant was switched on; a year later, sound-related activation is focused on a region close to the primary auditory cortex.

PLASTICITY SUBSEQUENT TO IMPLANTATION

Recent imaging studies show that cortical reorganisation can be observed in adults after implantation (Suarez *et al.*, 1999). These studies are mostly conducted in implanted post-lingually deaf adults, as pre-lingual deaf adults are no longer implanted and children cannot undergo scanning with radioactive tracers.

Reorganisation of the Primary Auditory Cortex

A reduction of both the number of activated regions in the whole brain and widespread activity within the primary auditory region have been observed when comparing data acquired one week after implantation and one year later in the same post-lingual patients (Fig. 8.1). Similar reductions of activation are shown in control subjects during explicit learning. They are associated with an increase in strength of the connectivity between regions implicated in the learning process (Buechel *et al.*, 1999). Improvement of synaptic efficiency in association with reduction of attentional effort when processing sounds may account for these observations in CI patients.

There is an apparent discrepancy between these observations and findings in animals showing an enlargement of cortical regions stimulated by implants (Klinke *et al.*, 1999). Such enlargements merely result from the absence of concurrent stimulation when using single-channel stimulation in congenitally deaf animals. With multichannel implants, as in post-lingual CI patients, the situation is closer to physiological conditions where competition for cortical space can occur within the primary auditory cortex due to concurrent stimulation of neighbouring electrodes and across auditory areas due to feedback connections from secondary and association areas.

Reorganisation of the Speech Perception System

To study the full range of adaptive plasticity, experimental design must go beyond mapping and address in detail the stimulus–response functions in areas where changes are expected. Many studies have described cerebral activation patterns in response to speech in post-lingual CI patients. Very few of them, however, have shown responses that are specific to speech in comparison to other sound categories and how these responses evolve over time after implantation.

As mentioned above, very soon after implantation words (contrasted with silence) are processed mostly by the contralateral association auditory cortex, whatever the side of implant. After a year of practice, activation specific to words (words > noises) appears in the same patients and progressively involves the classical left language regions. Yet, a clear left-sided activation may be observed only after rehabilitation in patients with very good performance. In these patients, activation patterns are very similar to those of normal hearing subjects, although less lateralised (Figs. 8.2 and 8.3).

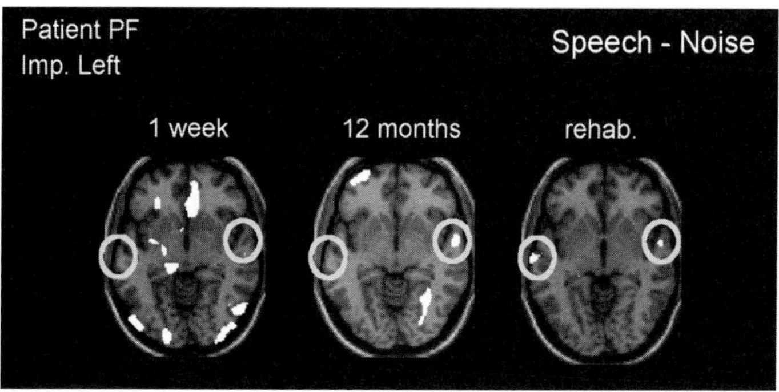

FIGURE 8.2
Evolution of speech-related activations in the auditory cortex in the same patient as in Fig. 8.1. At one week, no brain region is specifically associated with speech. After one year, speech recruits the auditory cortex contralateral to implant. After complete rehabilitation, speech activates only the classical superior temporal speech regions of the left hemisphere.

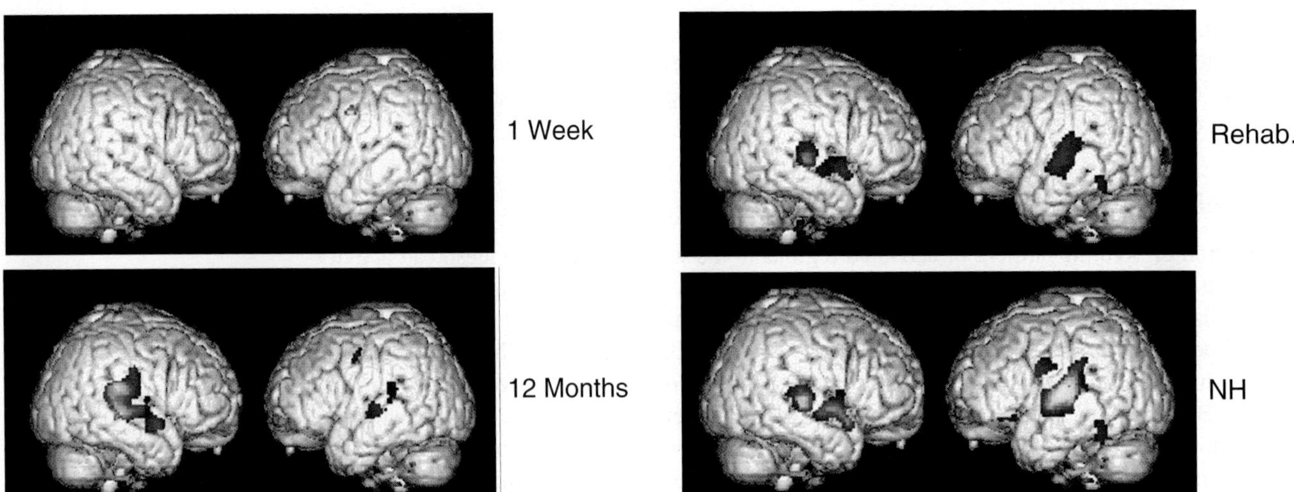

FIGURE 8.3
Cerebral activations with PET in groups of post-lingual cochlear implant patients tested at different stages of the rehabilitation process. The same four patients were tested during the first week after the implant switch-on and a year later. A group of six other patients were tested with an identical protocol after complete rehabilitation (Rehab.). The response patterns can be compared to normal-hearing subjects (NH). After several days of practice with the implant, speech does not produce specific cortical activation when contrasted with noises. After one year of practice, speech specifically involves peri-Sylvian regions, mostly in the right hemisphere (two of four patients were implanted on the left). In rehabilitated patients, the cortical pattern associated with speech is similar to normals, particularly in regard to restoration of the implication of the left hemisphere.

In a cross-sectional study involving post- and pre-lingual CI patients, Naito *et al.* (1997) did not observe a significant correlation between the relative increase in regional cerebral blood flow in left auditory association areas (BA21/22) in response to speech and the duration of practice with an implant. In the same cortical regions, a significant correlation with duration of implant utilisation was observed in post-lingual patients but only when meaningful stimuli (environmental sounds, words, and syllables) were contrasted with noises (Giraud *et al.*, 2001b). These two observations converge to suggest that the language system progressively learns to differentiate meaningful sounds from noises and that it probably does so by progressively reducing the entry of irrelevant inputs evoked by meaningless noises into the language system.

Several studies had previously shown that Wernicke's area was activated in post-lingual and even pre-lingual CI patients in response to speech (Okazawa *et al.*, 1996; Naito *et al.*, 1997); however, the specificity of the response was not clear. While studying the functional response properties of language-specific cortical regions and their plasticity, we demonstrated that Wernicke's area had broader response properties in rehabilitated post-lingual implant patients than in normal-hearing controls (Giraud *et al.*, 2001a) (Fig. 8.4). Wernicke's area responded selectively to words and syllables but not to environmental sounds and noises in controls (Giraud and Price, 2001), whereas in patients it also responded to nonverbal meaningful sounds (environmental sounds).

Altogether the studies suggest that deafness induces a loss of functional specialisation in auditory association areas. This process can be reversed by implantation. Some degree of specialisation is progressively reacquired but even in long-term rehabilitated CI patients remains cruder than in normal-hearing subjects. These findings confirm earlier observations made in CI patients that, unlike the obligatory recruitment of primary auditory cortex, recruitment of auditory association areas relies on experience and depends on the nature of the chronic auditory input.

Reorganisation in Multi-Modal Systems: Semantics, Memory, and Attention

Hard-wired reorganisation such as changes in functional specialisation of a given cortical region (remapping) is largely dependent on the nature of the afferent stimuli. It can be distinguished from other forms of adaptation that are more flexible and depend on task requirement (compre-

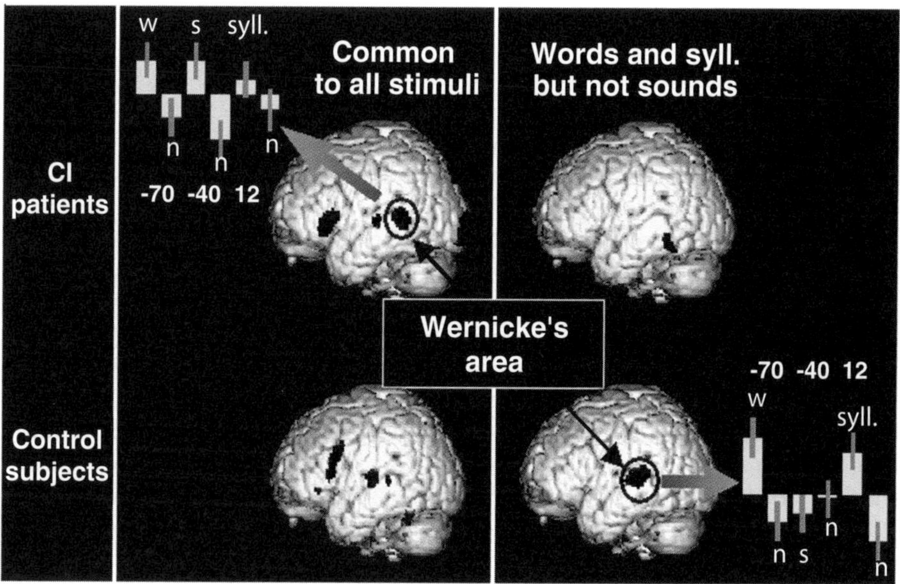

FIGURE 8.4
Wernicke's area (circle) has a finer functional specialisation in normal-hearing subjects than in rehabilitated post-lingual cochlear implant patients. This region is only recruited by speech in controls (w, words; syll, syllables) but also responds to environmental sounds (s) in cochlear implant patients. In both groups Wernicke's area does not respond to noices (n). (Adapted from Giraud *et al.*, 2001a.)

hension, repetition, passive listening) rather than on stimulus characteristics. This latter form of reorganisation implicates supramodal brain regions such as the semantic system and regions involved in memory and executive functions.

Several imaging studies have suggested that sound processing requires the involvement of larger cortical networks in CI users than in normal hearing subjects (Giraud *et al.*, 2000; Naito *et al.*, 2000). Wong *et al.* (1999) showed with PET that processing strategies in post-lingual CI patients differed from those in normal hearing subjects. These strategies involved brain regions outside the speech network, in particular the semantic system. We confirmed decreased responses in semantic regions in patients compared to control subjects (Giraud *et al.*, 2000) and sought to understand whether this indicated reduced semantics-related activations without changes in the response properties or alterations of the nature of the processes taking place in semantic regions (Giraud *et al.*, 2001a). An activation of the left anterior inferior temporal region was observed in normal-hearing subjects (Giraud and Price, 2001) but not consistently in CI patients. Decreased levels of activation and larger interindividual variability in CI patients than controls were also observed in the temporoparietal junction (BA21/39), another multimodal semantic region (Mummery *et al.*, 1998). No change in functional specialisation was associated with decreased activations in inferotemporal and temporoparietal semantic regions. We concluded that the same semantic regions are implicated in patients and controls, but their recruitment is less systematic in CI patients.

Semantic processing in post-lingual CI patients implicates more brain regions than in controls. We observed that meaningful sounds (words and environmental sounds) not only engaged semantic regions but also the parahippocampal gyrus, whereas meaningless sounds did not. In control subjects, no such activation was observed (Giraud *et al.*, 2001a). Activation of the parahippocampal region, a region that interfaces between perception and encoding of stimuli (Buffalo *et al.*, 1999; McDermott *et al.*, 1999; Rombouts *et al.*, 1999), suggests that mnemonic contributions to speech comprehension with an implant are important. This is not surprising since even very good implant performers compensate for acoustic ambiguities with an increased utilisation of contextual information (Wong *et al.*, 1999), which requires more internal rehearsing and more elaborate mnemonic operations.

Attention is another cognitive faculty that helps patients to increase the accuracy of comprehension when facing incomplete and ambiguous auditory stimuli. We observed that post-lingual rehabilitated patients recruit a set of regions classically involved in attention (Benedict *et al.*, 1998; Coull and Nobre, 1998; Rushworth *et al.*, 2001) in many auditory situations but also in the mere expectancy of auditory stimuli (Giraud *et al.*, 2000). Patients implanted on the left side showed a larger effect than the right implanted patients in the left lateral premotor and intraparietal regions when they were attending to speech. Activation of attentional regions reflects specific strategies to compensate for processing degraded speech signals with monaural stimulation (O'Leary *et al.*, 1996).

There is further evidence of enhanced attentional top-down mechanisms in sound processing in CI patients. When listening to sentences (contrasted with low-level auditory baselines), CI patients but not normal-hearing subjects recruited Heschl's gyrus. Recruitment of Heschl's gyrus is likely to correspond to top-down modulation of early auditory processing that is evoked by task demand. Greater activity in patients than in controls was observed in the lower brainstem at a location compatible with that of the superior olivary complex, during a task when speech stimuli were expected. This structure contains efferent neurons involved in low-level attentional mechanisms (Giard *et al.*, 1994) and in extraction of speech signals from background noise (*Giraud et al.*, 1997). As the olivo-cochlear neurons are no longer functional in CI patients, it is plausible to assume that top-down control should take place at the first stage where ascending auditory information can be modulated. These findings suggest that enhanced modulation via feedback loops also contributes to speech comprehension after cochlear implantation.

The conclusion of these studies is that patients resort to various neural strategies to access the meaning of sounds and achieve performance that are similar to those of controls. They recruit the semantic system in a less-specific and systematic way than controls but manage identical tasks by going through concurrent steps involving nonspecific cognitive networks such as those underlying attention and memory. The redistribution of cognitive resources in patients can be viewed as a form of cortical plasticity that does not entail alterations of functional neuroanatomy.

Cross-Modal Reorganisation

Several PET imaging studies have systematically pointed to an involvement of visual cortex in response to sounds in the absence of any visual stimulus (Young *et al.*, 1998; Giraud *et al.*, 2000, 2001a). We recently confirmed another form of postimplantation reorganisation that involves cortical regions beyond association areas and supramodal networks (Giraud *et al.*, 2001b). We found that visual cortex was activated by sounds as early as several days after the implant is switched on. Increased excitability of visual cortex by sounds does not merely reflect dependence on vision (in particular, lip-reading) during previous deafness; rather than attenuating after auditory restoration, the effect refines as a function of time from implantation (Fig. 8.5). The visual responses become increasingly selective to sounds that are likely to convey a meaning (words, syllables, and environmental sounds) and require complementary visual processing. Specific activation of the visual cortical response to meaning evolves in parallel with discrimination of noises from meaningful sounds in the association auditory cortex (BA42/22). No such evolution of neuronal response properties is observed in the primary auditory cortex, which remains sensitive to any kind of sound over time.

Parallel refinement of neural response properties in visual and auditory association areas can result from cross-modal learning. Similarly located activations in early visual cortex (B18, V2) were observed in response to pure tones after subjects had been trained to make specific audiovisual associations (*i.e.*, learned that tones signalled visual events) (McIntosh *et al.*, 1998). After such training, presentation of one stimulus alone raised the expectancy of the other and thus engaged the nonstimulated modality. These effects could be mediated by direct connections between auditory and visual association cortices or by higher order cortical areas. A regression analysis performed in CI patients showed that visual cortical activity correlated with that of superior parietal cortex (Giraud *et al.*, 2001b). This attentional region could relay cross-modal effects.

After implantation, patients learn to match new and ambiguous sounds with their visual source. As the main goal of patients' everyday training is speech comprehension, we hypothesised that visual activation should somehow be related to the visual support to speech, lip-reading. We observed a positive correlation between lip-reading abilities and visual cortical

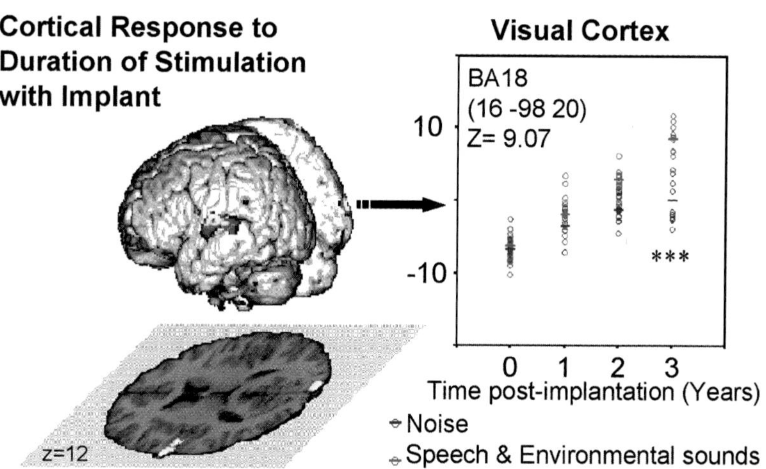

FIGURE 8.5
In post-lingual cochlear implants patients, the response of visual cortex to sounds evolves as a function of time after implantation in a stimulus-specific manner. Visual cortical activation was observed together with activation of auditory and superior parietal cortices. (Adapted from Giraud *et al.*, 2001b.)

recruitment; patients with the larger cerebral blood flow increases in this region were also those with the better lip-reading performances. As this observation seemed to contradict the intuitive idea that after implantation patients should rely less on lip-reading, we studied the evolution of lip-reading performance after implantation in 20 post-lingual patients. We observed an initial decrease of lip-reading performance just after implantation followed by a slight but significant improvement of performance, which parallels the refinement of the response properties in visual cortex.

As previously deduced from behavioural data in pre-lingual patients (Tyler *et al.*, 1997), these findings suggest that implantation promotes a mutual reinforcement of vision and hearing.

PLASTICITY AS A PREDICTOR OF THE OUTCOME OF IMPLANTATION

Aside from providing direct insights into the mechanisms of cortical plasticity, imaging techniques are expected to predict the outcome of implantation. Lee *et al.* (2001) recently demonstrated that speech perception after implantation was better if auditory cortex had been hypometabolic before implantation. Resting metabolic activity indicates to which extent deprived cortices have been taken over by competing synaptic inputs, a process that is detrimental to reconnecting the auditory signals to large-scale neural circuits. The study demonstrates a significant correlation between the degree of hypometabolism before implantation and the outcome of implantation. The study fits with former findings that showed (1) increased metabolic activity in the auditory cortices in cases of deafness of early onset and in the visual cortex of congenitally blind subjects (Catalan-Ahumada *et al.*, 1993), and (2) decreased metabolic activity in auditory cortex for post-lingual deafness of short duration (Ito *et al.*, 1993).

CONCLUSION

Brain imaging in cochlear implant patients has permitted identification and characterisation of different forms of brain plasticity associated with sensory deprivation and reafferentation and to delineation of the large-scale neuronal networks in which functional plasticity can operate. Cortical plasticity resulting from deafness generally spares primary auditory regions but affects post-processing cortices. The degree and nature of reorganisation in secondary and association auditory cortices depends on whether deafness occurred before or after critical stages in language development. In pre-lingual deaf subjects, hard-wired cross-modal connections preclude further participation of these regions in oral communication. In post-lingual deaf patients, cross-modal compensation is less dramatic and allows for functional recovery. Brain plasticity continues after implantation. As with deafness, the most important time-related changes are not observed in primary regions but rather in auditory association cortices, where modifications of the functional specialisation have been observed. Implantation also challenges supramodal cognitive resources which translates into a redistribution of the level of activity between brain regions involved in attention and memory and semantic processing. Repeated use of specific cognitive strategies by patients induces further cortical plasticity. The use of visual cues to compensate for missing auditory information progressively gives rise to stable and highly specialised cross-modal effects. The dynamics of these effects suggest that restoring auditory input yields a mutual reinforcement of vision and hearing rather than a return to segregation between the senses.

Acknowledgments

ALG is funded by the Alexander von Humboldt Stiftung.

References

Bavelier, D. and Neville, H. J. (2002, June). Cross-modal plasticity: where and how? *Nat. Rev. Neurosci.*, **3**(6), 443–452.

Bavelier, D., Tomann, A., Hutton, C., Mitchell, T., Corina, D., Liu, G., and Neville, H. (2000). Visual attention to the periphery is enhanced in congenitally deaf individuals. *J. Neurosci.*, **20**, 1–6.

Benedict, R. H. B., Lockwood, A. H., Shucard, J. L., Shucard, D. W., Wack, D., and Murphy, B. W. (1998). Functional neuroimaging of attention in the auditory modality. *NeuroReport*, **9**, 121–126.

Buechel, C., Coull, J. T., and Friston, K. J. (1999). The predictive value of changes in effective connectivity for human learning. Science, **283**,1538–1541.

Buffalo, E. A., Ramus, S. J., Clark, R. E., Teng, E., Squire, L. R., and Zola, S. M. (1999). Dissociation between the effects of damage to perirhinal cortex and area TE, *Learn. Mem.*, **6**, 572–599.

Catalan-Ahumada, M., Deggouj, N., De Volder, A., Melin, J., Michel, C., and Veraart, C. (1993). High metabolic activity demonstrated by positron emission tomography in human auditory cortex in case of deafness of early onset. *Brain Res.*, **623**, 287–292.

Coull, J. T. and Nobre, A. C. (1998). Where and when to pay attention: the neural systems for directing attention to spatial locations and to time intervals as revealed by both PET and fMRI. *J. Neurosci.*, **18**, 7426–7435.

Giard, M.-H., Collet, L., Bouchet, P., and Pernier, J. (1994). Auditory selective attention in the human cochlea. *Hear. Res.*, **33**, 353–356.

Giraud, A. L. and Price, C. J. (2001). The constraints functional neuroimaging places on classical models of auditory word processing. *J. Cogn. Neurosci.*, **13**, 754–765.

Giraud, A.-L., Garnier, S., Micheyl, C., Lina, G., Chays, A., and Chéry-Croze, S. (1997). Auditory efferents involved in speech-in-noise intelligibility. *NeuroReport*, **7**, 1779–1783.

Giraud, A. L., Truy, E., Frackowiak, R. S. J., Grégoire, M. C., Pujol, J. F., and Collet, L. (2000). Differential recruitment of the speech comprehension system in healthy subjects and rehabilitated cochlear implant patients. *Brain*, **123**, 1391–1402.

Giraud, A. L., Price, C. J., Graham, J. M., and Frackowiak, R. S. J. (2001a). Functional plasticity of language-related brain areas after cochlear implantation. *Brain*, **124**, 101–110.

Giraud, A. L., Price, C. J., Graham, J. M., Truy, E., and Frackowiak, R. S. J. (2001b). Cross-modal plasticity underpins recovery of language function after cochlear implantation. *Neuron*, **30**, 657–663.

Herzog, H., Lamprecht, A., Kuhn, A., Roden, W., Vosteen, K. H., and Feinendegen, L. E. (1991). Cortical activation in profoundly deaf patients during cochlear implant stimulation demonstrated by $H_2(15)O$ PET. *J. Comput. Assist. Tomogr.*, **15**, 369–375.

Ito, J., Sakakibara, J., Iwasaki, Y., and Yonekura, Y. (1993). Positron emission tomography of auditory sensation in deaf patients and patients with cochlear implants. *Ann. Otol. Rhinol. Laryngol.*, **102**, 797–801.

Klinke, R., Kral, A., Heid, S., Tillein, J., and Hartmann, R. (1999). Recruitment of the auditory cortex in congenitally deaf cats by long-term cochlear electrostimulation. *Science*, **285**, 1729–1733.

Lee, D. S., Lee, J. S., Oh, S. H., Kim, S. K., Kim, J. W., Chung, J. K., Lee, M. C., and Kim, C. S. (2001). Cross-modal plasticity and cochlear implants. *Nature*, **409**, 149–150.

McDermott, K. B., Ojemann, J. G., Petersen, S. E., Ollinger, J. M., Snyder, A. Z., Akbudak, E., Conturo, T. E., and Raichle, M. E. (1999). Direct comparison of episodic encoding and retrieval of words: an event-related fMRI study. *Memory* , **7**, 661–678.

McIntosh, A. R., Cabeza, R. E., and Lobaugh, N. J. (1998). Analysis of neural interactions explains the activation of occipital cortex by an auditory stimulus. *J. Neurophysiol.*, **80**, 2790–2796.

Mummery, C. J., Patterson, K., Hodges, J. R., and Price, C. J. (1998). Functional neuroanatomy of the semantic system, divisible by what? *J. Cogn. Neurosci.*, **10**, 766–777.

Naito, Y., Okazawa, H., Honjo, I., Hirano, S., Takahashi, H., Shiomi, Y., Hoji, W., Kawano, M., Ishizu, K., and Yonekura,

Y. (1995). Cortical activation with sound stimulation in cochlear implant users demonstrated by positron emission tomography. *Brain Res. Cogn. Brain Res.*, **2**, 207–14.

Naito, Y., Hirano, S., Honjo, I., Okazawa, H., Ishizu, K., Takahashi, H., Fujiki, N., Shiomi, Y., Yonekura, Y., and Konishi, J. (1997). Sound-induced activation of auditory cortices in cochlear implant users with post- and prelingual deafness demonstrated by positron emission tomography. *Acta Otolaryngol.*, **117**, 490–496.

Naito, Y., Tateya, I., Fujiki, N., Hirano, S., Ishizu, K., Nagahama, Y., Fukuyama, H., and Kojima, H. (2000). Increased cortical activation during hearing of speech in cochlear implant users. *Hear. Res.*, **143**, 139–146.

Neville, H. J. and Lawson, D. (1987a). Attention to central and peripheral visual space in a movement detection task: an event-related potential and behavioural study. I. Normal hearing adults. *Brain Res.*, **405**, 253–267.

Neville, H. J. and Lawson, D. (1987b). Attention to central and peripheral visual space in a movement detection task: an event-related potential and behavioural study. II. Congenitally deaf adults. *Brain Res.*, **405**, 268–283.

Neville, H. J. and Lawson, D. (1987c). Attention to central and peripheral visual space in a movement detection task. III. Separate effects of auditory deprivation and acquisition of a visual language. *Brain Res.*, **405**, 284–294.

Nishimura, H., Hashikawa, K., Doi, K., Iwaki, T., Watanabe, Y., Kusuoka, H., Nishimura, T., and Kubo, T. (1999). Sign language 'heard' in the auditory cortex. *Nature*, **397**, 116.

Nishimura, H., Doi, K., Iwaki, T., Hashikawa, K., Oku, N., Teratani, T., Hasegawa, T., Watanabe, A., Nishimura, T., and Kubo, T. (2000). Neural plasticity detected in short- and long-term cochlear implant users using PET. *NeuroReport*, **11**, 811–815.

O'Leary, D. S., Andreason, N. C., Hurtig, R. R., Hishwa, R. D., Watkins, G. L., Ponton, L. L., Rogers, M., Kirchner, P. T. (1996). A positron emission tomography study of binaurally and dichotically presented stimuli: effects of language and directed attention. *Brain Lang.*, **53**, 20–39.

Okazawa, H., Naito, Y., Yonekura, Y., Sadato, N., Hirano, S., Nishizawa, S., Magata, Y., Ishizu, K., Tamaki, N., Honjo, I., and Konishi, J. (1996). Cochlear implant efficiency in pre- and postlingually deaf subjects: a study with $H_2(15)O$ and PET. *Brain*, **119**, 1297–1306.

Petitto, L. A., Zatorre, R. J., Gauna, K., Nikelski, E. J., Dostie, D., and Evans, A. C. (2000). Speech-like cerebral activity in profoundly deaf people processing signed languages: implications for the neural basis of human language. *Proc. Natl. Acad. Sci. USA*, **95**, 13961–13966.

Ponton, C. W., Don, M., Waring, M. D., Eggermont, J. J., and Masuda, A. (1993). Spatio-temporal source modeling of evoked potentials to acoustic and cochlear implant stimulation. *Electroencephalogr. Clin. Neurophysiol.*, **88**, 478–493.

Rettenbach, R., Diller, G., and Sireteanu, R. (1999). Do deaf people see better? Texture segmentation and visual search compensate in adult but not in juvenile subjects. *J. Cogn. Neurosci.*, **11**, 560–583.

Rombouts, S. A., Scheltens, P., Machielson, W. C., Barkhof, F., Hoogenraad, F. G., Veltman, D. J., Valk, J., and Witter, M. P. (1999). Parametric fMRI analysis of visual encoding in the human medial temporal lobe. *Hippocampus*, **9**, 637–643.

Rushworth, M. F., Krams, M., and Passingham, R. E. (2001, July). The attentional role of the left parietal cortex: the distinct lateralization and localization of motor attention in the human brain. *J. Cogn. Neurosci.*, **13**(5), 698–710.

Suarez, H., Mut, F., Lago, G., Silveira, A., De Bellis, C., Velluti, R., Pedemonte, M., and Svirsky, M. (1999). Changes in the cerebral blood flow in postlingual cochlear implant users. *Acta Otolaryngol.*, **119**, 239–243.

Truy, E., Deiber, M. P., Cinotti, L., Mauguiere, F., Froment, J. C., and Morgon, A. (1995). Auditory cortex activity changes in long-term sensorineural deprivation during crude cochlear electrical stimulation: evaluation by positron emission tomography. *Hear. Res.*, **86**, 34–42.

Tyler, R. S., Fryauf-Bertschy, H., Kelsay, D. M., Gantz, B. J., Woodworth, G. P., and Parkinson, A. (1997). Speech perception by prelingually deaf children using cochlear implants. *Otolaryngol. Head Neck Surg.*, **117**, 180–187.

Wong, D., Miyamoto, R. T., Pisoni, D. B., Sehgal, M., and Hutchins, G. D. (1999). PET imaging of cochlear-implant and normal-hearing subjects listening to speech and nonspeech. *Hear. Res.*, **132**, 34–42.

Young, J. P., O'Sullivan, B. T., Gibson, W. P., Mitchell, T., Sanli, H., Withall, A., and Cervantes, R. (1998). Assessment of auditory cortical function in cochlear implant patients. *NeuroImage*, S384.

SECTION TWO

VISION AND VISUAL PERCEPTION

CHAPTER

9

Functional Specialisation in the Visual Brain: Probable and Improbable Visual Areas

INTRODUCTION

The foundation of much that is interesting and important in discoveries relating to the visual brain lies in its functional specialisation (Zeki, 1978; Zeki *et al.*, 1991). Indeed, the work of the past 10 years, especially in the human brain, has reinforced and extended this doctrine, derived from studies of the monkey brain in the 1970s. Before studies of monkey prestriate cortex were undertaken, the dominant view of how the visual brain is organised was that of Hubel and Wiesel (1977), whose brilliant studies had concentrated largely on one property, that of orientation selectivity. Sterling information was obtained about the specificity of connections in the visual brain, the columnar organisation of cells with common properties, the relationship of orientation columns to ocular dominance columns, and the relative contributions of nature and nurture to the functioning of the primary visual cortex, area V1. But, this work also led them to the somewhat erroneous conclusion that the visual brain is organised in a hierarchical fashion, with one area feeding another in succession and in the process generating areas with larger receptive fields and more complex properties. There are many features of brain organisation that such a postulated exclusive hierarchy fails to account for. Chief among these is the clinical picture, where damage to one area does not lead to total blindness but to an incapacity to perceive a specific attribute of the visual scene—for example, colour. Other features that we discuss below are the demonstrable perceptual hierarchy in vision, with different attributes being perceived at different times in a manner that no one had predicted, with colour being perceived before motion, which in turn is perceived before orientation (Moutoussis and Zeki, 1997a,b). Although no prediction in this regard was made from the principle of exclusive hierarchies, one would have expected all attributes of a certain complexity to be perceived at the same time, in relation to distance in time from stimulus appearance to processing. One would have expected, for example, that motion and orientation and colour would be processed simultaneously, as cells representing all categories are found in V1 and in V2. One would have also expected to find somewhere cells that are specific for orientation and colour and depth and motion and other attributes besides, but no such cells have been discovered, nor would one have predicted the observed chronoarchitecture of the visual brain, with different areas having different activity time courses (ATCs).

It is almost certain that this hierarchical concept developed largely (though not solely) because Hubel and Wiesel's earlier studies had been done mainly in the cat, an animal that, among other things, lacks what is commonly understood to be colour vision, with the consequence that no attention was paid to one of the most distinctive and easily separable attributes of vision. It is also partly the result of concentrating on orientation selectivity almost exclusively. This is probably why, in their early work, Hubel and Wiesel failed to recognise the functional specialisation that is such a distinctive feature of the visual brain, including even area 17 (V1). In fact, the subsequent studies of Livingstone and Hubel (1988) confirmed dramatically the presence of functional specialisation that had been predicted for V1 from a study of the specialisation of the areas to which V1 connects (Zeki, 1975). Much of the descriptions and theorising that comprise this and the following chapters of this section are therefore based on the concept of functional specialisation in the primate and especially the human visual brain.

In spite of the overwhelming evidence in its favour, there are still those who believe that the pursuit of functional specialisation in the visual brain is an outdated folly. They believe instead in what they call "multifunctionality." Schiller (1997), for example, writes: "Neurons become increasingly multifunctional as one ascends from peripheral to central structures in the nervous system; this is an especially notable property of cortical neurons" (a property that those who have recorded from directionally selective cells in V5 or orientation-selective cells in V3 or colour cells in V4 have searched for in vain). Schiller continues: "The process of *perceptual analysis* in the visual system is not to break down the visual scene into basic components. Such analysis is performed interactively by areas and neurons with multipurpose properties" (original emphasis). If true, then this is something that has been remarkable difficult to demonstrate with imaging experiments; indeed, imaging experiments collectively speak in favour of functional specialisation and against the doctrine of multifunctionality.

Multifunctionality, which is yesterday's hierarchy in disguise, is a view with which we do not therefore agree and will not pursue further in this essay. Of course, it is always possible to argue that the functional specialisation that has been so often demonstrated, especially by imaging experiments, is nothing more than the consequence of the technique employed. In physiology, conclusions are reached from single-cell recordings, either in the anaesthetised state, when everything else that is interesting is both dormant and isolated, or in the awake state, when a single attribute is selected. In anatomy, connections are studied that do not permit one to reach adequate conclusions about their dynamic state in the behaving organism. In imaging experiments, the experimenter formulates a hypothesis that he tests with highly selected and sometimes perhaps artificial stimuli, ones that the average individual is unlikely to encounter regularly, if at all, in daily existence. In real life, the argument may go, all these areas interact and the real analysis of the visual scene is thus performed interactively by the putatively ubiquitous "multipurpose neurons." Hence, if we could only image the activity in the brain during normal and complex viewing conditions, when the visual brain is stimulated with many attributes simultaneously we will find the activity in all these "specialised" areas to be highly correlated; it would then be difficult to be certain about the status of functional specialisation or draw any satisfactory conclusions about it. In fact, recent studies on the *chronoarchitecture* of the cerebral cortex show that it is in complex viewing conditions that the specialised areas are least correlated and therefore seem to be acting most autonomously, while the correlation between them is highest in quiescent states. This seemingly turns the above argument on its head. The best means of showing that the specialised areas are uncorrelated, and thus undifferentiated in terms of the time course of their activity, is in the quiescent state, when the brain is not stimulated.

The concept of functional specialisation in the visual brain is therefore central to the discussion that follows, where we explore its consequences. The reason for such a specialisation in the brain has been debated. One argument, true of almost any fact about the brain, is that it confers some evolutionary advantage. To the extent that this explains everything, it also explains nothing. We also do not find compelling the argument that functional specialisation is the consequence of a sort of evolutionary "economic housewife" attitude, designed to maintain the connections as short and therefore as economical as possible. Among the shortest connections in the brain are those between the blobs and the interblobs of V1 or between the thin stripes and interstripes of V2 (Rockland, 1985; Lund *et al.*, 1993). Yet, these connections do not erode the specialisation of cells in the compartments nor do they enhance multifunctionality. Even more, if the economic housewife argument were compelling, it would be difficult to see why the cortex wedges islands of wavelength-selective cells between non-wavelength-selective cells, making it necessary to have longer blob-to-blob connections than would otherwise be the case. On the other hand, longer connections, such as between V1 and V5, seem to enhance the specialisation of V5.

Given the apparent poverty of these arguments, we fall back on what seems to us to be the most convincing ones available currently. These are twofold: (1) that attributes of the visual world vary independently and hence must be independently represented, at least at some level (see below with respect to chronoarchitecture); and (2) that the requirements for constructing different attributes of the visual scene, such as colour or motion, are sufficiently different to require radically different machineries for their processing (Zeki, 1993). These differences are both of time and space. For colour, the brain must gauge the wavelength composition of the light coming from one patch and from spatially surrounding areas simultaneously in time; for motion, it is succession in time that is critical. We believe that these different requirements necessitate not only different cortical machineries, but also entail different processing times. These differences in processing times are what also lead to a temporal asynchrony in visual perception and to the distinctive chronoarchitecture of the cerebral cortex, both topics taken up below.

IMPROBABLE AREAS IN THE VISUAL BRAIN

The concept of functional specialisation is implicitly extended every time a new specialised area is discovered in the human brain, and there have been many such areas in the past 10 years, attesting to the health and vigour of our subject. But, every time a specific zone of the cortex is activated specifically by some visual stimuli and not others, one is faced with the question of whether to confer the status of an area on the active region. The apparently indiscriminate way in which cortical zones have been thus honoured makes it necessary to consider (or reconsider) the criteria that must be satisfied for conferring the status of an area on an active region of the cortex. Unless this is done, one could argue with varying degrees of plausibility that an active region is merely a subdivision of an area. In this regard, evidence derived from imaging experiments is not always easy to asses if not accompanied by mapping experiments, and many are not. What is clear is that the imaging community has been prepared to accept a great deal on faith, leading to quaint hypotheses about the way in which the human visual brain is organised. Any discussion of that subject must take into account the kind of evidence that our community has found acceptable enough to merit publication in journals of distinction and the extent to which that evidence is reliable. No discipline should be spared such an assault, and every discipline emerges healthier from it. The discussion that follows is not, however, an assessment of the merits of the techniques that are employed to analyse images of human brain activity. It is rather of the use that has been made of such techniques and of the paradigms submitted to them. It is above all a discussion of whether we should not demand more rigid proof before we accept hypotheses as established.

Criteria for Establishing a Visual Area

The right half of the visual field is represented in the left brain hemisphere, and vice versa, the two separate representations being unified by a commissure that links the two cerebral hemispheres, the corpus callosum (Fig. 9.1). An obvious criterion for conferring the status of a visual area on a region of cortex activated by visual stimuli is that it should have an independent and more or less complete map of the contralateral visual field, to include both the upper and

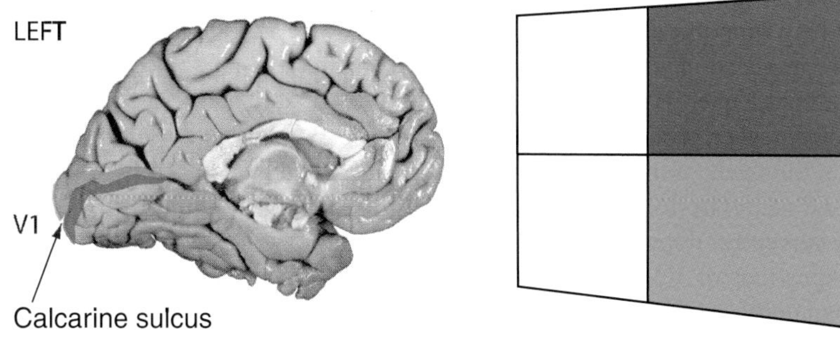

FIGURE 9.1
Representation of the right hemifield in the primary visual cortex, V1. The upper quadrant of the hemifield is represented below the calcarine sulcus, while the lower quadrant is represented above the calcarine sulcus.

lower quadrants. We say "more or less" because it is well known that a given part of the visual field may claim a disproportionately large or small space in terms of representation within an area, the expansion of the part of V1 representing the fovea being a well-known example. This primary criterion, of a more or less complete contralateral visual field representation, is relatively easy to establish, but the critical experiments are not always performed. There is, of course, no reason to suppose that the representation need always be restricted to the contralateral field; in some areas, of which V5 is an example, the ipsilateral field may be represented, as well (Tootell *et al.*, 1995, 1998). The ipsilateral representation in V5 appears to lag behind the contralateral representation by about 6 ms and is absent where the callosum is also absent (ffytche *et al.*, 1998). If confirmed, this would be the first example of what we shall call *chronotopography*, which we define as a temporal succession, however brief, in the representation of the two hemifields. To visual field representation may be added other features such as a distinct set of anatomical, including callosal, connections; identifiable and unique functional properties; and a distinctive architecture (Zeki, 1978), though the search for the latter has not always been fruitful. It is, of course, best if all criteria can be satisfied, but this is not in practice always possible, especially in the human brain.

In 1986, Van Essen's group (Burkhalter and Van Essen, 1986) proposed a radical departure. They had shown, they believed, that one of the areas constituting the primate visual brain, area V3, does not have a complete representation of the visual field, as had been supposed from earlier anatomical studies (Cragg, 1969; Zeki, 1969). Instead, they conceived of this area, which occupies a narrow strip anterior to area "VP" (Fig. 9.2), as being constituted of two different areas, a dorsal one called *V3* and a ventral one which they called *VP*, each representing one quadrant only of the contralateral hemifield. From this arose the strange concept of areas with quarterfield representations of the visual field. Kaas (1993) has referred to these areas as "improbable areas" because their presence implies that they register visual activity in one quadrant alone, without a corresponding area to register the same activity when it occurs in the other quadrant. This is odd; psychophysical experiments have shown that some attributes are more readily perceived when presented in one quadrant than in another (Rubin *et al.*, 1996; Gordon *et al.*, 1997) but none has ever shown that an attribute can only be perceived if presented in a given quadrant alone. In spite of this perceptual difficulty, such improbable areas have been widely, and unthinkingly, accepted by many, though not all, in the imaging community. If present, they would argue for a very distinctive feature of the organisation of the visual brain. The evidence in their favour, however, is so weak that it is surprising that they have gained any currency at all, let alone such wide currency.

The First Improbable Visual Area: "VP"

The first improbable area to be described is "VP", which is really the lower part of V3, but V3 was divided by Van Essen's group into two separate areas: V3 (representing lower visual fields) and "VP" (representing upper visual fields), even though the retinotopic map in ventral V3 ("VP"), in both the human (Sereno *et al.*, 1995; Shipp *et al.*, 1995; De Yoe *et al.*, 1996) and the monkey (Rosa *et al.*, 2000) is a mirror image of that in upper V3 (Fig. 9.2). The separation into two distinct areas was based on the supposition that lower V3, unlike its upper counterpart, not only does not receive a direct anatomical input from the primary visual cortex (area V1) but that it also has a high proportion of colour-selective cells (Burkhalter and Van Essen, 1986), unlike upper V3. The implication was obvious, that "VP" is an area registering activity in the upper contralateral quadrant alone, without a corresponding area to register the same activity (including, above all, colour) when it occurs in the lower contralateral quadrant, or leaving it to some other area to do so. Strangely, this radical idea was not challenged until recently, and then by neuroanatomists and neurophysiologists, not by many in the imaging community who seem to have embraced it fervently, if passively, judging by the multiplicity of publications that use the separate designations of V3 and "VP". This ready acceptance has encouraged a belief in the imaging community, or at least significant sections of it, that there may be other improbable areas in which one quadrant alone of the visual field is represented. Indeed, the precedence of "VP" has been used to erect other improbable areas. The evidence in favour of such a separation is therefore worth examining.

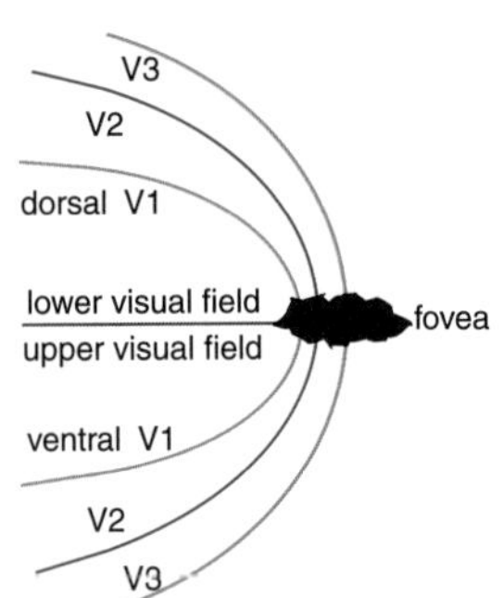

FIGURE 9.2
A schematic diagram of two topographically organised visual areas and their relation to area V1. Red lines show the horizontal meridian, green lines the vertical meridian. (Redrawn from Zeki, 1969.)

The Improbability of the Improbable VP

The notion that there is an asymmetrical anatomical input from V1 to upper and lower V3 was questioned years ago when Gattass *et al.* (1990) showed that there is a direct input from lower V1 to lower V3 in *Cebus*, and when detailed recording experiments showed that there is a continuous representation of visual fields in V3 from lower to upper quadrants as one proceeds dorsoventrally (Rosa *et al.*, 1988). Such findings, made in New World monkeys, have been substantially reinforced by more recent evidence (Lyon and Kaas, 2002) that in the macaque monkey, too, there is a direct input from V1 to V3. That study, with other supporting evidence (Lyon and Kaas, 2001), has led Lyon and Kaas to conclude that V3 is one continuous area, not two separate areas, and that it is characteristic of all primates. Thus, one of the main arguments for separating V3 into two areas, namely an asymmetry in anatomical input from V1, is no longer tenable.

The ready acceptance of such a subdivision in the macaque and its uncritical translation into the human brain, where the two corresponding areas have also been called V3 and "VP" by many, is especially surprising, as all human imaging experiments have shown that upper and lower parts of V3 are activated in the same way (Smith *et al.*, 1998; Press *et al.*, 2001), thus speaking against its separation into two areas, V3 and "VP". More significantly, no human imaging study has ever shown that human "VP" is specifically activated with colour, even when the question has been directly addressed (Wade *et al.*, 2002), although the supposed high concentration of colour cells in lower V3 was one of the main criteria used to separate it off into a separate area. The second criterion for separating V3 into two independent areas, namely an emphasis on colour in "VP", is thus also emaciated. The consensus of the *evidence* seems to be that there is no justification for separating V3 into two areas; V3 is instead one whole area, in which both upper and lower fields are represented, as was originally suggested and as recently strongly emphasised by Lyon and Kaas.

Another Improbable Area: V4v

One of the problems with unquestioning acceptance of the separation of V3 into two areas has been the implicit acceptance, which later became explicit, that there may be other such improbable cortical areas in which one quarter of the field alone is represented. The advent of the phase encoding method (Engel *et al.*, 1994) for mapping visual fields in human cerebral cortex revealed in some hands an area "V4v". The small "v" attached to V4 implied that it maps the upper contralateral quadrant only. No one seemed especially concerned that the same method did not reveal "V4d", the dorsal counterpart that should represent the inferior contralateral quadrant, presumably because of the implicit acceptance that improbable areas may, after all, exist. In fact, "V4v" was thought to be distinct from the human colour centre, area V4, in which both contralateral quadrants are topographically mapped (McKeefry and Zeki, 1997; Bartels and Zeki, 2000) (Fig. 9.3), and damage to which can lead to complete contralateral cerebral colour blindness (hemiachromatopsia) (Verrey, 1888). The confirmation by Hadjikhani *et al.* (1998) that both contralateral quadrants are topographically mapped within the ventrally located V4 reveals eloquently the confusion of experts and bystanders (Heywood and Cowey, 1998) alike, traceable in large measure to the blind acceptance of the concept of improbable areas. Hadjikhani *et al.* (1998) showed, like others before them (McKeefry and Zeki, 1997), that there is a complete representation of the contralateral hemifield within the colour center, V4. But, because of their belief in the existence of an area V4v, distinct from area V4 and representing the upper contralateral hemifield alone, they imagined that they had discovered "a new retinotopic area that we call 'V8'." This "previously undifferentiated cortical area … was consistently located just beyond the most anterior retinotopic area defined previously, area V4*v*" (my emphasis on the "v"). An examination of their results shows, however, that their "new" retinotopic area has in fact the same coordinates as our V4 and is thus nothing more than the rediscovery of a previously defined and named visual area. In spite of this, the claim that a "new" cortical area had been discovered was accepted uncritically (Fig. 9.4).

Heywood and Cowey (1998) wrote somewhat triumphantly that a "newly defined colour area" had been found and that it is this area, "V8", rather than "the favorite candidate, V4," when lesioned, produces cortical colour blindness, thus leading them unquestioningly to the view that

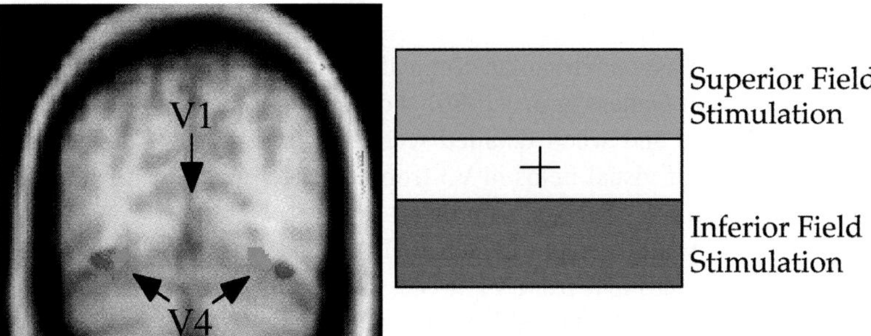

FIGURE 9.3
fMRI image of a coronal section of the visual brain showing activation in V4 produced by a colour Mondrian display. The activation shows the topography of V4, with superior visual field stimulation represented more laterally on the ventral surface of the brain and inferior visual field stimulation represented more medially. (From McKeefry D. and Zeki, S. M., *Brain*, 120, 2229–2242, 1997. With permission.)

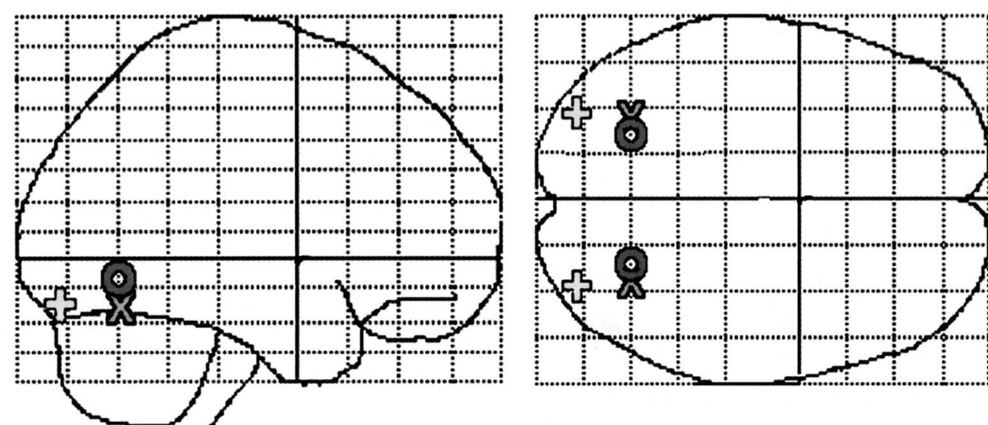

FIGURE 9.4
The locations of the three areas (as discussed in the text) in a glassbrain projection. The areas were located by using the Talairach coordinates of the three areas given in the paper by Hadjikhani *et al.* (1998). ○; s n s n n *et al.* *et al.* n y n **X** s n s n w n *et al.* n + s n s n y n *et al.* . ls . n . . *Eur. J. Neurosci.* . ss n.

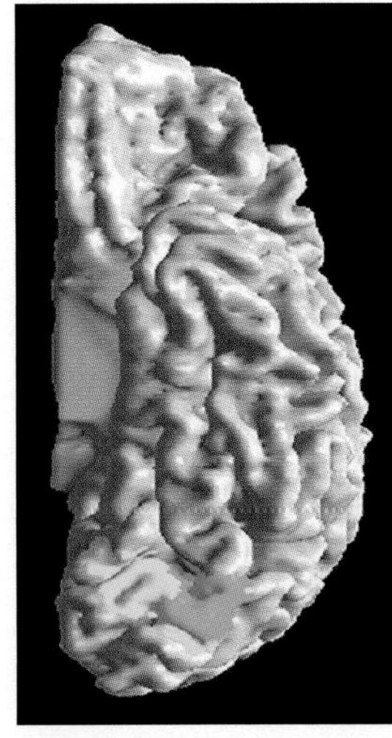

FIGURE 9.5
A ventral view of the left hemisphere.

"the *human* colour center is distinct from area V4." Note how, in this uncritical acceptance, the small "v" has been dropped from the equation. Had the small "v" been a part of the quote, one would have supposed that the "human colour center" lies in front of the improbable "V4v" but is coextensive with V4. This would, in turn, make it very difficult to argue in favour of a new area having been discovered. Of such power are the diminutive letters of the alphabet, especially when cleverly employed!

Does "V4v" Exist?

Tootell and Hadjikhani (2001) have since admitted that their "newly defined" and "previously undifferentiated" cortical area is in fact nothing more than the previously defined colour center but have pleaded that it should be called "V8" because the fourth visual map is constituted by their improbable area "V4v." Much, therefore, hinges on whether an improbable area such as "V4v" exists. We have not been able to find any evidence for a separate area "V4v", nor seemingly have others (*e.g.*, Kastner *et al.*, 1998). The question has been directly addressed by Wade *et al.* (2002) in the most detailed topographic studies of the human visual brain to date. They could not find a quarterfield representation corresponding to area "V4v". Instead, they found that V4 constitutes the fourth visual map, abuts V3, and corresponds to the colour centre of the human brain (Fig. 9.5). Thus, the argument for calling the colour centre "area V8" is etiolated. Given the evidence against a quarterfield representation constituting "V4v", it is up to its proponents and to those who believe in the existence of such improbable areas to demonstrate its existence convincingly and the existence of other improbable areas, or to withdraw it. The ready acceptance by many of the existence of an unproven "V4v", coming on top of the acceptance of the improbable "VP", naturally makes more emphatic questions about the quality of evidence that is deemed as proof of the existence of an area in human brain studies.

Precedence Is Finally Used Explicitly: The Case of KO

The acceptance of the improbable "V4v" was made possible by the implicit acceptance of the improbable "VP". But, the defunct and improbable "VP" has also been used explicitly as a precedent for yet another improbable area, "KO" (kinetic occipital), claimed to be "specialised for the processing of kinetic contours" (Van Oostende *et al.*, 1997). Attempts are currently being made to equate "KO" with dorsal V4 in the macaque ("V4d") (Tootell and Hadjikhani, 2001). The improbability of such an equation is reinforced by the improbability of the function imputed to "KO" from the evidence currently available (see below).

"V4d" is the part of area V4 in the macaque that represents lower visual fields. The equation of this part of macaque V4 alone with human "KO" implies that "KO" represents only lower contralateral visual fields. In fact, human mapping experiments are not compelling in this regard, and the experiments clearly have to be repeated. The evidence of Smith *et al.* (1998) that "KO" (which is better referred to as area V3B) represents only the lower contralateral visual field is not convincing, and their figures could equally well be interpreted to mean that V3A and V3B each contains a complete representation of the contralateral hemifield, though with an underemphasised representation of one quadrant. The evidence of Smith *et al.* is in any case contradicted by the work of Press *et al.* (2001) which shows a complete representation of the contralateral hemifield in V3B ("KO"). The equation of V3B with dorsal V4 ("V4d") alone, as proposed by Tootell and Hadjikhani (2001), would make of human V3B and monkey "V4d" improbable areas, when all the evidence suggests that macaque V4 has a complete map of the contralateral hemifield, "V4d" being nothing more than the dorsal part of V4 (Gattass *et al.*, 1990). In trying to understand why such claims have been so uncritically accepted, it becomes obvious that it is precedent rather than convincing evidence that has had a big role. Tootell and Hadjikhani (2001) have written that, "Although such 'separated' quarterfield representations are conceptually unsatisfying, they are not unprecedented: the quarterfield representations in macaque 'V3' and 'VP' have long been considered separate areas by some investigators, based on empirical differences between V3 and VP." But, there are also many who do not accept such improbable areas, and the weight of *evidence* is on their side.

The evidence in favour of V3B representing only the contralateral lower fields is therefore currently unconvincing. If eventually found to be true, then this would be the first area that registers activity in one quadrant of the visual field, leaving the same activity in the upper quadrant unregistered or registered in another area. What kind of activity might that be? This necessarily introduces another important topic, which is the quality of evidence that one is prepared to accept as indicative of a functional specialisation for an area. "KO", and its putative specialisation, illustrate the problem well, although "KO" may be just one example among others. Orban's group insisted that "KO" is "genuinely" specialised in the processing of kinetic contours (Orban *et al.*, 1995; Van Oostende *et al.*, 1997).

The idea that there are brain areas specialised for the processing of forms derived from motion was actually first posited by Gulyas *et al.* (1994), but it was based on a faulty analysis of their imaging data which has attracted criticism, making it questionable (Frackowiak *et al.*, 1996; Roland and Gulyas 1996). The evidence of Orban's group is not much more reliable. What if "KO", instead of being specialised for extracting contours from kinetic boundaries, is specialised for the extraction of boundaries, no matter how derived? A critical comparison, not done by Orban's group, is to study the activity in "KO" when contours are extracted from other attributes—for example, equiluminant colours. Equiluminant colours are especially interesting, as colour and motion seem to be the most easily separable from one another, perceptually, anatomically, physiologically, and in terms of their cortical representation. Studies that have undertaken such a comparison (Zeki *et al.*, 2003) show that "KO" is equally active when contours are extracted from equiluminant colours as when the same contours are extracted from kinetic contours; it is not, therefore, specialised in the processing of kinetic contours. Moreover, an independent

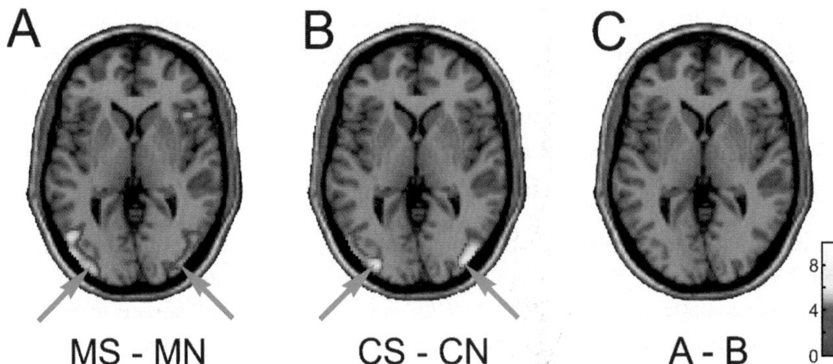

FIGURE 9.6
fMRI images of transverse sections of the brain. (A) Contrast of kinetic shapes versus kinetic non-shapes (MS – MN). (B) Contrast of colour shapes versus colour non-shapes (CS – CN). (C) Direct comparison of contrast shown in A with contrast shown in B (*i.e.*, interaction contrast [MS – MN] – [CS – CN]). Talairach coordinate z = +2. Arrows indicate position of area "KO" in each hemisphere. Statistical threshold $p < 0.05$, corrected. Scale shows relationship between colour and Z statistic. (From Zeki, S. M. *et al.*, *Cereb. Cortex*, in press. With permission.)

component analysis (Bell and Sejnowski, 1995) of the activity time course (ATC) in different visual areas when viewing complex scenes, shows that activity within "KO" correlates with that in V3 (Zeki *et al.*, 2003) (Fig. 9.6), suggesting that "KO" is part of the V3 family of areas, as was implied by Smith *et al.* (1998), who used the more neutral, and better, term of V3B to describe it. This makes more biological sense. An area that is specialised for an attribute, in this case for extraction of forms, should be able to do so regardless of how the forms are generated (Zeki and Shipp, 1988). There is much evidence from single-cell experiments in favour of this "cue invariance." Given that V3B is engaged when shapes are extracted from different sources, it is difficult to imagine that it does so for one quadrant of the visual field only, but that is precisely what would be the case if V3B represents one quadrant of the field of view only. Thus, not only is area V3B not specialised for kinetic contours, but it is also doubtful whether it is an improbable area, in the sense of representing lower contralateral visual fields alone.

It is a wonder that so fragile a concept as that of visual areas in which a quarter of the visual field alone is represented should have been so uncritically accepted for so many years and that so much should have been built on such a flimsy view. Of course, when the original concept collapses, the rest follows, as in a domino game. This is what we are witnessing today. The lesson to be learned from this is that we should demand a more critical assessment before accepting such concepts and also cease accepting the gratuitously proffered and uncritical opinion of the experts so unthinkingly. If there are such improbable areas, the case for them has to be made unequivocally.

CONCLUSION

It is therefore wise, in theorising about the cortex, to rely more on areas whose status is more certain. Of these, none doubts area V1. Areas V2 and V3 seem to be fairly robust but have not been studied in sufficient detail. Among the many other visual areas that have been discovered, the most robust so far have been area V5 and area V4, specialised respectively for motion and for colour. Given that these two attributes are also among the easiest to separate from one another psychophysically, and in terms of the anatomical mechanisms subserving them, we use them exhaustively, if not exclusively, in formulating our views about the functioning of the visual areas in relation to visual consciousness. Our approach is dictated in part by the results of our experiments and in part by our philosophical view that supposes that one of the primordial functions of the brain is to acquire knowledge and that knowledge can only be acquired in the conscious state. Hence, the study of consciousness is not some kind of optional extra, but an integral part of the study of the visual brain. Implicit in this view is an adherence to the doctrines of Schopenhauer and Kant, discussed elsewhere (Zeki, 1999), that all knowledge is subjective and that in seeking to understand how the brain acquires its knowledge we must seek to understand what limitations it imposes on the acquisition of knowledge and what formal contribution it makes to it.

The general view that we put forward here is that the brain areas that are specialised for processing different attributes are also specialised for perceiving those attributes; in other words, that a processing site is also a perceptual site. We have discussed at length elsewhere (Zeki, 1993; Zeki and Bartels, 1998, 1999) the clinical evidence that shows these specialised areas to be reasonably autonomous from one another. This is so because damage to one area alone, provided it is confined to that area, does not lead to total blindness but to an imperception of the attribute for which that area is specialised. Conversely, damage to much of the cortex, including area V1, does not lead to total blindness but to the capacity to experience certain specific visual attributes consciously, if the corresponding specialised visual area receives a visual input that bypasses V1 and is therefore intact. The above, together with the relatively new evidence that we review below, leads us to the conclusion that visual perception is not only distributed in space (functional specialisation) but also in time. Since to perceive something is to be conscious of it, we conclude further that there is no unique entity that we can call visual consciousness. Rather, visual consciousness consists of many specialised visual micro-consciousnesses, corresponding to the specialised areas, and that visual consciousness is therefore also distributed in space and in time.

References

Bartels, A. and Zeki, S. M. (2000). The architecture of the colour centre in the human visual brain: new results and a review. *Eur. J. Neurosci.*, **12**, 172–193.

Bell, A. J. and Sejnowski, T. J. (1995). An information maximisation approach to blind separation and blind deconvolution. *Neural Comput.*, **7**, 1129–1159.

Burkhalter, A. and Van Essen, D. C. (1986). Processing of colour, form and disparity information in visual areas VP and V2 of ventral extrastriate cortex in the macaque monkey. *J. Neurosci.*, **6**, 2237–2351.

Cragg, B. G. (1969).The topography of the afferent projections in circumstriate visual cortex studied by the Nauta method. *Vision Res.*, **9**, 733–747.

DeYoe, E. A., Carman, G. J., Bandettini, P., Glickman, S., and Wieser, J. *et al.* (1996). Mapping striate and extrastriate visual areas in human cerebral cortex. *Proc. Natl. Acad. Sci. USA*, **93**, 2382–2386.

Engel, S. A., Rumelhart, D. E., Wandell, B. A., Lee, A. T., and Glover, G. H. *et al.* (1994). fMRI of human visual cortex. *Nature*, **369**, 525.

ffytche, D. H., Howard, R. J., Brammer, M. J., David, A., Woodruff, P., and Williams, S. (1998). The anatomy of conscious vision: an fMRI study of visual hallucinations. *Nat. Neurosci.*, **1**, 738–742.

Frackowiak, R. S. J., Zeki, S. M., Poline, J. B., and Friston, K. J. (1996). A critique of a new analysis proposed for functional neuroimaging. *Eur. J. Neurosci.*, **8**, 2229–2231.

Gattass, R., Rosa, M. G. P., Sousa, A. P. B., Pinon, M. C. G., Fiorani, M., and Neuenschwander, S. (1990). Cortical steams of visual information processing in primates. *Brazilian J. Med. Biol. Res.*, **23**, 375–393.

Gordon, J., Shapley, R., Patel, P., Pastagia, J., and Truong, C. (1997). The lower visual field is better than the upper visual field at red/green recognition. *Invest. Ophthalmol. Visual Sci.*, **38**, 4199.

Gulyas, B., Heywood, C. A., Popplewell, D. A., Roland, P. E., and Cowey, A. (1994). Visual form discrimination from colour or motion cues: functional anatomy by positron emission tomography. *Proc. Natnl. Acad. Sci. USA,* **91**, 9965–9969.

Hadjikhani N., Liu, A. K., Dale, A., Cavanagh, P., and Tootell, R. B. H. (1998). Retinotopy and colour sensitivity in human visual cortical area V8. *Nat. Neurosci.*, **1**, 235–241.

Heywood, C. and Cowey, A. (1998). With colour in mind. *Nat. Neurosci.*, **1**, 171–173.

Hubel, D. H. and Wiesel, T. N. (1977). The Ferrier lecture. Functional architecture of macaque monkey visual cortex. *Proc. Roy. Soc. London Ser. B*, **198**, 1–59.

Kaas, J. H. (1993). The organisation of the visual cortex in primates: problems, conclusions and the use of comparative studies in understanding the human brain, in *The Functional Organisation of the Human Visual Cortex*, Gulyas, B., Ottoson, D., and Roland, P.E., Eds., pp. 1–11. Pergamon Press, Oxford.

Kastner, S., DeWeerd, P., Desimone, R., and Ungerleider, L. C. (1998). Mechanisms of directed attention in the human extrastriate cortex as revealed by functional MRI. *Science, 282*, 108–111.

Livingstone, M. S. and Hubel, D. H. (1988). Segregation of form, colour, movement, and depth: anatomy, physiology, and perception. *Science*, **240**, 740–749.

Lund, J. S., Yoshioka, T., and Levitt, J. B. (1993). Comparison of intrinsic connectivity in different areas of macaque monkey cerebral cortex. *Cereb. Cortex*, **3**, 148–62.

Lyon, D. C. and Kaas, J. H. (2001). Connectional and architectonic evidence for dorsal and ventral V3, and dorsomedial area in marmoset monkeys, *J. Neurosci.*, **2**, 249–261.

Lyon, D. C. and Kaas, J. H. (2002). Evidence for a modified V3 with dorsal and ventral halves in macaque monkeys. *Neuron*, **33**, 453–461.

McKeefry, D. and Zeki, S. M. (1997). The position and topography of the human colour centre as revealed by functional magnetic resonance imaging. *Brain*, **120**, 2229–2242.

Moutoussism, K. and Zeki, S. M. (1997a). A direct demonstration of perceptual asynchrony in vision. *Proc. Roy. Soc. London Ser. B*, **264**, 393–9.

Moutoussis, K. and Zeki, S. M. (1997b). Functional segregation and temporal hierarchy of the visual perceptive systems. *Proc. Roy. Soc. London Ser. B*, **264**, 1407–1414.

Orban, G.A., Dupont, P., DeBruyn, B., Vogels, R., Vandenberghe, R., and Mortelmans, L. (1995). A motion area in human visual cortex. *Proc. Natl. Acad. Sci. USA*, **92**, 993–997.

Press, W. A., Brewer, A. A., Dougherty, R. F., Wade, A. R., and Wandell, B. A. (2001). Visual areas and spatial summation in human visual cortex. *Vision Res.*, **41**, 1321–1332.

Rockland, K. S. (1985). A reticular pattern of intrinsic connections in primate area V2 (area 18). *J. Compar. Neurol.*, **235,** 467–478.

Roland, P. E. and Gulyas, B. (1996). Assumptions and validations of statistical tests for functional neuroimaging. *Eur. J. Neurosci.*, **8**, 2232–2235.

Rosa, M. P., Sousa, A. P. B., and Gattass, R. (1988). Representation of the visual field in the second visual area in the *Cebus* monkey. *J. Compar. Neurol.*, **275**, 326–345.

Rosa, M. P. G., Pinon, M. C., Gattass, R., and Sousa, A. P. B. (2000). 'Third tier' ventral extrastriate cortex in New World monkey, *Cebus apella*, *Exp. Brain Res.*, **132**, 287–305.

Rubin, N., Hakayama, K., and Shapley, R. (1996). Enhanced perception of illusory contours in the lower versus upper visual hemifields. *Science*, **271**, 651–653.

Schiller, P. H. (1997). Past and present ideas about how the visual scene is analyzed by the brain, in *Extrastriate Cortex in Primates*, Rockland, K.S., Kaas, J. H., and Peters, A., Eds., pp. 59–90. Plenum, New York.

Sereno, M. I., Dale, A. M., Reppas, J. B., Kwong, K. K., and Belliveau, J. W. *et al.* (1995). Borders of multiple visual areas in humans revealed by functional magnetic resonance imaging. *Science*, **268**, 889–893.

Shipp, S., Watson, J. D. G., Frackowiak, R. S. J., and Zeki, S. M. (1995). Retinotopic maps in human prestriate visual-cortex: the demarcation of areas V2 and V3. *NeuroImage*, **2**, 125–132.

Smith, A. T., Greenlee, M. W., Singh, K. D., Kraemer, F. M., and Hennig, J. (1998). The processing of first- and second-order motion in human visual cortex assessed by functional magnetic resonance imaging (fMRI). *J. Neurosci.*, **18**, 3816–3830.

Tootell, R. B. H., Reppas, J. B., Kwong, K. K., Malach, R., and Born, R. T. *et al.* (1995). Functional analysis of human MT and related visual cortical areas using magnetic resonance imaging. *J. Neurosci.*, **15**, 3215–3230.

Tootell, R. B. H., Mendola, J. D., Hadjikhani, N. K., Liu, A. K., and Dale, A. M. (1998). The representation of the ipsilateral visual field in human cerebral cortex. *Proc. Natl. Acad. Sci. USA*, **95**, 818–824.

Tootell, R. B. H. and Hadjikhani, N. (2001). Where is 'dorsal V4' in human visual cortex? Retinotopic, topographic and functional evidence, *Cereb. Cortex*, **11**, 298–311.

Van Oostende, S., Sunaert, S., Van Hecke, P., Marchal, G., and Orban, G. A. (1997). The kinetic occipital (KO) region in man: an fMRI study. *Cereb. Cortex*, **7**, 690–701.

Verrey D. (1888). Hémiachromatopsie droite absolue. Conservation partielle de la perception lumineuse et des formes. Ancien kyste hémorrhagique de la partie inférieure du lobe occipital gauche. *Archives D'Ophtalmologie (Paris)*, **8**, 289–300.

Wade, A. R., Brewer, A. A., Rieger, J. W., and Wandell, B. A. (2002). Functional measurements of human ventral occipital cortex: retinotopy and colour, *Philos. Trans. Roy. Soc. London B*, **357**(1424), 963–973.

Zeki, S. M. (1969). Representation of central visual fields in prestriate cortex of monkey. *Brain Res.*, **14**, 271–291.

Zeki, S, M. (1975). The functional organisation of projections from striate to prestriate visual cortex in the rhesus monkey. *Cold Spring Harbor Symp. Quant. Biol.*, **40**, 591–600.

Zeki, S. M. (1978). Functional specialisation in the visual cortex of the monkey. *Nature*, **274**, 423–428.

Zeki, S. (1993). *A Vision of the Brain*. Blackwell, Oxford, 366 pp.

Zeki, S. (1999). Splendours and miseries of the brain. *Philos. Trans. Roy. Soc. London B*, **354**, 2053–2065.

Zeki, S. and Bartels A. (1998). The autonomy of the visual systems and the modularity of conscious vision. *Philos. Trans. Roy. Soc. London B*, **353**, 1911–1914.

Zeki, S. and Bartels, A. (1999). Towards a theory of visual consciousness. *Consciousness and Cogn.*, **8**, 225–259.

Zeki, S. and Shipp, S. (1988). The functional logic of cortical connections, *Nature*, **335**, 311–317.

Zeki, S. Watson, J. D. G., Lueck, C. J., Friston, K. J., Kennard, C., and Frackowiak, R. S. J. (1991). A direct demonstration of functional specialisation in human visual cortex. *J. Neurosci.*, **11**, 641–649.

Zeki, S. Perry, R., and Bartels, A. (2003). The processing of kinetic contours in the brain. *Cereb. Cortex*, **13**, 189–202.

CHAPTER

10

Insights into Visual Consciousness

"A more precise knowledge and a firmer conviction of the wholly subjective nature of color contribute to a more profound comprehension of the Kantian doctrine of the likewise subjective, intellectual forms of all our knowledge, and so it affords a very suitable introductory course to philosophy." —Arthur Schopenhauer (1816), Über des Sehn und die Farbe: Eine Abhandlung [On Vision and Colors: An Essay]

The anatomical, physiological, and clinical evidence that we, and others, have gathered over the last quarter of a century, together with our more recent studies on perceptual asynchrony in vision and on the chronoarchitecture of the cerebral cortex, lead us to general views that we outline more explicitly below and which can be summarised as follows: The visual brain consists of several parallel, functionally specialised processing systems, each having several stages (*nodes*). The different systems terminate their tasks and reach a perceptual endpoint at different times; consequently, we perceive different attributes at different times with the result that visual perception is asynchronous. Because to perceive something is to be conscious of it, we are led ineluctably to the conclusion that, like the processing–perceptual nodes that are spatially distributed and require different times to bring their processing to a completion, so consciousness and the knowledge acquiring system of the visual brain to which they are tied are distributed in time and space.

THE DETERMINANTS OF VISUAL CONSCIOUSNESS

We put forward our view on visual consciousness with diffidence, acknowledging from the start that it is almost certainly incomplete and possibly even wrong, either wholly or in part. Yet, we have, collectively, gathered enough information about the visual pathways in the primate brain to make such speculations necessary and worthwhile for future experimentation. The view we put forward is deeply influenced by the philosophy of Kant and of Schopenhauer on the one hand and by the theory of functional specialisation in the visual brain on the other. The more recent demonstrations of a perceptual asynchrony in visual perception and of the chronoarchitecture of the cerebral cortex are now fundamental aspects of the theory of functional specialisation, and the results of these demonstrations must inevitably be woven not only into the theory of functional specialisation but also into what that theory naturally leads to: namely, a theory of visual consciousness. This article draws heavily on three previous ones (Zeki, 2001, 2002; Zeki and Bartels, 1999).

Had it not been our conviction that one of the primordial functions of the visual brain is the acquisition of knowledge about the world through the sense of vision, any discussion of visual consciousness would have been superfluous for us as mere anatomists and physiologists charting the organisation of the visual brain with our limited techniques. But our conviction has important consequences, for knowledge in any meaningful sense can only be acquired in the conscious state, and hence consciousness becomes an integral part of the study of the visual brain. We can then frame our question in the following way: What role does each cortical area play in the acquisition of knowledge and how does it contribute to the conscious state, without which we cannot acquire knowledge?

BRAIN CONCEPTS

A cornerstone of Kant's and Schopenhauer's philosophy is that to understand knowledge and its limits and to learn how we acquire it, it is necessary to inquire into the organ capable of acquiring knowledge and to understand the limits it imposes upon the acquisition of knowledge and the formal contribution that it makes to it, although both wrote in terms of the mind, not the brain. When Schopenhauer, in the opening quote, emphasised that all knowledge, of which colour constitutes an important example, is subjective and intellectual, he was emphasising that the mind (to us, the brain) imposes some concept upon the incoming signals, leading to an understanding (*Verstand*) which is the product of the application of the brain concept to the incoming signals. We can never know the "thing in itself" (*das Ding an sich*), because the only knowledge we have is elaborated through the medium of the mind (the brain) and its mechanisms, which are interposed between us and the "thing in itself." Kant wrote in his *Prologemena to Any Future Metaphysic* that, "Sensations without concepts are blind." An admirable illustration of this is the example of achromatopsia where, following a lesion in the V4 complex, the brain can no longer apply its concept of comparing the wavelength composition reflected from one part of the field of view with that reflected from large surrounding parts. It cannot, therefore, construct colours, with the consequence that the achromatopsic patient is blind to colours even though his retina and the pathways leading from it to the cortex are intact. Concepts here are to be thought of, therefore, as algorithms that the brain applies to the incoming signals. We can be a little more precise and say that, reflecting its functional specialisation, the visual brain applies different concepts (algorithms) in different areas to lead to an understanding of different attributes of the visual scene.

It is, of course, important to learn more about the details of the different algorithms applied in different visual areas. Progress in this area has been slow and what machine vision and computational neuroscience has provided as examples of algorithms, interesting though they are, are not necessarily the ones used by the brain. It is very likely that, in broad outline, the kind of algorithm that the brain uses to construct colours is similar to that proposed by Land (1974), but it is likely that the details vary significantly. The same is true for algorithms to construct motion or depth, or body language. Kant and Schopenhauer, ignorant at the time of facts about the brain that we now possess, tried to cast their questions about knowledge in very broad contexts; they inquired into the general rules that are applicable in the acquisition of *all* knowledge, and they tried to formulate rules about what they thought were innate, *a priori*, intuitions (namely, time and space) into which all sensory experience that leads to knowledge is read. Our horizon is far more limited; we inquire into such general rules that may be applicable in the acquisition of knowledge through the visual sense. We accept the Kantian doctrine of time and space as *a priori* intuitions, but we also suggest that, though factors of time and space are built into the machinery of every visual area, their characteristics differ from area to area (Zeki, 1999, 2001). It is sufficient here to mention the colour and motion systems to make this point. In the construction of colour, the colour system must compare *simultaneously* the wavelength composition of the light coming from one surface and that coming from surrounding surfaces. To undertake this comparison, two spatial extents must be compared simultaneously in time. With motion, it is the *successive* stimulation of two spatial points that is important, and the position of one point with respect to another is critical. It is possible, and even likely, that these different imperatives of time contribute to the distinctive activity time courses (ATCs) of different areas, and hence to the chronoarchitecture of the cerebral cortex that is discussed elsewhere in this book (see Chapter 13). It is also likely that these different imperatives contribute significantly to the observed asynchrony of visual perception. The differences in the spatial exigencies of different cortical areas are almost certainly contributed to by the finite receptive field sizes of different visual areas, the capacity of these fields being influenced (or not) by activity in surrounding or remotely located cells, characteristics of which there are many examples.

There is of course another element in the Kantian doctrine that all the systems must have in common—namely, the capacity to differentiate between the experiencing individual and what is occurring in the external environment. It is difficult to tell whether this is a characteristic that every area signals or contributes to, or whether it is a property signalled by some other, specialised area. But, in this search for universals and uniformities, it is interesting to inquire, even in the absence of any significant knowledge about the specialised concepts that the brain uses in its specialised areas, whether or not there is a general operation that the brain performs in every visual area, regardless of its specialisation. We believe that there is, and that it is *abstraction*.

ABSTRACTION AS A REPETITIVELY PERFORMED BRAIN OPERATION

By abstraction, we mean an emphasis on the general at the expense of the particular. The process entails the emphasis on a given attribute and indifference to other attributes. We have outlined above one of the reasons for this—namely, that different attributes vary independently in time. Another reason lies in the problem of knowledge; if knowledge of a particular attribute depended upon a single, particular, example, then we would have to have brains that are constructed otherwise. This has been emphasised by Frazer (1930) in his discussion of the Platonic doctrines. He writes:

> *...generalisation, while the highest power of the human intellect and a mark of its strength, is no less a mark of its weakness. Generalisation is but the compendious and imperfect way in which a finite mind grasps the infinity of the particulars. A mind that could grasp at once all particulars would not generalise ... if there is a mind which grasps the totality of things, it ... can have no need to have recourse to the summary which the limitation of our minds compels us to make use of.*

It is not difficult to discern this abstractive process in different visual areas. The cells of V5 are concerned principally with the direction of motion of a stimulus and care nothing about its colour and frequently about its precise shape, the response of many being optimal to spots moving in the appropriate direction. The consensus of evidence is that wavelength- or colour-selective cells are indifferent to the precise shape of a stimulus and to its direction of motion as well. Indeed, the colour center (the V4 complex) seems to construct colour in the abstract, leaving it to "higher" areas to be engaged when colour is a property of recognizable objects (Zeki and Marini, 1998; Bartels and Zeki, 2000). Equally, the consensus of opinion is that orientation-selective cells are indifferent to the colour of a stimulus, and commonly (though not always) indifferent to its direction of motion as well. Such examples may be multiplied for all known visual areas. Indeed, no one has yet succeeded in showing that the cells of an area respond to the attribute for which they are specialised only in a given set of conditions—for example, only to the face of a particular individual when viewed in a unique position and wearing a unique expression. We may thus say that the capacity to abstract at a certain level is an operation repetitively undertaken by each visual area in relation to the attribute for which it is specialised. Abstraction is, of course, the fundamental first step in the acquisition of knowledge, for without it the brain would be at the mercy of the particular and therefore hostage to the vagaries of the environment. We consider that this abstractive machinery is an innate characteristic of each visual area, although it can be disrupted by deprivation after birth, as the capacity to respond to lines of specific orientation appears to be genetically determined but lost if the brain is not exposed to the visual world at a critical time after birth (Hubel and Wiesel, 1977).

Hence, what we believe to be the innate "intuition" of abstraction, in addition to the Kantian innate "intuitions" of time and space, are characteristics of every visual area. These "intuitions" are part of the knowledge-acquiring machinery of each visual area and are critical in the application of the brain algorithm (the Kantian "concept") to the incoming signals. In short, each and every area of the visual brain has a knowledge-acquiring system of its own, tailored biologically to its needs and different in details from the knowledge-acquiring machinery of other visual areas. The knowledge-acquiring system of the visual brain is therefore spatially distributed between different visual areas. That this is so can also be inferred from the clinical evidence reviewed elsewhere (Zeki, 1997, 2001; Zeki and Bartels, 1999), which shows that lesions restricted to the territory of a specialised visual area result in an imperception in the visual attribute for which that area is specialised, without affecting other attributes significantly, if at all. Cerebral achromatopsia, akinetopsia, object agnosia, and prosopagnosia provide excellent examples. Perhaps the most dramatic examples come from patients who have been, for one reason or another, blinded completely by cerebral lesions and are yet able to perceive one attribute. The motion vision of the blind in the Riddoch syndrome (Zeki, 1991; Zeki and ffytche, 1998) provides a good example; when a visual area (in this case, V5) in a blind subject is disconnected from V1 and yet receives a visual input that bypasses V1 (through the pulvinar and the lateral geniculate nucleus), the subject consciously experiences the direction of motion of visual stimuli. The proponents of "blindsight," threatened by the importance of this demonstration for their theory and their view that activity in prestriate cortex is "unconscious" (Weiskrantz, 1990), fell back, after admitting that such patients can be conscious of the moving visual stimuli in their "blind" field, into arguing that what such subjects are aware of is not visual, as "conscious vision is not possible without V1" (Stoerig and Cowey, 1995). But, the recent compelling study of Stoerig and Barth (2001) has shown that subject GY, on whom the theory of "blindsight" rests very largely, is in fact conscious of a visual event in his blind field and that such "phenomenal" vision is therefore possible even in the absence of V1.

In fact, the concept of blindsight now has too many inconsistencies to deal with to be a viable alternative to the theory that we propose. Fundamental to the concept of "blindsight" has been the supposition that activity in the prestriate cortex is not conscious (Weiskrantz, 1990) and that the capacity to discriminate a visual stimulus without being conscious of it is the result of subcortical activity, while the cortex is involved whenever the subject is conscious of the stimulus. Neither of these suppositions turns out to be true. Indeed, the demonstration that subject GY is actually capable of discriminating what he is conscious of and incapable of discriminating what he is not conscious of (Zeki and ffytche, 1998), coupled to the demonstration that whether he is conscious or not depends upon the level of activity in the relevant visual areas of the brain, compromises the theory of blindsight significantly. We are thus left with a more realistic theory in terms of the known facts. Its tenets may be summarised as follows: (1) there is a tight correlation between correct discrimination and awareness, (2) activity in prestriate cortex have a conscious correlate even in the absence of V1, and (3) we seek an explanation in the difference between conscious and nonconscious states in terms of the level of activity at individual nodes of the visual brain, rather than supposing that in the first state activity is cortical while in the latter the subcortex alone is involved, as theories of blindsight have assumed. There is, in short, a profound difference between our view and that embodied in the theory of "blindsight."

An equally interesting example is provided by patients who, because of hypoxic episodes or heart attacks that have deprived the cortex of its blood supply, are blind but can perceive colours consciously. The important point here is twofold: First, activity in one system alone, the colour system, is relatively spared even in spite of severe damage to other systems and, second, the conscious visual percept may be mediated by area V1 alone. Collectively, the above evidence leads us to suppose that the perceptive systems, which are also perceptual systems, are more or less autonomous from one another (Zeki, 1998).

THE THEORY OF MICROCONSCIOUSNESSES

Given this apparent autonomy and given that the different visual areas have independent ATCs and reach perceptual stages at different times, as shown by the perceptual asynchrony in vision, we are naturally led to suppose that activity at each node of the visual "perceptual-processing" systems can have a conscious correlate, which we call a *microconsciousness* (Zeki and Bartels, 1999). Given the specialisation of the perceptual-processing systems, including their nodes, it is but one step from this to supposing that the microconsciousnesses are functionally specialised because they relate to the specialisation of the cells at that node. It would be difficult to conceive of the microconsciousness generated by the activity of cells in V5 to be related to colour or that generated by the activity of cells in V4 to be related to motion. Equally it would be difficult to imagine that the microconsciousness generated in V4 relates to faces or that generated in the fusiform face area to colours. Hence, visual consciousness is distributed in time and space, because spatially distributed specialised areas reach perceptual endpoints at different times. It follows from this that the knowledge-acquiring system of the brain is also distributed in time and space.

A significant aspect of the studies that have demonstrated a perceptual asynchrony in vision is the related demonstration of a *misbinding* in real time (Moutoussis and Zeki, 1997a,b) (see Chapter 12). This means, essentially, that the brain does not wait for an area to terminate its processing stages and reach a perpetual endpoint before binding it to the activity generated at other nodes. It shows that the brain binds together two attributes that it has already processed. If the two take different times to process, it binds the percepts that are already "available;" hence, because colour is processed and perceived before motion, at any give time t the brain binds the colour to what the motion system had completed processing, at time $t - 1$. The brain, therefore, misbinds in terms of veridical reality. From this, one can draw what seems to us to be an important conclusion—namely, that binding is post-conscious. The post-conscious binding that we speak of here is what we also refer to as *parallel binding*, to distinguish it from generative binding (Zeki and Bartels, 1999). Parallel binding refers to the coupling of the activity of cells within a single area or between areas. Unlike other theories, for example those of Crick and Koch (1990), Singer (1998) and Tononi and Edelman (1998), we do not suppose that communication between areas will result in a (micro-) conscious correlate, nor do we believe that this must necessarily entail the bringing together of the responses of two cells onto a third cell (but see below). Rather, we suppose that it is activity at the nodes that generates the microconsciousness, and it is the microconsciousnesses that are bound.

Kant and the Doctrine of Microconsciousness

Our concept of microconsciousnesses may fly in the face of the more general belief in the "unity of consciousness." The origins of this latter concept are not easy to trace, but the concept figures prominently in the writings of the illustrious Kant. Since formulating the theory of microconsciousness, we have come across passages from Kant that suggest to us that our formulation *may* not have been quite as alien to him as one may surmise from his emphasis on the unity of consciousness. It is difficult to be certain, because Kant's writings are so opaque, perhaps especially so to neurobiologists. It is always dangerous to give credit with hindsight, especially to those who were not explicit in their writings. Our reading of him may thus be overly generous in the light of what we have found and concluded. Kant's belief in the "unity of consciousness" does not preclude him from believing in microconsciousness, which is what we interpret his "empirical consciousness" to mean. For him, "perception is empirical consciousness," since "when appearance is combined with consciousness, it is called perception. Without the relation to an at least possible consciousness, appearance could never become for us an object of cognition, and hence would be nothing to us; and since appearance does not in itself have any objective reality and exists only in cognition, it would then be nothing at all" (Kant, *Critique of Pure Reason*, first ed., p. 120). He considered the relation between "empirical consciousness" and the unified, transcendental consciousness, to be of "great importance," even though its discussion is relegated to a footnote, albeit an extensive one . He wrote:

All presentations have a necessary reference to a ***possible*** *empirical consciousness. For if they did not have this reference, and becoming conscious of them were entirely impossible, then this would be tantamount to saying that they do not exist at all. But all empirical consciousness has a necessary reference to a transcendental consciousness (a consciousness that precedes all particular experience), viz., the consciousness of myself as original apperception. It is therefore absolutely necessary that in my cognition all consciousness belong to one consciousness (that of myself). ...The synthetic proposition that all the varied empirical*

> *consciousness must be combined in one single self-consciousness is the absolutely first and synthetic principle of our thought as such.* (Kant, Critique of Pure Reason, first ed., p. 117, footnote 138)

The emphasis in the original indicates a certain hesitation. This makes it obvious that he was thinking of the "unity of consciousness" in a very definitive way, preceding all experience and in reference to the experiencing person. But, he also saw that the "empirical consciousness" must be synthesised into "pure consciousness," a point repeatedly made in the *Critique*. In fact, he probably suspected that the various attributes must themselves be synthesised first before being synthesised into the "pure consciousness," although he could not have been aware of the principles of functional specialisation. He continues:

> *But because every appearance contains a manifold, so that different perceptions are in themselves encountered in the mind sporadically and individually, these perceptions need to be given a combination that in sense itself they cannot have. Hence there is in us an active power to synthesise this manifold* [which he calls "imagination"]. (Kant, Critique of Pure Reason, first ed., p. 120).

The unity that Kant speaks of can be translated to mean "aware of being aware," a unity that is not at all apparent to us except through the use of communication and especially language, nor it seems to other philosophers (*e.g.*, Dennett, 1991). In general, we are not aware of being aware; we are instead aware of particular events at particular instants, and more specifically of that which we are attending to at a given time. Even during linguistic communication, we are still not aware of being aware but are only aware of our interlocutor or the subject matter. We only become aware that our interlocutor is conscious in an inferential sense, in that he or she is conscious because he or she is able to conduct this conversation with us and could not do so unless conscious. But, the awareness of consciousness is elicited only when the question is framed. In common conversation, we are conscious of a few things only, and commonly of one thing at a time only. Hence, the synthetic unity into one overall consciousness, that of myself as the perceiving person, is not, we believe, a continuous prerequisite. But, this leaves us with the other synthesis, the capacity of the brain to integrate or bind all the different attributes (Kant's "manifold") that are perceived at different times, what Kant refers to as the "active power to synthesise this manifold."

Binding of Microconsciousnesses

Because of the perceptual asynchrony of vision and the misbinding that can be observed over very short presentations (Moutoussis and Zeki, 1997a,b), we think of this kind of binding, which we refer to as *parallel binding* and whose characteristics we have described elsewhere (Zeki and Bartels, 1999), as a post-conscious event, although the critical experiments to demonstrate this have not yet been done. The proposal nevertheless has a compelling logic. For activity at each node of a processing–perceptual system to have a perceptual (and therefore conscious) correlate confers advantages in that it increases the number of perceptual repertoires. This would be reduced if the processing systems had to report to a "terminal" station—either a common one or individual ones—for integration to occur. Such a hypothetical integration area would have to code in a perceptually explicit way the results of the processing at each node separately as well as in the required combinations. A more economical way would be to render the activity at each processing site perceptually explicit so that it can then be bound.

Others have suggested that what we call parallel, post-conscious binding facilitates figure/ground separation (binding within a node) or brings different visual attributes such as colour and motion together through the synchronous or oscillatory firing of cells in different nodes (Malsburg and Schneider, 1986; Engel *et al.*, 1999), a process regarded as necessary for generating conscious perception (Crick and Koch, 1990; Singer, 1998; Tononi and Edelman, 1998). But there seems to be no general agreement that synchronous or oscillatory firing in this context is of functional or perceptual relevance (Lamme and Spekreijse, 1998), nor is it known how the synchrony is generated—that is, whether it is of a top-down, bottom-up, or thalamo-cortical nature (Llinás *et al.*, 1998).

Each processing–perceptual system has a certain hierarchical structure, by which we mean that the visual attribute is processed at a more complex level at a given stage than at the antecedent one. The theory of multistage integration (Zeki, 1990, 1993; Bartels and Zeki, 1999) nevertheless supposes that there is no perceptual hierarchy in binding, since the perceptually explicit activity of cells at a relatively "low" level in one processing–perceptual system can be bound with the perceptually explicit activity of cells at a relatively "high" level of another, or the same, processing–perceptual system. A good example is provided by a green bus as it emerges from the shade into sunlight. The bus remains a bus and its colour remains green, but the intensity of the light and even its shade change. The recognition of the bus as a bus requires the activity of cells in an area at a high level in the visual pathways (the fusiform gyrus), but the recognition of a change in the shade of green, and in both the intensity and wavelength composition of the illuminating light, depends upon the activity of cells in V1, and possibly V2. A functional corollary of this is that at any given time, many functional units—consisting of stages at different levels of different processing systems—are formed dynamically, with the same stages constituting different units with other stages at another time. The functional units that are formed, therefore, criss-cross between different stages of different processing–perceptual systems (Zeki and ffytche, 1998). It remains open whether these functional units are defined by binding or whether the mere activity in an area is sufficient to make the generated percept part of our seemingly unified perception. They are in a dynamic state and the pattern of functional units formed between different stages of different processing–perceptual systems at any given time should be amenable to capture by imaging methods. The functional units formed will be further dynamically shaped by attentional and mnemonic factors. The notion of dynamically formed functional units that are unstable and subject to attentional and mnemonic factors is similar to the idea of *coalitions* proposed by Crick and Koch (2003), an idea to which we are obviously sympathetic.

We thus think of visual consciousness in terms of hierarchies. At the lowest level is the microconsciousness, of which awareness of colour and motion constitute good examples. But, because colour and motion are perceived at different times, with colour preceding motion, it follows that there is a temporal hierarchy at the level of the microconsciousnesses. The next step is the binding of the microconsciousnesses to constitute a macroconsciousness. Of necessity, this binding is a post- (micro-)conscious event. Examples are the binding of colour to motion. It is significant that binding between attributes (for example, colour to motion) takes a significantly longer time than binding within attributes (for example, up-down motion to left-right motion) (unpublished results from this laboratory). This in turn leads one to postulate a set of temporal hierarchies, in which the binding of one set of attributes leading to a given macroconsciousness may take longer than the binding of another set of attributes leading to another macroconsciousness, and the binding of several attributes may take longer still. The experiment has not been conducted yet, but such a result seems likely.

Micro- and macroconsciousnesses, with their individual temporal hierarchies, lead to the final, unified consciousness, that of myself as the perceiving person. To me, this and this alone qualifies as the unity of consciousness, and this alone can be described in the singular. Kant supposed that this "synthetic, transcendental" consciousness is present *a priori*—that is, before any experience is acquired. It is difficult to be conclusive in this regard, but it is worth pointing out that consciousness of oneself as the perceiving person amounts to being aware of being aware, and I believe that this requires communication with others and especially the use of language. It is also worth pointing out that the cortical programs to construct colour or visual motion must also be present before any experience is acquired and that all experience must therefore be read into these programs. It seems more likely that, ontogenetically, the microconsciousnesses precede the unified consciousness and that the programs for them are also present at birth. Hence, even though in adult life the unified consciousness sits at the apex of the hierarchy of consciousnesses, ontogenetically it is the microconsciousness that occupies this position.

There is currently a great deal of interest in searching for the neural correlate of consciousness. We believe that that search is bound to be elusive until one recognises that there are many consciousnesses, not one, and that the more proper search would be for the neural correlates of the consciousnesses. This shift in emphasis consists of nothing more than a shift from singular to plural, but it may constitute a major step in the quest for the neural substrate of consciousness(es).

References

Bartels, A. and Zeki, S. (2000). The architecture of the colour centre in the human visual brain: new results and a review. *Eur. J. Neurosci.*, **12**, 172–193.

Crick, F. and Koch, C. (1990). Towards a neurobiological theory of consciousness. *Semin. Neurosci.*, **2**, 263–275.

Crick, F. and Koch, C. (2003). *Nat. Neurosci.*, **6**, 119–126.

Dennett, D. (1991). *Consciousness Explained.* Little, Brown, Boston.

Engel, A. K., Fries, P., Roelfsema, P. R., König, P., and Singer, W. (1999). Temporal binding, binocular rivalry, and consciousness. *Conscious. Cogn.*, **8**, 155–158.

Frazer, J. G. (1930). *The Growth of Plato's Ideal Theory*. Macmillan, London.

Hubel, D. H. and Wiesel, T. N. (1977). The Ferrier lecture: functional architecture of macaque monkey visual cortex. *Proc. Roy. Soc. London Ser. B*, **198**, 1–59.

Kant, I. (1781/1787 [1996]). *Kritik der reinen Vernunft* [*Critic der reinen ßernunft*] (translated as *Critique of Pure Reason*, by W. S. Pluhar, Hacket Publishing, Indianapolis, IN).

Lamme, V. A. F. and Spekreijse, H. (1998). Neuronal synchrony does not represent texture segregation. *Nature*, **396**, 362–366.

Land, E. (1974). The retinex theory of colour vision. *Proc. Roy. Inst. Gr. Brit.*, **47**, 23–58.

Llinás, R., Ribary, U., Contreras, D., and Pedroarena, C. (1998). The neuronal basis for consciousness. *Philos. Trans. Roy. Soc. London B*, **353**, 1841–1849.

Malsburg, Cvd. and Schneider, W. (1986). A neural cocktail-party processor. *Biol. Cybernetics*, **54**, 29–40.

Moutoussis, K. and Zeki, S. (1997a). A direct demonstration of perceptual asynchrony in vision. *Proc. Roy. Soc. London Ser. B*, **264**, 393–399.

Moutoussis, K. and Zeki, S. (1997b). Functional segregation and temporal hierarchy of the visual perceptive systems. *Proc. Roy. Soc. London B*, **264**, 1407–1414.

Schopenhauer, A. (1854/1994). *Über das Sehn und die Farben: Eine Abhandlung* [*On Vision and Colours: An Essay*] (translated by E. J. F. Payne, Berg Publishers, Oxford).

Singer, W. (1998). Consciousness and the structure of neuronal representations. *Philos. Trans. Roy. Soc. London B*, **353**, 1829–1840.

Stoerig, P. and Barth, E. (2001). Low-level phenomenal vision despite unilateral destruction of primary visual cortex. *Conscious. Cogn.,* **10**, 574–587.

Stoerig, P. and Cowey, A. (1995). Visual perception and phenomenal consciousness. *Behav. Brain Res.*, **71**, 147–156.

Tononi, G. and Edelman, G. M. (1998). Consciousness and complexity. *Science*, **282**, 1846–1851.

Weiskrantz, L. (1990). The Ferrier lecture 1989: outlooks for blindsight—explicit methodologies for implicit processes. *Proc. Roy. Soc. London Ser. B*, **239**, 247–278.

Zeki, S. (1990). A theory of multi-stage integration in the visual cortex, in *The Principles of Design and Operation of the Brain*, Eccles, J. C. and Creutzfeldt, O., Eds., pp. 137–154. Vatican City: Pontifical Academy of Science.

Zeki, S. (1991). Cerebral akinetopsia (visual motion blindness): a review. *Brain*, **114**, 811–824.

Zeki, S. (1993). *A Vision of the Brain*. Blackwell, Oxford, 366 pp.

Zeki, S. (1997). The colour and motion systems as guides to conscious visual perception, in *Extrastriate Cortex in Primates*, Vol. 12, Rockland, K. S., Kaas, J. H., and Peters, A., Eds., pp. 777–809. Plenum, New York.

Zeki, S. (1998). Parallel processing, asynchronous perception and a distributed system of consciousness in vision. *Neuroscientist*, **4**, 365–372.

Zeki, S. (1999). Splendours and miseries of the brain. *Philos. Trans. Roy. Soc. London Ser. B*, **354**, 2053–2065.

Zeki, S. (2001). Localisation and globalisation in conscious vision. *Annu. Rev. Neurosci.*, **24**, 57–86.

Zeki, S. (2002). Improbable areas in the cerebral cortex. *Trends Cogn. Sci.*, **7**, 214–218.

Zeki, S. and Bartels, A. (1999). Towards a theory of visual consciousness. *Conscious. Cogn.*, **8**, 225–259.

Zeki, S. and ffytche, D. (1998). The Riddoch syndrome: insights into the neurobiology of conscious vision. *Brain*, **121**, 25–45.

Zeki, S. and Marini, L. (1998). Three cortical stages of colour processing in the human brain. *Brain*, **121**, 1669–1685.

CHAPTER

11

Processing Systems as Perceptual Systems

In the previous discussion of perceptual asynchrony in vision (Chapter 12), we have deliberately eschewed mention of particular areas in the brain. This is because, in the psychophysical experiments, we were studying the performance of a system, without relating the final percept to activity in any given area of the visual brain and less still to single cells within it. Yet, the question is not uninteresting and can be formulated thus: Is a processing site in the visual brain also a perceptual site, or is processing done at some node that is different from the node at which activity leads to conscious perception? If the latter is true, then a strong argument can be made that consciousness has a distinct and separate seat in the brain. The term "node" refers either to a whole area, such as V4 or V5, or to the functional subdivision of an area, such as the blobs and interblobs of V1, or the thin, thick, and interstripes of V2 (Zeki and Bartels, 1999). In the past (Zeki and Bartels, 1999), we assumed on the basis of clinical and imaging evidence that a processing site in the visual brain is also a perceptual site. We review this evidence briefly below and then examine the new and direct evidence to show that this is indeed so. Implicit in the term "processing" is the supposition that it is pre-perceptual, a means of getting to the final percept, whatever that may be. This supposition itself makes implicit assumptions that are worth discussing. The most obvious of these is that there are separate processing and perceptual systems, or at any rate that the processing stages antedate the perceptual ones. In anatomical and physiological terms, this implies that the processing system feeds the results of its operation into the perceptual system. This may be true within an individual node. The results of Logothetis and his colleagues (Logothetis, 1998) have shown, for example, that at each node there are cells whose responses correlate with perception and others whose responses do not, and it is plausible to suppose that, physiologically, the latter are the precursors of the former. Imaging evidence suggests that activity in an area (node) must reach a certain height for a conscious correlate to be generated (Zeki and ffytche, 1998) but does not tell us whether that height is due to the intensity of response of cells, the number recruited, or their synaptic activity. Evidence for the supposition that some nodes are purely processing ones and that they feed the results of their operations into other, purely perceptual, nodes does not exist. It would indeed be a somewhat inefficient way of encoding everything twice, once at the processing site and then again at the perceptual site. There is better evidence for our rival suggestion that the processing systems are also perceptual systems (Zeki, 1998), which leads us to speak of *processing–perceptual systems*.

IMAGING EVIDENCE TO EQUATE THE PROCESSING AND PERCEPTUAL SYSTEMS

Until the recent imaging experiments described below were undertaken, the most convincing, though still suggestive, experimental evidence for equating the processing with the perceptual system came from clinical and imaging studies and, more specifically, those using colour and motion vision. Colour is the end result of a complex series of operations; these depend on the physical properties of light and the surfaces reflecting it on the one hand and on the operations evolved by the brain to compare the relative efficiency of different surfaces for reflecting lights of different wavebands on the other (Land and McCann, 1971; Land, 1974; Zeki, 1985). The brain evidently computes the ratio of light of any given waveband reflected from one surface and from surrounding surfaces. Computational theories have proposed different implementations for these operations that allow the brain to "discount the illuminant," as Helmholtz (1911) put it, in order to construct constant colour that is independent of the wavelength composition coming from a single surface alone. The critical step in a colour-generating operation is thus ratio taking (Land, 1974; Courtney *et al.*, 1995), which enables the nervous system to compare the amount of light of a given waveband reflected from a given surface with the amount of light of the same waveband reflected from surrounding surfaces. In spite of changes in the wavelength composition of the illuminant, which entails a change in the absolute amounts of light of different waveband coming from every part of the scene, the ratios always remain the same; it is this operation that allows the nervous system to "discount the illuminant" and assign a constant colour to a surface.

The details of the neurophysiological implementation are not clear, but the colour pathways are relatively well understood and include the specialised compartments of areas V1 and V2, area V4, and further areas within the medial temporal cortex of both monkey and man (DeYoe and Van Essen, 1988; Livingstone and Hubel, 1988; Zeki and Shipp, 1988; Zeki and Marini, 1998). Damage to the human colour centre and, more specifically, to the V4 complex (Fig. 11.1) results in the syndrome of achromatopsia if the lesion is bilateral and hemiachromatopsia if it is unilateral. Interestingly, hemiachromatopsic patients are commonly unaware of their loss (Paulson *et al.*, 1994; our unpublished results), thus suggesting that the V4 complex itself is the conscious centre for colour. The V4 complex in fact consists of two areas, V4 and V4α (Bartels and Zeki, 2000). Of these, V4 has a distinct topographic organisation, whereas V4α does not

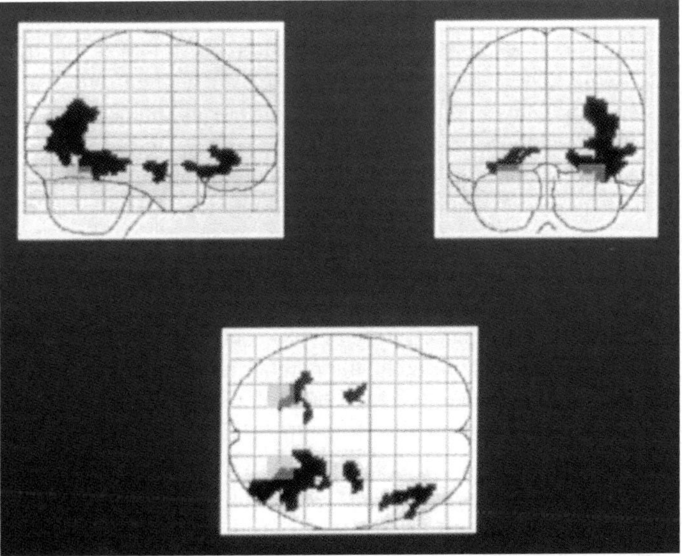

FIGURE 11.1
The group results of brain activation obtained when subjects compared normally coloured objects, such as red strawberries, with their black and white counterparts. Thresholded at $p < 0.0001$. The yellow squares represent the area of activation produced by comparing areas of activation produced by multicoloured Mondrian stimuli against their achromatic counterparts in the study of McKeefry and Zeki (1997).

appear to (McKeefry and Zeki, 1997; Bartels and Zeki, 2000),[1] and both appear to be involved in the processing of colours, be they of abstract or naturalistic scenes. Indeed, sophisticated new techniques, such as independent component analysis applied to functional magnetic resonance imaging (fMRI) data, show that the two areas can act as a functional unit (Bartels and Zeki, 2000; see following chapter). But, it is possible that the variation in the degree of severity resulting from lesions in the V4 complex (Damasio, 1985) is the consequence of unequal damage to this zone in different patients (Bartels and Zeki, 2000). If V1 and V2 were merely the processing stages and the V4 complex a mere perceptual one, then one would expect humans with total damage to V4 not to be able to experience colour at all, which is in fact what does happen. One can try to mimic the real world as far as possible experimentally by asking humans to view a multicoloured scene in which the wavelength composition of the light reflected from every part changes continuously, without changing the perceived colours (colour constancy), because the ratio of light of any given waveband reflected from one part and from adjacent parts remains constant. When, in imaging experiments, one compares the brain activity evoked by this highly demanding task for the colour system with the activity evoked when subjects view a multicoloured scene that does not change in wavelength composition, the maximal activity, which identifies the critical site of the operations undertaken to generate constant colours, occurs within the V4 complex (Bartels and Zeki, 2000). The ratio-taking operation would seem therefore to be localised to the V4 complex, the very area that, when damaged, results in achromatopsia. It involves areas V1 and V2 only minimally (this is in contrast to experiments that compare the brain activity produced by viewing coloured and black and white stimuli, when both V1 and V4 become strongly active (McKeefry and Zeki, 1996). This then suggests strongly that the processing site that is necessary for the generation of colours is the very site that, when damaged, leads to the syndrome of achromatopsia. It suggests, in summary, that the processing and perceptual sites are one and the same (Fig. 11.2).

If activity at a given node, of which V4 and V5 are examples, can lead to a conscious correlate, what about area V1? Because V1 is not directly connected to the frontal lobes, it has been suggested that we are not aware of what happens in V1, thus excluding V1 from direct involvement in conscious experience (Crick and Koch, 1995). This may well turn out to be so, and we have no compelling evidence against the suggestion; however, evidence in favour of the supposition that activity in V1 can have a conscious correlate in appropriate circumstances can to be found in electrophysiological experiments that have shown that within each area, including area V1, there are cells whose responses correlate with percepts (Logothetis, 1998). But, perhaps the most compelling, if not definitive, evidence comes from the study of a blind patient who was able to experience colour consciously.

It was Wechsler who, in 1933, described a remarkable case of carbon monoxide poisoning that had left its victim substantially blind without affecting his colour vision, or at any rate affecting it much less (Wechsler, 1933). This relative sparing of colour vision in patients blinded by hypoxia has been accounted for (Zeki, 1990) by supposing that the richer vasculature of the blobs of V1 (where wavelength-selective cells are concentrated) protects them from vascular insufficiency (Zheng *et al.*, 1991). Whatever the ultimate explanation may turn out to be, Wechsler's observation has been repeated several times (see Zeki, 1993, for a review), and there is little reason to doubt that hypoxic episodes, or cardiovascular attacks, can result in severe damage to the visual brain while sparing colour vision to a greater or lesser extent. This capacity has been studied in greater detail in a patient who had suffered a severe electric shock, with a consequent blindness that spared his colour vision (Humphrey *et al.*, 1995), which we account for, again, by the relative sparing of the more richly vascularised blobs of V1. Our further examination of him revealed that his colour vision (which, as described earlier, is completely

[1]The recently "discovered" "new" colour centre in the brain, termed "V8" (Hadjikhani *et al.*, 1998) is in fact nothing more than a rediscovery of V4, with which it shares the identical brain (Talairach) coordinates and hence does not provide any new insights into the conscious basis of colour vision, as assumed by Heywood and Cowey (1998). This "new" colour centre does not include V4α, which evidently was beyond the resolution of the techniques employed by Hadjikhani *et al.* (1998). On the other hand, we and others have found it difficult to confirm the existence of area "V4v" of Tootell and his colleagues (1996) reputedly representing upper visual fields only (see also Kastner *et al.*, 1998). The work of Wade *et al.* (2002) shows that there is no area "V4v" with a quarterfield representation only.

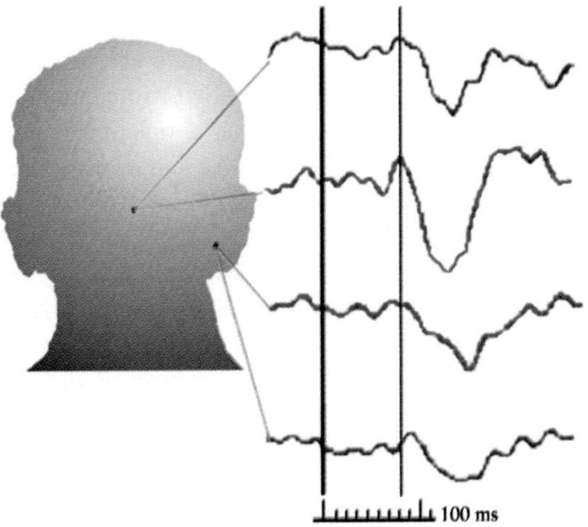

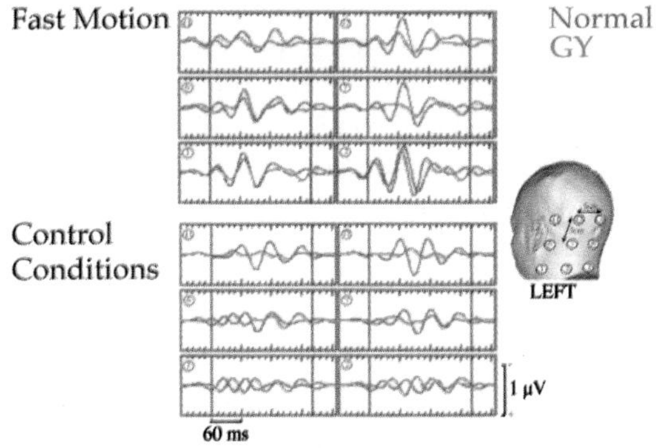

FIGURE 11.2
EEG traces recorded from normal subjects (red) and patient GY (green) while they were viewing fast-moving stimuli and control stimuli. Each box shows traces from one electrode location, which are numbered and shown in the diagram on the right. The two vertical lines within each box mark the stimulus onset and offset. (From ffytche, D. H. *et al.*, *Brain*, 119, 1971–1982, 1996. With permission.)

divorced from form vision in that he is not able to perceive the form of the colours which he describes correctly) is wavelength based. In other words, he is not able to construct constant colours. Imaging experiments show that, when he discriminates colours according to wavelength, the activity in his brain is located in area V1 (Zeki *et al.*, 1999). Even in spite of this, we are diffident about saying that activity in V1 has a conscious correlate, because we have no means of knowing what residual activity, which may have gone undetected in the functional magnetic resonance images, may have occurred elsewhere. The study raises interesting questions, in that the patient was able to categorise colours according to wavelength. If this is really due to activity in V1, then it provides some evidence in favour of the hypothesis of Walsh *et al.* (1992) regarding the capacity of the wavelength-selective cells of V1.

This evidence of the sparing of a given attribute (in this instance, colour) when all others are compromised complements the evidence on achromatopsia that shows a specific loss of colour when other faculties are either relatively or completely spared. Together, they amount to a further testament to the relative autonomy of the individual processing–perceptual systems.

THE MOTION VISION OF THE BLIND

Perhaps even more impressive than the colour studies are those relating to motion and specifically to the perception of motion in a visual field rendered blind by damage to area V1. These studies show that activity at a given station (or *node*) of a processing system (in this case, area V5) can have a conscious perceptual correlate, even if it is disconnected from antecedent cortical nodes. The experiment is a daring one, but it is a naturally occurring one, ready to be exploited after the infliction of accidental cerebral lesions. The specific question can be formulated thus: If visual input is forced into an intact cortical area that is disconnected from one of its (other) major sources of visual input (namely, V1), can activity in that area still lead to a conscious visual experience? An obvious choice is area V5, located in the prestriate cortex and receiving a dual visual input: the well-studied one through V1 and the much less well-studied one that reaches V5 through the superior colliculus and pulvinar (Cragg, 1969; Standage and Benevento, 1983) and also through the lateral geniculate nucleus (Fries, 1981; Yukie and Iwai, 1981), that is, a visual input that bypasses V1.

In fact, long before the presence and specialisation of V5 were established and the direct input to it determined anatomically, such an experiment (or more properly, observation) was made by George Riddoch (1917) who had studied soldiers blinded by lesions to V1 sustained during the Great War. He found that his patients, though blind when tested with static perimetry, were not so when tested with dynamic perimetry. Crucially, he repeatedly described his patients as being "conscious" of the motion, but not of much else besides (Riddoch, 1917). He explains, for example, that "patients with restricted visual fields from occipital wounds ... were immediately conscious of 'something' moving," but he also writes that conscious awareness was restricted to the perception of visual motion, the subjects being "...quite sure that neither shape nor colour could be attributed to [the movement], the nature of the movement being vague and shadowy" (Riddoch, 1917). His explanation for this phenomenon was improbable; he supposed that the mechanisms of visual motion within V1 were spared. This explanation was, and remains, so improbable that his work and conclusions were immediately dismissed by Holmes (1918) and relegated to oblivion for about 70 years (Zeki, 1991). But, more recent studies, especially on patient GY, confirm his observations. GY has been studied extensively for the syndrome of *blindsight*; indeed, his name is synonymous with the syndrome, and the syndrome itself is critically dependent upon GY. Our study of patient GY (Barbur *et al.*, 1993; Zeki, 1997), also blinded by a lesion to his occipital lobe sustained, significantly, during childhood showed that, just like the patients of Riddoch who had been studied within months after sustaining their injuries, GY could not discriminate accurately the direction of fast moving, high contrast, stimuli but he was also conscious of the direction of motion, in that he could describe it verbally. Interestingly, he first told us that the movement he saw was, like that of Riddoch's patients, that of shadows, similar to the perception of motion when a normal individual, with eyes closed, can perceive the shadow when a hand moves against daylight. Later, he described this percept as that of a dark shadow against a dark background and a "feeling" that something was moving. An examination of the literature on blindsight for other patients blinded by lesions in V1 shows similarly that they are commonly conscious of the visual stimuli presented to their blind fields (Zeki and ffytche, 1998). Sometimes subjects have a "feeling" but are "absolutely sure of it" (Weiskrantz, 1986); sometimes they see shadows or pinpoints of light (Weiskrantz, 1986; see Zeki and ffytche, 1998 for a review). It is worth emphasising that there is a very tight correlation in GY, as in normals studied with threshold stimuli, between awareness of a stimulus and its correct discrimination and, conversely, between lack of awareness and its incorrect discrimination (Zeki and ffytche, 1998). Imaging studies show that area V5 is active when GY is shown fast-moving stimuli which he can experience consciously (Zeki and ffytche, 1998). It would thus seem that preprocessing by area V1 is not a necessary precondition for the conscious experience of motion and that the notion that "conscious vision is not possible without V1" (Stoerig and Cowey, 1995; Stoerig, 1996) receives little support from these studies.

The studies reported above have forced a critical reevaluation of the syndrome of blindsight, whose proponents have now acknowledged that conscious vision without V1 is possible (Weiskrantz *et al.*, 1995). An endless number of papers have defended the syndrome of blindsight but, collectively, these justifications have not restored to the syndrome the credibility that it once had. We do not review these papers here (see Zeki and ffytche, 1998), but it is nevertheless worth drawing attention to a shift in the argument brought in to salvage whatever remains of the concept of blindsight. This can be summarised as follows: GY is indeed conscious when his blind field is appropriately stimulated, but his consciousness is not a visual consciousness. This argument has now been put to a final rest by the ingenious experiment of Stoerig and Barth

(2001), who have shown that GY's conscious experience is indeed visual. The title of their paper, which should be consulted for details, says it all: "Low-Level Phenomenal Vision Despite Unilateral Destruction of Primary Visual Cortex."

The ability of GY to experience consciously fast-moving visual stimuli presented to his blind field is almost certainly the consequence of the direct visual input to V5 that bypasses V1, mentioned above, an input curiously described, as it was not based on direct experimental evidence, as one "which may not reach consciousness" (Bullier *et al.*, 1994). Electroencephalographic experiments coupled with imaging ones have shown that this alternative pathway delivers signals from fast-moving ($>5° s^{-1}$) objects to V5, in GY just as in normals, whereas signals from slowly moving ($<5° s^{-1}$) objects are delivered to V5 through V1 (Beckers and Zeki, 1995; ffytche *et al.*, 1995, 1996) (Fig. 11.2). It is not surprising to find, therefore, that GY is able to experience consciously fast, but not slow, moving stimuli. We do not suppose that activity in V5 alone generates this conscious correlate. Imaging studies show that there are critical sites in the brain stem that are more active during conscious experience (Zeki and ffytche, 1998) and these may act as enabling systems—for example, through neuromodulation. The point we are making here is that to perceive fast motion and have a conscious experience of it does not require the mobilisation of nodes antecedent to V5 in the V1–V2–V5 pathway.

RESIDUAL PERCEPTUAL CAPACITIES REINFORCE THE VIEW THAT NODES ARE ALSO PERCEPTUAL SITES

Our supposition that perceptual sites are also processing sites would gain added weight if it can be shown that, with a lesion at a given node of a processing–perceptual system, a patient is not totally deprived of the capacity to experience the attribute for which that system is specialised, but instead has a residual perceptual capacity for that attribute which is a direct reflection of the physiological capacities of the nodes of the affected processing–perceptual system that are left intact by the lesion. It is now generally accepted that, because much of the visual input to the cerebral cortex passes through V1, lesions here usually, but not always (see below), result in total blindness. This is probably also true for V2 (Horton and Hoyt, 1991) which is interposed between V1 and the more specialised areas of the brain and which, like V1, has all the attributes of vision represented in it (Hubel and Livingstone, 1987; DeYoe and Van Essen, 1988; Zeki and Shipp, 1988). What is perhaps more interesting is to look at the perceptual capacities of patients in whom V1 and V2 are not totally destroyed but who have lesions in the areas of the prestriate cortex to which they project. If there is any substance to our supposition that activity at each node of a processing–perceptual system has a perceptual, and therefore conscious, correlate, then we should find that such patients are capable of a more elementary perceptual experience of the relevant attributes than normals but are nevertheless able to experience something of the relevant attribute. We have reviewed the clinical evidence in favour of our supposition in detail elsewhere (Zeki, 1993; Zeki and Bartels, 1999), and below we give only a brief recapitulation.

Given the organisation of the visual cortex at large, it could be expected that a patient with a relatively large lesion in the prestriate cortex that spares area V1 either partially or completely should be capable of a piecemeal analysis of his visual world. That this is so is suggested by our detailed analysis of the clinical evidence relating to object agnosia, prosopagnosia, akinetopsia, and achromatopsia (Zeki, 1993; Zeki and Bartels, 1999). It could also be expected that a patient with damage to the prestriate component of a given processing–perceptual system should be able to experience all attributes of the visual scene, save the one processed by the compromised system, as would a normal (Zeki and Bartels, 1999). But, one would also expect, if our hypothesis regarding processing–perceptual systems is correct, that such a patient would be able to experience something about the attribute processed by the damaged system, related to the physiological capacities of the undamaged nodes of that processing–perceptual system, meaning the physiological capacities of area V1 and possibly V2, which feed the specialised visual areas. This, too, is well illustrated by examples of visual object agnosia and prosopagnosia, two specialised systems that we have used specifically to provide direct evidence that processing systems are also perceptual systems, as well as by a study of the perceptual capacities of patients with akinetopsia or achromatopsia (for review, see Zeki and Bartels, 1999).

Further evidence in favour of our supposition comes indirectly from imaging experiments that have studied brain activity in conditions of "illusory" vision or hallucinations. Collectively, these reinforce the view that activity at a single node of a processing system can have a conscious correlate, without necessarily involving antecedent stages of the visual pathways. For example, the fast circular motion that is perceived by humans when viewing the static work of Leviant entitled *Enigma* correlates with the selective activation of one node of the motion processing system, area V5 (Zeki *et al.*, 1993) (Fig. 11.3), while the motion after-effect as well as mental imagery of motion correlate mainly with activation of V5 (Tootell *et al.*, 1995; Goebel *et al.*, 1998). Similarly, the perception of afterimages induced by colour correlates with the selective activation of one node of the colour processing system, the V4 complex (Sakai *et al.*, 1995), while viewing "illusory" Kanizsa triangles activates area V2 and V3 (Hirsch *et al.*, 1995; ffytche and Zeki, 1996). The latter is interesting in terms of physiology, for the evidence suggests that hallucinations constitute another condition that lends itself to isolating neural processing directly responsible for specific visual experiences. Patients suffering from the Charles Bonnet syndrome have visual hallucinations that can be rather restricted (*e.g.*, to the perception of objects, faces, colours, or textures). The brain activities during such hallucinations have been located in the regions in the visual cortex that are specialised for the corresponding attributes (ffytche *et al.*, 1998) without involving V1.

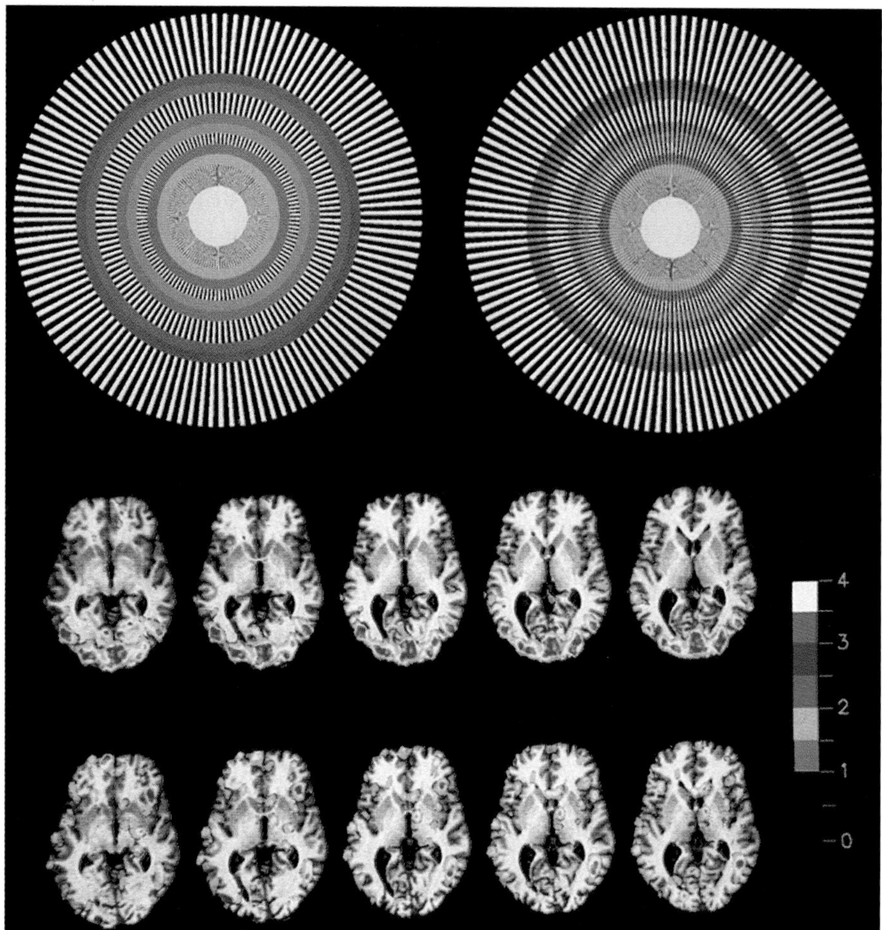

FIGURE 11.3

(Top) Two stimuli used in Zeki *et al.* (1993), based on Leviant's *Enigma*. When the centre is fixated, the illusory motion stimulus (left) results in the perception of rotatory motion, while the control stimulus (right) does not result in the perception of motion. (Bottom) Coregistered MRI and SPM images at successive 2-mm slices for a single subject. The upper row shows the result of comparing stationary and moving checkerboards; the lower row shows the result for the same slices comparing the illusory motion stimulus and its control. The colour scale to the right shows the Z values of the pixels.

A DIRECT DEMONSTRATION THAT PROCESSING SITES ARE ALSO PERCEPTUAL SITES

From the evidence detailed above, one obtains hints and suggestions, or hints followed by suggestions, but there are other studies that have left us uneasy about our interpretation. Chief among these are the compelling studies of Logothetis (1998) and his colleagues using binocular rivalry in the awake, behaving monkey and recording the activity of cells in different areas. The question asked in these experiments is: Are there cells in any visual area whose activity corresponds to the percept? The overall result has been that there are such cells in all areas, including even V1, but that their proportion increases as one samples from 'higher' areas. In fact, this is a result that is important for our theoretical formulations, and especially to our supposition that every node in the visual cortex is potentially a perceptual site (Zeki and Bartels, 1999). But, we needed to test our supposition in a different way, in an experiment designed to tap specifically a highly specialised area which could then be demonstrated to both process and perceive the specific stimulus. Equally informative have been the imaging experiments on bi- and multistable images (Kleinschmidt *et al.*, 1998; Lumer *et al.*, 1998). Unfortunately, they still left us with a puzzle. The switch in activity from one specialised area to another when the image shifted perceptually from, say, a face to a vase in the Rubin illusion, was also accompanied by activity in frontal and parietal cortex. This makes it difficult to equate processing with perception, as one could equally argue—especially in the absence of any temporal measurements—that it is processing in the frontoparietal system that determines what the subject perceives, tantamount to saying that the processing and the perceptual sites are different and that there is some kind of 'top-down' influence that dictates the percept. What is needed, then, is a more direct demonstration that the perceptual and processing sites are one and the same.

To our knowledge, the most compelling evidence that this is so comes from combined psychophysical imaging experiments that, instead of using binocular rivalry, have used binocular fusion (Moutoussis and Zeki, 2002). In these experiments, visual stimuli are delivered dichoptically in rapid and alternating succession to the eyes, with the consequence that there is no time for binocular rivalry to develop. If, say, the identical stimulus consisting of the outline of a house or face in red against a green background is delivered to both eyes, the two images will fuse and the subject will experience seeing a house (or face). If, on the other hand, the stimuli delivered to the two eyes are identical but of reverse colour contrast (*i.e.*, red outline against a green background to one eye and green outline against red background to the other), the subject will see a diffuse yellow, because of the fusion of the two images. One can then ask whether the same specific brain areas are activated when subjects perceive a house and when they do not. The answer (Fig. 11.4) is that it is the same areas that are activated, thus leading one ineluctably to the conclusion that processing areas are also perceptual areas. The difference between the two states, one in which subjects experience seeing a house (or face) and one in which they do not, is that the level of activity in the specific areas is higher in the former than in the latter state.

CONSCIOUS EXPERIENCE AS DEPENDENT UPON THE LEVEL OF ACTIVITY AT A NODE

In fact, the first direct experimental evidence in favour of such a suggestion came from a study of patient GY (Zeki and ffytche, 1998). Patient GY, recall, is usually aware of fast-moving stimuli and can discriminate their direction of motion correctly; however, he is not aware of slowly moving stimuli and cannot discriminate their direction of motion, or even their presence, correctly. When activity in his brain is imaged under these conditions, the contrast fast motion versus slow motion reveals activity in V5 alone. On the other hand, the contrast slow motion versus uniform grey (control) also reveals activity in V5 (Zeki and ffytche, 1998) (Fig. 11.5). In other words, the activity in V5 in the latter condition does not reach threshold levels to result in a conscious correlate. Therefore, "the switch from the unconscious to the conscious state correlates with the strength of activation in a given area" and leads to the supposition "of a positive relationship between cerebral activity in a specific visual area and awareness for a

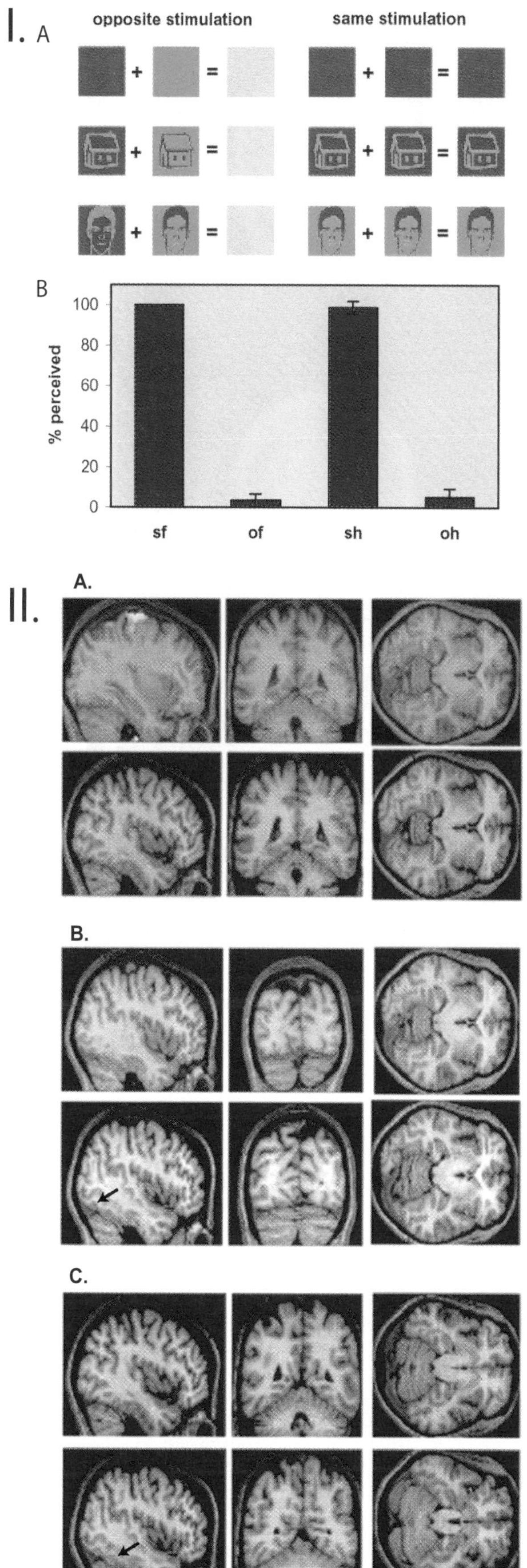

FIGURE 11.4

(I) (A) Schematic presentation of the stimulation method used in Moutoussiss and Zeki (2002). Pictures of houses, faces, and uniformly coloured controls were used. The input to the two eyes and the expected perceptual output (upper) and subjects' true psychophysical performance of the subjects (lower) are shown. Continuous fusion of the stimuli was achieved by using repetitive brief presentations. Dichoptic stimuli of opposite colour contrast between the two eyes were invisible (opposite stimulation), whereas identical stimuli of the same colour contrast were perceived the vast majority of the time (same stimulation). Control stimuli were never perceived, either as a face or a house. (B) The averaged performance of the seven subjects in the face/house/nothing discrimination task. The averaged percentage of the number of stimuli perceived is shown (of a total of 448 per subject per stimulus category) together with the standard error between the subjects. Abbreviations: sf, same faces; of, opposite faces; sh, same houses; oh, opposite houses. (II) Group results of brain regions showing stimulus-specific activation under conditions of same and opposite stimulation, revealing that such activation correlates with perceived and not-perceived conditions. (A, upper) The contrast same houses/same faces shows bilateral stimulus-specific activation in the parahippocampal gyrus (Talairach coordinates, 230, 244, 212 and 26, 244, 210). (A, lower) The contrast opposite houses/opposite faces shows unilateral stimulus-specific activation in the same region (238, 242, 210). (B, upper) The contrast same faces/same houses reveals stimulus-specific activation in a region of the fusiform gyrus (42, 282, 212). (B, lower) The contrast opposite faces/opposite houses reveals stimulus-specific activation in the same brain region (44, 274, 214), shown here by the arrow. (C, upper) The contrast same faces/same control when exclusively masked by the contrast same houses/same control revealed another region in the fusiform gyrus (238, 248, 218) showing face-specific activation. (C, lower) The same brain region in the opposite hemisphere (44, 256, 222) also shows much more significant face-specific activation under the contrast opposite faces/opposite houses; this area is shown by the arrow to distinguish it from the second area revealed by the same contrast.

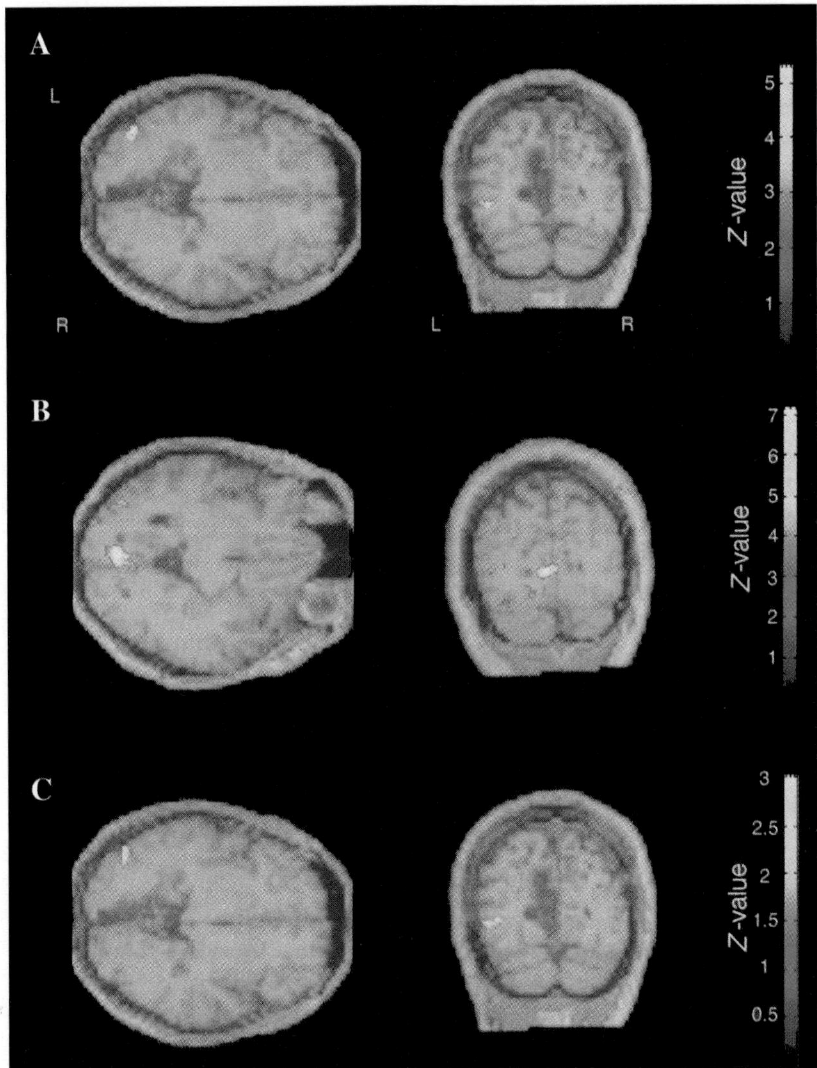

FIGURE 11.5
fMRI images of statistically significant increases in BOLD signal (shown in colour) superimposed on transverse and coronal sections of GY's brain. (A) The increases in cerebral activity comparing fast with slow motion in GY. (B) The increases in cerebral activity comparing fast with slow motion in a control subject. (C) The increases in cerebral activity comparing slow motion with an isoluminant grey control. (From Zeki, S. M. and ffytche, D., *Brain*, 121, 25–45, 1998. With permission.)

correspondingly specific visual attribute" (Zeki and ffytche, 1998). We do not know whether the excess activity in an area observed during conscious experience is due to the enhanced firing of cells that are also active in the unconscious (processing) state or whether it involves the recruitment of previously inactive cells. Whatever the reason for the heightened activity, it is interesting that our suggestion receives strong support from the imaging experiments of Rees *et al.* (2000) and Dehaene *et al.* (2001), both of whom report similar results.

THE PROBLEM OF INTEGRATION

Before the above psychophysical studies on perceptual asynchrony, the problem that functional specialisation creates in terms of bringing different visual attributes together with respect to time was not given much attention; however, the more general idea of integration (mostly spatial) has been puzzling scientists for a long time. If different visual attributes are processed by different specialised systems, how is it that the "output" of all these systems comes together for us to experience the single, unitary visual perception that we do? Early models of integration, influenced by the discovery of cells in the cortex having properties with a gradually increasing complexity, were based upon a hierarchical chain model of perception. The idea was that we have lower and higher processing levels within the visual system, with neuronal properties becoming more and more complex as one moves from the former to the latter (Hubel and Wiesel, 1977). Neurons with simple properties are the building blocks for more complex neurons having more sophisticated properties, which in turn are themselves the blocks for building neurons with even higher properties, and so on. At the end of this hierarchical chain one would then find the most sophisticated neurons, also known as "grandmother cells," that are able to signal the presence of very complicated images (instead of simply spots, lines, gratings, etc.) such as our grandmother. When the idea of functional specialisation matured, this serial hierarchical model was largely abandoned for a model consisting of several parallel pathways, each one responsible for the processing of a different visual attribute. The idea of a hierarchy and the build-up of more complex properties as one moves away from the retina still holds, but is now true within each parallel system separately. A new and challenging problem regarding integration thus arose, that of how does the output from all these different parallel pathways come together in order to give a unified rather than a segmented vision. An obvious solution would be that of convergence (*i.e.*, the existence of a single brain area to which all the higher areas of each parallel system would project). Anatomical studies, however, have revealed that no such area exists; therefore, the information from all the different functionally specialised systems does not eventually come together in a single place. The idea of integration through convergence has thus been largely abandoned, and a different solution needs to be found. Another possibility arose from the fact that the functionally specialised systems, although topographically segregated, do not remain absolutely isolated from one another. There are many instances in which cross-talk can occur between the different visual pathways. Considering areas such as V1 and V2 in which multiple visual attributes are represented in particular, the idea of different signals coming together in a single area where it would be "easier" for them to "communicate" (via stripe-to-stripe connections in area V2, for example) made such areas possible candidates for "integration." The problem, however, is that areas such as V2 are found quite early in the visual pathway, whereas integration is considered to take place more toward the end of the signal-processing chain. This problem can again be taken care of by considering the role of back projections from the higher areas, and in fact a lot of speculation on the role of back projections on integration has been made.

As a general rule, there are two basic common factors shared between all theories trying to solve the problem of integration. The first is that none has up to now given a satisfactory answer to the problem, and the second is that they all assume that such a thing as integration actually exists. This last view is challenged by the demonstration of temporally independent perceptual systems being present in the visual brain. The function of integration is supposed to be bringing together different visual attributes in the correct spatiotemporal order preconsciously. This is not what is happening, however, at least in terms of time. If each attribute is perceived independently and at its own time, perception is characterised by segregation rather than by integration. Perceptual asynchrony thus offers the possibility of a new, radical solution to the problem of integration—that is, the absence of integration. This idea is not as extreme as it may seem, nor are the problems it creates more complicated than the ones created if one accepts that there is integration. It assumes that the visual brain is made up of several independent systems and that our visual perception is a collection of the perceptions of all these systems. If one system is perceiving green and another system is perceiving upward motion, we are perceiving both because *we are* both these two systems. The same is true if we go beyond the limits of vision: We can hear, feel, touch, smell, move, think, etc.; there is no single part of the brain where all this is happening together. It is happening across the whole of our brain, and we are the integrated result of all these happenings but with no need for integration. Instead, temporal binding is important: things happening in the brain at the same time are bound with each other. There is thus a communication (a "connection") between the independent systems in terms of brain time, rather than in terms of axons and pathways.

This solution seems slightly metaphysical, and it might well be; however, until the mystery of consciousness is solved, the answer to the problems such an approach creates will have to wait as well. It is the personal taste of this chapter's authors to revisit the problem of integration in a more radical way. If this view seems extreme, the microconsciousness theory has a slightly different alternative to offer, that of perception without and before integration. Again, mutual integration between different processing systems is not necessary for the creation of a conscious percept, but there is post-conscious perceptual integration in terms of binding the conscious experiences generated in each system. A perceptual autonomy of not only the functionally specialised systems but also of the nodes of each system is supported by experiments and clinical studies, leading to the microconsciousness theory. We therefore speculate that each node of a functionally specialised system may have a conscious correlate, and integration may occur between the conscious correlates of any two (or more) nodes belonging to either the same or different processing–perceptual systems—the so-called theory of multistage integration (Zeki, 1990; Bartels and Zeki, 1998). In other words, if any binding occurs to give us our integrated image of the visual world, it must be a binding between microconsciousnesses generated at different nodes. Furthermore, because any two microconsciousnesses generated at any two nodes can be bound together, perceptual integration is post-conscious.

SUMMARY

The visual system is characterised by functional specialisation, an organisational principle dictating that each different visual attribute is processed by a different specialised system. This creates a problem concerning our subjective experience of a unified visual perception, including the time domain as well. Psychophysical experiments have demonstrated that different visual attributes are perceived at different times and independently from one another. This finding has extended functional specialisation to the perceptual domain as well, suggesting that each specialised system is not only a processing but also a perceptual system, able to reach conscious perception of its corresponding attribute. Integration at the processing level is thus not necessary; it can be thought of more as a temporal, post-conscious binding between the perceptual results of the independent systems. The question of whether and how this binding takes place remains mysterious, the answer hiding behind the ubiquitous mind-brain problem.

References

Barbur, J. L., Watson, J. D. G., Frackowiak, R. S. J., and Zeki, S. M. (1993). Conscious visual perception without V1. *Brain*, **116**, 1293–1302.

Bartels, A. and Zeki, S. (1998). The theory of multi-stage integration in the visual brain. *Proc. Roy. Soc. London Ser. B*, **265,** 2327–2332.

Bartels, A. and Zeki, S. (2000). The architecture of the colour centre in the human visual brain: new results and a review. *Eur. J. Neurosci.*, **12**, 172–193.

Beckers, G. and Zeki, S. (1995). The consequences of inactivating areas V1 and V5 on visual-motion perception. *Brain*, **118**, 49–60.

Bullier, J., Girard, P., and Salin, P. A. (1994). The role of area 17 in the transfer of information to extrastriate visual cortex, in *Cerebral Cortex.* Vol. 10. *Primary Visual Cortex in Primates*, Peters, A. and Rockland, K. S., Eds., pp. 301–330. Plenum, New York.

Courtney, S. M., Finkel, L. H., and Buchsbaum, G. (1995). A multistage neural network for colour constancy and colour induction. *IEEE Trans. Neural Networks*, **6**, 972–985.

Cragg, B. G. (1969). The topography of the afferent projections in circumstriate visual cortex studied by the Nauta method. *Vision Res.*, **9**, 733–747.

Crick, F. and Koch, C. (1995). Are we aware of neural activity in primary visual cortex? *Nature*, **375**, 121–123.

Damasio, A. R. (1985). Disorders of complex visual processing agnosias, achromatopsia, Balint's syndrome, and related difficulties of orientation and construction, in *Principles of Behavioural Neurology*, Mesulam, M. M., Ed., pp. 259–288. Davis, Philadelphia.

Dehaene, S., Naccache, L., Cohen, L., Bihan, D. L., Mangin, J. F. *et al.* (2001). Cerebral mechanisms of word masking and unconscious repetition priming. *Nat. Neurosci.*, **4**, 752–758.

DeYoe, E. A. and Van Essen, D. C. (1988). Concurrent processing streams in monkey visual cortex. *Trends Neurosci.*, **11**, 219–226.

ffytche, D. H. and Zeki, S. (1996). Brain activity related to the perception of illusory contours. *Neuroimage*, **3**, 104–108.

ffytche, D. H., Guy, C. N., and Zeki, S. (1995). The parallel visual motion inputs into areas V1 and V5 of human cerebral cortex. *Brain*, **18,** 1375–1394 .

ffytche, D. H., Guy, C. N., and Zeki, S. (1996). Motion specific responses from a blind hemifield. *Brain*, **119**, 1971–1982.

ffytche, D. H., Howard, R. J., Brammer, M. J., David, A., Woodruff, P., and Williams, S. (1998). The anatomy of conscious vision: an fMRI study of visual hallucinations. *Nat. Neurosci.*, **1**, 738–742.

Fries, W. (1981). The projection from the lateral geniculate nucleus to the prestriate cortex of the macaque monkey. *Proc. Roy. Soc. London Ser. B*, **213**, 73–80.

Goebel, R., Khorram Sefat, D., Muckli, L., Hacker, H., and Singer, W. (1998). The constructive nature of vision: direct evidence from functional magnetic resonance imaging studies of apparent motion and motion imagery. *Eur. J. Neurosci.*, **10**, 1563–1573.

Hadjikhani, N., Liu, A. K., Dale, A., Cavanagh, P., and Tootell, R. B. H. (1998). Retinotopy and colour sensitivity in human visual cortical area V8. *Nat. Neurosci.*, **1**, 235–241.

Helmholtz, Hv. (1911). *Handbuch der Physiologischen Optik*. Leopold Voss, Hamburg.

Heywood, C. and Cowey, A. (1998). With colour in mind. *Nat. Neurosci.*, **1**, 171–173.

Hirsch, J., Delapaz, R. L., Relkin, N. R., Victor, J., Kim, K. *et al.* (1995). Illusory contours activate specific regions in human visual cortex: evidence from functional magnetic resonance imaging. *Proc. Natl. Acad. Sci. USA*, **92**, 6469–6473.

Holmes, G. (1918). Disturbances of vision caused by cerebral lesions. *Br. J. Ophthalmol.*, **2**, 353–384.

Horton, J. C. and Hoyt, W. F. (1991). Quadrantic visual field defects: a hallmark of lesions in extrastriate (V2/V3) cortex. *Brain*, **114**, 1703–1718.

Hubel, D. H. and Livingstone, M. S. (1987). Segregation of form, colour and stereopsis in primate area 18. *J. Neurosci.*, **7**, 3378–3415.

Hubel, D. H. and Wiesel, T. N. (1977). The Ferrier lecture: functional architecture of macaque monkey visual cortex. *Proc. Roy. Soc. London Ser. B*, **198**, 1–59.

Humphrey, G. K., Goodale, M. A., Corbetta, M., and Aglioti, S. (1995). The McCollough effect reveals orientation discrimination in a case of cortical blindness. *Curr. Biol.*, **5**, 545–551.

Kastner, S., DeWeerd, P., Desimone, R., and Ungerleider, L. C. (1998). Mechanisms of directed attention in the human extrastriate cortex as revealed by functional MRI. *Science*, **282**, 108–111.

Kleinschmidt, A., Büchel, C., Zeki, S., and Frackowiak, R. S. J. (1998). Human brain activity during spontaneously reversing perception of ambiguous figures. *Proc. Roy. Soc. London Ser. B, Biol. Sci.*, **265**, 2427–2432.

Land, E. H. (1974). The retinex theory of colour vision. *Proc. Roy. Inst. Gr. Brit.*, **47**, 23–58.

Land, E. H. and McCann, J. J. (1971). Lightness and retinex theory. *J. Opt. Soc. Am.*, **61**, 1–11.

Livingstone, M. and Hubel, D. (1988). Segregation of form, colour, movement, and depth: anatomy, physiology, and perception. *Science*, 240, 740–749.

Logothetis, N. K. (1998). Single units and conscious vision. *Philos. Trans. Roy. Soc. London B*, **353**, 1801–18.

Lumer, E. D., Friston, K. J., and Rees, G. (1998). Neural correlates of perceptual rivalry in the human brain. *Science*, **280**, 1930–1934.

McKeefry, D. and Zeki, S. (1997). The position and topography of the human colour centre as revealed by functional magnetic resonance imaging. *Brain*, **120**, 2229–2242.

Moutoussis, K. and Zeki, S. (2002). The relationship between cortical activation and perception investigated with invisible stimuli. *Proc. Natl. Acad. Sci. USA*, **99**, 9527–9532.

Paulson, H. L., Galetta, S. L., Grossman, M., and Alavi, A. (1994). Hemiachromatopsia of unilateral occipitotemporal infarcts. *Am. J. Ophthalmol.*, **118**, 518–523.

Rees, G., Wojciulik, E., Clarke, K., Husain, M., Frith, C., and Driver, J. (2000). Unconscious activation of visual cortex in the damaged right hemisphere of a parietal patient with extinction. *Brain*, **123**, 1624–1633.

Riddoch, G. (1917). Dissociations of visual perception due to occipital injuries, with especial reference to appreciation of movement. *Brain*, **40**, 15–57.

Sakai, K., Watanabe, E., Onodera, Y, Uchida, I., Kato, H. *et al.* (1995). Functional mapping of the human colour centre with echo-planar magnetic resonance imaging. *Proc. Roy. Soc. London Ser. B*, **261**, 89–98.

Standage, G. P. and Benevento, L. A. (1983). The organisation of connections between the pulvinar and visual area MT in the macaque monkey. *Brain Res.*, **262**, 288–294.

Stoerig, P. (1996). Varieties of vision: from blind responses to conscious recognition. *Trends Neurosci.*, **19**, 401–406.

Stoerig, P. and Barth, E. (2001). Low-level phenomenal vision despite unilateral destruction of primary visual cortex. *Conscious. Cogn.*, **10**, 574–587.

Stoerig, P. and Cowey, A. (1995). Visual perception and phenomenal consciousness. *Behav. Brain Res.*, **71**, 147–156.

Tootell, R. B. H., Reppas, J. B., Dale, A. M., Look, R. B., Sereno, M. I. *et al.* (1995). Visual motion aftereffect in human cortical area MT revealed by functional magnetic resonance imaging. *Nature*, **375**, 139–141.

Tootell, R. B., Dale, A. M., Sereno, M. I., and Malach, R. (1996). New images from human visual cortex. *Trends in Neurosci.*, **19**, 481–489.

Wade, A. R., Brewer, A. A., Rieger, J. W., and Wandell, B. A. (2002). Functional measurements of human ventral occipital cortex, retinotopy and colour. *Philos. Trans. Roy. Soc. London B, Biol. Sci.*, **357**, 963–973.

Walsh, V., Kulikowski, J. J., Butler, S. R., and Carden, D. (1992). The effects of lesions of area V4 on the visual abilities of macaques, colour categorisation. *Behav. Brain Res.*, **52**, 81–89.

Wechsler, I. S. (1933). Partial cortical blindness with preservation of colour vision. *Arch. Ophthalmol.*, **9**, 957–965.

Weiskrantz, L. (1986). *Blindsight*. Oxford University Press, London.

Weiskrantz, L., Barbur, J. L., and Sahraie, A. (1995). Parameters affecting conscious versus unconscious visual discrimination with damage to the visual cortex (V1). *Proc. Natl. Acad. Sci. USA*, **92**, 6122–6126.

Yukie, M. and Iwai, E. (1981). Direct projection from the dorsal lateral geniculate nucleus to the prestriate cortex in macaque monkeys. *J. Comp. Neurol.*, **201**, 81–97.

Zeki, S. (1985). Colour pathways and hierarchies in the cerebral cortex, in *Central and Peripheral Mechanisms of Colour Vision*, Ottoson, D. and S Zeki, S. M., Eds., pp. 19–44. Macmillan, London.

Zeki, S. (1990). A century of cerebral achromatopsia. *Brain*, **113**, 1721–1777.

Zeki, S. (1991). Cerebral akinetopsia (visual motion blindness): a review. *Brain*, **114,** 811–824.

Zeki, S. (1993). *A Vision of the Brain*. Blackwell, Oxford.

Zeki, S. (1997). The colour and motion systems as guides to conscious visual perception, in *Extrastriate Cortex in Primates*, Vol. 12, Rockland, K. S., Kaas, J. H., and Peters, A., Eds., pp. 777–809, Plenum, New York.

Zeki, S. (1998). Parallel processing, asynchronous perception and a distributed system of consciousness in vision. *Neuroscientist*, **4,** 365–372.

Zeki, S. and Bartels, A. (1999). Towards a theory of visual consciousness. *Conscious. Cogn.*, **8**, 225–259.

Zeki, S. and ffytche, D. (1998). The Riddoch syndrome: insights into the neurobiology of conscious vision. *Brain*, **121**, 25–45.

Zeki, S. and Marini, L. (1998). Three cortical stages of colour processing in the human brain. *Brain*, **121**, 1669–1685.

Zeki, S. and Shipp, S. (1988). The functional logic of cortical connections. *Nature*, **335**, 311–317.

Zeki, S., Watson, J. D., and Frackowiak, R. S. (1993). Going beyond the information given, the relation of illusory visual motion to brain activity. *Proc. Roy. Soc. London Ser. B*, **252**, 215–222.

Zeki, S., Aglioti, S., McKeefry, D. and Berlucchi, G. (1999). The neurobiological basis of conscious colour perception in a blind patient. *Proc. Natl. Acad. Sci. USA*, **96**, 14124–14129.

Zheng, D., LaMantia, A. S., and Purves, D. (1991). Specialised vascularisation of the primate visual cortex. *J. Neurosci.*, **11**, 2622–2629.

C H A P T E R

12

The Asynchrony of Visual Perception

THE PROBLEM OF PROCESSING TIME: PERCEPTUAL ASYNCHRONY

The picture of both specificity and segregation—or functional specialisation (Zeki, 1974, 1975, 1978, 1980, 1993; Livingstone and Hubel, 1984a,b, 1987, 1988; DeYoe and Van Essen, 1985, 1988; Shipp and Zeki, 1985, 1989a,b, 1995; Zeki and Shipp, 1988, 1989; Zeki *et al.*, 1991; Nakamura *et al.*, 1993)—that is evident throughout the organisation of the visual system, from the very early to the very late stages, creates a problem (for the experimenter, not the brain): If different specialised systems process different attributes of the visual scene, do they all take the same amount of time to finish their job? "Finish their job" specifically refers to perception, the instant at which the subject becomes consciously aware of a colour, a shape, or some other attribute. Perception is perhaps not the only job of the visual system, but it is definitely one of its primordial jobs. The term *perception time* is used here to imply the time between the appearance of a stimulus in the field of view (on the screen in an experiment) and the moment[1] a human individual subjectively experiences this stimulus. Other names, such as *perceptual time*, *(total) processing time*, etc. can and sometimes are used, but a single term is used here to avoid complications.

As we define it, the term *perception time* is free from vague assumptions about the completion of brain processing, anatomical or physiological cell properties, the relationship between neural activity and perception, specific "perceptual" brain areas, etc. It is not, for example, defined as the time it takes for a percept to become established in a particular cortical area (whatever the latter may mean). Perception time is rather a property of the specialised system as a whole. In the context in which we use the term, the relation of perception time to things such as activity reaching certain levels, areas involved, back projections, oscillations and synchronisations, and so on is irrelevant. The important question is whether the perception time of different visual attributes is the same or different, given functional specialisation as the organising principle of the visual system in which each of the specialised systems is characterised by different properties, different types of neurons, different brain pathways, and so on.

[1]One assumption is made here—namely, that there is a certain point in time when perception takes place. Philosophical questions such as whether the time we attribute to an event is tied to the time at which the brain generates a representation of that event are not considered. The more simple idea that subjects believe things are happening at exactly the instance they perceive them (via some unknown type of neural activity) is adopted instead. In some cases, perception might be postponed, influenced, for example, by stimuli occurring afterwards, but once a conscious percept is formed it is also automatically given a point in time. A dissociation between the perception of the temporal order of events and the perception of events *per se* (Johnston and Nishida, 2001) is, in our belief, not a safe thought path to follow.

In addition, because different visual attributes are different in nature and can vary independently of one another, the job that each functionally specialised system has to do is unique and different from the ones that other specialised systems have to do. It is therefore difficult to suppose that different visual attributes will be perceived at exactly the same time interval after the appearance of the stimulus, although many in the past have written as if this was so. Synchronising all the different perceptions resulting from the separate processing of the different attributes of a stimulus would require some imaginary and highly complicated brain mechanism that is aware of all the detailed temporal differences in processing between the systems and is able perhaps to postpone the perception of some attributes until the processing of other attributes that take longer time is also ready to be perceived. In addition to the extreme complication of such a mechanism, it would also seem to be disadvantageous for the brain to delay a percept that can be made available at an earlier time. On the other hand, the idea of a perceptual asynchrony, with different visual attributes being perceived at different times, is daunting, contrary to any experience and intuition we may have about what is going on with respect to our perception.

At any rate, the question whether different attributes of a stimulus are perceived at exactly the same time after the appearance of the stimulus, or at different times, can be addressed in a relatively simple way: If attribute A is in general being perceived at time dt earlier than attribute B, then attribute B_1 presented on the screen at a given time t will not be perceived together with attribute A_1 also presented at time t, but with attribute A_2, which is presented at time $t + dt$. In other words, if the difference between the perception times of two attributes is exactly balanced by the difference between the times of occurrence of their presentation, visual attributes presented on the screen at different times should be perceived as presented at the same time. This idea has been tested by varying the colour of a set of moving dots on a computer monitor between red and green, while at the same time changing the direction of their motion between up and down (Moutoussis and Zeki, 1997a,b). Both the colour and the motion of the dots were thus dictated by identical square-wave oscillations, presented at various phase differences between them. Subjects were asked to report which motion/motion combination they believed took place most of the time on the screen (*i.e.*, to bind the two attributes with respect to their perceived appearance on the screen)—either red together with up and green together with down or vice versa. They were specifically instructed not to pay any attention to whether reversals in colour occurred at the same time as reversals in the direction of movement, what the colour of the dots was when they changed direction, what was their direction of motion when the colour changed, and so on. Binding the percepts of the two attributes was all they were asked to do.

If there is no perception time difference between colour and motion, then the perceptual experience of the subjects should follow exactly the (veridical) reality occurring on the computer screen; if, on the other hand, there is a perception time difference between colour and motion, the perception of the subjects should be different from the veridical reality on the screen. The results of such psychophysical experiments, comparing the perception of colour and motion, show that the latter is actually the case; colour was perceived by about 80 ms before motion; that is, the direction of motion was perceived together with the colour that took place on the screen 80 ms after that particular motion took place (Moutoussis and Zeki, 1997a,b). Although entirely consistent with the functional organisation of the visual brain and against the doctrine of exclusive hierarchies proposed by Hubel and Wiesel, this is still an astonishing result. The more general conclusion that the finding leads to, that different visual attributes are perceived at different times and thus independently of one another, is even more astonishing and counterintuitive.

The initial experiments were done with the same set of dots changing both colour and direction (Moutoussis and Zeki, 1997a). The reason was that different visual attributes belonging to the same object are normally thought to be integrated together, and this perhaps would be true for temporal integration as well. When the first set of experiments showed that this was not the case, it was clear that whether colour and motion belonged to the same or to different objects was irrelevant; the perception of each attribute was independent from the perception of the other in both cases (this incidentally constitutes an admirable example of what was mentioned earlier about the need for functional specialisation—namely, that two attributes belonging to the same object can vary independently). Indeed, when the experiments were repeated with colour stimulation in one half of the screen and motion stimulation in the other half (*i.e.*, each attribute this time belonging to a different object), results were identical with the ones in which colour and motion were bound to the same object (Moutoussis and Zeki, 1997b). The same temporal misbinding took place again, colour perception leading motion perception by the same amount of time. It thus became clear that "correct" temporal binding (*i.e.*, one corresponding to the veridical reality) is not what occurs in the brain over very brief time windows, but that what is perceptually bound instead is the independent percepts that each functionally specialised system produces during these brief time windows. These systems thus are not only processing but also perceptual systems, being able to give rise to the perception of their corresponding attribute independently and in their own time, even when this processing concerns the same object as that processed by another specialised system. Functional specialisation is in this way extended to the perceptual domain, and these experiments have revealed the segregated nature of conscious visual perception.

HOW SOLID IS THE PERCEPTUAL ASYNCHRONY RESULT/IDEA?

Some received the idea of different visual attributes being perceived at different times with both surprise and scepticism. A reflex reaction to the initial finding that colour is perceived before motion could be that it is a counterintuitive result. The reason for this might be that the motion system has been generally thought to be capable of faster processing than the colour system (Maunsel, 1999; Munk *et al.*, 1995; Raiguel *et al.*, 1989), just one step from the conclusion that motion should therefore be perceived before the colour. Such an argument, however, would miss the main point that there is asynchronous perception and would concentrate on a secondary finding, the fact that colour is faster, as if up to that moment it was common knowledge that motion is perceived before colour! The important question to ask is whether one attribute is perceived before the other, rather than which attribute is perceived before the other. Furthermore, predicting that motion should be perceived earlier is naïve, as it has never been possible to equate neural and perceptual events. For example, the fact that colour-specialised- thin CO stripes in V2 have longer activation latencies than motion-specialised thick stripes (Munk *et al.*, 1995) can in no way imply that motion is perceived before colour, as no one has succeeded in equating neural activation in either type of stripe with conscious visual experience. Perhaps the motion system is faster than the colour system because it has a more difficult task to achieve and thus more work to do, in which case a perceptual lag with respect to the colour system is explainable. Perhaps it is exactly because motion processing is more complicated than colour processing that the former is better equipped (in terms of conduction velocities required to reach the motion centre of the cortex from the retina) than the latter. One can go on speculating endlessly, but no concrete conclusion can be drawn as long as the mysterious relationship between neural activity and perception remains unsolved; however, the strength of the psychophysical method described above lies in the fact that it overrides all complicated brain processing mechanisms involved in perception and goes on to measure perception times directly, or, more precisely, perception time differences. No described scientific method is able to measure absolute perception times, because it is not yet possible to know when exactly a percept is formed. It is for this reason that scientists usually resort to other measures, reaction time being the most typical one.

Several studies have compared reaction times to motion and colour stimuli with varying results, depending upon the method. There is no way, however, in which information from these studies can be used to address the problem of differences in perception time, not to mention measuring perception time *per se*. The obvious reason is that nobody knows what elapses between sensory perception and motor reaction. This might differ between reactions to different visual attributes, so one cannot equate the perception-to-reaction time interval between, say, colour and motion, and thus estimate stimulation-to-perception differences based on stimulation-to-reaction data. It is not even true that the scheme stimulation–perception–reaction always holds; it is almost certain that stimulation–reaction shortcuts can in many cases bypass the stage of conscious perception. There is, for example, clear experimental evidence that the presence or absence of a difference in motion/motion reaction time measurements can depend on the motor task. Reaction time information thus has very little to offer the question of perception times, and any objections to perceptual asynchrony based on reaction time results are not convincing (Nishida and Johnston, 2002).

Because of the importance that we attach to the demonstration of perceptual asynchrony and because of its theoretical importance in learning how the visual brain functions and in formulating theories about visual consciousness, we address here some concerns regarding the experiments. One possible concern regarding the psychophysical results described above and the methods on which they are based, is that the demonstrated asynchrony is perhaps not a matter of perception *per se* but rather a matter of judgment of the time of occurrence of events (Nishida and Johnston, 2002). If so, the misjudgement reported does not necessarily reflect perception time differences, but could, for example, reflect the properties of a mechanism specialised in judging the temporal order of events. This does not, however, apply in our original perceptual asynchrony experiments, as subjects reported their perception online (*i.e.*, as the stimulus was still on the screen), and there was no limit to the duration of stimulus presentation. Subjects were directly reporting what they were (still) perceiving, and only when they had made up their mind did they choose to end the trial and respond. This method is very different from, say, single presentations, when a single colour and a single motion are flashed at various time offsets between them, and then subjects have to make a decision (with no stimulus present on the screen) based on memory, temporal order judgment, etc. (Viviani and Aymoz, 2001)—factors that might not always accurately reflect perception at the time of its occurrence. For example, post-prediction mechanisms can interact with temporal order judgments of single events, as shown in the flash-lag experiment of Eagleman and Sejnowski (2000). For the same reason, subjects were not asked in our experiments to report on the reversals of colour/motion (which are instantaneous events) but rather on their continuous motion/motion perception. The idea that the reported misbinding might reflect some "imperfections" of a hypothetical system responsible for subsequently determining the temporal properties of events is thus unsatisfactory, as online perception rather than perceived time of occurrence is under question.

Repeating these experiment by asking subjects to make temporal order judgments of the instances at which colour and motion changes occur, instead of reporting their combined motion/motion percept, can in some cases give misleading results. An ingenious way to avoid this problem altogether, providing further evidence in favour of the effect being a purely perceptual one, comes from combining such psychophysical studies with the colour-contingent motion after-effect (Arnold *et al.*, 2001). After watching a slowly rotating stimulus, a static stimulus appears to rotate in the opposite direction, and this after-effect can be made contingent on colour: If a particular colour is associated with a particular direction of rotation and another colour with the opposite direction (during the same adaptation period), a static pattern of either colour will appear to be rotating in a direction opposite to the one corresponding to that colour during the adaptation period. If colour states are correlated disproportionately with two directions of motion, the contingent motion after-effects observed are consistent, with the perceptual correlation between colour and motion being different from the physical correlation and with colour being perceived more quickly than motion. In other words, although subjects are not at all concerned with binding colour to motion directly, their reports on the motion after-effect are consistent with a perceptual misbinding as originally described.

If one assumes that what we actually perceive is not colour and motion, but rather colour and position, and therefore treats motion as a change of position over time rather than as an independent perception in itself, then a further objection to the psychophysical result described above can arise: Motion changes in this particular experiment are second-order temporal changes of the primary percept (position), whereas colour changes are first-order temporal changes. As far as both colour and motion perception are concerned, they can be described by two identical square-wave oscillations (up/down, green/red). But, if instead of motion we start thinking in terms of position, then the two oscillations are no longer identical, and this difference can now theoretically account for the reported "perception lag," especially if the task is to make temporal order judgments of changes (between two oscillations of a different type). In fact, one can make the position changes first order (here/there) and the colour changes second order (*e.g.*, gradually change in a sine-wave manner from green through yellow to red) and observe the reverse result on reports of when a change occurred (Nishida and Johnston, 2002). These manipulations, however, deviate significantly from the initial purpose of the experiment, which is to compare two different percepts each of which can have one of two values. If a sine wave is used to change the colour as described above, there are numerous colour percepts involved and naturally one cannot speak about specific colour perceptions *per se* any more. The interest is thus removed from the percept itself and transferred to the temporal characteristics of the stimulus; this is a totally different approach. But, motion perception is, as far as the brain is concerned, an independent entity, not the first derivative of position with respect to time. There can be motion perception without any perception of change in position (*e.g.*, random dot stimuli) or even without any physical change in position (*e.g.*, the well-known motion after-effect, Leviant illusion) (Zeki *et al.*, 1993). With respect to the brain, motion is thus just another sensation, just as are colour and form (Nakayama, 1985), so a change in motion perception from upward to downward is indeed (perceptually) a first-order change, just as a change of colour from red to green is.

Mechanistically speaking, one could still argue that, although two monitor frames are enough for a colour change to take place, three frames are necessary for a motion change. This possible 14-ms difference is much less than the 50 to 100 ms of reported perceptual asynchrony and is probably not at all part of the equation because, with the exception of the very first time glance at the stimulus, a single frame is enough to register that both the colour and direction of motion have changed. Furthermore, this misbinding method can be used to compare perception time differences between any two attributes, so the ambiguous motion can be left aside. When orientation is also included in such experiments, it is found to be perceived earlier than motion but later than colour (Moutoussis and Zeki, 1997b). The introduction of orientation not only generalises the finding of perceptual asynchrony beyond colour and motion but also serves as a good control for the method itself. Because only two attributes can be compared each time, the results of the three independent comparisons can be also compared between them to see if they make sense (if A before B and B before C, then A before C).

The currently available evidence leads us to accept the notion of a perceptual asynchrony in vision. This is consistent with the theory of functional specialisation in the visual brain, which it in fact consolidates. It allows us to inquire more closely into the nature of visual consciousness.

THE MICROCONSCIOUSNESS THEORY

If conscious visual perception is segregated, then consciousness itself is, by necessity, also segregated. The results of the psychophysical experiments described above inspired a new way of thinking about consciousness (Zeki and Bartels, 1999). The basic idea is that there is no single, integrated visual consciousness, but rather several different consciousnesses coexisting at the same time. In the light of this new way of thinking, previous knowledge is now approached from a different perspective. For example, clinical evidence shows that damage restricted to one system leads to an imperception in the attribute for which that system is specialised, not to global blindness, and, conversely, a system that is spared while all others are damaged can function more or less adequately (Zihl, 1983, 1991; Campion and Lato, 1985; Damasio, 1985; Blythe *et al.*, 1987; Hess *et al.*, 1989; Zeki, 1990, 1991; Ceccaldi *et al.*, 1992; Vaina, 1994; Kennard *et al.*, 1995; Zeki *et al.*, 1999). This is perhaps the most striking indication of a perceptual autonomy of different specialised systems and has not been given enough credit previously when considered to be just another manifestation of functional specialisation. However, after the psychophysical discovery of perceptual asynchrony, all these previous findings can be grouped together in what we now refer to as the *microconsciousness theory* (Zeki and Bartels, 1999). The realisation that there is no single consciousness in vision, but rather several microconsciousnesses emerging from the existence of several functionally specialised systems, is the driving force behind this theory. It goes beyond the psychophysical results described above and tries to relate the idea of multiple independent consciousnesses to well-known facts about the anatomy and physiology of the visual cortex. It states that the activity of cells in a given processing system is sufficient to create a conscious experience of the corresponding attribute without the necessity of interaction with activities of cells in other processing systems (which is not to say that other subcortical or cortical structures, such as the frontal lobes, may not be involved). The visual brain is thus composed of processing–perceptual systems, the neural activity in each of which can have a conscious correlate (microconsciousness) without the need for a central consciousness area. It is a challenging idea that we discuss at greater length in an ensuing chapter.

References

Arnold, D. H., Clifford, C. W. G., and Wenderoth, P. (2001). Asynchronus processing in vision: colour leads motion. *Curr. Biol.*, **11**, 596–600.

Blythe, I. M., Kennard, C., and Ruddock, K. H. (1987). Residual vision in patients with retrogeniculate lesions of the visual pathways. *Brain*, **10**, 887–905.

Campion, J. and Latto, R. (1985). Apperceptive agnosia due to carbon-monoxide poisoning: an interpretation based on critical band masking from disseminated lesions. *Behav. Brain Res.*, **15**, 227–240.

Ceccaldi, M., Mestre, D., Brouchon, M., Balzamo, M., and Poncet, M. (1992). Ambulatory autonomy and visual-motion perception in a case of almost total cortical blindness. *Rev. Nerurol. (Paris)*, **148**, 343–349.

Damasio, A. R. (1985). Disorders of complex visual processing agnosias, achromatopsia, Balint's syndrome, and related difficulties of orientation and construction, in *Principles of Behavioural Neurology*, Mesulam, M. M., Ed., pp. 259–288. Davis, Philadelphia.

DeYoe, E. A. and Van Essen, D. C. (1985). Segregation of efferent connections and receptive field properties in visual area 2 of the macaque. *Nature*, **317**, 58–61.

DeYoe, E. A. and Van Essen, D. C. (1988). Concurrent processing streams in monkey visual cortex. *Trends Neurosci.*, **11**, 219–226.

Eagleman, D. M. and Sejnowski, T. J. (2000). Motion integration and postdiction in visual awareness. *Science*, **287**, 2036–2038.

Hess, R. H., Baker, C. L., and Zihl, J. (1989). The 'motion-blind' patient: low level spatial and temporal filters. *J. Neurosci.*, **9**, 1628–1640.

Hubel, D. H. and Livingstone, M. S. (1987). Segregation of form, colour and stereopsis in primate area 18. *J. Neurosci.*, **7**, 3378–3415.

Johnston, A. and Nishida, S. (2001). Time perception: brain time or event time? *Curr. Biol.*, **11**, R427–R430.

Kennard, C., Lawden, M., Morland, A. B., and Ruddock, K. H. (1995). Colour identification and colour constancy are impaired in a patient with incomplete achromatopsia associated with prestriate cortical lesions. *Proc. Roy. Soc. London Ser. B, Biol. Sci.*, **260**, 169–175.

Livingstone, M. S. and Hubel, D. H. (1984a). Anatomy and physiology of a colour system in the primate visual cortex. *J. Neurosci.*, **4**, 309–356.

Livingstone, M. S. and Hubel, D. H. (1984b). Specificity of intrinsic connections in primate primary visual cortex. *J. Neurosci.*, **4** , 2830–2835.

Livingstone, M. S. and Hubel, D. H. (1988). Segregation of form, colour, movement, and depth: anatomy, physiology, and perception. *Science*, **240**, 740–749.

Maunsel, J. H. R., Ghose, G. M., Assad, J. A., McAdams, C. J., Boudreau, C. E., and Noeranger, B. D. (1999). Visual response latencies of magnocellular and parvocellular LGN neurons in macaque monkey. *Vis. Neurosci.*, **16**, 1–14.

Moutoussis, K. and Zeki, S. (1997a). A direct demonstration of perceptual asynchrony in vision. *Proc. Roy. Soc. London Ser. B*, **264**, 393–399.

Moutoussis, K. and Zeki, S. (1997b). Functional segregation and temporal hierarchy of the visual perceptive systems. *Proc. Roy. Soc. London Ser. B*, **264**, 1407–1414.

Munk, M. H. J., Nowak, L. G., Girard, P., Chounlamountri, N., and Bullier, J. (1995). Visual latencies in cytochrome oxidase bends of macaque area V2. *Proc. Natl. Acad. Sci. USA*, **92**, 988–992.

Nakamura, M., Gattass, R., Desimone, R., and Ungerleider, L. G. (1993). The modular organisation of projections from areas V1 and V2 to areas V4 and TEO in macaques. *J. Neurosci.*, **13**, 3681–3691.

Nakayama, K. (1985). Biological image motion processing: a review. *Vis. Res.*, **25**, 625–660.

Nishida, S. and Johnston, A. (2002). Marker correspondence, not processing latency, determines temporal binding of visual attributes. *Curr. Biol.*, **12**, 359–368.

Raiguel, S. E., Lagae, L., Culyas, B., and Orban, G. A. (1989). Response latencies of visual cells in macaque areas V1, V2 and V5. *Brain Res.*, **493**, 155–159.

Shipp, S. and Zeki, S. (1985). Segregation of pathways leading from area V2 to areas V4 and V5 of macaque monkey visual cortex. *Nature*, **315**, 322–325.

Shipp, S. and Zeki, S. (1989a). The organisation of connections between areas V5 and V1 in macaque monkey visual cortex. *Eur. J. Neurosci.*, **1**, 309–332.

Shipp, S. and Zeki, S. (1989b). The organisation of connections between areas V5 and V2 in macaque monkey visual cortex. *Eur. J. Neurosci.*, **1**, 333–354.

Shipp, S. and Zeki, S. (1995). Segregation and convergence of specialised pathways in macaque monkey visual cortex. *J. Anat.*, **187**, 547–562.

Vaina, L. M. (1994). Functional segregation of colour and motion processing in the human visual cortex: clinical evidence. *Cereb. Cortex*, **4**, 555–572.

Viviani, P. and Aymoz, C. (2001) Colour, form, and movement are not perceived simultaneously. *Vis. Res.*, **41**, 2909–2918.

Zeki, S. M. (1974). Functional organisation of a visual area in the posterior bank of the superior temporal sulcus of the rhesus monkey. *J. Physiol. London*, **236**, 549–573.

Zeki, S. M. (1975). The functional organisation of projections from striate to prestriate visual cortex in the rhesus monkey. *Cold Spring Harbor Symp. Quant. Biol.*, **40**, 591–600.

Zeki, S. M. (1978). Functional specialisation in the visual cortex of the monkey. *Nature*, **274**, 423–428.

Zeki, S. (1980). The responses of cells in the anterior bank of the superior temporal sulcus in macaque monkeys. *J. Physiol.*, **308**, 85.

Zeki, S. (1990). A century of cerebral achromatopsia. *Brain*, **113**, 1721–1777.

Zeki, S. (1991). Cerebral akinetopsia (visual motion blindness): a review. *Brain*, **114**, 811–824.

Zeki, S. (1993). *A Vision of the Brain*. Blackwell, Oxford.

Zeki, S. and Bartels, A. (1999). Towards a theory of visual consciousness. *Conscious. Cogn.*, **8**, 225–259.

Zeki, S. and Shipp, S. (1988). The functional logic of cortical connections. *Nature*, **335**, 311–317.

Zeki, S. and Shipp, S. (1989). Modular connections between areas V2 and V4 of macaque monkey visual cortex. *Eur. J. Neurosci.*, **1**, 494–506.

Zeki, S., Watson, J. D., Lueck, C. J., Friston, K. J., Kennard, C., and Frackowiak, R. S. (1991). A direct demonstration of functional specialisation in human visual cortex. *J. Neurosci.*, **11**, 641–649.

Zeki, S., Watson, J. D., and Frackowiak, R. S. (1993). Going beyond the information given: the relation of illusory visual motion to brain activity. *Proc. Roy. Soc. London Ser. B*, **252**, 215–222.

Zeki, S., Aglioti, S., McKeefry, D., and Berlucchi, G. (1999). The neurological basis of conscious colour perception in a blind patient. *Proc. Natl. Acad. Sci. USA*, **96**, 14124–14129.

Zihl, J., Von Cramon, D., and Mai, N. (1983). Selective disturbance of movement vision after bilateral brain damage. *Brain*, **106**, 313–340.

Zihl, J., Von Cramon, D., Mai, N., and Schmid, C. H. (1991). Disturbance of movement vision after bilateral posterior brain damage: further evidence and follow up observations. *Brain*, **114**, 2235–2252.

CHAPTER

13

The Chronoarchitecture of the Human Brain: Functional Anatomy Based on Natural Brain Dynamics and the Principle of Functional Independence

"Set the stone to the foundation mark, not the foundation mark to the stone."—Plutarch

CONCEPTUAL OVERVIEW

We consider here the extent to which the autonomy and functional specialisation of the cortical areas, as described in the previous and next chapters, can be demonstrated without *a priori* hypotheses about the functions of cortical areas. This leads us to propose a new approach to subdividing the cerebral cortex based on time. We refer to the resulting temporal architecture of the cerebral cortex as its *chronoarchitecture* (Bartels and Zeki, 2001; 2004b). As it is a consequence of the functional and structural organisation of the cortex, it does not reveal a cortical map that is distinct from that derived from anatomical tools or through classical functional mapping techniques. However, the latter two techniques depend critically on histological or molecular techniques that reveal features that are specific to each subdivision or on innovative stimulation techniques that have to be specific to each cortical subdivision. In contrast, *chronoarchitecture* relies only on one factor that is, as we will postulate, distinct to each functional and structural subdivision of the cortex, just like a fingerprint: the *activity time course* (ATC) obtained in natural conditions. We account for this by the *principle of functional independence*, which supposes that the separation of functionally specialised areas is an evolutionary consequence of the fact that *separate (internal and external) features vary independently over time*. Separate brain areas, therefore, process features that vary independently over time. The direct and logical consequence of this rule of functional independence is that functionally specialised cerebral modules will have ATCs that are, if not entirely independent, at least specific to each module, much like a fingerprint, when the brain is exposed to the natural environment that it evolved to deal with. We illustrate this by describing functional magnetic resonance imaging (fMRI) experiments in which we approximate natural viewing conditions through the free viewing of natural scenes (namely, the James Bond film *Tomorrow Never Dies*). To obtain the chronoarchitecture of the brain, we use a data-driven approach for our analysis—in this case, the independent component analysis (ICA) of Bell and Sejnowski (1995); this segregates areas from each other according to their differential ATCs. Despite the rapid dynamics of the complex stimuli and the slow nature of the blood-oxygen-level-dependent (BOLD) signal, distinct areas can be shown to have distinct ATCs which has allowed us to reveal a multitude of previously known and unknown areas and networks.

Chronoarchitectonic maps therefore mirror traditional ones, but as they collapse all the known and unknown functional and structural properties of cerebral architecture onto a single and measurable factor, they may be easier to derive, even for as yet uncharted regions. In addition, as the temporal fingerprint is a direct consequence of function, it also reflects functional similarity (or functional connectivity) and, as we will postulate, the strength of anatomical connections between areas as well.

The chronoarchitectonic approach therefore constitutes the logical development of one of the principal themes of cortical studies—namely, the attempt to identify distinct parts of the cerebral cortex and assign specific functions to each. It distinguishes and defines areas on the basis of the timing of activity in them in relation to the timing of activity in other areas, without *a priori* knowledge about anatomical location or function. Its weakness, which it shares with other anatomical mapping techniques (for example, the cyto- or myeloarchitectonic techniques), is that it does not allow one to infer specific functions for the areas that it maps or only partially by a correlation over time of the intensity of perceptual experience with that of brain activity (Bartels and Zeki, 2004a). Paradoxically, this may also be its strength, as it does not depend upon the simplistic and sometimes erroneous attribution of a single function.

Anatomical Maps: Structure Defines Function

It is almost a truism to say that, in the brain, structure defines function and function is defined by structure. Brains are not current von Neumann computers, in which multipurpose hardware is separated from specialised software; to the contrary, each patch of brain tissue has a specialised physical machinery for implementing a particular processing function. The only way to confer functional specificity on a particular area is to equip it with a distinct connectivity and a distinct internal physiology (which includes cellular composition, ionic mechanisms, and internal wiring). Biological systems do not use different structures to achieve the same function; rather, the contrary is true. Any anatomically distinct area must therefore also be functionally distinct. Statements such as: "The subdivision of the cerebral cortex into cytoarchitectonic areas does not imply, it is hardly necessary to state, a parcellation of cerebral function" (Talairach and Tournoux, 1988) highlight that an idea such as that outlined above, which was first formulated almost a century ago by Vogt and Vogt (1919), never comes along without persistent opposition.

The impetus for subdividing the cortex into histologically distinct parts and assigning special functions to them developed from Broca's (1861) discovery of a region important for articulate speech, together with the subsequent discovery by Fritsch (1870) of another, anatomically different and distinctive region that is critical in the production of willed movements. Together, these findings ushered in what Sholl (1967) has called an "era of feverish map making," during which anatomical methods were used to chart differences in the way that cells or fibres are arranged in different cortical areas. The former approach led to cytoarchitectonic maps of the cerebral cortex, while the latter yielded the myeloarchitectonic maps. Among the maps produced are those of Brodmann (1905), Campbell (1905), Vogt and Vogt (1919), von Economo and Koskinas (1925), and von Bonin and Bailey (1951). These maps are compatible because they chart the apparently immutable histological (and therefore functional) structure of the adult cortex. For this reason, they have been invaluable in past clinical, physiological, and imaging studies of the cerebral cortex and still act as templates for these. As the resolution of recent functional imaging techniques has in many cases gone beyond that of the histological maps, it would be desirable to find new methods to verify the functional subdivisions with anatomical methods. One way is likely to lie in the mapping of the distinct molecular properties on the cortical sheet, such as the expression of area-specific proteins. Such a *genoarchitecture* may reveal cortical subdivisions that go beyond the resolution of classical histological techniques and also that of functional imaging. Some first attempts of this approach seem promising, even though current studies represent only the embryonic stage of what has the potential to become an important field in neuroscience (Zilles and Clarke, 1997; Kim *et al.*, 2001; Ishibashi *et al.*, 2002). The additional potential of genoarchitecture to identify potential targets for drug action brings map making out of the passive observing state into the realm of clinical intervention. In addition it will no doubt shed some light on the evolutionary homology of areas across different species. One of the first, and most spectacular, examples of such molecular maps lies in the demonstration of the metabolic architecture in the primate visual areas V1 and V2 by staining for the metabolic enzyme cytochrome oxidase (Livingstone and Hubel, 1984; DeYoe and Van Essen, 1985; Shipp and Zeki, 1985; Hubel and Livingstone, 1987). In each area, the metabolic architecture reveals subdivisions that coincide with functional ones that are not apparent in the uniform cyto- or myeloarchitecture of each and which shows that V1 and V2 contain in fact separate interdigitating functional modules.

The maps derived from histological architectonic and molecular methods are blind with respect to function. Those who indulged in "feverish map making" were nevertheless satisfied that, in time, through clinical or experimental work, specific functions would be assigned to the areas that they charted, because of the doctrine that areas that differ in architecture will be found to differ in function (a doctrine, incidentally, to which no exception has yet been found). Similarly, chronoarchitectonic maps on their own do not assign functions to the subdivisions that they reveal. Instead, they look to other mapping methods and to clinical studies to complement their results functionally.

Myeloarchitecture: A Tool To Synchronise Different Percepts? The Hypothesis of Evolutionary Perceptual Synchronisation

Of the architectonic maps that have been produced, perhaps the most interesting from our present point of view is the myeloarchitectonic map. It charts the pattern of myelination in different cortical zones. This is fixed at birth in primary areas and matures in what Flechsig (1901) called the association cortex, probably reflecting the maturation of its function during development. Because conduction velocity is dependent upon fibre calibre and myelination, this should have, with hindsight, implied what brain studies have shown since—namely, that some areas have temporal properties different than others. A striking example is to be found in primate visual cortex, where the heavily myelinated area V5 is activated before area V1 by fast-moving stimuli (Beckers and Zeki, 1995; ffytche *et al.*, 1995). It is not entirely clear why some processing systems are equipped with faster processing powers than others. One of the most common explanations is that it is of advantage to react as quickly as possible to a moving threat, which would account for the high myelination of fibres that contribute to motion processing pathways, often referred to as the M-system as opposed to the P-system, which is more concerned with colours and object vision (Clarke and Miklossy, 1990). We propose here another explanation—namely, that a distinctive myelination is a consequence of evolutionary pressure to synchronise percepts that are created by different processing systems. This results in an apparent paradox: Earlier signal arrival times (conferred by heavier myelination and therefore faster conducting fibres) do not necessarily lead to a temporal advantage in perception. On the contrary, it seems that higher myelination and therefore speedier delivery of signals correlate with longer perceptual delays. A good example is to be found in what has been called the temporal hierarchy in perception (Moutoussis and Zeki, 1997a). Although electrophysiological inactivation (Beckers and Zeki, 1995; Schmolesky *et al.*, 1998) and electroencephalographic (ffytche *et al.*, 1995; Buchner *et al.*, 1997) methods show that signals from fast-moving stimuli ($>5° s^{-1}$) reach the cortex of V5 before colour signals reach V4 (Buchner *et al.*, 1994), perceptual experiments reveal that humans perceive colour before they perceive motion (Moutoussis and Zeki, 1997a; Arnold *et al.*, 2001; Viviani and Aymoz, 2001). The reasons for this precedence probably lie in the greater processing time needed to bring motion to a perceptual endpoint (that is, one that requires no further processing to create a conscious percept). Our hypothesis rests on the assumption that each cortical area is specialised not only to process a particular feature but also to generate a conscious percept for it, a *microconsciousness*. Any other assumption would have to imply that consciously perceived features are coded twice: once in the specialised area processing it and again in the place representing our conscious percept, which would be an unlikely waste of cortical resources. Thus, our conscious visual percept consists of several such microconsciousnesses, each generated by a different system (Zeki and Bartels, 1998, 1999a), leading us to perceive a given scene through several perceptual layers (Bartels and Zeki, 1998).

Time delays due to more or less complex processing demands that are inherent and specific to each part of the visual system can therefore, if not equalised, be cushioned and minimised by different degrees of myelination that speed up the delivery of signals to and within areas that have longer processing times. This accommodation may have been achieved to a degree that satisfied evolutionary pressure but did not escape the scrutiny of careful experimentation (Moutoussis and Zeki, 1997b; Arnold *et al.*, 2001; Viviani and Aymoz, 2001).

Our hypothesis of evolutionary perceptual synchronisation thus explains why a system with higher myelination and therefore faster processing resources still leads to relatively higher perceptual delays. Together, these psychophysical and anatomical findings imply that different cortical areas have ATCs that differ at any given moment and that these are specific to areas. We hypothesise that these temporal differences reflect inherent delays due to distinct processing demands, despite evolutionary attempts to compensate them by differential myelination. Thus we consider the myeloarchitectonic map to be the static reflection and precursor of our chrono-architectonic map. It is, in a sense, astonishing that the full implications of myeloarchitectonic maps were not seen before.

Functional Maps: The Limits of Human Imagination

As function is a direct consequence of structure, the existence of functionally specialised areas is a logical consequence of the *anatomical* parcellation of the cortex, or, rather, the biological necessity for functional specialisation imposes anatomically specialised machineries and hence anatomical parcellation. Unfortunately, the determination of function by modern imaging experiments is limited by human imagination, as such experiments map the hypotheses of human experimenters, with the consequence that nonspecific activation may be obtained that may involve several areas, or, alternatively, an area or areas may go undetected because the experiments have not been tailored to activate them. In contrast, anatomically generated maps are more "objective," but, unless coupled to functional or pathological studies, they are uncommonly dull. They rarely provide hints about the functions involved or the functional connections between areas.

Modern imaging techniques have opened a Pandora's box of what some rather disparagingly call "modern phrenology" and offer, in some regions of the cortex, a spatial resolution that is much superior to that provided by histological maps. Apart from the early visual areas V1, V2, and V3, which were first mapped by using retinotopic stimulation techniques (Engel *et al.*, 1994; Sereno *et al.*, 1995; Shipp *et al.*, 1995), all of the functionally specialised cortical areas in human have been identified by comparing the brain activity elicited during two or more stimulation conditions. If these conditions are well matched, with only one difference, a function may be assigned to the voxels whose activity survives the subtraction (Friston *et al.*, 1995a). An unavoidable problem with this approach is that the experimental conditions compared are chosen by the experimenter and not by the brain itself. We have a simple rule to which we know no exception: *Whenever there is a perceptual difference, there must be a difference in brain activity.* This rule applies almost invariably to brain imaging, even though the spatial and temporal resolution sets limits to it. A consequence of this is that one may therefore choose to compare any two situations, and in most cases find some brain regions that specifically respond to the difference. As the example of KO (kinetic occipital) demonstrates assigning a brain region a particular and unique function on the basis of limited observations may be quite wrong, as it is likely to respond to quite different experimental subtractions as well (Zeki *et al.*, 2003). Indeed, clinical studies show that brain regions that light up in imaging studies during a particular task are not always necessary for the performance of the task. Determining at which point to declare having found a brain area's "true" function is a difficult task, which requires much patience; not many areas have their functions completely and truly defined, the best two examples being areas V4 and V5, and even they may have functions beyond the ones assigned to them. In some cases, the experimental conditions chosen require the cooperation between different areas, which makes it difficult to segregate them even if they have very different functions. This is probably the case with the so-called "attentional network," which typically involves part of the parietal cortex and the frontal eye fields, areas that are rarely found to be activated separately, simply because we have not yet found the experimental conditions to separate them. It therefore makes much sense to complement current mapping techniques with other techniques that are not hypothesis driven but use markers that are inherent properties of cerebral areas, in this case their ATCs.

Chronoarchitecture and the Principle of Functional Independence: The External World, Its Independent Features, and Cerebral Organisation

"In fact, there are antipodes in one and the same city who go to sleep when the others get up..." —Seneca

A direct consequence of functional specialisation is that each brain area has a distinct ATC. The reasons that account for such differences on a scale of milliseconds have been outlined above and involve distinct input delays, processing speeds, and processing durations, as well as distinct molecular and cellular machineries available to each functional module and pathway. The same structural factors that differentiate cerebral subdivisions in the millisecond range may also contribute to temporal differences in the range of seconds. In the case of BOLD imaging, one such factor might, for example, lie in the density of vascularisation, which can be specific to different functional cortical subdivisions (Zheng *et al.*, 1991; Cavaglia *et al.*, 2001; Harrison *et al.*, 2002).

Yet, there is one additional marker, whose presence has been widely ignored so far. Like anatomical markers, it is independent of human hypotheses about function, yet present and distinct in all cerebral subdivisions. Like functional maps, it provides information about the functional proximity between different cerebral subdivisions. This marker is the ATC obtained during natural processing. This marker, by definition, differentiates functionally specialised cerebral subdivisions in time. We summarise it in the following principle: *The brain processes attributes in separate modules when they vary independently over time.* In other words, if one feature is invariably coupled with another, there is no need to distinguish between them at a neuronal level. We refer to this as to the *principle of functional independence*. It can be viewed in a strong and a weak form. The strong form is a hypothesis with regard to the evolution of the brain: The separation of functionally specialised areas is an evolutionary consequence of the fact that separate (internal and external) features vary independently over time. We use the term *independent* not in a mathematically strict form here, as it may include partial or full correlation during some periods. Features include external ones such as colour and motion and internal ones, such as feelings of thirst or anger. The weak form is a logical consequence of the strong form and concerns solely the dynamics of functionally specialised areas: When a brain is exposed to natural conditions, each functionally specialised area has an activity time course that is independent of that of other areas. We argue that the reason for this temporal segregation of distinct areas in the brain lies in the temporal independence of the features in the natural world; that is, they vary independently over time. Only features that vary independently from each other provide new information to the brain, and each requires processing by a specialised area. We do not imply that the latter are independent of each other, but clinical and functional evidence reveals that they have a remarkable degree of autonomy. Consistently co-occurring features contain the element of redundancy, as the appearance of one of several such features entirely predicts the remaining ones. Redundant features may therefore not be processed or may be processed only conjunctively in the same area.

For example, one could imagine a world in which each object is coupled to a unique colour (*e.g.*, all chairs are red and all tables are green). Seeing a colour is then equivalent to recognising an object, and the brain would hardly have developed two separate systems to achieve the task. Even if it had, the activity between the two would be indistinguishable during natural conditions, and neuroscientists would not have found out about the separation of the two. In our world, however, the colours of fruits vary and indicate their ripeness, motion occurs independently from colour, facial expressions vary independently of facial identities (usually), the colour of a surface is independent of its wavelength composition, etc. We are not aware of any exception to this principle, in that there are no two specialised brain areas that process two attributes that, in the world, are strongly correlated. This is likely to apply to other brain processes as well, such as those that evoke emotions, in that fear, anger, and affection, for example, can vary independently or in that goal-directed motor planning may be independent from the processing required to execute limb movements. This is not to say that any feature that varies independently in the environment is processed by dedicated cells or even areas but rather emphasises the converse: There are no two functionally specialised areas that do not process features that vary independently.

From this it follows that each functionally specialised brain area processes a feature that occurs independently over time compared to other features in the external world. The direct consequence of exposing the brain to the external world (or, put simply, to natural conditions) is that functionally specialised cerebral modules will have ATCs that are, if not entirely independent, at least specific to each module, much like a fingerprint. In our view, the principle of functional independence therefore has both an evolutionary and a dynamic aspect that share the same origin: Independently varying features require processing in separate modules, which explains why separate modules must, by definition, have independent ATCs. The principle of functional independence thus provides the basis for what has been termed the *autonomy* of different visual systems (Zeki and Bartels, 1998b).

There are several implications to this, which we address only briefly. One of these is that the more related two features are, the stronger the connections between the two corresponding processing areas are likely to be, such that the brain can take full advantage of the mutual information between them. In addition, the higher the correlation between two features, the higher the correlation between the ATCs of the two corresponding areas. For both these reasons, the correlation of ATCs of different areas is a direct indicator of the similarity of the features they process and at the same time reveals, we believe, the strength of anatomical connections between separate areas. There is, therefore, a direct link between the functional, structural, and temporal aspects of the brain. We propose that the temporal aspects can be used to reveal function and structure, and we refer to the product of such a temporal dissection of the brain as its chronoarchitecture (Bartels and Zeki, 2001; 2004b).

SPM VERSUS ICA: THE SENSE AND NO-SENSE OF DATA-DRIVEN fMRI ANALYSES

Theory

In the following we give a brief, intuitive methodological overview; the reader is referred to the specific literature for more detailed information.

There are basically two schools of fMRI time-series analysis methods, the first being based on hypothesis-driven inference and the second on data-driven exploration. Virtually all past and present imaging studies are based on the first method, in which activation elicited during different experimental conditions is compared usually by means of a multiple regression analysis (as for example implemented in statistical parametric mapping, or SPM; Friston *et al.*, 1995a), no matter whether the conditions have been presented as epochs or in event-related paradigms (Friston *et al.*, 1995a, 1998). This is probably the most powerful way to characterise brain dynamics elicited in controlled paradigms, especially as it does not necessarily require *a priori* knowledge of the expected hemodynamic response function. It is sufficient to know the on- and offsets of experimental conditions and, optionally, the values of a parametric correlate (Friston *et al.*, 1995a; Buchel *et al.*, 1998; Henson *et al.*, 2002).

A development that lies between data- and hypothesis-driven analyses is the correlation map, which maps the correlation coefficients across the entire brain to a particular "seed" voxel, which is determined using the traditional approach. Correlation maps based on resting-state activity have been shown to reveal functionally connected areas, especially when based on the low-frequency (<0.1 Hz) component of the ATCs (Biswal *et al.*, 1995; Arfanakis *et al.*, 2000; Cordes *et al.*, 2000, 2001; Hampson *et al.*, 2002). We use this approach below as an aid to verify and expand our ICA results, with the difference that our seeds are based on chronoarchitectonic subdivisions and ATCs derived from free viewing. The resulting correlation maps seem to capture functionally connected areas better than those obtained with the resting-state approach.

The second school represents the data-driven approach, which we have to rely on in order to reveal the chronoarchitecture of the brain. The strength and weakness of this approach lie in the fact that no *a priori* knowledge about the data is required; powerful computational tools segregate the data into meaningful segments, based entirely on the structure inherent to the data. The rules according to which the data are segmented depend on the algorithm used, of which there are many, each with its own merits and pitfalls. The ones most commonly applied to fMRI data are principal component analysis (PCA) and independent component analysis (ICA). The key weakness of PCA stems from its strength in other applications—namely, from its constraint to impose orthogonality upon its data projection. This has the consequence that a maximal amount of variance in the data is accounted for by the first component, while the last components account for virtually no variance. This stands in contrast to the organisation of the brain, in that each brain area occupies a similarly limited amount of space and therefore contributes similarly to the overall activity. In addition, ATCs of some areas may be correlated at times; any algorithm trying to segregate brain areas should therefore allow each component to account for a similar amount of the total variance and allow for partial correlation in time, which spatial ICA does.

Independent component analysis is an algorithm based on information theory that is capable of unmixing or decomposing any linear mixture of independent sources, which need not be known *a priori* (Bell and Sejnowski, 1995). The (mixed) data are iteratively fed through an unmixing matrix, which is adjusted such that the information in its output channels is maximised. This minimises the mutual information among them, thus rendering them independent of each other, which is the equivalent of recovering the original components if they were independent to start with. ICA and its derivatives may be applied to a variety of problems, including separation of mixed sounds such as speech. Perhaps its most successful application in neuroscience so far has been to separate sources in EEG data (Makeig *et al.*, 1997, 2002), as these applications actually facilitated new insights of neurobiological interest—for example, that event-related potentials are mainly generated by stimulus-induced phase resetting of ongoing brain processes rather than by stimulus-evoked brain events (Makeig *et al.*, 2002). McKeown *et al.* (1997, 1998b) were the first to apply spatial ICA to fMRI data, showing that ICA could isolate voxels whose time course correlated with their two task conditions and other voxels that represented artefacts. They also demonstrated that ICA is better in doing so than PCA. There have since been several other applications of ICA to fMRI data, and several optimisations of ICA to fMRI data have been proposed (McKeown, 2000b; Nakada *et al.*, 2000; Calhoun *et al.*, 2001a–c; Gu *et al.*, 2001; Nybakken *et al.*, 2002; Stone *et al.*, 2002; Suzuki *et al.*, 2002). On the whole, however, most of the recent fMRI/ICA literature has been concerned with problems associated with optimising the technique and showing that it works, a necessary step before it can be unleashed to reveal new insights about cortical function.

Experimental Comparison of ICA and SPM

In our hands, ICA applied to conventional fMRI datasets did equally well in identifying functionally activated areas as SPM (Zeki and Bartels, 1999b; Bartels and Zeki, 2000a,b), with SPM offering the advantage of sound statistical inference, easier data manipulation, and a choice of a variety of statistical contrasts. We illustrate the qualitative equivalence of ICA and SPM as applied to conventional epoch designs in Figs. 13.1 to 13.4, which show results from SPM and

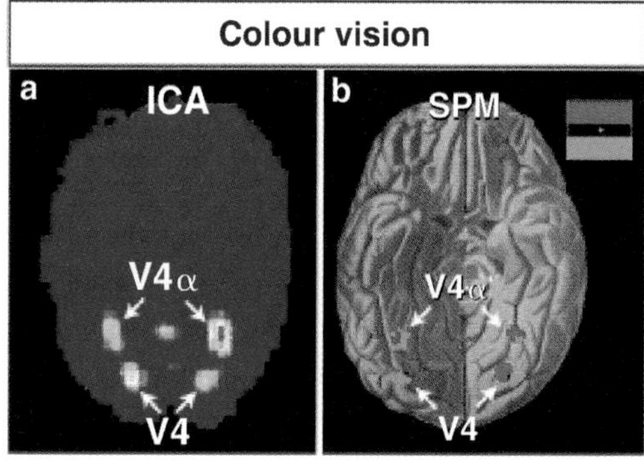

FIGURE 13.1
The colour-processing V4 complex in the human brain, revealed when subjects viewed coloured versus isochromatic stimuli in the lower or upper hemifield. (a) Independent component (IC) obtained by ICA (glass-brain view) containing the V4 complex in a single subject. (b) Composite image of SPM maps projected onto the ventral view of a human brain, showing colour-selective activity related to upper and lower hemifield stimulation (see inset for colour coding). (From Bartels, A. and Zeki, S. M., *Eur. J. Neurosci.*, 12, 172–193, 2000. With permission.)

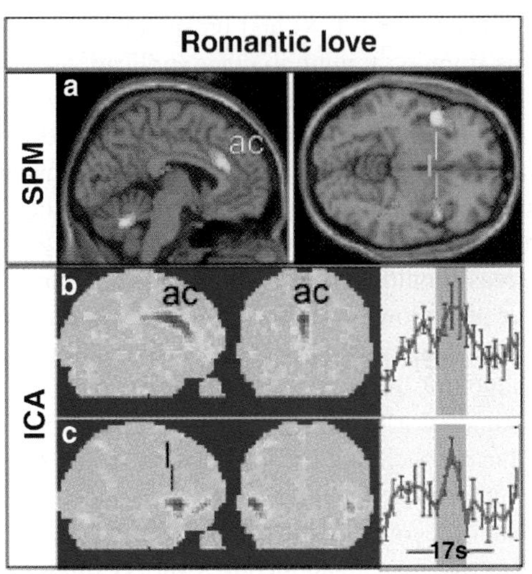

FIGURE 13.2
Activity related to the subjective experience of romantic love. The SPM group analysis shown in (a) revealed, among other areas, activity in a region within the anterior cingulate cortex (ac) and the middle insula (I). (b) and (c) ICA applied to single subjects isolated these areas in separate ICs, indicating specific activity time courses (ATCs) in each. ATCs are shown averaged across conditions, with the blue stripe indicating the love condition (error bars: s.e.m.). (From Bartels, A. and Zeki, S. M., *NeuroReport*, 11, 3829–3834. With permission.)

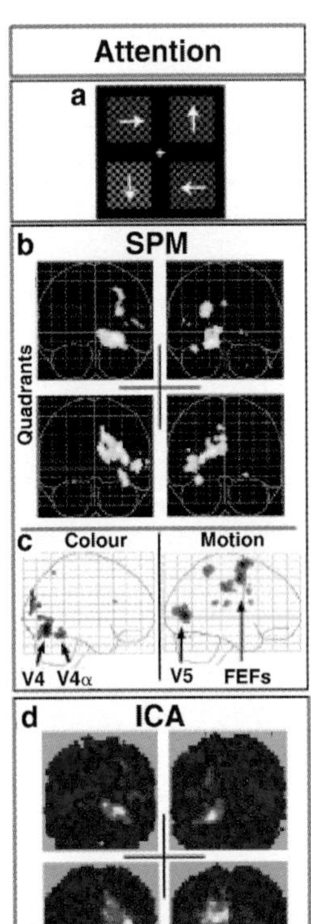

FIGURE 13.3
Attentional modulation of activity in the visual cortex. (a) Subjects fixated the middle of a screen while attending to either colour or motion in one of the four quadrants. SPM analysis: (b) Attention to different quadrants activated several visual areas in a retinotopic fashion, shown as coronal glass-brain views of a single subject arranged such that the one depicting attention to the top right is located in the top right, etc. (contrasts: attention to colour and motion in one quadrant versus attention to both attributes in the remaining three quadrants, $p < 0.05$, corrected). (c) Attention to colour or to motion reveals activity in V4 or in V5 (SPM contrasts: colour versus motion and vice versa). (d) ICA analysis (same subject as above); the ICs whose ATCs correlated most with the task conditions corresponded to the retinotopic attention maps shown in (b). (From Zeki, S. M. and Bartels, A., *Philos. Trans. Roy. Soc. London B*, 354, 1371–1382, 1999. With permission.)

ICA analyses obtained from four of our recent studies on colour vision, romantic love, spatial attention (Zeki and Bartels, 1999b; Bartels and Zeki, 2000a,b), and the relation of object recognition to motion (Bork and Zeki, 1998). It is obvious that ICA and SPM results are qualitatively equivalent, but SPM allowed us to attach significance values to its results. In addition, SPM made possible contrasts that revealed regions of activation that were not present in the ICA analysis; once an area has been "hijacked" in one independent component (IC), it does not usually occur again in another component. Our attention experiment serves as an example of this (Fig. 13.3). Subjects attended to either colour or motion in each of the four quadrants in turn, a total of eight conditions. The ICA analysis revealed in most subjects four primary ICs that represented activity associated with attention to each of the four quadrants and included the quadrantic representations of areas V1 to V4 and activity in V5. Almost identical activity patterns were revealed by SPM contrasts that compared attention to one quadrant versus attention to the remaining three (Fig. 13.3). SPM also allowed us to isolate activity in colour-selective V4 or in motion-selective V5 from activity in remaining visual areas (using the contrasts attention to colour versus attention to motion and vice versa) (Fig. 13.3). However, ICA only managed to isolate V5 in a separate IC but failed to isolate V4 on its own (Bartels, 2000; Bartels and Zeki, 2000a). In Fig. 13.4 we illustrate the performance of ICA compared to that of SPM in more detail. In this traditional epoch-design study intended for parametric statistical analysis, five subjects had viewed five types of stimuli arranged in repeated epochs of 30 s. The stimuli consisted of recognisable and scrambled objects, which could be either moving or stationary, and a blank screen (Bork and Zeki, 1998). An SPM analysis (Friston *et al.*, 1995b) showed that all non-blank stimuli activated the early visual areas V1/V2 (Fig. 13.4d), stimuli containing motion activated the V5 complex (Fig. 13.4e), and stimuli containing objects activated the object- and face-selective subdivisions of the lateral fusiform gyrus in the lateral occipital cortex (Fig. 13.4f), which is also known as the lateral occipital complex (LOC) (Malach *et al.*, 1995). ICA revealed the same subdivisions in the occipital lobe as SPM, with each in a separate independent component (Fig. 13.4a–c), thus showing that ICA can segregate regions that are commonly activated by stimulus epochs from whole brain activity. Each of these ICs had a time course that closely matched the BOLD time course of the hottest voxel revealed by SPM (Fig. 13.4d, left and right). Figure 13.5 illustrates the high reproducibility of these results when ICA is applied to separate subjects exposed to the same stimuli. It is, in the context of chronoarchitecture, important to note that the ATC in the distinct areas V1/V2 and in V5 correlate with the corresponding conditions, but that each has a distinct and specific waveform.

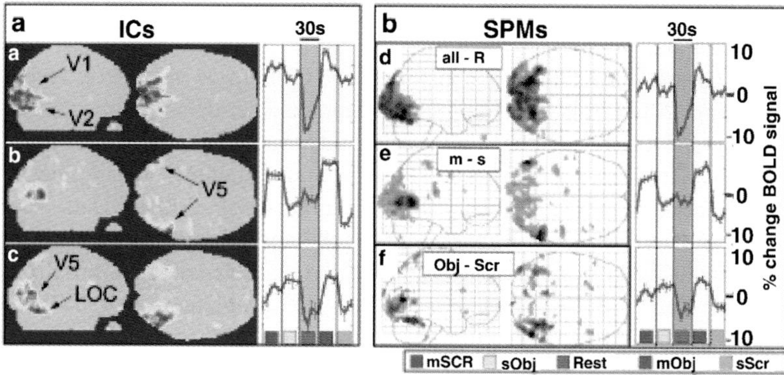

FIGURE 13.4
Comparison of an SPM and an ICA analysis of single subject data from a traditional epoch-design fMRI study on motion and object recognition. The three ICs obtained by ICA whose ATCs correlated most with the stimulus conditions revealed differential involvement of primary visual (a), visual-motion-selective (b), and object-selective (c) areas in different stimulus conditions, as is apparent in the ATCs shown to their right. ATCs of the ICs, (a) to (c), have arbitrary units and were averaged over the eight repeats of the conditions. (d) to (f) Statistical parametric maps (SPMs; $p < 0.001$, uncorrected) show the same cortical areas as revealed by ICA. BOLD signals taken from the most significant voxel are shown to the right of each SPM and are averaged over condition repeats (error bars: s.e.m.). mScr = moving scramble; sObj = static object; mObj = moving object; sScr = static scramble.

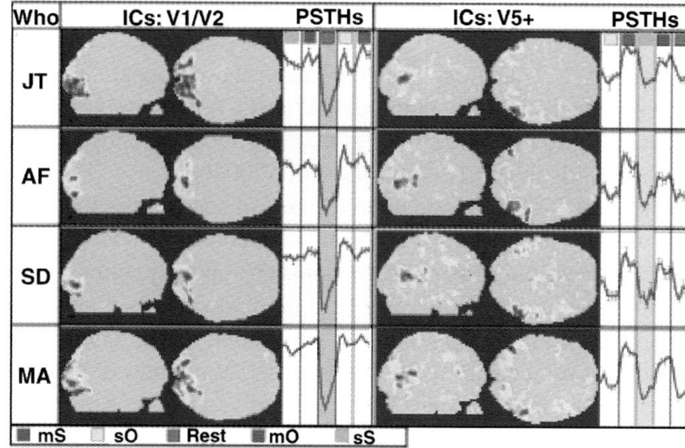

FIGURE 13.5
Consistency of ICA results across four subjects in the epoch-design experiment on motion and object recognition. For each subject, the ICs containing V1 (left) and V5 (right) are shown. These ICs had ATCs that correlated most with the task conditions. To the right of each IC the associated ATC is displayed, averaged over the eight stimulus conditions (peristimulus time histograms [PSTHs]). Note that ATCs are specific to the area and similar across subjects.

At the same time, such distinct temporal characteristics that are specific to areas should be a caveat to the still frequently used box-car regressors in SPM. These might, by accident, resemble better the specific ATC of one area than another, leading to apparent differences of activation in different areas, when in fact the difference may lie only in the activation waveform, not the activation intensity or significance.

ICA Applied to fMRI: A Solution in Search of a Problem?

We conclude, first, that spatial ICA applied to fMRI data is a powerful and reliable way of segregating temporally correlated voxels. It is, in fact, so successful in doing so that its results are qualitatively equivalent to those obtained using statistical mapping and may at times supersede them as it demonstrates specificity of activity in separate areas or correlations in networks of areas, rather than correlation with experimental tasks. Second, we conclude that, while the qualitative results of ICA and SPM are comparable, SPM offers the advantage of attaching significance values to its results. In addition, SPM allows for a multitude of statistical comparisons, which can reveal cortical preferences to particular stimuli that remain hidden to ICA in conventional paradigms.

Several other groups share this view (Friston, 1998; Calhoun *et al.*, 2001c; Nybakken *et al.*, 2002; Quigley *et al.*, 2002). It is therefore questionable whether data-driven approaches such as ICA will see a grand future in their application to conventional fMRI data unless they are improved and coupled with sound statistical tools. Some attempts toward the development of the latter have been made (McKeown, 2000a; Calhoun *et al.*, 2001a). Data-driven analysis techniques such as ICA are therefore best used for the analysis of uncontrolled experiments, rather than for the analysis of conventionally collected data, as has been proposed originally but is rarely ever done (McKeown *et al.*, 1998a). The problem is that truly uncontrolled experiments are extremely rare, as the timing of stimulation or the onset of spontaneous brain activity is usually accessible to the experimenter, even in experiments that do not fix such events *a priori* (*e.g.*, in the case of hallucinations or the reversal of visual illusions) (ffytche *et al.*, 1998; Kleinschmidt *et al.*, 1998; Lumer *et al.*, 1998). A potential, though rare, application of ICA might be on patients who are unable to report the onsets of spontaneous brain dysfunction.

In our view, hypothesis-driven analyses such as SPM are preferable for most imaging experiments. We see the key application of data-driven approaches such as ICA in the determination of the chronoarchitecture of the brain.

THE CHRONOARCHITECTURE OF THE BRAIN

According to the principle of functional independence, the chronoarchitecture of the human brain is revealed best by exposing it to natural conditions—only these are sufficiently complex and perceptually rich and have multiple attributes that vary independently to activate a multitude of areas, each in a characteristic way (Bartels and Zeki, 2004b).

With the confidence that ICA would be up to the task of segregating functionally specialised areas based solely on the characteristic ATCs of their constituent voxels, we embarked on experiments that are inaccessible to parametric statistics—namely, blind mapping of cerebral activity in free-viewing conditions. This was a first and undoubtedly crude attempt to map the chronoarchitecture of the brain. To approximate stimulation of the brain under more natural conditions, we asked eight subjects to freely view the first 22 minutes of the James Bond movie *Tomorrow Never Dies*. Two factors could potentially foil our approach. First, the brain was exposed to rapid, real-live stimuli, but we measured the slow BOLD response that has time constants in the range of several seconds, sampled at intervals of 3 to 4 seconds; therefore, there was a danger that all temporal variability of neural activity was smoothed out by the slow BOLD response, leading to a uniform and indistinguishable signal in all visual areas. Second, one would naturally expect from hypotheses such as those of Schiller (1997), which supposes that perceptual analysis "is performed interactively by areas and neurons with multipurpose properties" that, especially in natural conditions, the temporal characteristics of visual areas would be barely distinguishable, thus making it difficult to separate them on this basis. Our results showed that the first factor did not prohibit our approach and provided evidence against the supposition underlying the second factor. For reasons referred to below, the movie was interrupted every 2.5 or 3 minutes with a 30-s blank period, and, unless stated otherwise, the blank period and the 30 s following it were excluded from analyses involving time courses. For another experiment, the image was switched from colour to black and white every 30 s. The subsequent ICA analysis (involving 368 whole-brain images with ca. 60,000 voxels each per subject) revealed many areas in the visual and non-visual cortex, some of which have not been identified before. The ten areas that were identified most consistently in each subject are shown in Fig. 13.6, using results from a single subject. The areas are colour coded and superimposed on the individual's structural image. The areas shown in Fig. 13.6 correspond anatomically to V1 (foveal field representation), the anterior calcarine (presumably the peripheral field representation of V1/V2), ventral V2/V3, the colour-sensitive V4 complex, the motion-sensitive area V5, a posterior (LOp) and a lateral (LOl) subdivision of the object- and face-selective region in the fusiform gyrus (also known as lateral occipital complex, or LOC [Malach *et al.*, 1995] and a part

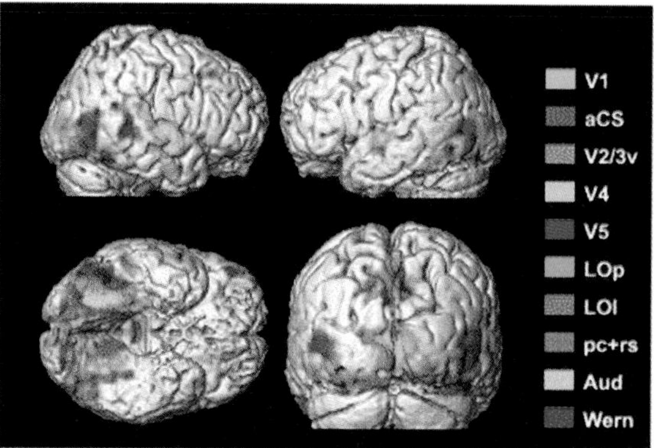

FIGURE 13.6
Ten chronoarchitectonically identified areas of a single subject who freely viewed the movie *Tomorrow Never Dies*. The regions were identified by ICA, colour-coded and superimposed onto the subject's brain. Each area had significant and specific inter-subject correlation with anatomically corresponding areas of the other subjects (see following figures). Abbreviations: aCS, ventral lip of the anterior calcarine sulcus; Aud, auditory cortex (BA41 and BA42); LOl, lateral part of the latero-occipital complex (LOC); LOp, posterior part of LOC; pc+rs, network containing precuneus (BA7) and retrosplenium (BA23 or BA30); Wern, Wernicke's area (BA22).

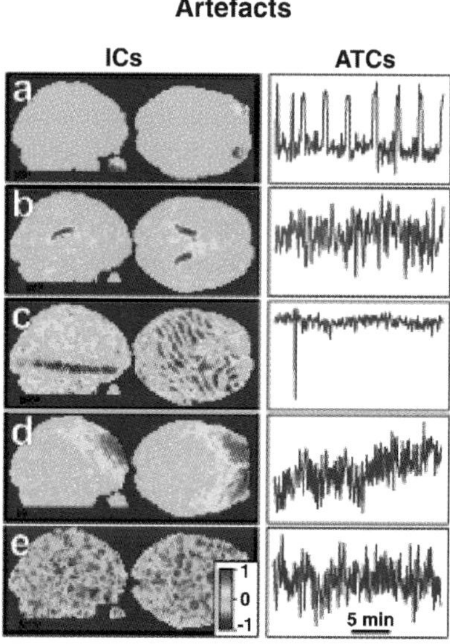

FIGURE 13.7
Representative artefacts together with their ATCs. (a) Eyes; ATCs reflect eye movements, which are reduced during the eight blank periods that interrupted the movie. (b) Part of the ventrikels; in each subject, the complete ventricals were isolated but fractionated into separate ICs. (c) Scanner-induced spike affecting only one slice at one point in time. (d) Movement artefact, affecting a large region on the surface of the brain, with a steadily increasing ATC. (e) Noise artefact; about 30% of ICs in an analysis contain this type of noise.

of it as fusiform face area, or FFA [Kanwisher *et al.*, 1997]), a parietal area in the precuneus, the auditory cortex, and a region corresponding to Wernicke's receptive speech area (Brodmann's area 22 [BA22]).

Revealing Functional Specificity by Correlations: Artefacts, Inter-Subject Correlations, and IC Rank Ordering

One of the problems in the interpretation of fMRI/ICA results is the identification of ICs that contain cortical or subcortical functional units and to separate them from potential artefacts, such as those induced by scanner noise, subject movement, breathing, or artery pulsation. Examples of some representative artefacts are shown in Fig. 13.7. This problem is especially acute in free-viewing experiments, as their uncontrolled nature makes it impossible to predict *a priori* the ATC of any area. One solution could lie on the temporal correlation of ATCs. Functionally corresponding areas in different subjects. We therefore propose as a method to detect functionally relevant ICs (*i.e.*, those whose ATCs are stimulus driven) to identify those whose ATCs correlate across several subjects.

We used two methods to test whether anatomically defined candidate regions, such as the eight ICs of all eight subjects containing the primary visual cortex (V1-ICs), had stimulus-driven (*i.e.*, common) activity:

1. *Inter-subject correlation.* The correlation coefficients between the $n*(n-1)/2$ inter-subject (n = number of subjects) pairs can be calculated and a t-test applied.
2. *Inter-subject IC rank ordering.* The ICs of each subject can be ordered according to the correlation coefficient of their ATC with the ATC of a candidate IC (*e.g.*, V1-IC) of another subject, and the position of each subject's candidate IC (*e.g.*, V1-IC) can be determined.

When repeated using the candidate IC (*e.g.*, V1-IC) of each subject, $n*(n-1)$ ranks are obtained, which we normalise to values from 0 to 100. A Kolmogoroff–Smirnoff test (a test not dependent on the normal distribution) can be used to establish whether the ranks obtained are higher than those expected for ATCs of random correlation, which would be equally distributed between 0 and 100. An advantage of inter-subject rank ordering compared to correlation is that it provides a relative measure, using the ICs within each subject as an internal control for unspecific correlations among all ICs.

We found that anatomically corresponding areas of different subjects had time courses that correlated, indicating a functional correspondence: The same stimulus activated distinct areas within each brain in a distinct way and consistently across separate brains. An empirical demonstration of this is given in Fig. 13.8, where time courses of anatomically corresponding ICs arbitrarily taken from the first three subjects are superimposed and shown along with the ICs. The latter contain cortical areas corresponding to the visual cortical areas V1, V4, and V5 and the auditory cortex. Each of these areas has a time course that is characteristic of it and preserved across subjects. This is quantified in Fig. 13.9 for the ten cortical areas shown in Fig. 13.6, which were identified in most subjects. Each of the anatomically corresponding areas in different subjects had significantly correlated ATCs across subjects ($p < 0.0001$, t-test on $n*(n-1)/2$ correlation coefficients, with n being the number of subjects having that area), indicating that

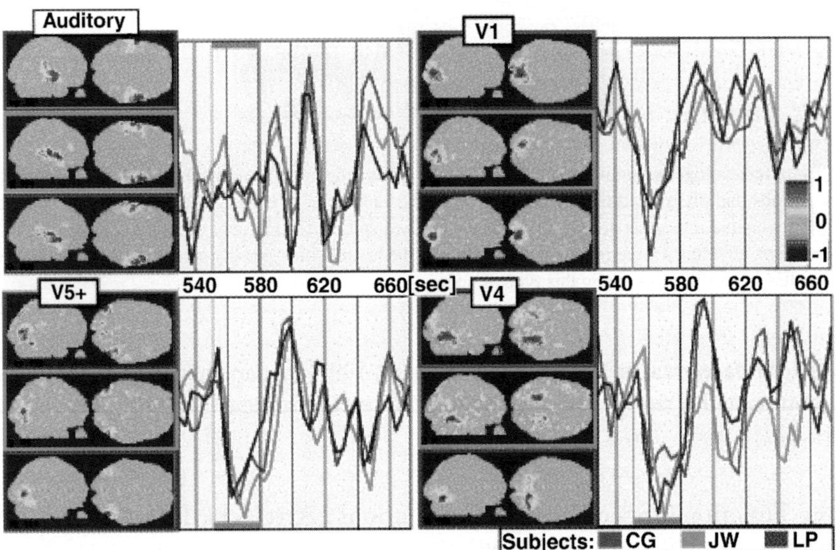

FIGURE 13.8
Free viewing of the movie elicited similar ATCs in anatomically corresponding areas in different brains. For four cortical regions (auditory cortex, V1, V5, and V4), the ICs of the first three participants in our study are shown, along with their superimposed ATCs (arbitrary units on the y-scale). The grey bars at the top and bottom indicate blank periods (black screen, no sound).

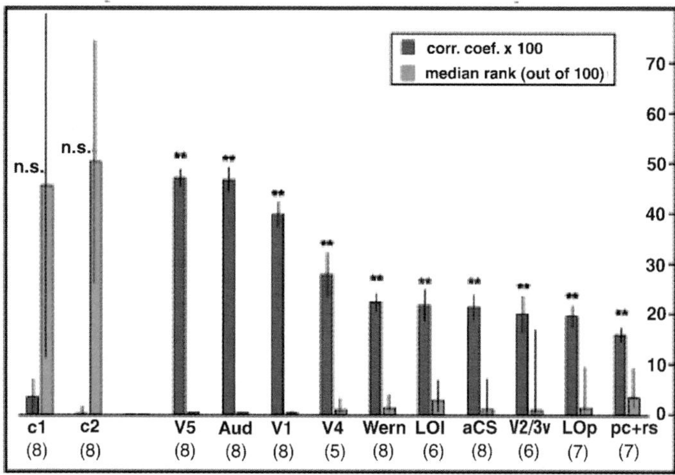

FIGURE 13.9
Anatomically corresponding areas had corresponding ATCs across subjects who viewed *Tomorrow Never Dies*. For each of the ten areas shown in Fig. 13.6, the mean inter-subject correlation coefficients ($r \pm$ s.e.m.) and the median inter-subject ranks (rank ± quartiles, normalised to 100) are shown. When, instead of anatomically corresponding areas, random areas out of the ten (control 1, c1) or any random IC (control 2, c2) were chosen, correlations were no longer different from zero, and ranks were not skewed toward zero. **: $p < 0.0001$ (t-test on correlation coefficients); $p < 10^{-13}$ (Kolmogoroff–Smirnoff test on ranks). See Fig. 13.6 for additional abbreviations; n, number of subjects with that area.

these areas were processing corresponding features of the movie. When the ATC of one subject's area was used to rank order all ICs of the remaining subjects, the anatomically corresponding areas of the latter appeared in the first ranks. Figure 13.9 shows the mean inter-subject correlations for the ATCs of these ten areas and their median inter-subject ranks. The controls show that this significant inter-subject correlation was abolished when areas that were compared did not correspond anatomically across subjects (control 1: $p = 0.26$, for each subject one of the above ten areas was randomly selected; control 2: $p = 0.50$, for each subject a random IC from all ICs was selected; for both controls, the results of 1000 combinations were averaged). Kolmogoroff–Smirnoff tests show that the distribution of rank orders is skewed toward the top ranks for each of the ten cortical areas ($p < 10^{-13}$, KS-test on $n*(n-1)$ ranks), while this was no longer significant in the controls (control 1: $p = 0.10$; control 2: $p = 0.43$). The high inter-subject correlations and low inter-subject rankings are therefore indicative of a common function of each of these anatomically corresponding areas. They cannot be accounted for by unspecific correlation of ATCs and must be due to area-specific processing that is similar in each subject. In Fig. 13.10, the correlation coefficients between these ten areas are shown, calculated within each brain. Most of these across-area/within brain correlations are lower than across-subject/within anatomically corresponding area correlations, and the highest within brain correlations do not reach the values of the highest across brain correlations. This highlights an astonishing degree of independence of the ATC of each area.

The above results show that when brains are exposed to natural conditions, functionally specialised areas have distinct ATCs that are characteristic of each area. These temporal characteristics are preserved across different subjects. ICA seems to be a sufficiently powerful tool to identify and segregate these areas based entirely on their distinct ATCs. In the next section we discuss whether free viewing really activates more areas distinctly than conventional fMRI paradigms.

Free Viewing Activates More Areas Differentially Than Traditional fMRI Paradigms

The more the number of areas that have characteristic ATCs, the more detailed will be the chronoarchitectonic maps. Above we hypothesised that, according to the principle of functional independence, exposure to natural conditions should activate more brain areas with more distinct

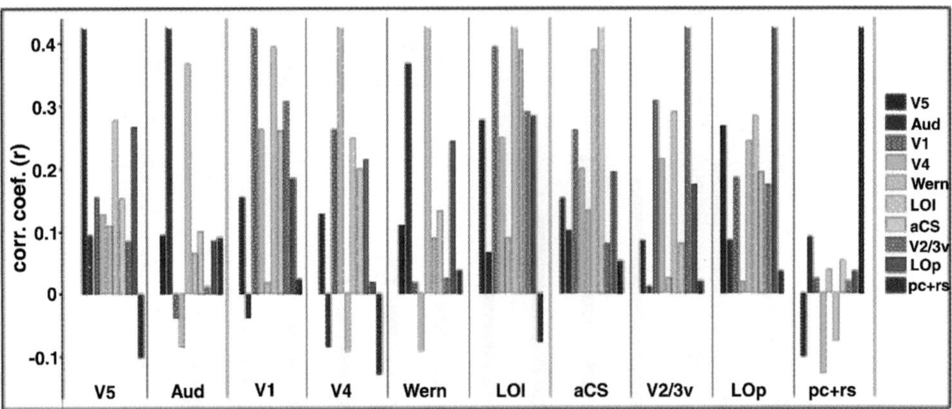

FIGURE 13.10
Median within-subject correlations between the ten areas of Fig. 13.6. For each of the ten areas shown in Fig. 13.6, the correlation coefficients with each of the other areas was calculated for each of the eight brains. Shown are the median values. See Fig. 13.6 for abbreviations.

ATCs than exposure to more simple stimuli. It was therefore crucial to determine whether the efficiency of free-viewing studies to activate a multitude of areas specifically is higher than that of epoch-design stimuli. We therefore compared the results obtained from our free-viewing study with those obtained from the more classical object-motion study. This was a conservative choice because, compared to other traditional fMRI studies, this study used a complex and perceptually rich stimulation; its moving-objects stimuli are in fact 6-s movie clips showing cars, people, or animals driving, cycling, or walking along streets, fields, and other complex scenes, and subjects were not constrained in their eye movements (Bork and Zeki, 1998, 2002). Our comparison therefore amounts to asking whether more complex stimuli activate more areas more differentially than less complex stimuli. To answer this, we calculated for each study the distribution of the *maximal intersubject correlations* of IC-ATCs (Fig. 13.11). This is obtained by identifying for a given IC the IC in each of the remaining subjects whose ATC correlates best with it. The average of each IC's best inter-subject correlations enters the distribution. This novel measure is more sensitive in revealing high inter-subject correlations than the distribution of all inter-subject correlations between ATCs of all ICs (Fig. 13.11, inset), which is dominated by a high number of low correlations. Both types of distributions indicate how many ICs have ATCs that correlate across subjects and therefore provide a measure for the number of stimulus-driven regions differentially activated in each study.

To obtain an equivalent comparison of the epoch study and the free-viewing one the latter was reanalysed such that both had the same number of scans and ICs per subject (200). The highly increased number of ICs with high inter-subject correlation (Fig. 13.11) in the free-viewing study (Fig. 13.11; two-sample Kolmogorov-Smirnov test: $p<10^{10}$) can only be explained by the fact that the more complex stimulus activated many more areas with different ATCs, and each in a distinct way but consistently across subjects. For data collected under different stimulation conditions but with the same technical and analytical parameters, such distributions reflect the effectiveness of the stimuli to differentially activate different areas. The above finding does not demonstrate that more areas are active during more complex tasks, but that more areas have differential and characteristic ATCs in natural conditions. This differential (or independent) activity in more areas during exposure to natural conditions is important for two reasons. First, it shows that area-specific ATCs can be obtained despite stimuli that are uncontrolled and whose dynamics are much more rapid than the measured BOLD signal. At the same time, it demonstrates that areas maintain a high degree of functional specificity in natural conditions, which is contrary to the view that many multipurpose areas process many features unspecifically in large cooperating networks (Schiller, 1996, 1997). Second, it is a necessary step in the experimental proof of the principle of functional independence, in that more areas obtain more characteristic ATCs in more natural conditions which can be accounted for by the independence of features that are processed by the brain in separate areas.

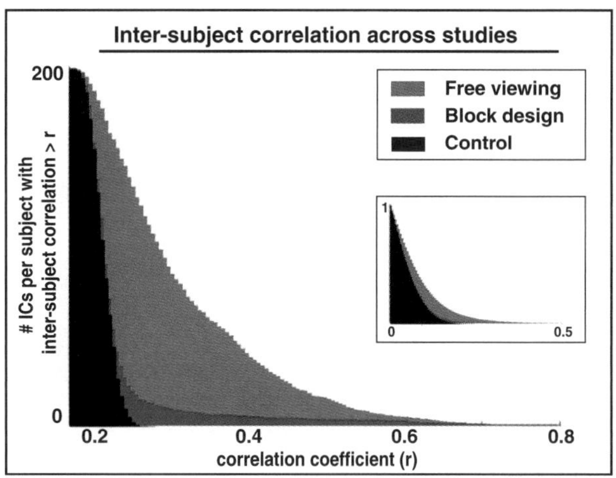

FIGURE 13.11
Free viewing activated more areas differentially than conventional epoch stimulation. Shown are the cumulative distribution of *maximal inter-subject correlations* among IC-ATCs and the normalized cumulative distribution of inter-subject-correlations (inset) (see text). Both indicate how many ICs have ATCs that correlate across subjects and therefore measure the number of stimulus-driven regions that were differentially activated in each study. **Red:** Free viewing data; **Blue:** Epoch data; **Black:** simulated random ATCs as a baseline (white noise convolved with the hemodynamic response function (HRF)). Data and analysis were equivalent in each study, with 200 ICs per subject.

Novel Areas and Networks Revealed by Chronoarchitectonic Maps

Using our approach of mapping the chronoarchitecture of the human brain, we identified some areas that have not been described, such as the anterior calcarine sulcus. We also found novel groups of areas, with highly correlated ATCs, the latter either due to related functional specialisations or strong anatomical connections, or both. In the following sections, a few of these findings are examined in more detail.

The Anterior Calcarine Sulcus

An area that showed suspiciously high inter-subject correlations and high IC rankings was one we were not familiar with from previous imaging studies. Its most significant voxels were distributed along the ventral lip of the anterior calcarine sulcus (aCS), which descends from the genu of the CS (ventral to the parieto-occipital sulcus, or POS) to a position ventral to the corpus callosum (just ventroposterior to the retrosplenial cortex, BA29 and BA30; see Figs. 13.12 and 13.15). Most likely, this region belongs anatomically to the striate cortex and presumably contains the representation of the far peripheral upper visual field of V1 and possibly V2; it has not been described in previous studies of the human visual brain. In the following, we refer to it as aCS. V1 and aCS had, consistently relatively distinct ATCs within each brain, but the ATCs of each were similar across brains (see Figs. 13.9 and 13.10).

If aCS represents the peripheral representation of V1 and possibly also V2, it might simply have escaped previous mapping procedures due to the limitation of the stimulation screens to the perifoveal region, with maximally 20 to 25° eccentricity. This "TV effect" has limited the stimulation of the ventral striate cortex in previous studies to reach an anterior limit close to the genu of the CS (Sereno *et al.*, 1995; Engel *et al.*, 1997; Tootell *et al.*, 1998). ICA detected this region, as well as the central field representation of V1, reliably in every subject and segregated the two in separate ICs. That the correlation of V1 and aCS across subjects was higher or equal to the correlation of the two areas within each subject indicates a distinct response to the same stimulus in each of the two areas. One reason for the common activity of aCS across subjects, despite its presumed visual field representation lying outside the stimulus screen, might lie in the diffuse feedback projections from higher areas, which are known to back-project to V1 in a much more diffuse way than the feed-forward connections that provide specific input to these higher areas (Zeki and Shipp, 1988). The explanation is unlikely to lie in common eye movements across subjects, which could have brought parts of the screen into the peripheral field of view, as our projection screen had a maximal eccentricity of about 15° (30° total horizontal

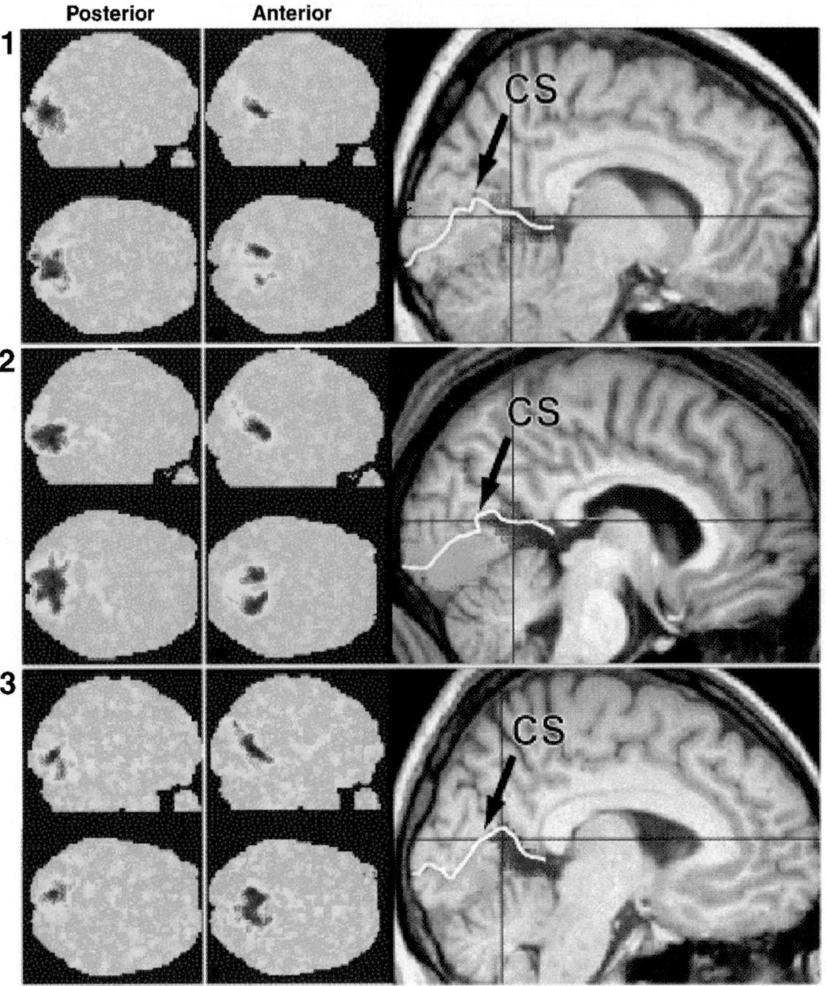

FIGURE 13.12
Activation in the anterior and posterior sections of the calcarine sulcus was isolated in separate ICs. Shown are the corresponding ICs of three subjects (1 to 3) in the form of glass-brain projections (sagittal and horizontal views) and sagittal sections of their structural scans (taken at $x = -8$, $x = -5$, and $x = -7$ mm, respectively) with the ICs superimposed (green = IC with posterior CS, red = IC with anterior CS). The calcarine sulcus has been redrawn with white for clarity.

extent). Even if subjects had fixated the edge of the screen, activity in V1 would not have spread anteriorly to the genu of the CS. Until the complete visual fields of V1 and V2, including their periphery, are mapped using retinotopic stimuli, we cannot exclude the possibility that aCS constitutes a separate area, distinct from V1 or V2. We are not unaware of the fact that Henschen (1910), to his dying day, insisted that central vision is represented in the anterior calcarine sulcus. Although his conclusions have been discounted through the pathological and perimetric studies of Inouye (1909), Holmes (1945), and others, it would be good to discount such a possibility through imaging studies as well.

V5 and the Lateral Occipital Complex (LOC)

The ICs containing an area in close proximity to that selective for visual motion, V5, had the most area-specific ATCs of all visual areas, and they achieved the highest inter-subject ranks and inter-subject correlations (see Fig. 13.9). In every subject, these ICs had a second set of significant voxels in the region of the lateral ventral occipital cortex (LOC) or fusiform face area (FFA) that has been associated with object- and face-selective responses (Malach *et al.*, 1995; Kanwisher *et al.*, 1997) (Fig. 13.13). The co-segregation of this region proximal to V5 (below referred to as 'V5', even though it may be part of a more dorsal subdivision of LOC that partially overlaps with *V5/MT* (Malach *et al.*, 1995; Kourtzi *et al.*, 2002; Downing *et al.*, 2001), and LOC suggests a particularly high correlation of activity between them during free viewing. To confirm

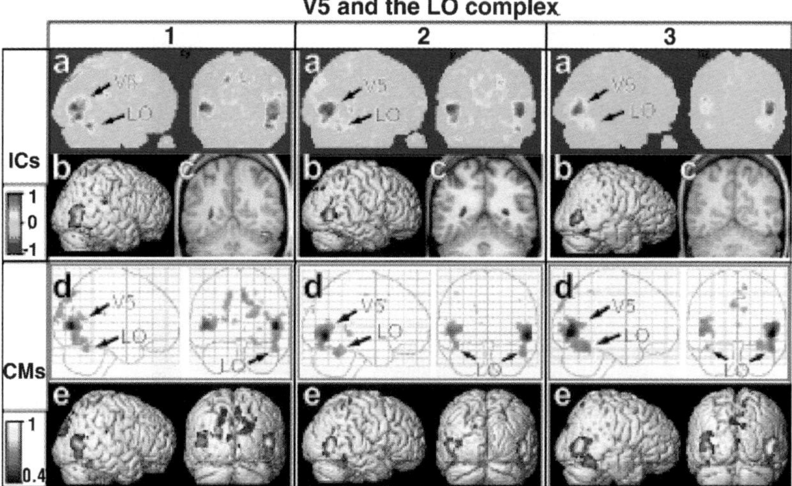

FIGURE 13.13
Correlated activity between V5 and LOC. Shown are the ICs, (a) to (c), and correlation maps (CMs), (d) and (e), of three subjects (1 to 3). The CMs show the correlation of the BOLD signal in the whole brain to that of the hottest voxel of the IC, which was located in right V5 in each subject. Raw IC glass-brain projections are shown in (a), along with rendered views (b) and on coronal sections (c) ($y = -54$, $y = -50$, $y = -59$ mm for subjects 1 to 3), the latter two thresholded at 30% activity. CMs are thresholded at a correlation coefficient (r) = 0.4, in both glass-brain (d) and rendered (e) views .

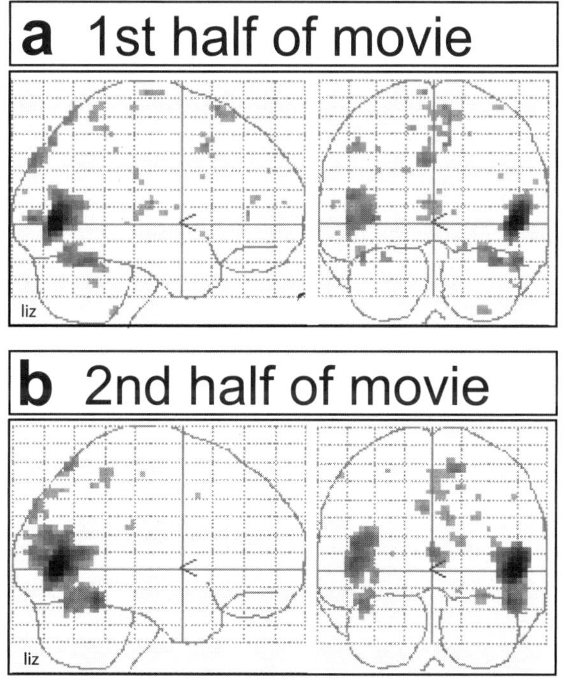

FIGURE 13.14
Results are independent of the stimulation in free viewing. CMs (shown as glass-brain projections and thresholded at r = 0.4) created for subject 3's right V5, based on (a) the first half of the movie and (b) the second half of the movie. Despite exposure to entirely different stimuli in the two halves, the CMs are indistinguishable.

this, and also to visualise the extent to which other areas in the brain correlated with activity in V5, we calculated the correlation coefficients between the BOLD signals of the most significant voxel in the V5-IC and all remaining voxels in the brain, thus creating correlation maps (CMs). The results were similar in all eight subjects; the CMs and ICs of three subjects are shown in Fig. 13.13. In all of the subjects, LOC is the area that has the strongest correlation and spatially the most extensive set of voxels correlating with activity in V5, and this bilaterally. The same result was found when only the first half or the second half of the movie were considered, which is shown in Fig. 13.14. This result leads us to conclude that the high correlation between V5 and

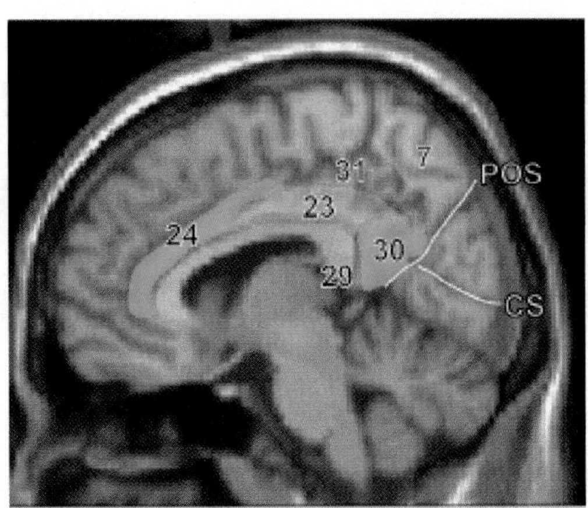

FIGURE 13.15
Schematic representation of the subdivisions of the posterior parietal cortex into distinct cytoarchitectonic maps according to Brodmann. Areas are superimposed onto a medial view of a template MRI structural scan, sectioned at x = 7 mm. BA29 and BA30 make up the retrosplenium, which is part of the posterior cingulate cortex including additionally BA23 and BA31. BA7 contains the precuneus. For anatomical orientation, the calcarine sulcus (CS) and the parieto-occipital sulcus (POS) have been outlined in white. The same colours were used repeatedly for purely graphical reasons.

LOC reflects a general property of these areas and is not specific to the stimulus used. Together with the evidence presented in the following sections, which invariably shows that areas that correlate in free viewing have strong anatomical connections, it suggests not only a functional link but also a strong anatomical link between V5 and LOC.

Area V5, classically referred to as a visual-motion selective area, has been implied in object recognition in the human by several previous studies. Kourtzi and Kanwisher (2000) have described that it is more active when subjects view static objects that imply motion than static objects that do not and, more recently, that human V5 has a general object selective response (Kourtzi *et al.*, 2002; Downing *et al.*, 2001). Our finding that V5 entertains its highest correlation of activity with the object-selective occipital ventral region in the LO complex (Malach *et al.*, 1995) confirms its involvement in object-related processing and even suggests an anatomical link between the two. The co-segregation of the two areas in a single component in each subject is testimony to the ability of such chronoarchitectonic maps to reveal inherent properties of brain organisation.

The Posterior Cingulate Cortex and Its Segregated Cooperation with the Parietal Cortex

The posterior cingulate cortex is subdivided on anatomical grounds into several structurally and functionally distinct subdivisions. Anatomically, the posterior cingulate cortex is comprised of Brodmann areas 23, 29, 30, and 31, and includes the retrosplenial cortex, which is located directly posterior to the corpus callosum and consists of BA29 and BA30. Figure 13.15 shows the approximate extent of these areas on a sagittal midline view of a structural MRI scan. Even though activated in a wide variety of studies, generally two classes of stimuli seem to activate two separate subdivisions in this region most consistently. BA23 and BA31, but not the retrosplenium, are involved in proprioception and visuospatial function in both monkeys and humans (Shima *et al.*, 1991; Richer *et al.*, 1993; Kawashima *et al.*, 1994). The retrosplenium (BA29 and BA30) is involved in episodic memory and spatial navigation, as is apparent from both imaging and clinical studies (see Maguire, 2001b, for a review). Its activation in emotional studies may be due to memory confounds (Maddock, 1999; Maguire, 2001b). We became interested in the posterior cingulate cortex because ICA dissected it into two separate compartments in almost every subject, contained in two separate ICs. One contained a region corresponding to posterior cingulate BA23, the other a region corresponding to the retrosplenial region BA29 and BA30, thus corresponding to the two functional subdivisions outlined above.

The first IC contained BA23 in the posterior cingulate cortex, the medial superior part of the precuneus (BA7), and, more faintly, the inferior parietal lobule (corresponding to BA40) bilaterally. Corresponding ICs in each subject had ATCs that correlated with a high significance and achieved high inter-subject ranks (see Fig. 13.9). ICs containing this network are displayed

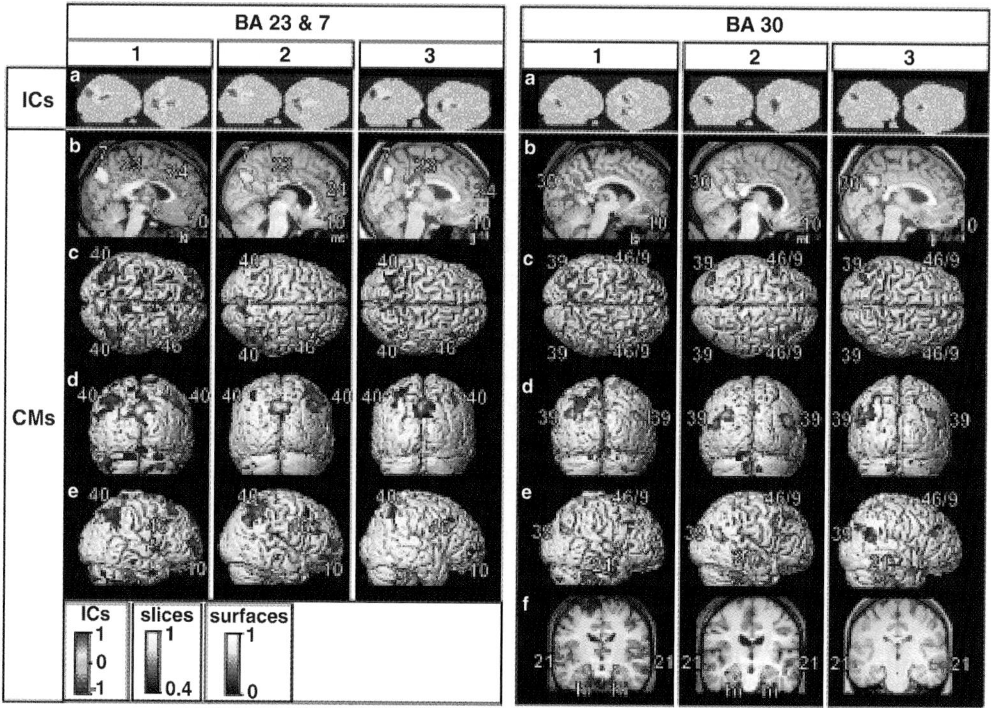

FIGURE 13.16
Two functional subdivisions in the posterior cingulate cortex, shown on three subjects (1 to 3). Left panel (BA23 and BA7): In each subject, the posterior cingulate BA23 and precuneus (BA7) were isolated in the same IC. Note the parietal cortex in both ICs and CMs. CMs reveal functional couplings with the inferior parietal lobule (BA40) and BA24 (anterior cingulate gyrus), BA46 (mid-dorsolateral prefrontal cortex), and BA10. Sagittal sections were taken at $x = 3, 4, 3$ mm. Right panel (BA30): The retrosplenial cortex (BA30) was isolated in a separate IC in each subject, and CMs show its correlations with the angular gyrus (BA39), BA46/9, the middle temporal gyrus (BA21), BA10, and the hippocampus (hi). Sagittal sections were taken at x = –7, 4, 3 mm, coronal sections at y = –14, –15, –25. Note the thalamic activation in both sections of subject 1.

in Fig. 13.16 for three subjects. Using the associated ATC of the ICs as seeds, CMs were computed to reveal correlations among the components of this network. The resulting CMs are shown for the same three subjects in Fig. 13.16 and reveal consistently the network highlighted in the ICs with the posterior cingulate cortex (BA23), the precuneus (BA7), and the inferior parietal lobule (BA40). In addition, the CMs contain consistently the anterior cingulate gyrus (BA24), as well as BA10 in the prefrontal cortex and, less consistently, various other frontal areas including BA46. This is in accord with the connectivity of these areas as shown in monkey. BA23 has direct anatomical connections with BA7, BA24, and the inferior parietal lobule (BA40) (Baleydier and Mauguiere, 1980; Pandya *et al.*, 1981; Vogt and Pandya, 1987; Cavada and Goldman-Rakic, 1989; Vogt *et al.*, 1992). The CMs seem therefore to reflect not only functional similarity but also anatomical connectivity.

Functionally, it is interesting to note that the network reported here, comprised of BA23, the precuneus, bilateral inferior parietal lobules, and medial prefrontal BA10, has been shown to commonly decrease activity in attention-demanding tasks. The location of these areas is compatible with the regions proposed to be responsible for a default mode of brain action: areas for which activity is high during resting but actively suppressed during demanding tasks (Raichle *et al.*, 2001; Greicius *et al.*, 2003). This interpretation is consistent with the correlation of this network with other areas found in this study. The IC containing this network was unique in that it had the lowest and partially negative correlations with the other ICs in the comparison (see Fig. 13.10).

The second IC contained a single region located in the retrosplenium, corresponding to the location of BA29 and BA30, referred to below as BA30. In addition, just as in the first IC, a faint region of bilateral activity can be discerned in the parietal cortex, but posterior to that found in the first IC. This IC was found in six out of the eight subjects but did not show consistent inter-subject correlations. However, the six subjects appeared to consist of two groups of three subjects, within whom inter-subject correlation and ranking achieved significance (correlations: $r = 0.13$ and 0.11, $p < 0.06$ and $p < 0.014$; median ranks = 3.3 and 8.4, $p < 0.001$ and $p < 10^{-4}$). We believe that all ICs represent the same functional area; their locations were identical in all subjects, as was their presumed connectivity as revealed by the CMs. The latter revealed a network that was distinct from the one uncovered with the first IC and is shown in Fig. 13.16. BA30 showed high correlations with the angular gyrus in the parietal cortex (BA39) bilaterally, with the mid-dorsolateral prefrontal region BA46/9 and with the middle temporal gyrus (BA21). Regions of the hippocampus, the superior temporal lobe, frontal regions such as BA10, and, in subject 1, some of the thalamic nuclei were also correlated, but not in every subject. Even though this catalogue of correlations might seem confusing, it makes sense: All of the regions listed above have direct anatomical connections with BA30 and all are known to be involved in processing associated with memory and navigation (Maguire, 2001a). BA30, therefore, seems to lie at the heart of this memory/navigation system, as was pointed out earlier by Maguire (2001a). In fact, the anatomical connections are summarised in the above publication in the following way which, when read while studying the CMs of Fig. 13.16, are almost a description of that figure: "The major reciprocal connections are between area 30 and mid-dorsolateral prefrontal cortex (areas 46, 9/46, and 9), and parahippocampal cortical areas … There are further connections with superior temporal sulcus and posterior parietal cortex, as well as with lateroposterior, laterodorsal and anterior thalamic nuclei. Thus the retrosplenial cortex is exceptionally well placed to contribute to the medial temporal lobe memory system as well as being a route through which prefrontal regions might interact with limbic areas" (Maguire, 2001a). We have gone into the details here to emphasise that, from a single study, the chronoarchitecture of the brain can reveal a family of areas with common functional concerns, which would require a number of hypothesis-led studies to reveal.

The two ICs containing these separate subregions within the posterior cingulate cortex performed obviously quite distinct functions, as one would expect from their distinct functional connectivity to other areas. The correlation between them was very low (median $r = 0.08$; quartiles, 0.02/0.20; $n = 5$).

In summary, the example we give here, of two functionally distinct subdivisions within the posterior cingulate cortex that coincide with anatomical and functional subdivisions known from earlier studies testifies to the power of the approach that we propose. Each of these distinct subdivisions entertains high temporal correlations with a distinct network of areas during free viewing, with whose components each has direct anatomical connections. Specifically, we have demonstrated that BA30 and BA23 are functionally connected to distinct parts in the parietal cortex which has not been shown before in the human brain and which probably has a counterpart in the monkey (Cavada and Goldman-Rakic, 1989). In addition, these results suggest that areas that correlate during free viewing are most likely directly connected anatomically, which adds an anatomical component to chronoarchitectonic maps.

Wernicke's Area, the Auditory Cortex, and Their Connectivity

In each subject ICA segregated a region in a separate IC that corresponded anatomically to Wernicke's receptive speech area (BA22) (Fig. 13.17) (Wernicke, 1874), with a highly significant inter-subject correlation of ($p < 10^{-12}$) (see Fig. 13.9). The ICs of five of the eight subjects contained, in addition to BA22, additional hot spots coinciding with presumptive Broca's area (BA44 and BA45) and with the premotor region of the frontal eye fields (BA6). Another IC contained the region corresponding to the auditory cortex (BA41 and BA42) in a separate IC in each subject. This IC showed no additional hot voxels outside of the auditory cortex, suggesting no strong cooperation with other areas. CMs based on the hottest voxels in Wernicke's BA22 and the auditory cortex revealed their functional connectivity. The former showed that BA22 is indeed highly correlated with premotor region BA6 and Broca's area, as suggested by the ICs, and in addition revealed its correlation with a parietal region (BA39). These correlations were also found in subjects in whom the IC contained BA 22 alone, and they are in accord with the anatomical connections known for BA22, which is connected with Broca's area (BA44 and BA45) and, less intensely, to parietal area BA39. Broca's area, in turn, has presumed connections to BA6 (Talairach and Tournoux, 1988). Both ICs and CMs showed bilateral activity and

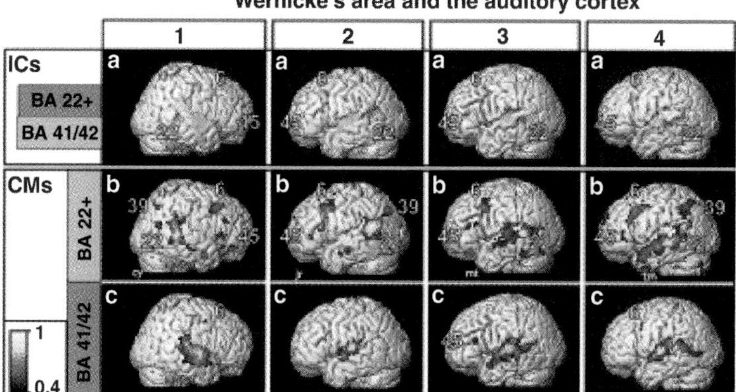

FIGURE 13.17
A dissection of Wernicke's speech area and the primary auditory cortex on the example of four subjects (1 to 4). (a) ICs are colour coded and superimposed on the subjects' structural renderings (green, IC containing auditory cortex; red, IC containing Wernicke's area [BA22]). ICs were thresholded at 30% activity. (b) and (c) CMs derived from seeds taken from the hottest voxels in either BA22 or auditory cortex reveal their functional connections, which correspond to anatomical ones.

correlations, even when the seed for the latter was chosen only from one hemisphere, which is compatible with many functional imaging studies on language showing a bilateral activation (Binder *et al.*, 2000). A recent study that localised Broca's area in a traditional fMRI paradigm and then created CMs based on "rest" conditions found correlations with BA6 and Wernicke's. Those results are compatible with ours and show that our approach is at least as powerful as the one that proposes to create CMs during the resting state (Biswal *et al.*, 1995; Hampson *et al.*, 2002).

Correlation maps based on the hottest voxel of the auditory cortex also revealed bilateral activity, but revealed at the same time a functional isolation of this area that was already suggested by the ICs: It lacked strong ($r > 0.4$) correlations with other cortical regions; weak correlations were present mainly with premotor area BA6 and Broca's BA44/45, which reached the threshold of $r > 0.4$ only in some of the subjects (Talairach and Tournoux, 1988). Surprisingly, CMs of BA22 and auditory cortex barely overlapped. Their mutual correlations were relatively low compared to the other areas revealed in their CMs (median $r = 0.37$; quartiles, 0.24, 0.45; $n = 8$).

In summary, our approach shows that Wernicke's area BA22 entertains high temporal correlations with parietal, premotor, and speech areas to which it is also anatomically connected and that the auditory cortex has correlations with premotor and speech areas with which it is anatomically connected. These results show once again that correlations between cortical areas during natural conditions can reveal their anatomical connectivity, even to areas that are anatomically remote.

Spinning all these results together leads us to formulate the following rule: *Areas that have high correlations between their ATCs obtained during natural viewing condition are likely to have direct anatomical connections. Conversely, areas that have weak or no temporal correlation are likely to have weak, indirect, or no connections.*

Dynamics in the Visual System During Free Viewing

Dynamics in and between visual areas have not been studied in the human brain when it is exposed to natural free-viewing conditions (Bartels and Zeki, 2004c). If perceptual analysis "…is performed interactively by areas and neurons with multipurpose properties" (Schiller, 1997) one would expect that correlations between visual areas would be very high during viewing, because then their multipurpose characteristics would be interactively engaged, while they would become low during quiescent states. We were therefore curious to learn more about the degree of correlation between visual areas during the presence and absence of natural stimuli and how these are affected by the sudden on- and offsets of the stimulus. We were especially

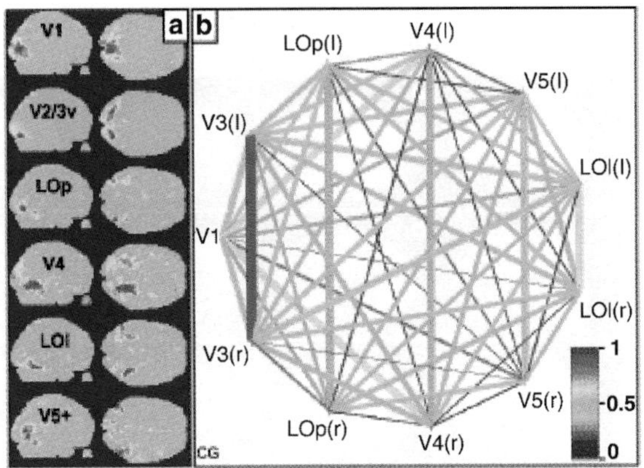

FIGURE 13.18
Correlations of BOLD signals between visual areas during free viewing of the movie. (a) Glass-brain views (lateral and transverse) of some visual ICs isolated from one subject. (b) Correlograms displaying the correlation (r) of BOLD signals between the most significant voxels of areas identified in (a).

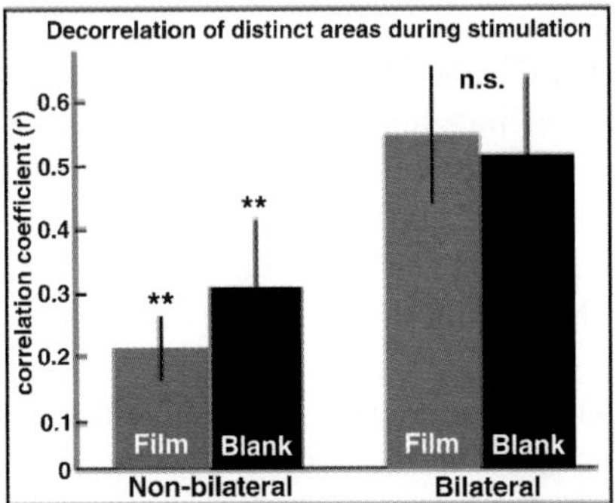

FIGURE 13.19
Stimulation leads to a decorrelation between different visual areas. The bars show the mean correlation coefficients (same data as in Fig. 13.20; subject weighted; ± standard deviation) of bilateral pairs of areas (known to have strong anatomical links and the same functional specialisation) and non-bilateral ones. Non-bilateral areas decorrelate during stimulation (paired t-test: $p < 0.008$, $n = 8$ subjects; $p < 10^{-20}$, $n = 1426$ pairs) compared to blank periods (last 15 s of blank periods), which is not true for bilateral areas. Even in the absence of stimulation, bilateral areas show a higher correlation than non-bilateral ones (two-sample t-test: $p < 0.002$, $n = 8$; $p < 10^{-6}$, $n_1 = 1426$, $n_2 = 75$).

interested to learn whether the correlations, which we take to imply functional connections, are maintained during periods of non-stimulation as well. In addition, it was interesting to see whether it would be possible to arrange the functional subdivisions revealed in the chronoarchitecture into a hierarchical tree that would group them with regard to their functional similarity and be indicative of the connections between them.

The first observation we made was that most visual areas were isolated by ICA in bilateral pairs (such as, for example, left and right V5, referred to below as bilateral or homologous areas), indicating that left and right hemispheric parts of the same area entertained a higher correlation among themselves than with other areas, illustrated in Fig. 13.18 by means of a correlogram showing the BOLD correlations between several visual areas of both hemispheres. Figure 13.19 quantifies this for the entire group, showing that bilateral areas in the two hemispheres have more than twice as high a correlation (mean: $r = 0.55 \pm 0.11$ std) than other pairs of areas (mean: $r = 0.22 \pm 0.05$ std) during viewing of the movie ($p < 10^{-6}$; $n = 8$). In addition, Fig. 13.19 shows that visual areas decorrelate in the presence of stimulation compared to the blank period; complex external stimulation appears to make their functional specificity (and differences) more apparent, in that areas assume ATCs that are more specific to them during stimulation than during rest (paired t-test: $p < 0.01$, $n = 8$ subjects; $p < 10^{-20}$, $n = 1501$ pairs of areas in all subjects). As expected for areas of the same specialisation, bilateral areas did not decorrelate in the presence of stimulation (in contrast to non-bilateral areas), as they share the same functional specialisa-

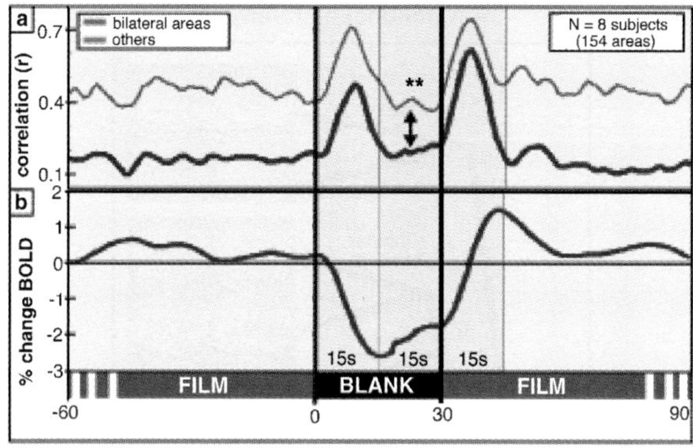

FIGURE 13.20
Event-related analysis of correlation and BOLD signal change among visual areas during movie and blank periods. (a) Mean correlation between all pairs of visual areas within subjects, averaged over all 8 subjects (154 areas in total). Correlation coefficients between pairs were calculated using a gliding window (size = 7 s) to obtain the instantaneous correlation coefficient at each time point of the session. Pairs included either only bilateral areas (red line) (*e.g.*, left/right V5) or only non-bilateral pairs (blue line) (*e.g.*, V1 versus V5), all within the same subject. The time series of these correlation coefficients were then cut up into the periods ±1 min around the eight 30-s blanks that interrupted the movie and were averaged, first within each subject, then across subjects (red line, bilateral pairs of areas, $n = 75$; blue line, all pairs excluding bilateral pairs, $n = 1426$). (b) mean BOLD signal of all 154 areas identified by ICA in the eight subjects, averaged (each subject with equal weight) and time-locked ±1 min around the blanks.

tion. Our finding that correlations between areas are lowest during movie viewing suggests that functionally specialised areas are most specific, and obviously least multifunctional, when engaged in processing. This is probably so because the optimal stimuli for each area, such as motion, colour, or faces, vary with a high degree of independence in the movie (Bartels and Zeki, 2004a). This specificity was reduced, and the cross-talk between areas increased, when they were not engaged in a specific processing task. Interestingly, in the absence of stimulation, the correlation between bilateral areas was still higher than that of non-bilateral pairs (last 15 s of blank, which is unaffected by the transition; $p < 0.0016$; two-sample t-test; $n = 8$). The latter effect can hardly be explained by common external stimulation and may be due either to imagery or to the strong interhemispheric connections between bilateral areas (Zeki, 1970; Pandya *et al.*, 1971; Clarke and Miklossy, 1990), which may synchronise the BOLD activity even in the absence of visual stimulation. If the latter is the case, the method of comparing correlations of ATCs in the absence and presence of stimulation may be used to detect strongly interconnected areas and to differentiate between connections that are always active and those that, though present, are in a dynamic state, that is to say only active when the task demands it (see Section 4).

We thus add three other rules: (1) Areas that remain highly correlated in the absence of stimulation are the most strongly and directly connected ones; (2) correlations between two areas may change depending on the task, implying a dynamism in connectivity; and (3) correlations between two areas decrease with increasing complexity of the stimuli that they are processing.

Figure 13.20 shows in an event-related fashion how BOLD signal and its correlation among visual areas is affected when the movie is interrupted by blank periods. During film viewing, the BOLD signal was high, while the correlation among visual areas was lowest. Blank periods led to a drop of BOLD by about 2% and a rise of the correlation. The latter effect was due to increased correlation among non-bilateral areas (see Fig. 13.19). Transitions from movie to blank and vice versa led to a steep rise of the correlations to about twice their normal value. Sharp transitions in stimulation, interestingly no matter whether onsets or offsets, thus lead to activity that is least area specific and therefore highly correlated across the cortex. This should be taken into account in conventional studies aiming to characterise dynamics between areas (Hampson *et al.*, 2002), as these seem to be unfavourably affected by stimuli involving such sharp, unnatural transitions.

Given the areas of an ICA-dissected human brain along with their activity time courses, it should therefore be possible to reveal the hierarchical organisation of their functional proximity, based on mutual correlations. To do so, we submitted ICs of each subject to a clustering

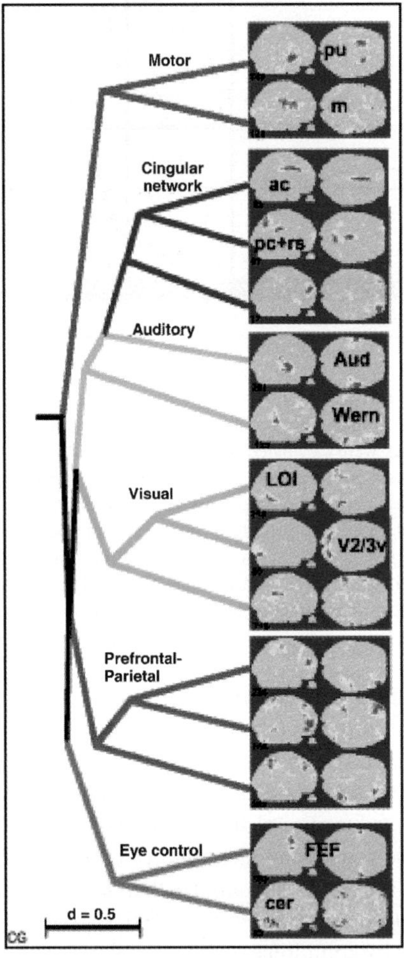

FIGURE 13.21
Hierarchical functional relationships between cortical areas revealed by the correlation of their ATCs. The chronodendrogram is the result of a clustering algorithm originally designed to build phylogenetic trees based on DNA similarity between related species (Felsenstein, 1981). Here, 15 representative ICs of subject 1 were used, and ICs were clustered based on the correlation coefficients matrix of their ATCs. Branches were subsequently coloured for graphical clarity. pu = putamen; m = molar cortex; FEF = frontal eye fields; cer = cerebellum; ac = anterior angulate.

algorithm, which grouped ICs in a hierarchical fashion using a distance matrix (d) based on the correlation (r) between their time courses: $d = (1 - |r|)$. This procedure, therefore, grouped areas according to their temporal and therefore functional similarity. We used a program originally designed to display the evolutionary phylogenetic relationship between different species, with a distance matrix based on DNA sequences (PHYLIP package, with the KITSCH algorithm to generate and draw the dendrograms (http://evolution.genetics.washington.edu/phylip.html; Felsenstein, 1981). Other clustering methods led to almost identical results.

In all subjects, functionally related areas were grouped in the same sub-branches of the resulting tree, and visual areas were segregated from other areas, as in the case shown. Figure 13.21 shows how some selected areas are temporally related in one subject. This method is useful for the identification of unexpected functional proximities between areas. In the case shown, we found the putamen to be highly correlated with the motor cortex; a subregion of the cerebellum to be grouped with the frontal eye fields, which are presumably both involved in eye-movement control; and the cingulate gyrus to be coactive with a bilateral region in the lateral prefrontal cortex. While correlations among members of each group were relatively high, correlations between different groups were too low to attribute significance to the order in which they appeared in such trees.

CONCLUSION

Cortical maps generated by the hypotheses of the experimenter may fall short in reflecting the true organisation of the human brain. Anatomical maps are more objective, as structural boundaries equal functional ones. Both maps rely however on specialised markers for each area, which may consist of unique stimuli or anatomical dyes. We have proposed here a new principle, the *principle of functional independence*. It states that feature independence in the external world led to the evolutionary segregation of areas that process them, and that therefore all functionally specialised modules have independent activity time courses when the brain is exposed to natural conditions. By definition, therefore, each functionally specialised module has an activity time course that is unique to it. We have shown that such temporal fingerprints of functionally distinct areas can be used to create a novel, time-based map of the cerebrum, which we call *chronoarchitecture*. Its creation requires the exposure of the brain to natural conditions, to ensure that distinct functions of cerebral modules are stimulated by complex and independent external features. We used independent component analysis to segregate the distinct cerebral modules based on their temporal differences. Our results show that the chronoarchitectonic map reveals the same subdivisions revealed by traditional functional imaging experiments and by anatomical methods, but that it can also reveal novel cortical subdivisions. In addition, our results show that the temporal similarity between chronoarchitectonically defined subdivisions reflect both their functional similarity and the strength of anatomical connections between them, which is a logical consequence of the principle of functional independence. We used this to map several novel networks of cooperating areas and a hierarchy of areas based on their temporal similarity.

We conclude that each functionally distinct area has a unique time signature that can be exploited to segregate it from others. The exposure of the brain to natural conditions facilitates this process by maximising the temporal differences between the areas. We confirmed this independently first by showing that, when the brain was freely viewing a movie, more areas were segregated by ICA than when the brain was exposed to a conventional paradigm, and, second, by the observation that visual stimulation leads to a decorrelation of activity (*i.e.*, an increase in specificity) in visual areas compared to the resting state.

The free-viewing conditions employed here reflect only one subset of natural conditions. As we constrained ourselves to describe areas whose activity was similar across different brains, we were limited to visual, parietal, and temporal areas. In each subject we also identified a multitude of areas whose activity was subject specific. These lay in cortical regions whose functions and functional subdivisions are less well understood, such as in frontal and prefrontal cortices. Different natural conditions that emphasise more emotive, mnemonic, and executive functions might synchronise these areas across subjects and allow their reliable characterisation better than the James Bond movie used here. Nevertheless, the fact that we mapped known and novel functional subdivisions even in the well-studied occipital brain shows that the chronoarchitectonic approach can guide the identification of unknown functional subdivisions in the human brain and that their activity time courses can provide clues about their functional proximity. Obviously, chronoarchitectonic mapping does not rely on ICA specifically, and future, better algorithms might improve the quality of the maps just as much as different stimulation techniques.

In summary, we have used the principle of functional independence to reveal the chronoarchitecture of the cerebral cortex, an architecture that reveals subdivisions that have different and independent activities throughout time in natural conditions. The underlying assumption is that areas that have differential activity time courses have different functions. Chronoarchitectonic maps reveal therefore fundamental organising principles of the human brain, based on inherent brain dynamics and independent of human hypotheses and artificial stimuli.

References

Arfanakis, K., Cordes, D., Haughton, V. M., Moritz, C. H., Quigley, M. A., and Meyerand, M. E. (2000). Combining independent component analysis and correlation analysis to probe interregional connectivity in fMRI task activation datasets. *Magn. Reson. Imaging*, **18**, 921–930.

Arnold, D. H., Clifford, C. W. G., and Wenderoth, P. (2001). Asynchronous processing in vision: colour leads motion. *Curr. Biol.*, **11**, 596–600.

Baleydier, C. and Mauguiere, F. (1980). The duality of the cingulate gyrus in monkey: neuroanatomical study and functional hypothesis. *Brain*, **103**, 525–554.

Bartels, A. (2000). The Modularity of Processing and Perception in the Visual Brain, Ph.D. thesis. University College London, U.K. (www.vislab.ucl.ac.uk).

Bartels, A. and Zeki, S. (2004a). Functional brain mapping during free viewing of natural scenes. *Hum. Brain Map*, in press.

Bartels, A. and Zeki, S. (2004b). The chronoarchitecture of the human brain, submitted.

Bartels, A. and Zeki, S. (2004c). Correlations during free viewing and rest as a guide to cortical connectivity, submitted.

Bartels, A. and Zeki, S. (2001). Chronoarchitecture: the dissection of the human brain into functional subdivisions by ICA analysis of fMRI data collected during free viewing of a movie. *Society for Neuroscience,* 620.15.

Bartels, A. and Zeki, S. (1998). The theory of multi-stage integration in the visual brain. *Proc. R. Soc. Lond. B.*, **265**, 2327–2332.

Bartels, A. and Zeki, S. (2000a). The architecture of the colour centre in the human visual brain: new results and a review. *Eur. J. Neurosci.*, **12**, 172–193.

Bartels, A. and Zeki, S. (2000b). The neural basis of romantic love. *NeuroReport*, **11**, 3829–3834.

Beckers, G. and Zeki, S. (1995). The consequences of inactivating areas V1 and V5 on visual-motion perception. *Brain*, **118**, 49–60.

Bell, A. J. and Sejnowski, T. J. (1995). An information maximisation approach to blind separation and blind deconvolution. *Neural Comput.*, **7**, 1129–1159.

Binder, J. R., Frost, J. A., Hammeke, T. A., Bellgowan, P. S., Springer, J. A., Kaufman, J. N., and Possing, E. T. (2000). Human temporal lobe activation by speech and nonspeech sounds. *Cereb. Cortex*, **10**, 512–528.

Biswal, B., Yetkin, F. Z., Haughton, V. M., and Hyde, J. S. (1995). Functional connectivity in the motor cortex of resting human brain using echo-planar MRI. *Magn. Reson. Med.*, **34**, 537–541.

Bork, A. C. and Zeki, S. M. (1998). The cortical site for the generation of forms from motion. *NeuroImage*, **7**, S329.

Broca, P. P. (1861). Perte de la parole, ramollisement chronique et destruction partielle du lobe antérieure gauche du cerveau. *Bulletin de la Société Anthropologique*, **2**, 235–238.

Brodmann, K. (1905). Beiträge zur histologischen Lokalisation der Grosshirnrinde. Dritte Mitteilung: Die Rindenfelder der niederen Affen. *J. Psychol. Neurol.*, **4**, 177–226.

Buchel, C., Holmes, A. P., Rees, G., and Friston, K. J. (1998). Characterizing stimulus–response functions using nonlinear regressors in parametric fMRI experiments. *NeuroImage*, **8**, 140–148.

Buchner, H., Weyen, U., Frackowiak, R. S. J., Romaya, J., and Zeki, S. (1994). The timing of visual-evoked potential activity in human area V4. *Proc. Roy. Soc. London Ser. B*, **257**, 99–104.

Buchner, H., Gobbele, R., Wagner, M., Fuchs, M., Waberski, T. D., and Beckmann, R. (1997). Fast visual evoked potential input into human area V5. *NeuroReport*, **8**, 2419–2422.

Calhoun, V. D., Adali, T., Pearlson, G. D., and Pekar, J. J. (2001a). A method for making group inferences from functional MRI data using independent component analysis. *Hum. Brain Mapping*, **14**, 140–151.

Calhoun, V. D., Adali, T., Pearlson, G. D., and Pekar, J. J. (2001b). Spatial and temporal independent component analysis of functional MRI data containing a pair of task-related waveforms. *Hum. Brain Mapping*, **13**, 43–53.

Calhoun, V. D., Adali, T., McGinty, V. B., Pekar, J. J., Watson, T. D., and Pearlson, G. D. (2001c). fMRI activation in a visual-perception task: network of areas detected using the general linear model and independent components analysis. *NeuroImage*, **14**, 1080–1088.

Campbell, A. W. (1905). *Histological Studies on the Localisation of Cerebral Function*. Cambridge University Press, Cambridge, U.K.

Cavada, C. and Goldman-Rakic, P. S. (1989). Posterior parietal cortex in rhesus monkey. I. Parcellation of areas based on distinctive limbic and sensory corticocortical connections. *J. Comp. Neurol.*, **287**, 393–421.

Cavaglia, M., Dombrowski, S. M., Drazba, J., Vasanji, A., Bokesch, P. M., and Janigro, D. (2001). Regional variation in brain capillary density and vascular response to ischemia. *Brain Res.*, **910**, 81–93.

Clarke, S. and Miklossy, J. (1990). Occipital cortex in man: organisation of callosal connections, related myelo- and cytoarchitecture, and putative boundaries of functional visual areas. *J. Comp. Neurol.*, **298**, 188–214.

Cordes, D., Haughton, V. M., Arfanakis, K., Wendt, G. J., Turski, P. A., Moritz, C. H., Quigley, M. A., and Meyerand, M. E. (2000). Mapping functionally related regions of brain with functional connectivity MR imaging. *Am. J. Neuroradiol.*, **21**, 1636–1644.

Cordes, D., Haughton, V. M., Arfanakis, K., Carew, J. D., Turski, P. A., Moritz, C. H., Quigley, M. A., and Meyerand, M. E. (2001). Frequencies contributing to functional connectivity in the cerebral cortex in 'resting-state' data. *Am. J. Neuroradiol.*, **22**, 1326–1333.

DeYoe, E. A. and Van Essen, D. C. (1985). Segregation of efferent connections and receptive field properties in visual area 2 of the macaque. *Nature*, **317**, 58–61.

Downing, P. E., Jiang, Y., Shuman, M., and Kanwisher, N. (2001). A cortical area selective for visual processing of the human body. *Science*, **293**, 2470–2473.

Engel, S. A., Rummelhart, D. E., Wandell, B. A., Lee, A. H., Glover, G. H., Chichilnisky, E.-J., and Shadlen, M. N. (1994). fMRI of human visual cortex. *Nature*, **369**, 525–525.

Engel, S. A., Glover, G. H., and Wandell, B. A. (1997). Retinotopic organisation in human visual cortex and the spatial precision of functional MRI. *Cereb. Cortex*, **7**, 181–192.

Felsenstein, J. (1981). Evolutionary trees from DNA sequences: a maximum likelihood approach. *J. Mol. Evol.*, **17**, 368–376.

ffytche, D. H., Guy, C. N., and Zeki, S. (1995). The parallel visual motion inputs into areas V1 and V5 of human cerebral cortex. *Brain*, **118**, 1375–1394.

ffytche, D. H., Howard, R. J., Brammer, M. J., David, A., Woodruff, P., and Williams S. (1998). The anatomy of conscious vision: an fMRI study of visual hallucinations. *Nat. Neurosci.*, **1**, 738–742.

Flechsig, P. (1901). Developmental (myelogenetic) localisation of the cerebral cortex in the human subject. *Lancet*, **2**, 1027–1029.

Friston, K. J. (1998). Modes or models: a critique on independent component analysis for fMRI. *Trends Cogn. Sci.*, **2**, 373–374.

Friston, K. J., Frith, C. D., Frackowiak, R. S. J., and Turner, R. (1995a). Characterizing dynamic brain responses with fMRI: a multivariate approach. *NeuroImage*, **2**, 166–172.

Friston, K. J., Holmes, A. P., Poline, J. B., Grasby, P. J., Williams, S. C. R., Frackowiak, R. S. J., and Turner, R. (1995b). Analysis of fMRI time-series revisited. *NeuroImage*, **2**, 45–53.

Friston, K. J., Fletcher, P., Josephs, O., Holmes, A., Rugg, M. D., and Turner, R. (1998). Event-related fMRI: characterizing differential responses. *NeuroImage*, **7**, 30–40.

Fritsch, G. and Hitzig, E. (1870). Über die elektrische Erregbarkeit des Grosshirns. *Archiv für Anatomie, Physiologie und wissenschaftliche Medizin*, **37**, 300–332.

Greicius, M. D., Krasnow, B., Reiss, A. L., and Menon, V. (2003). Functional connectivity in the resting brain: A network analysis of the default mode hypothesis. *Proc. Natl. Acad. Sci. U.S.A.*, **100**, 253–258.

Gu, H., Engelien, W., Feng, H., Silbersweig, D. A., Stern, E., and Yang, Y. (2001). Mapping transient, randomly occurring neuropsychological events using independent component analysis. *NeuroImage*, **14**, 1432–1443.

Hampson, M., Peterson, B. S., Skudlarski, P., Gatenby, J. C., and Gore, J. C. (2002). Detection of functional connectivity using temporal correlations in MR images. *Hum. Brain Mapping*, **15**, 247–262.

Harrison, R. V., Harel, N., Panesar, J., and Mount, R. J. (2002). Blood capillary distribution correlates with hemodynamic-based functional imaging in cerebral cortex. *Cereb. Cortex*, **12**, 225–233.

Henschen, S. E. (1910). Zentrale Sehstörungen. In: *Handbuch der Neurologie*, Lewandowsky, M., Ed., pp. 891–918, Springer-Verlag, Berlin.

Henson, R. N., Price, C. J., Rugg, M. D., Turner, R., and Friston, K. J. (2002). Detecting latency differences in event-related BOLD responses: application to words versus nonwords and initial versus repeated face presentations. *NeuroImage*, **15**, 83–97.

Holmes, G. (1945). The Ferrier Lecture: The organization of the visual cortex in man. *Proc. R. Soc. Lond. B*, **132**, 348–361.

Hubel, D. H. and Livingstone, M. S. (1987). Segregation of form, colour and stereopsis in primate area 18. *J. Neurosci.*, **7**, 3378–3415.

Inouye, T. (1909). Die Sehstörungen bei Schussverletzungen der Kortikalen Sehsphäre, nach Beobachtungen an Verwundeten der letzten japanischen Kriege. W. Engelmann, Leipzig.

Ishibashi, H., Hihara, S., Takahashi, M., Heike, T., Yokota, T., and Iriki A. (2002). Tool-use learning selectively induces expression of brain-derived neurotrophic factor, its receptor trkB, and neurotrophin 3 in the intraparietal multisensorycortex of monkeys. *Brain Res. Cogn. Brain Res.*, **14**, 3–9.

Kanwisher, N., McDermott, J., and Chun, M. M. (1997). The fusiform face area: a module in human extrastriate cortex specialised for face perception. *J. Neurosci.*, **17**, 4302–4311.

Kawashima, R., Roland, P. E., and O'Sullivan, B. T. (1994). Activity in the human primary motor cortex related to ipsilateral hand movements. *Brain Res.*, **663**, 251–256.

Kim, K.-H., Bartels, A., and Zeki, S. (2001). Differential gene expression of areas V4 and V5 in the visual cortices of human and macaque. *Soc. Neurosci.*, Abstract 286.15.

Kleinschmidt, A., Büchel, C., Zeki, S., and Frackowiak, R. S. J. (1998). Human brain activity during spontaneously reversing perception of ambiguous figures. *Proc. Roy. Soc. London Ser. B*, **265**, 2427–2422.

Kourtzi, Z. and Kanwisher, N. (2000). Activation in human MT/MST by static images with implied motion. *J. Cogn. Neurosci.*, **12**, 48–55.

Kourtzi, Z., Bulthoff, H. H., Erb, M., and Grodd, W. (2002). Object-selective responses in the human motion area MT/MST. *Nat. Neurosci.*, **5**, 17–18.

Livingstone, M. S. and Hubel, D. H. (1984). Anatomy and physiology of a colour system in the primate visual cortex. *J. Neurosci.*, **4**, 309–356.

Lumer, E. D., Friston, K. J., and Rees, G. (1998). Neural correlates of perceptual rivalry in the human brain. *Science*, **280**, 1930–1934.

Maddock, R. J. (1999). The retrosplenial cortex and emotion: new insights from functional neuroimaging of the human brain. *Trends Neurosci.*, **22**, 310–316.

Maguire, E. A. (2001a). The retrosplenial contribution to human navigation: a review of lesion and neuroimaging studies. *J. Psychol.*, **42**, 225–238.

Maguire, E. A. (2001b). The retrosplenial contribution to human navigation: a review of lesion and neuroimaging findings. *Scand. J. Psychol.*, **42**, 225–238.

Makeig, S., Jung, T. P., Bell, A. J., Ghahremani, D., and Sejnowski, T. J. (1997). Blind separation of auditory event-related brain responses into independent components. *Proc. Natl. Acad. Sci. USA*, **94**, 10979–10984.

Makeig, S., Westerfield, M., Jung, T. P., Enghoff, S., Townsend, J., Courchesne, E., and Sejnowski, T. J. (2002). Dynamic brain sources of visual evoked responses. *Science*, **295**, 690–694.

Malach, R., Reppas, J. B., Benson, R. R., Kwong, K. K., Jiang, H., Kennedy, W. A., Ledden, P. J., Brady, T. J., Rosen, B. R., and Tootell, R. B. H. (1995). Object-related activity revealed by functional magnetic resonance imaging in human occipital cortex. *Proc. Natl. Acad. Sci. USA*, **92**, 8135–8139.

McKeown, M. J. (2000a). Detection of consistently task-related activations in fMRI data with hybrid independent component analysis. *NeuroImage*, **11**, 24–35.

McKeown, M. J., Makeig, S., Brown, G. G., Jung, T. P., Kindermann, S. S., Bell, A. J., and Sejnowski, T. (1997). Analysis of fMRI data by decomposition into independent components. *Neurology*, **48**, 6056.

McKeown, M. J., Jung, T. P., Makeig, S., Brown, G., Kindermann, S. S., Lee, T. W., and Sejnowski, T. J. (1998a). Spatially independent activity patterns in functional MRI data during the Stroop colour naming task. *Proc. Natl. Acad. Sci. USA*, **95**, 803–810.

Moutoussis, K. and Zeki, S. M. (1997a). Functional segregation and temporal hierarchy of the visual perceptive systems. *Proc. Roy. Soc. London Ser. B*, **264**, 1407–1414.

Moutoussis, K. and Zeki, S. M. (1997b). A direct demonstration of perceptual asynchrony in vision. *Proc. Roy. Soc. London Ser. B*, **264**, 393–399.

Nakada, T., Suzuki, K., Fujii, Y., Matsuzawa, H., and Kwee, I. L. (2000). Independent component-cross correlation-sequential epoch (ICS) analysis of high field fMRI time series: direct visualisation of dual representation of the primary motor cortex in human. *Neurosci. Res.*, **37**, 237–244.

Nybakken, G. E., Quigley, M. A., Moritz, C. H., Cordes, D., Haughton, V. M., and Meyerand, M. E. (2002). Test-retest precision of functional magnetic resonance imaging processed with independent component analysis. *Neuroradiology*, **44**, 403–406.

Pandya, D. N., Karol, E. A., and Heilbronn, D. (1971). The topographical distribution of interhemispheric projections in the corpus callosum of the rhesus monkey. *Brain Res.*, **32**, 31–43.

Pandya, D. N., Van Hoesen, G. W., and Mesulam, M. M. (1981). Efferent connections of the cingulate gyrus in the rhesus monkey. *Exp. Brain Res.*, **42**, 319–330.

Quigley, M. A., Haughton, V. M., Carew, J., Cordes, D., Moritz, C. H., and Meyerand, M. E. (2002). Comparison of independent component analysis and conventional hypothesis-driven analysis for clinical functional MR image processing. *Am. J. Neuroradiol.*, **23**, 49–58.

Raichle, M. E., MacLeod, A. M., Snyder, A. Z., Powers, W. J., Gusnard, D. A., and Shulman, G. L. (2001). A default mode of brain function. *Proc. Natl. Acad. Sci. USA*, **98**, 676–682.

Richer, F., Martinez, M., Robert, M., Bouvier, G., and Saint-Hilaire, J. M. (1993). Stimulation of human somatosensory cortex: tactile and body displacement perceptions in medial regions. *Exp. Brain Res.*, **93**, 173–176.

Schiller, P. H. (1996). On the specificity of neurons and visual areas. *Behav. Brain Res.*, **76**, 21–35.

Schiller, P. H. (1997). Past and present ideas about how the visual scene is analysed by the brain, in *Extrastriate Cortex in Primates*, Rockland, K. S., Kaas, J. H., and Peters, A., Eds., pp. 59–90. Plenum, New York.

Schmolesky, M. T., Wang, Y., Hanes, D. P., Thompson, K. G., Leutgeb, S., Schall, J. D., and Leventhal, A. G. (1998). Signal timing across the macaque visual system. *J. Neurophysiol.*, **79**, 3272–3278.

Sereno, M. I., Dale, A. M., Reppas, J. B., Kwong, K. K., Belliveau, J. W., Brady, T. J., Rosen, B. R., and Tootell, R. B. H. (1995). Borders of multiple visual areas in humans revealed by functional magnetic resonance imaging. *Science*, **268**, 889–893.

Shima, K., Aya, K., Mushiake, H., Inase, M., Aizawa, H., and Tanji, J. (1991). Two movement-related foci in the primate cingulate cortex observed in signal-triggered and self-paced forelimb movements. *J. Neurophysiol.*, **65**, 188–202.

Shipp, S. and Zeki, S. M. (1985). Segregation of pathways leading from area V2 to areas V4 and V5 of macaque monkey visual cortex. *Nature*, **315**, 322–325.

Shipp, S., Watson, J. D. G., Frackowiak, R. S. J., and Zeki, S. M. (1995). Retinotopic maps in human prestriate visual-cortex: the demarcation of areas V2 and V3. *NeuroImage*, **2**, 125–132.

Sholl, D. A. (1967). *The Organisation of the Cerebral Cortex*. Hafner Publishing, New York.

Stone, J. V., Porrill, J., Porter, N. R., and Wilkinson, I. D. (2002). Spatiotemporal independent component analysis of event-related fMRI data using skewed probability density functions. *NeuroImage*, **15**, 407–421.

Suzuki, K., Kiryu, T., and Nakada, T. (2002). Fast and precise independent component analysis for high field fMRI time series tailored using prior information on spatiotemporal structure. *Hum. Brain Mapping*, **15**, 54–66.

Talairach, J. and Tournoux, P. (1988). *Co-Planar Stereotaxic Atlas of the Human Brain*. Thieme, Stuttgart.

Tootell, R. B., Hadjikhani, N. K., Vanduffel, W., Liu, A. K., Mendola, J. D., Sereno, M. I., and Dale, A. M. (1998). Functional analysis of primary visual cortex (V1). in humans. *Proc. Natl. Acad. Sci. USA*, **95**, 811–817.

Viviani, P. and Aymoz, C. (2001). Colour, form and movement are not perceived simultaneously. *Vision Res.*, **41**, 2909–2918.

Vogt, B. A. and Pandya, D. N. (1987). Cingulate cortex of the rhesus monkey. II. Cortical afferents. *J. Comp. Neurol.*, **262**, 271–289.

Vogt, B. A., Finch, D. M., and Olson, C. R. (1992). Functional heterogeneity in cingulate cortex: the anterior executive and posterior evaluative regions. *Cereb. Cortex*, **2**, 435–443.

Vogt, C. and Vogt, O. (1919). Allgemeinere Ergebnisse unserer Hirnforschung. Vierte Mitteilung. Die physiologische Bedeutung der architektonischen Rindenfelderung auf Grund neuer Rindenreizungen. *J. Psychol. Neurol.*, **25**, 399–462.

von Bonin, G. and Bailey, P. (1951). *The Isocortex of Man*. University of Illinois Press, Urbana.

von Economo, C., and Koskinas, G. (1925). Individuelle und physiologische Bedeutung der Areale, in *Die Cytoarchitektonik der Hirnrinde des erwachsenen Menschen*. Springer-Verlag, Berlin.

Wernicke, C. (1874). *Der aphasische Symptomencomplex*. Cohn & Weigert, Breslau.

Zeki, S. (1970). Interhemispheric connections of prestriate cortex in the monkey. *Brain Res.*, **19**, 63–75.

Zeki, S. and Bartels, A. (2003). The processing of kinetic contours in the brain. *Cereb. Cortex*, **13**, 189–202.

Zeki, S. and Bartels, A. (1998). The asynchrony of consciousness. *Proc. Roy. Soc. London Ser. B*, **265**, 1583–1585.

Zeki, S. and Bartels, A. (1998) The autonomy of the visual systems and the modularity of conscious vision. *Phil. Trans. R. Soc. Lond. B*, **353**, 1191–1914.

Zeki, S. and Bartels, A. (1999a). Toward a theory of visual consciousness. *Conscious Cogn.*, **8**, 225–259.

Zeki, S. and Bartels, A. (1999b). The clinical and functional measurement of cortical (in-) activity in the visual brain, with special reference to the two subdivisions (V4 and V4α) of the human colour centre. *Philos. Trans. Roy. Soc. London B*, **354**, 1371–1382.

Zeki, S. and Shipp, S. (1988). The functional logic of cortical connections. *Nature*, **335**, 311–317.

Zheng, D., LaMantia, A. S., and Purves, D. (1991). Specialised vascularisation of the primate visual cortex. *J. Neurosci.*, **11**, 2622–2629.

Zilles, K. and Clarke, S. (1997). Architecture, connectivity, and transmitter receptors of human extrastriate visual cortex: comparison with nonhuman primates, in *Extrastriate Cortex in Primates*, Rockland, K. S., Kaas, J. H., and Peters, A., Eds., pp. 673–742. Plenum, New York.

CHAPTER

14

Unilateral Neglect and the Neuroanatomy of Visuospatial Attention

INTRODUCTION

Unilateral neglect is one of the most complex and fascinating of neurological syndromes in that it challenges our most fundamental beliefs about the way in which the human brain functions (Robertson and Marshall, 1993; Driver and Mattingley, 1998; Driver and Vuilleumier, 2001). Patients with this condition will typically fail to notice events or objects lying to their left, usually as a result of a lesion of the right parietal cortex that involves the right supramarginal gyrus (SMG) (Vallar and Perani, 1986). They may ignore anyone standing to their left, fail to look after the left side of their own bodies, and leave uneaten any food lying on the left side of their plate. Although these patients may have a small visual field defect in the left inferior quadrant, they can usually see things in their left visual field if their attention is actively drawn to them. Their behaviour can be contrasted with that of a patient with a left homonymous hemianopia (blindness in the left visual field of both eyes), who will typically overcome their inability to see objects on the left simply by moving their eyes around and will not neglect the left side of space.

As our understanding of this condition has progressed, it has become apparent that this is not a single syndrome but an umbrella term for a number of dissociable conditions relating to the patient's representation of space (Stone *et al.*, 1998). It would be impossible to review the entire syndrome in the course of a single article. Here we focus entirely on one aspect of visual neglect—namely, the apparent abnormality in the allocation of visuospatial attention which appears to be a part of the syndrome. We are deliberately ambiguous in referring to the deficit as being to the left side (in most patients), without defining what the deficit is to the left of, to avoid the complex issues of the multiple coordinate frames within which neglect can operate (Driver and Halligan, 1991) and discussion of the gradient of neglect (Kinsbourne, 1970). We concentrate instead on a paradox that arises from the asymmetry of the lesions that cause visual neglect and a possible resolution that is offered by the functional imaging literature on visuospatial attention in normal subjects (Perry and Zeki, 2000). The other components of the neglect syndrome and other conceptual frameworks have been covered extensively elsewhere (Robertson and Marshall, 1993; Mesulam, 1999).

NEGLECT AS A DEFICIT OF VISUOSPATIAL ATTENTION

What, then, is the basis of considering neglect as a disorder of visuospatial attention? This concept was originally based on the simple clinical observation that patients are apparently unaware of visual stimuli at a given location under some circumstances, but not in others. The simplest example, easily demonstrated at the bedside, is a component of the syndrome known as *extinction*. Typically, the patient is asked to look straight ahead into the examiner's eyes, and the examiner extends his hands into the right and left side of the patient's visual periphery. When the examiner moves the fingers of one or other hand, the patient reports which one has moved, either by saying "right" or "left" or by pointing to the correct side. In this way, the examiner can establish that both hands fall within the patient's intact visual field and that the patient understands the task. Now the examiner moves the fingers of both hands simultaneously. A normal patient will simply report that both sides have moved, even if this was unexpected. The patient with extinction, however, will only report movement on the intact side, apparently ignoring movement on the affected side (usually the left side). A similar phenomenon can often be demonstrated in the somatosensory system, when both of the patient's hands are tapped simultaneously, demonstrating *tactile extinction*.

These tests establish that the patient can perceive a stimulus on the affected side, but that they do so only in certain perceptual circumstances. The name *extinction* implies that a stimulus on the intact side can extinguish one on the affected side. As far as the stimulus on the affected side is concerned, what has changed from the unextinguished context to the extinguished one? Presumably, there is some resource available when the stimulus is presented alone (no extinction), but which is drained from the affected side by the stimulus on the intact side (extinction). Perceptual resources that can shift without any external evidence of the change (such as eye movements) tend to be labelled by the umbrella term *attention*. Functional imaging studies have shown that, in patients with visual extinction, the "extinguished" stimulus is represented in early visual cortex (Rees *et al.*, 2000; Vuilleumier *et al.*, 2001). Thus, activity in these areas may not be sufficient to lead to visual awareness; activity that corresponds to attention, possibly in parietal cortex, is also required (Rees, 2001).

So far, we have used the word *attention* to mean a resource that is variably applied to the internal representation of a particular location in space, resulting in perception of a stimulus there under some circumstances and failure of perception in others. The word *attention*, however, has been used in many different ways in the psychophysical literature, and there is a danger that the same word may be used for several quite distinct physiological phenomena, incorrectly implying a unitary mechanism. Posner and colleagues have developed an experimental method that defines very precisely a type of visuospatial attention, which we will call *Posner attention*. A brief description of their method is warranted here, as this technique has been used both in normal subjects and in neglect patients, and in what follows we will use the word *attention* to refer to this well-defined psychophysical phenomenon.

Posner's (1980) method required a normal subject to press a button as quickly as possible after the onset of a visual target, which could appear in either of two boxes, one on each side of the fixation point. In some trials, called *valid cue trials*, one of these boxes became brighter just before the target appeared inside it, in which case subjects responded to the target more quickly. The reduced reaction time was attributed to attention being shifted toward the cued box, just in time for the appearance of the target. In *invalid cue trials*, the brightening of the box on one side preceded the appearance of the target in the box on the other side, resulting in slower detection, presumably because the subject's attention was directed toward the wrong side in these trials.

In these experiments, therefore, attention is a resource that is variably applied to the internal representation of a particular spatial location, resulting in more rapid detection at that location. Recently, this type of attention has been characterised as a spotlight that can be directed to any location within the visual field at will, with the result that perceptual performance improves at that location. A number of functional imaging studies have charted the relationship between the topographical characteristics of this spotlight and corresponding local increases in activity in early visual areas (Kastner *et al.*, 1998; Tootell *et al.*, 1998; Brefczynski and DeYoe, 1999).

Is the attention that normal subjects can direct toward a particular location, in anticipation of a target appearing there, the same as the attention that appears to be lacking in the affected field of a neglect patient? The evidence available suggests that it is. Posner *et al.* (1984) showed that neglect patients were particularly slow to detect targets in their neglected field when their attention was first invalidly cued into their intact field. These patients therefore appeared to be deficient in their ability to redirect Posner attention toward the target once it had been sent in the wrong direction. This study provides a bridge between the clinical literature on neglect patients, much of which is purely descriptive, and the extensive psychophysical and functional imaging literature on Posner attention in normal subjects (Corbetta, 1998). In the current discussion, we will adopt the simple view that one of the reasons why neglect patients do not respond to stimuli on their neglected side is that their ability to shift Posner attention to this side is severely impaired, resulting in a failure to detect stimuli here. Once again, although we are concentrating on this aspect of neglect, we do not intend to imply that a deficit of visuospatial attention captures the whole pathology of the neglect syndrome.

THE RIGHT SUPRAMARGINAL GYRUS AND THE PARADOX OF NEGLECT

The deficit of visuospatial attention exhibited by neglect patients, taken together with the observation that patients with lesions including the right supramarginal gyrus often exhibit neglect (Vallar and Perani, 1986), leads naturally to the conclusion that this region of cortex plays a special role in the allocation of spatial attention. But, there is immediately a problem here. If the right SMG performs this function for the whole of visual space, then why does a lesion here lead to such an asymmetrical deficit, with neglect of one side (or in one direction) and not the other? On the other hand, if the right SMG performs this function for the left (contralateral) side of space, as the neglect syndrome seems to imply, then where is the structure that performs an equivalent function for the right side of space? The left supramarginal gyrus does not offer itself as a good candidate. Lesions here do not result in persistent neglect, but rather in a quite different combination of deficits (Gerstmann's syndrome) (Critchley, 1966). Indeed, no lesion typically produces severe and persistent right-sided neglect.

Currently the most popular explanation for this asymmetry is the hypothesis that the right parietal cortex is involved in shifting attention bilaterally, but the left parietal cortex can only shift attention to the right (Heilman and Valenstein, 1979; Weintraub and Mesulam, 1987; Mesulam 1999). According to this explanation, shifts of attention to the left can only be mediated by the right parietal lobe; therefore, damage here results in left neglect. By contrast, shifts of attention to the right can be mediated by either parietal lobe, so unilateral damage does not usually result in neglect of the right half of space. Throughout this review, we will continue to return to this influential hypothesis, which we designate the BIRCOL hypothesis (BIlateral representation in the Right parietal cortex, COntralateral representation in Left parietal cortex).

A PROBLEM FOR THE BIRCOL HYPOTHESIS

Leaving aside specific anatomical theories for a moment, there are two possible general explanations for the marked difference in prevalence between neglect of the left side of space and neglect of the right side (*i.e.*, in the total number of patients exhibiting these phenomena at any given time). One is that the incidence of left-sided neglect (*i.e.*, the number of new cases arising in a given year) may be higher than that of right-sided neglect. Alternatively, the incidence may be similar, but right-sided neglect may recover far more quickly than left-sided neglect, leaving an excess of left neglect patients. Stone *et al.* (1991) have shown that the latter explanation is correct. Forty-four consecutive patients who suffered acute hemispheric stroke were examined three days after. Of these, 55% showed left-sided neglect on a line-cancellation task (see above), but almost as many (42%) showed right-sided neglect, so the incidence of neglect on the two sides does not appear to be very different. When both groups of patients were reexamined three months after their strokes, however, 33% still had left-sided neglect, but not a single patient showed right-sided neglect by this time (Stone *et al.*, 1991). The main reason, therefore, why so few right hemineglect patients are found on the wards is that recovery from right-sided neglect tends to be very rapid.

These clinical observations cast considerable doubt on the BIRCOL hypothesis. If the right hemisphere can shift attention in either direction, even in the normal brain, then why should patients with left parietal lesions experience rightward neglect at the acute stage? Surely the intact right parietal cortex should still be able shift attention to the right. From the clinical evidence alone, one might argue that the right hemisphere only has the *potential* to mediate ipsilateral attention shifts, and that this potential is unmasked by damage to the left parietal cortex. In this case, though, we should not observe bilateral responses in the right parietal cortex of the normal brain, but, as reviewed in the next section, this is what functional imaging studies have shown. In spite of these objections, however, the BIRCOL hypothesis has remained the most popular explanation for the asymmetry of the neglect syndrome. In particular, several functional imaging studies have been interpreted as supporting this model, so it is to these that we will turn next.

EPOCH-BASED FUNCTIONAL IMAGING STUDIES OF VISUOSPATIAL ATTENTION

If the BIRCOL hypothesis were true, at least in its simplest formulation, then one would expect to be able to demonstrate the proposed asymmetry in the functional anatomy of visuospatial attention in the normal brain. Attention shifts to the left should only engage the right parietal cortex, whereas attention shifts to the right should produce bilateral parietal activity; however, the results from positron emission tomography (PET) and, more recently, functional magnetic resonance imaging (fMRI) have not been so straightforward.

One way of studying the functional anatomy of the spatial attention system in the normal brain is to allow subjects to do what they would normally do when their attention is drawn to a stimulus in peripheral vision, which is to look at it. The rapid eye movement that is used to bring an object of interest to the centre of vision is called a *saccade*. A disadvantage of studying saccades is that one cannot easily dissociate brain activity related to the capture of attention by the visual stimulus from activity related to the mechanics of making an eye movement. The preferred method for studying the system of visuospatial attention, therefore, has been to require subjects to make a 'covert' shift of spatial attention, *i.e.*, to move their attention to a stimulus in peripheral vision without moving their eyes.

There are numerous functional imaging studies of saccades and plenty of others deal with covert attention shifts, so surely an abundance of evidence should be available to test the BIRCOL hypothesis. In fact, almost none of the studies address this question, and the reason for this is a technical one. Until very recently, all functional imaging studies utilised an epoch-based design. In the context of saccades, the experiment would typically consist of a number of experimental epochs during which subjects continuously performed saccades for 30 s or so and another series of epochs during which subjects were at rest. Brain activity was then compared between these two conditions. Presumably it was not considered practical to require subjects to make a series of rightward saccades for the entire 30 s, without any return saccades to bring the gaze back to the centre. As a consequence, all block-design studies of saccades, and almost all studies of covert attention, have pooled leftward and rightward shifts (saccades: Melamed and Larsen, 1979; Fox *et al.*, 1985; Paus *et al.*, 1993, 1995; Petit *et al.*, 1993, 1996, 1997; Anderson *et al.*, 1994; Nakashima *et al.*, 1994; O'Driscoll *et al.*, 1995; O'Sullivan *et al.*, 1995; Darby *et al.*, 1996; Müri *et al.*, 1996; Sweeney *et al.*, 1996; Bodis-Wollner *et al.*, 1997; Corbetta *et al.*, 1998; Law *et al.*, 1998; Luna *et al.*, 1998) (covert attention shifts: Vandenberghe *et al.*, 1996; Coull and Nobre, 1998; Gitelman *et al.*, 1999; Kim *et al.*, 1999).

Only two epoch-based studies of covert attention have addressed the question of the laterality of the areas involved: Corbetta *et al.* (1993) and Nobre *et al.* (1997). Corbetta *et al.* (1993) required subjects to shift their attention covertly between locations in one or other visual field during PET scanning. They also attempted a partial dissociation between leftward and rightward shifts within each visual hemifield, but no difference was found between them. The visual field within which the shifts were made, however, did have an effect on the pattern of results. At first sight the prediction from the clinical literature, alluded to above, appeared to be borne out by the data. The left superior parietal lobule (SPL) was mainly involved for shifts within the right visual field (RVF). The right SPL, however, appeared to be involved in shifts into either visual hemifield. A relatively posterior locus showed greater responses during shifts within the left visual field (LVF), whereas another locus, slightly more anterior, showed greater responses during shifts within RVF. These were qualitative comparisons: the responses related to LVF and RVF shifts were not directly compared with each other. These authors concluded that, in accordance with the BIRCOL hypothesis, the right SPL contributes to attention shifts within either visual hemifield.

Nobre *et al.* (1997), also using PET scanning, designed epochs during which subjects repeatedly shifted their attention into and out of one or other visual hemifield (interspersed with occasional shifts into the opposite hemifield). Once again, there was no direct comparison of responses from the RVF with those from the LVF. The results, however, were broadly consistent with those of Corbetta *et al.* (1993). The left parietal cortex was only engaged by shifts into the RVF. The right parietal cortex, however, appeared to be involved in shifting attention into either visual hemifield; however, Nobre *et al.* (1997) did not find the spatial segregation of the RVF and LVF responses within the right parietal cortex that Corbetta *et al.* (1993) had observed.

It would have been easy to conclude from these two papers that the problem of the right parietal bias for lesions causing hemineglect was now solved, with the functional imaging data coming out in clear support of the BIRCOL hypothesis. However, several nagging difficulties remained. Firstly, none of the studies of saccades or covert attention shifts showed a clear role for the region of cortex most frequently implicated in neglect, on the surface of the right *inferior* parietal lobule (Vallar and Perani, 1986). This may even have raised some doubts about the true location and extent of the lesions causing neglect, as these had been inferred from computed tomography (CT) scans which is much more difficult than an equivalent study using MRI would be. Secondly, as mentioned in the previous section, if the normal right parietal cortex can shift attention in either direction, then why do patients with left parietal lesions experience rightward neglect at all, even transiently (Stone *et al.*, 1991)? Surely the intact right hemisphere should immediately be capable of shifting attention to the right in these patients.

Finally, the simplest interpretation of the BIRCOL hypothesis raises a conceptual difficulty. If the two parietal lobes perform essentially the same operations and if the right hemisphere alone can perform these operations for left-sided locations, then why are these same operations duplicated across both hemispheres when applied to right-sided locations? A slight modification of the original BIRCOL hypothesis avoids this difficulty. Perhaps there are two distinct operations (or sets of operations) that are damaged in neglect. One of them might be distributed across the hemispheres in the usual contralaterally biased fashion. The other may be unique to the right hemisphere, which therefore undertakes this function for both sides of space. This modification, arising from an attempt to find a plausible implementation of the BIRCOL hypothesis, foreshadows the conclusions from event-related studies, which will lead us to consider an alternative hypothesis.

AN EVENT-RELATED FUNCTIONAL MRI STUDY OF VISUOSPATIAL ATTENTION

The epoch-based approach to functional imaging, initially using PET and subsequently using fMRI, has allowed an explosion of fascinating studies of the normal human brain. The development of event-related fMRI (Boynton *et al.*, 1996; Josephs *et al.*, 1997; Friston *et al.*, 1998; Rosen *et al.*, 1998), however, allowed new questions to be addressed using fMRI. In the present context, the signal related to a saccade or shift of attention to the left could easily be dissociated from the return shift to the right. One might reasonably have expected this technique to yield cleaner information about the functional anatomy of the system for spatial attention, perhaps confirming the pattern of laterality suggested by the studies of Corbetta *et al.* (1993) and Nobre *et al.* (1997).

The results obtained from event-related fMRI therefore came as something of a surprise. Far from confirming the BIRCOL hypothesis, they seemed to tell a completely different story. Perry and Zeki (2000) and Corbetta *et al.* (2000) used event-related fMRI to compare saccades and covert attention shifts within the same experiment. Both groups found that covert shifts activated the frontoparietal network, which is familiar from the epoch-based studies mentioned in the previous section (see Fig. 14.1); however, these studies also showed a highly significant cluster on the surface of the right inferior parietal lobule, in the supramarginal gyrus (R SMG in

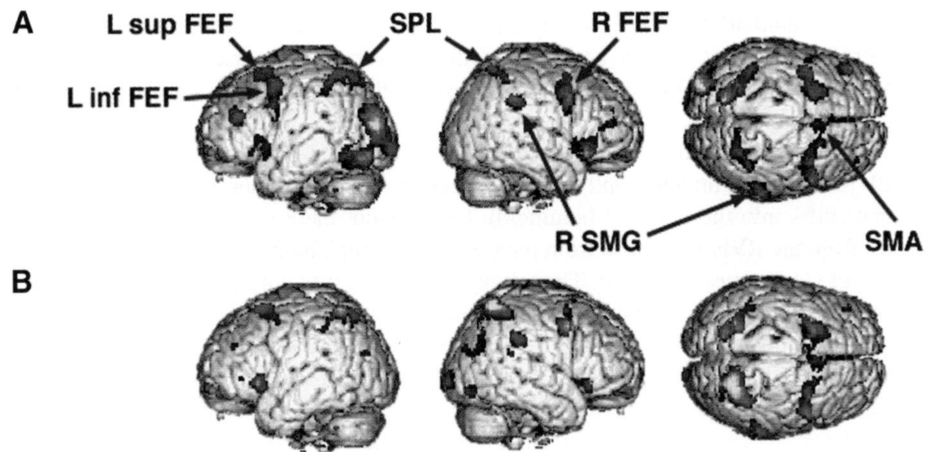

FIGURE 14.1
Areas active during covert attention shifts to the right (panel A) and to the left (panel B), as shown by functional MRI. Colours indicate degree of statistical significance, from low significance in red to high significance in yellow. Height threshold $p < 0.001$, uncorrected. Abbreviations: L sup FEF, superior locus of left frontal eye field; L inf FEF, inferior locus of left frontal eye field; SPL, superior parietal lobule; R FEF, right frontal eye field; R SMG, right supramarginal gyrus; SMA, supplementary motor area. (From Perry, R. J. and Zeki, S. M., *Brain*, **123**, 2273–2288, 2000. With permission.).

Fig. 14.1). This cluster was quite distinct from those in the intraparietal sulcus (IPS) and the SPL, and activity at this location had not appeared in most previous studies of spatial attention in the normal brain. In retrospect, a review of the epoch-based studies of attention shows that in one PET study (Coull and Nobre, 1998) there was a response in the right SMG, but this activity was not significant at the corrected level, so the authors did not emphasise it at the time.

The right SMG location reported by Perry and Zeki (2000) and Corbetta *et al.* (2000) coincided precisely with the region implicated in studies of neglect. Furthermore, as would be anticipated from the clinical literature, no activity was seen at a corresponding location in the left hemisphere. These event-related fMRI studies therefore provided a much stronger bridge between clinical and functional imaging studies. Why this area has not shown up in numerous previous studies of saccades or covert attention shifts is not yet clear, but we will return to this issue in the next section.

Perry and Zeki (2000) were able to take advantage of their event-related design to examine the laterality of the attention system, examining the signal related to outward shifts (in this case, to the right and into the RVF [Fig. 14.1A] or to the left and into the LVF [Fig. 14.1B]) without contamination of the signal by return shifts. The activity in the SPLs, extending down into the IPS, showed significantly greater responses to contralateral stimuli than to ipsilateral ones. The top-view brains to the right in Fig. 14.1 illustrate this point: rightward shifts (Fig. 14.1A) produced more significant activity (shown by more yellow) in the left SPL, whereas leftward shifts (Fig. 14.1B) elicited more significant activity in the right SPL. This pattern was already suggested by the distribution of activity in Corbetta *et al.* (1993), although in their study responses to LVF and RVF shifts were not compared directly. The contralateral bias of the parietal cortex was expected from physiological studies in non-human primates. These show that, while the receptive fields of parietal neurons often cross the midline, they are invariably centred in the contralateral visual hemifield (Yin and Mountcastle, 1977; Motter and Mountcastle, 1981).

One of the interesting characteristics of the right SMG, shown in Fig. 14.1, is that the responses from the RVF (Fig. 14.1A) and LVF (Fig. 14.1B) appear to be identical in this area (Perry and Zeki, 2000). The most obvious interpretation, in line with the BIRCOL hypothesis (in the modified form mentioned at the end of the previous section), is that this area mediates shifts into either visual field. However, if the right SMG carries a topographic map of space (*i.e.*, a map in which space in the visual scene is represented as space across the cortical surface), then even if the whole of visual space were represented within one hemisphere one would expect to see at least some segregation of LVF and RVF responses, rather than the complete overlap that is actually observed. An alternative interpretation seemed much more likely, that the right SMG does not contain a topographic map at all.

Sereno *et al.* (2001) have recently confirmed the contralateral bias of the SPLs. These authors used retinotopic mapping methods inspired by those originally used in early visual areas (Sereno *et al.*, 1995; DeYoe *et al.*, 1996) and showed that an area of the SPL, extending from the cortical surface into the medial bank of the IPS, carries a topographic map of contralateral visual space. Although they described this map as retinotopic, a craniotopic coordinate system was not ruled out, as the starting position of the subject's eyes was always the same. In support of the conclusions of Perry and Zeki (2000), the study by Sereno *et al.* (2001) showed no evidence of a similar topographic map in the right SMG.

AN ALTERNATIVE TO THE BIRCOL HYPOTHESIS

Regardless of whether the right SMG carries representations of both sides of visual space (as implied by the BIRCOL hypothesis) or whether, as seems more likely, the contribution of this area is a non-topographic one, these results pose a problem in trying to explain the syndrome of neglect. How can damage to a region that gives similar responses to right- and left-sided stimuli result in left hemineglect?

The functional imaging studies, taken together with the study of Stone *et al.* (1991) described earlier, suggest an appealing resolution of this difficult paradox (Perry and Zeki, 2000) that relies on the idea that there may be at least two components of visuospatial neglect (Robertson, 1993). The contralateral bias of both SPLs suggests that a lesion of either SPL should result in an immediate contralateral spatial deficit, as is observed acutely in stroke patients (Stone *et al.*, 1991). The SPLs (including the IPS component of these clusters) would therefore be the anatomical substrate for the spatial component of neglect. The right SMG, on the other hand, is hypothesised to have a non-topographic (possibly even non-spatial) role, which is essential for the rapid recovery of the spatial deficit. It is highly unlikely that left SPL/IPS lesions involve the right SMG, so recovery from these is excellent. Right SPL/IPS lesions, on the other hand, often extend into the right SMG, resulting in a lasting deficit. We designate this model the NORICS hypothesis (NOn-topographic representation in Right Inferior parietal cortex; Contralateral representation in Superior parietal cortex).

The NORICS hypothesis allows us to make a very simple prediction. If the right SMG subserves a non-topographic function, which does not discriminate between the right and left sides of space, we would suggest that lesions that are restricted to this region of cortex should not cause the highly asymmetrical deficit of neglect. This prediction is not contradicted by the current clinical literature: The right inferior parietal lobule has been identified as the area that is *common* to the lesions causing neglect, but all of the lesions have spread beyond this region. Lesions causing neglect are usually large, so it may be difficult to test our prediction; however, suggestive evidence for this idea is found in a study of global versus local processing by Robertson *et al.* (1988), described in more detail later on. These authors selected a group of six patients with lesions mostly involving the right inferior parietal lobule but with relative sparing of the right SPL. They mention in their Methods section that only one of these patients showed any evidence of neglect at the time of testing (at least a year after the damage occurred), and even in this case the neglect was very mild. Whether more of these patients showed neglect at the acute stage is not known.

NON-TOPOGRAPHIC COMPONENTS OF NEGLECT

If the operations performed by the right SMG are not topographically mapped across this region of cortex, what might these operations be? An obvious possibility is that they are not spatial operations at all. Although this may seem an odd claim in view of the highly spatial nature of the neglect deficit, the NORICS hypothesis would suggest that this syndrome only results when there is concurrent damage to the spatial mechanisms of the SPL and IPS, as well as the right

SMG. Here, we briefly discuss one putative non-spatial function that we will refer to as *alerting*. Alternatively, the SMG might be the site of a mechanism that performs a spatial function, but the afferent connections of this area may allow exactly the same group of neurons to perform this local spatial function anywhere in the visual field. If the function of these neurons is not tied to a particular location in space, then no fixed topography would be expected in the right SMG. The example mentioned here is a deficit in switching between local and global processing, which has been proposed as a component of neglect (Robertson and Eglin, 1993).

Alerting

A first approach to trying to narrow down the possible functions of the right SMG is to inquire why this region has only appeared weakly, or not at all, in so many epoch-based studies of visuospatial attention. Admittedly, the reason may simply be technical: Possibly the positive blood-oxygen-level-dependent (BOLD) response here is followed by an equally large negative undershoot, so that a train of responses here does not produce the change in baseline required in epoch-based studies. A more interesting possibility, however, is that stimuli in event-related studies can be made much less predictable than in epoch studies. In an epoch-based study, most or all of the stimuli presented during a given epoch are of the same type, as far as the analysis is concerned. Thus, if one is interested in contrasting responses to rightward and leftward shifts in attention in an epoch-based study, then some epochs must consist mainly of rightward shifts, and others mainly of leftward shifts (Corbetta *et al.*, 1993). The direction of most of the shifts required is therefore predictable once the epoch is underway, and few if any events occur at unexpected locations. In an event-related study, by contrast, the direction of shift for each trial can be made entirely unpredictable. Could it be that the right SMG performs a function that is only accessed when events occur at unexpected locations?

Support for this idea comes from the study of Corbetta *et al.* (2000), who took advantage of the event-related fMRI method to dissociate out responses during different components of the Posner task described earlier. The main response of the right SMG appeared to be related to the appearance of a target rather than to the appearance of a cue, and the largest target-related response occurred during invalid trials. Thus, the right SMG does appear to be particularly responsive to visual events at unexpected locations. One might speculate that, when a sudden or salient event occurs at an unexpected location, there may be a non-spatial alerting response that speeds up the appropriate deployment of spatial attention. This alerting signal may be available beyond the visual domain, as the right SMG also appears to respond to novel stimuli in auditory or tactile channels (Downar *et al.*, 2000).

If such a non-spatial alerting response is the main impetus for recovery from the spatial deficit in neglect, then this may explain why patients with right-sided lesions tend to have persistent neglect, whereas those with left-sided lesions have transient neglect (Stone *et al.*, 1991). While patients with lesions of the left parietal cortex may initially have difficulty in orienting to right-sided stimuli, the intact right SMG may alert them to the fact that there is a new stimulus somewhere that requires their attention. Every time this happens, there will be a tendency to keep searching until this stimulus is found, and eventually this search will extend into the neglected right side of space. Repeated exposure to such stimuli may be the impetus for recovery from the spatial deficit. Most neglect patients with right-sided lesions, however, will have lost this alerting mechanism. When a stimulus appears to the left, their spatial mechanisms fail to locate them and, furthermore, the impaired right SMG fails to alert them to the fact that anything is wrong. Here, there is no impetus to recovery and the spatial deficit persists.

If the failure of an alerting mechanism contributes to the deficit in neglect, then one might expect that the severity of neglect should be reduced if the patient is alerted to the presence of a stimulus by some other means. This is exactly what was found by Robertson *et al.* (1998), who tested eight neglect patients with right hemisphere lesions, most of which involved the right inferior parietal lobule. These authors used a task in which patients were shown a series of trials in which two horizontal bars appeared, one on each side of fixation. They had to judge which bar appeared first. Each patient showed a bias, in that bars on the left were judged to have appeared later than they actually did with respect to those on the right. The size of this bias was used as an index of the severity of neglect. On trials where patients were alerted to the imminent appearance of the first bar by a 300-ms tone burst, presented centrally, the bias was significantly reduced. Thus, their spatial (rightward) bias was partially overcome by a non-spatial alerting signal. Possibly this auditory signal replaced the non-spatial function that had previously been performed automatically by the right SMG.

Global Versus Local Processing

A failure of global processing has also been proposed as a contributory factor in neglect (Robertson and Eglin, 1993). When we look at a tree, we can either attend to the overall shape of the tree (its global aspect) or we can attend to an individual leaf (one of the local elements making up the tree). Robertson *et al.* (1988) tested the ability of patients with lesions in the region of the right or left temporo-parietal junctions (TPJs) to detect targets at the global or local levels. Most of these lesions encroached on the SMG, which lies immediately above the right TPJ (see Fig. 14.1). These authors used Navon letters (Navon, 1977), stimuli in which 12 to 14 identical small capital letters are arranged in the shape of one large capital letter. Subjects can read either the letter presented at the global level or that presented (multiply) at the local level. When patients were shown a series of Navon letters, they had to press a button whenever they detected target letters (S or H), but they were instructed to ignore distracter letters (A or E). Across several conditions, patients with lesions involving the right TPJ tended to spot targets at the local level more rapidly than those at the global level. Although this was a rather weak effect in the whole group and only became significant in a subgroup analysis, the authors interpreted it as showing that an area near the right TPJ plays a part in global processing. By contrast, patients with lesions of the left superior temporal gyrus were much slower at spotting a target at the local level, suggesting that this region is important for local processing.

Fink *et al.* (1997) tested the hypothesis that the right TPJ might be involved in global processing, using PET imaging in normal subjects. From the clinical literature one might have expected that the right TPJ would be one area that would appear in an analysis comparing attention to the global level directly with attention to the local level, but instead this analysis revealed a significant cluster in right prestriate cortex. However, in an experiment where subjects had to switch between the global and local levels at varying intervals, activity in the right TPJ showed a positive correlation with length of interval. These authors therefore suggested that this region is involved in sustained attention to one or other perceptual level. It is not clear yet how this observation relates to the clinical study of Robertson *et al.* (1988), but a speculative unifying explanation might be that in the normal brain, attention to global stimuli is the default condition, and only when attention must be held at the global level in spite of local distractions does the right TPJ come into play.

Although the evidence at present is somewhat confusing, it does seem possible that a region near the right TPJ is involved in global processing, although it is too early to say what this role might be. Judging from the Fink *et al.* (1997) study, this global processing area is probably not the same as that found in the studies of covert attention by Perry and Zeki (2000) and Corbetta *et al.* (2000). Activity related to sustained global/local attention (Fink *et al.*, 1997) appears to lie relatively posteriorly, possibly in the angular gyrus, whereas covert attention shifts engage a more anterior area in the right SMG (Coull and Nobre, 1998; Corbetta *et al.*, 2000; Perry and Zeki, 2000).

Even if there are separate areas involved in alerting and in global processing, these are sufficiently close neighbours on the cortical surface that most lesions affecting one will affect the other. So, might disruption of global processing also have a part to play in the neglect syndrome? Robertson and Eglin (1993) have suggested that neglect may arise because of a failure of global processing, resulting from damage to the right parietal lobe. This hypothesis relies on the observation that even in normal subjects there is a slight rightward bias of spatial attention (Reuter-Lorenz *et al.*, 1990). Patients with defective global processing, it is argued, are forced to shift their attention laboriously between multiple local elements in a visual display. This deficit hugely increases the attentional load, thereby exaggerating the normal physiological rightward bias (Robertson and Eglin, 1993).

One problem with this hypothesis, however, is that, of the patients studied by Robertson *et al.* (1988) who were believed to have a deficit of global processing, all but one had no evidence of neglect at the time of testing, as mentioned earlier. In spite of these difficulties, however, Robertson and Eglin (1993) use the example of global versus local processing to reinforce the important point that the asymmetry of neglect may represent hemispheric specialisation for a function that interacts with spatial attention rather than for spatial attention *per se*.

Conceptually, one might imagine that there is a relationship between these two proposed functions of the right inferior parietal lobule. If there is an alerting mechanism that indicates the onset of a new or salient stimulus, without specifying the location of that stimulus, an appropriate response might well be to zoom attention out to the global scale, to maximise the chance of detecting the new stimulus.

CONCLUSION

The advent of techniques for mapping activity in the human brain provided an exciting opportunity to test the leading explanation for the asymmetry of neglect, which we have called the BIRCOL hypothesis. The results were more difficult to interpret than had perhaps been expected. The neglect literature appeared to implicate the right inferior parietal lobule in spatial attention shifts, whereas epoch-based functional imaging studies showed attention-related activity in the superior parietal lobules and the intraparietal sulcus. More recently, event-related studies have shown the expected inferior parietal activity but have raised a new problem: If this area is involved in shifting attention bilaterally, then how can a lesion here produce a unilateral deficit? These problems have forced us to adopt a new hypothesis, which we call the NORICS hypothesis. Here, the spatial component of neglect is explained by damage to topographically mapped areas in the superior parietal lobule and the intraparietal sulcus, whereas the persistence of right-sided neglect reflects the additional loss of a non-topographic function, possibly that of alerting, which results in poor recovery from the spatial deficit. The NORICS hypothesis appears to us to provide a better explanation for a wide range of experimental observations and in particular provides a new and appealing explanation for the observation that leftward neglect is much more prevalent than rightward neglect.

References

Anderson, T. J., Jenkins, I. H., Brooks, D. J., Hawken, M. B., Frackowiak, R. S. J., and Kennard, C. (1994). Cortical control of saccades and fixation in man: a PET study. *Brain*, **117**, 1073–1084.

Bodis-Wollner, I., Buchner, S. F., Seelos, K. C., Paulus, W., Reiser, M., and Oertel, W. H. (1997). Functional MRI mapping of occipital and frontal cortical activity during voluntary and imagined saccades. *Neurology*, **49**, 416–420.

Boynton, G. M., Engel, S. A., Glover, G. H., and Heeger, D. J. (1996). Linear systems analysis of functional magnetic resonance imaging data in human V1. *J. Neurosci.*, **16**, 4207–4221.

Brefczynski, J. A. and DeYoe, E. A. (1999). A physiological correlate of the 'spotlight' of visual attention. *Nat. Neurosci.*, **2**, 370–374.

Corbetta, M. (1998). Frontoparietal cortical networks for directing attention and the eye to visual locations: identical, independent or overlapping neural systems? *Proc. Natl. Acad. Sci. USA*, **95**, 831–838.

Corbetta, M., Miezin, F. M., Shulman, G. L., and Peterson, S. E. (1993). A PET study of visuospatial attention. *J. Neurosci.*, **13**(3), 1202–1226.

Corbetta, M., Akbudak, E., Conturo, T. E., Snyder, A. Z., Ollinger, J. M., Drury, H. A., Linenweber, M. R., Petersen, S. E., Raichle, M. E., Van Essen, D. C., and Shulman, G. L. (1998). A common network of functional areas for attention and eye movements. *Neuron*, **21**, 761–773.

Corbetta, M., Kincade, M. J., Ollinger, J. M., McAvoy, M. P., and Schulman, G. L. (2000). Voluntary orienting is dissociated from target detection in human posterior parietal cortex. *Nat. Neurosci.*, **3**, 292–297.

Coull, J., and Nobre, A. C. (1998). Where and when to pay attention: the neural systems for directing attention to spatial locations and to time intervals as revealed by both PET and fMRI. *J. Neurosci.*, **18**(18), 7426–7435.

Critchley, M. (1966). The enigma of Gerstmann's syndrome. *Brain*, **89**, 183–198.

Darby, D. G., Nobre, A. C., Thangaraj, V., Edelman, R., Mesulam, M.M., and Warach, S. (1996). Cortical activation in the human brain during lateral saccades using EPISTAR functional magnetic resonance imaging. *NeuroImage*, **3**, 53–62.

DeYoe, E. A., Carman, G. J., Bandettini, P., Glickman, S., Wieser, J., Cox, R., Miller, D., and Neitz, J. (1996). Mapping striate and extrastriate visual areas in human cerebral cortex. *Proc. Natl. Acad. Sci. USA*, **93**, 2382–2386.

Downar, J., Crawley, A. P., Mikulis, D. J., and Davis, K. D. (2000). A multimodal cortical network for the detection of changes in the sensory environment. *Nat. Neurosci.*, **3**(3), 277–283.

Driver, J. and Halligan, P. W. (1991). Can visual neglect operate in object-centred coordinates? An affirmative single-case study. *Cogn. Neuropsychol.*, **8**, 475–496.

Driver, J. and Mattingley, J. B. (1998). Parietal neglect and visual awareness. *Nat. Neurosci.*, **1**, 17–22.

Driver, J. and Vuilleumier, P. (2001). Perceptual awareness and its loss in unilateral neglect and extinction. *Cognition*, **79**, 39–88.

Fink, G. R., Halligan, P. W., Marshall, J. C., Frith, C. D., Frackowiak, R. S J., and Dolan, R. J. (1997). Neural mechanisms involved in the processing of global and local aspects of hierarchically organised visual stimuli. *Brain*, **120**, 1779–1791.

Fox, P. T., Fox, J. M., Raichle, M. E., and Burde, R. M. (1985). The role of cerebral cortex in the generation of voluntary saccades: a positron emission tomographic study. *J. Neurophysiol.*, **54**, 348–369.

Friston, K. J., Fletcher, P., Josephs, O., Holmes, A., Rugg, M. D., and Turner, R. (1998). Event-related fMRI: characterising differential responses. *NeuroImage*, **7**, 30–40.

Gitelman, D. R., Nobre, A. C., Parrish, T. B., LaBar, K. S., Kim, Y.-H., Meyer, J. R., and Mesulam, M.-M. (1999). A large-scale distributed network for covert spatial attention: further anatomical delineation based on stringent behavioural and cognitive controls. *Brain*, **122**, 1093–1106.

Heilman, K. M. and Valenstein, E. (1979). Mechanisms underlying hemispatial neglect. *Ann. Neurol.*, **5**, 166–170.

Josephs, O., Turner, R., and Friston, K. (1997). Event-related fMRI. *Hum. Brain Mapping*, **5**, 243–248.

Kastner, S., De Weerd, P., Desimone, R., and Ungerleider, L. G. (1998). Mechanisms of directed attention in the human extrastriate cortex as revealed by functional MRI. *Science*, **282**, 108–111.

Kim, Y.-H., Gitelman, D. R., Nobre, A. C., Parrish, T. B., LaBar, K. S., and Mesulam, M.-M. (1999). The large scale neural network for spatial attention displays multifunctional overlap but differential asymmetry. *NeuroImage*, **9**, 269–277.

Kinsbourne, M. (1970). A model for the mechanism of unilateral neglect of space. *Trans. Am. Neurol. Assoc.*, **95**, 143–146.

Law, I., Svarer, C., Rostrup, E., and Paulson, O. B. (1998). Parieto-occipital cortex activation during self-generated eye movements in the dark. *Brain*, **121**, 2189–2200.

Luna, B., Thulborn, K. R., Strojwas, M. H., McCurtain, B. J., Berman, R. A., Genovese, C. R., and Sweeney, J. A. (1998). Dorsal cortical regions subserving visually guided saccades in humans: an fMRI study. *Cereb. Cortex*, **8**, 40–47.

Melamed, E. and Larsen, B. (1979). Cortical activation pattern during saccadic eye movements in humans: localisation by focal cerebral blood flow increases. *Ann. Neurol.*, **5**, 79–88.

Mesulam, M.-M. (1999). Spatial attention and neglect: parietal, frontal and cingulate contributions to the mental representation and attentional targeting of salient extrapersonal events. *Philos. Trans. Roy. Soc. London B, Biol. Sci.*, **354**, 1325–1346.

Motter, B. C. and Mountcastle, V. B. (1981). The functional properties of the light-sensitive neurons of the posterior parietal cortex studies in waking monkeys: foveal sparing and opponent vector organisation. *J. Neurosci.*, **1**, 3–26.

Müri, R. M., Iba-Zizen, M. T., Derosier, C., Cabanis, E. A., and Pierrot-Deseilligny, C. (1996). Location of the human posterior eye field with functional magnetic resonance imaging. *J. Neurol. Neurosurg. Psychiatry*, **60**, 445–448.

Nakashima, Y., Momose, T., Sano, I., Katayama, S., Nakajima, T., Niwa, S-I., and Matsushita, M. (1994). Cortical control of saccade in normal and schizophrenic subjects: a PET study using a task-evoked rCBF paradigm. *Schizophrenia Res.*, **12**, 259–264.

Navon, D. (1977). Forest before trees: the precedence of global features in visual perception. *Cogn. Psychol.*, **9**, 353–383.

Nobre, A. C., Sebestyen, G. N., Gitelman, D. R., Mesulam, M.-M., Frackowiak, R. S. J., and Frith, C. D. (1997). Functional localisation of the system for visuospatial attention using positron emission tomography. *Brain*, **120**, 515–533.

O'Driscoll, G. A., Alpert, N. M., Matthysse, S. W., Levy, D. L., Rauch, S. L., and Holzman, P. S. (1995). Functional neuroanatomy of antisaccade eye movements investigated with positron emission tomography. *Proc. Natl. Acad. Sci. USA*, **92**, 925–929.

O'Sullivan, E. P., Jenkins, I. H., Henderson, L., Kennard, C., and Brooks, D. J. (1995). The functional anatomy of remembered saccades: a PET study. *NeuroReport*, **6**, 2141–2144.

Paus, T., Petrides, M., Evans, A. C., and Meyer, E. (1993). Role of the human anterior cingulate cortex in the control of oculomotor, manual, and speech responses: a positron emission tomography study. *J. Neurophysiol.*, **70**, 453–469.

Paus, T., Marrett, S., Worsley, K. J., and Evans, A. C. (1995). Extraretinal modulation of cerebral blood flow in the human visual cortex: implications for saccadic suppression. *J. Neurophysiol.*, **74**, 2179–2183.

Perry, R. J. and Zeki, S. M. (2000). The neurology of saccades and covert shifts in spatial attention. An event-related fMRI study. *Brain*, **123**, 2273–2288.

Petit, L., Orssaud, C., Tzourio, N., Salamon, G., Mazoyer, B., and Berthoz, A. (1993). PET study of voluntary saccadic eye movements in humans: basal ganglia-thalamocortical system and cingulate cortex involvement. *J. Neurophysiol.*, **69**, 1009–1017.

Petit, L., Orssaud, C., Tzourio, N., Crivello, F., Berthoz, A., and Mazoyer, B. (1996). Functional anatomy of prelearned sequence of horizontal saccades in humans. *J. Neurosci.*, **16**, 3714–3726.

Petit, L., Clark, V. P., Ingelholm, J., and Haxby, J. V. (1997). Dissociation of saccade-related and pursuit-related activation in human frontal eye fields as revealed by fMRI. *J. Neurophysiol.*, **77**, 3386–3390.

Posner, M. I. (1980). Orienting of attention. *Q. J. Exp. Psychol.*, **32**, 3–25.

Posner, M. I., Walker, J. A., Friedrich, F. J., and Rafal, R. D. (1984). Effects of parietal injury on covert orienting of attention. *J. Neurosci.*, **4**, 1863–1874.

Rees, G. (2001). Neuroimaging of visual awareness in patients and normal subjects. *Curr. Opin. Neurobiol.*, **11**, 150–156.

Rees, G., Wojciulik, E., Clarke, K., Husain, M., Frith, C., and Driver, J. (1999). Unconscious activation of visual cortex in the damaged right hemisphere of a parietal patient with extinction. *Brain*, **123**, 1624–1633.

Reuter-Lorenz, P. A., Kinsbourne, M., and Muscovitch, M. (1990). Hemispheric control of spatial attention. *Brain Cogn.*, **12**, 240–266.

Robertson, I. H. (1993). The relationship between lateralised and non-lateralised attentional deficits in unilateral neglect, in *Unilateral Neglect: Clinical and Experimental Studies*, Robertson, I. H. and Marshall, J. C., Eds., pp. 257–275. Lawrence Erlbaum, Hove, U.K.

Robertson, L. C. and Eglin, M. (1993). Attentional search in unilateral visual neglect, in *Unilateral Neglect: Clinical and Experimental Studies*, Robertson, I. H. and Marshall, J. C., Eds. Lawrence Erlbaum, Hove, U.K.

Robertson, I. H. and Marshall, J. C., Eds. (1993). *Unilateral Neglect: Clinical and Experimental Studies*. Lawrence Erlbaum, Hove, U.K.

Robertson, I. H., Lamb, M. R., and Knight, R. T. (1988). Effect of lesions of temporal-parietal junction on perceptual and attentional processing in human. *J. Neurosci.*, **8**, 3757–3769.

Robertson, I. H., Mattingley, J. B., Rorden, C., and Driver, J. (1998). Phasic alerting of neglect patients overcomes their spatial deficit in visual awareness. *Nature*, **395**, 169–172.

Rosen, B. R., Buckner, R. L., and Dale, A. M. (1998). Event-related functional MRI: past, present and future. *Proc. Natl. Acad. Sci. USA*, **95**, 773–780.

Sereno, M. I., Dale, A. M., Reppas, J. B., Kwong, K. K., Belliveau, J. W., Brady, T. J., Rosen, B. R., and Tootell, R. B. (1995) Borders of multiple visual areas in humans revealed by functional MRI. *Science*, **268**, 889–893.

Sereno, M. I., Pitzalis, S., and Martinez, A. (2001). Mapping of contralateral space in retinotopic coordinates by a parietal cortical area in humans. *Science*, **294**(5545), 1350–1354.

Stone, S. P., Wilson, B., Wroot, A., Halligan, P. W., Lange, L. S., Marshall, J. C., and Greenwood, R. J. (1991). The assessment of visuo-spatial neglect after acute stroke. *J. Neurol. Neurosurg. Psychiatry*, **54**, 345–350.

Stone, S. P., Halligan, P. W., Marshall, J. C., and Greenwood, R. J. (1998). Unilateral neglect: a common but heterogeneous syndrome. *Neurology*, **50**, 1902–1905.

Sweeney, J. A., Mintun, M. A., Kwee, S., Wiseman, M. B., Brown, D. L., Rosenberg, D. R., and Carl, J. R. (1996). Positron emission tomography study of voluntary saccadic eye movements and spatial working memory. *J. Neurosci.*, **75**(1), 454–468.

Tootell, R. B. H., Hadjikhani, N. E., Hall, K., Marrett, S., Wim Vanduffel, W., Vaughan, J. T., and Dale, A. M. (1998). The retinotopy of visual spatial attention, *Neuron*, **21**, 1409–1422.

Vallar, G. and Perani, D. (1986) The anatomy of unilateral neglect after right hemisphere stroke lesions: a clinical CT scan correlation study in man. *Neuropsychologia*, **24**, 609–622.

Vandenberghe, R., Dupont, P., De Bruyn, B., Bormans, G., Michiels, J., Mortelmans, L., and Orban, G. A. (1996). The influence of stimulus location on the brain activation pattern in detection and orientation discrimination: a PET study of visual attention. *Brain*, **119**, 1263–1276.

Vuilleumier, P., Sagiv, N., Hazeltine, E., Poldrack, R. A., Swick, D., Rafal, R. D., and Gabrieli, J. D. (2000). Neural fate of seen and unseen faces in visuospatial neglect: a combined event-related MRI and event-related potential study. *Proc. Natl. Acad. Sci. USA*, **98**, 3495–3500.

Weintraub, S. and Mesulam M.-M. (1987). Right cerebral dominance in spatial attention: further evidence based on ipsilateral neglect. *Arch. Neurol.*, **44**, 621–625.

Yin, T. C. T. and Mountcastle, V. B. (1977). Visual input to the visuomotor mechanisms of the monkey's parietal lobe. *Science*, **197**, 1381–1383.

SECTION THREE

HIGHER COGNITIVE FUNCTIONS

C H A P T E R

15

Mechanisms of Attention

WHAT IS ATTENTION?

Much valuable work still needs to be done constructing maps of the relationships between cognitive processes and brain function. Nevertheless, it is universally acknowledged that we must eventually go beyond mapping. We must use functional imaging to elucidate the mechanisms that underlie cognitive processes. So far, it is in studies of attention that the most progress has been made in this endeavour.

The particular aspect of attention we are concerned with here is that defined by William James (1890): "Every one knows what attention is. It is the taking possession of the mind, in clear and vivid form, of one out of what seem several simultaneous possible objects or trains of thought. Focalisation, concentration, of consciousness are of its essence. It implies withdrawal from some things in order to deal effectively with others." This definition of attention emphasises selection. Many stimuli impinge on our senses, but only a few are selected to be the focus of attention. The rest are rejected. Attention is the mechanism by which this selection is achieved. Attention to a stimulus has effects in three related domains: The attended stimulus occupies the foreground of our conscious experience, it affects our behaviour more than unattended stimuli, and it elicits greater changes in neural activity than unattended stimuli.

How does one stimulus rather than another get selected to be the focus of attention?

"Some are born great, some achieve greatness, and some have greatness thrust upon them." —William Shakespeare *(Twelfth Night)*

Stimuli become the focus of our attention in the same ways that Shakespeare described for greatness. Some stimuli, such as large, bright, flashing objects, will by their very nature attract our attention. Other stimuli become attention grabbing through a process of learning. For example, after much experience our attention will become captured by the alarm emitted by our motorcycle when it is kicked by a passing Professor of Neurology. Finally, some stimuli become the focus of our attention because the experimenter demands it ("attend to the red letters and ignore the green figures").

The aim of functional imaging studies of attention is to uncover the neural mechanisms by which this attentional selection is achieved. Imaging studies of attention have two major advantages over studies of other cognitive processes. First, there is a theory of selection (the biased competition model of Desimone and Duncan, 1995) which applies at both the cognitive and the physiological level. Second we already know enough about where sensory signals are processed in the brain to constrain our studies of attention to particular brain regions. We can therefore study how signal processing in these regions is modified by attention.

AN ATTENDED STIMULUS ELICITS MORE NEURAL ACTIVITY

Event-Related Potentials (ERPs)

Our basic assumption is that there is competition between stimuli for processing by the nervous system. The stimulus that wins this competition elicits more neural activity and becomes the focus of attention. This phenomenon was first demonstrated in humans through evoked potentials extracted from electrical activity measured from the surface of the scalp. Immediately after an auditory stimulus, such as a tone, there is a change in brain activity. This evoked response can be revealed by time-locked averaging. Stimuli in different modalities are associated with different patterns of activity. The early components (~0–10 ms for auditory stimuli) of this activity are generated in the brain stem, while later components (~10–200 ms) probably arise in primary sensory cortex. The form of the early components is almost entirely determined by the nature of the eliciting stimulus (*e.g.*, intensity); however, the form of the later components can also be altered by the prior state of the subject even though the stimuli presented in the two states are physically identical. In particular, the N100 component of the auditory evoked potential (a negative potential occurring ~100 ms after the eliciting stimulus) is altered by whether or not the subject is attending to the eliciting stimulus (Hillyard *et al.*, 1995). In the most commonly used design, a series of tones is presented fairly rapidly (~200-ms inter-stimulus interval) to the left and the right ear. The subject is asked to attend to one ear in order to detect target tones that differ slightly from non-target tones in pitch or intensity. Tones in the attended ear elicit larger N100 responses than tones in the non-attended ear. This is an example of a top-down effect in attention. The attentive state of the subject, usually determined by instructions from the experimenter, has modulated the response of the brain to an auditory stimulus. This is an example of a mental state modifying physiology.

Attention to Features

One of the earliest functional imaging studies replicated this result and showed, in addition, that the increase in neural activity could be localised to the brain region in which the attended feature was processed. Corbetta and colleagues (1990) showed volunteers a complex visual display and asked them to attend to colour, movement, or shape. Even though the visual display was the same in each condition, the pattern of brain activity altered depending on the direction of attention. When attention was directed toward colour, greater activity was seen in the lingual gyrus; when attention was directed toward motion, greater activity was seen at the junction of occipital, temporal, and parietal cortex. These areas had previously been identified as being specialised for the processing of these visual features, with the colour area labelled V4 and the motion area labelled V5 (MT) by analogy with the monkey (Allman and Kaas, 1971; Zeki, 1974).

This observation has been replicated in a number of subsequent studies using fMRI. These studies have concentrated on visual motion because the visual motion area, V5 (MT), is easy to localise and reasonably circumscribed (Watson *et al.*, 1993). O'Craven *et al.* (1997) showed volunteers displays containing both moving and stationary dots. When attention was directed to the moving dots, greater activity was observed in V5 (MT). Beauchamp *et al.* (1997) showed volunteers a central fixation point surrounded by an annulus containing moving coloured points. Attention to the speed of the points was associated with greater activity in V5 (MT) than attention to the colour of the points. Büchel *et al.* (1998) showed volunteers moving dots, and attention to this motion increased activity in V5 (MT). Enhancement, to a lesser extent, was also seen in earlier visual processing areas (V1/V2 border).

Viewing movement for a sufficient period of time produces a motion after-effect when the movement ceases (Aristotle, 300 BC, reprinted 1931). The experience of this after-effect is associated with increased activity in V5 (Tootell *et al.*, 1995). The motion after-effect is enhanced (lasts longer) when volunteers attend to the movement during the induction period (Chaudhuri, 1991; Shulman, 1991). Huk and colleagues (2001) showed that changes in attention could explain the enhanced activity in V5 (MT) seen when volunteers experience a motion after-effect. The motion after-effect is inherently attention grabbing, and it is this shift of attention toward motion that causes the increased activity in V5 (MT).

Attention to Spatial Location

A ubiquitous paradigm in attention research involves directing the volunteer's attention to a particular position in space. When visual stimuli are used, this shift in attention is usually covert. In other words, the volunteers are not allowed to move their eyes but must continue to fixate centrally. The earliest study using such a paradigm was by Corbetta *et al.* (1993); however, this study was designed to identify areas involved in the control of attention (frontal and parietal cortex) rather than to study the effects of attention on the visual areas where the targets were processed. Heinze *et al.* (1994) took electroencephalograms (EEGs) readings and recorded blood flow (using positron emission tomography, or PET) while volunteers attended to stimuli in the left or right visual field. They observed enhanced processing in the fusiform gyrus contralateral to the attended stimulus. Their EEG data suggested that theses effects were occurring ~100 ms after stimulus onset. This experiment was repeated using functional magnetic resonance imaging (fMRI) (Mangun *et al.*, 1998). The results replicated the previous study and demonstrated that the effects were sufficiently robust to be seen in single subjects. Attentional modulation was seen in posterior fusiform and middle occipital gyri in the hemisphere contralateral to the attended visual stimuli.

In most of these early studies, the effects of attention were observed at late stages of visual processing such as V4 and V5 (MT). This is consistent with electrophysiological studies in monkeys where attentional effects in V1 are smaller and more difficult to elicit than in later processing areas (*e.g.*, Haenny and Schiller, 1988); however, there are now several imaging studies showing robust effects of attention in human primary visual cortex. Watanabe and colleagues (1998) presented volunteers with moving wedges. In contrast to passive viewing, attention to one side of the wedge was associated with increased activity in V1. Brefczynski and DeYoe (1999) showed volunteers a complex stimulus composed of many segments containing coloured lines. Attention to a particular segment was associated with increased activity in visual areas corresponding to the retinotopic location of that segment. The largest effect was seen in V4, an area specialised for the processing of colour and orientation; however, effects were also seen in earlier stages of visual processing, including V1. Similar results have obtained by Somers *et al.* (1999), who presented a central target surrounded by an annulus and required volunteers to attend (covertly) to the central target or the annulus. Attention was associated with increased activity in many visual areas including V1. This modulation was spatially specific to the retinotopic representations of the attended location. Of particular interest is the observation that, in the regions representing the unattended location, there was a decrease in activation relative to a passive viewing condition (see also Smith *et al.*, 2000). This means that when volunteers were attending to the annulus there was a complex annulus-shaped window of attention. This is not compatible with a simple "spotlight" model of spatial attention (Posner *et al.*, 1980) and suggests that, in this paradigm at least, attention is object based (Duncan, 1980).

Attention to Objects

There is also direct evidence of increased activity associated with attention to objects. Wojciulik *et al.* (1998) showed volunteers a series of complex displays, each containing two faces and two houses. Attention to the faces rather than the houses was associated with greater activity in the fusiform gyrus in a region previously shown to respond to the presentation of faces (the fusiform face area, or FFA) (Puce *et al.*, 1995; Kanwisher *et al.*, 1997). Rees *et al.* (1999) showed volunteers a series of line drawings and letter strings that appeared superimposed at fixation. The volunteers had to attend to either the line drawings or the letter strings while performing a difficult sequential matching task. Real words were embedded in the series of letter strings, and these words elicited activity in posterior basal temporal cortex in an area known to be more responsive to words than letter strings (the word form area, or WFA) (Price, 1998). This activity only appeared when the volunteers were attending to the letter strings. When they attended to the line drawings, they were apparently unaware of the presentation of the words and no activity could be detected in the word form area (see Fig. 15.1).

This last experiment is concerned with competition between different objects in the same location. Competitive effects can also be shown when similar objects are presented in different

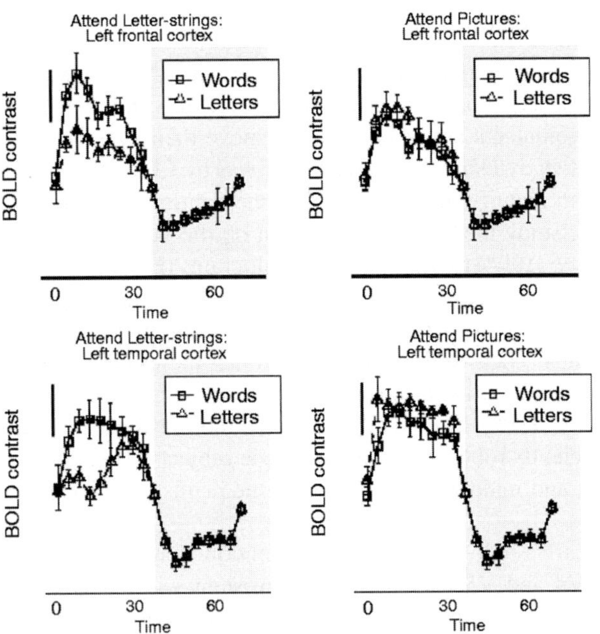

FIGURE 15.1
Time course of activity in left frontal (upper panels, coordinates –39, 6, 27) and left posterior basal temporal cortex (lower panels, visual word area, coordinates –39, –36, –24). All four panels use the same plotting conventions. Average BOLD contrast evoked at each locus is plotted as a function of time, collapsing across epochs and participants. Note that the areas for which the time courses are shown were identified as those areas showing a maximal simple main effect of words under attention to letters. Unshaded areas represent scans acquired in the experimental conditions, and shaded areas represent those acquired during the passive fixation baseline. Error bars indicate interparticipant standard error and the dark scale bar represents a 0.5% BOLD signal change. Activity evoked when the letter stream contained meaningful words is plotted with black squares and a solid line, and activity when the same stream included only meaningless letter strings is plotted with triangles and a dotted line. (From Rees, G. *et al.*, 1999. With permission.)

locations. Fink *et al.* (2000) showed volunteers visual characters presented unilaterally or bilaterally. Characters in one hemifield were reported less accurately when competing characters appeared in the other hemifield. In addition, there was greater activity in areas of striate and extrastriate cortex evoked by stimuli presented without competing characters in the other hemifield.

It is in the nature of objects that they consist of a collection of features. A typical visual object might be defined by a combination of colour, shape, and movement. These features are processed in different parts of the visual system (Zeki, 1974). Does attention to just one feature of an object lead to increased activity in all the regions that analyse other features of that object? O'Craven *et al.* (1999) showed volunteers complex stimuli consisting of a face transparently superimposed on a house, with one object moving and the other stationary. In different conditions, the volunteers attended to the face, the house, or the motion. When volunteers attended to motion, there was increased activity in V5 (MT), but, in addition, if it was the face that was moving, there was also increased activity in the fusiform face area. This result is also consistent with attention being object based. Attention to one aspect of an object leads automatically to enhanced processing of other aspects of that object. This result demonstrates that attention involves cooperation as well as competition.

COMPETITION AND COOPERATION

We have reviewed some of the many studies demonstrating that attention is associated with an increase in activity in the brain region concerned with the processing of whatever it is that is being attended to (feature, location, or object). There is also some evidence for a reduction of activity when attention is withheld. These results are consistent with the idea that attention involves a competitive process. We are then naturally led to ask the question, "Where does this competition take place?" For competition to occur there must be a location at which signals from the competing features or objects interact. Likewise, there must be a location in which signals from different features can interact so that cooperation can occur. In order to identify these sites of competitive or cooperative interaction we also need some indication that such interactions are occurring.

Competition Within Receptive Fields

In the monkey, competition can occur within the receptive field of a single cell. If two objects fall within the same receptive field, then less activity is elicited than would occur if a single object were presented. Attention to one of the two objects overcomes this suppressive effect (Moran and Desimone, 1985). This observation is consistent with a simple mechanism, analogous to lateral inhibition, in which all the objects falling in the receptive field mutually inhibit each other. The result of this competition is that the difference in output signal between the winner and the losers is enhanced (Lee *et al.*, 1999), while at the same time the overall activity in the region is reduced. In this case, the sign of competition within a brain region is reduced activity.

Kastner *et al.* (1998) used fMRI to see whether the same processes could be detected in the human brain. Volunteers were required to attend to one of a number of visual stimuli, which were either close together or far apart. When the stimuli were close together, there was reduced activity in visual processing areas (V1, V2, V4, TEO). In the monkey, the receptive fields of cells get bigger as we move from early (V1) to late (IT) stages of visual processing. This was reflected in the fMRI study by the observation that the reduction in activity that occurred when stimuli were close together was greatest in TEO and least in V1 (Kastner *et al.*, 2001).

Competition (and Cooperation) Between Distant Locations

In most studies of attention, however, the competing (or cooperating) signals are being processed in distinct, segregated regions. This applies for features (colour [V4] versus motion [V5]), locations (left versus right hemifields), and objects (fusiform face area versus parahippocampal place area). In these cases, is there a direct interaction between the two processing regions or is the interaction mediated by a third, multi-modal region? There is considerable evidence to suggest that competition and cooperation are mediated by a third region located in parietal cortex. Whether the exact location of this third region depends upon the nature of the competing or cooperating signals remains to be determined.

Corbetta *et al.* (1995) used a visual search task in which targets were defined by the conjunction of colour and motion. In comparison to searches based on colour or motion alone, the conjunction search activated a region of superior parietal cortex. The authors suggest that activity in this location is linked with attention to spatial location because an influential theory (Treisman and Gelade, 1980) has proposed that detection of feature conjunctions requires attention to a specific spatial location; however, attention to spatial locations does not seem to be necessary for the observation of activity in this region of parietal cortex (see below). We propose that this region is more generally involved when there is an interaction between modalities, with position in space being one of the many possible modalities.

The parietal activity observed in this study was revealed by contrasting a task in which there was cooperation between colour and motion with tasks in which no such cooperation was required. In principle, it should be possible to use the same strategy to identify regions involved in competition; however, in the various studies reviewed in the first section of this chapter, such a comparison was not possible. For example, an experiment might contrast attending to colour with attending to motion. In this case, competition is happening in both tasks. The comparison of the two tasks reveals activity associated with signals that have won the competition. If there is a change in activity related simply to the occurrence of competition, then that change will be present in both tasks and will not be revealed in the comparison. If selective attention always involves competition, then the activity associated with this competition can only be revealed by contrast with a comparison task in which no selective attention is required. Such comparisons will always be problematic. The stimulus presentation could be changed so that competing stimuli were no longer present. In this case, any changes in activity might be due to changes in stimulation rather than changes in competition. Volunteers might be asked to view the display passively, but in this case execution of a response as well as competition has been removed. Volunteers might be told to ignore the competing stimuli in the periphery and to base their responses on some central feature. In this case, selective attention is still required although in a much easier form. Bearing in mind these problems it is nevertheless striking that studies adopting these various approaches obtain consistent results.

Coull and Frith (1998) contrasted attention (and also working memory) to spatial locations and to objects. Volunteers saw a sequence of digits that appeared in eight different spatial locations and had to attend to a particular digit or a particular location. In the working memory version, they had to detect sequences of digits or locations. The non-attentive control condition was rest with eyes closed. Intraparietal sulcus (IPS), superior parietal lobule, and premotor cortex were all activated during attention to a location *and* during attention to an object, although more so for spatial attention. In addition, these areas were activated during both the attention task and the working memory task, although more so in the working memory task. A second experiment was performed in which the volunteers attended to objects (@, %, ?, &c.) which appeared centrally in order to further reduce the spatial component of the task. For this task, IPS and premotor cortex were also activated, but not superior parietal lobule. These results suggest that IPS has a role whether competition is between spatial locations or objects. On the other hand, superior parietal lobule may be more specifically concerned with competition between spatial locations.

The classic paradigm invented by Posner (1980) has been used in many imaging studies in which attention is directed toward locations in space where certain objects may appear (see review by Corbetta, 1998). Volunteers fixate centrally and are presented with cues that indicate whether the target will be on the left or the right. For ~80% of trials the cue is valid. For these trials, reaction times for target detection are faster than with neutral or invalid cues. Coull and Nobre (1998) used an ingenious variation of this task in which the cues could also indicate locations in time (early or late) as well as space (left or right). Common areas of activity were observed bilaterally in parietal cortex for attention to locations in time as well as space, although there were also interesting differences in the patterns of activation associated with the two tasks.

Fink *et al.* (1997) contrasted space-based and object-based attention. Volunteers attended to either one side of space (left or right hemifield) or one side of an object. In either case, activations associated with attention were observed in parietal cortex. Vandenberghe *et al.* (1997) required volunteers to attend to features of objects in the left or right visual field. Activity was seen in parietal cortex when the volunteers attended to a single feature in one hemifield. This activity was enhanced when they attended to two features of an object in the one hemifield.

Culham *et al.* (1998) used an interesting task in which volunteers had to track a subset of moving targets (Pylyshyn and Storm, 1988). Volunteers viewed a display of nine green bouncing balls. At the start of each trial some of these balls briefly turned red to indicate that these were the targets. Volunteers then had to follow the movements of these target balls while maintaining fixation. In this task there is cooperation between the movement and position of the target balls and competition from the non-targets. Attentive tracking was associated with activity in a number of regions of parietal cortex (SPL, IPS, IPL). The same regions were also activated in an attention-shifting task. Frontal regions were also activated. Other studies (Culham *et al.*, 2001; Jovicich *et al.*, 2001) have used versions of this paradigm in order to identify sources of top-down signals, but these will discussed in a later section.

The main aim of this section has been to identify regions where signals interact, as such interactions are an essential component of selective attention; however, in the studies reviewed so far the comparison condition has usually been passive viewing. Thus, in addition to the cooperation and competition between signals, the attentive conditions have also involved the top down processes through which the volunteers were able to direct their attention as required by the experimenter and make appropriate responses when a target was detected. Given all these requirements, the reader will not be surprised to learn that a number of premotor and prefrontal areas were activated in addition to the parietal areas we have listed. What then is the justification for assuming that it is these parietal areas that are concerned with interactions between competing and cooperating signals and not the frontal areas? There is extensive evidence from neurophysiological studies in monkeys that the parietal cortex contains a number of multimodal regions where such interactions can take place (Andersen *et al.*, 1997). In addition, there are imaging studies in which competition and cooperation occurs between signals without any top-down processes being involved. In these studies, activity is seen in parietal cortex, but not in frontal cortex. We shall return to the problem of top-down processes in the last section of this chapter.

Macaluso and his colleagues (2000a,b) have performed a number of studies aimed at identifying multimodal processing areas concerned with vision and touch. In one study (Macaluso *et al.*, 2000a) volunteers received bilateral stimulation in either vision *or* touch and were required to detect targets on one side or the other. Two areas were identified that responded to both vision and touch and showed greater activity for rightward versus leftward directed attention: left intraparietal sulcus and left occipitotemporal junction. In a second experiment it was found that the response of the parietal area to touch only occurred when the volunteers' eyes were open so that they could see the hand being touched. This latter result suggests that this area is not only multimodal in the sense of responding to both vision and touch, but is also concerned with interactions between these signals.

In a second study (Macaluso *et al.*, 2000b), interaction between vision and touch during attention was studied explicitly. Volunteers received bilateral visual stimulation and were required to detect targets on the left or the right. Unlike the previous study, irrelevant touches also occurred. Sometimes a touch occurred at the same location as the visual target and sometimes on the opposite side. As has been observed previously, responses to visual targets were faster when there was a coincident touch. Underlying this behavioural effect greater activity was elicited in visual cortex by a target in the presence of a coincident touch (Fig. 15.2). The area of visual cortex showing this modulation is unimodal and receives no direct inputs from tactile receptors. The modulation by touch seen in this experiment must therefore derive from back projections from multimodal regions. Analysis of functional connectivity revealed two parietal regions that might be the source of these signals. Activity in these regions showed a greater correlation with activity in the visual area in the presence of coincident touch.

This observation confirms the idea that certain regions of parietal cortex have a role in the interaction between signals that underlies attention. In addition, the observation makes an important point about the nature of top-down processes. At the physiological level, the effect of touch on activity in visual cortex was top-down because it depended upon back-projections from parietal cortex; however, at the psychological level the effect of touch was bottom-up. The tactile signal was entirely uninformative about when or where a visual signal would occur so there was nothing to be gained by directing attention toward touch. Furthermore, the volunteer could not anticipate when a tactile stimulus would coincide with a visual target. The interaction between touch and vision was a process that happened automatically when a tactile stimulus happened to coincide with a visual target.

A similar point can be made from the observation of Calvert *et al.* (2000) concerning the combination of vision and hearing in speech perception. Volunteers experienced semantically congruent or incongruent audiovisual speech or each modality in isolation. It is well established that congruent audiovisual speech is easier to understand, while discordant input creates problems for understanding. Here, again, at the psychological level this is a bottom-up effect that occurs automatically. Activity parallel with the behavioural observations was observed in left superior temporal sulcus. Activity in this region was greater in the congruent condition and reduced in the incongruent condition.

MECHANISMS FOR CONTROLLING COMPETITION

On the basis of the various studies reviewed in the last section we can conclude that parietal cortex contains a number of multimodal regions in which competition and cooperation occurs between many different kinds of signal. How do these interactions permit one signal or group of signal to win the competition and become the focus of attention? A simple mechanism in which each competing signal inhibits all the others (analogous to lateral inhibition) will allow the strongest signal to win the competition and pass on for further processing. The study by Kastner *et al.* (1998) provides some evidence for such a mechanism when the competing stimuli are all

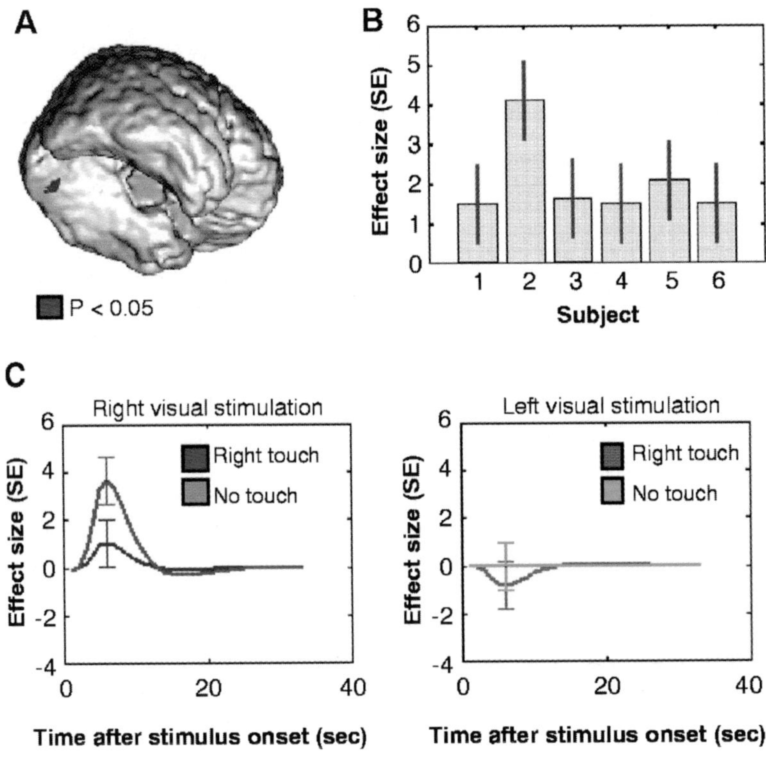

FIGURE 15.2
Cross-modal effects in the left lingual gyrus. An interaction between side of the visual stimulation and the presence of right somatosensory input was detected in the left lingual gyrus. We found signal amplification when the right visual stimulus was coupled with the right tactile stimulation. (A) Group results of activation rendered on the brain surface. (B) Size of the interaction effect for each subject (with standard error, SE). The search volume for each subject-specific maximum was restricted to the same region as for the group effect (*i.e.*, areas showing a main effect of side of the visual stimulation). The plotted effect is the weighted sum of parameter estimates from the multiple regression. For the interaction shown, this weighting corresponds to participants receiving right visual stimuli with right tactile stimuli versus those without right touch minus participants receiving left visual stimuli with right tactile stimuli versus those without. All effects are scaled to SE units. (C) Estimated signal in the cluster showing significant amplification of response to right visual stimuli by right touch. The shape of the curves reflects the function used to fit the data. The effect size (scaled to SE units) is the sum of the parameter estimates for the six participants for each of the four events. For each event type, the parameters were estimated by fitting the mean signal across the activated voxels. (From Macaluso, E. *et al.*, 2000b. With permission.)

in the visual modality and close together. This mechanism is sufficient for situations in which attention is directed in a bottom-up manner, such that a stimulus that is intrinsically salient will attract our attention. However, in most studies, attention is directed in a top-down manner. We ignore the intrinsically salient stimulus and attend to something that would not naturally attract our attention. Our attention is directed wilfully in that sense that we are doing what the experimenter has told us to do rather than simply reacting to the stimuli that impinge upon us. In Desimone and Duncan's model, this wilful direction of attention is achieved by a biasing signal. This is a top-down signal that boosts the activity associated with the feature or object to which we have decided to attend.

Modulating Activity in Stimulus Processing Sites

We have already reviewed a number of studies in which the stimulus input did not change, but the activity in feature processing areas was increased when attention was directed at that feature. This increase in activity in the absence of any change in stimulus input is the mark of top-down effects. In principle, there are two ways in which this increase in activity could happen (*e.g.*, see Rees and Frith, 1998). First, the top-down signal might cause an increase in *gain* in the region. In this case, when attention is directed toward it, a stimulus would elicit greater than usual activity in the relevant region (Fig. 15.3). Second, the top-down signal might cause an increase

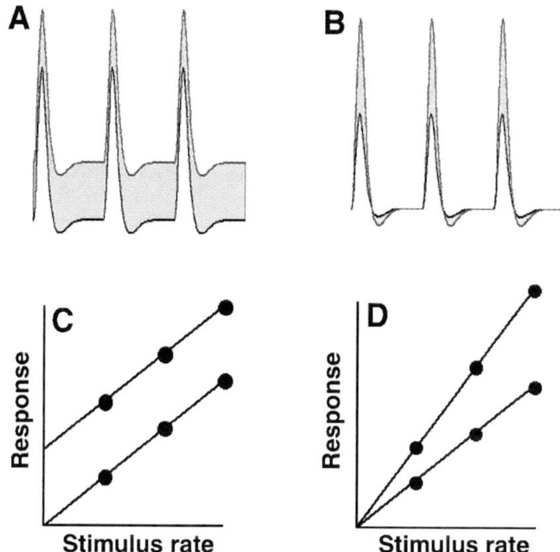

FIGURE 15.3
Theoretical illustration of bias and gain control mechanisms of attention. (A) and (B) Schematic illustration of how stimulus-evoked neural activity (red) might be modulated (grey) by an attentional signal. This modulation could take the form of (A) an additive bias signal or (B) a true modulation of stimulus-evoked responses. (C) and (D) Varying the rate at which stimuli are presented produces a monotonic relationship between the evoked response (per unit time) and the frequency of presentation. The attentional effects (A, B) can now be distinguished by their effects on intercept (A, C) or slope (B, D) of this relationship. (From Rees, G. and Frith, C. D., 1998. With permission.)

in *base level* activity. In this case, there would be greater activity in the region during attention even before any stimulus arrived (Fig. 15.3). It is also possible, of course, that both mechanisms could operate.

Positron emission tomography was used in an attempt to distinguish between these possibilities by varying the rate of presentation of stimuli (tones) (Frith and Friston, 1996). Assuming that each stimulus elicits the same increase in neural activity (and, hence, blood flow), then the increase in activity with increasing rate of presentation (the slope) is a measure of the activity elicited by each stimuli. If attention to the stimuli increases the gain of the system, then this slope should increase. If attention alters base level activity, the slope will remain the same (Fig. 15.3). Activity in auditory cortex was strongly correlated with rate of presentation of the tones; however, attention to the tones did not change the slope of this relationship; during attention, the activity in this region increased a similar amount whatever the rate of presentation. This observation implies that there was a change in baseline activity, but not in gain. This result contrasts with EEG studies. These have consistently shown that attention to a tone increases the amplitude of the response elicited by that tone in auditory cortex, indicating a change in gain (Hillyard *et al.*, 1973). One possible explanation for this discrepancy is that attention increases the synchrony of the activity in this region. An increase in the synchrony of firing would increase the amplitude of the evoked potential even though the total activity had not changed. The observation that activity in the thalamus was correlated with rate of presentation of the tones, but only when attention was directed towards them, would be consistent with the idea that the thalamus has a role in synchronising activity in regions currently involved in processing signals that are the focus of attention.

The observation that top-down processes controlling attention produce a shift in baseline activity in stimulus-processing regions implies that this change in activity would be observed even in the absence of any relevant stimulus. This possibility can be examined more directly using event-related fMRI. Kastner *et al.* (1999) asked volunteers to covertly attend to a particular location in a visual scene. They demonstrated that there were increases in activity in extrastriate cortex associated with directing attention to a particular location even when no visual stimulus actually occurred in that location. Chawla *et al.* (1999) asked volunteers to attend to moving or coloured stimuli and measured baseline activity and stimulus evoked activity separately. Baseline activity in motion- and sensitive-sensitive areas of extrastriate cortex was enhanced by selective attention to these attributes, even in the absence of moving or coloured stimuli. When a relevant stimulus was presented, there was a further enhancement of activity produced by the attended feature. In a computational simulation, these authors showed that in principle changes in background activity in the absence of stimulation could produce such changes in activity evoked by an attended feature of a subsequent visual stimulus (Chawla *et al.*, 2000). They therefore concluded that attention modulates sensitivity of neural populations to inputs by changing background activity.

Modulating Connectivity with Stimulus Processing Sites

We have reviewed the evidence that one effect of the biasing signal associated with top-down control of attention is to increase activity in the sites at which the attended signal is being processed. This implies that transmission of information about an attended attribute (*e.g.*, colour) is enhanced while transmission of information about other attributes (*e.g.*, motion) is reduced. We could put this another way and say that *connectivity* between early visual processing regions where both colour and motion signals are processed and the colour-processing region V4 is increased while connectivity between early visual areas and the motion-processing region V5 (MT) is reduced. In principle, it is possible to measure such changes in connectivity by looking at the correlation between patterns of activity over time in different brain regions. Functional MRI is particularly suitable for this purpose because many observations are available for calculating such correlations.

In a series of papers, Friston and colleagues (Büchel and Friston, 1997; Büchel *et al.*, 1999; Friston and Büchel, 2000) have investigated the changes in connectivity between brain regions that associated with selective attention. Of particular relevance here is the study by Friston and Büchel (2000) in which volunteers were asked to attend to visual motion. During attention to visual motion, they observed that connectivity between V2 and V5 was enhanced.

Friston and Büchel also obtained evidence that this change in connectivity was driven by signals from parietal cortex; however, we shall return to this evidence in the next section. For the moment, we conclude that top-down modulation of stimulus processing sites during selective attention increases baseline activity in these sites and increases the connectivity of these sites with earlier, less specialised stimulus processing areas. We shall now consider the nature and source of the top-down signals upon which wilful selective attention depends.

TOP-DOWN BIASING SIGNALS AND THE VOLUNTARY CONTROL OF ATTENTION

So far we have discussed the sites in the brain at which selective attention operates. Sites are brain regions where the signals, which define the focus of attention, are processed. If we are attending to colour, then the site will be the colour processing area, V4. If we are attending to faces, then the site will be the face area in the fusiform gyrus (fusiform face area, or FFA). Sites can be identified because they are activated by the appropriate stimulus even in the absence of attention. V4 will be activated if volunteers passively view stimuli in which colour changes occur while all other attributes remain constant (Zeki and Marini, 1998). The same area is activated if the stimulus remains constant, but the volunteer attends to colour (Corbetta *et al.*, 1990). Likewise, the FFA is more activated if volunteers passively view a sequence of different faces rather than a sequence of different places or objects (Puce *et al.*, 1995; Kanwisher *et al.*, 1997). Even more strikingly, the FFA is activated if there is change from one face to another that the volunteer does not even notice (Beck *et al.*, 2001; see Chapter 16). In the case of wilful attention, this increase in activity in the site is the result of biases caused by a top-down signal. We now want to consider the nature of wilful attention and ways of identifying the source of this top-down signal.

Wilful Attention

Wilful attention is required most obviously in situations where the stimulus at the focus of our attention is not intrinsically salient. It is difficult for me to attend to the writing of this section of the chapter when, as is all too frequently the case, my colleagues in the next room are engaged in loud competition regarding their physical prowess in various domains. In an experimental context, it is difficult to ignore the large flashing stimuli and wait for the small dim ones. In circumstances like these, voluntary attention requires mental effort. For this reason, we like to use the term *wilful attention*. Effort is required to carry on performing the task. We would much prefer to relax, stop thinking about what we are doing, and behave in an entirely automatic, stimulus-driven manner. But, if we do this, we will respond to the wrong stimuli.

Two principles emerge from this characterisation of wilful attention. First, there is the need for prior knowledge. We need to know which kind of stimuli we should attend to and which kind of responses we should make, in advance of the appearance of any stimuli. Second, there is the necessity to maintain this knowledge in mind for the duration of the experiment. The process by which we maintain task priorities in mind is as good a definition as any of working memory. To put this in slightly more physiological terms, wilful attention requires two processes. First, there is the need to alter connectivity in order to enhance responses to certain kinds of signals and to link these signals to certain kinds of responses. Second, there is the need to maintain this altered connectivity in the face of competition from other, better-established patterns. Is it possible to identify the brain regions involved in these processes?

To anticipate our conclusions from reviewing the many studies on this topic, activity in parietal and frontal cortex has been consistently observed during tasks requiring wilful attention, and these areas overlap with those active during traditional working memory tasks; however, we believe that a distinction can be made concerning the roles of parietal and frontal cortex. Parietal cortex contains multimodal regions in which interactions can occur between signals from distant processing sites. Such interactions occur whether or not attention is wilfully directed. Parietal cortex also contains the regions where stimuli are linked with appropriate responses by eye or limb. In contrast, frontal regions have a specific and necessary role in wilful attention. It is these regions that initiate and maintain the patterns of connectivity needed for any particular case of wilful attention.

Much of the evidence that a frontoparietal network is involved in attention comes from the studies we have already mentioned using the covert attention task developed by Posner. Contrasting performance of this task with passive viewing of the same stimuli has consistently revealed activity in a network of frontal and parietal areas (Corbetta *et al.*, 1995, Coull *et al.*, 1996, Culham *et al.*, 1998).

Evidence that there is a hierarchy of control within this system comes from the studies of Friston and his colleagues to which we have already referred. In all these studies volunteers were required to attend to visual motion and this attentive condition was compared with a non-attentive condition involving identical stimulation. In the attentive condition Büchel *et al.* (1998) observed activity in striate (V1/V2 border), extrastriate (V3a, V5), parietal, and frontal cortex. In terms of our terminology, the striate and extrastriate cortical regions are likely to be sites as they respond to visual motion even during passive viewing. The parietal and frontal regions are more likely to be sources of top-down signals, because these areas only respond to visual motion when this is being made the focus of attention. Friston and Büchel (2000) investigated changes of connectivity within this network of areas. During attention, the response of V5 (MT) to "driving" inputs from V2 was increased and this modulation was driven by activity in (posterior) parietal cortex. Finally, Büchel and Friston (1997) showed that connectivity between posterior parietal cortex and V5 (MT) was modulated by activity in prefrontal cortex. These observations imply a hierarchy of control. During wilful attention to visual motion, signals from prefrontal cortex cause enhanced connectivity between parietal cortex and V5 (MT), perhaps biasing activity related to visual motion in a particular spatial location (see Fig. 15.4). In turn, this increases connectivity between early visual areas and V5 (MT) so that signals about visual motion are enhanced relative to signals about other attributes. In the remainder of this section, we shall consider the precise roles of these parietal and frontal areas in the control of selective attention.

Top-Down Signals in the Absence of Wilful Attention

We have already discussed the study by Macaluso *et al.* (2000b) that demonstrated that irrelevant, but coincident, tactile stimuli could enhance responses to visual stimuli in unimodal

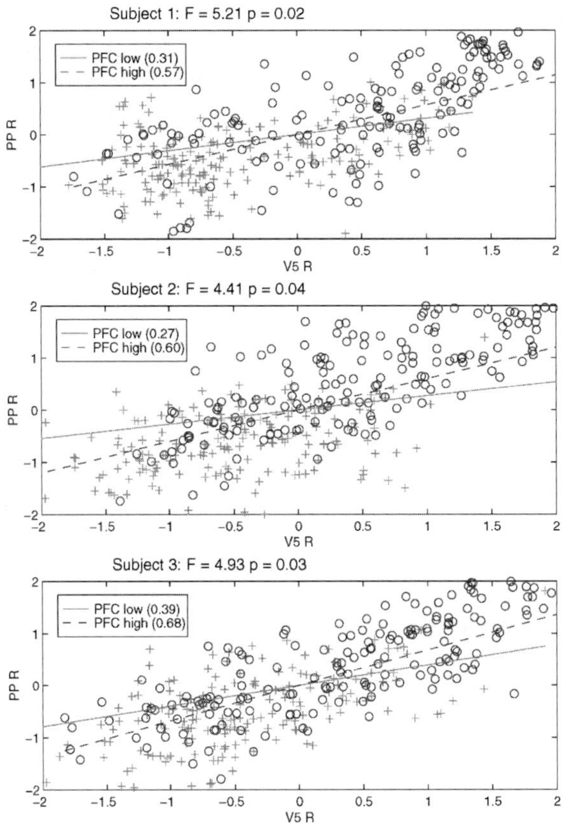

FIGURE 15.4
Regression between V5 and parietal cortex (PP) as a function of activation in prefrontal cortex (PFC). This demonstrates the modulatory effect of the PFC on the connection between V5 and PP for three subjects attending to visual motion. All observations were divided into two groups: one with observations in which PFC activity is high, and one in which PFC activity is low. The graphs show separate regression curves for both groups. The F statistics and associated p values reflect the significance of the interaction term (V5 × PFC), in the presence of the two main effects (V5 and PFC) of the following regression model: PP = b1 V5 + b2 PFC + b3 V5 × PFC. (From Büchel, C. and Friston, K., 1997. With permission.)

visual areas. An analysis of connectivity suggested that this enhancement is mediated by back projections from multimodal parietal areas that receive signals from somatosensory areas. In this experiment, volunteers wilfully attended to visual signals occurring in particular spatial locations; however, they were not wilfully directing their attention to the tactile stimuli, as these were uninformative and were as likely to occur in the same location or in the opposite location as the visual target. Nevertheless, the enhancement of the visual response by a tactile cue was the result of a top-down biasing signal arising in parietal cortex. We propose that these top-down signals with an origin in parietal cortex occur whenever there is competition or cooperation between stimuli in different domains, whether or not attention is being directed wilfully. For wilful attention, additional activity in prefrontal cortex is required. Unfortunately most experimental paradigms do not allow us to make this distinction; however, a few studies are consistent with the conclusion that parietal cortex is involved in multimodal interactions rather than wilful attention.

It is well known that lesions of the right inferior parietal cortex can lead to unilateral left-sided neglect (Vallar and Perani, 1986). A patient with neglect will apparently not notice visual events occurring in his left hemifield. This applies to unexpected and salient events and is not, therefore, a specific problem with wilful attention. Indeed, if patients are put into an attentive and alert state by the presentation of a warning sound before visual stimulation, their neglect can sometimes be overcome (Robertson *et al.*, 1998). Visual extinction is one component of the neglect syndrome and is also commonly associated with right parietal damage (for a review, see Driver and Mattingley, 1998). Patients with this disorder are aware of a stimulus in the left hemifield as long as it is presented on its own, but if two stimuli are presented simultaneously, one on the left and one on the right, then the patient will only see the one on the right. In this case, the one on the left is said to have been extinguished. Rees *et al.* (2000) showed that these extinguished stimuli still elicit activity in striate and extrastriate cortex in the right hemisphere. Furthermore, when the stimuli were faces, activity could be detected in the right fusiform face area (Rees *et al.*, 2002). Similar results have been obtained from another patient by Vuilleumier *et al.* (2001). These studies show that activity in visual processing regions is not sufficient to attract attention and suggest that parts of parietal cortex are needed in addition. This notion is reinforced by the observation by Vuilleumier *et al.* (2001) that successful detection of the left-sided target during bilateral stimulation was associated with enhanced connectivity between right visual areas and the intact, left parietal cortex.

Downar *et al.* (2000) explicitly studied involuntary attention to events in three different modalities using visual, auditory, and tactile stimuli. The stimuli were presented in different modalities and spatial locations and subjects were asked to passively observe the stimuli. The quality of the stimulation in each modality changed intermittently, and brain responses to these stimulus transitions were determined. In addition to the expected unimodal areas, they identified multimodal areas that responded to stimulus changes in all three modalities. These areas were primarily in the right hemisphere and included the temporoparietal junction. Corbetta *et al.* (2000) also observed activation of the right temporoparietal junction when a visual target appeared at an unattended location. Marois *et al.* (2000b) also observed activation of the temporoparietal junction in response to infrequent oddball changes from a standard stimulus whether these changes were in identity or spatial location, or both. These results are consistent with the idea that activity in parietal cortex (at least in the region of the temporoparietal junction) is necessary if attention is to be involuntarily drawn to multimodal changes in stimulation. It has been proposed that these inferior temporoparietal regions form part of a right-lateralised network that is not involved in top-down selection but instead is specialised for the detection of behaviourally relevant stimuli, particularly when they are salient or unexpected (Corbetta and Shulman, 2002).

Identifying the Source of Top-Down Biasing Signals

We have already discussed criteria for identifying brain sites at which top-down attentional signals have their effect. First, a site is activated by certain kinds of signal (*e.g.*, visual motion or faces) whether or not attention is directed toward these signals. Second, directing attention toward these signals further increases activation even though there has been no change in the signal. To identify the source of the top-signals associated with attention a different set of criteria are required.

Anticipatory Activity

In order to direct attention to towards some signal we need to know in advance what that signal will be. Thus, the presence of activity prior to the occurrence of a signal is taken to be a sign that top-down biasing is in operation; however, we have already reviewed the evidence that anticipatory activity of this kind can be observed in stimulus processing sites (*e.g.*, V5 (MT) in the study by Chawla *et al.*, 1999). To be identified as a *source* of a top-down signal we would therefore want to see anticipatory activity in an area that was not involved in sensory processing. Some studies have explicitly or implicitly used these criteria for identifying sources of top-down signals. Kastner *et al.* (1999) observed activity in anticipation of a visual stimulus at a peripheral location. We have already mentioned the activity in visual areas, but there were even stronger increases of activity in frontal and parietal areas that the authors suggest were the source of a top-down biasing signal. Corbetta *et al.* (2000) also observed activation of the intraparietal sulcus when a location was attended before visual-target presentation.

Sustained Activity

Analogous to the criterion of anticipatory activity is the criterion of sustained activity. If the volunteer does not know precisely when the relevant stimulus will appear then the top-down biasing signal must be present throughout the period of attention. Thus, the region that is the source of this signal will show sustained activity throughout the period and, in contrast to a stimulus processing site, will not show stimulus-elicited changes in activity. Rees *et al.* (1996) used the method of varying stimulus rate to distinguish sustained from stimulus-elicited activity during attention. When volunteers had to detect conjunctions of colour and form as opposed to detection of changes in a single feature, sustained activity was seen in premotor cortex (BA8). Presence of sustained activity has also been widely used as a criterion for identifying regions involved in maintenance functions in working memory. For example, Rowe *et al.* (2000, 2001) required volunteers to keep in mind spatial locations for variable amounts of time. Two brain regions showed sustained activity during this interval: premotor cortex (BA8) and IPS.

Task-Independent Activity

If the top-down biasing signals associated with wilful attention derive from a common source then activity should be seen in this source (or sources) whatever the precise form of the attentional task. This is in contrast to sites, which will be strongly task dependent since their location will be determined by the nature of the sensory signals that have to be processed. Wojciulik and Kanwisher (1999) used three very different visual attention tasks contrasted with easier versions of the same tasks. Two parietal areas were activated in all three tasks (note that the functional imaging scans covered only parietal and occipital cortex, so they could not detect any activity in frontal cortex). Coull and Frith (1998) observed common activity bilaterally in IPS and in premotor cortex for attention to spatial locations and attention to objects presented centrally.

Load-Dependent Activity

A number of groups (Culham *et al.*, 2001; deFockert *et al.*, 2001; Jovicich *et al.*, 2001) have suggested that areas directly involved in attentional processes (sources of top-down signals in our terminology) will show increasing activity as a function of attentional load. Load is related to the mental effort needed to stay on task. In the study of Jovicich *et al.*, attentional load was operationally defined as the number of targets that the subject was asked to track. Using this task, they identified a number of parietal and frontal areas in which activity was strongly correlated with increasing load. In contrast, frontal eye field (FEF) and parietal area 7 showed no change in activity with load although these areas did show greater activity than during a passive viewing task.

Using these various criteria for identifying the sources of top-down signals studies has consistently revealed activation in various frontal and parietal regions; however, the precise function of these regions remains unknown. Does function relate to the domain in which the competition for attention is occurring? For example, is it possible that different regions are required for modulating competition between modalities (*e.g.*, sight versus sound) as opposed to competition within modalities (*e.g.*, visual motion versus visual form)? Or perhaps function relates to the type of process engaged, so that one region might be required for inhibiting irrelevant stimuli, while another is required for maintaining task priorities in the context of low arousal. These questions are very similar to those we ask about the role of prefrontal cortex in Chapter 18. Clearly, the mechanisms underlying wilful selective attention are a subset of executive functions. As with all other executive functions, we are not going to be able to answer these questions until we have a much more information as to what these functions are in mechanistic terms.

MECHANISMS OF TOP-DOWN BIAS IN SELECTIVE ATTENTION

The biased competition model, around which we have constructed this chapter, states that a stimulus gains our attention by winning a competition with other stimuli. In wilful attention, a biasing signal is used to increase the chances that a particular stimulus will win this competition; however, this model is not specific about the nature of the competition or the level at which it occurs, nor does the model say anything precise about how the biasing signal modulates the competition.

Early and Late Selection

A long-standing debate in cognitive psychology has concerned the level at which competition occurs. On the one hand, experiments demonstrated early selection. So, for example, signals in an attended ear might be heard while any information about signals in the other, unattended ear would be lost (Treisman and Geffen, 1967). In this case, selection has occurred at an early stage of auditory processing. On the other hand, there were other experiments demonstrating late selection. For example, calling the volunteer's name in the unattended ear would be noticed and produce a response, indicating that unattended signals were still being processed up to the level of semantics (Corteen and Wood, 1972). The evidence we have already reviewed from imaging studies demonstrates that, at the physiological level, both early and late selection can occur. (Although, interestingly, these demonstrations are all in the visual domain, while the classic behavioural studies were largely in the auditory domain.)

A number of studies have shown that wilful selective attention can modulate activity in primary visual cortex (V1) at the earliest stage of cortical processing (Gandhi *et al.*, 1999; Somers *et al.*, 1999; Watanabe, 1998). By the time you read this chapter, we would not be surprised if even earlier modulation had not been demonstrated (O'Connor *et al.*, 2002, note added in press). On the other hand, studies of change blindness (Beck *et al.*, 2001) and neglect (Rees *et al.*, 2000, 2002; Vuillumieur *et al.*, 2001) have shown that unattended visual stimuli can be processed at least up to the level where they have been classified as faces rather than other kinds of object.

Perceptual Load

It was already known from ingenious behavioural studies that the nature of an attentive task can alter the level at which selection occurs (see Lavie, 1995, for a review). Tasks with a low perceptual load (*e.g.*, deciding whether a word is in upper or lower case) are compatible with late selection of unattended stimuli. On the other hand, tasks with high perceptual load (*e.g.*, deciding how many syllables a word has) are associated with early selection of unattended stimuli. Rees *et al.* (1997) studied activity in V5 (MT) produced by irrelevant visual motion. When the perceptual load of the primary visual task (see above) was low, the irrelevant motion elicited marked activity in V5. When the perceptual load of the primary task was high, then the irrelevant motion did not elicit any activity in V5 (MT) above that seen in a condition in which there was no visual motion (see Fig. 15.5). This study shows that when the primary visual task has a high load processing of irrelevant visual stimuli ceases at an early stage in the visual processing stream.

This study implies three things. First, the strength of the top-down signal increases with the difficulty (at least in terms of perceptual load) of the task for which selective attention is required. Second, selective attention specifically attenuates activity elicited by irrelevant stimuli (rather than, or as well as, increasing activity elicited by attended stimuli; see also the studies by Somers *et al.*, 1999, and Smith *et al.*, 2000, reviewed earlier in this chapter). Third, we cannot choose not to process irrelevant stimuli. If the task we have chosen to do does not use up our perceptual capacity, then irrelevant stimuli will be processed whether we like it or not. This point was already made by Lavie's behavioural studies. With a low load task, irrelevant stimuli do not just elicit neural activity, but they can also interfere with task performance. There is a sense, then, in which selective attention cannot be wilful. We can wilfully choose to perform a particular task, but the extent to which we can ignore irrelevant stimuli is wholly determined by the nature of the task being executed. No wonder the brain regions implicated in the top-down modulation of attention are identical to those implicated in executive processes.

The effect of a high-load task on the processing of irrelevant stimuli implies that there is a limited capacity system for perceptual processing. Other stimuli will simply not be processed once this capacity is filled, whether or not they are relevant. The attentional blink seems to be an example of this effect (Broadbent and Broadbent, 1987). This is the observation that there is a transient, but severe, impairment in the ability to see the second of two targets that are close together in time. This effect, which lasts about 400 ms, is particularly marked when the detection

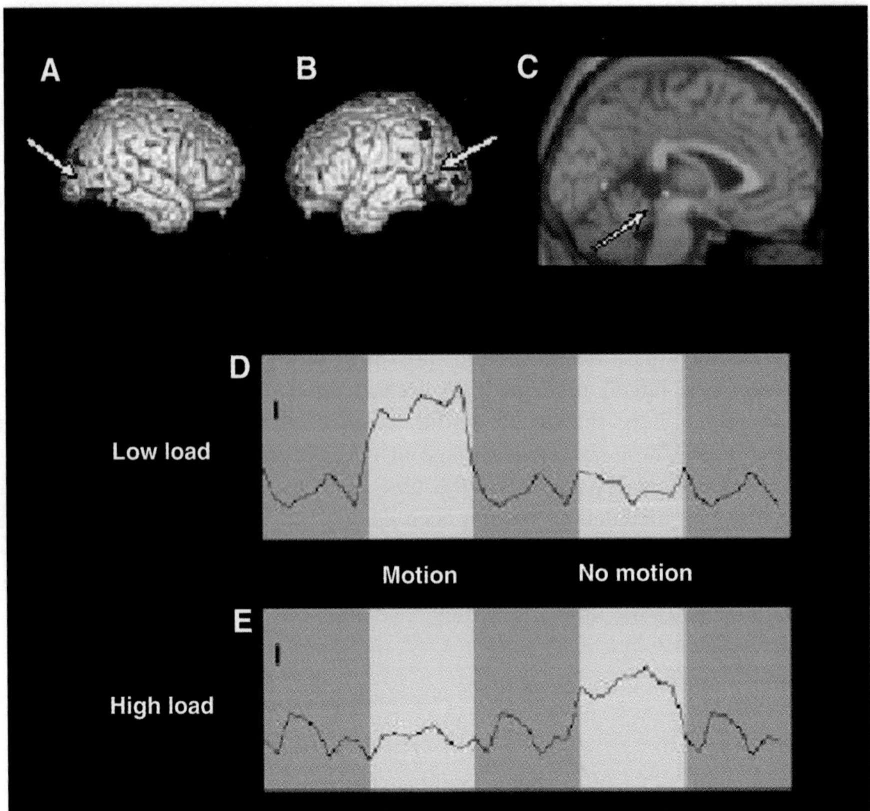

FIGURE 15.5
(A) and (B) Lateral views of the right and left hemispheres of a T1-weighted-volume, rendered anatomical image that conforms to the stereotactic space of Talairach and Tournoux. Superimposed in red are areas where brain activity in the group of participants showed the predicted interaction between the effects of visual motion and linguistic processing load. The locations of the right and left V5 complex activity are indicated by the arrows. (C) A sagittal slice through the same canonical anatomical image, on which is superimposed the location of activity in the SC (arrow) that is due to the interaction of visual motion and linguistic processing load. (D) and (E) Mean activity over all participants and replications of each experimental condition taken from the left V5 complex area. Activity during baseline periods (dark grey shading) is shown alternating with that during experimental conditions (light grey shading). The order in which the conditions are displayed is illustrative and does not correspond to that used in the experiment (order of conditions was counterbalanced across participants). The scale bar represents a value of 0.1% BOLD signal change. (From Rees, G. *et al.*, 2001. With permission.)

of the first target is made difficult by the presence of distracters. In a series of experiments, Marois *et al.* (2000a,b) showed that, in target detection tasks that induce an attentional blink, there was greater activity in the same intraparietal and frontal cortex regions previously associated with attentional control (IPS and PMC).

In both the studies we have just reviewed, the irrelevant visual stimuli were in the same modality as the attentional task. Rees *et al.* (2001) investigated the effect of load on the processing of irrelevant visual motion when the primary task was in the auditory modality. Volunteers either detected loud voices among quiet voices (low load) or two-syllable words among one- and three-syllable words (high load). In this experiment, the load of the auditory task had no effect on the processing of irrelevant visual motion either in terms of activity in V5 (MT) or in terms of the length of the visual motion after-effect. Behavioural studies have also noted this lack of a load effect across modalities (Soto-Faraco, 2002; but see Berman and Colby, 2002). This result suggests that perceptual capacity is modality specific, so that, for example, filling the capacity in the visual domain has no effect on the auditory domain. This is consistent with claims that the attentional blink also is modality specific (Duncan *et al.*, 1997). Shulman *et al.* (1997) reached similar conclusions on the basis of a meta-analysis of several studies of visual attention. They concluded that there was little evidence for attenuation of activity in early stages of auditory or somatosensory processing during attention to the visual modality. Experiments

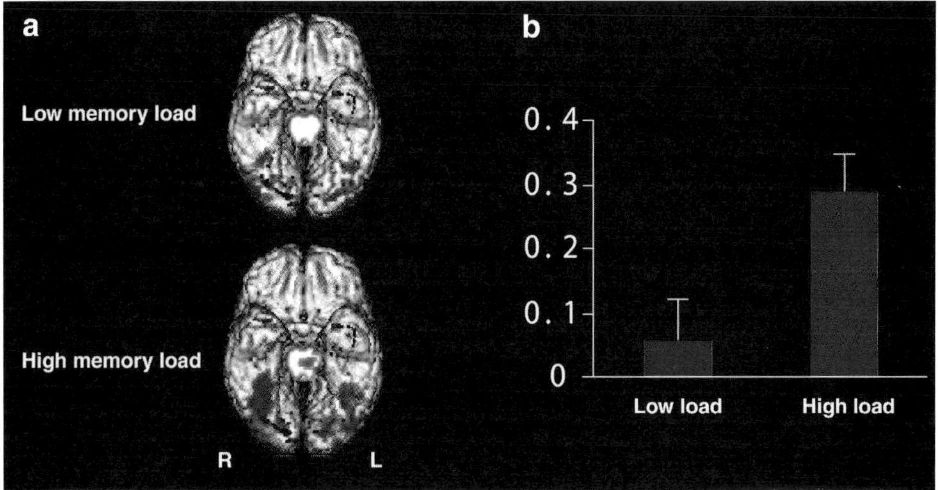

FIGURE 15.6
Distracter-related activity in high versus low working memory. (A) Two views of the ventral surface of a template brain on which are superimposed loci where activity was significantly greater in the presence than in the absence of distractor faces under conditions of low working memory load (top) and high working memory load (bottom). A threshold of $Z = 3.10$ (corresponding to $p = 0.001$, uncorrected) is used for display purposes. (B) Mean distracter-related activity (percent signal change for face presence minus face absence) for the maxima of the interaction in the right fusiform gyrus (36, −64, −16), plotted separately for low and high working memory load. Data are averaged across participants. Error bars represent interparticipant standard error. (From deFockert, J. *et al.*, 2001. With permission.)

contrasting attentional competition within and between modalities would be extremely interesting, as the evidence so far suggests that different mechanisms may be involved. Perhaps competition between modalities only occurs at a relatively late stage of processing.

The Role of Working Memory in Attention

We have repeatedly noted the correspondences between selective attention and working memory both in terms of brain regions activated (frontal and parietal) and cognitive processes engaged (keeping in mind task priorities). deFockert *et al.* (2001) directly studied the effect of working memory load on selective attention. They argued that, if selective attention engages the same processes as do working memory tasks, then performance of a working memory task should interfere with the ability to selectively attend. In order to engage their working memory, volunteers were given a string of digits to hold in mind while they performed an additional, unrelated task. They had to decide whether names presented successively belonged to politicians or pop stars, while an irrelevant face distracter was presented. When the working memory load was high the irrelevant distracters caused greater interference effects on performance of the selective attention task and elicited greater activity in the fusiform face area (see Fig. 15.6). This result shows that the process that attenuates responses to irrelevant distracters cannot be fully engaged by a selective attention task if a traditional working memory task is already being performed. We assume, therefore, that one of the processes common to selective attention and working memory has the role of attenuating responses to irrelevant stimuli. Because, in this experiment, the attention task was visual while the working memory task was usually considered to be auditory/verbal (even though the letters were presented visually), we speculate this process for attenuating responses to irrelevant stimuli operates across modalities.

We presume that the source of the attenuating signal must arise in a brain region that is activated by the high-load working memory task. Three regions were activated more for the high-load than the low-load working memory task: prefrontal cortex (BA44), premotor cortex (BA8), and superior parietal lobule (BA7). The activation in Broca's area (left BA44) probably relates specifically to the need to keep a sequence of digits in mind, a requirement that is likely to have engaged the articulatory loop; however, the premotor and parietal activations are in locations similar to those seen in many studies of attention and working memory. Indeed, the location of the premotor activation (BA8) is almost identical to that reported in studies of Rowe *et al.* (2000, 2001), where sustained activity was seen during the performance of a very different working memory task involving spatial material.

Intention and Attention

Lavie's studies of the effects of load on attention show that the focus of attention is determined by the nature of the task the volunteer intends to perform. Some aspects of this focus are explicit—for example, when the volunteer has been instructed to monitor the RED letter strings; however, there are also implicit effects of intention that determine whether or not stimuli will be attended to. Whenever we perform an attentional task, a number of sensory changes will result directly from performance of the task. If we move our eyes to fixate the target of attention, then there will be dramatic changes in stimulation of many retinal locations. If we press a button to indicate that we have detected the target, then there will be tactile stimulation of our finger. If we give a verbal response, then there will be auditory stimulation from the sound of our own voice. These stimuli are entirely uninformative and can be predicted on the basis of our intended actions. The brain activity elicited by these stimuli is minimal. In these cases, the response to the stimuli has been attenuated because their occurrence can be predicted. This is another example of a top-down effect at the physiological level with no equivalent top-down process at the psychological level.

Fink *et al.* (1997) contrasted attention to spatial locations and attention to parts of objects. In one condition, as in most studies of this kind, the volunteers had to maintain their gaze on the centre of the display; however, a second condition was included in which they were allowed to move their eyes at will. In this condition, all the volunteers made saccadic eye movements when the stimuli were presented. This condition was therefore associated with movements of stimuli across the retina. However, while there was significantly more activity in V1 in the condition with eye movements, there was no detectable difference in activity in any other visual area including V5 (MT) the visual motion area.

Curio *et al.* (2000) used magnetoencephalography (MEG) to show that we do not respond to the sound of our own voice. When volunteers heard a sequence of speech sounds consisting of repetitions of the vowel /a/ interspersed with the occasional /ae/, the odd-ball stimulus elicited a characteristic evoked potential. However, if the volunteer repeatedly said the syllable /ga/ aloud, then there was no special response when he infrequently said /ba/. The same effect occurs if the sound is self-produced much more indirectly. Schafer and Marcus (1973) used EEG to measure auditory evoked potentials to tones. In one condition, the volunteers generated the tones themselves by pressing a button. In this case, the amplitude of the evoked potential was much reduced in comparison to tones that were occurring randomly and not under the control of the volunteer. Blakemore *et al.* (1998a) repeated this experiment using PET. Activity in auditory cortex was reduced when the tones were predictable, either because they occurred regularly or because they were generated by the volunteer pressing a button.

The same results have been demonstrated in the tactile domain. Blakemore *et al.* (1998b) showed that self-generated tactile stimuli activate primary and secondary somatosensory cortex far less than the same stimulus applied by someone else. In this experiment, the volunteer stimulated the palm of his left hand with a tickling stick held in his right hand. It has also been found that an active arm movement elicits less activity in parietal cortex than the same movement made passively (Weiller *et al.*, 1996; Blakemore *et al.*, 2003). It is generally believed that the attenuation of these self-generated sensory signals is achieved through a system that predicts the sensory consequences of movements on the basis of the commands sent to the motor system. It is also believed that the cerebellum has a major role in the development of this forward model. Results from the few relevant imaging studies are consistent with this belief (Blakemore *et al.*, 1999b, 2001).

All of these studies show that the sensory stimulation generated by our own actions are automatically attenuated and thereby largely eliminated from attention. Presumably these effects can be overridden, such as when we use our fingers to feel the roughness of a surface, but we are not aware of any experiments on this topic.

BEYOND THE BIASED COMPETITION MODEL

The biased competition model has provided a very useful framework, not only for structuring this chapter but also for guiding neuroimaging studies of selective attention in many different laboratories; however, at least in the form we have presented it here, the biased competition model is underspecified. It states that there are bottom-up processes that determine which stimulus will win the competition for attention, but it does not say anything about the intrinsic properties of the stimulus that wins. The model states that there is a top-down biasing signal that modifies the competition, but it does not say anything about the nature of this top-down signal. Now that so many imaging experiments have been performed, is it possible to use all these observations to flesh out the model a little? In the last section of this chapter, we will make some suggestions that go slightly beyond the biased competition model.

The Distinction Between Bottom-Up and Top-Down Processes

As we have already noted, the distinction between bottom-up and top-down processes can be made at the level of physiology and at the level of psychology, but these two ways of making the distinction need not correspond. At the physiological level, the distinction is made in terms of the direction of flow of neural signals. Bottom-up signals go from primary sensory areas to secondary sensory areas and so on. Top-down signals go in the opposite direction and are sometimes referred to as reentrant or feedback signals. Anatomically, the majority of reciprocal connections between cortical areas are symmetric with regard to the cortical layers in which connections originate and terminate. This has led to the hypothesis of an anatomical hierarchy, with some connections representing forward (ascending) connections while their reciprocal counterparts represent feedback pathways (Felleman and Van Essen, 1991; but see Young, 1992). At the psychological level, bottom-up processes are determined solely by the current stimuli or, in other words, they are stimulus driven. Top-down processes involve more than the current stimuli but have two forms that we might refer to as weak and strong. If there is an effect of recently acquired knowledge on the way stimuli are processed, then this would be an example of a weak top-down process. This is an example of the prior state of the volunteer altering the way in which the stimulus is processed; however, this effect might occur automatically without the volunteer intending it or even being aware of it. We would therefore reserve the use of the term *strong top-down processes* for situations in which the volunteer deliberately and consciously adopts a particular state (or *script*, to use the term of Jack and Roepstorff, 2002), usually on the basis of instructions from the experimenter. In this case, the top-down signal flows from the experimenter (via the homunculus).

It is clear that the distinction in cognitive terms need not coincide with the distinction in physiological terms. When there is competition or cooperation between signals processed in distant sites and processing is modified in one site by what is happening in the other, this must be due to a top-down, reentrant signal. Direct evidence for such an effect comes from the study by Macaluso *et al.* (2000a). In this example, activity in a visual area was modified by the occurrence of a tactile stimulus via top-down signals from a parietal area. At the cognitive level, no top-down processes were involved as there was no prior knowledge available to modify the processing of the visual stimulus. We cannot therefore always map top-down processes at the cognitive level onto reentrant signals at the physiological level.

Nevertheless, we can speculate that another kind of mapping is possible. The deliberate deployment of attention is robustly associated with activity in parietal and frontal cortex. However, activity in parietal cortex is also found when prior knowledge is automatically applied and, in the experiment of Macaluso *et al.*, even where there was no prior knowledge. Furthermore, the studies of Büchel and Friston suggest that parietal cortex is below prefrontal cortex in a hierarchy of control. We are therefore led to the hypothesis that strong top-down processes are specifically associated with frontal, and more probably prefrontal activity. In other words, strong top-down processes at the psychological level map onto reentrant signals arising from prefrontal cortex.

The Role of Information in Bottom-Up Competition

We have just defined bottom-up processes (at the psychological level) as being concerned solely with the current stimuli and being independent of the state of our volunteer. In this case, there should be some intrinsic property that predicts which stimuli will win and which will lose the competition for attention. What property is it that determines that some stimuli are more salient than others?

We have observed that self-generated stimuli hardly ever win the competition. The mechanism by which self-generated sensory signals are attenuated depends upon prediction. The forward model predicts what sensory signals will occur and precisely when they will arrive (Blakemore *et al.*, 1999a). In terms of information theory, the occurrence of a predictable stimulus provides no information. We already knew what was going to happen. Such stimuli do not attract our attention. Conversely, an unexpected event provides much information. Such stimuli do attract our attention. All other things being equal, when many stimuli are impinging upon us, it will be the one carrying the highest information that will win the competition, elicit the most activity, and reach the forefront of our attention. This happens because the brain is continually trying to predict what will happen next. If we knew about the mechanisms underlying these predictions, it should be possible to compute the information provided by a stimulus and thus predict the likelihood that it will attract attention. Much of the brain's predictions operate over rather short periods of time. Sudden changes in stimulus intensity (*e.g.*, visual transients) are noticed because they violate short-term expectations that stimulation will remain as they were. Very slow changes will not attract our attention and may remain undetected in the absence of prior knowledge (Simons *et al.*, 2000). Precisely because it is slow the change can be predicted by the brain and therefore does not carry information.

The odd-ball paradigm is particularly suited to analysis in terms of information. The information carried by the odd-ball stimulus will depend upon its frequency relative to the standard. Low-frequency odd-balls elicit greater activity (*e.g.*, Braver *et al.*, 2001); however, the information carried by the odd-ball will also vary from moment to moment depending on how long it is since the last odd-ball occurred. This variation also effects elicited activity (Huettel *et al.*, 2002). We suggest therefore, that one factor that determines the salience of a stimulus, the bottom-up factor, is the amount of information that it carries. This is consistent with recent observations that single-unit activity in monkey V1 reflects both behavioural evidence and higher order perceptual saliency (Lee *et al.*, 2002)

The Role of Value in Top-Down Control

So far we have suggested that bottom-up attentional effects can be explained in terms of expectation. We can also think about top-down (willed) attentional effects in terms of expectations. We have already concluded that top-down attentional biasing is not the result of deciding to attend selectively to something; rather, it the result of deciding (or being instructed) to perform a task. The top-down biasing results from the task instructions (or the *script*, to use Jack and Roepstorff's term). The script tells the volunteer what to expect and what to do. The script specifies that some stimuli are important while others should be ignored. It specifies that there are certain responses that should be used while others should not be used. It specifies the meaning of the responses that should be used (*e.g.*, pressing the left button means a red light has been seen).

The importance of expectations in the operation of top-down biases is illustrated by an experiment in which volunteers were not fully informed (Frith and Allen, 1983). They were told to press a button whenever the word *PRESS* appeared on a computer screen. They were also told that the word *READY* would appear and remain on the screen for 10 seconds immediately prior to the word *PRESS*. The volunteers were not told that irrelevant tones would also occur. The first time that an irrelevant tone occurred while the word *READY* was on the screen the majority of the volunteers pressed the button. This erroneous response never happened again, presumably because tones were then added to the script as possible events that should be ignored.

How does the expectation created by the script for task performance relate to information? Because both the relevant and the irrelevant stimuli are equally expected and often equally frequent, they do not differ in information. Instead, they differ in value. If we were teaching a monkey to do the task, then responses to relevant stimuli would be rewarded while responses to irrelevant stimuli would not. Our instructions to the volunteer permit the instant attachment of value to the relevant stimuli. The value of a stimulus depends upon the context in which it is occurring, or, in other words, on the script currently in operation. In animals, stimuli acquire value by a slow process of learning in which neurotransmitters such as dopamine and subcortical regions such as the basal ganglia play a key role (see Schultz, 1998, for a review). One of the major questions that cognitive brain imagers must address concerns how verbal instructions (and self-generated scripts) can so readily short-circuit this slow learning process.

How Salience Depends on Both Information and Value

Value is independent of information, but, whether a stimulus is salient (*i.e.*, whether or not it will capture our attention), depends on the combination of value and information. In change blindness experiments, the volunteer anticipates that changes will occur and puts high value on these changes, but the information in the changes is too low, relative to the visual transients associated with the blank screen or other salient changes, to capture attention. During inattentional blindness experiments, a change fails to attract attention for opposite reasons. The student is so intent on explaining to the stranger how to get to the psychology department that the identity of the stranger has no value to her. The replacement of the stranger by someone else does not attract her attention (Simons, 2000). In this example, the information in the change is high, but the value placed upon the change by the current script is low. The change does not capture attention. But, this experiment only works once; the next time the student has a new script: "Always be on your guard against psychologists," which alters the value of irrelevant changes. Another key question for cognitive imagers to address concerns the mechanism by which information and value interact to determine the salience of a stimulus.

The Implementation of Top-Down Control

This aspect of attention is a component of the executive systems discussed in Chapter 18 and all the evidence points to a key role for frontal cortex, with parietal cortex in a subsidiary position. In a typical experiment, the top-down control is needed to apply and maintain the task priorities or script. We have already mentioned three distinct requirements: (1) assigning value to stimuli (*i.e.*, specifying categories of relevant and irrelevant stimuli), (2) assigning value to responses (*i.e.*, specifying categories of appropriate and inappropriate responses), and (3) assigning meanings to the appropriate responses. In animal experiments, the monkey learns through rewards to assign values to particular stimuli in particular contexts. In human studies, the instructions given by the experimenter determine the script adopted by the volunteer and this effectively generates an instant and arbitrary context for the experiment. At least part of the work done by prefrontal cortex is necessary to maintain this arbitrary, self-imposed context against competition from older, better-established scripts. Whichever region is involved in this maintenance is at the top of the hierarchy of control. Below this level are the regions with similar roles applied in more specific domains such as maintaining the relative values of stimuli or responses for the duration of the experiment. It is likely that these roles can be assigned to specific regions of frontal cortex, as we hint at in Chapter 18. For example, dorsolateral prefrontal cortex may be necessary for designating and maintaining appropriate and inappropriate responses. So, can the region at the top of the hierarchy be identified with the homunculus? It has the desirable property of not needing to be very clever, because all it needs to decide is, "Shall I do what the experimenter wants or not?" To which we reply, "Are you feeling lucky, homunculus?"

References

Allman, J. M. and Kaas, J. H. (1971). A representation of the visual field in the posterior third of the middle temporal gyrus of the owl monkey (*Aotus trivirgatus*). *Brain Res.*, **31**, 85–105.

Andersen, R. A. (1997). Multimodal integration for the representation of space in the posterior parietal cortex. *Philos. Trans. Roy. Soc. London B, Biol. Sci.*, **352**, 1421–1428.

Aristotle. (1931). *The Works of Aristotle*. Volume III. *Parva Naturalia: De Somniis*, Ross, W. D., Ed. (translated by J. I. Beare). Clarendon, Oxford.

Beauchamp, M. S., Cox, R. W., and DeYoe, E. A. (1997). Graded effects of spatial and featural attention on human area MT and associated motion processing areas. *J. Neurophysiol.*, **78**, 516–520.

Beck, D., Rees, G., Frith, C. D., and Lavie, N. (2001). Neural correlates of change detection and change blindness. *Nat. Neurosci.*, **4**, 645–650.

Berman, R.A. and Colby C. (2002). Auditory and visual attention modulate motion processing in area MT+. *Cogn. Brain Res.*, **14**, 64–74.

Blakemore, S. J., Rees, G., and Frith, C. D. (1998a). How do we predict the consequences of our actions? A functional imaging study. *Neuropsychologia*. **36**, 521–529.

Blakemore, S. J., Wolpert, D. M., and Frith, C. D. (1998b). Central cancellation of self-produced tickle sensation *Nat. Neurosci.*, **1**, 635–640.

Blakemore, S. J., Frith, C. D., and Wolpert, D. M. (1999a). Spatio-temporal prediction modulates the perception of self-produced stimuli. *J. Cogn. Neurosci.*, **11**, 551–559.

Blakemore, S. J., Wolpert, D. M., and Frith, C. D. (1999b). The cerebellum contributes to somatosensory cortical activity during self-produced tactile stimulation. *NeuroImage*, **10**, 448–459.

Blakemore, S. J., Frith, C. D., and Wolpert, D. M. (2001). The cerebellum is involved in predicting the sensory consequences of action. *NeuroReport*, **12**, 1879–1884.

Blakemore, S. J., Oakley, D., and Frith, C. (2003). Delusions of alien control in the normal brain. *Neuropsychologia*, **41**, 1058–1067.

Braver, T. S., Barch, D. M., Grey, J. R., Molfese, D. L., and Snyder, A. (2001). Anterior cingulate cortex and response conflict: effects of frequency, inhibition and errors. *Cereb. Cortex*, **11**, 825–836.

Brefczynski, J. A. and DeYoe, E. A. (1999). A physiological correlate of the 'spotlight' of visual attention. *Nat. Neurosci.*, **2**, 370–374.

Broadbent, D. E. and Broadbent, M. H. P. (1987). From detection to identification: response to multiple targets in rapid serial visual presentation. *Percept. Psychophys.*, **42**, 105–113.

Büchel, C. and Friston, K. J. (1997). Modulation of connectivity in visual pathways by attention: cortical interactions evaluated with structural equation modelling and fMRI. *Cereb. Cortex*, **7**, 768–778.

Büchel, C., Josephs, O., Rees, G., Turner, R., Frith, C. D., and Friston, K. J. (1998). The functional anatomy of attention to visual motion: a functional MRI study. *Brain*, **121**, 1281–1294.

Büchel, C., Coull, J. T., and Friston, K. J. (1999). The predictive value of changes in effective connectivity for human learning. *Science*, **283**(5407), 1538–1541.

Calvert, G. A., Campbell, R., and Brammer, M. J. (2000). Evidence from functional magnetic resonance imaging of crossmodal binding in the human heteromodal cortex. *Curr. Biol.*, **10**, 649–657.

Chaudhuri, A. (1991). Modulation of the motion aftereffect by selective attention. *Nature*, **344**, 60–62.

Chawla, D., Rees, G., and Friston, K. J. (1999). The physiological basis of attentional modulation in extrastriate visual areas. *Nat. Neurosci.*, **2**, 671–676.

Chawla, D., Lumer, E. D., and Friston, K. J. (2000). Relating macroscopic measures of brain activity to fast, dynamic neuronal interactions. *Neural Comput.*, **12**, 2805–2821.

Corbetta, M. and Shulman, G. L. (1998). Human cortical mechanisms of visual attention during orienting and search. *Philos. Trans. Roy. Soc. London B, Biol. Sci.*, **353**(1373), 1353–1362.

Corbetta, M. and Shulman, G. L. (2002). Control of goal-directed and stimulus-driven attention in the brain. *Nat. Rev. Neurosci.*, **3**, 201–215.

Corbetta, M., Miezin, F. M., Dobmeyer, S., Shulman, G. L., and Petersen, S. E. (1990). Attentional modulation of neural processing of shape, colour, and velocity in humans. *Science*, **248**, 1556–1559.

Corbetta, M., Shulman, G. L., Miezin, F. M., and Petersen, S. E. (1995). Superior parietal cortex activation during spatial attention shifts and visual feature conjunction. *Science*, **270**, 802–805.

Corbetta, M., Kincade, J. M., Ollinger, J. M., McAvoy, M. P., and Shulman, G. L. (2000). Voluntary orienting is dissociated from target detection in human posterior parietal cortex. *Nat. Neurosci.*, **3**, 292–297.

Corteen, R. S. and Wood, B. (1972). Autonomic responses to shock associated words. *J. Exp. Psychol.*, **94**, 308–313.

Coull, J. T. and Frith, C. D. (1998). Differential activation of right superior parietal cortex and intraparietal sulcus by spatial and nonspatial attention. *NeuroImage*, **8**(2).:176–87.

Coull, J. T. and Nobre, A. C. (1998). Where and when to pay attention: the neural systems for directing attention to spatial locations and to time intervals as revealed by both PET and fMRI. *J. Neurosci.*, **18**, 7426–7435.

Culham, J. C., Brandt, S. A., Cavanagh, P., Kanwisher, N. G., Dale, A. M., and Tootell, R. B. (1998). Cortical fMRI activation produced by attentive tracking of moving targets. *J. Neurophysiol.*, **80**(5), 2657–2670.

Culham, J. C., Cavanagh, P., and Kanwisher, N. G. (2001). Attention response functions: characterising brain areas using fMRI activation during parametric variations of attentional load. *Neuron*, **32**, 737–745.

Curio, G., Neuloh, G., Numminen, J., Jousmaki, V., and Hari, R. (2000). Speaking modifies voice-evoked activity in the human auditory cortex. *Hum. Brain Mapping*, **9**(4), 183–191.

deFockert, J., Rees, G., Frith, C. D., and Lavie, N. (2001). The role of working memory in the control of attention. *Science*, **291**, 1803.

Desimone, R. and Duncan, J. (1995). Neural mechanisms of selective visual attention. *Annu. Rev. Neurosci.*, **18**, 193–222.

Downar, J., Crawley, A. P., Mikulis, D. J., and Davis, K. D. (2000). A multimodal cortical network for the detection of changes in the sensory environment. *Nat. Neurosci.*, **3**(3), 277–283.

Driver, J. and Mattingley, J. B. (1998). Parietal neglect and visual awareness. *Nat. Neurosci.*, **1**, 17–22.

Duncan, J. (1980). The locus of interference in the perception of simultaneous stimuli. *Psychol. Rev.*, **87**(3), 272–300.

Duncan, J., Martens, S., and Ward, R. (1997). Restricted attentional capacity within but not between sensory modalities. *Nature*, **387**(6635), 808–810.

Felleman, D. J. and Van Essen, D. C. (1991). Distributed hierarchical processing in the primate cerebral cortex. *Cereb. Cortex*, **1**, 1–47.

Fink, G. R., Dolan, R. J., Halligan, P. W., Marshall, J. C., and Frith, C. D. (1997). Space-based and object-based visual attention: shared and specific neural domains. *Brain*, **120**, 2013–2028.

Fink, G. R., Driver, J., Rorden, C., Baldeweg, T., and Dolan, R. J. (2000). Neural consequences of competing stimuli in both visual hemifields: a physiological basis for visual extinction. *Ann. Neurol.*, **47**(4), 440–446.

Friston, K. J. and Büchel, C. (2000). Attentional modulation of effective connectivity from V2 to V5 (MT) in humans. *Proc. Natl. Acad. Sci. USA*, **97**(13), 7591–7596.

Frith, C. D. and Friston, K. J. (1996). The role of the thalamus in "top down" modulation of attention to sound. *NeuroImage*, **4**(3, Pt. 1), 210–215.

Gandhi, S. P., Heeger, D. J., and Boynton, G. M. (1999). Spatial attention affects brain activity in human primary visual cortex. *Proc. Natl. Acad. Sci. USA*, **96**(6), 3314–3319.

Haenny, P. E. and Schiller, P. H. (1988). State dependent activity in monkey visual cortex. I. Single cell activity in V1 and V4 on visual tasks. *Exp. Brain Res.*, **69**, 225–244.

Heinze, H. J., Mangun, G. R., Burchert, W., Hinrichs, H., Scholz, M., Munte, T. F., Gos, A., Scherg, M., Johannes, S., Hundeshagen, H. *et al.* (1994). Combined spatial and temporal imaging of brain activity during visual selective attention in humans. *Nature*, **372**(6506), 543–546.

Hillyard, S. A., Hink, R. F., Schwent, V. L., and Picton T. W. (1973). Electrical signs of selective attention in the human brain. *Science*, **182**, 177–180.

Hillyard, S. A., Mangun, G. R., Woldorff, M. G., and Luck, S. J. (1995). Neural systems mediating selective attention, in *The Cognitive Neurosciences*, Gazzaniga, M. S., Ed., pp. 665–680. MIT Press, Cambridge, MA.

Huettel, S. A., Mack, P. B., and McCarthy, G. (2002). Perceiving patterns in random series: dynamic processing of sequence in prefrontal cortex. *Nat. Neurosci.*, **5**, 485–490.

Huk, A. C., Ress, D., and Heeger, D. J. (2001). Neuronal basis of the motion aftereffect reconsidered. *Neuron*, **32**(1), 161–172.

Jack, A. I. and Roepstorff, A. (2002). Retrospection and cognitive brain mapping: from stimulus–response to script–report. *Trends Cogn. Sci.*, **6**(8), 333–339.

James, W. (1890/1976). *The Principles of Psychology*. Harvard University Press, Cambridge, MA.

Jovicich, J., Peters, R. J., Koch, C., Braun, J., Chang, L., and Ernst, T. (2001). Brain areas specific for attentional load in a motion-tracking task. *J. Cogn. Neurosci.*, **13**(8), 1048–1058.

Kanwisher, N., McDermott, J., and Chun, M. M. (1997). The fusiform face area: a module in human extrastriate cortex specialised for face perception. *J. Neurosci.*, **17**, 4302–4311.

Kastner, S., De Weerd, P., Desimone, R., and Ungerleider, L. G. (1998). Mechanisms of directed attention in the human extrastriate cortex as revealed by functional MRI. *Science*, **282**, 108–111.

Kastner, S., Pinsk, M. A., De Weerd, P., Desimone, R., and Ungerleider, L. G. (1999). Increased activity in human visual cortex during directed attention in the absence of visual stimulation. *Neuron*, **22**, 751–761.

Kastner, S., De Weerd, P., Pinsk, M. A., Elizondo, M. I., Desimone, R., and Ungerleider, L. G. (2001). Modulation of sensory suppression: implications for receptive field sizes in the human visual cortex. *J. Neurophysiol.*, **86**, 1398–1411.

Lavie, N. (1995). Perceptual load as a necessary condition for selective attention. *J. Exp. Psychol. Hum. Percept. Perform.*, **21**, 451–468.

Lee, D. K., Itti, L., Koch, C., and Braun, J. (1999). Attention activates winner-take-all competition among visual filters. *Nat. Neurosci.*, **2**, 375–381.

Lee, T. S., Yang, C. F., Romero, R. D., and Mumford, D. (2002). Neural activity in early visual cortex reflects behavioural experience and higher-order perceptual saliency. *Nat. Neurosci.*, **5**, 589–597.

Macaluso, E., Frith, C., and Driver, J. (2000a). Selective spatial attention in vision and touch: unimodal and multimodal mechanisms revealed by PET. *J. Neurophysiol.*, **83**, 3062–3075.

Macaluso, E., Frith, C. D., and Driver, J. (2000b). Modulation of human visual cortex by crossmodal spatial attention. *Science*, **289**, 1206–1208.

Mangun, G. R., Buonocore, M. H., Girelli, M., and Jha, A. P. (1998). ERP and fMRI measures of visual spatial selective attention. *Hum. Brain Mapping*, **6**(5–6), 383–389.

Marois, R., Chun, M. M., and Gore, J. C. (2000a). Neural correlates of the attentional blink. *Neuron*, **28**, 299–308.

Marois, R., Leung, H. C., and Gore, J. C. (2000b). A stimulus-driven approach to object identity and location processing in the human brain. *Neuron*, **25**, 717–728.

Moran, J. and Desimone, R. (1985). Selective attention gates visual processing in the extrastriate cortex. *Science*, **229**, 782–784.

O'Connor, D. H., Fukui, M. M., Pinsk, M. A., and Kastner, S. (2002). Attention modulates responses in the human lateral geniculate nucleus. *Nat. Neurosci.*, **5**, 1203–1209.

O'Craven, K. M., Rosen, B. R., Kwong, K. K., Treisman, A., and Savoy, R. L. (1997). Voluntary attention modulates fMRI activity in human MT-MST. *Neuron*, **18**, 591–598.

O'Craven, K. M., Downing, P. E., and Kanwisher, N. (1999). fMRI evidence for objects as the units of attentional selection. *Nature*, **401**, 584–587.

O'Regan, J. K., Rensink, R. A., and Clark, J. J. (1999). Change-blindness as a result of 'mudsplashes' [letter]. *Nature*, **398**, 34.

Posner, M. I. (1980). Orienting of attention. *Q. J. Exp. Psychol.*, **32**, 3–25.

Price, C. J. (1998). The functional anatomy of word comprehension and production. *Trends Cogn. Sci.*, **2**, 281–288.

Puce, A., Allison, T., Gore, J. C., and McCarthy, G. (1995). Face-sensitive regions in human extrastriate cortex studied by functional MRI. *J. Neurophysiol.*, **74**, 1192–1199.

Pylyshyn, Z. W. and Storm, R.W. (1988). Tracking multiple independent targets: evidence for a parallel tracking mechanism. *Spatial Vis.*, **3**(3), 179–197.

Rees, G. and Frith, C. D. (1998). How do we select perceptions and actions? Human brain imaging studies. (1998). *Philos. Trans. Roy. Soc. London B*, **353**, 1283–1293.

Rees, G., Frith, C. D., and Lavie, N. (1997). Modulating irrelevant motion perception by varying attentional load in an unrelated task. *Science*, **278**, 1616–1619.

Rees, G., Russell, C., Frith, C. D., and Driver, J. (1999). Inattentional blindness versus inattentional amnesia for fixated but ignored words. *Science*, **286**, 2504–2507.

Rees, G., Wojciulik, E., Clarke, K., Husain, M., Frith, C., and Driver, J. (2000). Unconscious activation of visual cortex in the damaged right hemisphere of a parietal patient with extinction. *Brain*, **123**, 1624–1633.

Rees, G., Frith, C., and Lavie, N. (2001). Perception of irrelevant visual motion during performance of an auditory attention task. *Neuropsychologia*, **39**, 937–949.

Rees, G., Wojciulik, E., Clarke, K., Husain, M., Frith, C. D., and Driver J. (2002). Neural correlates of conscious and unconscious vision in parietal extinction. *Neurocase*, **8**, 387–393.

Rensink, R. A., O'Regan, J. K., and Clark, J. J. (1997). To see or not to see: the need for attention to perceive changes in scenes. *Psychol. Sci.*, **8**, 368–373.

Robertson, I. H., Mattingley, J. B., Rorden, C., and Driver, J. (1998). Phasic alerting of neglect patients overcomes their spatial deficit in visual awareness. *Nature*, **395**, 169–172.

Rock, I. and Gutman, D. (1981). The effect of inattention on form perception *J. Exp. Psychol.Hum. Percept. Perform.*, **7**, 275–285.

Rowe, J. B. and Passingham, R. E. (2001). Working memory for location and time: activity in prefrontal area 46 relates to selection rather than maintenance in memory. *NeuroImage*, **14**, 77–86.

Rowe, J. B., Toni, I., Josephs, O., Frackowiak, R. S., and Passingham, R. E. (2000). The prefrontal cortex: response selection or maintenance within working memory? *Science*, **288**, 1656–1660.

Schafer, E. W. and Marcus, M.M. (1973). Self-stimulation alters human sensory brain responses. *Science*, **181**(95), 175–177.

Schultz, W. (1998). Predictive reward signal of dopamine neurons. *J. Neurophysiol.*, **80**(1), 1–27.

Shulman, G. L. (1991). Attentional modulation of mechanisms that analyse rotation in depth. *J. Exp. Psychol. Hum. Percept. Perform.*, **17**, 726–737.

Shulman, G. L., Corbetta, M., Buckner, R. L., Raichle, M. E., Fiez, J. A., Miezin, F. M., and Petersen, S. E. (1997). Top-down modulation of early sensory cortex. *Cereb. Cortex*, **7**(3), 193–206.

Smith, A. T., Singh, K. D., and Greenlee, M. W. (2000). Attentional suppression of activity in the human visual cortex. *NeuroReport*, **11**(2), 271–277.

Simons, D. J. (2000). Attentional capture and inattentional blindness. *Trends Cogn. Sci.*, **4**(4), 147–155.

Simons, D. J., Franconeri, S. L., and Reimer, R. L.(2000). Change blindness in the absence of a visual disruption. *Perception*, **29**(10), 1143–1154.

Somers, D. C., Dale, A. M., Seiffert, A. E., and Tootell, R. B. (1999). Functional MRI reveals spatially specific attentional modulation in human primary visual cortex. *Proc. Natl. Acad. Sci. USA*, **96**, 1663–1668.

Soto-Faraco, S. and Spence, C. (2002). Modality-specific auditory and visual temporal processing deficits. *Q. J. Exp. Psychol.*, **55A**(1), 5–22.

Tootell, R. B., Reppas, J. B., Dale, A. M., Look, R. B., Sereno, M. I., Malach, R., Brady, T. J., Rosen, B. R. (1995). Visual motion aftereffect in human cortical area MT revealed by functional magnetic resonance imaging. *Nature*, **375**, 139–141.

Treisman, A. and Geffen, G. (1967). Selective attention: perception or response? *Q. J. Exp. Psychol.*, **19**, 1–18.

Treisman, A. and Gelade, G. (1980). A feature-integration theory of attention. *Cogn. Psychol.*, **12**, 97–136.

Treue, S. and Maunsell, J. H. (1996). Attentional modulation of visual motion processing in cortical areas MT and MST. *Nature*, **382**(6591), 539–541.

Vallar, G. and Perani, D. (1986). The anatomy of unilateral neglect after right-hemisphere stroke lesions: a clinical/CT-scan correlation study in man. *Neuropsychologia*, **24**, 609–622.

Vandenberghe, R., Duncan, J., Dupont, P., Ward, R., Poline, J. B., Bormans, G., Michiels, J., Mortelmans, L., and Orban, G. A. (1997). Attention to one or two features in left or right visual field: a positron emission tomography study. *J. Neurosci.*, **17**, 3739–3750.

Vuilleumier, P., Sagiv, N., Hazeltine, E., Poldrack, R., Rafal, R., and Gabrieli, J. (2001). The neural fate of seen and unseen faces in visuospatial neglect: a combined event-related fMRI and ERP study of visual extinction. *Proc. Natl. Acad. Sci. USA*, **98**, 3495–3500.

Watanabe, T., Sasaki, Y., Miyauchi, S., Putz, B., Fujimaki, N., Nielsen, M., Takino, R., and Miyakawa, S. (1998). Attention-regulated activity in human primary visual cortex. *J. Neurophysiol.*, **79**, 2218–2221.

Watson, J. D., Myers, R., Frackowiak, R. S., Hajnal, J. V., Woods, R. P., Mazziotta, J. C., Shipp, S., and Zeki, S. (1993). Area V5 of the human brain: evidence from a combined study using positron emission tomography and magnetic resonance imaging. *Cereb. Cortex*, **3**, 79–94.

Weiller, C., Juptner, M., Fellows, S., Rijntjes, M., Leonhardt, G., Kiebel, S., Muller, S., Diener, H. C., Thilmann, A. F. (1996). Brain representation of active and passive movements. *NeuroImage*, **4**,105–110.

Wojciulik, E. and Kanwisher, N. (1999). The generality of parietal involvement in visual attention. *Neuron*, **23**, 747–764.

Wojciulik, E., Kanwisher, N., and Driver, J. (1998). Covert visual attention modulates face-specific activity in the human fusiform gyrus: fMRI study. *J. Neurophysiol.*, **79**(3), 1574–1578.

Young, M. P. (1992). Objective analysis of the topological organisation of the primate cortical visual system. *Nature*, **358**, 152–155.

Zeki, S. M. (1974). Functional organisation of a visual area in the posterior bank of the superior temporal sulcus of the rhesus monkey. *J. Physiol (London)*, **236**, 549–573.

Zeki, S. M. and Marini, L. (1998). Three cortical stages of colour processing in the human brain. *Brain*, **121**, 1669–1685.

Zeki, S. M., Watson, J. D., Lueck, C. J., Friston, K. J., Kennard, C., and Frackowiak, R. S. (1991). A direct demonstration of functional specialisation in human visual cortex. *J. Neurosci.*, **11**, 641–649.

CHAPTER

16

The Neural Correlates of Consciousness

AN EXPERIMENTAL FRAMEWORK

In the first edition of this book there was a final chapter on the future of imaging in which use of the word *consciousness* was strictly avoided until the very last sentence. Now that we have moved into a new millennium it has no longer been so easy to resist the *Zeitgeist*. That single sentence has become a whole chapter.

It is remarkable how willing neuroscientists have become to speculate about the biological basis of consciousness (Edelman, 1989; Crick, 1994), and philosophers who once dominated this topic increasingly defer to neuroscience data when discussing the nature of consciousness (Dennett, 1991; Churchland, 1993). From both sides of the debate we are told that questions about the neural basis of consciousness can be answered through experimentation. In this chapter, we shall try to make as clear as possible the assumptions that underlie such experiments and indicate the areas where progress is likely to be made in respect to functional imaging. We will, however, only consider the problem of the *association* between consciousness and neural activity. We have no idea how consciousness emerges from the physical activity of the brain and we do not know whether consciousness can emerge from non-biological systems, such as computers. Nevertheless, we believe that systematic exploration of the neural correlates of consciousness will increase our understanding of the nature and purpose of consciousness.

At this point the reader will expect to find a careful and precise definition of consciousness. You will be disappointed. Consciousness has not yet become a scientific term that can be defined in this way. Currently we all use the term *consciousness* in many different and often ambiguous ways. Precise definitions of different aspects of consciousness will emerge through an iterative process from the kinds of experiments we discuss in this chapter. No doubt some of these definitions will have a rough correspondence to some of the ways we use the term at the moment, but to make precise definitions at this stage is premature.

Rather than a precise definition we shall adopt William James' approach and claim that we all know what consciousness is. We all have first-hand knowledge of what it is like to be conscious, as opposed to not being conscious (as in deep, dreamless sleep). We all know that when we are conscious we experience something; our consciousness has phenomenal content. When consciousness is absent, then phenomenal content is also absent. (Whether, on the other hand, we can be conscious without having any experience is more controversial.) A major feature of our conscious experience is that the phenomenal content of this experience is constantly changing. Yet, at the same time, our sense of our self, the person having the experience, remains constant.

Questions about the neural correlates of consciousness are essentially questions about the relationships between mental states (states of consciousness) and neural states (states of the brain). A fundamental assumption is that for every mental state there is an associated neural state. We also assume that mental states are completely determined by neural states. In other words, it is impossible for there to be a change of mental state without a corresponding change in neural state. On the other hand, as we shall see, it *is* possible for there to be a change in neural state without a change in mental state.

Levels Versus Contents of Consciousness

A useful distinction can be made between factors influencing the overall level of consciousness and those determining its content. The level of consciousness is associated with arousal. It varies continuously from deep dreamless sleep, through drowsiness to alert wakefulness. As we shall see, quite circumscribed brain lesions can lead to severe restrictions in the level of consciousness, such as coma and persistent vegetative state. The level of consciousness can also be altered by exogenous substances, such as anaesthetics and psychoactive drugs (Kihlstrom *et al.*, 1990).

The other major aspect of consciousness is the content of subjective experience (*i.e.*, what one is conscious of). This is determined by the interaction between exogenous factors derived from our environment and endogenous factors such as attention. The contents of consciousness include percepts of the objects around us, memories of past events, and intentions concerning future actions. The contents of consciousness can vary quite independently of the level of consciousness. Specific brain lesions can alter the contents of consciousness without having any effects on the level of consciousness. For example, after posterior lesions patients can sometimes lose awareness of colour, while the awareness of other aspects of the world remains normal.

On the other hand, the level of arousal has a major influence on the contents of consciousness. On the whole, as arousal increases the extent and quality of conscious experience also increases; however, very high levels of arousal can be associated with impoverished contents of consciousness (Easterbrook, 1959). Of particular interest is the dream state characterised by vivid polymodal sensory experience (Hobson, 1988). As suggested by Llinas and Pare (1991), insights into the nature of consciousness can be gained by analysis of the similarities and differences between waking and dreaming and between these states and slow wave sleep. Both dreaming and wakefulness are endowed with subjective experience, although the former is dissociated from awareness of external (and internal) sensory events.

Conscious and Unconscious Processes

Many people have worried about how it is possible to relate the physical activity in neurons to the mental activity that forms the contents of consciousness. They question whether it is possible even in principle to link physical and mental entities. There is, however, a simple way in which activity in neurons fulfils the same function as the contents of consciousness.

The contents of consciousness have a special relation to things in the world. When I consciously perceive an object (such as a line), I have a mental representation of that line and its properties, such as its orientation. My mental representation of the line stands for the real line in the world outside. Mental representations can also stand for things that are not currently in the world outside. When I remember something, I have a mental representation of a past event. When I imagine something, I have a mental representation of something that could occur in the outside world. When I have the intention to perform some action, I have a mental representation of a future state of the world. But, neuroscientists also talk about representations in relation to activity in neurons. For example, the activity in a single cell in the visual cortex might be said to represent the orientation of a line falling in the receptive field of that cell. This is a neural representation of something in the outside world. Evidence for even more abstract kinds of neural representation have been claimed: "The role of the prefrontal cortex in visual attention is to provide neural representations of to-be-attended information" (Miller and Desimone, 2000). Given that the term *representation* can be applied to both mental and physical activity, we have the possibility of a simple link between neural activity and the contents of consciousness. The content of consciousness is determined by whatever is represented in the currently active neurons.

However, just because there is activity in a neuron representing orientation, it does not follow that there is also a mental representation of line orientation. Indeed, much of the work showing that activity in particular neurons represents particular properties of the visual world was carried out in anaesthetised animals (Fujita *et al.*, 1992). From our experiences as anaesthetised humans we infer that these animals had no conscious experience associated with the neural activity. With humans we can obtain direct evidence that neural activity representing some aspect of the outside world does not necessarily lead to consciousness of that aspect.

The most striking examples of such dissociation come from studies of patients with lesions. For example, the patient DF (Milner and Goodale, 1995) has visual form agnosia. She cannot perceive what shape objects have and is unable to report the orientation of a line; yet, she is able to use visual information about shape and orientation to make appropriate reaching and grasping movements. When making such movements there must be neural activity in her brain that represents shape and orientation; furthermore, this neural activity influences her behaviour, but, for her, there is no corresponding mental representation.

In normal subjects, appropriate behaviour in the absence of conscious perception can be observed in masking experiments. The introduction of a mask (for example, a face with a neutral expression) a few tens to hundreds of milliseconds after presentation of a stimulus (such as a face with an angry expression) can abolish the subjective perception of the stimulus; yet, autonomic and motor responses to aspects of the stimulus may still be possible (Ohman and Soares, 1994). The volunteer reports seeing only a face with a neutral expression, but the autonomic response elicited by the angry face is still present. In this paradigm, it should be possible to show that the presence of a certain kind of neural activity predicts autonomic and motor responses. Using masking it has been shown, for example, that activity in the amygdala changes with changes in facial expression of which the subject is unaware (Morris *et al.*, 1998).

From these observations and many other experiments (Milner and Rugg, 1992) it follows that there are two classes of cognitive process. There are those cognitive processes that occur in the absence of any conscious experience, and there are those cognitive processes that are associated with conscious experience. It is probable that the unconscious processes are in the majority (Nisbett and Wilson, 1977; Bargh and Chartrand, 1999). A major assumption of the program for identifying the neural correlates of consciousness is that there is a qualitative difference between neural activity associated with conscious and unconscious processes. Our key question, which remains unanswered as yet, is "What is special about the neural activity that leads to conscious experience?" But, before this question can be addressed, we need to consider how to measure conscious experience.

Indices of Conscious Experience

This discovery of unconscious processes has the important implication that we cannot infer that someone is conscious of something in the environment simply because this thing influences their behaviour. Neither neural activity nor behaviour is a sufficient indicator of conscious experience.

Verbal Reports

So how do we know about the contents of consciousness? The most direct way is by verbal report. I learn about your current mental representations from what you tell me about your perceptions, memories, and intentions. You can describe the colour of an object, rate the intensity of a sensation, report whether one experience is the same or different from another. Such reports depend upon a shared communication system such as language. Except when, for some reason, you decide to lie to me, this system works well. After all, outside the laboratory such reporting is the basis of human communication. This communication system is constantly tuned to maintain the successful sharing of experience. I validate my understanding of your report by matching your description to my experience.

Behavioural Reports

We do not need to use language to report our mental experiences. Gestures and movements can be made with a deliberate communicative intent. In many experiments, the observer will indicate that he sees something by pressing a button. In this case, a behavioural response (the button press) is a report in the sense that it means something; observer and experimenter have agreed, prior to the experiment, that a button press will mean that the stimulus has been perceived. More complex behavioural reports can be agreed upon. For example, in an experiment on binocular rivalry (see below), the observer can press the left button for one percept and the right button for the other. The advantage of a behavioural report is that it can be used in situations where verbal report is not possible. A patient in the locked-in state can indicate his or her wishes only by minimal movements of the eyes (Gallo and Fontanarosa, 1989). The same procedure can be used in studies of animals. In a binocular rivalry experiment, a monkey can be trained to press the left button for one percept and the right button for the other (Leopold and Logothetis, 1996).

However, in certain circumstances, these nonverbal reports can be ambiguous. In a forced-choice experiment, the volunteer, whether human or monkey, must always give a response; for example, the volunteer might be required to report whether the stimulus was on the left or the right by pressing the left or the right button. But, in some trials, he is not conscious of any stimulus. In these trials, he has to guess. In other words, his choice of which button to press is, as far as he is aware, not based on any aspect of the stimulus. Nevertheless, these guesses may sometimes be better than chance. In these cases, there is a discrepancy between the button press and the verbal report. In guessing trials we would be looking at an unconscious processing system, while in the other trials we would be looking at a conscious processing system. But, how do we know which are the guessing trials? This problem is particularly difficult for studies with monkeys. We would argue that the communication system incorporated in the nonverbal report was inadequate in this example because the volunteer was not given the means to indicate that he was not aware of any stimulus. A "report" button might be added so that the monkey (or the human) can indicate when he was not aware of the stimulus (Cowey and Stoerig, 1995; Hampton, 2001).

Identifying the Neural Correlates of the Contents of Consciousness

In our search for the neural correlates of consciousness we aim to identify the kind of neural activity that has a formal relationship with subjective reports about consciousness and its contents (*i.e.*, mental representations). There are two parts to this aim. The first part is to identify neural activity that is related to mental representations. We are searching for situations in which changes in neural activity predict changes in mental representation and conversely. We can predict either the direction of the change or the time at which the change occurs. For example, in a study of sensory thresholds, the presence (or absence) of a certain pattern of neural activity would predict the presence (or absence) of a particular mental representation. The time at which the change in neural activity occurred would also predict the time of the change of mental representation. It should be noted, however, that for this prediction it is not necessary for the changes in the two domains to occur at the same time. It is merely necessary that an early change in the neural activity is associated with an early change in the mental representation. Prediction is still possible if there is a systematic time difference between the changes in the two domains.

It is also necessary to show that these relationships are not simply the concomitant consequence of changes in stimulation or changes in behaviour. The most direct way of "partialling out" these unwanted effects is to keep them constant, hence the emphasis on paradigms in which, for example, subjective experience changes while stimulation remains constant.

The second part of our aim is to show that neural activity associated with mental representations is qualitatively different from other kinds of neural activity. To achieve this aim it is necessary to identify neural correlates of changing stimulation and changing behaviour that occur in the absence of changes in mental representations. Comparison of these different kinds of neural activity will demonstrate that a certain pattern or type of neural activity is uniquely associated with mental representations: the neural signature of consciousness.

A Taxonomy of Experimental Paradigms for Studying Consciousness

In Tables 16.1 and 16.2 we have made an attempt to systematise the experimental paradigms relevant to three hypothetical types of neural activity (see also Frith *et al.*, 1999). We have associated these with three kinds of psychological processes: those concerned with the present

TABLE 16.1 Experimental Paradigms for Studying the Neural Correlates of Consciousness in Normal States

	Perception	Memory	Action
Subjective experiences changes, stimulation and/or behaviour constant	Activity assiociated with multi-stable perception (Lumer *et al.* 1998; Kleinschmidt *et al.* 1998, Portas *et al.*, 2000)	Activity associated with episodic recall (Rugg *et al.*, 1998)	Activity associated with awareness of intentions (Libet *et al.*, 1983; Haggard *et al.*, 2002)
Stimulation changes, subjective experience remains constant	Activity elicited by undetected stimulus changes (He *et al.*, 1996; (Beck *et al.*, 2001)	Activity elicited by unrecognised old items (Rugg *et al.*, 1998)	Activity associated with stimuli eliciting action without awareness (Dehaene *et al.*, 1998)
Behaviour changes, subjective experience remains constant	Activity associated with stimuli eliciting correct guesses (Pierce and Jastrow, 1885; Elliott and Dolan, 1998)	Activity associated with implicit learning (Hazeltine *et al.*, 1997)	Activity associated with implicit motor behaviour (Rosetti, 1998)

TABLE 16.2 Experimental Paradigms for Studying the Neural Correlates of Consciousness in Abnormal States

	Perception	Memory	Action
Subjective experiences changes, stimulation and/or behaviour constant	Activity associated with hallucinations (Dierks *et al.*, 1999; McGonigle *et al.*, 2002; Shergill *et al.*, 2001)	Activity associated with confabulation (Burgess and Shallice, 1996)	Activity associated with delusions of control (Spence *et al.*, 1997; Blakemore *et al.*, 2003)
Stimulation changes, subjective experience remains constant	Activity elicited by neglected stimuli (Rees *et al.*, 2000; Vuilleumier *et al.*, 2001).	Activity elicited by old items in cases of amnesia (Costello *et al.*, 1998; Diamond *et al.*, 1996)	Activity associated with stimuli eliciting unintended actions (Lhermitte, 1983)
Behaviour changes, subjective experience remains constant	Activity associated with Correct reaches in form agnosia (Milner and Goodale, 1995)	Activity associated with implicit learning in amnesia (Knowlton *et al.*, 1992)	Activity associated with Anarchic hand movements (Marchetti and Della Salla, 1998)

(perception and imagery), those concerned with the past (memory), and those concerned with the future (intentions and actions). These tables provide the basis of a program for the development of experimental studies of the neural correlates of consciousness. Because studies of neurological cases and other disorders associated with abnormal mental states continue to play such a major role in the identification of the neural correlates of consciousness we have included a second table specifically for such studies. Functional imaging has played and will continue to play a major role in identifying the neural correlates of consciousness. In the rest of this chapter, we discuss some of these studies and the implications of their results.

LEVELS OF CONSCIOUSNESS

Arousal and Attention

Our level of consciousness is closely associated with our level of arousal. Furthermore, the ability to deploy our attention in order to determine the contents of our consciousness also depends upon our level of arousal. From studies on animals a number of subcortical structures have been identified that play a role in maintaining arousal. Multiple ascending activating systems located in the upper brain stem, basal forebrain, and posterior hypothalamus promote and maintain wakefulness by acting on the thalamus and/or the cortex. The small size of many of the relevant nuclei makes it difficult for functional imaging to reveal activation specifically related to level of consciousness/arousal, but results obtained so far are consistent with animal studies (see below).

Arousal becomes increasingly difficult to maintain after sleep deprivation. When attention has to be deployed in a state of sleep deprivation, the frontal cortex is more activated (Drummond *et al.*, 2000). In another study of sleep deprivation greater activity was observed in the thalamic system when attention had to be maintained (Portas *et al.*, 1998). These studies suggest that some kind of compensatory mechanism provides for acceptable levels of attention when the endogenous level of arousal is too low; however, high levels of attention cannot be sustained for long when the intrinsic level of arousal is low. When sleep pressure builds up beyond a certain limit performance declines (Horne, 1978), and the brain shows a decreased activation of thalamic and cortical regions (Thomas *et al.*, 2000).

Several positron emission tomography (PET) investigations, as well as the functional magnetic resonance imaging (fMRI) study by Portas *et al.* (1998), suggest that the thalamo-cortical system plays a major role in the interaction between attention and arousal in humans (Kinomura *et al.*, 1996; Coull *et al.*, 1997; Sturm *et al.*, 1999). Tonic activity in this system is also directly correlated with the electroencephalogram (EEG) activity present during waking (Steriade and McCarley, 1990).

Waking, Sleeping, and Dreaming

Comparison of waking and sleeping is an obvious way to identify neural correlates of levels of consciousness. It used to be thought that sleep was a state during which we lose contact with the environment and enter a state of oblivion. Now an increasing number of studies are showing that sleep is anything but a passive state. Our sleeping brains not only are capable of producing the rich mental activity we experience during dreams but can also process auditory information (Bastuji *et al.*, 1995; Perrin *et al.*, 1999; Portas *et al.*, 2000a; Czisch *et al.*, 2002), consolidate memories (Maquet *et al.*, 2000; Louie and Wilson, 2001; Stickgold *et al.*, 2001), maintain a temporal reference (Hawkins, 1989), act according to plans (LaBerge and Rheingold, 1997), and retain the conditioning effects of subliminal perceptions (Hennevin *et al.*, 1998). Hence, sleep must be characterised, not by a lack of cognitive processes, but by cognitive processes specific to sleep that have hardly yet been studied. Many of these processes are not associated with conscious experience, but those associated with dreams are associated with a special kind of conscious experience that is not directly linked to environmental stimuli and is largely outside voluntary control.

On the basis of measures of EEG and electromyogram (EMG) sleep can be divided into several clear stages. For simplicity we shall only consider two of these stages: non-rapid eye movement (NREM) sleep and rapid eye movement (REM) sleep (for a review of human sleep staging, see Rechtschaffen and Kales, 1968).

NREM Sleep

Non-rapid eye movement sleep is characterised by highly synchronous activity over the whole brain. Typical EEG patterns are spindles, K complexes, and delta waves. This synchronised activity is associated with a shift of large distributed neuronal populations in the brain from the tonic discharge pattern present during waking to a burst-mode activity appearing during sleep (Steriade *et al.*, 1993). Global cerebral blood flow (Madsen, *et al.*, 1991b) and glucose metabolism are reduced dramatically during NREM sleep (Buchsbaum *et al.*, 1989; Maquet *et al.*, 1990). Brain areas that consistently show specific deactivation during NREM sleep are the brainstem, the thalamus and orbitofrontal cortex, the basal forebrain, the anterior cingulate cortex, the basal ganglia, and the precuneus (Maquet *et al.*, 1996; Braun *et al.*, 1997; Hofle *et al.*, 1997; Maquet *et al.*, 1997; Andersson *et al.*, 1998; Kajimura *et al.*, 1999).

The deactivation of the brainstem, thalamus, and basal forebrain during NREM sleep can be related to their role in controlling arousal; however, this is not the case for orbitofrontal and anterior cingulate cortex, basal ganglia, and precuneus. The basal ganglia may play an active role in sleep-state modulation via their outflow to the wake-relating cholinergic neurons of the midbrain reticular formation (Inglis and Winn, 1995). Alternatively, the basal ganglia deactivation might be a consequence of frontal and thalamic demodulation of these nuclei (Maquet *et al.*, 1997). Reduced activity in anterior cingulate may be related to its role in controlling attention, as attention to external cues is virtually abolished during sleep. Deactivation of the precuneus has also been observed in other altered forms of consciousness including hypnosis (Maquet *et al.*, 1999) and coma (Laureys *et al.*, 1999); however, the precise function of this region remains unknown.

Despite the low level of brain activity associated with NREM sleep, external stimuli are still processed. A recent fMRI study (Portas *et al.*, 2000a) showed that two different types of auditory stimuli (a "beep" and someone calling the subject's own name) presented during NREM sleep produced bilateral activation of the thalamus, primary auditory cortex, and the caudate nucleus. During waking the same areas were activated, but the activity in the thalamus was greater and there was additional activity in prefrontal, parietal, and cingulate cortex. The study of Portas *et al.* indicates that external stimuli find their way to primary sensory cortices during sleep without eliciting conscious experience. The deactivation of association cortex may prevent the further processing necessary for awareness. Other functional imaging studies have shown that the wave of deactivation observed in NREM sleep affects association cortex more than unimodal cortex (Braun *et al.*, 1997; Andersson *et al.*, 1998; Kajimura *et al.*, 1999). It is interesting to note that middle-latency evoked potentials (mainly generated in primary auditory cortex and thalamus) are largely eliminated during NREM sleep (Erwin and Buchwald, 1986). The presence of neural activity (as indicated by the blood-oxygen-level-dependent [BOLD] signal) in the absence of an evoked potential might indicate that, during NREM sleep, neural activity elicited by external stimuli is not synchronised. The BOLD signal relates to any increase of neural activity, while evoked potentials can be detected only when this neural activity is synchronised.

Even though during NREM sleep "messages sent to cortical cells are reduced in terms of firing rate and frequency range, such messages are not deprived of information content and the analysis of complex sounds remains possible" (Edeline *et al.*, 2000). This is confirmed by the study of Portas *et al.* (2000a) that showed that presentation of the subject's own name during NREM sleep elicited greater activity in the left amygdala and prefrontal cortex than presentation of a simple "bleep." This observation implies the existence of a functional network capable of detecting and facilitating the processing of emotionally relevant stimuli (*e.g.*, one's own name) without awareness during sleep.

REM Sleep

In one particular stage of sleep, the EEG shows the low voltage and fast activity characteristic of waking, but muscle tone is actively inhibited and behavioural sleep persists. Stereotypic bursts of saccadic eye movements called *rapid eye movements* occur, giving this state the name REM sleep. In 90 to 95% of cases, arousal during REM sleep yields reports of dreaming. Dreams are characterised by vivid hallucinatory imagery usually in the visual domain and illusions of motion. Awakening during non-REM sleep yields reports of sensation and motion in only 5 to 10% of cases, and these reports describe experiences of considerably reduced intensity. Thus, although experiences are occasionally reported in stages of sleep other than REM, these are more like thoughts and do not have the vivid quality of dreams. Dreaming resembles waking consciousness in that both involve mental representations. Dreaming differs from waking consciousness in that the dreamer has no insight (except at the moment of waking) and regards the dream events as completely real. Dreaming also differs from waking consciousness in that memory of the dream fades rapidly and is lost unless rehearsed immediately upon waking. Within 5 minutes of the termination of a period of REM sleep awakening yields no report of dreaming and it is estimated that there is amnesia (in the sense of a lack of episodic memory) for over 95% of dreams. What we do remember of our dreams derives mainly from those fragments dwelt upon immediately after waking (Hobson, 1988).

The thalamocortical system is highly activated during REM sleep at a similar or higher level than during waking (Llinas and Ribary, 1993). Functionally, REM sleep is characterised by high cerebral energy requirements (Maquet *et al.*, 1990) and blood flow (Madsen *et al.*, 1991a; Madsen and Vorstrup, 1991; Lenzi *et al.*, 1999). Two PET studies showed activation of the mesopontine tegmentum during REM sleep (Maquet *et al.*, 1996; Braun *et al.*, 1997) consistent with the presence of REM-on cells in this area (El Mansari *et al.*, 1989; Kayama *et al.*, 1992). Other areas more active during REM than NREM sleep include thalamic nuclei, limbic and paralimbic areas, amygdaloid complex, the hippocampal formation, and anterior cingulate cortex. Posterior cortices in temporo-occipital areas are also activated. By contrast, the dorsolateral prefrontal and parietal cortex as well as the posterior cingulate and precuneus are the least active brain regions (Maquet *et al.*, 1996; Braun *et al.*, 1997; Nofzinger *et al.*, 1997; Braun *et al.*, 1998; Lovblad *et al.*, 1999).

The role of the amygdala during REM sleep has often been associated with the emotion and stress sometimes experienced during dreaming (Maquet and Franck, 1997). Fear-related emotions are significantly more frequent in dream reports than in waking event reports (Fosse *et al.*, 2001).

The increased activity in the hippocampus during REM sleep may be related to memory consolidation (Louie and Wilson, 2001). The neurochemical changes that occur across sleep/wake states and especially the cholinergic changes that occur in the hippocampus during REM sleep might provide a mechanism by which sleep modulates specific cellular synaptic communication involved in hippocampus-dependent memory storage (Graves *et al.*, 2001). Maquet *et al.* (2000) found that recent experience affects the pattern of brain activity during the following REM sleep periods. They showed that the brain areas in which activity was elicited by performance of a serial choice reaction time task were consistently reactivated during periods of REM sleep during the night following practice of the task. This reactivation may relate to the consolidation in memory of what has been learned about a task, as sleep deprivation interferes with such learning (Maquet, 2001; Stickgold *et al.*, 2001).

It has been suggested that the activation of the occipital cortex during REM sleep may relate to the vivid visual imagery often experienced during dreaming. This activation, in combination with the deactivation of frontal and parietal association cortices (Maquet *et al.*, 1996; Braun *et al.*, 1997, 1998; Nofzinger *et al.*, 1997) may account for some of the characteristic features of dreams such as lack of insight, distortion of time perception, and amnesia on waking. Schwartz and Maquet (2002) have made the interesting suggestion that some of the bizarre features of dreams resemble the experiences of patients with circumscribed brain lesions. For example, a common feature of dream experience is a mismatch between the identity of the character seen in the dream and that character's physical appearance: "I had a talk with your colleague (in my dream), but she looked different, much younger, like someone I went to school with, perhaps a 13-year-old girl." This resembles the experience of patients with Frégoli syndrome, in which an unknown person is recognised as a familiar person despite the lack of any obvious physical resemblance (Forstl *et al.*, 1991). Frégoli syndrome is associated with temporal and frontal lesions. It has been suggested that Frégoli syndrome is generated by simultaneous activation of high-order associative areas of the temporal lobes that store information about personal identities and the fusiform face area, responsible for the identification of visual facial features (Puce *et al.*, 1996; Kanwisher *et al.*, 1997). At the same time, there is an absence of selective reciprocal constraints and monitoring from prefrontal regions (Ellis and Young, 1990). Schwartz and Maquet (2002) suggest that the combination of high activity in temporo-occipital regions with low activity in dorsolateral prefrontal cortex (DLPFC) might be functionally equivalent to the effect of lesions that lead to disorders of conscious perception like Frégoli syndrome.

Further studies of dream experiences and comparisons of these with waking experiences will be very important for gaining a better understanding of the neural correlates of consciousness; however, the next step will be to develop techniques for using event-related fMRI to characterise brain activity associated with individual dream experiences.

Abnormal States of Consciousness

Non-rapid eye movement sleep is not the only state in which the brain remains active in the absence of conscious experience. After certain kinds of brain damage, patients may enter comatose or vegetative states (VSs) in which there appears to be a complete absence of consciousness. In the long term, functional neuroimaging studies of such patients may gain clinical significance and provide useful information for the diagnosis, prognosis, and management of these patients.

In particular, it would be desirable to find a reliable neural signature of consciousness that would distinguish the comatose or VS patient from the patient with locked-in syndrome. The latter patient is fully conscious but is unable to reveal his state because he has no way of communicating. We will not deal with these issues here because, in our view, the available data cannot yet be used for these purposes.

Coma is the consequence of major cerebral insults (traumatic or non traumatic) and indicates a serious dysfunction of the brainstem and diencephalic activating structures or of widespread bilateral lesions in the cerebral hemispheres (Plum and Posner, 1980). By definition, comatose patients cannot be aroused (due to their impaired state of vigilance) and are consequently unaware. *Vegetative state*, a term first coined by Jennet and Plum (1972), most often follows a period of coma. After a period of several days to a few weeks, activity resumes in brainstem and diencephalic structures such that clinical signs of arousal are observed. Furthermore, patients go through a cycle of sleeping and waking. In contrast, cortical function remains severely deteriorated and no sign of awareness can be reliably detected. Vegetative patients appear to be awake but are nevertheless unaware of their external (and, hence, internal) world. *Minimally conscious state* refers to patients who are no longer comatose or vegetative but remain severely disabled. These patients are unable to follow instructions reliably. They cannot communicate but demonstrate inconsistent behavioural evidence of awareness of their environment. They may follow instructions for a few minutes but then lapse once again into a state of apparent unawareness (Giacino *et al.*, 2002).

Clinical practice reveals how difficult it is to recognise unambiguous signs of conscious perception of the environment and of the self in these patients. Objective assessment of residual brain function in severely brain-injured patients is difficult because motor responses may be limited or inconsistent. This problem is reflected in frequent misdiagnoses of vegetative state, minimally conscious state, and locked-in syndrome (Childs and Mercer, 1996). In addition, consciousness is not an all-or-none phenomenon but appears as a continuum between different pathological conditions (Plum and Posner, 1980). There is also a theoretical limitation to the establishment of a purely clinical diagnosis, as it relies solely on inferences that conscious experience in another person is present or absent (Jennett and Plum, 1972). Functional neuroimaging cannot replace the clinical assessment of patients with altered states of consciousness. Nevertheless, it can describe objectively how deviant from normal is the cerebral activity and its regional distribution, at rest and under various conditions of stimulation. We hope that the use of functional neuroimaging will substantially increase our understanding of severely brain-injured patients.

The Neuronal Loss Hypothesis

A straightforward hypothesis suggests that the extensive and severe neuronal loss in the brains of VS patients is causally related to their loss of consciousness (Kinney and Samuels, 1994). Recently, Rudolf *et al.* (2000) semiquantitatively estimated the cerebral uptake of ^{11}C-flumazenil, a benzodiazepine antagonist used as a neuronal marker in nine VS patients studied early in their evolution. The cortical ^{11}C-flumazenil uptake was only 4.5 times higher than in the white matter, a figure comparable to acute stroke and suggestive of substantial neuronal loss. These results corroborate the postmortem pathological findings in cerebral cortex (Kinney and Samuels, 1994). In keeping with the neuronal loss hypothesis, cerebral glucose metabolism (Levy *et al.*, 1987; Momose *et al.*, 1989; DeVolder *et al.*, 1990; Tommasino *et al.*, 1995; Plum *et al.*, 1998; Laureys *et al.*, 2000c) and cerebral blood flow are invariably reported to be dramatically decreased in VS patients, typically 40 to 60% below normal values; however, the low cerebral glucose metabolism could indicate: (1) a severe reduction of the number of viable neurons, (2) a decreased energy metabolism in viable neurons, or (3) a combination of both.

Residual Cerebral Reactivity to External Stimuli

More recently, with the advent of PET-$H_2{}^{15}O$ studies, several groups have considered the possibility that the remaining cerebral neuronal populations could remain reactive to external stimulations. In a postencephalomyelitis VS patient (who subsequently recovered consciousness), the presentation of familiar faces (as compared to scrambled images) elicited activation of the right fusiform gyrus and extrastriate areas 18 and, 19 (Menon *et al.*, 1998). Similarly, in a posttraumatic VS patient, the anterior cingulate, the right middle temporal, and the right premotor cortices were more activated by a story told by the patient's mother than by the presentation of non-words (de Jong *et al.*, 1997). In a recent prospective study, five postanoxic/ischaemic VS patients were submitted to monaurally presented clicks (Laureys *et al.*, 2000a). In the same experimental session, their cerebral glucose metabolism was also measured in the resting state. The patient data were compared to normal control populations studied in the same conditions. In control subjects, the auditory stimuli were related to an activation of the transverse temporal gyrus and the adjacent superior temporal gyri on both sides and of the contralateral lateral superior temporal and temporoparietal cortices. A conjunction analysis showed that, in the VS patients, as in the normal subjects, the transverse and the adjacent superior temporal gyri were activated on both sides. This activation persisted despite a substantial (more than 60%) decrease in the patients' local glucose metabolism. In contrast, the group of VS patients versus controls by condition interaction (auditory stimulation versus rest) showed that the contralateral temporoparietal cortex was significantly less activated in VS patients than in control subjects. Likewise, under noxious stimulation, primary sensory cortex was activated in 15 VS patients as in normal subjects, whereas the secondary somatosensory area was significantly less activated in VS patients than in normal control subjects (Laureys *et al.*, 2003).

These observations suggest that, in postanoxic/ischaemic VS patients, primary sensory cortices are more likely than the adjacent associative cortices to show a persistent response to external stimulation. This stands in contrast with the results of Menon *et al.* (1998) and de Jong *et al.* (1997), showing the activation of associative cortices. These apparently discrepant results could be explained by the difference in experimental design: Menon *et al.* (1998) and de Jong *et al.* (1997) used complex stimuli, whereas Laureys *et al.* (2000a) used basic auditory (clicks) and somatosensory (electrical) stimuli (Laureys *et al.*, 2003). Furthermore, it is likely that the topography of the lesions may vary from patient to patient.

Functional Connectivity

At this stage, we must acknowledge that it is not known whether these residual activations can lead to conscious perception. Furthermore, if consciousness is subtended by large-scale cerebral networks, the description of cerebral integration would certainly provide further insight on how external stimuli are processed in VS patients and whether such processing can lead to conscious perception. Two groups independently suggested that even if some brain areas remain able to process information, they might not operate properly because they are disconnected, and thus isolated, from other brain areas (Plum *et al.*, 1998; Laureys *et al.*, 1999). In combination with the neuronal loss, impairment of connectivity would be one important factor that renders VS patients unconscious. Impairment of functional connectivity was shown between the thalamus and some associative cortical areas (Laureys *et al.*, 2000b), as well as between cortical regions (Laureys *et al.*, 1999). A cascade of disconnections were also demonstrated along the processing streams of auditory (Laureys *et al.*, 2000a) and noxious inputs (Laureys *et al.*, 2003) when the patient was submitted to external stimuli. Although no definitive conclusion can be drawn from these data, it seems likely that the loss of functional connectivity hampers conscious perception.

Residual Brain Plasticity in VS Patients

It could be argued that the alteration of functional connectivity is due to the neuronal loss itself; no normal functional connections can be expected after a massive neuronal destruction. Although this reasoning is possibly true for many VS patients, it cannot explain how it is that cerebral functional connectivity can normalise when the patient recovers consciousness. It was recently shown that functional connectivity between the thalamic nuclei and several associative cortical areas, significantly reduced in the vegetative state, is restored after recovery of consciousness (Laureys *et al.*, 2000b) (Fig. 16.1). This single-case observation supports the hypothesis that the remaining neurons can resume a normal function if their functional interrelations are restored, eventually leading to the reemergence of consciousness. Thus, while neuronal loss is certainly of primary importance in the lack of consciousness in VS patients, it seems that, at least in some cases, brain plasticity can permit the remaining neurons to resume normal functional connections and eventually normal function (Laureys *et al.*, 2000b).

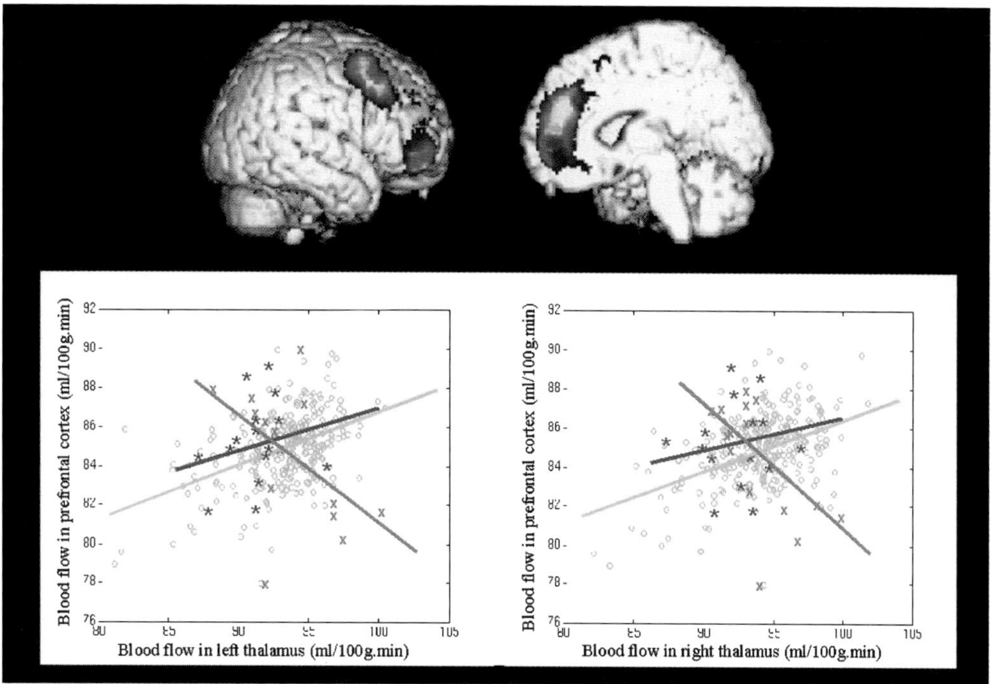

FIGURE 16.1
(Top) Brodmann's areas 8, 10, 9, and 24/32, in which functional connectivity with both thalami was different from controls when the patient was in a vegetative state; these differences were not apparent when he recovered consciousness. Shown on a surface-rendered, normalised MRI (display thresholded at $p < 0.001$, uncorrected). (Bottom) Regression between activity in both thalami and right prefrontal cortex (area 10) in controls (green open circles) compared with patient in vegetative state (red crosses) and after recovery (blue asterisks). Modulation between thalami and frontal cortex is impaired during vegetative state and is no longer different from controls after recovery. (From Laureys, S. *et al.*, 2000a. With permission.)

Some Sets of Cerebral Areas Seem Critical for Consciousness To Arise

The brain areas that in VS have the lowest cerebral glucose metabolism and regain a more normal metabolic level after recovery of consciousness are mainly located in the polymodal associative cortex of the frontal, parietal and temporal lobes (Brodmann's areas 8, 9, 10, 44, 45, 40, mesial 7 and 31) (Laureys *et al.*, 2000b). It is worthwhile remembering that very similar brain areas are also more active in wakefulness than in sleep in normal subjects (Maquet, 2000). The results of these independent studies of VS patients and sleeping normal subjects suggest that these cortical regions are probably intimately related to conscious processes. There are hints from these studies that an adequate level of consciousness requires the viability of a certain subset of brain regions and also requires interactions among these regions and between these regions and the thalamus.

THE CONTENTS OF CONSCIOUSNESS

Even when we are fully conscious in the sense of being wide awake, the contents of our consciousness can vary dramatically. Our senses are constantly bombarded with multiple stimuli, but at any time we are only conscious of a small fraction of these. How are the contents of our consciousness determined?

The neural correlates of the contents of consciousness have been studied most extensively in the visual system. The primate visual system is organised in a distributed fashion, with different aspects of the visual scene analysed in different cortical areas (Zeki, 1978; Felleman and Van Essen, 1991). A prominent clinical finding in humans is that damage to cortical areas containing neurons that represent particular features of the visual environment leads to a corresponding deficit in the contents of consciousness. Thus, damage to V5 (MT) leads to akinetopsia (the inability to see movement; Zihl *et al.*, 1983) and damage to different areas of the fusiform gyrus may cause prosopagnosia (the inability to recognise faces) or achromatopsia (the inability to see colour; Damasio *et al.*, 2000). These findings suggest that activity in a functionally specialised cortical area is required to evoke consciousness of the attribute analysed in that area.

Neuroimaging data are consistent with this idea. Patients with schizophrenia who experience visual and auditory hallucinations show activity in modality-specific cortex during hallucinatory episodes (Silbersweig *et al.*, 1995; Dierks *et al.*, 1999). Similarly, patients with damage to the peripheral visual system who experience hallucinations with specific phenomenal content show activity in functionally specialised areas of visual cortex corresponding to the content of their hallucinations (ffytche *et al.*, 1998).

In normal subjects, visual imagery activates category-specific areas of visual cortex (D'Esposito *et al.*, 1997; Goebel *et al.*, 1998a; Howard *et al.*, 1998; O'Craven and Kanwisher, 2000). Contingent after-effects based on colour or motion activate either V4 (Sakai *et al.*, 1995; Hadjikhani *et al.*, 1998; Barnes *et al.*, 1999) or V5 (MT) (Tootell *et al.*, 1996; Culham *et al.*, 1998; He *et al.*, 1998), respectively, and the time course of such activation reflects phenomenal experience (Tootell *et al.*, 1996; He *et al.*, 1998). Perception of illusory or implied motion in a static visual stimulus results in activation of V5 (MT) (Zeki *et al.*, 1993; Kourtzi and Kanwisher, 2000), whereas perception of illusory contours activates extrastriate cortex (Hirsch *et al.*, 1995; ffytche and Zeki, 1996). Differential activity in word-processing areas is present when subjects are consciously aware of the meaning of visually presented words and absent when they are not (Rees *et al.*, 1999). Common to all these experimental paradigms are changes in subjects' phenomenal experience without corresponding physical stimulus changes. Altered brain activity is observed in areas of the brain known to contain neurons whose stimulus specificities encompass the attribute represented in consciousness.

Binocular rivalry provides a powerful experimental paradigm with which to study the neural correlates of visual awareness (Leopold and Logothetis, 1999). When dissimilar images are presented to the two eyes, they compete for perceptual dominance. Each image is visible in turn for a few seconds while the other is suppressed. Because perceptual transitions between each monocular view occur spontaneously without any change in the physical stimulus, neural correlates of consciousness may be distinguished from neural correlates attributable to stimulus characteristics. In human primary visual cortex (V1), fluctuations in activity are about half as large as those evoked by real stimulus alternation (Polonsky *et al.*, 2000). However, further along the ventral stream, responses in the fusiform face area (FFA) during rivalry are larger than those in VI and equal in magnitude to responses evoked by real alternation of stimuli (Tong *et al.*, 1998). This suggests that neural competition during rivalry has been resolved by these later stages of visual processing and that activity in FFA therefore reflects the contents of consciousness rather than the retinal stimulus. Qualitatively, these observations are compatible with findings in monkeys demonstrating that the majority of neurons in inferior temporal cortex show responses that reflect the monkey's percept rather than the retinal stimulus (Logothetis and Schall, 1989; Leopold and Logothetis, 1996). However, there are also important quantitative discrepancies, as the modulation of the fMRI signal in human V1 is somewhat stronger than expected from investigations in monkey (Tootell *et al.*, 1996; Polonsky *et al.*, 2000). This discrepancy emphasises the desirability of understanding the relationship between the neural correlates of consciousness measured with different techniques and in different species (Rees *et al.*, 2000), a process that will be facilitated by the use of fMRI in non-human primates (Logothetis *et al.*, 1999).

Necessary and Sufficient Correlates of Consciousness in Ventral Visual Cortex

The data discussed above suggest that, for a visual feature to be represented in consciousness, activity must be present in the relevant functionally specialised area of ventral visual cortex; however, although activation of extrastriate cortex may be necessary for consciousness, this activity is not sufficient. When volunteers incorrectly report the absence of a visual stimulus, activity may nevertheless be seen in both primary (Ress *et al.*, 2000) and extrastriate (Kastner *et al.*, 1999) visual cortex. In FFA, changes in the identity of a face stimulus evoke activity even when the subject is blind to the change (Beck *et al.*, 2001). Masked words of which a subject is

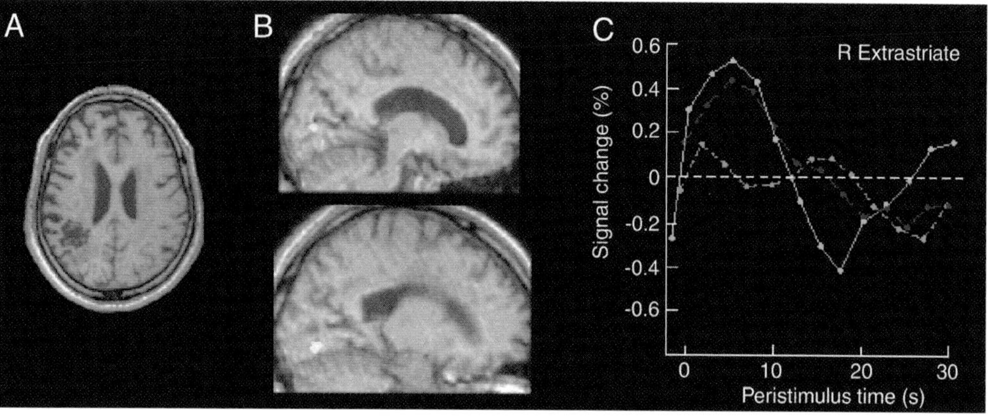

FIGURE 16.2
Activation of ventral visual cortex is not sufficient for awareness. (a) An axial slice of a T1-weighted anatomical magnetic resonance image shows a right parietal lesion in the patient under study. Clinically, the patient showed left visual extinction to bilateral simultaneous stimulation. (b) Activation is evoked by an unseen extinguished left-visual-field stimulus in right primary visual cortex (upper panel) and early extrastriate cortex (lower panel). Activations are displayed on a sagittal slice through an anatomical image of the patient's damaged right hemisphere. (c) Activation in these extrastriate right hemisphere areas (R Extrastriate) produced by an extinguished left-visual-field stimulus (solid line) has a time course similar to that evoked by a seen unilateral left-visual-field stimulus (long dashes). A seen unilateral right-visual-field stimulus (short dashes) produces little ipsilateral activation. (From Rees, G., 2001. With permission.)

unaware nevertheless evoke activity in the ventral visual pathway (Dehaene *et al.*, 2001). After damage to primary visual cortex, activity in ventral visual cortex need not necessarily lead to visual awareness (Sahraie *et al.*, 1997; Goebel *et al.*, 1998b; though see Barbur *et al.*, 1993). These findings complement recent work addressing the neural correlates of visual extinction, a common component of the neglect syndrome following right parietal damage (Driver and Mattingley, 1998). Patients with visual extinction show deficient awareness for contralesional visual stimuli, particularly when a competing stimulus is also present ipsilesionally. Extinction illustrates that visual awareness can be lost even when V1 is intact. Two recent neuroimaging studies show that areas of both primary and extrastriate visual cortex that are activated by a seen left-visual- field stimulus are also activated by an unseen and extinguished left-visual-field stimulus (Rees *et al.*, 2000; Vuilleumier *et al.*, 2001) (Fig. 16.2).

Indeed, the unconscious processing of an extinguished face stimulus extends even to the FFA (Rees *et al.*, 2000). Thus, the presence of activity in these areas is not sufficient to evoke awareness following right parietal damage. However, on trials when one patient (correctly) reports seeing bilateral stimulation, awareness is specifically associated with covariation of activity in a distributed network involving primary visual cortex, inferior temporal cortex, and areas of prefrontal and left parietal cortex (Vuilleumier *et al.*, 2001). This observation represents direct evidence that awareness may be specifically associated with covariation between visual cortex and nonvisual areas of cortex, complementing earlier studies showing similar distributed interactions associated with consciousness in normals (Dolan *et al.*, 1997; Lumer and Rees, 1999; McIntosh *et al.*, 1999).

The mere presence of activity in ventral visual cortex, therefore, does not automatically lead to consciousness, and the sufficient conditions that lead to visual awareness remain under active empirical investigation. The two main possibilities are not mutually exclusive. First, some form of interaction between activity in the ventral visual cortex and nonvisual areas may be required. This has been proposed on theoretical grounds (Crick and Koch, 1995), and some empirical evidence supporting this notion has already been presented. Second, some particular property of activity within a ventral visual area may be sufficient. Which property is relevant remains a matter of controversy. One possibility is that activity greater than some threshold may be sufficient to support awareness. Consistent with this, conscious recognition of objects shows a strong correlation with fMRI signal strength in object-responsive regions of visual cortex (Grill-Spector *et al.*, 2000). A minimum duration of neural activity might be required for conscious experience (Libet *et al.*, 1964). For example, patients experiencing visual hallucinations show a

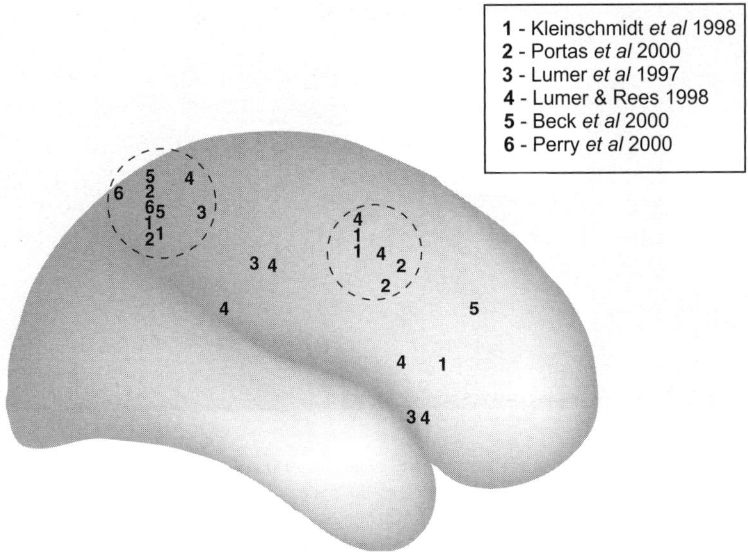

FIGURE 16.3
Parietal and prefrontal correlates of consciousness. Areas of parietal and prefrontal cortex showing activation during several studies of conscious perception are plotted as a lateral through projection. Each number is placed at the center of a cluster of activation; where loci from the same study overlapped, they have been omitted for clarity. Prominent clustering of activations in superior parietal and premotor cortex is apparent. (From Rees, G., 2001. With permission.)

rise in fMRI signal in visual cortex some time before they report the presence of the hallucination (ffytche *et al.*, 1998). Alternatively, a specific form of neural activity such as recurrent processing or synchrony might be required (von der Malsburg, 1981; Engel *et al.*, 1991; Lamme and Roelfsema, 2000). Finally, it should be acknowledged that awareness might depend on a type of neural activity to which neuroimaging measures are insensitive. For example, fMRI is relatively insensitive to the fine-grained time course of neural activity. Thus, if awareness depends on synchrony of neural firing (von der Malsburg, 1981; Engel *et al.*, 1991), then fMRI may be insensitive to such changes. It may be relevant to this point to remember that middle-latency-evoked potentials to auditory stimuli during NREM sleep are dramatically reduced in comparison to waking, while fMRI responses show much less change. This would be consistent with a specific reduction in the synchrony of firing when these stimuli are processed without awareness. Of course, it is possible that this change in synchrony in primary auditory cortex with awareness is the result of reentrant signals from higher regions.

Parietal and Prefrontal Correlates of Consciousness

The clinical observation that disturbances of visual awareness may follow parietal damage provides evidence for a contribution of dorsal cortical areas to consciousness. Several other lines of evidence have supported this notion. In monkeys, chronic blindness follows a massive cortical ablation that spares most of the modality-specific visual cortex, but not parietal and frontal areas (Nakamura and Mishkin, 1986). Furthermore, anatomical and electrophysiological studies show that parietal and prefrontal cortex are reciprocally connected and act together with visual cortex (Friedman and Goldman-Rakic, 1994). Direct evidence in normal humans for parietal and prefrontal correlates of consciousness has come from recent studies of bistable perception. Brain activity during spontaneous fluctuations in awareness has been examined both for binocular rivalry and for a variety of bistable figures (Kleinschmidt *et al.*, 1998; Lumer *et al.*, 1998; Lumer and Rees, 1999). Unlike the rivalry studies discussed previously (Tong *et al.*, 1998; Polonsky *et al.*, 2000) these studies focused on activity that was time-locked to the transitions between different perceptual states. Cortical regions for which activity reflects perceptual transitions include ventral extrastriate cortex and also parietal and frontal regions previously implicated in the control of spatial attention (Lumer *et al.*, 1998). However, whereas extrastriate areas are also engaged by nonrivalrous perceptual changes, activity in frontal and parietal cortex is specifically associated with the perceptual alternations during rivalry. Similar parietal and frontal regions are active during perceptual transitions occurring while viewing a range of bistable figures such as the Necker cube and Rubins face/vase (Kleinschmidt *et al.*, 1998) and during stereo pop-out, as compared to those regions active during stable viewing (Portas *et al.*, 2000b). In addition, these areas of frontal and parietal cortex are activated when subjects become consciously aware of the presence of a change in a visual scene, compared to when they are change blind (Beck *et al.*, 2001). Finally, parietal cortex is specifically active during perceptual binding of colour and motion during object recognition (Perry and Zeki, 2000).

Despite varied paradigms and types of visual stimulation, the anatomical location of the areas involved in these studies is remarkably consistent, with a prominent focus in superior parietal cortex. These observations suggest the existence of a general mechanism in frontal and parietal cortex that is specifically related to visual consciousness and active during transitions between different types of perceptual experience (Fig. 16.3). Although frontal and parietal areas play a prominent role in the organisation of behaviour, their involvement in rivalry is independent of motor report (Lumer and Rees, 1999). During binocular rivalry, activity is coordinated between ventral visual areas, parietal areas, and prefrontal areas in a way that is not linked to external motor or sensory events but instead varies in strength with the frequency of perceptual events. Similarly to the work discussed earlier (Dolan *et al.*, 1997; Vuilleumier *et al.*, 2001), this suggests that functional interactions between visual and frontoparietal cortex may make an important contribution to consciousness.

The majority of studies of the neural correlates of consciousness have concerned the visual system; however, similar results have been obtained in studies of other modalities. We have already mentioned the study by Portas *et al.* (2000a) that contrasted conscious and unconscious processing of auditory stimuli by scanning volunteers when awake and when in NREM sleep. Auditory cortex was activated in both states, but when the volunteers were awake additional activity was seen in parietal and frontal cortex. Rosen *et al.* (1996) studied a group of patients with silent myocardial ischaemia who showed all the usual physiological effects (ischaemic electrocardiographic changes) after treatment with dobutamine but with the complete absence of severe chest pain experienced by most patients suffering from angina pectoris, as well as a group of patients who did experience the chest pains. During an ischaemic incident, both groups showed activity in brainstem regions associated with the processing of pain signals, but only the group who experienced the pain showed activity in frontal cortex.

Substantive and Transitive States of Mind

If activity in parietal and frontal cortex makes a contribution to visual experience, what is the nature of that contribution? It is striking to note that the studies reviewed here all focus on transitions between experiences with different types of phenomenal content. James (1890) made a phenomenal distinction between the experience of rapid changes in perceptual awareness (transitive states) and stable contemplation (substantive states). Both are part of our everyday experience of the visual environment (stream of consciousness). One may speculate that the neural correlates of conscious experience in parietal cortex (see Fig. 16.3) are thus, more specifically, correlates of transitive states. The anatomical loci associated with these correlates substantially overlap with areas previously associated with covert spatial attention (Corbetta *et al.*, 1995). Indeed, the deployment of spatial attention and the phenomenal experience of binocular rivalry both entail the suppression of visual information from conscious perception. Monocular stimuli become periodically invisible during rivalry; sensory events associated with unattended (or neglected) stimuli have a diminished impact on awareness. Both phenomena may call on common neural machinery in frontoparietal cortex that is involved in the selection of neuronal activity leading to visual awareness.

If the Jamesian phenomenological distinction between substantive and transitive states is acknowledged, then it is possible that the maintenance of a conscious perceptual state may involve different cortical mechanisms to those involved in generating transitions (Portas *et al.*, 2000b). Sustained perceptual experience is an obvious feature of consciousness, but such experience is inconsistent with the idea that the basic neural machinery of the brain is designed

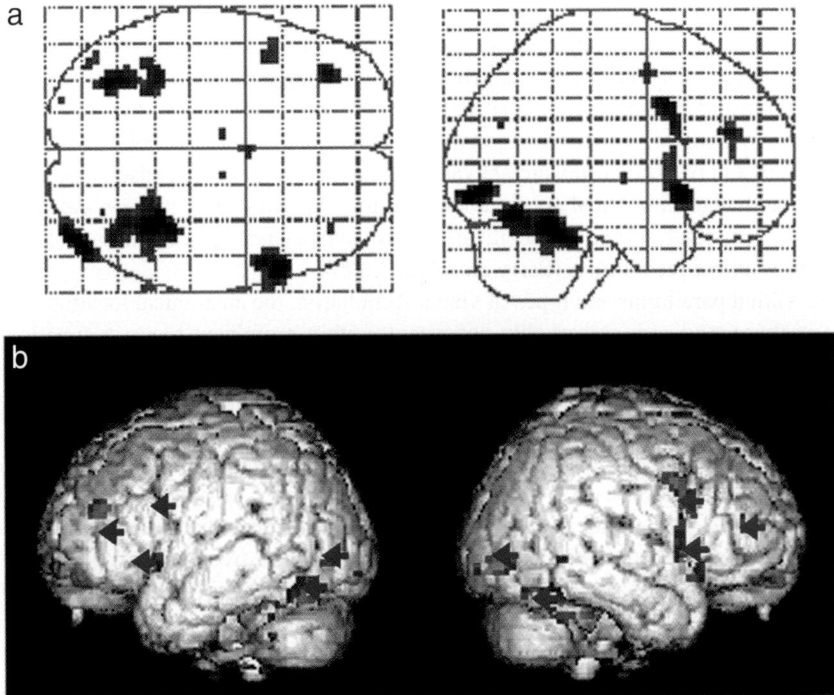

FIGURE 16.4
Brain activity associated with maintenance of a conscious perceptual state overlaps with that associated with working memory. (a) Activation map associated with stable face perception during binocular rivalry is shown as a through-projection onto a horizontal (left) and lateral (right) representation of standard stereotactic space. Activation in FFA is apparent, consistent with previous observations (Tong, *et al.*, 1998). Note the absence of activity in parietal cortex, where prominent activation is instead seen during rivalrous transitions (see Fig. 16.3). (b) The same activation map is now rendered on a template brain volume that has been transformed into standardized stereotactic space. Left and right lateral views are shown on the left and right of the figure, respectively. Blue arrows indicate the locations of areas that show sustained activity in a face working-memory task (Courtney *et al.*, 1997). Data from Kleinschmidt *et al.*, (1998) and Lumer (2000). (From Rees, G., 2001. With permission.)

to represent only the unexpected (Friston, 2002). For a percept to be sustained it would be necessary to fill in the lost information or override rapid attenuation of activity when stimulation remains constant. Such mechanisms might depend on top-down signals from high-level brain regions. Future work in this area may prove rewarding, as there are tantalising indications that such mechanisms do exist. When the stereo image in the experiment of Portas *et al.* (2000b) popped out, this event was associated with transient activity in frontal and parietal cortex; however, in the subsequent period in which perception of the same image was sustained, activity was seen in different regions of prefrontal cortex and in the hippocampus. Thus, sustaining a visual percept recruits different anatomical loci from those associated with immediate conscious recognition. Similarly, regions of brain activation in frontal and parietal cortex associated with transient selection of an item from spatial working memory differ from those associated with sustained maintenance of items in working memory (Rowe *et al.*, 2000). Finally, data from binocular rivalry studies are also consistent with an anatomical distinction between activity related to transitions and that related to the maintenance of a conscious state. Brain areas activated (Lumer *et al.*, 1998; Lumer, 2000) during epochs of sustained face perception (rather than transition-related activity discussed previously) include the FFA, as previously demonstrated (Tong *et al.*, 1998); however, in addition, several prefrontal areas show greater activity during sustained face perception. There is a remarkable overlap (Fig. 16.4) between these loci and those previously implicated in maintaining working memory for faces in a delayed match-to-sample task (Courtney *et al.*, 1997). Such evidence is preliminary, but nevertheless one may speculate that the Jamesian phenomenological distinction between transitive and substantive states of mind is mirrored by the involvement of distinct regions of dorsal and ventral frontoparietal cortex associated with attention and working memory.

ACTION AND INTENTION

Conscious and Unconscious Processes in the Control of Action

Will is the sense of being in control of our own actions and is a major component of consciousness (along with emotion and cognition), but, as with sensory processing, most of the processes by which we control our actions do not enter consciousness. A number of studies have shown that we can all make rapid and accurate grasping movements without being aware of the information that is being used to control these movements (Pisella *et al.*, 2000). In some cases, we are not even aware of having made the movement.

A series of experiments from Jeannerod's group have demonstrated dissociations between behaviour and awareness in normal volunteers making rapid grasping movements. Corrections to the trajectory of a movement made in response to target movements occur several hundred milliseconds in advance of reported awareness of target movement (Castiello *et al.*, 1991). Fourneret and Jeannerod (1998) required subjects to move their hands forward in order to draw a vertical line on a computer screen. The subjects could not see their hands and so could not see that a distortion had been introduced by the computer. Thus, in one condition, in order to draw the vertical line on the screen, subjects had to move their hand, not forward, but 10° to the left. In other conditions, different degrees and directions of distortion were applied. The striking result was that subjects were not aware that they were not making the movements that they saw on the screen. If they were asked to repeat a movement, then, even in the absence of visual feedback, they made a straightforward movement rather then the deviant one that they had just performed. It would seem that as long the intended goal is obtained (in this case, drawing a straight forward line), unexpected sensory feedback does not reach awareness.

Knoblich and Kircher (personal communication) have recently carried out a similar study. Subjects were instructed to draw circles with a pen, which they saw reproduced by a moving dot. Parametric degrees of velocity change were introduced between a subject's movement and its visual consequences (the movement of the dot), and subjects were instructed to lift the pen as soon as they detected a change. The results clearly demonstrated that subjects tended to compensate for the velocity changes well before they were aware of the discrepancy and lifted the pen.

Neural Correlates of Awareness of Action

The relationship of neural activity in the motor system to the timing of the awareness of intentions has been studied extensively. Libet *et al.* (1983) have shown that the brain activity that precedes a voluntary movement (the EEG readiness potential) can be detected well in advance of reports of awareness of the intention to move. This pioneering study illustrates the advantages of studying the motor system because correlations can be explored between the times at which mental and physical events occur. Haggard and Eimer (1999) have presented data suggesting that the time of awareness of initiating a movement correlates with the time at which the late lateralised component of the readiness potential begins (probably reflecting the time at which the exact movement is specified), but not with the beginning of the early phase of the readiness potential. Studies that combine the high spatial resolution of fMRI and the high temporal resolution of EEG should be able to locate the brain regions associated with these various potentials.

Ii is easy to imagine making movements without producing any overt behaviour, and this mental activity can have detectable consequences. First, mental practice of various motor tasks can lead to a significant improvement in subsequent performance (for a review, see Feltz and Landers, 1983). Mental training affects various outcomes of motor performance such as muscular strength (Yue and Cole, 1992), movement speed (Pascual-Leone *et al.*, 1995), and temporal consistency (Vogt, 1995). Second, prolonged performance of tasks in the imagination can lead to significant physiological changes. Subjects who performed or mentally simulated leg exercise had increased heart rates and respiration rates in both conditions (Decety *et al.*, 1991).

Changes in brain activity associated with movements made in the imagination can readily be detected using brain imaging. Decety *et al.* (1994) asked subjects to imagine grasping three-dimensional objects presented to them. Stephan *et al.* (1995) compared execution of a sequence of joystick movements with imagining making such a sequence. These studies showed that the brain regions activated during motor imagery are a subset of those activated during motor execution.

Jeannerod (1994) has argued that motor imagery is closely related to motor preparation. Preparing to make a movement and holding it in readiness while waiting for a signal to release the movement engages the same processes as those involved in imagining making that movement. Functional imaging studies of motor preparation and motor imagery highlight activity in anterior cingulate cortex (ACC), anterior supplementary motor cortex (SMA), inferior lateral premotor cortex, and inferior parietal lobe (Decety *et al.*, 1994; Stephan *et al.*, 1995; Krams *et al.*, 1998). A recent fMRI study that directly compared brain activity during imagining and executing hand movements showed that, although the networks are partially overlapping, several regions are more engaged by imagination (Gerardin *et al.*, 2000). These included bilateral premotor, prefrontal and SMA regions, and left posterior parietal areas. Because these areas are engaged by motor preparation and motor imagery, it is seems likely that they are involved with representations of intended and predicted movements. It has been argued that covert attention (that is, attending to a particular object without actually moving the eyes or hands toward it) is equivalent to mentally reaching for that object with the eyes (foveation) or the hand (Rizzolatti *et al.*, 1987; Corbetta, 1998). During the performance of covert attention tasks, activity is observed in areas that overlap with those seen during motor imagery tasks: anterior cingulate cortex, SMA, lateral premotor cortex (frontal eye fields), and intraparietal sulcus (Corbetta *et al.*, 1993; Nobre *et al.*, 1997).

Another way to isolate the neural correlates of consciousness of action is to try to keep the action the same while varying awareness of it. In one study by Jueptner *et al.* (1997), volunteers learned a choice reaction time task in which there were four stimuli corresponding to four keys. The stimuli came on in a sequence, which repeated exactly every eight trials. As subjects learned this sequence, their responses became faster. After many minutes of practice, they could perform this task without attending to their actions. That their actions were automatic was confirmed by showing that they could do something else at the same time without reaction times being slowed (Passingham, 1996). At the beginning of practice, much activity was observed in frontal cortex, but this activity returned to resting levels once the task had become automatic. After their performance had become automatic, volunteers were also scanned in a condition where they were instructed to think about their performance. In comparison to performance without thought, activity was seen in anterior cingulate cortex (18 10 28, posterior rostral cingulate zone) and in dorsolateral prefrontal cortex. Similar results have been obtained when the comparison is made between learning motor tasks with and without awareness (Grafton *et al.*, 1995; Hazeltine *et al.*, 1997). Awareness that one is learning a skill is also associated with activity in anterior cingulate cortex.

Haggard and Magno (1999) have shown that transcranial magnetic stimulation (TMS) over this brain region delays the initiation of a response and the awareness of initiating that response equally. In contrast, TMS over primary motor cortex delays the initiation of the response more than the awareness of the initiation. Haggard *et al.* (2002) showed that awareness of TMS-caused involuntary movements is delayed compared to awareness of voluntary movements. The sensory consequences of voluntary movements are perceived as being closer in time to the movement than they actually are; this binding effect is reversed when the movement is involuntary. Anterior cingulate cortex is activated not only during awareness of our own actions but also possibly in a slightly more anterior region (anterior rostral cingulate zone) when we are aware of other features of our mental state, including pain (Rainville *et al.*, 1997), thoughts (McGuire *et al.*, 1996), and emotions (Lane *et al.*, 1997).

Phantom Limbs

Abnormal awareness of the state of the motor system in the absence of sensory input or motor output occurs in cases of phantom limbs, but as yet few studies have explored the neural correlates of these experiences, as they are difficult to control. McGonigle *et al.* (2002) investigated a patient who intermittently experiences a phantom left arm in addition to her normal arm.

This phantom appears about 90 seconds after a movement of the real left arm and occupies the position previously occupied by that arm. Looking at the left arm or moving it again eliminates the experience of the phantom (Hari *et al.*, 1998). Because the appearance and disappearance of the phantom could be reasonably well controlled it was possible to perform an event-related fMRI study identifying neural activity specifically associated with experience of the phantom (Fig. 16.5). Only one region could be identified that was robustly associated with the presence of the phantom. This was a region of SMA contralateral to the phantom in the anterior part of SMA proper, as defined by Pickard and Strick (1996). Why activity in this region should be linked with the experience of the *previous* position of the arm remains unclear; however, this result shows that activity in what is traditionally considered a motor area can determine the

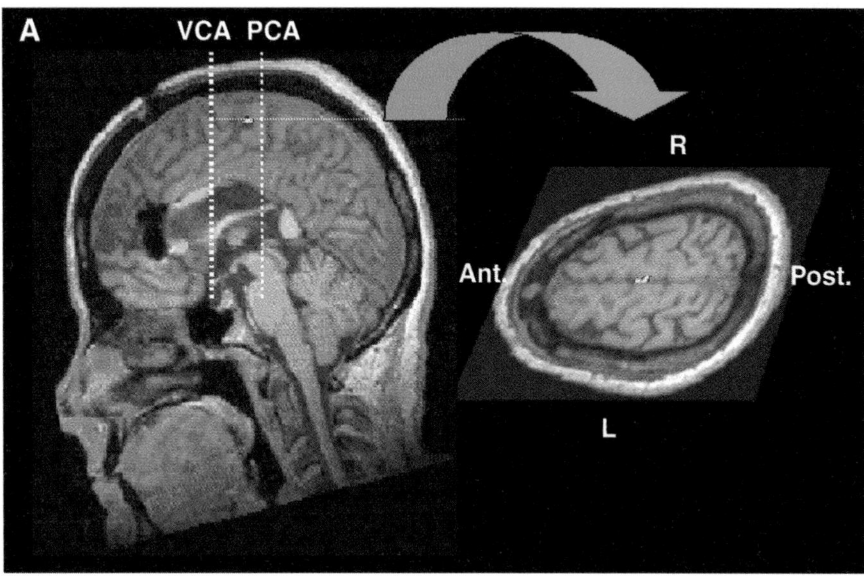

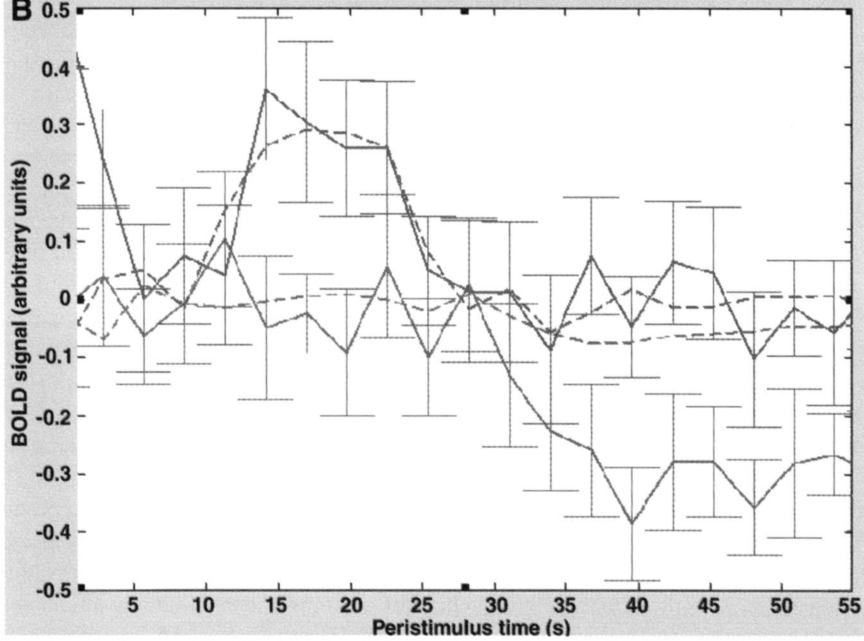

FIGURE 16.5
(A) Sagittal slice (2 mm thick) of the patient's structural scan showing the location of the significant SMA cluster (9 voxels, $t = 5.11$, $P < 0.012$ corrected for multiple comparisons). (B) BOLD signal change at peak voxel of SMA cluster. The blue trace shows activity during 'phantom on' periods. The red trace shows activity during 'phantom off' periods. The error bars show the standard error of the mean around each time point. The traces are shown as a function of peristimulus time. (From McGonigle, D. J., *et al.*, 2002. With permission.)

contents of consciousness. The studies reviewed here consistently relate consciousness of intended actions (and even past actions) to activity in regions of the motor system, especially midline structures such as ACC and SMA; however, we do not yet know whether activity in these areas is necessary or sufficient for experiencing our own actions.

Being in Control

Although we are only conscious of some aspects of our motor system, we are strongly aware of being in control of our actions. Our sense of being in control derives from the experience that our actions are caused by our intentions. In the simple task used by Libet *et al.* (1983), we have the urge to lift our finger and, as a result, we lift it. When we make a movement that we did not intend, we experience a loss of control. Wegner (2002) has persuasively argued that this experience of causation is based on the temporal contingency between the intention and the action. We first have the intention and then, shortly afterwards, the action occurs. Because of this close contingency we believe that we caused the action; however, this belief can sometimes be false. If a volunteer finds her hand moving shortly after having the thought of moving her hand, then she believes that she initiated the movement herself even though the movement was actually caused by someone else (Wegner and Wheatley, 1999). In other circumstances, the reverse error can occur; the volunteer makes the movement, but falsely attributes the cause of this movement to someone else. Thus, in a sense our experience of controlling our own actions is illusory. All we can actually experience is the contingency between the intention and the action. As we have already mentioned, our awareness of intentions, actions, and their consequences seems to be associated with systematic distortions of timing. When we feel that we are in control of our actions and their consequences, the various events are experienced as being closer together in time. When our actions are involuntary and events occur that are not perceived as caused, then the various events seem further apart in time (Haggard *et al.*, 2002), but which comes first? Does the experience of being an agent arise more easily because the time between intention and action is reduced? Or does the time seem reduced because we experience the intention as causing the action?

Whatever the direction of causality, our sense of being in control depends upon being aware of the contingency between the intention and the action and between the action and its consequence. Does our experience of being in control arise from a kind of Pavlovian conditioning by which an unconditioned stimulus (UCS, the action) becomes associated with a conditioned stimulus (CS, the intention)? At first sight it might seem far-fetched to relate a low-level conditioning process to the conscious experience of being in control; however, it has recently been shown that a certain form of Pavlovian conditioning, *trace conditioning*, seems only to occur when the subject is conscious of the contingency between the UCS and the CS. The special feature of the trace conditioning paradigm is that there is a temporal gap between the end of the CS and the beginning of the UCS, so that a memory trace of the CS has to be carried across the interval. The hippocampus appears to play an important role in this kind of learning (Clark and Squire, 1998; Büchel *et al.*, 1999). Perhaps this result relates to the observation discussed earlier in this chapter where we presented some preliminary evidence that maintaining sustained consciousness of a percept depends on a neural system distinct from that involved in attention switches and may involve the hippocampus (Portas *et al.*, 2000b). This sustaining of consciousness is particularly relevant to our sense of ourselves, not only as agents but also as permanent entities in an otherwise changing world.

Contingency implies prediction. The experience of an intention to act allows us to predict that the action will shortly occur, but we can also make more specific predictions about the sensory consequences of the action. We have already discussed in Chapter 15 the observation that activity associated with the sensory consequences of our movements is greatly attenuated. The subjective experience of self-generated sensations is also greatly attenuated, and this attenuation is reduced if distortions are introduced so that predictions about the sensory consequences of our actions are no longer fulfilled (Blakemore *et al.*, 1999). If tactile stimulation is applied to the palm of the hand, then activity is elicited in the contralateral primary somatosensory area (SI) and bilateral secondary somatosensory area (SII); however, if the volunteer applies the same tactile stimulation to her own palm, then this activity is dramatically reduced, in line with the reduction in reported sensation (Blakemore *et al.*, 1998) (Fig. 16.6). This is another example of conscious experience changing while sensory input remains constant, suggesting that these regions may have a special role in the experience of tactile stimulation. However, in addition to the change in tactile experience, there is also the change in the experience of being in control through making a movement. Can we identify distinct neural correlates of these different aspects of the experience of action?

If our arm is passively moved up and down, there is no direct tactile stimulation as in the tickling experiment we have just considered; nevertheless, there are clearly sensory consequences of the passive movement associated with the changes in muscle tension and sensed changes in joint positions. In comparison to the same movements made actively, passive arm movements are associated with greater activity in inferior parietal cortex (parietal-operculum) (Weiller *et al.*, 1996). Presumably, when the movement is made actively, the sensory signals arriving in inferior parietal cortex can be predicted and therefore attenuated. In a recent experiment, we attempted to isolate the sense of being in control from the performance of active movements (Blakemore *et al.*, 2003). Highly susceptible volunteers were hypnotised and scanned in three conditions. In one condition, their arm was passively moved up and down. In the second, they moved their arm actively in the same way. In the critical third condition, they were given the hypnotic suggestion that their arm would be moved up and down passively, as in the first condition. In this condition, the volunteers were making active arm movements but experienced them as passive. With passive movements, as in the experiment by Weiller *et al.* (1996), greater activity was seen in inferior parietal lobe (parietal-operculum). Greater activity was also seen in the insula and the cerebellum; however, greater activity was also seen in these regions when the volunteers experienced their movements as passive even though they were active. This suggests that activity in these areas is specifically associated with the experience of passivity.

A posterior superior region in the parietal cortex was also activated in a study in which volunteers were scanned while moving a joystick that moved a cursor on a screen. In one condi-

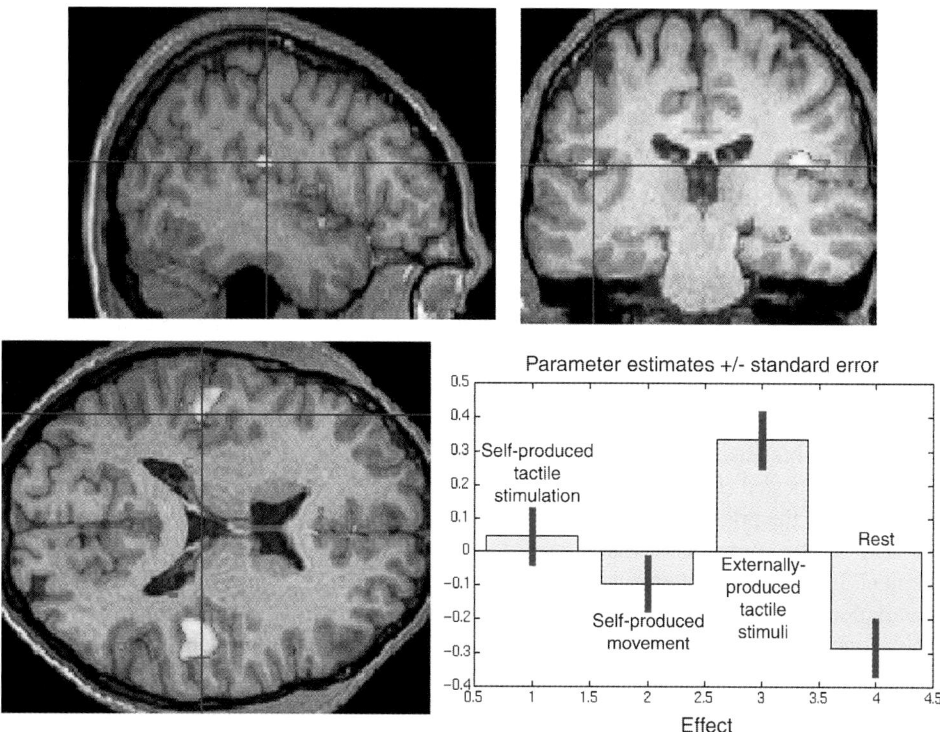

FIGURE 16.6

The lower right hand panel shows the parameter estimates of the BOLD signal in bilateral secondary somatosensory cortex ($P < 0.05$ corrected for multiple comparisons). Activity during self-produced tactile stimulation is attenuated in comparison with externally produced tactile stimulation. The remaining panels show the activity superimposed on a standard structural scan (From Blakemore, S.-J. *et al.*, 1998. With permission.)

tion, the movement of the cursor was controlled by the volunteer, while in another condition the movement was controlled by the experimenter (Farrer and Frith, 2002). The condition in which the volunteer moved but saw movements made by another was associated with greater activity in inferior parietal cortex.

Activity has also been observed in inferior parietal cortex in a number of studies in which volunteers watch the movements of others in order to imitate them (Decety *et al.*, 1997; Grezes and Costes, 1998; Decety *et al.*, 2002). The same region is also activated when volunteers imagine that movements are being made (Ruby and Decety, 2001). There is also a difference depending on whether the volunteer imagines himself or the experimenter making the movements. Imagining that the movement is made by someone else elicits greater activity in right inferior parietal cortex (probably Brodmann's area 39), while imagining one's self making the movement elicits greater activity in left inferior parietal cortex at a more anterior location (BA40). The relevance of these differences in laterality remains to be determined. Nevertheless, a number of studies suggest that the feeling of controlling one's actions is associated with a reduction of activity in right inferior parietal cortex. We shall return to a consideration of the precise role of this region after considering some studies of abnormalities in the experience of the control of action.

Abnormalities in the Experience of Control

Various abnormalities in the experience of control can occur. Patients suffering from the anarchic hand syndrome have a hand (usually the hand contralateral to damage in SMA) that acts without their control. In some cases, the actions of this hand seem to be elicited by the sight of nearby objects. For example, the hand may grasp doorknobs or pick up a pencil and scribble with it (Goldberg *et al.*, 1981). The patient is aware that the hand is carrying out actions that she has not intended and will try to prevent the hand from moving.

Patients with utilisation behaviour show a very similar pattern except that both hands may be involved (Lhermitte, 1983). This disorder is associated with large lesions of frontal cortex often involving medial regions. As with the anarchic hand, the actions performed by the patient can be elicit by the presentation of objects. If the patient sees a pair of spectacles he will put them on, and if he sees a glass of water he will drink from it; however, unlike the patient with an anarchic hand, the patient with utilisation behaviour does not recognise that his actions are inappropriate (and presumably unintended). Rationalisations are produced to explain his behaviour ("I thought you wanted me to do that"). We have suggested that these patients are no longer aware of their prior intentions and therefore cannot recognise that their actions are unintended (Frith *et al.*, 2000). The use of functional imaging with such patients could be very informative about the neural correlates of our experience of actions and intentions.

Many patients with schizophrenia describe passivity experiences in which actions, thoughts, or emotions are made for them by some external agent rather than by their own will: "My fingers pick up the pen, but I don't control them; what they do has nothing to do with me" or "The force moved my lips, and I began to speak; the words were made for me" (Mellors, 1970). In most cases, the actions made when the patient feels that he is being controlled by alien forces are not discrepant with his intentions.

We have suggested (Frith *et al.*, 2000) that this experience of alien control arises from a lack of awareness of the predicted limb position. The patient is aware of his goal, of the intention to move and of the movement having occurred, but he is not aware of having initiated the movement. It is as if the movement, although intended, has been initiated by some external force. In a variation on this theme Spence (1996) has suggested that the problem has to do with the timing of awareness. Spence suggests that a delusion of control occurs when the awareness of the sensory consequences of the movement precedes the awareness of initiating the movement. This is in the opposite order of the normal experience of our own agency. We suggest that, in the presence of delusions of control, the patient is not aware of initiating a movement, as this depends upon awareness of the predicted consequences of the movement. For reasons that remain to be determined, this awareness of the predicted consequences is not available.

There is nothing obviously abnormal in the motor control of these patients. This observation suggests that accurate representations of predicted states are available and used by the motor system; however, these representations are not available to awareness. A number of experiments confirm that there are subtle problems consistent with a lack of awareness of predicted actions. Patients with delusions of control fail to make rapid error corrections based on awareness of discrepancies between intended and predicted limb positions, although they have no difficulty correcting errors based on visual feedback about actual limb positions (Malenka *et al.*, 1982; Frith and Done, 1989). These patients have difficulty distinguishing between correct visual feedback about the position of their hand and false feedback when the image of the hand they see is in fact that of another person attempting to make the same movements as the patient (Daprati *et al.*, 1997). The perception of self-produced stimulation is not attenuated relative to externally produced stimulation in patients with passivity symptoms and/or auditory hallucinations (Blakemore *et al.*, 2000).

Spence *et al.* (1997) used brain imaging to identify brain activity associated with the experience of delusions of control. They scanned schizophrenic patients with and without such delusions while they performed a response selection task. The presence of delusions of control was associated with overactivity in right inferior parietal cortex. We suggest that this overactivity reflects a heightened response to the sensory consequences of the movements the patients were making during scanning. Normally, activity associated with sensory stimulation is much reduced if this stimulation is the direct consequence of our own movements (Blakemore *et al.*, 1998; Curio *et al.*, 2000). This is because the sensory consequences of our movements can be predicted. In the presence of delusions of control, modulation of sensory areas based on such predictions fails, and the regions are overactive. Although the patient is making an active movement, the brain activity resembles that seen with passive arm movements (Weiller *et al.*, 1996), and the associated experience is of a passive movement. We have already seen that greater activity is also seen in this area when normal volunteers attribute actions to others rather than themselves.

Schizophrenic patients do not have any fundamental problems with the control of their actions. The problem lies in their awareness of control; therefore, it seems unlikely that the brain abnormality associated with delusions of control is located in parietal cortex, where the overactivity is observed. Damage to this region is more likely to produce movement problems such as dyspraxia. It is more likely that the damage involves the system that normally modulates activity at this site such as dorsolateral prefrontal cortex. Spence *et al.* (1997) observed underactivity in DLPFC in schizophrenic patients relative to controls, but this was not specifically related to the presence of delusions of control. Nevertheless, when patients who had delusions of control recovered, activity in DLPFC normalised along side the normalisation of activity in inferior parietal cortex. Fletcher *et al.* (1999) provide direct evidence of abnormal modulation of long-range cortico-cortical connections in patients with schizophrenia and suggest that the anterior cingulate has a key role in this system by modulating the effect that DLPFC has on posterior regions.

The Role of Frontal and Parietal Cortex in the Experience of Being in Control

One broad conclusion we might reach on the basis of the material reviewed above is that activity in frontal regions (in particular ACC and SMA) is associated with awareness of movement intentions, whereas parietal activity (especially in inferior parietal cortex) is associated with awareness of the sensory consequences of movement. There is good evidence that when we initiate a movement what we are aware of is the intended movement and the predicted sensory consequences. We are only aware of the actual sensory consequences when things go wrong. The feeling of being in control arises precisely when all our predictions and expectations about our movements are fulfilled. In this case, what we are aware of is a series of motor intentions. This awareness is associated with activity in medial frontal regions. When things go wrong we, quite correctly, feel that we are not in control of our movements and the associated activity will be seen in areas such as the inferior parietal cortex that are concerned with the sensory consequences of movement. The overactivity in the parietal cortex of patients with schizophrenia is associated with the experience that they are not in control of their actions.

The experience of being in control is closely related to the experience of being an agent. It is not just that we predict what is gong to happen; we *cause* what is gong to happen. For a discussion of whether this experience is an illusion, see Wegner (2002). Wegner argues that the only data available to the motor control system concerns contingency: Our acts follow our intentions to act. However, this is nothing but correlation and, as all psychology students know, correlation does not mean causation. Wegner shows how easy it is in the laboratory to fool people into believing that intentions have caused actions when this is not in fact the case.

We are not only aware of our own agency, but also of agency in others. There is a clear difference in the experience of interacting with another agent as opposed to an inanimate object or a machine (Gallagher *et al.*, 2003). There is speculation that the brain mechanisms that allow us to experience our own agency must somehow be related to the mechanisms that permit us to experience agency in others. As with ourselves, another agent performs actions that can be predicted from intentions. However, before we can confirm that the actions we are observing were predicted by intentions, we must have some way of knowing what another's intentions might be. A number of studies (for a review, see Frith 2001; also see Chapter 18) have observed that an area of medial prefrontal cortex (paracingulate cortex) is activated when we try to make explicit inferences about the intentions of others. This region is immediately adjacent (anterior and inferior) to the region that is more active when we attend to our own actions. This provides very indirect evidence that the brain systems that support our awareness of the mental states of others may be linked to the systems that support awareness of our own motor control system.

WHAT KINDS OF REPRESENTATIONS ARE NEEDED TO SUPPORT AWARENESS?

One the prime goals of studies of the neural correlates of consciousness is to demonstrate a qualitative difference between the neural activity supporting conscious as opposed to unconscious representations. This goal has, to a large extent, been achieved. Activity in certain discrete brain regions seems to be necessary for conscious experience, and thalamo-cortical connectivity seems to be necessary for normal conscious wakefulness, but these observations do not increase our understanding of the nature and function of consciousness. The observation that activity associated with consciousness occurs in one brain area rather than another does not in itself tell us anything special about consciousness. We want to know if there is something special about the activity that occurs in these regions. Do the neurons in these regions perform a special kind of computation or do they represent information in a special way?

It is well established that the same information is represented repeatedly in the brain, but in different forms. This principle is most obvious when we consider the position of an object in space. In the early visual system, the position of this object is represented in retinotopic coordinates. In these areas, the neural representation of the object will change if we move our eyes; however, many other coordinate systems are used, and there is some evidence that the parietal cortex has a role in making translations between different coordinate systems (Buneo *et al.*, 2002). For example, there are regions that code positions of objects in terms of head coordinates and in terms of shoulder coordinates. Of particular interest are regions, such as the hippocampus, where *allocentric* coordinates are used (O'Keefe and Nadel, 1978). In such regions, the neural representation of the position of an object remains the same wherever we are in relation to it. In other words, the position is coded in absolute spatial terms.

Each of these coordinate systems can be used for controlling different movements. We can compute the eye movement needed to foveate an object on the basis of retinotopic coordinates, but if we want to reach and grasp an object with our hand then shoulder-centred coordinates would be more useful for computing the required arm movement. Is there a particular form of representation that would be most useful for *conscious* experience of our movements? Jeannerod (1999) has suggested that conscious judgment about a movement requires a different form of representation than that needed for comparisons of predictions and outcomes within the motor system. Following Barresi and Moore (1996), he suggests that conscious judgments about movements require *third-person* information, while control of movement depends upon private *first-person* information. An example of this private, first-person information would be the representation of a reaching movement in egocentric, shoulder-centred coordinates. But, why should conscious judgment about movements require third-person information, and what kind of representation does such information require? Our own approach to this question (Frith, 1995) has been to consider the close relationship between consciousness and reportability. The only way we can know about someone else's consciousness is because they tell us about it. Indeed, the only experiences we can share with others are conscious experiences. For this sharing to be successful, we have to present our experience in a form that is accessible to someone else. One such form would be in terms of the *allocentric* representations we have already discussed in relation to describing the positions of objects in space. In order to tell someone else where an object is we cannot use an egocentric representation ("it's to the left"). We need to use allocentric representations that work equally well from the other's (or any) viewpoint ("it's north of the oak tree"). On this basis, we would predict that the inferior parietal activity associated with observation of the actions of others reflects the activation of allocentric representations of movements. The same would apply to the representations supported by mirror neurons. These are cells that become active, not only when we ourselves make an action but also when we observe someone else make the same action. Thus, the action is represented in a form that is independent of the view of the person acting.

Awareness and the Representations of Objects

In an earlier part of this chapter, we discussed visual consciousness—that is, the awareness of visually presented objects. We presented evidence that visual awareness is associated with activity in areas in the ventral stream that are specialised in representing the feature or object of which we are aware (*e.g.*, V4 for colour, FFA for faces). From our argument from reportability we would expect these representations that support awareness to be independent of viewpoint. Just as with actions, if we want to tell other people about the objects we have seen then we should do so in a form that is independent of our own particular viewpoint; however, in the case of objects, this form of representation is also useful for identifying the objects. We need to be able to recognise that this is the same object even when we see it from an unusual view. Thus, the kind of representation in the ventral stream that helps us to recognise objects would also be useful for sharing our experience of objects with others. This position is similar to that of Milner and Goodale (1995), who suggest that we are aware of information in the ventral stream that has to do with recognising and remembering things while we are not aware of information in the dorsal stream that has to do with reaching and grasping. Viewer-independent representations are useful for visual features as well as objects. As Zeki (1983) has shown, activity in V4 represents colour, not wavelength of light. In other words, V4 represents an object as red even when it is illuminated in yellow or green light. Here, again, we have a representation that is independent of point of view. Perhaps we can make a strong prediction: For neural activity to be a correlate of conscious experience, that activity must represent the object of the experience in a viewer-independent code.

CONCLUSIONS

In a short time remarkable progress has been made in identifying the neural correlates of consciousness. Studies of normal sleep and of patients in abnormal states of arousal suggest that activity in cortico-thalamic circuitry is necessary for any kind of conscious experience. A number of areas in sensory (especially visual) cortex have been identified where activity is necessary for the conscious experience of particular objects and features; however, this activity is not sufficient for conscious experience of these objects and features. Additional activity is also required in frontal and parietal regions.

Studies of awareness of action have identified regions in the medial motor system where activity is associated with awareness of current and intended actions, while regions of inferior parietal cortex display activity associated with the awareness of whether actions are our own or someone else's. Activity in these regions is associated with the experience of being an agent and being in control of what we are doing.

Our knowledge about the neural correlates of various aspects of consciousness has greatly increased. Yet, on the other hand, this knowledge hardly goes beyond correlation. Why do only some brain regions display activity that is associated with consciousness? Why does activity in frontal and parietal regions need to be added to activity in earlier sensory processing areas for conscious experience to emerge? Does this coordinated activity actually create conscious experience and, if so, how?

As yet we have only the sketchiest answers to these questions. The ideas about reportability and viewer-independent representations provide an independent means of defining a class of neurons (in terms of how they represent things) that might have a special relationship with conscious experience. We could take the reportability argument further and suggest that, for conscious experience, it is not sufficient for there to be viewer-independent representations. It is also necessary for the motor components of the report to be prepared—that is, the words or the nonverbal gestures that could be used to communicate the experience. Perhaps the activity seen in frontal and parietal cortex represents report preparation. There are many objections to this argument. First, we all have conscious experiences that just cannot be reported. A trivial armchair example concerns the enormous detail that I have available in my visual image of the world. There is simply too much available ever to be reportable. At the empirical level we have the observations of Lumer and Rees (1999) that, even when volunteers do not have to report binocular rivalry changes, activity is still seen in the entire system, including frontal and parietal cortex. We could argue that the subjects were covertly reporting the changes to themselves, but this seems like a Freudian manoeuvre that renders the original hypothesis no longer testable.

One problem is that, while we have evidence about activity that is necessary for conscious experience, we know nothing about what activity is sufficient for conscious experience. Our hunch is that the next stage of progress is likely to derive from further studies of awareness of the motor system (*i.e.*, self-awareness) and awareness of other people. The major advantage of consciousness is that it allows interactions between brains. Because we are conscious we can describe and thereby share our experiences, and, yet, in the vast majority of the experiments described in this chapter, the volunteers were isolated as far as possible from interaction with other people. It is foolish to imagine that we can solve the problem of consciousness by studying brains in isolation.

References

Andersson, J., Onoe, H., Hetta, J., Lindstrom, K., Valind, S., Lilja, A., Sundin, A., Fasth, K. J., Westerberg, C., Broman, J. E., Watanabe, Y., and Langstrom, B. (1998). Brain networks affected by synchronised sleep visualised by positron emission tomography. *J. Cerebral Blood Flow Metab.*, **18**, 701–715.

Barbur, J. L., Watson, J. D., Frackowiak, R. S., and Zeki, S. (1993). Conscious visual perception without V1. *Brain*, **116**, 1293–1302.

Bargh, J. A. and Chartrand, T. L. (1999). The unbearable automaticity of being. *Am. Psychol.*, **54**, 462–479.

Barnes, J., Howard, R. J., Senior, C., Brammer, M., Bullmore, E. T., Simmons, A., and David, A. S. (1999). The functional anatomy of the McCollough contingent colour after-effect. *NeuroReport*, **10**(1), 195–199.

Barresi, J. and Moore, C. (1996). Intentional relations and social understanding. *Behav. Brain Sci.*, **19**, 107–154.

Bastuji, H., Garcialarrea, L., Franc, C., and Mauguiere, F. (1995). Brain processing of stimulus deviance during slow-wave and paradoxical sleep: a study of human auditory-evoked responses using the oddball paradigm. *J. Clin. Neurophysiol.*, **12**(2), 155–167.

Beck, D. M., Rees, G., Frith, C. D., and Lavie, N. (2001). Neural correlates of change detection and change blindness. *Nat. Neurosci.*, **4**(6), 645–650.

Blakemore, S.-J., Wolpert, D. M., and Frith, C. D. (1998). Central cancellation of self-produced tickle sensation. *Nat. Neurosci.*, **1**, 635–640.

Blakemore, S.-J., Frith, C. D., and Wolpert, D. M. (1999). Spatio-temporal prediction modulates the perception of self-produced stimuli. *J. Cogn. Neurosci.*, **11**, 551–559.

Blakemore, S.-J., Smith, J., Steel, R., Johnstone, E. C., and Frith, C. D. (2000). The perception of self-produced sensory stimuli in patients with auditory hallucinations and passivity experiences: evidence for a breakdown in self-monitoring. *Psychol. Med.*, **30**, 1131–1139.

Blakemore, S.-J., Oakley, D. A., and Frith, C. D. (2003). Delusions of alien control in the normal brain. *Neuropsychologia*, **41**, 1058–1067.

Braun, A. R., Balkin, T. J., Wesensten, N. J., Carson, R. E., Varga, M., Baldwin, P., Selbie, S., Belenky, G., and Herscovitch, P. (1997). Regional cerebral blood flow throughout the sleep-wake cycle. *Brain*, **120**, 1173–1197.

Braun, A. R., Balkin, T. J., Wesensten, N. J., Carson, R. E., Varga, M., Baldwin, P., Selbie, S., Belenky, G., and Herscovitch, P. (1998). Dissociated pattern of activity in visual cortice and their projections during human rapid eye-movement sleep. *Science*, **279**, 91–95.

Büchel, C., Dolan, D. J., Armony, J. L., and Friston, K. J. (1999). Amygdala–hippocampal involvement in human aversive trace conditioning revealed through event-related functional magnetic resonance imaging. *J. Neurosci.*, **19**(24), 10869–10876.

Buchsbaum, M. S., Gillin, J. C., Wu, J., Hazlett, E., Sicotte, N., Dupont, R. M., and Bunney, W. E. (1989). Regional cerebral glucose metabolic rate in human sleep assessed by positron emission tomography. *Life Sci.*, **45**, 1349–1356.

Buneo, C. A., Jarvis, M. R., Batista, A. P., and Andersen, R. A. (2002). Direct visuomotor transformations for reaching. *Nature*, **416**(6881), 632–636.

Burgess, P. W. and Shallice, T. (1996). Confabulation and the control of recollection. *Memory*, **4**, 1–53.

Castiello, U., Paulignan, Y., and Jeannerod, M. (1991). Temporal dissociation of motor responses and subjective awareness. *Brain*, **114**, 2639–2655.

Childs, N. L. and Mercer, W. N. (1996). Misdiagnosing the persistent vegetative state: misdiagnosis certainly occurs. *Br. Med. J.*, **313**(7062), 944.

Churchland, P. S. (1993). *Neurophilosophy: Towards a Unified Science of Mind and Brain.* MIT Press, Cambridge, MA.

Clark, R. E. and Squire, L. R. (1998). Classical conditioning and brain systems: the role of awareness. *Science*, **280**, 77–81.

Corbetta, M. (1998). Frontoparietal cortical networks for directing attention and the eye to visual locations: identical, independent, or overlapping neural systems? *Proc. Natl. Acad. Sci. USA*, **95**(3), 831–838.

Corbetta, M., Miezin, F. M., Shulman, G. L., and Petersen, S. E. (1993). A PET study of visuospatial attention. *J. Neurosci.* **13**(3), 1202–1226.

Corbetta, M., Shulman, G. L., Miezin, F. M., and Petersen, S. E. (1995). Superior parietal cortex activation during spatial attention shifts and visual feature conjunction. *Science*, **270**(5237), 802–805.

Costello, A., Fletcher, P. C., Dolan, R. J., Frith, C. D., and Shallice, T. (1998). The origins of forgetting in a case of isolated retrograde amnesia following a haemorrhage: evidence from functional imaging. *Neurocase*, **4**(6), 437–446.

Coull, J. T., Frith, C. D., Dolan, R. J., Fraclowiak, R. S. J., and Grasby, P. M. (1997). The neural correlates of the noradrenergic modulation of human attention, arousal and learning. *Eur. J. Neurosci.*, **9**, 589–598.

Courtney, S. M., Ungerleider, L. G., Keil, K., and Haxby, J. V. (1997). Transient and sustained activity in a distributed neural system for human working memory. *Nature*, **386**, 608–611.

Cowey, A. and Stoerig, P. (1995). Blindsight in monkeys. *Nature*, **373**, 247–249.

Crick, F. (1994). *The Astonishing Hypothesis.* Macmillan, London.

Crick, F. and Koch, C. (1995). Are we aware of neural activity in primary visual cortex? *Nature*, **373**, 121–123.

Culham, J. C., Brandt, S. A., Cavanagh, P., Kanwisher, N. G., Dale, A. M., and Tootell, R. B. (1998). Cortical fMRI activation produced by attentive tracking of moving targets. *J. Neurophysiol.*, **80**(5), 2657–2670.

Curio, G., Neuloh, G., Numminen, J., Jousmaki, V., and Hari, R. (2000). Speaking modifies voice-evoked activity in the human auditory cortex. *Hum. Brain, Mapping*, **9**(4), 183–191.

Curran, T., Schacter, D. L., Johnson, M. K., and Spinks, R. (2001). Brain potentials reflect behavioural differences in true and false recognition. *J. Cogn. Neurosci.*, **13**(2), 201–216.

Czisch, M., Wetter, T. C., Kaufmann, C., Pollmacher, T., Holsboer, F., and Auer, D. P. (2002). Altered processing of acoustic stimuli during sleep: reduced auditory activation and visual deactivation detected by a combined fMRI/EEG study. *NeuroImage*, **16**(1), 251–258.

Damasio, A. R., Tranel, D., and Rizzo, M. (2000). Disorders of complex visual processing, in *Principles of Cognitive and Behavioural Neurology*, Mesulam, M.-M., Ed., pp. 332–372. Oxford University Press, London.

Daprati, E., Franck, N., and Georgieff, N. (1997). Looking for the agent: an investigation into consciousness of action and self-consciousness in schizophrenic patients. *Cognition*, **65**, 71–86.

Decety, J., Jeannerod, M., Germain, M., and Pastene, J. (1991). Vegetative response during imagined movement is proportional to mental effort. *Behav. Brain Res.*, **42**, 1–5.

Decety, J., Perani, D., Jeannerod, M., Bettinardi, V., Tadary, B., Woods, R., Mazziotta, J. C., and Fazio, F. (1994). Mapping motor representations with PET. *Nature*, **371**, 600–602.

Decety, J., Grezes, J., Costes, N., Perani, D., Jeannerod, M., Procyk, E., Grassi, F., and Fazio, F. (1997). Brain activity during observation of actions: influence of action content and subject's strategy. *Brain*, **120**, 1763–1777.

Decety, J., Chaminade, T., Grezes, J., and Meltzoff, A. N. (2002). A PET exploration of the neural mechanisms involved in reciprocal imitation. *NeuroImage*, **15**(1), 265–272.

Dehaene, S., Naccache, L., Le Clec, H. G., Koechlin, E., Mueller, M., Dehaene-Lambertz, G., van de Moortele, P. F., and Le Bihan, D. (1998). Imaging unconscious semantic priming. *Nature*, **395**(6702), 597–600.

Dehaene, S., Naccache, L., Cohen, L., Le Bihan, D., Mangin, J.-F., Poline, J.-B., and Rivière, D. (2001). Cerebral mechanisms of word masking and unconscious repetition priming. *Nat. Neurosci.*, **4**, 752–758.

de Jong, B. M., Willemsen, A. T., and Paans, A. M. (1997). Regional cerebral blood flow changes related to affective speech presentation in persistent vegetative stat. *J. Neurol. Neurosurg.*, **99**, 213–216.

Dennett, D. (1991). *Consciousness Explained.* Penguin Books, London.

D'Esposito, M., Detre, J. A., Aguirre, G. K., Stallcup, M., Alsop, D. C., Tippet, L. J., and Farah, M. J. (1997). A functional MRI study of mental image generation. *Neuropsychologia*, **35**, 725–730.

DeVolder, A. G. *et al.* (1990). Brain glucose metabolism in postanoxic syndrome: positron emission tomographic study. *Arch. Neurol.*, **47**, 197–204.

Diamond, B. J., Mayes, A. R., and Meudell, P. R. (1996). Autonomic and recognition indices of memory in amnesic and healthy control subjects. *Cortex*, **32**, 439–459.

Dierks, T., Linden, D. E. J., Jandl, M., Formisano, E., Goebel, R., Lanfermann, H., and Singer, W. (1999). Activation of Heschl's gyrus during auditory hallucinations. *Neuron*, **22**(3), 615–621.

Dolan, R. J., Fink, G. R., Rolls, E., Booth, M., Holmes, A., Frackowiak, R. S., and Friston, K. J. (1997). How the brain learns to see objects and faces in an impoverished context. *Nature*, **389**, 596–599.

Driver, J. and Mattingley, J. B. (1998). Parietal neglect and visual awareness. *Nat. Neurosci.*, **1**(1), 17–22.

Drummond, S. P. A., Brown, G. G., Christian Gillin, J., Stricker, J. L., Wong, E. C., and Buxton, R. B. (2000). Altered brain response to verbal learning following sleep deprivation. *Nature*, **403**(6770), 605–606.

Easterbrook, J. A. (1959). The effect of emotion on cue utilisation and the organisation of behaviour. *Psychol. Rev.*, **66**, 183–201.

Edeline, J. M., Manunta, Y., and Hennevin, E. (2000). Auditory thalamus neurons during sleep: changes in frequency selectivity, threshold, and receptive field size. *J. Neurophysiol.*, **84**(2), 934–952.

Edelman, G. M. (1989). *The Remembered Present*. Basic Books, New York.

El Mansari, M., Sakai, K., and Jouvet, M. (1989). Unitary characteristics of presumptive cholinergic tegmental neurons during the sleep-waking cycle in freely moving cats. *Exp. Brain Res.*, **76**(3), 519–529.

Elliott, R. and Dolan, R. J. (1998). Neural response during preference and memory judgments for subliminally presented stimuli: a functional neuroimaging study. *J. Neurosci.* **18**(12), 4697–4704.

Ellis, H. D., and Young, A. W. (1990). Accounting for delusional misidentifications. *Br. J. Psychiatry*, **157**, 239–248.

Engel, A. K., Konig, P., Kreiter, A. K., and Singer, W. (1991). Interhemispheric synchronisation of oscillatory neuronal responses in cat visual cortex. *Science*, **252**, 1177–1179.

Erwin, R. and Buchwald, J. S. (1986). Midlatency auditory evoked-responses: differential effects of sleep in the human. *Electroencephalogr. Clin. Neurophysiol.*, **65**(5), 383–392.

Farrer, C. and Frith, C. D. (2002). Experiencing oneself vs. another person as being the cause of an action: the neural correlates of the experience of agency. *NeuroImage*, **15**(3), 596–603.

Felleman, D. J. and Van Essen, D. C. (1991). Distributed hierarchical processing in the primate cerebral cortex. *Cereb. Cortex*, **1**(1), 1–47.

Feltz, D. L. and Landers, D. M. (1983). The effects of mental practice on motor skill learning and performance: a meta-analysis. *J. Sports Psychol.*, **5**, 27–57.

ffytche, D. H. and Zeki, S. (1996). Brain activity related to the perception of illusory contours. *NeuroImage*, **3**(2), 104–108.

ffytche, D. H., Howard, R. J., Brammer, M. J., David, A., Woordruff, P., and Williams, S. (1998). The anatomy of conscious vision: an fMRI study of visual hallucinations. *Nat. Neurosci.*, **1**, 738–742.

Fletcher, P., McKenna, P. J., Friston, K. J., Frith, C. D., and Dolan, R. J. (1999). Abnormal cingulate modulation of fronto-temporal connectivity in schizophrenia. *NeuroImage*, **9**, 337–342.

Forstl, H., Almeida, O. P., Owen, A. M., Burns, A., and Howard, R. (1991). Psychiatric, neurological and medical aspects of misidentification syndromes: a review of 260 cases. *Psychol. Med.*, **21**(4), 905–910.

Fosse, R., Stickgold, R., and Hobson, J. A. (2001). The mind in REM sleep: reports of emotional experience. *Sleep* **24**(8), 947–955.

Fourneret, P. and Jeannerod, M. (1998). Limited conscious monitoring of motor performance in normal subjects. *Neuropsychologia*, **36**, 1133–1140.

Friedman, H. R. and Goldman-Rakic, P. S. (1994). Coactivation of prefrontal cortex and inferior parietal cortex in working memory tasks revealed by 2DG functional mapping in the rhesus monkey. *J. Neurosci.*, **14**, 2775–2788.

Friston, K. J. (2002). Beyond phrenology: what can neuroimaging tell us about distributed circuitry. *Ann. Rev. Neurosci.*, **25**, 221–250.

Frith, C. D. (1995). Consciousness is for other people. *Behav. Brain Sci.*, **18**, 682–683.

Frith, C. D. and Done, D. J. (1989). Experiences of alien control in schizophrenia reflect a disorder in the central monitoring of action. *Psychol. Med.*, **19**, 359–363.

Frith, C. D., Perry, R., and Lumer, E. (1999). The neural correlates of conscious experience: an experimental framework. *Trends Cogn Sci.*, **3**, 105–114.

Frith, C. D., Blakemore, S.-J., and Wolpert, D. M. (2000). Abnormalities in the awareness and control of action. *Philos. Trans. Roy. Soc. London B*, **355**, 1771–1788.

Frith, U. (2001). Mind blindness and the brain in autism. *Neuron*, **32**(6), 969–979.

Fujita, I., Tanaka, K., Ito, M., and Cheng, K. (1992). Columns for visual features of objects in monkey inferotemporal cortex. *Nature*, **360**(6402), 343–346.

Gallagher, H. L., Jack, A. I., Roepstorff, A., and Frith, C. D. (2002). Imaging the intentional stance. *NeuroImage.*, **16**, 968–976.

Gallo, U. E. and Fontanarosa, P. B. (1989). Locked-in syndrome: report of a case. *Am. J. Emerg. Med.*, **6**, 581–583.

Gerardin, E., Sirigu, A., Lehericy, S., Poline, J. B., Gaymard, B., Marsault, C., Agid, Y., and Le Bihan, D. (2000). Partially overlapping neural networks for real and imagined hand movements. *Cereb. Cortex*, **10**(11), 1093–1104.

Giacino, J. T., Ashwal, S., Childs, N., Cranford, R., Jennett, B., Katz, D. I., Kelly, J. P., Rosenberg, J. H., Whyte, J., Zafonte, R. D., and Zasler, N. D. (2002). The minimally conscious state: definition and diagnostic criteria. *Neurology*, **58**(3), 349–353.

Goebel, R., Khorram-Sefat, D., Muckli, L., Hacker, H., and Singer, W. (1998a). The constructive nature of vision: direct evidence from functional magnetic resonance imaging studies of apparent motion and motion imagery. *Eur. J. Neurosci.*, **10**, 1563–1573.

Goebel, R., Stoerig, P., Muckli, L., Zanella, F. E., and Singer, W. (1998b). Ipsilesional visual activation in ventral extrastriate cortex in patients with blindsight. *Soc. Neurosci. Abstr.*, **24**, 1508.

Goldberg, G., Mayer, N. H., and Toglia, J. U. (1981). Medial frontal cortex and the alien hand sign. *Arch. Neurol.*, **38**, 683–686.

Grafton, S. T., Hazeltine, E., and Ivry, R. (1995). Functional mapping of sequence learning in normal humans. *Hum. Brain Mapping*, **1**, 221–234.

Graves, L., Pack, A., and Abel, T. (2001). Sleep and memory: a molecular perspective. *Trends Neurosci.*, **24**(4), 237–243.

Grezes, J. and Costes, N. (1998). Top-down effect of strategy on the perception of human biological motion: a PET investigation. *Cogn. Neuropsychol.*, **15**(6–8), 553–582.

Grill-Spector, K., Kushnir, T., Hendler, T., and Malach, R. (2000). The dynamics of object-selective activation correlate with recognition performance in humans. *Nat. Neurosci.*, **3**(8), 837–843.

Hadjikhani, N., Liu, A. K., Dale, A. M., Cavanagh, P., and Tootell, R. B. H. (1998). Retinotopy and colour sensitivity in human visual cortical area V8. *Nat. Neurosci.*, **1**(3), 235–241.

Haggard, P., Clark, S., and Kalogeras, J. (2002). Voluntary action and conscious awareness. *Nat. Neurosci.*, **5**(4), 382–385.

Haggard, P. and Eimer, M. (1999). On the relation between brain potentials and awareness of voluntary movements. *Exp. Brain Res.*, **126**, 128–133.

Haggard, P. and Magno, E. (1999). Localising awareness of action with transcranial magnetic stimulation. *Exp. Brain Res.*, **127**, 102–107.

Hampton, R. R. (2001). Rhesus monkeys know when they remember. *Proc. Natl. Acad. Sci. USA*, **98**, 5359–5362.

Hari, R., Hänninen, R., Mäkinen, T., Jousmäki, V., Forss, N., Seppä, M., and Salonen, O. (1998). Three hands: fragmentation of human bodily awareness. *Neurosci. Lett.*, **240**, 131–134.

Hawkins, J. (1989). Sleep disturbance in intentional self-awakenings: genetic-genetic and transient factors. *Percept. Motor Skills*, **69**(2), 507–510.

Hazeltine, E., Grafton, S. T., and Ivry, R. (1997). Attention and stimulus characteristics determine the locus of motor-sequence encoding: a PET study. *Brain*, **120**, 123–140.

He, S., Cohen, E. R., and Hu, X. P. (1998). Close correlation between activity in brain area MT/V5 and the perception of a visual motion aftereffect. *Curr. Biol.*, **8**(22), 1215–1218.

Hennevin, E., Maho, C., and Hars, B. (1998). Neuronal plasticity induced by fear conditioning is expressed during paradoxical sleep: evidence from simultaneous recordings in the lateral amygdala and the medial geniculate in rats. *Behav. Neurosci.*, **112**(4), 839–862.

Hirsch, J., Delapaz, R. L., Relkin, N. R., Victor, J., Kim, K., Li, T., Borden, P., Rubin, N., and Shapley, R. (1995). Illusory contours activate specific regions in human visual cortex: evidence from functional magnetic resonance imaging. *Proc. Natl. Acad. Sci. USA*, **92**(14), 6469–6473.

Hobson, J. A. (1988). *The Dreaming Brain*. Basic Books, New York.

Hofle, N., Paus, T., Reutens, D., Fiset, P., Gotman, J., Evans, A. C., and Jones, B. E. (1997). Regional cerebral blood flow changes as a function of delta and spindle activity during slow wave sleep in humans. *J. Neurosci.*, **17**, 4800–4808.

Horne, J. A. (1978). A review of the biological effects of total sleep deprivation in man. *Biol. Psychol.*, **7**(1–2), 55–102.

Howard, R. J., ffytche, D. H., Barnes, J., McKeefry, D., Ha, Y., Woodruff, P. W., Bullmore, E. T., Simmons, A., Williams, S. C., and David, A. S. (1998). The functional anatomy of imagining and perceiving colour. *NeuroReport*, **9**, 1019–1023.

Inglis, W. L. and Winn, P. (1995). The pedunculopontine tegmental nucleus: where the striatum meets the reticular formation. *Progr. Neurobiol.*, **47**, 1–29.

James, W. (1890). *The Principles of Psychology*. Harvard University Press, Boston, MA.

Jeannerod, M. (1994). The representing brain: neural correlates of motor intention and imagery. *Behav. Brain Sci.*, **17**, 187–202.

Jeannerod, M. (1999). To act or not to act: perspectives on the representation of actions. *Q. J. Exp. Psychol., Ser. A*, **52**, 981–1020.

Jennett, B. and Plum, F. (1972). Persistent vegetative state after brain damage: a syndrome in search of a name. *Lancet*, **1**, 734–737.

Jueptner, M., Stephan, K. M., Frith, C. D., Brooks, D. J., Frackowiak, R. S., and Passingham, R. E. (1997). Anatomy of motor learning. I. Frontal cortex and attention to action. *J. Neurophysiol.*, **77**, 1313–1324.

Kajimura, N., Uchiyama, M., Takayama, Y., Uchida, S., Uema, T., Kato, M., Sekimoto, M., Watanabe, T., Nakajima, T., Horikoshi, S., Ogawa, K., Nishikawa, M., Hiroki, M., Kudo, Y., Matsuda, H., Okawa, M., and Takahashi, K. (1999). Activity of midbrain reticular formation and neocortex during the progression of human non-rapid eye movement sleep. *J. Neurosci.*, **19**(22), 10065–10073.

Kanwisher, N., McDermott, J., and Chun, M. M. (1997). The fusiform face area: a module in human extrastriate cortex specialised for face perception. *J. Neurosci.*, **17**(11), 4302–4311.

Kastner, S., Pinsk, M. A., De Weerd, P., Desimone, R., and Ungerleider, L. G. (1999). Increased activity in human visual cortex during directed attention in the absence of visual stimulation. *Neuron*, **22**(4), 751–761.

Kayama, Y., Ohta, M., and Jodo, E. (1992). firing of 'possibly' cholinergic neurons in the rat laterodorsal tegmental nucleus during sleep and wakefulness. *Brain Res.*, **569**(2), 210–220.

Kihlstrom, J. F., Schacter, D. L., Cork, R. C., Hurt, C. A., and Behr, S. E. (1990). Implicit and explicit memory following surgical anesthesia. *Psychol. Sci.*, **1**, 303–306.

Kinney, H. C. and Samuels, M. A. (1994). Neuropathology of the persistent vegetative state: a review. *J. Neuropathol. Exp. Neurol.*, **53**, 548–558.

Kinomura, S., Larsson, J., Gulyas, B., and Roland, P. E. (1996). Activation by attention of the human reticular formation and thalamic intralaminar nuclei. *Science*, **271**(5248), 512–515.

Kleinschmidt, A., Buchel, C., Zeki, S., and Frackowiak, R. S. J. (1998). Human brain activity during spontaneously reversing perception of ambiguous figures. *Proc. Roy. Soc. London Ser. B, Biol. Sci.*, **265**, 2427–2433.

Knowlton, B. J., Ramus, S. J., and Squire, L. R. (1992). Intact artificial grammar learning in amnesia: dissociation of abstract knowledge and memory for specific instances. *Psychol. Sci.*, **3**, 172–179.

Kourtzi, Z. and Kanwisher, N. (2000). Activation in human MT/MST by static images with implied motion. *J. Cogn. Neurosci.*, **12**(1), 48–55.

Krams, M., Rushworth, M. F. S., Deiber, M.-P., Frackowiak, R. S. J., and Passingham, R. E. (1998). The preparation, execution and suppression of copied movements in the human brain. *Exp. Brain Res.*, **120**, 386–398.

LaBerge, S. and Rheingold, H. (1997). *Exploring the World of Lucid Dreaming*. Ballantine Books, New York.

Lamme, V. A. and Roelfsema, P. R. (2000). The distinct modes of vision offered by feedforward and recurrent processing. *Trends Neurosci.*, **23**, 571–579.

Lane, R. D., Fink, G. R., Chua, P. M. L., and Dolan, R. J. (1997). Neural activation during selective attention to subjective emotional responses. *NeuroReport*, **8**, 3969–3972.

Laureys, S., Goldman, S., Phillips, C., Van Bogaert, P., Aerts, J., Luxen, A., Franck, G., and Maquet, P. (1999). Impaired effective cortical connectivity in vegetative state: preliminary investigation using PET. *NeuroImage*, **9**, 377–382.

Laureys, S., Faymonville, M. E., Degueldre, C., Del Fiore, G., Damas, P., Lambermont, B., Janssens, N., Aerts, J., Franck, G., Luxen, A., Moonen, G., Lamy, M., and Maquet, P. (2000a). Auditory processing in the vegetative state. *Brain*, **123**, 1589–1601.

Laureys, S., Faymonville, M. E., Luxen, A., Lamy, M., Franck, G., and Maquet, P. (2000b). Restoration of thalamocortical connectivity after recovery from persistent vegetative state. *Lancet*, **355**(9217), 1790–1791.

Laureys, S., Faymonville, M. E., Moonen, G., Luxen, A., and Maquet, P. (2000c). PET scanning and neuronal loss in acute vegetative state. *Lancet*, **355**(9217), 1825–1826.

Laureys, S., Faymonville, M. E., Peigneux, P., Damas, P., Lambermont, B., Del Fiore, G., Degueldre, C., Aerts, J., Luxen, A., Franck, G., Lamy, M., Moonen, G., and Maquet, P. (2002). Cortical processing of noxious stimuli in the persistent vegetative state. *NeuroImage.*, **17**(2), 732–741.

Lenzi, P., Zoccoli, G., Walker, A. M., and Franzini, C. (1999). Cerebral blood flow regulation in REM sleep: a model for flow-metabolism coupling. *Arch. Ital. Biol.*, **137**(2–3), 165–179.

Leopold, D. A. and Logothetis, N. K. (1996). Activity changes in early visual cortex reflect monkeys' percepts during binocular rivalry. *Nature*, **379**, 549–553.

Leopold, D. A. and Logothetis, N. K. (1999). Multistable phenomena: changing views in perception. *Trends Cogn. Sci.*, **3**, 254–264.

Levy, D. E. *et al.* (1987). Differences in cerebral blood flow and glucose utilisation in vegetative versus locked-in patients. *Ann. Neurol.*, **22**, 673–682.

Lhermitte, F. (1983). 'Utilisation behaviour' and its relation to lesions of the frontal lobes. *Brain*, **106**, 237–255.

Libet, B., Wright, E. W. J., Delattre, L., Levin, G., and Feinstein, B. (1964). Production of threshold levels of conscious sensation by electrical stimulation of human somatosensory cortex. *J. Neurophysiol.*, **27**, 546–578.

Libet, B., Gleason, C. A., Wright, E. W. J., and Pearl, D. K. (1983). Time of conscious intention to act in relation to onset of cerebral activity (readiness potential): the unconscious initiation of a freely voluntary act. *Brain*, **106**(SEP), 623–642.

Llinas, R. R. and Pare, D. (1991). On dreaming and wakefulness. *Neuroscience*, **44**, 521–535.

Llinas, R. R, and Ribary, U. (1993). Coherent 40-Hz oscillation characterises dream state in humans. **90**(5), 2078–2081.

Logothetis, N. K. and Schall, J. D. (1989). Neuronal correlates of subjective visual perception. *Science*, **245**(4919), 761–763.

Logothetis, N. K., Guggenberger, H., Peled, S., and Pauls, J. (1999). Functional imaging of the monkey brain. *Nat. Neurosci.*, **2**, 555–562.

Louie, K. and Wilson, M. A. (2001). Temporally structured replay of awake hippocampal ensemble activity during rapid eye movement sleep. *Neuron*, **29**(1), 145–156.

Lovblad, K. O., Thomas, R., Jakob, P. M., Scammell, T., Bassetti, C., Griswold, M., Ives, J., Matheson, J., Edelman, R. R., and Warach, S. (1999). Silent functional magnetic resonance imaging demonstrates focal activation in rapid eye movement sleep. *Neurology*, **53**(9), 2193–2195.

Lumer, E. D. (2000). Binocular rivalry and human visual awareness, in *Neural Correlates of Consciousness: Conceptual and Empirical Questions*, Metzinger, T., Ed. pp. 231–240, MIT Press, Cambridge, MA.

Lumer, E. D. and Rees, G. (1999). Covariation of activity in visual and prefrontal cortex associated with subjective visual perception. *Proc. Natl. Acad. Sci. USA*, **96**(4), 1669–1673.

Lumer, E. D., Friston, K. J., and Rees, G. (1998). Neural correlates of perceptual rivalry in the human brain. *Science*, **280**(5371), 1930–1934.

Madsen, P. L. and Vorstrup, S. (1991). Cerebral blood flow and metabolism during sleep. *Cerebrovasc. Brain Metab. Rev.* **3**(4), 281–296.

Madsen, P. L., Holm, S., Vorstrup, S., Friberg, L., Lassen, N. A., and Wildschiodtz, G. (1991a). Human regional cerebral blood flow during rapid-eye-movement sleep. *J. Cereb. Blood Flow Metab.*, **11**(3), 502–507.

Madsen, P. L., Schmidt, J. F., Wildschiodtz, G., Friberg, L., Holm, S., Vorstrup, S., and Lassen, N. A. (1991b). Cerebral O_2 metabolism and cerebral blood flow in humans during deep and rapid-eye-movement sleep. *J. Appl. Physiol.*, **70**(6), 2597–2601.

Malenka, R. C., Angel, R. W., Hamptom, B., and Berger, P. A. (1982). Impaired central error correcting behaviour in schizophrenia. *Arch. Gen. Psychiatry*, **39**, 101–107.

Maquet, P. (2000). Functional neuroimaging of normal human sleep by positron emission tomography. *J. Sleep Res.*, **9**(3), 207–231.

Maquet, P. (2001). The role of sleep in learning and memory. *Science*, **294**(5544), 1048–1052.

Maquet, P. and Franck, G. (1997). REM sleep and the amygdala. *Mol. Psychiatry*, **2**, 195–196.

Maquet, P., Dive, D., Salmon, E., Sadzot, B., Franco, G., Poirrier, R., and Franck, G. (1990). Cerebral glucose utilisation during sleep-wake cycle in man determined by positron emission tomography and [^{18}F]-2-fluoro-2 deoxy-D-glucose method. *Brain Res.*, **513**, 136–143.

Maquet, P., Aerts, J., Delfiore, G., Degueldre, C., Luxen, A., and Franck, G. (1996). Functional neuroanatomy of human rapid-eye-movement sleep and dreaming. *Nature*, **383**, 163–166.

Maquet, P., Degueldre, C., Delfiore, G., Aerts, J., Peters, J. M., Luxen, A., and Franck, G. (1997). Functional neuroanatomy of human slow wave sleep. *J. Neurosci.*, **17**, 2807–2812.

Maquet, P., Faymonville, M. E., Degueldre, C., Delfiore, G., Franck, G., Luxen, A., and Lamy, M. (1999). Functional neuroanatomy of hypnotic state. *Biol. Psychiatry*, **45**(3), 327–333.

Maquet, P., Laureys, S., Peigneux, P., Fuchs, S., Petiau, C., Phillips, C., Aerts, J., Del Fiore, G., Degueldre, C., Meulemans, T., Luxen, A., Franck, G., Van der Linden, M., Smith, C., and Cleeremans, A. (2000). Experience-dependent changes in cerebral activation during human REM sleep. *Nat. Neurosci.*, **3**(8), 831–836.

Marchetti, C. and Della Salla, S. (1998). Disentangling the alien and anarchic hand. *Cogn. Neuropsychiatry*, **3**, 191–208.

McGonigle, D. J., Hänninen, R., Salenius, S., Hari, R., Frackowiak, R. S. J., and Frith, C. D. (2002). Whose arm is it anyway?: an fMRI case study of a somatoform disorder. *Brain*, **125**(6), 1265–1274.

McGuire, P. K., Paulesu, E., Frackowiak, R. S. J., and Frith, C. D. (1996). Brain activity during stimulus independent thought. *NeuroReport*, **7**, 2095–2099.

McIntosh, A. R., Rajah, M. N., and Lobaugh, N. J. (1999). Interactions of prefrontal cortex in relation to awareness in sensory learning. *Science*, **284**, 1531–1533.

Mellors, C. S. (1970). First-rank symptoms of schizophrenia. *Br. J. Psychiatry*, **117**, 15–23.

Menon, D. K., Owen, A. M., Williams, E. J., Minhas, P. S., Allen, C. M. C., Boniface, S. J., and Pickard, J. D. (1998). Cortical processing in persistent vegetative state. *Lancet*, **352**, 200.

Miller, E. K. (2002). The neural basis of the top-down control of visual attention in the prefrontal cortex. In: *Control of Cognitive Processes: Attention and Performance 18*, Monsell, S. and Driver, J., Eds., pp. 511–534, MIT Press, Cambridge.

Milner, A. D. and Goodale, M. A. (1995). *The Visual Brain in Action*. Oxford University Press, London.

Milner, A. D. and Rugg, M. D., Eds. (1992). *The Neuropsychology of Consciousness*. Academic Press, London.

Momose, T. *et al.* (1989). Effect of cervical spinal cord stimulation (cSCS) on cerebral glucose metabolism and blood flow in a vegetative patient assessed by positron emission tomography (PET) and single photon emission computed tomography (SPECT). *Radiat. Med.*. **7**, 243–246.

Morris, J., Ohman, A., and Dolan, R. J. (1998). Conscious and unconscious emotional learning in the human amygdala. *Nature*, **393**, 467–470.

Nakamura, R. K. and Mishkin, M. (1986). Chronic 'blindness' following lesions of nonvisual cortex in the monkey. *Exp. Brain Res.*, **63**(1), 173–184.

Nisbett, R. E. and Wilson, T. D. (1977). Telling more than we can know: verbal reports on mental processes. *Psychol. Rev.*, **84**, 231–259.

Nobre, A. C., Sebestyen, G. N., Gitelman, D. R., Mesulam, M. M., Frackowiak, R. S., and Frith, C. D. (1997). Functional localisation of the system for visuospatial attention using positron emission tomography. *Brain*, **120**(Pt. 3), 515–533.

Nofzinger, E. A., Mintun, M. A., Wiseman, M. B., Kupfer, D. J., and Moore, R. Y. (1997). Forebrain activation in REM sleep: an FDG PET study. *Brain Res.*, **770**, 192–201.

O'Craven, K. M. and Kanwisher, N. (2000). Mental imagery of faces and places activates corresponding stimulus-specific brain regions. *J. Cogn. Neurosci.*, **12**, 1013–1023.

Ohman, A. and Soares, J. J. F. (1994). Unconscious anxiety: phobic responses to masked stimuli. *J. Abnormal Psychol.*, **103**, 231–240.

O'Keefe, J. and Nadel, L. (1978). *The Hippocampus as a Cognitive Map*. Oxford University Press, London.

Pascual-Leone, A., Dang, N., Cohen, L. G., Brasil-Neto, J., Cammarota, A., and Hallett, M. (1995). Modulation of motor responses evoked by transcranial magnetic stimulation during the acquisition of new fine motor skills. *J. Neurophysiol.*, **74**, 1037–1045.

Passingham, R. E. (1996). Attention to action. *Philos. Trans. Roy. Soc. London B, Biol. Sci.*, **351**, 1423–1432.

Perrin, F., Garcia-Larrea, L., Mauguiere, F., Bastuji, H. A., and Gallagher, H. L. (1999). Differential brain response to the subject's own name persists during sleep. *Clin. Neurophysiol.*, **110**(12), 2153–2164.

Perry, R. J. and Zeki, S. (2000). Integrating motion and colour within the visual brain: an fMRI approach to the binding problem. *Soc. Neurosci. Abstr.*, **26**, 250.

Picard, N. and Strick, P. L. (1996). Motor areas of the medial wall: a review of their location and functional activation. *Cereb. Cortex*, **6**, 342–353.

Pierce, C. S. and Jastrow, J. (1885). On small differences in sensation. *Memoirs Natl. Acad. Sci.*, **3**, 75–83.

Pisella, L., Gréa, H., Tilikete, C., Vighetto, A., Desmurget, M., Rode, G., Boisson, D., and Rossetti, Y. (2000). An 'automatic pilot' for the hand in human posterior parietal cortex: toward reinterpreting optic ataxia. *Nat. Neurosci.*, **3**, 729–736.

Plum, F. and Posner, J. (1980). *The Diagnosis of Stupor and Coma*. Davis, Philadelphia.

Plum, F., Schiff, N., Ribary, U., and Llinas, R. (1998). Coordinated expression in chronically unconscious persons. *Philos. Trans. Roy. Soc. London B*, **353**(1377), 1929–1933.

Polonsky, A., Blake, R., Braun, J., and Heeger, D. J. (2000). Neuronal activity in human primary visual cortex correlates with perception during binocular rivalry. *Nat. Neurosci.*, **3**(11), 1153–1159.

Portas, C. M., Rees, G., Howseman, A. M., Josephs, O., Turner, R., and Frith, C. D. (1998). A specific role for the thalamus in mediating the interaction of attention and arousal in humans. *J. Neurosci.*, **18**(21), 8979–8989.

Portas, C. M., Krakow, K., Allen, P., Josephs, O., Armony, J. L., and Frith, C. D. (2000a). Auditory processing across the sleep-wake cycle: simultaneous EEG and fMRI monitoring in humans. *Neuron*, **28**(3), 991–999.

Portas, C. M., Strange, B. A., Friston, K. J., Dolan, R. J., and Frith, C. D. (2000b). How does the brain sustain a visual percept? *Proc. Roy. Soc. London Ser. B, Biol. Sci.*, **267**(1446), 845–850.

Puce, A., Allison, T., Asgari, M., Gore, J. C., and McCarthy, G. (1996). Differential sensitivity of human visual cortex to faces, letterstrings, and textures: A functional magnetic resonance imaging study. *J. Neurosci.*, **16**(16), 5205–5215.

Rainville, P., Duncan, G. H., Price, D. D., Carrier, B., and Bushnell, M. C. (1997). Pain effect encoded in human anterior cingulate, but not somatosensory cortex. *Science*, **277**, 968–971.

Rechtschaffen, A. and Kales, A. (1968). *A Manual Standardised Terminology, Techniques and Scoring System for Sleep Stages of Human Subjects*, U.S. Department of Health, Washington, D.C.

Rees, G. (2001). *Curr. Opinion Neurobiol.*, **11**, 150–156.

Rees, G., Russell, C., Frith, C. D., and Driver, J. (1999). Inattentional blindness versus inattentional amnesia for fixated but ignored words. *Science*, **286**(5449), 2504–2507.

Rees, G., Wojciulik, E., Clarke, K., Husain, M., Frith, C., and Driver, J. (2000). Unconscious activation of visual cortex in the damaged right hemisphere of a parietal patient with extinction. *Brain*, **123**(Pt. 8), 1624–1633.

Ress, D., Backus, B. T., Heeger, D. J., and Gallagher, H. L. (2000). Activity in primary visual cortex predicts performance in a visual detection task. *Nat. Neurosci.*, **3**, 940–945.

Rizzolatti, G., Riggio, L., Dascola, I., and Umilta, C. (1987). Reorienting attention across the horizontal and vertical meridians: evidence in favour of a premotor theory of attention. *Neuropsychologia*, **25**, 31–40.

Rosen, S. D., Paulesu, E., Nihoyannopoulos, P., Tousoulis, D., Frackowiak, R. S. J., Frith, C. D., Jones, T., and Camici, P. G. (1996). Silent ischemia as a central problem: regional brain activation compared in silent and painful myocardial ischemia. *Ann. Intern. Med.*, **124**, 939–949.

Rossetti, Y. (1998). Implicit short-lived motor representations of space in brain damaged and healthy subjects. *Consciousness Cogn.*, **7**(7), 520–558.

Rowe, J. B., Toni, I., Josephs, O., Frackowiak, R. S. J., and Passingham, R. E. (2000). The prefrontal cortex: response selection or maintenance within working memory? *Science*, **288**, 1656–1660.

Ruby, P. and Decety, J. (2001). Effect of subjective perspective taking during simulation of action: a PET investigation of agency. *Nat. Neurosci.*, **4**(5), 546–550.

Rudolf, J., Sobesky, J., Grond, M., and W.D., H. (2000). Identification by positron emission tomography of neuronal loss in acute vegetative state. *Lancet*, **355**, 115–116.

Rugg, M. D., Mark, R. E., Walla, P., Schloerscheidt, A. M., Birch, C. S., and Allan, K. (1998). Dissociation of the neural correlates of implicit and explicit memory. *Nature*, **392**(6676), 595–598.

Sahraie, A., Weiskrantz, L., Barbur, J. L., Simmons, A., and Williams, S. C. R. (1997). Pattern of neuronal activity associated with conscious and unconscious processing of visual signals. *Proc. Natl. Acad. Sci. USA*, **94**(17), 9406–9411.

Sakai, K., Watanabe, E., Onodera, Y., Uchida, I., Kato, H., Yamamoto, E., Koizumi, H., and Miyashita, Y. (1995). Functional mapping of the human colo center with echo-planar magnetic resonance imaging. *Proc. Roy. Soc. London Ser. B, Biol. Sci.*, **261**(1360), 89–98.

Schwartz, S. and Maquet, P. (2002). Sleep imaging and the neuropsychological assessment of dreams. *Trends Cogn. Sci.*, **6**(1), 23–30.

Shergill, S. S., Cameron, L. A., Brammer, M. J., Williams, S. C. R., Murray, R. M., and McGuire, P. K. (2001). Modality specific neural correlates of auditory and somatic hallucinations. *J. Neurol. Neurosurg. Psychiatry*, **71**(5), 688–690.

Silbersweig, D. A., Stern, E., Frith, C., Cahill, C., Holmes, A., Grootoonk, S., Seaward, J., McKenna, P., Chua, S. E., Schnorr, L. *et al.* (1995). A functional neuroanatomy of hallucinations in schizophrenia. *Nature*, **378**(6553), 176–179.

Spence, S. A. (1996). Free will in the light of neuropsychiatry. *Philos. Psychiatry Psychol.*, **3**, 75–90.

Spence, S. A., Brooks, D. J., Hirsch, S. R., Liddle, P. F., Meehan, J., and Grasby, P. M. (1997). A PET study of voluntary movement in schizophrenic patients experiencing passivity phenomena (delusions of alien control). *Brain*, **120**, 1997–2011.

Stenberg, G., Lindgren, M., Johansson, M. Olsson, A., and Rosen, I. (2000). Semantic processing without conscience identification: Evidence from event-related potentials, *J. Exp. Psychology-Learning Memory and Cognition*, **26**(4), 973–1004.

Stephan, K. M., Fink, G. R., Passingham, R. E., Silbersweig, D., Ceballos-Bauman, A. O., Frith, C. D., and Frackowiak, R. S. J. (1995). Functional anatomy of the mental representation of upper extremity movements in healthy subjects. *J. Neurophysiol.*, **73**, 373–386.

Steriade, M. and McCarley, R. W. (1990). *Brainstem Control of Wakefulness and Sleep*. Plenum, New York.

Steriade, M., McCormick, D. A., and Sejnowski, T. J. (1993). Thalamocortical oscillations in the sleeping and aroused brain. *Science*, **262**(5134), 679–685.

Stickgold, R., Hobson, J. A., Fosse, R., and Fosse, M. (2001). Sleep, learning, and dreams: off-line memory reprocessing. *Science*, **294**(5544), 1052–1057.

Sturm, W., de Simone, A., Krause, B. J., Specht, K., Hesselmann, V., Radermacher, I., Herzog, H., Tellmann, L., Muller-Gartner, H. W., and Willmes, K. (1999). Functional anatomy of intrinsic alertness: evidence for a fronto-parietal-thalamic-brainstem network in the right hemisphere. *Neuropsychologia*, **37**(7), 797–805.

Thomas, M., Sing, H., Belenky, G., Holcomb, H., Mayberg, H., Dannals, R., Wagner, H., Thorne, D., Popp, K., Rowland, L., Welsh, A., Balwinski, S., and Daniel Redmond, D. (2000). Neural basis of alertness and cognitive performance impairments during sleepiness. I. Effects of 24 h of sleep deprivation on waking human regional brain activity *J. Sleep Res.*, **9**(4), 335–358.

Tommasino, C. *et al.* (1995). Regional cerebral metabolism of glucose in comatose and vegetative state patients. *J. Neurosurg. Anesthesiol.*, **7**, 109–116.

Tong, F., Nakayama, K., Vaughan, J. T., and Kanwisher, N. (1998). Binocular rivalry and visual awareness in human extrastriate cortex. *Neuron*, **21**(4), 753–759.

Tootell, R. B., Reppas, J. B., Dale, A. M., Look, R. B., Sereno, M. I., Malach, R., Brady, T. J., and Rosen, B. R. (1996). Visual motion aftereffect in human cortical area MT revealed by functional magnetic resonance imaging. *Nature*, **375**(6527), 139–141.

Vogt, S. (1995). On relations between perceiving, imagining and performing in the learning of cyclical movement sequences. *Br. J. Psychol.*, **86**, 191–216.

von der Malsburg, C., Ed. (1981). *The Correlation Theory of Brain Function.* Max Planck Institute for Biophysical Chemistry, Gottingen.

Vuilleumier, P., Sagiv, N., Hazeltine, E., Poldrack, R., Rafal, R., and Gabrieli, J. (2001). The neural fate of seen and unseen faces in visuospatial neglect: a combined event-related fMRI and ERP study of visual extinction. *Proc. Natl. Acad. Sci. USA*, **98**, 3495–3500.

Wegner, D. M. (2002). *The Illusion of Conscious Will.* MIT Press, Cambridge, MA.

Wegner, D. M. and Wheatley, T. (1999). Apparent mental causation: sources of the experience of will. *Am. Psychol.*, **54**, 480–492.

Weiller, C., Juptner, M., Fellows, S., Rijntjes, M., Leonhardt, G., Kiebel, S., Muller, S., Diener, H. C., and Thilmann, A. F. (1996). Brain representation of active and passive movements. *NeuroImage*, **4**(2), 105–110.

Yue, G. and Cole, K. J. (1992). Strength increases from the motor program: comparison of training with maximal voluntary and imagined muscle contractions. *J. Neurophysiol.*, **67**, 1114–1123.

Zeki, S. M. (1978). Functional specialisation in the visual cortex of the rhesus monkey. *Nature*, **274**, 423–428.

Zeki, S. M. (1983). The relationship between wavelength and colour studied in single cells of monkey striate cortex. *Progr. Brain Res.*, **58**, 219–227.

Zeki, S. M., Watson, J. D. G., and Frackowiak, R. S. J. (1993). Going beyond the information given: the relation of illusory visual motion to brain activity. *Proc. Roy. Soc. London Ser. B, Biol. Sci.*, **252**(1335), 215–222.

Zihl, J., Von Cramon, D., and Mai, N. (1983). Selective disturbance of movement vision after bilateral brain damage. *Brain*, **106**(JUN), 313–340.

CHAPTER

17

Functional Imaging of Cognitive Psychopharmacology

INTRODUCTION

The majority of chapters in this volume are based on the idea of neuro*anatomical* segregation of function. In this chapter, however, we are concerned with neuro*chemical* functional specialisation. In other words, a particular cognitive process may be linked not only to a certain network of brain areas but also to a particular neurochemical system. Moreover, through a marriage of techniques, functional neuroimaging can provide us with the ability to localise psychopharmacological effects to discover which neurochemical in which brain area(s) is associated with a specific cognitive function.

The notion of neurochemical functional specificity has been around for decades, with the majority of work being conducted in animals; however, in recent years pharmaceutical agents targeted at individual neurotransmitter systems (*e.g.*, the noradrenergic system) or even at specific neurotransmitter receptors (*e.g.*, the $\alpha 2$ adrenoceptor) have been made available for use in healthy volunteers. For the most part, studies in humans complement already-established findings in rats or monkeys. For example, the well-known role of dopamine (DA) in working memory function as measured by the delayed-response task in monkeys (for a review, see Goldman-Rakic, 1987) has been confirmed in studies of human subjects (Luciana *et al.*, 1992; Müller *et al.*, 1998); however, the human literature has lagged behind the animal research in one key area: anatomical localisation. Through the use of targeted neurotoxic lesions or intracerebral drug injections in animals, it is possible to shut down or stimulate neurochemical functioning in discrete and localised brain regions and so make the link between function, pharmacology, and anatomy. For example, the dopaminergic modulation of working memory is thought to occur primarily in the prefrontal cortex (Goldman-Rakic, 1987). With the advent of functional neuroimaging techniques such as positron emission tomography (PET) and functional magnetic resonance imaging (fMRI), we can now safely parallel this line of research in human subjects. Among the advantages of psychopharmacological functional imaging studies is the ability to study the neurochemical bases of a wider and more sophisticated range of cognitive processes than are displayed by an animal. In addition, the procedure is clearly much less invasive than animal lesion studies, and the number of hours spent training subjects is dramatically shortened.

Briefly, the technique requires subjects to perform cognitive tasks in the scanner in the presence or absence (usually placebo) of a psychoactive agent. A direct comparison of task-induced brain activity between drug and placebo sessions can then reveal whether the drug has modulated activity in some, or all, of the task-related brain areas. Put simply, this neurochemical influence manifests itself as an attenuation or enhancement of activity that is already ongoing due to performance of the task. Thus, we measure the *modulatory* effects of pharmacological agents on cognitive brain systems, rather than their ability to excite or inhibit neural tissue *de novo*.

GENERAL METHODOLOGY

Mechanisms of Neuromodulation

A neurotransmitter or psychoactive drug can exert its effect on neuronal activity in one of two ways. In both cases, the substance (or "ligand") binds to a suitable receptor, located on the cell membrane; however, the physical properties of the receptor itself then dictate the way in which the cell responds. The first, most common, receptor mechanism is direct and fast acting (on the order of milliseconds). Binding of neurotransmitters such as glutamate, acetylcholine, or γ-amino butyric acid (GABA) to this receptor directly alters cell membrane permeability, allowing ions, such as sodium or chloride, to enter the neuron (the ion channel is part of the same macromolecule as the receptor). The ion influx triggers an action potential and excites or inhibits neuronal activity according to specific properties of the neurotransmitters (*e.g.*, inhibitory GABA or excitatory acetylcholine). The second receptor mechanism is slower acting (seconds to minutes) and longer lasting and is seen with neuromodulatory neurotransmitters, such as the monoamines (dopamine, noradrenaline, serotonin), acetylcholine, and GABA (although note that acetylchloline and GABA are not purely neuromodulatory, as their receptors may also comprise ligand-gated ion channels, functioning directly to alter cell permeability as described above). Neuromodulators exert their effects on neuronal activity indirectly via intracellular second messenger systems such as calcium or cAMP (cyclic 3,5-adenosine monophosphate). Once the neuromodulator has bound to a suitable receptor on the neuron, second messengers initiate a biochemical cascade that alters the responsiveness of the neuron to extrinsic chemical or physiological factors. Neuronal responsivity can be modulated presynaptically by altering the synthesis and/or release of neurotransmitters or postsynaptically by changing the excitability of postsynaptic neurons. The modulatory effects of these neuromodulators have important implications for cognition and, more specifically, for functional neuroimaging, as the effects of a drug could differ in the face of (task-induced) increases or decreases in local neuronal activity. In order to image the psychopharmacological effects of neuromodulatory drugs, two complementary methods are available: receptor binding studies or functional activation studies. Each of these is discussed in turn.

Radioligand Receptor Binding Studies (PET and SPECT)

In these studies, the binding density of radioactively labelled tracers are measured with either positron emission tomography (PET) or single-photon-emission computed tomography (SPECT). By labelling a drug that binds to particular receptor types (*e.g.*, ^{11}C-raclopride binds specifically to dopaminergic D2 receptors), the functioning of a specific neurotransmitter system can be compared across groups. Typically, a patient group is compared to a control group and regional differences in binding density are reported. For example, binding of the D1 receptor antagonist ^{11}C-NNC 112 was recently reported to be increased in the dorsolateral prefrontal cortex of unmedicated schizophrenics compared to controls and was correlated with poor performance on a test of verbal working memory (Abi-Dargham *et al.*, 2002). Similarly, striatal uptake of ^{18}F-fluorodopa (which indexes DA neuron density rather than binding to a particular receptor) is decreased in patients with Parkinson's disease compared to controls and is shown to inversely correlate with severity of motor symptoms and disease duration (for reviews, see Brooks, 2000; Thobois *et al.*, 2001). In both of these examples, abnormal receptor binding is used as an index of neurotransmitter dysfunction in the patient group. However, the link between pharmacology and cognition is rather indirect (correlative); patients are scanned during a resting state, and cognitive performance is measured separately. Koepp *et al.* (1998) have pioneered a more behaviourally satisfying approach by directly comparing degree of receptor binding *during* performance of a cognitive task compared to a control task. During the cognitive task, radioligand binding was significantly reduced, thus providing the first evidence of task-induced ligand displacement. This method is clearly a valid and exciting complement to conventional functional activation studies.

Functional Activation Studies (PET and fMRI)

In functional activation studies, the effects of neuromodulatory agents on levels of $H_2{}^{15}O$ (PET) or blood-oxygen-level-dependent (BOLD) contrast (fMRI) are measured in one cognitive condition compared to another. These studies identify brain regions and/or networks for which the cognition-related activity changes following drug administration; however, they do not pinpoint the site of direct drug effect in the same way as radioligand studies, as overall changes in cortical activity may occur downstream from the initial site of action. Typically, and most efficiently, a factorial design is employed with drug administration and task performance as the factors of interest (see Fig. 17.1). Within the constraints of this experimental design, all drug-induced changes are relative to the prevailing cognitive context and do *not* index the direct or primary effects of a drug on local neural activity. By examining the differential effects of a drug during one task condition compared to another, the effects of the drug on noncognitive physiological factors (*e.g.*, vasculature) are averaged out. In other words, the factorial design provides an index of how *task-associated* activity is modulated by the drug, not how brain activity in general is modulated by the drug.

The question of whether to test drug effects within or between subjects is a fundamental issue in cognitive psychopharmacology and is just as pertinent to functional neuroimaging studies as to behavioural ones. With the advent of fMRI and consequently the ability to test the same subject on many separate occasions, placebo-controlled, double-blind, within-subject, counterbalanced designs (in which the subject acts as his or her own control, being tested both with and without drug) are preferable in terms of sensitivity. With this design, particularities of individual brain anatomy and the subjects' behavioural tendencies are equated across drug and no-drug sessions. However, care must be taken with these designs to ensure that there are no psychological or pharmacological carryover effects. For example, a suitable pharmacodynamic wash-out period between drug and placebo sessions must be respected. Furthermore, some psychological research questions preclude the use of within-subject designs—for example, learning or conditioning experiments in which repeated exposure to the same stimuli produces alterations in task performance which could be confounded with drug effects; in such cases, between-group comparisons are required.

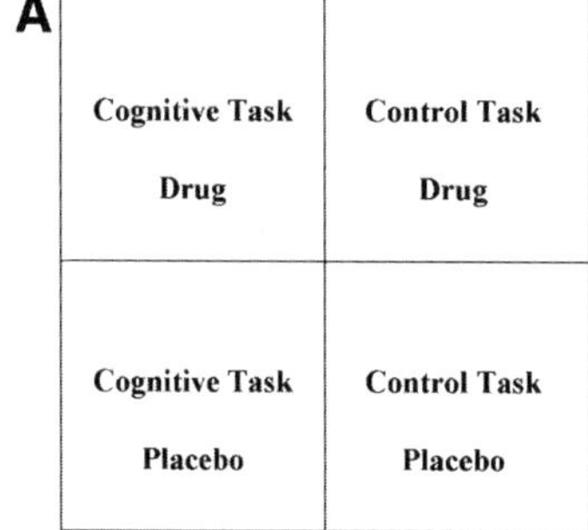

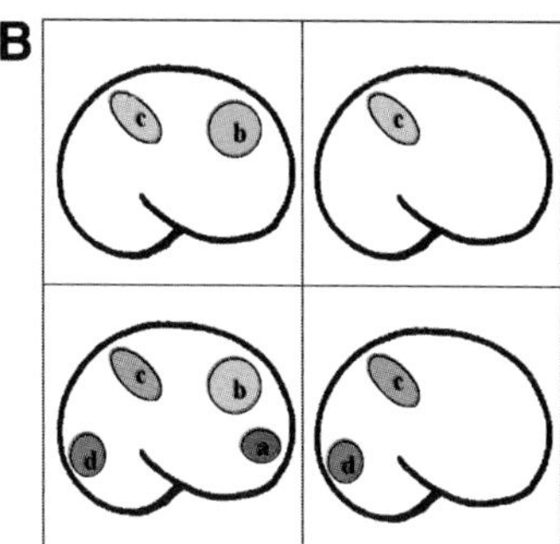

FIGURE 17.1
(Left) A typical 2 × 2 factorial design employed in psychopharmacological imaging experiments, with one pharmacological factor and one cognitive factor yielding four separate conditions. (Right) Hypothetical brain activations produced by each of the four conditions. In this example, the drug affects activation in area *c* equally across both cognitive conditions, representing a global (noncognitive) effect of the drug on brain activity. The drug affects area *b* during the cognitive task only, however, representing a *functionally selective* neurochemical modulation of one of the neuroanatomical substrates of this cognitive process.

Specificity

One of the most thorny problems when interpreting the results of psychopharmacological studies, either behavioural or neuroimaging, is specificity of effect. In other words, are the observed effects specific for a particular class of drug (neurochemical specificity), are they selective for a particular process or task (cognitive specificity), or are they specific to a particular brain region (anatomical specificity). Specificity can be demonstrated by varying one of these three components while keeping the other two fixed. A lack of specificity would suggest that observed drug effects derive from more general consequences of drug administration, such as the sedative/excitatory properties of the drug, the vascular effects of the drug on global blood flow or neurovascular coupling, or the anxiogenic quality of the drug administration itself. In functional neuroimaging experiments, *cognitive* specificity can be demonstrated by measuring brain activity during the task of interest and comparing it to activity during a control task. For example, in Fig. 17.1, the drug attenuates activity in areas *b* and *c* during the cognitive task but only in area *c* during the control task; therefore, nonspecific drug effects on area *c* could be interpreted as noncognitive effects on, for example, global blood flow. However, the drug effect on area *b* during the cognitive task only suggests that this region plays a fundamental role in the neurochemical modulation of the cognitive process of interest. Similarly, *anatomical* specificity can be demonstrated by a selective modulation of the neuroanatomical network normally activated by the task. In Fig. 17.1, the task normally activates regions *a*, *b*, *c*, and *d*; of these regions, the drug modulates activity in areas *b* and *c* only. It is therefore unlikely that the drug is merely exerting a tonic modulatory effect by adding an inhibitory or excitatory bias to the entire set of task-related activations. Finally, *neurochemical* specificity can be demonstrated by including a comparison drug state in the design, as well as the placebo control. Referring to Fig. 17.1, if drug X selectively modulates activity in area *b* (as illustrated) as compared to placebo, but drug Y selectively modulates activity in area *a*, then it is unlikely that modulation of task-associated brain activity is a general consequence of, for example, the shared sedative side-effects of the drugs. Rather, the particular neurochemical properties of drug X are essential for producing the effect in area *b*.

A great number of pharmacological neuroimaging studies have been conducted in the past decade. To facilitate ease of reading and pertinence to this volume as a whole, we limit our discussion to studies of a cognitive nature only and, more specifically, restrict our discussion to those that have explicitly manipulated neurotransmitter function by external administration of a neuromodulatory drug. A notable exception to this are radioligand task-induced displacement studies (Koepp *et al.*, 1998).

DOPAMINE (DA)

Projection System and Receptor Types

The dopaminergic system is comprised of three anatomically separate projection pathways, each originating from midbrain nuclei. The first of these is the *mesostriatal system*, which originates in the pars compacta of the substantia nigra and projects to the dorsal striatum (caudate-putamen). The second pathway, the *mesolimbic system*, originates in the ventral tegmental area (VTA) and innervates the ventral striatum of the basal ganglia (nucleus accumbens, olfactory tubercle, and ventromedial head of the caudate nucleus) as well as certain limbic structures. Finally, the *mesocortical pathway*, also originating from the VTA, projects to frontal and cingulate cortex. In comparison to the widespread innervation patterns of both the noradrenergic and serotonergic systems, the dopaminergic system has a much more discrete area of innervation concentrated in the striatum and anterior cortex. The two main DA receptors are D1 and D2, although D3, D4, and D5 receptors have also been characterised. Receptors of the D1 type are located postsynaptically, while D2 receptors are located both pre- and postsynaptically, with the presynaptic receptor functioning as an autoreceptor to regulate DA synthesis and release. Dopaminergic D1 and D2 receptors are both present in extremely high concentrations in the striatum of rat and human brains; however, they are differentially distributed in the primate frontal cortex, with high levels of D1 receptors in this region and relatively low levels of D2 (Cortés *et al.*, 1989; Camps *et al.*, 1989; Goldman-Rakic *et al.*, 1990).

Functional Specialisation

In functional terms, the dopaminergic system is perhaps one of the most-studied neurotransmitter systems in cognitive psychopharmacology. This is almost certainly due to its well-documented and prominent role in disorders such as schizophrenia and Parkinson's disease, and a variety of methodological techniques have been used to explore the link between dopamine and cognitive dysfunction. For example, neuropsychological studies in patients have provided a means of examining cognitive and motor impairments associated with chronic and endogenous dopaminergic imbalance, while psychopharmacological studies in healthy volunteers examine deficits associated with acute perturbation of the dopamine system via externally administered dopaminergic agents. More specifically, anatomical specificity of dopaminergic effect has been demonstrated by behavioural studies of animals with neurotoxic lesions (e.g., 6-OHDA or MPTP, which impair dopamine function locally), by intracerebral drug injections, or by using electrophysiological single-unit recording techniques. Using a variety of these techniques, neurotoxic dopaminergic lesions of *dorsal* striatum (*i.e.*, caudate nucleus) have been shown to selectively impair motor performance (Amalric and Koob, 1987; Robbins and Everitt, 1992), while electrophysiological recording of *ventral* striatum (*i.e.*, nucleus accumbens) reveal dopaminergic neural activity selectively associated with reward (Schultz *et al.*, 1993; Schultz, 1997). The dopaminergic system of the prefrontal cortex, on the other hand, has been strongly associated with working memory function (Brozoski *et al.*, 1979; Sawaguchi and Goldman-Rakic, 1991; Roberts *et al.*, 1994; Williams and Goldman-Rakic, 1995).

Functional Neuroimaging

One of the earliest functional neuroimaging studies of the catecholaminergic modulation of cognition was conducted in schizophrenics performing the Wisconsin card sort test (WCST) (Daniel *et al.*, 1991). During task performance, SPECT measures of left dorsolateral prefrontal cortex activity were increased in patients given dextroamphetamine but not in those given placebo. Furthermore, increases in prefrontal activity were correlated with drug-induced improvements in task performance. These results suggest that both behavioural and anatomical indices of prefrontal dysfunction in schizophrenia are reversible by catecholaminergic stimulation. A similar conclusion was reached in a later PET study, which examined the effects of the relatively selective dopamine agonist apomorphine on prefrontal function in schizophrenic patients (Dolan *et al.*, 1995, Fletcher *et al.*, 1996). Compared to controls, schizophrenic patients failed to activate anterior cingulate cortex during performance of a verbal fluency task; however, infusion of apomorphine increased task-induced anterior cingulate activity in schizophrenics, thus normalising their frontal brain activity. Intriguingly, there were no effects of apomorphine on verbal fluency-related activity in control subjects (Fletcher *et al.*, 1996). This contrasts with the results of Grasby *et al.* (1992), who examined dopaminergic modulation of memory-associated areas in healthy volunteers. Using a task of verbal episodic recall, they observed attenuation of task-induced activity in left dorsolateral prefrontal cortex by apomorphine. To reconcile these findings, Fletcher *et al.* (1996) suggested that verbal fluency activates prefrontal cortex to a lesser extent than episodic recall, thus precluding observation of a dopaminergic modulation. In other words, dopaminergic modulation of brain function is highly task-dependent. This observation is echoed in the results of Mattay *et al.* (1996). In healthy volunteers, dextroamphetamine increased left prefrontal cortex activity during performance of the WCST (thus replicating the result of Daniel *et al.*, 1991, in a different subject population) while activity in the right hippocampus was increased during performance of Raven's progressive matrices.

At least two recent studies have examined the neuroanatomical substrates of the catecholaminergic modulation of working memory (WM). Using the nonselective catecholaminergic agents methylphenidate or dextroamphetamine, these studies found drug-induced changes in activity of dorsolateral prefrontal cortex during spatial or verbal WM task performance respectively (Mattay *et al.*, 2000; Mehta *et al.*, 2000). Paradoxically, these changes were observed in left prefrontal cortex for the spatial WM task and right prefrontal cortex for the verbal task. The existing literature would predict exactly the opposite pattern of effect (Smith and Jonides,

1998). Another intriguing distinction between the two studies was the direction of effect each stimulant exerted. While both drugs improved performance, methylphenidate decreased prefrontal activity (Mehta *et al.*, 2000), but dextroamphetamine increased it (Matta *et al.*, 2000). Mehta *et al.* (2000) suggest that their prefrontal decreases could, in fact, reflect increased WM efficiency following drug administration: methylphenidate could have increased processing of signals and reduced processing of noise, resulting in a net reduction in neural activity. Common to both studies, on the other hand, was the behavioural observation that greater drug-induced improvements in WM performance were evident in subjects who had lower baseline WM capacity (Kimberg *et al.*, 1997). Mattay *et al.* (2000) further noted drug-induced *impairments* of performance in subjects with *high* baseline WM capacity. This effect is reminiscent of the oft-cited, inverted-U-shaped relationship between catecholamine activity and performance (for a review, see Arnsten, 1998), such that too much or too little noradrenaline or dopamine degrades performance, with intermediate levels producing optimal task performance. Mattay *et al.* (2000) suggested that administration of dextroamphetamine to subjects with high-baseline WM capacity may have pushed them toward the hypercatecholaminergic extremity of the inverted-U-shaped curve, thus impairing performance. The inverted-U-shaped relationship between catecholamines and performance has often been invoked to explain apparently incongruous behavioural results; however, it may also clarify the differences in directionality of prefrontal activity in these two functional imaging studies. Although Mattay *et al.* (2000) noted increases in both prefrontal activity and WM performance when averaging across all subjects, the prefrontal changes were considerably greater in subjects whose performance actually deteriorated with drug infusion (*i.e.*, those with a high-baseline WM capacity). In other words, *increases* in prefrontal activity may be particularly related to performance *decreases*. This inverse relationship between activity and performance is consistent with the results of Mehta *et al.* (2000), who found methylphenidate-induced decreases in prefrontal activity alongside increases in performance.

As well as modulation of prefrontal activity, Mehta *et al.* (2000) noted a drug-induced attenuation of activity in left superior parietal cortex. The authors were careful (rightly so) not to discuss the results of their methylphenidate study in terms of either noradrenergic or dopaminergic effect. However, an interesting follow-up study, using more selective catecholaminergic drugs, may perhaps examine whether the parietal effects were noradrenergic in origin, and the frontal effects dopaminergic. Although Mattay *et al.* (2000) suggested that the dextroamphetamine effects were entirely dopamine based, this drug does not act selectively on the dopaminergic system.

Kimberg *et al.* (2001), on the other hand, used bromocriptine, a selective D2 dopamine receptor agonist, in their fMRI study of verbal WM, WCST performance, and motor function. Bromocriptine attenuated activity in left posterior parietal cortex (in the region of the intraparietal sulcus) during verbal WM, in left anterior insula during WCST, and in left visual cortex during the motor reaction time task. It enhanced motor task-related activity in an extremely small region of right premotor cortex. Importantly, Kimberg *et al.* (2001) used the same "n-back" verbal WM task as Mattay *et al.* (2000). Although both tasks activated right prefrontal cortex (in the region of BA9), there was no modulation of this area by bromocriptine (Kimberg *et al.*, 2001). This suggests that the modulation of activity in this region by dextroamphetamine was not mediated by D2 receptors (Mattay *et al.*, 2000). The possibility remains, of course, that dextroamphetamine modulated prefrontal function via an effect on D1 receptors (Muller *et al.*, 1998); however, a non-dopaminergic effect on noradrenergic function cannot be ruled out.

A clinical counterpart to these WM studies has recently been conducted in patients with Parkinson's disease (Cools *et al.*, 2002). Patients were scanned in the presence (ON) or absence (OFF) of L-dopa medication while performing a spatial WM task and a sophisticated planning task. Abstinence from L-dopa medication (OFF) increased activity in right dorsolateral prefrontal cortex during both spatial WM and planning tasks. A *post hoc* comparison to age-matched controls showed that L-dopa normalised prefrontal function by bringing its activity down to control levels. In other words, there was no significant difference in right prefrontal activity between controls and patients on L-dopa medication, but it was significantly increased in patients off medication. In a similar study, Mattay *et al.* (2002) also observed increases in WM-associated areas (during WM performance), including prefrontal and parietal cortices, in patients off the medication. Interestingly, however, there was a corresponding increase in activity of motor areas (during motor task performance) in patients on the medication. The opposing effects of dopaminergic manipulations on working memory systems and motor systems complement previous findings in animals. For example, 6-OHDA lesions of monkey prefrontal cortex depleted this region of dopamine and impaired performance on a test of spatial WM, but also concurrently increased dopamine levels in dorsal striatum and improved performance on a test of attentional set shifting (Roberts *et al.*, 1994).

Striatal dopamine function was also the focus of the ground-breaking radioligand displacement study by Koepp *et al.* (1998). Healthy volunteers were scanned twice, once during a quiet resting state and once during performance of a video game that taxed both motor and reward processes. Binding density of ^{11}C raclopride (a selective D2 agonist) was significantly reduced in both dorsal and ventral striatum during performance of the game compared to rest. This suggests that binding of *endogenous* dopamine (competing with ^{11}C raclopride for D2 receptors) was increased. As striatal binding potential also correlated with performance, the authors concluded that ligand displacement provides an effective means of indexing the neuroanatomical bases of dopaminergic function by indirectly measuring endogenous task-induced dopamine release. A preliminary report by Zald *et al.* (2002) shows that ^{11}C-raclopride can be used to distinguish cognitive processes more selectively. As compared to a sensorimotor control task, both predictable and unpredictable reward reduced ^{11}C-raclopride binding in dorsal, but not ventral, striatum; however, this effect was greater for predictable, rather than unpredictable, reward conditions. Another very recent study has used ligand displacement to examine the dopaminergic basis of food motivation in food-deprived humans (Volkow *et al.*, 2002). ^{11}C-raclopride binding was significantly altered in dorsal, but not ventral, striatum and correlated with self-reports of hunger. The authors concluded dopamine in the dorsal striatum is implicated in an aspect of food motivation distinct from its role in mediating reward (which would occur via the ventral striatum). Finally, a clinical application of this method by Ouchi *et al.* (2002) demonstrated decreased ^{11}C-raclopride binding in dorsal striatum during performance of a simple motor task in the hemisphere contralateral to motor execution in healthy volunteers, but in the ipsilateral hemisphere of Parkinson's disease patients. These changes correlated inversely with performance, and the authors suggest this hemispheric difference may account, in part, for coordination problems in patients.

NORADRENALINE (NA)

Projection System and Receptor Types

The central noradrenergic system has two distinct projection systems: the ventral noradrenergic bundle (VNAB), associated mainly with sexual and feeding behaviours, and the ascending dorsal noradrenergic bundle (DNAB) of the locus ceruleus (LC) system, implicated in a variety of cognitive functions. The LC innervates a widespread area of the brain, with its largest projections being to the hippocampus and neocortex (Ungerstedt, 1971). Noradrenaline has been shown to follow a general anterior–posterior gradient of both tissue concentration and density of innervation, with high levels being recorded in most areas of the frontal cortex; however, the peak noradrenergic concentrations and highest density of noradrenergic innervation occur in the somatosensory cortex of the parietal lobe (Brown *et al.*, 1979; Levitt *et al.*, 1984). Foote and Morrison (1987) have also reported high concentrations of noradrenaline in the inferior parietal cortex. The four main subtypes of noradrenergic receptor in the brain are $\alpha 1$, $\alpha 2$, $\beta 1$, and $\beta 2$. All of these are primarily postsynaptic receptors except for the $\alpha 2$ receptor, which can be located both pre- and postsynaptically, as well as on the LC neurons themselves. The presynaptic and LC receptors act as autoreceptors, attenuating noradrenergic activity via a negative feedback mechanism when stimulated.

Functional Specialisation

Early electrophysiological studies in rats demonstrated a link between activity of the noradrenergic system and an increase in the signal-to-noise ratio of evoked responses (Foote *et al.*, 1975; Segal and Bloom, 1976). Later, in monkeys, phasic LC activity was shown to increase to targets, but not distracters, during performance of a visual odd-ball target detection task (Aston-Jones *et al.*, 1994), although this response was evident only when tonic LC activity was at an intermediate level, corresponding to intermediate levels of arousal (Rajkowski *et al.*, 1998). The selectivity of this phasic LC response supports behavioural evidence across species, that acute effects of noradrenergic manipulations on attentional function depend upon the underlying (or tonic) level of arousal of the subject (for a review, see Coull, 2001). The noradrenergic α2 receptor system in particular has been implicated in the interaction between arousal and attention. Alpha-2 receptors have also been implicated in working memory function in monkeys, but this appears to be a localised function of α2 receptors in prefrontal cortex and, perhaps even more specifically, of the α2A receptor subtype (Arnsten *et al.*, 1996). Finally, the noradrenergic β receptor system has been implicated in emotional long-term memory, with the beta-blocker propanolol impairing memory for emotive, but not neutral, stimuli (Cahill *et al.*, 1994; Stegeren *et al.*, 1998).

Functional Neuroimaging

Results from one of our own PET studies (Coull *et al.*, 1997) suggest that arousal level interacts with the effects of noradrenaline (NA) on neuroanatomical, as well as behavioural, indices of performance. We compared the effects of clonidine on neural correlates of attentional performance to those of a resting baseline. Contrary to expectation, clonidine did not modulate attention-related regional activity but did selectively attenuate activity in both the thalamus and the LC during the rest condition (Fig. 17.2a). We suggested that this result fits with previous behavioural evidence that arousal level interacts with effects of NA on cognitive performance, as the cognitive tasks appeared to have been sufficiently arousing to counteract the drug effects on

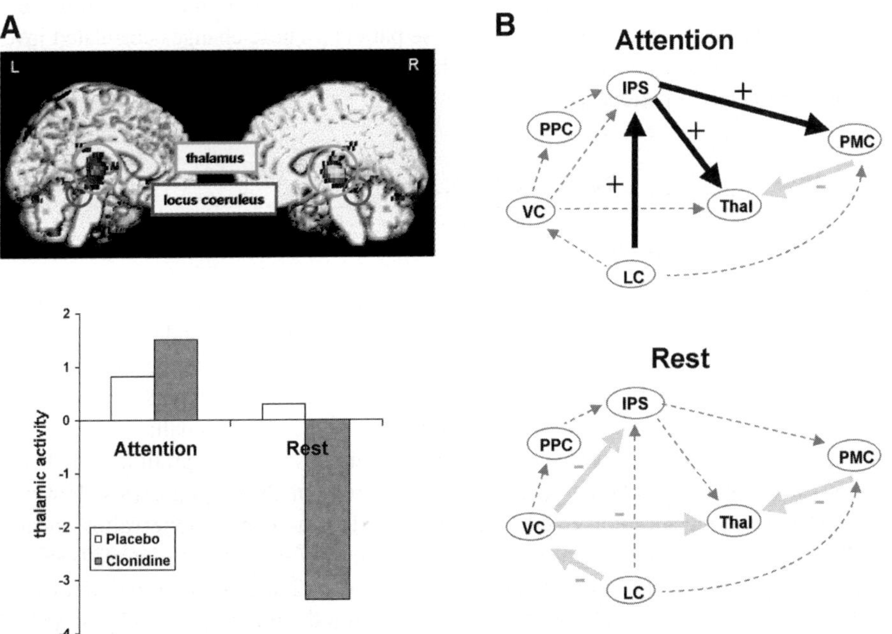

FIGURE 17.2
(a) As compared to placebo, the α2 adrenoceptor agonist clonidine selectively modulated activity in thalamus and locus ceruleus during the rest condition only. Midsaggittal brain templates show areas of drug-induced attenuations in activity, while the plot shows differential thalamic responses to placebo and clonidine during rest compared to an attentional task. Thalamic activity is measured from the site of maximal change (x, y, z = 12, −20, 4), and values represent the difference between baseline activity and that following placebo or drug administration (Coull *et al.*, 1997). (b) Clonidine-induced changes in measures of effective connectivity relative to placebo. Drug effects are strikingly different depending on whether the subject is performing an attentional task or resting quietly. In general, clonidine significantly increases (+, black lines) cross-talk between attention-associated regions during performance of the attentional task, but reduces (–, grey lines) inter-region cross-talk during rest. Dashed lines represent no significant difference between placebo and clonidine (Coull *et al.*, 2000).

thalamic and brainstem activity. This study suggested that both thalamus and LC provide important neuroanatomical substrates for the α2 modulation of the interaction between attention and arousal. A follow-up analysis of this dataset (Coull *et al.*, 2000), using measures of effective connectivity, examined the effects of clonidine on the cross-talk *between* regions rather than drug effects on relative activity *within* a specified region. Effective connectivity allowed us to measure changes in the functional strength of a putative anatomical connection (Friston, 1994; Horowitz *et al.*, 1999) under different pharmacological states. Compared to placebo, we observed that administration of clonidine significantly increased cross-talk between attention-related regions during attentional task performance but reduced the cross-talk between brain regions during the rest condition (Fig. 17.2b). There were no significant effects of the drug on task performance. We suggested, therefore, that during task performance, and in order to maintain optimal performance in the face of clonidine administration, the functional cross-talk between attention-related brain regions (frontal and parietal cortices, thalamus, and LC) had to increase in order to compensate for the potentially deleterious effects of the drug. Indeed, a significant correlation showed that the more task performance deteriorated with clonidine, the more parietal activity increased in compensation. These results are suggestive of a retaliatory response of the brain to neurochemical challenge, rather than a direct effect of the drug on the connections themselves. Furthermore, they illustrate the effect of clonidine on a network of areas that interact dynamically with one another in order to optimise behaviour under differing levels of arousal.

A very recent fMRI study from our group was designed to identify the brain areas underlying the relationship between the effects of α2 agents on attentional performance and the subjects underlying level of arousal (Coull *et al.*, 2003). We examined the brain regions differentially modulated by the α2 agonist dexmedetomidine during performance of an attentional task in the presence (noise condition) or absence (quiet condition) of loud white noise. We used both placebo and the sedative agent midazolam as control drug states. Compared to placebo, midazolam impaired accuracy during noise and quiet conditions equally, but dexmedetomidine impaired performance during the quiet condition only (Fig. 17.3a). In other words, the presence of loud white noise attenuated the detrimental effect of dexmedetomidine on attentional performance. This behavioural effect was accompanied by a dexmedetomidine-related increase in left pulvinar activity during the noise, but not quiet, condition (Fig. 17.3b). Several functional imaging studies have already associated activity in mid- to posterior regions of the thalamus with arousal (Kinomura *et al.*, 1996) or with the interaction between attention and arousal (Portas *et al.*, 1998); therefore, dexmedetomidine-related increases in pulvinar activity during the noise condition may reflect an interaction between increased tonic levels of arousal and an attenuation in the phasic effects of the drug on performance.

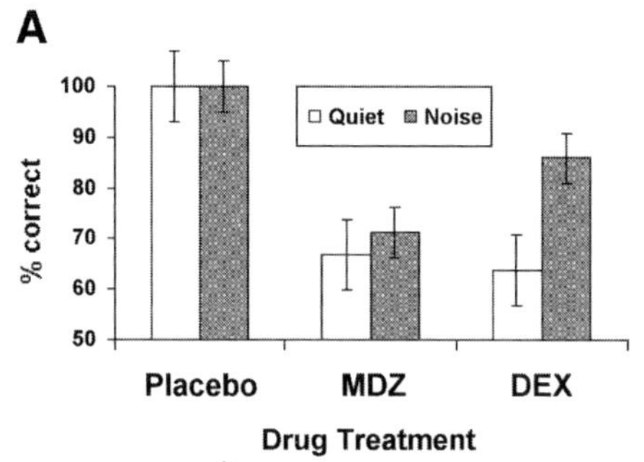

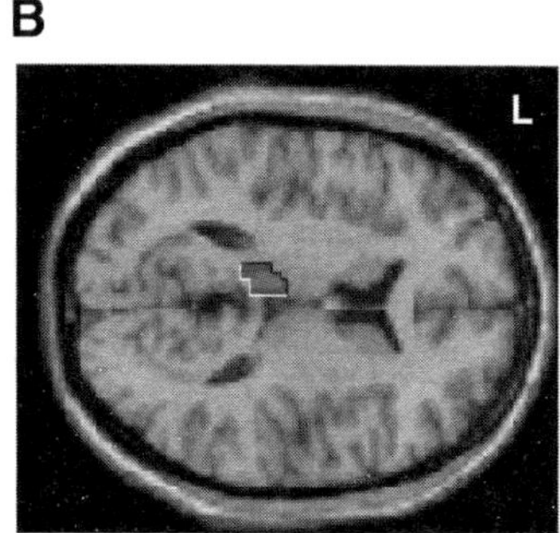

FIGURE 17.3
(a) As compared to placebo, both the α2 adrenoceptor agonist dexmedetomidine and the benzodiazepine midazolam impair attentional performance in *quiet* testing conditions. Simultaneous presentation of loud white *noise*, however, significantly attenuates the deleterious effects of dexmedetomidine on attention, resulting in near-normal levels of performance. Conversely, the midazolam-induced impairment is not modulated by presentation of noise, and subjects perform equally badly in quiet and noisy conditions. (b) Dexmedetomidine selectively increases activity in the left pulvinar nucleus of the thalamus during noisy, but not quiet, conditions.

A number of studies suggest that α2 agents may have a specific effect on spatial aspects of attention. The α2 antagonist idazoxan narrowed the focus of selective spatial attention (Smith *et al.*, 1992), while clonidine infusion broadened it (Coull *et al.*, 1995). Clonidine was also shown to facilitate the disengagement of spatial attention, as measured by the Posner covert spatial orienting of attention task (Clark *et al.*, 1989). In an fMRI study, Coull *et al.* (2001) examined the neuroanatomical substrates of the effects of α2 agents on spatial attention in healthy volunteers. Clonidine significantly affected spatial orienting performance, with a concomitant attenuation of right superior parietal cortex activity. Other regions of the spatial orienting network were unaffected by clonidine administration, suggesting that the right superior parietal cortex is particularly implicated in the modulation of spatial attention by α2 agents. In the same study, we also showed that clonidine-induced impairments of temporal aspects of attention were associated with attenuation of activity in left prefrontal cortex and insula, and clonidine-induced impairments of alerting effects were associated with attenuation of activity in left inferior parietal cortex. In other words, clonidine does not just attenuate activity in the brain as a whole but has regional and localised effects depending on the cognitive context.

The effects of α2 adrenoceptor agents on another aspect of spatial cognition, spatial WM, has been investigated in monkeys by Avery *et al.* (2000). The noradrenergic α2 system, most probably via a postsynaptic α2A receptor mechanism, has been heavily implicated in WM function in monkeys (Arnsten *et al.*, 1996; Arnsten, 1998). In particular, the α2 receptors of the prefrontal cortex are thought to underlie this effect (Arnsten and Goldman-Rakic, 1985). Avery *et al.* (2000) collected SPECT measures of regional activity from monkeys performing a spatial delayed response task. Compared to placebo, the α2A agonist guanfacine improved task performance and increased activity in dorsolateral prefrontal cortex. These two effects were correlated. In addition, guanfacine had no effect on activity in a control area of temporal cortex; however, the authors did not include a control task in their design and admit that modulation of prefrontal cortex by guanfacine may not be selective for WM. In humans, Swartz *et al.* (2000) compared the modulatory effects of guanfacine on delayed and immediate matching to sample tasks. Drug effects in volunteers were compared to patients with frontal (FLE) or temporal lobe epilepsy (TLE), whose epileptogenic zones were aligned to the left hemisphere. Guanfacine improved performance of the delayed task across all subject groups, but the neuroimaging results differentiated subject groups. In healthy volunteers, guanfacine increased regional cerebral blood flow (rCBF) in left premotor cortex; however, in patients with FLE, there was no effect of the drug in premotor cortex in either hemisphere, while in patients with TLE the guanfacine effect was restricted to the right premotor cortex. The authors conclude the reorganisation of the effects of guanfacine on task-related activity in patients was mediated by a direct drug effect on frontal cortex in FLE patients but by an indirect effect, via contributing brain structures, in TLE patients. The results of this ambitious study are disappointing in that guanfacine modulated premotor cortex rather than dorsolateral prefrontal cortex, as would be predicted by the animal literature (Arnsten, 1998); although in humans, a premotor area of superior frontal cortex (BA8) (Passingham, 1993) is activated by WM tasks (Courtney *et al.*, 1998), particularly the maintenance component (Rowe *et al.*, 2000).

Modulation of dorsolateral prefrontal cortex was observed in a PET study of the modulatory effects of clonidine in healthy volunteers versus depressed patients (Fu *et al.*, 2001). During performance of a sustained attention task, clonidine decreased rCBF in superior dorsolateral prefrontal cortex (BA10) in healthy controls but increased activity in the same area in depressed patients. The authors suggest these opposing effects reflect a presynaptic effect of clonidine in healthy subjects, but a postsynaptic one in patients. In support of this, presynaptic α2 adrenoceptor function has been shown to be compromised in depression (Ordway *et al.*, 1994; Schatzberg and Schildkraut, 1995).

In conclusion, presynaptic effects of α2 adrenoceptor agents may reflect modulation of the interaction between arousal and attention via an action on the thalamus, while postsynaptic effects may reflect modulation of processes dependent on prefrontal function, such as working memory. As mentioned previously, β adrenergic receptors have been linked to emotional long-term memory. A very recent fMRI study by Strange *et al.* (submitted) has shown that increased amygdala activity during encoding of emotional material and increased hippocampal activity during retrieval of emotional material are abolished by the β-blocker propanolol.

SEROTONIN (5-HT)

Projection System and Receptor Types

As with the noradrenergic system, serotonergic innervation of the brain is widespread. The median and dorsal raphé nuclei of the brainstem provide the major source of serotonergic neurons in the central nervous system and are systematically organised so as to differentially innervate discrete regions of the brain. Specifically, ascending pathways from the dorsal raphé project mainly to the frontal cortex and striatum, while projections from the median raphé innervate mainly the hippocampus and septum. There are at least 14 receptor subtypes, ranging from 5-HT1 to 5-HT7 receptors (Barnes and Sharp, 1999; Meneses *et al.*, 1999). The functional significance of each of these receptor subtypes is still under discussion.

Functional Specialisation

Evidence for a specific role of serotonin in memory and learning is promising but rather inconsistent (Altman and Normile, 1988; McEntee and Crook, 1991; Gower, 1992; Meneses, 1999). A general consensus from the animal literature appears to be that, while stimulation of serotonergic activity often impairs these processes (McEntee and Crook,1991), a reduction in serotonergic function does not always facilitate memory or learning (Gower, 1992). This is further complicated by the contrasting mnemonic properties of drugs acting at different receptor subtypes (Buhot *et al.*, 2000). In humans, there is a distinct lack of specific receptor agents with which to examine mnemonic function; therefore, a more general serotonergic manipulation that is often used is a low-tryptophan drink which reduces levels of central 5-HT function by depleting tryptophan, a precursor of serotonin. Memory studies using this manipulation have shown impairments on learning and long-term memory consolidation, with no effect on shorter-term episodic recall or recognition (Parks *et al.*, 1993; Riedel *et al.*, 1999; Schmitt *et al.*, 2000).

In addition to its role in memory function, the serotonergic system has been implicated in processes of response inhibition or impulse control (Linnoila *et al.*, 1983; Evenden, 1999). In rats, serotonergic depletion or 5-HT2 receptor stimulation produced premature (or impulsive) responding in a choice reaction-time task (Harrison *et al.*, 1997; Koskinen *et al.*, 2000). Infusion of 5-HT1A and 5-HT1B receptor agonists and 5-HT2 antagonists impaired measures of latent inhibition in the rat (Cassaday *et al.*, 1993), a paradigm in which preexposure to a stimulus alone retards learning of it being paired with another item. In other words, an inability to inhibit the initial (non)response interferes with acquisition of a new pairing. Similarly in humans, tryptophan depletion impaired the ability to reverse learned stimulus–reward associations, with no effect on episodic memory encoding or attentional set-shifting (Parks *et al.*, 1993; Rogers *et al.*, 1999; Rubinsztein *et al.*, 2001). Tryptophan depletion also attenuated the deleterious effects of spatially incompatible stimulus–response relationships in a speeded reaction-time task (Coull *et al.*, 1995). Finally, one of the first studies in humans to suggest a role for 5-HT in response inhibition used the Stroop colour-word task, in which competing response tendencies must be inhibited in order to perform efficiently. Ingestion of a low-tryptophan drink improved the ability of schizophrenic patients to perform the task by reducing colour-word interference (Rosse *et al.*, 1992). These results are all suggestive of a role for serotonin in the inhibitory control of behaviour.

Functional Neuroimaging

A PET study of the serotonergic modulation of learning and memory using the 5-HT1A agonist buspirone found drug-induced attenuation of activity in retrosplenial brain areas of healthy volunteers performing a verbal learning task (Grasby *et al.*, 1992). Conversely, the dopaminergic agonist apomorphine was found to attenuate task-induced increases in activity of left dorsolateral prefrontal cortex. The authors concluded that because the retrosplenial area is densely connected to the hippocampus, their results could indicate a role for serotonin in human mnemonic function subserved by parahippocampal, rather than frontal, brain areas. It is pertinent to note that lesions of the retrosplenial cortex have also been reported to produce deficits in reversal learning in animals (Berger *et al.*, 1986), suggesting serotonergic modulation of this region may also contribute to the effects of serotonergic agents on response inhibition.

A very recent fMRI study has directly examined the neuroanatomical substrates of the serotonergic modulation of response inhibition using a Go/NoGo task (Anderson *et al.*, 2002). Healthy volunteers were scanned following administration of either placebo or *m*CPP (*m*-chlorophenylpiperazine), a 5-HT2 receptor agonist. In a direct comparison of NoGo to Go trials, *m*CPP enhanced NoGo-related activity in right lateral orbitofrontal cortex as compared to saline. Drug-related activity enhancements were also noted in medial visual cortex and right-sided temporal and parietal cortices and caudate nucleus. The authors interpret these results as representing a serotonergic modulation of impulse control via lateral orbitofrontal cortex, an area that has often been implicated in response inhibition.

Serotonergic modulation of higher cognitive processes, such as executive function, was demonstrated by Morris *et al.* (1999) using a verbal fluency task. PET measurements of fluency-associated activity in left anterior cingulate were attenuated by tryptophan depletion in healthy volunteers. Serotonergic modulation of motor processes have also been examined recently. The selective serotonin reuptake inhibitor paroxetine modulated activity in primary motor and sensorimotor areas, including S1, M1, and SMA, during performance of a motor task, as compared to rest (Loubinoux *et al.*, 2002); however, the significance of either of these findings for the functional specialisation of the serotonin system is more difficult to reconcile with the existing behavioural literature, which emphasises a role for 5-HT in either memory and learning or response inhibition (impulsivity).

ACETYLCHOLINE (ACH)

Projection System and Receptor Types

Cholinergic cell groups also send widespread projections to the entire cortex, suggesting a global modulation of cortical information processing by acetylcholine (Ach). Two groups of cholinergic projection neurons are found: (1) the basal forebrain cholinergic neurons (including nucleus basalis, medial septum, and diagonal band of Broca) which innervate the cerebral cortex and hippocampus, and (2) the brainstem cholinergic neurons (including laterodorsal and pedunculopontine tegmental nuclei) that primarily innervate the thalamus. Additionally, there are cholinergic interneurons in striatal areas (Cooper *et al.*, 1996). Cholinergic neurotransmission can occur through different types of muscarinic or nicotinic receptor and is terminated through action of acetylcholinesterases. Both types of receptors are heterogeneously distributed. In the human brain, high concentrations of muscarinic cholinergic M2 receptors are found in subcortical areas such as the thalamus and the caudate/putamen. In the cortex, M2 receptors are highly concentrated in primary sensory areas including somatosensory, auditory, and visual areas (Zilles and Palomero-Gallagher, 2001). Nicotinic receptors are highly concentrated in the thalamus. Cortical areas show low receptor concentrations, with the exception of sensorimotor areas (Zilles *et al.*, 2002). Cortical ACh is hypothesised to facilitate neuronal responsiveness and plasticity (Rasmusson, 2000) and may be mediated specifically through muscarinic receptors (Sato *et al.*, 1987a; Metherate and Ashe, 1991). Evidence of long-lasting changes in neuronal reactivity due to ACh were first shown by Krnjevic and Phillis (1963), and several other studies have confirmed this facilitative role of basal forebrain ACh upon responses to visual (Sato *et al.*, 1987b), auditory (Metherate and Ashe, 1991), or somatosensory (Tremblay *et al.*, 1990) stimulation. Additionally, further studies have shown that, rather than globally enhancing cerebral responses to sensory stimulation, ACh specifically facilitates responses to behaviourally relevant stimuli (Ashe *et al.*, 1989), suggesting that cortical ACh enhances the ability to detect and select salient stimuli for further processing (Sarter and Bruno, 1997).

Functional Specialisation

Psychopharmacological studies have postulated a role of cholinergic neurotransmission in attention, learning, and memory: a hypothesis supported by the finding that cognitive deficits in Alzheimer's disease are concomitant with a loss of cholinergic markers (Perry *et al.*, 1981).

In humans and animals, blockade of cholinergic muscarinic receptors (*e.g.*, with scopolamine) or lesions of cholinergic basal forebrain neurons were found to impair performance in a variety of attention and learning paradigms (for reviews, see Hagan and Morris, 1988; Fibiger, 1991; Blokland, 1996). Conversely, enhancing the availability of acetylcholine (*e.g.*, with physostigmine) reverses lesion- and pharmacologically induced deficits and improves cognitive function in patients with Alzheimer's disease (Hagan, 1994). Thus, scopolamine-induced amnesia has long been used as an experimental model for cognitive changes that occur with aging and Alzheimer's disease. Newer evidence suggests however that ACh seems to be more specifically involved in attentional processes rather than in learning and memory (for a review, see Blokland, 1996).

In humans, drug-induced cognitive impairments are easily obtained with parenteral administration of scopolamine doses from 0.4 to 0.6 mg, especially in the elderly (Curran *et al.*, 1991b; Molchan *et al.*, 1992; Vitiello *et al.*, 1997; Little *et al.*, 1998). Drugs used to investigate experimentally increased cholinergic neurotransmission, on the other hand, are mainly acetylcholinesterase inhibitors, such as physostigmine. Acetylcholinesterase inhibitors increase the action of acetylcholine by preventing its breakdown and thus affect both muscarinic and nicotinic cholinergic receptors. Alternatively, cognitive effects of increased cholinergic neurotransmission can be investigated by stimulating either muscarinic or nicotinic receptors selectively with receptor agonists such as nicotine. Though improvements of cognitive processes after cholinergic stimulation have been reported (Davis and Mohs, 1982; Wesnes and Warburton, 1984; Levin, 1992; Nordberg, 1993; Hagan, 1994), the effects are often small and less consistent than memory impairments observed with anticholinergic drugs (Parnetti *et al.*, 1997). Indeed, there are even indications that a highly overactive cholinergic system can induce attentional dysfunctions (Sarter, 1994).

Functional Neuroimaging

The majority of neuroimaging studies with a challenge to the cholinergic system investigate the neuronal basis of pharmacologically induced memory impairments and improvements. Furthermore, because cholinergic stimulation seems beneficial in some patients with Alzheimer's disease, several neuroimaging studies have investigated effects of acetylcholinesterase inhibitors on blood flow, metabolism, or cholinergic receptor binding in Alzheimer's disease patients. The latter type of study is not covered in this chapter (for a review, see Nordberg, 1999).

The first psychopharmacological neuroimaging study tackling the cholinergic system was performed by Cohen *et al.* (1994) with flurodeoxyglucose (FDG)-PET. Volunteers performed an auditory discrimination task under scopolamine or placebo. Scopolamine induced significant behavioural impairments and reduced metabolic activity in the thalamus. Several other areas were also found to be affected, including a reduction of activity in the cingulate and an increase of activity in basal ganglia. The authors speculate that the regional distribution of the effects of scopolamine is consistent with a cholinergic role in sensory aspects of attention. A very recent PET study (Mentis *et al.*, 2001) also showed that simple sensory processing-related activity can be cholinergically modulated. Elderly volunteers were exposed to a pattern-flash stimulus under placebo, physostigmine, or a combination of physostigmine and scopolamine. Physostigmine decreased activity in occipital and inferior parietal cortex. The addition of scopolamine reversed decreases in activity in occipital but not inferior parietal cortex, suggesting that task-dependent occipital activity is regulated by cholinergic muscarinic receptors (Mentis *et al.*, 2001). The authors further speculate that parietal effects might be explained by nicotinic action. Given the low density of nicotinic receptors in human parietal cortex, however, a direct action on nicotinic receptors in this brain area is unlikely (Zilles *et al.*, 2002).

The effects of cholinergic drugs on higher cognitive processes, such as learning and memory, have been investigated by several authors using functional neuroimaging. Cerebral correlates of the memory-impairing effects of scopolamine on verbal memory were studied by Grasby *et al.* (1995). Subjects received either drug or placebo and were presented with auditory word lists, either short (control) or long (memory), that they were required to remember and immediately recall. Behaviourally, the drug reduced the number of words recalled from the long list. Memory-induced increases in activity were attenuated by scopolamine in left and right prefrontal cortex and anterior cingulate, suggesting that the memory-impairing action of scopolamine might be due to disturbances in activity in these brain regions. Note, however, that the authors were not able to differentiate between encoding and retrieval. A recent fMRI study by Sperling *et al.* (2002) also showed a reduction of inferior prefrontal task-related activity during face–name association learning under scopolamine. Additionally, reduced activations were found in fusiform cortex and hippocampus. These scopolamine-induced neuronal deficits were concomitant with impaired face recognition. A slightly different approach to localising the amnesic effects of cholinergic blockade was taken by Rosier *et al.* (1999). Subjects had to perform an object-recognition task where encoding and retrieval were separated by three days. Scopolamine was administered during encoding, whereas PET measurements were performed during recognition testing three days later. Scopolamine induced behavioural impairments and decreased blood flow in left fusiform gyrus that correlated with behavioural performance. Increases in activity were found in the thalamus and bilateral intraparietal cortex. Even though the authors were not able to investigate the effects of scopolamine on encoding, the advantage of such an approach is to measure drug-related deficits without the confounding effects of drug action on cerebral blood flow. Behavioural and cerebral effects of increased cholinergic neurotransmission in a working memory task have been studied in several experiments by Furey and colleagues (1997) using physostigmine. In a first PET study, participants performed a WM task for faces. Reaction times improved over scans under physostigmine, indicating improved recognition. The drug reduced task-related increases in right inferior temporal/cerebellar cortex and prefrontal cortex. Furthermore, the magnitude of rCBF reduction in prefrontal cortex correlated with decreased reaction times. The study shows that stimulation of cholinergic neurotransmission, which has been shown to improve working memory, modulates activity in a brain region (prefrontal cortex) known to be activated under WM conditions. The somewhat counterintuitive result of reduced prefrontal activity during physostigmine was interpreted by authors as the effect of reduced effort needed to perform the task during physostigmine. It is not clear, however, how this relates to reduced task-related frontal activations found after blocking cholinergic neurotransmission with scopolamine (Grasby *et al.*, 1995; Sperling *et al.*, 2002). A second analysis of the data (Furey *et al.*, 2000a) investigated correlations of reaction times with rCBF under physostigmine. This analysis yielded positive correlations between reaction times and rCBF in right frontal cortex, left temporal cortex, anterior cingulate, and left hippocampus and a negative correlation in medial occipital visual cortex. Because PET studies are not able to investigate different stages of working memory tasks within a block, Furey *et al.* (2000b) performed a further fMRI experiment. Using the same task, several extrastriate regions and the intraparietal sulcus showed increased responses to faces under physostigmine. These responses were bigger during the encoding phase than during retrieval. The authors suggest that improved working memory under physostigmine is due to increased perceptual processing of relevant stimuli. A recent study in our lab extended these findings to a case of selective attention to emotional and neutral faces. In a 2×2 factorial design, subjects viewed fearful or neutral faces which were either at an attended location or not. When compared to placebo, physostigmine enhanced activations to all attended faces by recruitment of additional fusiform areas and induced differential activity in left mid-fusiform to emotional as compared to neutral faces. Furthermore, stimulus-related physostigmine effects were observed in frontoparietal areas. These findings suggest that cholinergic enhancement may bias processing specifically towards biologically significant stimuli.

The role of nicotinic neurotransmission on cognitive function was investigated in two studies, both differentiating between smokers on the one hand and either ex- or non-smokers on the other. Ernst *et al.* (2001) investigated the effects of nicotine on WM. A two-back WM task was used, and subjects received either nicotine gum or placebo. The only common effect to smokers and ex-smokers was a reduction of cingulate activity after ingestion of nicotine, and several differences were found between the smokers and ex-smokers. Compared to placebo, smokers showed reductions of brain activity under nicotine during task performance, while ex-smokers showed increases in prefrontal cortex and left and right inferior parietal areas. Because the behavioural effects of nicotine were only evident in smokers, it is not clear whether the differential cerebral effects of the drug in these two groups are due to altered sensitivity of cholinergic receptors in smokers or to different behavioural outcomes of nicotine administration. Effects of nicotine on cingulate activity were also found by Ghatan *et al.* (1998). Volunteers performed a visuospatial planning task under placebo or nicotine infusion. The main effect of nicotine in smokers and non-smokers was a decrease in rCBF in anterior cingulate cortex and cerebellum and an increase in the parieto-occipital region. In smokers, a task by drug interaction was investigated and yielded increased task-related activity in left occipito-temporal region after nicotine. These results, however, are difficult to interpret because the design and infused dose were different for smokers and non-smokers and no behavioural effects were obtained with nicotine.

Psychopharmacological studies have often tried to dissociate cholinergic effects in explicit and implicit learning paradigms. While cholinergic modulation of explicit memory has frequently been shown behaviourally (Caine *et al.*, 1981; Frith *et al.*, 1984; Nissen *et al.*, 1987; Rusted and Warburton, 1988; Curran *et al.*, 1991a), cholinergic effects on implicit learning are controversial. Several studies in our group have tried to investigate a possible cholinergic modulation of neuronal and behavioural correlates of implicit learning (Thiel *et al.*, 2001, 2002a–c). A first experiment investigated repetition priming, a basic learning mechanism that is concomitant with decrement in extrastriate responses to repeated stimuli (repetition suppression). Prior to the study, volunteers were given placebo, scopolamine, or lorazepam (see GABAergic systems for lorazepam effects). In a word-stem completion paradigm, scopolamine attenuated the behavioural expression of priming and its neuronal correlates (repetition suppression in left extrastriate, left middle frontal, and left inferior frontal cortices) (see Fig. 17.4). Note that scopolamine also affected repetition-related cingulate activity, which is in line with reductions of activity in this brain region in explicit learning paradigms (Grasby *et al.*, 1995).

Similar results were obtained in a face priming task, where scopolamine seemed to attenuate repetition suppression in right fusiform cortex, indicating that cholinergic systems influence the neuronal plasticity necessary for repetition priming. Because ACh seemed to modulate plasticity evident in priming paradigms, we further asked whether cholinergic modulation of learning-related plasticity is also evident in other implicit learning paradigms. Animal evidence suggests that cholinergic cortical projections are important for modulating learning-related auditory cortex plasticity in aversive conditioning paradigms (Weinberger, 1997). Based on the animal evidence, we designed a psychopharmacological fMRI study able to address cholinergic modulation of plasticity in the human brain. We used a conditioning paradigm where subjects were presented with high (1600-Hz) and low (400-Hz) tones, one of which was conditioned by pairing with an electrical shock (Thiel *et al.*, 2002a). Prior to presentation, subjects were given either placebo or scopolamine. Learning-related plasticity, expressed as a conditioning-specific

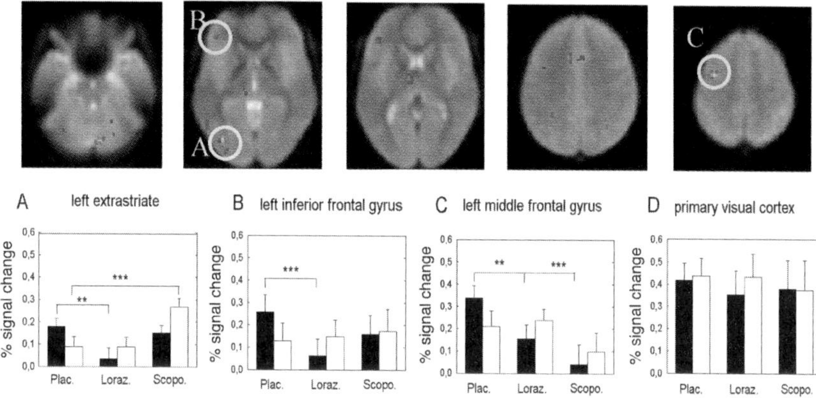

FIGURE 17.4

Drug modulation of activity in a word stem completion paradigm. (Top) Activated regions show impaired repetition suppression under scopolamine and lorazepam (*i.e.*, a drug by repetition suppression interaction) and include, among others, left inferior frontal cortex, left extrastriate cortex, and left middle frontal cortex. (Bottom) Plots of percent signal change (mean and S.E.M.). Compared to placebo, lorazepam reduced activations to new words in all three brain regions. In contrast, scopolamine showed increased activations to old words compared to placebo in extrastriate cortex. Note that the voxel in primary visual cortex shows neither repetition suppression nor an effect of drug. $^{***}p < .001$, $^{**}p < .05$ ANOVAs followed by *post hoc* Tukeys tests comparing activations to new and old words between placebo and drug groups. (From Thiel, C. M. *et al.*, *J. Neurosci.*, 21, 6846–6852, 2001. With permission.)

enhanced cerebral response in auditory cortex was evident under placebo but not under scopolamine (Fig. 17.5). These findings are supported by a wealth of animal literature and nicely illustrate that psychopharmacological approaches in neuroimaging are able to extend findings based on animal research to the human brain. Further evidence for cholinergic modulation of auditory cortex plasticity comes from three PET studies investigating eye-blink conditioning (Schreurs *et al.*, 1997). Two of these studies were performed without a drug challenge, whereas the second was done under scopolamine (but not placebo controlled). When the authors compared activations during conditioning with pseudoconditioning in scopolamine subjects with those from the previous nonpharmacological PET studies (Molchan *et al.*, 1994), they were not able to reproduce the conditioning-associated activations in auditory cortex. This suggests again that cholinergic blockade might have abolished plastic changes in auditory cortex (although the authors themselves did not interpret the findings in this respect).

To further investigate a facilitating role of ACh in auditory cortex during conditioning, we conducted a follow-up study using the same paradigm and a physostigmine infusion to enhance Ach (Thiel *et al.*, 2002c). Contrary to our expectations, it was found that physostigmine reduced conditioning-specific activity. This was due to increased activations to the irrelevant unconditioned stimulus (CS-). The findings are difficult to reconcile with the above-mentioned results of Furey (1997, 2000) and might be due to several factors (for further discussion, see Thiel *et al.*, 2002c). Nevertheless they are worth mentioning in that they show that benefits of cholinergic enhancement might depend on several factors, including, for example, elevation of ACh to an optimal level and precise timing of such elevated neurotransmitter levels. These factors could be especially critical when trying to improve stimulus processing in *healthy* humans. Thus, while cholinergic enhancement is clearly beneficial in states of reduced cholinergic activity, such as in Alzheimer's disease, it might have adverse effects when optimal ACh levels

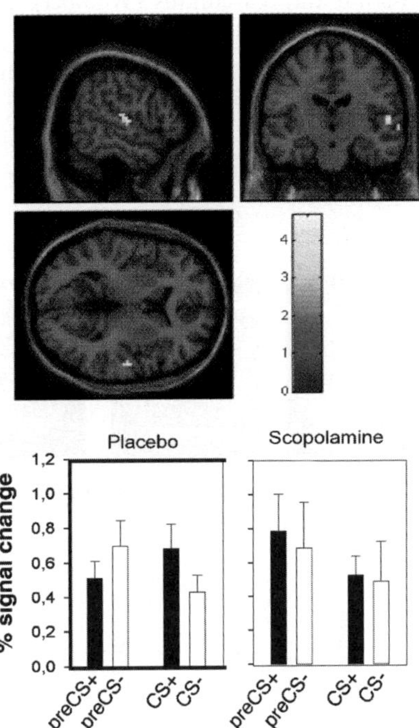

FIGURE 17.5
(Top) Cholinergic modulation of conditioning-related activity in auditory cortex. Activations represent a group (placebo versus scopolamine) by time (preconditioning versus conditioning) and by conditioning (CS+ versus CS–) interaction. Significant differences indicating a higher time by conditioning interaction in placebo compared to scopolamine subjects were found in the right auditory cortex. (Bottom) Plots of percent signal change (mean and S.E.M.). Note the increase in right auditory cortex activation to the CS+ (black symbols) when comparing preconditioning with the conditioning phase and the decrease in activation for the CS– (white symbols) in the placebo group, while scopolamine subjects showed decreases in activations for the CS+. (Results of the low tone group modified from Thiel *et al.*, 2002b.)

are already present. This is supported by *in vitro* evidence for decreased ACh release in normal brain tissue when a cholinesterase inhibitor is applied as opposed to increased ACh release in brains of Alzheimer's disease patients (Nordberg *et al.*, 1989).

In summary, effects of cholinergic drugs on brain areas associated with specific cognitive functions has almost exclusively focused on learning and memory. Even though the effects were dependent on the respective tasks and paradigms, several commonalities are found across studies. When looking at explicit learning paradigms, several studies have found effects in prefrontal cortex and anterior cingulate. The direction of these frontal cortical changes were, however, always activity reductions, no matter whether the action of the drug was an attenuation (Cohen *et al.*, 1994; Grasby *et al.*, 1995; Thiel *et al.*, 2001) or stimulation (Ghatan *et al.*, 1998; Furey *et al.*, 2000b; Ernst *et al.*, 2001) of cholinergic neurotransmission. Another commonality found in many of these studies was the effects of cholinergic drugs on brain areas involved in relatively early steps of stimulus processing such as extrastriate areas, for example (Furey *et al.*, 2000b; Mentis *et al.*, 2001; Thiel *et al.*, 2001). These findings are in line with the suggestion that cortical ACh modulates the general efficacy of cortical information processing (Sarter and Bruno, 1997). Given this evidence and behavioural studies that have suggested for a while that cholinergic systems are involved in attention rather than learning (Blokland, 1996), it is remarkable that only very recently has research started to focus on cholinergic modulation of neuronal correlates of attentional functions (Lawrence *et al.*, 2002; Bentley *et al.*, 2003).

GABA (BENZODIAZEPINES)

Projection System and Receptor Types

The amino acid GABA (γ-aminobutyric acid) is the major inhibitory neurotransmitter in the central nervous system and exerts a crucial role in regulating brain excitability. Indeed, around 40% of all central nervous system neurons utilise GABA as their primary neurotransmitter. In contrast to the far-reaching actions of the monoaminergic and cholinergic cortical projection systems, GABA is primarily involved in mediating inhibition within intrinsic circuits and maintaining local neuronal dynamics (Elliott *et al.*, 2000). The three types of GABA receptors are GABA-A, GABA-B, and GABA-C. GABA-A receptors are frequently studied and constitute a heterogeneous family of multi-subunit receptor channels that are targets for many drugs including benzodiazepines, barbiturates, and anaesthetics (McKernan and Whiting, 1996). Benzodiazepines have been the focus of many psychopharmacological studies because they include some of the most widely prescribed psychotropic drugs, such as diazepam (valium). These drugs act through displacement of an endogenous inhibitor at GABA-A receptors, thus potentiating the action of tonically released GABA (for reviews, see Paul, 1995; Cooper *et al.*, 1996). GABA-A receptors are found in extremely high concentrations throughout the human cortex (Zilles *et al.*, 2002). In rats it was shown that one benzodiazepine binding GABA-A receptor is localised on interneurons in hippocampus and cortex and on cerebral Purkinje cells. Other benzodiazepine receptors are found on hippocampal pyramidal cells or on cholinergic and monoaminergic neurons where they regulate neurotransmitter turnover (McKernan and Whiting, 1996).

Functional Specialisation

Enhancement of GABA-A-mediated inhibition with benzodiazepines can lead to a variety of cognitive and emotional effects. Neuroimaging studies involving challenges to the GABAergic system have thus investigated neuronal correlates of benzodiazepine action. Benzodiazepines are prescribed for their sedative, hypnotic, and anxiolytic effects, but they also exhibit muscle relaxant, anticonvulsant, and amnestic properties. The amnestic properties have contributed to the use of these drugs (alongside muscarinic antagonists) as pharmacological models of memory dysfunction (Barbee, 1993). Well-documented acquisition deficits are seen following administration of different benzodiazepines (Ghoneim *et al.*, 1984; Rodrigo and Lusiardo, 1988; Hennessey *et al.*, 1991), which are thought to underlie the benzodiazepine-induced anterograde amnesic state, whereby conversion of memories from short-term memory to long-term memory is impaired (Curran, 1986, 1991). Less commonly, diazepam-induced memory impairments have also been interpreted in terms of central executive dysfunction (Rusted *et al.*, 1991; Coull *et al.*, 1995a). Interestingly, a dissociation in the cognitive effects of two different benzodiazepines (namely, lorazepam and diazepam) has often been described. While both drugs impair explicit memory, only lorazepam affects implicit memory (Legrand *et al.*, 1995). Studies with lorazepam have furthermore shown that the drug affects perceptual integration, and it was suggested that GABA-A-mediated inhibition may represent a candidate for generating synchronisation and binding at the network level (Elliott *et al.*, 2000; Beckers *et al.*, 2001).

Functional Neuroimaging

Functional neuroimaging studies have mainly investigated benzodiazepine modulation in relation to memory encoding. Because encoding-related activity has been found in non-pharmacological studies within the prefrontal cortex, it was hypothesised that memory impairing effects of benzodiazepines might be localised in this brain region. A successful demonstration of the prefrontal actions of the drug during memory encoding and furthermore a dissociation of these effects from impairments of executive function was given by Coull *et al.* (1999). Following a factorial design, with memory encoding and stimulus ordering (executive task) as factors, subjects performed four different tasks involving visually presented letter strings. Independent of task, diazepam increased activity in extrastriate cortex and decreased activity in prefrontal and temporal cortices. Task by drug interactions showed that diazepam attenuated activity in left dorsal prefrontal cortex during memory encoding and in left frontal operculum during ordering, suggesting different cerebral loci for the effects of diazepam on tasks involving executive function and episodic memory.

Using two other benzodiazepines (midazolam and triazolam) and also a verbal encoding task, neither Bagary *et al.* (2000) nor Mintzer *et al.* (2001) were able to show drug-induced attenuations of frontal cortical activity even though the drugs induced memory deficits. In the study by Bagary *et al.* (2000), subjects performed three tasks involving orally presented words that had to be remembered (encoding) or not remembered (implicit processing) and a motor control condition. Even though midazolam decreased rCBF independently in several regions, including temporal, prefrontal, and parieto-occipital areas, the drug did not affect frontal cortical activations when encoding was compared with implicit processing. The study by Mintzer *et al.* (2001) compared semantic with orthographic encoding and found attenuation of activity in right anterior cingulate, right cerebellum, and left precuneus after triazolam. These regions have been previously shown to be relevant for encoding and other cognitive functions. Note, however, that none of these areas was active when the task was performed under placebo. Attenuation of inferior prefrontal activations was found in a recent fMRI study investigating the effects of lorazepam on face–name association learning (Sperling *et al.*, 2002). Further lorazepam-induced, encoding-related activity changes were evident in fusiform cortex and hippocampus. A benzodiazepine modulation of fusiform activity is further supported by evidence of Rosier *et al.* (1997). Volunteers received diazepam during encoding of abstract shapes. As previously (see prior section discussing the cholinergic system), cerebral correlates of drug effects were not studied during encoding but three days later during recognition when drug-induced impairments were evident.

Behavioural effects of benzodiazepines in explicit learning paradigms are well documented and are generally similar for different types of benzodiazepines. In contrast, only lorazepam has been shown to reliably induce impairments of implicit memory. We investigated the effects of lorazepam on implicit learning in two repetition priming paradigms with event-related fMRI (Thiel *et al.*, 2001, 2002b) (see also section on cholinergic systems). Our results showed that in a word-stem completion paradigm lorazepam impaired behavioural and neuronal indices of repetition priming in left extrastriate, left middle frontal, and left inferior frontal cortices (Thiel *et al.*, 2001) (see Fig. 17.4). In contrast, when using a face repetition paradigm, neither the behavioural nor the neuronal indices of priming were impaired with lorazepam (Thiel *et al.*, 2002b). Independent of priming, the drug did, however, attenuate left fusiform activity to presentation of faces, which is in line with effects reported by Sperling *et al.* (2002) and Rosier *et al.* (1997). Benzodiazepine-induced deactivations in temporal and parieto-occipital regions were also found by Bagary *et al.* when comparing an implicit word-processing condition with a motor control task, even though the drug did not impair implicit memory significantly (Bagary *et al.*, 2000).

Because both benzodiazepines and antimuscarinic drugs induce learning and memory impairments, some of the above studies have compared cholinergic and GABAergic modulation of cognitive function in the same paradigm. Rosier *et al.* (1997 and 1999) showed a similar reduction of fusiform activity after diazepam and scopolamine during shape recognition (Rosier *et al.*, 1997). Sperling *et al.* (2002) also found an overlap of lorazepam- and scopolamine-induced activity reductions during encoding of face–name associations which were evident in fusiform, hippocampus, and inferior prefrontal cortex (Sperling *et al.*, 2002). Although there is a considerable overlap of affected brain regions and cognitive deficits between these two classes of drugs and animal evidence shows a close interaction between cholinergic and GABAergic systems, a modification of cholinergic function does not provide a complete account of the behavioural effects of benzodiazepines. (Preston *et al.*, 1989).

One of our own psychopharmacological neuroimaging studies now provides the first hints for a possible neuronal differentiation between lorazepam and scopolamine. While both drugs impaired response suppression in the same brain regions, the pattern of these impairments might differ, especially in extrastriate cortex (Thiel *et al.*, 2001) (see Fig. 17.4). Further studies that investigate commonalities and differences between various drugs are clearly needed to investigate the interaction of different neurotransmitter systems in cognitive function. This approach is common to psychopharmacological animal studies (and also several human psychopharmacological studies) but has barely been applied to neuroimaging.

Even though benzodiazepines are prescribed for treatment of anxiety, and several neuroimaging studies have shown changes in benzodiazepine receptors in anxiety (for reviews, see Nutt and Malizia, 2001), only a few studies have investigated the effects of benzodiazepines in cognitive tasks relating to emotion. Using FDG-PET and administering two doses of diazepam, Wit *et al.* (1991) scanned subjects while they performed a visual monitoring task and completed a mood questionnaire. Behavioural effects of the drug were modest, and the neuronal effect (which was not analysed task dependently) was an nonspecific activity reduction. The second study was also not able to obtain any effects on behavioural or neuronal measures following administration of diazepam when examining drug effects on phobogenic stimulation in spider phobics (Fredrikson *et al.*, 1995). The first evidence for task- and brain-region-specific effects of lorazepam on emotion was reported only recently (Northoff *et al.*, 2002). In a combined magnetoencephalography (MEG)/fMRI study, Northoff *et al.* examined the effects of the benzodiazepine during processing of emotional pictures and found that lorazepam decreased and increased orbitofrontal activity to negative and positive emotional pictures, respectively.

In summary, studies of the effects of benzodiazepines on brain mechanisms involved in higher cognitive functions have almost exclusively focused on modulation of learning and memory. While two studies have shown a reduction of learning-related frontal activations (Coull *et al.*, 1999; Sperling *et al.*, 2002), two other studies were not able to replicate these findings (Bagary *et al.*, 2000; Mintzer *et al.*, 2001). Apparently, more reliably obtained are the drug-induced attenuations of fusiform activity, which have been found with two different benzodiazepines in three different paradigms (Rosier *et al.*, 1997; Sperling *et al.*, 2002; Thiel *et al.*, 2002b). Future neuroimaging studies should extend the range of cognitive functions studied. Because benzodiazepines are used for treatment of anxiety, psychopharmacological neuroimaging studies that investigate their effects in relation to emotion might be promising and clinically important. Another issue that might be worth investigating with neuroimaging are the effects of benzodiazepine on perceptual integration, which has been shown in several psychopharmacological studies (Wagemans *et al.*, 1998; Elliott *et al.*, 2000) and might be due to an action of benzodiazepines in fusiform cortex. Finally, because there are many available benzodiazepines (differing pharmacodynamics and possible receptor binding), a comparison of neuronal effects of different types of benzodiazepines might be useful. Functionally, such an approach could also help in understanding why, behaviourally, only lorazepam has shown reliable impairments of implicit memory.

CONCLUSIONS

Functional neuroimaging is a useful tool for psychopharmacology research as it enables anatomical localisation of specific neuromodulatory drug effects on human cognitive processes. In addition, by extrapolating from associated neuropsychological and neuroimaging literature, it can help interpret the functional significance of the effects of a drug on a particular task. For example, if a drug is known to impair performance of the WCST task, and drug-induced modulations of lateral orbitofrontal cortex but not dorsolateral prefrontal cortex are observed, then we may infer that the drug impairs performance of this task via an effect on response inhibition rather than WM. Psychopharmacological manipulation is a useful tool for functional neuroimaging research as it provides us with functional neurochemical "lesions" that may provide a way of informing cognitive theories of functional segregation. And, finally, the inclusion of a neurochemical manipulation in a functional neuroimaging study adds a third dimension to theories of functional segregation. We can examine the relationship between cognition, anatomy, *and* neurochemistry. This enables identification not only of the brain region selectively associated with a process of interest, but also of the neurochemical in this region that is capable of modulating the cognitive process.

References

Abi-Dargham, A., Mawlawi, O., Lombardo, I., Gil, R., Martinez, D., Huang, Y., Hwang D.-R., Keilp, J., Kochan, L., van Heertum, R., Gorman J., and Laruelle, M. (2002)., Prefrontal dopamine D1 receptors and working memory in schizophrenia. *J.Neurosci.*, **22**, 3708–3719.

Altman, H. J. and Normile, H. J. (1988). What is the nature of the role of the serotonergic nervous system in learning and memory: prospects for development of an effective treatment strategy for senile dementia., *Neurobiol. Aging*, **9**, 627–638.

Amalric, M. and Koob, G. F. (1987). Depletion of dopamine in the caudate nucleus but not in nucleus accumbens impairs reaction-time performance in rats. *J. Neurosci.*, **7**, 2129–2134.

Anderson, I. M., Clark, L., Elliott, R., Kulkarni, B., Williams, S. R., and Deakin, J. F. W. (2002). 5-HT2 receptor activation by *m*-chlorophenylpiperazine detected in humans with fMRI. *NeuroReport*, **13**, 1547–1551.

Arnsten, A. F. T. (1998). Catecholamine modulation of prefrontal cortical cognitive function. *Trends Cogn. Sci.*, **2**, 436–447.

Arnsten, A. F. T. and Goldman-Rakic, P. S. (1985). Alpha-2 adrenergic mechanisms in prefrontal cortex associated with cognitive decline in aged nonhuman primates. *Science*, **230**, 1273–1276.

Arnsten, A. F. T., Steere, J. C., and Hunt, R. D. (1996)., The contribution of α2-noradrenergic mechanisms to prefrontal cortical cognitive function: potential significance for attention-deficit hyperactivity disorder. *Arch. Gen. Psychol.*, **5**, 448–455.

Ashe, J. H., McKenna, T. M., and Weinberger, N. M (1989). Cholinergic modulation of frequency receptive fields in auditory cortex. II. Frequency-specific effects of anticholinesterases provide evidence for a modulatory action of endogenous ACh. *Synapse*, **4**, 44–54.

Aston-Jones, G., Rajkowski, J., Kubiak, P., and Alexinsky, T. (1994)., Locus coeruleus neurons in monkey are selectively activated by attended cues in a vigilance task. *J. Neurosci.*, **14**, 4467–4480.

Avery, R. A., Franowicz, J. S., Studholme, C., van Dyck, C. H., and Arnsten, A. F. T. (2000). The alpha-2A-adrenoceptor agonist, guanfacine, increases regional cerebral blood flow in dorsolateral prefrontal cortex of monkeys performing a spatial working memory task. *Neuropsychopharmacology*, **23**, 240–249.

Bagary, M., Fluck, E., File, S. E., Joyce, E., Lockwood, G., and Grasby, P. (2000). Is benzodiazepine-induced amnesia due to deactivation of the left prefrontal cortex? *Psychopharmacolology*, **150**, 292–299.

Barbee, J. G. (1993)., Memory, benzodiazepines, and anxiety: integration of theoretical and clinical perspectives. *J. Clin. Psychiatry*, **54**(suppl.), 86–97.

Barnes, N. M. and Sharp, T. (1999). A review of central 5-HT receptors and their function. *Neuropharmacology*, **38**, 1083–1152.

Beckers, T., Wagemans, J., Boucart, M., and Giersch, A. (2001). Different effects of lorazepam and diazepam on perceptual integration. *Vision Res.*, **41**, 2297–2303.

Bentley, P., Vuilleumier, P., Thiel, C. M., Driver, J., and Dolan, R. J. (2003). Effects of attention and emotion on face repetition, priming and their, modulation by cholinergic enhancement. *J. Neurophysiol.*, **90**, 1171–1181.

Berger, T W., Weikart, C., L., Bassett, J. L., and Orr, W. B. (1986). Lesions of the retrosplenial cortex produce deficits in reversal learning of the rabbit nictitating membrane response: implications for potential interactions between hippocampal and cerebellar brain systems. *Behav. Neurosci.*, **100**, 802–809.

Blokland, A. (1996). Acetylcholine: a neurotransmitter for learning and memory? *Brain Res. Rev.*, **21**, 285–300.

Brooks, D. J. (2000). PET studies and motor complications in Parkinson's disease. *Trends Neurosci.*, **23**, S101–S108.

Brown, R. M., Crane, A. M., and Goldman, P. S. (1979). Regional distribution of monoamines in the cerebral cortex and subcortical structures on the rhesus monkey: concentrations *in vivo* synthesis rates. *Brain Res.*, **168**, 133–150.

Brozoski, T J., Brown, R., Rosvold, H. E., and Goldman, P. S. (1979). Cognitive deficit caused by regional depletion of dopamine in prefrontal cortex of rhesus monkeys. *Science*, **205**, 929–931.

Buhot, M. C., Martin, S., and Segu, L. (2000). Role of serotonin in memory impairment. *Ann. Med.*, **32**, 210–221.

Cahill, L., Prins, B., Weber, M., and McGaugh, J. L. Beta-adrenergic activation and memory for emotional events. *Nature*, **371**, 702–704.

Caine, E.D., Weingartner, H., Ludlow, C.L., Cudahy, E.A., and Wehry, S. (1981). Qualitative analysis of scopolamine-induced amnesia., *Psychopharmacology*, **74**, 74–80.

Camps, M., Cortés, R., Gueye, B., Probst A., and Palacios, J. M. (1989). Dopamine receptors in human brain: autoradiographic distribution of D2 sites. *Neuroscience*, **28**, 275–290.

Cassaday, H. J., Mitchell, S. N., Williams, J. H., Gray, J. A. (1993). 5,7-Dihydroxytryptamine lesions in the fornix-fimbria attenuate latent inhibition. *Behav. Neural Biol.*, **59**, 194–207.

Clark, C. R., Geffen, G. M. and Geffen, L. B. (1989). Catecholamines and the covert orientation of attention in humans. *Neuropsychologia*, **27**, 131–139.

Cohen, R.M., Gross, M., Semple, W. E., Nordahl, T. E., and Sunderland, T. (1994). The metabolic brain pattern of young subjects given scopolamine. *Exp. Brain Res.*, **100**, 133–143.

Cools, R., Stefanova, E., Barker, R. A., Robbins, T. W., and O.wen, A. M. (2002). Dopaminergic modulation of high-level cognition in Parkinson's disease: the role of the prefrontal cortex revealed by PET. *Brain*, **125**, 584–594.

Cooper, J. R., Bloom, F. E., and Roth, R. H. (1996). *The Biochemical Basis of Neuropharmacology*, pp. 194–225. Oxford University Press, London.

Cortés, R., Gueye, B., Pazos, A., Probst A., and Palacios, J. M. (1989). Dopamine receptors in human brain: autoradiographic distribution of D1 sites. *Neuroscience*, **28**, 263–273.

Coull, J. T. (2001). Modulation of attention by noradrenaline α2-agents varies according to arousal level. *Drug News Perspect.*, **14**, 1–14.

Coull, J. T., Jones, M. E. P., Egan, T., Frith, C. D., and Maze, M. (2003). Noradrenergic á2 attetional effects vary with arousal level: modulation of the thalamic pulvinar in heatlhy humans. *NeuroImage*, **19**(1), 531.

Coull, J. T., Sahakian, B. J., Middleton, H. C., Young, A. H., Park, S. B., McShane, R. H., Cowen, P. J., and Robbins, T. W. (1995). Differential effects of clonidine, haloperidol, diazepam and tryptophan depletion on focused attention and attentional search. *Psychopharmacology*, **121**, 222–230.

Coull, J. T., Frith, C. D., Dolan, R. J., Frackowiak, R. S., and Grasby, P.M. (1997). The neural correlates of the noradrenergic modulation of human attention, arousal and learning. *Eur. J., Neurosci.*, **9**, 589–598.

Coull, J. T., Frith, C. D., and Dolan, R. J. (1999). Dissociating neuromodulatory effects of diazepam on episodic memory encoding and executive function., *Psychopharmacology*, **145**, 213–222.

Coull, J. T., Buchel, C., Friston, K J., and Frith, C. D. (2000). Noradrenergically mediated plasticity in a human attentional neuronal network. *NeuroImage*, **10**, 705–715.

Coull, J. T., Nobre, A. C., and Frith, C. D. (2001). The noradrenergic alpha2 agonist clonidine modulates behavioural and neuroanatomical correlates of human attentional orienting and alerting. *Cereb. Cortex*, **11**, 73–84.

Courtney S. M., Petit, L., Maisog, J. M., Ungerleider, L. G., and Haxby, J. V. (1998). An area specialised for spatial working memory in human frontal cortex. *Science*, **279**, 1347–1351.

Curran, H.V., Pooviboonsuk, P., Dalton, J. A., and Lader, M. H. (1991a). Differentiating the effects of centrally acting drugs on arousal and memory: an event-related potential study of scopolamine, lorazepam and diphenhydramine. *Psychopharmacology*, **135**, 27–36.

Curran, H. V., Schifano, F., and Lader, M. H. (1991b). Models for memory dysfunction? A comparison of the effects of scopolamine and lorazepam on memory, psychomotor performance and mood. *Psychopharmacology*, **103**, 83–90.

Daniel, D. G., Weinberger, D. R., Jones, D. W., Zigun, J. R., Coppola, R., Handel, S., Bigelow, L B., Goldberg, T E., Berman, K. F., and Kleinman, J. E. (1991). The effect of amphetamine on regional cerebral blood flow during cognitive activation in schizophrenia. *J. Neurosci.*, **11**, 1907–1917.

Davis, K. L. and Mohs, R. C. (1982). Enhancement of memory processes in Alzheimer's disease with multiple-dose intravenous physostigmine. *Am. J. Psychiatry*, **139**, 1421–1424.

de Wit, H., Metz, J., Wagner, N., and Cooper, M. (1991). Effects of diazepam on cerebral metabolism and mood in normal volunteers. *Neuropsychopharmacology*, **5**, 33–41.

Dolan, R. J., Fletcher, P., Frith, C. D., Friston, K. J., Frackowiak, R. S. J., and Grasby, P. M. (1995). Dopaminergic modulation of impaired cognitive activation in the anterior cingulate cortex in schizophrenia., *Nature*, **378**, 180–182.

Elliott, M. A., Becker, C., Boucart, M., and Muller, H. J. (2000). Enhanced GABA(A) inhibition enhances synchrony coding in human perception, *NeuroReport*, **11**, 3403–3407.

Ernst, M., Matochik, J. A., Heishman, S. J., Van Horn, J. D., Jons, P. H., Henningfield, J. E., and London, E. D. (2001). Effect of nicotine on brain activation during performance of a working memory task. *Proc. Natl. Acad. Sci. USA*, **98**, 4728–4733.

Evenden, J. L. (1999). Impulsivity: a discussion of clinical and experimental findings. *J. Psychopharmacol.*, **13**, 180–192.

Fibiger, H. C. (1991). Cholinergic mechanisms in learning, memory and dementia: a review of recent evidence. *TINS*, **14**, 220–223.

Fletcher, P. C., Frith, C. D., Grasby, P. M., Friston, K. J., and Dolan, R. J. (1996). Local and distributed effects of apomorphine on fronto-temporal function in acute unmedicated schizophrenia. *J. Neurosci.*, **16**, 7055–7062.

Foote, S. L. and Morrison, J. H. (1987). Extrathalamic modulation of cortical function. *Ann. Rev., Neurosci.*, **19**, 67–95.

Foote, S. L., Aston-Jones, G., and Bloom, F. E. (1975). Impulse activity of locus coeruleus neurons in awake rats and monkeys is a function of sensory stimulation and arousal. *Proc. Natl. Acad. Sci. USA*, **77**, 3033–3037.

Fredrikson, M., Wik, G., Annas, P., Ericson, K., and Stone-Elander, S. (1995). Functional neuroanatomy of visually elicited simple phobic fear: additional data and theoretical analysis. *Psychophysiology*, **32**, 43–48.

Friston, K. J. (1994). Functional and effective connectivity in neuroimaging: a synthesis. *Hum. Brain Mapping*, **2**, 56–78.

Frith, C. D., Richardson, J. T., Samuel, M., Crow, T. J., and McKenna, P. J. (1984). The effects of intravenous diazepam and hyoscine upon human memory. *Q. J. Exp. Psychol. A*, **36**, 133–144.

Fu, C. H. Y., Reed, L. J., Meyer, J. H., Kennedy, S., Houle, S., Eisfield, B. S., and Brown, G. M. (2001). Noradrenergic dysfunction in the prefrontal cortex in depression: an ^{15}O H_2O PET study of the neuromodulatory effects of clonidine. *Biol. Psychiatry*, **49**, 317–325.

Furey, M. L., Pietrini, P., Haxby, J. V., Alexander, G. E., Lee, H. C., VanMeter, J., Grady, C. L., Shetty, U., Rapoport, S. I., Schapiro, M. B., and Freo, U. (1997). Cholinergic stimulation alters performance and task-specific regional cerebral blood flow during working memory. *Proc, Natl. Acad. Sci. USA*, **94**, 6512–6516.

Furey, M. L., Pietrini, P., Alexander, G. E., Schapiro, M. B., and Horwitz, B. (2000a). Cholinergic enhancement improves performance on working memory by modulating the functional activity in distinct brain regions: a positron emission tomography regional cerebral blood flow study in healthy humans. *Brain Res. Bull.*, **51**, 213–218.

Furey, M. L., Pietrini, P., and Haxby, J. V. (2000b). Cholinergic enhancement and increased selectivity of perceptual processing during working memory. *Science*, **290**, 2315–2319.

Ghatan, P.H., Ingvar, M., Eriksson, L., Stone-Elander, S., Serrander, M., Ekberg, K., and Wahren, J. (1998). Cerebral effects of nicotine during cognition in smokers and non-smokers. *Psychopharmacology*, **136**, 179–189.

Goldman-Rakic, P. S. (1987). Circuitry of the primate prefrontal cortex and the regulation of behaviour by representational memory, in *Handbook of Physiology* . Vol. V. *The Nervous System of the Brain,* Section 1, Part 1, *Higher Functions of the Brain*, Plum, F., Ed., American Physiological Society, Bethesda, MD.

Goldman-Rakic, P. S., Selemon, L. D., and Schwartz, M. L. (1984). Dual pathways connecting the dorsolateral prefrontal cortex with the hippocampal formation and parahippocampal cortex in the rhesus monkey. *Neuroscience*, **12**, 719–743.

Goldman-Rakic, P. S., Lidow, M. S., and Gallager, D. W. (1990). Overlap of dopaminergic, adrenergic and serotonergic receptors and complemantarity of their subtypes in primate prefrontal cortex. *J. Neurosci.*, **10**, 2125–2138.

Gower, A. J. (1992). 5-HT receptors and cognitive function, in *Central 5-HT Receptors and Psychotropic Drugs*, Marsden, C. A. and Heal, D. J., Eds., pp. 239–259. Blackwell Scientific, Oxford.

Grasby, P. M., Friston, K. J., Bench, C. J., Frith, C. D., Paulesu, E., Cowen, P. J., Liddle, P. F., Frackowiak, R. S. J., and Dolan, R. (1992). The effect of apomorphine and buspirone on regional cerebral blood flow during the performance of a cogntive task: measuring neuromodulatory effects of psychotropic drugs in man. *Eur. J. Neurosci.*, **4**, 1203–1212.

Grasby, P. M., Frith, C. D., Paulesu, E., Friston, K. J., Frackowiak, R. S., and Dolan, R. J. (1995). The effect of the muscarinic antagonist scopolamine on regional cerebral blood flow during the performance of a memory task. *Exp. Brain Res.*, **104**, 337–348.

Hagan, J. J. (1994). The status of the cholinergic hypothesis of dementia, in *Anti-Dementia Agents: Research and Prospects for Therapy,* Nicholson, C. D., Ed., pp. 85–138. Academic Press, London.

Harrison, A. A., Everitt, B. J., and Robbins, T. W. (1997). Central 5-HT depletion enhances impulsive responding without affecting the accuracy of attentional performance: interactions with dopaminergic mechanisms. *Psychopharmacology*, **133**, 329–342.

Horwitz, B., Tagamets, M. A., and McIntosh, A. R. (1999). Neural modelling, functional brain imaging, and cognition. *Trends Cogn. Sci.*, **3**, 91–98.

Kimberg, D. Y., Aguirre, G. K., Lease, J., and D'Esposito, M. (2001). Cortical effects of bromocriptine, a D2 dopamine receptor agonist, in human subjects, revealed by fMRI. *Hum. Brain Mapping*, **12**, 246–257.

Kinomura, S., Larsson, J., Gulyas B., and Roland, P. E. (1996). Activation by attention of the human reticular formation and thalamic intralaminar nuclei. *Science*, **271**, 512–515.

Koepp, M. J., Gunn, R. N., Lawrence, A. D., Cunningham, V. J., Dagher, A., Jones, T., Brooks, D. J., Bench, C. J., and Grasby, P. M. (1998). Evidence for striatal dopamine release during a video game. *Nature*, **393**, 266–268.

Koskinen, T., Ruotsalainen, S., Puumala, T., Lappalainen, R., Koivisto, E., Mannisto, P. T., and Sirvio, J. (2000). Activation of 5-HT2A receptors impairs response control of rats in a five-choice serial reaction time task. *Neuropharmacology*, **39**, 471–481.

Krnjevic, K. and Phillis, J. W. (1963). Acetylcholine-sensitive cells in the cerebral cortex. *J. Physiol.*, **166**, 296–327.

Lawrence, N. S., Ross, T. J., and Stein, E. A. (2002). Cognitive mechanisms of nicotine on visual attention. *Neuron*, **36**, 539–348.

Legrand, F., Vidailhet, P., Danion, J. M., Grange, D., Giersch, A., van der Linden, M., and Imbs, J. L. (1995). Time course of the effects of diazepam and lorazepam on perceptual priming and explicit memory. *Psychopharmacology*, **118**, 475–479.

Levin, E. D. (1992). Nicotinic systems and cognitive function. *Psychopharmacology*, **108**, 417–431.

Levitt, P., Rakic, P., and Goldman-Rakic, P. S. (1984). Region-specific distribution of catecholamine afferents in primate cerebral cortex: a fluorescence histochemical analysis. *J. Comp. Neurol.*, **227**, 23–36.

Linnoila, M., Virkkunen, M., Scheinin, M., Nuutila, A., Rimon, R., and Goodwin, F. K. (1983). Low cerebrospinal fluid 5-hydroxyindoleacetic acid concentration differentiates impulsive from nonimpulsive violent behaviour. *Life Sci.*, **33**, 2609–2614.

Little, J. T., Johnson, D. N., Minichiello, M., Weingartner, H., and Sunderland, T. (1998). Combined nicotinic and muscarinic blockade in elderly normal volunteers: cognitive, behavioural, and physiologic responses. *Neuropsychopharmacology*, **19**, 60–69.

Loubinoux, I., Pariente, J., Boulanouar, K., Carel, C., Manelfe, C., Rascol, O., Celsis, P., and Chollet, F. (2002). A single dose of the serotonin neurotransmission agonist paroxetine enhances motor output: double-blind, placebo-controlled, fMRI study in healthy subjects. *NeuroImage*, **15**, 26–36.

Luciana, M., Depue, R. A., Arbisi, P., and Leon, A. (1992). Facilitation of working memory in humans by a D2 dopamine receptor agonist. *J. Cogn. Neurosci.*, **4**, 58–68.

Mattay, V. S., Berman, K. F., Ostrem, J. L., Esposito, G., Van Horn, J. D., Bigelow, L. B., and Weinberger, D. R. (1996). Dextroamphetamine enhances 'neural-network-specific' physiological signals: a positron emission tomography rCBF study. *J., Neurosci.*, **16**, 4816–4822.

Mattay, V. S., Callicott, J. H., Bertolino, A., Heaton, I., Frank, J. A., Coppola, R., Berman, K F., Goldberg, T. E., and Weinberger, D. R. (2000). Effects of dextroamphetamine on cognitive performance and cortical activation. *NeuroImage*, **12**, 268–275.

Mattay, V. S., Tessitore, A., Callicott, J. H., Bertolino, A., Goldberg, T. E., Chase, T. N., Hyde, T. M., and Weinberger, D. R. (2002). Dopaminergic modulation of cortical function in patients with, Parkinson's disease. *Ann. Neurol.*, **51**, 156–164.

McEntee, W. J. and Crook, T. H. (1991). Serotonin, memory, and the aging brain., *Psychopharmacology*, **103**, 143–149.

McKernan, R.M. and Whiting, P. J. (1996). Which $GABA_A$-receptor subtypes really occur in the brain? [see comments]. *Trends Neurosci.*, **19**, 139–143.

Mehta, M. A., Owen, A. M., Sahakian, B. J., Mavaddat, N., Pickard, J. D., and Robbins, T. W. (2000). Methylphenidate enhances working memory by modulating discrete frontal and parietal lobe regions in the human brain. *J. Neurosci.*, **20**, R651–R656.

Meneses, A. (1999). 5-HT system and cognition. *Neurosci. Biobehav. Rev.*, **23**, 1111–1125.

Mentis, M. J., Sunderland, T., Lai, J., Connolly, C., Krasuski, J., Levine, B., Friz, J., Sobti, S., Schapiro, M., and Rapoport, S. I. (2001). Muscarinic versus nicotinic modulation of a visual task: a pet study using drug probes. *Neuropsychopharmacology*, **25**, 555–564.

Metherate, R. and Ashe, J. H. (1991). Basal forebrain stimulation modifies auditory cortex responsiveness by an action at muscarinic receptors. *Brain Res.*, **559**, 163–167.

Mintzer, M. Z., Griffiths, R. R., Contoreggi, C., Kimes, A. S., London, E. D., and Ernst, M. (2001). Effects of triazolam on brain activity during episodic memory encoding: a PET study. *Neuropsychopharmacology*, **25**, 744–756.

Molchan, S. E., Martinez, R. A., Hill, J. L., Weingartner, H. J., Thompson, K., Vitiello, B., and Sunderland, T. (1992). Increased cognitive sensitivity to scopolamine with age and a perspective on the scopolamine model. *Brain Res. Rev.*, **17**, 215–226.

Molchan, S. E., Sunderland, T., McIntosh, A. R., Herscovitch, P., and Schreurs, B. G. (1994). A functional anatomical study of associative learning in humans. *Proc. Natl. Acad. Sci. USA*, **91**, 8122–8126.

Morris, J. S., Smith, K. A., Cowen, P. J., Friston, K. J., and Dolan, R. J. (1999). Covariation of activity in habenula and dorsal raphe nuclei following tryptophan depletion. *NeuroImage*, **10**, 163–172.

Müller, U., von Cramon, D. Y., and Pollmann, S. (1998). D1 versus D2 receptor modulation of visuospatial working memory in humans. *J. Neurosci.*, **18**, 2720–2728.

Nissen, M. J., Knopman, D. S., and Schacter, D. L. (1987). Neurochemical dissociation of memory systems. *Neurology*, **37**, 789–794.

Nordberg, A. (1993). *In vivo* detection of neurotransmitter changes in Alzheimer's disease. *Ann. N.Y. Acad. Sci.*, **695**, 27–33.

Nordberg, A. (1999). PET studies and cholinergic therapy in Alzheimer's disease. *Rev. Neurol.*, **155**(Suppl, 4), S53–S63.

Nordberg, A., Nilsson-Hakansson, L., Adem, A., Lai, Z., and Winblad, B. (1989). Multiple actions of THA on cholinergic neurotransmission in Alzheimer brains. *Prog. Clin. Biol. Res.*, **317**, 1169–1178.

Northoff, G., Witzel, T., Richter, A., Gessner, M., Schlagenhauf, F., Fell, J., Baumgart, F., Kaulisch, T., Tempelmann, C., Heinzel, A., Kotter, R., Hagner, T., Bargel, B., Hinrichs, H., Bogerts, B., Scheich, H., and Heinze, H. J. (2002). GABA-ergic modulation of prefrontal spatio-temporal activation pattern during emotional processing: a combined fMRI/MEG study with placebo and lorazepam. *J. Cogn, Neurosci.*, **14**, 348–370.

Nutt, D. J. and Malizia, A. L. (2001). New insights into the role of the GABA(A)-benzodiazepine receptor in psychiatric disorder. *Br. J. Psychiatry*, **179**, 390–396.

Ordway, G. A., Widdowson, P. S., Smith, K. S., and Halaris, A. (1994). Agonist binding to alpha-2 adrenoceptors is elevated in the locus coeruleus from victims of suicide. *J. Neurochem.*, **63**, 617–624.

Ouchi, Y., Yoshikawa, E., Futatsubashi, M. O., Kada, H., Torizuka, T., and Sakamoto, M. (2002). Effect of simple motor performance on regional dopamine release in the striatum in Parkinson's disease patients and healthy subjects: a positron emission tomogrpahy study. *J. Cereb. Blood Flow Metab.*, **22**, 746–752.

Park, S. B., Coull, J., T., McShane, R. H., Young, A. H., Sahakian, B. J., Robbins, T W., and Cowen, PJ (1994). Tryptophan depletion in normal volunteers produces selective impairments in learning and memory. *Neuropharmacology*, **33**, 575–588.

Parnetti, L., Senin, U., and Mecocci, P. (1997). Cognitive enhancement therapy for Alzheimer's disease: the way forward. *Drugs*, **53**, 752–768.

Passingham, R. (1993). The frontal Lobes and Voluntary Action, pp. 103–123. Oxford University Press, London.

Paul, S. E. (1995). GABA and glycine, in *Psychopharmacology: The Fourth Generation of Progress*, Bloom, F. E. and Kupfer, D. J., Eds., Raven Press, New York.

Perry, E. K., Blessed, G., Tomlinson, B. E., Perry, R. H., Crow, T. J., Cross, A. J., Dockray, G. J., Dimaline, R., and Arregui, A. (1981). Neurochemical activities in human temporal lobe related to aging and Alzheimer-type changes. *Neurobiol. Aging*, **2**, 251–256.

Portas, C. M., Rees, G., Howseman, A. M., Josephs, O., Turner R., and Frith, C. D. (1998). A. specific role for the thalamus in mediating the interaction of attention and arousal in humans. *J. Neurosci.*, **18**, 8979–8989.

Rajkowski, J., Kubiak, P., Ivanova S., and Aston-Jones, G. (1998). State-related activity, reactivity of locus coeruleus neurons in behaving monkeys. *Adv. Pharmacol.*, **42**, 740–744.

Rasmusson, D. D. (2000). The role of acetylcholine in cortical synaptic plasticity. *Behav. Brain Res.*, **115**, 205–218.

Riedel, W. J., Klaassen, T., Deutz, N. E., van Someren, A., and van Praag, H. M. (1999). Tryptophan depletion in normal volunteers produces selective impairment in memory consolidation. *Psychopharmacology*, **141**, 362–369.

Robbins, T. W. and Everitt, B. J. (1992). Functions of dopamine in the dorsal and ventral striatum. *Semin. Neurosci.*, **4**, 119–127.

Roberts, A. C., De Salvia, M. A., Wilkinson, L. S., Collins, P., Muir, J. L., and Robbins, T. W. (1994). 6-Hydroxy-dopamine lesions of the prefrontal cortex in monkeys enhance performance on an analogue of the Wisconson card sort, test: possible interactions with subcortical dopamine. *J. Neurosci.*, **14**, 2531–2544.

Rogers, R. D., Blackshaw, A. J., Middleton, H. C., Matthews, K., Hawtin, K., Crowley, C., Wallace, C., Deakin, J. F., Sahakian, B. J., and Robbins, T. W. (1999). Tryptophan depletion impairs stimulus–reward learning while methyl-phenidate disrupts attentional control in healthy young adults: implications for the monoaminergic basis of impulsive behaviour. *Psychopharmacology*, **146**, 482–491.

Rosier, A. M., Cornette, L., Dupont, P., Bormans G., Michiels, J., Mortelmans, L., and Orban, G. A. (1997). Positron-emission tomography imaging of long-term shape recognition challenges. *Proc. Natl. Acad. Sci. USA*, **94**, 7627–7632.

Rosier, A. M., Cornette, L., Dupont, P., Bormans, G., Mortelmans, L., and Orban, G. A. (1999). Regional brain activity during shape recognition impaired by a scopolamine challenge to encoding. *Eur. J., Neurosci.*, **11**, 3701–3714.

Rosse, R. B., Schwartz, B. L., Zlotolow, S. R. D., Banay-Schwartz, M., Trinidad, A. C., Peace, T. D., and Deutsch, S. I. (1992). Effect of a low-tryptophan diet as an adjuvant to conventional neuroleptic therapy in schizophrenia. *Clin. Neuropharmacol.*, **15**, 129–141.

Rowe, J. B., Toni, I., Josephs, O., Frackowiak, R. S. J., and Passingham, R. E. (2000). The prefrontal cortex: response selection or maintenance within working memory? *Science*, **288**, 1556–1560.

Rubinsztein, J. S., Rogers, R. D., Riedel, W. J., Mehta, M. A., Robbins, T. W., and Sahakian, B. J. (2001). Acute dietary tryptophan depletion impairs maintenance of 'affective set' and delayed visual recognition in healthy volunteers. *Psychopharmacology*, **154**, 319–326.

Rusted, J. M. and Warburton, D. M. (1988). The effects of scopolamine on working memory in healthy young volunteers. *Psychoparmacology*, **96**, 145–152.

Sarter, M. (1994). Neural mechanisms of the attentional dysfunctions in senile dementia and schizophrenia: two sides of the same coin? *Psychopharmacology*, **114**, 539–550.

Sarter, M. and Bruno, J. P. (1997). Cognitive functions of cortical acetylcholine: toward a unifying hypothesis. *Brain Res. Rev.*, **23**, 28–46.

Sato, H., Hata, Y., Masui, H., and Tsumoto, T. (1987a). A. functional role of cholinergic innervation to neurons in the cat visual cortex. *J. Neurophysiol.*, **58**, 765–780.

Sato, H., Hata, Y., Masui, H., and Tsumoto, T. (1987b). A. functional role of cholinergic innervation to neurons in the cat visual cortex. *J. Neurophysiol.*, **58**, 765–780.

Sawaguchi, T. and Goldman-Rakic, P. S. (1994). The role of D1-dopamine receptor in working memory: local injections of dopamine antagonists into the prefrontal cortex of rhesus monkeys performing an oculomotor delayed-response task. *J. Neurophysiol.*, **71**, 515–528.

Schmitt, J. A., Jorissen, B. L., Sobczak, S., van Boxtel, M. P., Hogervorst, E., Deutz, N. E., and Riedel, W. J. (2000). Tryptophan depletion impairs memory consolidation but improves focused attention in healthy young volunteers. *J. Psychopharmacol.*, **14**, 21–29.

Schreurs, B. G., McIntosh, A. R., Bahro, M., Herscovitch, P., Sunderland, T., and Molchan, S. E. (1997). Lateralisation and behavioural correlation of changes in regional cerebral blood flow with classical conditioning of the human eyeblink response. *J. Neurophysiol.*, **77**, 2153–2163.

Schultz, W. (1997). Dopamine neurons and their role in reward mechanisms. *Curr. Opin. Neurobiol.*, **7**, 191–197.

Schultz, W., Apicella, P., and Ljungberg, T. (1993). Responses of monkey dopamine neurones to reward and conditioned stimuli during successive steps of learning a delayed response task. *J. Neurosci.*, **13**, 900–913.

Segal, M. and Bloom, F. E. (1976). The action of norepinephrine in the rat hippocampus. IV. The effects of locus coeruleus stimulation on evoked hippocampal unit activity. *Brain Res.*, **107**, 513–525.

Smith A. P. and Nutt, D. (1996). Noradrenaline and attention lapses. *Nature*, **380**, 291.

Smith, A. P., Wilson, S. J., Glue, P., and Nutt, D. J. (1992). The effects and after effects of the α2-adrenoceptor antagonist idazoxan on mood, memory and attention in normal volunteers. *J. Psychopharmacol.*, **6**, 376–381.

Smith, E. E. and Jonides, J. (1998). Neuroimaging analyses of human working memory. *Proc. Natl. Acad. Sci. USA*, **95**, 12061–12068.

Sperling, R., Greve, D., Dale, A., Killiany, R., Holmes, J., Rosas, H. D., Cocchiarella, A., Firth, P., Rosen, B., Lake, S., Lange, N., Routledge, C., and Albert, M. (2002). Functional, MRI detection of pharmacologically induced memory impairment. *Proc. Natl. Acad. Sci. USA*, **99**, 455–460.

Stegeren, A. H., Everaerd, W., Cahill, L., McGaugh, J. L., and Gooren, L. J. (1998). Memory for emotional events: differential effects of centrally versus peripherally acting beta-blocking agents. *Psychopharmacology*, **138**, 305–310.

Swartz, B. E., Kovalik, E., Thomas, K., Torgersen D., and Mandelkern, M. A. (2000). The effects of an alpha-2 adrenergic agonist, guanfacine, on rCBF in human cortex in normal controls and subjects with focal epilepsy. *Neuropsychopharmacology*, **23**, 263–275.

Thiel, C. M., Henson, R. A., Morris, J. S., Friston, K. J., and Dolan, R. J. (2001). Pharmacological modulation of behavioural and neuronal correlates of repetition priming. *J. Neurosci.*, **21**, 6846–6852.

Thiel, C. M., Friston, K. J., and Dolan, R. J. (2002a). Cholinergic modulation of experience-dependent plasticity in human auditory cortex. *Neuron*, **35**, 567–574.

Thiel, C. M., Henson, R. N. A., and Dolan, R. J. (2002b). Scopolamine but not lorazepam impairs face repetition priming: a psychopharmacological fMRI study. *Neuropsychopharmacology*, **27**, 282–292.

Thiel, C. M., Bentley, P., and Dolan, R. J. (2002c). Effects of cholinergic enhancement on conditioning-related responses in human auditory cortex. *Eur. J. Neurosci.*, **16**, 2199–2206.

Thobois, S., Guillouet S., and Brouselle, E. (2001). Contributions of, PET and SPECT to the understanding of the pathophysiology of, Parkinson's Disease., *Neurophysiol. Clin.* **31**, 321–340.

Tremblay, N., Warren, R. A., and Dykes, R. W. (1990). Electrophysiological studies of acetylcholine and the role of the basal forebrain in the somatosensory cortex of the cat. II. Cortical neurons excited by somatic stimuli. *J. Neurophysiol.*, **64**, 1212–1222.

Ungerstedt, U. (1971). Stereotaxic mapping of the momoamine pathways in the rat brain. *Acta Phys. Scand.*, **367**(suppl.), 1–49.

Vitiello, B., Martin, A., Hill, J., Mack, C., Molchan, S., Martinez, R., Murphy, D. L., and Sunderland, T. (1997). Cognitive and behavioural effects of cholinergic, dopaminergic, and serotonergic blockade in humans. *Neuropsychopharmacology*, **16**, 15–24.

Volkow, N. D., Wang, G. J., Fowler, J. S., Logan, J., Jayne, M., Franceschi, D., Wong, C., Gatley, S. J., Gifford, A., N., Ding, Y. S., and Pappas, N. (2002). 'Nonhedonic' food motivation in humans involves dopamine in the dorsal striatum and methylphenidate amplifies this effect. *Synapse*, **44**, 175–180.

Wagemans, J., Notebaert, W., and Boucart, M. (1998). Lorazepam but not diazepam impairs identification of pictures on the basis of specific contour fragments. *Psychopharmacology*, **138**, 326–333.

Weinberger, N. M. (1997). Learning-induced receptive field plasticity in the primary auditory cortex. *Semin. Neurosci.*, **9**, 59–67.

Wesnes, K. and Warburton, D. M. (1984). Effects of scopolamine and nicotine on human rapid information processing performance. *Psychoparmacologia*, **82**, 147–150.

Williams, G. V. and Goldman-Rakic, P. S. (1995). Modulation of memory fields by dopamine D1 receptors in prefrontal cortex. *Nature*, **376**, 572–575.

Zald, D. H., El-Deredy, W., Boileau, I., Gunn, R., McGlone, F., Dichter G., and Dagher, A. (2002). Measurement of dopamine release during expecetd and unexpected reward, paper presented at the NeuroImage Human Brain Mapping 2002 meeting, Sendai, Japan.

Zilles, K. and Palomero-Gallagher, N. (2001). Cyto-, myelo-, and receptor architectonics of the human parietal cortex., *NeuroImage*. **14**, S8–20.

Zilles, K., Schleicher, A., Palomero-Gallagher, N., and Amunts, K. (2002). Quantitative analysis of cyto- and receptorarchitecture of the human brain, in *Brain Mapping: The Methods*, Toga, A. W. and Mazziotta, J. C., Eds., Academic Press, San Diego.

CHAPTER

18

Mechanisms of Control

Questions about neural basis of executive control have tended to become synonymous with questions about the functional anatomy of the prefrontal cortex; however, in whatever form they have been asked these questions still remain unanswered. We have still not identified specific executive functions that can be associated with discrete brain systems. We have still not succeeded in carving up human prefrontal cortex into its functional components. This is not for want of trying. In this chapter, we are concerned mainly with functional imaging studies, rather than results from lesion studies with monkeys or neurological patients. Even so, there are many more relevant functional imaging studies than it will be possible to review here. We therefore concentrate on a limited number of themes that illustrate different approaches to the study of control mechanisms. Of course, we all know that the prefrontal cortex does not act by itself. The executive properties of this region emerge through interactions with other brain areas; however, in this chapter we are largely concerned with attempts to assign specific control functions to different regions of prefrontal cortex. First, we consider some claims about why it has proved so difficult to anatomise prefrontal function.

THE PROBLEMS OF EXPLORING THE FUNCTIONAL ANATOMY OF THE EXECUTIVE SYSTEM

To be brief, the problem with prefrontal cortex is that no obvious mapping has been found between subregions and function. Different tasks activate the same subregions and, in consequence, many different functions have been assigned to the same subregion. Different subregions are activated by the same task, so different functions cannot be assigned. This is in marked contrast to studies of posterior regions, where specific regions can be associated with motion perception, face perception, and so on.

Can Prefrontal Cortex Be Subdivided?

At the heart of the functional brain imaging research program is the belief that different cortical regions have different functions. This belief is based on Korbinian Brodmann's (1909) demonstration that the cortex can be divided into distinct areas on the basis of cytoarchitecture. An area defined in this way has distinctly, although subtly, different local neural circuitry from adjacent regions. In addition, each region receives inputs and sends outputs to particular distant regions. Given these structural differences, it is reasonable to infer that each region defined in this way is performing different computations on different signals. It is the nature of the computations and source of the signals on which they are performed that determine the function of the region.

Prefrontal cortex is no different from other cortical regions in that it consists of a number of distinct Brodmann areas (Fig. 18.1). More recent studies using far more sophisticated methods have confirmed and elaborated Brodmann's original observations (Petrides and Pandya, 1994; Rajkowska and Goldman-Rakic, 1995). In terms of structure, then, there is no reason to think that prefrontal cortex acts as a whole and does not contain subregions with distinct functions.

Is the Location of Subregions Too Variable?

In order to assign a function to a particular region on the basis of functional brain imaging it is necessary to show that the region has the same function in different people. But, if the precise position of this region were highly variable from one person to another, then it would not be possible to identify the common region of activation. This is essentially a technical problem. When it becomes possible to study cytoarchitecture *in vivo*, this problem will be resolved. We have no intention, however, of waiting for these technical advances, as there is little evidence to suggest that prefrontal cortex is dramatically more variable than other cortical regions. Several studies are available that can be used to make probabilistic estimates from Talairach coordinates of the most likely brain region that has been activated in terms of Brodmann areas and sulcal

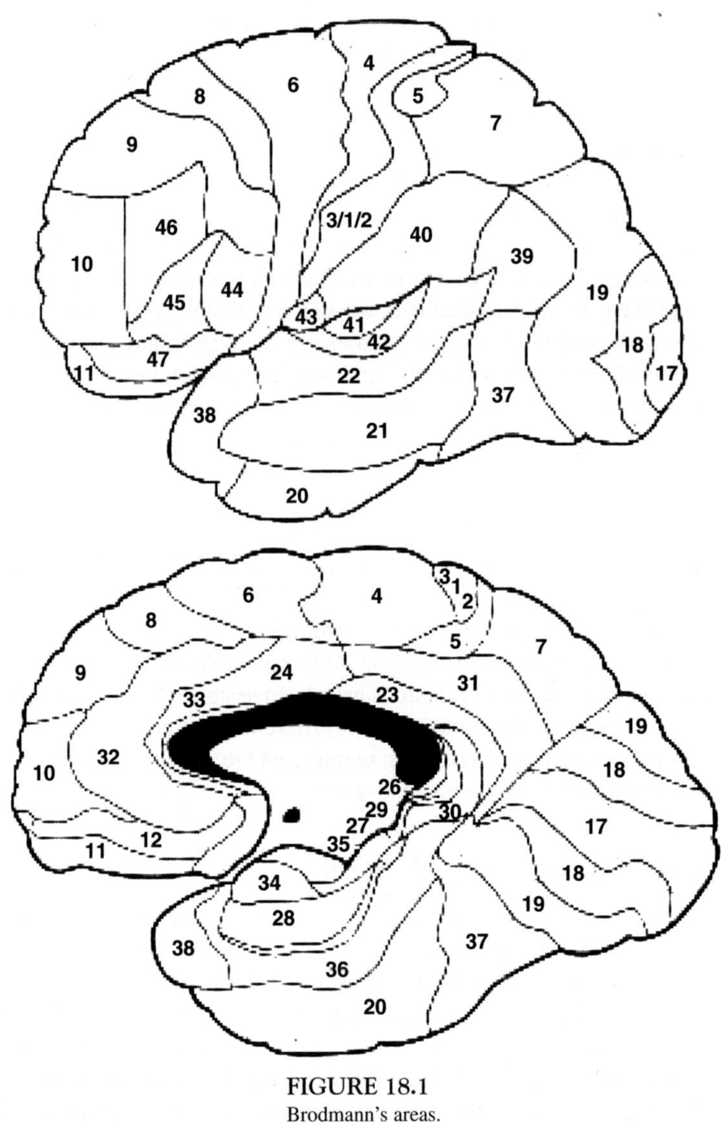

FIGURE 18.1
Brodmann's areas.

landmarks (Rajkowska and Goldman-Rakic 1995; Amunts *et al.*, 1999; Tomaiuolo *et al.*, 1999; Chiavaras *et al.*, 2001).

How Can We Specify the Functions of Prefrontal Cortex?

So far we have considered the anatomical problems that confront the student of prefrontal function. Assuming that distinct subregions of prefrontal cortex can be defined in anatomical terms, the problem remains of assigning functions to these regions. We believe that the failure to make progress in our understanding of prefrontal cortex arises from the problem of specifying these functions. This specification has to be an iterative process. We have to guess what the function might be, design our experiment accordingly, and then modify our description of the function on the basis of the results. This approach applies whether we are studying patients with lesions, recording from single cells in monkeys, or scanning human volunteers.

The Executive Role of Prefrontal Cortex

The first guess as to the function of frontal cortex that we are aware of was made by the Swedish mystic, Emmanuel Swedenborg. Around 1740, he wrote, "If this portion of the cerebrum … is wounded then the internal senses—imagination, memory, thought—suffer; the very will is blunted. …This is not the case if the injury is in the back part of the cerebrum" (quoted in Gross, 1998). However, systematic studies of the effects of lesions in prefrontal cortex did not begin until the middle of the 20th century. From many such studies (Milner, 1963; Luria 1966; Shallice 1988), the idea was developed that prefrontal cortex was an "executive system" (Baddeley, 1986); in other words, our prefrontal cortex is a system for selecting and carrying through actions. More posterior parts of the cortex provide the information needed for selecting the most appropriate action and the means for performing that action. Such an executive system will be most active in novel circumstances and has many components, such as planning, allocating resources, selecting responses, maintaining priorities, and monitoring task performance. On the basis of these formulations, many tasks have been developed that are sensitive to prefrontal lesions. Given this success in specifying a function of prefrontal cortex as a whole, the way forward seemed clear. The different subregions of prefrontal cortex would subserve the different components of executive function such as those listed above; however, we must remember that these terms (monitoring, manipulation, etc.) are just working hypotheses about possible functions of prefrontal cortex. We might, for example, perform a study in which we found that some precise prefrontal region was activated by both manipulation and monitoring as defined in the task we were using. We should not conclude that the function of this region was to perform both monitoring and manipulation. Rather, we should conclude that we needed to define a single new function that underlay both monitoring and manipulation. In order to define such functions, we need to think in terms of computations (Shallice, 1988; Cohen *et al.*, 1996; Dehaene *et al.*, 1998) rather than necessarily vague verbal labels.

Guessing Function from Anatomical Connections

Another source of evidence for guessing the functions of prefrontal subregions comes directly from anatomy (Rushworth, 2000). For example, dorsolateral prefrontal cortex (DLPFC; BA9/46) is interconnected mainly with what can loosely be termed "motor" structures. These include the parietal lobe, the premotor cortex (including supplementary motor area, or SMAs), and motor regions of anterior cingulate cortex. In contrast, ventrolateral prefrontal cortex (VLPFC; BA45/47) has strong connections with visual and auditory areas in the temporal cortex and with perirhinal regions involved in the representation of objects based on signals from many modalities. These observations link DLPFC and VLPFC, respectively, with the dorsal and ventral visual streams (Ungerleider *et al.*, 1982). Therefore, we might expect that DLPFC should be concerned with movement guidance (*e.g.*, selecting responses), while VLPFC should be concerned with object identification (Milner and Goodale, 1995). Similar arguments have advanced about subdivisions of orbital and medial prefrontal cortex (Barbas *et al.*, 1999; Price 1999).

THE EVIDENCE FOR FUNCTIONAL SPECIALISATION IN PREFRONTAL CORTEX

Lesion studies have only provided weak support for these conjectures, but there are many excuses for this. In human studies, the lesions tend to be large and are rarely restricted to specific subregions. In monkeys, the prefrontal cortex is far less developed, and many high-level executive functions may not be in the animals' behavioural repertoire. Such excuses are not available for functional imaging studies. The resolution available (especially for functional magnetic resonance imaging, or fMRI) is quite sufficient to distinguish activity in different prefrontal subregions. The executive tasks that volunteers can perform in the scanning environment are limited only by the imagination of the experimenter. In the short history of functional brain imaging, such tasks have already varied from remembering the positions of dots to solving deep problems in moral philosophy. Nevertheless, the results of these many studies have not led to much agreement about what the functions of prefrontal subregions might be.

The frequently published meta-analysis by Duncan and Owen (2000) nicely illustrates both the success and failure of this functional imaging program. These authors carefully selected 20 imaging studies involving tasks that emphasised four different components of executive function: (1) suppression of inappropriate responses, (2) coping with novelty, (3) maintaining items in working memory, and (4) recognising objects from inadequate information. In each study, the critical comparison was with an easier version of the experimental task. Thus, the activations revealed by this comparison should reveal the regions engaged by the major component of the task. The results of this meta-analysis are shown in Fig. 18.2. Three areas have been activated: the superior part of anterior cingulated cortex (ACC) and the posterior parts of DLPFC and VLPFC. On the one hand, these results give strong evidence of segregation within prefrontal cortex; orbital frontal cortex and more anterior parts of medial prefrontal cortex were not activated by any of the tasks. On the other hand, there was complete overlap between activations associated with all the tasks in the areas that were activated. The implication is that all three areas are equally involved in a number of different components of executive function, and the functions of these areas are equivalent. Later in this chapter we consider the function of anterior medial prefrontal cortex; however, the majority of imaging studies of prefrontal cortex are concerned with the kinds of tasks entered into Duncan and Owen's meta-analysis, and most of the arguments have revolved around the functions of DLPFC, VLPFC, and ACC. Is it possible that these regions do not have different functions?

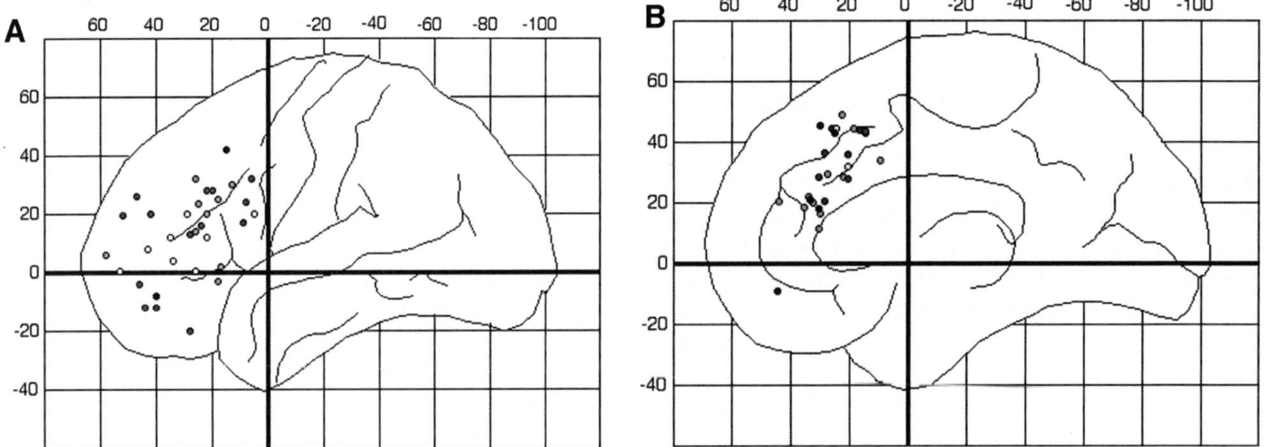

FIGURE 18.2
Frontal activations associated with four different executive functions (redrawn from data provided by John Duncan). Lateral and medial surfaces of the human brain are shown in standard Talairach space. (A) Activations in left lateral frontal cortex. (B) Activations in medial frontal cortex.

Do the Functions of Prefrontal Subregions Vary To Suit the Circumstances?

One proposal has been that the functions of some prefrontal subr[illegible] continually modified to suit the current circumstances (for a review, see Duncan, 2001) [illegible] comes from a working memory study in which monkeys ha[illegible] location of an object (Rao *et al.*, 1997). Many neurons were f[illegible] that carried information about both identity and location. The [illegible] when the task requirements switched from identity to locati[illegible] properties, discarding identity information and taking up lo[illegible] tions fit with the idea that the prefrontal cortex supports a "g[illegible] a "working memory" (Baddeley, 1986) in which is maintai[illegible] performance of the current task (Dehaene *et al.*, 1998). Th[illegible] relevant stimuli, specifications of stimuli that should be i[illegible] responses, and so on. In this case, the precise function of p[illegible] task that is currently being performed. The implication for [illegible] will activate the same prefrontal areas. The only variation w[illegible] activate larger areas. This is in effect a more localised version of [illegible] brain acts as a whole and exhibits equipotentiality.

How Should Function Be Specified?

We believe that this proposal is an example of cowardice in the face of complexity: "Prefro[illegible] cortex is very complex. It acts as whole and it is not possible to analyse it into component parts." The problem is difficult, but that is no reason to cease trying to solve it. Advances may be slow, but they will come through simplification of the complex whole into its components. One approach is to reconsider how to specify the function of an area. In posterior regions, function can be specified in terms of the kind of information that is represented. Thus, there are regions that represent motion or colour (Zeki, 1978), faces, or places (Kanwisher *et al.*, 1997). Following this approach it has been suggested that prefrontal regions can be distinguished as representing information about objects or information about locations (Goldman-Rakic, 1987). This distinction does not seem to work very well (Rao *et al.*, 1997; Nystrom *et al.*, 2000). An alternative is that the distinction is in terms of processes (*e.g.*, maintenance of information versus manipulation of information [Petrides 1996] or error correction versus monitoring [Carter *et al.*, 1998]). Once we think in terms of processes, there are limitless possibility for specification as we increase the abstractness at which the process is described. We shall discuss some of the processes that have been proposed later in this chapter, but first let us consider at least two more basic reasons specifically related to process specification that may contribute to the failure of imaging studies to reveal a functional anatomy for prefrontal cortex.

All Tasks Are Dirty

One thing we can be sure of is that the function of prefrontal cortex is not to perform the Wisconsin Card Sorting test or the Stroop test. The functions of prefrontal cortex will have to be described in terms of cognitive processes, not in terms of tasks. One danger is that tasks can sometimes be treated as if they were cognitive processes. The Wisconsin Card Sorting test is clearly a task, but working memory is often treated as if it were a single process when it is in fact a type of task that involves many processes. The problem for identifying brain areas associated with processes is that all tasks are dirty. There is no task that taps a single executive process. Successful performance of any task engages many processes. For example, the simple frontal test of verbal fluency (saying all the words you can think of beginning with the letter S, Benton 1968) requires accessing a store of words, developing a strategy for finding suitable words, rejecting unsuitable words, keeping track of the words given so far, saying the word, and so on. When this test is used to examine a patient with a lesion, a large battery of additional tests are given to demonstrate that many of these component processes are intact. In an imaging study, control tasks have to be devised to isolate the component process of interest. The complexity of executive tasks renders this procedure much more difficult. For example, the strategy of making the task more difficult may simply engage a larger number of component processes. From this point of view, difficult tasks may be less informative for identifying component processes. A single imaging experiment with a small number of conditions may not provide enough information to reach any clear conclusions.

All People Are Different

A basic requirement of an imaging experiment is that all volunteers have performed the tasks in the same way. In other words, they have all engaged the same cognitive processes. It is of the nature of executive tasks that we cannot take this assumption for granted. The first problem relates to novelty and practice. Executive processes are engaged by novel situations. With sufficient experience, most situations become routine and executive processes are no longer required. A number of experiments (Raichle *et al.*, 1994; Jueptner *et al.*, 1997) have shown that activation of frontal cortex can fall to zero (*i.e.*, to resting levels) after a task has been practiced sufficiently. Any study of an executive task must take account of changes that may occur with practice and possible differences in the experience volunteers bring to the study.

The second problem concerns differences in strategy. Complex tasks can be approached in different ways. For example, in the verbal fluency tasks we have already discussed, one volunteer might just wait for words to pop into his head, while another goes systematically through the alphabet (Sa..., Sc..., Se..., etc.) in order to find words. These two people are clearly engaging different processes in order to perform the same task. Careful analysis of performance can reveal the presence of these different strategies, but a much more direct route is to ask the volunteers to describe what they were doing (Sperling and Speelman, 1970). Post-scan debriefing should be a mandatory requirement of functional imaging studies, especially if executive functions are being studied. Given the small groups typically used in imaging experiments, we would prefer it if all volunteers applied the same strategies; unfortunately, the more tightly a task is constrained to eliminate the possibility of adopting different strategies, the less it has the properties of an executive task.

All these difficulties make it more difficult to identify specific cognitive functions for subregions of prefrontal cortex. Nevertheless, the challenge remains to develop theories of what these functions might be and to design experiments that can isolate these functions. We hope that readers of this chapter will go back to their scanners determined to do better than we have.

IMAGING FRONTAL TASKS

An obvious starting point for imaging studies of prefrontal function is to use those tasks that are known to be sensitive to frontal lobe damage; however, immediately we are faced with the problem of exploring the cognitive components associated with task performance in order to devise suitable control tasks. A task that is sensitive to frontal lobe damage may not necessarily be the best starting point for identifying the cognitive processes that map most naturally onto prefrontal functions

The Wisconsin Card Sorting Test

The Wisconsin Card Sorting test (WCST) is widely considered to be the task most sensitive to frontal lobe lesions (Milner, 1963). In this test, the patient is presented with a pack of cards. On each card is drawn a set of collared shapes (two blue triangles, three red circles, etc.) and the patient has to sort the cards into groups. The task is inherently ambiguous because the colour of the objects on the cards or their shape or their number can be used for sorting. At any time only one of these dimensions is valid for sorting and the patient has to discover by trial and error which dimension is currently valid. Once the patient has learned the rule, the experimenter switches to another dimension and the patient has to discover this new dimension. Patients with frontal lesions have difficulty switching to a new dimension because they tend to go on sorting on the basis of the previously correct dimension even though they are told their choices are wrong (Milner, 1963). This is obviously a complex task that engages many cognitive processes. Furthermore, different processes are involved at different stages. The most critical stage is when the experimenter chooses a new dimension for sorting. At this stage, the subject has to detect the change and respond appropriately.

The WCST was one of the first executive tasks to be used in an imaging experiment (Weinberger *et al.*, 1986). In comparison to simple unambiguous control tasks, such as choice reaction time, performance of the WCST activates large areas of prefrontal cortex, especially DLPFC. To take such studies any further it necessary to isolate some of the cognitive components of the WCST. One strategy is to design variations of the basic task (which is a form of visual discrimination learning) with different kinds of shift. The shift from sorting by the dimension of colour to sorting by shape or number is sometimes described as an extra-dimensional (ED) shift. Using positron emission tomography (PET) Rogers *et al.* (2000) contrasted ED shifts with intradimensional (ID) shifts (*e.g.*, still sorting by colour, but with new colours). Extradimensional shifts were associated with greater activity in left anterior PFC (BA10) and right DLPFC (BA9/46). In addition, ED shifts were associated with *reduced* activity in visual processing areas (BA17 and BA37). This latter observation reminds us that prefrontal cortex does not act on its own. It achieves its effects by modulating activity in more posterior regions (see Chapter 15).

Another strategy has been to use event-related fMRI to isolate different stages in the performance of the task. Monchi *et al.* (2001) used this technique to distinguish the time at which the subjects received feedback about their previous choice from the time at which they made their next choice. DLPFC (BA9/46) showed increased activity at the time feedback was received, whether this was positive or negative. In contrast, VLPFC (BA47/12) showed increased activity only at the time negative feedback was received. Such feedback indicates the need for a shift in responding and a reclassification of stimulus features. Konishi *et al.* (1999) isolated WCST trials on which set shifting was required and compared these with no-go trials in a Go/NoGo task. In both cases, activity was observed in the posterior part of the inferior frontal sulcus predominantly in the right hemisphere (BA44/45). This observation suggests that activity in this region in the WCST is associated with the requirement to inhibit responses based on the dimension that is no longer correct.

These attempts to dissect the WCST into different cognitive components have identified at least three different regions of PFC that seem to have different functions, but it is still not clear precisely what these functions are, and, in the absence of direct comparisons within studies, we can not be sure that these really are distinct regions.

The Tower of London Task

The Tower of London (TOL) task (Shallice 1982) emphasises the processes involved in planning ahead. The patient is presented with three coloured balls arranged on three rods. His task is to rearrange the balls into a new configuration specified by the experimenter. Possible moves are severely restricted because only one ball can be moved at a time and must be placed on a rod before the next move can be made. Planning ahead is required for this task because obvious moves may have to be delayed to make other necessary rearrangements. Many measures of performance can be taken, such as the number of moves taken and the time to complete the rearrangement. A computerised version of this task has been used to demonstrate a characteristic pattern of impaired performance in patients with frontal lesions (Robbins, 1996).

Dagher *et al.* (1999) used PET in a study in which the difficulty of the TOL task was systematically varied by varying the number of moves needed to solve a problem. In areas concerned with visual processing and with movement execution, activity did not vary with difficulty. In DLPFC and ACC, by contrast, activity increased with increasing difficulty. The authors concluded that these latter areas are involved in planning; however, this task involves many processes in addition to planning. In particular, the subject must try out possible moves in his head, a procedure that requires working memory. With more moves, there will be a greater working memory load.

Rowe, J. B. *et al.* (2001) used PET in an attempt to isolate the planning component from the working memory component by devising a control task in which the volunteer generated moves without being constrained by a final goal. In this study, planning was defined as "the process of evaluating which of a number of possible paths will lead to a *prespecified* goal." The traditional planning version of the task activated DLPFC, but so did the control task. No additional activity was detected in DLPFC that could be related to planning. The authors concluded that DLPFC is involved in generating, selecting, and remembering mental moves but not in planning. Perhaps their definition of planning was so restrictive that no cognitive process was left to be revealed.

The Stroop Task

The Stroop task (Stroop, 1935) emphasises processes required to resolve conflict. In the traditional form of the task, the subject is presented with a list of words and has to name the colour of the ink in which the word is written. If the words are incongruent colour names (*e.g.*, the word RED is written in green ink), then the naming time is greatly increased in comparison to naming the ink colour in neutral words or letter strings. The problem for the subject is to inhibit the strong tendency to read the colour word rather than name the colour of the ink. Patients with frontal lesions have difficulty with this task (Perret, 1974). This task has been used extensively in imaging studies. One of the very earliest brain imaging studies demonstrated activity in ACC when performing this task (Pardo *et al.*, 1990). This was a PET experiment in which activity could only be studied in blocks of trials; however, the same results have been obtained in event-related fMRI studies in which it is possible to look at individual trials on which conflict occurs (Leung *et al.*, 2000). This observation has led to the suggestion that ACC has a special role in tasks in which conflicts must be resolved, and many subsequent experiments have tried to elucidate precisely what this role might be. Many experiments have gone beyond the standard Stroop task and attempted to specify the cognitive processes that are involved in the resolution of conflict, at the same time trying to link these processes to anterior cingulate cortex. We consider these attempts later in this chapter.

The Limited Value of Studying Frontal Tasks

The attempts to use functional imaging to study frontal tasks reveal how limited such studies must be. The immediate problem is to devise suitable control tasks. The design of such tasks depends critically on an analysis of the cognitive components of the frontal task. We have to define such components to subtract them or vary them systematically. Consideration of the components in frontal tasks is a useful starting point, but having defined the components it is nearly always possible to devise simpler and better tasks for further exploration of these components. A good example of this approach is the study of intra- and extradimensional shifts by Rogers *et al.* (2000). We shall return to studies directed at cognitive components rather than tasks later in this chapter.

The Restricting Nature of Frontal Tasks

Another problem is that we gain a very restricted view of executive function if we only study tasks already developed by neuropsychologists. There are at least three problems. First, large areas of human endeavour are not probed by these tasks. For example, much of our time, effort and emotion involve interactions with other people. Discovering secret agendas and getting our own way at home and in committees are problems that must engage high-level cognitive processes. Yet, until very recently, neuropsychologists had no tasks that tapped such processes. In the next section, we review evidence that medial prefrontal cortex has a special role in certain aspects of social interaction.

The second problem is that most frontal tasks are very artificial. Tasks like the WCST are typical laboratory tasks that have little relation to anything we do in our everyday lives. Yet, unlike other laboratory tasks, they do not have the advantage of isolating discrete processes. It is well established that patients with large frontal lesions can perform many frontal tasks such as the WCST normally while being clearly impaired in their everyday lives. The use of more realistic tasks (such as going shopping on Lambs Conduit Street) can uncover these problems. It is important to use realistic as well as laboratory-based tasks in order to identify the full range of executive processes. In a later section of this chapter, we consider scanning studies of navigation tasks presented in as realistic a fashion as the scanning environment allows.

The third problem concerns the *a priori* assumption that executive processes are frontal. Activity in prefrontal cortex may well be necessary for executive functions to be engaged, but it is clearly not sufficient. Would it not be better to describe executive functions in terms of distributed systems in which some prefrontal region is just one component of many? Imaging studies are particularly suited to identifying extended systems of brain regions. In the next two sections, we describe tasks (involving mentalising and navigation, respectively) that clearly engage distributed systems of this kind.

INTERACTING MINDS: A SPECIAL ROLE FOR MEDIAL PREFRONTAL CORTEX?

The meta-analysis by Duncan and Owen (2000) showed that typical executive tasks characteristically activate many, but not all, areas of prefrontal cortex. In this section, we focus on one of the regions that did not appear in this meta-analysis. The implication is that this region, the medial prefrontal cortex around the paracingulate sulcus, is not involved in traditional executive tasks (Duncan, 2001). One aspect of human behaviour that sets us apart from other primates is our superior social abilities. The most exceptional of these must be our ability to explain or predict the behaviour of others, almost as if we can read their minds. This ability is often referred to as having a "theory of mind" or *mentalising*. Our ability to mentalise is an automatic, high-level, and, almost without exception, human function (Heyes, 1998). In these circumstances, we can have no data from animal studies directly relevant to the brain systems underlying mentalising ability. The development of this ability is believed to be determined by an innate cognitive mechanism (Leslie, 1987) possibly dedicated and domain specific (Fodor, 1992; Leslie and Thaiss, 1992). Evidence from studies of autism support this theory. Autism is a biologically based disorder that appears to be characterised by a selective impairment in theory of mind (Frith, 2001).

Mentalising with Stories and Cartoons

In a number of studies using tasks that have been developed and validated with autistic people, we have examined the neural substrates of mentalising ability. Using PET, Fletcher *et al.* (1995b) scanned volunteers while they read and answered questions about short stories. In one type of story (theory of mind stories), the behaviour of the protagonists could only be explained on the basis of their (false) beliefs. In a second type of story, the events could be understood on the basis of physical causality or general knowledge. In this instance, the beliefs and intentions of the characters were irrelevant. A third condition consisted of unlinked sentences. This condition acted as a control for reading, attention to sentence meaning, memory, and question answering. Comparison of activation during theory-of-mind stories versus the "physical-causality stories revealed task-specific activation in the left medial prefrontal gyrus (peaking in BA8 Talairach coordinates: −12, 36, 36) and the anterior cingulate cortex, as well as increased activation of the posterior cingulate cortex and the inferior parietal lobe on the right. However, only the left medial prefrontal activation was found to be unique to mentalising.

Happé *et al.* (1996) repeated this study on high-functioning autistic individuals diagnosed with Asperger's syndrome. Scanning patients who are unable to perform the task is meaningless; however, a small minority of autistic individuals are able to pass standard false belief tests. It is believed that this ability does not originate from the same automatic and innate mechanism as normal volunteers but may reflect a general purpose reasoning and learned process. This is highlighted by their poorer performance on more naturalistic mentalising tests (Happé, 1993). The pattern of activity was the same as in the Fletcher *et al.* (1995b) study with one exception, although differences in activation between conditions was smaller in the Asperger's syndrome group. The exceptional activation was in the medial prefrontal region. The Asperger's syndrome group activated an adjacent but more ventral area of the medial prefrontal cortex, BA9/10. The control subjects also activated this region but to a far lesser extent. BA9 has been implicated in imaging studies of general cognitive ability and particularly problem solving (Dolan *et al.*, 1992), which fits with the idea that individuals with Asberger's syndrome apply a general-purpose reasoning mechanism when tackling theory of mind tests.

Gallagher *et al.* (2000) compared the same story comprehension task with an equivalent nonverbal task that involved understanding the joke in captionless cartoons. Once again, theory-of-mind cartoons, in which one of the characters holds a false belief, were compared with physical-causality cartoons and a lower level control of jumbled line drawings. The aims of this study were to examine anatomical convergence between mentalising tasks presented in different modalities while exploiting the superior spatial resolution of fMRI compared to PET. A conjunction analysis of the verbal and nonverbal mentalising conditions showed considerable overlap in brain activation specifically in the medial prefrontal cortex, which was pinpointed to be the anterior paracingulate cortex (–10, 48, 12). Activation was also seen in the temporo-parietal junctions, particularly on the right and in the temporal poles bilaterally; however, these regions were also activated during the physical causality tasks, although to a lesser extent. Thus, they were not uniquely involved in mentalising.

We have found a similar pattern of activation in another study (Castelli *et al.*, 2000) in which volunteers were scanned using PET while watching silent computer-presented animations. The characters in the animations were simple geometrical shapes whose movement patterns selectively evoked mental state attribution (coaxing, teasing) or simple action description, either goal directed (fighting, following) or random, based entirely on their kinematic properties (Heider and Simmel, 1944). The mental state attribution condition was compared with the random action and again we activated the medial prefrontal cortex, slightly more anteriorly than in previous studies (–6, 58, 32). A number of other regions were also activated, including the right temporoparietal junction demonstrated by Gallagher *et al.* (2000), basal temporal cortex, and the occipital cortex. The goal-directed condition elicited intermediary activity in the same network of regions when compared to the random sequence. From the above results, we infer that these regions form a network for processing information about intentions driving behaviour.

The medial prefrontal activation seen by both Fletcher *et al.* (1995b) and Gallagher *et al.* (2000) has been observed in other theory-of-mind imaging studies. Goel *et al.* (1995) used PET to scan adults engaged in a complex task in which subjects had to model the knowledge and inference of another mind concerning the function of unfamiliar and familiar objects. They found widespread activation associated with this task, including activation of left medial frontal lobe and left temporal lobe. Using a nonverbal comic strip adaptation of the story comprehension paradigm, Brunet *et al.* (2000) found bilateral activations in the anterior cingulate cortex and the right anterior paracingulate (4, 56, 44) to be associated with attribution of intentions. They also found bilateral temporal activation to be associated with the involvement of characters but not specifically mentalising.

Online Mentalising

All of the above studies have employed "offline" tasks requiring the volunteer to consider a scenario and retrospectively explain the behaviour of the person or persons involved. In a more recent study, Gallagher *et al.* (2002), using PET, used an "online" paradigm that allowed tight control of other cognitive demands. Volunteers played a computerised version of the children's game "stone, paper, scissors." In the mentalising condition, volunteers believed they were playing against the experimenter and thus adopted what Dennett (1996) describes as an "intentional stance," which is to treat a system as a rational entity, attributing to it beliefs and goals. In the comparison condition, volunteers believed they were playing against a computer which used a rule-based strategy and thus treated their opponent as an entity without intentions or desires. In fact, in both instances during the critical scan window, they played against a random sequence. The only difference between the conditions was the attitude, or stance, adopted by the volunteer. In a third condition, the subjects were told they were playing against a random sequence. We inferred that the rule-solving condition engaged the same higher cognitive processes as the mentalising condition, with the exception of the Mentalising component. Fewer cognitive processes were involved in the random generation condition, although these were all engaged in the rule solving. Thus, the random generation acted as a low level control. The main comparison of the mentalising condition versus rule solving showed only one region of significant activation; the anterior paracingulate cortex bilaterally (8, 54, 12) (Fig. 18.3). No

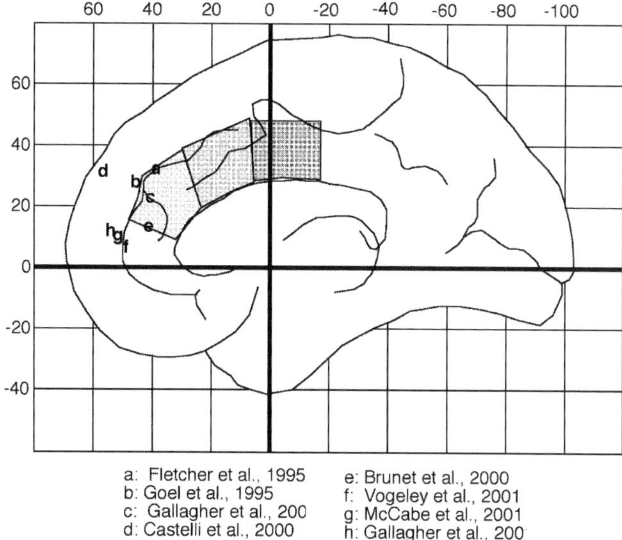

FIGURE 18.3
Locations of medial frontal activity associated with mentalising. The medial surface of the human brain is shown in standard Talairach space. The shaded areas indicate the divisions of anterior cingulated cortex proposed by Picard and Strick (1996).

further regions appeared even when the statistical threshold was lowered to $p = 0.1$. This is consistent with the previous studies of mentalising, although, unlike the studies that have also activated a range of additional regions of the brain, this was the *only* region to be activated in association with mentalising.

Similar results were reported by McCabe *et al.* (2001), who used an online task that involved anticipating the behaviour of another player; however, unlike the study of the "stone, paper, scissors" game, the task was cooperative rather than competitive. In the critical comparison, McCabe *et al.* also observed activity in anterior paracingulate cortex at coordinates very similar to those observed in the present study (5, 52, 10).

The Role of the Temporoparietal Junction

The absence of activity in any other region is striking, because in all the other studies of mentalising reviewed above activity was also seen in two other regions: temporoparietal junction and temporal pole; however, this activity does not seem to be uniquely associated with mentalising. The temporoparietal region has also been activated in imaging studies involving the perception of biological motion (Bonda *et al.*, 1996; Calvert *et al.*, 1997; Grezes *et al.*, 1998; Puce, 1998; Grezes *et al.*, 1999). This area seems to be activated when the behaviour of an agent is explicitly observed or described. In most theory-of-mind studies, mental states are inferred on the basis of this behaviour. In the "stone, paper, scissors" study, however, no behaviour was observed or described. All that the volunteers knew about their opponents were their previous moves. As a result, no biological motion was seen or implied by pictures or verbal descriptions.

Mentalising and Executive Function

That prefrontal cortex has a necessary role in mentalising has been confirmed by recent neuropsychological studies (Channon, 2000; Rowe, A. D. *et al.*, 2001; Stuss *et al.*, 2001). In particular, patients with bilateral medial frontal lesions have been shown to be impaired on tasks of detecting deception (Stuss *et al.*, 2001). Patients with autism, like patients with frontal lobe lesions, typically have difficulties with executive tasks as well as mentalising. It has therefore been argued that the performance of mentalising tasks depends upon executive functions (Russell, 1997). For example, in a task involving false beliefs there is a conflict between the false belief and the true state of affairs. Holding both of these in mind and resolving the conflict might require executive processes similar to those involved in Stroop tasks. Nevertheless, performance of mentalising tasks can clearly be dissociated from performance of typical executive tasks. In the study by Rowe, A. D. *et al.* (2001), the patients with frontal lesions performed worse than controls on both mentalising and executive tasks; however, after covarying out executive performance, there was still a significant impairment in theory of mind performance. Single case studies have also revealed that double dissociation is possible between mentalising and executive performance. Fine *et al.* (2001) describe a patient with congenital amygdala damage who is impaired on mentalising tasks but not on executive tasks, while Blair and Cipolloti (2000) describe a patient with orbital-frontal damage who is impaired on executive tasks but not on mentalising tasks.

What Is the Role of This Region of Medial Prefrontal Cortex?

These results suggest that either this region of PFC either does not have an executive function as traditionally conceived or it has a domain-specific executive function restricted to social interactions; however, the precise function of this region (anterior paracingulate cortex, bordering on the anterior cingulate) remains unknown. The region is clearly anterior to the region of the anterior cingulate (rCZp) concerned with conflict monitoring (for a meta-analysis, see Barch *et al.*, 2001), which we will discuss in more detail later in this chapter; however, adjacent regions of the paracingulate cortex have been activated in studies that required volunteers to reflect on their own inner states. Tasks requiring such self-reflection include visual self-recognition (Kircher *et al.*, 2000), memory for autobiographical events (Maguire and Mummery 1999; Maguire *et al.*, 2000b), monitoring one's own speech (McGuire *et al.*, 1996), monitoring one's own thoughts (McGuire *et al.*, 1996a), being tickled (Blakemore *et al.*, 1998), perceiving pain (Rainville *et al.*, 1997), and monitoring one's own emotional responses (Lane *et al.*, 1997; Gusnard *et al.*, 2001). Additionally, medial prefrontal areas have been shown to be active during metaphor comprehension (Bottini *et al.*, 1994), which according to some theorists requires recognition of the speaker's intentions (Sperber and Wilson, 1995). Taken together, these results suggest that this circumscribed region of anterior paracingulate cortex is involved in the representation of mental states of the self as well as those of others.

A System for Social Cognition?

Although paracingulate cortex seems to have a special role in mentalising, several other brain regions have been activated when volunteers perform mentalising tasks. These may form part of a network dedicated to social cognition (Frith, 2001). One structure that has been repeatedly implicated is the amygdala (Baron-Cohen *et al.*, 2000). We have already referred to the patient studied by Fine *et al.* (2001) who was severely impaired in his ability to represent mental states, yet showed normal executive functioning. This patient suffered early or congenital left amygdala damage. Baron-Cohen *et al.* (1999) reported activation in the left amygdala (in addition to medial prefrontal activation) during a task in which normal volunteers were required to infer the mental state of an individual from the expression of their eyes. They also found significantly less amygdala activation when adults with high functioning autism and Asperger's syndrome performed the same task. Some neuroanatomical studies of autism, postmortem (Bauman and Kemper, 1994) and *in vivo* (Abell *et al.*, 1999), have found abnormalities in the amygdala complex. Neuroimaging studies have demonstrated a role for the amygdala in processing facial expressions (Morris *et al.*, 1996), monitoring gaze (Wicker *et al.*, 1998; Kawashima *et al.*, 1999), and perceiving biological motion (Bonda *et al.*, 1996). These are all tasks with an obvious social component. In all the studies of mentalising reviewed above, activity was observed in the temporal poles. This activity was adjacent to and in some cases spread into the amygdala (see review by Frith, 2001).

We have already discussed a third area, the temporoparietal junction at the posterior end of the superior temporal sulcus (STS), which is also frequently activated when volunteers perform mentalising tasks. These three regions, paracingulate cortex, temporal pole, and posterior STS, may form a brain system with a special role in social cognition. A fourth region, orbitofrontal cortex, has also been frequently been implicated in social cognition (Adolphs, 1999) but does not seem to be involved in mentalising. The precise role of the medial frontal region in social cognition remains unclear. Is this region necessary for representing mental states whether of the self or of other people? To answer such questions, we need to develop a cognitive account of how mental states are represented so that much more precise experiments can be conducted.

Prior to the first imaging studies in 1995 we had no reason to suspect that specific regions of prefrontal cortex would be involved in mentalising. Furthermore, it is still not clear whether this role has any family resemblance to the kinds of executive functions attributed to other prefrontal regions.

KNOWING ONE'S PLACE: BRAIN SYSTEMS FOR NAVIGATING IN SPACE AND TIME

While mentalising seems to be a uniquely human ability, the ability to navigate through space is an attribute of nearly all animals; nevertheless, there are aspects of navigation that involve high-level cognitive functions. For example, in humans the ability to mentally represent the events that happen to us as we move around in the environment is fundamental to normal functioning in everyday life. The consequences of losing these representations or access to them through brain injury or disease can be devastating. Representing where we are and how we got there in both physical and social space, as well as planning and executing future actions, draws heavily on the storehouse of our prior experiences. Neuropsychological evidence for the importance of the human medial temporal region, and the hippocampus in particular, in mnemonic processing has accumulated over many decades from studies of patients with brain lesions. While numerous neuroimaging studies have examined different aspects of memory (for reviews of functional neuroimaging studies that have activated the hippocampal region, see Desgranges *et al.*, 1998; Lepage *et al.*, 1998; Schacter and Wagner, 1999), the memory for experiences gleaned from living in the real world has been less commonly studied using neuroimaging. More complex and realistic stimuli undoubtedly present a challenge for neuroimaging both in terms of experimental execution and data interpretation. Such studies, however, provide the means for tapping into the true (real-world) context for the remembering brain.

Considering first navigation through space, this is not typically thought of as a frontal function, yet executive processes are clearly involved. We have to plan our route. We have to keep track of where we have been so far in order to know in what direction to go next. We have to be able to suppress habitual behaviour to take account of recent changes in our environment. Does navigation use an executive system that involves prefrontal cortex?

In non-human animals, there is very strong evidence that the hippocampus is particularly important for navigation. The discovery of *place cells* (pyramidal cells in the rat hippocampus with location-specific activity; (O'Keefe and Dostrovsky, 1971) provided physiological grounding for the study of navigation. Since then, a vast literature of physiological, lesion, and pharmacological studies points to an intimate link between the rodent or small mammal hippocampus and navigation. Examining the neural basis of navigation in humans using functional neuroimaging has necessitated the use of novel paradigms to preserve ecological validity while facilitating experimental control. Studies have included paradigms where a town layout was learned from watching film footage of travel through it (Maguire *et al.*, 1996), taxi drivers generated and described routes though London (Maguire *et al.*, 1997), or subjects recalled a route learned in the real world before scanning (Ghaem *et al.*, 1997). Another increasing popular means to examine navigation during neuroimaging is to use virtual-reality paradigms. In one such study, subjects were scanned using PET while they performed retrieval tasks in a complex virtual-reality town (see Fig. 18.4A) which they had spent some time learning prior to scanning (Maguire *et al.*, 1998). During scanning, subjects found their way to specified destinations in the town using internal representations built up during learning. This resulted in activation of the right hippocampus during successful trials when compared with unsuccessful trials. In addition, there was a significant correlation between blood flow changes in the right hippocampus and the accuracy of navigation—the more accurate the path taken to the goal place, the more active the right hippocampus (Fig. 18.4B), in line with rodent models of hippocampal function. Overall, the functional neuroimaging evidence seems to implicate the medial temporal region in humans in navigation, and the right hippocampus in particular. Recent evidence from structural neuroimaging using voxel-based morphometry in London taxi drivers has also confirmed this right hippocampal navigation role in humans (Maguire *et al.*, 2000).

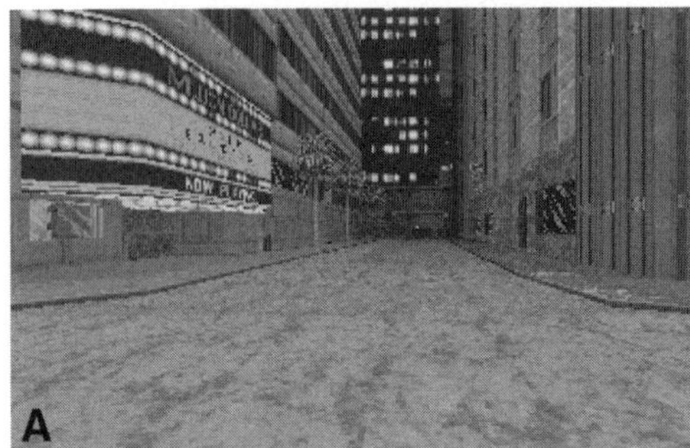
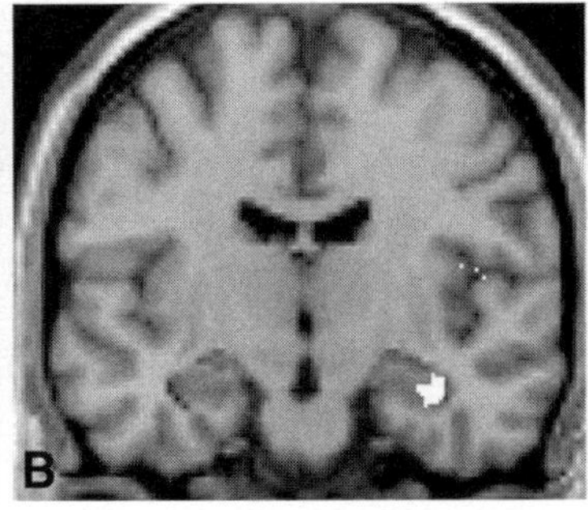
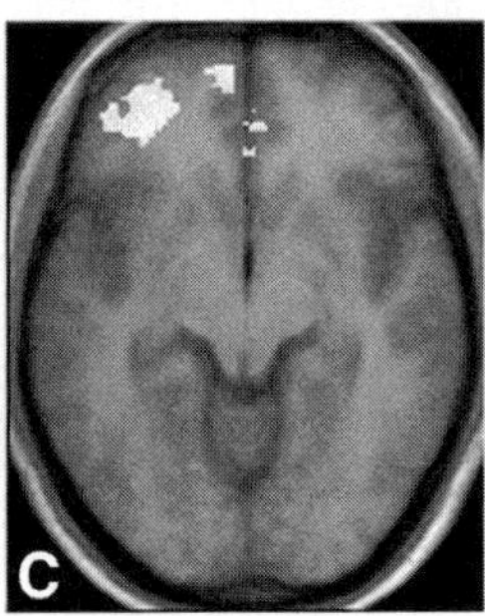

FIGURE 18.4
Navigating in virtual reality. (A) A view in the virtual reality town. (B) Activity in the right hippocampus associated with accuracy of navigation. (C) Activity in left prefrontal cortex associated with taking detours. (Data from Maguire, E. A. *et al.*, 1998.)

Thus, the right hippocampus in humans seems to closely parallel that in animals with its involvement in spatial representations. But what about prefrontal cortex? In the same virtual reality town (Maguire *et al.*, 1998), the left frontal cortex was active when roads were blocked in the virtual town and subjects were required to plan and execute a detour strategy in order to reach the goal destination (Fig. 18.4C). In another study involving a virtual-reality, maze-like environment, Grön *et al.* (2000) compared men and women. They found that men activated their left hippocampus more than women, while women activated right frontal and parietal areas more than men during navigation. Women have been noted in previous behavioural studies to rely on landmarks to aid navigation more than males, who are more likely to navigate using cardinal directions (Sandstrom, 1998). The right prefrontal activation in women may reflect a greater use of working memory in order to have immediate access to salient landmarks in line with this strategy. Findings such as these suggest that prefrontal areas may not be involved in the basic processes of navigation, but rather have a more general role in using and manipulating the representations encoded and stored more posteriorly in the brain.

Navigation is, of course, just one form of representation. There are many other varieties of memory often noted in the literature (see Chapter 25), and one general distinction that is often made is in terms of events and facts (often termed *episodic* and *semantic memory*). Autobiographical events have occurred in a particular place at a particular time, whereas facts comprise general knowledge not tied to any one specific episode (Tulving, 1983; for a review of autobiographical memory and functional neuroimaging, see Maguire, 2001). In recent fMRI studies, the neural bases for recollecting real-world memories were of four types: autobiographical events, public events, autobiographical facts, and general knowledge (Maguire *et al.*, 2000b). The autobiographical events and public events were those that subjects recalled over a time scale ranging from a couple of weeks prior to scanning to over 20 years or more ago (Maguire *et al.*, 2001a).

A common memory retrieval network comprised of medial and left lateral cortical and limbic areas was found to support the recollection of each memory type. Although all brain regions in the network were involved in memory retrieval, some regions within this network showed a clear preference for certain memory types. The left hippocampus (Fig. 18.5A) and medial frontal cortex (Fig. 18.5B) were most responsive to the retrieval of autobiographical event memories. The modulation of hippocampal activity by the memory for personal events in particular suggests that it is this aspect of memory retrieval that might critically depend on the hippocampus and is impaired with hippocampal pathology (Vargha-Khadem *et al.*, 1997). In the previous section of this chapter, we have shown that medial prefrontal cortex seems to be involved in the representation of mental states. In the case of autobiographical memory, this region may have been involved in representation of the mental state experienced by the volunteer when the memory was laid down. The only other prefrontal activity observed in these sorts of studies was a more ventrolateral prefrontal region on the right (Maguire *et al.*, 2001a). This region was most active during retrieval of recent memories and showed decreased activation the more remote the memories become over 20 or more years. This was in contrast to the hippocampus, where there was no modulation in relation to age of memory. The prefrontal finding may reflect the degree

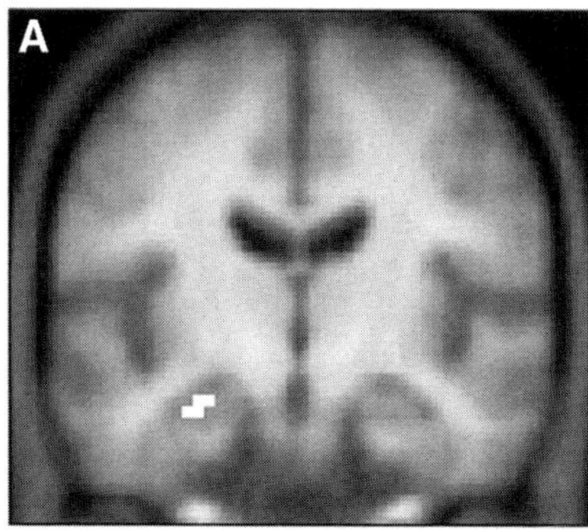

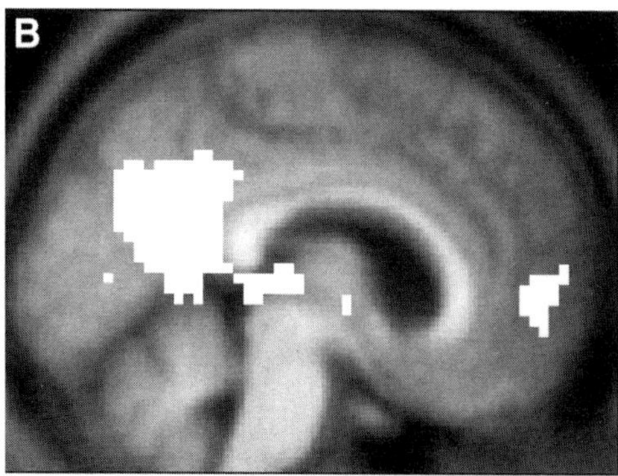

FIGURE 18.5
Some of the brain regions activated during the recall of autobiographical memories. (A) Left hippocampus. (B) Medial perfrontal cortex (and precuneaus). (Data from Maguire, E. A. *et al.*, 2002b.)

of integration of the memory trace with relevant contextual information, with more active integration occurring the more recently acquired the memory.

The overall lack of prefrontal activations in the real-world memory tasks outlined above stands in contrast to neuroimaging studies that employ conventional laboratory stimuli (*e.g.*, learning word lists or word pairs). In the latter sort of study, prefrontal activity abounds (for a review, see Fletcher and Henson, 2001 and Chapter 26) with much debate about the relative contributions of different subregions. A recent study where autobiographical events and virtual reality were combined may provide some insights into this puzzling disparity. Virtual autobiographical events were experienced while subjects followed a prescribed route through the virtual-reality town and, along the way, repeatedly met two characters who gave them different objects in two different places (Burgess *et al.*, 2001). Each receipt of an object comprised an event the memory for which was subsequently probed in a forced choice recognition test during fMRI scanning. The aspect of the event that the subjects were required to remember was indicated by a word presented underneath the objects—for example, *place* required them to remember which of the two objects they received in that place, thus testing memory for the spatial context of an event; *first* asked which object had been received before the other, thus testing memory for the temporal context of an event; and *person* asked which object they received from that person.

Recall of several aspects of the context of the events was associated primarily with activation of the left hippocampus and other regions similar to those noted in the retrieval of autobiographical events noted above. Interestingly, and unlike the studies employing real-world stimuli, retrieval of the virtual events activated seven well-circumscribed prefrontal areas: anterior cingulate and bilateral dorsolateral, ventrolateral, and anterior prefrontal cortex (Fig. 18.6). The areas have a close correspondence to the areas classically activated in previous studies of episodic retrieval of laboratory stimuli, although they are not usually all activated in the same study. For example, a recent conjunction analysis of four studies (Lepage *et al.*, 2000) identifies almost identical regions to six of the seven activated (the exception being left ventrolateral prefrontal cortex). Why the sudden emergence of the prefrontal cortex? One possible explanation concerns the similarity of the events used in the virtual reality study (and in conventional experiments on memory), both to each other and of their contexts (all 16 events involving one of two people and one of two places within a short space of time). This contrasts with the rich diversity and temporal separation of autobiographical events (*e.g.*, being at a wedding or going to the dentist). Thus, much of the prefrontal involvement in the VR episodic memory task might reflect processes required to overcome the interference caused by the similarity of the events and their context. This would be consistent with comparisons of frontal and temporal lesions, implicating the medial temporal lobes in the storage of episodic memory and the frontal lobes in the use of organisational strategies in encoding and retrieval (Frisk and Milner, 1990; Incisa della Rocchetta and Milner, 1993; Gershberg and Shimamura, 1995; Smith *et al.*, 1995; Owen *et al.*, 1996; Kopelman and Stanhope, 1998), including those relating to interference (Incisa della Rocchetta and Milner, 1993; Smith *et al.*, 1995).

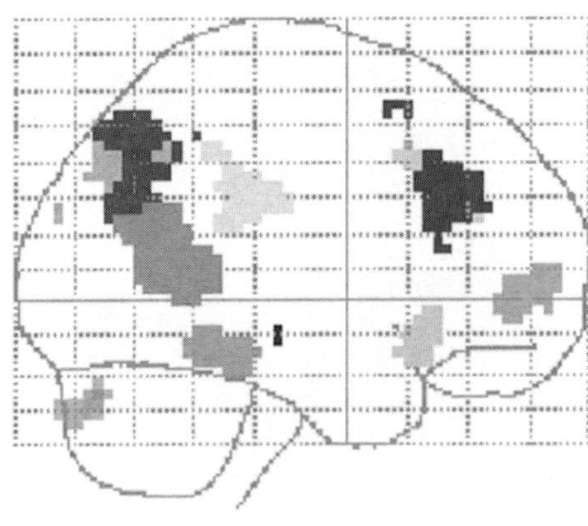

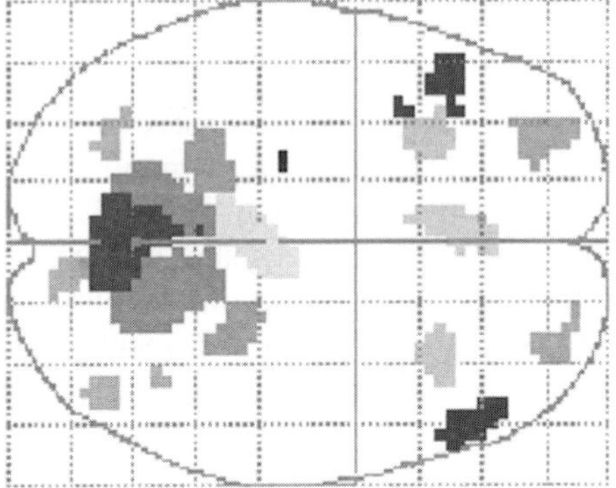

FIGURE 18.6
Significant activations associated with autobiographical retrieval of virtual events are shown on a glass brain. Activity can be seen in anterior cingulate and bilateral dorsolateral, ventrolateral, and anterior prefrontal cortex. (Data from Burgess, N. *et al.*, 2001.)

The sorts of studies reviewed here have provided useful insights into the role of the human hippocampus in navigation and episodic memory and suggest possibly differential contributions of the left and right hippocampi that require further investigation. These paradigms have also been useful in assessing the functional integrity of residual brain tissue, particularly hippocampal, in memory-impaired patients (Maguire *et al.*, 2001b). In addition, effective connectivity analyses (see Chapter 51) of the autobiographical-events neuroimaging data have provided a means of probing representations at the systems level and how this may be disrupted in situations of pathology (Maguire *et al.*, 2000b, 2001b).

The studies also suggest that many aspects of navigation in space and time can occur without involvement of prefrontal cortex. When prefrontal regions are involved, their function resembles that seen across a wide range of tasks. Thus, DLPFC seems to be involved when alternative routes have to selected, VLPFC is involved in monitoring retrieval of recent episodic memories, and medial frontal cortex is involved when remembering past states of the self. Studies of important everyday skills such as navigation and mentalising are vital for identifying extended brain systems, but in order to identify roles for the components of these systems, whether these components are in prefrontal cortex or elsewhere, we must try to isolate fundamental cognitive processes. In the rest of this chapter we consider the attempts that have been made to specify such components in ACC and DLPFC.

ANTERIOR CINGULATE CORTEX: RESPONSE CONFLICT OR RESPONSE PREPARATION?

It is important to remember that the ACC is a large region (Fig. 18.7) that probably has many different functions. The most posterior part of it (the cingulate motor area, or caudal cingulate zone [cCZ]; Picard and Strick 1996; Paus *et al.*, 1998) is part of the motor system and, in the

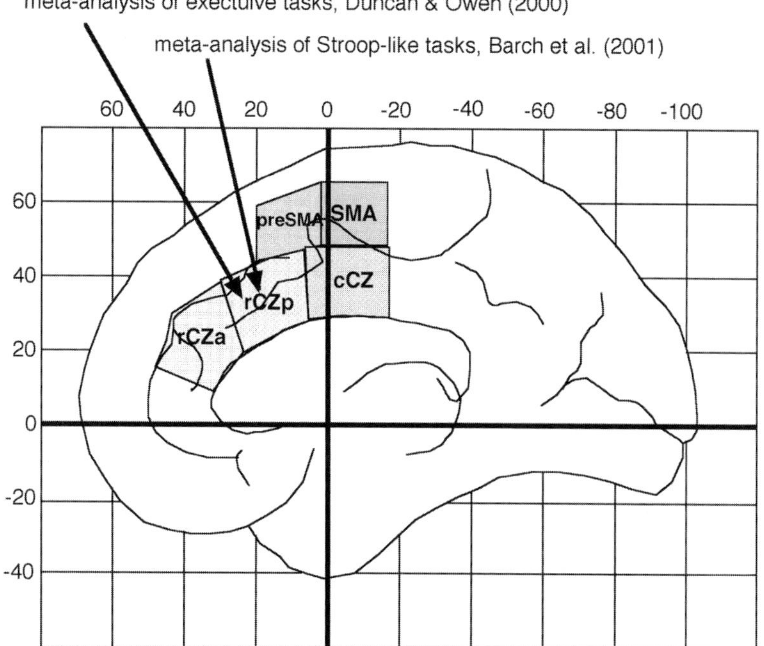

FIGURE 18.7
Subregions of anterior cingulate cortex showing points of maximum activation in executive tasks. The medial surface of the brain is shown in standard Talairach space.

monkey at least, sends projections directly to spinal chord. In most studies using Stroop-like tasks, activation is observed in a region of ACC immediately anterior to this (posterior rostral cingulate zone [rCZp]; see meta-analysis by Barch *et al.*, 2001). ACC continues around the front of the corpus callosum and then underneath it. These most inferior regions seem to play a role in the processing of emotion (Bush *et al.*, 2000).

From an anatomical point of view, ACC is part of the motor system and is likely therefore to have a role in high-level motor control. In an influential early study, Paus *et al.* (1993) showed that ACC (along with DLPFC) was more active in tasks that involved novel stimulus–response pairings which were opposite to those previously practiced by the volunteers. For example, volunteers might practice pressing their left finger to a red light and their right finger to a green light. They would then be scanned with the instruction to press with their left finger to the green light. To perform this task, the subjects had to attend to their actions and inhibit prepotent responses. ACC activation was observed for three different response modalities, and there was some evidence that the different modalities mapped onto slightly different regions of ACC. The regions activated are close to those seen in Stroop tasks (Barch *et al.*, 2001). Whether there are somatotopic mappings within these more anterior regions of ACC remains unclear. On the basis of meta-analyses of large numbers of studies, Paus *et al.* (1998) and Picard and Strick (1996) claimed that there was somatotopy, but Barch *et al.* (2001) deny this. Comparisons across studies can be misleading. Highly significant within-subject effects could be entirely invisible in between-subject comparisons. On the other hand, differences between studies could result from unidentified procedural variations rather than the difference of interest. Barch *et al.* (2001) compared two response modalities (manual and vocal) and two processing domains (spatial and verbal) in the same study. rCZp activation was clearly present when subjects were presented with Stroop-like tasks (*e.g.*, pressing the left button when the word RIGHT appears to the left of fixation) for both response modalities and for both processing domains. However, it was the same regions that were activated by the different modalities and the different domains.

From their meta-analysis of a very large number of studies, Barch *et al.* (2001) provided mean Tallairach coordinates that clearly fall in rCZp (3, 19, 35). This provides a useful anchor point for considering the various claims made for the precise role of ACC in Stroop-like tasks. At the broadest level of specification this region of ACC seems to be involved in the resolution of conflict. As we have already seen, it does not seem to matter whether this conflict is between verbal responses, manual responses, or oculo-motor responses (Barch *et al.*, 2001). Conflict in the semantic domain between items being retrieved from episodic memory (Herrmann *et al.*, 2001) also elicits activity in this area (6, 22, 43). However, the claim that even conflict at the meta-cognitive level associated with tip-of-the-tongue phenomena in memory retrieval (Maril *et al.*, 2001) activates the same region is less convincing. The area activated in this study (–6, 39, 21) is more anterior and inferior and lies in the anterior rostral cingulate zone (rCZa). It is very close to the region activated when volunteers have irrelevant thoughts during scanning (McGuire *et al.*, 1996a). This is the area we have already suggested has a special role in representing mental states. Tip-of-the-tongue experiences are concerned precisely with close monitoring of our current mental state.

Stimulus Conflict or Response Conflict?

Zysset *et al.* (2001) have made the strong claim that ACC activation is associated only with conflict at the level of response selection and not at the level of stimulus selection (sometimes called *interference*). They used an ingenious task in which stimulus conflict had to be resolved in order to select a response, while there was no response conflict. They report no increase in activity in ACC in incongruent trials relative to congruent and neutral trials; however, they do report highly significant activation in preSMA (1, 26, 42). These coordinates are right on the edge of rCZp and fall within the area defined in the meta-analysis of Barch *et al.* (2001). Other studies reporting almost identical coordinates have assigned them to ACC rather than preSMA (4, 25, 43) (Carter *et al.*, 1998).

To be convinced about the critical difference between activity in rCZp and preSMA, we would want to see a direct comparison of tasks with and without response conflict in the same volunteers. Van Veen *et al.* (2001) used the flanker task devised by Eriksen and Eriksen (1974) to partially separate stimulus and response conflict. In addition to standard congruent and incongruent conditions, the study included a condition in which there was conflict at stimulus level, but not at the response level. Activity was observed in ACC (–3, 32, 31) in association with response conflict, but not stimulus conflict. This activity is more anterior and inferior to that in many previous reports; it falls into the region referred to by Pickard and Strick as the rostral cingulate zone, anterior part (rCZa).

A study by Banich *et al.* (2000) is also consistent with the suggestion that activity in ACC is not elicited when conflict occurs only at the level of the stimulus. In this study, volunteers had to monitor Stroop-like stimuli for rare targets that never actually occurred. As a result, responses were not actually made. When incongruent trials were compared with neutral trials, no activity was observed anywhere in ACC (or SMA) even though quite a liberal statistical criterion was used.

The conflict associated with the traditional Stroop task is very striking. Volunteers immediately recognise this as the kind of tricky task beloved of psychologists; however, activity in rCZp is also elicited by tasks in which the response conflict is far less obvious. Braver *et al.* (2001) hypothesised that any task in which one response was less frequent than another would elicit activity in this area whenever the less frequent response had to be performed. This expectation harks back to the original study by Paus *et al.* (1993) in which activity was observed in ACC when responses had to be made that were incompatible with some prevailing prepotent response tendency. Making an infrequent response goes against the tendency associated with the frequent response.

Using event-related fMRI, Braver et al. (2001) showed that rCZp was activated by infrequent responses, whether these occurred in the context of a Go/NoGo task (with the NoGo trials being infrequent), an odd-ball target detection task, or a two-choice reaction time task in which one stimulus was less frequent. Note that in the Go/NoGo task and the odd-ball task the conflict arises from competition between the generation of a single response and the suppression of that response, rather than competition between multiple alternate responses. Activity was observed in rCZp both for the commission of an infrequent response (odd-ball task) and the omission of an infrequent non-response (Go/NoGo task). It is also important to note that, in the study of Braver *et al.*, activity in rCZp was not observed for NoGo trials when these were as frequent as Go trials, confirming the study of Konishi *et al.* (1999) in which NoGo and Go trials were also equally frequent.

These observations suggest that activity in rCZp is associated with making low-frequency responses rather than inhibition, although the activity did seem to be somewhat enhanced when low frequency occurred in the context of response inhibition (disjunction test; see Braver *et al.*, 2001). In the original Stroop task, both these processes coincide as the volunteer must inhibit reading the colour word while making the far less frequent response (in everyday life) of naming the ink colour.

Conflict Monitoring or Conflict Resolution?

The results discussed so far still leave open the question of the role of ACC (rCZp) in situations of response conflict. One possibility is that rCZp activity is elicited by the occurrence of errors as these are more likely to occur in situations of response conflict; however, on the basis of a series of elegant event-related fMRI experiments, Carter and his colleagues (1998) concluded that ACC is involved in the monitoring of response conflict, rather than simply detecting errors. They observed that activity in rCZp (4, 25, 43) was higher on trials on which errors occurred, but also that it was equally high on response conflict trials on which no errors occurred. This suggests that the activity relates to the conflict (*i.e.*, potential for error) rather than errors *per se*. The same result has been obtained by Ullsperger and von Cramon (2001), at almost identical coordinates (4, 28, 42); however, these authors refer to the region as pre-SMA. The region lies on the border between ACC and prefrontal cortex. In an adjacent, more inferior region (7, 19, 30) which clearly falls in ACC (rCZp), Ullsperger and von Cramon identified an area that was more active during error trials, but not during high-conflict trials associated with correct responses.

If the activity in rCZp relates to the potential for response conflict, rather than the detection of errors, there are two distinct possibilities for its precise role. First, it may simply monitor the potential for conflict, sending signals indicating that steps need to be taken to resolve this conflict. Second it may initiate and sustain the executive processes required for resolving response conflict. This distinction is very similar to that between bottom-up and top-down processes discussed in the chapter on attention. If rCZp activity initiates and sustains executive processes, then activity would be related to *expectation* of response conflict. The activity would be tonic rather than phasic and elicited in association with individual trials on which conflict occurred. The activity would occur prior to the occurrence of responses. We have already mentioned the study by Banich *et al.* (2000) in which volunteers were anticipating response conflict although none actually occurred. The failure to observe activity in ACC on incongruent trials in this study would suggest that this region does not have a role in initiating and sustaining processes need to resolve response conflict. Botvinick *et al.* (1999) used a very different paradigm in which executive processes were engaged on a trial-by-trial basis. They also concluded that ACC (–2, 31, 29; a peak that falls slightly anterior to rCZp) was involved with monitoring conflict rather than implementing executive processes.

Response Conflict or Response Preparation?

Our discussion of the role of ACC (rCZp) derives from the original studies of the Stroop task, which linked this region with conflict, but there is whole body of work relating to working memory tasks that has also implicated this region. This illustrates another problem with attempts to assign functions to frontal regions on the basis of brain imaging studies. Careful arguments are developed on the basis of one large body of work, while the results of another large body of work using different types of task are ignored. Most of the argument relating to working memory has concerned the role of different regions of lateral prefrontal cortex. As a result, studies of this task have often not been considered relevant to discussion of the role of ACC. Petit *et al.* (1998) provide a very useful review of activations observed in ACC (and SMA) in working memory tasks. They also provide a useful diagram of the different regions of the medial wall in Talairach coordinates. It is clear from this review that rCZp has been activated in many working memory tasks. Using event-related fMRI, Petit *et al.* (1998) showed that there is sustained activity in rCZp (and also preSMA) during working memory for both spatial positions (1, 15, 36) and faces (–1, 16, 33). This is clearly the same region as that revealed by the meta-analysis of Barch et *al.*

(2001) of studies involving response conflict (3, 19, 35). Because the same region was activated whether remembering faces or positions, Petit *et al.* suggest this activity is associated with response preparation. In the control tasks, the volunteers knew in advance exactly which response they would have to make, while in both the working memory tasks they had to prepare to make a left or a right button press. Petit *et al.* do not link the activity in rCZp to response conflict but to some form of high-level response preparation. Perhaps activity in this region (and preSMA) relates to response preparation when the response can only be partially specified in advance (*i.e.*, preparation to make a left *or* a right button press). In this formulation, the key process is not monitoring conflict between responses but preparation for multiple response possibilities. We might speculate that, as we move toward the posterior along the medial wall, intended responses are represented in a more and more specific form.

Another body of work implicating ACC concerns implicit and explicit motor control. Jueptner *et al.* (1997) required volunteers to learn a short sequence of key presses until this task could be performed without attention. They then investigated which brain areas became more activated when the volunteers deliberately thought about which key they would be pressing next in the sequence. When attending to their actions in this way, activity was seen in ACC (18, 10, 28) and DLPFC. This task can be seen as involving conflict between the response currently being performed and the one that is going to be performed next. Indeed, there is small, but significant increase in reaction time when volunteers have to attend to responses in a well-learned sequence; however, the same pattern of activity is observed when explicit sequence learning is compared with implicit sequence learning. In an implicit sequence learning task, volunteers are unaware that there is a consistent sequence of key presses, but nevertheless show decreases in reaction time with practice. This implicit sequence learning occurs in the absence of activity in ACC and DLPFC. Only when subjects are aware that there is sequence to be learned does activity appear in ACC and DLPFC (Grafton *et al.*, 1995; Hazeltine *et al.*, 1997). Presumably this knowledge allows volunteers to prepare their response in advance and thus respond more quickly. These observations are consistent with a formulation in terms of response preparation rather than response conflict.

A Localiser Task?

We have concluded that ACC (or rather rCZp) is involved with the representation of response in a rather abstract form. However, it is clear that there are many alternative formulations in the literature. One problem concerns the precise area we are considering. Is it ACC or preSMA? This problem relates to our discussion at the beginning of this chapter: Is it possible to divide ACC in discrete functional components or does it act as a whole? Our review of the various studies of ACC clearly reveals that many of these have successfully shown adjacent areas to have different functions (Ullsperger and von Cramon 2001). On the other hand, comparison across studies leads to great confusion as to whether the regions activated are the same or different. This problem is only going to be resolved if we can develop localiser tasks analogous to those used for the visual system to identify the FFA or V5. If different studies use the same localiser task, it will be much easier to conclude that the same region is being considered. One possible localiser for activations in ACC would be one of the odd-ball tasks used by Braver *et al.* (2001).

Is Activity in ACC Uniquely Related to Response Preparation?

So far we have restricted our discussion of the Stroop task solely to the ACC. This illustrates another common problem in brain imaging studies. A careful argument is proposed about the function of a particular area without considering the possibility that another area may show precisely the same pattern of activity across tasks. Does the evidence for the role of ACC in monitoring response conflict apply equally well to any other area? There are certainly some studies in which the pattern of activity in ACC is very similar to that observed in DLPFC (Paus *et al.*, 1993); however, in many other experiments this is clearly not the case. For example, in the study of Braver *et al.* (2001), while activity was elicited in rCZp for infrequent responses in all three task contexts, the pattern in other brain regions was different. Activity in right DLPFC was significantly greater for the Go/NoGo task than for the odd-ball task or the CRT task. In the study by Banich *et al.* (2000) in which volunteers developed an attentional set for coping with conflict but did not have to respond, activity was seen in DLPFC and in VLPFC but not in ACC. These results and others have led to the suggestion that the initiation and sustaining of executive processes required to deal with conflict are associated with lateral prefrontal cortex. We consider the precise role of DLPFC in the next section.

DORSOLATERAL PREFRONTAL CORTEX AND RESPONSE SELECTION

In the early days of functional imaging every task seemed to activate dorsolateral prefrontal cortex (DLPFC), and every experimenter was happy to define a different role for this region. For example, it was proposed that DLPFC was critical for willed action (Frith *et al.*, 1991), for working memory (Petrides *et al.*, 1993), or for semantics (Petersen *et al.*, 1988). The tasks used in these studies were complex and involved many processes. Inevitably the selection of one of these processes to be associated with DLPFC was somewhat arbitrary. We now have evidence from a whole range of tasks and also from studies in which the parameters of one task have been systematically varied. We have already discussed some of the attempts to distinguish the role of ACC from DLPFC. Many studies have systematically searched for differences between DLPFC, VLPFC, and other prefrontal regions. Are we any nearer to a precise definition in cognitive terms of a role for DLPFC?

Word Generation Studies

The task of word generation has been widely used in functional imaging. Some experiments involve the traditional verbal fluency tasks used by neuropsychologists (*e.g.*, produce as many words beginning with S or as many animals as possible; Benton, 1968) while others use versions of the "verb for noun" task introduced by Petersen *et al.* (1988) in which subjects must generate a verb that goes with a noun (*e.g.*, cake: eat, knife: cut). The pattern of activation produced by these tasks is relatively robust when compared with baseline tasks such as word repetition. Increased activity is typically seen in left DLPFC, Broca's area, and anterior cingulate cortex. The precise pattern of activity will, necessarily, depend upon the control task used in the comparison. For example, when compared to rest, word generation is associated with an increase in temporal lobe areas, while, when compared to word repetition, there is a relative decrease in these areas (Warburton *et al.*, 1996).

In Fig. 18.8 and Table 18.1 we summarise data from seven studies of word generation that all used the same PET camera and the same method of analysis. In the four experiments described

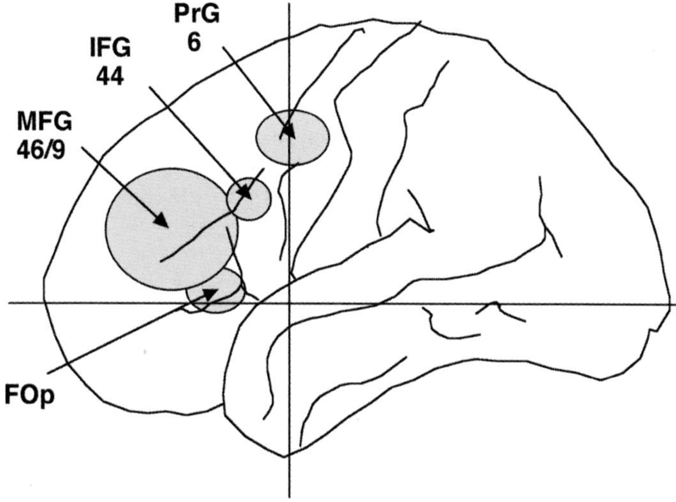

FIGURE 18.8
Areas of frontal cortex where activity is associated with word generation. (PrG, precentral gyrus, IFG, inferior frontal gyrus; MFG, middle frontal gyrus; Fop, frontal operculum.) (From Frith, C. D., 2000. With permission.)

TABLE 18.1 Means and Standard Deviations for Locations of Peak Activations and Number of Studies in Which Activations Were observed in Each Region

	Talairach Coordinates			
Brain Region	*x* **Mean (SD)**	*y* **Mean (SD)**	*z* **Mean (SD)**	**Number of Studies**
Anterior cingulate (BA32/6)	3 (6)	15 (8)	46 (7)	6
Frontal operculum	39 (4)	21 (4)	4 (3)	6
Precentral gyrus (BA6)	39 (4)	1 (5)	44 (4)	3
Inferior frontal gyrus (BA44)	38 (4)	12 (3)	28 (3)	5
Middle frontal gyrus	38 (7)	32 (7)	21 (8)	6

Note: On the basis of the coordinates of the peak activations in frontal cortex listed in seven independent experiments on word generation, five distinct areas could be identified: (1) *Anterior cingulate cortex*, supplementary motor area (BA32/6); all the peaks in this region were within 12 mm from the midline ($|x|$), and all other activations were at least 26 mm from the midline. (2) *Frontal operculum*; all the peaks in this region were inferior to 10 mm above the line joining the anterior and posterior commissures ($z < 10$), and all other activations were superior to this level. (3) *Precentral gyrus* (BA6); all the peaks in this region were less than 5 mm in front of the origin defined by the anterior commissure ($y < 5$), and all other activations were more anterior. (4) *Inferior frontal gyrus* (BA44); all the peaks in this region lay between 5 mm and 18 mm in front of the origin ($18 : y > 5$). (5) *Middle frontal gyrus* (BA46/9); all the peaks in this region lay more than 20 mm in front of the origin ($y > 18$).

Source: Data from Warburton *et al.* (1996; four experiments), Frith *et al.* (1991), Friston *et al.* (1993), and Spence *et al.* (1998).

by Warburton *et al.* (1996), volunteers silently generated words. In the verb generation task (experiments 1, 2, and 3), subjects heard six concrete nouns per minute and generated as many verbs as possible for each noun (*e.g.*, apple: eat, pick, slice, peel). In the noun generation task (experiment 3), they generated basic-level nouns appropriate to superordinate nouns (*e.g.*, furniture: table, chair, stool, cabinet). In experiment 4, the verb generation task was carried out in German by German volunteers. In all these experiments, control data were available for rest. Additional comparison tasks included detecting verb–noun matches (experiment 1), listening to nouns (experiment 2), and subvocal repetition of heard pseudo-words (experiment 4). In the studies by Frith *et al.* (1991), Friston *et al.* (1993), and Spence (1998), volunteers generated aloud words beginning with specified letters which were cued at a fixed rate (one word for each cue heard). In the baseline task, volunteers repeated the letter cues rather than generating new words. In the latter two studies, there were data from six generation scans and six repetition scans for each volunteer. This summary is restricted to activity observed in the frontal lobes.

The size of the five regions shown in Fig. 18.8 are determined by the standard deviation of the mean peak of activity across the studies. Each axis of the ellipse is 4 SDs. The large region centred on Brodmann areas 46/9 probably includes distinct subregions, but these could not be resolved in the studies reviewed here. What might be the roles of these five regions? On the basis of lesion studies, we would expect the frontal operculum to have a specific role in the production of speech (Dronkers, 1996). The regions listed as being in BA44 and BA6 are part of premotor cortex and therefore likely to be involved in high-level aspects of movement production (Passingham, 1997). The large area listed as being in BA46/9 is the region of DLPFC that is widely believed to have a key role in planning and executive control (Luria, 1966; Goldman-Rakic, 1987; Fuster, 1989). We have already discussed possible roles for ACC; in this section, we concentrate on DLPFC but indicate in which circumstances the pattern activity in ACC diverges from that seen in DLPFC.

Modality of Response

If DLPFC has a role in high-level executive function, we would expect activation in this region for response generation tasks whatever the modality of the response. In addition to the experiment on word generation, the study of Frith *et al.* (1991) included a separate experiment in which volunteers generated a sequence of random finger movements by lifting either the first or second finger of the left hand in response to a tactile pacing signal. This task was characterised as involving willed action, as a volunteer had to decide for himself which finger to lift on each trial. This task was contrasted with one in which the choice of response was determined by an external signal; on each trial, the volunteer simply lifted the finger that was touched. The willed action task produced activation in DLPFC (–35, 39, 21) close to the area that was activated during word generation. A number of other studies have also shown that DLPFC is activated when volunteers have to select for them selves among different hand and arm movements. Deiber *et al.* (1991) compared selecting between four different movements of a joystick with repeating the same movement on every trial and observed activation in DLPFC (–34, 32, 28; 34, 36, 28). Jueptner *et al.* (1997) compared selecting four different button presses with a well-learned sequence of presses and also observed activity in DLPFC (–28, 42, 16; 22, 26, 24). Jahanshahi *et al.* (1995) showed that DLPFC was also active (30, 40, 24) when volunteers had to select when to make a hand movement rather than which movement to make.

These various studies imply that left DLPFC activation during self-generated response selection may arise regardless of response modality; however, the verbal and the motor tasks used differ in ways other than response modality. In the finger lifting task, only two basic responses were possible: moving the first or second finger. In the word generation task, a different response had to be produced on every trial. Spence *et al.* (1998) looked for an effect of response modality in two much more comparable tasks. The first was a standard joystick task in which the volunteer had to produce a series of movements using the right hand in four different directions in response to a pacing tone. In the second, the volunteer had to produce a random series of mouth movements by saying the two syllables "lah" and "bah" in random order, again in response to a pacing tone. In both paradigms the control tasks were to produce a prespecified stereotyped sequence of joystick or mouth movements. For both response modalities an area of activity was seen in left DLPFC (hand: –38, 32, 36; mouth: –30, 42, 24). When both tasks were entered into the same analysis there was a main effect of condition (self-generated versus stereotyped sequences) in DLPFC (–40, 30, 32), but no interaction with response modality.

There were marked differences between the tasks in the pattern of brain activity in more posterior regions. For example, the joystick task generated activity in the parietal cortex while the mouth task did not. The only difference in the frontal regions, however, was that joystick movements and finger movements were associated with bilateral activation of DLPFC and premotor cortex, while for mouth movements and word generation the activity was restricted to the left DLPFC and the left frontal operculum.

These results suggest that DLPFC (and ACC) have a general role in tasks involving the generation of response sequences that is independent of response modality. At first sight, it might also seem that activity in this region is also independent of the number of responses available for selection; however, this is probably a false impression. When producing a long sequence of two finger movements in accordance with instructions to do so randomly we probably do not choose just one response at a time, but rather a short subsequence of movements that passes some criterion for randomness. The number of possible such subsequences could be quite large. For example, if we were just choosing two finger movements, there are 16 different sequences of four movements. We also need to keep track of where we are in the current subsequence and which subsequences have been produced already, just as we need to keep track of the words that have been produced so far in a word generation task. These considerations indicate a number of possible roles for DLPFC. Among these are (1) generating candidate responses or response sequences, (2) checking suitability of responses, (3) keeping track of what has happened so far, or (4) high-level coordination of all of these different task components. Keeping track of what has happened so far is one of the important roles of working memory, a process that many believe is instantiated in DLPFC (Goldman-Rakic, 1995).

Transient or Sustained Activity?

If the role of DLPFC in these response generation tasks is to maintain in working memory the sequence of responses given so far, then we would expect to see sustained activity in this region in between the production of each response. This prediction is best tested using event-related fMRI in which the pattern of haemodynamic activity associated with a single trial in different brain regions can be observed directly. Rowe *et al.* (2000) and Rowe and Passingham (2001) report a pair of elegant experiments in which event-related fMRI was used to investigate activity associated with working memory for locations in space and time. In the second of these studies, volunteers saw a sequence of events in which a single red dot appeared successively in three different positions on a monitor. There was then a variable delay during which volunteers attempted to remember the sequence that had occurred. After the delay a number appeared on the monitor (*e.g.*, 2) and the volunteer moved a cursor to the position on the screen that had been occupied by the dot on its second appearance. In the control task, there was nothing to be remembered during the interval and at the end of the delay the volunteer simply moved the cursor to the position indicated on the monitor.

Sustained activity that varied with the length of the delay was observed in superior frontal sulcus bilaterally (BA8: study 1, [–22, 8, 60] and [24, 4, 54]; study 2, [–18, 0, 56] and [28, 8, 60]) and in intraparietal cortex. Sustained activity could not be detected in DLPFC; however, transient activity in DLPFC was associated with the selection of the appropriate response at the end of the delay period (BA46: study 1, [42, 38, 28] and [30, 28, 40]; study 2, [42, 38, 30] and [–48, 32, 18]). Rowe *et al.* concluded that, rather than maintaining items in working memory, the role of DLPFC (BA46) is to select items from working memory. This implies a very general role in selection for this region that applies to items in memory as well as to overt responses in different modalities.

In the tasks used by Rowe *et al.*, simple maintenance of material in working memory did not activate DLPFC. Previous studies have observed sustained activity in this region during working memory tasks; however, it seems likely that in these studies more than simple maintenance processes were required. In some studies, volunteers were explicitly instructed to rehearse the items they were holding in memory (Courtney *et al.*, 1997). In tasks involving verbal material it is likely that volunteers will rehearse the material even without instruction, particularly if the material approaches or exceeds the capacity of working memory (Rypma and D'Esposito, 1999). In these examples, some sort of manipulation of the material in working memory was involved in addition to maintenance.

Dual Task Interference

However, we are not justified in concluding that the activity in DLPFC can be related solely to some sort of response selection process. A major requirement for an executive system is the ability to choose relevant processes and allocate appropriate resources when those currently engaged can no longer cope with the task at hand. Such a high-level process would be engaged at certain points in a response generation task, particularly when the task is difficult or very novel, but studies in which difficulty is related to the need for dual-task performance suggest that DLPFC does not have such a role.

Jahanshahi *et al.* (2000) looked at the effects of rate in a response generation task. Volunteers were required to generate random sequences of numbers at six different rates with counting aloud at the same rates as the control task. Marked linear effects of rate were seen in auditory cortex and in motor cortex and cerebellum for both conditions. During random number generation, there was greater activity in DLPFC and premotor (bilaterally) and anterior cingulate cortex. However, activity in these areas did not increase with increasing rate. Indeed, at the two highest rates (1 number per second and 2 numbers per second) there was a significant decrease in activity in DLPFC, but not in ACC (See Fig. 18.9a). This effect was manifest in brain activity as an interaction between task and rate (*i.e.*, a decrease in activity at high rates for the random number generation task while there was no change in the counting task). This interaction effect was seen in DLPFC (–34, 40, 24), but not in any of the other frontal areas associated with random number generation.

At the highest rates of performance of the random number generation task there was a reduction in the randomness of the response sequence produced (see Fig. 18.9b). This took the form of an increase in the number of response pairs which consisted of adjacent numbers (1/2, 5/6, etc.) and a reduction in the number of response pairs that were 2 apart (1/3, 5/7, etc.). There was also a negative correlation between randomness (as defined above) and activity in left DLPFC (–52, 34, 18).

We do not believe that a high-level executive role is compatible with the reduction of activity in this region and the associated decrease in randomness seen at the highest rates of responding. Jahanshahi *et al.* (2000) interpret this as reflecting interference between the task of random

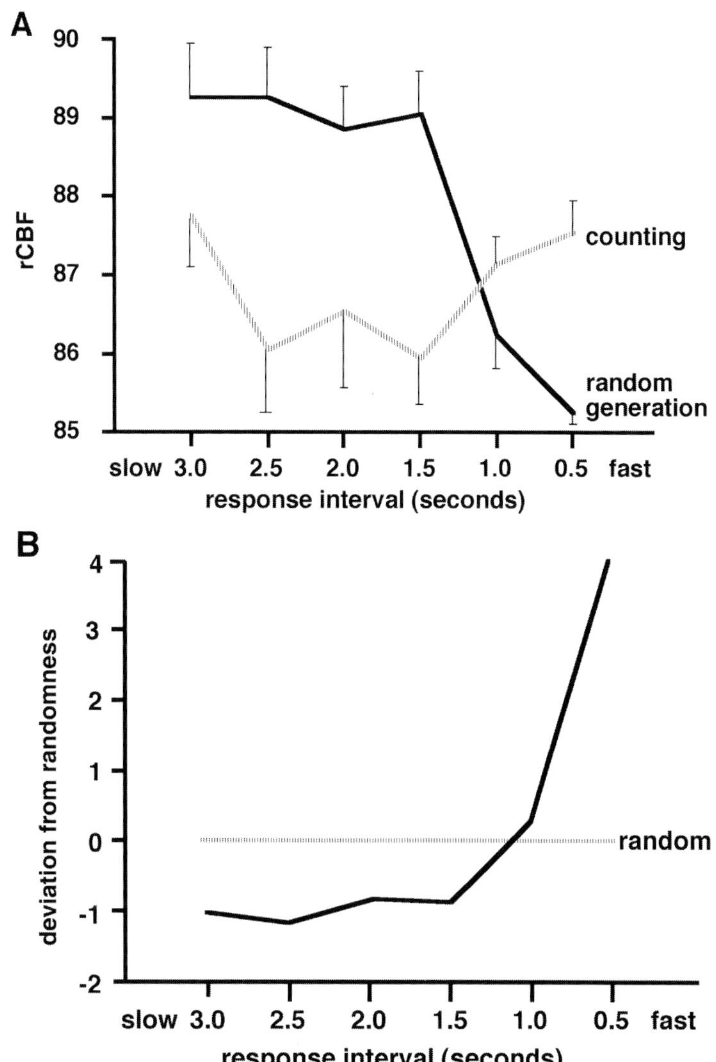

FIGURE 18.9
DLPFC and random number generation. (A) Blood flow in DLPFC at different rates of counting and random number generation. Activity is reduced when random numbers have to be generated rapidly. (B) Randomness of number sequences generated at different rates. There is a reduction of randomness at high rates. (From Frith, C. D., 2000. With permission.)

generation and the need to produce responses rapidly. At high rates, a volunteer may find that the time has come to make a response before a suitable response has been chosen. For that time his attempt to produce a suitably random response has to be abandoned so that a response can be made even though it is not ideal. This is precisely the point at which a high-level executive decision has to be made about priorities; yet, activity in DLPFC decreased. It therefore seems unlikely that this region has a high-level executive role.

Goldberg *et al.* (1998) have shown a similar effect with dual task interference on the Wisconsin Card Sorting task. Performance of a shadowing task while sorting produced an impairment of performance and a reduction of the activity in DLPFC associated with sorting. This effect was revealed as an significant interaction in DLPFC: (card sorting – control) > [(card sorting + shadowing) – (control + shadowing)]; –52, 28, 16). The same effect was also observed by Fletcher *et al.* (1995a) in a study of memory acquisition. A secondary choice reaction time task impaired memory performance and reduced the activity in left DLPFC associated with memory acquisition. Here, again, there was a significant interaction in left DLPFC: (memory – control) > [(memory + RT task) - RT task)]; –48, 34, 8). Different results were obtained by D'Esposito *et al.* (1995) who observed increases in activity in DLPFC when two tasks had to be performed at once; however, in this study, when the two tasks were performed simultaneously the decrements in performance were not large and it is not clear whether or not they were significant. There was no detectable activity in DLPFC in this study when the two tasks were performed separately. Perhaps the increased activity associated with dual task performance reflected the need to apply novel response selection processes when the two tasks were combined. In the studies of Jahanshahi *et al.* (2000) and Goldberg *et al.*, (1998), activity in ACC did not decrease during the interfering conditions, while in the study of Fletcher *et al.* (1995a) ACC was the only area to show an increase in activity during the dual task condition. This is additional evidence that ACC has a function distinct from that of DLPFC.

When several processes are competing for limited resources, there is a need for some higher level executive system to make appropriate allocations. The greater the competition, the harder this executive will have to work. The observation of reduced activity in DLPFC coupled with impaired performance suggests that this region is concerned with a lower level process that receives insufficient resources at high levels of competition. What sort of low-level executive process might be subserved by DLPFC? My subjective experience of trying to generate random numbers at too high a rate is as follows. At the moment that I have to make the next response, I have not had time to think of an item that I consider sufficiently random. I am forced, therefore, to produce one of the unsuitable items that happens to be available. This is likely to be a recently emitted item or one that has been primed by the last response (*i.e.*, the next number in a counting sequence). I do not totally give up, however. I continue to try to find a "random" response for each trial and the sequence I produce does not become completely stereotyped. Given this scenario, the volunteer might well be aware that his responses are not ideal. Perhaps activity in DLPFC is necessary to prevent the production of inappropriate responses and has to be reduced when an inappropriate response has to be emitted because there is not time to complete the selection process. Another low-level process that might be instantiated in DLPFC could be keeping track of the responses selected so far. In the random number generation task, a reduction in randomness would occur if the volunteer could not keep track of recent selections. In this case, the volunteer would not be aware that his responses were not random. Which of these alternative accounts is correct could be addressed by asking volunteers about their experience of doing the task and their confidence in the randomness of their responses.

Contextual Constraint

There is evidence, however, that DLPFC is active in response selection tasks even when there is no requirement to keep track of previous responses. Nathaniel-James *et al.* (1997) studied word generation using the sentence completion task developed by Burgess and Shallice (1996). In this task, the volunteer is shown a sentence with the last word missing. In one version of the task, he must generate the word that best fits the sentence. In the other version, he must generate a word that does *not* fit the sentence. Both versions of this task, especially the latter, are performed badly by patients with frontal lobe lesions (Burgess and Shallice, 1996). When normal volunteers perform this task, much activity is observed in left DLPFC for both versions compared to rest or to reading sentences in which the last word is supplied. Nathaniel-James & Frith (2002) have examined the effect of the constraint supplied by the sentence on the pattern of activity. Six levels of constraint were used derived from the Bloom and Fischler (1980) sentence completion norms. An example of high constraint would be "He posted the letter without a ________" (99% of subjects gave "stamp") and an example of low constraint would be "The police had never seen a man so ________" (14 different responses were given; the most frequent—"drunk"—was given by only 9% of subjects). Volunteers were asked to give a good completion or an inappropriate completion at each of the six levels of constraint. When the six inappropriate completions were compared with the six appropriate completions activity was observed in left DLPFC. There was no effect of constraint in the inappropriate condition, but when volunteers had to give an appropriate completion there was more activity in DLPFC under conditions of low constraint. This latter effect appeared as a significant interaction between task and the linear component of constraint in left DLPFC (–32, 58, 26).

In both the situations in which DLPFC was activated (low constraint and inappropriate completions), it was necessary to select between a number of possible responses; however, these conditions are also more difficult than the high constraint condition and volunteers took longer to produce their responses. Is it the lack of constraint on response selection that leads to the activity in DLPFC or is it some more general problem associated with the difficulty of the task? In a study by Desmond *et al.* (1998), volunteers had to generate words on the basis of word stems that could have either few or many completions. For example, the stem MOV– can only be completed as the word MOVE (or morphemically related words), while the stem MOR– has many possible completions (MORAL, MORBID, MORE, MORTAL, etc.). fMRI was used to contrast activity elicited by stems with many or few possible completions. In contrast to the sentence completion task, this word stem completion task is more difficult when the stem has few rather than many possible completions. Nevertheless, the many completion condition (*i.e.*, the less constrained condition) produced greater activity in the left DLPFC (–25, 44, 27). Clearly, it is the lack of constraint and not the difficulty of the task that leads to activity in DLPFC.

In these completion tasks there is no requirement to keep track of the sequence of responses, thus this component of working memory is not involved. In addition, volunteers cannot prepare and hold their response in advance. Clearly, working memory is required to keep in mind the current instructions (whether the response should be appropriate or inappropriate, for example); however, this requirement is independent of constraint. In combination with the various studies already considered, the results from these studies of the effects of response constraint strongly suggest that DLPFC activation is greater in situations in which the volunteer must select one from many rather than few alternatives. One possible formulation of the common feature of all the tasks reviewed here would be the need to create and sustain an arbitrary category of responses appropriate for the task in hand. This process includes the requirement to suppress responses outside the arbitrary category. For example, when generating words starting with a certain letter it is necessary to suppress semantic associations, and when generating random sequences of finger movements it is necessary to suppress sequences such as LLLL or LRLR. In these tasks it is the "sculpting" of the response space normally achieved by external context that has to be self-generated. This proposal is similar to that of Cohen *et al.* (1997) who give DLPFC a role in sustaining contextual information.

Other Characterisations of the Function of DLPFC

One important component of the executive system that is likely to be involved in response generation tasks is monitoring. We have suggested that DLPFC is not involved in monitoring in the sense of keeping track of the responses produced so far; however, monitoring might be required prior to each individual response to check that an appropriate response is being selected. Such a process might have to work harder when many rather than few responses are available for selection. We suspect that monitoring in this sense is closely related to the notion of response sculpting as both are mechanisms for ensuring that the correct response is selected; however, it might be possible to choose between these formulations by studying what happens when response selection breaks down at high rates of performance. If this was due to the failure of a monitor system, then presumably the volunteer would not be able to indicate which of his responses were inappropriate. On the other hand, if the "response sculpting" mechanism failed then the volunteer would know that incorrect responses were being made.

In this section, we have concentrated largely on tasks involving response selection; however, it is well established that activation in DLPFC is also elicited by working memory tasks. Such tasks involve many processes, leaving open the question of which particular process is relevant to the activity in DLPFC. We have already discussed the evidence from Rowe, J. B. *et al.* (2000) that DLPFC is not involved in maintaining items in working memory but is engaged when items have to be selected from working memory. However, a number of amateurs of DLPFC have speculated that this region is involved during the manipulation of items in working memory (Petrides, 1996). What precisely is meant by manipulation? A working memory task popular with brain imagers and that requires manipulation is the *n*-back task, in which the volunteer sees a sequence of letters and has to detect whether the currently presented item is the same as the item presented *n* trials previously. To do this, the volunteer must keep the last *n* items in memory and continuously update which is the target item. It is only the target items to which the volunteer must respond. This continuous updating involves creating new and arbitrary stimulus–response relationships. Clearly, the manipulation of items in working memory involved in the *n*-back task can be seen in terms very similar to the response sculpting process that we suggest is required for the performance of response generation tasks.

Wagner *et al.* (2001) studied a working memory task in which volunteers had to hold in mind three words and then reorder them in terms of their desirability (*e.g.*, LUCK, CURE, GLORY). This was contrasted with a task in which three words simply had to be rehearsed. The semantic comparisons and manipulation of order (which the authors strangely label "monitoring") required by the experimental task was associated with activity in right DLPFC (37, 25, 37; 37, 41, 28), while activity in right VLPFC (–43, 34, 12) was already seen in the task which only required rehearsal, without manipulation. These observations are consistent with the suggestion from the studies by Rowe J. B. *et al.* (2000) and Rowe and Passingham (2001) that DLPFC is involved when items have to be selected from working memory. Reordering the items in terms of desirability requires the repeated selection of items from the working memory pool.

A more detailed analysis of the various working memory tasks that activate DLPFC supplemented by the use of new tasks concerned with particular components of working memory is needed to determine whether our formulation of the function of DLPFC in response generation can also be applied to other working memory tasks.

Achievement of Response Selection

How does DLPFC influence response selection across different modalities? We have previously suggested (Friston *et al.*, 1991) that DLPFC modulates activity in those posterior brain regions where responses relevant to the task are represented. In word generation tasks, activity is seen in the temporal lobe (Warburton *et al.*, 1996), while in tasks requiring the movement of a joystick (Spence, 1998) or the fingers (Frith *et al.*, 1991), activity is seen in parietal cortex. Whether this activity is seen as an increase or a decrease seems to depend critically on the control task. With word generation, there is an increase of activity in temporal lobe relative to rest but a decrease relative to word repetition. This is the case even when the generation and repetition are silent (Warburton *et al.*, 1996, experiment 4), thus the activity does not reflect a response to external inputs from the volunteer's own voice. The situation is much less clear in relation to the parietal activity seen in the limb movement tasks. Decreases were seen when self-generated finger movements were compared to repetition (Frith *et al.*, 1991), but increases were seen for the equivalent comparison on the joystick task (Spence 1998).

We have suggested that the relative decreases seen in temporal cortex during word generation reflect a modulation of the region by signals from DLPFC which permit self-generated response selection to occur (Friston *et al.*, 1991). The appropriate responses emerge through the suppression of the very much greater number of inappropriate responses leading to an overall reduction of activity. In terms of our formulation, the decrease could represent the self-generated sculpting of the response space imposed by DLPFC. The manipulation of response rate during word generation sheds some light on the precise nature of the modulation (unpublished PET data). In temporal cortex, we observed a highly significant effect of rate on activity. This effect has been observed in a number of studies and we have suggested that it is a reflection of the transient increase in activity associated with each trial. This activity is presumably associated with stimulus analysis and/or responses production (Rees and Frith, 1998). Because the location of the activity lies in Wernicke's area, we suggest that the rate effect observed in temporal cortex in the word generation task reflects transient activity associated with the selection of each word. In addition, there was an effect of task on the activity in this area. This effect did not alter the slope of the line relating activity and task rate (*i.e.*, there was no significant difference in the slopes of the lines between the two conditions); however, the intercept was shifted down so that there was a general reduction of activity in word generation task compared to the word repetition task.

Because there was no significant change in slope, the transient activity associated with each response was not affected by the task. The change in intercept suggests that there was a tonic change in activity. This implies that there was a reduction of activity in this area during the word generation task even when no responses were being generated. This is consistent with a top-down mechanism whereby a form of bias is imposed on the relevant population of cells by the task set, analogous to the bias proposed to underlie stimulus selection in the model of Desimone and Duncan (1995). Here also there are similarities with the computational model put forward by Cohen *et al.* (1996)

Does DLPFC (BA46) Have a Specific Role in Response Selection?

By identifying a series of different circumstances in which DLPFC (BA46) is activated in association with response selection we have tried to derive a single cognitive function for this region. The evidence suggests, first, that DLPFC is not at the apex of an action control system, as the process instantiated there competes for resources with other processes. Second, it appears that DLPFC is not solely involved in keeping track of response sequences, as it is activated in tasks in which keeping track of responses is not required (*e.g.*, the stem completion task of Desmond *et al.*, 1998). We suggest that DLPFC is most likely involved in defining a set of responses suitable for the task and biasing these for selection, when external inputs do not automatically achieve such selection. This function resembles that component of Shallice's Supervisory Attentional System (Shallice, 1988, chap. 14) which modulates the lower level contention-scheduling system.

It is important to break this executive system into such low-level components because it will then lose its mystical and homuncular nature. Nevertheless, the formulation we have put forward remains very crude. A major problem stems from the fact that most of our discussion has been restricted to consideration of DLPFC in isolation. Only when we can discuss in truly mechanistic terms how it interacts with other areas will we begin to gain a proper understanding of its role in executive function.

Our formulation of the function of DLPFC (BA46) as *sculpting the response space* combines two of the various approaches we discussed at the beginning of this chapter. Sculpting is a process like monitoring, but this process is restricted to the limited domain of responses (or possibly actions). This is consistent with the argument from anatomy that DLPFC has particularly strong connections with the "action system" in the parietal lobe. From this perspective we could develop the somewhat grandiose speculation that sculpting is a general prefrontal function that is applied to different domains by different subregions. For example, we have argued elsewhere that orbital frontal cortex has the function of *sculpting the reward space* (Elliott *et al.*, 2000) through its connections with posterior reward systems such as the amygdala. The reader could derive mild entertainment by seeing how far the systematic application of this idea can explain the function of all prefrontal regions.

CONCLUSION

It is our hope that the reader will have found this chapter highly unsatisfactory. We have considered some topics in great detail while at the same time failing to discuss a number of other important studies. We have drawn conclusions about the role of certain regions through careful selection of the evidence. Our grasp of anatomy has been distinctly shaky. We hope the reader will not make the same mistakes. If we are to understand the role of prefrontal cortex in higher cognitive functions we need to take into account a much wider range of evidence. We need to be much more precise in our characterisation of cognitive functions. We need to be much more accurate in our localisation of brain activity. It is up to you.

References

Abell, F., Krams, M., Ashburner, J., Passingham, R., Friston, K., Frackowiak, R. S. J., Happe, F., Frith, C. D., and Frith, U. (1999). The neuroanatomy of autism: a voxel-based whole brain analysis of structural scans. *NeuroReport,* **10**, 1647–1651.

Adolphs, R. (1999). Social cognition and the human brain. *Trends Cogn. Sci.,* **3**(12), 469–479.

Amunts, K., Schleicher, A., Burgel, U., Mohlberg, H., Uylings, H. B. M., and Zilles, K. (1999). Broca's region revisited: cytoarchitecture and intersubject variability. *J. Compar. Neurol.,* **412**(2), 319–341.

Baars, B. J. (1988). *A Cognitive Theory of Consciousness*. Cambridge University Press, New York.

Baddeley, A. D. (1986). *Working Memory*. Clarendon Press, Oxford.

Banich, M. T., Milham, M. P., Atchley, R. A., Cohen, N. J., Webb, A., Wszalek, T., Kramer, A. F., Liang, Z. P., Barad,

V., Gullett, D., Shah, C., and Brown, C. (2000). Prefrontal regions play a predominant role in imposing an attentional 'set': evidence from fMIRI. *Cogn. Brain Res.,* **10**(1–2), 1–9.

Barbas, H., Ghashghaei, H., Dombrowski, S. M., and Rempel-Clower, N. L. (1999). Medial prefrontal cortices are unified by common connections with superior temporal cortices and distinguished by input from memory-related areas in the rhesus monkey. *J. Compar. Neurol.,* **410**(3), 343–367.

Barch, D. M., Braver, T. S., Akbudak, E., Conturo, T., Ollinger, J., and Snyder, A. (2001). Anterior cingulate cortex and response conflict: effects of response modality and processing domain. *Cereb. Cortex,* **11**(9), 837–848.

Baron-Cohen, S., Ring, H. S. W., Bullmore, E., Brammer, M., Simmons, A., and Williams, S. (1999). Social intelligence in the normal and autistic brain: an fMRI study. *Eur. J. Neurosci.,* **11**, 1891–1898.

Baron-Cohen, S., Ring, H. A., Bullmore, E. T., Wheelwright, S., Ashwin, C., and Williams, S. C. R. (2000). The amygdala theory of autism. *Neurosci. Biobehav. Rev.,* **24**, 355–364.

Bauman, M. L. and Kemper, T. L. (1994). Neuroanatomic observations of the brain in autism, in *The Neurobiology of Autism*. Bauman, M. L. and Kemper, T. L., Eds., pp. 119–145. Johns Hopkins Press, Baltimore, MD.

Benton, A. L. (1968). Differential behavioural effects in frontal lobe disease. *Neuropsychologia,* **6**, 53–60.

Blair, R. J. R. and Cipolotti, L. (2000). Impaired social response reversal: a case of 'acquired sociopathy'. *Brain,* **123**: 1122–1141.

Blakemore, J.-S., Wolpert, D. M., and Frith, C. D. (1998). Central cancellation of self-produced tickle sensation. *Nat. Neurosci.,* **1**, 635–639.

Bloom, P. A. and Fischler, I. (1980). Completion norms for 329 sentence contexts. *Memory Cogn.,* **8**, 631–642.

Bonda, E., Petrides, M., Ostry, D., and Evans, A. (1996). Specific involvement of human parietal systems and the amygdala in the perception of biological motion. *J. Neurosci.,* **16**: 3737–3744.

Bottini, G., Corcoran, R., Sterzi, R., Paulesu, E., Schenone, P., Scarpa, P., Frackowiak, R. S. J., and Frith, C. D. (1994). The role of the right hemisphere in the interpretation of figurative aspects of language: a positron emission tomography activation study. *Brain,* **117**, 1241–1253.

Botvinick, M., Nystrom, L. E., Fissell, K., Carter, C. S., and Cohen, J. D. (1999). Conflict monitoring versus selection-for-action in anterior cingulate cortex. *Nature,* **402**, 179–181.

Braver, T. S., Barch, D. M., Gray, J. R., Molfese, D. L., and Snyder, A. (2001). Anterior cingulate cortex and response conflict: effects of frequency, inhibition and errors. *Cereb. Cortex,* **11**(9), 825–836.

Brodmann, K. (1909). *Vergleichende Lokalisationslehre der Großhirnrinde in ihren Prinzipien dargestellt auf Grund des Zellenbaues*. Barth, Leipzig.

Brunet, E., Sarfati, Y., Hardy-Bayle, M.-C., and Decety, J. (2000). A PET investigation of the attribution of intentions with a nonverbal task. *NeuroImage,* **11**, 157–166.

Burgess, N., Maguire, E. A., Spiers, H., and O'Keefe, J. (2001). A temporoparietal and prefrontal network for retrieving the spatial context of life-like events. *NeuroImage,* **14**, 439–453.

Burgess, P. W. and Shallice, T. (1996). Response suppression, initiation and strategy use following frontal lobe lesions. *Neuropsychologia,* **34**, 263–273.

Bush, G., Luu, P., and Posner, M. I. (2000). Cognitive and emotional influences in anterior cingulate cortex. *Trends Cogn. Sci.,* **4**(6), 215–222.

Calvert, G. A., Bullmore, E. T., Brammer, M. J., Campbell, R., Williams, S. C., McGuire, P. K., Woodruff, P. W., Iverson, S. D., and David, A. S. (1997). Activation of auditory cortex during silent lipreading. *Science,* **276**, 593–596.

Carter, C. S., Braver, T. S., Barch, D. M., Botvinick, M. M., Noll, D., and Cohen, J. D. (1998). Anterior cingulate cortex, error detection, and online monitoring of performance. *Science,* **280**, 747–749.

Castelli, F., Happé, F., Frith, U., and Frith, C. D. (2000). Movement and mind: a functional imaging study of perception and interpretation of complex intentional movement patterns. *NeuroImage,* **12**, 314–325.

Channon, S. (2000). The effects of anterior lesions on performance on a story comprehension test: left anterior impairment on theory of mind-type task. *Neuropsychologia,* **38**(7), 1006–1017.

Chiavaras, M. M., LeGoualher, G., Evans, A., and Petrides, M. (2001). Three-dimensional probabilistic atlas of the human orbitofrontal sulci in standardised stereotaxic space. *NeuroImage,* **13**(3), 479–496.

Cohen, J. D., Braver, T. S., and O'Reilly, R. C. (1996). A computational approach to the prefrontal cortex. *Philos. Trans. Roy. Soc. London B,* **351**, 1515–1527.

Cohen, J. D., Perlstein, W. M., Braver, T. S., Nystrom, L. E., Noll, D. C., Jonides, J., and Smith, E. E. (1997). Temporal dynamics of brain activation during a working memory task. *Nature,* **386**, 604–608.

Courtney, S. M., Ungerleider, L. G., Keil, K., and Haxby, J. V. (1997). Transient and sustained activity in a distributed neural system for human working memory. *Nature,* **386**, 608–611.

Dagher, A., Owen, A. M., Boecker, H., and Brooks, D. J. (1999). Mapping the network for planning: a correlational PET activation study with the Tower of London task. *Brain,* **122**(10), 1973–1987.

Dehaene, S., Kerszberg, M., and Changeux, J. P. (1998). A neuronal model of a global workspace in effortful cognitive tasks. *Proc. Natl. Acad. Sci. USA,* **95**(24), 14529–14534.

Deiber, M.-P., Passingham, R. E., Colebatch, J. G., Friston, K. J., Nixon, P. D., and Frackowiak, R. S. J. (1991). Cortical areas and the selection of movement. *Exp. Brain Res.,* **84**, 393–402.

Dennett, D. C. (1996). *Kinds of Minds*. Basic Books, New York.

Desgranges, B., Baron, J.-C., and Eustache, F. (1998). The functional neuroanatomy of episodic memory: the role of the frontal lobes, the hippocampal formation, and other areas. *NeuroImage,* **8**, 198–213.

Desimone, R. and Duncan, J. (1995). Neural mechanisms of selective visual attention. *Ann. Rev. Neurosci.,* **18**, 193–222.

Desmond, J. E., Gabrieli, J. D. E., and Glover, G. H. (1998). Dissociation of frontal and cerebellar activity in a cognitive task: evidence for a distinction between selection and search. *NeuroImage,* **7**, 368–376.

D'Esposito, M., Detre, J. A., Alsop, D. C., Shin, R. K., Atlas, S., and Grossman, M. (1995). The neural basis of the central executive system of working memory. *Nature,* **378**, 279–281.

Dolan, R. J., Bench, C. J., Brown, R. G., Scott, L. C., Friston, K. J., and Frackowiak, R. S. J. (1992). Regional cerebral blood flow abnormalities in depressed patients with cognitive impairment. *J. Neurol. Neurosurg. Psychiatry,* **55**: 768–773.

Dronkers, N. F. (1996). A new brain region for coordinating speech articulation. *Nature,* **384**, 159–161.

Duncan, J. (2001). An adaptive coding model of neural function in prefrontal cortex. *Nat. Rev. Neurosci.,* **2**(11), 820–829.

Duncan, J. and Owens, A. M. (2000). Dissociative methods in the study of frontal lobe function, in *Control of Cognitive Processes*, Vol. XVIII, Monsell, S. and Driver, J., Eds., pp. 567–576. MIT Press, Cambridge, MA.

Elliott, R., Dolan, R. J., and Frith, C. D. (2000). Dissociable functions in the medial and lateral orbitofrontal cortex: evidence from human neuroimaging studies. *Cereb. Cortex,* **10**, 308–317.

Eriksen, B. A. and Eriksen, C. W. (1974). Effects of noise letters upon the identification of a target letter in a nonsearch task. *Percept. Psychophys.,* **16**(1), 143–149.

Fine, C., Lumsden, J., and Blair, R. J. R. (2001). Dissociation between theory of mind and executive functions in a patient with early left amygdala damage. *Brain,* **124**, 287–298.

Fletcher, P. C. and Henson, R. N. (2001). Frontal lobes and human memory: insights from functional neuroimaging. *Brain,* **124**: 849–881.

Fletcher, P. C., Frith, C. D., Grasby, P., Shallice, T., Frackowiak, R. S. J., and Dolan, R. J. (1995a). Brain systems for encoding and retrieval of auditory-verbal memory. *Brain,* **118**, 401–416.

Fletcher, P. C., Happé, F., Frith, U., Baker, S. C., Dolan, R. J., Frackowiak, R. S. J., and Frith, C. D. (1995b). Other minds in the brain: a functional imaging study of theory of mind in story comprehension. *Cognition,* **57**, 109–128.

Fodor, J. A. (1992). A theory of the child's theory of mind. *Cognition,* **44**, 283–296.

Frisk, V., and Milner, B. (1990). The role of the left hippocampal region in the acquisition and retention of story content. *Neuropsychologia*, **28**, 349–359.

Friston, K. J., Frith, C. D., Liddle, P. F., and Frackowiak, R. S. J. (1991). Investigating a network model of word generation with positron emission tomography. *Proc. Roy. Soc. London Ser. B,* **244**, 101–106.

Friston, K. J., Frith, C. D., Liddle, P. F., and Frackowiak, R. S. J. (1993). Functional connectivity: the principal-component analysis of large (PET) data sets. *J. Cereb. Blood Flow Metab.,* **13**, 5–14.

Frith, C. D. (2000). The role of dorsolateral prefrontal cortex in the selection of action as revealed by functional imaging, in: *Control of Cognitive Processes*, Vol. XVIII, Monsell, S. and Driver, J., Eds., pp. 544–565. MIT Press, Cambridge, MA.

Frith, C. D., Friston, K. J., Liddle, P. F., and Frackowiak, R. S. J. (1991). Willed action and the prefrontal cortex in man: a study with PET. *Proc. Roy. Soc. London Ser. B,* **244**, 241–246.

Frith, U. (2001). Mind blindness and the brain in autism. *Neuron,* **32**(6), 969–979.

Fuster, J. M. (1989). *The Prefrontal Cortex.* Raven Press, New York.

Gallagher, H. L., Happe, F., Brunswick, N., Fletcher, P. C., Frith, U., and Frith, C. D. (2000). Reading the mind in cartoons and stories: an fMRI study of theory of mind in verbal and nonverbal tasks. *Neuropsychologia,* **38**, 11–21.

Gallagher, H. L., Jack, A. I., Roepstorff, A., and Frith, C. D. (2002). Imaging the intentional stance. *NeuroImage*, **16**, 814–821.

Gershberg, F. B., and Shimamura, A. P. (1995). Impaired use of organizational strategies in free recall following frontal lobe dam-age. *Neuropsychologia*, **33**, 1305–1333.

Ghaem, O., Mellet, E., Crivello, F., Tzourio, N., Mazoyer, B., Berthoz, A., and Denis, M. (1997). Mental navigation along memorised routes activates the hippocampus, precuneus, and insula. *NeuroReport,* **8**, 739–744.

Goel, V., Grafman, J. N. S., and Hallett, M. (1995). Modelling other minds. *NeuroReport,* **6**, 1741–1746.

Goldberg, T. E., Berman, K. F., Fleming, K., Ostrem, J., Van Horn, J. D., Esposito, G., Mattay, V. S., Gold, J. M., and Weinberger, D. R. (1998). Uncoupling cognitive workload and prefrontal cortical physiology. *NeuroImage,* **7**, 296–303.

Goldman-Rakic, P. S. (1987). Circuitry of primate prefrontal cortex and regulation of behaviour by representational knowledge, in *Handbook of Physiology: The Nervous System*, Mountcastle, V. B., Ed., p. 5. Williams & Wilkins, Baltimore, MD.

Goldman-Rakic, P. S. (1995). Architecture of the prefrontal cortex and the central executive. *Ann. N.Y. Acad. Sci.,* **769**, 71–83.

Grafton, S. T., Hazeltine, E., and Ivry, R. (1995). Functional mapping of sequence learning in normal humans. *Hum. Brain Mapping,* **1**, 221–234.

Grezes, J., Costes, N., and Decety, J. (1998). Top-down effect of strategy on the percption of human biological motion: a PET investigation. *Cogn. Neuropsychol.,* **15**, 553–582.

Grezes, J., Costes, N., and Decety, J. (1999). The effects of learning and intention on the neural network involved in the perception of meaningless actions. *Brain,* **122**, 1875–1887.

Grön, G., Wunderlich, A. P., Spitzer, M., Tomczak, R., and Riepe, M. W. (2000). Brain activation during human navigation: gender-different neural networks as substrate of performance. *Nat. Neurosci.,* **3**, 404–408.

Gross, C. G. (1998). *Brain, Vision, Memory: Tales in the History of Neuroscience*. MIT Press, Cambridge, MA.

Gusnard, D. A., Akbudak, E., Shulman, G. L., and Raichle, M. E. (2001). Medial prefrontal cortex and self-referential mental activity: relation to a default mode of brain function. *Proc. Natl. Acad. Sci. USA,* **98**(7), 4259–4264.

Happé, F. G. E. (1993). Communicative competence and theory of mind in autism: a test of relevance theory. *Cognition,* **48**, 101–119.

Happé, F. G. E., Ehlers, S., Fletcher, P., Frith, U., Johansson, M., Gillberg, C., Dolan, R. J., Frackowiak, R. S. J., and

Frith, C. D. (1996). Theory of mind in the brain: evidence from a PET scan study of Asperger syndrome. *NeuroReport,* **8**, 197–201.

Hazeltine, E., Grafton, S. T., and Ivry, R. (1997). Attention and stimulus characteristics determine the locus of motor-sequence encoding: a PET study. *Brain,* **120**, 123–140.

Heider, F. and Simmel, M. (1944). An experimental study of apparent behaviour. *Am. J. Psychol.,* **57**, 243–259.

Herrmann, M., Rotte, M., Grubich, C., Ebert, A. D., Schiltz, K., Munte, T. F., and Heinze, H. J. (2001). Control of semantic interference in episodic memory retrieval is associated with an anterior cingulate-prefrontal activation pattern. *Hum. Brain Mapping,* **13**(2), 94–103.

Heyes, C. M. (1998). Theory of mind in nonhuman primates. *Behav. Brain Sci.,* **21**, 101–134.

Incisa della Rochetta, A., and Milner, B. (1993). Strategic search and retrieval inhibition: The role of the frontal lobes. *Neuropsychologia*, **31**, 503–524.

Jahanshahi, M., Jenkins, I. H., Brown, R. G., Marsden, C. D., Passingham, R. E., and Brooks, D. J. (1995). Self-initiated vs. internally triggered movements. *Brain,* **118**, 913–933.

Jahanshahi, M., Dirnberger, G., Fuller, R., and Frith, C. D. (2000). The role of dorsolateral prefrontal cortex in random number generation. *NeuroImage,* **12**, 713–725.

Jueptner, M., Stephan, K. M., Frith, C. D., Brooks, D. J., Frackowiak, R. S. J., and Passingham, R. E. (1997). Anatomy of motor learning: I. Frontal cortex and attention to action. *J. Neurophysiol.,* **77**, 1313–1324.

Kanwisher, N., McDermott, J., and Chun, M. M. (1997). The fusiform face area: a module in human extrastriate cortex specialised for face perception. *J. Neurosci.,* **17**(11), 4302–4311.

Kawashima, R., Sugiura, M., Kato, T., Nakamura, A., Hatano, K., Ito, K., Fukuda, H., Kojima, S., and Nakamura, K. (1999). The human amygdala plays an important role in gaze monitoring. *Brain,* **122**, 779–783.

Kircher, T. T. J., Senior, C., Phillips, M. L., Rabe-Hesketh, S., Benson, P. J., Bullmore, E. T., Brammer, M., Simmons, A., Bartels, M., and David, A. S. (2000). Recognizing one's own face. *Cognition*, **78**, 1–15.

Konishi, S., Kawazu, M., Uchida, I., Kikyo, H., Asakura, I., and Miyashita, Y. (1999). Contribution of working memory to transient activation in human inferior prefrontal cortex during performance of the Wisconsin Card Sorting test. *Cereb. Cortex,* **9**(7), 745–753.

Kopelman, M. D., and Stanhope, N. (1998). Recall and recognition memory in patients with focal frontal, temporal lobe and dience-phalic lesions. *Neuropsychologia*, **36**, 785–795.

Lane, R. D., Fink, G. R., Chua, P. M., and Dolan, R. J. (1997). Neural activation during selective attention to subjective emotional responses. *NeuroReport,* **8**, 3969–3972.

Lashley, K. S. (1929). *Brain Mechanisms and Intelligence*. University of Chicago Press, Chicago.

Lepage, M., Habib, R., and Tulving, E. (1998). Hippocampal PET activations of memory encoding and retrieval: the HIPER model. *Hippocampus,* **8**, 313–322.

Leslie, A. M. (1987). Pretense and representation in infancy: the origins of theory of mind. *Psychol. Rev.,* **94**, 412–426.

Leslie, A. M. and Thaiss, L. (1992). Domain specificity in conceptual development: neuropsychological evidence from autism. *Cognition,* **43**, 225–251.

Leung, H. C., Skudlarski, P., Gatenby, J. C., Peterson, B. S., and Gore, J. C. (2000). An event-related functional MRI study of the Stroop colour word interference task. *Cereb. Cortex,* **10**, 552–560.

Luria, A. R. (1966). *Higher Cortical Functions in Man*. Tavistock, London.

Maguire, E. A. (2001). Neuroimaging studies of autobiographical event memory. *Philos. Trans. Roy. Soc. London, Biol. Sci.,* **356**, 1441–1451.

Maguire, E. A. and Mummery, C. J. (1999). Differential modulation of a common memory retrieval network revealed by positron emission tomography. *Hippocampus,* **9**, 54–61.

Maguire, E. A., Frackowiak, R. S. J., and Frith, C. D. (1996). Learning to find your way: a role for the human hippocampal formation. *Proc. Roy. Soc. London Ser. B,* **263**, 1745–1750.

Maguire, E. A., Frackowiak, R. S. J., and Frith, C. D. (1997). Recalling routes around london: activation of the right hippocampus in taxi drivers. *J. Neurosci.,* **17**, 7103–7110.

Maguire, E. A., Burgess, N., Donnett, J. G., Frackowiak, R. S. J., Frith, C. D., and O'Keefe, J. (1998). Knowing where, and getting there: a human navigation network. *Science,* **280**, 921–924.

Maguire, E. A., Gadian, D. G., Johnsrude, I. S., Good, C. D., Ashburner, J., Frackowiak, R. S. J., and Frith, C. D. (2000a). Navigation-related structural change in the hippocampi of taxi drivers. *Proc. Natl. Acad. Sci. USA,* **97**, 4398–4403.

Maguire, E. A., Mummery, C. J., and Buchel, C. (2000b). Patterns of hippocampal-cortical interaction dissociate temporal lobe memory subsystems. *Hippocampus,* **10**, 475–482.

Maguire, E. A., Henson, R. N. A., Mummery, C. J., and Frith, C. D. (2001a). Activity in right prefrontal cortex, but not hippocampus, varies parametrically with the increasing remoteness of memories. *NeuroReport,* **12**, 441–444.

Maguire, E. A., Vargha-Khadem, F., and Mishkin, M. (2001b). The effects of bilateral hippocampal damage on fMRI regional activations and interactions during memory retrieval. *Brain,* **124**, 1156–1170.

Maril, A., Wagner, A. D., and Schacter, D. L. (2001). On the tip of the tongue: an event-related fMRI study of semantic retrieval failure and cognitive conflict. *Neuron,* **31**(4), 653–660.

McCabe, K., Houser, D., Ryan, L., Smith, V., and Trouard, T. (2001). A functional imaging study of cooperation in two-person reciprocal exchange. *Proc. Natl. Acad. Sci. USA,* **98**, 11832–11835.

McGuire, P. K., Paulesu, E., Frackowiak, R. S. J., and Frith, C. D. (1996a). Brain activity during stimulus independent thought. *NeuroReport,* **7**, 2095–2099.

McGuire, P. K., Silbersweig, D. A., and Frith, C. D. (1996b). Functional neuroanatomy of verbal self-monitoring. *Brain,* **119**, 907–917.

Milner, A. D. and Goodale, M. A. (1995). *The Visual Brain in Action*. Oxford University Press, London.

Milner, B. (1963). Effects of different brain lesions on card sorting. *Arch. Neurol.,* **9**, 90–100.

Monchi, O., Petrides, M., Petre, V., Worsley, K., and Dagher, A. (2001). Wisconsin card sorting revisited: distinct neural circuits participating in different stages of the task identified by event-related functional magnetic resonance imaging. *J. Neurosci.,* **21**(19), 7733–7741.

Morris, J., Frith, C. D., Perrett, D., Rowland, D., Young, A., Calder, A., and Dolan, R. J. (1996). A differential neural response in the human amygdala to fearful and happy facial expressions. *Nature,* **383**, 812–815.

Nathaniel-James, D. A., Fletcher, P., and Frith, C. D. (1997). The functional anatomy of verbal initiation and suppression using the Hayling test. *Neuropsychologia,* **35**, 559–566.

Nathaniel-James, D. A. and Frith, C. D. (2002). The role of the dorsolateral prefrontal cortex: evidence from the effects of contextual constraint in a sentence completion task. *NeuroImage.* **16**, 1094–1102.

Nystrom, L. E., Braver, T. S., Sabb, F. W., Delgado, M. R., Noll, D. C., and Cohen, J. D. (2000). Working memory for letters, shapes, and locations: fMRI evidence against stimulus-based regional organisation in human prefrontal cortex. *NeuroImage,* **11**(5), 424–446.

O'Keefe, J. and Dostrovsky, J. (1971). The hippocampus as a spatial map: preliminary evidence from unit activity in the freely-moving rat. *Brain Res.,* **34**, 171–175.

Owen, A. M., Morris, R. G., Sahakian, B. J., Polkey, C. E., and Robbins, T. W. (1996). Double dissociations of memory and executive functions in working memory tasks following frontal lobe excisions, temporal lobe excisions or amygdalo-hippocampectomy in man. *Brain,* **119**, 1597–1615.

Pardo, J. V., Pardo, P. J., Janer, K. W., and Raichle, M. E. (1990). The anterior cingulate cortex mediates processing selection in the Stroop attentional conflict paradigm. *Proc. Natl. Acad. Sci. USA,* **87**(1), 256–259.

Passingham, R. E. (1997). Functional organisation of the motor system, in *Human Brain Function.* Frackowiak, R. S. J., Friston, K. J., Frith, C. D., Dolan, R. J., and Mazziotta, J. C., Eds., pp. 243–274. Academic Press, San Diego.

Paus, T., Petrides, M., Evans, A. C., and Meyer, E. (1993). Role of the human anterior cingulate cortex in the control of oculomotor, manual, and speech responses: a positron emission tomography study. *J. Neurophysiol.,* **70**(2), 453–469.

Paus, T., Kosci, L., Caramanos, Z., and Westbury, C. (1998). Regional differences in the effects of task difficulty and motor output on blood flow response in the human anterior cingulate cortex. *NeuroReport,* **9**, 35–45.

Perret, E. (1974). The left frontal lobe in man and the suppression of habitual responses in verbal categorical behaviour. *Neuropsychologia,* **12**, 342–345.

Petersen, S. E., Fox, P. T., Posner, M. I., Mintun, M., and Raichle, M. E. (1988). Positron emission studies of the cortical anatomy of single-word processing. *Nature,* **331**, 585–589.

Petit, L., Courtney, S. M., Ungerleider, L. G., and Haxby, J. V. (1998). Sustained activity in the medial wall during working memory delays. *J. Neurosci.,* **18**(22), 9429–9437.

Petrides, M. (1996). Specialised systems for the processing of mnemonic information within the primate frontal cortex. *Philos. Trans. Roy. Soc. London B, Biol. Sci.,* **351**(1346), 1455–1461.

Petrides, M. and Pandya, D., N. (1994). Comparative architectonic analysis of the human and the macaque frontal cortex, in *Handbook of Neuropsychology*, Vol. 1, Boller, F. and Graffman, J., Eds., pp. 17–58. Elsevier, New York.

Petrides, M., Alivisatos, B., Meyer, R., and Evans, A. C. (1993). Functional activation of the human frontal cortex during the performance of verbal working memory tasks. *Proc. Natl. Acad. Sci. USA,* **90**, 878–882.

Picard, N. and Strick, P. L. (1996). Motor areas of the medial wall: a review of their location and functional activation. *Cereb. Cortex,* **6**(3), 342–353.

Price, J. L. (1999). Prefrontal cortical networks related to visceral function and mood. *Ann. N.Y. Acad. Sci.,* **877**, 383–396.

Puce, A., Allison, T., Bentin, S., Gore, J.C., and McCarthy, G. (1998). Temporal cortex activation in humans viewing eye and mouth movements. *J. Neurosci.,* **18**, 2188–2199.

Raichle, M. E., Fiez, J. A., Videen, T. O., MacLoed, A. M., Pardo, J. V., Fox, P. T., and Petersen, S. E. (1994). Practice related changes in human brain functional anatomy during nonmotor learning. *Cereb. Cortex,* **4**, 8–26.

Rainville, P., Duncan, G.H., Price, D.D., Carrier, B., and Bushnell, M.C. (1997). Pain affect encoded in human anterior cingulate but not somatosensory cortex. *Science,* **277**, 968–971.

Rajkowska, G. and Goldman-Rakic, P. S. (1995). Cytoarchitectonic definition of prefrontal areas in the normal human cortex. 2. Variability in locations of areas 9 and 46 and relationship to the Talairach coordinate system. *Cereb. Cortex,* **5**(4), 323–337.

Rao, S. C., Rainer, G., and Miller, E. K. (1997). Integration of what and where in the primate prefrontal cortex. *Science,* **276**(5313), 821–824.

Rees, G. and Frith, C. D. (1998). How do we select perceptions and actions? Human brain imaging studies. *Philos. Trans. Roy. Soc. London B, Biol. Sci.,* **353**, 1283–1293.

Robbins, T. W. (1996). Dissociating executive functions of the prefrontal cortex. *Philos. Trans. Roy. Soc. London B, Biol. Sci.,* **351**(1346), 1463–1470.

Rogers, R. D., Andrews, T. C., Grasby, P. M. B., and Robbins, T. W. (2000). Contrasting cortical and subcortical activations produced by attentional-set shifting and reversal learning in humans. *J. Cogn. Neurosci.,* **12**(1), 142–162.

Rowe, A. D., Bullock, P. R., Polkey, C. E., and Morris, R. G. (2001). Theory of mind impairments and their relationship to executive functioning following frontal lobe excisions. *Brain,* **124**, 600–616.

Rowe, J. B. and Passingham, R. E. (2001). Working memory for location and time: activity in prefrontal area 46 relates to selection rather than maintenance in memory. *NeuroImage,* **14**, 77–86.

Rowe, J. B., Toni, I., Josephs, O., Frackowiak, R. S. J., and Passingham, R. E. (2000). The prefrontal cortex: response selection or maintenance within working memory? *Science,* **288**, 1556–1560.

Rowe, J. B., Owen, A. M., Johnsrude, I. S., and Passingham, R. E. (2001). Imaging the mental components of a planning task. *Neuropsychologia,* **39**(3), 315–327.

Rushworth, M. F. S. (2000). Anatomical and functional subdivision within the primate lateral prefrontal cortex. *Psychobiology,* **28**(2), 187–196.

Russell, J. (1997). How executive disorders can bring about an inadequate 'theory of mind,' in *Autism As an Executive Disorder*, Russell, J., Ed., pp. 256–304. Oxford University Press, New York.

Rypma, B. and D'Esposito, M. (1999). The roles of prefrontal brain regions in components of working memory: effects of memory load and individual differences. *Proc. Natl. Acad. Sci. USA,* **96**, 6558–6563.

Sandstrom, N. J., Kaufman, J., and Huettel, S.A (1998). Males and females use different distal cues in a virtual environment navigation task. *Cogn. Brain Res.,* **6**, 351–360.

Schacter, D. L. and Wagner, A. D. (1999). Medial temporal lobe activations in fMRI and PET studies of episodic encoding and retrieval. *Hippocampus,* **9**, 7–24.

Shallice, T. (1982). Specific impairments of planning. *Philos. Trans. Roy. Soc. London B, Biol. Sci.,* **298**, 199–209.

Shallice, T. (1988). *From Neuropsychology to Mental Structure*. Cambridge University Press, Cambridge, U.K.

Smith, M. L., Leonard, G., Crane, J., and Milner, B. (1995). The effects of frontal- or temporal-lobe lesions on susceptibility to interference in spatial memory. *Neuropsychologia*, **33**, 275–285.

Spence, S. A., Hirsch, S.R., Brooks, D.J., and Grasby, P.M (1998). Prefrontal cortex activity in people with schizophrenia and control subjects. *Br. J. Psychiatry,* **172**, 316–323.

Sperber, D. and Wilson, D. (1995). *Relevance: Communication and Cognition*. Blackwell, Oxford.

Sperling, G. and Speelman, I. (1970). Acoustic similarity and auditory short-term memory: experiments and a model, in *Models of Human Memory*, Norman, D. A, Ed., Academic Press, San Diego.

Stroop, J. (1935). Studies of interference in serial verbal reactions. *J. Exp. Psychol.,* **18**, 643–662.

Stuss, D. T., Gallup, G. G., and Alexander, M. (2001). The frontal lobes are necessary for theory of mind. *Brain,* **124**, 279–286.

Tomaiuolo, F., MacDonald, J. D., Caramanos, Z., Posner, G., Chiavaras, M., Evans, A. C., and Petrides, M. (1999). Morphology, morphometry and probability mapping of the pars opercularis of the inferior frontal gyrus: an *in vivo* MRI analysis. *Eur. J. Neurosci.,* **11**(9), 3033–3046.

Tulving, E. (1983). *Elements of Episodic Memory*. Clarendon Press, London.

Ullsperger, M. and von Cramon, D. Y. (2001). Subprocesses of performance monitoring: a dissociation of error processing and response competition revealed by event-related fMRI and ERPs. *NeuroImage,* **14**(6), 1387–1401.

Ungerleider, L. G. and Mishkin, M. (1982). Two cortical visual systems, in *Analysis of Visual Behaviour*. Ingle, D. J., Goodale, M. A., and R. J. W. Mansfield, R. J. W., Eds., pp. 549–558. MIT Press, Cambridge, MA.

van Veen, V., Cohen, J. D., Botvinick, M. M., Stenger, V. A., and Carter, C. S. (2001). Anterior cingulate cortex, conflict monitoring, and levels of processing. *NeuroImage,* **14**(6), 1302–1308.

Vargha-Khadem, F., Gadian, D. G., Watkins, K. E., Connolly, A., Van Paesschen, W., and Mishkin, M. (1997). Differential effects of early hippocampal pathology on episodic and semantic memory. *Science,* **277**, 376–380.

Wagner, A. D., Maril, A., Bjork, R. A., and Schacter, D. L. (2001). Prefrontal contributions to executive control: fMRI evidence for functional distinctions within lateral prefrontal cortex. *NeuroImage,* **14**(6), 1337–1347.

Warburton, E., Wise, R. J. S., Price, C. J., Weiller, C., Hadar, U., Ramsay, S., and Frackowiak, R. S. J. (1996). Noun and verb retrieval by normal subjects. *Brain,* **119**, 159–179.

Weinberger, D. R., Berman, K. F., and Zec, R. F. (1986). Physiological dysfunction of dorsolateral prefrontal cortex in schizophrenia. 1. Regional cerebral blood-flow evidence. *Arch. Gen. Psychiatry,* **43**(2), 114–124.

Wicker, B., Michel, F., Henaff, M., and Decety, J. (1998). Brain regions involved in the perception of gaze: a PET study. *NeuroImage*, **8**, 221–227.

Zeki, S. M. (1978). Functional specialisation in the visual cortex of the rhesus monkey. *Nature,* **274**, 423–428.

Zysset, S., Muller, K., Lohmann, G., and von Cramon, D. Y. (2001). Color-word matching Stroop task: separating interference and response conflict. *NeuroImage,* **13**(1), 29–36.

SECTION FOUR

EMOTION AND MEMORY

CHAPTER

19

Functional Neuroanatomy of Human Emotion

INTRODUCTION

Emotion is central to human experience. It colors how we perceive the world and influences our decisions, actions, and memories. Without emotion, without feelings of pleasure, pride, anger, grief, and jealousy, our mental life would be reduced to cold, cognitive information processing. The fleeting, subjective nature of emotional states makes them less than ideal objects for psychological or neuroscientific study. Emotional responses are more difficult to categorise and quantify than sensory, motor, or mnemonic processes. Consequently, emotion is either ignored by psychologists and neuroscientists or treated merely as an unwelcome source of noise or bias in relation to "normal" cognitive function. There has recently been renewed interest in the neural basis of emotion and its relationship to cognitive function and behaviour (Damasio, 1994, 1999; LeDoux, 1996). This chapter reviews recent findings in the neuroscientific study of emotion focusing on data from human functional neuroimaging experiments. We begin with a brief historical overview of theories of emotion.

THEORETICAL APPROACHES TO EMOTION

Philosophical and Psychological Theories

Since Plato (360 B.C.), a tradition in Western thought contrasts the animal, reflexive *body* with the uniquely human, rational *mind* or *soul*. Rene Descartes (1641) (Fig. 19.1a) concluded that, "It is certain that ... my mind, by which I am what I am, is entirely and truly distinct from my body, and may exist without it." This philosophical dualism has had a profound impact on metapsychological theories of emotion and the mind. Freud's model of mental structure in which an unconscious *id* (representing innate instincts and desires) is contrasted with a conscious *ego* and *superego* (representing the individual's interaction with the external world and society) embodies an essentially dualist philosophical position (Breuer and Freud, 1895). More recent controversies concerning the primacy of cognition and emotion have also been influenced by dualistic approaches to the mind (Lazarus, 1984; Zajonc, 1984). The philosophical and psychological split between mind and body, cognition and emotion, has had important consequences for neural theories of emotion, which are considered below.

Neuropsychological Theories

One of earliest and most influential accounts of the neural basis of emotion is that of William James (1884) (Fig. 19.1b). According to this "peripheralist" theory, emotion is the perception of

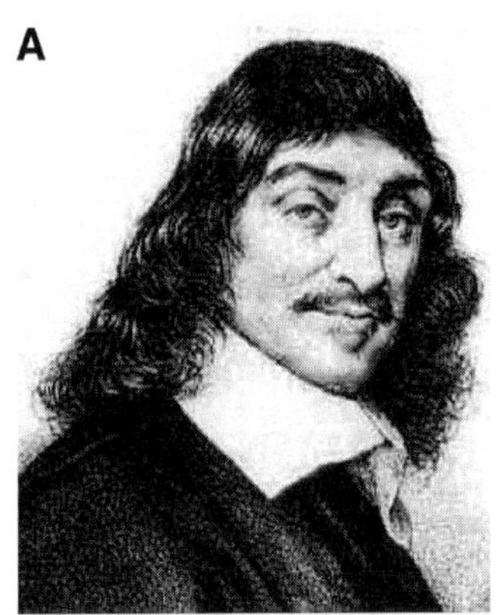

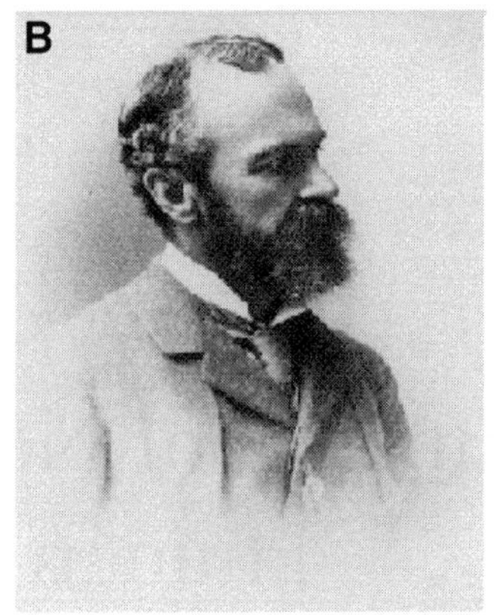

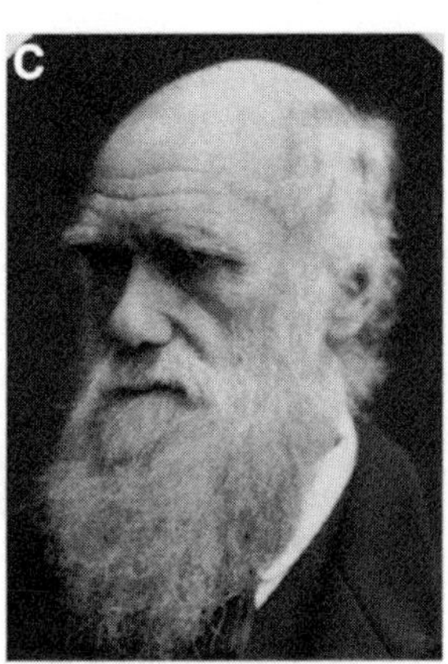

FIGURE 19.1
(a) Rene Descartes (1596–1650); (b) William James (1842–1910); (c) Charles Darwin (1809–1882).

specific bodily changes, automatically elicited by appropriate stimuli. Thus, rather than our heart pounding because we feel afraid, we feel afraid *because* our heart is pounding. Within this account, the particular emotion we feel depends on a central representation of the pattern of stimulation in the peripheral autonomic nervous systems and not on emotion-specific processes in the central nervous system. Damasio (1994) has recently proposed a modified peripheralist theory in which emotional stimuli elicit bodily states ("somatic markers") whose central representation contributes to decision making. An important feature of James' theory is that it emphasises the automatic, involuntary nature of emotional responses; however, the theory has been criticised for failing to explain how emotional stimuli are initially processed and evaluated prior to evoking bodily responses. It has also been questioned whether the peripheral changes elicited by emotional stimuli are sufficiently distinct to account for the entire range of experienced emotion or feelings.

In the first half of the 20th century, James' peripheralist approach was challenged by experimental findings in animals. Bard (1929) demonstrated that rage reactions in cats are disrupted by brain lesions that include hypothalamus. If hypothalamus is spared, however, rage reactions can still be elicited even when the entire cerebral cortex is removed (Bard, 1929). On the basis of these observations, Cannon (1929) proposed a "centralist" theory of emotion in which thalamus mediates emotional perception and hypothalamus mediates emotional expression. Papez (1937) expanded this circuit by adding structures such as hippocampus and the mammillary bodies. A primary role for hippocampus in emotion was proposed on the basis of pathological changes seen in the brains of individuals who had died of rabies; rabies patients typically experience intense affective symptoms, such as fear (Papez, 1937). Papez' emotional circuit was subsequently adopted by Maclean (1949), who incorporated his own clinical observations and Freudian metapsychological structuralism into a "limbic" theory of emotion. Maclean's limbic theory emphasised a central role for hippocampus as the "emotional keyboard" (Maclean, 1949).

It is notable that although "centralist" theories locate emotional processes in the central nervous system, they nevertheless embody an anatomical segregation from non-emotional cognitive functions. Thus, emotion is thought to be located in the primitive, unconscious, visceral brain, whereas cognition resides in the more recently evolved cerebral neocortex. Although the limbic system approach to emotion continued to be influential in the 20th century, evidence has mounted that key structures in these models (*e.g.*, hippocampus) have little role in emotional processing *per se*. Consequently, the usefulness of the limbic approach to understanding emotion is increasingly questioned (LeDoux, 1996).

Evolutionary Theories

An increasingly influential approach to understanding the role of emotion and its neural organisation has its intellectual basis in evolutionary biology. Darwin (1872) (Fig. 19.1c), in one of his most accessible works, proposed that emotions are evolutionarily determined, stereotyped behaviour patterns. Rather than being an interference to rational, purposeful behaviour (as is implied in dualistic, cognitive accounts of the mind), emotion is viewed as critical for survival. The adaptive value of emotional responses is implicit in their universality, innateness, and conservation across species (Ekman, 1982). To illustrate the overriding power of emotion on behaviour, Darwin (1872) recounted: "I put my face close to the thick glass-plate in front of a puff-adder in the Zoological Gardens, with the firm determination of not starting back if the snake struck at me; but, as soon as the blow was struck, my resolution went for nothing, and I jumped a yard or two backwards with astonishing rapidity. *My will and reason were powerless against the imagination of a danger which had never been experienced.*" Darwin's anecdote strikingly illustrates the automatic, reflexive nature of emotional responses, particularly in relation to threats and dangers in the environment. It is in relation to this aspect of emotional processing, fear responses, that the greatest progress has been made in understanding the neural basis of emotion. In both animals and humans, the amygdala, a small nucleus in the medial temporal lobe, is a critical component of the brain's fear circuitry.

FUNCTIONAL SEGREGATION OF EMOTIONAL PROCESSING

Amygdala

Anatomy and Physiology

The amygdala is an heterogeneous structure that, in primates, consists of at least 13 anatomically and functionally distinct subnuclei (Amaral *et al.*, 1992). In addition to its complex internal structure, the amygdala has extensive external anatomical connections (Amaral and Price, 1984; Amaral, 1985, 1992; Russchen *et al.*, 1985). This extrinsic connectivity gives the amygdala the potential to integrate sensory information from all modalities and to influence autonomic and motor output systems. Sensory afferents project mainly to the lateral nucleus of the amygdala and arrive via parallel routes; for example, in addition to sensory inputs from high-level areas of temporal lobe, there is evidence for direct subcortical projections from auditory and visual thalamic nuclei (Jones and Burton, 1976; LeDoux, 1984; Linke *et al.*, 1999, 2000; Wilhelmi *et al.*, 2001).

Electrophysiological studies in animals indicate both modality-specific and multimodal cells in amygdala, supporting a proposal that amygdala is involved in cross-modal integration of biologically salient stimuli (*e.g.*, the sight and taste of food) (Nishijo *et al.*, 1988, 1998). The lateral nucleus sends projections to medial and basal subnuclei for further processing of sensory inputs (Pitkanen and Amaral, 1998). Intrinsic connections from medial and basal nuclei pass to the main output region of the amygdala, the central nucleus (Savander *et al.*, 1996).

Amygdala efferents project to widespread regions of the brain, including hypothalamus, basal forebrain, entorhinal cortex, ventral striatum, cingulate gyrus, orbitofrontal cortex, and brainstem autonomic centers (Amaral *et al.*, 1992). The nucleus reticularis pontis caudalis (NRPC), a brainstem nucleus involved in the acoustic startle reflex, receives a direct amygdala projection (Rosen *et al.*, 1991). Significantly, potentiation of acoustic startle by fear-conditioned stimuli is abolished by lesions of the amygdala (Davis, 1992; Hitchcock and Davis, 1991). Amygdala efferents also project back to early sensory processing regions (*e.g.*, occipitotemporal and insula cortices) from which the amygdala receives inputs (Amaral *et al.*, 1992). It has been suggested that these feedback connections may enable amygdala to modulate early sensory processing, thus enhancing the neural representation of biologically significant stimuli (Morris *et al.*, 1998a; Rolls and Treves, 1998).

Animal Studies

Kluver and Bucy (1939) reported the behavioural effects of bilateral ablation of the temporal lobe (including amygdala) in rhesus monkeys. Compared with controls, postoperative monkeys were tame and placid, no longer showing fear or anger responses. Weiskrantz (1956), using more restricted lesions in monkeys, identified the amygdala as the critical structure in these behavioural changes (*e.g.*, absence of fear responses). Electrical stimulation of the amygdala, on the other hand, whether in monkey, rat, lizard, or human, consistently evokes fear responses

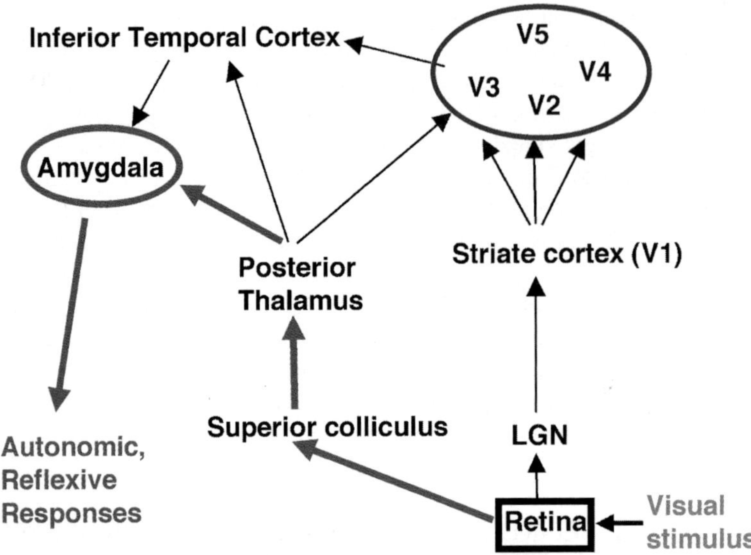

FIGURE 19.2
Parallel visual pathways in the primate brain. The geniculostriate visual pathway, which provides the main input to visual cortical areas V1, V2, V3, etc., is indicated by thin black arrows. An extrageniculostriate visual pathway, comprised of superior colliculus, posterior visual thalamus, and amygdala is indicated by thick red arrows.

(Greenberg *et al.* 1984; Halgren *et al.* 1978; LeDoux, 1987). Animal research also shows that the amygdala, in addition to responding to *innately* fearful stimuli, is involved in *learning* about threats and dangers in the environment (Blanchard and Blanchard, 1972; LeDoux, 1996). Animal lesion experiments using fear conditioning paradigms have shown that destruction of the amygdala prevents the learning of temporal associations between neutral and aversive stimuli (LeDoux, 1996).

The crucial importance of direct thalamo-amygdala pathways in emotional processing has been demonstrated in animal lesion studies (Iwata *et al.*, 1986; LeDoux *et al.*, 1984). The projection from medial geniculate nucleus to amygdala can mediate auditory fear conditioning despite removal of auditory neocortex (LeDoux *et al.*, 1984). There is also evidence of a subcortical pathway for *visual* signals to reach amygdala independently of visual neocortex (Fig. 19.2). Superior colliculus, which receives a direct retinal input, projects to the pulvinar and adjacent extrageniculate visual nuclei in the posterior thalamus (Benvenuto and Fallon, 1972; Linke *et al.*, 1999). Posterior thalamus, in turn, sends direct projections to lateral nucleus of amygdala (Jones and Burton, 1976; Linke *et al.*, 1999, 2000; Wilhelmi *et al.*, 2001) (Fig. 19.2). Anatomical tracing studies have shown that thalamo-amygdaloid projection neurons receive direct synaptic connections from superior colliculus cells, supporting the proposal of a colliculo-thalamo-amygdala visual pathway (Linke *et al.*, 1999) (Fig. 19.2). It has been suggested that subcortical sensory pathways subserve low-resolution, automatic processing of emotional stimuli leading to reflexive, automatic responses, while more detailed analysis of the same stimuli, involving (in humans) semantic and verbal categorisation, requires sensory neocortex (LeDoux, 1996) (Fig. 19.2).

Fear and Threat Perception

Advances in elucidating emotion circuitry in animals have benefited from the use of experimental protocols with simple, standardised stimuli (*e.g.*, fear conditioning with auditory tones and foot shocks) and readily measurable behavioural responses (*e.g.*, changes in heart rate, freezing). Investigation of emotional processing in the human brain has similarly been aided by the use of standardised stimuli, most notably emotional facial expressions (Ekman and Friesen, 1976) (Fig. 19.3a). Behavioural research on basic emotional facial expressions has broadly supported the proposal of innate, evolutionarily determined mechanisms that respond in an automatic and stereotyped way to a limited class of emotional stimuli (Darwin, 1872; Ekman, 1972; Ohman and Mineka, 2001; Seligman, 1971). One of the most striking demonstrations

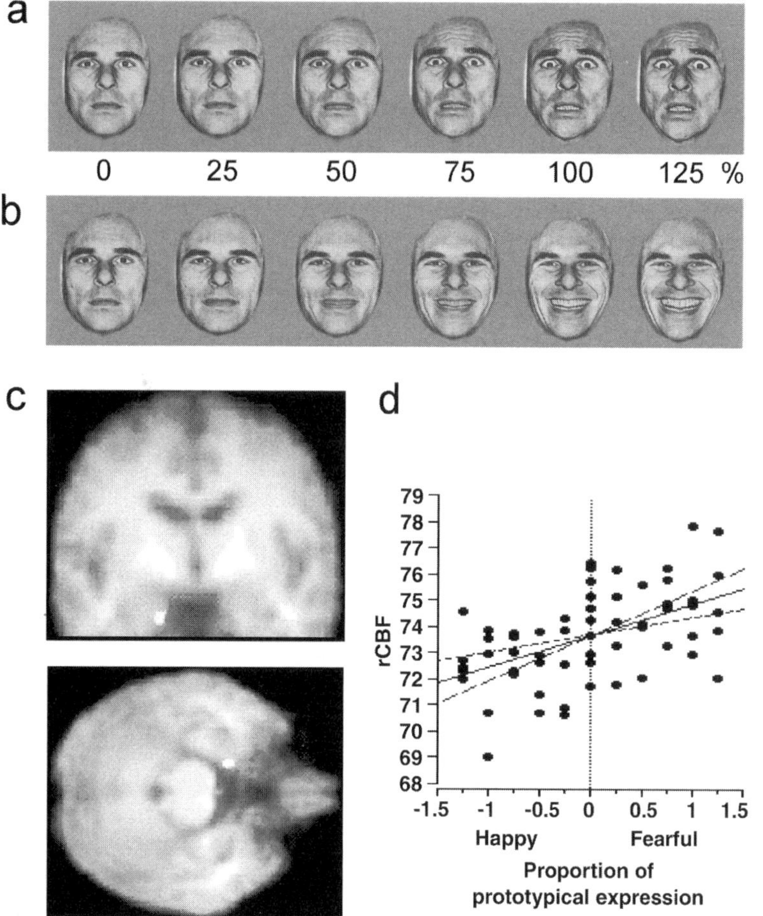

FIGURE 19.3
Morphed emotional expressions. In both (a) and (b), the 0% face is the neutral prototype. The 100% face is the prototype for fearful (a) and happy (b) expressions. The other faces were produced by computer graphical manipulation. (c) A statistical parametric map showing a significant activation in left amygdala in the contrast of fearful minus happy conditions; an uncorrected p value of 0.001 was used as the threshold for the contrast. (d) A plot of regional cerebral blood flow in left amygdala as a function of the proportion of happy or fearful prototypes in the morphed emotional expression; the 100% happy face is given a value of −1, the 100% fearful face is +1, and the neutral face is 0.

of this segregation in emotional sensory processing comes from neuropsychological studies of patients with restricted bilateral amygdala damage (Adolphs *et al.*, 1994; Calder *et al.*, 1996). These patients, who perform normally on a wide range of psychological tasks, show a specific and profound deficit in the recognition of fearful facial expressions (Adolphs *et al.*, 1994; Calder *et al.*, 1996) (see Fig. 19.8).

Following neuropsychological observations implicating the amygdala in fearful face perception (Adolphs *et al.*, 1994; Calder *et al.*, 1996), several functional neuroimaging studies reported selective amygdala responses to fearful faces in intact, healthy subjects (Breiter *et al.*, 1996; Morris *et al.*, 1996) (Fig. 19.3). Morris *et al.* (1996) found that fearful faces evoked left, but not right, amygdala activity, while Breiter *et al.* (1996) reported left > right amygdala responses to fearful expressions. Other functional neuroimaging studies have also reported left lateralised amygdala responses during explicit processing of fearful faces (Killgore and Yergulun-Todd, 2001; Philips *et al.*, 2001; Thomas *et al.*, 2001, Vuilleumier *et al.*, 2001; Wright *et al.*, 2001). These neuroimaging studies, showing *lateralisation* of amygdala responses to fearful faces, contrast with neuropsychological data that indicate that *bilateral* amygdala lesions are necessary for deficits in fear perception (Adolphs *et al.*, 1994; Calder *et al.*, 1996). It is likely, therefore, that in addition to lateralised specialisation, there is redundancy of function between left and right amygdala.

Functional neuroimaging data have shown that amygdala responses to fearful faces tend to diminish with repeated presentations (Breiter *et al.*, 1996; Philips *et al.*, 2001; Wright *et al.*, 2001). Intriguingly, several studies report lateralised differences in time-dependent responses to fearful faces, with more rapid decreases in right than left amygdala (Philips *et al.*, 2001; Wright *et al.*, 2001). Wright *et al.* (2001) suggest that right amygdala forms part of a "dynamic emotional stimulus detection system," whereas left amygdala is specialised for "sustained stimulus evaluations." This putative specialisation of left amygdala may result from its more extensive connectivity to frontal and temporal regions in the dominant (left) hemisphere engaged in verbal and semantic processing. By contrast, emotional stimuli presented in implicit, nonverbal paradigms (*e.g.*, using backward masking) have been reported to evoke differential responses in right amygdala (Critchley *et al.*, 2002; Morris *et al.*, 1998c). It is possible that sex-dependent differences in lateralisation of language processing (Kansaku *et al.*, 2000; Kansaku and Kitazawa, 2001) are related to reported differences in lateralisation of amygdala activity between male and female subjects (Cahill *et al.*, 2001; Killgore and Yurgelun-Todd, 2001).

The question of whether amygdala responses to fear-related stimuli generalise to sensory modalities other than vision has been addressed in behavioural and neuroimaging studies. A neuropsychological study of a patient with bilateral amygdala damage reported a selective recognition deficit for fearful vocalisations (Scott *et al.*, 1997); however, this finding has not been replicated by other studies of patients with restricted bilateral amygdala damage (Adolphs and Tranel, 1999; Anderson and Phelps, 1998). It is notable that the patient investigated by Scott *et al.* (1997) had lesions that extended beyond the amygdala, suggesting that neural processing of fearful vocalisations may be more distributed than for fearful facial expressions and that damage restricted to amygdala may be less critical. Significantly, functional neuroimaging studies have reported that fearful vocalisations activate several other brain regions (*e.g.*, ventral prefrontal cortex, temporal cortex, and anterior insula), in addition to amygdala (Phillips *et al.*, 1998a; Morris *et al.*, 1999b).

Studies in monkeys and humans suggest that fear in facial expressions is conveyed principally by the eyes (de Bonis, 2000; Emery, 2000). This proposal has been investigated in a functional neuroimaging study using "chimerical" emotional faces, in which fearful eyes were combined with neutral mouths and vice versa (Morris *et al.*, 2002) (Fig. 19.4). Fearful eyes alone were sufficient to elicit increased responses in right amygdala, superior colliculus, and posterior thalamus (Fig. 19.4). No increased responses were observed to fearful mouths alone; however, a distinct, segregated response to canonical fearful faces (*i.e.*, fearful eyes *and* mouth) was observed in left amygdala (Fig. 19.4); therefore, this finding suggests that, whereas right amygdala responds to a specific feature (*i.e.*, eyes) in a fearful expression, left amygdala responds to the overall configuration or conjunction of features.

The coactivation of superior colliculus, posterior thalamus, and right amygdala by fearful eyes (Morris *et al.*, 2002) is in agreement with the proposal that these structures constitute a parallel subcortical visual pathway that is able to process emotionally salient stimuli independently of visual neocortex. Because superior colliculus, posterior thalamus, and right amygdala were activated by fearful eye (but *not* fearful mouth) chimerical faces, the low-resolution representation in this subcortical pathway would appear to be particularly sensitive to eyes. It is notable that a simple direct stare is a potent threatening stimulus in monkeys and, in certain situations, in humans (Emery, 2000). It has been reported that neutral faces evoke greater amygdala responses with direct eye gaze than when gaze is averted (Kawashima *et al.*, 1999).

Although fearful faces have proved to be one of the most reliable and effective stimuli in eliciting amygdala responses, other emotional expressions, including sad (Blair *et al.*, 1999; Schneider *et al.*, 1997), angry (Hariri *et al.*, 2000), and disgusted (Gorno-Tempini, 2001), have been reported to evoke increased amygdala activity. Interestingly, neutral faces have also been reported to evoke increased amygdala responses compared to happy faces (Morris *et al.*, 1996). Neutral > happy amygdala responses may reflect the mildly unsettling nature of unsmiling, neutral faces or may be the result of happy faces providing a positive "no threat" signal that produces a decrease in tonic amygdala activity.

Increased amygdala responses are also elicited by faces that subjects rate as "untrustworthy" (Winston *et al.*, 2002). Here, subjects' ratings of untrustworthiness were positively correlated with ratings of anger and negatively correlated with ratings of happiness in the faces (Winston

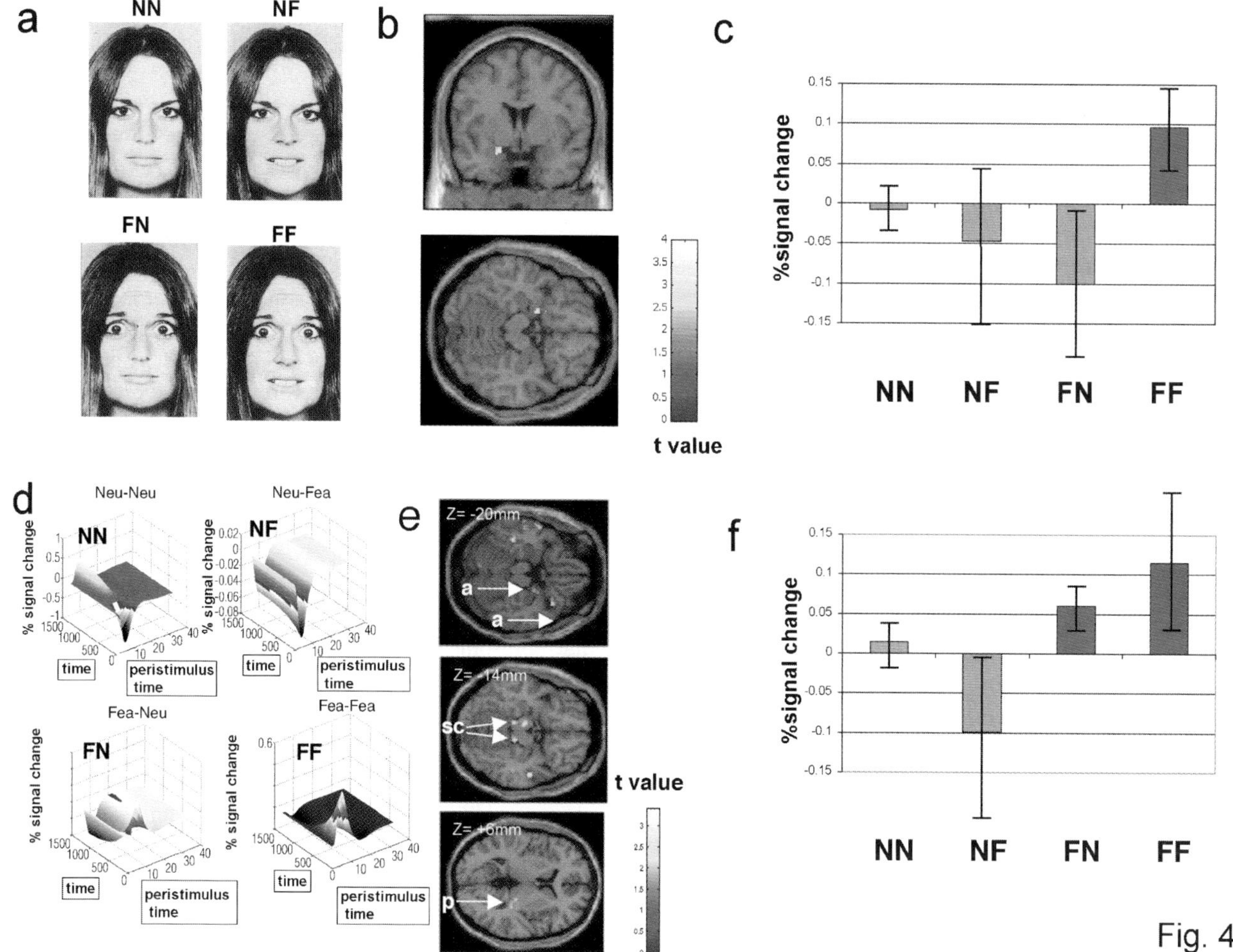

FIGURE 19.4
(a) Prototypical and chimerical faces. FF and NN are prototypical faces (fearful and neutral, respectively). FN is a chimerical face in which the upper half (eyes) is derived from the fearful prototype and the lower half (mouth) from the neutral prototype. NF is a chimerical face with neutral upper half and fearful lower half. (b) A statistical parametric map (SPM) showing an increased response in left anterior amygdala to prototypical faces (FF) compared to all other conditions (NN, FN, and NF faces). The SPM is displayed on orthogonal sections of a canonical MRI centered on the maximal voxel in left amygdala ($x = -22$, $y = 4$, $z = -20$). A p value of 0.01 (uncorrected) was used as the threshold for displaying the contrast. (c) A graphical representation of mean BOLD (blood-oxygen-level-dependent) fMRI signal change (as a percentage of global mean intensity) at the maximal left amygdala voxel ($x = -22$, $y = 4$, $z = -20$) in all four conditions; bars represent 2 standard errors. (d) Three-dimensional plots of time-dependent changes in event-related hemodynamic responses in all four chimeric conditions. Time-dependent changes in response were modeled by an exponential function with a time constant one quarter of the session length in right amygdala ($x = 22$, $y = -4$, $z = -20$). (e) A statistical parametric map showing regions of right amygdala (a), superior colliculus (sc), and posterior thalamus (p), where responses showed a time-dependent interaction in the comparison of fearful eye (FF and FN) and neutral eye (NF and NN) conditions; the SPM is displayed on transverse sections ($z = -20$ mm, -14 mm, and $+6$ mm) of a canonical MRI; and $p = 0.01$ (uncorrected) was used as the threshold for displaying the contrast. (f) A graphical representation of parameter estimates for time-dependent changes in response at the maximal superior colliculus voxel ($x = -12$, $y = -28$, $z = -14$) in all four conditions; bars represent 2 standard errors.

et al., 2002). Several studies have also reported increased amygdala responses in white American subjects viewing pictures of unfamiliar black (African-American) faces (Hart *et al.*, 2000; Phelps *et al.*, 2000); however, increased amygdala activity was not seen when white Americans viewed familiar, positively regarded black (African-American) faces, suggesting that the response is a learned, culturally specific phenomenon and does not reflect innate processes (Phelps *et al.*, 2000).

Both animal and human data support the proposal that amygdala mediates the detection and evaluation of potential threats and dangers in the environment. Thus, increased amygdala responses have been observed to both the innate, direct threat signal represented by fearful expressions (Morris *et al.*, 1996) and the more subtle, indirect threat posed by "untrustworthy" individuals (Winston *et al.*, 2002); however, amygdala responses to potential threat or harm are not restricted to faces or people. Functional neuroimaging studies have shown that non-facial stimuli, including threatening words (Isenberg *et al.*, 1999), aversive tastes (O'Doherty *et al.*, 2001; Zald *et al.*, 2002), and aversive odors (Royet *et al.*, 2000; Zald and Pardo, 1997) also evoke increased amygdala responses. Thus, any stimulus (in any modality) that is perceived as a potential danger can evoke increased amygdala responses.

Animal data indicate that, in addition to responding to aversive or threatening stimuli, the amygdala also responds to appetitive stimuli such as food (Sanghera *et al.*, 1979). An appetitive role for amygdala in human emotional perception is supported by functional neuroimaging data showing increased amygdala responses to a pleasant (glucose) taste (O'Doherty *et al.*, 2001); however, in subsequent functional neuroimaging studies, both O'Doherty *et al.* (2002) and Zald *et al.* (2002) failed to observe increased amygdala responses to pleasant (sucrose or glucose) solutions. It is also notable that increased amygdala responses have not been observed to other positive stimuli such as pleasant pictures (Paradiso *et al.*, 1999) and attractive faces (Nakamura *et al.*, 1998). O'Doherty *et al.* (2002) have commented that the previously reported amygdala activation to pleasant taste (O'Doherty *et al.*, 2001) may have resulted from the blocked design of the previous study producing reward expectancy. Compared to human amygdala processing of threatening and aversive stimuli, therefore, the nature of amygdala responses to primary appetitive stimuli remains uncertain (see below for discussion of amygdala and appetitive conditioning).

Fear Conditioning

The range of dangers and threats that confront an organism is subject to change. Adaptive behaviour requires an ability to learn about potentially harmful (and rewarding) stimuli and modify behavioural responses appropriately. This type of learning can be described as emotional learning and has been studied in animals using aversive (fear) and appetitive conditioning techniques. The most significant progress in determining the underlying neural circuitry has been made in fear conditioning (LeDoux, 1996; LeDoux *et al.*, 1984, 1990; Weinberger, 1995).

Results of human lesion studies (Bechara *et al.*, 1995; LaBar *et al.*, 1995) agree with animal data (LeDoux, 1996), indicating medial temporal lobe (particularly the amygdala) involvement in fear conditioning. Early functional neuroimaging studies of fear conditioning, however, observed learning-related responses in thalamus, anterior cingulate, orbitofrontal cortex, and sensory cortical areas but *not* in amygdala (Fredrikson *et al.*, 1995; Hugdahl *et al.*, 1995). Subsequent studies did show learning-dependent amygdala activity in terms of a correlation with acquired autonomic responses (Furmark *et al.*, 1997) or conditioning-related thalamic responses (Morris *et al.*, 1997). Among the problems faced by these early positron emission tomography (PET) studies of emotional learning was the effect of repeated, blocked presentation of stimuli, leading to expectancy confounds, coupled with an inability to index temporal changes in responses to conditioned stimuli.

The advent of mixed-trial, event-related fMRI protocols (Friston *et al.*, 1998) helped to overcome the methodological and technical limitations inherent in blocked PET experiments. Consequently, event-related fMRI studies of fear conditioning reported differential amygdala responses to aversively conditioned stimuli (CS+) relative to non-conditioned stimuli (CS–) (Buchel *et al.*, 1998; LaBar *et al.*, 1998) (Fig. 19.5). One advantage of event-related fMRI time series is that changes in condition-specific responses can be modeled across time. Both Buchel *et al.* (1998) and LaBar *et al.* (1998) showed that conditioning-related amygdala responses are best characterised by time × condition interactions in which initially increased CS+ responses progressively decrease across time relative to CS– responses. *Mean* CS+ > CS– responses were observed in anterior cingulate and anterior insula (Buchel *et al.*, 1998). The dynamic, time-dependent nature of amygdala activation provides further explanation for the failure of simple subtractive PET analyses to detect learning-related amygdala responses. Buchel *et al.* (1999) showed that rapidly adapting amygdala and hippocampal activity is also involved in aversive "trace" conditioning (in which a temporal delay occurs between the offset of the conditioned stimulus (CS+) and the unconditioned stimulus (UCS).

Phelps *et al.* (2001) investigated a non-conditioning form of fear learning in which subjects were verbally informed about an association between a neutral stimulus and an aversive event but never actually experienced the pairing. Left dorsal amygdala and left insula cortex showed increased responses to stimuli verbally associated with the aversive event. Although human

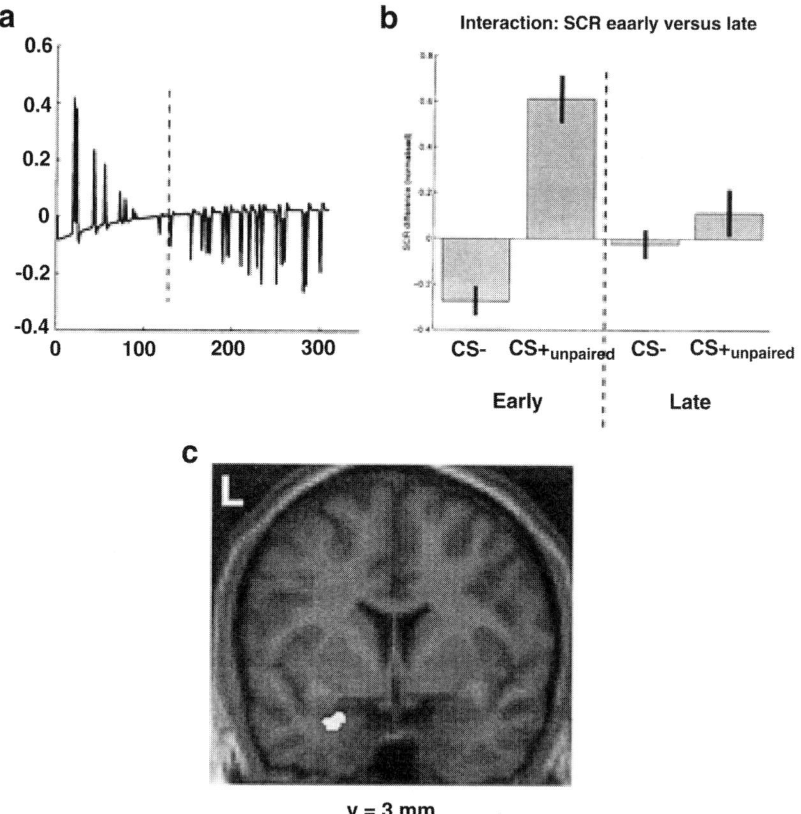

FIGURE 19.5
Rapid habituation of amygdala responses to CS+ (unpaired) stimuli. (a) The fitted response for CS+ events (unpaired with UCS) in a single subject in left amygdala. Responses evoked by CS+ (unpaired) stimuli are initially positive and then decrease to become deactivations (relative to baseline) after 120 scans (8.2 min). (b) The differences in SCR responses comparing the first 8 min to the last 12 min of the conditioning phase. The difference between SCR elicited by CS+ (unpaired) versus CS– is larger for the first 8 min of the experiment. This interaction is significant ($t[18] = 2.5$, $p < 0.05$). The vertical dashed lines in (a) indicate the cutoff between early and late (117 volumes = 8 min) used for the SCR interaction analysis shown in (b). (c) Activation of the left amygdala ($Z = 4.6$). overlaid on a template T1 MRI. Statistical inference is based on the difference between the time by condition interaction shown in (a) relative to responses evoked by CS– stimuli.

lesion studies (Bechara *et al.* 1995) indicate that amygdala is not critical for the acquisition of this type of "cognitive" fear learning, the neuroimaging data of Phelps *et al.* (2001) suggest that amygdala is nevertheless involved in emotional responses consequent upon such learning. The findings also accord with a proposal that lateralisation of amygdala activity is related to hemispheric dominance for language (see above).

Animal studies indicate that amygdala, in addition to its critical role in aversive (fear) conditioning, contributes to appetitive conditioning (Gallagher *et al.*, 1990; Parkinson *et al.*, 2000). The failure of patients with amygdala damage to show normal preference conditioning for visual stimuli paired with a food reward suggests that human amygdala has a role in appetitive learning (Johnsrude *et al.*, 2000). Further evidence for such a role comes from a human functional neuroimaging study that reported responses in posterior dorsal amygdala and the dopaminergic ventral tegmental area (VTA) to a visual cue predicting receipt of a pleasant sweet taste (O'Doherty *et al.*, 2002). It remains unclear, however, whether aversive and appetitive learning processes operate in a segregated, parallel fashion within the amygdala or whether they form part of a single process mediating the acquired "behavioural salience" of stimuli.

Functional neuroimaging studies showing amygdala involvement in the modulation of memory by appetitive stimuli (Hamann *et al.*, 1999; Morris *et al.*, 2001a) and conditioning-related modulation of sensory cortex (Armony and Dolan, 2001; Morris *et al.*, 2001) are discussed in the section on functional integration, and the role of amygdala in reversal fear conditioning (Morris and Dolan, 2002) is discussed in the section on orbitofrontal cortex (see below).

Unconscious Fear Processing

A common feature in the theoretical approaches arising from Darwin, Freud, and James is that emotional processes occur automatically, without conscious, cognitive mediation. James (1885), for example, in an insight that parallels Darwin's account of the snake at the zoo, proposed that emotional responses "follow directly the perception of the exciting fact." James was not able to explain, however, why certain stimuli (and not others) should elicit emotional responses. More recent investigations employing the evolutionary concept of "preparedness" and the presentation of biologically salient stimuli outside of conscious awareness have revisited this issue.

Seligman (1970) proposed that certain objects such as spiders and snakes have a genetically predetermined or "prepared" ability to elicit fearful behaviour as a result of their threat to our distant ancestors' survival. "Prepared" fear learning is postulated to be rapid, automatic, persistent (resistant to extinction), and independent of conscious cognitive processing. Behavioural studies conducted by Ohman and his colleagues have provided empirical support for Seligman's preparedness theory (Ohman *et al.* 1978; Ohman and Soares, 1993, 1998). These authors showed that when potentially phobic stimuli (*e.g.*, snakes and spiders) are aversively conditioned by being paired with an electric shock, autonomic responses to these conditioned "prepared" stimuli show resistance to extinction compared to non-phobic stimuli (*e.g.*, flowers and mushrooms) (Ohman *et al.* 1978; Ohman and Soares, 1993).

If a target visual stimulus is shown for < 40 ms and is immediately followed by a masking stimulus, subjects typically report seeing the mask but not the target; however, when aversively conditioned fear-relevant visual stimuli (*e.g.*, snakes or angry faces) are masked, they continue to elicit enhanced autonomic responses even though they are not consciously perceived (Ohman and Soares, 1993). By contrast, fear-*irrelevant* stimuli, such as flowers or happy faces, do not elicit increased autonomic responses when aversively conditioned and masked (Ohman and Soares, 1993). These behavioural results accord with the idea that "prepared" stimuli are processed by an automatic, pre-attentive neural system that can function independently from explicit attentional processes (Ohman and Mineka, 2001).

Functional neuroimaging experiments have used backward masking techniques in order to manipulate subjects' awareness of fear-related stimuli and identify neural structures mediating unconscious fear processing. Whalen *et al.* (1999b) observed enhanced responses in bilateral amygdala (right > left) to fearful faces masked with neutral faces. Subjects who passively viewed the faces during scanning were subsequently asked if they remembered seeing any emotional expressions; none of the subjects included in the study reported seeing fearful or happy faces. Although subjects' memory, rather than their awareness of the face stimuli was measured in this experiment, the results strongly suggest that *innate* fear-related stimuli can be processed by the amygdala without being consciously perceived.

Morris *et al.* (1998c) conducted a functional neuroimaging experiment that combined visual backward masking and aversive (fear) conditioning in order to measure neural responses related to non-conscious fear learning (Fig. 19.6). Angry faces were paired with an aversive UCS (loud noise) to produce fear conditioning. The conditioned angry faces were then presented backwardly masked by neutral faces. The subjects' explicit task was to detect (via button presses) any occurrence of the target angry faces. The masked conditioned angry faces elicited increased skin conductance responses, thereby providing evidence of emotional learning, even though subjects failed to detect any target presentations (*i.e.*, subjects were aware only of the neutral masks). Despite the subjects' lack of awareness, enhanced neural responses to the masked conditioned angry faces were observed in right ventral amygdala. By contrast, *unmasked* presentations of conditioned angry faces elicited increased responses in *left*, but not right, amygdala. A formal test of the interaction between conditioning and masking showed that masking significantly enhanced right amygdala responses to the fear conditioned faces.

The masking-dependent lateralisation of amygdala activity observed by Morris *et al.* (1998c) is in agreement with other neuropsychological studies of emotional processing. Several behavioural studies have shown a right hemisphere advantage for processing emotional facial expressions (DeKosky *et al.* 1980; Gazzaniga, 1983; Gur *et al.*, 1994). Moreover, a study of

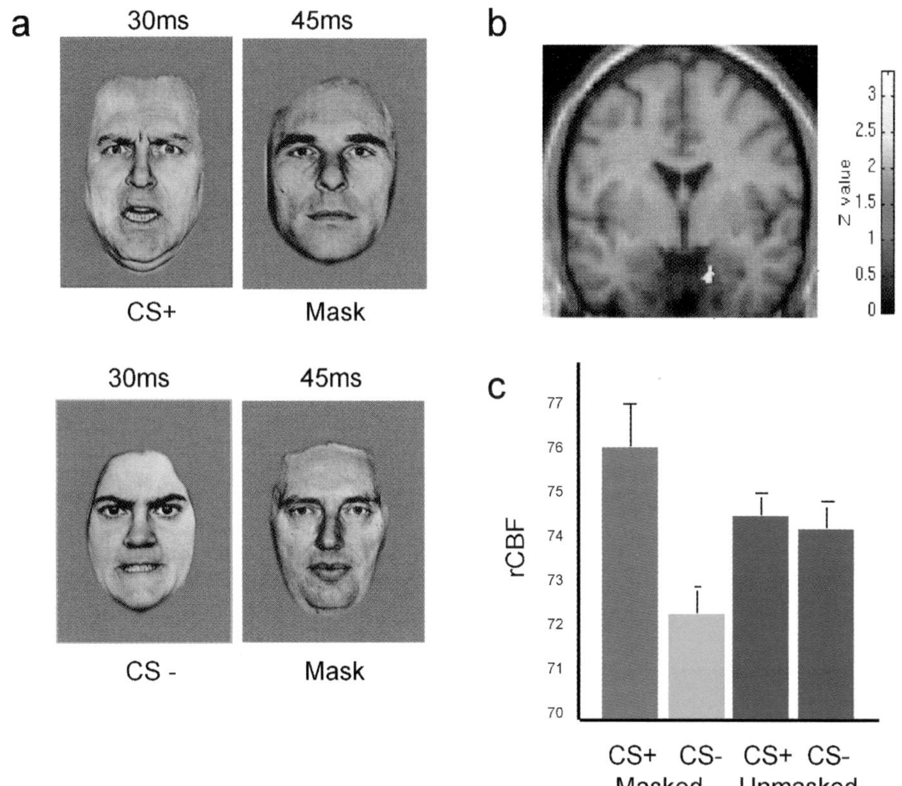

FIGURE 19.6
Masked fear conditioning. (a) Angry faces either previously paired with noise (CS+) or never previously paired with noise (CS–) were backwardly masked by neutral faces. The target angry faces were displayed for 30 ms and immediately followed by the 45-ms neutral masks. (b) A statistical parametric map (SPM) showing activation in the region of the right amygdala in the contrast of masked CS+ and CS– angry faces. An uncorrected threshold of $p = 0.01$ was used for display of the contrast. The SPM is displayed on a coronal slice ($y = -2$ mm) of a canonical MRI image. (c) A graphical display of the mean regional cerebral blood flow at the maximal voxel of activation in the right amygdala ($x = -18$, $y = -2$, $z = -28$). Bars represent 2 standard errors. In the unmasked conditions, the order of the angry and neutral faces was reversed so that the neutral face was displayed first for 30 ms and was immediately followed by 45-ms angry faces.

"split-brain" patients found that emotional visual stimuli presented to the right hemisphere elicited *greater* autonomic responses when masked than when unmasked (Ladavas *et al.*, 1993). Because masking represents a degradation of stimulus quality, right-sided lateralisation of responses to masked angry faces may reflect greater sensitivity of facial expression processing in the right hemisphere. However, because unmasking *abolished* differential responses in right amygdala and resulted in *decreased* autonomic responses to emotional stimuli in the study by Ladavas *et al.* (1993), increased sensitivity cannot be the sole factor. An alternative interpretation might be that explicit, *controlled* processing (located primarily in left hemisphere) modulates or inhibits concurrent *automatic* processes (located primarily in right hemisphere) in order to prevent potential response conflicts. Disruption of explicit (conscious) processing (for example, by backward masking), releases implicit (non-conscious) processes from ongoing inhibitory modulation, resulting in enhanced responses.

Learning theorists have presumed that the formation of stimulus associations requires explicit, controlled processing normally associated with conscious awareness (Dawson and Schell, 1985; Lovibond and Shanks, 2002; Ohman, 1979). However, several pyschophysiological experiments have challenged this assumption, by showing that backwardly masked, fear-relevant, "prepared" stimuli (*e.g.*, snakes, spiders, angry faces) can be associated with aversive stimuli (as indexed by differential autonomic responses), even though awareness of the association is prevented by masking (Esteves and Ohman, 1994; Ohman and Soares, 1998). Such "learning without awareness" does *not* seem to occur, however, for fear-irrelevant stimuli (*e.g.*, flowers or happy faces) (Esteves and Ohman, 1994; Ohman and Soares, 1998).

Morris *et al.* (2001) investigated the neural basis of implicit fear conditioning in a functional neuroimaging experiment in which a masked angry face was paired with an aversive UCS (loud noise). Subjects were unaware of the occurrence of the masked angry face and of its association with the noise UCS. Subsequent unmasked presentation of the implicitly conditioned angry face elicited increased responses in left amygdala, pulvinar, and extrastriate cortex. These results indicate that emotional learning without awareness is associated with differential neural activity not only in amygdala and thalamus but also in sensory neocortex. The data also highlight that *explicit* (non-masked) presentations of fear-conditioned stimuli evoke increased *left* amygdala responses even when fear conditioning has been acquired implicitly (non-consciously).

Although a subcortical visual pathway to amygdala has been described anatomically (Jones and Burton, 1976; Linke *et al.*, 1999, 2000; Wilhelmi *et al.*, 2001) (Fig. 19.2), a functional role for this pathway in fear processing has not been demonstrated in animals. However, a colliculo-thalamo-amygdala visual pathway mediating fear conditioning in human subjects is suggested in a connectivity analysis of functional neuroimaging data related to processing of masked fear-conditioned faces (Morris *et al.*, 1999a) (Fig. 19.7). The premise here is that brain regions forming a functional cooperative network will display covariation of activity during processing of relevant stimuli (Friston *et al.*, 1997). Right amygdala responses to masked fear-conditioned

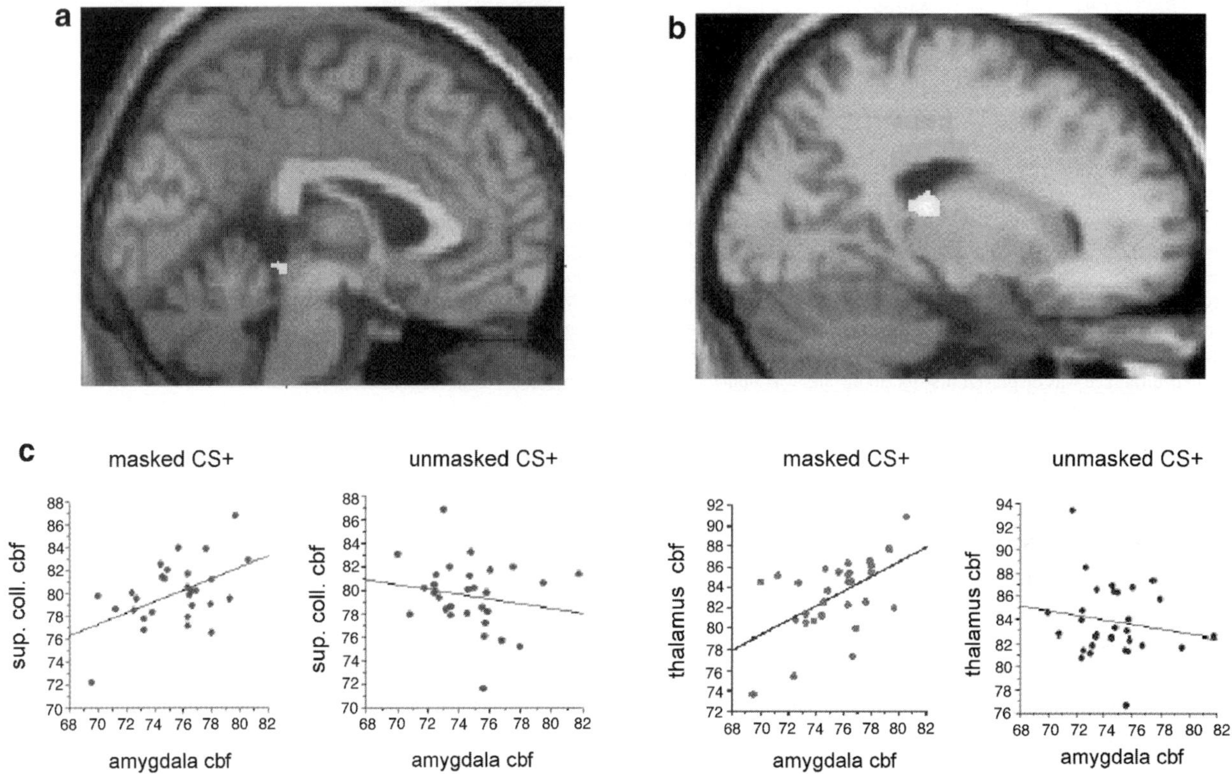

FIGURE 19.7

(a) A statistical parametric map (SPM) showing a region of right pulvinar that exhibits a positive covariation with the right amygdala specifically during presentation of the masked ("unseen") CS+ faces. The region of covariation in the pulvinar is displayed on a sagittal section of a canonical structural MRI centered on the maximal voxel in the right pulvinar ($x = 18$, $y = -28$, $z = 12$). (b) A statistical parametric map showing a region in the superior colliculus that exhibits a positive covariation with the right amygdala specifically during presentation of masked ("unseen") CS+ faces. The analysis and threshold used were the same as in (a). The region of covariation in the superior colliculus is displayed on a sagittal section ($y = 0$) of a canonical structural MRI. (c) Graphical displays showing bivariate regression plots of right amygdala and right pulvinar activity. The graph on the left plots rCBF (in mL/dL/min) in the maximal right amygdala voxel ($x = 18$, $y = -2$, $z = -28$) and maximal right pulvinar voxel ($x = 18$, $y = -28$, $z = 12$) during presentation of the masked ("unseen") CS+ faces. The graph on the right plots rCBF values for the same voxels in the unmasked ("seen") condition. Regression lines have been fitted to the data. (d) Graphical displays showing bivariate regression plots of activity in right amygdala and superior colliculus. The graph on the left plots rCBF (in mL/dL/min) in the maximal right amygdala voxel ($x = 18$, $y = -2$, $z = -28$). and maximal collicular voxel ($x = 0$, $y = -36$, $z = -8$) during presentation of the masked ("unseen") CS+ faces. The graph on the right plots rCBF values for the same voxels in the unmasked ("seen") condition. Regression lines have been fitted to the data.

faces (Morris *et al.*, 1998c) (Fig. 19.6) when used as a covariate of interest showed positive covariation with superior colliculus and right posterior thalamus. By contrast, bilateral regions of fusiform cortex covaried *negatively* with right amygdala during processing of masked fear-conditioned faces.

Patients with damage to primary visual cortex display residual visual abilities (*e.g.*, accurate detection and localisation of moving or flashing stimuli), despite lacking conscious visual awareness in their blind field (Poppel *et al.*, 1973; Weiskrantz *et al.*, 1974). It has been suggested that the colliculo-pulvinar visual pathway may mediate this non-conscious perception or *blindsight* (Weiskrantz *et al.* 1974; Zihl and von Cramon, 1979b), thus providing an intriguing parallel with the colliculo-thalamo-amygdala pathway proposed to mediate responses to masked fear-related stimuli (Morris *et al.*, 1998c, 1999a). This analogy between blindsight and visual backward masking is supported by human psychophysical data (Meeres and Graves, 1990) and electrophysiological experiments in monkeys (Macknik and Livingstone, 1998). Transient neural responses in monkey V1 (striate cortex), normally occurring immediately after the offset of a target stimulus, are inhibited by masks that render the target invisible to human subjects (Macknik and Livingstone, 1998). The disruption of these transient V1 after-discharges by visual backward masking may constitute, therefore, a temporary functional equivalent of the permanent loss of visual awareness seen after striate cortex lesions.

The functional analogy between blindsight and visual backward masking is also supported by behavioural data obtained in patient GY, who has a right hemianopia following early damage to his left occipital lobe (Fig. 19.8a). GY, who displays residual visual abilities typical of blindsight (Barbur *et al.* 1980; Blythe *et al.* 1987), also demonstrates above-chance discrimination of emotional expressions presented in his blind field (de Gelder, 1999). In a functional neuroimaging study, Morris *et al.* (2001) investigated whether this non-conscious discrimination of emotional stimuli displayed by GY is mediated by a colliculo-thalamo-amygdala pathway, bypassing damaged striate cortex. GY was shown lateralised presentations of fearful and happy expressions in his blind (right) and intact (left) hemifields. Fearful faces presented in the intact hemifield elicited left amygdala responses. Fearful faces presented in the blind hemifield evoked bilateral amygdala responses (Fig. 19.8). When amygdala responses were used as a covariate of interest (Friston *et al.*, 1997), a condition-specific covariation of activity between amygdala, pulvinar, and superior colliculus was evident, again supportive of the idea that a subcortical colliculo-pulvinar pathway conveys visual signals to amygdala independently of visual cortex.

In a second functional neuroimaging experiment, GY was presented with an aversively conditioned angry face in either his blind or intact hemifield (Morris *et al.*, 2001). Bilateral (right > left) amygdala responses were elicited when the conditioned angry face was presented in his blind hemifield. Blind hemifield presentation of CS+ faces also evoked increased responses in superior colliculus. In a further analysis, right amygdala activity was used as a covariate of interest to test for psychophysiological interactions with other structures (Friston *et al.*, 1997). A positive covariation between amygdala and pulvinar activity was identified during "blind" presentation of CS+ faces. These data provide further evidence, therefore, that superior colliculus, pulvinar, and amygdala can mediate aversive conditioning of "prepared" visual stimuli, even in the absence of primary visual cortex.

Orbitofrontal Cortex

Anatomy

The cortex on the ventral (orbital) surface of the frontal lobe is highly developed in primates and is comprised of Area 11 rostrally, Area 12 laterally, Area 13 caudally, and Area 14 medially (Carmichael and Price, 1994; Chiavaras and Petrides, 2000). The main thalamic input into orbitofrontal cortex is from the magnocellular (medial) part of the mediodorsal nucleus, which itself receives inputs from temporal lobe structures, including amygdala (Krettek and Price, 1974, 1977). Caudal orbitofrontal cortex receives a direct projection from amygdala, as well as olfactory, gustatory, somatosensory, and visual inputs (Carmichael and Price, 1995b). Medial and lateral orbitofrontal cortex receives direct inputs from anterior cingulate (Carmichael and Price, 1995a). Orbitofrontal cortex has outputs to basal ganglia, hypothalamus, and brainstem and also sends projections back to inferior temporal cortex, amygdala, and anterior cingulate

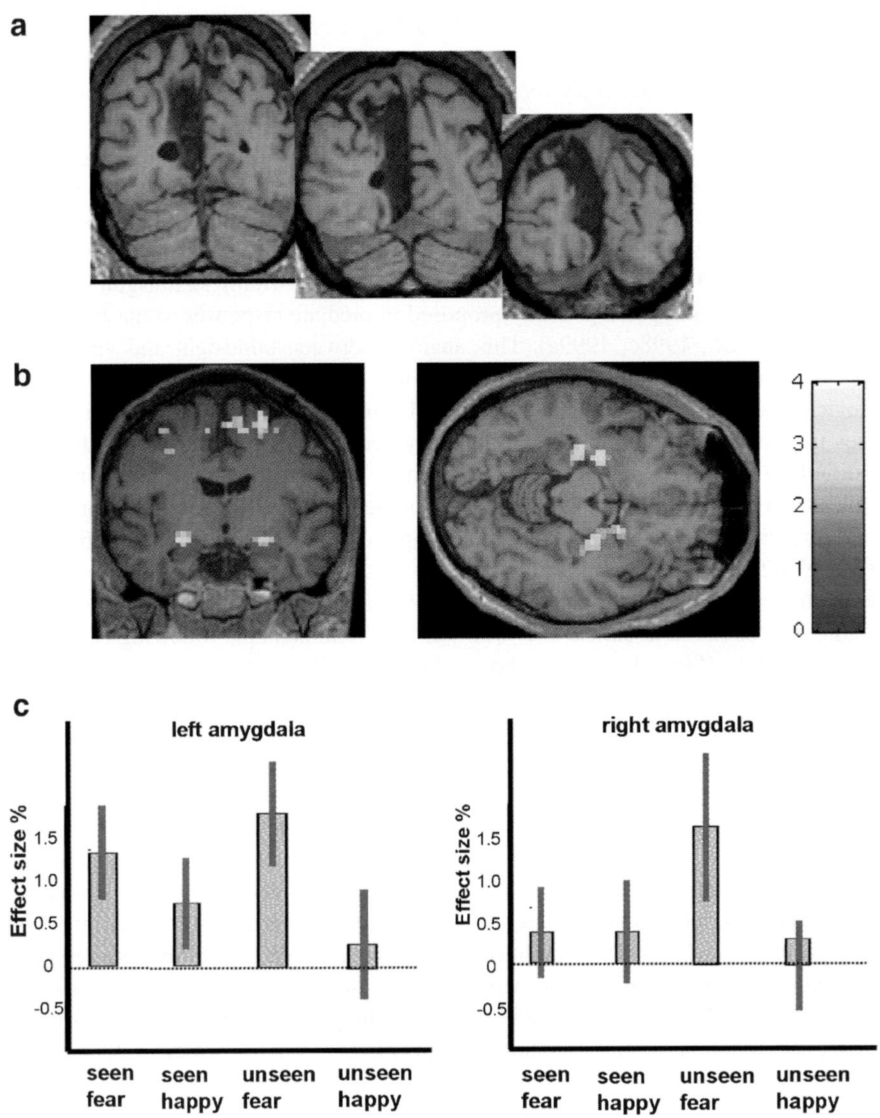

FIGURE 19.8
(a) Patient GY's left occipital lesion; three-dimensional structural MRI of GY's brain illustrates left occipital damage; a horizontal cut-away, 6 mm above the anterior–posterior commissure (AC–PC) axis, is shown. Coronal sections of GY's structural MRI shows extent of striate cortex lesion (74, 78, and 82 mm posterior to the anterior commissure). (b) A statistical parametric map (SPM) showing bilateral increased amygdala responses (indicated by arrows) to fearful faces (compared to happy faces) presented in the right (blind) hemifield. Amygdala activations are projected onto a transverse section of GY's structural MRI centered on the maximal voxel in right amygdala (located 22 mm to the right of midline, 0 mm posterior and 10 mm inferior to anterior commissure). A threshold of $p < 0.01$ (uncorrected) was used to display the contrast. (c) Graphical display of parameter estimates for both right and left amygdala responses to "seen" fearful and happy faces (*i.e.*, presented in intact visual field) and "unseen" fearful and happy faces (*i.e.*, presented in blind visual field).

(Cavada *et al.*, 2000). The anatomical connectivity of orbitofrontal cortex gives it the potential, like amygdala, to integrate sensory information from diverse sources, to modulate sensory and other cognitive processing via feedback connections, and, finally, to influence motor and autonomic output responses.

Reward, Reversal, and Extinction

Animal Lesions and Electrophysiology Animals with lesions to ventral prefrontal (orbitofrontal) cortex show changed behaviour toward both aversive and appetitive stimuli; for example, lesioned monkeys exhibit less aggressive behaviour toward humans, and snakes and are less likely to refuse foods such as meat (Butter et al., 1969a,b, 1970). Orbitofrontal lesions in animals also disrupt reward learning, especially in paradigms involving changes in reinforcement contingencies. In particular, animals with damage to orbitofrontal cortex show deficits in reversal learning in that they continue to respond to stimuli previously associated with reward rather than switching responses to currently reinforced stimuli. Animals with orbitofrontal lesions also show abnormal extinction of learned responses, evident in persistent responding to stimuli that no longer predict food delivery (Butter, 1969; Jones and Mishkin, 1972).

Electrophysiological recordings in monkeys have shown that cells in orbitofrontal cortex respond to rewarding or reinforcing stimuli such as the sight, taste, and smell of food (Rolls *et al.*, 1989; Thorpe *et al.* 1983). Reward-related orbitofrontal responses are dependent on monkeys' motivational state (*e.g.*, level of hunger or satiety) (Rolls *et al.*, 1989; Thorpe *et al.* 1983). Selective satiation of a particular food results in decreased orbitofrontal responses to that food, leaving responses to other, non-satiated foods unaffected (Critchley and Rolls, 1996). Monkey orbitofrontal cells have also been found to be responsive to reversal of reinforcement contingencies in visual and olfactory discrimination paradigms (Rolls *et al.*, 1996; Thorpe *et al.*, 1983). Amygdala cells, however, unlike those in orbitofrontal cortex, do not show reversal of discriminatory responses in similar paradigms (Sanghera *et al.*, 1979). Thus, one account of these findings is that amygdala is critically involved in initial acquisition of emotional learning, whereas orbitofrontal cortex is involved in dynamic reassessment and relearning of emotional associations (Rolls, 1999).

Human Neuropsychology and Functional Neuroimaging Damage to human OFC produces a characteristic clinical syndrome of irresponsible, disinhibited behaviour and childish, fatuous affect (Eslinger and Damasio, 1985). Behavioural studies have shown that patients with orbitofrontal damage are impaired on emotional visual discrimination reversal tasks (Rolls *et al.*, 1994). Compared with other brain-damaged controls, orbitofrontal patients continue to respond to target stimuli after reinforcement contingencies are reversed (*i.e.* when responding to the targets has negative rather than rewarding consequences) (Rolls *et al.*, 1994). Similarly, in gambling tasks, patients with orbitofrontal damage are impaired in altering their behaviour in response to changes in reward expectation (Bechara *et al.*, 1997).

Human neuroimaging experiments have reported increased activity in orbitofrontal cortex to primary reinforcing stimuli, such as pleasant touch (Francis *et al.*, 1999), pleasant sounds (Blood and Zatorre, 2001), pleasant and aversive taste (O'Doherty *et al.*, 2001), and food odor (O'Doherty *et al.*, 2000). However, as in the monkey, human orbitofrontal responses to food stimuli are decreased by satiety (O'Doherty *et al.*, 2000 Morris *et al.*, 2001). These data indicate that orbitofrontal cortex cells respond to the reinforcement value of stimuli, rather than their specific physical characteristics (see Chapter 22).

The role of human orbitofrontal cortex in emotional learning reversal has been investigated in an event-related functional magnetic resonance imaging (fMRI) study (Morris and Dolan, 2003) (Fig. 19.9). In the initial phase of the experiment, subjects were repeatedly shown pictures of two faces. One of the faces (A, CS+) was immediately followed by a loud (>90-dB) aversive noise for 33% of the presentations; the other face (B, CS−) was never followed by the noise. The initial phase was followed seamlessly by three other phases: (1) a repeat phase, in which face A continued to be paired with the noise (A, CS+; B, CS−); (2) a reversal phase in which face B (and not face A) was followed by noise (B, CS+; A, CS−); and (3) a new phase in which two new faces (C and D) were shown, one of which (C) was paired with noise for 33% of trials (C, CS+; D, CS−). During acquisition of conditioning, in the initial and repeat phases, face A (CS+) evoked increased responses in amygdala (Fig. 19.9a). In the reversal phase, face A (new CS−, old CS+) continued to elicit increased responses in amygdala, while face B (new CS+, old CS−) elicited increased activity in orbitofrontal cortex (Fig. 19.9b). These data agree with the idea that amygdala and orbitofrontal cortex have distinct roles in emotional learning; that is, amygdala is crucial for acquisition and retention of emotional associations (LeDoux, 1996), and orbitofrontal cortex is involved in rapid and flexible modification of emotional responses that reflect changing stimulus contingencies (Rolls, 1999).

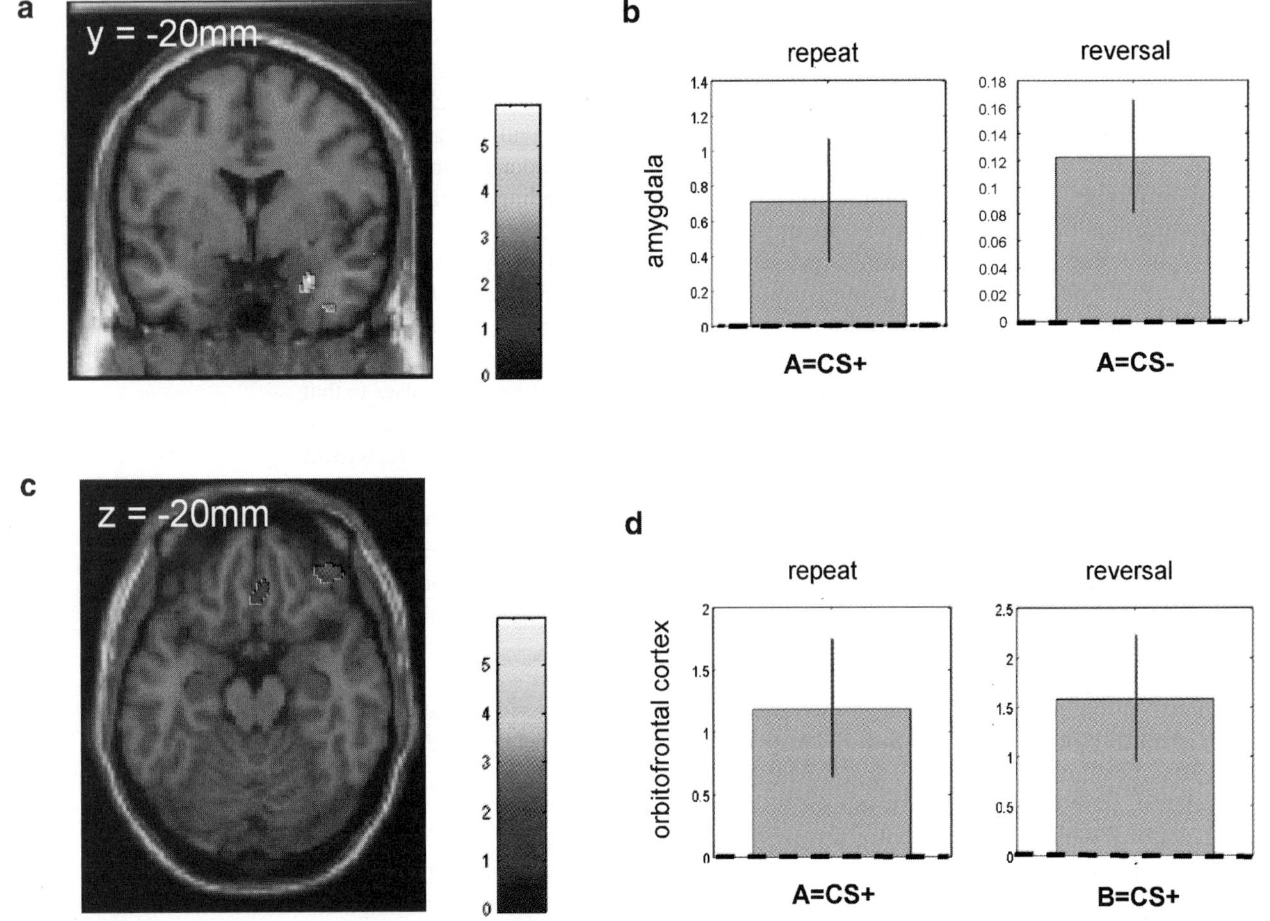

FIGURE 19.9
(a) A statistical parametric map (SPM) indicating medial and lateral regions of right orbitofrontal cortex ([$x = 4$, $y = 38$, $z = -14$] and [$x = 42$, $y = 44$, $z = -16$]) that have increased responses to the CS+ face in both repeat and reversal phases of a reversal fear conditioning paradigm, irrespective of the identity (*i.e.*, A or B) of the face. (b) A graphical display showing parameter estimates for the response to the CS+ face (relative to CS–). in the repeat and reversal phases in the lateral orbitofrontal region displayed in (a). (c) An SPM showing a ventral region of right amygdala ($x = 30$, $y = 2$, $z = -26$) with increased responses to the CS+ (face A) in the repeat phase of a reversal fear conditioning paradigm that persists in the reversal phase (*i.e.*, when face A becomes the CS–). (d) A graphical display showing parameter estimates for the response to the CS+ face (relative to CS–) in the repeat and reversal phases in the right ventral amygdala region displayed in (c).

Insula

Anatomy and Physiology

Insula cortex is a multimodal sensory region with visceral, gustatory, somatosensory, visual, and auditory afferents and reciprocal connections to amygdala, hypothalamus, cingulate gyrus, and orbitofrontal cortex. In addition to its role in interoceptive representation and autonomic control (Oppenheimer *et al.*, 1992; Small *et al.*, 1999), the insula has also been implicated in the acquisition of inhibitory avoidance behaviour (Bermudez-Rattoni *et al.*, 1991). It has been postulated that the insula functions as a multimodal integration cortex that coordinates sensorimotor responses to noxious or unexpected stimuli (Augustine, 1996).

Disgust and Other Visceral Processing

A patient with a selective lesion of insula cortex has been reported to show impaired recognition and experience of disgust for both facial and vocal expressions (Calder *et al.*, 2000). Several functional neuroimaging studies of healthy subjects have also reported increased insula responses to facial expressions of disgust (Phillips *et al.*, 1997, 1998a,b; Sprengelmeyer *et al.*, 1998). However, increased insula activity has also been reported in relation to sadness (Lane *et al.*, 1997), fear (Morris *et al.*, 1996), fear conditioning (Buchel *et al.*, 1998; Critchley *et al.*,

2002), instructed fear (Phelps, *et al.*, 2001), the experience of phobic symptoms (Rauch *et al.*, 1995), hunger and satiety states (Morris and Dolan, 2001; Tatarini *et al.*, 1999), perception of noxious stimuli (Casey *et al.*, 1994; Derbyshire *et al.*, 1994), and explicit facial emotion categorisation (George *et al.*, 1993; Gorno-Tempini *et al.*, 2001). Although the insula may exhibit functional specialisation for disgust (Calder *et al.*, 2001), its role in emotional processing is not restricted to one particular emotion. Critchley *et al.* (2002) have suggested that insula may play a crucial role in mediating the influence of peripheral autonomic arousal on consciously experienced emotional states (see Chapter 20), a suggestion that would accord with a role for this region in subjective aspects of emotion (*i.e.*, "feeling" states).

Anterior Cingulate

Anatomy and Physiology

The cingulate gyrus is a cytoarchitecturally distinct band of cortex forming the dorsal part of Broca's *grande lobe limbique* (1878). Animal data indicate that cingulate cortex is functionally heterogeneous, comprised of different subregions (Bussey *et al.*, 1997; Devinsky *et al.*, 1995; Vogt *et al.*, 1992). One model of its functional parcellation involves a distinction between cognitive and affective zones. An *affective* ventral subdivision of anterior cingulate (comprised of Brodmann's areas 25, 32, 33) has connections to amygdala, nucleus accumbens, orbitofrontal cortex, anterior insula, and autonomic brainstem regions (Devinsky *et al.*, 1995). A more dorsal *cognitive* subdivision (comprising caudal areas 24′ and 32′ and cingulate motor area) has anatomical connections with parietal cortex, posterior cingulate, supplementary motor area, and dorsolateral prefrontal cortex (Devinsky *et al.*, 1995). The anatomical connectivity of anterior cingulate makes it well placed to evaluate the behavioural relevance of stimuli and influence autonomic and motor responses.

Emotional Monitoring

Cingulate cortex has long been implicated in emotional processing. In light of the affective consequences of cingulate lesions, Papez (1937) concluded that, "The cortex of the cingular gyrus may be looked on as the receptive organ for the experiencing of emotion." Cingulate cortex is also implicated in emotional responses. Smith (1945) reported that electrical stimulation of anterior cingulate cortex in macaque monkeys produces changes in heart rate, blood pressure, and respiration, in addition to eliciting vocalisations and facial expressions. Functional neuroimaging data indicate a wide role for anterior cingulate cortex in emotional processing. Anterior cingulate responses have been reported to facial expressions of emotion, including fear and anger (Blair *et al.*, 1998; George *et al.*, 1993; Morris *et al.*, 1996), emotional pictures (Lane *et al.*, 1997), emotional words (George *et al.*, 1994; Whalen *et al.*, 1998a), fear-conditioned stimuli (Buchel *et al.*, 1998; Knight *et al.*, 1999; LaBar *et al.*, 1998), cardiovascular arousal (Critchley *et al.*, 2000b), painful stimuli (Talbot *et al.*, 1991), pain intensity (Buchel *et al.*, 2001), pain affect (Rainville *et al.*, 1997), and pain expectation (Sawamoto *et al.*, 2000).

Functional neuroimaging studies have implicated dorsal anterior cingulate in (non-emotional) cognitive tasks involving stimulus selection and response competition (Carter *et al.*, 2000; Nobre *et al.*, 1997; see Chapters 15 and 19 on selective attention in this volume). Similarly, selectively attending to subjective emotional states (Lane *et al.*, 1997) or being presented with a response conflict in an emotional Stroop task (George *et al.*, 1994; Whalen *et al.*, 1998a) has also been shown to activate anterior cingulate, although more ventrally than for non-emotional cognitive tasks. Accordingly, one function of ventral anterior cingulate may be to monitor and evaluate external stimuli (especially when aversive or painful) and select appropriate responses with respect to ongoing emotional priorities and goals (Davidson *et al.*, 2002; Rolls, 1998).

Affective Disorder

Several lines of evidence support a critical role for anterior cingulate in regulating mood states as well as emotional and social behaviour. In animals (especially mammals), anterior cingulate lesions disrupt a range of social behaviours, including maternal and play responses (Slotnick, 1967; Murphy *et al.*, 1981). Patients with acquired anterior cingulate lesions typically display apathy, amotivation, and relative insensitivity to pain (Cohen *et al.*,1999; Degos *et al.*, 1993).

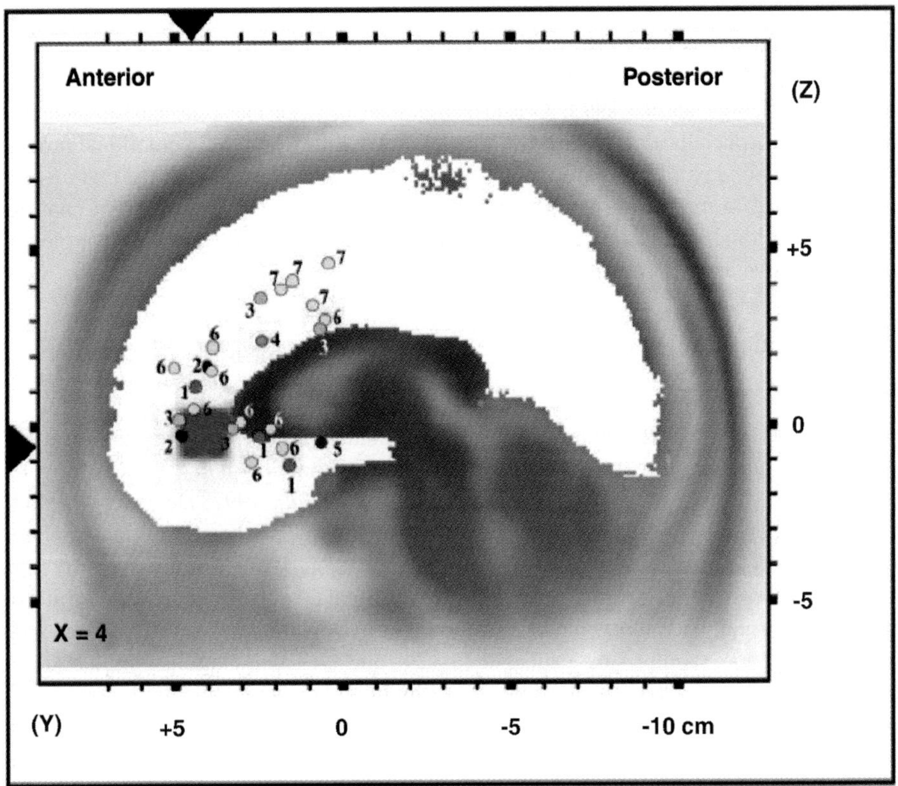

FIGURE 19.10
Summary of functional brain imaging studies of anterior cingulate cortex (ACC) involvement in depression as well as during various cognitive and affective task manipulations. Foci of ACC activation or deactivation were registered to a common stereotaxic brain atlas (Talairach and Tournoux, 1988) and plotted on a sagittal brain slice (anterior part of the head to the left). The large red area and the black triangles show the location of the ACC cluster found to be associated with degree of treatment response in Pizzagalli *et al.* (2001): 1, Studies of depressed subjects that showed pretreatment hyperactivity among patients who responded to treatment; 2, posttreatment decreased activity in responders; 3, hypoactivity in depressed subjects; 4, increased activity with remission of depression; 5, decreased activity with remission of depression. Studies involving emotional (6) and cognitive (7) tasks in nonpsychiatric subjects are also reported. Coordinates are in millimeters (Talairach and Tournoux, 1988), with the origin at the anterior commissure. (From Davidson *et al.*, 2002. With permission.)

Functional neuroimaging studies of patients with affective disorders have found abnormal activity in both anterior cingulate and adjacent subgenual prefrontal cortex (Bench *et al.*, 1992; Blumberg *et al.*, 2000; Drevets *et al.*, 1997; Mayberg *et al.*, 1994; Smith *et al.*, 1997) (Fig. 19.10). Resting state activity in dorsal and subgenual anterior cingulate is typically decreased in depressed patients (Bench *et al.*, 1992; Drevets *et al.*, 1997) and increased in patients during manic episodes (Blumberg *et al.*, 2000). Remission of depression is associated with increased resting state activity in dorsal anterior cingulate (Bench *et al.*, 1995; Mayberg *et al.*, 1999). Activity in a rostral region of anterior cingulate (Brodmann's area 24) predicts the response of depressed patients to treatment, with responders reported to have hyperactivity in this region (Pizzagalli *et al.*, 2001).

Other regions reported to have abnormal activity in depression include amygdala and orbitofrontal cortex, both of which are extensively connected to anterior cingulate (Drevets, 1999). Amygdala activity is elevated in depression and correlates positively with depression severity (Drevets, 1999). Remission of depression, by contrast, is associated with decreases in amygdala activity (Drevets *et al.*, 1997, 2002). The opposing patterns of depression-related activity observed in amygdala and prefrontal regions has led to the suggestion that amgydala is normally subject to inhibitory modulation by cingulate and orbitofrontal cortex (Drevets, 1999). It is proposed that in depression prefrontal modulation of amygdala is disrupted, leading to abnormal processing of emotional stimuli (Drevets, 1999). One difficulty with this proposal is the lack of neuropsychological evidence indicating a role for amygdala in mood regulation.

The principal source of cerebral serotonin is the dorsal raphe nucleus (Tork and Hornung, 1990). Animal experiments indicate that the activity of serotonergic neurons in the dorsal raphe is modulated by projections from the habenula nucleus in the epithalamus (Wang and Aghajanian, 1977). Because the habenula itself receives a major input from serotonergic projection regions (*i.e.*, anterior cingulate, amygdala, and orbitofrontal cortex), it represents a critical point of convergence in a feedback loop regulating cerebral serotonin levels (Reisine *et al.*, 1982; Sutherland, 1982; Wang and Aghajanian, 1977). A role for habenula in the etiology of affective disorder is supported by several animal experiments (Caldecott-Hazard, 1988; Amat *et al.*, 2001). Data from a human functional neuroimaging study employing tryptophan depletion also indicates a critical role for habenula in the development of depression (Morris *et al.*, 1999c). Covariation between habenula and dorsal raphe activity was found to correlate positively with the severity of depressive symptoms induced by tryptophan depletion (Morris *et al.*, 1999c). This finding emphasises that an account of how the brain mediates emotion and other complex behaviours requires an understanding of *functional connectivity* between anatomically segregated brain areas.

FUNCTIONAL INTEGRATION OF EMOTIONAL PROCESSING

A striking characteristic of emotion-related brain regions (particularly amygdala) is the extensive reciprocal anatomical connectivity they display with other brain areas involved in sensory, motor, and non-emotional cognitive functions (Amaral *et al.*, 1992). Emotion-related regions also have important anatomical connections with neuromodulatory systems (*e.g.*, cholinergic nucleus basalis of Meynert, serotonergic dorsal raphe, and dopaminergic ventral tegmentum). Moreover, emotion-related brain regions such as amygdala are rich in receptors for circulating hormones such as glucocorticoids, adrenaline, and estrogen (Krezel *et al.*, 2001; McGaugh *et al.*, 2000; Osterlund *et al.*, 2000). This complex neuroanatomical organisation suggests that emotional processing cannot simply be conceptualised as an encapsulated module in a hierarchical sequence of discrete cognitive processes. Comprehensive models of emotional processing, therefore, need to account for the dynamic interaction of emotion with other sensory, motor, and cognitive functions. Empirical data relating to the functional integration of emotional processing in the brain are considered below.

Emotional Modulation of Sensory Processing

In addition to receiving multiple sensory inputs, the amygdala sends efferent fibers back to early sensory areas of the brain (Amaral *et al.*, 1992). Intriguingly, whereas the visual cortical input to amygdala derives primarily from anterior temporal regions, amygdala efferents project back to much earlier visual areas, including V1, from which amygdala does not receive a direct input (Amaral *et al.*, 1992). Amygdala is therefore well placed to integrate biologically salient emotional signals from multiple sensory modalities and modulate ongoing sensory processing via direct feedback and other modulatory connections (*e.g.*, via the cholinergic nucleus basalis of Meynert). It has been suggested that one function of this feedback to sensory regions may be to enhance perception of behaviourally relevant stimuli (*e.g.*, potential threats and dangers) (Amaral *et al.*, 1992; Rolls, 1992).

Visual

Several human neuroimaging studies have reported emotional modulation of visual cortical responses (Dolan *et al.*, 1996; Fredrikson *et al.*, 1993; Lane *et al.*, 1999; Lang *et al.*, 1998; Morris *et al.*, 1998a, 2001). The neural mechanisms underlying this phenomenon are still uncertain; however, evidence that modulatory interactions with amygdala may be involved has been provided by analyses of neuroimaging data testing for psychophysiological interactions (Friston *et al.*, 1997). Increased covariation of response between amygdala and extrastriate cortical regions is seen during processing of fearful as opposed to happy faces (Morris *et al.*, 1998a). This finding indicates that following activation of amygdala by fearful facial expressions, feedback from amygdala to visual cortex enhances ongoing perceptual processing. Similar findings have been reported by Rotshtein *et al.* (2001), who found increased covariation between amygdala and lateral occipital complex during processing of unpleasant and bizarre faces, and by George *et al.* (2001), who reported increased covariation between amygdala and fusiform gyrus during processing of direct (as opposed to indirect) eye gaze. The data from George *et al.* (2001) not only support a modulatory role for amygdala in regard to visual cortical processing of faces but also concur with evidence that the amygdala's response to fear (and threat) in faces is dependent principally on the eyes (Morris *et al.*, 2002).

Further evidence implicating amygdala in modulation of sensory processing is provided by a behavioural study of patients with restricted amygdala damage (Andersen and Phelps, 2001). In an attentional blink task, healthy subjects showed enhanced perception of aversive words compared to emotionally neutral words. Patients with damage to left (but not right) amygdala failed to show this emotional enhancement of visual perception for words (Andersen and Phelps, 2001). In addition to providing support to the proposal that amygdala is critical for emotional modulation of perceptual processing (LeDoux, 1996; Morris *et al.*, 1998a; Rolls and Treves, 1998), the data from Andersen and Phelps (2001) provide further evidence concerning lateralisation of amygdala function where the left amygdala, due to its greater connectivity with language-related brain areas, tends to have greater involvement in explicit, cognitive, verbal tasks (Andersen and Phelps, 2001; Morris *et al.*, 1996; Phelps *et al.*, 2001).

Auditory

Nonverbal emotional vocalisations have been shown to evoke differential responses in amygdala, insula, caudate, temporal, and orbitofrontal cortices (Morris *et al.*, 1999b; Phillips *et al.*, 1998a). Morris *et al.* (1999b), showed a fear-specific psychophysiological interaction between amygdala and insula responses; that is, they demonstrated that fearful vocalisations change the covariation of activity between insula and amygdala (Friston *et al.*, 1997). This finding indicates that perception of fearful vocalisations involves a functional *interaction* between amygdala and insula and not simply separate, distinct responses in these two structures. A similar fear-specific psychophysiological interaction was observed between amygdala and a pontine region in the brainstem, the nucleus reticularis pontis caudalis (NRPC), which has been implicated in mediating the acoustic startle reflex (Davis, 1992; Rosen *et al.*, 1991). Animal studies have shown that fear-related potentiation of acoustic startle depends on a direct projection from amygdala to NRPC (Davis, 1992; Hitchcock and Davis, 1991). The data from Morris *et al.* (1999b) indicate that a similar functional network may also operate in humans.

Animal electrophysiological experiments have shown that fear conditioning induces rapid and long-lasting receptive field plasticity in auditory cortical cells (Weinberger, 1995). In guinea pigs, pairing an auditory tone (CS+) of a specific frequency with an aversive UCS (*e.g.*, electric shock) produces increased auditory cortex responses to the CS+ frequency and decreased responses to other frequencies (Bakin and Weinbeger, 1990). This retuning of the brain by fear conditioning occurs very rapidly (after 5 to 10 trials) and persists for at least 8 weeks (Weinberger *et al.*, 1993). Conditioning-dependent auditory receptive field plasticity is expressed under deep general anesthesia, indicating that it is not related to changes in arousal or attention (Lennartz and Weinberger, 1992). Animal electrophysiological studies have shown the critical importance of amygdala (Armony *et al.*, 1998; Quirk *et al.*, 1997) and the cholinergic nucleus basalis of Meynert (Bakin and Weinberger, 1996; Kilgard and Mezernich, 1998) in the development of learning-related changes in auditory responses.

Human functional neuroimaging studies also provide evidence for amygdala and nucleus basalis involvement in fear-conditioned changes in auditory responses (Morris *et al.*, 1998b; Thiel *et al.*, 2002). Aversive (fear) conditioning of high- and low-frequency tones produces learning-related modulation of responses in orbitofrontal cortex, basal forebrain, and tonotopic auditory cortex (Morris *et al.*, 1998b). A regression analysis of neuroimaging data from Morris *et al.* (1998b) revealed a positive covariation between auditory cortex and amygdala responses, consistent with animal data implicating amygdala in learning-related auditory cortex plasticity (Armony *et al.*, 1998; Quirk *et al.*, 1997). An event-related fMRI study using a similar conditioning paradigm has shown that the expression of learning-related auditory cortex responses is prevented by prior administration of the anticholinergic scopolamine (Thiel *et al.*, 2002). These data agree, therefore, with animal studies indicating a critical role for the cholinergic nucleus basalis of Meynert in learning-related auditory cortex plasticity (Bakin and Weinberger, 1996; Kilgard and Mezernich, 1998).

Cross-Modal

A role for amygdala in cross-modal sensory integration was proposed after surgical amygdala lesions in monkeys were found to impair intermodal but not intramodal performance on a delayed non-match to sample task (Murray and Mishkin, 1985). However, subsequent excitotoxic lesion studies indicated the involvement of adjacent perirhinal cortex, rather than amygdala in sensory–sensory associative learning, suggesting that previously reported deficits on cross-modal tasks were probably due to inadvertent damage to perirhinal cortex during surgical removal of amygdala (Goulet and Murray, 2001). Nevertheless, while amygdala does not appear to be necessary for learning associations about the *physical* features of stimuli, other lesion studies indicate that an intact amygdala *is* crucial for intermodal associative learning involving the biological "value" of stimuli (Malkova *et al.*, 1997). Thus, performance in second-order conditioning and reinforcer devaluation tasks is disrupted by lesions of the basolateral nucleus of amygdala but not by damage to perirhinal cortex (Hatfield *et al.*, 1996; Thornton *et al.*, 1998).

Human neuroimaging studies have implicated amygdala in the acquisition of associations between behaviourally salient stimuli of different modalities (*e.g.*, emotional faces and loud, aversive noises) (Buchel *et al.*, 1998; Morris *et al.*, 1998c). Intriguingly, cross-modal, learning-related responses are observed not only in amygdala but also in unimodal sensory cortex (Armony and Dolan, 2001; Morris *et al.*, 2001). Morris *et al.* (2001) observed that a fear-conditioned visual stimulus (*i.e.*, an emotional face previously implicitly paired with a loud noise) modulated neural activity not only in amygdala and face-related fusiform gyrus but also in primary auditory cortex. An attentional explanation for the modulation of auditory cortex by the facial stimulus is excluded by the implicit nature of the association between face and noise. Modulation of activity in auditory cortex has also been observed with an aversive visual context, a background screen of a particular color associated with delivery of a noise UCS (Armony and Dolan, 2001). One interpretation of these findings is that the visual CS+ (or aversive context) accesses a representation of the auditory UCS, resulting in modulation of sensory processing specific to the UCS modality (*i.e.*, auditory cortex). Amygdala is ideally placed to mediate cross-modal, learning-dependent modulation of sensory processing observed in these studies (Armony and Dolan, 2001; Morris *et al.*, 2001), as it is implicated in the formation of CS–UCS associations (LeDoux, 1996) and has extensive reciprocal connections with both auditory and visual sensory systems (Amaral *et al.*, 1992).

Human behavioural and electrophysiological studies have shown that when visual and auditory emotional stimuli (*e.g.*, an emotional facial expression and a voice with an emotional tone) are presented concurrently, automatic (pre-attentive) cross-modal binding of the affective information occurs very early in perceptual processing (de Gelder, 1999; Pourtois *et al.*, 2000). The neural basis of this cross-modal emotional integration was investigated in a functional neuroimaging study in which fearful and happy faces were presented to subjects concurrently with sentences spoken in either a fearful or a happy tone (Dolan *et al.*, 2001). Enhanced responses to fearful faces in both amygdala and face-related fusiform gyrus were decreased by the concurrent presentation of happy voices (Dolan *et al.*, 2001), underlining the potential role of amygdala in cross-modal integration of emotionally salient sensory information and in emotional modulation of responses in unimodal sensory cortex.

Emotional Modulation of Memory

Intense emotional experiences (*e.g.*, one's own wedding day) are more likely to be remembered than non-emotional, neutral events. Animal experiments indicate that the enhancing effect of emotional arousal on performance in memory tasks is dependent on the release of stress hormones such as adrenaline and corticosterone (Gold and van Buskirk, 1975; Micheau *et al.*, 1981). Animal studies also show that amygdala, in particular the basolateral nucleus, is critically involved in mediating the enhancing effect of adrenaline and corticosterone on memory performance (Liang *et al.*, 1986; Roozendaal and McGaugh, 1996; for a review, see McGaugh *et al.*, 2000).

Studies of human subjects using arousing, emotional stimuli indicate that similar neural mechanisms of emotional modulation of memory operate in the human brain. In healthy volunteers, the adrenergic blocker propanolol selectively impairs memory of emotionally arousing events compared to neutral events (Cahill *et al.*, 1994). On the other hand, patients with bilateral amygdala lesions fail to show emotional enhancement of memory exhibited by intact subjects (Cahill *et al.*, 1995). In a PET study, healthy subjects were tested on their recall of emotional (aversive) and neutral film clips (Cahill *et al.*, 1996). Right amygdala activity during viewing (encoding) of the films positively correlated with the number of emotional films recalled, but not with the number of recalled neutral clips (Cahill *et al.*, 1996). Constraints in the design of the PET experiment meant that the correlation between amygdala activity during encoding and subsequent memory recall reported by Cahill *et al.* (1996) depended on inter-subject variability; however, a subsequent event-related fMRI study also found a positive association between amygdala activity and emotionally enhanced recall on a within-subject basis (Canli *et al.*, 2001).

The animal and human studies described above indicate the critical role of amygdala in emotional enhancement of memory during *encoding*; however, other functional neuroimaging studies suggest that amygdala activity may also be critical for *retrieval* of emotionally salient items (Dolan *et al.*, 2000; Maratos et al, 2001). Increased responses in left amygdala were found in subjects performing a memory recognition task on emotional pictures (Dolan *et al.*, 2000). Increased amygdala responses were not observed with the same stimuli during another, nonmnemonic, cognitive task, indicating that the amygdala response was specifically related to memory retrieval (Dolan *et al.*, 2000). Recognition of words previously presented in an emotionally negative context is also associated with increased left amygdala activity (Maratos *et al.*, 2001). Other brain regions activated by episodic retrieval of emotional context include hippocampus, posterior cingulate, and prefrontal cortex (Maratos *et al.*, 2001).

The amygdala also appears to be critical for enhanced memory of pleasant or appetitive stimuli (Hamann *et al.*, 1999; Morris *et al.*, 2001). Hamann *et al.* (1999) reported that bilateral amygdala activity positively correlated with enhanced memory for both pleasant and aversive stimuli, but not for "interesting," emotionally unarousing stimuli. In a further analysis, Hamann *et al.* (1999) found a significant correlation between amygdala and hippocampal activity, supporting the proposal that emotional modulation of memory involves amygdala–hippocampal interactions (McGaugh *et al.*, 2000). In another functional neuroimaging study, Morris *et al.* (2001) presented pictures of food and non-food (household) items to subjects while they were in fasting or sated states (Fig. 19.11). Subjects subsequently performed a recognition memory task on each stimulus category during PET neuroimaging. Recognition memory was significantly enhanced for food but *not* household items in the fasting state. Neuroimaging data showed that left amygdala responses positively correlated with memory for food, but not household items (Fig. 19.11a). Further analysis of the data identified a significant psychophysiological interaction (food versus non-food) between amygdala and orbitofrontal cortex responses consistent with the idea that emotional (and motivational) modulation of memory for appetitive stimuli involves an interaction between amygdala and orbitofrontal cortex (Fig. 19.11b). This proposal is also supported by animal lesion data showing that surgical disconnection of amygdala and orbitofrontal cortex, a procedure that otherwise leaves these structures intact, disrupts the ability of monkeys to adjust behaviour following devaluation of a food reward (Baxter *et al.*, 2000).

CONCLUSION

Over the past decade, functional neuroimaging studies have made significant contributions to our understanding of the neural organisation of human emotion. In particular, neuroimaging experiments have demonstrated the importance of functional *integration* of emotional and non-emotional processes in the brain (*e.g.*, as exemplified by emotional enhancement of memory and perception), as well as functional *specialisation* of distinct brain regions (*e.g.*, amygdala responses to fearful faces). The neuroscientific investigation of emotion has been hindered in

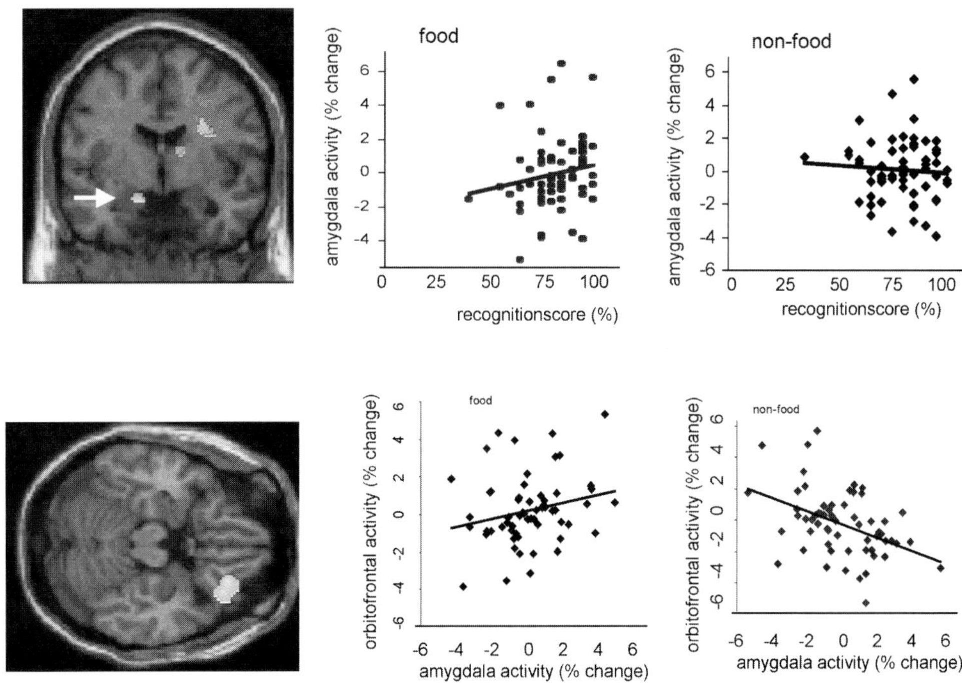

FIGURE 19.11
(a) A statistical parametric map (SPM) showing a left amygdala activation ($x = -14$, $y = -4$, $z = -20$) that covaried positively with memory for food items but negatively with memory for non-food. Left amygdala is indicated by a white arrow. Activations are displayed on a coronal MRI section from a representative subject. (b) Plots of left amygdala activity in food and non-food conditions with respect to recognition score. Activity is shown in terms of percentage signal change, and linear regression lines have been fitted to the data. (c) An SPM showing a psychophysiological interaction between right orbitofrontal cortex and left amygdala rCBF. Measures of rCBF in maximal amygdala voxel ($x = -14$, $y = -4$, $z = -20$) were used as a covariate of interest in a condition-dependent regression analysis. The orbitofrontal activation is displayed on a coronal MRI section from a representative subject. (d) Plots of right orbitofrontal activity in food and non-food conditions with respect to left amygdala activity. Activations are shown in terms of percentage signal change, and linear regression lines have been fitted to the data.

the past by a philosophical dualism that tended to emphasise the separation of affective and cognitive processes. The revival of evolutionary, comparative approaches (Darwin, 1872; Ekman, 1982; LeDoux, 1996) has enabled emotion and cognition to be viewed from a common neurobiological perspective rather than from the separate domains of metapsychology and cognitive psychology.

The concept of *value-dependent neural selection* (Friston *et al.*, 1994) (Fig. 19.12) has proved valuable in modelling emotional processes in the brain, as it combines an evolutionary perspective with an explicit account of both functional integration and functional segregation. Friston *et al.* (1994) proposed that the brain contains a "value" system that is activated by evolutionarily determined, "innate" cues. Critical anatomical components of the value system would include amygdala and the cholinergic nucleus basalis of Meynert. Neuromodulatory outputs from value systems facilitate synaptic plasticity in widespread brain regions including, crucially, sensory areas. Thus, if a particular stimulus regularly occurs during activation of the value system (*e.g.*, sight of a particular food with a pleasant taste), connectivity between the sensory processing of that stimulus and the value system will be enhanced. In this way, a previously novel or neutral stimulus is able to gain access to the value system and thus acquire value. The concept of value-dependent neural selection has close parallels with animal models of learning-related auditory receptive field plasticity (Weinberger, 1995) (Fig. 19.7) and has proved useful in interpreting the results of human functional neuroimaging experiments on auditory conditioning (Morris *et al.*, 1997).

The interaction of hormonal, neurochemical, genetic and developmental factors in the neural processing of emotion is now being addressed in a more detailed and systematic way. Animal studies have demonstrated, for example, that amygdala modulates the response of

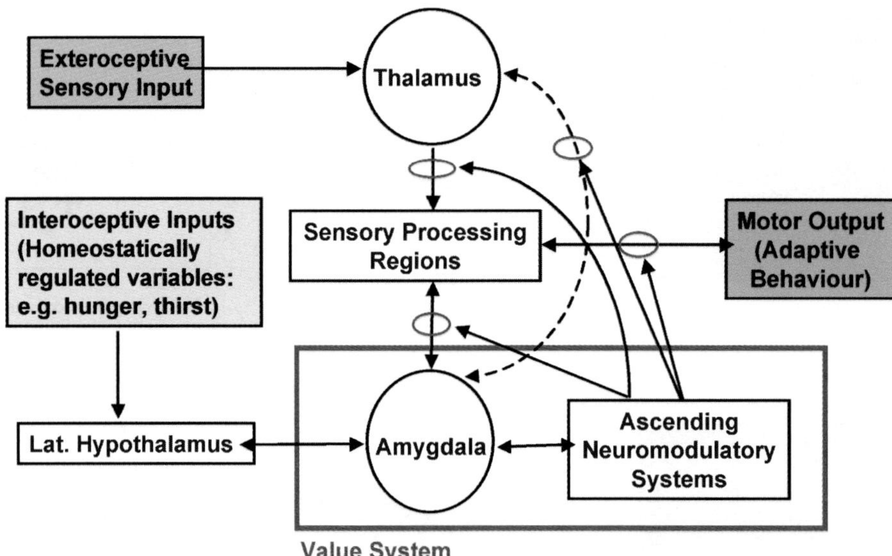

FIGURE 19.12
Value-dependent neural selection. Evolutionarily determined value systems in the brain selectively increase the probability of adaptive behaviours by modulating synaptic changes in the circuits relevant to those behaviours. The amygdala and associated neuromodulatory systems, by virtue of their connectivity with widely distributed brain regions, are well suited to mediate value-dependent modulation (red circles). The neural value system responds to evolutionarily important (innate) cues, but if value-dependent modulation is extended to the inputs of the value-system itself, then previously neutral cues are able to acquire value through a process of (emotional) learning. The receptive field plasticity observed in both human and animal studies of emotional learning is predicted by this synthetic neural model. (Adapted from Friston *et al.*, 1994.)

the hypothalamic–pituitary–adrenal axis to immune challenges, thus providing a possible mechanism for emotional states to influence pathophysiological processes (Xu *et al.*, 1999). Human functional neuroimaging data, on the other hand, have linked a particular variant of a serotonin transporter gene to enhanced amygdala responses to fearful and angry faces, thus providing a possible neurogenetic basis for individual differences in anxiety traits (Hariri *et al.*, 2002). Advances in our knowledge of the human genome (Lander *et al.*, 2001) will undoubtedly make the combination of molecular genetics and functional neuroimaging a powerful tool in the investigation of the neural basis of human emotion.

References

Adolphs, R. and Tranel, D. (1999). Intact recognition of emotional prosody following amygdala damage. *Neuropsychologia*, **37**, 1285–1292

Adolphs, R., Tranel, D., Damasio, H., and Damasio, A. R. (1994). Impaired recognition of emotion in facial expressions following bilateral damage to the human amygdala. *Nature*, **372**, 669–672.

Amaral, D. G. (1986). Amygdalohippocampal and amygdalocortical projections in the primate brain. *Adv. Exp. Med. Biol.*, **203**, 3–17.

Amaral, D. G. and Price, J. L. (1984). Amygdalo-cortical projections in the monkey (*Macaca fascicularis*). *J. Comp. Neurol.*, **230**, 465–496.

Amaral, D. G., Price, J. L., Pitkanen, A., and Carmichael, S. T. (1992). Anatomical organisation of the primate amygdaloid complex, in *The Amygdala: Neurobiological Aspects of Emotion, Memory and Mental Dysfunction*, Aggleton, J. P., Ed., pp. 1–66. Wiley-Liss, New York.

Amat, J., Sparks, P. D., Matus-Amat, P., Griggs, J., Watkins, L. R., and Maier, S. F. (2001). The role of the habenular complex in the elevation of dorsal raphe nucleus serotonin and the changes in the behavioural responses produced by uncontrollable stress. *Brain Res.*, **917**, 118–126.

Anderson, A. K. and Phelps, E. A. (2001). Lesions of the human amygdala impair enhanced perception of emotionally salient events. *Nature*, **411**, 305–309.

Armony, J. L. and Dolan, R. J. (2001). Modulation of auditory neural responses by a visual context in human fear conditioning. *NeuroReport*, **12**, 3407–3411.

Armony, J. L., Quirk, G. J., and LeDoux, J. E. (1998). Differential effects of amygdala lesions on early and late plastic components of auditory cortex spike trains during fear conditioning. *J. Neurosci.*, **18**, 2592–2601.

Augustine, A. R. (1996). Circuitry and functional aspects of the insular lobe in primates including humans. *Brain Res. Rev.*, **22**, 229–244.

Baird, A. A., Gruber, S. A., Fein, D. A., Maas, L. C., Steingard, R. J., Renshaw, P. F., Cohen, B. M., and Yurgelun-Todd, D. A. (1999). Functional magnetic resonance imaging of facial affect recognition in children and adolescents. *J. Am. Acad. Child Adolesc. Psychiatry*, **38**, 195–199.

Bakin, J. S. and Weinberger, N. M. (1990). Classical conditioning induces CS-specific receptive field plasticity in the auditory cortex of the guinea pig. *Brain Res.*, **536**, 271–286.

Bakin, J. S. and Weinberger, N. M. (1996). Induction of a physiological memory in the cerebral cortex by stimulation of the nucleus basalis. *Proc. Natl. Acad. Sci. USA*, **93**, 11219–24.

Barbur, J. L., Ruddock, K. H., and Waterfield, V. A. (1980). Human visual responses in the absence of the geniculo-calcarine projection. *Brain*, **103**, 905–928.

Bard, P. (1929). The central representation of the sympathetic system: as indicated by certain physiological observations. *Arch. Neurol. Psychiatry*, **22**, 230–246.

Baxter, M. G., Parker, A., Lindner, C. A. A., Izquierdo, A. D., and Murray, E. A. (2000). Control of response selection by reinforcer value requires interaction of amygdala and orbitofrontal cortex. *J. Neurosci.*, **20**, 4311–4319.

Bechara, A., Tranel, D., Damasio, H. Adolphs, R., Rockland, C., and Damasio, A. R. (1995). Double dissociation of conditioning and declarative knowledge relative to the amygdala and hippocampus in humans. *Science*, **269**, 1115–1118.

Bechara, A. Damasio, H. Tranel, D., and Damasio. A. R. (1997). Deciding advantageously before knowing the advantageous strategy. *Science*, **275**, 1293–1295.

Bench, C. J., Friston, K. J., Brown, R. G., Scott, L. C., Frackowiak, R. S., and Dolan, R. J. (1992). The anatomy of melancholia: focal abnormalities of cerebral blood flow in major depression. *Psychol. Med.*, **22**, 607–615.

Bench, C. J., Frackowiak, R. S., and Dolan, R. J. (1995). Changes in regional cerebral blood flow on recovery from depression. *Psychol. Med.*, **25**, 247–261

Bermudez-Rattoni, F., Introini-Collison, I. B., and McGaugh, J. L. (1991). Reversible lesions of the insular cortex by tetrodotoxin produce retrograde and anterograde amnesia for inhibitory avoidance and spatial learning. *Proc. Natl. Acad. Sci. USA*, **88**, 5379–5382.

Berns, G. S., McClure, S. M., Pagnoni, G., and Montague, P. R. (2001). Predictability modulates human brain response to reward. *J. Neurosci.*, **21**, 2793–2798.

Bevenuto, L. A. and Fallon, J. H. (1975). The ascending projections of the superior colliculus in the rhesus monkey (*Macaca mulatta*). *J. Comp. Neurol.*, **160**, 339–362.

Birbaumer, N., Grodd, W., Diedrich, O., Klose, U., Erb, M., Lotze, M., Schneider, F., Weiss, U., and Flor, H. (1998). fMRI reveals amygdala activation to human faces in social phobics. *NeuroReport*, **9**, 1223–1226.

Blair, R. J., Morris, J. S., Frith, C. D., Perrett, D. I., and Dolan, R. J. (1999). Dissociable neural responses to facial expressions of sadness and anger. *Brain* **122**, 883–893.

Blanchard, D. C. and Blanchard, R. J. (1972). Innate and conditioned reactions to threat in rats with amygdaloid lesions. *J. Comp. Physiol. Psychol.*, **81**, 281–290.

Blood, A. J., Zatorre, R. J. (2001). Intensely pleasurable responses to music correlate with activity in brain regions implicated in reward and emotion. *Proc. Natl. Acad. Sci. USA*, **98**, 11818–118123.

Blumberg, H. P., Stern, E., Martinez, D., Ricketts, S., de Asis, J., White, T., Epstein, J., McBride, P. A., Eidelberg, D., Kocsis, J. H., and Silbersweig, D. A. (2000). Increased anterior cingulate and caudate activity in bipolar mania. *Biol. Psychiatry*, **48**, 1045–1052.

Blythe, I. M., Kennard, C., and Ruddock, K. H. (1987). Residual vision in patients with retrogeniculate lesions of the visual pathways. *Brain*, **110**, 887–905.

Breiter, H. C., Etcoff, N. L., Whalen, P. J., Kennedy, D. N., Rauch, S. L., Buckner, R. L., Strauss, M. M., Hyman, S. E., and Rosen, B. R. (1996). Response and habituation of the human amygdala during visual processing of facial expression. *Neuron*, **2**, 875–887.

Breiter, H. C., Gollub, R. L., Weisskoff, R. M., Kennedy, D. N., Makris, N., Berke, J. D., Goodman, J. M., Kantor, H. L., Gastfriend, D. R., Riorden, J. P., Mathew, R. T., Rosen, B. R., and Hyman, S. E. (1997). Acute effects of cocaine on human brain activity and emotion. *Neuron*, **19**, 591–611.

Bremner, J. D., Innis, R. B., Salomon, R. M., Staib, L. H., Ng, C. K., Miller, H. L., Bronen, R. A., Krystal, J. H., Duncan, J., Rich, D., Price, L. H., Malison, R., Dey, H., Soufer, R., and Charney, D. S. (1997). Positron emission tomography measurement of cerebral metabolic correlates of tryptophan depletion-induced depressive relapse. *Arch. Gen. Psychiatry*, **54**, 364–374.

Breuer, J. and Freud, S. (1895/2000). *Studies on Hysteria*. Basic Books Classics, New York.

Broca, P. (1878). Anatomie comparee des circonvolutions cerebrales. Le grand lobe limbique et la scissure limbique dans la serie des mammiferes. *Revue Anthropologique*, **I**, 385–498.

Buchanan, T. W., Lutz, K., Mirzazade, S., Specht, K., Shah, N. J., Zilles, K., and Jancke, L. (2000). Recognition of emotional prosody and verbal components of spoken language: an fMRI study. *Brain Res. Cogn Brain Res.*, **9**, 227–238.

Buchel, C., Morris, J., Dolan, R. J., and Friston, K. J. (1998). Brain systems mediating aversive conditioning: an event-related fMRI study. *Neuron*, **20**, 947–957.

Buchel, C., Dolan, R. J., Armony, J. L., and Friston, K. J. (1999). Amygdala–hippocampal involvement in human aversive trace conditioning revealed through event-related functional magnetic resonance imaging. *J. Neurosci.*, **19**, 10869–10876.

Buchel C, Bornhovd, K., Quante, M., Glauche, V., Bromm, B., and Weiller, C. (2002). Dissociable neural responses related to pain intensity, stimulus intensity, and stimulus awareness within the anterior cingulate cortex: a parametric single-trial laser functional magnetic resonance imaging study. *J. Neurosci.*, **22**, 970–976.

Bullmore, D., Perrett, I., Rowland, D., Williams, S. C., and Gray, J. A. David, A. S. (1997). A specific neural substrate for perceiving facial expressions of disgust. *Nature*, **389**, 495–498.

Bussey, T. J., Everitt, B. J., and Robbins, T. W. (1997). Dissociable effects of cingulate and medial frontal cortex lesions on stimulus-reward learning using a novel Pavlovian autoshaping procedure for the rat: implications for the neurobiology of emotion. *Behav. Neurosci.*, **111**, 908–919.

Butter, C. M. (1969). Perseveration in extinction and in discrimination reversal tasks following selective prefrontal ablations in *Macaca mulatta*. *Physiol. Behav.*, **4**, 163–171.

Butter, C. M., McDonald, J. A., and Snyder, D. R. (1969a). Orality, preference behaviour and reinforcement value of non-food object in monkeys with orbital frontal lesions. *Science*, **164**, 1306–1307.

Butter, C. M., Snyder, D. R., and McDonald, J. A. (1969b). Effects of orbitofrontal lesions on aversive and aggressive behaviours in rhesus monkeys. *J. Comp. Physiol. Psychol.*, **72**, 132–144.

Cahill, L. and McGaugh, J. L. (1998). Mechanisms of emotional arousal and lasting declarative memory. *Trends Neurosci.*, **21**, 294–299.

Cahill, L., Babinsky, R., Markowitsch, H. J., and McGaugh, J. L. (1995). The amygdala and emotional memory. *Nature*, **377**, 295–296.

Cahill, L., Haier, R. J., Fallon, J., Alkire, M. T., Tang, C., Keator, D., Wu, J., and McGaugh, J. L. (1996). Amygdala activity at encoding correlated with long-term, free recall of emotional information. *Proc. Natl. Acad. Sci. USA*, **93**, 8016–8021.

Cahill, L., Haier, R. J., White, N. S., Fallon, J., Kilpatrick, L., Lawrence, C., Potkin, S. G., and Alkire, M. T. (2001). Sex-related difference in amygdala activity during emotionally influenced memory storage. *Neurobiol. Learn. Mem.*, **75**, 1–9.

Caldecott-Hazard, S., Mazziotta, J., and Phelps, M. (1988). Cerebral correlates of depressed behaviour in rats, visualised using ^{14}C-2-deoxyglucose autoradiography. *J. Neurosci.*, **8**, 1951–1961.

Calder, A. J., Keane, J., Manes, F., Antoun, N., and Young, A. W. (2000). Impaired recognition and experience of disgust following brain injury. *Nat. Neurosci.*, **3**, 1077–1078.

Calder, A. J., Lawrence, A. D., and Young, A. W. (2001). Neuropsychology of fear and loathing. *Nat. Rev. Neurosci.*, **2**, 352–363.

Cancelliere, A. E. and Kertesz, A. (1990). Lesion localisation in acquired deficits of emotional expression and comprehension. *Brain Cogn.*, **13**, 133–147.

Canli, T., Zhao, Z., Brewer, J., Gabrieli, J. D., and Cahill, L. (2000). Event-related activation in the human amygdala associates with later memory for individual emotional experience. *J. Neurosci.*, **20**(RC99), 1–5

Canli, T., Zhao, Z., Desmond, J. E., Kang, E., Gross, J., and Gabrieli, J. D. (2001). An fMRI study of personality influences on brain reactivity to emotional stimuli. *Behav. Neurosci.*, **115**, 33–42.

Cannon, W. B. (1927). The James–Lange theory of emotion: a critical examination and an alternative theory. *Am. J. Psychol.*, **39**, 106–124.

Carmichael, S. T. and Price, J. L. (1994). Architectonic subdivision of the orbital and medial prefrontal cortex in the macaque monkey. *J. Comp. Neurol.*, **346**, 366–402.

Carmichael, S. T. and Price, J. L. (1995a). Limbic connections of the orbital and medial prefrontal cortex in macaque monkeys. *J. Comp. Neurol.*, **363**, 615–641.

Carmichael, S. T. and Price, J. L. (1995b). Sensory and premotor connections of the orbital and medial prefrontal cortex of macaque monkeys. *J. Comp. Neurol.*, **363**, 642–664.

Carter, C. S., Macdonald, A. M., Botvinick, M., Ross, L. L., Stenger, V. A., Noll, D., and Cohen, J. D. (2000). Parsing executive processes: strategic vs. evaluative functions of the anterior cingulate cortex. *Proc. Natl. Acad. Sci. USA*, **97**, 1944–1948.

Casey, B. J. (2001). Amygdala response to facial expressions in children and adults. *Biol. Psychiatry*, **49**, 309–316.

Casey, K. L. *et al.* (1994). Positron emission tomographic analysis of cerebral structures activated specifically by repetitive noxious heat stimuli. *J. Neurophysiol.*, **71**, 802–807.

Cavada, C., Company, T., Tejedor, J., Cruz-Rizzolo, R. J., and Reinoso-Suarez, F. (2000). The anatomical connections of the macaque monkey orbitofrontal cortex: a review. *Cereb. Cortex*, **10**, 220–242.

Chiavaras, M. M. and Petrides, M. J. (2000). Orbitofrontal sulci of the human and macaque monkey brain. *J. Comp. Neurol.*, **422**, 35–54.

Cohen, R. A., Kaplan, R. F., Moser, D. J., Jenkins, M. A., and Wilkinson, H. (1999). Impairments of attention after cingulotomy. *Neurology*, **53**, 819–24.

Critchley, H. D. and Rolls, E. T. (1996). Hunger and satiety modify responses in the primate orbitofrontal cortex: analysis in an olfactory discrimination task. *J. Neurophysiol.*, **75**, 1659–1672.

Critchley, H. D., Daly, E., Phillips, M., Brammer, M., Bullmore, E., Williams, S., Van Amelsvoort, T., Robertson, D., David, A., and Murphy, D. (2000a). Explicit and implicit neural mechanisms for processing of social information from facial expressions: a functional magnetic resonance imaging study. *Hum. Brain Mapping*, **9**, 93–105.

Critchley, H. D., Corfield, D. R., Chandler, M. P., Mathias, C. J., and Dolan, R. J. (2000b). Cerebral correlates of autonomic cardiovascular arousal: a functional neuroimaging investigation in humans. *J. Physiol.*, **523**, 259–270.

Critchley, H. D. *et al.* (2002). Fear conditioning in humans: the influence of awareness and autonomic arousal on functional neuroanatomy. *Neuron*, **33**, 653–663.

Damasio, A. (1994). *Descartes' Error*. Avon Books, New York.

Damasio, A. (1999). *The Feeling of What Happens*. Harcourt Brace, New York.

Darwin, C. (1872/1965). *The Expression of the Emotions in Man and Animals*. University of Chicago Press, Chicago.

Davidson, R. J., Pizzagalli, D., Nitschke, J. B., and Putnam, K. (2002). Depression: perspectives from affective neuroscience. *Annu. Rev. Psychol.*, **53**, 545–574.

Davis, M. (1992). The amygdala and conditioned fear, in *The Amygdala: Neurobiological Aspects of Emotion, Memory and Mental Dysfunction*, Aggleton, J. P., Ed., pp. 255–306. Wiley-Liss, New York.

Dawson, M. E. and Schell, A. M. (1995). Information processing and human autonomic classical conditioning. *Adv. Psychophysiol.*, **1**, 89–109.

de Gelder, B. Recognising emotions by ear and eye, in: Lane, R. and Nadel, L. eds Cognitive Neuroscience of Emotions. Oxford: Oxfrod University Press, 1999 pp84–105.

Degos, J. D., da Fonseca, N., Gray, F., and Cesaro, P. (1993). Severe frontal syndrome associated with infarcts of the left cingulate gyrus and the head of the right caudate nucleus a clinical pathological case. *Brain*, **116**, 1541–1548.

DeKosky, S. T., Heilman, K. M., Bowers, D., and Valenstein, E. (1980). Recognition and discrimination of emotional faces and pictures. *Brain Lang.*, **9**, 206–214.

Delgado P. L., Charney D. S. , Price L. H. , Aghajanian G. K., Landis H., and Heninger G. R. Serotonin function and the mechanism of antidepressant action. Reversal of antidepressant-induced remission by rapid depletion of plasma tryptophan. *Arch. Gen. Psychiatry*, 1990 **47**, 411–8.

Derbyshire S. W., Jones A. K., Devani P., Friston K. J., Feinmann C., Harris M., Pearce S., Watson J. D., and Frackowiak, R. S. J. Cerebral responses to pain in patients with atypical facial pain measured by positron emission tomography. J Neurol Neurosurg Psychiat 1994; **57**, 1166–72.

Descartes, R. Meditations on First Philosophy. 1641/1996. Cambridge University Press.

Devinsky, O., Morrell, M. J., and Vogt, B. A. (1995). Contributions of anterior cingulate cortex to behaviour. *Brain*, **118**, 279–306.

Dolan, R. J., Fletcher, P., Morris, J., Kapur, N., Deakin, J. F., and Frith, C. D. (1996). Neural activation during covert processing of positive emotional facial expressions. *NeuroImage*, **4**, 194–200.

Dolan, R. J., Lane, R., Chua, P., and Fletcher, P. (2000). Dissociable temporal lobe activations during emotional episodic memory retrieval. *NeuroImage*, **11**, 203–209.

Drevets, W. C. (1999). Prefrontal cortical-amygdalar metabolism in major depression. *Ann. N.Y. Acad. Sci.*, **877**, 614–637.

Drevets, W. C., Price, J. L., Simpson, J. R., Jr., Todd, R. D., Reich, T., Vannier, M., and Raichle, M. E. (1997). Subgenual prefrontal cortex abnormalities in mood disorders. *Nature*, **386**, 824–827.

Drevets, W. C., Price, J. L., Bardgett, M. E., Reich, T., Todd, R. D., and Raichle, M. E. (2002). Glucose metabolism in the amygdala in depression: relationship to diagnostic subtype and plasma cortisol levels. *Pharmacol. Biochem. Behav.*, **71**, 431–447.

Ekman, P. (1982). *Emotion in the Human Face*. Cambridge University Press, Cambridge, U.K.

Ekman, P. and Friesen, W. V. (1976). *Pictures of Facial Affect*. Consulting Psychologists Press, Palo Alto, CA.

Elliott, R., Baker, S. C., Rogers, R. D., O'Leary, D. A., Paykel, E. S., Frith, C. D., Dolan, R. J., and Sahakian, B. J. (1997). Prefrontal dysfunction in depressed patients performing a complex planning task: a study using positron emission tomography. *Psychol. Med.*, **27**, 931–942.

Eslinger, P. and Damasio, A. (1985). Severe disturbance of higher cognition after bilateral frontal lobe ablation: patient EVR. *Neurology*, **35**, 1731–1741.

Esteves, F. and Ohman, A. (1994). Nonconscious associative learning: Pavlovian conditioning of skin conductance responses to masked fear-relevant facial stimuli. *Psychophysiology*, **31**, 375–385.

Esteves, F., Dimberg, U., and Ohman, A. (1994). Automatically elicited fear: conditioned skin conductance responses to masked facial expressions. *Cogn. and Emotion* **9**, 99–108.

Francis, S., Rolls, E. T., Bowtell, R., McGlone, F., O'Doherty, J., Browning, A., Clare, S., and Smith, E. (1999). The representation of pleasant touch in the brain and its relationship with taste and olfactory areas. *NeuroReport*, **10**, 453–459.

Fredrikson, M., Wik, G., Greitz, T., Eriksson, L., Stone-Elander, S., Ericson, K., and Sedvall, G. (1993). Regional cerebral blood flow during experimental phobic fear. *Psychophysiology*, **30**, 126–130.

Fredrikson, M., Wik, G., Fischer, H., and Andersson, J. (1995). Affective and attentive neural networks in humans: a PET study of Pavlovian conditioning. *NeuroReport*, **7**, 97–101.

Friston, K. J., Tononi, G., Reeke, G. N., Jr., Sporns, O., and Edelman, G. M. (1994). Value-dependent selection in the brain: simulation in a synthetic neural model. *Neuroscience*, **59**, 229–243.

Friston, K. J., Buechal C., Fink, G., Morris, J. S., Rolls, E. T., and Dolan, R. J. (1997). Psychophysiological and modulatory interactions in neuroimaging. *Neuroimage* **6**, 218–229.

Friston, K. J., Fletcher, P., Josephs, O., Holmes, A., Rugg, M. D., and Turner, R. (1998). Event-related fMRI: characterising differential responses. *NeuroImage*, **7**, 30–40.

Furmark, T., Fischer, H., Wik, G., Larsson, M., and Fredrikson, M. (1997). The amygdala and individual differences in human fear conditioning. *NeuroReport*, **8**, 3957–3960.

Gallagher, M. S., Graham, P. W., and Holland, P. C. (1990). The amygdala central nucleus and appetitive Pavlovian conditioning: lesions impair one class of conditioned behaviour. *J. Neurosci.*, **10**, 1906–1911.

Gazzaniga, M. S. and Smylie, C. S. (1983). Facial recognition and brain asymmetries: clues to underlying mechanisms. *Annals of Neurologyl* **13**, 536–540.

George, M. S., Ketter, T. A., Gill, D. S., Haxby, J. V., Ungerleider, L. G., Herscovitch, P., and Post, R. M. (1993). Brain regions involved in recognising facial emotion or identity: an oxygen-15 PET study. *J. Neuropsychiatry Clin. Neurosci.*, **5**, 384–394.

George, M. S., Ketter, T. A., Parekh, P. I., Rosinsky, N., Ring, H., Casey, B. J. *et al.* (1994). Regional brain activity when selecting a response despite interference: an $H_2{}^{15}O$ PET study of the Stroop and the emotional Stroop. *Hum. Brain Mapping*, **1**, 194–209.

George, M. S., Parekh, P. I., Rosinsky, N., Ketter, T. A., Kimbrell, T. A., Heilman, K. M., Herscovitch, P., and Post, R. M. (1996). Understanding emotional prosody activates right hemisphere regions. *Arch. Neurol.*, **53**, 665–670.

George, N., Driver, J., and Dolan, R. J. (2001). Seen gaze-direction modulates fusiform activity and its coupling with other brain areas during face processing. *NeuroImage*, **13**, 1102–1112.

Gold, P. E. and Van Buskirk, R. B. (1975). Facilitation of time-dependent memory processes with posttrial epinephrine injections. *Behav. Biol.*, **13**, 145–153.

Gorno-Tempini, M. L., Pradelli, S., Serafini, M., Pagnoni, G., Baraldi, P., Porro, C., Nicoletti, R., Umita, C., and Nichelli, P. (2001). Explicit and incidental facial expression processing: an fMRI study. *NeuroImage*, **14**, 465–473.

Goulet, S. and Murray, E. A. (2001). Neural substrates of crossmodal association memory in monkeys: the amygdala versus the anterior rhinal cortex. *Behav. Neurosci.*, **115**, 271–284.

Gray, J. A. and Brammer, M. J. (2001). Time courses of left and right amygdalar responses to fearful facial expressions. *Hum. Brain Mapping*, **12**, 193–202.

Greenberg, N., Scott, M., and Crews, D. (1984). Role of the amygdala in the reproductive and aggressive behaviour of the lizard. *Physiology and behaviour*, **32**, 147–151.

Gur, R. C., Skolnick, B. E., and Gur, R. E. (1994). Effects of emotional discrimination tasks on cerebral blood flow: regional activation and its relation to performance. *Brain and Cognition* **25**, 271–286.

Halgren, E., Babb, T. L., Rausch, R., and Crandall, P. H. (1978). Mental phenomena evoked by electrical stimulation of the human hippocampal formation and amygdala. *Brain*, **101**, 83–117.

Hamann, S. B., Ely, T. D., Grafton, S. T., and Kilts, C. D. (1999). Amygdala activity related to enhanced memory for pleasant and aversive stimuli. *Nat. Neurosci.*, **2**, 289–293.

Hariri, A. R., Bookheimer, S. Y., and Mazziotta, J. C. (2000). Modulating emotional responses: effects of a neocortical network on the limbic system. *NeuroReport*, **11**, 43–48.

Hariri, A. R., Mattay, V. S., Tessitore, A., Kolachana, B., Fera, F., Goldman, D., Egan, M. F., and Weinberger, D. R. (2002). Serotonin transporter genetic variation and the response of the human amygdala. *Science*, **297**, 400–403.

Hatfield, T., Han, J. S., Conley, M., Gallagher, M., and Holland, P. (1996). Neurotoxic lesions of basolateral, but not central, amygdala interfere with Pavlovian second-order conditioning and reinforcer devaluation effects. *J. Neurosci.*, **16**, 5256–5265.

Heninger, G. R., Charney, D. S., and Sternberg, D. E. (1984). Serotonergic function in depression: prolactin response to intravenous tryptophan in depressed patients and healthy subjects. *Arch. Gen. Psychiatry*, **41**, 398–402.

Hitchcock, J. M. and Davis, M. (1991). Efferent pathway of the amygdala involved in conditioned fear as measured with the fear-potentiated startle paradigm. *Behav. Neurosci.*, **105**, 826–842.

Hornak, J., Rolls, E. T., and Wade, D. (1996). Face and voice expression identification in patients with emotional and behavioural changes following ventral frontal lobe damage. *Neuropsychologia*, **34**, 247–261.

Hugdahl, K., Berardi, A., Thompson, W. L., Kosslyn, S. M., Macy, R., Baker, D. P., Alpert, N. M., and LeDoux, J. E. (1995). Brain mechanisms in human classical conditioning: a PET blood flow study. *NeuroReport*, **6**, 1723–1728.

Hume, D., Iversen, S. D., and Mishkin, M. (1970). Perseverative interference in monkey following selective lesions of the inferior prefrontal convexity. *Exp. Brain Res.*, **11**, 376–386.

Iwata, J., LeDoux, J. E., Meeley, M. P., Arneric, S., and Reis, D. J., (1986). Intrinsic neurons in the amygdaloid field projected to by the medial geniculate body mediate emotional responses conditioned to acoustic stimuli. *Brain Res.*, **383**, 195–214.

James, W. (1884). What is an emotion? *Mind*, **9**, 188–205.

Johnsrude, I. S., Owen, A. M., White, N. M., Zhao, W. V., and Bohbot, V. (2000). Impaired preference conditioning after anterior temporal lobe resection in humans. *J. Neurosci.*, **20**, 2649–2656.

Jones, B. and Mishkin, M. (1972). Limbic lesions and the problem of stimulus-reinforcement associations. *Exp. Neurol.*, **36**, 362–377.

Kansaku, K. and Kitazawa, S. (2001). Imaging studies on sex differences in the lateralisation of language. *Neurosci. Res.*, **41**, 333–337.

Kansaku, K., Yamaura, A., and Kitazawa, S. (2000). Sex differences in lateralisation revealed in the posterior language areas. *Cereb. Cortex*, **10**, 866–872.

Kesler-West, M. L., Andersen, A. H., Smith, C. D., Avison, M. J., Davis, C. E., Kryscio, R. J., and Blonder, L. X. (2001). Neural substrates of facial emotion processing using fMRI. *Brain Res. Cogn Brain Res.*, **11**, 213–226.

Kilgard, M. P. and Merzenich, M. M. (1998). Cortical map reorganisation enabled by nucleus basalis activity. *Science*, **279**, 1714–1718.

Killgore, W. D. and Yurgelun-Todd, D. A. (2001). Sex differences in amygdala activation during the perception of facial affect. *NeuroReport*, **12**, 2543–2547.

Killgore, W. D., Oki, M., and Yurgelun-Todd, D. A. (2001). Sex-specific developmental changes in amygdala responses to affective faces. *NeuroReport*, **12**, 427–433.

Kluver, H. and Bucy, P. C. (1939). Preliminary analysis of the functions of the temporal lobes in monkeys. *Arch. Neurol. Psychiat.*, **42**, 979–1000.

Knight, D. C., Smith, C. N., Stein, E. A., and Helmstetter, F. J. (1999). Functional MRI of human Pavlovian fear conditioning: patterns of activation as a function of learning. *NeuroReport*, **10**, 3665–3670.

Krettek, J. E. and Price, J. L. (1974). A direct input from amygdala to the thalamus and the cerebral cortex. *Brain Res.*, **67**, 169–174.

Krettek, J. E. and Price, J. L. (1977). The cortical projections of the mediodorsal nucleus and adjacent thalamic nuclei in the rat. *J. Comp. Neurol.*, **171**, 157–192.

Krezel, W., Dupont, S., Krust, A., Chambon, P., and Chapman, P. F. (2001). Increased anxiety and synaptic plasticity in estrogen receptor beta-deficient mice. *Proc. Natl. Acad. Sci. USA*, **98**, 12278–12282.

LaBar, K. S., LeDoux, J. E., Spencer, D. D., and Phelps, E. A. (1995). Impaired fear conditioning following unilateral temporal lobectomy in humans. *J. Neurosci.*, **15**, 6846–6855.

LaBar, K. S., Gatenby, J. C., Gore, J. C., LeDoux, J. E., and Phelps, E. A. (1998). Human amygdala activation during conditioned fear acquisition and extinction: a mixed trial study. *Neuron*, **20**, 937–945.

Ladavas, E., Cimatti, D., Del Pesce, M., and Tuozzi, G. (1993). Emotional evaluation with and without conscious stimulus identification: evidence from a split-brain patient. *Cogn. Emotion*, **7**, 95–114.

Lander, E. S. *et al.* (2001). Initial sequencing and analysis of the human genome. *Nature*, **409**, 860–921.

Lane, R. D., Reiman, E. M., Ahern, G. L., Schwartz, G. E., and Davidson, R. J. (1997). Neuroanatomical correlates of happiness, sadness, and disgust. *Am. J. Psychiatry*, **154**, 926–933.

Lang, P. J., Bradley, M. M., Fitzsimmons, J. R., Cuthbert, B.N., Scott, J. D., Moulder, B., and Nangia, V. (1998). Emotional arousal and activation of the visual cortex: an fMRI analysis. *Psychophysiology*, **35**, 199–210.

Lazarus, R. S. (1984). On the primacy of affect. *Am. Psychol.*, **39**, 124–129.

LeDoux, J. E. (1987). Emotion, in *Handbook of Physiology*, Section 1, *The Nervous System*, Vol. 5, *Higher Functions of the Brain*, Plum, F., Ed., pp. 419–460. American Physiological Society, Bethesda, MD.

LeDoux, J. E. (1996). *The Emotional Brain*. Simon & Shuster, New York.

LeDoux, J. E., Sakaguchi, A., and Reis, D. J. (1984). Subcortical efferent projections of the medial geniculate nucleus mediate emotional responses conditioned to acoustic stimuli. *J. Neurosci.*, **4**, 683–698.

LeDoux, J. E., Cicchetti, P., Xagoraris, A., and Romanski, L. M. (1990). The lateral amygdaloid nucleus: sensory interface of the amygdala in fear conditioning. *J. Neurosci.*, **10**, 1062–1069.

Lennartz, R. C. and Weinberger, N. M. (1992). Frequency-specific receptive field plasticity in the medial geniculate body induced by pavlovian fear conditioning is expressed in the anesthetised brain. *Behav. Neurosci.*, **106**, 484–497.

Liang, K. C., Juler, R. G., and McGaugh, J. L. (1986). Modulating effects of posttraining epinephrine on memory: involvement of the amygdala noradrenergic system. *Brain Res.*, **368**, 125–133.

Linke, R., de Lima, A. D., Scwegler, H., and Pape, H.-C. (1999). Direct synaptic connections of axons from superior colliculus with identified thalamo-amygdaloid projection neurons in the rat: possible substrates of a subcortical visual pathway to the amygdala. *J. Comp. Neurol.*, **403**, 158–170.

Linke, R., Braune, G., and Schwegler, H. (2000). Differential projection of the posterior paralaminar thalamic nuclei to the amygdaloid complex in the rat. *Exp. Brain Res.*, **134**, 520–532.

Lovibond, P. F. and Shanks, D. R. (2002). The role of awareness in Pavlovian conditioning: empirical evidence and theoretical implications. *J. Exp. Psychol. Anim. Behav. Proc.*, **28**, 3–26.

Macknik, S. L. and Livingstone, M. S. (1998). Neuronal correlates of visiblility and invisibility in the primate visual system. *Nat. Neurosci.*, **1**, 144–149.

Maclean, P. D. (1952). Some psychiatric implications of physiological studies on frontotemporal portion of limbic system (visceral brain). *Electroencephalogr. Clin. Neurophysiol.*, **4**, 407–418.

Malkova, L., Gaffan, D., and Murray, E. A. (1997). Excitotoxic lesions of the amygdala fail to produce impairment in visual learning for auditory secondary reinforcement but interfere with reinforcer devaluation effects in rhesus monkeys. *J. Neurosci.*, **17**(15), 6011–6020.

Maratos, E. J., Dolan, R. J., Morris, J. S., Henson, R. N., and Rugg, M. D. (2001). Neural activity associated with episodic memory for emotional context. *Neuropsychologia*, **39**, 910–920.

Mayberg, H. S., Lewis, P. J., Regenold, W., and Wagner, H. N., Jr. (1994). Paralimbic hypoperfusion in unipolar depression. *J. Nucl. Med.*, **35**, 929–934.

Mayberg, H. S., Liotti, M., Brannan, S. K., McGinnis, S., Mahurin, R. K., Jerabek, P. A., Silva, J. A., Tekell, J. L., Martin, C. C., Lancaster, J. L., and Fox, P. T. (1999). Reciprocal limbic-cortical function and negative mood: converging PET findings in depression and normal sadness. *Am. J. Psychiatry*, **156**, 675–682.

McGaugh, J. L., Ferry, B., Vazdarjanova, A., and Roozendaal, B. (2000). Amygdala: role in modulation of memory storage, in *The Amygdala: A Functional Analysis*, Aggleton, J. P., Ed., pp. 391–423, Oxford University Press, London.

Meeres, S. L. and Graves, R. E. (1990). Localisation of unseen visual stimuli by humans with normal vision. *Neuropsychologia*, **28**, 1231–1237.

Micheau, J., Destrade, C., Soumireu-Mourat, B. (1981). Intraventricular corticosterone injection facilitates memory of an appetitive discriminative task in mice. *Behav. Neural Biol.*, **31**, 100–104.

Morris, J. S. and Dolan, R. J. (2003). Orbitofrontal and amygdala responses during fear reversal learning. *NeuroImage*, submittted.

Morris, J. S., Frith, C. D., Perrett, D. I., Rowland, D., Young, A. W., Calder, A. J., and Dolan, R. J. (1996). A differential neural response in the human amygdala to fearful and happy facial expressions. *Nature*, **383**, 812–815.

Morris, J. S., Friston, K. J., and Dolan, R. J. (1997). Neural responses to salient visual stimuli. *Proc. Roy. Soc. London Ser. B*, **264**, 760–775.

Morris, J. S., Friston K. J., Buechal C., Frith, C. D., Young, A. W., Calder, A. J., and Dolan, R. J. (1998a). A neuromodulatory role for the human amygdala in processing emotional facial expressions. *Brain*, **121**, 47–57.

Morris, J. S., Friston, K. J., and Dolan, R. J. (1998b). Experience-dependent modulation of tonotopic neural responses in human auditory cortex. *Proc. Roy. Soc. London Ser. B, Biol. Sci.*, **265**, 649–657.

Morris, J. S., Ohman, A., and Dolan, R. J. (1999a). A subcortical pathway to the right amygdala mediating "unseen" fear. *Proc. Natl. Acad. Sci. USA*, **96**, 1680–1685.

Morris, J. S., Scott, S. K., and Dolan R. J. (1999b). Saying it with feeling: neural responses to emotional vocalisations. *Neuropsychologia*, **37**, 1155–1163.

Morris, J. S., Ohman, A., Dolan, R. J. (1998c). Conscious and unconscious emotional learning in the human amygdala. *Nature*, **393**, 467–470.

Morris, J. S., Smith, K. A., Cowan, P. J., Friston, K. J., and Dolan, K. J., (1999c). Covariation of activity in habenuia and dorsal raphé nuclei following tryptophan depletion. *NeuroImage*, **10**, 163–172.

Morris, J. S., Buechel, C., and Dolan, R. J. (2001a). Parallel neural responses in amygdala subregions and sensory cortex during implicit aversive conditioning. *NeuroImage*, **13**, 1044–1052.

Morris, J. S. and Dolan, R. J. (2001b). Involvement of human amygdala and orbitofrontal cortex in hunger-enhanced memory for food stimuli. *J. Neurosci.*, **21**, 5304–5310.

Murphy, M. R., MacLean, P. D., and Hamilton, S. C. (1981). Species-typical behaviour of hamsters deprived from birth of the neocortex. *Science*, **213**, 459–461.

Murray, E. A. and Mishkin, M. (1985). Amygdalectomy impairs crossmodal association in monkeys. *Science*, **228**, 604–606.

Nakamura, K., Kawashima, R., Nagumo, S., Ito, K., Sugiura, M., Kato, T., Nakamura, A., Hatano, K., Kubota, K., Fukuda, H., and Kojima, S. (1998). Neuroanatomical correlates of the assessment of facial attractiveness. *NeuroReport*, **9**, 753–757.

Nishijo, H., Ono, T., and Nishino, H. (1988). Topographic distribution of modality-specific amygdalar neurons in alert monkey. *J. Neurosci.*, **8**, 3556–3569.

Nishijo, H., Uwano, T., Tamura, R., and Ono, T. (1998). Gustatory and multimodal neuronal responses in the amygdala during licking and discrimination of sensory stimuli in awake rats. *J. Neurophysiol.*, **79**, 21–36.

Nobre, A. C., Sebestyen, G. N., Gitelman, D. R., Mesulam, M. M., Frackowiak, R. S., and Frith, C. D. (1997). Functional localisation of the system for visuospatial attention using positron emission tomography. *Brain*, **120**, 515–533.

O'Doherty, J., Rolls, E. T., Francis, S., Bowtell, R., McGlone, F., Kobal, G., Renner, B., and Ahne, G. (2000). Sensory-specific satiety-related olfactory activation of the human orbitofrontal cortex. *NeuroReport*, **11**, 893–897.

O'Doherty, J., Rolls, E. T., Francis, S., Bowtell, R., and McGlone, F. (2001). Representation of pleasant and aversive taste in the human brain. *J. Neurophysiol.*, **85**, 1315–1321.

O'Doherty, J. P., Deichmann, R., Critchley, H. D., and Dolan, R. J. (2002). Neural responses during anticipation of a primary taste reward. *Neuron*, **33**, 815–826.

Ohman, A. (1979). The orienting response, attention, and learning: an information processing perspective, in *The Orienting Reflex in Humans*, Kimmel, H. D., Van Olst, E. H., and Orlebeke, J. F., Eds., pp. 443–472. Lawrence Erlbaum, Hillsdale, NJ.

Ohman, A. and Mineka, S. (2001). Fears, phobias, and preparedness: toward an evolved module of fear and fear learning. *Psychol. Rev.*, **108**, 483–522.

Ohman, A. and Soares, J. J. F. (1993). On the automaticity of phobic fear: conditioned skin conductance responses to masked phobic stimuli. *J. Abnorm. Psychol.*, **102**, 121–132.

Ohman, A. and Soares, J. J. F. (1998). Emotional conditioning to masked stimuli: expectancies for aversive outcomes following non-recognised fear-relevant stimuli. *J. Exp. Psychol. Gen.*, **127**, 69–82.

Ohman, O., Friedrikson, M., and Hugdahl, K. (1978). Orienting and defensive responding in the electrodermal system: palmar-dorsal differences and recovery rate during conditioning to potentially phobic stimuli. *Psychophysiology*, **15**, 93–101.

Oppenheimer, S. M., Gelb, A., Girvin, J. P., and Hachinski, V. (1992). Cardiovascular effects of human insula cortex stimulation. *Neurology*, **42**, 1727–1732.

Osterlund, M. K., Keller, E., and Hurd, Y. L. (2000). The human forebrain has discrete estrogen receptor alpha messenger RNA expression: high levels in the amygdaloid complex. *Neuroscience*, **95**, 333–342.

Papez, J. W. (1937). A proposed mechanism for emotion. *Arch. Neurol. Psychiatry*, **38**, 725–743.

Paradiso, S., Johnson, D. L., Andreasen, N. C., O'Leary, D. S., Watkins, G. L., Ponto, L. L., and Hichwa, R. D. (1999). Cerebral blood flow changes associated with attribution of emotional valence to pleasant, unpleasant, and neutral visual stimuli in a PET study of normal subjects. *Am. J. Psychiatry*, **156**, 1618–1629.

Parkinson, J. A., Robbins, T. W., and Everitt, B. J. (2000). Dissociable roles of the central and basolateral amygdala in appetitive emotional learning. *Eur. J. Neurosci.*, **12**, 405–413.

Petrides, M. (1999). Human cortical gustatory areas: a review of functional neuroimaging data. *NeuroReport*, **10**, 7–14.

Phelps, E. A., O'Connor, K. J., Gatenby, J. C., Gore, J. C., Grillon, C., and Davis, M. (2001). Activation of the left amygdala to a cognitive representation of fear. *Nat. Neurosci.*, **4**, 437–441.

Phillips, M. L., Young, A. W., Scott, S. K., Calder, A. J., Andrew, C., Giampietro, V., Williams, S. C., Bullmore, E. T., Brammer, M., and Gray. J. A. (1998a). Neural responses to facial and vocal expressions of fear and disgust. *Proc. Roy. Soc. London Ser. B, Biol. Sci.*, **265**, 1809–1817.

Phillips, M. L., Young, A. W., Senior, C., Brammer, M., Andrew, C., Calder, A. J., Sprengelmeyer, E. T. R., Rausch, M., Eysel, U. T., and Przuntek, H. (1998b). Neural structures associated with recognition of facial expressions of basic emotions. *Proc. Roy. Soc. London Ser. B, Biol. Sci.*, **265**, 1927–1923.

Phillips, M. L., Bullmore, E. T., Howard, R., Woodruff, P. W., Wright, I. C., Williams, S. C., Simmons, A., Andrew, C., Brammer, M., and David, A. S. (1998c). Investigation of facial recognition memory and happy and sad facial expression perception: an fMRI study. *Psychiatry Res.*, **83**(3), 127–138.

Philips, M. L., Young, A. W., Senior, C., Brammer, M., Andrew, C., Calder, A. J., Bullmore, E. T., Perrett, D. I., Rowland, D., Williams, S. C., Gray, J. A., and David, A. S. (1997). A specific neural substrate for perceiving facial expressions of disgust. *Nature*, **389**, 495–498.

Pitkanen, A. and Amaral, D. G. (1998). Organisation of the intrinsic connections of the monkey amygdaloid complex: projections originating in the lateral nucleus. *J. Comp. Neurol.*, **398**, 431–458.

Pizzagalli, D., Pascual-Marqui, R. D., Nitschke, J. B., Oakes, T. R., Larson, C. L., Abercrombie, H. C., Schaefer, S. M., Koger, J. V., Benca, R. M., and Davidson, R. J. (2001). Anterior cingulate activity as a predictor of degree of treatment response in major depression: evidence from brain electrical tomography analysis. *Am. J. Psychiatry*, **158**, 405–415.

Plato. (1993). *Phaedo*, Rowe, C. J., Ed. Cambridge University Press, Cambridge, U.K.

Poppel, E., Held, R., and Frost, D. (1973). Residual visual function after brain wounds involving the central visual pathways in man. *Nature*, **243**, 295–296.

Pourtois, G., de Gelder, B., Vroomen, J., Rossion, B., and Crommelinck, M. (2000). The time-course of intermodal binding between seeing and hearing affective information. *NeuroReport*, **11**, 1329–1333.

Quirk, G. J., Armony, J. L., and LeDoux, J. E. (1997). Fear conditioning enhances different temporal components of tone-evoked spike trains in auditory cortex and lateral amygdala. *Neuron*, **19**, 613–624.

Rainville, P., Duncan, G. H., Price, D. D., Carrier, B., and Bushnell, M. C. (1997). Pain affect encoded in human anterior cingulate but not somatosensory cortex. *Science*, **277**, 968–971.

Rauch, S. L. *et al.* (1995). A positron emission tomographic study of simple phobic symptom provocation. *Arch. Gen. Psychiatry*, **52**, 20–28.

Reisine, T. D., Soubrie, P., Artaud, F., Glowinski, J. (1982). Involvement of lateral habenula-dorsal raphe neurons in the differential regulation of striatal and nigral serotonergic transmission cats. *J. Neurosci.*, **2**, 1062–1071.

Rolls, E. T. (1999). *The Brain and Emotion*. Oxford University Press, London.

Rolls, E. T. and Treves, A. (1998). *Neural Networks and Brain Function*. Oxford University Press, London.

Rolls, E. T., Sienkiewicz, Z. J., and Yaxley, S. (1989). Hunger modulates the responses to gustatory stimuli of single neurons in the orbitofrontal cortex of the macaque monkey. *Eur. J. Neurosci.*, **1**, 53–60.

Rolls, E. T., Hornak, J., Wade, D., and McGrath, J. (1994). Emotion-related learning in patients with social and emotional changes associated with frontal lobe damage. *J. Neurol. Neurosurg. Psychiatry*, **57**, 1518–1524.

Rolls, E. T., Critchley, H. D., Mason, R., and Wakeman, E. A. (1996). Orbitofrontal cortex neurons: role in olfactory and visual association learning. *J. Neurophysiol.*, **75**, 1970–1981.

Roozendaal, B. and McGaugh, J. L. (1996). Amygdaloid nuclei lesions differentially affect glucocorticoid-induced memory enhancement in an inhibitory avoidance task. *Neurobiol. Learn. Mem.*, **65**(1), 1–8.

Rosen, J. B., Hitchcock, J. M., Sananes, C. B., Miserendino, M. J., and Davis, M. (1991). A direct projection from the central nucleus of the amygdala to the acoustic startle pathway: anterograde and retrograde tracing studies. *Behav. Neurosci.*, **105**, 817–825.

Rotshtein, P., Malach, R., Hadar, U., Graif, M., and Hendler, T. (2001). Feeling or features: different sensitivity to emotion in high-order visual cortex and amygdala. *Neuron*, **32**, 747–757.

Royet, J. P., Zald, D., Versace, R., Costes, N., Lavenne, F., Koenig, O., and Gervais, R. (2000). Emotional responses to pleasant and unpleasant olfactory, visual, and auditory stimuli: a positron emission tomography study. *J. Neurosci.*, **20**, 7752–7759.

Russchen, F. T., Bakst, I., Amaral, D. G., Price, J. L. (1985). The amygdalostriatal projections in the monkey: an anterograde tracing study. *Brain Res.*, **329**, 241–257.

Sanghera, M. K., Rolls, E. T., and Roper-Hall, A. (1979). Visual responses of neurons in the dorsolateral amygdala of the alert monkey. *Exp. Neurol.*, **63**, 610–626.

Savander, V., Go, C. G., Ledoux, J. E., and Pitkanen, A. (1996). Intrinsic connections of the rat amygdaloid complex: projections originating in the accessory basal nucleus. *J. Comp. Neurol.*, **374**, 291–313.

Sawamoto, N., Honda, M., Okada, T., Hanakawa, T., Kanda, M., Fukuyama, H., Konishi, J., and Shibasaki, H. (2000). Expectation of pain enhances responses to nonpainful somatosensory stimulation in the anterior cingulate cortex and parietal operculum/posterior insula: an event-related functional magnetic resonance imaging study. *J. Neurosci.*, **20**, 7438–7445.

Schneider, F., Grodd, W., Weiss, U., Klose, U., Mayer, K. R., Nagele, T., and Gur, R. C. (1997). Functional MRI reveals left amygdala activation during emotion. *Psychiatry Res.*, **76**, 75–82.

Schneider, F., Habel, U., Kessler, C., Salloum, J. B., and Posse, S. (2000). Gender differences in regional cerebral activity during sadness. *Hum. Brain Mapping*, **9**, 226–238.

Scott, S. K., Young, A. W., Calder, A. J., Hellawell, D. J., Aggleton, J. P., Johnson, M. (1997). Impaired auditory recognition of fear and anger following bilateral amygdala lesions. *Nature*, **385**, 254–257.

Seligman, M. E. P. (1971). Phobias and preparedness. *Behav. Ther.*, **2**, 307–320.

Slotnick, B. M. (1967). Disturbances of maternal behaviour in the rat following lesions of the cingulate cortex. *Behaviour*, **2**, 204–236.

Small, D. A., Zald, D. H., Jones-Gotman, M., Zatorre, R. J., Pardo, J. V., Frey, S., and Petrides, M. (1999). Human cortical gustatory areas: a review of functional neuroimaging data. *NeuroReport*, **10**, 7–14.

Smith, K. A., Fairburn, C. G., and Cowen, P. J. (1997). Relapse of depression after rapid depletion of tryptophan. *Lancet*, **349**, 915–919.

Smith, K. A., Morris, J. S., Friston, K. J., Cowen, P. J., and Dolan, R. J. (1999). Brain mechanisms associated with depressive relapse and associated cognitive impairment following acute tryptophan depletion. *Br. J. Psychiatry*, **174**, 525–529.

Smith, W. (1945). The functional significance of the rostral cingular cortex as revealed by its responses to electrical stimulation. *J. Neurophsyiol.*, **8**, 241–255.

Sprengelmeyer, R., Rausch, M., Eysel, U. T., and Przuntek, H. (1998). Neural structures associated with recognition of facial expressions of basic emotions. *Proc. Roy. Soc. London Ser. B, Biol, Sci.*, **265**, 1927–1931.

Stanley, M. and Mann, J. J. (1983). Increased serotonin-2 binding sites in frontal cortex of suicide victims. *Lancet*, **1**(8318), 214–216.

Sutherland, R. J. (1982). The dorsal diencephalic conduction system: a review of the anatomy and functions of the habenular complex. *Neurosci. Biobehav. Rev.*, **6**, 1–13.

Talbot, J. D., Marrett, S., Evans, A. C., Meyer, E., Bushnell, M. C., and Duncan, G. H. (1991). Multiple representations of pain in human cerebral cortex. *Science*, **251**, 1355–1358.

Tataranni, P. A., Gautier, J.-F., Chen, K., Ueker, A., Bandy, D., Salbe, A. D., Pratley, R. E., Lawson, M., Reiman, E. M., and Ravussin, E. (1999). Neuroanatomical correlates of hunger and satiation in humans using positron emission tomography. *Proc. Natl. Acad. Sci. USA*, **96**, 4569–4574.

Thiel, C. M., Friston, K. J., and Dolan, R. J. (2002). Cholinergic modulation of experience-dependent plasticity in human auditory cortex, *Neuron*, **35**, 567–574.

Thornton, J. A., Malkova, L., and Murray, E. A. (1998) Rhinal cortex ablations fail to disrupt reinforcer devaluation effects in rhesus monkeys (*Macaca mulatta*). *Behav. Neurosci.*, **112**, 1020–1025.

Thorpe, S. J., Rolls, E. T., and Maddison, S. (1983). Neuronal activity in the orbitofrontal cortex of the behaving monkey. *Exp. Brain Res.*, **49**, 93–115.

Tork, I. and Hornung, J.-P. (1990). Raphe nuclei and the serotonergic system, in *The Human Nervous System*, Paxinos, G., Ed., pp. 1002–1022. Academic Press, San Diego.

Ungerleider, L. G., Galkin, T. W., and Mishkin, M. (1983). Visuotopic organisation of projections from striate cortex to inferior and lateral pulvinar in rhesus monkey. *J. Comp. Neurol.*, **217**, 137–157.

Vogt, B. A., Finch, D. M., and Olson, C. R. (1992). Functional heterogeneity in cingulate cortex: the anterior executive and posterior evaluative regions. *Cereb. Cortex*, **2**, 435–443.

Vuilleumier, P., Armony, J. L., Driver, J., and Dolan, R. J. (2001). Effects of attention and emotion on face processing in the human brain: an event-related fMRI study. *Neuron*, **30**, 829–841.

Wang, R. Y. and Aghajanian, G. K. (1977). Physiological evidence for habenula as major link between forebrain and midbrain raphe. *Science*, **197**, 89–91.

Weinberger, N. M. (1995). Retuning the brain by fear conditioning, in *The Cognitive Neurosciences*, Gazzaniga, M. S., Ed., pp. 1071–1089. MIT Press, Cambridge, MA.

Weiskrantz, L. (1956). Behavioural changes associated with ablation of the amygdaloid complex in monkeys. *J. Comp. Physiol. Psychol.*, **49**, 381–391.

Weiskrantz, L., Warrington, E. K., Sanders, M. D., and Marshall, J. (1974). Visual capacity in the hemianopic field following a restricted occipital ablation. *Brain*, **97**, 709–728.

Whalen, P. J., Bush, G., McNally, R. J., Wilhelm, S., McInerney, S. C., Jenike, M. A., and Rauch, S. L. (1998a). The emotional counting Stroop paradigm: a functional magnetic resonance imaging probe of the anterior cingulate affective division. *Biol. Psychiatry*, **44**, 1219–1228.

Whalen, P. J., Rauch, S. L., Etcoff, N. L., McInerney, S. C., Lee, M. B., and Jenike, M. A. (1998b). Masked presentations of emotional facial expressions modulate amygdala activity without explicit knowledge. *J. Neurosci.*, **18**, 411–418.

Wilhelmi, E., Linke, R., de Lima, A. D., and Pape, H. C. (2001). Axonal connections of thalamic posterior paralaminar nuclei with amygdaloid projection neurons to the cholinergic basal forebrain in the rat. *Neurosci. Lett.*, **315**, 121–124.

Winston, J. S., Strange, B. A., O'Doherty, J., and Dolan, R. J. (2002). Automatic and intentional brain responses during evaluation of trustworthiness of faces. *Nat. Neurosci.*, **5**, 277–283.

Wright, C. I., Fischer, H., Whalen, P. J., McInerney, S. C., Shin, L. M., and Rauch, S. L. (2001). Differential prefrontal cortex and amygdala habituation to repeatedly presented emotional stimuli. *NeuroReport*, **12**, 379–383.

Xu, Y., Day, A., and Buller, K. M. (1999). The central amygdala modulates hypothalamic–pituitary–adrenal axis responses to systemic interleukin-1β administration. *Neuroscience*, **94**, 175–183.

Young, A. W., Aggleton, J. P., Hellawell, D. J., Johnson, M., Broks, P., and Hanley, J. R. (1995). Face processing impairments after amygdalotomy. *Brain*, **118**, 15–24.

Zajonc, R. B. (1984). On the primacy of affect, in *Approaches to Emotion*, Scherer, K. R. and Ekman, P., Eds., pp. 259–270. Lawrence Erlbaum, Hillsdale, NJ.

Zald, D. H. and Pardo, J. V. (1997). Emotion, olfaction, and the human amygdala: amygdala activation during aversive olfactory stimulation. *Proc. Natl. Acad. Sci. USA*, **94**, 4119–4124.

Zald, D. H., Hagen, M. C., and Pardo, J. V. (2002). Neural correlates of tasting concentrated quinine and sugar solutions. *J. Neurophysiol.*, **87**, 1068–1075.

Zihl, J. and von Cramon, D. (1979). The contribution of the 'second visual system' to directed visual attention in man. *Brain*, **102**, 835–856.

CHAPTER

20

Central Representation of Autonomic States

OVERVIEW

Self-regulation is a basic principle in the physiological organisation of complex organisms. A hierarchy of homeostatic mechanisms regulates and optimises internal organismic states within and across organ systems. At the top of this hierarchy, the coordinated control of organ systems is mediated in the short term by peripheral neural activity and in the longer term by humoral agents. Together, these major regulatory systems integrate bodily states with environmental and motivational demands.

The systemwide coordination of bodily organs is mediated neurally via the autonomic nervous system, which innervates the pupils, skin, cardiovascular system, lungs, and gastrointestinal and genitourinary tracts, thereby providing input into every major bodily system (Brading, 1999). Functionally, the autonomic nervous system mediates both continuous control of autoregulatory "vegetative" processes and dynamic modification of these homeostatic functions to facilitate the execution of behavioural repertoires and responses to environmental contingencies. Autonomic activity is, as a consequence, continuously modulated to reflect the physical, cognitive, and emotional/motivational state of an organism. Feedback is fundamental to homeostatic autonomic control. On one level, there is continuous monitoring of basic homoeostatic processes and, on another, there is context-specific representation of bodily responses (arousal states) during behaviour (Damasio, 1994, 1999). In humans, these central representations of autonomic states interact and influence emotional experience and cognition. The focus of this chapter is to provide an account of cerebral control of autonomic processes based upon evidence acquired through human functional neuroimaging. The prime emphasis is on mapping brain activity relating to cardiovascular and electrodermal activity, indices of bodily states of autonomic arousal.

BACKGROUND

Autonomic nervous activity is often conceptualised as being independent of volitional control and largely a self-adjusting system that operates outside of awareness. Aside from the intrinsic innervation of the gastrointestinal tract, neuronal regulation of bodily states is achieved for the most part by balance of activity within sympathetic and parasympathetic autonomic subdivisions, as first proposed by Langley (1898, 1921). Sympathetic activity facilitates motor action by increasing cardiac output by dilating vessels of the musculature and reducing blood supply to the gut. In contrast, parasympathetic activity promotes more recuperative vegetative functions including reducing heart rate, lowering of blood pressure, and slowing gut motility.

Bodily states of arousal associated with survival behaviours (*e.g.*, fight and flight responses) are therefore characterised by increased sympathetic activity and, in most instances, decreased parasympathetic activity. Notably, although most organs are regulated by sympathetic and parasympathetic nerves acting in apposition, eccrine sweat glands lack a parasympathetic supply.

A context-dependent modulation of peripheral autonomic activity is fundamental to understanding the close interaction between emotion and arousal states. Automatic elicitation of (preparatory) arousal states (*e.g.*, for fight or flight) may be intrinsically coupled with subjective emotional experience (James, 1894), and the context in which autonomic arousal is experienced may influence the quality of an accompanying affect (Schachter and Singer, 1962). Autonomic bodily changes are proposed to be the basis of subjective "feeling states" which are important influences on cognitive process such as decision making (Damasio, 1994, 1999). Many autonomic responses, particularly as manifest in the skin (sweating, piloerection, vasomotor changes), also contribute to emotional expression and social signalling that guide inter-individual interactions (Darwin, 1998). The isolated sympathetic innervation of sweat glands, reflected in measures of electrodermal activity (EDA), is closely associated with emotional arousal states. EDA, as a result, is widely used as a sensitive index of automatic implicit emotional processing (Venables and Christie, 1980; Fowles *et al.*, 1981; Bouscein, 1992; Dawson, *et al.*, 2000).

PERIPHERAL ANATOMY

In the periphery, sympathetic (with origins in thoraco-lumbar spinal segments) and parasympathetic (with origins in cranial nerve motor nuclei and sacral spinal segments) outflows are anatomically segregated. In the spinal cord, descending sympathetic axons synapse with preganglionic sympathetic cell bodies located in the intermediolateal column of thoraco-lumbar spinal segments (T1–L2). The preganglionic neurons project in an ipsilateral distribution to the two chains of sympathetic ganglia that lie in parallel with the spine, extending from upper cervical to sacral regions. In these ganglia, preganglionic fibres synapse in an approximate dermatomal fashion, and unmyelinated postganglionic fibres enter adjacent spinal nerves eventually to innervate effector organs. In addition to chains of sympathetic ganglia, some preganglionic fibres synapse in separate cervical or abdominal ganglia, while others travel directly to the adrenal medulla. Acetylcholine is the neurotransmitter at synapses within the sympathetic ganglia. The majority of postganglionic sympathetic synapses use noradrenaline as the principal transmitter (exceptions include the innervation of sweat glands and vasodilatation of muscle vessels mediated cholinergically (Sato, 1977; Anderson *et al.*, 1989; Brading, 1999).

In contrast, craniosacral parasympathetic efferents originate in motor nuclei of cranial nerves III, VII, IX, and X (vagus) as well as from sacral spinal segments. Preganglionic fibres travel to ganglia in or adjacent to the effector organ, where short postganglionic fibres innervate the relevant target tissue. Acetylcholine is the neurotransmitter at both ganglionic and effector synapses. Most peripheral bodily organs receive their parasympathetic innervation via the vagus nerve. Parasympathetic fibres within oculomotor (III), facial (VII), and glossopharyngeal (IX) cranial nerves mediate pupil and salivary gland responses, and sacral parasympathetic fibres innervate distal bowel and urogenital systems (Brading, 1999).

CENTRAL ANATOMY

Homeostatic autonomic control is supported by a functional organisation of nuclei within hypothalamus, pons, and medulla. Posterior and lateral hypothalamic nuclei influence sympathetic function via brainstem centres such as tegmentum, raphé, periaqueductal grey, paraventricular, parabrachial, and medial reticular nuclei. The anterior hypothalamus influences parasympathetic efferent responses in medullary nuclei (nucleus ambiguus and dorsal motor nucleus of the vagus, Edinger-Westphal nucleus, and salivatory nucleus). Afferent visceral information is represented in the nucleus of the solitary tract and in hypothalamic nuclei that lie in close proximity to these efferent autonomic centres. Regions such as central amygdaloid nucleus, bed nucleus of the stria terminalis, and locus coeruleus also contribute to autonomic control and project directly to brainstem autonomic nuclei and sympathetic cell bodies in the spinal cord (Willette *et al.*, 1984, Bennarroch, 1997; Blessing, 1997; Collins, 1999; Spyer, 1999). These descending connections are ipsilateral (Davidson and Koss, 1975).

Higher brain regions also influence the homeostatic mechanisms governed by hypothalamic and brainstem nuclei. Thus, autonomic responses can be evoked or modulated by stimulation of cortical and subcortical regions including: (1) insula (implicated in somatic and visceral representations) (Oppenheimer and Cechetto, 1990); (2) motor cortex, neostriatum, and cerebellum (involved in initiation and control of limb movements) (Kaada, 1951; Delgado, 1960; Bradley *et al.*, 1987; 1991; Angyan, 1994; Lin and Yang, 1994); (3) amygdala and hippocampus (involved in emotion perception, threat responses, and episodic memory) (Kaada, 1951; Gelsema *et al.*, 1989); and (4) anterior cingulate and ventromedial prefrontal (areas implicated in attention, motivation, and decision-making) (Kaada, 1951; Buchanan *et al.*, 1985; Neafsey, 1990). Neuronal electrophysiological recordings also indicate that many putative *efferent* autonomic centres also receive afferent information concerning peripheral autonomic states (Cechetto and Saper, 1987; reviewed in Cechetto and Saper, 1990).

Human evidence also points to a role for higher brain centres in autonomic control and contextual generation of autonomic arousal states. Stimulation of the insula (Oppenheimer *et al.*, 1992), medial prefrontal cortex/anterior cingulate (Pool and Ransohoff, 1949), and medial temporal lobe (Fish *et al.*, 1993) elicit changes in blood pressure and heart rate (which may be accompanied by subjective mood changes). Right-sided stimulation of insula increases heart rate and blood pressure, suggesting lateralisation of higher sympathetic control (Oppenheimer *et al.*, 1992). Stimulation of limbic areas (*i.e.*, amygdala, hippocampus, and cingulate) produces strong ipsilateral EDA responses (Mangina and Buezeron-Mangina, 1996). By contrast, orbitofrontal damage reduces anticipatory arousal to emotive stimuli (Damasio *et al.*, 1990), while lesions of the amygdala block EDA responses that accompany conditioning (Bechara *et al.*, 1995). Lesions, particularly on the right to lateral prefrontal cortex, ventral, and medial prefrontal cortex, anterior cingulate, and parietal lobe, also diminish EDA (Oscar Berman and Gade, 1979; Zoccolotti *et al.*, 1982; Tranel and Damasio, 1994; Zahn *et al.*, 1999; Tranel, 2000). Furthermore, autonomic dysfunction in neurodegenerative conditions, such as diffuse Lewy body disease, multiple system atrophy, Huntington's disease, and perhaps Parkinson's disease (Mathias and Bannister, 1999), points to a contribution to human autonomic control from structures such as basal ganglia and cerebellum. It should be noted that the nature of lesion studies and neurodegenerative diseases involving heterogeneous distributions of pathology, as well as the diffuse nature of pathophysiological process in neurological diseases, renders it difficult to make strong inferences regarding the contribution of distinct regions to higher autonomic control in humans (Fig. 20.1).

AROUSAL, EMOTION, AND COGNITION

The notion of nonspecific autonomic arousal states characterised by increased sympathetic drive and decreased parasympathetic drive is a useful heuristic, although dissociable patterns of activity may be evident within both sympathetic and parasympathetic autonomic axes (Morrison, 2001; Porges, 1995) and varied patterns of autonomic activity may accompany different emotions (Collett *et al.*, 1997). The autonomic arousal concept, usually indexed by EDA or cardiovascular changes, underlies many psychophysiological observations relating to emotion, cognition, and bodily state.

The close relationship between arousal states and emotion was first formally embodied within the James–Lange theory (James, 1894), which proposed that arousal and emotion were equivalent. Cannon (1927), however, argued that visceral changes were nonspecific, insensitive, and too slow to account for emotional experience. Instead, the Cannon–Bard theory (Cannon, 1929) proposed that emotive stimuli produce synchronous activation of autonomic arousal (perhaps as an epiphenomenon) and subjective emotional feeling states; however, the importance of peripheral arousal states to emotional perception was never fully dismissed. Schachter and Singer (1962) provided evidence for arousal-induced emotion where the nature of the emotion (positive or negative) was determined by contextual factors of a social or cognitive nature. More

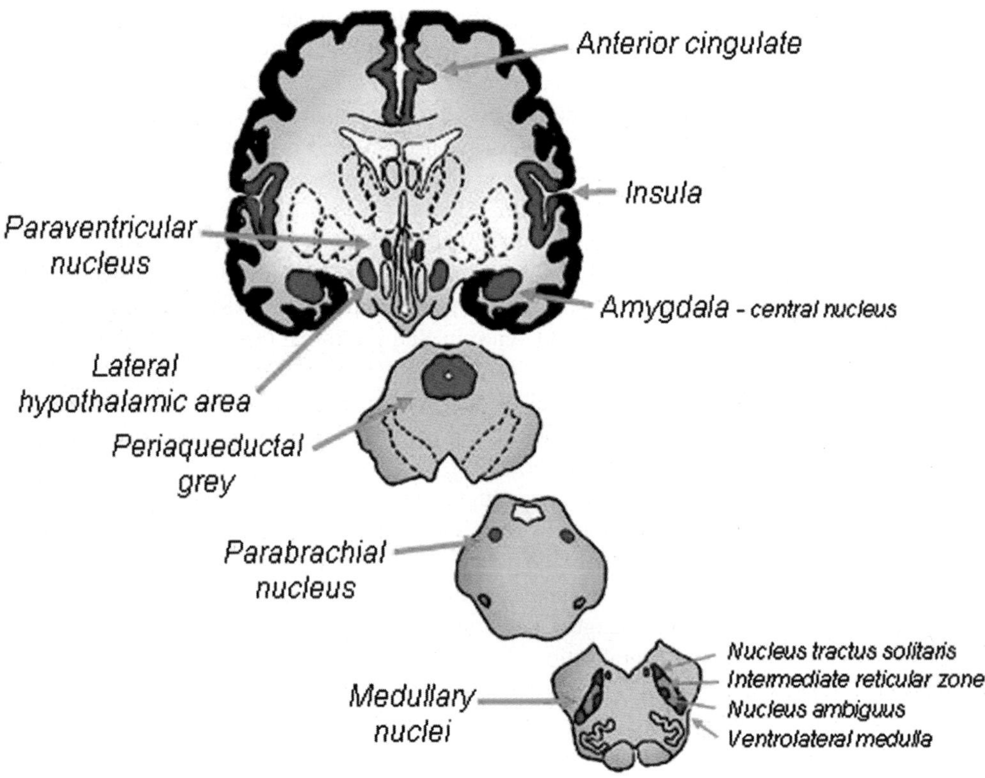

FIGURE 20.1
Brain regions implicated in autonomic control. Summary figure of principal brain areas implicated in autonomic control. The anatomical locations of these regions are shown in red.

recently, Damasio has revived many aspects of the James–Lange argument, formulating the notion of *somatic markers* (Damasio *et al.*, 1990, 1991; Damasio, 1994). Somatic markers describe states of autonomic arousal (indexed by EDA), the central representation of which biases behaviour and guides strategic decision-making. Within this hypothesis a particular emphasis is placed on the role of ventromedial prefrontal (orbitofrontal) cortex in the generation and representation of these bodily states. Crucially, ventromedial prefrontal cortex and amygdala in medial temporal lobe are implicated in both autonomic control (see above) and emotion (LeDoux, 1992; Rolls, 1996). Thus, damage to these regions may result in disturbed social and emotional behaviour, associated with abnormalities in strategic decision making (Damasio *et al.*, 1990; Shallice and Burgess, 1991; Bechara *et al.*, 1997; Adolphs *et al.*, 1998). Patients with ventromedial prefrontal damage persist with maladaptive behavioural patterns despite consequential punishing outcomes (Bechara *et al.*, 1997, 1999). In decision-making tasks, these patients do not generate normal anticipatory arousal when taking risks in contrast to the anticipatory arousal seen in normal subjects (Damasio *et al.*, 1990; Bechara *et al.*, 1996, 1997). The somatic marker hypothesis proposes that arousal states prospectively guide decision making, and in their absence ventromedial prefrontal patients persist with punishing maladaptive behaviours.

With amygdala damage, autonomic responses are reduced during anticipation, punishment, threat, and fear conditioning (Bechara *et al.*, 1999) but are preserved to basic stimuli, such as loud noises (Tranel and Damasio, 1989; Zahn *et al.*, 1999; Tranel, 2000). These findings suggest that the amygdala is involved in generating arousal to stimuli for which motivational meaning is acquired through experience and learning. The amygdala is also implicated in the emotional enhancement of memory, whereby events and stimuli with strong emotional content or context are remembered better than unemotional material. The central idea here is that arousal associated with sympathetic activity modulates amygdalo-hippocampal activity, thereby enhancing memory consolidation (Cahill, 1997; Cahill and McGaugh, 1998). These studies highlight the interaction between autonomic arousal states and cognitive and emotional functioning. They also point to the potential confound of ascribing cognitive functions to activated brain regions without considering that the activity may also reflect generation and/or representation of arousal states, a byproduct of many cognitive acts.

Observed psychological sequellae of systemic illness provide evidence that primary abnormalities of bodily states may predispose to precipitate and maintain psychopathology. An extension of the theoretical models described above is the proposition that control of peripheral autonomic arousal may underlie individual psychological profiles and contribute to the expression of psychiatric disorders. There is considerable evidence for this proposition. Personality traits, representing pervasive behavioural styles that can be traced to infantile temperament (Rutter, 1987), are associated with differences in autonomic tone and responsivity (Kamanda *et al.*, 1992; Stifter and Jain, 1996). Aggressive and antisocial acts have been reported to be more frequent in adults who exhibited low autonomic arousal as children (Hodgins *et al.*, 1996; Raine, 1996, Scarpa *et al.*, 1997), leading to speculation that developmental thresholds for stimulating autonomic responses prospectively influence adult behaviour. Such reasoning has also been applied to models of psychopathy (Mawson and Mawson, 1977). There is also evidence to suggest that the autonomic coordination of bodily responses with environmental challenges and intentional behaviours is basic to cognitive and emotional maturation. Abnormalities in autonomic function are associated with many causes of mental impairment, including Down's syndrome (Sacks and Smith, 1989; Ferri *et al.*, 1998), fragile X (Boccia and Roberts, 2000), and Rett's syndrome (Julu *et al.*, 1997); however, congenital primary autonomic failure does not necessarily predispose to mental impairment (Welton *et al.*, 1979; Mathias and Bannister, 1999).

Many studies have reported abnormalities in autonomic responses in autism, a developmental disorder characterised by deficits in social and emotional development (Porges, 1976; Palkovitz and Wiesenfeld, 1980; Zahn *et al.*, 1987). Hirstein *et al.* (2001) observed a close relationship between autonomic responsiveness and stereotyped behaviours in autistic children and postulated a primary autonomic basis to the symptomatology of autism. Among acquired psychiatric disorders, the psychological manifestations of schizophrenia may have a basis in a lack of integration among peripheral levels of bodily arousal, cognitive states, and emotional behaviour. For example, this lack of integration could account for the experience of delusional moods and feelings of control, as well as unstable representations of self. Autonomic abnormalities have been observed in schizophrenic patients (Zahn *et al.*, 1987; Hultman and Ohman, 1989) and may in fact predict impending psychotic relapse (Dawson *et al.*, 1994; Hazlett *et al.*, 1997). Among affective disorders, anxiety disorders are most closely related to autonomic hyperresponsiveness. Situational autonomic hyperactivity appears to be a crucial factor in fear conditioning and related learning mechanisms that underlie the pathogenesis and maintenance of anxiety symptoms in panic disorders, phobias, and posttraumatic stress disorder (PTSD). Thus, many effective behavioural therapies are focused on diminishing involuntary autonomic arousal through exposure and habituation. It is also of interest that much overlap exists between *neurological* conditions such as neurocardiogenic (vasovagal syncope) and essential hyperhydrosis (a sweating disorder) and *psychological* conditions such as blood/needle phobia and social anxiety (Mathias and Bannister, 1999). In contrast to the generalised increases in bodily arousal associated with anxiety or manic exuberance (Metzger *et al.*, 1999), major depression is often associated with selective blunting of autonomic responses (Guinjoan *et al.*, 1995).

The above observations highlight a close interaction between autonomic activity and psychological status; however, dysfunction in the integration of bodily arousal with cognitive and emotional behaviours has rarely been considered as an important contributory factor to psychopathological processes. The usefulness to psychophysiologists of autonomic indices as objective indicators of attention and emotion in healthy subjects may underlie a more general cultural reluctance to attribute a causal relationship between bodily states and background psychological states.

NEUROIMAGING EVIDENCE

Correlates of Cardiovascular Arousal

Functional neuroimaging is now a major neuroscientific tool for investigating *in vivo* human brain function. Relatively few functional imaging studies have examined central autonomic control and representation. More frequently, autonomic indices, such as EDA, have been used within the context of functional imaging paradigms as an index of emotional processing and learning—for example, to index the acquisition or expression of fear conditioning (Buchel *et al.*, 1998; Morris *et al.*, 1998).

Emotional, cognitive and motor behaviours may induce different degrees of arousal depending on the specific task demands (Fig. 20.2). Many (blocked) studies comparing activity during a difficult (cognitive or motor) task with an easier control condition may unintentionally elicit activity reflecting autonomic states. Similar caveats apply to studies of emotional processing. Notably, activity in regions such as anterior cingulate and insula cortices (putative centres of autonomic control) is frequently observed in neuroimaging experiments where stress or effort are crucial and often uncontrolled variables (Paus *et al.*, 1998).

A general approach to relate peripheral autonomic responses to regional brain activity has involved scanning subjects performing specific tasks (autonomic function tests often being used clinically) that engender cardiovascular autonomic responses (*e.g.*, increases in heart rate and blood pressure). These tasks include the Valsalva manoeuvre (breathing against a closed glottis), isometric handgrip exercise, deep inspiration, mental stress (arithmetic), and cold pressor tests. In one such functional magnetic resonance imaging (fMRI) study, King *et al.* (1999) reported increased activity in anterior and posterior insula, medial prefrontal cortex, and ventroposterior thalamus during respiratory, Valsalva, and exercise challenge. Similarly, a subsequent fMRI study (Harper *et al.*, 2000) described activity increases in ventral and medial prefrontal cortex,

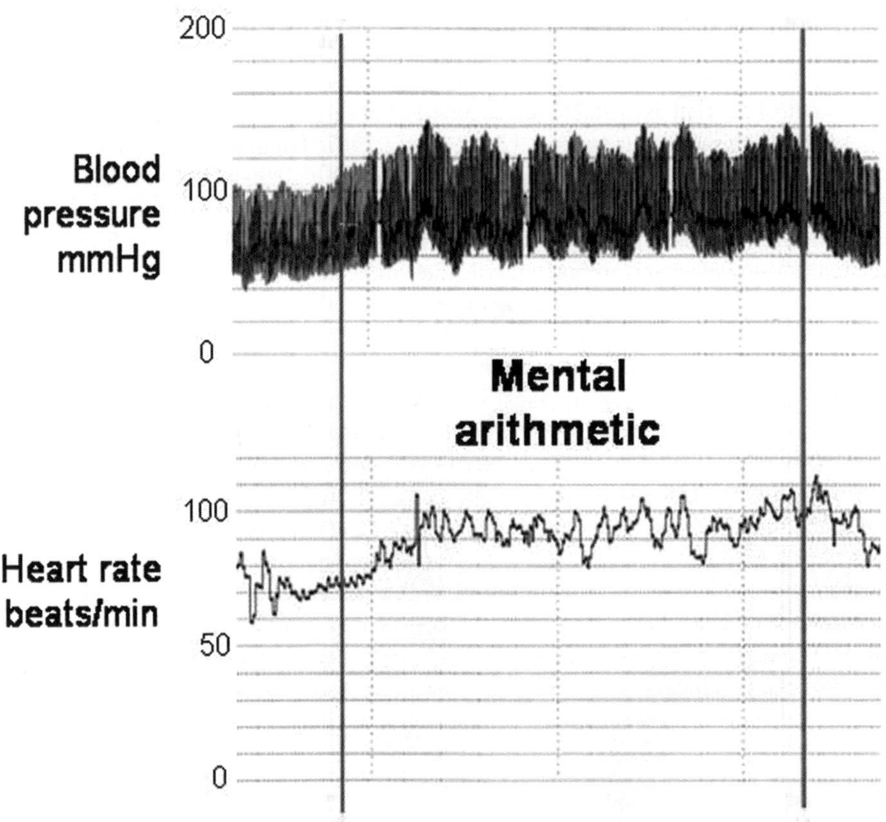

FIGURE 20.2
Cardiovascular response to cognitive stress. Example Portapres2 trace of beat-to-beat blood pressure and heart rate changes in a healthy young individual during performance of a mental arithmetic task. The subject performed serial subtractions of 7 from 400 out loud in front of the examining scientist. This exercise produced robust increases in heart rate and blood pressure over the task period (between the red lines), which were also accompanied by increased ventilation reflected in variability of the heart rate.

anterior cingulate, insula, medial temporal lobe, medial thalamus, cerebellum midbrain, and pons during cold pressor challenge and performance of Valsalva manoeuvres.

In one of our early studies of central autonomic control (Critchley *et al.*, 2000a), we used positron emission tomography (PET) to examine brain activity during cardiovascular arousal induced by mental or physical effort. Activity in these states was compared with activity associated with low-grade, effortless control tasks. In this study, we scanned healthy subjects (mean age, 35), all of whom experienced increased heart rates and blood pressures when performing effortful compared to control tasks (Fig. 20.3). To relate regional brain activity to cardiovascular arousal, we first tested for activity common to effortful task performance, independent of whether the subject was performing mental arithmetic or isometric exercise (Price and Friston, 1997). In this analysis, we observed increased activity in right anterior cingulate, dorsal pons, and midline cerebellum. To further characterise autonomic-related regional brain activity, the measured increases in heart rate and blood pressure during each individual scan were entered as covariates of interest into the analysis. Activity in right anterior cingulate, right insula, and pons covaried with increases in blood pressure and heart rate independent of task modality (shown by using a conjunction analyses to determine activity common to exercise and arithmetic conditions) (Fig. 20.3). This study suggested that cortical regions such as anterior cingulate are important for integrating cognitive and volitional behaviours when engaged in effortful tasks, with peripheral states of cardiovascular arousal. The study also suggested laterality of sympa-

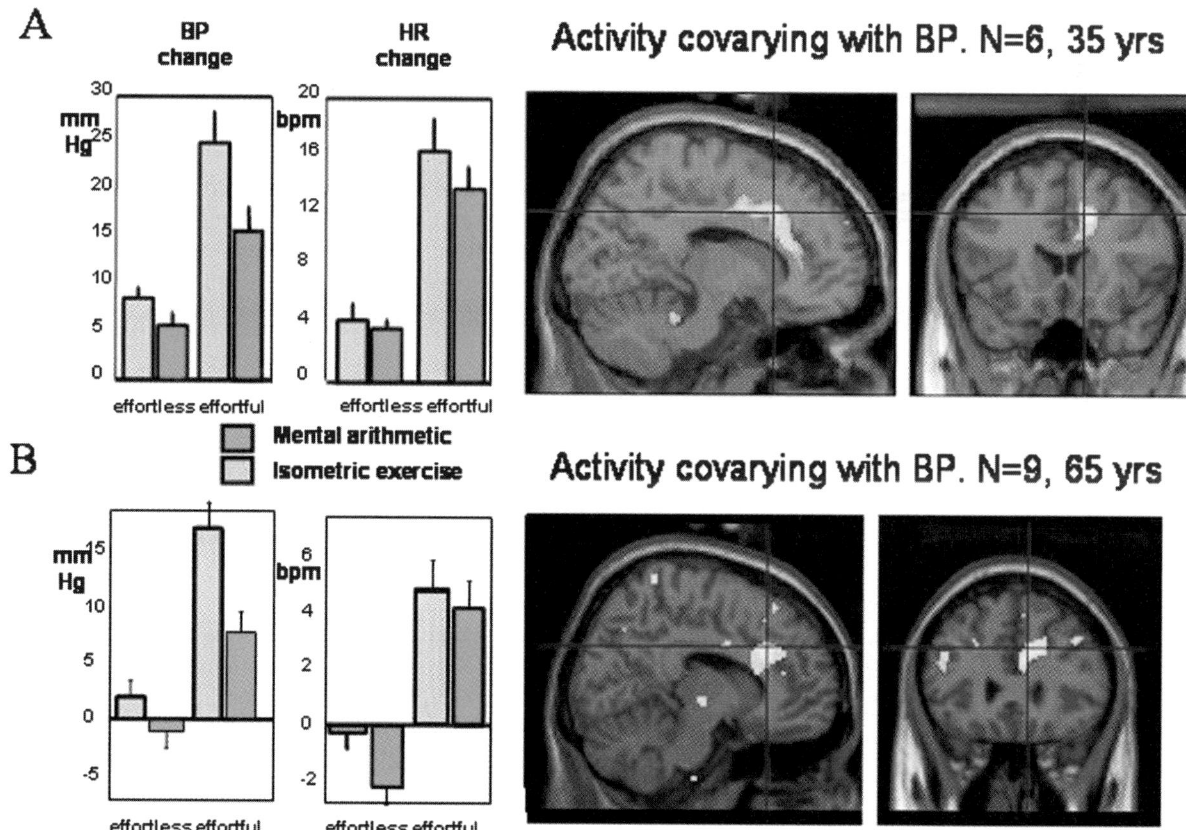

FIGURE 20.3

PET investigations of cardiovascular arousal. (A) Six healthy subjects, mean age 35 yr, were scanned using $H_2{}^{15}O$ PET during performance of effortful mental arithmetic (covert serial subtractions) and isometric handgrip exercise (30% of grip strength sustained over 3 minutes, performed with right hand) and during corresponding effortless control conditions (covert counting and minimal grip). The bar charts to the left illustrate mean changes in blood pressure and heart rates during each task, showing cardiovascular arousal during cognitive and physical effort. On the right, activity covarying with increases in blood pressure during both mental arithmetic and exercise is plotted on a parasagittal and coronal sections of a template brain, illustrating increases in right anterior cingulate activity with increasing blood pressure, independent of task modality. (B) A repetition of this PET study was conducted in an older age group. Nine healthy subjects, mean age 65 yr, were scanned as above. As with the younger subjects, mental and physical effort increased blood pressure and heart rates, and increases in blood pressure were associated with enhanced right anterior cingulate activity, independent of whether the pressor response resulted from exercise or cognitive work.

thetic responses to the right hemisphere which accords with an earlier proposal based upon stimulation of human insular cortices (Oppenheimer *et al.*, 1992). This relationship between anterior cingulate activity and increases in blood pressure was later confirmed in a replication of this study within an older group (mean age, 65) of healthy subjects (Fig. 20.3).

In an extension of this basic approach to mapping brain activity relating to cardiovascular arousal, we used the superior temporal resolution associated with fMRI (Critchley *et al.*, 2003). In this study, during simultaneous acquired electrocardiography (ECG) measures, we scanned subjects while they performed repetitions of motor and cognitive tasks chosen to induce variability in heart rate across the study session. In the motor tasks, subjects performed isometric handgrip squeezes, either squeezing for 6 s then relaxing for 6 s or squeezing for 11 s and relaxing for 11 s, repeated over 3-min blocks. The cognitive tasks took the form of an *n*-back working memory task, in which subjects monitored serial presentations of letters, responding in the low-demand, one-back sessions to immediate repetitions of stimuli and in the high-demand, two-back task to repetitions of letter stimuli separated by an interposing letter. Heart rate variability (HRV) was derived from R-wave intervals of the ECG. Further indices reflecting sympathetic and parasympathetic modulation of heart rate were derived using power spectral analyses of R–R interbeat intervals. In this procedure, which has become standard in clinical autonomic practice and research, the spectral power of HRV at high frequency (0.15–0.50 Hz) is closely related to parasympathetic nervous control of the heart, whereas low-frequency spectral power (0.05–0.15 Hz) predominantly reflects sympathetic activity.

Changes in HRV (increases or decreases) were associated with covariation of activity in anterior/mid-cingulate cortex, somatomotor cortex, and insulae that partially overlapped with regions activated by the cognitive and physical challenges (Fig. 20.4). Moreover, increases in the low-frequency, sympathetic component of HRV was associated with increased cingulate, somatomotor, and insular activity. This finding contrasts with increases in activity relating purely to parasympathetic components of HRV observed in anterior temporal lobe (uncal regions bilaterally) and basal ganglia. Some overlap in regions showing covariation with sympathetic and parasympathetic components of HRV was observed in somatomotor cortex and medial parietal lobe. These findings support findings from our previous study that indicated that activity within anterior and mid-cingulate cortex is associated with control of cardiovascular autonomic arousal, particularly by the sympathetic axis of the autonomic nervous system.

Electrodermal Arousal

Electrodermal activity is not confounded by changes in parasympathetic activity and has been extensively used to objectively index attention and emotion in psychophysical experiments (Venables and Christie, 1980; Fowles *et al.*, 1981; Bouscein 1992; Ohman and Soares, 1993; Dawson, *et al.*, 2000). Functional neuroimaging studies of fear conditioning and subjective affective experience (Buchel *et al.*, 1998; Morris *et al.*, 1998; Chua *et al.*, 1999; Lane *et al.*, 1999) have also used EDA as an objective measure of emotional processing and observed activity within amygdala, insula, or anterior cingulate that was at least partly related to EDA. However, the first neuroimaging study to directly explore the relationship between EDA and brain activity was that of Fredrikson *et al.* (1998). These investigators used PET neuroimaging and continuous electrodermal recording to identify changes in brain activity relating to EDA arousal, while subjects were presented with intrinsically emotive stimuli, including skin shocks and videos of snakes. Stimuli evoking strong EDA responses were associated with modulation of activity in motor cortex, anterior and posterior cingulate, right insula, right inferior parietal lobe, and extrastriate visual cortex. In fact, positive correlations were observed between with EDA and activity in cingulate and motor cortices, and decreased correlations were found in insula, parietal, and visual cortex. This study suggested a distributed neural system governing electrodermal arousal within human brain and highlighted involvement of regions such as anterior cingulate cortex in EDA responses. In a similar fMRI experiment, Williams and colleagues (2000) examined processing of visual stimuli during simultaneous EDA monitoring. Stimuli producing strong EDA responses evoked increased activity (relative to those that did not) in ventromedial prefrontal cortex, anterior cingulate, and medial temporal lobe.

In one of our own experiments, we used fMRI (Critchley *et al.*, 2000b) to index brain activity

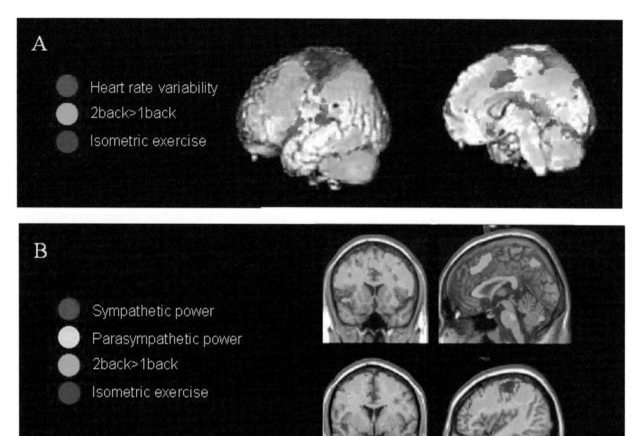

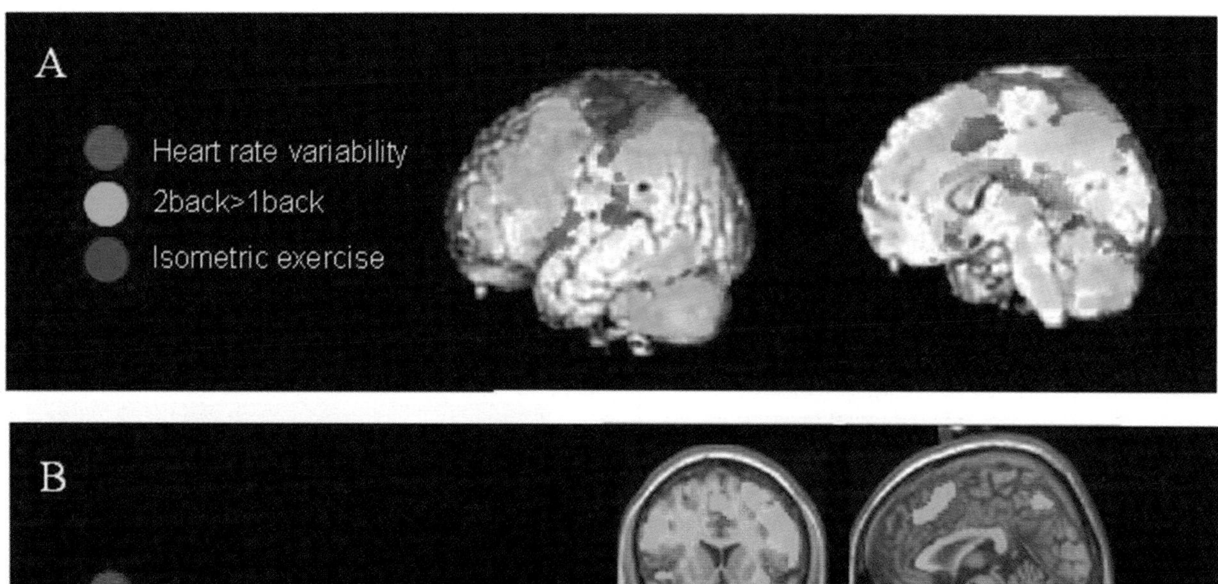

FIGURE 20.4
Regional activity during fMRI study of heart rate variability. Preliminary data from an fMRI study of five subjects is presented. Subjects were scanned while performing handgrip squeeze exercises and cognitive tasks of different degrees of mental effort (one-back and two-back working memory tasks) during simultaneous electrocardiography. (A) Group data are mapped onto a rendered template brain. Significant activity increases related to cognitive effort (two-back versus one-back tasks), are plotted in green, and activity related to the exercise conditions (primarily left somatomotor cortex) is plotted in blue. Activity related to increases or decreases in heart rate variability (F-contrast) is shaded in red, and is particularly apparent in anterior/mid-cingulate (overlapping with cognitive activity), somatomotor cortex (overlapping with motor activity), secondary somatosensory cortex, and insulae. (B) Regressors reflecting sympathetic and parasympathetic components of the autonomic control of heart rate were derived using power spectral analysis of heart rate variability. Activity associated with increased sympathetic power was observed in regions including anterior/mid-cingulate cortex and insulae (shown in red). Activity related to parasympathetic power (shown in yellow) was less evident (the regressor had been orthogonalised with the regressor for sympathetic activity), but was observed in regions including bilateral medial temporal lobe (unci) and basal ganglia. Significant group data are plotted on coronal and parasagittal sections of a template brain, with cognitive activity (two-back versus one-back) shown in green, and motor activity in blue.

relating to EDA fluctuations evoked naturalistically by performance of a cognitive gambling task. On each trial of a gambling task, subjects saw a pair of playing cards and had to make a two-choice button press decision to win (or lose) money. Visual feedback of overall winnings, and whether the correct response had been made was given after each response (Elliott *et al.*, 2000) (Fig. 20.5). Task-performance-evoked, subject-specific EDA fluctuations were used as covariates of interest in two sets of analyses. First, the EDA trace over the course of the experiment was used as a regressor of interest to examine brain activity covarying with this peripheral measure of arousal. Second, distinct peaks in the EDA trace were used to identify activity related to generation and feedback re-representation of discrete EDA responses. Task-specific variability was excluded by entering appropriate regressors derived from the feedback given to the subject. EDA fluctuation over the course of the experiment was associated with increased activity in bilateral ventromedial prefrontal cortex, right insula/orbitofrontal cortex, right inferior parietal cortex, and extrastriate visual cortex. Prior to discrete EDA responses, increased activity within left ventromedial prefrontal cortex, extrastriate cortex, and cerebellum suggests that these

A Visual presentation during task

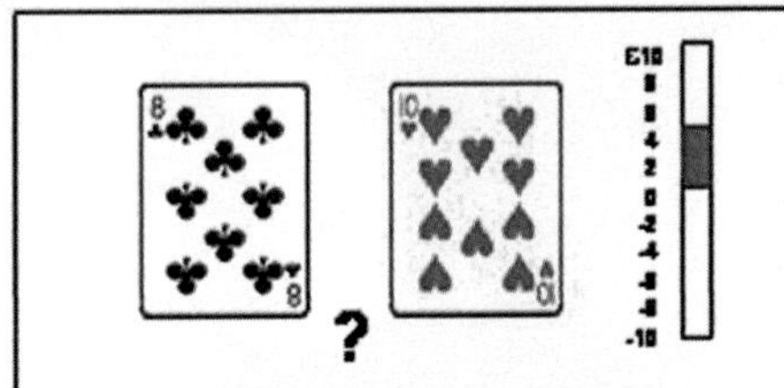

B Random function determining winnings

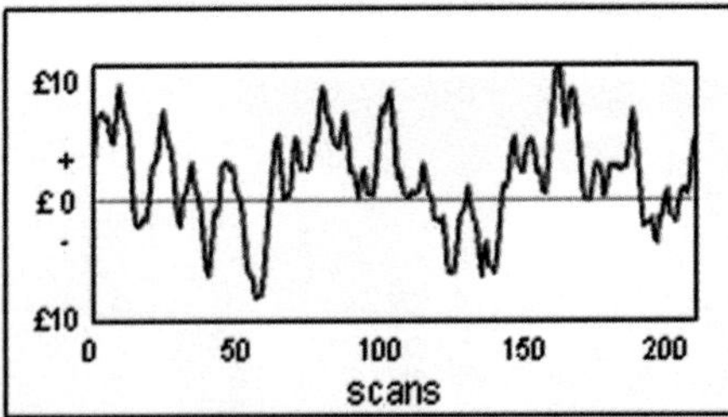

C EDA in one individual during task

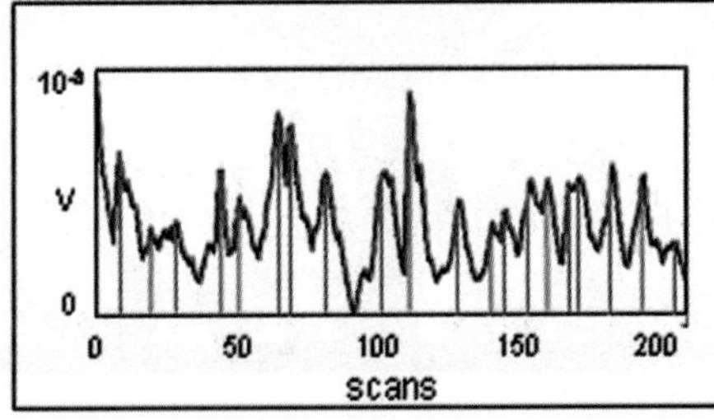

D Activity covarying with EDA

Right anterior insula / orbitofrontal cortex

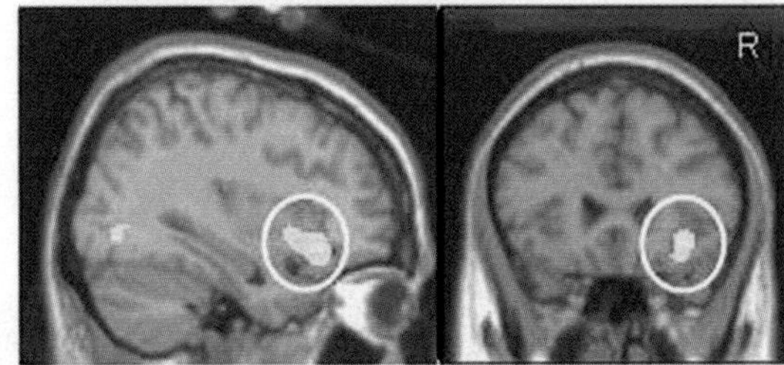

Bilateral ventromedial prefrontal cortex

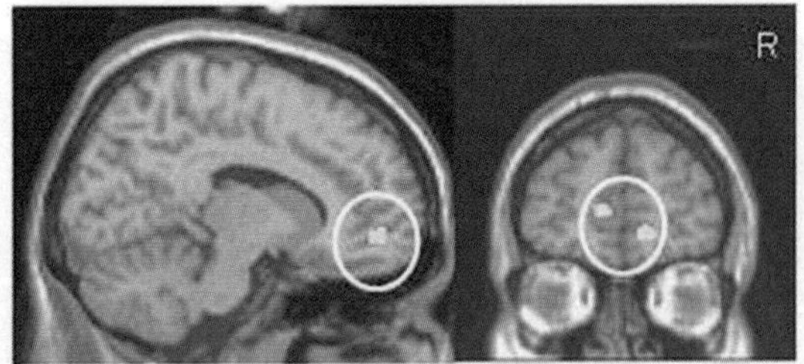

Inferior parietal lobe and extrastriate cortex

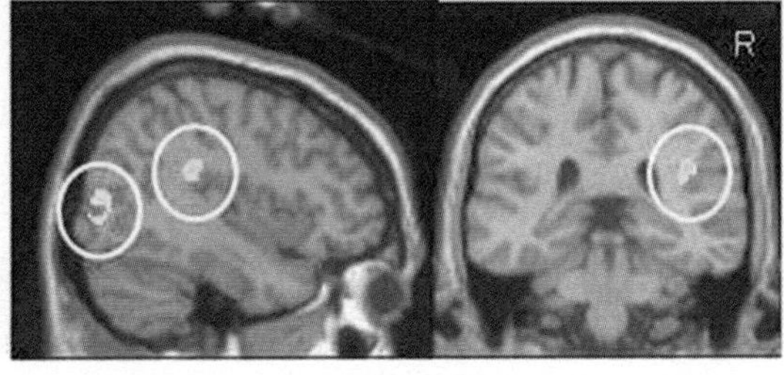

FIGURE 20.5
Regional activity relating to EDA during gambling task performance. (A) Six subjects were scanned using fMRI while performing a decision-related gambling task. In individual trials, the subject was presented with pairs of playing cards and was required to respond to one or the other in order to win money. Immediate feedback was given (tick/cross replacing the question mark) that indicated if the subject had won or lost money, and the level of overall winnings was modified accordingly. (B) Unknown to the subject, feedback (wins/losses) on any particular trial was predetermined by a binomial random walk. (C) Performing the task produced individualised fluctuations in EDA recorded throughout the task (black line). In a covariance analysis these continuous data were used to examine activity covarying with EDA. Also, peaks in EDA responses were identified (illustrated in red) and used in an event-related analysis. (D) Brain regions covarying with EDA; significant group activity is mapped on parasagittal and coronal sections of a template brain and is observed in anterior insula and ventromedial prefrontal cortices, extrastriate visual cortex, and right parietal lobe.

regions preferentially contribute to EDA generation. Conversely, following individual EDA responses, the greater right medial prefrontal cortex activity suggests that this region is important for representation of peripheral EDA arousal. These observations suggest a partial segregation, even within ventromedial prefrontal cortex, of regional brain activity supporting generation and representation of EDA.

The observation that ventromedial prefrontal activity contributes to generation and representation of EDA responses during decision-making gambling task performance is important because of its consistency with both the reported effects of prefrontal lesions on generation of EDA responses (Tranel and Damasio, 1994; Bechara *et al.*, 1996; Zahn *et al.*, 1999) and the proposed modulation of these areas during motivational decision making by EDA-related arousal (Damasio, 1994; Bechara *et al.*, 1996, 1997). The study also showed activity in regions such as inferior parietal lobule and extrastriate visual cortex associated with EDA. These areas are critical to directing visual attention, and the imaging findings suggest that sympathetic arousal and attention may share a common neural substrate; however, the study only dealt with the mechanisms by which cognitive or emotional responses are integrated with EDA arousal and notably failed to demonstrate anterior cingulate activity in association with EDA, in contrast to other observations (Tranel and Damasio, 1994; Fredikson *et al.*, 1998; Williams *et al.*, 2000).

These latter issues were addressed in a further fMRI study that examined how arousal, indexed by EDA, may influence regional brain activity during anticipation of a rewarding or punishing outcome (Critchley *et al.*, 2001a). A second gambling task was designed in which the subject had to guess, when presented with one playing card (face value between 1 and 10), if the face value of the next card presented would be higher or lower. Correct decisions were associated with financial gain, and wrong decisions with financial loss. These decisions were therefore associated with different but predictable risks that were a function of the face value of the cue card. Although the subjects responded as soon as they saw the first card, the second card (indicating if the subject had won or lost) was presented after a fixed delay period. The question addressed here was how sympathetic arousal (indexed by EDA) and the risk-value of each decision modulated brain activity during anticipation of the outcome. During the anticipatory delay period, anterior cingulate and dorsolateral prefrontal cortex activity varied parametrically with the degree of anticipatory EDA response. Activity in anterior cingulate and insula cortex was influenced by risk, and a conjunction analysis confirmed that anterior cingulate cortex was the only area to be modulated by both risk and arousal (Fig. 20.6).

Damage to both dorsolateral prefrontal and anterior cingulate cortices have previously been observed to diminish the EDA response magnitude (Zahn *et al.*,1999; Tranel, 2000). The neuroimaging findings strongly implicate anterior cingulate cortex in the integration of cognitive processes (for example, processing risk and expectancy) with EDA and other bodily states of

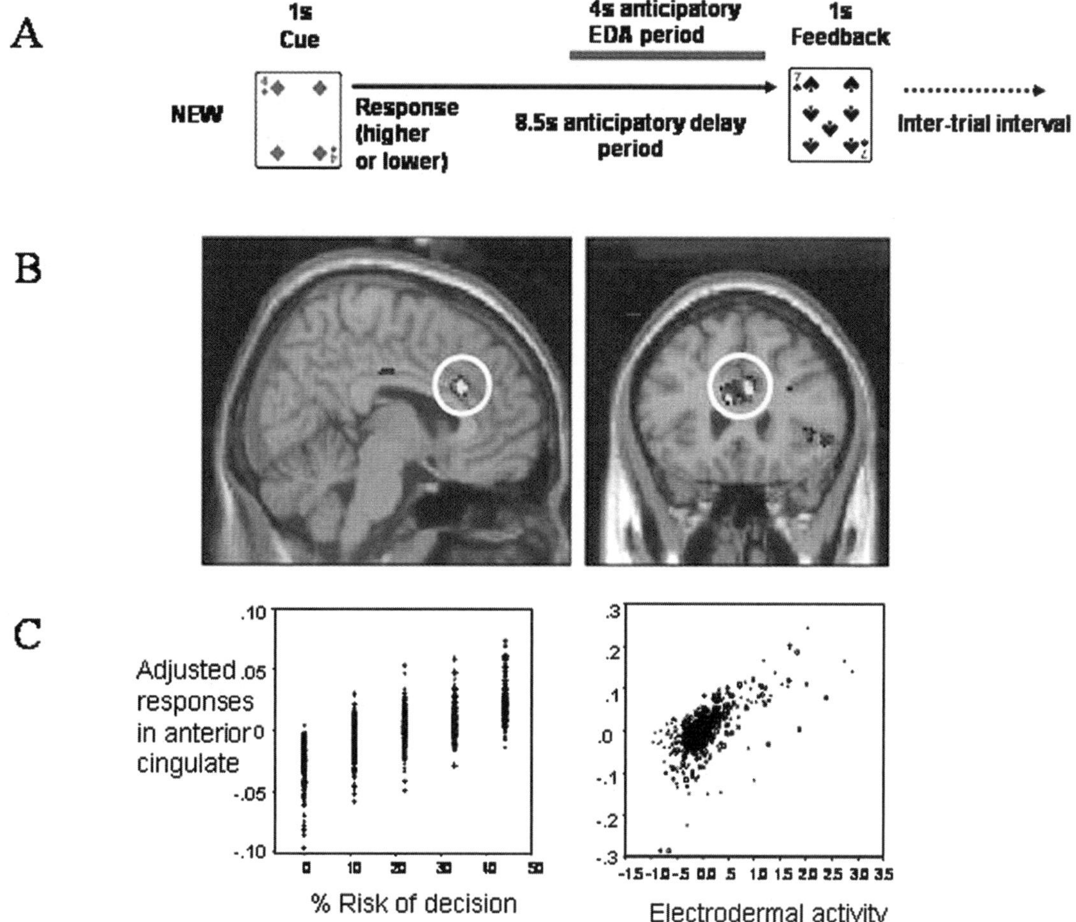

FIGURE 20.6
Modulation of delay-period activity by risk and anticipatory arousal indexed by EDA. (A) Diagram of individual trial. Subjects made a response to a cue card, judging if next (feedback) card would be higher or lower. Activity during the delay period before outcome was examined for modulation by riskiness of decision and by anticipatory EDA response (mean EDA in 4 s prior to outcome feedback). (B) and (C) Activity within anterior cingulate was modulated as function of both risk and EDA.

arousal. The role of the dorsolateral prefrontal activation in these studies may reflect a more selective relationship between contextual control of bodily arousal during cognitive processing of information about expectation, action, and experience.

Volitional Regulation of Autonomic Responses

In a further neuroimaging study, we examined the functional neuroanatomy by which conscious psychological processes may influence EDA (Critchley *et al.*, 2001b). Although autonomic processes such as EDA are generally beyond conscious influence, biofeedback relaxation techniques can enable subjects to gain control over autonomic responses. Prior to PET scanning, we trained subjects in performance of a biofeedback relaxation task in which EDA was used as an index of sympathetic arousal and was continuously visible in the form of a thermometer. As a subject relaxed and the level of EDA arousal decreased, there was a parallel decrease in the column height of the thermometer until the column eventually reached the "bulb" (which served as a fixed endpoint). Subjects were trained to relax rapidly and effectively using this EDA biofeedback task. During PET scanning, subjects performed repetitions of four different tasks: (1) biofeedback relaxation, where the subjects aimed to relax and decrease the column height while receiving accurate EDA feedback; (2) attempted relaxation with false feedback, where the display column fluctuated randomly; (3) no relaxation with EDA biofeedback, where subjects attempted to stem any downward drift in their EDA level; and (4) attempting not to relax while watching a false, randomly fluctuating display (Fig. 20.7). EDA was recorded during all experimental tasks, whether or not it contributed to the visual feedback. The main effect of subjects attempting to relax and reduce EDA arousal was associated with increased activity in anterior cingulate, inferior parietal cortex, and globus pallidus. Integration of the intention to relax with feedback of subjects' EDA levels (*i.e.*, the interaction between true versus false EDA biofeedback and relaxation versus no relaxation), was associated with increased activity in ventromedial prefrontal cortex, anterior cingulate, and cerebellar vermis. Finally, activity in medial temporal lobe involving the uncus, just anterior to the amygdala, reflected the rate of decrease in EDA-indexed arousal across all experimentally tasks (Fig. 20.6). Together, these observations implicate brain regions such as ventromedial prefrontal cortex and anterior cingulate in integration of bodily arousal with cognitive processes (intention to relax). Interestingly, in contrast to studies of sympathetic arousal (Critchley *et al.*, 2000a,b), activity during performance of relaxation tasks was greater in the left hemisphere than the right. Also, the observation that activity in the uncus is associated with sympathetic relaxation suggests a mechanism by which relaxation strategies may therapeutically influence brain regions mediating fear and stress responses, such as the adjacent amygdala.

We subsequently developed a similar biofeedback relaxation task for fMRI that utilised the higher spatial and enhanced temporal resolution of this technique to delineate a matrix of regional brain activity relating to volitional decreases in electrodermal activity and examine in more detail the neuroanatomy supporting cognitive influences on autonomic responses (Critchley *et al.*, 2002). We obtained fMRI measures in 17 subjects to assess brain activity relating biofeedback relaxation in which a visual index of electrodermal arousal was modulated by accuracy (addition of random noise) or sensitivity (by scalar adjustments of feedback). Performance of biofeedback relaxation tasks activated a central autonomic matrix, including insula, cingulate, thalamus, hypothalamus, and brainstem, as well as somatosensory cortex, dorsolateral prefrontal cortex, and extrastriate cortical area V5. Noisy feedback to subjects was associated with increased activity in anterior cingulate, amygdala, and V5. Activity within the anterior insula was not only modulated by both the accuracy and sensitivity of feedback but also reflected an interaction between these qualities of feedback. Thus, the increased insular response to noise in the feedback signal was modulated by the perceptual qualities (sensitivity) of the feedback. These findings highlight neural substrates supporting integration of perceptual processing, interoceptive awareness, and intentional modulation of bodily states of arousal. In particular, our findings suggest that activity in anterior cingulate mediates the intentional drive to decrease sympathetic activity, whereas insula activity may support *sensory* integration of interoceptive and external information about bodily states, a process that is likely to be closely related to "feeling states" and interoceptive awareness.

A PET study of biofeedback relaxation

Relaxation x feedback interaction

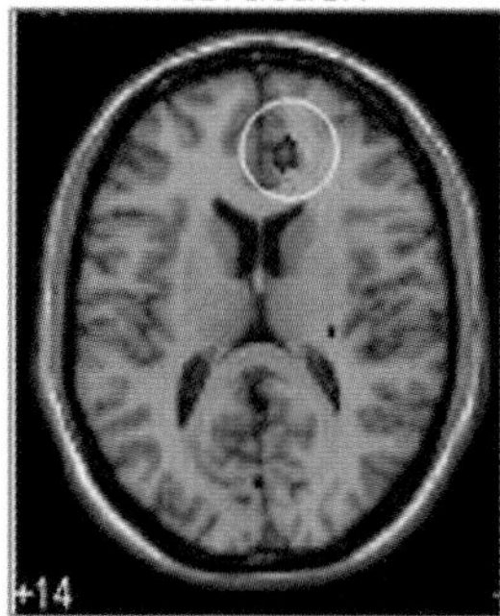

Activity covarying with *rate* of electrodermal relaxation

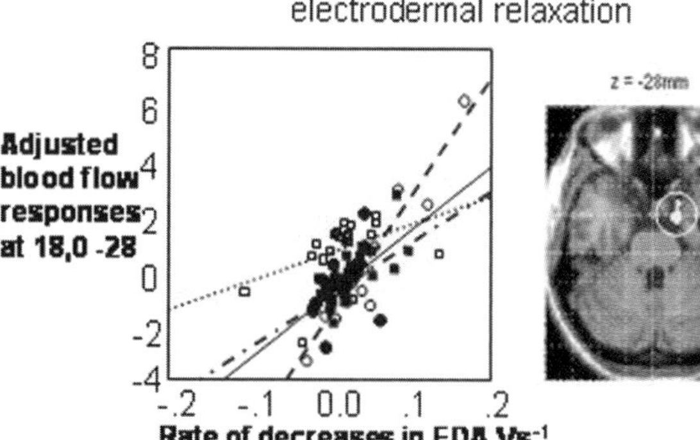

B fMRI study of biofeedback relaxation

Main effect of performing EDA biofeedback relaxation task

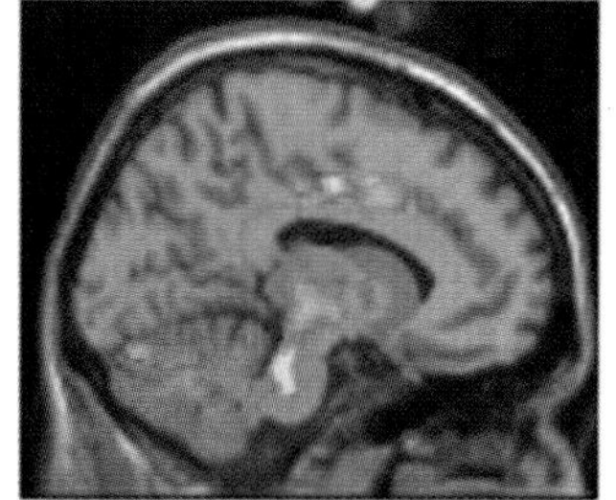

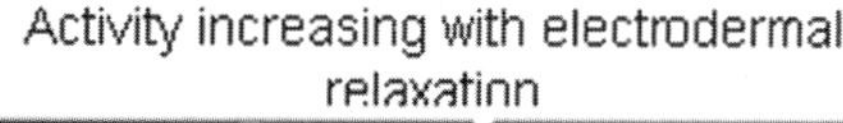

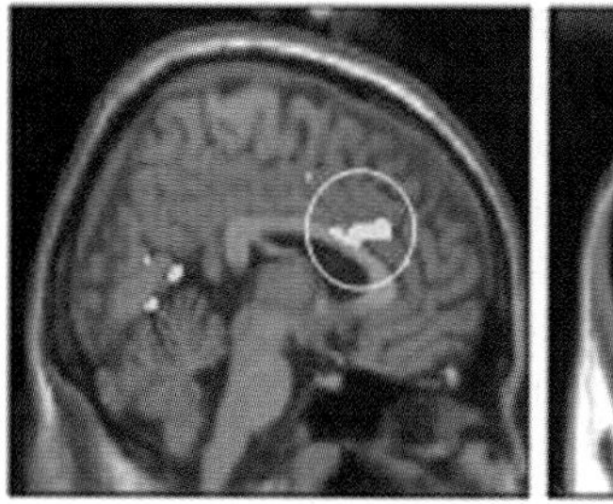

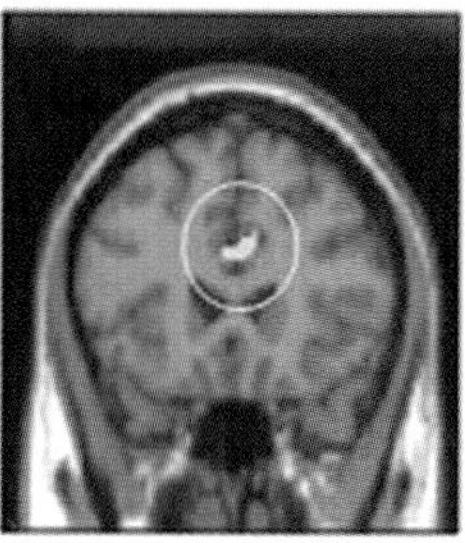

FIGURE 20.7
Regional activity relating to EDA biofeedback relaxation tasks. (A) PET study: Subjects were scanned using $H_2{}^{15}O$ PET during relaxation or no-relaxation conditions with or without biofeedback. EDA was continuously monitored during the experiment and used as the signal for biofeedback in half the tasks. The interaction of the intentional relaxation with the presence of feedback, reflecting biofeedback relaxation *per se*, was associated with activity in anterior cingulate cortex. The location of this activity, on an axial section of a template brain, is depicted on the left. Activity relating to rates of EDA relaxation, independent of which condition was performed, was observed in the right uncus anterior to the amygdala. The relationship between adjusted blood flow within this region and the rates of relaxation is plotted next to the location of this effect depicted on a template brain. (B) fMRI study: Subjects were scanned while performing biofeedback relaxation tasks, which differed either in the sensitivity or the in the accuracy of the feedback signal. Compared to rest, performance of biofeedback tasks was associated with activity in a distributed network of cortical, subcortical, and brainstem regions, including many putative autonomic control centres. The figure to the left shows group activity plotted on a parasagittal section of a template brain, illustrating involvement of cingulate, thalamus, hypothalamus pons, and cerebellum in biofeedback task performance. The figure to the right illustrates increased activity within anterior cingulate cortex in association with decreasing EDA arousal across the whole experiment.

Patient Studies

All the studies described above, conducted in healthy subjects, relied on cognitive physical or emotional drive to produce associated changes in peripheral autonomic activity. Rather than interpreting these changes as epiphenomena, irrelevant to observed brain activity, our approach has involved an exploration of how these bodily changes relate directly to regional activity. It is also relevant to note that individual differences exist in the efficacy of emotional or psychological stimuli in triggering autonomic responses. Patient groups, such as those with phobias and anxiety-related disorders, may demonstrate chronic changes in autonomic arousal, circumscribed precipitants to autonomic responses, or exaggerated autonomic responses to mundane stimuli; however, very few studies have utilised such patient groups as a hyperreactivity model for investigation of central autonomic control. Nevertheless, many studies conducted on such patients have observed increases in limbic and paralimbic activity during provocation of anxiety symptoms overlapping with regions now more directly implicated in autonomic control (McGuire *et al.*, 1994; Fredrikson *et al.*, 1997; Rauch *et al.*, 1997).

Neurological patient groups can provide potentially greater insights into the central physiology of human autonomic regulation. Critical to understanding central mechanisms for generation and re-representation of states of autonomic arousal is the ability to dissect afferent and somataesthetic components of autonomic control. There is clear evidence from animal studies for feedback mechanisms of autonomic control at the level of brainstem (Willette *et al.*, 1984; Bennarroch, 1997; Blessing, 1997; Collins, 1999; Spyer, 1999). Such feedback loops are at the foundation of theoretical models of emotion (James, 1894; Damasio, 1994) and even consciousness (Damasio, 1999). The core idea here is that feedback representations of visceral and somatomotor activity may give emotional colour to ongoing experience and support a bedrock representation of the "self." Patients with discrete lesions to efferent or efferent limbs of these control loops consequently provide insights into the dynamics of autonomic regulation and the wider influences of bodily responses on emotion and cognition.

Methodologically, experimental lesions of human autonomic feedback loops present a number of problems. For neuroimaging experiments, the ideal is a reversible peripheral lesion that blocks autonomic nervous activity at the level of autonomic effectors or that blocks afferent information about (autonomic) bodily responses prior to this information reaching the central nervous system. Central lesions to putative autonomic centres would themselves provide corollary support for inferences made from imaging experiments of peripheral lesions.

Several possible approaches can provide a lesion model of autonomic control. Drugs such as peripherally acting beta-adrenoreceptor blockers diminish cardiovascular sympathetic responses and do not affect cerebral circulation directly (Olesen, 1986). This approach has the advantage of being acute, reversible, and applicable to healthy volunteers in repeated-measures experimental designs. Disadvantages are that parasympathetic bodily responses are preserved (including the parasympathetic withdrawal component of cardiovascular arousal) and EDA is unaffected. Notably, beta-blockade has not been used to examine autonomic control in functional imaging studies to date. Patient groups with spinal cord transections or peripheral autonomic neuropathy may provide powerful clinical lesion models. High spinal cord transections, above the level of sympathetic outflow, effectively uncouple peripheral sympathetic responses from central drive and block spinal transmission of somatoaesthetic information. However, vagal efferent (parasympathetic) control and afferent viscerosensory information are preserved. Again, functional imaging has not yet been applied to examine central autonomic control and representation in the context of high spinal cord lesions.

Patients with selective autonomic failure, as manifest in the rare syndrome of pure autonomic failure (PAF) prove a unique group to examine central autonomic control. Whereas peripheral autonomic neuropathy is associated with a variety of disease processes, selective peripheral lesions of the autonomic nervous system are rare. We have studied patients with PAF who have an acquired selective peripheral autonomic denervation affecting postganglionic sympathetic and parasympathetic neurons but who have no central neurological pathology (Mathias and Bannister, 1999; Mathias, 2000). Using the same experimental PET design as the earlier investigation of autonomic centres of cardiovascular arousal, we examined regional activity in PAF patients and matched controls during the performance of cognitive and physical stressor tasks. By virtue of the diagnosis of PAF, differences in regional brain activity between patients and controls must be consequent to absent feedback of autonomic bodily changes normally accompanying effortful behaviour. We envisaged decreased activity in PAF subjects within brain regions mapping autonomic arousal and perhaps increases within regions generating autonomic arousal states. An interesting initial observation was increased pontine activity across effortful and effortless cognitive and physical tasks in PAF patients (Fig. 20.8). In the previous study of young healthy controls, activity in this region was observed during performance of effortful pressor tasks associated with increases in cardiovascular arousal. This newer finding in PAF patients suggests that above and beyond the generation of arousal patterns during effort, the dorsal pontine region is responsible for continuous, autoregulatory efferent control of autonomic responses. In this role, pontine activity is governed by afferent feedback and is largely independent of higher cognitive or physical drive. Reduced activity across all tasks was observed in regions including insula and primary somatosensory cortex, consistent with the notion that these areas are primarily involved with the continuous mapping of bodily states (Fig. 20.8).

A Main effect of peripheral autonomic failure

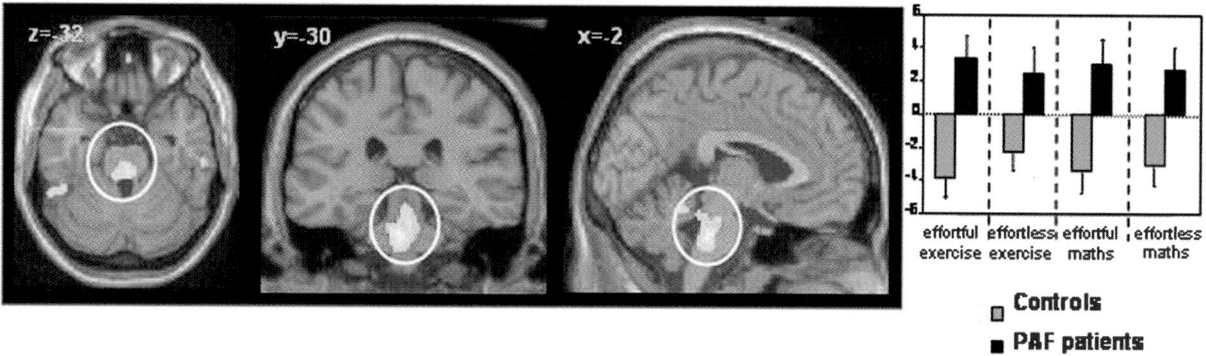

B Interaction of diagnosis with effort

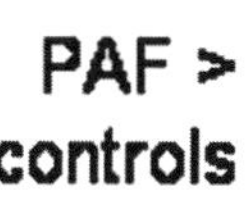

z = 34mm

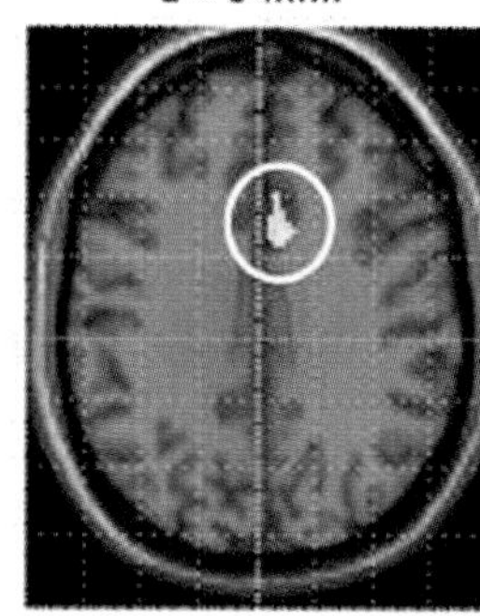

controls > PAF

z = 36mm

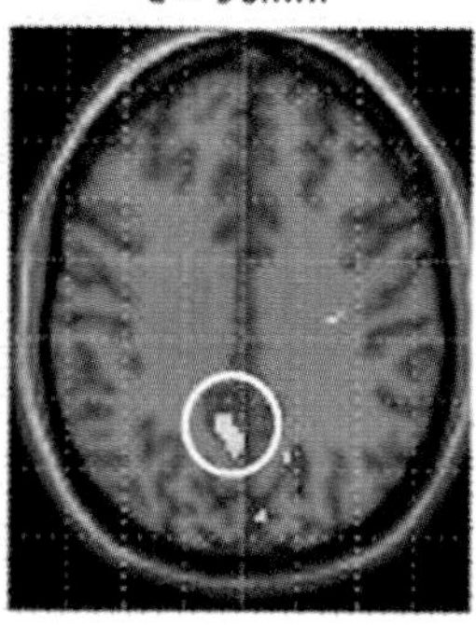

FIGURE 20.8
Regional activity differences in patients with pure autonomic failure (PAF). Patients with PAF, (a peripheral autonomic denervation,) and matched controls were scanned using PET during performance of effortful cognitive (mental arithmetic) and physical (isometric exercise) stress tasks and low-grade, effortless, control conditions. Consistent with their diagnosis, PAF subjects did not show significant increases in blood pressure or heart rate. (A) Independent of task, PAF patients showed significantly increased blood flow relative to controls in dorsal pons, consistent with increased autoregulatory activity in the absence of continuous negative feedback of autonomic responses. The figure plots this group difference in activity on axial coronal and parasagittal sections of a template brain, together with bar graphs of the adjusted blood flow responses for the four task conditions for the patient groups. (B) In the absence of autonomic responses during effortful cognitive and physical behaviours, patients with PAF had significantly greater activity than controls in right anterior cingulate (beyond that seen in association with autonomic arousal (see Figure 20.3B), suggestive of a context-specific increase in activity in the absence of negative feedback of autonomic arousal. In contrast, decreased activity in posterior cingulate/medial parietal cortex was observed in PAF patients during effortful behaviour, independent of task modality. The anatomical locations of these second-order differences are illustrated on axial sections of a template brain.

Of particular interest were brain areas that showed context-dependent changes in activity; that is, distinct brain areas showed differences between PAF patients and controls during physical and mental effort (accompanied by autonomic arousal in controls) but not during effortless tasks. In the previous PET study we observed right anterior cingulate activity covarying with increases in cardiovascular arousal in young controls (mean age, 35). In the present study, the same effect was observed in older controls (mean age, 65) (Fig. 20.3). It was therefore surprising to observe significantly greater right anterior cingulate activity in PAF patients, who generated no cardiovascular arousal, compared to matched healthy controls. Importantly, this observation was in keeping with the notion that anterior cingulate activity is responsible for context-specific autonomic modulation of bodily states to meet behavioural demands (Fig. 20.8). Thus, performance of effortful tasks increases the intact drive to modulate bodily arousal in the PAF patients. In healthy subjects, these context-specific autonomic responses negatively feedback to regulate efferent sympathetic drive, whereas in PAF subjects there is no such feedback and the peripheral autonomic drive from anterior cingulate cortex is consequently greater.

Lesion Studies of Central Autonomic Control

Many of the above neuroimaging investigations implicate anterior/ mid-cingulate cortex in autonomic control, particularly in the contextual generation of states of bodily arousal in response to task demands. An implication of this is that lesions affecting anterior cingulate cortex would be associated with abnormal autonomic responses during volitional or emotional behaviours. As described in the introduction, particular brain lesions are known to affect autonomic responsiveness, and reductions in EDA are reported following damage to regions including anterior cingulate (Tranel and Damasio, 1989; Zahn *et al.*, 1999; Tranel, 2000). To date, we have studied three patients with lesions primarily involving anterior cingulate cortex (Fig. 20.9). On a battery of autonomic function tests, conducted in the Autonomic Unit at the National Hospital for Neurology and Neurosurgery, all three subjects demonstrated abnormalities in cardiovascular

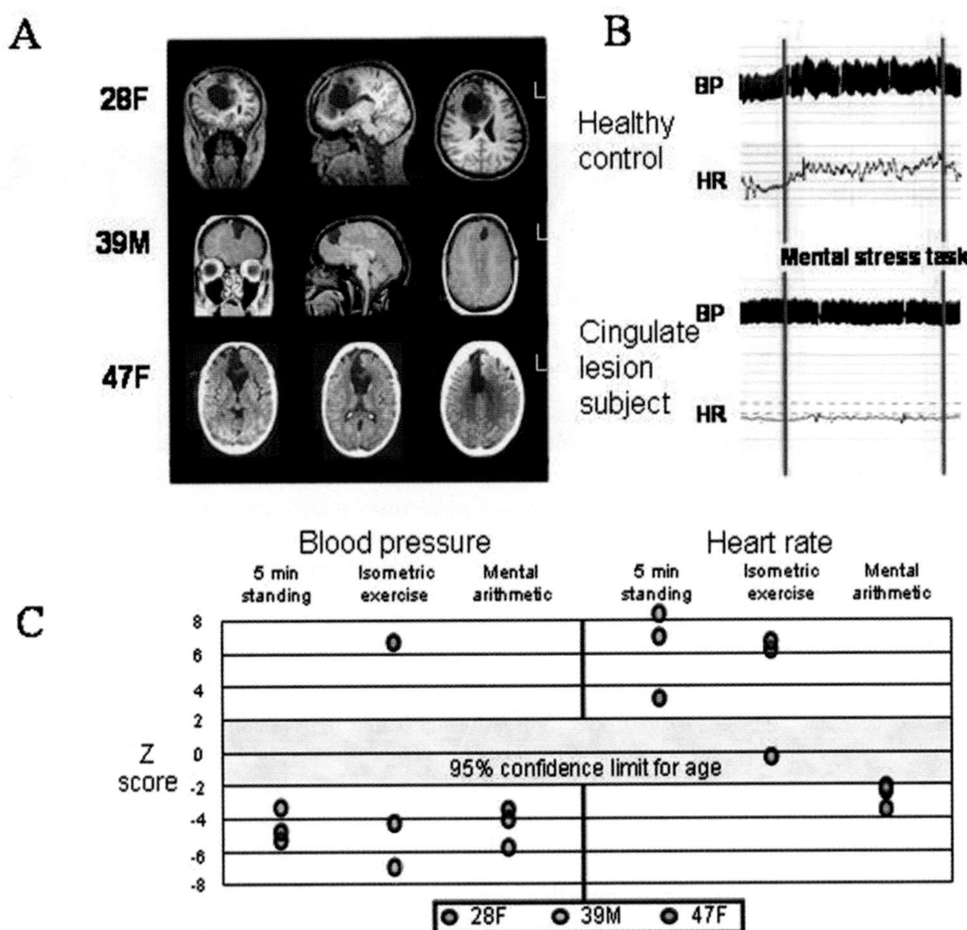

FIGURE 20.9

Lesions to the anterior cingulate cortex. (A) Three subjects with brain lesions involving anterior cingulate cortex underwent autonomic function tests. The location of each subject's lesion is shown on structural MRI scans. Clinical neuropsychometric evaluation of these subjects revealed no significant deficits including performance of standard executive function tasks. (B) On the basis of functional imaging, context-specific abnormalities in autonomic arousal were predicted during effortful behaviour, particularly during cognitive stress tasks. This figure illustrates the absence of cardiovascular arousal during (normal) performance of a serial subtraction mental arithmetic task in one of the anterior cingulate lesion subjects, below the blood pressure and heart rate responses of a healthy subject performing the same task. Brief calibration artifacts of the Portapres2 apparatus are apparent on these traces. (C) Deviations from normative blood pressure and heart rate responses for the three subjects are illustrated on a plot of Z-scores. Normative data were derived from 147 healthy subjects tested in the same manner (Mathias and Bannister, 1999). All three cingulate patients showed significantly reduced cardiovascular arousal during mental arithmetic stress testing, consistent with predictions. On effortful isometric exercise, all three showed abnormalities, with an exaggerated blood pressure response in one. Interestingly, abnormalities were also observed on postural testing, with a failure of cingulate patients to increase blood pressure rapidly on standing, resulting in a compensatory tachycardia.

arousal responses to volitional behaviours such as isometric exercise and mental arithmetic. Interestingly, the normal blood pressure changes to orthostatic challenge were also diminished. All three subjects had decreases in blood pressure in response to standing, with compensatory increases in heart rate. These observations not only validate our inferences about the role of anterior cingulate cortex activity associated with integration of autonomic arousal with during volitional and effortful behaviour, but also, interestingly, suggest that its role in autonomic regulation extends to a lower level (postural challenge) than that anticipated by our studies.

Further work is required to examine how autonomic abnormalities impact emotional and perhaps cognitive experiences. Despite an absence of gross neuropsychological deficits in the three patients with anterior cingulate lesions or indeed in PAF patients, there may still be subtle changes in subjective emotional experience, as some early data have suggested to be the case in PAF patients (Critchley *et al.*, 2001c). Our observations in anterior cingulate patients provide powerful support for the proposal that behaviourally driven changes in bodily states are initiated in part at the level of anterior cingulate cortex, but further studies are required to obtain a mechanistic understanding of the contribution of regions such as insula and somatosensory cortex, implicated in representations of changes in bodily states to cognitive and emotional processing.

CONCLUSIONS

Peripheral autonomic responses and the central representation of changes in bodily arousal are dynamically integrated with brain processes underlying emotion, cognition, and physical behaviour. The characterisation of the complexities of central autonomic control is necessary for a comprehensive systems-level understanding of human brain function. Interest in this area is increasing, much of it driven by experimental and theoretical advances in emotion research. The studies described above represent early inroads into mapping autonomic-related regional activity and its integration with behaviour. Already findings from these studies have important experimental and clinical implications. For example, the observation of an association between activity in anterior cingulate cortex and generation of autonomic states raises important issues with respect to interpretation of its role in a range of functional neuroimaging experiments involving cognitive paradigms.

Increasing availability of detailed physiological recordings during functional magnetic resonance imaging and methodological developments in both the acquisition and analyses of functional imaging data will help elucidate the distributed dynamics of autonomic control with the inclusion of hypothalamic and brainstem regions that have hitherto been poorly visualised. Key questions regarding human autonomic control remain. First, there is the issue of how efferent autonomic control is centrally organised in terms of organ specificity (skin, heart, or gut, perhaps at an autoregulatory level) or behavioural specificity (emotions, escape, anticipation). The neuroanatomical dissociation of different components within autonomic axes (*e.g.*, EDA from cardiovascular sympathetic control) also requires further investigation, as does the question of lateralisation of arousal-related responses in cerebral cortex and descending pathways. The dissociation of brain areas involved in generating autonomic arousal from feedback information about bodily state remains an important goal that may only be achieved through studies involving patient groups with discrete autonomic or sensory lesions. Probably the most important area to be addressed remains a characterisation of neural processes supporting the contextual integration of autonomic bodily states with behaviour.

The interdependence of bodily autonomic states with cognitive, emotional, and physical processes has implications beyond the design and interpretation of neuroimaging studies. Whereas human neuropsychology has hitherto embraced a dualist model of brain and body, important theoretical models (Damasio, 1994, 1999) argue that brain function in isolation cannot provide a comprehensive explanation for either subjective experience or observable motivational behaviours. Likewise, purely cognitive neuropsychological approaches underestimate the biological, especially bodily, contribution to high-level behaviours. The fact that all cognitive states are to a greater or lesser degree yoked to autonomic states means that a comprehensive account of cognition must necessarily also involve an account of autonomic control.

References

Adolphs, R., Tranel, D., and Damasio, A. R. (1998). The human amygdala in social judgment. *Nature*, **393**, 470–474.

Anderson, C. R., McLachlan, E. M., and Srb-Christie, O. (1989). Distribution of sympathetic preganglionic neurons and monoaminergic nerve terminals in the spinal cord of the rat. *J. Comp. Neurol.*, **283**, 269–284.

Angyan, L. (1994). Somatomotor and cardiorespiratory responses to basal ganglia stimulation in cats. *Physiol. Behav.*, **56**, 167–173.

Bechara, A., Tranel, D., Damasio, H., Adolphs, R., Rockland, C., and Damasio, A. (1995). Double dissociation of conditioning and declarative knowledge relative to the amygdala and hippocampus in humans. *Science*, **267**, 1115–1118.

Bechara, A., Tranel, D., Damasio, H., and Damasio, A. R. (1996). Failure to respond autonomically to anticipated future outcomes following damage to prefrontal cortex. *Cereb. Cortex*, **6**, 215–225.

Bechara, A., Damasio, H., Tranel, D., and Damasio, A. R. (1997). Deciding advantageously before knowing the advantageous strategy. *Science*, **275**, 1293–1295.

Bechara, A., Damasio, H., Damasio, A. R., and Lee, G. P. (1999). Differential contributions of the human amygdala and ventromedial prefrontal cortex to decision-making. *J. Neurosci.*, **19**, 5473–5481.

Bennarroch, E. E. (1997). Functional anatomy of the central autonomic network, in *Central Autonomic Network: Functional Organisation and Clinical Correlations*, Bennarroch, E. E., Ed., pp. 29–60. Futura Publishing, Armonk, NY.,.

Blessing, W. W. (1997). Inadequate frameworks for understanding bodily homeostasis. *Trends Neurosci.*, **20**, 235–239.

Boccia, M. L. and Roberts, J. E. (2000). Behaviour and autonomic nervous system function assessed via heart period measures: the case of hyperarousal in boys with fragile X syndrome. *Behav. Res. Meth. Instrum. Comput.*, **32**, 5–10.

Bouscein, W. (1992). *Electrodermal Activity*. Plenum, New York.

Brading, A. (1999). *The Autonomic Nervous System and Its Effectors*, Blackwell Scientific, Oxford.

Bradley, D. J., Ghelarducci, B., and Spyer, K. M. (1991). The role of the posterior cerebellar vermis in cardiovascular control. *Neurosci. Res.*, **12**, 45–56.

Buchanan, S. L., Valentine, J., and Powell, D. A. (1985). Autonomic responses are elicited by electrical stimulation of the medial but not lateral frontal cortex in rabbits. *Behav. Brain Res.*, **18**, 51–62.

Buchel, C., Morris, J., Dolan, R., and Friston, K. (1998). Brain systems mediating aversive conditioning: an event-related fMRI study. *Neuron*, **20**, 947–957.

Cahill, L. (1997). The neurobiology of emotionally influenced memory implications for understanding traumatic memory. *Ann. N.Y. Acad. Sci.*, **821**, 238–246.

Cahill, L,. and McGaugh, J. L. (1998). Mechanisms of emotional arousal and lasting declarative memory. *Trends Neurosci.*, **21**, 294–249.

Cannon, W. B. (1927). The James–Lange theory of emotions. *Am. J. Psychol.*, **39**, 115–124.

Cannon, W. B. (1929). *Bodily Changes in Pain, Hunger, Fear and Rage: An Account of Recent Research into the Function of Emotional Excitement*, 2nd ed., Appleton, New York.

Cechetto, D. F,. and Saper, C. B. (1987). Evidence for a viscerotopic sensory representation in the cortex and thalamus in the rat. *J. Comp. Neurol.*, **262**, 27–45.

Cechetto, D. R,. and Saper, C. B. (1990). Role of the cerebral cortex in autonomic function, in *Central Regulation of Autonomic Functions*, Loewy, A. D. and Spyer, K. M., Eds., pp. 208–223. Oxford University Press, London.

Chua, P., Krams, M., Toni, I., Passingham, R., and Dolan, R. (1999). A functional anatomy of anticipatory anxiety. *NeuroImage*, **9**, 563–571.

Collet, C., Vernet-Maury, E., Delhomme, G., and Dittmar, A. (1997). Autonomic nervous system response patterns specificity to basic emotions. *J. Auton. Nerv. Syst.*, **12**, 45–57.

Collins, K. J. (1999). Temperature regulation and the autonomic nervous system, in *Autonomic Failure: A Textbook of Clinical Disorders of the Autonomic Nervous System*. 4th ed., Mathias, C. J. and Bannister, R., Eds., pp. 169–195.Oxford University Press, London..

Critchley, H. D., Corfield, D. R., Chandler, M. P., Mathias, C. J., and Dolan, R. J. (2000a). Cerebral correlates of autonomic cardiovascular arousal: a functional neuroimaging investigation. *J. Physiol. London*, **523**, 259–270.

Critchley, H. D., Elliot, R., Mathias, C. J., and Dolan, R. J. (2000b). Neural activity relating to the generation and representation of galvanic skin conductance response: a functional magnetic imaging study. *J. Neurosci.*, **20**, 3033–3040.

Critchley, H. D., Mathias, C. J., and Dolan, R. J. (2001a). Neural activity relating to reward anticipation in the human brain. *Neuron*, **29**, 537–545.

Critchley, H. D., Melmed, R. N., Featherstone, E., Mathias, C. J., and Dolan, R. J. (2001b). Brain activity during biofeedback relaxation: a functional neuroimaging investigation. *Brain*, **124**, 1003–1012.

Critchley, H. D., Mathias, C. J., and Dolan, R. J. (2001c). Neural correlates of first and second-order representation of bodily states. *Nat. Neurosci.*, **2**, 207–212.

Critchley, H. D., Melmed, R. N., Featherstone, E., Mathias, C. J., and Dolan, R. J. (2002). Volitional control of autonomic arousal: a functional magnetic resonance study. *NeuroImage*, **16**, 909–919.

Critchley, H. D., Mathias, C. J., Josephs, O., O'Doherty, J., Zanini, S., Dewar, B. K., Cipolotti, L., Shallice, T., and Dolan, R. J. (2003). Human cingulate cortex and autonomic control: converging neuroimaging and clinical evidence. *Brain*, **216** (epub).

Damasio, A. R. (1994). *Descartes' Error: Emotion, Reason and the Human Brain*. Grosset Putnam, New York.

Damasio, A. R. (1999). *The Feeling of What Happens: Body and Emotion in the Making of Consciousness*. Harcourt Brace, New York.

Damasio, A. R., Tranel, D., and Damasio, H. C. (1990). Individual with sociopathic behaviour caused by frontal damage fail to respond autonomically to social stimuli. *Behav. Brain Res.*, **41**, 81–894.

Damasio, A. R., Tranel, D., and Damasio, H. C. (1991). Somatic markers and the guidance of behaviour: theory and preliminary testing, in *Frontal Lobe Function and Dysfunction*, Levin, H. S., Eisenberg, H. M., and Benton, L. B., Eds., chpt. 11. Oxford University Press, New York.

Darwin, C. (1998). In *The Expression of the Emotions in Man and Animals*, 3rd ed., Ekman, P., Ed., Oxford University Press, London.

Davison, M. A,. and Koss, M. C. (1975). Brainstem loci for activation of electrodermal response in the cat. *Am. J. Physiol.*, **229**, 930–934.

Dawson, M. E., Nuechterlein, K. H., Schell, A. M., Gitlin, M., and Ventura, J. (1994). Autonomic abnormalities in schizophrenia: state or trait indicators? *Arch. Gen. Psychiatry*, **51**, 813–824.

Dawson, M. E., Schell, A. M., and Filion, D. L. (2000). The electrodermal system, in *Handbook of Psychophysiology*, 2nd ed., Cacioppo, J. T., Tassinary, L. G., and Berntson, G. C., Eds., pp. 200–223. Cambridge University Press, Cambridge, U.K. .

Delgado, J. M. (1960). Circulatory effects of cortical stimulation. *Physiol. Rev.*, **40**,(Suppl. 4), 146–178.

Elliott, R., Friston, R. J., and Dolan, R. J. (2000). Dissociable responses associated with reward, punishment and risk-taking behaviour. *J. Neurosci.*, **20**, 6159–6165.

Ferri, R., Curzi-Dascalova, L., Del Gracco, S., Elia, M., Musumeci, S. A., and Pettinato, S. (1998). Heart rate variability and apnea during sleep in Down's syndrome. *J. Sleep Res.*, **7**, 282–287.

Fish, D. R., Gloor, P., Quesney, F. L., and Olivier, A. (1993). Clinical responses to electrical brain stimulation of temporal and frontal lobes in patients with epilepsy: pathophysiological implications. *Brain*, **116**, 397–414.

Fowles, D. C., Christie, M. J., Edelberg, R., Grings, W. W., Lykken, D. T., and Venables, P. H. (1981). Publication recommendations for electrodermal measurements. *Psychophysiology*, **18**, 232–239.

Fredrikson, M., Fischer, H., and Wik, G. (1997). Cerebral blood flow during anxiety provocation. *J. Clin. Psychiatry*, **58**(Suppl. 16), 16–21.

Fredrikson, M., Furmark, T., Olsson, M. T, Fischer, H., Andersson, J., and Langstrom, B. (1998). Functional neuroanatomical correlates of electrodermal activity: a positron emission tomographic study. *Psychophysiolgy*, **35**, 179–185.

Gelsema, A. J., Agarwal, S. K., and Calaresu, F. R. (1989). Cardiovascular responses and changes in neural activity in the rostral ventrolateral medulla elicited by electrical stimulation of the amygdala of the rat. *J. Autonomic Nerv. Syst.*, **27**, 91–100.

Guinjoan, S. M., Bernabo, J. L., and Cardinali, D. P. (1995). Cardiovascular tests of autonomic function and sympathetic skin responses in patients with major depression. *J. Neurol. Neurosurg. Psychiatry*, **59**, 299–302.

Harper, R. M., Bandler, R., Spriggs, D., and Alger, J. R. (2000). Lateralised and widespread brain activation during transient blood pressure elevation revealed by magnetic resonance imaging. *J. Comp. Neurol.*, **417**, 195–204.

Hazlett, H., Dawson, M. E., Schell, A. M., and Nuechterlein, K. H. (1997). Electrodermal activity as a prodromal sign in schizophrenia. *Biol. Psychiatry*, **41**, 111–113.

Hirstein, W., Iversen, P., and Ramachandran, V. S. (2001). Autonomic responses of autistic children to people and objects. *Proc. Roy. Soc. London Ser. B, Biol. Sci.*, **268**, 1883–1888.

Hodgins, S., Mendick, S. A., Brennan, P. A., Schulsinger, F., and Engberg, M. (1996). Mental disorder and crime: evidence from a Danish birth cohort. *Arch. Gen. Psychiatry*, **53**, 489–496.

Hultman, C. M,. and Ohman, A. (1998). Perinatal characteristics and schizophrenia: electrodermal activity as a mediating link in a vulnerability–stress perspective. *Int. J. Dev. Neurosci.*, **16**, 307–316.

James, W. (1894). Physical basis of emotion. *Psychol. Rev.*, **1**, 516–529, (reprinted in *Psychol. Rev.*, **101**, 205–210, 1994).

Julu, P. O., Kerr, A. M., Hansen, S., Apartopoulos, F., and Jamal, G. A. (1997). Functional evidence of brain stem immaturity in Rett syndrome. *Eur. Child Adolesc. Psychiatry*, **6**,(Suppl. 1), 47–54.

Kaada, B. R. (1951). Somato-motor, autonomic and electrocorticographic responses to electrical stimulation of rhinencephalic and other structures in primates, cat and dog. *Acta Physiol. Scand.*, **24**,(Suppl. 83), 1–285.

Kamada, T., Miyake, S., Kumashiro, M., Monou, H., and Inoue, K. (1992). Power spectral analysis of heart rate variability in type As and type Bs during mental workload. *Psychosom. Med.*, **54**, 462–470.

Kimble, D. P., Bagshaw, M. H., and Pribram, K. H. (1965). The GSR of monkeys during orienting and habituation after selective partial ablations of the cingulate and frontal cortex. *Neuropsychologia*, **3**, 121–128.

King A,. B., Menon, R. S., Hachinski, V., and Cechetto, D. F. (1999). Human forebrain activation by visceral stimuli. *J. Comp. Neurol.*, **413**, 572–582.

Lane, R. D., Chua, P. M., and Dolan, R. J. (1999). Common effects of emotional valence arousal and attention on neural activation during visual processing of pictures. *Neuropsychologia*, **37**, 989–997.

Langley, J. N. (1898). On the union of cranial autonomic (visceral) fibres with the nerve cells of the superior cervical ganglion. *J. Physiol.*, **23**, 240–270.

Langley, J. N. (1921). *The Autonomic Nervous System, Part 1*. Heffer, Cambridge, U.K.

LeDoux, J. E. (1921). Emotion and the amygdala, in *The Amygdala*, Aggleton, J. P., Ed., pp. 339–351. Wiley-Liss, New York.

Lencz, T., Raine, A., and Sheard, C. (1996). Neuroanatomical bases of electrodermal hypo-responding: a cluster analytic study. *Int. J. Psychophysiol.*, **22**,(3), 141–153.

Lin, M. T. and Yang, J. J. (1994). Stimulation of the nigrostriatal dopamine system produces hypertension and tachycardia in rats. *Am. J. Physiol.*, **266**, H2489–H2496.

Mangina, C. A. and Beuzeron-Mangina, J. H. (1996). Direct electrical stimulation of specific human brain structures and bilateral electrodermal activity. *Int. J. Psychophysiol.*, **22**, 1–8.

Mathias, C. J. (2000). Disorders of the autonomic nervous system, in *Neurology in Clinical Practice*, Bradley, W. G., Daroff, R., B., Fenichel, G. M,. *et al.*, Eds., pp. 2131–2165. Butterworth-Heinemann, Woburn, MA..

Mathias, C. J. and Bannister, R., Eds. (1999). *Autonomic Failure: A Textbook of Clinical Disorders of the Autonomic Nervous System*, 4th ed., pp. 169–195. Oxford University Press, London..

Mawson, A. R. and Mawson, C. D. (1977). Psychopathy and arousal: a new interpretation of the psychophysiological literature. *Biol. Psychiatry*, **12**, 49–74.

McGuire, P. K., Bench, C. J., Frith, C. D., Marks, I. M., Frackowiak, R. S., and Dolan, R. J. (1994). Functional anatomy of obsessive-compulsive phenomena. *Br. J. Psychiatry*, **164**, 459–468.

Metzger, L. J., Orr, S. P., Berry, N. J., Ahern, C. E., Lasko, N., B., and Pitman, R. K. (1999). Physiologic reactivity to startling tones in women with posttraumatic stress disorder. *J. Abnorm. Psychol.*, **108**, 347–352.

Morris, J. S., Ohman, A., and Dolan, R. J. (1998). Conscious and unconscious emotional learning in the human amygdala. *Nature*, **393**, 467–470.

Morrison, S. F. (2001). Differential control of sympathetic outflow. *Am. J. Regul. Integr. Comp. Physiol.*, **281**, R683–R698.

Neafsey, E. J. (1990). Prefrontal cortical control of the autonomic nervous system: anatomical and physiological observations. *Progr. Brain Res.*, **85**, 147–165.

Ohman, A. and Soares, J. J. (1993). On the automatic nature of phobic fear: conditioned electrodermal responses to masked fear-relevant stimuli. *J. Abnorm. Psychol.*, **102**, 121–132.

Olesen, J. (1986). Beta-adrenergic effects on cerebral circulation. *Cephalalgia*, **6**(Suppl. 5), 41–46.

Oppenheimer, S. M. and Cechetto, D. F. (1990). Cardiac chronotropic organisation of the rat insular cortex. *Brain Res.*, **533**, 66–72.

Oppenheimer, S. M., Gelb, A., Girvin, J. P., and Hachinski, V. C. (1992). Cardiovascular effects of human insular cortex stimulation. *Neurology*, **42**, 1727–1732.

Oscar-Berman, M,. and Gade, A. (1979). Electrodermal measures of arousal in humans with cortical or subcortical brain damage, in *The Orientating Reflex in Humans*, Kimmel, H. *et al.*, Eds., pp. 665–676. Lawrence Erlbaum, Hillsdale, NJ.

Palkovitz, R. J. and Wiesenfeld, A. R. (1980). Differential autonomic responses of autistic and normal children. *J. Autism Dev. Disord.*, **10**, 347–360.

Paus, T., Koski, L., Caramanos, Z., and Westbury, C. (1998). Regional differences in the effects of task difficulty and motor output on blood flow response in the human anterior cingulate cortex: a review of 107 PET activation studies. *NeuroReport*, **9**, R37–R47.

Pool, J. L. and Ransohoff, J. (1949). Autonomic effects on stimulating the rostral portion of the cingulate gyri in man. *J. Neurophysiol.*, **12**, 385–392.

Porges, S. W. (1976). Peripheral and neurochemical parallels of psychopathology: a psychophysiological model relating autonomic imbalance to hyperactivity, psychopathy, and autism. *Adv. Child Dev. Behav.*, **11**, 35–65.

Porges, S. W. (1995). Orienting in a defensive world: mammalian modification of our evolutionary heritage. A polyvagal theory. *Psychophysiology*, **32**, 301–318.

Price, C. J. and Friston, K. J. (1997). Cognitive conjunction: a new approach to brain activation experiments. *NeuroImage*, **5**, 261–270.

Raine, A. (1996). Autonomic nervous system factors underlying disinhibited, antisocial, and violent behaviour: biosocial perspectives and treatment implications. *Ann. N.Y. Acad. Sci.*, **794**, 46–59.

Rauch, S. L., Savage, C. R., Alpert, N. M., Fischman, A. J., and Jenike, M. A. (1997). The functional neuroanatomy of anxiety: a study of three disorders using positron emission tomography and symptom provocation. *Biol. Psychiatry*, **42**, 446–452.

Rolls, E. T. (1996). The orbitofrontal cortex. *Philos. Trans. Roy. Soc. London B, Biol. Sci.*, **351**, 1433–1443.

Rutter, M. (1987). Temperament, personality and personality disorder. *Br. J. Psychiatry*, **150**, 443–458.

Sacks, B. and Smith, S. (1989). People with Down's syndrome can be distinguished on the basis of cholinergic dysfunction. *J. Neurol. Neurosurg. Psychiatry*, **52**, 1294–1295.

Sato, K. (1977). The physiology, pharmacology, and biochemistry of the eccrine sweat gland. *Rev. Physiol. Biochem. Pharmacol.*, **79**, 51–131.

Scarpa, A., Raine, A., Venables, P. H., and Mednick, S. A. (1997). Heart rate and skin conductance in behaviourally inhibited Mauritian children. *J. Abnorm. Psychol.*, **106**, 182–190.

Schachter, S. and Singer, J. E. (1962). Cognitive, social and pysiological determinants of emotional state. *Psychol. Rev.*, **69**, 379–399.

Shallice, T. and Burgess, P. W. (1991). Deficits in strategy application following frontal lobe damage in man. *Brain*, **114**, 727–741.

Spyer, K. M. (1999). Central nervous control of the cardiovascular system, in *Autonomic Failure: A Textbook of Clinical Disorders of the Autonomic Nervous System*, Mathias, C. J. and Bannister, R., Eds., pp. 45–55. Oxford University Press, London. .

Stifter, C. A. and Jain, A. (1996). Psychophysiological correlates of infant temperament: stability of behaviour and autonomic patterning from 5 to 18 months. *Dev. Psychobiol.*, **29**, 379–391.

Tranel, D. and Damasio, H. (1989). Intact electrodermal skin conductance responses after bilateral amygdala damage. *Neuropsychologia*, **27**, 381–390.

Tranel, D. and Damasio, H. (1994). Neuroanatomical correlates of electrodermal skin conductance responses, *Psychophysiology*, **31**, 427–438.

Tranel, D. (2000). Electrodermal activity in cognitive neuroscience: neuroanatomical and neuropsychological correlates, in *Cognitive Neuroscience of Emotion*, Lane, R. D. and Nadel, L., Eds., pp. 192–224. Oxford University Press, London.

Venables, P. H. and Christie, M. J. (1980). Electrodermal activity, in *Techniques in Psychophysiology*, Martin, I. and Venables, P. H., Eds., pp. 3–67. Wiley, New York.

Vissing, S. F., Scherrer, U., and Victor, R. G. (1991). Stimulation of skin sympathetic nerve discharge by central command: differential control of sympathetic outflow to skin and skeletal muscle during static exercise. *Circ. Res.*, **69**, 228–238.

Welton, W., Clayson, D., Axelrod, F. B., and Levine, D. B. (1979). Intellectual development and familial dysautonomia. *Pediatrics*, **63**, 708–712.

Willette, R. N., Punnen, S., Krieger, A. J., and Sapru, H. N. (1984). Interdependence of rostral and caudal ventrolateral medullary areas in the control of blood pressure. *Brain Res.*, **321**, 169–174.

Williams, L. M., Brammer, M. J., Skerrett, D., Lagopolous, J., Rennie, C., Kozek, K., Olivieri, G., Peduto, T., and Gordon, E. (2000). The neural correlates of orienting: an integration of fMRI and skin conductance orienting. *NeuroReport*, **11**, 3011–3015.

Zahn, T. P., Rumsey, J. M., and Van Kammen, D. P. (1987). Autonomic nervous system activity in autistic, schizophrenic, and normal men: effects of stimulus significance. *J. Abnorm. Psychol.*, **96**, 135–144.

Zahn, T. P., Grafman, J., and Tranel, D. (1999). Frontal lobe lesions and electrodermal activity: effects of significance. *Neuropsychologia*, **37**, 1227–1241.

Zoccolotti, P., Scabini, D., and Violani, C. (1982). Electrodermal responses in patients with unilateral brain damage. *J. Clin. Neuropsychol.*, **4**, 143–150.

CHAPTER

21

Reciprocal Links Between Emotion and Attention

INTRODUCTION

Emotion and attention represent fundamental human psychological processes that influence perception, action, and conscious experience. At any point in time, humans are confronted with a myriad of simultaneous competing environmental stimuli but have a limited processing capacity. The brain must meet the challenge of detecting and representing only those stimuli most relevant for ongoing behaviour and survival.

It is likely that attentional mechanisms evolved to enable the brain to regulate its sensory inputs so as to afford such selective perceptual processing and goal-oriented action. A large body of work suggests that attention is necessary for an explicit representation of even basic stimulus properties in conscious awareness and to allow rapid and accurate discrimination among current sensory events (Posner and Petersen, 1990). Without selective attention, stimuli may escape conscious awareness or fail to enter working memory (Mack and Rock, 1998). However, there is evidence that a degree of stimulus processing can still take place independent of attention and awareness, and this pre-attentive processing may serve to preferentially guide attention to salient events (Merikle *et al.*, 2001). From an adaptive–evolutionary perspective, it can be assumed that emotion has a privileged role in biasing the allocation of attentional resources toward events with particular significance for an organism's motivational state.

In this chapter, we review evidence from human functional neuroimaging investigation indicating that dedicated brain systems are specifically tuned to process emotional information. In particular, we address how emotional processing can interact with attentional systems, focusing on the neural mechanisms by which emotion can affect the allocation of attention, as well as the degree to which selective attention in turn influences emotional processing.

Converging data from human functional imaging in healthy subjects, neuropsychological studies of brain-damaged patients, and monkey neurophysiology indicate that selective attentional mechanisms rely on a complex neural network predominantly centred on parietal, frontal, and cingulate cortices that are in turn intimately connected with subcortical structures such as thalamus, basal ganglia, and basal forebrain nuclei (Mesulam, 1999; Posner and Petersen, 1990). This distributed attentional system can control conscious perception by regulating information processing in modality-specific areas (see Chapter 15), thereby enhancing the neural representation of relevant stimuli and suppressing irrelevant representations. Brain systems implicated in emotional processing are anatomically distinct but nevertheless show important overlaps with classic attentional networks. For instance, the prefrontal cortex, anterior cingulate cortex, striatum, thalamus, and cholinergic basal forebrain nuclei are all implicated in both attentional and emotional processes, as are early sensory-specific pathways which offer a common input to both attentional and emotional control mechanisms. These overlapping sites provide a number of potential nodes for convergence between emotion and attention that might contribute either to the selection or suppression of salient environmental stimuli.

While evidence indicates considerable overlap between systems subserving attention and emotion, there remains the possibility that anatomically distinct routes might allow emotional information to be extracted with substantial independence from voluntary attention, and prior to access into conscious awareness. Thus, behavioural and neuroimaging evidence indicate that affectively significant events can be detected even without awareness of their occurrence (see Chapter 19). Such unconscious or "pre-attentive" analysis of emotional value might enable an individual to respond to affectively relevant stimuli, regardless of ongoing cognitive processing and current allocation of attention. In keeping with this, we will outline a view suggesting that emotion and attention constitute two independent though highly interacting neural systems that exert dissociable regulatory influences at several different stages of cortical processing, from elaborating sensory inputs through to preparing response outputs.

BACKGROUND: BEHAVIOURAL AND NEUROPSYCHOLOGICAL FINDINGS

A variety of psychophysical studies have suggested that emotional signals can influence cognition, particularly attention. Only a brief overview will be given here (for extended reviews, see Öhman *et al.*, 2000; Robinson, 1998). Thus, many studies examining the cognitive consequences of emotion have adapted paradigms extensively used in the literature on attention, such as visual search (Eastwood *et al.*, 2001; White, 1995), exogenous orienting (Mogg *et al.*, 1994, 1997; Stormark *et al.*, 1999), inattentional blindness (Anderson and Phelps, 2001; Mack and Rock, 1998), or Stroop interference (Mathews and Klug, 1993). In classic visual search tasks, the time to detect a specified target typically increases in direct proportion to the number of irrelevant distracters, indicating serial attentive processing of every stimuli in the display, unless the discrimination of targets from distracters occurs in early parallel processing stages that are independent of attention. In the latter case, attention is automatically drawn to the target ("pop-out") and detection time can be independent of distracter number. Several search experiments have shown more rapid detection of emotional stimuli among neutral distracters than vice versa, with a relatively flat or much shallower search rate as a function of the number of distracters. Such attentional benefits in search experiments have been reported when targets were faces with positive or negative expressions (Eastwood *et al.*, 2001; Hansen and Hansen, 1988; Öhman *et al.*, 2001b; White, 1995), spiders (Kindt and Brosschot, 1997), or snakes (Öhman *et al.*, 2001a). These effects suggest that the emotional value of stimuli can be perceived by some rapid pre-attentive route that then facilitates focal attention to the location of an emotional target more efficiently than to a neutral target. The most consistent capture of attention by emotion is usually found with negatively valenced or fear-related stimuli (Öhman *et al.*, 2000), and search rate slopes seem shallower for schematic faces with a negative/angry than a positive/happy expression (Eastwood *et al.*, 2001). Moreover, the superiority of emotional targets is enhanced for fearful or angry faces in anxious individuals and for feared stimuli in phobic subjects (Öhman *et al.*, 2000). However, some studies in normal subjects do not find significant pop-out effects for emotional faces in visual searches (Nothdurft, 1993).

Another strategy has examined the effect of emotional versus neutral cues on spatial orienting of attention toward peripheral visual targets, following the classical paradigm developed by Posner *et al.* (1982). Orienting is typically faster to targets appearing on the same side as an emotional cue (*e.g.*, faces, spiders, threat words, conditioned shapes) and slower to those appearing on the opposite side (Armony and Dolan, 2002; Bradley *et al.*, 1999; Mogg *et al.*, 1994, 1997; Stormark *et al.*, 1999). In some cases, disengaging from invalid cues to reorient elsewhere appears to be especially slow when such invalid cues are emotional, suggesting that attention is not only captured but also tends to dwell longer on emotional stimuli (Fox, 2000). Similar effects can occur even when emotional cues are masked and not consciously perceived (Bradley *et al.*, 1997a). Again, these influences of emotion on attentional orienting are modulated by anxiety or phobic traits in the participants (Bradley *et al.*, 1999; Mogg *et al.*, 1994).

Enhanced detection of emotional faces has also been found in conditions where normal subjects must focus their attention to one location so that they will usually remain blind to stimuli presented at another unattended location (Mack and Rock, 1998). Similarly, the perception of words with aversive meaning is less disrupted relative to that of neutral words when attentional resources are limited, as during the attentional blink subsequent to discriminating successive targets in a rapid serial visual stream (Anderson and Phelps, 2001). Likewise, patients with unilateral spatial neglect and visual extinction after focal brain damage may suffer from an abnormal spatial bias in attention and fail to perceive a stimulus in their contralesional hemifield in the presence of a simultaneous stimulus on the ipsilesional side. However, this contralesional deficit is much less severe for faces with happy or angry versus neutral emotional expressions (Vuilleumier and Schwartz, 2001a) or for spiders versus flowers (Vuilleumier and Schwartz, 2001b). These findings suggest that processing of emotional stimuli occurs prior to selective attention and that this pre-attentive processing may serve to enhance stimulus detection. On the other hand, a recent study (Anderson and Phelps, 2001) has revealed that a resistance of aversive words to extinction from awareness during the attentional blink is not observed in patients with lesions in the amygdala, a structure critically implicated in emotion and fear processing (Armony and LeDoux, 2000), suggesting that a modulation of attention and awareness may arise from a specialised neural mechanism related to affective processing.

SEGREGATED AND INTEGRATED SYSTEMS FOR EMOTIONAL PROCESSING

Before discussing reciprocal interactions between emotion and attention, we briefly review recent data concerning the neural basis of emotional processing (see also Chapter 19). It seems reasonable to conjecture that different types of emotions, associated with distinct experiential qualities, are mediated, at least partly, by separate neural systems. Moreover, each type of emotion can be elicited by different cues in different sensory modalities. Accordingly, functional neuroimaging studies have used a wide variety of stimuli and procedures to investigate affective responses produced by external stimuli or internal states. Stimuli employed in these studies have included human faces with specific expressions (*e.g.*, fear, happiness, or disgust), words with emotional meaning (*e.g.*, sex or death), pictures with emotionally laden content (complex scenes or film clips with views of accidents, mutilation, spiders, etc.), or, more rarely, auditory words or voices with affective tones. Other studies have focused on somatosensory sensation using painful stimulation. This line of research has begun to delineate a number of brain areas engaged in emotional processing, although the precise function of individual regions is still unclear. Some regions may show an apparent selectivity for certain types of emotion or for certain classes of stimuli, whereas others may show more general responses to different types of emotion and different types of stimuli; however, a considerable heterogeneity across studies precludes definitive conclusions.

Many neuroimaging studies have examined differential brain activity in response to faces conveying distinct emotional expressions. Facial expressions provide a valuable tool to assess neural systems involved in affective processing because they constitute a crucial signal for social communication, and their recognition is universal and presumed to rely on hard-wired neuronal circuits (Ekman and Oster, 1979; Öhman *et al.*, 2000). The best identified emotion circuit is that mediating processing of fearful facial expressions and other non-facial, threat-related stimuli, where there is a high degree of convergence between human functional neuroimaging and neuropsychological investigations (Calder *et al.*, 2001). These data also accord with findings from animal physiology and computational modelling perspectives (Armony and LeDoux, 2000; LeDoux, 1996). Fear, a crucial emotion for adaptive and survival behaviour, is also likely to have privileged links with neural systems of attention governing perception and action (Armony and LeDoux, 2000).

A key structure implicated in fear processing is the amygdala, a heterogeneous collection of nuclei in anterior medial temporal lobe (Armony and LeDoux, 2000; LeDoux, 1996). Functional imaging studies such as those by Breiter *et al.* (1996), Morris *et al.* (1996), and Thomas *et al.* (2001) have consistently observed an activation of the amygdala when subjects are shown faces with a fearful expression, compared to neutral faces (see Chapter 19), a finding consistent with deficits in recognising fearful expressions after amygdala damage (Calder *et al.*, 2001). The amygdala is also activated by fearful voices (Morris *et al.*, 1999; Phillips *et al.*, 1998b), pictures of threatening scenes (Irwin *et al.*, 1996; Lane *et al.*, 1997c, 1999), threat-related words (Isenberg *et al.*, 1999; Tabert *et al.*, 2001), and elementary visual or auditory stimuli with acquired aversive value due to Pavlovian conditioning (Buchel and Dolan, 2000; Buchel *et al.*, 1998, 1999; LaBar *et al.*, 1998). Fearful faces and other threat-related stimuli also activate anterior and posterior cingulate cortices (Maddock, 1999; Morris *et al.*, 1996, 1998a), inferior prefrontal cortices (Kesler-West *et al.*, 1999; Morris *et al.*, 1996, 1998a; Sprengelmeyer *et al.*, 1998; Whalen *et al.*, 1998b), and orbitofrontal cortices (Armony and Dolan, 2002; Sugase *et al.*, 1999; Vuilleumier *et al.*, 2001b); however, many of the latter areas are also activated by other categories of facial emotional expression suggesting that these may have a more general function in emotional behaviour rather than perceptual processing of signals representing fear *per se*.

The amygdala has also been activated by faces with other negative expressions such as anger (Critchley *et al.*, 2000; Hariri *et al.*, 2000) or sadness (Blair *et al.*, 1999). Processing angry faces increases activity in anterior cingulate and lateral prefrontal cortices (Blair *et al.*, 1999; Kesler-West *et al.*, 1999; Sprengelmeyer *et al.*, 1998), as well as orbitofrontal cortices (Blair *et al.*, 1999). By contrast, sad faces activate anterior and medial temporal regions (Blair *et al.*, 1999; George *et al.*, 1995), although in other studies they do not produce significant effects compared to neutral faces (Kesler-West *et al.*, 2001). On the other hand, happy faces activate orbitofrontal (Kesler-West *et al.*, 2001; Morris *et al.*, 1996, 1998a), inferior prefrontal (Dolan *et al.*, 1996; Phillips *et al.*, 1998a), and anterior cingulate cortices (Dolan *et al.*, 1996; Phillips *et al.*, 1998a). In a few studies, a response in the amygdala to happy or highly arousing positive stimuli has been reported (Garavan *et al.*, 2001; Phillips *et al.*, 1998a). Thus, across studies, there is considerable variability in the reported activations for angry, sad, and happy emotion in faces.

By contrast, facial expressions of disgust are associated with a more reliable pattern of activation, evoking consistent activity in insula and basal ganglia (caudate and putamen) in addition to inferior prefrontal and lateral temporal cortex (Phillips *et al.*, 1997, 1998b; Sprengelmeyer *et al.*, 1998). This role of insula and basal ganglia in mediating the perception of disgust is also in accord with the deficits reported following focal lesions in these regions (Calder *et al.*, 2001).

Functional neuroimaging studies have also revealed that some brain areas respond to emotional more than neutral stimuli, regardless of emotion or stimulus type. These include regions in temporal, orbitofrontal, prefrontal, and cingulate cortices, as well as ventral parts of basal ganglia, thalamus, or upper brainstem (Blair *et al.*, 1999; Critchley *et al.*, 2000; George *et al.*, 1995; Lane *et al.*, 1997c; Morris *et al.*, 1998a; Northoff *et al.*, 2000; Paradiso *et al.*, 1999; Phillips *et al.*, 1998b; Sprengelmeyer *et al.*, 1998; Thomas *et al.*, 2001; Vuilleumier *et al.*, 2001b). These areas might constitute final converging nodes for the processing of emotional stimuli in general (Sprengelmeyer *et al.*, 1998) or mediate nonspecific arousing effects. It is interesting to note that some of these same areas are also implicated in attentional and cognitive executive control processes. Thus, it has been suggested that prefrontal regions are in a position to enhance the representation of stimuli that are currently most relevant and inhibit those that are irrelevant, while cingulate regions may control the selection of appropriate motor action (Bush *et al.*, 2000; Posner and Petersen, 1990). A general response to a variety of emotional stimuli might therefore reflect neural mechanisms that have the capacity to influence ongoing processing and elicit appropriate behaviour based on affective cues or priorities. Also, nonspecific increases in activity are often found in visual cortical areas in response to visual emotional stimuli, suggesting enhanced sensory processing of affectively significant events (see below). Thus, at least some of the neural systems activated by emotion might not be necessary for the detection and evaluation of salient stimuli *per se*, but instead play a crucial role in adjusting the allocation of attentive and cognitive resources to the presence of such stimuli.

HOW ATTENTION INFLUENCES EMOTIONAL PROCESSING: AUTOMATIC VERSUS DELIBERATE PROCESSING OF EMOTIONAL STIMULI

A critical aspect of adaptive behaviour is the necessity to monitor the environment and detect potentially significant stimuli (*e.g.*, emotional) even when these are unexpected and hence not currently task relevant or are outside the focus of attention. Automatic emotional processing could provide the organism with a capacity to interrupt ongoing activities and redirect attentional resources toward unforeseen threats. In support of this idea, behavioural studies provide evidence that detection of emotional stimuli (particularly threat-related stimuli) occurs rapidly and automatically (Globisch *et al.*, 1999; Mogg *et al.*, 1997), even when stimuli are initially presented at unattended locations or outside awareness (Bradley *et al.*, 1997b; Mogg and Bradley, 1999; Stormark *et al.*, 1999), as reviewed above. Other behavioural findings in healthy subjects (Schweinberger and Soukup, 1998) and neuropsychological dissociations (Calder *et al.*, 2001) in relation to face processing also suggest that emotional expressions are analysed through specialised pathways, independent from those involved in the analysis of identity and other non-emotional facial features (*e.g.*, speech lip cues).

It is noteworthy that neuroimaging studies examining responses to emotional stimuli have employed experimental conditions where the emotional significance of stimuli had no bearing with the subjects' actual task. For example, faces with fearful expressions activate the amygdala and related brain structures, even when subjects were primarily asked to attend to the gender of the faces in order to make female/male judgments (Morris *et al.*, 1996, 1998a; Phillips *et al.*, 1997, 1998b; Sprengelmeyer *et al.*, 1998; Vuilleumier *et al.*, 2001b). This suggests that emotional features can be extracted from the stimuli even though these are not relevant to the gender decision task. Likewise, emotional effects produced by facial expressions of anger (Blair *et al.*, 1999; Sprengelmeyer *et al.*, 1998), sadness (Blair *et al.*, 1999), disgust (Phillips *et al.*, 1997, 1998b; Sprengelmeyer *et al.*, 1998), and happiness (Morris *et al.*, 1996, 1998a; Phillips *et al.*, 1998a) were also obtained when subjects made gender decision on the faces, without explicitly attending to the facial expressions *per se*. One study (Dolan *et al.*, 1996) also showed that during a delayed match-to sample memory task requiring subjects to hold a face identity in mind over a 45-second interval, neural activity was greater for happy than neutral faces in the fusiform and inferior frontal cortex, as well as anterior cingulate and thalamic regions. This again suggests that the emotional salience of faces was represented despite being irrelevant to the task.

Such effects, however, do not provide a direct demonstration that emotional expression is automatically processed without attention, because the differential emotional responses observed in these tasks could result from deliberate attentional and/or strategic factors. Several recent studies have addressed this issue by systematically comparing the effects of the same emotional stimuli across different task conditions. This approach has allowed a more direct assessment of whether some emotional effects may reflect mandatory responses, occurring independently of task or attention.

Task-Dependent Responses to Emotional Faces

Critchley *et al.* (2000) used fMRI to compare intentional ("explicit") and incidental ("implicit") processing of emotional faces. Subjects were presented with blocks of mixed angry and happy faces, alternating with blocks of neutral faces, while they judged either the gender (male versus female) or expression (neutral versus emotional) of each face. A main effect of emotion, independent of task (*i.e.*, evoked by the mixed angry and happy, compared to neutral faces during both judgment conditions) was found in visual areas including fusiform and peristriate cortex, middle temporal gyrus, and retrosplenial cortex, as well as in the vicinity of the posterior amygdala/superior hippocampal junction and pulvinar nucleus of the thalamus (all in left hemisphere). Activity in bilateral posterior amygdala/hippocampal regions was specifically increased during gender versus emotional judgements (*i.e.*, when emotional expressions were incidental to the task). A similar increase for incidental emotional stimuli was also found in left insula, left inferior prefrontal cortex, and bilateral anterior putamen. By contrast, intentional processing of emotion enhanced activity in left middle temporal gyrus, bilateral fusiform regions, and left posterior putamen. These findings suggest that explicit visual analysis of emotional traits may engage specific processes in middle temporal gyrus and fusiform cortex (see Fig. 21.1), consistent with the properties of neurons found in temporal lobe regions by neurophysiology studies in the monkey (Hasselmo *et al.*, 1989; Perrett *et al.*, 1992). On the other hand, fusiform cortex and limbic areas such as the reported amygdala/hippocampal regions and

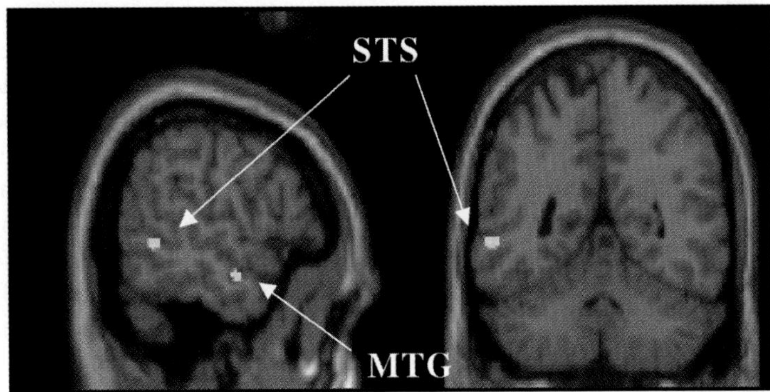

FIGURE 21.1
Explicit attention to faces with emotional expression (fearful versus neutral) may specifically increase activation in the superior temporal sulcus (STS), here in the left hemisphere (–56, –50, –2). A second peak is also seen in anterior middle temporal gyrus (–54, –14, –16). (Unpublished fMRI data.)

retrosplenial areas might be involved in incidental detection of emotional stimuli. However, limitations of this blocked study include not only a relatively imprecise anatomical localisation of the reported amygdala effects but also the failure to distinguish stimulus-driven responses from top-down modulations due to task set and the impossibility of differentiating effects of angry (aversive) and happy (positive) emotions. Furthermore, a true obligatory implicit processing of emotion should occur equally when subjects voluntarily attend to, or ignore, the expression in faces.

A similar approach was used in another blocked fMRI study by Naramuto *et al.* (2001). These authors compared the effect of matching pairs of faces based on emotional expression (happy, sad, or fearful) versus identity, and found that the intentional emotional task selectively increased activity in the right superior temporal sulcus. Matching the two faces' identity versus matching the shape of the faces' contour increased activity in bilateral fusiform regions. The right superior temporal region in this study (coordinates: $x = -49$, $y = -42$, $z = 4$) was relatively homologous to the temporal area on the left side (–55, –52, 10) previously reported in the Critchley *et al.* (2000) study. However, here again, any difference between distinct emotion types could not be assessed because the pairs of faces were presented in blocks mixing happy and sad expressions or mixing happy and fearful expressions. Notably no activation differences were found in a contrast between these blocks. Given that there were no blocks with neutral faces alone, Naramuto *et al.* (2001) could not assess effects due to obligatory processing of emotion, as this could have occurred for all three expressions when subjects were matching identity or when they were matching expression. Another limitation in this study was that analyses were restricted to a few regions of interest in fusiform and temporal cortex, previously defined by a preferential activation for all faces versus scrambled stimuli.

Gorno-Tempini *et al.* (2001) used functional magnetic resonance imaging (fMRI) in a paradigm similar to Critchley *et al.* (2000), in which single faces were shown each in turn. Processing of happy and disgust facial expressions were compared during either gender or emotional classification tasks. Faces were presented in blocks with a majority of happy faces, a majority of disgust faces or neutral faces alone. In contrast to previous findings (Morris *et al.*, 1996; Phillips *et al.*, 1997; Sprengelmeyer *et al.*, 1998), no brain region was found to exhibit a significant response to emotional expressions independent of task (for both happiness and disgust). However, the right caudate, right thalamus, and left amygdala were more activated by disgust versus happy faces during the emotion classification task (relative to the gender decision task). Conversely, bilateral orbitofrontal cortex showed activation to happy relative to disgust faces that was greater during the emotion classification task; however, the authors did not report whether emotional versus neutral expressions produced significant effects during the incidental (gender) conditions. While activity in the reported areas might be modulated by intentional attention to emotionality of the faces, other areas might possibly show distinct effects that are specific to such "incidental" conditions (see Critchley *et al.*, 2000).

On the other hand, this study identified brain regions showing a main effect of intentional emotional processing. Activity in the right inferior and precentral frontal gyri, anterior insula, and right fusiform cortex was greater when subjects judged expression (irrespective of emotion type) as compared to gender. No effect was found in the superior temporal cortex, although bilateral increases in the latter regions were observed in a contrast of all faces (neutral or emotional) versus scrambled non-face stimuli ([56, –60, 8] and [–60, –60, 8]); however, the observed involvement of frontal areas converges with previous PET studies reporting similar results during deliberate processing of facial emotion. For example, selective increases have been observed in bilateral inferior frontal and right anterior cingulate cortex when subjects matched faces based on their expression versus identity (George *et al.*, 1993), while increases also occurred in inferior frontal gyrus when subjects judged emotional valence (positive or negative) of facial expression versus attractiveness (Nakamura *et al.*, 1999).

In a similar vein, Hariri *et al.* (2000) compared the effect of judging emotion from either faces or verbal labels in a blocked fMRI design. Subjects were shown a target face (with fearful or angry expression) and had to match the expression of this face either to one of two other simultaneously presented faces or to one of two simultaneously presented words (*afraid* or *angry*). Fearful and angry faces were always mixed. Compared to a simple shape-matching control task, the perceptual matching of emotional faces activated the right fusiform cortex, right thalamus, and bilateral amygdala; whereas, the linguistic matching of a verbal label with expression activated the right fusiform cortex and right inferior frontal cortex. The authors interpreted their results as indicating a suppression of the amygdala and thalamus response to emotional stimuli during the cognitive linguistic task, perhaps mediated by increased right frontal activity; however, there were at least two majors confounds in this study. A decrease in amygdala responses might simply be due to the fact that only one emotional face per trial was presented in the linguistic condition versus a total of three faces per trial for the perceptual matching. Moreover, at least one fearful face was bound to appear on each trial in the perceptual matching, compared to only half of the trials in the linguistic condition, and these more frequent fearful expressions were likely to elicit the most effective responses in the amygdala.

A similar problem concerns a recent positron emission tomography (PET) study (Liberzon *et al.*, 2000) examining how cognitive task instructions could modulate the response to emotional non-face stimuli. The same pictures with aversive content (eliciting fear or disgust) or neutral content were shown first during an emotional rating phase, then a second time mixed with new face exemplars during a memory recognition phase. Right amygdala and thalamic increases for emotional compared to neutral pictures were found only during emotional rating, together with a left middle frontal response. However, because half of the pictures during the memory recognition task were repeated from the rating phase, these decreased emotional effects were potentially confounded with habituation versus novelty factors known to influence medial temporal lobe activity. In another PET study (Lane *et al.*, 1999), amygdala responses to arousing (both pleasant and unpleasant) stimuli were not modulated by attentional distraction during a dual task.

Alternatively, a modulation of amygdala responses to aversive stimuli by task demands might occur only for complex pictures in which the emotional content derives from a specific combination of elements in the context represented by the scene and not for fearful faces that constitute more special, biologically salient stimuli. Such a dissociation has indeed been suggested by a recent fMRI study (Keightley *et al.*, 2000) showing that intentional (explicit) versus incidental (implicit) emotional processing tasks increased amygdala activation for negative scenes but did not change the effect of negative faces. Moreover, the main effect of intentional versus incidental emotional tasks activated middle temporal gyri and orbitofrontal cortex bilaterally for faces alone but not for scenes (the latter elicited more activity in right superior prefrontal and occipital areas).

In sum, converging evidence suggests that selective attention to, and explicit categorisation of, emotional traits in faces can specifically activate middle or superior temporal cortical areas (Critchley *et al.*, 2000; Gorno-Tempini *et al.*, 2001; Keightley *et al.*, 2000; Narumoto *et al.*, 2001). This area (Fig. 21.1) might correspond to neurons in superior temporal sulcus that respond to facial expression in monkeys (Hasselmo *et al.*, 1989; Sugase *et al.*, 1999). Such regions might preferentially encode changeable aspects of faces such as expression, gaze, or speech mouth cues (Haxby *et al.*, 2000), in contrast to ventral temporal regions in the fusiform cortex that are more concerned with invariant facial features related to identity. In addition, selective attention to emotionality in faces can also activate inferior dorsolateral frontal regions (George *et al.*, 1993; Gorno-Tempini *et al.*, 2001; Narumoto *et al.*, 2001), possibly implicated in more cognitive or attentional components of the task. It is unclear if the same frontal regions are also activated by emotional scenes (Keightley *et al.*, 2000). Alternatively, such frontal effects might reflect activation of premotor cortex controlling facial movements, possibly reflecting responses in "mirror" neurons involved in both motoric encoding of self facial expressions and perceptual recognition of others' facial expressions (Dimberg *et al.*, 2000). In this regard, it would be of interest to investigate the overlap between activity elicited by perceptual discrimination of facial expressions in conspecifics and self-generated facial movements. Also, it remains to be established whether the superior temporal and inferior frontal cortices are similarly engaged by all types of facial emotion and whether different emotions produce specific hemispheric asymmetries, as suggested by the findings of Critchley *et al.* (2000) and Naramuto *et al.* (2001). On the other hand, the current neuroimaging studies do not provide clear evidence as to whether neural responses elicited by specific emotional stimuli are always obligatory, occurring regardless of task, or can be modulated by selective attention and task demands. Deliberate attention seems capable of influencing the response to some facial expressions—for instance, to happiness (*e.g.*, in orbitofrontal cortex) and disgust (*e.g.*, in basal ganglia)—but there is no convincing evidence that such an influence can also modulate the response to highly salient emotional expressions such as fearful faces (*e.g.*, in amygdala). Indeed, some facial expressions might constitute unique, biologically prepared cues that are more effective in eliciting obligatory emotional responses than complex scene pictures (Keightley *et al.*, 2000; Öhman *et al.*, 2000). Any modulation for other simple non-facial but strongly threat-related stimuli (*e.g.*, a fear-conditioned colour) is still open to inquiry. Indeed, an obligatory processing of fear-related cues (but not necessarily of any other emotional cues), independent of voluntary attention, would be consistent with a special status of fear processing pathways in the brain (Armony and LeDoux, 2000; LeDoux, 1996; Robinson, 1998) and previous findings that fear-conditioned stimuli can elicit both behavioural responses (Öhman *et al.*, 2000) and amygdala activation (Morris *et al.*, 1998b) without awareness of the eliciting event.

Effects of Spatial Attention on Emotional Face Processing

In an event-related fMRI study, Vuilleumier *et al.* (2001b) manipulated the effect of emotion and the effect of spatial attention in a systematic manner to examine how neural responses to fearful expression in faces were influenced by whether these faces were relevant for the task at hand and in the focus of attention, as opposed to task irrelevant and outside the focus of attention. On each trial, subjects were briefly shown two faces and two houses, arranged in a cross-format, with the pair of faces either horizontally or vertically aligned (and, consequently, the pair of houses either vertically or horizontally aligned, respectively; see Fig. 21.2A). The two faces had a fearful expression on half of the trials but a neutral expression on the other half. Subjects maintained eye fixation at the centre. During some blocks of trials, subjects were instructed to concentrate only on the two horizontal stimuli and judged whether they were the same or different pictures (*i.e.*, two same versus different faces, or two same versus different houses); during other blocks, they had to concentrate on the two vertical pictures and similarly judged whether these were the same or different. Thus, on any given trial, subjects could see two faces at task-relevant locations, with either a neutral or fearful expression, or equally often they could see two houses at task-relevant locations, with faces at ignored locations having either a neutral or fearful expression. In this way, the neural response to fearful emotional expression could be compared directly for faces in the focus of attention and faces outside the focus of attention. Importantly, the event order was fully randomised, so that subjects could neither predict the relevant stimulus category nor facial expression.

As expected, based on previous studies (Corbetta *et al.*, 1990; Wojciulik *et al.*, 1998), spatial attention strongly modulated extrastriate visual areas. Bilateral fusiform cortex (*i.e.*, the so-called fusiform face area) showed an increased activity when faces appeared at the relevant locations (Fig. 21.2B,C), whereas parahippocampal cortex (*i.e.*, the so-called place area) showed

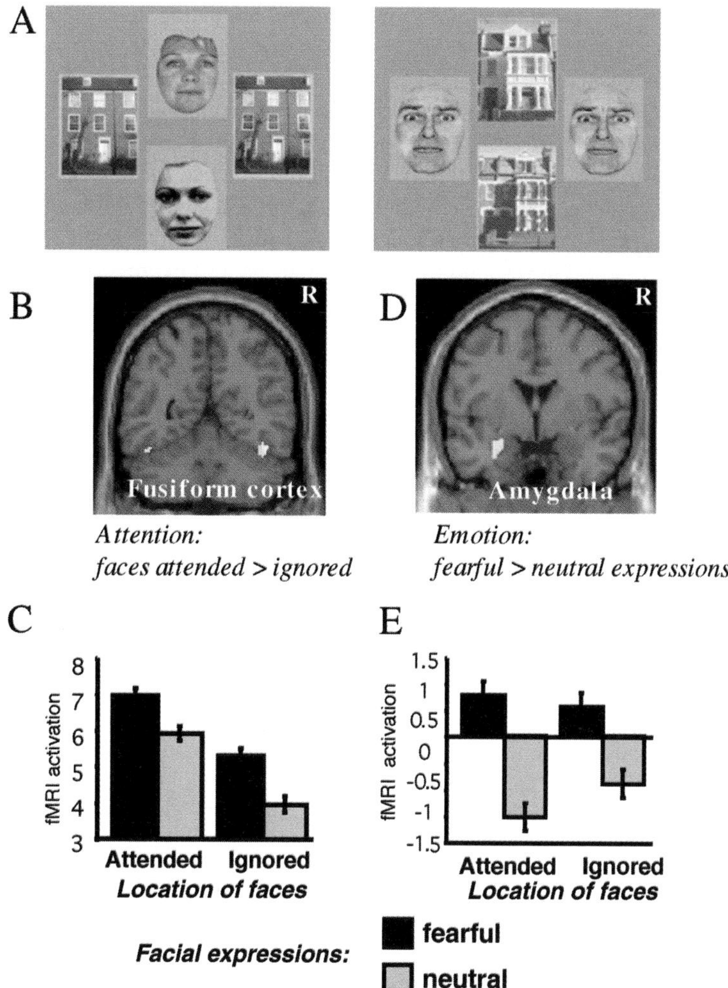

FIGURE 21.2
Distinct effects of emotion and attention on visual responses. (A) Examples of stimuli. On each trial, subjects were briefly shown two houses and two faces (with either fearful or neutral expression) but concentrated only on two prespecified locations(either horizontal or vertical) to make same/different judgments about the stimuli presented there. (B) Face-specific areas in fusiform cortex showed increased activity bilaterally when faces were presented at the attended locations (as opposed to houses). (C) Fusiform activity was also increased when fearful (as opposed to neutral) faces were presented, but this effect was independent from the effect of attention (*i.e.*, it occurred even when faces appeared at the ignored locations). (D) and (E) Left amygdala showed increased activity when fearful (versus neutral) faces were presented, regardless of whether faces were presented inside or outside the focus of attention. (fMRI data from Vuilleumier *et al.*, 2001b.)

an increased activity when houses appeared at the relevant locations, regardless of expression. Note that such increases were purely attributable to spatial attention, as the visual displays were in fact identical across all conditions. Critically, a left amygdala response to fearful compared to neutral faces occurred regardless of whether the faces were at the relevant/attended locations or at the irrelevant/unattended locations (Fig. 21.2D,E), demonstrating that fear processing in the amygdala was obligatory and unaffected by the same modulation of spatial attention that strongly influenced the fusiform response to faces. Note also that facial expression was never relevant to the task and thus was processed incidentally in all conditions.

Another remarkable finding in this study was that activity in the fusiform cortex was enhanced for fearful compared to neutral faces (Fig. 21.2C). This enhancement occurred both when the faces were at the relevant/attended locations or at the irrelevant/unattended locations. Moreover, this enhancement was specific to the face area in fusiform cortex but did not affect the place area in parahippocampal cortex. An explanation for this effect of emotional expression on fusiform activity is that it may reflect influences from amygdala feedback connections onto extrastriate cortex, which exert modulatory influences enhancing the visual processing of emotionally relevant stimuli (Amaral *et al.*, 1992; Sugase *et al.*, 1999). A modulation of the fusiform gyrus as a function of fearful facial expression was similarly reported in a previous PET study (Morris *et al.*, 1998a). Importantly, the new findings from this event-related fMRI study (Vuilleumier *et al.*, 2001b) suggest that the effect of emotion on visual cortex is independent of, and additive to, the effect of spatial attention. We will return to this issue below.

Finally, the systematic 2×2 (attention × emotion) factorial design of this study also allowed a direct assessment of the effect of spatial attention on emotional processing (Fig. 21.3). Thus, some brain areas were found to respond to fearful versus neutral expressions specifically when the faces appeared at the relevant/attended locations. These areas included early visual areas in striate cortex, medial temporal pole, and caudal parts of the anterior cingulate cortex (all in the left hemisphere). Such effects might reflect increased alertness, arousal, or awareness of emotional cues (Bush *et al.*, 2000; Lane *et al.*, 1997a). Conversely, some brain areas responded to fearful more than neutral expressions, specifically when the faces appeared at the irrelevant/ignored locations. These latter regions included orbitofrontal cortex, ventral caudate nucleus, and caudal parts of the anterior cingulate (all in the right hemisphere). These effects might reflect mechanisms monitoring currently unattended sensory inputs and adjusting behavioural response according to task demands when emotionally salient information must be ignored (Robbins and Everitt, 1996; Rolls, 1996).

A further fMRI study (Pessoa *et al.*, 2001) manipulated spatial attention toward or away from faces that had a fearful, happy, or neutral expression. In some blocks, subjects had to attend to centrally presented faces to judge their gender; in other blocks, they had to attend to two bar segments simultaneously presented in peripheral fields on each side of the central face and judge whether these bars had the same or different orientation. Fearful expressions activated the amygdala more than neutral or happy expressions, both when the face was selectively attended and when the bars were attended (*i.e.*, with faces now ignored). On the other hand, amygdala activity increased with attention to the face compared to the bars, but this occurred for all faces regardless of their emotional valence, although this effect was apparently greater for fearful than

A *Greater fear responses with attention*

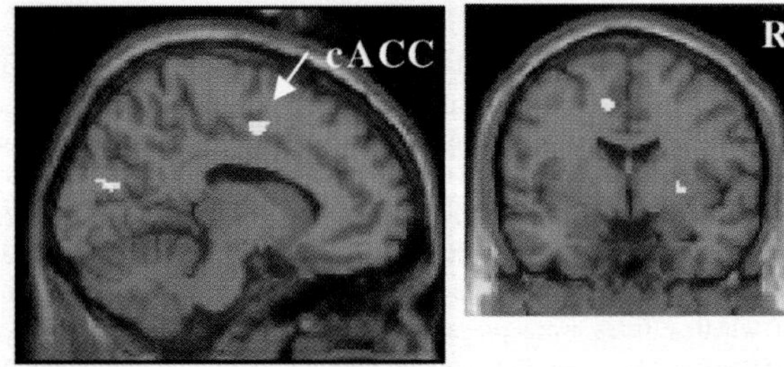

B *Greater fear responses with inattention*

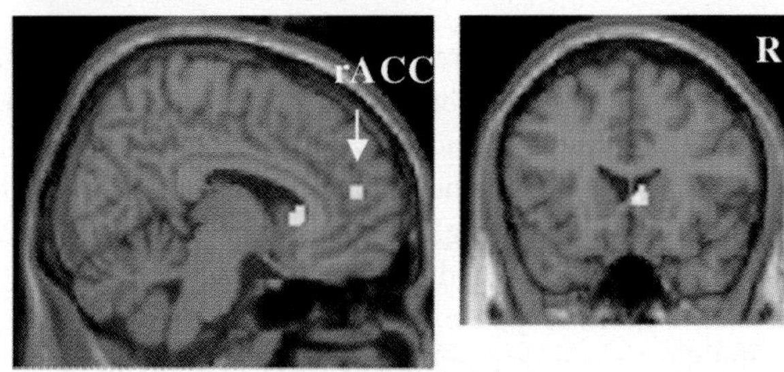

FIGURE 21.3
Effects of spatial attention on emotional responses. (A) The caudal region of left anterior cingulate cortex (cACC) (−10, −2, 48), as well as left primary visual cortex and right putamen, showed increased responses to fearful versus neutral faces specifically with attention to the faces (relative to attention to other locations occupied by houses). (B) Conversely, the rostral region of right anterior cingulate cortex (rACC) (8, 50, 16), as well as ventral caudate and orbitofrontal cortex (not shown), responded more to fearful versus neutral faces when attention was focused away from the faces (and directed to houses instead). (fMRI data from Vuilleumier *et al.*, 2001b.)

happy and neutral faces. The same pattern was also found in fusiform cortex. However, the attended stimulus category was fully predictable on each trial, and, given the general enhancement to all facial expressions, it is unclear from this study whether attention truly increased stimulus-driven responses to emotional cues or instead increased baseline activity in the amygdala through strategic top-down influences (Phelps *et al.*, 2001). Nevertheless, these results are consistent with an extraction of fear-related cues in faces even without selective attention to expression.

Direct support for emotional face processing occurring without attention also comes from a study in a right-parietal-damaged patient with left spatial neglect and visual extinction (Vuilleumier *et al.*, 2001a). This neurological disorder is characterised by a failure to direct attention to the side of space opposite the lesion (*i.e.*, to the left, in this case). In many instances, the patient remains unaware of a stimulus occurrence in the left visual field (LVF) when presented with a simultaneous competing stimulus stimuli in the right visual field (RVF), although the patient can detect the same left-sided stimulus when presented alone (Driver and Vuilleumier, 2001). Event-related fMRI was obtained in this left extinction patient (Fig. 21.4A), while pictures of fearful faces, neutral faces, or houses were briefly shown in the RVF, LVF, or both fields simultaneously (BS). On the critical BS trials, a face with either a fearful or neutral expression appeared in LVF, together with a house in RVF (Fig. 21.4B). The left-side faces were extinguished from the patient's awareness in 65% of BS trials. This design allowed a systematic 2×2 factorial analysis of critical BS trials, separately examining the effect of emotional expression (fearful versus neutral) and perception (conscious awareness versus extinction) of left-side faces, similar to the factorial design of our previous study in normal subjects (Vuilleumier *et al.*, 2001b). Results revealed that awareness relative to extinction of LVF faces increased bilateral fusiform activity (while extinguished faces in LVF produced covert activation in striate and extrastriate areas compared to trials with a house alone in RVF). However, fearful faces activated the left amygdala and bilateral orbitofrontal areas both when seen and when extinguished (Fig. 21.4C,D). Thus, amygdala responses to fearful faces did not significantly differ between conscious awareness and extinction, despite the strong increase in fusiform cortex activity associated with awareness. These findings parallel those in normal subjects (Vuilleumier *et al.*, 2001b) and converge with previous reports of an amygdala response to masked emotional stimuli in normals (Morris *et al.*, 1998b; Whalen *et al.*, 1998b).

In addition, fusiform activity also showed an additional modulation by fearful expression independent of awareness or extinction (Fig. 21.4D), again consistent with our proposal of feedback influences from automatically elicited amygdala responses on visual cortical processing (Morris *et al.*, 1998a; Sugase *et al.*, 1999). This modulation might represent the neural substrate of an enhanced capture of attention by emotional stimuli as previously observed in behavioural studies of patients with neglect and extinction (Vuilleumier and Schwartz, 2001a,b). Consequently, this finding supports our results in normal subjects, suggesting that an emotional modulation of fusiform is independent of spatial attention mechanisms (presumably damaged in neglect and extinction).

It is of interest that unconscious processing of threatening faces has also been shown in patient GY with blindsight (see Chapter 19). It remains a goal for future research to determine whether emotional processing can exhibit a similar independence from voluntary spatial attention for other categories of stimuli, including events with acquired aversive value due to past experience, such as occurs with fear conditioning, or facial expressions other than fear. One possibility is that that such pre-attentive emotional processing might occur only for threat-related information (Armony and LeDoux, 2000; Robinson, 1998).

Effects of Attention on Non-Visual Emotional Processing

Much less is known about emotional responses to auditory stimuli and any effect of attention on such responses. While human-related sounds activate specific areas in lateral temporal cortex, compared to non-human sounds (Belin *et al.*, 2000), nonverbal affective relative to neutral vocalisations increase activity in left middle temporal gyrus, anterior insula, ventral prefrontal cortex, and right caudate nucleus (Morris *et al.*, 1999). Fearful voices evoke specific effects in amygdala compared to other (happy, sad, disgust, neutral) expressions (Dolan *et al.*, 2001;

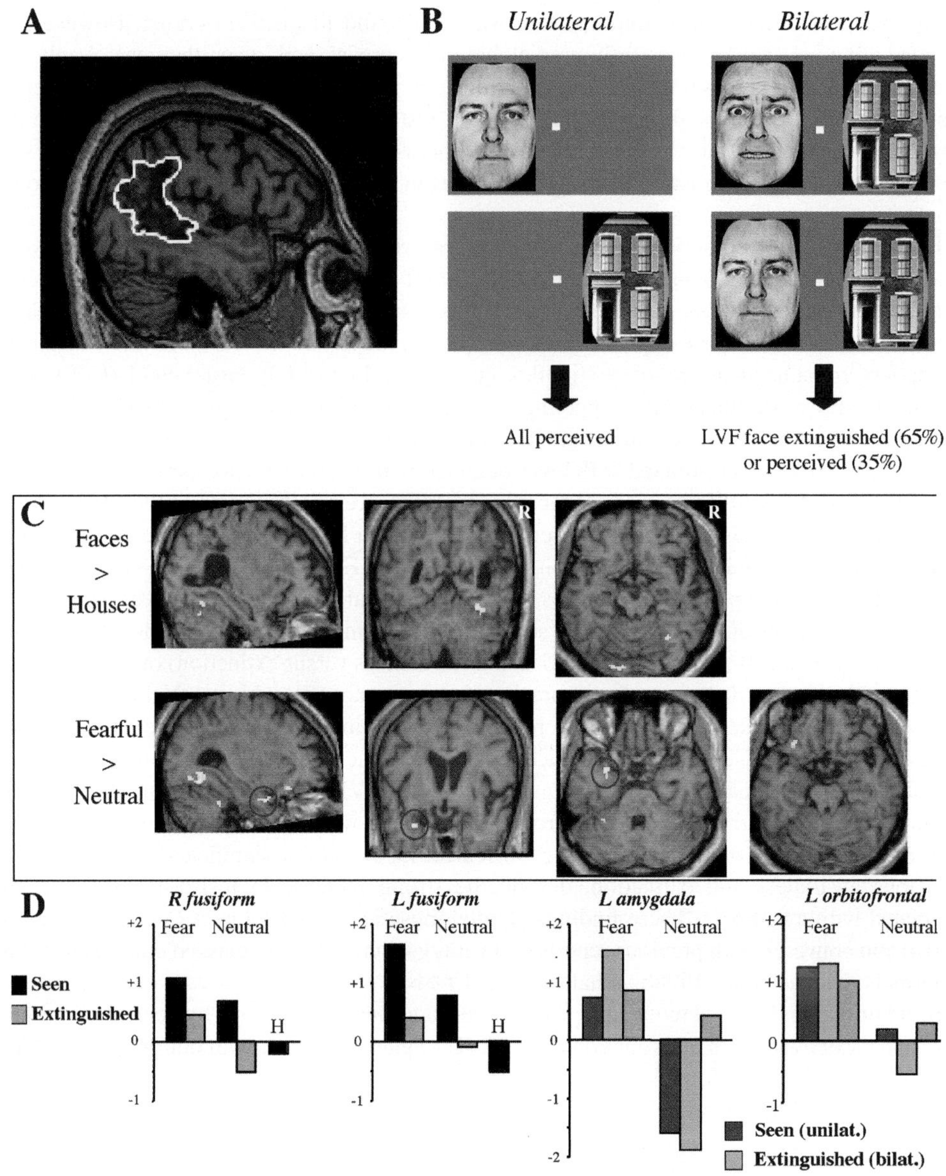

FIGURE 21.4
Fear processing with and without awareness in a patient with left spatial neglect and visual extinction. (A) Focal right parietal damage in the patient. (B) Example of stimuli. Faces or houses were presented unilaterally in either the right (RVF) or left (LVF) visual field. Faces had either a neutral or fearful expression. The critical stimuli were bilateral trials with a face in the LVF and house in RVF, in which the left-sided face was extinguished from the patient's awareness on many trials (65%) and consciously seen only on a few trials (35%). (C) Activation by seen faces, as opposed to seen houses, was observed in the right fusiform cortex (irrespective of emotional expression and field), and activation by fearful compared to neutral faces was observed in the left amygdala (red circle), as well as orbitofrontal and fusiform cortex. (D) Size of activation across stimulus conditions for the regions shown above. Fusiform activity increased when faces were consciously perceived, irrespective of expression, but also increased when faces were fearful, irrespective of awareness. Left amygdala and orbitofrontal cortex responded to fearful faces both when consciously perceived and extinguished. The left amygdala also showed a weak response to neutral faces when these were extinguished but no response to neutral faces when these were consciously seen. (fMRI data from Vuilleumier *et al.*, *Neuropsychologia*, 2002.)

Morris *et al.*, 1999; Phillips *et al.*, 1998b). Both laughing and crying also activate bilateral amygdala and insula regions (Sander and Scheich, 2001).

In the fMRI study by Sander and Scheich (2001), amygdala responses to laughing and crying were independent of attention to emotion, occurring regardless of whether subjects had to passively listen to stimuli, monitor rare changes in sound pitch, or concentrate on affective meaning and self-generate the corresponding emotion. By contrast, insula responses to crying were modulated by attention to self-generated emotion. Another PET study (Imaizumi *et al.*, 1997) also found task-dependent increases in insula, inferior frontal gyrus, and cerebellum when subjects classified emotional tones of words spoken by different actors, whereas activity increased in bilateral temporal poles and right superior frontal gyrus when subjects identified different actors' voices. This study did not include neutral tones and did not examine any possible differential effects between distinct emotion types (happy, angry, surprise, disgust).

Finally, an fMRI study (Jancke *et al.*, 2001) showed that responses to dichotic words with and without emotional content increase activity in contralateral auditory cortex with selective spatial attention to one ear, whereas a greater right-side response in superior temporal sulcus and inferior frontal gyrus, possibly attributed to emotion words, was not affected by spatial attention or by task demands (*i.e.*, involving discrimination of phonetic or affective cues in the words). However, this study did not directly compared emotional versus neutral words, and focused only on a few selected regions of interest.

EFFECTS OF ATTENTION ON EMOTIONAL EXPERIENCE

Another kind of modulation is that exerted on emotional processes, in a top-down manner, when subjects direct attention to their internal affective states or feelings. It is beyond the scope of this chapter to review in detail the functional neuroimaging work related to this issue, but some results from this research provide interesting insights into neural mechanisms by which cognitive processes regulate emotional responses.

Selective attention to subjective emotional experience can be induced through different methods, with or without external stimulation. In several PET studies, subjects were presented with emotional faces (George *et al.*, 1995; Schneider *et al.*, 1995) or emotional film clips (Beauregard *et al.*, 1998; Lane *et al.*, 1997b, 1998; Reiman *et al.*, 1997) and asked to enter into the corresponding feeling states or to evaluate the degree of their own affective reactions to each stimulus. A consistent finding is that attention to self-experienced emotion increases activity in rostral anterior cingulate cortex (ACC) and adjacent medial frontal cortex (BA9). Other common areas of increased activity are found in bilateral insula, anterior temporal lobe, and subcortical structures such as thalamus and basal ganglia. A similar pattern (Fig. 21.5A) was found when making emotional versus spatial judgements on static emotional pictures (Lane *et al.*, 1997a) or when viewing pictures associated with emotionally evocative versus neutral captions (Teasdale *et al.*, 1999).

Other PET studies have examined the effect of evoking emotional representations without external stimuli—for instance, through intentional recall of personally experienced episodes (Damasio *et al.*, 2000; Lane *et al.*, 1997b; Pardo *et al.*, 1993; Reiman *et al.*, 1997), imagination of action plans in emotional versus neutral situations (Partiot *et al.*, 1995), or mental visualisation of aversive versus neutral pictures (Kosslyn *et al.*, 1996). Again, these various tasks produce consistent activation in medial prefrontal cortex and insula. Visualising aversive stimuli also enhanced cerebral blood in early visual cortex (BA17 and 18) relative to neutral stimuli (Kosslyn *et al.*, 1996). Differential effects associated with specific emotions (*e.g.*, sadness, happiness, or disgust) were found in orbitofrontal areas (Lane *et al.*, 1997b; Pardo *et al.*, 1993; Reiman *et al.*, 1997) and various subcortical regions (Damasio *et al.*, 2000). Altogether, these results suggest a general role of ACC and insula in volitional self-generation of emotion and conscious emotional experience.

A notable feature of many of these studies (Damasio *et al.*, 2000; Reiman *et al.*, 1997; Teasdale *et al.*, 1999) is an absence of significant modulation in the amygdala for purely mental evocations of affective states, including evocations of fear-related or aversive information; however, evocation of fear-related memories induces significant increases in regions such as the insula and midbrain (*e.g.*, Damasio *et al.*, 2000). This might reflect an amygdala involvement specifically in response to exteroceptive signals but not to purely endogenously driven cognitive or recall processes (Damasio *et al.*, 2000; Drevets and Raichle, 1998; Reiman *et al.*, 1997; Teasdale *et al.*, 1999). In other words, the functions of the amygdala may relate to perceptual processing of emotional stimuli and the generation of automatic and obligatory behavioural responses but have little to do with the elaboration of emotional experiences *per se*. This suggests

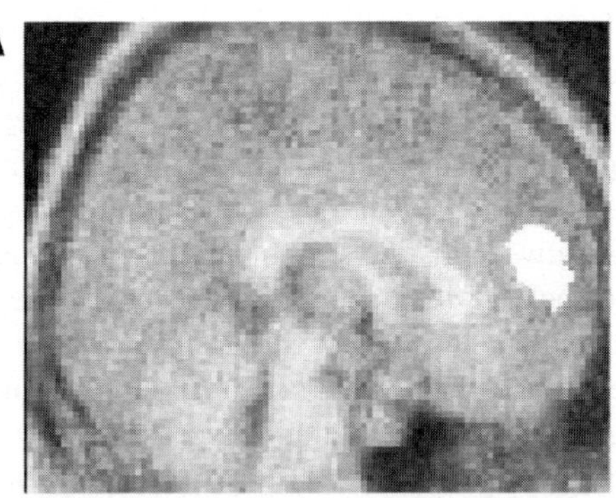

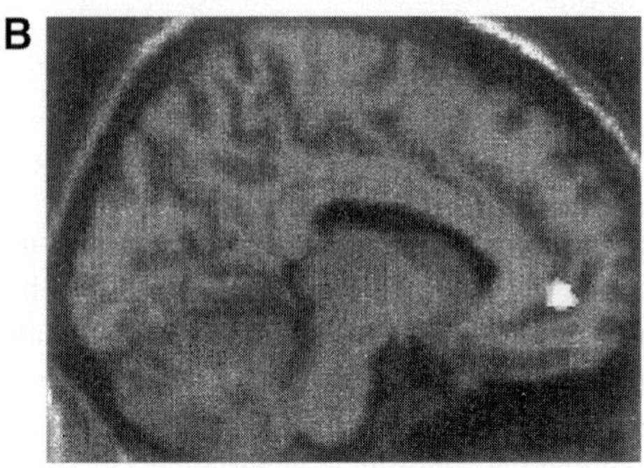

FIGURE 21.5
Regions in anterior cingulate cortex (ACC) that are modulated by attention to emotion. (A) Rostral regions in ACC and medial prefrontal cortex (peak: 0, 50, 16) show increased activity when subjects attentively judged their subjective feelings elicited by emotional pictures as compared to when they judged only spatial features of the pictures (indoor/outdoor). (PET data from Lane *et al.*, 1997.) (B) Subgenual region in ACC (peak: –6, 36, –3) showing increased activity in a Go/NoGo task when the targets (for Go responses) are words with emotional content, as compared to words with a neutral content. (fMRI data from Elliott *et al.*, 2000.)

a crucial distinction in neural systems mediating what has been termed *emotion generation* compared to those mediating the experience of feeling states (Damasio, 1999).

Nevertheless, both subjective feelings states and amygdala activation elicited by an external perceptual event can be modulated by cognitive factors and expectations that contribute to an aversive evaluation of incoming stimuli. For example, it has been demonstrated (Phelps *et al.*, 2001) that the occurrence of a cue that was expected to be paired with an electrical shock after verbal instructions (but actually never experienced with any shock) is sufficient to activate the amygdala, as well as the insula, ACC, and striatum. This result provide a demonstration that some forms of aversive reaction and learning in response to external events can be modulated by higher order cognitive representations and anticipatory attention.

HOW EMOTION INFLUENCES ATTENTION: ENHANCEMENT VERSUS INTERFERENCE EFFECTS ON COGNITIVE PERFORMANCE

An important role of basic emotions is to regulate an organism's state by influencing current sensory processing and preparing specific behavioural responses to meet environmental challenges. Thus, the consequences of elicitation of an emotion include a wide range of vegetative, sensorimotor, and cognitive mechanisms that can provoke a more detailed stimulus analysis, enhance the representation of relevant stimuli, suppress irrelevant information, increase speed of processing, or facilitate the resolution of conflict between competing alternatives (Armony and LeDoux, 1997; Armony *et al.*, 1997). From this perspective, it might be expected that emotional signals can affect the allocation of attentional resources in order either to facilitate performance in a current task or to interrupt ongoing activity and redirect attention towards a more relevant event. Several imaging studies have specifically examined how emotional signals influence attentional, perceptual, and cognitive processes, even in conditions where emotion is not directly relevant to the task goals.

Modulation of Cortical Sensory Processing by Emotion

As already mentioned, a common finding in neuroimaging studies is an increased activation of sensory cortical areas in response to stimuli with emotional significance, as compared to neutral stimuli. Thus, emotional facial expressions enhance activity in inferior temporal and fusiform areas involved in visual analysis and identification of objects and faces. Such increases in fusiform cortex have most consistently been reported for fearful faces (Breiter *et al.*, 1996; Morris *et al.*, 1996, 1998a; Vuilleumier *et al.*, 2001b) and happy faces (Breiter *et al.*, 1996). Similarly, complex visual scenes with aversive compared to neutral contents increase activation of striate and extrastriate cortex, including medial and lateral occipital cortex (Lane *et al.*, 1997c, 1999; Lang *et al.*, 1998; Teasdale *et al.*, 1999), lingual and inferior temporal gyri (Fredrikson *et al.*, 1993; Taylor *et al.*, 2000; Teasdale *et al.*, 1999; Wik *et al.*, 1993), and occasionally more anterior (Lane *et al.*, 1999) or lateral (Kosslyn *et al.*, 1996; Taylor *et al.*, 2000) areas of temporal neocortex. Fewer studies have found such increases for pleasant pictures (Lane *et al.*, 1998, 1999; Simpson *et al.*, 2000).

Enhanced visual responses have also been observed for stimuli with acquired aversive value following Pavlovian fear conditioning (*e.g.*, previous exposure paired with an unpleasant loud noise or electric shock) (Armony and Dolan, 2002; Buchel *et al.*, 1998). In these studies, the same stimuli were counterbalanced across conditions so as to be either fear conditioned (CS+) or neutral (CS–) in different subjects. This suggests that the enhanced visual responses is unlikely to be simply due to differences in low-level visual features of the stimuli. Other studies have attempted to match featural and semantic complexities of neutral and emotional pictures (Lane *et al.*, 1999; Taylor *et al.*, 2000) or have kept facial features constant but changed their affective meaning by inverting them (Rotshtein *et al.*, 2001). These studies nonetheless report a selective modulation of visual cortex activity by emotional stimuli. Moreover, such effects cannot be explained by differential eye-movement scanning patterns (Lane *et al.*, 1999; Lang *et al.*, 1998; Vuilleumier *et al.*, 2001b). Altogether, these findings provide direct support for the idea that emotional significance augments the analysis of sensory inputs at early stages of cortical processing.

Emotion might have modulatory effects on sensory object processing in a number of ways. One possibility is that any enhancement reflects a direct interaction with mechanisms of attention, whereby the perceived affective or arousing value of stimuli can elicit more selective focusing and greater recruitment of cognitive resources through top-down influences mediated by, for example, frontoparietal and thalamic systems (Armony and LeDoux, 2000; Mesulam, 1999). A. substantial body of evidence including neurophysiology in monkeys and functional imaging data in humans indicate that these attentional networks play a critical role in modulating sensory cortical areas at various stages of processing in order to enhance the representation of relevant objects, features, or locations, at the expense of irrelevant ones (Corbetta *et al.*, 1990; Posner and Petersen, 1990). Frontoparietal attentional systems might receive direct inputs from regions concerned with ascertaining the motivational significance of stimuli, such as, for example, through reciprocal connections with anterior and posterior cingulate cortices, basal forebrain nuclei (Maddock, 1999; Mesulam, 1999; Posner and Petersen, 1990), or orbitofrontal areas (Armony and Dolan, 2002; Rolls, 1996). Inputs from these regions might in turn serve to modulate the response to emotional stimuli.

Some evidence suggests, however, that a modulation of sensory cortices by emotion might be mediated by distinct processes, independent of other mechanisms of attention mediated by the classic frontoparietal networks. Thus, in the study by Vuilleumier *et al.* (2001) discussed above, activity in the fusiform cortex showed an enhanced activity for fearful compared to neutral faces regardless of whether these appeared at the relevant/attended locations or at the irrelevant/ attended locations (Fig. 21.2C), suggesting that this modulation by emotion was independent of the modulation by voluntary spatial attention (and in fact strictly additive to it). A similar modulation of fusiform cortex by emotion was independent of awareness in the patient with spatial neglect in whom parietal cortical systems of attention are damaged (Fig. 21.4C,D). Therefore, top-down signals onto sensory cortices might involve direct feedback connections from regions that are primarily concerned with the detection and evaluation of affective stimuli, such as amygdala and orbitofrontal cortex. In particular, as already described, the amygdala sends re-entrant projections to all levels of the ventral visual processing stream, from early striate cortex to late higher order areas in extrastriate temporal cortex (Amaral *et al.*, 1992). These inputs might directly act to enhance sensory processing of stimuli once their emotional value is detected in the amygdala (Anderson and Phelps, 2001).

We have investigated a potential role for the amygdala in influencing visual cortical activity in an event-related fMRI study in patients with amygdala damage (Vuilleumier *et al.*, 2002). This study used the same 2×2 factorial paradigm as the above experiment by Vuilleumier *et al.* (2001), in which fearful or neutral faces are presented at either task-relevant/attended locations or task-irrelevant/ignored locations (see Fig. 21.2A). Two groups of patients who had medial temporal lobe sclerosis and epilepsy were compared; one had both amygdala and hippocampal damage (H+A+), whereas the other had hippocampal damage only, without amygdala damage (H+A–), as determined from an abnormal T2 signal on structural MRI, using the fast-FLAIR (fluid-attenuated inversion recovery), dual-echo sequence (Woermann *et al.*, 2001). These patients were also compared to a group of healthy, age- and education-matched controls (H–A–). The critical results concerned areas showing a main effect of fearful versus neutral faces, regardless of attention. Consistent with the previous findings in young healthy subjects (Vuilleumier *et al.*, 2001b), such an effect of emotion was found in inferior temporal and fusiform cortex in normal controls and in patients with hippocampal damage only (H+A–); however, the patients with *amygdala* damage (H+A+) did not exhibit increased activity in response to fearful faces in their *intact* visual cortex (Fig. 21.6B). By contrast, the main effect of attention to faces versus houses showed a similar pattern of fusiform modulation in all three groups (Fig. 21.6A). This finding converges with results from a PET study (Morris *et al.*, 1998b) demonstrating that neural activity in extrastriate visual cortex shows condition-specific covariation with amygdala responses to facial expressions, suggesting significant functional connections between these areas. Similarly, recent single-cell recordings in the monkey visual cortex have revealed that face-selective neurons exhibit enhanced responses to emotional faces as compared to neutral ones, with a latency 50 ms longer than the initial discriminatory response to faces versus shapes, consistent with feedback modulation from other areas involved in emotional evaluation (Sugase *et al.*, 1999).

Subcortical neurotransmitter pathways might provide an alternative source of modulation to that provided by re-entrant amygdala-extrastriate connections. Cholinergic neurons in the basal forebrain receive prominent inputs from the amygdala and orbitomedial frontal cortex (Holland and Gallagher, 1999; Sarter and Bruno, 2000) and in turn project widely to the cortex, including posterior parietal areas involved in shifts of attention and early sensory cortical areas (Robbins, 1997; Sarter and Bruno, 2000). Animal studies have suggested that the basal forebrain cholinergic pathways may contribute to shifting attentional focus, enhancing signal to noise and prolonging neuronal responses to stimuli (Robbins, 1997). In fact, direct electrical stimulation of the amygdala evokes neocortical activation mediated by acetylcholine (Kapp *et al.*, 1994). The cholinergic system is thus well positioned to mediate both attentional and emotional modulation of cortical processing.

In an event-related fMRI study (Bentley *et al.*, in press), we have investigated this issue by again using the same factorial experiment (Vuilleumier *et al.*, 2001b) as described above (Fig. 21.2) to examine the effect produced by injection of a pro-cholinergic drug (physostigmine) versus placebo. Results from this study suggest that cholinergic modulation enhances the effect of attention on fusiform cortex, with greater responses to task-relevant faces after injection of drug than that observed after placebo. This would be consistent with an improved selectivity of attention and better filtering-out of irrelevant house distracters cortex (Furey *et al.*, 2000; Sarter and Bruno, 2000). A response to fearful faces was not affected by cholinergic stimulation in the amygdala itself but was associated with increased activity in left fusiform and inferior occipital cortex (though lessening over time). Increased effects of emotion were also found in bilateral prefrontal regions, particularly when fearful faces occurred at attended locations and

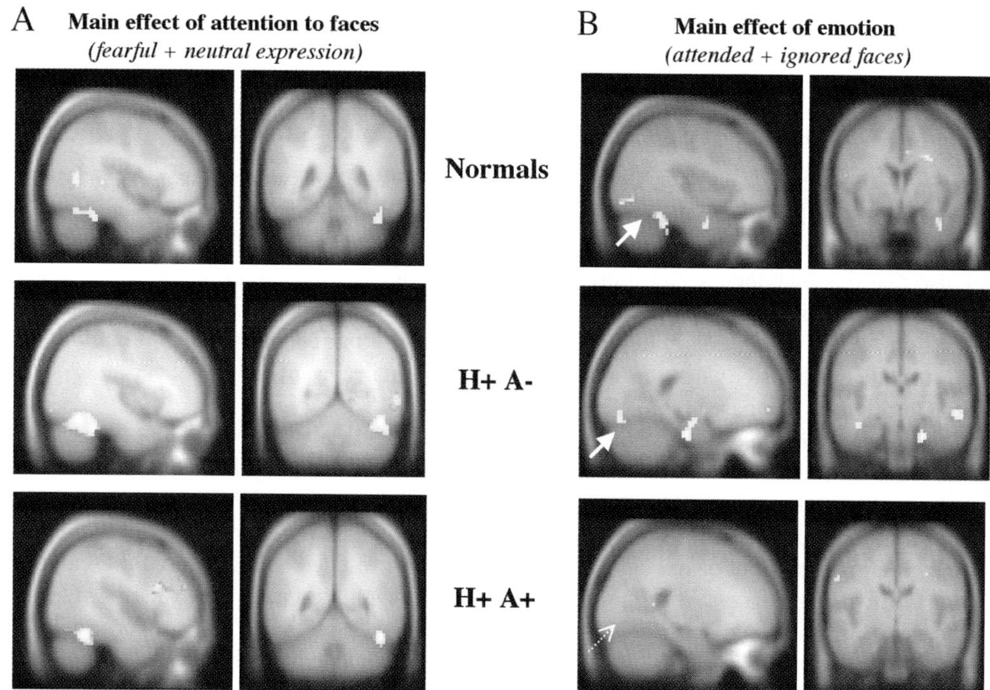

FIGURE 21.6
Remote effects of amygdala damage on visual cortical response to fearful faces; same experimental paradigm as in Vuilleumier *et al.* (2001b) (see Fig. 21.2A). Preliminary results in a group of patients with epilepsy and medial temporal lobe sclerosis (all left-sided) involving *only* the hippocampus and sparing the amygdala (H+A–, $n = 14$) or involving *both* the hippocampus *and* amygdala (H+A+, $n = 9$). Normal controls were a group of healthy relatives matched for age and education ($n = 10$). (A) Selective attention to faces versus houses increased fusiform activity in all three groups. (B) An increase produced by fearful versus neutral faces irrespective of attention was found in visual cortical areas (arrows) in healthy subjects as well as in patients with hippocampal damage only (H+A–) but not in patients with amygdala damage (H+A+). Note that visual cortex was similarly intact in all groups. (Unpublished fMRI data.)

in bilateral orbitofrontal cortex when fearful faces occurred at ignored locations. Such effects might reflect a greater distraction by emotional stimuli due to cholinergic modulation, requiring a subsequent engagement of frontal regions for monitoring potential response conflicts and adjusting ongoing goal-directed behaviour.

Finally, noradrenergic neurotransmitters might constitute another potential route through which emotional arousal influences cortical processing and redirection of attention. Arousal mechanisms implicate the locus coeruleus in the brain stem which receives substantial inputs from the amygdala and, in turn, sends extensive projections to the forebrain neocortex thought to regulate selective attention and attentional shifting (Aston-Jones *et al.*, 2000; Robbins, 1997). In keeping with this, a PET study by Lane *et al.* (1999) suggested that arousal can increase activation in visual cortex during exposure to emotional pictures, with the site of such effects overlapping with those due to selective attention and emotional valence. A. 3×2×2 factorial design was employed in which subjects were required to memorise different blocks of pleasant, unpleasant, or neutral scenes, each including either low- or high-arousal stimuli. Pictures were shown during either a low-load or high-load distracting auditory task. Extensive extrastriate visual areas showed a common effect for each of these three factors, with similar increases in right medial occipital cortex and anterior temporal cortex produced by emotional valence (unpleasant > pleasant > neutral), arousal (high > low), and selective attention (low > high distraction); however, a potential limitation of this study was that the different conditions were blocked, and common visual increases could potentially have resulted from changes in attentional set. Higher arousal also enhanced activity in right medial frontal regions, in the same way as greater selective attention did, suggesting an additional modulation of behavioural output and perhaps experiential stages of emotional processing. These frontal effects of arousal seem consistent with animal studies indicating that connections between locus coeruleus and anterior cingulate cortex may be important in regulating attentional shifts and behavioural flexibility (Aston-Jones *et al.*, 2000).

Involuntary Orienting of Spatial Attention to Emotional Stimuli

Neuroimaging studies converge with behavioural studies in normal subjects (Mogg *et al.*, 1994; Öhman *et al.*, 2001b) and neglect patients (Vuilleumier and Schwartz, 2001a,b) to suggest not only that some emotional information can be "automatically" analysed even without attention but also that this may then serve to prioritise orienting of attention toward emotionally salient stimuli. Thus, spatial attention can be preferentially drawn to the location of emotional stimuli, with visual search (Eastwood *et al.*, 2001) or detection of a peripheral target (Stormark *et al.*, 1999) usually being faster when the target is preceded by an irrelevant emotional cue at the same spatial location, as compared to another location.

The mechanisms underlying such reflexive shifts of attention to emotional cues have been examined in an event-related fMRI experiment (Armony and Dolan, 2002) using a prototypical paradigm of spatial orienting (Gitelman *et al.*, 1999; Posner *et al.*, 1982). Subjects performed a simple task requiring them to detect, as quickly as possible, a small peripheral dot that could appear either in their right or left visual field. The dot was preceded by a very brief presentation (50 ms) of two angry faces at each location (Fig. 21.7A), with the faces being totally irrelevant to the task. Critically, only one of these faces (conditioned stimulus, CS+) was occasionally paired with an unpleasant, loud, white-noise burst noise (unconditioned stimulus, US). This procedure is known to induce a strong aversive affect toward the CS+ through classical Pavlovian fear conditioning, an effect known to involve enhanced amygdala activity as demonstrated in numerous animal studies (LeDoux, 1996) and neuroimaging studies (Buchel and Dolan, 2000). The critical experimental trials were those where the conditioned face (CS+) was presented on one side with the neutral face (CS–) on the other side (without the noise). Response times were found to be much slower when the target dot appeared on the side opposite the CS+ (incongruent trials) than when it coincided with the side of the CS+ (congruent trials), suggesting that spatial attention was indeed captured by the CS+ and had to be shifted contralaterally on incongruent trials. By contrast, attention was equally divided between the two hemifields on trials where the CS+ or CS– were presented on both sides.

Bilateral activation in the amygdala and fusiform cortex was observed for trials with CS+ faces, as compared to trials with only CS– faces (Fig. 21.7D), demonstrating reliable fear conditioning. Importantly, in contrast to trials with bilaterally divided attention, those with a unilateral CS+ capturing attention activated an extensive network including intraparietal sulcus, frontal eye field, anterior cingulate/supplementary motor cortex, and lateral orbitofrontal cortex in both hemispheres (Fig. 21.7B). Moreover, trials in which the CS+ was presented in the left visual field produced a greater parietal activation in the right hemisphere, whereas right-field presentations of the CS+ activated both left and right parietal cortices. These findings reveal a striking overlap between activations evoked by a lateralised CS+ and frontoparietal systems known to play a key role in spatial orienting of attention (Gitelman *et al.*, 1999; Posner and Petersen, 1990), consistent with the idea that an enhanced saliency of emotional events can trigger shifts of attention toward their location within the environment.

Notably, the only difference between the emotional orienting effects found here and spatial orienting effects found in attentional studies was an additional bilateral activation in lateral orbitofrontal cortex (Fig. 21.7C). As lateral orbitofrontal cortex is reciprocally connected to posterior parietal areas and frontal eye fields, this region might provide a crucial interface between emotional and attentional processes, specifically those involved in the modulation of spatial orienting by the affective value of sensory stimuli (Armony and Dolan, 2002).

Similarly, an earlier PET study (Fredrikson *et al.*, 1995) found that pictures of snakes previously conditioned by pairing with electric shocks, compared to the same pictures before conditioning, evoked increased activity in the cortical attentional networks, including bilateral parietal, left prefrontal, and anterior and posterior cingulate cortex. In addition, subcortical activations were found in ventromedial thalamus, hypothalamus, and central grey of the midbrain. Altogether, such findings demonstrate that emotional fear responses involved distributed neural networks concerned with attentive and autonomic functions.

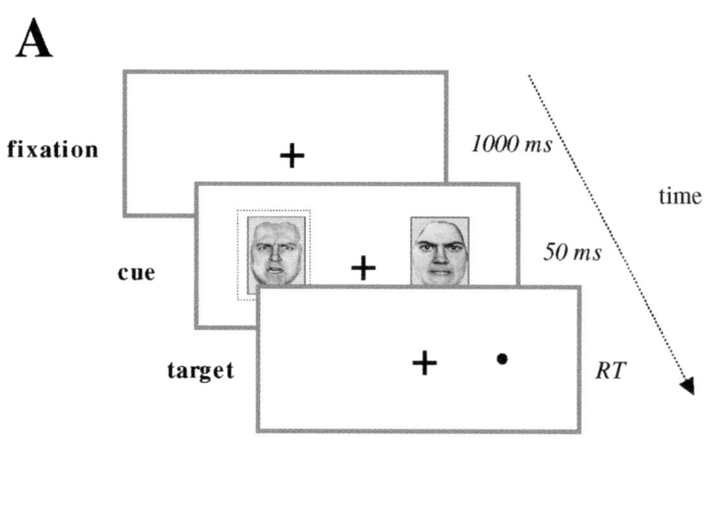

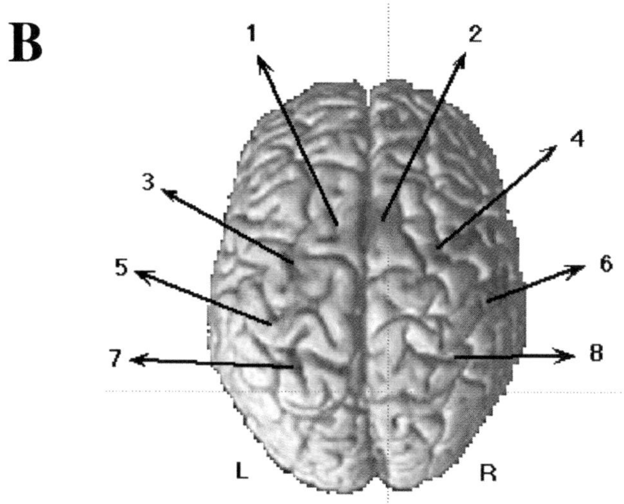

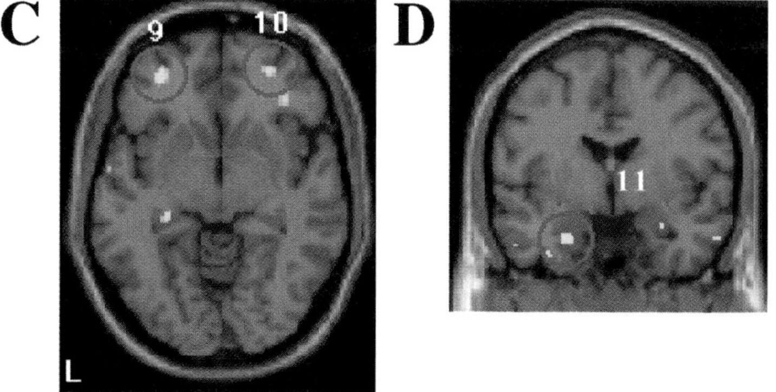

FIGURE 21.7
Effects of emotion on orienting of spatial attention. (A) Illustration of stimuli and task. On each trial, subjects had to detect a peripheral dot in the right or left visual field, preceded by a pair of angry faces. Only one face (CS+) is fear-conditioned by occasional pairing with a loud noise on trials where this face appears alone on both sides. On critical trials, the CS+ face (illustrated by dashed red lines) appears in one hemifield together with a CS– face in the other hemifield. Although task irrelevant, the CS+ faces produce a bias in spatial attention toward their location and slow the detection of target dots appearing on the opposite side. (B) and (C) Cortical regions showing increased activation on trials with a unilateral CS+ face capturing attention to one side, relative to trials with attention bilaterally divided to both sides (*i.e.*, two CS+ or two CS– faces). Nomenclature: 1, left SMA/anterior cingulate; 2, right SMA/anterior cingulate; 3, left frontal eye fields; 4, right frontal eye fields; 5, left anterior IPS/precentral sulcus; 6, right anterior IPS/precentral sulcus; 7, left intraparietal sulcus; 8, right intraparietal sulcus; 9, left orbitofrontal cortex; 10, right orbitofrontal cortex; 11, left amygdala. Note that the network of areas with such responses to a lateralised emotional cue is strikingly similar to the distributed neural system known to be implicated in spatial orienting of attention (B) but included additional activation in lateral orbitofrontal cortex (C). (D) The left amygdala was activated by all trials with CS+ faces versus CS– faces, indicating reliable fear conditioning. (fMRI data from Armony and Dolan, 2002.)

Modulation of Executive Control by Emotion

Emotional information can also affect the control of goal-directed action and its response preparation stages. Brain structures involved in basic emotional processing (such as the amygdala) have direct output projections toward motor systems that can mediate the expression of behavioural reactions, such as approach or avoidance. While simple and stereotyped reaction may be controlled by subcortical circuits (such as basal ganglia and central grey in brainstem), other flexible cognitive adjustments engage specific structures in prefrontal cortex.

Elliott *et al.* (2000) used fMRI to investigate the effect of emotion on selective attention to action using a Go/NoGo paradigm. Subjects were shown series of words, briefly presented each in turn, and had to respond only to relevant target words in the series, based either on their orthographic form (plain or italic text) or their emotional meaning (sad or happy), while the emotional meanings of irrelevant distracter words were also varied (neutral or opposite emotion). Selective attention to word meaning versus orthographic form activated left inferior frontal gyrus and left dorsal ACC, irrespective of whether word meaning was emotional or neutral, consistent with a general role of these regions in semantic and executive control. By contrast, selective detection of emotionally valenced targets, compared to neutral targets, activated the right rostral subgenual ACC and the right insula, as well as the left hippocampal region, regardless of the emotional valence of the targets (sad or happy). These regions were considered to represent an interface between cognition and emotion, involved when behavioural responses must be guided by emotional cues. Indeed, it has been proposed that rostral ACC (Fig. 21.5B) might particularly be important for regulating response selection mechanisms in the presence of affective and motivational signals (Bush *et al.*, 2000). On the other hand, Elliott *et al.* (2000) found no differential effects due to the emotional valence of task-irrelevant distracters when subjects selectively responded only to neutral targets among the word stream. This suggests that the processing of sad and happy emotional meaning in the words did not occur automatically in such conditions, but rather depended on top-down control due to the task set. It remains a goal for future studies to see whether a more obligatory emotional response to distracters would be obtained in such a Go/NoGo task with negative words that have stronger aversive meaning or with biologically more relevant stimuli, such as emotional faces.

Other investigators (Whalen *et al.*, 1998a), using fMRI, have examined the interference effects of emotional word meaning on responses in the Stroop task, where different aspects of the stimulus compete to determine behaviour. In such emotional Stroop tasks, interference is typically elicited by irrelevant emotional versus neutral meaning of printed words for which the colour must be read aloud. In the emotional Stroop variant used by Whalen *et al.* (1998), subjects had to count the number of negative (or neutral) words presented on the screen. Blocks with negative words increased activity in the left rostral/pregenual ACC compared to blocks with neutral words, as well as in the left superior parietal cortex. This finding again suggests that a distracting effect due to irrelevant emotional content might specifically engage executive control mechanisms mediated by rostral ACC. Interestingly, in the same subjects, a non-emotional variant of this Stroop task (*i.e.*, the counting of number-words) activated more dorsal regions in ACC, suggesting a differential role in the control of interference based on more abstract cognitive representations (Bush *et al.*, 1998). However, all subjects had performed the cognitive before the emotional Stroop and exhibited significant response time costs only in the cognitive version, so that the difference between emotional and cognitive interference across these two studies (Bush *et al.*, 1998; Whalen *et al.*, 1998a) might be confounded with practice or difficulty.

Emotional processing may also reduce activity in some cortical areas that mediate higher level cognitive and attentional functions, not only compared to active performance of a cognitive task but also compared to passive resting state (Drevets and Raichle, 1998; Shulman *et al.*, 1997; Whalen *et al.*, 1998a). Such decreases have been reported in several PET studies for dorsal regions in ACC and dorsolateral prefrontal cortex (Drevets and Raichle, 1998), as well as inferior medial prefrontal cortex (Sheline *et al.*, 2000; Simpson *et al.*, 2001a). This has usually been interpreted as reflecting an interference caused by emotion on ongoing cognitive processes, which are transiently suppressed by concurrent affective states. Likewise, left prefrontal and ACC activation during a verbal fluency task is reduced by manipulations of mood states (*i.e.*, induced depression or elation) that concomitantly increase activity in orbitofrontal cortex (Baker *et al.*, 1997). In contrast, it has been proposed that during the performance of various cognitive or attentional tasks on neutral stimuli (*e.g.*, verbal fluency or visual discriminations), a similar reciprocal suppression of activity may occur in brain areas that are normally implicated in emotional processing, including the amygdala, rostral ACC, and orbitofrontal cortex (as well as in some other regions, such as the cuneus and posterior cingulate) (Drevets and Raichle, 1998; Shulman *et al.*, 1997; Whalen *et al.*, 1998a). Also, activity in inferior medial prefrontal cortex is reduced only when a task is well practiced and provokes no anxiety (Simpson *et al.*, 2001a,b). It has been hypothesised that such changes in emotion-related areas during cognitive tasks might reflect a reduction in spontaneous motivational and affective evaluation of environmental and bodily states during the performance of attentionally demanding cognitive processes (Drevets and Raichle, 1998), at least as long as these are carried out in a relatively neutral context or concern relatively neutral material. Such decreases may not be seen when similar cognitive tasks are performed on surface features of emotionally valenced pictures (Simpson *et al.*, 2000). Moreover, as we have described above, a number of behavioural (Anderson and Phelps, 2001; Mathews and Klug, 1993) and imaging (Armony and Dolan, 2002; Vuilleumier *et al.*, 2001b) results indicate that performing an attentionally demanding cognitive task in the presence of either relevant or irrelevant emotional stimuli (most typically threat-related) can still engage processes responsible for the evaluation of affective significance in stimuli (*e.g.*, in amygdala, rostral ACC, or orbitofrontal cortex). Overall, this would be consistent with a key role of these structures in monitoring incoming inputs for salient stimuli through attention-independent channels and then regulating the allocation of attentional resources to achieve priority goals, being turned down in a safe context but kicking in to interrupt higher order cognitive processes in the face of potential threat signals.

MODULATION OF MEMORY BY EMOTION

Attention not only governs the selection of information for conscious perception and goal-directed action but also enhances the formation of memory traces for later recall. Emotion again bears much resemblance to attention in this respect, as a large body of behavioural work has shown that stimuli with affective value, or stimuli presented in an emotional context, tend to be subsequently remembered much better than neutral stimuli. Several recent functional neuroimaging studies have begun to reveal the neural substrates of such emotional effects on memory (Cahill *et al.*, 1996; Hamann *et al.*, 1999; Maratos *et al.*, 2001), but it is beyond the scope of this chapter to review this emerging literature. Note that an emotional modulation of memory can occur both at encoding and retrieval stages (Dolan *et al.*, 2000; Taylor *et al.*, 1998) and might partly result from mechanisms reviewed above that intensify the sensory processing and enhance the allocation of attention toward emotionally relevant stimuli. In addition, there might be further mechanisms specifically related to memory consolidation that are directly modulated by brain areas involved in emotional and arousal processes, as has been proposed for the amygdala (Cahill *et al.*, 1996; Hamann *et al.*, 1999). As for the modulation of attention, the modulation of memory by emotion might thus implicate multiple, reciprocally interacting pathways between the amygdala or related structures, on the one hand, and distant areas in sensory cortices, prefrontal cortex, and hippocampus, on the other hand.

CONCLUSION

Attention and emotion share many reciprocal links. Thus, both attention and emotion involve distributed neural networks of highly interactive cortical and subcortical brain regions that are in a position to regulate processes related to perception, action, and memory. Likewise, both attention and emotion are intimately associated with conscious experience. Whereas attentional processes may control selective processing of sensory events that ultimately determine the content of conscious awareness, emotional processes may operate without attention or without awareness but can nonetheless influence the allocation of attention and hence readily permeate or intrude into awareness. It also remains possible that distinct stimuli and different kinds of emotion might engage unique neural systems that in turn exert distinct effects on attentive and cognitive processes. Stimuli with intrinsic biological value (*e.g.*, faces) or special affective significance (*e.g.*, threat-related) might have a particular status in such interactions between emotion and attention. Thus, the fear system provides a dedicated neural system for mediating fast and automatic responses to signals of potential danger, with the amygdala being activated by fear-related stimuli regardless of whether attention is directed to other features or other locations in space. This in turn allows for a direct feedback modulation on visual cortices which can be preserved after damage to parietal systems of attention (as in neglect patients) but lost after damage to the amygdala itself (as in epileptic patients).

Moreover, reciprocal interactions between emotion, attention, and cognition have potentially important implications for understanding a number of psychiatric diseases. An abnormal modulation of attention by emotion, mood, or past affective experiences has now been observed by both behavioural and imaging studies in a variety of conditions, including anxiety, phobia, posttraumatic stress disorder, obsessive–compulsive disorder, depression, or schizophrenia. More generally, the study of such interactions between emotional and attentional–cognitive processes also raises the general question of individual differences and of their underlying neural substrates. This constitutes a new challenge for cognitive neuroscience, which can now be powerfully addressed by neuroimaging research.

Finally, new insights into the neural underpinnings of reciprocal interactions between emotion and attention emphasise a dynamic interplay between distinct areas, organised as extended system networks, that are engaged in reciprocal exchanges of information. Such a perspective on brain function clearly goes beyond views of a strictly modular specialisation of subcomponents and purely feedforward processing of information, as traditionally considered by cognitive neuroscience research.

References

Amaral, D. G., Price, J. L., Pitkänen, A., and Carmichael, S. T. (1992). Anatomical organisation of the primate amygdaloid complex, in The *Amygdala: Neurobiological Aspects of Emotion, Memory and Mental Dysfunction*. Aggleton J., Ed., pp. 1–66. Wiley-Liss, New York.

Anderson, A. K. and Phelps, E. A. (2001). Lesions of the human amygdala impair enhanced perception of emotionally salient events. *Nature*, **411**, 305–309.

Armony, J. L. and LeDoux, J. E. (1997). How the brain processes emotional information. *Ann. N.Y. Acad. Sci.*, **821**, 259–270.

Armony, J. L. and Dolan, R. J. (2002). Modulation of spatial attention by fear-conditioned stimuli: an event-related fMRI study. *Neuropsychologia*, **40**, 817–826.

Armony, J. L. and LeDoux, J. E. (2000). How danger is encoded: towards a systems, cellular, and computational understanding of cognitive-emotional interactions in fear, in *The New Cognitive Neurosciences*, Gazzaniga, M. S., Ed., pp. 1067–1080. MIT Press, Cambridge, MA.

Armony, J. L., Servan-Schreiber, D., Cohen, J. D., and LeDoux, J. E. (1997). Computational modelling of emotion: explorations through the anatomy and physiology of fear conditioning. *Trends in Cogn. Sci.*, **1**, 28–34.

Aston-Jones, G., Rajkowski, J., and Cohen, J. (2000). Locus coeruleus and regulation of behavioural flexibility and attention. *Prog. Brain Res.*, **126**, 165–182.

Baker, S. C., Frith, C. D., and Dolan, R. J. (1997). The interaction between mood and cognitive function studied with PET. *Psychol. Med.*, **27**, 565–578.

Beauregard, M., Leroux, J. M., Bergman, S., Arzoumanian, Y., Beaudoin, G., Bourgouin, P. *et al.* (1998). The functional neuroanatomy of major depression: an fMRI study using an emotional activation paradigm. *NeuroReport*, **9**, 3253–3258.

Belin, P., Zatorre, R. J., Lafaille, P., Ahad, P., and Pike, B. (2000). Voice-selective areas in human auditory cortex. *Nature*, **403**, 309–312.

Bentley P., Thiel C., Vuilleumier P., Driver J., and Dolan, R. J. Cholinergic enhancement modulates neural correlates of selective attention and emotional processing. *NeuroImage*, in press.

Blair, R. J., Morris, J. S., Frith, C. D., Perrett, D. I., and Dolan, R. J. (1999). Dissociable neural responses to facial expressions of sadness and anger. *Brain*, **122**, 883–893.

Bradley, B. P., Mogg, K., and Lee, S. C. (1997a). Attentional biases for negative information in induced and naturally occurring dysphoria. *Behav. Res. Ther.*, **35**, 911–927.

Bradley, B. P., Mogg, K., Millar, N., Bonham-Carter, C. *et al.* (1997b). Attentional biases for emotional faces. *Cogn. Emot.*, **11**, 25–42.

Bradley, B. P., Mogg, K., White, J., Groom, C., and de Bono, J. (1999). Attentional bias for emotional faces in generalised anxiety disorder. *Br. J. Clin. Psychol.*, **38**, 267–278.

Breiter, H. C., Etcoff, N. L., Whalen, P. J., Kennedy, W. A., Rauch, S. L., Buckner, R. L. *et al.* (1996). Response and habituation of the human amygdala during visual processing of facial expression. *Neuron*, **17**, 875–887.

Buchel, C. and Dolan, R. J. (2000). Classical fear conditioning in functional neuroimaging. *Curr. Opin. Neurobiol.*, **10**, 219–223.

Buchel, C., Morris, J., Dolan, R. J., and Friston, K. J. (1998). Brain systems mediating aversive conditioning: an event-related fMRI study. *Neuron*, **20**, 947–957.

Buchel, C., Dolan, R. J., Armony, J. L., and Friston, K. J. (1999). Amygdala-hippocampal involvement in human aversive trace conditioning revealed through event-related functional magnetic resonance imaging. *J. Neurosci.*, **19**, 10869–10876.

Bush, G., Whalen, P. J., Rosen, B. R., Jenike, M. A., McInerney, S. C., and Rauch, S. L. (1998). The counting Stroop: an interference task specialised for functional neuroimaging–validation study with functional MRI. *Hum. Brain Mapping*, **6**, 270–282.

Bush, G., Luu, P., and Posner, M. I. (2000). Cognitive and emotional influences in anterior cingulate cortex. *Trends Cogn. Sci.*, **4**, 215–222.

Cahill, L., Haier, R. J., Fallon, J., Alkire, M. T., Tang, C., Keator, D. *et al.* (1996). Amygdala activity at encoding correlated with long-term, free recall of emotional information. *Proc. Natl. Acad. Sci. USA*, **93**, 8016–8021.

Calder, A., Lawrence, A., and Young, A. (2001). Neuropsychology of fear and loathing. *Nat. Rev. Neurosci.*, **2**, 352–363.

Corbetta, M., Meizin, F. M., Dobmeyer, S., Shulman, G. L., and Petersen, S. E. (1990). Selective attention modulates neural processing of shape, color and velocity in humans. *Science*, **248**, 1556–1559.

Critchley, H., Daly, E., Phillips, M., Brammer, M., Bullmore, E., and Williams, S. *et al.* (2000). Explicit and implicit neural mechanisms for processing of social information from facial expressions: a functional magnetic resonance imaging study. *Hum. Brain Mapping*, **9**, 93–105.

Damasio, A. R. (1999). *The Feeling of What Happens: Body and Emotion in the Making of Consciousness*. Harcourt Brace, New York.

Damasio, A. R., Grabowski, T. J., Bechara, A., Damasio, H., Ponto, L. L., Parvizi, J. *et al.* (2000). Subcortical and cortical brain activity during the feeling of self-generated emotions. *Nat. Neurosci.*, **3**, 1049–1056.

Dimberg, U., Thunberg, M., and Elmehed, K. (2000). Unconscious facial reactions to emotional facial expressions. *Psychol. Sci.*, **11**, 86–9.

Dolan, R. J., Fletcher, P., Morris, J., Kapur, N., Deakin, J. F., and Frith, C. D. (1996). Neural activation during covert processing of positive emotional facial expressions. *NeuroImage*, **4**, 194–200.

Dolan, R. J., Lane, R., Chua, P., and Fletcher, P. (2000). Dissociable temporal lobe activations during emotional episodic memory retrieval. *NeuroImage*, **11**, 203–209.

Dolan, R. J., Morris, J. S., andde Gelder, B. (2001). Crossmodal binding of fear in voice and face. *Proc. Natl. Acad. Sci. USA*, **98**, 10006–10010.

Drevets, W. C. and Raichle, M. E. (1998). Reciprocal suppression of regional cerebral blood flow during emotional versus higher cognitive processes: implications for interactions between emotion and cognition. *Emot. Cogn.*, **12**, 353–385.

Driver, J. and Vuilleumier, P. (2001). Perceptual awareness and its loss in unilateral neglect and extinction. *Cognition*, **79**, 39–88.

Eastwood, J. D., Smilek, D., and Merikle, P. M. (2001). Differential attentional guidance by unattended faces expressing positive and negative emotion. *Percept. Psychophys.*, **63**, 1004–1013.

Ekman, P. and Oster, H. (1979). Facial expressions of emotion. *Ann. Rev. Psychol.*, **30**, 527–554.

Elliott, R., Rubinsztein, J. S., Sahakian, B. J., and Dolan, R. J. (2000). Selective attention to emotional stimuli in a verbal go/no-go task: an fMRI study. *NeuroReport*, **11**, 1739–1744.

Fox E., Russo, R., Bowles, R. J., and Dutton, K. (2000). Do threatening stimuli draw or hold visual attention in subclinical anxiety? *J. Exp. Psychol.*, **130**, 681–700.

Fredrikson, M., Wik, G., Greitz, T., Eriksson, L., Stone-Elander, S., Ericson, K. *et al.* (1993). Regional cerebral blood flow during experimental phobic fear. *Psychophysiology*, **30**, 126–130.

Fredrikson, M., Wik, G., Fischer, H., and Andersson, J. (1995). Affective and attentive neural networks in humans: a PET study of Pavlovian conditioning. *NeuroReport*, **7**, 97–101.

Furey, M. L., Pietrini, P., Alexander, G. E., Schapiro, M. B., and Horwitz, B. (2000). Cholinergic enhancement improves performance on working memory by modulating the functional activity in distinct brain regions: a positron emission tomography regional cerebral blood flow study in healthy humans. *Brain Res. Bull.*, **51**, 213–218.

Garavan, H., Pendergrass, J. C., Ross, T. J., Stein, E. A., and Risinger, R. C. (2001). Amygdala response to both positively and negatively valenced stimuli. *NeuroReport*, **12**, 2779–2783.

George, M. S., Ketter, E. A., Gill, D. S., Haxby, J. V., Ungerleider, L. G., Herscovitch, P. *et al.* (1993). Brain regions involved in recognising facial emotion or identity: an oxygen-15 PET study. *J. Neuropsychiatry and Clin. Neurosci.*, **5**, 384–394.

George, M. S., Ketter, T. A., Parekh, P. I., Horwitz, B., Herscovitch, P., and Post, R. M. (1995). Brain activity during transient sadness and happiness in healthy women, **112**, 383–390.

Gitelman, D. R., Nobre, A. C., Parrish, T. B., LaBar, K. S., Kim, Y. H., Meyer, J. R. *et al.*, (1999). A large-scale distributed network for covert spatial attention: further anatomical delineation based on stringent behavioural and cognitive controls. *Brain*, **122**, 1093–1106.

Globisch, J., Hamm, A. O., Esteves, F., and Öhman, A. (1999). Fear appears fast: temporal course of startle reflex potentiation in animal fearful subjects. *Psychophysiology*, **36**, 66–75.

Gorno-Tempini, M. L., Pradelli, S., Serafini, M., Pagnoni, G., Baraldi, P., Porro, C. *et al.* (2001). Explicit and incidental facial expression processing: an fMRI study. *NeuroImage*, **14**, 465–473.

Hamann, S. B., Ely, T. D., Grafton, S. T., and Kilts, C. D. (1999). Amygdala activity related to enhanced memory for pleasant and aversive stimuli. *Nat. Neurosci.*, **2**, 289–293.

Hansen, C. H. and Hansen, R. D. (1988). Finding the face in the crowd: an anger superiority effect. *J. Personality Social Psychol.*, **54**, 917–924.

Hariri, A. R., Bookheimer, S. Y., and Mazziotta, J. C. (2000). Modulating emotional responses: effects of a neocortical network on the limbic system. *NeuroReport*, **11**, 43–48.

Hasselmo, M. E., Rolls E T., and Baylis, G. C. (1989). The role of expression and identity in the face-selective responses of neurons in the temporal visual cortex of the monkey. *Behav. Brain Res.*, **32**, 203–218.

Haxby, J. V., Hoffman, E. A., and Gobbini, M. I. (2000). The distributed human neural system for face perception. *Trends Cogn. Neurosci.*, **4**, 223–232.

Holland, P. C. and Gallagher M. (1999). Amygdala circuitry in attentional and representational processes. *Trends Cogn. Sci.*, **3**, 65–73.

Imaizumi, S., Mori, K., Kiritani, S., Kawashima, R., Sugiura, M., Fukuda, H. *et al.* (1997). Vocal identification of speaker and emotion activates different brain regions. *NeuroReport*, **8**, 2809–2812.

Irwin, W., Davidson, R. J., Lowe, M. J., Mock, B. J., Sorenson, J. A., and Turski, P. A. (1996). Human amygdala activation detected with echo-planar functional magnetic resonance imaging. *Psychiatry Res.*, **67**, 135–143.

Isenberg, N., Silbersweig, D., Engelien, A., Emmerich, S., Malavade, K., Beattie, B. *et al.* (1999). Linguistic threat activates the human amygdala. *Proc. Natl. Acad. Sci. USA*, **96**, 10456–10459.

Jancke, L., Buchanan, T. W., Lutz, K., and Shah, N. J. (2001). Focused and nonfocused attention in verbal and emotional dichotic listening: an fMRI study. *Brain Lang.*, **78**, 349–363.

Kapp, B. S., Supple, W. F., and Whalen, P. J. (1994). Effects of electrical stimulation of the amygdaloid central nucleus on neocortical arousal in the rabbit. *Behav. Neurosci.*, **108**, 81–93.

Keightley, M. L., Grady, C. L., Graham, S., Winocur, G., and Mayberg, H. S. (2000). Separate brain systems for emotional processing of faces and pictures. *SFN Abstracts*, 755.16.

Kesler-West, M. L., Andersen, A. H., Smith, C. D., Avison, M. J., Davis, C. E., Avison, R. G. *et al.* (1999). A functional magnetic resonance imaging (fMRI) study of the perception of emotional facial expressions. *J. Cogn. Neurosci.*, **11**(Suppl.), 82.

Kesler-West, M. L., Andersen, A. H., Smith, C. D., Avison, M. J., Davis, C. E., Kryscio, R. J. *et al.* (2001). Neural substrates of facial emotion processing using fMRI. *Brain Res. Cogn. Brain Res.*, **11**, 213–226.

Kindt, M. and Brosschot, J. F. (1997). Phobia-related cognitive bias for pictorial and linguistic stimuli., *J. Abnormal Psychol.*, **106**, 644–648.

Kosslyn, S. M., Shin, L. M., Thompson, W. L., McNally, R. J., Rauch, S. L., Pitman, R. K. *et al.* (1996). Neural effects of visualising and perceiving aversive stimuli: a PET investigation. *NeuroReport*, **7**, 1569–1576.

LaBar, K. S., Gatenby, J. C., Gore, J. C., LeDoux, J. E., and Phelps, E. A. (1998). Human amygdala activation during conditioned fear acquisition and extinction: a mixed-trial fMRI study. *Neuron*, **20**, 947–957.

Lane, R. D., Fink G. R., Chau, P. M., Dolan, R. J. (1997a). Neural activation during selective attention to subjective emotional responses. *NeuroReport*, **8**, 3969–3972.

Lane, R. D., Reiman, E M., Ahern, G. L., Schwartz, G. E., and Davidson, R. J. (1997b). Neuroanatomical correlates of happiness, sadness, and disgust. *Am. J. Psychiatry*, **154**, 926–933.

Lane, R. D., Reiman, E. M., Bradley, M. M., Lang, P. J., Ahern, G. L., Davidson, R. J. *et al.* (1997c). Neuroanatomical correlates of pleasant and unpleasant emotion. *Neuropsychologia*, **35**, 1437–1444.

Lane, R. D., Reiman, E. M., Axelrod, B., Yun, L. S., Holmes, A., and Schwartz, G. E. (1998). Neural correlates of levels of emotional awareness: evidence of an interaction between emotion and attention in the anterior cingulate cortex., *J. Cogn. Neurosci.*, **10**, 525–535.

Lane, R. D., Chua, P. M., and Dolan, R. J. (1999). Common effects of emotional valence, arousal and attention on neural activation during visual processing of pictures. *Neuropsychologia*, **37**, 989–997.

Lang, P. J., Bradley, M. M., Fitzsimmons, J. R., Cuthbert, B. N., Scott, J. D., Moulder, B. *et al.* (1998). Emotional arousal and activation of the visual cortex: an fMRI analysis. *Psychophysiology*, **35**, 199–210.

LeDoux, J. E. (1996). *The Emotional Brain*. Simon & Schuster, New York.

Liberzon, I., Taylor, S. F., Fig, L. M., Decker, L. R., Koeppe, R. A., and Minoshima, S. (2000). Limbic activation and psychophysiologic responses to aversive visual stimuli, interaction with cognitive task. *Neuropsychopharmacology*, **23**, 508–516.

Mack, A. and Rock, I. (1998). *Inattentional Blindness*. MIT Press, Cambridge, MA.

Maddock, R. J. (1999). The retrosplenial cortex and emotion: new insights from functional neuroimaging of the human brain. *Trends Neurosci.*, **22**, 310–316.

Maratos, E. J., Dolan, R. J., Morris, J. S., Henson, R. N., and Rugg, M. D. (2001). Neural activity associated with episodic memory for emotional context. *Neuropsychologia*, **39**, 910–920.

Mathews, A. and Klug, F. (1993). Emotionality and interference with color-naming in anxiety. *Behav. Res. Ther.*, **31**, 57–62.

Merikle, P., Smilek, D., and Eastwood, J. D. (2001). Perception without awareness: perspectives from cognitive psychology. *Cognition*, **79**, 115–134.

Mesulam, M. M. (1999). Spatial attention and neglect: parietal, frontal and cingulate contributions to the mental representation and attentional targeting of salient extrapersonal events. *Philos. Trans. Roy. Soc. London B, Biol. Sci.*, **354**, 1325–1346.

Mogg, K. and Bradley, B. P. (1999). Orienting of attention to threatening facial expressions presented under conditions of restricted awareness. *Cogn. Emot.*, **13**, 713–740.

Mogg, K., Bradley, B. P., and Hallowell, N. (1994). Attentional bias to threat: roles of trait anxiety, stressful events, and awareness. *Q. J. Exp. Psychol. A*, **47**, 841–864.

Mogg, K., Bradley, B. P., de Bono, J., and Painter, M. (1997). Time course of attentional bias for threat information in non-clinical anxiety. *Behav. Res. Ther.*, **35**, 297–303.

Morris, J. S., Frith, C. D., Perrett, D. I., Rowland, D., Young, A. W., Calder, A. J. *et al.* (1996). A differential neural response in the human amygdala to fearful and happy facial expressions. *Nature*, **31**, 812–815.

Morris, J. S,, Friston, K. J., Buchel, C., Frith, C. D., Young, A. W., Calder, A. J. *et al.* (1998a). A neuromodulatory role for the human amygdala in processing emotional facial expressions. *Brain*, **121**, 47–57.

Morris, J. S., Öhman A., and Dolan, R. J. (1998b). Conscious and unconscious emotional learning in the human amygdala. *Nature*, **393**, 476–470.

Morris, J. S., Scott, S. K., and Dolan, R. J. (1999). Saying it with feeling: neural responses to emotional vocalisations. *Neuropsychologia*, **37**, 1155–1163.

Nakamura, K., Kawashima, R., Ito, K., Sugiura, M., Kato, T., Nakamura, A. *et al.* (1999). Activation of the right inferior frontal cortex during assessment of facial emotion. *J. Neurophysiol.*, **82**, 1610–1614.

Narumoto, J., Okada, T., Sadato, N., Fukui, K., and Yonekura, Y. (2001). Attention to emotion modulates fMRI activity in human right superior temporal sulcus. *Brain Res. Cogn. Brain Res.*, **12**, 225–231.

Northoff, G., Richter, A., Gessner, M., Schlagenhauf, F., Fell, J., Baumgart, F. *et al.* (2000). Functional dissociation between medial and lateral prefrontal cortical spatiotemporal activation in negative and positive emotions: a combined fMRI/MEG study. *Cereb Cortex.*, **10**, 93–107.

Nothdurft, H. C. (1993). Faces and facial expressions do not pop out. *Perception*, **22**, 1287–1298.

Öhman, A. and Flykt A. (2000). Unconscious emotion: evolutionary perspectives, psychophysiological data, and neuropsychological mechanisms, in *Cognitive Neuroscience of Emotion*, Lane, R. D. and Nadel, L., Eds., pp. 296–327. Oxford University Press, New York.

Öhman, A., Flykt A., and Esteves F. (2001a). Emotion drives attention: detecting the snake in the grass., *J. Exp. Psychol. Gen.*, **130**, 466–478.

Öhman, A., Lundqvist, D., and Esteves, F. (2001b). The face in the crowd revisited: a threat advantage with schematic stimuli., *J. Personality Soc. Psychol.*, **80**, 381–396.

Paradiso, S., Johnson, D. L., Andreasen, N. C., O'Leary, D. S., Watkins, G. L., Ponto, L. L. *et al.* (1999). Cerebral blood flow changes associated with attribution of emotional valence to pleasant, unpleasant, and neutral visual stimuli in a PET study of normal subjects. *Am. J. Psychiatry*, **156**, 1618–1629.

Pardo, J. V., Pardo, P. J., and Raichle, M. E. (1993). Neural correlates of self-induced dysphoria. *Am. J. Psychiatry*, **150**, 713–719.

Partiot, A., Grafman, J., Sadato, N., Wachs, J., and Hallett, M. (1995). Brain activation during the generation of non-emotional and emotional plans. *NeuroReport*, **6**, 1397–1400.

Perrett, D. I., Hietanen, J. K., Oram, M. W., and Benson, P. J. (1992). Organisation and functions of cells responsive to faces in the temporal cortex. *Philos. Trans. Roy. Soc. London B, Biol. Sci.*, **335**, 23–30.

Pessoa, L., McKenna, M., Gutierrez, E., and Ungerleider, L. G. (2002). Neural processing of emotional faces require attention. *PNAS*, **99**, 11458–11463.

Phelps, E. A., O'Connor, K. J., Gatenby, J. C., Gore, J. C., Grillon, C., and Davis, M. (2001). Activation of the left amygdala to a cognitive representation of fear. *Nat. Neurosci.*, **4**, 437–441.

Phillips, M. L., Young, A. W., Senior, C., Brammer, M., Andrew, C., Calder, A. J. *et al.* (1997). A specific neural substrate for perceiving facial expressions of disgust. *Nature*, **389**, 495–498.

Phillips, M. L., Bullmore, E. T., Howard, R., Woodruff, P. W., Wright, I. C., Williams, S. C. *et al.* (1998a). Investigation of facial recognition memory of happy and sad facial expression perception: an fMRI study. *Psychiatry Res.*, **83**, 127–138.

Phillips, M. L., Young, A. W., Scott, S. K., Calder, A. J., Andrew, C., Giampietro, V. *et al.* (1998b). Neural responses to facial and vocal expressions of fear and disgust. *Proc. Roy. Soc. London Ser. B, Biol. Sci.*, **265**, 1809–1817.

Posner, M. I. and Petersen S. (1990). The attention system of the human brain. *Ann. Rev. Neurosci.*, **13**, 25–42.

Posner, M. I., Cohen, Y., and Rafal, R. (1982). Neural systems control of spatial orienting. *Philos. Trans. Roy. Soc. London B, Biol. Sci.*, **298**, 187–198.

Reiman, E. M., Lane, R. D., Ahern, G. L., Schwartz, G. E., Davidson, R. J., Friston, K. J. *et al.* (1997). Neuroanatomical correlates of externally and internally generated human emotion. *Am. J. Psychiatry*, **154**, 918–925.

Robbins, T. W. (1997). Arousal systems and attentional processes. *Biol. Psychol.*, **45**, 57–71.

Robbins, T. W. and Everitt, B. J. (1996). Neurobehavioural mechanisms of reward and motivation. *Curr. Opin. Neurobiol.*, **6**, 228–236.

Robinson, M. D. (1998). Running from William James' bears: a review of preattentive mechanisms and their contributions to emotional experience. *Emot. Cogn.*, **12**, 667–696.

Rolls, E. T. (1996). The orbitofrontal cortex. *Philos. Trans. Roy. Soc. London B, Biol. Sci.*, **351**, 1433–1443.

Rotshtein, P., Malach, R., Hadar, U., Graif, M., and Hendler, T. (2001). Feeling or features: different sensitivity to emotion in high-order visual cortex and amygdala. *Neuron*, **32**, 747–757.

Sander, K. and Scheich, H. (2001). Auditory perception of laughing and crying activates human amygdala regardless of attentional state. *Brain Res. Cogn. Brain Res.*, **12**, 181–198.

Sarter, M. and Bruno, J. P. (2000). Cortical cholinergic inputs mediating arousal, attentional processing and dreaming: differential afferent regulation of the basal forebrain by telencephalic and brainstem afferents. *Neuroscience*, **95**, 933–952.

Schneider, F., Gur, R. E., Mozley, L. H., Smith, R. J., Mozley, P. D., Censits, D. M. *et al.* (1995). Mood effects on limbic blood flow correlate with emotional self-rating: a PET study with oxygen-15 labeled water. *Psychiatry Res.*, **61**, 265–283.

Schweinberger, S. R. and Soukup, G. R. (1998). Asymmetric relationships among perceptions of facial identity, emotion, and facial speech. *J. Exp. Psychol. Hum. Percept. Perform.*, **24**, 1748–1765.

Sheline, Y. I., Berger, K. L., Snyder, A., Ollinger, J., Barch, D., and Mintun, M. (2000). fMRI study using masked fearful emotional faces deactivates inferior medial prefrontal cortex [abstract]. *Soc. Neurosci.*, Abstr. 403.5.

Shulman, G. L., Corbetta, M., Buckner, R. L., Fiez, J. A., Miezen, F. M., Raichle, M. E. *et al.* (1997). Common blood flow changes across visual tasks. II. Decreases in cerebral cortex, *J. Cogn Neurosci.*, **9**, 648–663.

Simpson, J. R., Jr., Ongur, D., Akbudak, E., Conturo, T. E., Ollinger, J. M., Snyder, A. Z. *et al.* (2000). The emotional modulation of cognitive processing: an fMRI study. *J. Cogn Neurosci.*, **12**, 157–170.

Simpson, J. R., Jr., Drevets, W. C., Snyder, A. Z., Gusnard, D. A., and Raichle, M. E. (2001a). Emotion-induced changes in human medial prefrontal cortex. II. During anticipatory anxiety. *Proc. Natl. Acad. Sci. USA*, **98**, 688–693.

Simpson, J. R., Jr., Snyder, A. Z., Gusnard, D. A., and Raichle, M. E. (2001b). Emotion-induced changes in human medial prefrontal cortex. I. During cognitive task performance. *Proc. Natl. Acad. Sci. USA*, **98**, 683–687.

Sprengelmeyer, R., Rausch, M., Eysel, U. T., and Przuntek, H. (1998). Neural structures associated with recognition of facial expressions of basic emotions. *Proc. Roy. Soc. London Ser. B, Biol. Sci.*, **265**, 1927–1931.

Stormark, K. M., Hugdahl, K., and Posner, M. I. (1999). Emotional modulation of attention orienting: a classical conditioning study. *Scand. J. Psychol.*, **40**, 91–99.

Sugase, Y., Yamane, S., Ueno, S., and Kawano, K. (1999). Global and fine information coded by single neurons in the temporal visual cortex. *Nature*, **400**, 869–873.

Tabert, M. H., Borod, J. C., Tang, C. Y., Lange, G., Wei, T. C., Johnson, R. *et al.* (2001). Differential amygdala activation during emotional decision and recognition memory tasks using unpleasant words: an fMRI study. *Neuropsychologia*, **39**, 556–573.

Taylor, S. F., Liberzon, I., Fig, L. M., Decker, L. R., Minoshima, S., Koeppe, R. A. (1998). The effect of emotional content on visual recognition memory: a PET activation study. *NeuroImage*, **8**, 188–197.

Taylor, S. F., Liberzon I., and Koeppe, R. A. (2000). The effect of graded aversive stimuli on limbic and visual activation. *Neuropsychologia*, **38**, 1415–1425.

Teasdale, J. D., Howard, R. J., Cox, S. G., Ha, Y., Brammer, M. J., Williams, S. C. *et al.* (1999). Functional MRI study of the cognitive generation of affect. *Am. J. Psychiatry*, **156**, 209–215.

Thomas, K. M., Drevets, W. C., Whalen, P. J., Eccard, C. H., Dahl, R. E., Ryan, N. D. *et al.* (2001). Amygdala response to facial expressions in children and adults. *Biol. Psychiatry*, **49**, 309–316.

Vuilleumier, P. and Schwartz, I. (2001a). Emotional facial expressions capture attention. *Neurology*, **56**, 153–158.

Vuilleumier, P. and Schwartz, S. (2001b). Beware and be aware: capture of attention by fear-relevant stimuli in patients with unilateral neglect. *NeuroReport*, **12**, 1119–1122.

Vuilleumier, P., Armony, J. L., Driver, J., and Dolan, R. J. (2001a). Amygdala activation by seen and unseen fearful faces in unilateralspatial neglect: event-related fMRI. *NeuroImage*, **13**, S482.

Vuilleumier, P., Armony, J. L., Driver, J., and Dolan, R. J. (2001b). Effects of attention and emotion on face processing in the human brain: an event-related fMRI study. *Neuron*, **30**, 829–841.

Vuilleumier, P., Armony, J. L., Clark, K., Husack, M., Driver, J., and Dolan, R. J. (2002). Neural response to emotional faces with and without awareness: event-related fMRI in a paretal with visual extinction and spatial neglect. *Neuropsychologia*, **40**, 2156–2166.

Vuilleumier, P., Richardson, M., Armony, J., Driver, J., Duncan, J., and Dolan, R. J. Remote effects of amygdala lesions on processing of emotional faces in visual cortex, in preparation.

Whalen, P. J., Bush, G., McNally, R. J., Wilhelm, S., McInerney, S. C., Jenike, M. A. *et al.* (1998a). The emotional counting Stroop paradigm: a functional magnetic resonance imaging probe of the anterior cingulate affective division. *Biol. Psychiatry*, **44**, 1219–1228.

Whalen, P. J., Rauch, S. L., Etcoff, N. L., McInerney, S. C., Lee, M. B., and Jenike, M. A. (1998b). Masked presentations of emotional facial expressions modulate amygdala activity without explicit knowledge. *J. Neurosci.*, **18**, 411–418.

White, M. (1995). Preattentive analysis of facial expressions of emotion. *Cogn. Emot.*, **9**, 439–460.

Wik, G., Fredrikson, M., Ericson, K., Eriksson, L., Stone-Elander, S., Greitz, T. (1993). A functional cerebral response to frightening visual stimulation. *Psychiatry Res.*, **50**, 15–24.

Woermann, F. G., Steiner, H., Barker, G. J., Bartlett, P. A., Elger, C. E., Duncan, J. S. *et al.* (2001). A fast FLAIR dual-echo technique for hippocampal T2 relaxometry: first experiences in patients with temporal lobe epilepsy. *J. Magn. Reson. Imaging*, **13**, 547–552.

Wojciulik, E., Kanwisher, N., and Driver, J. (1998). Covert visual attention modulates face-specific activity in the human fusiform gyrus: fMRI study. *J. Neurophysiol.*, **79**, 1574–1578.

CHAPTER

22

Brain Systems Mediating Reward

INTRODUCTION

Reward is one of the most powerful influences driving animal behaviour; the vast majority of behaviours are driven by a need to access rewards and avoid punishments. The basic physiological rewards of food, drink, and the drive to propagate the species (encompassing sexual and parental behaviour) are fundamental primary reinforcers. Drugs, which exert direct or indirect neurochemical effects on reward systems, also serve as primary rewards in both animals and humans. In humans, particularly, motivating rewards may also take a variety of more abstract forms. For example, we are strongly motivated by social reinforcers: the desire to please others or achieve social status and success. These considerations make it clear that understanding reward processes is central to any neurobiological account of human behaviour.

Reward processes are probably one of the most fully characterised aspects of animal behaviour. In humans, by contrast, reward processes are less well understood. One reason is that the basic experience of reward is not a process that can be easily quantified in an objective manner. This contrasts with processes such as memory and attention, where objective paradigms to measure function have been developed and used in psychological and neuropsychological contexts. Furthermore, many seminal animal studies of reinforcement have depended on electrophysiological measurement of neuronal firing in response to rewards. It is only with the advent of neuroimaging techniques, providing an analogous tool for direct measurement of brain activity, that the study of human reward processes has become feasible.

This chapter begins with a brief review of an extensive animal literature on which many functional neuroimaging paradigms in humans have been based. Although there have been relatively few human neuropsychological studies of reward processing, a number of important recent studies are reviewed. The prime focus of the chapter, however, is neuroimaging evidence that has begun to dissociate different roles for component structures within human reward systems. Both positron emission tomography (PET) and functional magnetic resonance imaging (fMRI) have been used to characterise responses to primary reinforcers, particularly drugs of abuse, as well as responses to secondary cues that are associated with primary rewards. These findings, and their implications for normal and abnormal human reward systems, are discussed. Practical and methodological considerations, however, have meant that many studies have assessed human reward processing by exploiting the importance of social reinforcers. A particular potent social reinforcer in Western society is money. Financial reinforcement is a strong behavioural motivator, as well as being a stimulus that lends itself to systematic experimental control. Models of reward processing that depend on winning and losing money have therefore become crucial tools for imaging reward processes, and a number of such studies are considered. Their results have important implications for our understanding of differential functional roles within reward systems.

ANIMAL MODELS

Introduction

Aspects of reward processing have been much more widely studied in experimental animals than in humans. Thus, much of the theoretical framework underpinning recent functional neuroimaging advances is derived directly from an extensive animal literature. It is therefore appropriate to begin this chapter with a brief summary of pertinent findings, although a comprehensive review of animal reward processing is beyond the scope of this volume.

Rewards that serve as primary reinforcers, such as food or water, elicit autonomic (unconditioned) responses in animals. If these primary reinforcers are paired with originally neutral stimuli, such as lights or tones, animals will learn stimulus-reinforcement associations and the predictive stimuli will elicit conditioned responses. Animals can also learn to associate particular actions with primary reinforcers, exhibiting instrumental learning or operant conditioning. When conditioned stimuli or instrumental responses cease to be paired with reinforcing stimuli, animals will rapidly cease to respond to them, displaying extinction. These concepts are at the heart of classic and contemporary animal leaning theory (Rescorla and Wagner, 1972; Dickinson, 1980; Mackintosh, 1983; Balleine and Dickinson, 1998).

These reward-related behaviours suggest that the mammalian brain must be capable of a number of distinct types of reward processing. Clearly, there must be neuronal responses to primary reinforcers that mediate the experience of rewards. There must also be neurons capable of coding predictive relations among stimuli, responses, and rewards, as well as coding the motivational significance or value of rewards and anticipation of reward.

Neuronal Basis of Reward Processing in Animals

The seminal studies of Olds and Milner (1954) used the intercranial self-stimulation (ICSS) paradigm to demonstrate regions of the rat brain mediating reward functions. Critical reward sites included the midbrain dopaminergic system projecting from the ventral tegmental area (VTA) to the nucleus accumbens (NAcc) and regions of the prefrontal cortex. This system has therefore been characterised as a neurochemical substrate of reward (Wise and Rompre, 1989), playing a key role in responses to natural reinforcers as well as the reinforcing effects of drugs of abuse (Koob and Le Moal, 1997; Wise, 1998).

The Dopamine Hypothesis of Reward

The dopamine hypothesis of reward remains influential, although it has undergone refinement in recent years (Spanagel and Weiss, 1999). These refinements suggest that the specific role of mesolimbic dopamine neurons may be in the acquisition of reward-related behaviours, rather than subjective responses to rewards *per se*. Thus, the precise role of dopamine in reward remains controversial. It should be noted that reward is not a unitary function, and its components can be dissociated and characterised in a number of ways. Berridge and Robinson (1998) extensively review the literature and conclude that the role of dopamine is not in mediating the hedonic pleasure of rewards ("liking" rewards) or in mediating the predictive associations in reward learning (learning new likes and dislikes); rather, they propose that the key role of dopamine is in mediating incentive salience ("wanting" rewards).

A different, and influential, theory of the role of dopamine in reward is that of Schultz (Schultz, 1998; Schultz *et al.*, 2000). Based on substantial empirical evidence, this theory emphasises the role of dopamine in reward prediction, where the firing of dopamine neurons to rewards is modulated by the predictability of those rewards. Thus, during associative learning, the response of dopamine neurons transfers from the primary reward to conditioned stimuli predictive of reward occurrence (Schultz *et al.*, 1993). Dopaminergic responses to actual rewards are more pronounced when they are unpredictable (Mirenowicz and Schultz, 1994; Schultz *et al.*, 1997). This dopaminergic coding of reward predictability is interpreted in terms of an error signal, which is critical in learning associations between conditioned stimuli and rewards.

Neuroanatomy of Reward

The neuroanatomical literature on reward processing in animals has also become increasingly refined. The ventral striatum, particularly the NAcc, remains the structure most reliably linked to reward-related processes (Wise, 1980; Robbins and Everitt, 1992; 1996; Schultz *et al.*, 1993; Stern and Passingham, 1996). Midbrain regions of VTA and substantia nigra (Ljungberg *et al.*, 1992; Schultz, 1997) are also crucially involved, as are the amygdala (Cador *et al.*, 1989; Everitt and Robbins, 1992) regions of the basal forebrain (Arvanitogiannis *et al.*, 1996) and orbitofrontal cortex (OFC) (for a review, see Rolls, 1999, 2000). Recent advances have allowed differential roles of these regions, and indeed within these regions, to be identified (Fig. 22.1).

Striatal neurons fire in response to actual reinforcers but also show sustained activity during the anticipation of rewards (Schultz *et al.*, 1992; Hollerman and Schultz, 1998), suggesting that these neurons have access to stored representations of reward. A striatal response during the preparation, initiation, and execution of movements is also dependent on rewards (Schultz *et al.*, 2000). Kalives and Nakamura (1999) propose that the NAcc acts as in integration site for reward processing. Projections from the NAcc to the VTA produce a prediction error signal that codes novelty mismatch between predictors and rewards, in line with the theory of Schultz, discussed above. Projections from the NAcc to the amygdala mediate the response to conditioned rewards, while projections to prefrontal regions mediate the integration of reward with experience and the shaping of behavioural responses. A key role for the amygdala in reward conditioning has been emphasised in a number of recent studies (Hatfield *et al.*, 1996; Killcross *et al.*, 1997; Schoenbaum *et al.*, 1998; Holland and Gallagher, 1999). Specifically, these studies implicate the basolateral nucleus of the amygdala in associative learning, in contrast to the central nucleus, which is proposed to fulfil an orienting function.

The OFC has been suggested to play an important evaluative role in reward processing. Although caudal regions of the OFC code physical attributes of rewarding stimuli (*e.g.*, taste and

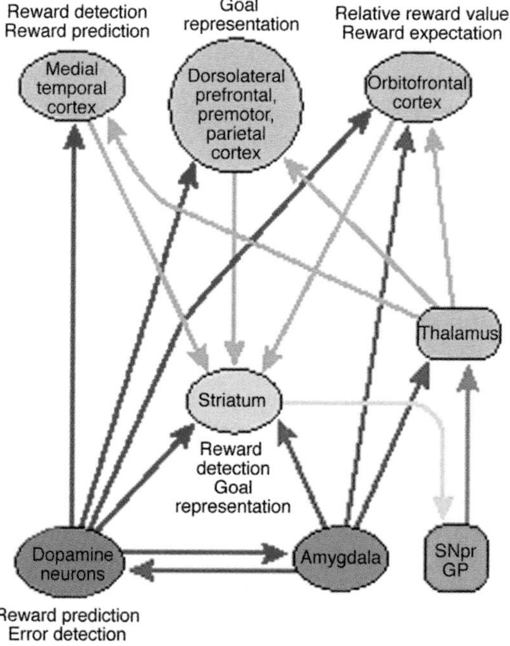

FIGURE 22.1
Reward processing and the brain. Many reward signals are processed by the brain, including those that are responsible for the detection of past rewards, the prediction and expectation of future rewards, and the use of information about future rewards to control goal-directed behaviour. SNpr, substantia nigra pars reticulata; GP, globus pallidus. (From Schultz, W. *et al.*, *Cereb. Cortex*, 10, 272–283, 2000. With permission.)

smell; see Rolls, 1999, 2000), more rostral regions also play a role in mediating reward preference (Tremblay and Schultz, 1999). Certain OFC responses to gustatory rewards subside as an animal reaches satiation, leading to the suggestion that OFC neurons code the relative, rather than the absolute, value of rewards (Watanabe, 1999). This can be interpreted as a role for the OFC in representing the motivational or incentive value of rewarding stimuli (Schoenbaum *et al.*, 1998; Gallagher *et al.*, 1999; Baxter *et al.*, 2000). Further, lesions to the orbitofrontal cortex in monkeys result in perseverative responding in monkeys performing simple reversal tasks (Iversen and Mishkin, 1970; Dias *et al.*, 1996), deficits that can be interpreted as a failure to respond to changes in reinforcement contingencies. These much more flexible responses to predictive or rewarding stimuli, dependent on their current value to the animal, are an important component of higher order reward processing essential for adaptive behaviour in both animals and humans.

NEUROPSYCHOLOGY/BEHAVIOURAL STUDIES IN HUMANS

Introduction

Deficits in reward-related processing are not commonly reported as a consequence of neurological damage or disorder. This may relate to the fact that patients with selective damage to subcortical regions involved in reward processing are rare. Lesions to prefrontal components of reward circuitry have been more commonly reported. Damasio (1994) provides a detailed account of a patient with extensive damage to the orbitofrontal cortex who shows pronounced difficulties with real-life decision making, in spite of intact intellectual function. Social decision making critically depends on assessing the value, in incentive terms, of possible outcomes of behaviour, and these deficits can therefore be thought of as a failure of high-level reward processing. Rolls *et al.* (1994) also report profound deficits in social behaviour resulting from orbitofrontal damage. Patients with neurological and psychiatric diseases may also have deficits in reward-related processing. Thus, Fibiger (1984) and Cummings (1993) argue that the high incidence of anhedonia and depression in patients with Parkinson's disease may be mediated by dysfunction in dopaminergic reward systems. Aspects of primary depression can also be characterised in terms of reinforcement deficits (Lewinsohn, 1974, 1979; Murphy *et al.*, 1998). Another class of psychiatric disorder that can be theoretically related to reward processing deficits is substance abuse (Grant *et al.*, 1999; Jentsch and Taylor, 1999), as many abused substances directly or indirectly stimulate dopaminergic reward systems.

While the phenomenology of certain symptoms seen in patient groups can be related to deficits in reward processing, the neuropsychology of reward-related functions has been under-explored compared to other cognitive domains. A number of important avenues of empirical study have advanced our understanding in recent years and provide the basis for experimental hypotheses underpinning functional neuroimaging research.

Reward Conditioning and Amygdala Lesions

A paradigm that has been adapted directly from the animal literature to examine human reward systems is conditioned preference. Normal volunteers have been shown to develop a conditioned preference for initially neutral stimuli predictive of rewards (Niedenthal, 1990; Baeyens *et al.*, 1993; Todrank *et al.*, 1995; Johnsrude *et al.*, 1999). Until recently there has been little investigation of the neural substrates underlying these behavioural effects. Johnsrude *et al.* (2000) used a preference conditioning paradigm to assess performance in a group of patients with unilateral anterior temporal lobe resections. These patients had amygdala lesions as well as variable degrees of hippocampal and parahippocampal damage. Patients with unilateral frontal lobe lesions were also assessed, using a paradigm adapted from classic tasks in the animal literature. Subjects were presented with abstract patterns in the context of an irrelevant working memory task, and these patterns were paired with food reward on a variable percentage of trials. Subjects were then given a forced choice preference test.

In the preference judgment phase of the experiment, normal subjects displayed a marked preference for the pattern paired most frequently with reward. Interestingly, the working memory context had largely masked any explicit learning of contingencies; subjects attributed their preferences to physical properties of the stimuli rather than the conditioning effects of reward. Patients with unilateral frontal damage showed an impairment on the working memory task used to mask the conditioning procedure but established normal conditioned preferences for rewarded patterns. Conversely, the patients with amygdala and medial temporal lesions performed normally on the working memory task but showed severe impairments of preference conditioning. This clear double dissociation between working memory and the acquisition of stimulus–reward associations is consistent with the animal evidence implicating the amygdala and related structures in reward conditioning. Although both neuropsychological and neuroimaging studies have examined fear conditioning in humans (Bechara *et al.* 1995; LaBar *et al.*, 1995, 1998; Buechel *et al.*, 1998; Morris *et al.*, 1998), this is among the first neuropsychological studies to assess the neural basis of reward conditioning.

Gambling Models of Decision Making

Introduction

The basic concepts of gambling models in neuropsychology are that subjects must apply a degree of probabilistic reasoning to a situation where the goal of their performance is to maximise receipt of financial rewards. An influential series of neuropsychological studies by Damasio and colleagues have used such a gambling task, with symbolic (play money) financial rewards and penalties. The basic experimental layout is as follows. Subjects must choose, on a series of trials, between high- and low-risk decks of cards, although at the outset of the task they do not know which decks are which. The high-risk decks offer a prospect of immediate large rewards but carry a cost of even larger long-term penalties. The low-risk decks offer smaller immediate rewards but even smaller long-term penalties. Thus, over a series of trials, subjects can maximise their overall rewards by choosing cards from the low-risk rather than the high-risk decks. This task was designed as a model for real-life decision-making situations where subjects must assess the risks associated with certain courses of action against the potential benefits of those actions. The processing of the relative values of possible rewarding and punishing outcomes is an important component of reaching these decisions. Control subjects performing this task gradually learn the contingencies and then choose the low-risk decks on the majority of trials. Interestingly, they still occasionally opt for the high-risk decks, gambling on a favourable outcome. This suggests that the process of taking a risk has its own intrinsic reward value.

Deficits in Patients with Orbitofrontal Lesions

Patients with lesions of the orbitofrontal cortex show pronounced impairments in real-life decision making, in the context of otherwise preserved intellectual abilities (Damasio, 1994). Using the gambling model, Bechara *et al.* (1994) demonstrated significant impairments in patients with orbitofrontal lesions. The patients continued to opt for high-risk decks, suggesting they were guided by the prospect of immediate short-term gains at the expense of detrimental long-term consequences. Strikingly, the ability of the patients to understand and accurately describe the contingencies governing the task was uncompromised. Despite this, they failed to actually use their knowledge to guide behaviour, an apparent dissociation between understanding the contingencies and ability to make appropriate behavioural responses that has also been reported by Rolls (1996). The authors tested their hypothesis that ventromedial patients exhibit a "myopia for the future" using a variant of the paradigm where the punishment was immediate but the reward was delayed (Bechara *et al.*, 2000). Thus, the advantageous decks had high immediate punishments but even higher long-term rewards, while the disadvantageous decks had low immediate punishments but even lower long-term rewards. The orbitofrontal patients were as impaired on this variant of the task as the original task, opting for the decks with lower immediate punishment, even though these were not the advantageous decks in the longer term. Thus, the original deficit in these patients cannot be explained by either hypersensitivity to reward or hyposensitivity to punishment (either of which would predict a reduced impairment on the new variant of the task) but reflects a genuine insensitivity to future consequences. Further, neither decreasing the delayed punishment in the original task, nor increasing the delayed reward in the variant shifted the behaviour of the patients toward a more advantageous strategy.

Insensitivity to future consequences, rather than hypersensitivity to reward, following OFC damage is also in accord with animal literature implicating this region in higher level representational aspects of reward processing.

In addition to these behavioural abnormalities, Bechara *et al.* (1996, 2000) also reported abnormalities in anticipatory skin conductance responses (SCRs) in patients with orbitofrontal lesions performing the gambling paradigms. Control subjects show elevated SCRs not only in response to receiving rewards and punishments but also *prior* to making high-risk choices. The former response was intact in the patients, but the latter, anticipatory response was abolished. Again, this argues against either hypersensitivity to reward or hyposensitivity to punishment because the SCR responses to the actual reinforcers were normal. Patients with bilateral damage to the amygdala were also found to be impaired on the gambling task (Bechara *et al.*, 1999) and failed to show anticipatory SCRs to risky choices; however, unlike patients with ventromedial frontal damage, the amygdala patients also failed to show the normal elevation of SCRs in response to the actual receipt of rewards and punishments (Fig. 22.2).

The authors interpreted this finding in terms of different roles for the amygdala and OFC in reward-guided decision making. The amygdala is hypothesised to play a key role in ascribing affective attributes to stimuli, consistent with evidence that amygdala damage impairs the acquisition of aversive conditioning in humans (Bechara *et al.* 1995; La Bar *et al.*, 1995, 1998; Morris *et al.*, 1998). By contrast, signals arising from orbitofrontal cortex are hypothesised to be involved in generating autonomic reactions associated with the anticipation of reward and punishment but may be less important in their actual experience.

A study by Rogers *et al.* (1999b) also reported deficits on a gambling task in patients with orbitofrontal lesions. In this task, subjects had to make probabilistic judgments to accumulate reward points. Subjects were presented with ten boxes, some red and some blue, and were told that a token was hidden in one of them. One part of the task was to guess whether the token is hidden in a red or a blue box. Subjects also had to stake a proportion of their accumulated points on the outcome of each trial, providing an assessment of both their confidence in the judgment they were making and their willingness to take risks. The proportions of red and blue boxes changed across trials, and normal confidence in judgment changed accordingly. For example, in a situation with nine red boxes and one blue box, subjects could be more confident than in a situation with six red boxes and four blue boxes. Patients with ventromedial prefrontal lesions were differentially impaired relative to controls and to patients with dorsolateral lesions on all aspects of this task.

Studies by Rolls and colleagues (1994) have also reported a spectrum of social behavioural abnormalities in patients with orbitofrontal damage. The specific form of associated neuropsychological deficit reported by this group was in stimulus-reinforcement learning, an impairment that correlated with behavioural abnormalities in patients. In particular, these patients were impaired on reversal learning and extinction, a finding directly analogous to deficits reported following OFC lesions in animals (Iversen and Mishkin, 1970; Dias *et al.*, 1996). Specifically, when these patients learned a set of stimulus–reinforcement contingencies, they were inflexible in adapting their behaviour to a change in contingencies. Like patients studied by Damasio and colleagues, these patients also demonstrated an inability to use reward and contingency information to guide behaviour. Both research groups have interpreted their findings in terms of an insensitivity to reinforcement cues resulting from OFC damage. This suggests a crucial role for this region in the modulation of action and behaviour by potential rewards.

Deficits Associated with Parkinson's Disease and Depression

Deficits in reversal learning in a probabilistic reasoning task have been reported in patients with Parkinson's disease (Swainson *et al.*, 2000), specifically in patients with moderate to severe disorder and therefore taking higher levels of L-DOPA medication. The authors relate these deficits to impaired dopamine function in this patient group. Further evidence that dopamine-mediated reward systems are abnormal in Parkinson's disease comes from a study by Charbonneau *et al.* (1996), showing that medicated patients are more impaired on an incentive learning task than an associative learning task without incentives. However, patients with Parkinson's disease have not been found to be impaired on the Bechara/Damasio gambling task, in contrast to a group of patients with Huntington's disease who did show risky decision making (Stout *et al.*, 2001).

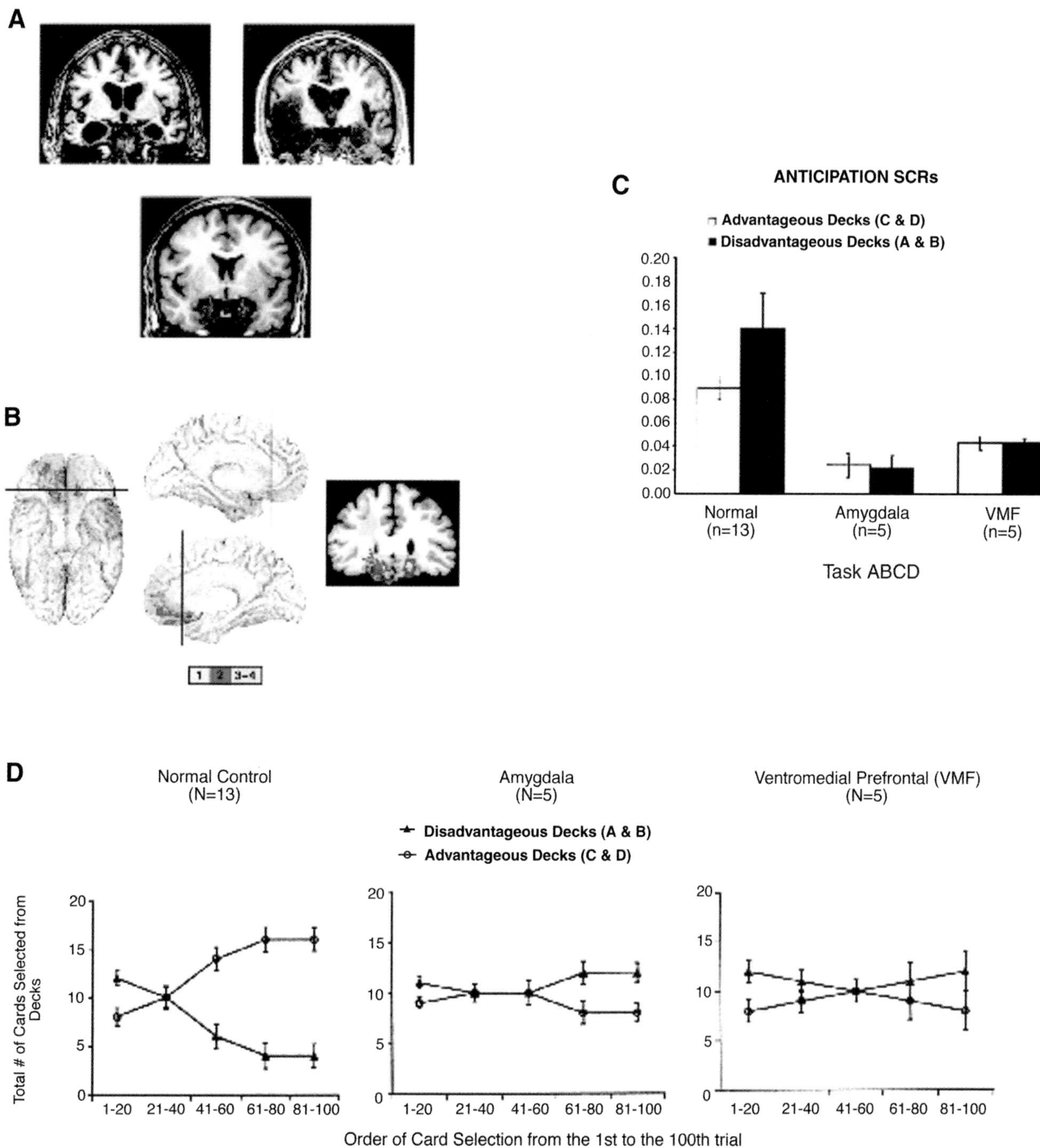

FIGURE 22.2

Effects of amygdala and orbitofrontal lesions on gambling. (A) Bilateral amygdala lesions; coronal sections through the amygdala from three patients showing complete bilateral destruction of the amygdala. (B) Bilateral ventromedial frontal lesions; shown are mesial and inferior views of the overlap of lesions from four VMF patients. (C) Means ± SEM of anticipatory SCRs (μS/s) generated by controls, amygdala, or VMF patients in association with the advantageous decks (C and D, white columns) versus the disadvantageous decks (A and B, black columns). (D) Means ± SEM of the total number of cards selected from the advantageous versus the disadvantageous decks in each block of 20 cards, which were made by normal controls and by patients with bilateral amygdala or VMF cortex lesions. (From Bechara, A. *et al.*, *J. Neurosci.*, 19, 5473–5581, 1999. With permission.)

Patients with primary depression have not, to our knowledge, been assessed on the Bechara/Damasio task, but evidence suggests that this group has deficits in gambling-type situations. Pacini *et al.* (1998) studied the performance of a subclinically depressed group on a ratio bias paradigm. This paradigm is based on the phenomenon that normal subjects will judge the probability of an event occurring as higher if it is presented as a ratio of two large numbers rather than two small numbers. Thus, 10-in-100 odds are reliably judged better than 1-in-10 odds. More strikingly, 8- or 9-in-100 odds will also be judged better than 1-in-10, although this is objectively not the case (Denes-Raj *et al.*, 1994). Pacini *et al.* (1998) used a version of this paradigm, where subjects were asked to choose between two displays of counters: one with 100 counters, of which 7, 9, or 10 were red, and one with only 10 counters, 1 of which was red. This was done under two incentive conditions—$0.10 and $2, which represented the amount won if a red counter was subsequently drawn by the experimenter. In the low-incentive condition, depressed patients performed *better* than controls (the so-called "depressive realism" effect); however, in the high-incentive condition, control performance improved significantly while depressed performance did not. This suggests that depressed patients fail to modulate performance in response to incentives, an effect also reported in a different context by Elliott *et al.* (1997a). Here, depressed patients failed to use feedback information (a form of reinforcement) to modify performance on a complex planning task. An influential behavioural theory of depression proposed by Lewinsohn (1974, 1979) suggests that depressed patients may show either, or both, a reduced capacity to experience reward or a reduction in reward-seeking behaviour. The latter possibility would be consistent with a deficit in responding to behavioural incentives in these laboratory situations.

Deficits in Drug Abusers

Several studies have used delay discounting procedures to study reward-related deficits in drug abusers. The premise of these tasks is that subjects must choose between an immediate small reward and a delayed but larger reward. Varying the delay shows that the subjective value of the rewards decreases as a function of increasing delay (Green *et al.*, 1994). Substance abusers have been shown to discount the value of delayed rewards more rapidly than controls; that is, the length of delay that they tolerate in order to obtain the larger reward is shorter. This effect has been shown in heroin addicts (Madden *et al.*, 1997) and problem drinkers (Vuchinich and Simpson, 1998). A similar pattern of deficit was reported in a mixed group of substance abusers (Petry and Casarella, 1999), a study that also reported a significant interaction with gambling behaviour. Substance-abusing subjects with co-morbid gambling problems thus showed even more rapid discounting of delayed rewards than non-gambling substance abusers.

Experimental gambling tasks have also been used in neuropsychological studies of drug abusers. Performance of the Bechara gambling task has been shown to be impaired in people dependent on cocaine (Grant *et al.*, 1997), opiates (Petry *et al.*, 1998), and alcohol (Mazas *et al.*, 2000). Rogers *et al.* (1999b) also reported deficits on their task in chronic amphetamine and opiate abusers. The decisions involved in these tasks are crucially dependent on judgments about the potential reward values of possible outcomes; therefore, these findings suggest that an impairment in reward-related processing may be a correlate of long-term drug use. Like orbitofrontal patients, substance abusers also show impairments in real-life decision making; indeed, the tendency to choose an immediate reward (of a drug) in spite of detrimental long-term consequences can be thought of as the defining behaviour of substance abusers. Bechara *et al.* (2000) have suggested that the apparent similarities in behaviour, both real-life and neuropsychological, of orbitofrontal patients and substance abusers may in fact be mediated by different underlying deficits. A number of authors have argued that the aberrant drug-seeking behaviour in drug abusers may reflect a hypersensitivity to reward (Grant *et al.* 1999; Jentsch and Taylor, 1999) rather than an insensitivity to future consequences. This is a hypothesis that is testable neuropsychologically (for example, by using variants of the gambling task). Further, functional imaging provides the potential to assess this hypothesis at a neuronal level.

NEUROIMAGING OF RESPONSES TO PRIMARY REINFORCERS

Introduction: Problems and Issues

In much of the animal electrophysiological literature studying reward processing, the rewards used are either appetising food or drink or drugs of abuse. Neuroimaging methods offer us, in some respects, a human analogue of animal electrophysiology; therefore, using these techniques to examine responses to primary reinforcers is a fertile ground for comparative studies. Studies of ingestive behaviour in humans are problematic, however, because the motor components of eating and drinking result in significant correlated head movements that render the data extremely difficult to interpret.

Drug studies also pose a number of problems. It is obviously only ethical in humans to study drugs of abuse in already-addicted subjects. While neuroimaging studies of substance abusers have been informative (see below), there is always a caveat that we are potentially studying the response of brains rendered abnormal through prolonged exposure to psychoactive substances. At a technical level, there is also a problem in dissociating physiological effects of the drug on the vasculature from subjective effects on reward pathways. This is particularly an issue in fMRI. However, in spite of these practical concerns, a number of neuroimaging studies of the effects of primary reinforcers have been performed.

Taste/Smell Studies

Rather than studying subjects actually consuming food rewards, an alternative approach has been to use tastes and smells associated with food reinforcement to elicit reward-related responses. It could be argued that taste and smell have no primary reward value and are therefore conditioned rather than unconditioned reinforcers; however, the linkage is undeniably very strong, and taste, at least, has been conceptualised by some as a primary rather than conditioned reinforcer; a pleasant taste is rewarding independent of the physiological value of the food to which it relates. An fMRI study of taste stimuli (Rolls *et al.*, 1997) demonstrated neuronal responses in the insula (primary taste cortex) and medial OFC in response to the taste of glucose. The orbitofrontal region also responded to the smell of vanilla. As discussed above, there are both taste and olfactory receptors in posterior OFC regions; however, evidence that OFC also mediates the reinforcing aspect of these sensory stimuli comes from an fMRI study of satiety by O'Doherty *et al.* (2000). The reward value of a food decreases when it is eaten to satiety, and this decrease is greater than that for other foods, an effect known as *sensory-specific satiety*. O'Doherty *et al.* scanned subjects before and after eating a large meal and found that the OFC response to the odour of a food eaten to satiety decreased, whereas there was no similar decrease in response to the odour of a food not eaten in the meal. These results implicate the OFC cortex in sensory-specific satiety and suggest that reinforcing, rather than sensory or discriminative, properties of stimuli are represented in this region.

Small *et al.* (2001) studied a similar phenomenon in subjects eating chocolate to beyond satiety during PET scanning. They found differential patterns of activation associated with chocolate when it was rated as pleasant and when it was related as unpleasant (due to feelings of satiety). Of particular note was a dissociation of OFC function, with medial regions showing more activation to chocolate rated as pleasant and lateral regions showing activation to chocolate rated as unpleasant. The authors interpreted this as evidence for functional segregation of the neural representation of reward and punishment within the OFC.

Food reinforcement has also been used in a human analogue of Schultz's seminal electrophysiological studies of anticipation and expectancy of food reward. O'Doherty *et al.* (2002) have used fMRI to look at neural responses associated with anticipation of a pleasant taste. They reported responses in midbrain, amygdala, striatum, and orbitofrontal cortex during expectation of a fully predictable pleasant taste reward. The midbrain, striatal, and amygdala response were *not* seen when the reward itself was experienced, as Schultz's animal findings would predict. Only a right lateral OFC focus (Fig. 22.3) responded to experience as well as expectation of reward.

Studies with Drugs of Abuse

Cocaine Studies

Both PET and fMRI have been used to study the primary reward responses associated with cocaine reinforcement in drug addicts. In an fMRI study of the effects of acute cocaine infusions in cocaine abusers, Breiter *et al.* (1997) reported neuronal responses associated with different aspects of cocaine reinforcement. Subjects were scanned following both cocaine and a control infusion of saline, with 5 min of scanning pre-infusion and 13 min post-infusion. During

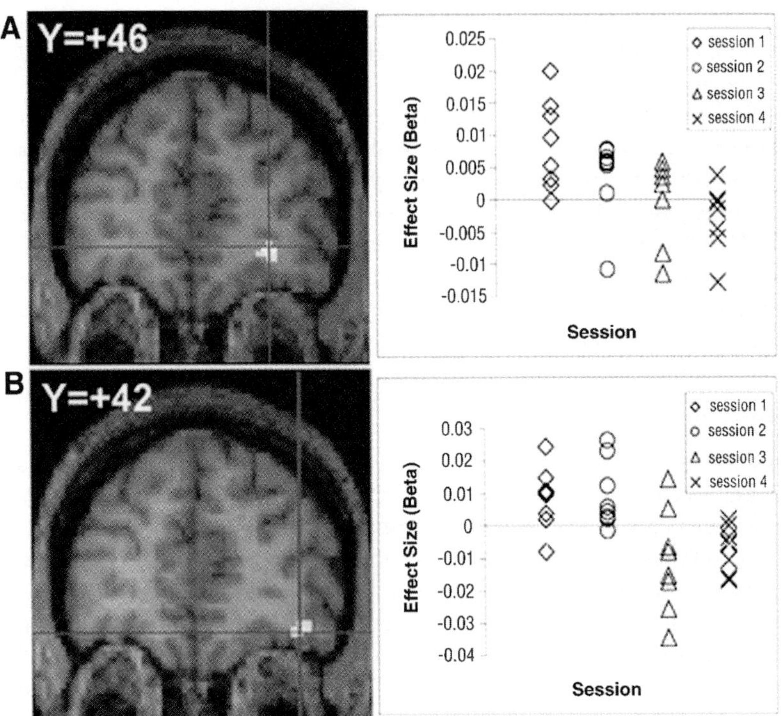

FIGURE 22.3
Orbitofrontal responses to anticipation and experience of pleasant taste. Activation in orbitofrontal cortex (on left of figure) attenuated by the fourth session during (A) anticipation of glucose reward, and (B) receipt of taste reward. The effect size (values) for individual subjects across four sessions are plotted (right). Note that these values show a decreasing trend in most subjects from session 1 to session 4. (From O'Doherty, J. *et al.*, *NeuroReport*, 11, 893–897, 2000. With permission.

scanning, they reported subjective response to the infusions on visual analogue scales. The four scales used were for "rush," "high," "low," and "craving," and subjects rated their feelings on each scale once every minute. Subjective ratings for high and rush peaked rapidly 1 to 3 min after infusion, while ratings for low and craving peaked later, 11 to 12 min after infusion.

Cocaine relative to saline produced focal neuronal responses in regions that included ventral tegmental area, nucleus accumbens, caudate, putamen, basal forebrain, insula, hippocampus, parahippocampal gyrus, cingulate, and lateral prefrontal cortex. A decrease in blood-oxygen-level-dependent (BOLD) signal was observed in temporal pole, amygdala, and medial prefrontal cortex. This pattern of neuronal responses was seen reliably on retest in a subset of subjects. BOLD signal in ventral tegmental area, basal forebrain, caudate, cingulate, and some lateral prefrontal regions correlated with subjective ratings of rush, peaking within 3 min of infusion. Signal change in nucleus accumbens, parahippocampal gyrus, and other lateral prefrontal regions correlated with craving, peaking toward the end of the 13-min post-infusion scanning period. The amygdala signal and subjective ratings of craving were negatively correlated (Fig. 22.4).

While this study clearly demonstrates responses in primary reward circuitry associated with acute effects of cocaine, a number of interpretational challenges are posed by the data. The authors' *a priori* hypothesis was that accumbens response would be associated with the acute euphoric effects of cocaine and therefore correlate with subjective ratings of "rush" and "high." Instead, the accumbens response correlated more closely with subjective craving, although it was also seen during the early rush period. This suggests a complex role for the nucleus accumbens in mediating not only consummatory aspects of reward, as indexed by "rush," but also incentive aspects, as indexed by "craving."

A follow-up study by the same group (Breiter *et al.*, 1998) used a cardiac gating procedure to determine whether artefacts associated with heart-rate changes may have affected the previous data. Cardiac gating also compensated for movement artefact in the brain stem, allowing the authors to assess cocaine-dependent changes in this region. Many of the key findings of the

a

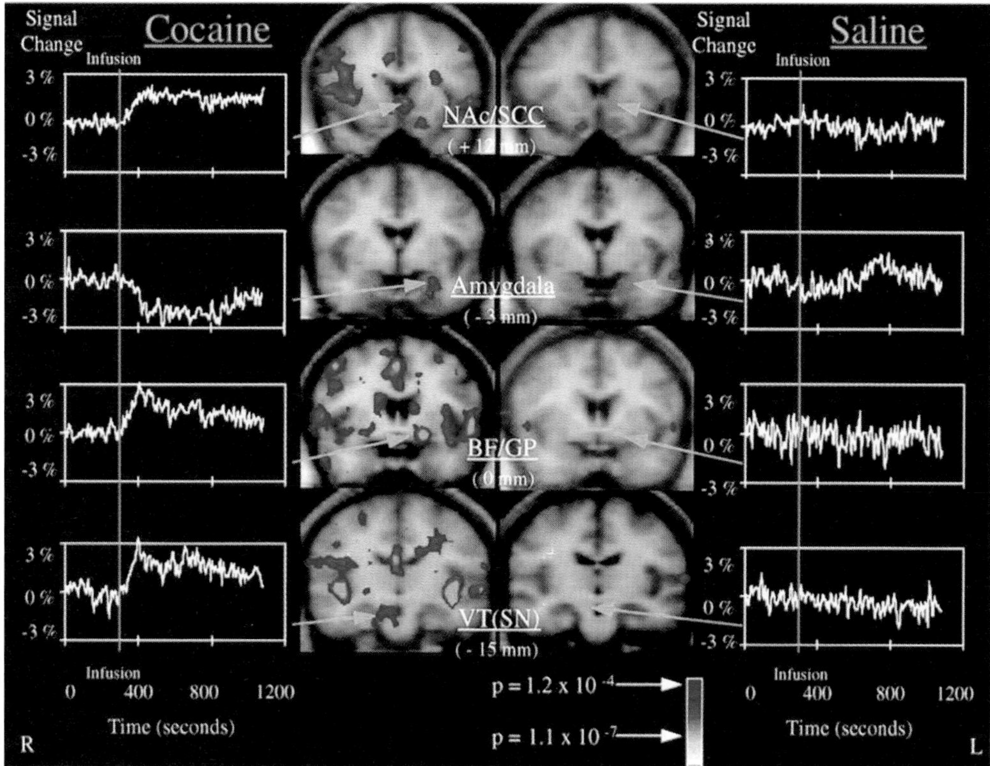

FIGURE 22.4
Regions responding to acute infusion of cocaine relative to saline. Images of subcortical brain regions showing significant fMRI signal changes after cocaine, but not after saline, infusions. On the left are Kolmogorov–Smirnov (KS) statistical maps at four coronal levels of pre- versus post-infusion time points for the average fMRI data from ten subjects who received cocaine. These KS statistical maps are overlaid on corresponding greyscale average structural maps. Activations with positive signal change include the NAc/SCC, BF/GP, and VT, while activations with negative signal change include the amygdala. The signal intensity versus time graph for the activations (for all voxels with $p < 10^{-6}$ within the named region) is placed next to each image. On the right are identical slice planes overlaid with the KS statistical map for the saline infusion; the saline signal intensity versus time graphs for the same anatomic regions active during cocaine are placed next to the saline images to demonstrate the absence of comparable change. (From Breiter, H. C. *et al.*, *Neuron*, 19, 591–611, 1997. With permission.)

earlier study were replicated, with the cardiac gating approach adding validity to the ventral tegmental signal as well as allowing identification of further brainstem changes in the dorsal raphe. This raphe signal suggests that serotonin as well as dopamine may be mediating the acute effects of cocaine. Interestingly, in this study the amygdala signal was positive rather than negative, which is more consistent with previous studies; however, the authors note pronounced individual heterogeneity, complicating the picture further. Across their two studies, five people had negative amygdala changes, four had no change, and eight had positive changes. It is also important to note that these were studies of cocaine abusers and it is entirely possible that the normal amygdala response to reinforcing stimuli may have been affected by cocaine abuse. A series of studies by Volkow and colleagues (1990, 1992, 1997, 1999) have characterised a number of long-term functional changes associated with cocaine abuse, including significant reductions of D2 dopamine receptors in frontostriatal circuits. These long-term changes, as a consequence of cocaine abuse, may account for some of the apparent anomalies in the studies of acute cocaine effects in abusers.

Alcohol Studies

Ingvar *et al.* (1998) investigated the effect of 0.07% alcohol (a moderate dose) on regional cerebral blood flow using three-dimensional butanol ^{15}O PET in non-alcoholic volunteers.

Alcohol increased regional cerebral blood flow in the brainstem, medial temporal lobes, and anterior cingulate cortex, but it had no effect on the neocortical activation patterns in response to cognitive challenge tasks. Thus, a moderate dose of alcohol selectively activated cerebral reward systems without influencing cortical cognitive systems.

The interactions between the effects of alcohol and cocaine have also been studied. Volkow *et al.* (2000) reported a blunting of regional brain glucose metabolism, measured with FDG PET, in response to intoxication with alcohol in a group of cocaine-abusing subjects. Specifically, attenuated response was observed in the cingulate, orbitofrontal, and medial prefrontal cortices and the amygdala, hippocampus, and parahippocampal gyrus. The authors interpreted their findings in terms of dopaminergic effects. These limbic and prefrontal regions receive dopamine projections that are sensitive to the normal effects of alcohol. In cocaine abusers, decreased sensitivity of dopamine cells (Volkow *et al.*, 1997) may result in the decreased metabolic response to alcohol.

Nicotine Studies

Stein *et al.* (1998) performed an fMRI study of the effects of intravenous nicotine in a group of active cigarette smokers. An initial injection of saline was followed by a series of nicotine injections at steadily increasing doses over 1-min periods. Dose-dependent increases of neuronal response were seen in the nucleus accumbens, amygdala, anterior cingulate, and other prefrontal regions. Thus, although the neuropharmacology of nicotine is clearly different from alcohol or cocaine, it stimulates overlapping regions of reward circuitry.

Drug-Related Cues

The studies discussed above provide evidence that drugs of abuse produce functional changes in human reward circuitry; however, the use of infusions or injections of actual drugs raises a number of practical and interpretational problems. In fMRI studies, particularly, the effects of drugs on global metabolism and the vasculature can potentially confound the interpretation of results. Although there have been ingenious attempts to overcome these problems, as discussed above, an alternative approach that obviates these criticisms is to look at neuronal responses to drug-related cues. These cues are effectively conditioned stimuli that drug users have learned to associate with the primary reinforcing effects of drugs.

A PET study by Sell *et al.* (1999) assessed activations in a group of heroin addicts following injection of either placebo or heroin, in response to video stimuli. Two types of video were used: a drug video showing drug-related situations and a neutral video with no references to drug-taking behaviour. Both heroin itself and heroin-related cues produced activations in midbrain regions, specifically the periaqueductal grey extending to the ventral tegmental area. This suggests that cue-elicited responses to drug-related stimuli can produce neuronal responses similar to those of the actual drug. The authors also used a psychophysiological interaction procedure (as discussed in Section 2 of this book) to show that activations of the anterior cingulate, amygdala, basal forebrain, and lateral prefrontal cortex, specific to salient visual cues, were seen when, and only when, brainstem activation was high. This is consistent with the theory that modulatory afferents from midbrain regions enhance responses to incentive stimuli in its projection regions.

The drug-related video also exerted a significant influence on subjective ratings of the urge to use heroin (Sell *et al.*, 2000). These "urge to use" measures were correlated with activations in the precuneus, implicated in retrieval from episodic memory, and insula cortex, implicated in affective processing. Actual injections of heroin produced significant increases in a subjective rating of "feeling high," and the experience of this high correlated with increased blood flow in hippocampal regions.

Cue-related activation of similar regions has been reported in studies of cocaine-abusing subjects, using both PET (Grant *et al.*, 1996; Childress *et al.*, 1999; Wang *et al.*, 1999, Kilts *et al.*, 2001) and fMRI (Maas *et al.*, 1998). Activations of lateral and medial prefrontal cortex, anterior cingulate, amygdala, insula, and OFC have all been reported that correlate with cue-induced craving. There are some subtle differences in the neural substrates of cue-induced craving for cocaine and craving induced by the drug itself. For example, Breiter *et al.* (1997) reported a negative association between amygdala response and cocaine reinforcement, while a *positive* correlation has been reported between amygdala activity and cue-elicited craving (Grant *et al.*, 1996; Childress *et al.*, 1999). This may, in part, reflect the pronounced individual variation in amygdala response, as discussed by Breiter *et al.* (1998). Further, activation of the nucleus accumbens, which correlates strongly with responses to the actual drug, has not been associated with cue-induced responses. These discrepancies suggest important differences between cue-elicited craving and cocaine-elicited craving. To some extent, these may reflect a difference between primary and secondary reinforcement, as the cues are secondary reinforcers that subjects have learned to associate with drug reward. As discussed above, the animal literature suggests that different components of reward circuitry respond differentially to primary and secondary reinforcers. For example, amygdala lesions have been shown to abolish conditioned responses while leaving responses to primary reinforcers intact. This may be consistent with a greater positive association between amygdala response and cue-elicited craving; however, these issues require further investigation.

FINANCIAL REWARD AND GAMBLING

Introduction

As discussed previously, gambling models have been used to look at decision making, risk taking, and reward in neuropsychological contexts. The emphasis of a number of these studies was on the decision-making aspect, although reward information critically informed the decisions made. In the neuroimaging context, gambling-type models have been adapted to allow us to focus on the responses to financial rewards. Money cannot be described as a primary reinforcer in any classic sense, as it has no intrinsic physiological value; however, it has enormous social value and is clearly a strong behavioural motivator in most modern societies. Gambling paradigms are readily adaptable for use as cognitive activation paradigms; they can be computerised, and various parameters (size of reward, probability of reward, etc.) can be systematically varied to study the functional correlates of different psychological components.

One of the first studies of financial reward was a PET study (Thut *et al.*, 1997) that compared financial reward with a simple "OK" reinforcer. Subjects performed a cognitive task (delayed Go/NoGo) under the two conditions. In half the blocks, subjects were rewarded with money; in the other half, they were simply told "OK". Financial reward was associated with elevated rCBF in midbrain, thalamus, dorsolateral prefontal cortex (DLPFC), and OFC. This study provides clear evidence that financial reward influences neuronal response on the basis of its reward value rather than just its informational properties. This section of the chapter examines the literature on neuroimaging of financially rewarded paradigms in some detail.

Ligand-Binding PET, Dopamine, and Reward

As discussed, the role of dopamine in reward has been well-established in animal studies. The imaging studies of drug effects are entirely consistent with dopaminergic projection systems mediating reward function in humans. A study by Koepp *et al.* (1998) provides clear evidence that dopamine transmission is also important in mediating response to financial reinforcement. This study used PET with the radioligand carbon 11 raclopride, which binds to striatal dopamine receptors. Reduced levels of raclopride binding result from an elevation of dopamine release in response to some psychological or pharmacological manipulation. In this study, subjects performed a financially rewarded video game during scanning, and the decreased raclopride binding in the striatum provided clear evidence of increased dopamine release in response to this task. The effect was most pronounced in the ventral portion of the striatum, incorporating nucleus accumbens (Fig. 22.5).

The magnitude of the effect was of the same order as the effect seen following intravenous amphetamine (Breier *et al.*, 1997) and is therefore indicative of significant increases in dopamine transmission. Although this study and technique provide a high degree of neurochemical specificity, the use of a single complex task means that the results cannot be unequivocally attributed to effects of the financial rewards. The motor demands of the task and stimulus novelty may also have contributed to the increased dopamine release, and it is noteworthy that both

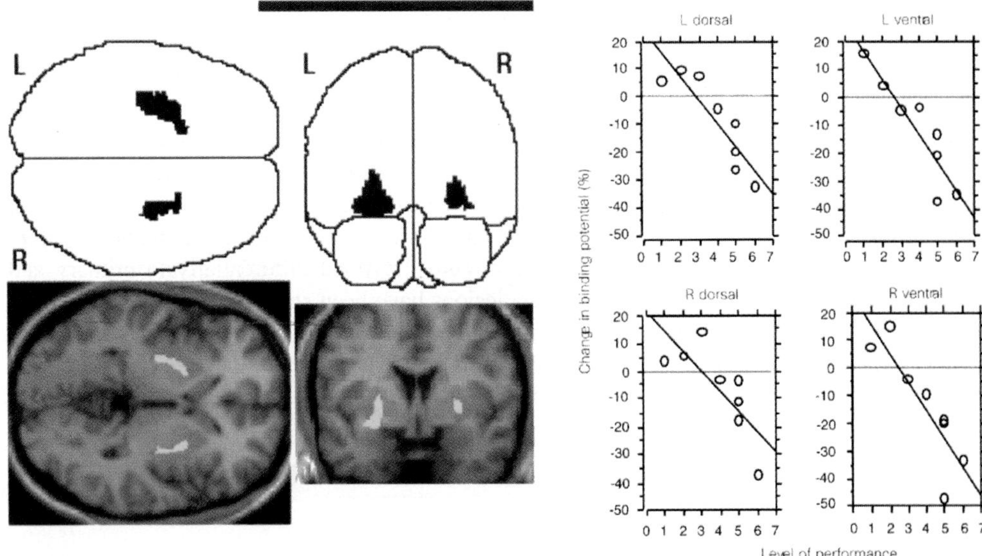

FIGURE 22.5
Carbon 11 raclopride in ventral striatum during rewarded videogame. Shown are regions of the brain in which there was a statistically significant correlation between reduced [^{11}C] raclopride binding potential and task performance; such a correlation was more pronounced in the ventral striatum To the left is shown percentage change in [^{11}C] raclopride binding potential between task and baseline conditions, plotted against performance level. A significant inverse correlation is seen in all striatal regions (Spearman rank correlation coefficients for left and right ventral and left dorsal striatum: $r = -0.86$, $p = 0.017$; for right dorsal striatum: $r = -0.83$, $p = 0.020$). (From Koepp, M. J. *et al.*, *Nature*, 393, 266–268, 1998. With permission.)

motor behaviour and stimulus novelty are associated with dopamine transmission. Also, while the presence of financial rewards in the task doubtless plays some role in the observed effect, it is not possible to dissociate the separable components of reward responses, such as anticipation of reward, incentive motivation by reward, and the actual experience of reward. Other PET and fMRI experiments have attempted to explore dissociable roles for these processes.

fMRI Studies of Experiencing Financial Rewards

Delgado *et al.* (2000) performed an event-related fMRI study to examine the neuronal responses to receiving financial rewards and punishments. In their paradigm, subjects were presented with a series of computerised cards on which they knew a number from 1 to 9 would appear. At a prompt, they had to guess whether the number would be greater or less than 5. Correct and incorrect guesses were financially rewarded and penalised, and on trials where the number 5 appeared a neutral stimulus indicated that the subject had neither won nor lost. Differential neuronal responses to reward and punishment were observed in the striatum. Response in the dorsal striatum, and specifically the caudate, was sustained after receipt of a reward but decreased sharply after punishment. A similar pattern of response was observed in the ventral striatum, and in both regions the intensity of response increased over time. These findings are entirely consistent with the animal literature reviewed above relating striatal function to the actual experience of rewards. The study also reported significant neuronal responses in the medial temporal lobe, although the authors were unable to localise this to a particular structure. The imaging sequence in this study was chosen to focus on basal ganglia regions and therefore did not address hypotheses about, for example, prefrontal regions.

In a similar study (Elliott *et al.*, 2000), we assessed responses to winning and losing money and also considered the dissociation of these reward-related responses with respect to psychological context. Subjects performed a series of trials in which they had to guess which of two "naturalistic" playing card stimuli presented on a computer screen was correct. They were instructed that on each trial the computer had randomly selected one stimulus as correct, and the task was simply guessing against the computer. For each correct guess, subjects won £1, and for each incorrect guess, they lost £1. Cumulative rewards were displayed throughout at the side of the screen; in some phases of the experiment subjects had overall winnings, and in other phases they had overall losses. Unknown to subjects, the sequence of wins and losses was predetermined, regardless of which playing card stimulus they actually chose. The haemodynamic response in this study was modelled using regressors based on the overall height of the reward bar and the interaction between the height of the bar and its rate of change of height. This enabled us to assess neuronal responses to increasing reward level and to high levels of reward occurring in the context of increasing reward (a "winning streak" in lay terms). We also examined regions that responded *both* to winning and losing streaks—the stages of the experiment where subjects felt the greatest excitement associated with the experience of gambling. Each successive choice in these latter situations was associated with a subjectively increased expectation that the subject's "luck was about to change," an expectation that was independent of the valence of current experience (*i.e.*, whether subjects were winning or losing).

Neuronal responses that correlated positively with the height of the reward bar were observed in a midbrain region close to the substantia nigra and a region of ventral striatum. This region was shown to correspond to the nucleus accumbens in a subset of subjects by co-registration with their individual structural scans; thus, higher levels of financial reward were associated with responses in the ascending dopamine projection systems mediating primary reward responses in experimental animals. By contrast, reward in the context of a winning streak was associated with enhanced responses in ventral pallidum, thalamus, and subgenual cingulate cortex (Fig. 22.6).

A negative relationship between reward level and neuronal response was observed in bilateral hippocampus, a response that was further enhanced in the context of a losing streak. Regions responsive to both winning and losing streaks included head of caudate, insula, and posterior lateral OFC cortex bilaterally. A number of possible roles for these regions would be consistent with this finding. It is possible that these regions mediate the autonomic experience of excitement associated with the gambling situation, which may in itself be reinforcing. The OFC may also be involved in mediating an expectation of an imminent change in stimulus–reward associations. As discussed above, lesions to OFC in both animals and humans result in impaired

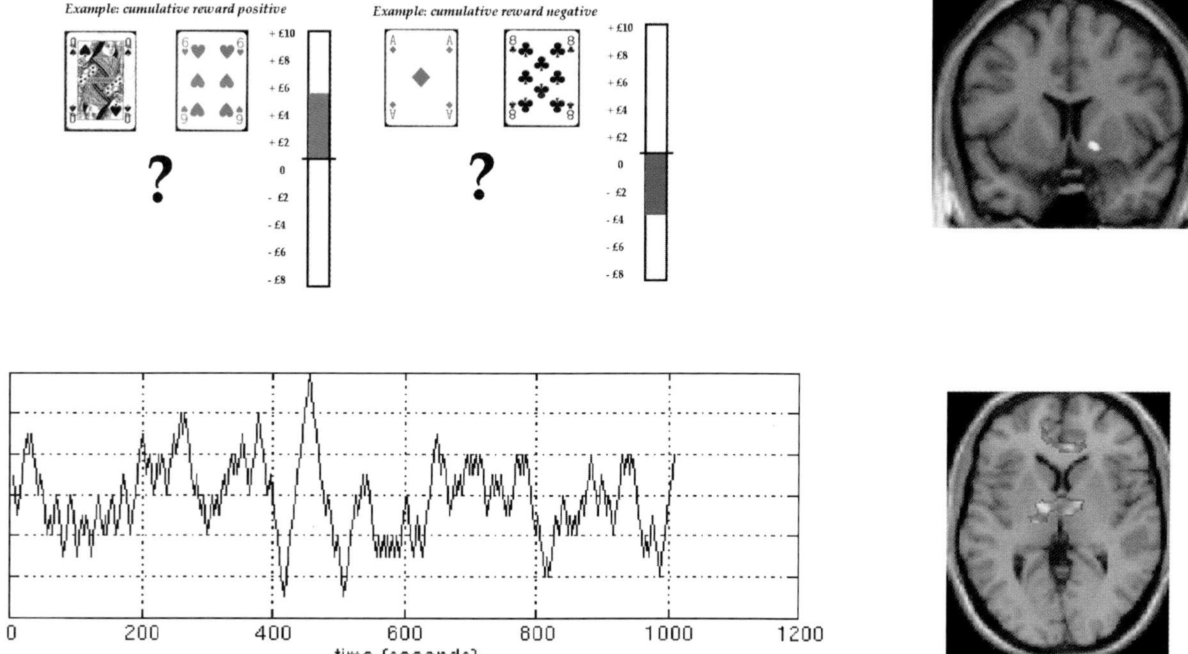

FIGURE 22.6
Event-related responses to changing reward levels. The simple gambling task is shown top right and the binomial random walk function determining the sequence of wins and losses is shown below. To the right are the neuronal responses in ventral striatum to reward level and in globus pallidus, thalamus, and subgenual cingulate to winning streaks. (From Elliott, R. *et al.*, *J. Neurosci.*, 20, 6159–6165, 2000. With permission.)

reversal learning, where the relationships between stimuli and rewards or punishments shift. It is likely that on a winning or losing streak, subjects may be anticipating such a shift.

A specific role for OFC (both medial and lateral regions) in the expectation of reward during performance of a gambling task was reported by Breiter *et al.* (2001). This study used a gambling task with two distinct phases: expectancy and outcome. Neural responses were observed in regions including the extended amygdala, ventral striatum, and hypothalamus, as well as the OFC, with a tendency toward right lateralisation (consistent with the right lateralised Nacc response described by Elliott *et al.*, 2000). The authors noted that most regions in their study responded in both the expectancy and the outcome stages, unlike the taste reward study of O'Doherty *et al.* (2002) discussed above; however, there is a crucial difference between these studies. In a gambling task, the outcome is never fully predictable, unlike O'Doherty's taste rewards. It is plausible that subcortical responses to rewarding outcomes are only abolished when those outcomes become fully predictable, in line with the electrophysiological findings of Schultz and colleagues.

fMRI Studies of Incentive

The incentive value of financial reward was studied using fMRI by Knutson *et al.* (2000), based on paradigms used in animal studies by Schultz and colleagues (see above). Using an event-related design, they presented subjects with a series of visual stimuli in a reaction time task. Different coloured stimulus were used to predict, after a variable delay interval, the brief presentation of a white target stimulus to which subjects were required to respond as quickly as possible. This simple task was first presented under a control condition where there were no financial consequences for a given response. Subjects then performed the task under reward and punishment conditions, presented in a counterbalanced order. In the reward condition, 20% of cues predicted that the response during subsequent presentation of the white target would be financially rewarded. In the punishment condition, 20% of cues predicted that a failure to respond during subsequent presentation of the white target would be financially penalised. The task was calibrated individually for each subject so that they succeeded on approximately 60% of trials.

The haemodynamic responses under these conditions were modelled using regressors based on "incentive" trials (those with cues predictive of reward and punishment) compared to "non-incentive" trials. These regressors actually conflated responses during the delay period and responses to both the targets and the subsequent feedback about winning or losing; however, the differential effect of incentives during the delay period was clearly a significant factor driving neuronal responses, and the authors interpreted their findings in terms of incentive-driven behaviour.

Neuronal responses to the reward incentive trials, relative to non-incentive trials, were observed in the caudate, putamen, mesial prefrontal cortex, and left motor cortex. Interestingly, the same regions responded on the punishment incentive trials, and punishment-specific responses were seen in the thalamus, anterior cingulate, and (at a lower significance threshold) the mid-brain and locus coeruleus. The authors interpret their findings as consistent with roles for striatal and medial frontal circuitry in mediating incentive driven behaviour. The study is also consistent with findings from the animal literature that the same regions that mediating responses to reward also mediate responses to escapable or avoidable stress (Ravard *et al.*, 1990; Salomone *et al.*, 1994). Although there is a chance of punishment in the negative incentive condition in this study, that punishment can be avoided by appropriate behaviour (responding quickly enough). This is an example of the interesting reciprocal relations between reward and punishment, where an expected reward that is not received may actually be experienced as a form of punishment. Conversely, an expected punishment that is not experienced may be experienced as a form of reward.

These findings suggest that the dorsal striatum may play a subtly different role from the ventral striatum in human reward processing. As discussed previously, ventral striatum critically mediates the actual response to a reward. Knutson *et al.* (2000) report dorsal striatum response in an incentive condition when subjects are preparing to execute the movement that will elicit the reward (or avoidance of punishment). This is consistent with the proposed role of the striatum in the initiation of reward-related movements (Schultz 2000) and suggests that it is specifically dorsal striatal regions that fulfil this function.

Further evidence that dorsal regions of the striatum play a particular role in reward-related action rather than simple response to reward comes from a recent fMRI study of the modulation of reward processing by the requirement to work for reward (Elliott *et al.*, unpublished observations). In this blocked fMRI design, subjects performed a simple target detection task. They were told that certain target stimuli (defined by colour) required responses with a button press, while other stimuli that did not. They were also told that targets may or may not be rewarded; thus, subjects performed under four conditions:

Targets requiring responses (rewards)
Targets requiring responses (no rewards)
Targets not requiring responses (rewards)
Targets not requiring responses (no rewards)

This is a factorial design, and the critical analysis is of the interaction between the movement and reward factors, examining not only the main effects of reward or movement but also, most crucially, the modulation of one by the other. The requirement to make a response caused a significant enhancement of neuronal response to reward in regions including the dorsal striatum. Again this suggests that this region mediates the generation of incentive driven action. Interestingly, the reverse side of the interaction—representing responses to reward that were enhanced in the *absence*, relative to the presence, of an eliciting movement—was associated with enhanced neuronal response in regions that included medial OFC (Fig. 22.7). This OFC response may reflect the putative role for this region in associative learning. With no intervening response, the association between predictive stimulus and reward is stronger and the response of this region is augmented. It should be noted that both striatal and OFC responses are seen in *both* reward conditions in this study but are selectively augmented under the different response conditions, again indicating dissociable roles for these regions in reward processing.

Functional Imaging Studies of Gambling

The studies described above do not involve an explicit role for contingency judgment, which is central to many experimental gambling tasks. Although the paradigm used by Elliott *et al.* (2000) uses gambling-type stimuli, the 50:50 contingencies mean that reward expectancy is objectively set at chance. An event-related fMRI approach that manipulated outcome contingency was taken in a study by O'Doherty *et al.* (2001). This study also differs from the studies described previously in that, like the Bechara/Damasio task, it used symbolic rather than actual monetary rewards. The paradigm was based on a standard reversal learning task, such that subjects had to choose between two stimuli on a series of trials. Responses to reward and punishment were compared during an acquisition and a reversal stage. In the acquisition stage, one of the stimuli was associated with large rewards on 70% of trials and small punishments on 30% of trials, while the other was associated with large punishments on 60% of trials and small rewards on 40% of trials. In the reversal stage, these contingencies were switched. The subjects' task was to

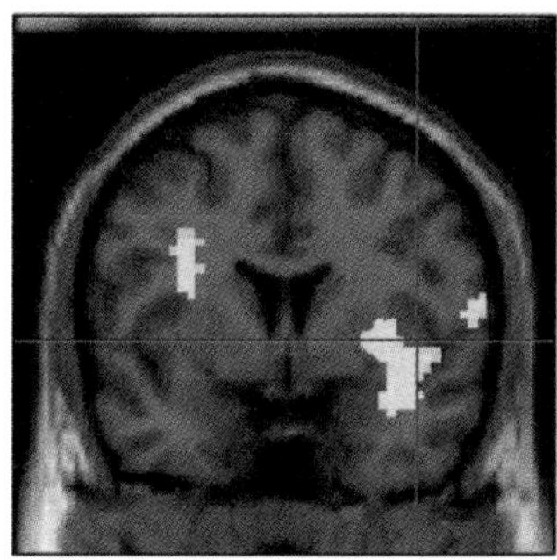

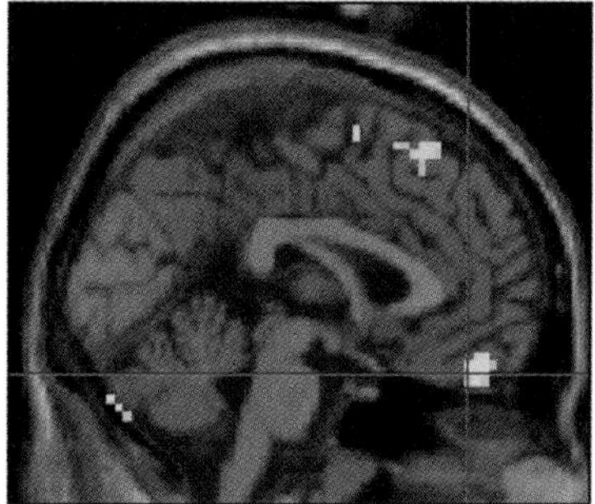

FIGURE 22.7
Shown are the elevated neuronal response to reward in the dorsal striatum when subjects must execute a movement to obtain the reward and the elevated neuronal response in the OFC when the reward is directly predicted by the stimulus with no intervening reward (Elliott, R. *et al.*, unpublished results).

try to respond to the more profitable stimulus throughout; thus, the appropriate response to the reversal of contingencies was to switch responding to the other stimulus. The findings of this study revealed interesting dissociations within the OFC. Medial OFC response was associated with the experience of reward relative to punishment, irrespective of the stage of the experiment. Further, neuronal activity in this region correlated significantly with the magnitude of the experienced reward. Corresponding neuronal responses to punishment, relative to reward, were observed in the anterior lateral OFC, and again this response was significantly correlated with the magnitude of punishment. This finding is consistent with the PET activation in response to chocolate reported by Small *et al.* (2001) and discussed above. It seems that for both food and financial reinforcement there is a dissociation between medial OFC response to reward and lateral OFC response to punishment. Other prefrontal responses were also noted in this study, including a medial prefrontal response to reward. It should be noted that the imaging sequence used was designed to focus on the OFC, minimising the signal dropout problems associated with this region; therefore, it is not clear whether more extensive posterior and subcortical response may have been observed had the sequence allowed whole brain coverage.

Recent fMRI data (Elliott *et al.*, unpublished observations), using whole brain imaging with a parametric design and a rewarded target detection task, also identified OFC as the region where there is a significant relationship between response and reward size. By contrast, the study by Elliott *et al.* (2000) suggests that increasing magnitude of reward is associated with neuronal response in the ventral striatum. There are several possible reasons for the discrepancy between these findings. In the Elliott *et al.* (2000) study, each individual reward had the same value; therefore, the total amount won reflects the number of rewarding events experienced. The studies by O'Doherty *et al.* (2001) and Elliott *et al.* (unpublished data) use variable magnitudes of individual reward events. As discussed earlier, the animal literature implicates OFC in mediating representations of reward values, while the ventral striatum responds to actual experiences of reward. It is plausible that the ventral striatum selectively codes the number of rewarding events, while the OFC selectively codes the value of each event. Another difference is that the probability of reward was set at chance in the study of Elliott *et al.* (2000), while the other studies used rewards that were relatively more predictable. It may be that the ventral striatum responds to more unpredictable rewards while the OFC responds when rewards can be predicted to a certain extent.

An explicit study of the modulatory effect of changing the probability of a rewarding outcome was by Rogers *et al.* (1999a). This was a $H_2{}^{15}O$ PET study that focused on differential responses to choosing between different reward and probability scenarios. The experimental paradigm used involved presenting subjects with a series of choices between an unlikely, but large, reward and a more likely, but smaller, reward. Resolving this conflict was associated with activations in the inferior and orbitofrontal cortices, incorporating medial regions (BA10) and both anterior (BA11) and posterior (BA47) lateral regions. These findings are consistent with those of O'Doherty *et al.* (2001b), as well as the neuropsychological studies discussed above that critically implicate OFC regions in decision-making behaviour involving the weighing up of risks and possible outcomes. Again, the rewards used here were abstract in nature (subjects win points rather than actual money) which provides further support for the hypothesis that OFC fulfils an abstract representational function in reward processing.

Neuroimaging of Reward Expectation

In electrophysiological studies in animals, measures of delay activity in the interval between a predictive stimulus, or response, and a reward are taken as an index of reward expectancy functions. An event-related fMRI study of delay activity in humans was carried out by Critchley *et al.* (2001). This study specifically examined neuronal responses between reward-related decisions and their subsequent outcomes. The paradigm was a simple card-playing task where subjects were presented with a playing card and had to predict whether the next card in the series would be higher in value. This paradigm incorporated a parametric variation in uncertainty because subjects could be more confident of their prediction if the presented card was very high or low in value than if it was a mid-value card. After an 8.5-s delay, subjects were told whether or not their prediction was correct and given a corresponding financial reward or penalty. Neuronal responses were measured during the delay interval, as were skin conductance responses to provide an index of arousal.

Delay-related neuronal responses were seen in the OFC bilaterally, medial PFC, temporal pole, and right parietal cortex. The anticipatory responses in OFC and anterior cingulate were modulated by uncertainty, showing increased response as the degree of uncertainty, or risk, increased. The anterior cingulate response was also modulated by increased arousal, as was response in the dorsolateral PFC. The authors propose that the OFC activity mediates outcome expectancy, which relates to reward expectancy. It is interesting to note that the focus of OFC response in this study was lateral rather than occurring in the medial region that has previously been more closely associated with risk-taking behaviour. Similar lateral rather than medial foci were observed in the card-playing study of Elliott *et al.* (2000), specifically in the context of either a winning or a losing streak. This was interpreted as possibly reflecting an anticipatory phenomenon where subjects expected contingencies to shift at any moment. O'Doherty *et al.* (2001a) observed lateral OFC response associated with expectation of fully predictable food reward. It is therefore possible that lateral regions of OFC play a particular role in anticipatory aspects of reward processing in humans, although this hypothesis has little firm basis in the animal literature. The differential roles of lateral and medial OFC in reward processing clearly require further clarification. An important caveat to recognise here is that OFC is a region particularly prone to susceptibility artefact and signal dropout in fMRI; therefore, the failure of studies to observe neuronal response in this region may not reflect a true absence of involvement.

SOCIAL REINFORCEMENT

As discussed earlier, financial reward can be thought of as a particular form of social reinforcement, but there are many other social reinforcers that provide a clear incentive motivating human behaviour. The desire to please others, to gain respect, or to be esteemed within society are all powerful forces determining our behavioural choices. In fact, the desire for some form of social reinforcement can outweigh the desire for primary reinforcement in certain situations, as any dieter will testify. Much of the reward research described above has a clear theoretical basis in the animal literature. By moving into the realms of social reinforcement, functional imaging can potentially offer insights into more uniquely human experience.

One simple form of social reinforcement is being congratulated on successful performance. In a PET study of the effects of performance feedback (Elliott *et al.*, 1997b), we found that performance of cognitive tasks was significantly modulated by the presence compared to the absence of performance feedback. Feedback took the form of a large tick or cross, accompanied by the words "you are right" or "you are wrong." There were no differences in the activations associated with positive and negative feedback, but the presence compared to the absence of feedback was associated with activation of the caudate nucleus. Two different tasks were used in this study: a complex planning task based on the Tower of London (Shallice, 1982) and a simple, six-choice guessing task. A further activation in medial OFC was associated with feedback in the guessing but not the planning task. This is consistent with the neuropsychological and imaging evidence (reviewed above) that the OFC is particularly involved in situations where information about potential reinforcement is used to guide decision making. There was no explicit reward in this study, but the feedback provided a form of abstract social reinforcement, as well as the only means by which subjects could evaluate their performance, as there was no absolute criterion by which responses could be judged correct or incorrect.

A recent unpublished fMRI study looked at the differences between congratulatory social reinforcement and financial reward (Longe *et al.*, unpublished observations). In this study, subjects were told to respond to occasional target stimuli in a stream of distracters as quickly as possible. If they responded faster than a (fictional) mean response speed allegedly obtained from pilot data, they would be rewarded; if they responded slower, they would be penalised. In one condition, the reinforcement was financial (a symbolic representation of +£ or –£, indicating success or otherwise). In the other condition, the reinforcement was a happy or a sneering face, accompanied by the messages *well done!* or *too slow!*, respectively. The social condition was associated with enhanced response in medial prefrontal regions (anterior cingulate, anterior medial prefrontal cortex, and medial orbitofrontal cortex), as well as medial temporal lobe regions, including the amygdala. By contrast, financial reinforcement was associated with more significant neuronal response in parietal and dorsolateral prefrontal regions. These differences were seen even when the event related responses to the rewarding stimuli were excluded from the analysis, suggesting that the differences do not simply reflect face-processing responses.

This dissociation can potentially be interpreted in terms of a conceptual distinction between the value of a reward and its role as a behavioural goal. In animals, OFC responds preferentially to rewards that are more valuable to the animal. It may be that, given the relatively small sums of money used here, the social reinforcement of a smiling face has more intrinsic value to the subjects. It certainly has more immediacy in that subjects must wait until after scanning for the financial reward to become tangible. Conversely, the financial reward may be a more powerful behavioural goal over the course of the experiment; under the financial condition, the subjects are responding with the specific behavioural aim of winning as much as possible. A related possibility is that the OFC/amygdala and DLPFC/parietal cortex preferentially code the hedonic and the informational value of rewards respectively. Smiling faces may produce a more basic hedonic response, while financial rewards may be more salient informational stimuli to guide behavioural modification. It is entirely consistent with the known functions of the medial OFC and right DLPFC that these regions should differentially subserve these conceptually separate responses to reward information.

We also performed a conjunction analysis to identify those regions that responded to *both* social and financial reinforcers, relative to a no-reinforcement condition. The main region involved was the OFC. A *post hoc* event-related analysis suggested a dissociation between medial and lateral OFC foci, with a medial region responding to both social and financial rewards, while a right lateral OFC region responded to both social and financial punishments (see Fig. 22.8). This dissociation is similar to that reported by O'Doherty *et al.* (2001b) for abstract symbolic reinforcers. It is interesting to note that the medial OFC responds to both social and financial rewards, as revealed by the conjunction analysis, but more strongly to the social rewards, as revealed by the comparison.

The study discussed above used faces as a symbolic social reinforcer, in comparison to a symbolic financial reinforcer. Recent studies have looked explicitly at the reward values of different faces. Kampe *et al.* (2001) reported that viewer-rated attractiveness of an unfamiliar face was associated with increased activation in the ventral striatum. Strikingly, this increased response was seen *only* if the direction of eye gaze of the attractive face was toward the subject. If the face was directing eye gaze away from the subject, response in the ventral striatum decreased. The authors suggest that activation of reward circuitry is important in the initiation of social interaction. The gender specificity of this effect was clearly demonstrated by Aharon *et al.* (2001), who showed that, although heterosexual males rated both beautiful male and beautiful female faces as aesthetically attractive, a differentially enhanced response in the ventral striatum was observed only to beautiful female faces. This suggests a reward value of beauty that is distinct from aesthetic judgment and is presumably important in social relationships.

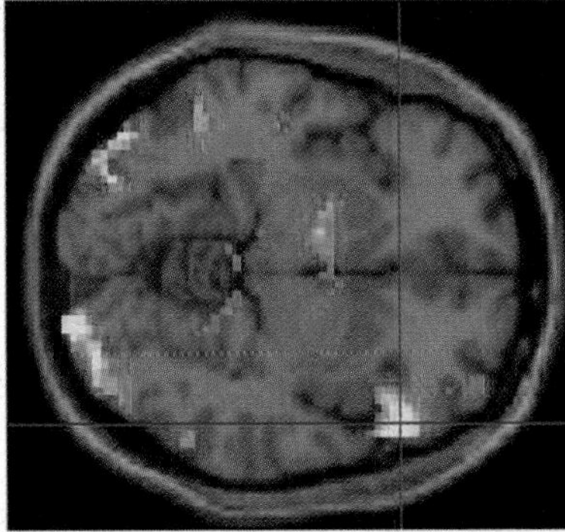
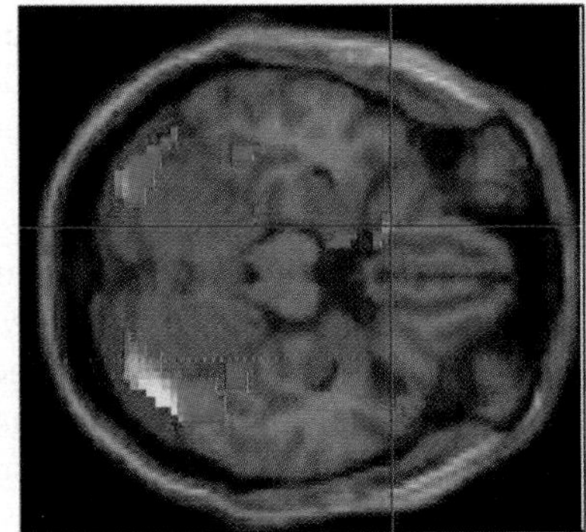

FIGURE 22.8
Medial OFC responses to both social and financial rewards and lateral OFC responses to both social and financial punishments (Longe, O. A. *et al.*, unpublished results).

Another potential form of social reinforcement is performing better than our peers in a competitive context. Studies discussed above have considered winning in the context of winning money; however, winning can also involve outperforming other people. This was explicitly exploited by Zalla *et al.* (2000), who studied the brain responses to winning and losing in a fictitious cognitive tournament. Subjects performed a simple target detection task requiring them to respond as quickly as possible to a prespecified target stimulus. Subjects were provided with feedback (using the verbal stimuli "WIN" or "LOSE") to inform them whether their responses were faster or slower than those of other subjects in the study. A control stimulus of "NEXT" was also used, and the proportion of informative feedback (WIN/LOSE) relative to uninformative feedback (NEXT) was varied parametrically in different task blocks. Although subjects believed they were competing in a real tournament and that the feedback received was genuinely contingent on response speed, there was actually no tournament and the experiment was completely fixed such that subjects received the same feedback regardless of actual performance.

The study was designed to assess neuronal responses to winning and losing, measured in terms of changing frequency of the WIN and LOSE trials. Response in the left amygdala was associated with increasing frequency of win trials, while response in the right amygdala correlated with increasing frequency of lose trials. This dissociation comparing left- and right-sided responses is consistent with previous evidence for lateralised response to positive and negative emotional states, with left hemisphere regions responding to positive states and right hemisphere regions to negative (Sackheim *et al.*, 1982; Davidson, 1995; Canli *et al.*, 1998). However, not all studies of the neural basis of emotional processing have supported claims of valence-specific laterality (see Chapter 19), so this interpretation remains speculative. It is, nonetheless, an intriguing finding.

One of the interesting anomalies in neuroimaging studies of reward to date is the lack of consistency with which an amygdala response is observed. In the animal literature, the amygdala has been repeatedly demonstrated to be a core component of reward processing systems, particularly those implicated in appetitive and aversive conditioning. Neuropsychological evidence also implicates the amygdala in conditioning in humans (Johnsrude *et al.*, 2000); however, relatively few of the functional imaging studies of reward have activated this region. Zalla *et al.* (2000) suggested that the amygdala response observed in this study may reflect the social context of the task. The subjects here believed they were competing against one another and would be ranked on the basis of their performance. This explicitly competitive context may have increased the emotional arousal and motivational salience associated with the reinforcing stimuli.

The study also reported OFC responses to increased frequency of winning. The response described here is in the lateral region of the OFC cortex, which O'Doherty *et al.* have associated with *losing* money. Further, Zalla *et al.* (2000) report responses in striatal regions associated with increasing frequency of losing, and again this finding is inconsistent with evidence implicating the striatum, especially ventral regions, in the processing of reward. One interpretation of these contradictory findings is that the social competitive context of the task alters the motivational qualities of the stimuli and the emotional responses to them. It should be noted that although the words "win" and "lose" were used here, subjects were not actually winning or losing anything in this experiment; the motivation was simply outperforming other people. This may represent a conceptually different form of winning, and this issue requires further consideration.

CONCLUSIONS AND FUTURE DIRECTIONS

The functional imaging of reward processing has lagged behind that of other cognitive domains; however it is currently one of the most exciting avenues of neuroimaging research, particularly with the advent of increasingly sophisticated event-related fMRI methodology. Event-related approaches are allowing investigators to explicitly test, in humans, hypotheses derived from the extensive electrophysiological literature in animals. Evidence to date suggests that critical regions in animal reward pathways are also implicated in human responses to both physiologically salient rewards, such as food and drugs, and to more abstract and social reinforcers, such as money.

As in animals, the striatum is at the hub of human reward processing systems. The ventral part of this region, including the nucleus accumbens, responds to the actual experience of reward, in financial reward studies as well as those using psychoactive drugs. The dorsal striatum appears to play a rather different role, mediating the use of reward representations to generate goal-directed behaviour; thus, this region has been reported in studies of incentive responses and in situations where an actual reward is elicited by a specific behavioural response (analogous to instrumental conditioning in animals). These striatal responses are presumably driven by dopaminergic projections from the midbrain, and the development of the carbon 11 raclopride technique has allowed this process to be studied explicitly (Koepp *et al.*, 1998). Further research is needed to combine the neurochemical sophistication of ligand-binding PET techniques with activation paradigms that can dissociate different components of reward-related processing.

The amygdala is also a key region in animal reward systems, responding particularly to conditioned reinforcers in associative learning contexts. This region has been less reliably activated in reward-related neuroimaging studies. Amygdala responses have been reported in studies using reinforcing drugs, or cues associated with them, and also where face stimuli are used as rewards. The amygdala also responds in the context of social competition; however, its role in mediating financial reward remains unclear. It is possible that amygdala responses are more pronounced when the primary reinforcer has physiological salience, as in the drug studies, and that money is too abstract a form of reward to elicit responses. This account would not be entirely supported by the animal literature; the role of the basolateral amygdala in conditioned reinforcement strongly suggests that this region has access to abstract representations of reward. Another possibility is that the amygdala response is maximal as conditioned associations are being learned, and this learning occurs so rapidly in humans that any amygdala signal is too transient to be detectable in neuroimaging. Even in event-related designs, observable responses to particular types of stimuli are only obtained across a number of actual instances and, if amygdala responses only occur on the first few trials, the cumulative BOLD signal may be undetectable. It is also possible that amygdala response is only seen in situations where the affective salience is maximised (drug cues, faces, or competitive social contexts), and it is this affective response, rather than an associative learning response, that is being observed. Further evidence is needed to clarify the role of the amygdala in human reward processing.

Finally, prefrontal regions play an important role in reward processing. Schultz (2000) proposes that DLPFC is particularly implicated in goal-directed behaviour, and there is some evidence to support this notion in the imaging data, particularly in the studies comparing financial and social reinforcement (Thut *et al.*, 1997; Elliott *et al.*, unpublished observations). Not all financial reward studies have reported DLPFC activity. A possible reason for this discrepancy is that, in a number of the studies described, goal-directed behaviour is a common feature of the different conditions; that is, subjects were constantly planning and executing behaviours in an attempt to elicit rewards and/or avoid penalties. The contrasts between different incentive values, different contingencies, and so on may not reveal differential functions for the DLPFC when the general context of goal-directed behaviour remains constant.

A more reliably activated region in these imaging studies is the OFC. In spite of the technical problems obtaining detectable BOLD signal from the orbital regions, many of the studies discussed have reported OFC responses. In general terms, this region appears to play a role in the more abstract representation of value, being involved when rewards are symbolic or social as well as when they are more tangible. The region may also play a key role in the flexible monitoring of contingency, weighing the value of an outcome against the likelihood of its occurrence in order to decide the best course of action. This evaluative role under conditions of uncertainty critically underpins much of our social behaviour, as is evident from the social problems of patients with damage to this region. An outstanding issue raised by the literature discussed above concerns the relative roles of the medial and lateral OFC, as there are apparent discrepancies between studies. Elliott *et al.* (2000b) have suggested that medial OFC plays a particular role in mediating stimulus–reward associations while lateral OFC is involved in the suppression of previously rewarded responses. Although much of the data reviewed here can be accommodated by this formulation, several studies suggest a further anticipatory role for the lateral OFC. In some contexts, this may reflect an anticipation of the need to suppress responses as contingencies change. However, this argument cannot readily account for the modulation of delay by uncertainty reported by Critchley *et al.* (2001) or the association between lateral OFC activity and winning in a competition (Zalla *et al.*, 2000). The role of this region in reward processes therefore requires further clarification.

This discussion has focused on dissociable roles for ventral and dorsal striatum, amygdala, and prefrontal regions in human reward processing, although there are obviously a number of other interconnected regions involved. Further elaboration of these interacting roles represents an important challenge for neuroimaging over the next few years. An understanding of human reward processing has potentially crucial implications for a number of neurological and psychiatric disorders, which are characterised by impairments in reinforcement processing.

References

Aharon, I., Etcoff, N., Ariely, D., Chabris, C. F., O'Connor, E., and Breiter, H. C. (2001). Beautiful faces have variable reward value: fMRI and behavioural evidence. *Neuron*, **32**, 537–551.

Arvanitogiannis, A., Waraczynski, M., and Shizgal P. (1996). Effects of excitotoxic lesions of the basal forebrain on MFB self-stimulation. *Physiol. Behav.*, **59**, 795–906.

Baeyens, F., Hermans, D., and Eelen, P. (1993). The role of CS-US contingency in human evaluative conditioning. *Behav. Res. Ther.*, **31**, 731–737.

Balleine, B. W. and Dickinson, A. (1998). Goal-directed instrumental action: contingency and incentive learning and their cortical substrates. *Neuropharmacology*, **37**, 407–419.

Baxter, M. G., Parker, A., Lindner, C. C., Izquierdo, A. D., and Murray, E. A. (2000). Control of response selection by reinforcer value requires interaction of amygdala and orbitofrontal cortex. *J. Neurosci.*, **20**, 4311–4319.

Bechara, A., Damasio, A. R., Damasio, H., and Anderson, S. W. (1994). Insensitivity to future consequences following damage to human prefrontal cortex. *Cognition*, **50**, 7–15.

Bechara, A., Tranel, D., Damasio, H., Adolphs, R., Rockland, C., and Damasio, A. R. (1995). Double dissociation of conditioning and declarative knowledge relative to the amygdala and hippocampus in humans. *Science*, **269**, 1115–1118.

Bechara, A., Tranel, D., Damasio, H., and Damasio, A. R. (1996). Failure to respond autonomically to anticipated future outcomes following damage to the prefrontal cortex. *Cereb. Cortex*, **6**, 215–225.

Bechara, A., Damasio, H., Damasio, A. R., and Lee, G. P. (1999). Different contributions of the human amygdala and ventromedial prefrontal cortex to decision making. *J. Neurosci.*, **19**, 5473–5581.

Bechara, A., Tranel, D., and Damasio, H. (2000). Characterisation of the decision-making deficit of patients with ventromedial prefrontal lesions. *Brain*, **123**, 2189–2202.

Berridge, K. C. and Robinson, T. E. (1998). What is the role of dopamine in reward: hedonic impact, reward learning, or incentive salience? *Brain Res. Rev.*, **28**, 309–369.

Breier, A., Su, T. P., Saunders, R., Carson, R. E., Kolachana, B. S., de Bartolomeis, A., Weinberger, D. R., Weisenfeld, N., Malhotra, A. K., Eckelman, W. C., and Pickar, D. (1997). Schizophrenia is associated with elevated amphetamine-induced synaptic dopamine concentrations: evidence from a novel positron emission tomography method. *Proc. Natl. Acad. Sci. USA*, **94**, 2569–2574.

Breiter, H. C., Gollub, R. L., Weisskoff, R. M., Kennedy, D. N., Makris, N., Berke, J. D., Goodman, J. M., Kantor, H. L., Gastfriend, D. R., Riorden, J. P., Mathew, R. T., Rosen, B. R., and Hyman, S. E. (1997). Acute effects of cocaine on human brain activity and emotion. *Neuron*, **19**, 591–611.

Breiter, H. C., Gollub, R. L., Edminster, W., Talavage, T., Makris, M., Melcher, J., Kennedy, D., Kantor, H., Elman, I., Riorden, D., Gastfriend, T., Campbell, M., Foley, R. M., Weisskoff, R. M., and Rosen, B. R. (1998). Cocaine induced brainstem and subcortical activity observed through fMRI with cardiac gating. *Proc. Int. Soc. Magn. Reson. Med.*, **1**, 499.

Breiter, H. C., Aharon, I., Kahneman, D., Dale, A., and Shizgal, P. (2001). Functional imaging of neral responses to expectancy and experience of monetary gains and losses. *Neuron*, **30**, 619–639.

Buechel, C., Morris, J., Dolan, R. J., and Friston, K. J. (1998). Brain systems mediating aversive conditioning: an event-related fMRI study. *Neuron*, **20**, 947–957.

Cador, M., Robbins, T. W., and Everitt, B. J. (1989). Involvement of the amygdala in stimulus-reward associations: interaction with ventral striatum. *Neuroscience*, **30**, 77–86.

Canli, T., Desmond, J. E., Zhao, Z., Glover, G., and Gabrieli, J. D. (1998). Hemispheric asymmetry for emotional stimuli detected with fMRI. *NeuroReport*, **9**, 3233–3239.

Charbonneau, D., Riopelle, R. J., and Beninger, R. J. (1996). Impaired incentive learning in treated Parkinson's disease. *Can. J. Neurol. Sci.*, **23**, 271–278.

Childress, A. R., Mozley, P. D., McElgin, W., Fitzgerald, J., Reivich, M., and O'Brien, C. P. (1999). Limbic activation during cue-induced cocaine craving. *Am. J. Psychiatry*, **156**, 11–18.

Critchley, H. D., Mathias, C. J. and Dolan, R. J. (2001). Neural activity in the human brain relating to uncertainty and arousal during anticipation. *Neuron*, **29**, 537–545.

Cummings, J. L. (1993). Depression and Parkinson's disease: a review. *Am. J. Psychiatry*, **150**, 843–834.

Damasio, A. R. (1994). *Descartes' Error*. Putnam, New York.

Davidson, R. J. (1995). Asymmetric brain function, emotion and affective style, in *Brain Asymmetry*, Davidson, R. J. and Hugdahl, K., Eds., pp 361–87. MIT Press, Cambridge, MA.

Delgado, M. R., Nystrom, L. E., Fissell, C., Noll, D. C., and Fiez, J. A. (2000). Tracking the haemodynamic response to reward and punishment in the striatum. *J. Neurophysiol.*, **84**, 3072–3077.

Denes-Raj, V. and Epstein, S. (1994). Conflict between intuitive and rational processing: when people behave against their better judgment. *J. Personality and Soc. Psychol.*, **66**, 819–829.

Dias, R., Robbins, T. W., and Roberts, A. C. (1996). Dissociation in prefrontal cortex of affective and attentional shifts. *Nature*, **380**, 69–72.

Dickinson, A. (1980). *Contemporary Animal Learning Theory*, Cambridge University Press, Cambridge, U.K.

Elliott, R., Sahakian, B. J., Herrod, J. J., Robbins, T. W., and Paykel, E. S. (1997a). Abnormal response to negative feedback in unipolar depression: evidence for a disease-specific impairment. *J. Neurol. Neurosurg. Psychiatry*, **63**, 74–82.

Elliott, R., Frith, C. D., and Dolan, R. J. (1997b). Differential neural response to positive and negative feedback in planning and guessing tasks. *Neuropsychologia,* **15**, 1395–1404.

Elliott, R., Friston, K. J., and Dolan, R. J. (2000a). Dissociable neural responses associated with reward, punishment and risk-taking behaviour. *J. Neurosci.*, **20**, 6159–6165.

Elliott, R., Frith, C. D., and Dolan, R. J. (2000b). Dissociable functions in the medial and lateral orbitofrontal cortex: evidence from human neuroimaging studies *Cereb. Cortex,* **10**, 308–317.

Everitt, B. J. and Robbins, T. W. (1992). Amygdala–ventral striatum interactions and reward-related processes, in *The Amygdala*, Aggleton, J. P., Ed., pp. 401–429, John Wiley & Sons, New York.

Fibiger, H. C. (1984). The neurobiological substrates of depression in Parkinson's disease: a hypothesis. *Can. J. Neurol. Sci.*, **11**, 1105–1107.

Gallagher, M., McMahan, R. W., and Schoenbaum, G. (1999). Orbitofrontal cortex and representation of incentive value in associative learning. *J. Neurosci.*, **19**, 6610–6614.

Grant, S., London, E., Newlin, D., Villemagne, V., Liu, X, Contoreggi, C., Phillips, R., and Margolin, A. (1996). Activation of memory circuits during cue-elicited cocaine craving. *Proc. Natl. Acad. Sci USA*, **93**, 12040–12045.

Grant, S., Contoreggi, C., and London, E. D. (1997). Drug abusers show impaired performance on a test of orbitofrontal function. *Soc. Neurosci. Abstr.*, **23**, 1943.

Green, L., Fristoe, N., and Myerson J. (1994). Temporal discounting and preference reversals in choice between delayed outcomes. *Psychonomic Bull. Rev.*, **1**, 383–389.

Hatfield, T., Han, J.-S., Conley, M., Gallagher, M., and Holland, P. (1996). Neurotoxic lesions of basolateral, but not central, amygdala interfere with Pavlovian second-order conditioning and reinforcer devaluation effects. *J. Neurosci.*, **16**, 5256–52665.

Holland, P. C. and Gallagher, M. (1999). Amygdala circuitry in attentional and representational processes. *Trends Cogn. Sci.*, **3**, 65–73.

Hollerman, J. R. and Schultz, W. (1998). Dopamine neurons report an error in the temporal prediction of reward during learning. *Nat. Neurosci.*, **1**, 304–309.

Ingvar, M.,Ghatan, P. H., Wirsen-Meurling, A., Risberg, J., Von Heijne, G., Stone-Elander, S., and Ingvar, D. H. (1998). Alcohol activates the cerebral reward system in man. *J. Studies Alcohol*, **59**, 258–269.

Iversen, S. and Mishkin, M. (1970). Perseverative interference in monkey following selective lesions of the inferior prefrontal convexity. *Exp. Brain Res.*, **11**, 376–386.

Jentsch, J. D. and Taylor, J. R. (1999). Impulsivity resulting from frontostriatal dysfunction in drug abuse: implications for the control of behaviour by reward-related stimuli. *Psychopharmacology*, **146**, 373–390.

Johnsrude, I. S., Owen, A. M., Zhao, W. V., and White, N. M. (1999). Conditioned preference in humans: a novel experimental approach. *Learning Motiv.*, **30**, 250–264.

Johnsrude, I. S., Owen, A. M., White, N. M., Zhao, W. V., and Bohbot, V. (2000). Impaired preference conditioning after anterior temporal lobe resection in humans. *J. Neurosci.*, **20**, 2649–2656.

Kalivas, P. W., and Nakamura, M. (1999). Neural systems for behavioural activation and reward. *Curr. Opin. Neurobiol.*, **9**, 223–227.

Kampe, K. K., Frith, C. D., Dolan, R. J., and Frith, U. (2001). Reward value of attractiveness and gaze. *Nature*, **413**, 589.

Killcross, S., Robbins, T. W., and Everitt, B. J. (1997). Different types of fear-conditioned behaviour mediated by separate nuclei within the amygdala. *Nature*, **388**, 377–380.

Kilts, C. D., Schweitzer, J. B., Quinn, C. K., Gross, R. E., Faber, T. L., Muhammed, F., Ely, T. D., Hoffman, J. M., and Drexler, K. P. (2001). Neural activity related to drug craving in cocaine addiction. *Arch. Gen. Psychiatry*, **58**, 342–344.

Koepp, M. J., Gunn, R. N., Lawrence, A. D., Cunningham, V. J., Dagher, A., Jones, T., Brooks, D. J., Bench, C. J., and Grasby, P. M. (1998). Evidence for striatal dopamine release during a video game. *Nature*, **393**, 266–268.

Koob, G. F. and Le Moal, M. (1997). Drug abuse: hedonic homeostatic dysregulation. *Science*, **278**, 52–58.

Knutson, B., Westdorp, A., Kaiser, E., and Hommer, D. (2000). fMRI visualisation of brain activity during a monetary incentive delay task. *NeuroImage*, **12**, 20–27.

LaBar, K. S., LeDoux, J. E., Spencer, D. D., and Phelps, E. A. (1995). Impaired fear conditioning following unilateral temporal lobectomy in humans. *J. Neurosci.*, **15**, 6846–655.

LaBar, K. S., Gatenby, J. C., Gore, J. C., LeDoux, J. E., and Phelps, E. A. (1998). Human amygdala activation during conditioned fear acquisition and extinction: a mixed trial fMRI study. *Neuron*, **20**, 937–945.

Lewinsohn, P. M. (1974). A behavioural approach to depression, in *The Psychology of Depression: Contemporary Theory and Research*, Friedman, R. J. and Katz, M. M., Eds., pp. 157–185. Winston/Wiley, New York.

Lewinsohn, P. M., Youngren, M. A., and Grosscup, S. J. (1979). Reinforcement and depression, in *The Psychobiology of Depressive Disorders*, Depue, R. A., Eds., pp. 291–316. Academic Press, New York.

Ljungberg, T., Apicella, P., and Schultz, W. (1992). Responses of monkey DA neurons during learning of behavioural reactions. *J. Neurophysiol.*, **67**, 145–163.

Maas, L. C., Lukas, S. E., Kaufman, M. J., Weiss, R. D., Daniels, S. L., Rogers, V. W., Kukes, T. J., and Renshaw, P. F. (1998). Functional magnetic resonance imaging of human brain activation during cue-induced cocaine craving. *Am. J. Psychiatry*, **155**, 124–126.

Mackintosh, N. J. (1983). *Conditioning and Associative Learning*. Oxford University Press, London.

Madden, G. J., Petry, N. M., Badger, G. J., and Bickel, W. K. (1997). Impulsive and self-control choices in opioid-dependent patients and non-drug-using control participants: drug and monetary rewards. *Exp. Clin. Psychopharmacol.*, **5**, 256–263.

Mazas, C. A., Finn, P. R., and Steinmetz, J. E. (2000). Decision-making biases, antisocial personality and early-onset alcoholism. *Alcohol Clin. Exp. Res.*, **24**, 1036–1040.

Mierencowicz, J. and Schultz, W. (1994). Importance of unpredictability for reward responses in primate dopamine neurons. *J. Neurophysiol.*, **72**, 1024–1027.

Morris, J. S., Ohman, A., and Dolan, R. J. (1998). Conscious and unconscious emotional learning in the human amygdala. *Nature*, **393**, 467–470.

Murphy, F. C., Sahakian, B. J., and O'Carroll, R. E. (1998). Cognitive impairments in depression: psychological models and clinical issues, in *New Models for Depression: Advances in Biological Psychiatry*, Vol 19, Ebert, D. and Ebmeier, K. P., Eds., pp. 1–33, Karger, Basel, Switzerland.

Niedenthal, P. M. (1990). Implicit perception of affective information. *J. Exp. Social Psychol.*, **26**, 505–527.

O'Doherty, J., Rolls, E. T., Francis, S., Bowtell, R., McGlone, F., Kobal, G., Renner, B., Ahne, G. (2000). Sensory-specific satiety-related olfactory activation of the human orbitofrontal cortex, *NeuroReport*, **11**, 893–897.

O'Doherty, J. P., Kringelbach, M. L., Rolls, E. T., Hornak, J., and Andrews, C. (2001). Abstract reward and punishment in the human orbitofrontal cortex. *Nat. Neurosci.*, **4**, 95–102.

O'Doherty, J. P., Deichmann, R., Critchley, H. D., and Dolan, R. J. (2002). Neural responses during anticipation of a primary taste reward. *Neuron*, **33**, 815–826.

Olds, J. and Milner, P. M. (1954). Positive reinforcement produced by electrical stimulation of septal area and other regions of rat brain. *J. Comp. Physiol. Psychol.*, **47**, 419–427.

Pacini, R., Muir, F., and Epstein, S. (1998). Depressive realism from the perspective of cognitive-experiential self theory. *J. Personality Soc. Psychol.*, **74**, 1056–1068.

Petry, N. M. and Casarella, T. (1999). Excessive discounting of delayed rewards in substance abusers with gambling problems. *Drug Alcohol Depend.*, **56**, 25–32.

Petry, N. M., Bickel, W. K., and Arnett, M. (1998). Shortened time horizons and insensitivity to future consequences in heroin addicts. *Addiction*, **93**, 729–738.

Ravard, S., Carnoy, P., Herve, D., Tassin, J., Theibot, M., and Soubrie, P. (1990). Involvement of prefrontal dopamine neurones in behavioural blockade by controllable vs. uncontrollable negative events in rats. *Behav. Brain Res.*, **37**, 9–18.

Rescorla, R. A. and Wagner, A. R. (1972). A theory of Pavlovian conditioning: variations in the effectiveness of reinforcement and non-reinforcement, in *Classical Conditioning.* II. *Current Research and Theory*, Black, A. H. and Prokasy, W. F., Eds., pp. 64–69. Appleton-Century-Crofts, New York.

Robbins, T. W. and Everitt, B. J. (1992). Functions of dopamine in the dorsal and ventral striatum. *Semin. Neurosci.*, **4**, 119–127.

Robbins, T. W. and Everitt, B. J. (1996). Neurobiobehavioural mechanisms of reward and motivation. *Curr. Opin. Neurobiol.*, **6**, 228–236.

Rogers, R. D., Owen, A. M., Middleton, H. C., Williams, E. J., Pickard, J. D., Sahakian, B. J. and Robbins, T. W. (1999a). Choosing between small likely rewards and large, unlikely rewards activates inferior and orbital prefrontal cortex. *J. Neurosci.*, **19**, 9029–9038.

Rogers, R. D., Everitt, B. J., Baldacchino, A., Blackshaw, A. J., Swainson, R., Wynne, K., Baker, N. B., Hunter, J., Carthy, T., Booker, E., London, M., Deakin, J. F. W., Sahakian, B. J., and Robbins, T. W. (1999b). Dissociable deficits in the decision-making cognition of chronic amphetamine abusers, opiate abusers, patients with focal damage to prefrontal cortex, and tryptophan-depleted normal volunteers: evidence for monoaminergic mechanisms. *Neuropsychopharmacology*, **20**, 322–339.

Rolls, E. T. (1996). The orbitofrontal cortex. Phil. Trans. R. Soc. Lond., B., **351**:1433–1444.

Rolls, E. T. (1999). The Brain and Emotion. Oxford University Press, Oxford UK.

Rolls, E. T. (2000). The Orbitofrontal Cortex and reward. Cerebral Cortex **10**, 284–94.

Rolls, E. T., Hornak J., Wade, D., and McGrath, J. (1994). Emotion-related learning in patients with social and emotional changes associated with frontal lobe damage. *J. Neurol. Neurosurg. Psychiatry*, **57**, 1518–1524.

Rolls, E. T., Francis, S., Bowtell, R., Browning, D., Clare, S., Smith, T. *et al.* (1997). Taste and olfactory activation of the orbitofrontal cortex. *NeuroImage*, **5**, S199.

Sackeim, H. A., Greenberg, M. S., Weiman, A. L., Gur, R. C., Hungerbuhler, J. P., and Geschwind, N. (1982). Hemispheric asymmetry in the expression of positive and negative emotions: neurologic evidence. *Arch. Neurol.*, **39**, 210–218.

Salomone, J. D. (1994). The involvement of nucleus accumbens dopamine in appetitive and aversive motivation. *Behav. Brain Res.*, **61**, 117–133.

Schoenbaum, G., Chiba, A. A., and Gallagher, M. (1998). Orbitofrontal cortex and basolateral amygdala encode expected outcomes during learning. *Nat. Neurosci.*, **1**, 155–159.

Schultz, W. (1997). Dopamine neurons and their role in reward mechanisms. *Curr. Opin. Neurobiol.*, **7**, 191–197.

Schultz, W. (1998). Predictive reward signal of dopamine neurons. *J. Neurophysiol.*, **80**, 1–27.

Schultz, W., Apicella, P., Scarnati, E., and Ljungberg, T. (1992). Neuronal activity in monkey ventral striatum related to the expectation of reward. *J. Neurosci.*, **12**, 4595–4610.

Schultz, W., Apicella, P., Ljungberg, T., Romo, R., and Scarnati, E. (1993). Reward-related activity in the monkey striatum and substantia nigra. *Prog. Brain Res.*, **99**, 227–235.

Schultz, W., Dayan, P., and Read-Montague, P. R. (1997). A neural substrate of prediction and reward. *Science*, **275**, 1593–1599.

Schultz, W., Tremblay, L., and Hollerman, J. R. (2000). Reward processing in primate orbitofrontal cortex and basal ganglia. *Cereb. Cortex*, **10**, 272–283.

Sell, L. A., Morris, J., Bearn, J., Frackowiak, R. S. J., Friston, K. J., and Dolan, R. J. (1999). Activation of reward circuitry in human opiate addicts. *Eur. J. Neurosci.*, **11**, 1042–1048.

Sell, L. A., Morris, J. S., Bearn, J., Frackowiak, R. S. J., Friston, K. J., and Dolan, R. J. (2000). Neural responses associated with cue-evoked emotional states and heroin in opiate addicts. *Drug Alcohol Depend.*, **60**, 207–216.

Shallice, T. (1982). Specific impairments in planning. *Philos. Trans. Roy. Soc. London B*, **298**, 199–209.

Small, D. M., Zatorre, R. J., Daghar, A., Evans, A. C., and Jones-Gotman, M. (2001). Changes in brain activity related to eating chocolate: from pleasure to aversion. *Brain*, **124**, 1720–133.

Spanagel, R. and Weiss, F. (1999). The dopamine hypothesis of reward: past and current status. *Trends Neurosci.*, **22**, 521–527.

Stein, E. A., Pankiewicz, J., Harsch, H. H., Cho, K. K., Fukker, S. A., Hoffman, R. G., Hawkins, M., Rao, S. M., Bandettini, P. A., and Bloom, A. S. (1998). Nicotine-induced limbic-cortical activation in the human brain: a functional MRI study. *Am. J. Psychiatry*, **155**, 1009–1015.

Stern, C. E. and Passingham, R. E. (1996). The nucleus accumbens in monkeys (*Macaca fascicularis*). II. Emotion and motivation. *Behav. Brain Res.*, **75**, 179–193.

Stout, J. C., Rodawalt, W. C., and Siemers, E. R. (2001). Risky decision making in Huntington's disease. *J. Int. Neuropsychol. Soc.*, **7**, 92–101.

Swainson, R., Rogers, R. D., Sahakian, B. J., Summers, B. A., Polkey, C. E., Robbins, T. W. (2000). Probabilistic learning and reversal deficits in patients with Parkinson's disease or frontal or temporal lobe lesions: possible adverse effects of dopaminergic medication. *Neuropsychologia*, **38**(5), 596–612.

Thut, G., Schultz, W., Roelcke, U., Nienhusdmeier, M., Missimer, J., Maguire, R. P., and Leenders, K. L. (1997). Activation of human brain by monetary reward. *NeuroReport*, **8**, 1225–1228.

Todrank, J., Byrnes, D., Wrzesniewski, A., and Rozin, P. (1995). Odors can change preferences for people in photographs: a cross-modal evaluative conditioning study with olfactory USs and visual CSs. *Learning Motiv.*, **26**, 116–140.

Tremblay, L. and Schultz, W. (1999). Relative reward preference in primate orbitofrontal cortex. *Nature*, **398**, 704–708.

Volkow, N. D., Fowler, J. S., Wolf, A. P., Schlyer, D., Chyng-Yann, S., Alpert, R., Dewey, S., Logan, J., Bendriem, B., and Christman, D. (1990). Effects of chronic cocaine abuse on postsynaptic dopamine receptors. *Am. J. Psychiatry*, **147**, 719–724.

Volkow, N. D., Hitzemann, R., and Wang, G.-J. (1992). Long-term frontal brain metabolic changes in cocaine abusers. *Synapse*, **11**, 184–190.

Volkow, N. D., Wang G.-J., Fowler, J. S., Logan, J., Gatley, S. J., Pappas, N., Hitzemann, R., Chen, A. D., and Pappas, N. (1997). Decreased striatal dopaminergic responsivity in detoxified cocaine abusers. *Nature*, **386**, 830–833.

Volkow, N. D., Fowler, J. S., and Wang, G.-J. (1999). Imaging studies on the role of dopamine in cocaine reinforcement and addiction in humans. *J. Psychopharmacol.*, **13**, 337–345.

Volkow, N. D., Wang, G. J., Fowler, J. S., Franceschi, D., Thanos, P. K., Wong, C., Gatley, S. J., Ding, Y.-S., Molina, P., Schlyer, D., Alexoff, D., Hitzemann, R., and Pappas, N. (2000). Cocaine abusers show a blunted response to alcohol intoxication in limbic brain regions. *Life Sci.*, **66**, 161–167.

Vuchinich, R. E. and Simpson, C. A. (1998). Hyperbolic temporal discounting in social drinkers and problem drinkers. *Exp. Clin. Psychopharmacol.*, **6**, 292–305.

Wang, G. J., Volkow, N. D., Fowler, J. S., Cervany, P., Hitzemann, R. J., Pappas, N. R., Wong, C. T., and Felder, C. (1999). Regional brain metabolic activation during craving elicited by recall of previous drug experiences. *Life Sci.*, **64**, 775–784.

Watanabe, M. (1999). Attraction is relative not absolute. *Nature*, **398**, 661–662.

Wise, R. A. (1980). The dopamine synapse and the notion of 'pleasure centres' in the brain. *Trends Neurosci.*, **3**, 91–94.

Wise, R. A. (1998). Drug activation of brain reward pathways. *Drug Alcohol Depend.*, **51**, 13–22.

Wise, R. A. and Rompre, P.-P. (1989). Brain dopamine and reward. *Annu. Rev. Psychol.*, **40**, 191–225.

Zalla, T., Koechlin, E., Pietrini, P., Basso, G., Aquino, P., Sirigu, A., and Grafman, J. (2000). Differential amygdala responses to winning and losing: a functional magnetic resonance imaging study in humans. *Eur. J. Neurosci.*, **12**, 1764–1770.

CHAPTER

23

Implicit Memory

INTRODUCTION

Implicit Versus Explicit Memory

This chapter is concerned with imaging studies of *implicit memory*; the next chapter is concerned with *explicit memory*. These terms were introduced by Graf and Schacter (1985) and are used in the present context to refer to the phenomenological experience of whether memory retrieval is accompanied by conscious awareness of the past (explicit memory) or is not (implicit memory). This distinction is based primarily on studies of the amnesic syndrome that suggest that amnesic patients can show effects of prior experience in their behaviour, even when they are not apparently aware of the prior experience. For example, many studies have shown that, when asked to identify a fragmented word, amnesic patients are more likely to identify such words if they have seen them previously in a "study" phase (Warrington and Weiskrantz, 1974). This "priming" effect is typically as large as that seen in healthy controls; however, when the patients are given the same type of word fragments, but this time asked to use them as cues to recall the corresponding word from a study phase, they are much worse than controls (Graf *et al.*, 1984). Thus, the patients are said to have intact implicit memory but impaired explicit memory. The dissociation between implicit and explicit memory is further supported by functional dissociations in healthy individuals, such as differential effects of study processing (Jacoby and Dallas, 1981) and retention interval (Tulving *et al.*, 1982).

Implicit memory is normally associated with *indirect* memory tasks (such as the word identification task described above), in which no reference is made to the previous experience (Richardson-Klavehn and Bjork, 1988). This is in contrast with *direct* memory tasks (such as recall and recognition), which refer participants to previous experiences. However, it is important to distinguish between the type of memory retrieval (implicit/explicit), its hypothetical underlying neural basis, and the type of tests used to measure memory (Schacter and Tulving, 1994). For example, even though an indirect test does not refer participants to a previous experience, participants may voluntarily, or involuntarily, recollect that experience. Conversely, unconscious forms of memory may influence performance on a direct memory task. In other words, direct or indirect memory tests are not necessarily "pure" in the sense that performance on either could involve a mixture of both implicit and explicit memory. That is, people may consciously recall some aspects of a prior episode, but not other aspects that nonetheless affect their behaviour. As a consequence, considerable effort has been devoted to developing methods that dissociate implicit and explicit contributions to memory tasks (Hayman and Tulving, 1989; Jacoby *et al.*, 1993; Richardson-Klavehn and Gardiner, 1995; Schacter *et al.*, 1989). Few imaging studies to date have achieved this dissociation, however; thus, it must be kept in mind that the brain activations discussed in this and the subsequent chapter may reflect contributions of implicit, explicit, or both types of memory.

This chapter is confined to imaging studies directed at one example of implicit memory, *repetition priming*; likewise, the subsequent chapter is confined to one example of explicit memory, *recognition memory*. The reason for restricting interest to these two examples is that the paradigms used to investigate them are similar, facilitating their comparison. In both cases, the basic contrast is between repeated and initial presentations of stimuli within the experimental context. In the context of priming, these conditions are often referred to as *primed* and *unprimed*, respectively; in the context of recognition memory, the conditions are often called *old* and *new*, respectively. More generally, the two conditions will be termed *repetition* and *control* conditions, and the subtraction of the positron emission tomography (PET)/functional magnetic resonance imaging (fMRI) data for repetition conditions from those for control conditions will be termed the *repetition effect*.

In some cases, the control condition consists of the initial presentations of the same stimulus, perhaps in a separate study phase; in other cases, the control condition consists of different stimuli that were not presented previously. In some cases, the stimuli in the repetition condition are not repeated exactly; instead, the repetition pertains to a common referent of the stimulus. For example, the primed stimulus in a priming paradigm (the *target*) may only be semantically related to a previous stimulus (the *prime*), or the words in a recognition memory test may be studied visually but tested auditorily. The important difference between the two paradigms is whether the test instructions are indirect (*e.g.*, "does this stimulus depict an animate object?," with the behavioural measure of priming being a shorter response time) or direct (*e.g.*, "did you see this stimulus in the study phase?," with the behavioural measure of recognition being response accuracy).

One potential generalization that has emerged from imaging studies of these two paradigms is that priming is associated with a reduced haemodynamic response for repetition versus control conditions (a negative repetition effect, or *repetition suppression*), whereas recognition memory is associated with an increased response for the repetition condition (a positive repetition effect, or *repetition enhancement*). One purpose of this chapter, however, is to argue that this generalization is likely to be too simplistic.

Given the plethora of recent imaging studies on memory, even when restricted to repetition priming and recognition memory, the reviews in both chapters must also be selective. Thus, both chapters concentrate on studies performed at the Wellcome Department of Imaging Neuroscience (for more comprehensive reviews of priming, see Henson, in press; Schacter and Buckner, 1998).

Repetition Priming

This chapter concentrates on PET and fMRI studies of priming. As stated above, repetition priming has been associated with a reduction in the haemodynamic response. Furthermore, this repetition suppression is normally restricted to regions that are generally responsive to the stimuli used (*e.g.*, regions activated by repeated and control stimuli versus a low-level baseline such as fixation) (Schacter and Buckner, 1998). A simple interpretation of this finding is that the suppression reflects facilitated processing of a repeated stimulus (the target) due to performance of the same processes in the recent past (on the prime)—the "hot tubes" or "greased tracks" metaphors. A second observation is that repetition effects are often seen in multiple brain regions, suggesting that several stages in the processing pathway between stimulus and response can be facilitated (one or all of which may contribute to the behavioural measure of priming). Indeed, the amount of behavioural priming may depend on the degree of overlap between the pathways used for prime and target—the "component process" view of priming (Henson, in press; Witherspoon and Moscovitch, 1989). A third observation is that repetition effects are not seen in all regions associated with processing stimuli in the task. For example, repetition effects are not normally seen in early visual regions or late motor regions in visual-motor priming paradigms. This suggests that not all component processes between stimulus and response are facilitated by repetition. The computational properties of a process that determine whether it can be significantly facilitated by repetition is an important, though as yet unresolved, question. (A *process* in the current context is assumed to be a mapping or transformation between two representations, at least one of which is stimulus-specific.) The next section focuses on examples of face priming. One important conclusion resulting from these studies is that priming may also be associated with a response increase (repetition enhancement) under some conditions.

SUPPRESSION VERSUS ENHANCEMENT: FACE PRIMING

A series of three experiments have explored effects of face repetition during indirect tasks, using various manipulations of the face images and/or face familiarity. The focus of these experiments has been on the lateral midfusiform, a region widely implicated in face processing (Kanwisher *et al.*, 1997). As can be seen in Fig. 23.1, the pattern of repetition effects in this region across the three studies is complex and appears to contain discrepancies (*e.g.*, opposite interactions between face familiarity and repetition in the George *et al.*, 1999, and Henson *et al.*, 2000, studies). However, there are important differences between the stimuli used, and the complex pattern can be explained by a combination of two assumptions (Henson, in press).

The first assumption is that, when the same process occurs on initial and repeated presentations of a stimulus, a region subserving that process will show repetition suppression; however, when priming causes a process to occur on repeated presentations that did not occur on initial presentations, the region will show repetition enhancement. This assumption applies, in principle, to any form of priming. The second assumption, which is specific to face priming studies, is that the particular processes subserved by the right lateral midfusiform include both face perception (*i.e.*, discrimination of faces from non-face visual objects) and face recognition (*i.e.*, discrimination between familiar and unfamiliar faces).

Participants in the PET study of Dolan *et al.* (1997) passively viewed binarised images of either unfamiliar faces or objects, which were difficult to perceive as such on their initial presentation. When these degraded images were repeated following intervening presentation of an intact, greyscale version of each image (Fig. 23.1A), a greater number were reported to give a clear percept (though not when irrelevant images intervened, indicating stimulus-specific priming rather than a general practice effect). Greater responses to primed than unprimed face

	Unprimed	Primed		Repetition effect
A. Dolan et al (1997)				
Perception	X	√	=>	enhancement
Recognition	X	X		
B. George et al (1999)				
Perception	√	√	=>	suppression
Recognition	X	X		
Perception	√	√		
Recognition	X	√	=>	enhancement
C. Henson et al (2000)				
Perception	√	√		
Recognition	X	√	=>	enhancement
Perception	√	√		
Recognition	√	√	=>	suppression

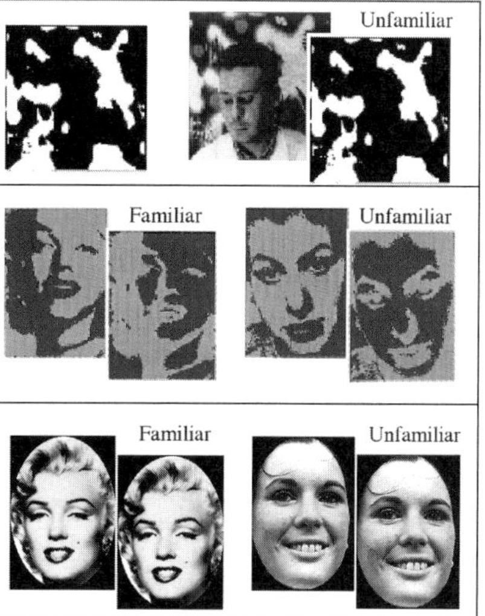

FIGURE 23.1
Schematic of the hypothetical processes of perception and recognition occurring for unprimed and primed face presentations across the studies of (A) Dolan *et al.* (1997), B) George *et al.* (1999), and (C) Henson *et al.* (2000). Examples of the stimuli used in each study are shown on the right. A combination of these two processes, together with a simple hypothesis about their hemodynamic correlates (see text), can explain the complex pattern of repetition effects across the three studies.

images were observed in a right midfusiform region (+44, –38, –28). This repetition enhancement can be attributed to a new process of face perception that occurred more often for repeated than initial image presentations.

Participants in the blocked fMRI study of George *et al.* (1999) viewed two-tone images of either famous or unfamiliar faces (Fig. 23.1B), monitoring for a rare target stimulus (not of interest). For the positive images, the shading provided by the light/dark tones was sufficient to identify the famous faces. For the negative images, the contrast polarity of the tones was reversed, producing faces that were difficult to identify (only ~20% of famous face negatives were identified). Identification of famous negatives was made easier (~45% identified) when they were primed by positive images of the same face. Greater bilateral midfusiform responses (*e.g.*, +46, –54, –12) were seen for blocks of famous negatives that were preceded by positive versions (primed) than for blocks of famous negatives that were not (unprimed). In contrast, these regions exhibited decreased responses to blocks of unfamiliar negatives that were preceded by positive versions, relative to blocks of unfamiliar negatives that were not.

An important difference between the George *et al.* (1999) and Dolan *et al.* (1997) studies is that the two-tone images of George *et al.* were perceived as faces, unlike (initial presentations of) the binarised images of Dolan *et al.* Thus, in the George *et al.* study, face perception occurred for both primed and unprimed face negatives, and the repetition of this process explains the repetition suppression for primed unfamiliar negatives. For the famous negatives, however, additional face recognition was more likely for primed than unprimed blocks. Assuming that the fusiform response increase due to face recognition was sufficient to outweigh the decrease due to repeated face perception, the repetition enhancement for famous negatives is consistent with the present hypothesis.

Participants in the third study of Henson *et al.* (2000) again performed an indirect target-monitoring task, this time while viewing intact images of famous and unfamiliar faces, each of which was presented twice in a randomised, event-related fMRI design (Fig. 23.1C). The right midfusiform (+45, –57, –24) evidenced an interaction between face familiarity and repetition, with repetition suppression for famous faces but repetition enhancement for unfamiliar faces.

An important difference between the famous faces of George *et al.* (1999) and Henson *et al.* (2000) is that the intact famous faces of Henson *et al.* could be recognized on initial presentations, unlike the unprimed famous negatives of George *et al.* Thus, face recognition (and perception) occurred in the Henson *et al.* study for both initial and repeated presentations of famous faces, explaining the associated fusiform repetition suppression. To explain the repetition enhancement for unfamiliar faces, Henson *et al.* (2000) assumed that a single presentation of an intact unfamiliar face was sufficient to form a new, structural representation of that face, such that it can be recognized (as familiar) when repeated.* This additional process of face recognition on repeated but not initial presentations of unfamiliar faces can then explain the repetition enhancement.

The assumption that initial presentations of unfamiliar stimuli can, under some conditions, form a new structural representation is consistent with the perceptual representation system (PRS) hypothesis of Schacter (1990). Indeed, this assumption also allows the present hypothesis to explain the repetition effects observed in a PET study of Schacter *et al.* (1995). This study used two-dimensional drawings of abstract (unfamiliar) objects, which either could or could not exist in three dimensions (possible or impossible objects, respectively). Behavioural experiments have shown that only the possible objects can be primed (Cooper *et al.*, 1992), leading to the hypothesis that new structural representations are only formed in the PRS for objects that are structurally coherent. Consistent with this, Schacter *et al.* (1995) only found a fusiform repetition effects for possible objects. Importantly, this repetition effect was a repetition enhancement. This pattern can be explained if, in addition to perception (of a three-dimensional object) that occurs on both first and second presentations of possible objects, the new structural representation allows

* This representation was assumed to be perceptual in nature (*e.g.*, a new face recognition unit; Goshen-Gottstein and Ganel, 2000) and clearly would not have the same semantic associations as those for famous faces, though it might be sufficient for an explicit recognition memory decision (which is well above chance under these conditions; Henson *et al.*, 2002). Note that such representations were less likely to be formed for the two-tone images in the George *et al.* (1999) study, for which explicit recognition was likely to be poor.

recognition of repeated presentations as individual objects (analogous to the above argument for unfamiliar faces in Henson *et al.*, 2000). For impossible objects on the other hand, perception (of a three-dimensional object) cannot occur on either first or second presentations, so the fusiform is not activated, and neither repetition suppression nor repetition enhancement result.

Fusiform repetition enhancement has not always been found for unfamiliar faces (Henson *et al.*, 2002, 2003) or unfamiliar possible objects (van Turennout *et al.*, 2000; Vuilleumier *et al.*, 2002). This may reflect additional sensitivity of repetition effects to the task (Henson *et al.*, 2002) or the repetition lag (Henson *et al.*, 2000). What is found consistently is an interaction between familiarity and repetition in the midfusiform, with greater repetition suppression for familiar than unfamiliar stimuli. Repetition suppression for unfamiliar stimuli is seen in more posterior visual regions, such as lateral occipital cortex (Henson *et al.*, 2002; van Turennout *et al.*, 2000; Vuilleumier *et al.*, 2002). This suppression may reflect repetition of earlier visual processes common to familiar and unfamiliar stimuli.

In summary, a simple hypothesis—that repetition suppression occurs when the same process is performed on initial and repeated presentations, whereas repetition enhancement occurs when a new process occurs on repetition—can explain quite a complex pattern of fusiform repetition effects in indirect memory tasks using faces. In the case of the right midlateral fusiform, these processes are assumed to include both face perception and face recognition. This secondary assumption receives independent support from other contrasts in these studies, such as the greater response to primed faces than primed objects in the Dolan *et al.* (1997) study (*i.e.*, face perception), greater responses to unprimed positive than unprimed negative images of famous faces in the George *et al.* (1999) study (face recognition), and greater responses to initial presentations of famous than initial presentations of unfamiliar faces in the Henson *et al.* (2000) study (face recognition). These processes may in fact generalize to other types of visual object (including, for example, familiar and unfamiliar symbols; Henson *et al.*, 2000). The extent to which this hypothesis extends to other priming paradigms remains to be tested.

VISUAL OBJECT PRIMING: PRIMING AS A TOOL

If one assumes that repetition of the same process on initial and repeated stimulus presentations produces a response decrease, then this repetition suppression can be used as a tool to investigate the nature of the processes performed in different brain regions. This logic has been applied most extensively to visual object processing, by testing whether repetition suppression generalizes across various changes in the visual stimulus. For example, if a region shows equivalent levels of repetition suppression for objects depicted from either the same or different viewpoint, then the processes subserved by that region can be assumed to operate over view-independent (or object-based) representations. More generally, the logic is that, if region R shows reduced repetition suppression to a target that differs from the prime only on dimension D, then the processes subserved by region R are sensitive to dimension D. This is analogous to the way that behavioural priming has been used to investigate different stages in object processing (Biederman and Cooper, 1991).

Moreover, it has been claimed that such an approach is particularly useful in neuroimaging because it offers greater spatial resolution (Grill-Spector *et al.*, 1999; Naccache and Dehaene, 2001). The argument behind this "hyper-resolution" is that a voxel sampled by fMRI or PET may contain a mixture of neurons with different selectivities (Fig. 23.2A). Though the spatial distribution of neural firing within that voxel may distinguish two stimuli, the mean level of activity may not. However, if these neurons fire less vigorously following prior presentation of the same stimulus (*i.e.*, habituate or adapt), the mean activity levels will differ, and the region will show repetition suppression effects that are detectable with fMRI or PET.

This logic was first used by Grill-Spector *et al.* (1999) in a blocked fMRI paradigm. The response in the lateral occipital complex (LOC), which includes lateral occipital and posterior fusiform regions, decreased as the frequency of object repetition within a block increased (a technique they called "fMR adaptation"). The degree to which this adaptation was sensitive to variations in the repeated objects was used to isolate the representational level of different regions within LOC. For example, a more anterior part of LOC (in posterior fusiform gyrus and

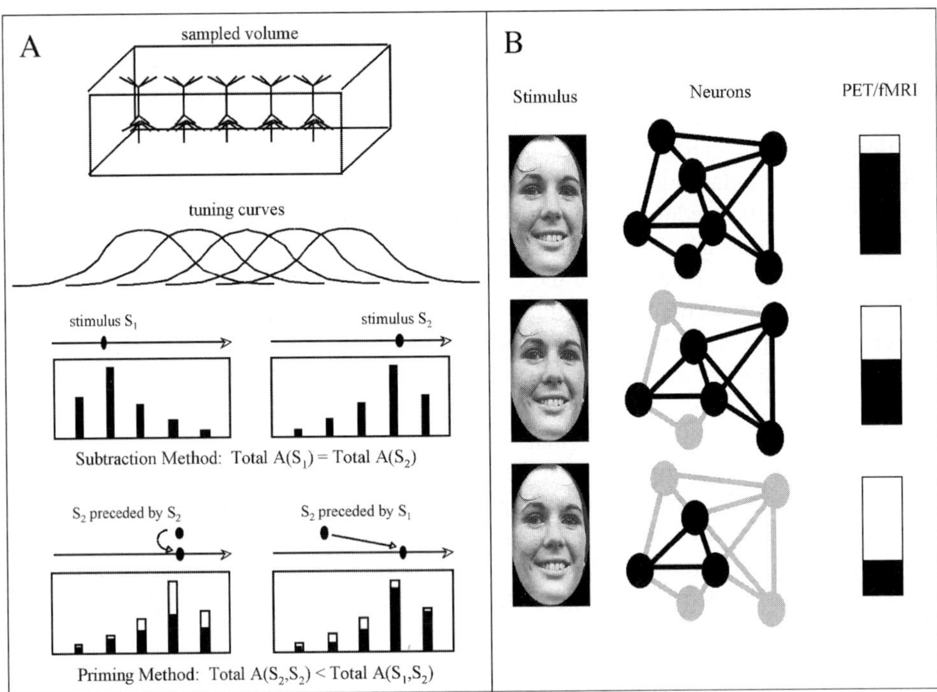

FIGURE 23.2
(A) Schematic of hyper-resolution argument of Grill-Spector *et al.* (1999) and Naccache and Dehaene (2001). Automatic, neuron-specific adaptation may reveal hemodynamic differences in an image voxel that encompasses many neurons with different tuning curves, even when a conventional subtraction of two different stimuli may not. (Adapted from Naccache and Dehaene, 2001.) (B) Sharpening theory of Wiggs and Martin (1998) in which repetition of a stimulus (left column) produces stimulus-specific response suppression in some neurons (grayed out in middle column), which "drop out" of the stimulus representation, and a decrease in the hemodynamic response (repetition suppression; right column).

occipitotemporal sulcus) was invariant to the size and location of the object but not to the illumination or viewpoint of the object, implicating this region in non-retinotopic but view-based (rather than fully object-based) representations.

One problem with the approach of Grill-Spector *et al.* (1999), in which the size of the stimulus set is varied across blocks, is that participants are likely to anticipate different frequencies of repetitions (particularly if a direct memory task such as a "one-back task" is used). In such cases, any adaptation may simply reflect decreases in attention. Moreover, the relationship between multiple, short lag repetitions and the single, long-lag repetition used in typical priming experiments needs to be established (immediate repetition, in particular, may be a special case; Bentin and Moscovitch, 1988; Nagy and Rugg, 1989). Indeed, it may be useful to distinguish neural *adaptation*, which is likely under the short-lag, high-frequency repetition conditions of the Grill-Spector *et al.* (1999) paradigm, from neural *response suppression*, which occurs after a single presentation and can be long lasting.

Event-related fMRI paradigms allow repeated and nonrepeated stimuli to be randomly intermixed such that participants cannot anticipate repetitions. Kourtzi and Kanwisher (2000), for example, compared event-related responses to pairs of trials in which either the same or different objects were depicted, and they varied the order of such trial pairs unpredictably. The immediate repetition in this particular design may still represent a special case, however. An event-related approach to long-lag priming was taken by Vuilleumier *et al.* (2002). The aim of this study was to simultaneously examine effects of viewpoint changes and size changes on visual object processing. Participants made object decisions regarding real or nonsense objects (Fig. 23.3A), reaction times for which showed priming in all cases. However, although the magnitude of the priming effect for objects was independent of size changes, it was greater for objects repeated in the same than different view (Tarr *et al.*, 1998).

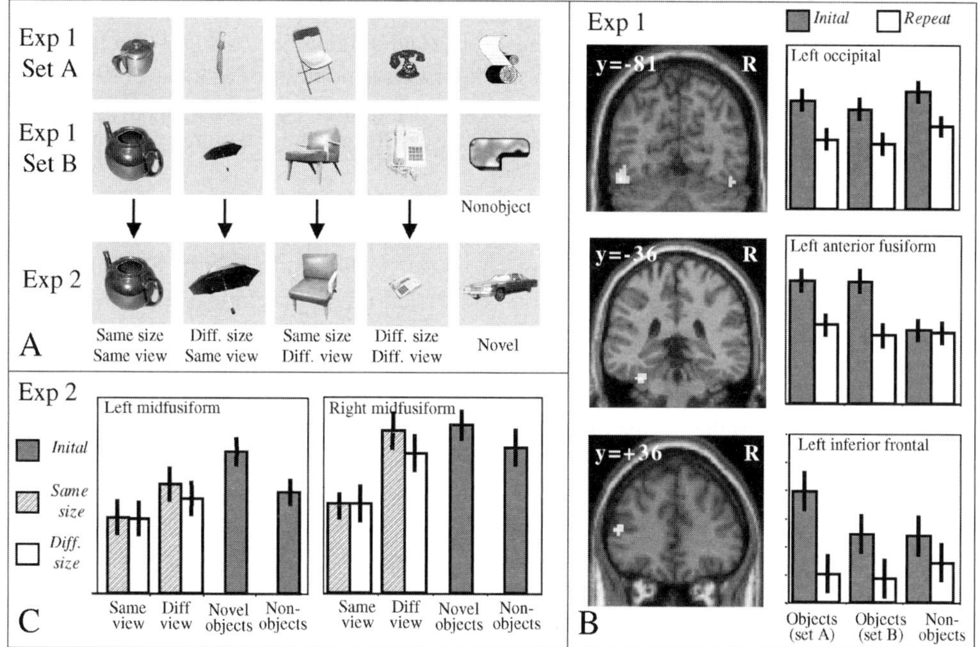

FIGURE 23.3
(A) Stimuli and conditions in Vuilleumier *et al.* (2002). Sets A and B contained different exemplars of a category with the same basic-level name. In Experiment 1, set A was presented before set B, such that the first presentation of a set B object was preceded by a different exemplar with the same name. In Experiment 2, objects from one or other set in Experiment 1 were repeated in either the same or different size and from the same or different viewpoint, together with novel objects not seen in Experiment 1. Non-objects were present in both experiments, and participants performed an object/non-object decision. (B) Canonical response parameter estimates in Experiment 1 from left occipital cortex (top) showing repetition suppression for both objects and non-objects, from left anterior fusiform (middle) showing repetition suppression for objects only, and from left inferior frontal cortex (bottom) in which first presentations of set B objects showed repetition suppression relative to first presentations of set A objects. (C) Canonical response parameter estimates in Experiment 2 from left and right midfusiform regions; left midfusiform showed repetition suppression across different sizes and different views, whereas right midfusiform showed repetition suppression only across same views.

Bilateral lateral occipital regions (*e.g.*, –48, –75, –3) showed similar levels of repetition suppression for both real and nonsense objects (Fig. 23.3B). This is consistent for a role of these regions in general shape extraction, prior to object recognition (Malach *et al.*, 1995). Bilateral middle (*e.g.*, +42, –57, –18) and left anterior (–33, –36, –27) fusiform, however, showed greater repetition suppression for real than nonsense objects, suggesting a role in object recognition.*

Despite the fact that early retinotopic regions showed greater responses to large than small objects, as expected, such size changes did not interact with repetition effects in any brain region. This suggests that object repetition effects only emerge after location-invariant (non-retinotopic) representations have been accessed. View changes, on the other hand, revealed an interesting lateralization of fusiform responses. Whereas right midfusiform showed an interaction between view changes and repetition effects, with greater repetition suppression for same than different views, the left midfusiform showed similar levels of repetition suppression for same and different views (Fig. 23.3C). In other words, the left fusiform exhibited view invariance, whereas the right fusiform exhibited view specificity.

This hemispheric lateralization is not unprecedented. Koutstaal *et al.* (2001) compared repetition effects across same and different exemplars of the same object category (with the same name). They found a greater effect of exemplar change in right than left fusiform. This reflected repetition suppression for both same and different exemplars in the left fusiform, but only for same exemplars in the right fusiform. In other words, it appeared that the right fusiform treated

* Unlike Schacter *et al.* (1995), no repetition enhancement was found for nonsense objects in the present study (even though the nonsense objects were still possible three-dimensional structures). The nature of fusiform repetition effects for unfamiliar objects remains unclear.

different exemplars (*e.g.*, two different umbrellas) as different objects, whereas the left fusiform treated them as the same object. Koutstaal *et al.* (2001) and Vuilleumier *et al.* (2002) related their fusiform laterality effects to the hemispheric specialization hypothesis of Marsolek (1995). This hypothesis is based on behavioural priming effects using split-visual-field presentation and postulates that the right hemisphere retains specific visual-form representations, whereas the left hemisphere retains more abstract representations.

The Vuilleumier *et al.* (2002) study, however, also included a manipulation of same versus different exemplars and did not find the same results at Koutstaal *et al.* (2001). Although the left fusiform generalized over different views of an object, it did not appear to generalize over different exemplars of the same object category. Only a left inferior prefrontal region (−48, +36, +12) showed repetition suppression across different exemplars (from set A to set B in Fig. 23.3B; see legend), probably reflecting facilitation of verbal processes related to object naming. The reason for the apparent discrepancy between the Vuilleumier *et al.* and Koutstaal *et al.* studies is unclear but may relate to the degree of visual similarity between the different exemplars of the same category (for further discussion, see Vuilleumier *et al.*, 2002).

In summary, the results of studies like that of Vuilleumier *et al.* (2002) are converging on a hierarchical model of visual object processing in which object representations become more abstracted from posterior to anterior occipital/temporal regions and possibly more abstracted in left than right hemispheres. Early retinotopic regions do not appear to show repetition effects. Rather, lateral occipital regions appear to support the earliest stage at which repetition effects emerge, and these appear to arise from size-invariant, but not view-invariant, representations that are independent of long-term object experience (*i.e.*, are equivalent for familiar and unfamiliar objects). More anterior fusiform regions appear to support long-term knowledge of familiar objects, which appears to be view-independent in the left fusiform and view-dependent in the right fusiform. Later stages of object naming can also show repetition effects that engage components of the language system, including left inferior frontal cortex.

VERBAL PRIMING: PRIMING AS A TOOL

The same logic of using repetition effects to map functional anatomy has also been used in imaging studies of language. Behavioural priming effects across various changes in letter case, word form, or modality, for example, have been used for many years to argue for separate stages of orthographic, morphological, phonological, and/or lexicosemantic processing. A preliminary study of word repetition effects was performed by Henson (2001). Initial and repeated presentations of words and pseudo-words were randomly intermixed in an event-related fMRI design. Of particular interest was the interaction between lexicality and repetition, which was seen in a left anterior temporal region (−36, −6, −33), with repetition suppression for words, and repetition enhancement for pseudo-words. This region may support processing of visual word forms (or even abstract lexical representations), although other properties unique to the words (*e.g.*, semantics) cannot be ruled out (see below).

Other imaging studies have examined *semantic priming*, which refers to the facilitation (or inhibition) of the processing of the meaning of a target stimulus by a preceding prime. Semantic priming tends to be short lived, restricted to immediate prime-target presentations. At least two potential contributions to semantic priming have been proposed: automatic spreading of activation in a semantic network (Collins and Loftus, 1975) and strategic/attentional effects (Posner and Snyder, 1975).

Mummery *et al.* (1999) varied the proportion of semantically related prime targets across PET scans (from 0 to 100%) in order to study semantic priming within a lexical decision task. Increasing this proportion is believed to increase the relative contribution of strategic effects (Neely, 1991). Consistent with this hypothesis, the amount of priming (per target) increased as the proportion of related prime-target pairs increased. The responses in a left anterior temporal region (−40, −4, −28), close to that in Henson (2001), decreased as the proportion increased from 0 to 75%, but increased from 75 to 100%. Though difficult to interpret unambiguously, one explanation for this pattern is a combination of an automatic semantic process producing the decrease (due to increasing levels of repetition suppression as the incidence of repeated semantic processing within the scan increased) that is offset by a strategic effect at the highest proportion of related pairs (producing the response increase, perhaps due to nonspecific enhancement of semantic processing in that region).

In a subsequent study, Rossell *et al.* (2003) used event-related fMRI to compare prime-target stimulus onset asynchonies (SOAs) of 200 ms versus 1000 ms in a lexical decision task. Automatic processes in semantic priming are assumed to dominate at short prime-target SOAs (<250 ms), whereas strategic effects are assumed to become more important at longer SOAs (Neely, 1991). The only region showing repetition suppression was in left anterior temporal cortex (−40, +14, −24), slightly anterior to that observed by Mummery *et al.* (1999). This supports a role for this region in semantic processing; however, the amount of repetition suppression did not interact with SOA, leaving its precise role unclear.

The left anterior temporal cortex (−42, 0, −30) also showed repetition suppression for blocks of sentences with the same versus different syntactic forms in a study by Nopponey and Price (submitted). A behavioural experiment confirmed priming of such sentences in the form of shorter reading times for same versus different syntactic forms. This *syntactic priming* could not reflect word-specific semantic priming, as the sentences contained different content words, but could reflect facilitation of sentence-level semantic integration (*e.g.*, the assignment of thematic roles to sentence arguments). The above priming studies thus represent important inroads into the functional anatomy of semantic processing and suggest future studies that may further refine the nature of the semantic processing (*e.g.*, by factorially varying same versus different content words and same versus different syntactic frames).

In summary, by assuming that repetition suppression is as a signature of repeated processing, the investigation of various stimulus manipulations on the amount of repetition suppression offers a potentially powerful means of mapping different stages in stimulus-processing. An alternative approach is to keep the stimulus constant while varying the relationship between the tasks performed on prime and target (*i.e.*, varying the manner in which the prime and target are processed; see Henson, in press). In both cases, however, before a brain region evidencing repetition suppression can be associated with a particular process, precautions must be taken to rule out other psychological processes, such as explicit memory or attention, that may also covary with the stimulus/task manipulations in that region.

NEURAL MECHANISMS OF REPETITION SUPPRESSION

A potential neural analogue of the repetition suppression observed with fMRI and PET is *response suppression* (Desimone, 1996) or *decremental responses* (Brown and Xiang, 1998). These terms refer to a decrease in the firing rate of neurons, typically recorded in inferior temporal regions of the non-human primate, following repetition of a stimulus. The decreased firing rate is not nonspecific habituation, because it occurs after a single exposure to a stimulus and does not affect the firing rate to other stimuli for which the neuron is responsive. (This stimulus-specific suppression thus represents a slightly different conception of the neuron-specific habituation assumed by Grill-Spector *et al.*, 1999; see Fig. 23.3A.) Moreover, it can last hours or days and through numerous intervening stimuli, although the longevity of the effect typically decreases from anterior (*e.g.*, 24 hr in perirhinal cortex, 10 min in area TE) to posterior regions, sometimes not surviving a single intervening stimulus in occipital-temporal regions (Brown and Xiang, 1998).

Wiggs and Martin (1998) extended this phenomenon to human imaging findings on priming. They proposed that repeated processing of a stimulus produces a "sharpening" of its cortical representation, whereby neurons coding features unnecessary for processing that stimulus respond less (*i.e.*, exhibit response suppression). This results in a decrease in the mean firing rate of a population of neurons, hence a decrease in the haemodynamic response from that region of cortex (Fig. 23.2B). This "sparser" representation then allows (somehow) faster/more accurate behavioural responses.

Though offering an attractive link between these different levels of neuroscience, there are potential complications to this simple mapping. For example, the association of neuronal response suppression with priming is yet to be established in non-human primates, as the same phenomenon (when observed in perirhinal cortex) has been interpreted in terms of explicit recognition memory (Brown and Xiang, 1998; see next chapter). One possibility is that the same neural signal of decreased firing rates is used for different purposes in different brain regions. Second, a mechanistic account is needed to explain how sparser representations allow faster/more accurate processing (*i.e.*, priming). Third, the limited duration of neural response suppression in posterior occipito-temporal regions (Baylis and Rolls, 1987) is unlikely to account for the haemodynamic repetition suppression observed across days in those regions in humans (van Turennout *et al.*, 2000). Fourth, such a theory would not appear to be able to explain the greater fusiform repetition suppression effects for familiar than unfamiliar stimuli, as the opposite interaction would be predicted by the Wiggs and Martin (1998) theory—namely, greater repetition suppression for unfamiliar than familiar stimuli (given that the latter are already likely to have sparse representations) (Li *et al.*, 1993). See Henson and Rugg (2002) for further discussion of these issues.

Two further questions concern the relationship between neural firing rates and haemodynamic responses (aside from the physiological relationship between action potentials, local field potentials, and blood-oxygen-level-dependent [BOLD] responses) (Logothetis *et al.*, 2001). Even with event-related fMRI, it must be remembered that the haemodynamic response effectively integrates several seconds of neural/synaptic activity. This means that a decrease in the magnitude of the haemodynamic response may not reflect decreased neural firing rates *per se*, but a shortened duration of neural/synaptic activity. One way to try to distinguish these possibilities is to test for differences in the peak latency, as well as magnitude, of the event-related BOLD response. Henson and Rugg (2001) found that repetition of famous faces not only decreased the peak magnitude of the BOLD impulse response in a right fusiform region but also decreased its peak latency (though not onset latency). The most parsimonious account of this combined change in BOLD magnitude and peak latency is that repetition reduced the duration of underlying neural/synaptic activity. At least one reason for a reduced duration of neural activity, in an alternative mechanism of repetition suppression, is a decreased "settling" time in an attractor neural network, following short-term weight changes associated with processing of the prime. Such networks have been applied successfully to priming data (Plaut and Shallice, 1993).

A final question concerns the onset latency of repetition effects. Neural response suppression can be very rapid, with the shortest differential latency in perirhinal neurons equalling their visual response latency (70 to 80ms) and estimates of the mean population latency being as short as 150 ms (Ringo, 1996). These estimates have been used to argue that response suppression (even in anterior temporal regions) is a local effect, too rapid for reentrant (or top-down) influences (Brown and Xiang, 1998). These latencies are shorter than the latencies of stimulus repetition effects measured with event-related potentials (ERPs) in humans, which typically onset at 250 to 300 ms (Rugg and Doyle, 1994). (Earlier repetition effects of 100 to 200 ms have been reported in some ERP studies, but usually for immediate repetition; Nagy and Rugg, 1989, though for exceptions see George *et al.*, 1997; Tsivilis *et al.*, 2001.) Human intracranial ERP recordings in inferior temporal regions, for example, show early face-specific potentials, onsetting 150 to 200 ms after the stimulus, but provide no evidence that these potentials are sensitive to repetition of faces; such effects only emerge 250 to 300 ms after the stimulus (Puce *et al.*, 1999).

These ERP data therefore raise the possibility that haemodynamic repetition suppression in humans involve later (*e.g.*, reentrant) effects.* Indeed, in an exciting study that used fMRI data to constrain the source of magnetoencephalography (MEG) priming-related effects in a semantic decision task to words (Dale *et al.*, 2000), an initial wave of activity had spread to temporal, parietal, and even frontal regions by 185 ms. The earliest repetition effect, however, emerged in a left anterior inferior temporal region at 250 ms and was strongest at 385 ms. These data reinforce the possibility that priming effects do not necessarily arise in a "first pass" through the neural circuitry and that effects in posterior regions include top-down influences from more anterior regions.

One possibility is that repetition effects in a region reflect changes in the prediction error fed back from higher levels in a processing pathway (Friston, 2003). According to this model,

*As with any imaging study, it must be remembered that, just because activations occur in brain regions associated with "early" stages of visual processing, this does not mean that differences in the underlying neural activity occur early in time.

stimulus processing modifies the strengths of recurrent synaptic connections between different levels of a neural hierarchy, which in turn affect the dynamics of each level in settling on an interpretation (*e.g.*, recognition) of a stimulus. In the case of repetition suppression, an increase in the synaptic efficacy of feedforward and feedback connections between two layers, following initial presentation of a stimulus, decreases the error in the lower level between its bottom-up (stimulus-related) and top-down (prediction-related) inputs when that stimulus is repeated. This reduced error may result in more rapid stimulus recognition and a reduced haemodynamic response in the lower region. The important perspective offered by this model is that priming reflects interactions between different brain regions. The specific regions will then depend on the set of component processes engaged by the stimulus and task.

PHARMACOLOGICAL CHALLENGES

The cholinergic system influences neural plasticity and has been shown to modulate explicit memory (*e.g.*, Curran *et al.*, 1998; see also Chapter 17, this volume). Its role in implicit memory is more controversial, because the administration of a cholinergic blocker (such as the drug scopolamine, an acetylcholine antagonist) has not been found to affect measures of priming in some studies (Schifano and Curran, 1994; though see below). Furthermore, scopolamine does not appear to affect the neural phenomenon of response suppression (Miller and Desimone, 1993). By contrast, modulations of the GABAergic system (by the drug lorazepam, for example, a GABA agonist) do affect priming (Vidailhet *et al.*, 1999).

Thiel *et al.* (2001) examined the effects of both scopolamine and lorazepam on repetition suppression in an event-related fMRI study of word-stem completion. Both drugs were found to reduce behavioural measures of priming, consistent with previous studies using lorazepam, but contrary to previous studies using scopolamine. This suggests that cholinergic blockage can impair some forms of priming (one reason why such an effect was not seen in previous studies may be that they used smaller doses of scopolamine). Both drugs also reduced the amount of repetition suppression in left extrastriate occipital cortex (−36, −75, −6) and left inferior (−45, +39, −9) and posterior (−39, −3, 54) frontal cortex (Fig. 23.4A), regions associated with word-stem priming in the placebo group and in previous studies (*e.g.*, Buckner *et al.*, 2000).*

The reason for the reduced repetition suppression under the drugs was a reduced response to unprimed stems relative to the placebo group (except for the extrastriate region in the scopolamine group; Fig. 23.4A). This suggests that the drugs impaired initial processing of the stimuli, perhaps impairing the registration of stimulus information and so not affecting the response when the stimuli were repeated. The failure to find an effect of scopolamine on neural measures of response suppression (Miller and Desimone, 1993) may reflect differences between the haemodynamic and neural indices or differences in the experimental paradigms (*e.g.*, the task, or the repetition lag).

Thiel *et al.* (2002) examined effects of the same drugs within a face-priming paradigm. Participants made speeded familiarity decisions regarding familiar and unfamiliar faces, half of which had been presented in a previous study phase. In this case, reduced priming, in the form of decreased reaction times (RTs) for familiar but not unfamiliar faces, was found with scopolamine, but not with lorazepam. A right fusiform region (+30, −45, −30) showed similar familiarity-by-repetition interactions in the placebo and lorazepam groups, with greater repetition suppression for familiar than unfamiliar faces, but this interaction was not significant in the scopolamine group (Fig. 23.4B), although no interactions between the scopolamine and placebo groups reached significance, either. These data support those of Thiel *et al.* (2001) in suggesting that cholinergic blockage can attenuate priming. They also suggest that the effect of GABAergic modulation on priming (at least with lorazepam) may depend on the specific priming task (*e.g.*, identification versus production tasks) (Gabrieli *et al.*, 1999).

* It is possible that scopolamine affects arousal and/or explicit memory in this paradigm. However, the priming effects did not correlate with various measures of sedation or with global haemodynamic estimates. Moreover, a concurrent manipulation of the degree of semantic processing at study (which improves explicit memory, see next chapter) did not interact with the amount of priming. This argues against explicit memory contamination of the behavioural measures (though it remains possible that differences in explicit memory contaminated the haemodynamic measures).

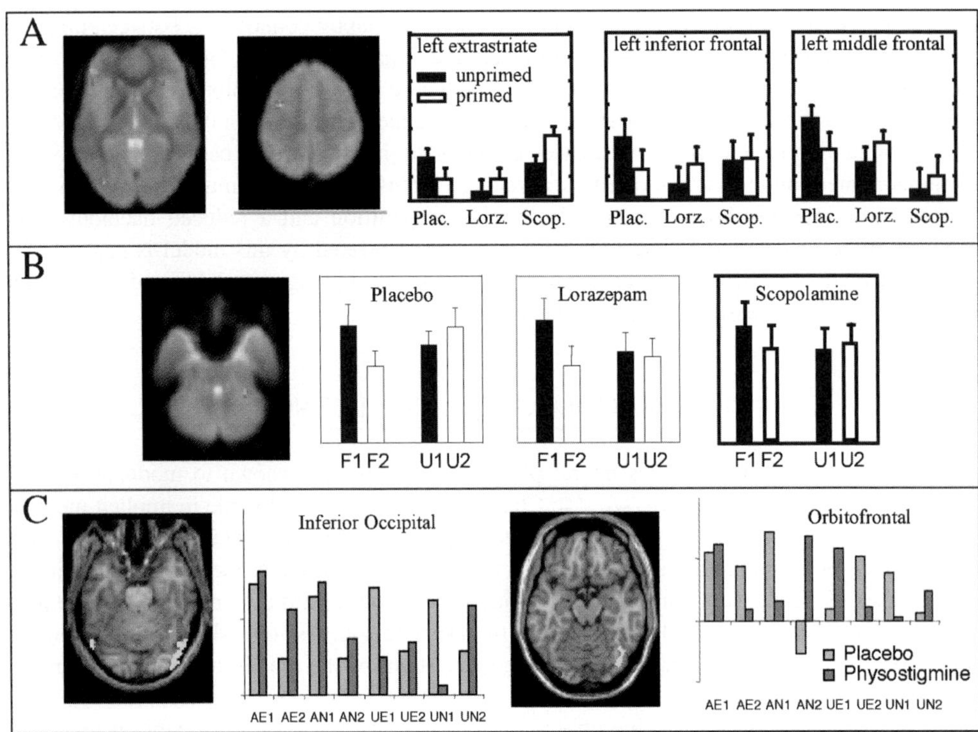

FIGURE 23.4
(A) Left extrastriate, inferior frontal, and dorsal frontal regions from Thiel *et al.* (2001), together with canonical response parameter estimates to unprimed and primed word stems in placebo, lorazepam, and scopolamine groups. (B) Right midfusiform from Thiel *et al.* (2002), together with canonical response parameter estimates to first and second presentations of familiar (F1 and F2) and unfamiliar (U1 and U2) faces in the placebo, lorazepam and scopolamine groups. (C) Right inferior occipital and orbitofrontal regions from Bentley *et al.* (2003), together with canonical response parameter estimates in the eight experimental conditions (A, attended; U, unattended; N, neutral, E, emotional; 1, first face-pair presentation; and 2, second face-pair presentation) for the placebo and physostigmine groups.

Thiel *et al.* (2002) performed a further behavioural study on an independent group of participants, in which scopolamine was administered after the study phase. In this case, priming did not differ significantly from a placebo group. This supports the assumption that cholinergic blockade affects the acquisition rather than expression of priming.

A study by Bentley *et al.* (2003) examined the effects of physostigmine, a cholinesterase inhibitor (*i.e.*, having effects broadly complementary to those of scopolamine). This study also manipulated the factors of attention and emotion in a face/house matching paradigm. Two pairs of stimuli were presented simultaneously, one pair above or below a central fixation point (vertical locations) and the other pair left or right of fixation (horizontal locations). In each trial, one stimulus pair consisted of the same or different (unfamiliar) faces, and the other consisted of the same or different (unfamiliar) houses. Prior to a block of trials, participants were cued to respond "same" or "different" to the two stimuli appearing in either the vertical or horizontal locations. In this way, covert spatial attention could be directed toward either faces or houses.

The critical stimuli were the face pairs, which repeated across two to five intervening trials (the repetition factor). Each face pair also consisted of either neutral or fearful faces (the emotion factor) and could occur in either attended or unattended locations (the attention factor). Note that either both presentations of a face pair were attended or both presentations were unattended. For the placebo group, reaction times showed priming for neutral but not fearful faces when attended (for unattended faces, reaction times pertain to match decisions for the houses, for which the notion of priming is unclear). The lack of priming for fearful faces may reflect automatic orienting or attentional capture that counteracts any facilitation due to prior processing. This interaction between repetition and emotion for attended faces was absent in the physostigmine group, however.

A right occipital region (+40, –78, –18) in the placebo group showed repetition suppression for both attended and unattended face pairs, regardless of face emotion (Fig. 23.4C). Interestingly, a parahippocampal region (–22, –32, –10) showed repetition enhancement for unattended faces (*i.e.*, when houses were task relevant), possibly reflecting reduced interference from "distracting" faces. Assuming that the paradigm was successful in abolishing attention to task-irrelevant locations (as suggested by Vuilleumier *et al.*, 2001), the occipital findings suggest that some brain regions can show automatic repetition suppression in the absence of top-down modulation. (Note that these lateral occipital repetition suppression effects for unfamiliar faces resemble those found by Henson *et al.*, 2002, and are posterior to the fusiform regions that did appear sensitive to top-down modulation in that study.) Under physostigmine, however, repetition suppression in these regions was only found for attended faces. Indeed, a left occipital region (–34, –68, –22; not shown) showed greater repetition suppression under physostigmine than under placebo, but only for attended faces. This is consistent with the suggestion that cholinergic enhancement selectively facilitates processing of attended stimuli (Sarter *et al.*, 2001).

An interaction between repetition and emotion for attended (but not unattended) faces was found in right lateral orbitofrontal cortex (+38, +38, –14) for the placebo group, with greater suppression for neutral than fearful faces (Fig. 23.4C), paralleling the behavioural data. This interaction appeared to reverse under physostigmine, however, with greater relative repetition suppression for emotional faces. This is consistent with cholinergic enhancement of the processing of emotional stimuli (Holland and Gallagher, 1999).

In summary, pharmacological manipulations, such as those that affect the cholinergic system, can be shown to interact with behavioural measures of priming and their putative underlying haemodynamic correlates. The interactions are complex, depending on the specific priming task, levels of attention, valence of the stimuli, and probably factors such as dose levels and time of administration. Nonetheless, pharmacological manipulations may offer one way to dissociate implicit and explicit contributions to repetition effects and also provide an important means to get at the mechanisms underlying neural (and haemodynamic) repetition effects, particularly in conjunction with artificial neural network models (Sohal and Hasselmo, 2000).

CONCLUSION

This chapter has described studies selected from the Wellcome Department of Imaging Neuroscience that combine functional imaging with the behavioural phenomenon of repetition priming. Several themes have been discussed: (1) a simple hypothesis that distinguishes repetition suppression and repetition enhancement, using face priming as an example; (2) the use of repetition suppression as a tool for functional mapping, illustrated with examples from visual object and verbal semantic priming; (3) possible neural mechanisms underlying haemodynamic repetition effects; and (4) the value of pharmacological manipulations.

Several caveats remain to be addressed. Foremost, no imaging study to date has ruled out explicit memory contamination of repetition effects (except for studies of masked priming; see, for example, Dehaene *et al.*, 2001, which may represent a special case; Henson, 2003). Some simple precautions to minimize explicit memory include the use of speeded responses, switching the task performed on prime and target (also ruling out facilitation of low-level response contingencies), and experimental manipulations known to reduce explicit memory encoding (*e.g.*, divided attention at study). However, even though explicit memory may be shown not to contribute to a concurrent behavioural measure of priming (*e.g.*, if speeded decisions to a target are too fast for recollection to play a role), because PET and fMRI average activity over seconds, the resulting haemodynamic changes may include effects of processes operating subsequent to the behavioural response, such as incidental recollection of the prime. A better solution is to use paradigms in which explicit memory for repetition is also measured (Schott *et al.*, 2002), or even to use direct memory paradigms (*e.g.*, focusing on old items that are "missed" in a recognition memory task; see next chapter). The scanning of amnesic patients (or normal participants under the influence of certain drugs) may be another way to minimize explicit memory, provided priming is still intact.

A second caveat is the question of cause and effect. Reduced responses to repeated stimuli in regions of interest may be an effect, rather than the cause, of behavioural priming effects. Repetition suppression in the fusiform, for example, may reflect diminished attention to the stimulus or shortened gaze duration, as a consequence of priming-related facilitation in other brain regions. Questions like these are difficult to answer with imaging techniques alone and would benefit from concurrent demonstrations of reduced priming in patients with damage to the region of interest (Keane *et al.*, 1995) or following transcranial magnetic stimulation (TMS) of that region. Another approach is to use haemodynamic data to help localize MEG/EEG effects and argue for cause or effect on the basis of temporal precedence in the time course of repetition effects.

Acknowledgments

This work is funded by Wellcome Trust Fellowship 060924. The author would like to thank Paul Bentley, Ray Dolan, Pia Rotshtein, Mick Rugg, Tim Shallice, and Christiane Thiel for useful discussions.

References

Baylis, G. C. and Rolls, E. T. (1987). Responses of neurons in the inferior temporal cortex in short term and serial recognition memory tasks. *Exp. Brain Res.*, **65**, 614–622.

Bentin, S. and Moscovitch, M. (1988). The time course of repetition effects for words and unfamiliar faces. *J. Exp. Psychol. Gen.*, **117**, 148–160.

Bentley, P., Vuilleumier, P., Thiel, C. M., Driver, J., and Dolan, R. J. (2003). Effects of attention and emotion on repetition priming and their modulation by cholinergic enhancement, *J. Neurophysiol.*, **90**, 1171–1181.

Biederman, I. and Cooper, E. E. (1991). Evidence for complete translational and reflectional invariance in visual object priming. *Perception*, **20**, 585–593.

Brown, M. W. and Xiang, J. Z. (1998). Recognition memory: neuronal substrates if the judgement of prior occurrence. *Progr. Neurobiol.*, **55**, 149–189.

Buckner, R. L., Koutstaal, W., Schacter, D. L., and Rosen, B. R. (2000). Functional MRI evidence for a role of frontal and inferior temporal cortex in amodal components of priming. *Brain*, **123**(Pt. 3), 620–640.

Collins, A. M. and Loftus, E. F. (1975). A spreading-activation theory of semantic processing. *Psychol. Rev.*, **82**, 407–428.

Cooper, L. A., Schacter, D. L., Ballesteros, S., and Moore, C. (1992). Priming and recognition of transformed three-dimensional objects: effects of size and reflection. *J. Exp. Psychol. Learn. Mem. Cogn.*, **18**, 43–57.

Curran, H. V., Pooviboonsuk, P., Dalton, J. A., and Lader, M. H. (1998). Differentiating the effects of centrally acting drugs on arousal and memory: an event-related potential study of scopolamine, lorazepam and diphenhydramine. *Psychopharmacol. (Berlin)*, **135**, 27–36.

Dale, A. M., Liu, A. K., Fischl, B. R., Buckner, R. L., Belliveau, J. W., Lewine, J. D., and Halgren, E. (2000). Dynamic statistical parametric mapping: combining fMRI and MEG for high-resolution imaging of cortical activity. *Neuron*, **26**, 55–67.

Dehaene, S., Naccache, L., Cohen, L., Bihan, D. L., Mangin, J. F., Poline, J. B., and Riviere, D. (2001). Cerebral mechanisms of word masking and unconscious repetition priming. *Nat. Neurosci.*, **4**, 752–758.

Desimone, R. (1996). Neural mechanisms for visual memory and their role in attention. *P.N.A.S.*, **93**, 13494–13499.

Dolan, R. J., Fink, G. R., Rolls, E., Booth, M., Holmes, A., Frackowiak, R. S. J., and Friston, K. J. (1997). How the brain learns to see objects and faces in an impoverished context. *Nature*, **389**, 596–599.

Friston, K. J. (2003). Functional integration and inference in the brain. *Progr. Neurobiol.*, **68**, 113–143.

Gabrieli, J. D., Vaidya, C. J., Stone, M., Francis, W. S., Thompson-Schill, S. L., Fleischman, D. A., Tinklenberg, J. R., Yesavage, J. A., and Wilson, R. S. (1999). Convergent behavioural and neuropsychological evidence for a distinction between identification and production forms of repetition priming. *J. Exp. Psychol. Gen.*, **128**, 479–498.

George, N., Jemel, B., Fiori, N., and Renault, B. (1997). Face and shape repetition effects in humans: a spatio-temporal ERP study. *NeuroReport*, **8**, 1417–1423.

George, N., Dolan, R. J., Fink, G. R., Baylis, G. C., Russell, C., and Driver, J. (1999). Contrast polarity and face recognition in the human fusiform gyrus. *Nat. Neurosci.*, **2**, 574–580.

Goshen-Gottstein, Y. and Ganel, T. (2000). Repetition priming for familiar and unfamiliar faces in a sex-judgment task: evidence for a common route for the processing of sex and identity. *J. Exp. Psychol. Learn. Mem. Cogn.*, **26**, 1198–1214.

Graf, P. and Schacter, D. (1985). Implicit and explicit memory for new associations in normal and amnesic subjects. *J. Exp. Psychol. Learn. Mem. Cogn.*, **11**, 501–518.

Graf, P., Squire, L. R., and Mandler, G. (1984). The information that amnesic patients do not forget. *J. Exp. Psychol. Learn. Mem. Cogn.*, **10**, 164–178.

Grill-Spector, K., Kushnir, T., Edelman, S., Avidan, G., Itzchak, Y., and Malach, R. (1999). Differential processing of objects under various viewing conditions in the human lateral occipital complex. *Neuron*, **24**, 187–203.

Hayman, C. A. and Tulving, E. (1989). Contingent dissociation between recognition and fragment completion: the method of triangulation. *J. Exp. Psychol. Learn. Mem. Cogn.*, **15**, 228–240.

Henson, R. N. (2001). Repetition effects for words and nonwords as indexed by event-related fMRI: a preliminary study. *Scand. J. Psychol.*, **42**, 179–186.

Henson, R. N. A. (in press). Neuroimaging studies of priming.

Henson, R. N. A. (2004). Explicit memory, in *Human Brain Function*, 2nd ed., Frackowiak, R. S. J., Ed., Academic Press, San Diego.

Henson, R. N. A. and Rugg, M. D. (2001). Effects of stimulus repetition on latency of the BOLD impulse response. *NeuroImage*, **13**, 683.

Henson, R. N. A. and Rugg, M. D. (2002). Neural response suppression, haemodynamic repetition effects, and behavioural priming. *Neuropsychologia*, **41**, 263–270.

Henson, R. N., Shallice, T., and Dolan, R. (2000). Neuroimaging evidence for dissociable forms of repetition priming. *Science*, **287**, 1269–1272.

Henson, R. N., Shallice, T., Gorno-Tempini, M. L., and Dolan, R. J. (2002). Face repetition effects in implicit and explicit memory tests as measured by fMRI. *Cereb. Cortex*, **12**, 178–186.

Henson, R. N., Goshen-Gottstein, Y., Ganel, T., Otten, L. J., Quayle, A., and Rugg, M. D. (2003). Electrophysiological and haemodynamic correlates of face perception, recognition and priming. *Cereb. Cortex*, **13**, 793–825.

Holland, P. C. and Gallagher, M. (1999). Amygdala circuitry in attentional and representational processes. *Trends Cogn. Sci.*, **3**, 65–73.

Jacoby, L. L. and Dallas, M. (1981). On the relationship between autobiographical memory and perceptual learning. *J. Exp. Psychol. Gen.*, **110**, 306–340.

Jacoby, L. L., Toth, J. P., and Yonelinas, A. P. (1993). Separating conscious and unconscious influences of memory: measuring recollection. *J. Exp. Psychol. Gen.*, **122**, 139–154.

Kanwisher, N., McDermott, J., and Chun, M. M. (1997). The fusiform face area: a module in human extrastriate cortex specialised for face perception. *J. Neurosci.*, **17**, 4302–4311.

Keane, M. M., Gabrieli, J. D., Mapstone, H. C., Johnson, K. A., and Corkin, S. (1995). Double dissociation of memory capacities after bilateral occipital-lobe or medial temporal-lobe lesions, *Brain*, **118**, 1129–1148.

Kourtzi, Z. and Kanwisher, N. (2000). Cortical regions involved in perceiving object shape. *J. Neurosci.*, **20**, 3310–3318.

Koutstaal, W., Wagner, A. D., Rotte, M., Maril, A., Buckner, R. L., and Schacter, D. L. (2001). Perceptual specificity in visual object priming: functional magnetic resonance imaging evidence for a laterality difference in fusiform cortex. *Neuropsychologia*, **39**, 184–199.

Li, L., Miller, E. K., and Desimone, R. (1993). The representation of stimulus familiarity in anterior inferior temporal cortex. *J. Neurophysiol.*, **69**, 1918–1929.

Logothetis, N. K., Pauls, J., Augath, M., Trinath, T., and Oeltermann, A. (2001). Neurophysiological investigation of the basis of the fMRI signal. *Nature*, **412**, 150–157.

Malach, R., Reppas, J. B., Benson, R. R., Kwong, K. K., Jiang, H., Kennedy, W. A., Ledden, P. J., Brady, T. J., Rosen, B. R., and Tootell, R. B. (1995). Object-related activity revealed by functional magnetic resonance imaging in human occipital cortex. *Proc. Natl. Acad. Sci. USA*, **92**, 8135–8139.

Marsolek, C. J. (1995). Abstract visual-form representations in the left cerebral hemisphere. *J. Exp. Psychol. Hum. Percept. Perform.*, **21**, 375–386.

Miller, E. K. and Desimone, R. (1993). Scopolamine affects short-term memory but not inferior temporal neurons. *NeuroReport*, **4**, 81–84.

Mummery, C. J., Shallice, T., and Price, C. J. (1999). Dual-process model in semantic priming: a functional imaging perspective. *NeuroImage*, **9**, 516–525.

Naccache, L. and Dehaene, S. (2001). The priming method: imaging unconscious repetition priming reveals an abstract representation of number in the parietal lobes. *Cereb. Cortex*, **11**, 966–974.

Nagy, M. E. and Rugg, M. D. (1989). Modulation of event-related potentials by word repetition: the effects of inter-item lag. *Psychophysiology*, **26**, 431–436.

Neely, J. H. (1991). Semantic priming effects in visual word recognition: a selective review of current findings and theories, in *Basic Processes in Reading: Visual Word Recognition*, Besner, D. and Humphreys, G., Eds., Lawrence Erlbaum, Hillsdale, NJ.

Noppeney, U. and Price, C. J. (2003). An fMRI study of synactic adaptation, submitted.

Plaut, D. C. and Shallice, T. (1993). Perseverative and semantic influences on visual object naming errors in optic aphasia: a connectionist account. *J. Cogn. Neurosci.*, **5**, 89–117.

Posner, M. I. and Snyder, C. R. R. (1975). Facilitation and inhibition in the processing of signals, in *Attention and Performance V*, Rabbitt, P. and Dornic, F., Eds., Academic Press, New York.

Puce, A., Allison, T., and McCarthy, G. (1999). Electrophysiological studies of human face perception. III. Effects of top-down processing on face-specific potentials. *Cereb. Cortex*, **9**, 445–458.

Richardson-Klavehn, A. and Bjork, R. A. (1988). Measures of memory. *Annu. Rev. Psychol.*, **39**, 475–543.

Richardson-Klavehn, A. and Gardiner, J. M. (1995). Retrieval volition and memorial awareness in stem completion: an empirical analysis. *Psychol. Res.*, **57**, 166–178.

Ringo, J. L. (1996). Stimulus specific adaptation in inferior temporal and medial temporal cortex of the monkey. *Behav. Brain Res.*, **76**, 191–197.

Rossell, S., Price, C. J., and Nobre, A. C. (2003). The anatomy and time course of semantic priming investigated by fMRI and ERPs. *Neuropsychologia*, **33**, 111–119

Rugg, M. D. and Doyle, M. C. (1994). Event-related potentials and stimulus repetition in direct and indirect tests of memory, in *Cognitive Electrophysiology*, Heinze, H. J., Munte, T., and Mangun, G. R., Eds., pp. 124–148. Birkhauser, Boston.

Sarter, M., Givens, B., and Bruno, J. P. (2001). The cognitive neuroscience of sustained attention: where top-down meets bottom-up. *Brain Res. Brain Res. Rev.*, **35**, 146–160.

Schacter, D. L. (1990). Perceptual representation systems and implicit memory. *Ann. N.Y. Acad. Sci.*, **608**, 543–567.

Schacter, D. L. and Buckner, R. L. (1998). Priming and the brain. *Neuron*, **20**, 185–195.

Schacter, D. L. and Tulving, E. Eds. (1994). *Memory Systems 1994*. MIT Press, Cambridge, MA.

Schacter, D. L., Bowers, J., and Booker, J. (1989). Intention, awareness and implicit memory: the retrieval intentionality criterion, in *Implicit Memory: Theoretical Issues*, Lewandowsky, S., Dunn, J. C., and Kirsner, K., Eds., pp. 47–465. Lawrence Erlbaum, Hillsdale, NJ.

Schacter, D. L., Relman, E., Uecker, A., Polster, M. R., Yun, L. S., and Cooper, L. A. (1995). Brain regions associated with retrieval of structurally coherent visual information. *Nature*, **376**, 587–590.

Schifano, F. and Curran, H. V. (1994). Pharmacological models of memory dysfunction? A comparison of the effects of scopolamine and lorazepam on word valence ratings, priming and recall. *Psychopharmacol. (Berlin)*, **115**, 430–434.

Schott, B., Richardson-Klavehn, A., Heinze, H. J., and Duzel, E. (2002). Perceptual priming versus explicit memory: dissociable neural correlates at encoding. *J. Cogn. Neurosci.*, **14**, 578–592.

Sohal, V. S. and Hasselmo, M. E. (2000). A model for experience-dependent changes in the responses of inferotemporal neurons. *Network*, **11**, 169–190.

Tarr, M. J., Williams, P., Hayward, W. G., and Gauthier, I. (1998). Three-dimensional object recognition is viewpoint dependent. *Nat. Neurosci.*, **1**, 275–257.

Thiel, C. M., Henson, R. N. A., Morris, J. S., Friston, K. J., and Dolan, R. J. (2001). Pharmacological modulation of behavioural and neuronal correlates of repetition priming. *J. Neurosci.*, **21**, 6846–6852.

Thiel, C. M., Henson, R. N., and Dolan, R. J. (2002). Scopolamine but not lorazepam modulates face repetition priming: a psychopharmacological fMRI study. *Neuropsychopharmacology*, **27**, 282–292.

Tsivilis, D., Otten, L. J., and Rugg, M. D. (2001). Context effects on the neural correlates of recognition memory: an electrophysiological study. *Neuron*, **31**, 497–505.

Tulving, E., Schacter, D., and Stark, H. (1982). Priming effects in word-fragment completion are independent of recognition memory. *J. Exp. Psycho. Learn. Mem. Cogn.*, **8**, 336–341.

van Turennout, M., Ellmore, T., and Martin, A. (2000). Long-lasting cortical plasticity in the object naming system. *Nat. Neurosci.*, **3**, 1329–1334.

Vidailhet, P., Danion, J. M., Chemin, C., and Kazes, M. (1999). Lorazepam impairs both visual and auditory perceptual priming. *Psychopharmacology (Berl)*, **147**, 266–73.

Vuilleumier, P., Armony, J. L., Driver, J., and Dolan, R. J. (2001). Effects of attention and emotion on face processing in the human brain: an event-related fMRI study. *Neuron*, **30**, 829–841.

Vuilleumier, P., Henson, R. N., Driver, J., and Dolan, R. J. (2002). Multiple levels of visual object constancy revealed by event-related fMRI of repetition priming. *Nat. Neurosci.*, **5**, 491–499.

Warrington, E. K. and Weiskrantz, L. (1974). The effect of prior learning on subsequent retention in amnesic patients. *Neuropsychologia*, **12**, 419–428.

Wiggs, C. L. and Martin, A. (1998). Properties and mechanisms of perceptual priming. *Curr. Opin. Neurobiol.*, **8**, 227–233.

Witherspoon, D. and Moscovitch, M. (1989). Stochastic independence between two implicit memory tests. *J. of Exp. Psychol. Learn. Mem. Cogn.*, **15**, 22–30.

CHAPTER

24

Explicit Memory

INTRODUCTION

The previous chapter focused on neuroimaging studies of repetition priming, a form of implicit memory. This chapter concerns imaging studies of recognition memory, a form of explicit memory (see Chapter 23 for definitions of these terms). The haemodynamic correlates of recognition memory are indexed by the same basic repetition effect as are the correlates of repetition priming—namely, the difference between repeated ("old") and initial ("new") presentations of a stimulus within an experimental context. The difference is that recognition memory is tested by a direct memory task, in which participants discriminate old from new stimuli (as distinct from the indirect tasks discussed previously). Like the previous chapter, this chapter is selective in focusing on recognition memory (as distinct from other tests of explicit memory, such as recall) and also in focusing only on studies performed at the Wellcome Department of Imaging Neuroscience (for more comprehensive reviews, see Buckner and Wheeler, 2001; Desgranges *et al.*, 1998; Fletcher and Henson, 2001; Rugg, 2002).

INTRODUCTION: RECOGNITION MEMORY

Whereas repetition priming has typically been associated with a reduced haemodynamic response for repetition versus control conditions (repetition suppression), recognition memory has typically been associated with an increased response for repetition conditions (repetition enhancement, or an "old/new" effect). As with priming, however, this generalisation may not always hold. The old/new effect is normally conditioned on correct recognition memory judgments—namely, the difference between *hits* (old stimuli called "old"), *correct rejections* (new stimuli called "new"), excluding *misses* (old stimuli called "new"), and *false alarms* (new stimuli called "old"). This is the case for all the event-related studies described below.

Recognition memory has traditionally been conceptualised in terms of signal-detection theory (Green and Swets, 1966), in which stimuli are assumed to have a continuous range of strengths in memory. Old and new stimuli are represented by two overlapping distributions along this continuum, with the central tendency of old stimuli being greater than that of new stimuli. The difference in these central tendencies is called the *discriminability*. Participants are assumed to place a decision boundary somewhere on the continuum, called the *response criterion*, which they use to categorise stimuli as either old or new. The strength of an old or new item relative to this criterion determines whether it becomes a hit, miss, correct rejection, or false alarm (Fig. 24.1). Estimates of the discriminability (*e.g.*, d') and response criterion (*e.g.*, β) can be

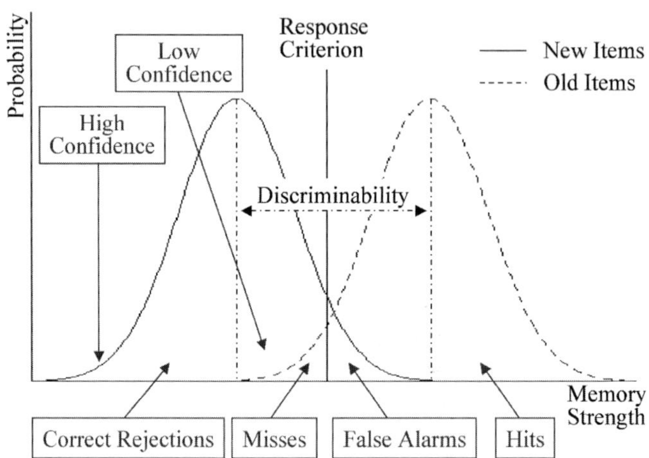

FIGURE 24.1
Schematic of signal detection theory, together with classification of recognition decisions (boxed labels).

obtained by various methods, although a summary measure such as (pH – pFA), the proportion of old words that are hits minus the proportion of old words that are false alarms, is often a satisfactory index of memory accuracy.

Though the signal detection model can explain some important results in recognition memory, many researchers have argued that it is insufficient (Mandler, 1980). Consequently, dual-process models have been developed that propose two distinct contributions to recognition memory: *recollection* and *familiarity* (both examples of explicit memory). Recollection refers to retrieval of the specific event in the past in which a stimulus was presented (*e.g.*, time and place) and is associated with episodic memory. Familiarity, on the other hand, is associated with a feeling that a stimulus has been experienced before, in the absence of memory for the context in which that stimulus occurred. Recollection is often viewed as multidimensional and effortful; familiarity is often viewed as a unidimensional quantity and relatively automatic. In some models, familiarity is equated with the memory strength in signal detection theory, whereas recollection is modelled as an independent, all-or-none occurrence (Yonelinas *et al.*, 1996). The precise manner in which familiarity and recollection combine in a recognition memory judgment —in an independent, redundant, or exclusive manner—remains controversial, however (Knowlton and Squire, 1995).

The next section covers the old/new effects observed in simple yes/no recognition memory tests, including early positron emission tomography (PET) studies. The Familiarity Versus Recollection section deals with variants of recognition memory tests, in which decisions are augmented by indications of the subjective experience or confidence accompanying each decision, or which are conditional on a requirement to retrieve some aspect of the study episode (referred to as tests of *source memory*). These variants have been used in attempts to dissociate the neural correlates of recollection and familiarity. The New/Old Effects section discusses new/old effects (or repetition suppression) in recognition memory tests. Finally, the Subsequent Memory Effects section discusses a slightly different topic that does not concern repetition effects *per se* but rather studies of memory encoding that examine responses to initial presentations of stimuli that predict subsequent memory when those stimuli are repeated.

BASIC OLD/NEW EFFECTS

Early PET and functional magnetic resonance imaging (fMRI) studies of recognition memory, before the advent of event-related fMRI, investigated old/new effects by comparing blocks in which a high proportion of stimuli were old with blocks in which a low proportion were old. For example, the PET study of Rugg *et al.* (1996) used this method to compare blocks of 80, 20, and 0% studied words. In a control task, participants distinguished between two symbol strings, with the proportion of target strings varying in the same ratios. Regions in which the response increased with the proportion of old items in the memory task, having covaried out the proportion of targets in the control task, included bilateral anterior prefrontal cortex ([+38, +48, +8] and [–30, +46, –4]), right dorsolateral prefrontal cortex (+42, +22, +28), and medial prefrontal cortex (+4, +20, +48). In a similar comparison of 0 and 80% studied words, Rugg *et al.* (1998a) found old/new effects in right anterior prefrontal (+32, +50, +18), left lateral parietal (–36, –80, +40), and medial parietal cortex (–2, –74, +36).

There are a number of reasons, however, why such blocked repetition effects are difficult to interpret. People are known to be sensitive to event probabilities (Fitzgerald and Picton, 1981). Thus, even though attempts can be made to disguise the old/new ratio manipulation (*e.g.*, by having more balanced old/new ratios during run-in periods before and/or after each block), participants are likely to notice that they have made one response more often than the other during the last few trials. A low incidence of old responses during a 20%-old block, for example, may lead participants to question their memory and perhaps adjust their response criterion accordingly (to be more lenient). This means that any differences between the mean haemodynamic responses during blocks of different ratios may reflect differences in expectances or strategies, rather than old/new memory effects *per se*.

These problems are not so acute for event-related fMRI studies, in which old and new stimuli are randomly intermixed (in equal proportions), and the mean stimulus-locked responses are compared directly. Indeed, such methods can be used to test directly the interaction between probability effects and old/new effects. Herron *et al.* (in press), for example, compared the event-related repetition effect for old versus new words for three sessions with different old/new ratios (75:25, 50:50, or 25:75). Whereas lateral and medial parietal regions showed repetition enhancement that appeared to be independent of the probability of old items, several prefrontal regions showed an interaction between old/new ratios and repetition. Indeed, some of these prefrontal regions showed a switch from repetition enhancement under the low old/new ratio to repetition suppression under the high old/new ratio. In other words, the responses in these regions were greater for the rarer type of item. Though the reason for this crossover interaction is unclear (it could relate to the fact that participants were informed of the ratio manipulation, which may cause them to treat the rarer items as the targets; see Wagner *et al.*, 1998a), it provides strong evidence for strategic effects in such designs and so questions the results from previous blocked studies. The data also promote a general picture of automatic retrieval effects in posterior regions and strategic (task-dependent) post-retrieval effects in frontal regions.

Nonetheless, despite the fact that a number of event-related fMRI studies of yes/no recognition memory have used unequal old/new proportions and that some of the associated prefrontal activations may relate to post-retrieval decision processes, a consistent pattern of regions showing old/new effects has emerged (Rugg and Henson, 2002). Maratos *et al.* (2001), for example, found a network of regions showing repetition enhancement, including left anterior prefrontal cortex (–20, +64, +12), left parahippocampal cortex (–16, –28, –8), posterior cingulate (+4, –54, +18), precuneus (–6, –58, +36), and bilateral lateral parietal cortex ([–36, –62, +56] and [+34, –68, +40]), even though the old/new ratio was 3:1. Interestingly, this retrieval success network was common to three types of old words (negative, positive, or neutral) that had been studied in the context of sentences describing emotionally negative, positive, or neutral situations, respectively. Emotional modulation of repetition effects, which probably reflected episodic retrieval of the associated study sentence, was also observed in regions including left amygdala, right dorsolateral prefrontal cortex, and posterior cingulate for negative emotions and orbitofrontal, right anterior prefrontal, and left anterior temporal cortex for positive emotions.

RECOLLECTION VERSUS FAMILIARITY

Other studies have used variants of the basic yes/no recognition memory task. Henson *et al.* (1999b), for example, asked participants to make a three-way decision regarding old and new words: *remember*, *know*, or *new*. This remember–know (R–K) distinction was proposed by Tulving (1985) to capture the subjective difference between recalling a prior episode (*e.g.*, what occurred before or after a studied item) and a feeling of "oldness" in the absence of memory for a specific occurrence (a phenomenological distinction that might map onto the hypothetical

REMEMBER - KNOW

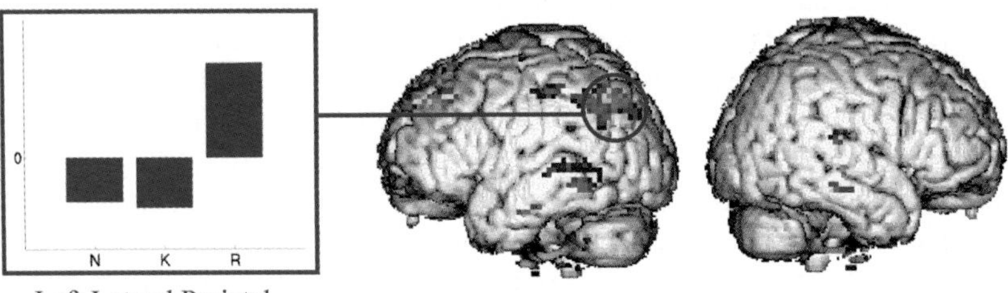

Left Lateral Parietal

KNOW - REMEMBER

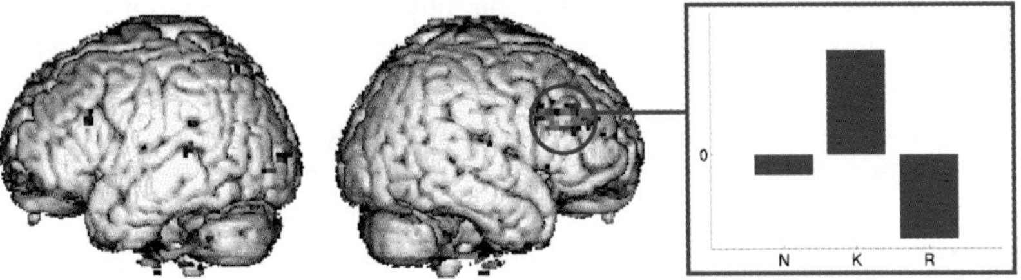

Right Dorsal Prefrontal

FIGURE 24.2
Data from Henson *et al.* (1999b) showing regions with greater event-related responses to correct remember (R) than correct know (K) decisions to old words (top row), and the opposite pattern of greater event-related responses to K than R decisions (bottom row). Data are rendered onto the lateral surfaces of a canonical brain. N, correct rejections of new words. Zero level is the average across all three response categories.

processes of recollection and familiarity). Note that these decisions are assumed to be qualitatively, and not simply quantitatively, different (though see Donaldson, 1996). Thus, while people are normally confident of their R judgments, they can still be highly confident of their K judgments, too (Gardiner *et al.*, 1994). In the Henson *et al.* (1999b) study, although the (pH – pFA) rate for K judgments was less than that for R judgments, it was still greater than zero (under various scoring assumptions), indicating that K judgments were not mere guesses.

Collapsing across R and K judgments produced old/new effects similar to those described in the previous section. Direct comparisons of correct R versus correct K judgments (Fig. 24.2) revealed greater responses for R judgments in regions including left anterior superior prefrontal (–21, +54, +39), lateral parietal (–57, –51, +39), and posterior cingulate (0, –30, +36) regions and greater responses for K judgments in regions including right dorsolateral prefrontal cortex (+51, +30, +27), anterior cingulate (–12, +9, +36), and dorsal precuneus (–12, –60, +57). The former results suggest that the anterior prefrontal, lateral parietal, and posterior cingulate regions showing old/new effects in simple yes/no recognition memory tests represent (processes contingent on) recollection of the study episode.* Given their somewhat contextually impoverished study phases, the source information associated with recollection in these experiments is most likely to be internal source (Johnson *et al.*, 1993), such as semantic associations made to the words presented at study.

According to a dual-process model, the relative increases for K judgments might implicate right prefrontal and anterior cingulate cortices in support of a familiarity process; however, this type of inference depends on assumptions about how the hypothetical constructs of recollection and familiarity relate to R and K judgments—for example, whether they are independent, redundant, or exclusive (Knowlton and Squire, 1995). The preferred interpretation of Henson

* Another study using the R–K paradigm by Eldridge *et al.* (2000) reported similar regions showing greater responses to R than K judgments but additional repetition enhancement in the hippocampus, although (pH – pFA) for K judgments was close to zero, at least under exclusivity or independence scoring assumptions, suggesting that many K judgments were guesses.

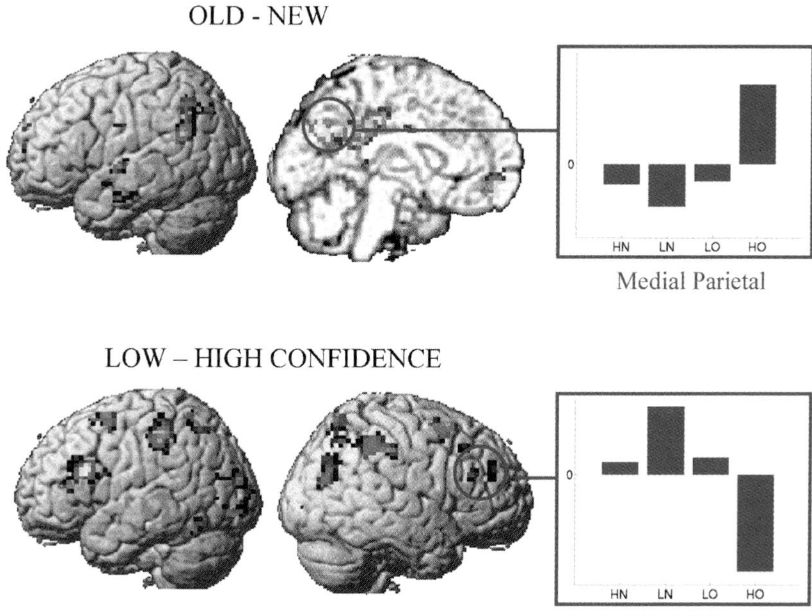

FIGURE 24.3
Data from Henson *et al.* (2000) showing regions with greater event-related responses to hits (old) than correct rejections (new), collapsed across confidence rating (top row), and greater event-related responses to correct low than high confidence responses, collapsed across old/new (bottom row). HN, high-confidence new response; LN, low-confidence new response; LO, low-confidence old response; HO, high-confidence old response. Zero level is the average across all four response categories.

et al. (1999b) was that the right prefrontal and anterior cingulate activations reflect increased post-retrieval *monitoring* (Henson *et al.*, 1999a; Shallice *et al.*, 1994) for K than R judgments. In other words, when a word seems familiar, but one cannot remember the specific episode in which it was studied, one attempts additional verification of the retrieved information before reaching a decision. This is consistent with the observation of longer response times for K than R judgments in this study. The familiarity signal itself is assumed to arise elsewhere (such as perirhinal cortex; see New/Old Effects section).

This hypothesis was tested in a subsequent study by Henson *et al.* (2000), which used confidence judgments, rather than R–K judgments. For each word, participants made a four-way decision of *confident old*, *unconfident old*, *unconfident new*, or *confident new*. Appealing to a signal detection model, the authors reasoned that low-confidence judgments (which are close to the response criterion; see Fig. 24.1) should require greater monitoring than high-confidence judgments, regardless of whether those judgments are old or new. Consistent with this hypothesis, the right dorsolateral prefrontal region identified in their previous study (Henson *et al.*, 1999b) showed a main effect of low versus high confidence, reinforcing its role in post-retrieval monitoring rather than memory *per se*. Regions showing a main effect of old versus new words included the usual network of left anterior prefrontal (–21, +63, +21), posterior cingulate (+3, –42, +21), precuneus (0, –69, +33), and left lateral parietal cortex (–48, –57, +48). The posterior cingulate/precuneus regions showed a particularly large response to high-confidence old judgments, consistent with a role for these regions in recollection (Fig. 24.3).

In another study attempting to isolate recollection, Cansino *et al.* (2002) used pictures rather than words, presented in one of four spatial quadrants at study. At test, a source memory task was used in which participants made a five-way decision to indicate whether the pictures were new or old and, if old, in which spatial location they occurred at study. Over 60% of responses to old words represented a correct source judgment, so that most could be associated with recollection, given that the chance rate was 25%. Regions showing increased responses associated with recollection included left anterior prefrontal (–10, +58, +32), right lateral parietal (+62, –34, +24), left parahippocampal (–14, –44, –4) and right hippocampal formation (+26, –16, –14). The left anterior prefrontal finding is consistent with that of Henson *et al.* (1999b), supporting a role of this region in recollection; the right rather than left parietal finding may reflect a different type of source memory (*e.g.*, spatial, rather than verbal associations). The reverse contrast of incorrect versus correct source judgments revealed bilateral dorsolateral prefrontal ([+44, +30, +40] and [–36, –36, +36]) and intraparietal sulcus ([+28, –56, +46] and [–24, –66, +40]). The dorsolateral finding is consistent with the K–R findings of Henson *et al.* (1999b), supporting a role for this region in post-retrieval monitoring when source information is elusive.

Rugg *et al.* (2003) required source memory judgments for words presented in one of two colours and in one of two spatial locations. In this case, an exclusion task was used (Jacoby *et al.*, 1993), in which participants pressed one key if a test word was presented in a specific study context (*e.g.*, red and left of fixation)—the so-called *targets*—and pressed another key if a test word was studied in a different context, was studied but the context forgotten, or was new—the *non-targets*. The data from this task were compared with those from a standard yes/no recognition task (or inclusion task), in which one key was pressed for old words (regardless of source) and another key for new words.* Analysis was restricted to prefrontal cortex. Regions showing old/new effects common to both the inclusion and exclusion tasks included bilateral anterior prefrontal cortex ([–45, +48, +6] and [+39, +60, –3]). Note that these old/new effects also included greater responses to correctly excluded non-targets than correct rejections in the exclusion task, even though both conditions were associated with the same key press (*i.e.*, controlling for target detection or response selection effects). A region in the right dorsolateral prefrontal cortex (+48, +42, +24) showed a greater (and delayed) response to hits in the exclusion task than to hits in the inclusion task. Because the exclusion but not inclusion task requires verification of the spatial/colour source associated with old items, this dorsolateral prefrontal response is again consistent with a role for this region in post-retrieval monitoring (in that monitoring can operate over either recollected or familiarity-driven information).

In summary, a number of recent event-related fMRI studies of recognition memory have identified a common set of regions showing basic old/new effects (repetition enhancement). These include regions of left and right anterior and dorsolateral prefrontal cortex and in lateral and medial parietal cortices. Furthermore, some of these regions appear to covary with recollection (as operationalised by R judgments, high-confidence judgments, or correct source judgments), particularly in left anterior prefrontal, left lateral parietal, and posterior cingulate cortices. Responses in other regions, such as dorsolateral prefrontal cortex, seem better explained in terms of post-retrieval decision processes. These responses may therefore vary with the specific type of decision required or with where subjects place their response criterion. An important consequence of the latter is that these regions may show either an old/new or a new/old effect, depending on whether the response criterion is closer to the central tendency of the old or new distribution, respectively.

These prefrontal and parietal old/new effects, however, are not those that might be expected from neuropsychological studies of amnesia, which strongly implicate medial temporal lobe (MTL) structures in explicit memory. The failure to find MTL old/new effects in many of the above studies (with the exception of parahippocampal old/new effects in Maratos *et al.*, 2001, and Cansino *et al.*, 2002) could simply reflect reduced sensitivity within the MTL. Alternatively, the lack of old/new differences might reflect the involvement of MTL in both the encoding of new items and the retrieval of old items, such that there is no net repetition effect. However, preliminary results (below) suggest that some MTL structures do show repetition effects, but these are new/old effects, rather than old/new effects.

NEW/OLD EFFECTS

Surprisingly, few of the above studies considered regions that showed a reduced response for old relative to new words (*i.e.*, repetition suppression). In a meta-analysis, Henson *et al.* (2003) found a region in right anterior MTL (+22, –6, –28), more likely in perirhinal cortex than

* In attempt to control for differences in nonspecific difficulty between the inclusion and exclusion tasks, an orthogonal manipulation of study list length was used. This manipulation did not interact with any of the other contrasts.

hippocampus, that showed a new/old effect common to four different experiments. The effect was found regardless of whether the stimuli were words or pictures or whether the memory test was direct or indirect. Furthermore, the effect did not appear sensitive to whether a source memory judgment to the old stimuli was correct or incorrect (Cansino *et al.*, 2002) or whether the task did or did not require source retrieval (Rugg *et al.*, 2003). These findings suggest that this new/old effect is independent of recollection but are consistent with a familiarity signal (at least within a redundancy or independence dual-process model).

This anterior MTL repetition suppression could, however, also reflect priming (at a high level of the visual processing pathway) i.e., be an implicit memory effect. This possibility cannot be refuted by the imaging data. Nonetheless, there is strong evidence from lesion (Meunier *et al.*, 1993) and electrophysiological studies (Brown and Xiang, 1998) in animals for a role of perirhinal cortex in explicit recognition memory. Moreover, human lesion studies (Hamann and Squire, 1997) suggest that MTL damage that includes perirhinal cortex does not affect perceptual priming. Thus, the anterior MTL repetition suppression is likely to reflect a familiarity signal that is used for explicit recognition memory judgments.

Interestingly, the response to old items in these MTL regions was a deactivation relative to the interstimulus (fixation) baseline. This is not a conceptual problem, as it is possible that repetition of a stimulus produces a sparse pattern of neural firing, in which only a small subset of neurons fire, while the rest are suppressed below spontaneous firing levels (as found in some single-cell studies of human MTL; see Fried *et al.*, 2002). More puzzling is the fact that new items did not appear to activate this region above interstimulus baseline. This is certainly a problem for a priming account in which repetition suppression is attributed to the facilitation of a process occurring on first presentations of a stimulus (in which case one might expect significant response to new items versus baseline; see Chapter 23).

The association of anterior MTL cortex with a familiarity signal is consistent with the theory of Aggleton and Brown (1998). These authors used data from human and nonhuman lesions to argue that the recollection and familiarity processes assumed by dual-process models are supported by dissociable structures within MTL: with a hippocampal-anterior thalamic circuit associated with recollection and a perirhinal-medial dorsal thalamic circuit associated with familiarity. In a *post hoc* observation, Rugg (personal communication) found a significant interaction in the Cansino *et al.* (2002) study between correct and incorrect source judgments and two MTL regions. The right anterior cortical region (+22, –6, –28) identified in the meta-analysis of Henson *et al.* (2003) showed equivalent decreases for correct and incorrect source judgments relative to correct rejections, whereas a slightly more posterior and superior region, most likely in the right hippocampus (+26, –16, –14), showed less of a decrease for correct than incorrect source judgments. Though this single dissociation clearly requires replication, it supports the anatomical realisation of recollection and familiarity suggested by Aggleton and Brown (1998)' although it is less clear why the hippocampal response for correct source judgments, while above that for incorrect source judgments, was still below that for correct rejections of new items.

SUBSEQUENT MEMORY EFFECTS

This final section is not concerned with repetition effects *per se*, but rather with differences between items at study according to whether or not they are later remembered, the so-called *subsequent memory effect*. In this paradigm, participants are scanned at study (rather than test) while performing a task on presented items. After a short delay, they are given a memory test (usually a recognition memory test with concurrent confidence or source judgments), which is used to sort items at study into those remembered and those forgotten. The memory test is normally unexpected (*i.e.*, participants are not aware during study that their memory for the items will be tested later). Note that a similar logic could be used for priming (*i.e.*, to identify regions that predict the size of the subsequent priming effect), as has been done with event-related potentials (ERPs) (Schott *et al.*, 2002).

Imaging studies of subsequent memory effects generally find greater responses to remembered than forgotten items in ventral prefrontal ([–45, +24, –6] in Henson *et al.*, 1999b;

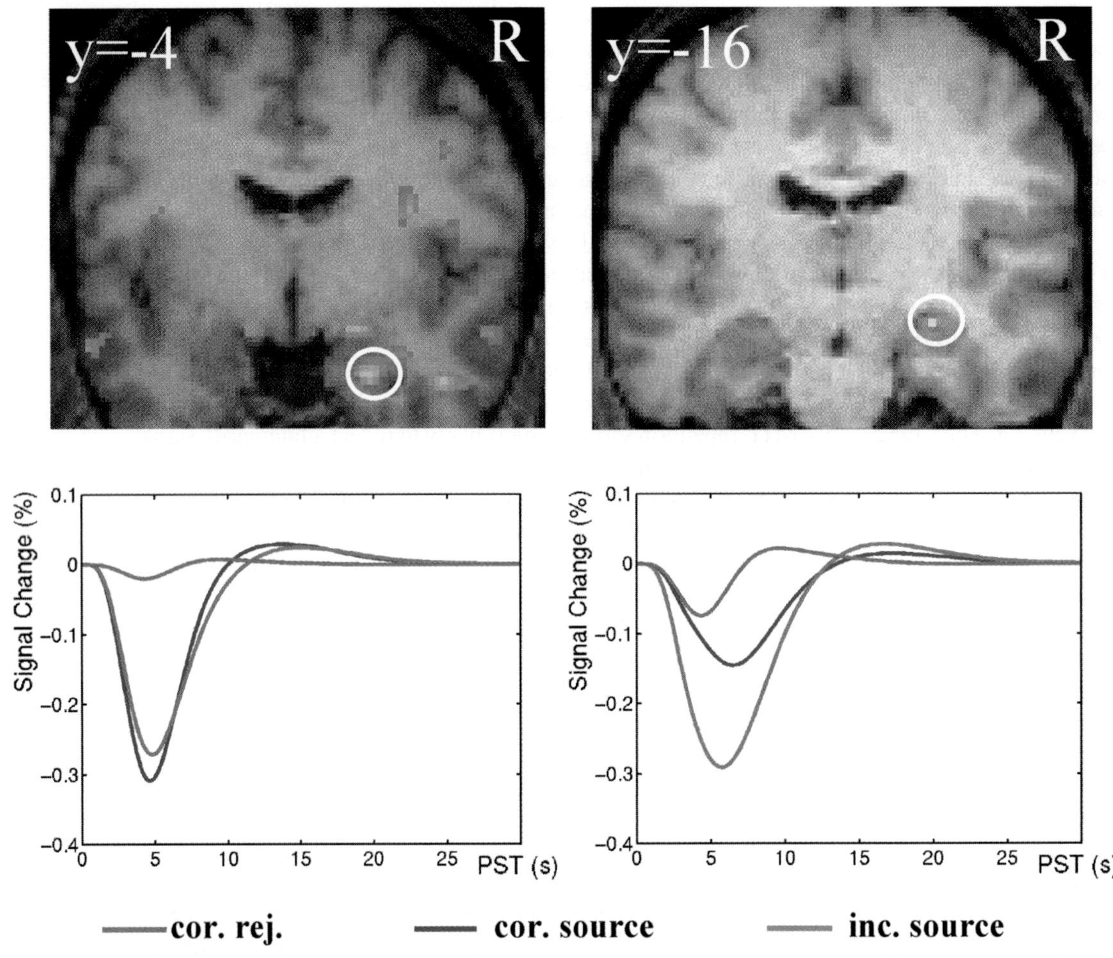

FIGURE 24.4
Coronal sections through a canonical brain from Cansino *et al.* (2002), showing regions in anterior medial temporal cortex (left) and hippocampus (right). Below each region is the best-fitting canonical response for correct rejections of new items (red), old items given the correct source (blue), and old items given the incorrect source (green).

[–36, +36, –9] in Otten *et al.*, 2001) and midfusiform cortices ([–38, –54, –12] in Cansino *et al.*, 2002; [–48, –54, –18] in Otten *et al.*, 2001), often stronger on the left with words. However, it is important to note that these effects are normally only seen for items subsequently recognised with high confidence (Otten *et al.*, 2001; Wagner *et al.*, 1998b), with R judgments (Brewer *et al.*, 1998; Henson *et al.*, 1999b), or with correct source judgments (Cansino *et al.*, 2002). Thus, these regions seem specifically to predict subsequent recollection (or episodic retrieval) rather than subsequent familiarity.* This is consistent with a study that focused on the MTL (Strange *et al.*, 2002), in which regions of left hippocampus (–22, –26, –16) and left perirhinal cortex (–30, –4, –36) predicted subsequent free recall of items from short lists of intentionally studied words. The relationship between this perirhinal encoding effect at study and the perirhinal familiarity effect at test remains to be determined.

One important question is whether these regions predict subsequent recollection regardless of the study task (as would be the case if they were part of a specialised memory system, the so-called *structuralist* perspective; see Schacter and Tulving, 1994), or whether different regions predict recollection under different study and/or test tasks (a *proceduralist* perspective; see Kolers and Roediger, 1984). Otten *et al.* (2001) examined the role of the study task by asking participants to make either semantic or orthographic decisions about words. The semantic deci-

* Note that these effects are unlikely to reflect random variations in attention or arousal at study, given that reaction times to perform the study task do not typically differ for words later remembered and words later forgotten (Otten *et al.*, 2001).

sion was whether the word referred to an animate or inanimate entity; the orthographic decision was whether the first and last letters of the word were in alphabetical order. A left ventral prefrontal region (–45, +24, –6) and a left anterior hippocampal region (–27, –15, –12) predicted subsequent memory under both the semantic and orthographic tasks. This could be taken as support for the structuralist view that there exists a specialised memory system (in the MTL) that, via interactions with ventral prefrontal cortex, allows successful memory regardless of study task.

In a subsequent study, however, Otten and Rugg (2001) compared subsequent memory effects under a semantic task with those under a phonological study task. The semantic decisions were again animate/inanimate; the phonological decision was whether the word contained an odd or even number of syllables. In this case, a double dissociation was found between left ventral prefrontal (–51, +18, +15) and medial prefrontal (–3, +48, +33) regions that showed greater subsequent memory effects under the semantic than phonological task, and left intraparietal (–39, –45, +51), left fusiform (–42, –48, –15), and left occipital (–24, –75, +33) regions that showed a subsequent memory effect for the phonological but not semantic study task (Fig. 24.4). These data therefore support the proceduralist view that regions predicting memory encoding vary with the study task. In other words, memory is a by-product of the particular processes performed on an item at study.

Thus, some support can be found for both the structuralist and the proceduralist views. One possibility is that the components of an episodic memory are stored across different cortical regions (the specific components being those that are emphasised by the study task), but, in order to bind these components together, they must be associated with an index to that memory stored in the MTL (which represents a specialised memory system).

Another interesting question is whether there are variations in people's psychological state that predict subsequent memory (Rugg and Wilding, 2000), in addition to variations in their responses to individual stimuli. Otten *et al.* (2002) addressed this question using alternating epochs (blocks) of either a semantic or phonological study task (as in Otten and Rugg, 2001). Each epoch of 83 s contained 12 words. By randomly varying the time between words, the correlation between the epoch-related (or state-related) and event-related (or item-related) regressors was reduced to an extent that each effect could be estimated with reasonable efficiency (Chawla *et al.*, 1999). The item-related effects replicated those of Otten and Rugg (2001). More interestingly, a few regions showed a state-related effect that varied linearly with the number of words remembered within each epoch (even though differential item effects had been removed). For the semantic task, these regions were in left ventral prefrontal cortex (–48, +18, +3) and precuneus (–3, –60, +30); for the phonological task, there was one region in dorsal

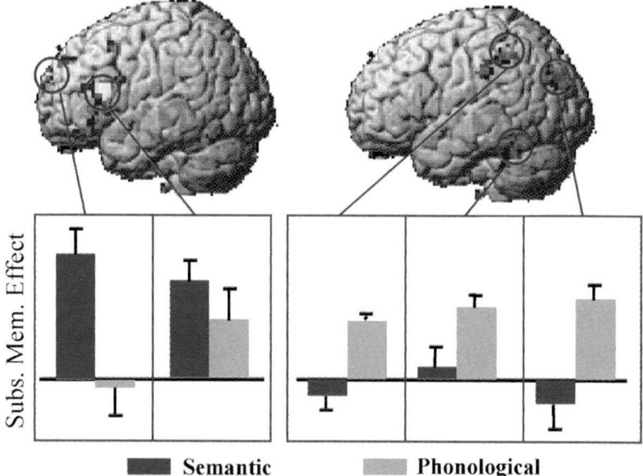

FIGURE 24.4
Regions from Otten and Rugg (2001) showing differential subsequent memory effects during a semantic task and during a phonological task. Bars show differences between canonical response parameter estimates for subsequently remembered versus subsequently forgotten items for each region for the semantic task (blue) and phonological task (green).

precuneus (0, −54, +60). These state-related encoding effects may reflect, for example, variations across epochs in strategies or levels of sustained attention. Only the left ventral prefrontal region also showed an item-related subsequent memory effect. Interestingly, the state-related activity in this region correlated negatively with subsequent memory, unlike the positive correlation of its item-related activity. One possibility is that a trade-off occurred between the cognitive processes underlying the two effects. These data clearly force further theorising about the nature of different processes that engender good memory.

A final important question is whether the same regions that predict subsequent recollection also reflect that recollection at test (as might be expected from a neural *transfer appropriate processing* account; see Blaxton *et al.*, 1996). In the only two studies to compare imaging data acquired at study and test, the regions predicting subsequent recollection and the regions showing recollection-dependent responses did not overlap (Cansino *et al.*, 2002; Henson *et al.*, 1999b). This lack of overlap suggests that the cortical regions predicting subsequent recollection may have more to do with the types of working memory operations that lead to better memory (*e.g.*, organisation; see Wagner *et al.*, 1999), rather than the types of contextual information associated with those memories (contrary to the componential view of episodic memories outlined above); however, further studies are necessary to examine the question of study–test interactions in more detail.

CONCLUSION

The most robust repetition effects in recognition memory tests are found in cortical regions, including prefrontal cortex and lateral and medial parietal cortices. Some of these, particularly left anterior prefrontal, left lateral parietal, and posterior cingulate, appear to respond most vigorously in association with recollection (at least for words). These activations may reflect reinstatement of study context in working memory. Other prefrontal activations (particularly in dorsolateral regions) are more likely to relate to post-retrieval monitoring of retrieved information (in order, for example, to make a confidence judgment). In other words, these prefrontal activations may reflect decision processes required by recognition memory tasks, rather than memory *per se*. This is particularly apparent in the study of Herron *et al.* (in press), in which some prefrontal old/new effects can become new/old effects simply by varying the proportion of old items.

Activation of MTL regions, as would be expected for neuropsychological studies of amnesia, are less robust. Nonetheless, one interesting pattern beginning to emerge is the association of familiarity with anterior MTL cortex (particularly perirhinal cortex) and association of recollection with the hippocampal formation, as predicted by the model of Aggleton and Brown (1998). An example of this pattern arises in the single dissociation of the Cansino *et al.* (2002) study, although further studies are required to explicitly test this *post hoc* observation. One elaboration of this dual-process view is that perirhinal cortex codes the *recency* of perceiving a stimulus (conforming to the memory strength continuum of signal-detection models), whereas hippocampus associates that stimulus with the spatiotemporal context in which it was perceived.

Other imaging studies have examined encoding into memory by investigating the brain regions that predict subsequent recognition memory (particularly subsequent recollection). These regions may depend on the type of processes performed at study, consistent with a proceduralist account of memory; however, studies have also identified MTL regions that predict subsequent memory across a range of tasks, consistent with the structuralist view of a specialised memory system. An appealing hypothesis is that episodic memories consist of a number of components that relate to the particular stimulus attributes elaborated at study (depending on the study task) and hence engage different cortical regions according to those attributes (*e.g.*, the semantic or phonological properties of words). However, a necessary condition for these components to bind together in a single episodic memory may be that they are associated with an index represented in the MTL.

One important avenue for future research will be to relate findings using direct memory tasks with the findings in analogous paradigms using indirect memory tasks (described in Chapter 23). In particular, there is a need to dissociate the contributions of implicit and explicit memory to both types of test. For example, as discussed here, the perirhinal new/old effects could represent a form of implicit memory (*i.e.*, the repetition suppression often associated with priming). One way to test this is to perform a recognition memory test that produces sufficient numbers of recognition misses. If the perirhinal cortex response covaries with the participant's memory judgment (*i.e.*, is deactivated, with respect to correct rejections, for hits and possibly false alarms but not for misses), then that response is more likely to represent a familiarity signal used in recognition memory (Rugg *et al.*, 1998b). If, however, its response to hits and misses is similar (and different from that to correct rejections and possibly false alarms)—in other words, the response covaries with the objective fact of whether or not the item was repeated—then that response is more likely to represent an implicit form of memory. Alternatively, one could examine these responses as a function of various manipulations known to affect explicit or implicit memory differently (*e.g.*, changes in study–test modality), or in patients with impaired recognition memory or impaired priming (see Conclusion section of Chapter 23). Now that studies of repetition priming and of recognition memory have produced a number of robust findings, future studies might benefit from more careful comparison of repetition effects across these two types of memory test. In any case, the extant data promise an exciting future.

Acknowledgments

This work is funded by Wellcome Trust Fellowship 060924. The author would like to thank Mick Rugg and Ray Dolan for many useful discussions.

References

Aggleton, J. P. and Brown, M. W. (1998). Episodic memory, amnesia, and the hippocampal-anterior thalamic axis. *Behav. Brain Sci.*, **22**, 425–444.

Blaxton, T. A., Bookheimer, S. Y., Zeffiro, T. A., Figlozzi, C. M., Gaillard, W. D., and Theodore, W. H. (1996). Functional mapping of human memory using PET: comparisons of conceptual and perceptual tasks. *Can. J. Exp. Psychol.*, **50**, 42–56.

Brewer, J. B., Zhao, Z., Desmond, J. E., Glover, G. H., and Gabrieli, J. D. E. (1998). Making memories: brain activity that predicts how well visual experience will be remembered. *Science*, **281**, 185–187.

Brown, M. W. and Xiang, J. Z. (1998). Recognition memory: neuronal substrates if the judgement of prior occurrence. *Prog. Neurobiol.*, **55**, 149–189.

Buckner, R. L. and Wheeler, M. E. (2001). The cognitive neuroscience of remembering. *Nat. Neurosci. Rev.*, **2**, 624–634.

Cansino, S., Maquet, P., Dolan, R. J., and Rugg, M. D. (2002). Brain activity underlying encoding and retrieval of source memory. *Cereb. Cortex*, **12**, 1048–1056.

Chawla, D., Rees, G., and Friston, K. J. (1999). The physiological basis of attentional modulation in extrastriate visual areas. *Nat. Neurosci.*, **2**, 671–676.

Desgranges, B., Baron, J.-C., and Eustache, F. (1998). The functional neuroanatomy of episodic memory: the role of the frontal lobes, the hippocampal formation, and other areas. *NeuroImage*, **8**, 198–213.

Donaldson, W. (1996). The role of decision processes in remembering and knowing. *Memory Cogn.*, **24**, 523–533.

Eldridge, L. L., Knowlton, B. J., Furmanski, C. S., Bookheimer, S. Y., and Engel, S. A. (2000). Remembering episodes: a selective role for the hippocampus during retrieval. *Nat. Neurosci.*, **3**, 1149–1152.

Fitzgerald, P. G. and Picton, T. W. (1981). Temporal and sequential probability in evoked potential studies. *Psychophysiology*, **18**, 141.

Fletcher, P. C. and Henson, R. N. (2001). Frontal lobes and human memory: insights from functional neuroimaging. *Brain*, **124**, 849–881.

Fried, I., Cameron, K. A., Yashar, S., Fong, R., and Morrow, J. W. (2002). Inhibitory and excitatory responses of single neurons in the human medial temporal lobe during recognition of faces and objects. *Cereb. Cortex*, **12**, 575–584.

Gardiner, J. M., Gawlik, B., and Richardson-Klavehn, A. (1994). Maintenance rehearsal affects knowing not remembering: elaborative rehearsal affects remembering not knowing. *Psychonomic Bull. Rev.*, **1**, 107–110.

Green, D. M. and Swets, J. A. (1966). *Signal Detection Theory and Psychophysics*. Wiley, New York.

Hamann, S. B. and Squire, L. R. (1997). Intact perceptual memory in the absence of conscious memory. *Behav. Neurosci.*, **111**, 850–854.

Henson, R. N. A. (2004). Implicit memory, in *Human Brain Function*, 2nd ed., Frackowiak, R. S. J., Ed., Academic Press, San Diego.

Henson, R. N. A., Shallice, T., and Dolan, R. J. (1999a). Right prefrontal cortex and episodic memory retrieval: a functional MRI test of the monitoring hypothesis. *Brain*, **122**, 1367–1381.

Henson, R. N. A., Rugg, M. D., Shallice, T., Josephs, O., and Dolan, R. (1999b). Recollection and familiarity in recognition memory: an event-related fMRI study. *J. Neurosci.*, **19**, 3962–3972.

Henson, R. N. A., Rugg, M. D., Shallice, T., and Dolan, R. J. (2000). Confidence in recognition memory for words: dissociating right prefrontal roles in episodic retrieval. *J. Cogn. Neurosci.*, **12**, 913–923.

Henson, R. N. A., Cansino, S., Herron, J. E., Robb, W. G. K., and Rugg, M. D. (2003). A familiarity signal in human anterior medial temporal cortex? *Hippocampus*, **13**, 259–262.

Herron, J., Henson, R. N. A., and Rugg, M. D. (in press). Probability effects on the neural correlates of retrieval success: an fMRI study. *NeuroImage*.

Jacoby, L. L., Toth, J. P., and Yonelinas, A. P. (1993). Separating conscious and unconscious influences of memory: measuring recollection. *J. Exp. Psychol. Gen.*, **122**, 139–154.

Johnson, M. K., Hashtroudi, S., and Lindsay, D. S. (1993). Source monitoring. *Psychol. Rev.*, **114**, 3–28.

Knowlton, B. J. and Squire, L. R. (1995). Remembering and knowing: two different expressions of declarative memory. *J. Exp. Psychol. Learn. Memory Cogn.*, **21**, 699–710.

Kolers, P. A. and Roediger, H. L. (1984). Procedures of mind. *J. Verbal Learn. Verbal Behav.*, **23**, 425–449.

Mandler, G. (1980). Recognising: the judgement of previous occurrence. *Psychol. Rev.*, **87**, 252–271.

Maratos, E. J., Dolan, R. J., Morris, J. S., Henson, R. N., and Rugg, M. D. (2001). Neural activity associated with episodic memory for emotional context. *Neuropsychologia*, **39**, 910–920.

Meunier, M., Bachevalier, J., Mishkin, M., and Murray, E. A. (1993). Effects on visual recognition of combined and separate ablations of the entorhinal and perirhinal cortex in rhesus monkeys. *J. Neurosci.*, **13**, 5418–5432.

Otten, L. J. and Rugg, M. D. (2001). Task dependency of the neural correlates of episodic encoding as measured by fMRI. *Cereb. Cortex*, **11**, 1150–1160.

Otten, L. J., Henson, R. N., and Rugg, M. D. (2001). Depth of processing effects on neural correlates of memory encoding: relationship between findings from across- and within-task comparisons. *Brain*, **124**, 399–412.

Otten, L. J., Henson, R. N., and Rugg, M. D. (2002). State-related and item-related neural correlates of successful memory encoding. *Nat. Neurosci.*, **28**, 28.

Rugg, M. D. (2002). Functional imaging of memory, in *Handbook of Memory Disorders*, 2nd ed., Baddeley, A. D., Kopleman, M. D., and Wilson, B. A., Eds., pp. 57–80. John Wiley & Sons, Chichester.

Rugg, M. D. and Henson, R. N. A. (2002). Episodic memory retrieval: an (event-related) functional neuroimaging perspective, in *The Cognitive Neuroscience of Memory Encoding and Retrieval*, Parker, A. E., Wilding, E. L., and Bussey, T., Eds., pp. 3–37, Psychology Press, Hise.

Rugg, M. D. and Wilding, E. L. (2000). Retrieval processing and episodic memory. *Trends Cogn. Sci.*, **4**, 108–115.

Rugg, M. D., Fletcher, P. C., Frith, C. D., Frackowiak, R. S. J., and Dolan, R. J. (1996). Differential activation of the prefrontal cortex in successful and unsuccessful memory retrieval. *Brain*, **119**, 2073–2083.

Rugg, M. D., Fletcher, P. C., Allan, K., Frith, C. D., Frackowiak, R. S. J., and Dolan, R. J. (1998a). Neural correlates of memory retrieval during recognition memory and cued recall. *NeuroImage*, **8**, 262–273.

Rugg, M. D., Mark, R. E., Walla, P., Schloerscheidt, A. M., Birch, C. S., and Allan, K. (1998b). Dissociation of the neural correlates of implicit and explicit memory. *Nature*, **392**, 595–598.

Rugg, M. D., Henson, R. N., and Robb, W. G. (2003). Neural correlates of retrieval processing in the prefrontal cortex during recognition and exclusion tasks. *Neuropsychologia*, **41**, 40–52.

Schacter, D. L. and Tulving, E. Eds., (1994). *Memory Systems 1994*, pp. 1–38. MIT Press, Cambridge, MA.

Schott, B., Richardson-Klavehn, A., Heinze, H. J., and Duzel, E. (2002). Perceptual priming versus explicit memory: dissociable neural correlates at encoding. *J. Cogn. Neurosci.*, **14**, 578–592.

Shallice, T., Fletcher, P., Frith, C. D., Grasby, P., Frackowiak, R. S. J., and Dolan, R. J. (1994). Brain regions associated with acquisition and retrieval of verbal episodic memory. *Nature*, **368**, 633–635.

Strange, B. A., Otten, L. J., Josephs, O., Rugg, M. D., and Dolan, R. J. (2002). Dissociable human perirhinal, hippocampal, and parahippocampal roles during verbal encoding. *J. Neurosci.*, **22**, 523–528.

Tulving, E. (1985). Memory and consciousness. *Can. Psychol.*, **26**, 1–12.

Wagner, A. D., Desmond, J. E., Glover, G. H., and Gabrieli, J. D. E. (1998a). Prefrontal cortex and recognition memory: functional-MRI evidence for context-dependent retrieval processes. *Brain*, **121**, 1985–2002.

Wagner, A. D., Schacter, D. L., Rotte, M., Koustaal, W., Maril, A., Dale, A. M., Rosen, B. R., and Buckner, R. L. (1998b). Building memories: remembering and forgetting of verbal experiences as predicted by brain activity. *Science*, **21**, 188–191.

Wagner, A. D., Koutstaal, W., and Schacter, D. L. (1999). When encoding yields remembering: insights from event-related neuroimaging. *Philos. Trans. Roy. Soc. London B, Biol. Sci.*, **354**, 1307–1324.

Yonelinas, A. P., Dobbins, I., Szymanski, M. D., Dhaliwal, H. S., and King, L. (1996). Signal-detection, threshold, and dual-process models of recognition memory: ROCs and conscious recollection. *Conscious. Cogn.*, **5**, 418–441.

CHAPTER

25

Prefrontal Cortex and Long-Term Memory Encoding and Retrieval

INTRODUCTION

The application of functional neuroimaging techniques to human long-term memory has created a growing interest in the contribution of frontal lobe function to these processes. The near ubiquitous activation of lateral prefrontal cortices during memory encoding and retrieval tasks has been surprising given that prior neuropsychological studies have placed a major emphasis on the importance of medial temporal cortices. Thus, there seems to be a degree of disagreement between findings from functional neuroimaging and neuropsychology with respect to the brain structures contributing to long-term memory function. The question explored in this chapter concerns the nature of frontal lobe contribution to long-term memory and, while we do address the specific disagreements with findings from lesion studies, we suggest that areas of apparent inconsistency most likely reflect the fact that functional neuroimaging is concerned with the transient processes that occur at encoding or retrieval. Thus, by their nature they are perhaps likely to emphasise frontal involvement whereas the more slowly evolving process that constitutes memory consolidation is less amenable to functional neuroimaging.

The growing body of work implicating frontal cortex in memory encoding and retrieval provides a considerable challenge in understanding prefrontal activations in terms of processes. In view of the uncertainty surrounding the precise nature of the cognitive processes upheld by frontal cortex (FC), the experiments discussed here are considered in terms of the tasks used rather than with a strict adherence to a particular cognitive framework. An attempt will be made, however, to consider emergent patterns, from both memory encoding and retrieval studies, in terms of a tentative regional parcellation of function. This parcellation will then be examined in terms of existing models of functional topography within the prefrontal cortex. The emphasis is on verbally based memory but consideration is given to effects of material types (*i.e.*, verbal or non-verbal), particularly with reference to observation of lateralisation in frontal activations.

The chapter is divided into three parts. The first and second parts consider existing encoding and retrieval studies, respectively. The third attempts to draw together findings from both stages and to consider the extent to which common or analogous processes are associated with overlapping frontal activations.

BRAIN ACTIVATIONS ASSOCIATED WITH EPISODIC MEMORY ENCODING

Because memory encoding occurs irrespective of whether or not subjects are aware that their memory will be later tested (and, indeed, irrespective of whether or not their memory *is* later tested), the definition of an encoding study is complex. At the outset, it is important to consider what, precisely, is meant by the term *encoding*. It may, to some extent, be satisfactory to suggest that encoding processes (or processes that promote encoding) are reflected in subsequent retrieval measures. That is, we recognise that they have been operative when we test whether material is subsequently recalled. This description is, however, circular and incomplete. A number of factors influence retrieval, not all of which occur at the encoding stage, and this should caution against defining encoding processes purely in these terms. Moreover, such a description may fail to address the true nature of the encoding processes. Many cognitive operations may correlate with subsequent retrieval abilities, but this does not necessarily make them encoding operations. Undoubtedly, careful observations of how different cognitive operations performed on study material influence the extent to which that material is later recalled will be most valuable. We must nevertheless acknowledge that differential brain activations may reflect the different nature of these cognitive operations and may be interpretable only indirectly in terms of memory encoding. An alternative approach, and one that it has been possible to exploit fully only with the introduction of event-related fMRI, has been to define an encoding-related brain activation according to whether or not it is predictive of subsequent retrieval. In addition, the brain regions that are predictive of subsequent retrieval success may be compared across different task settings. As we will discuss, this approach too produces ambiguity because it may prove difficult to specify the processes occurring during the study phase that are predictive of subsequent success during the test phase.

Two classes of imaging study have explored the neuronal correlates of memory encoding. The first has sought to influence the likelihood with which an item will subsequently be retrieved (and thereby, presumably, influence the extent to which encoding processes are operative) by changing the processing requirements. This approach was largely adopted due to limitations imposed by the necessity of blocked experimental designs. It has been superseded (at least in studies in which memory encoding is directly under study) by an alternative approach—that of using subsequent memory measures to separate successful from unsuccessful encoding events within the setting of an event-related fMRI design. This broad division in experimental approach is used here to structure our consideration of the neuroimaging data.

Manipulating Encoding Through Manipulating Task Requirements.

The classic levels-of-processing approach to memory encoding (Craik and Lockhart, 1972) formed the basis for one of the earliest studies applying neuroimaging directly to encoding processes (Tulving *et al.*, 1994a). Because semantic processing engenders high levels of subsequent memory, Tulving *et al.* suggested that comparison of a semantic with a non-semantic processing task should identify systems that include brain areas associated with the encoding process. Because this effect occurs in the absence of any explicit attempt on the part of the subject to memorise material, a corollary of this approach is that language studies, in which encoding processes might be emphasised by the inclusion of semantic processing demands, should also be considered as encoding studies. An early positron emission tomography (PET) study of encoding showed that processing of words according to their meaning rather than their constituent letters produced higher levels of subsequent retrieval and of left FC activation (Kapur *et al.*, 1994). Further, Shallice *et al.* (1994) showed that left frontal activation accompanied the encoding of verbal paired associates (compared to a passive listening task) and that, when a concurrent motor distracting task was carried out, this produced an attenuation of the left frontal activation and a reduction in subsequent retrieval scores.

The above findings suggest that left FC activity may be an important accompaniment to cognitive operations that promote successful verbal encoding. The precise nature of these cognitive operations has been the subject of many subsequent functional neuroimaging studies of memory. The important observation that successful encoding with semantic processing (Craik and Lockhart, 1972) has provided the theoretical basis for a number of neuroimaging studies exploring, both directly and indirectly, episodic encoding. Several theoretical positions that have been taken are briefly described below, and the evidence in support of them is considered.

Left FC Activation at Encoding Reflects the Retrieval of Semantic Information

Tulving and colleagues (1994a), drawing on the levels-of-processing theory (Craik and Lockhart, 1972), together with a number of observations made in functional imaging studies

(Petersen *et al.*, 1988; Raichle *et al.*, 1994), suggested that the left FC activation reflected retrieval of semantic attributes. This account also suggested that lateralisation of frontal activations might reflect encoding and retrieval of verbal material, an observation that will be considered in more detail later in this chapter.

In support of the idea of semantic retrieval, many studies of semantic verbal processing have observed activation in a number of areas of left FC (Binder *et al.*, 1997; Gabrieli *et al.*, 1998; Poldrack *et al.*, 1999). This is also the case when pictorial material is presented (Vandenberghe *et al.*, 1996; Wiggs *et al.*, 1999). Moreover, Demb *et al.* (1995) produced evidence that this left FC activation does not reflect non-specific task difficulty. However, this general view that left FC participates in semantic retrieval is not universally held. Price and colleagues (Price, *et al.*, 1997) suggested that activity in left FC reflects nonspecific effects of g response-production control rather than semantic processing *per se*. In support of this, view, Frith *et al.* (1991) showed that internally generated movements are accompanied by widespread left FC activation. The question of whether the left frontal participation in retrieval (or maintenance, selection, control, or organisation; see below) is specific to semantic material is unresolved at present, but we suggest that this question may require a high degree of anatomical spatial resolution to address satisfactorily. This possibility is highlighted in one of the more thorough attempts to resolve the issue where it has been suggested that left ventrolateral frontal cortex (VLFC) may be divided into a posterior region, the activation of which reflects phonological processing, and an anterior region reflecting semantic processing (Poldrack *et al.*, 1999).

Left FC Activation at Encoding Reflects Maintenance of Semantic Information

Goldman-Rakic (1998) has suggested that different regions of FC subserve working memory for different domains. Gabrieli and colleagues (1998) used an ingenious experimental approach that proposed that, while left FC activation reflects semantic processing of verbal material, it is concerned with the maintenance of semantic material in working memory rather than with the retrieval of that material. This suggestion was based upon the observation that word stem completion tasks (*e.g.*, when a subject sees a three-letter stem and has to complete it to make a word) using stems that offer many possible completions (*e.g.*, STA...) produce higher left FC activation than those offering fewer possibilities (*e.g.*, PSA...). The logic is that the retrieval demands would be greater for the latter but that more possible responses would be available (and held online in semantic working memory) for the former.

Left FC Activation at Encoding Reflects Selection of Semantic Information

The evidence from Gabrieli's study is open to another interpretation: that left FC activation in encoding tasks reflects the fact that subjects have to select from competing semantic information, a view that Thompson-Schill and colleagues have put forward compellingly (1997). Gabrieli and colleagues acknowledged this and expressed reservations as to whether maintenance processes could ever satisfactorily be separated from selection processes. While, in our view, no functional imaging study has yet unambiguously achieved this separation, there is perhaps evidence in favour of a view that left FC activation at encoding reflects, in part, selection processes. For example, in a PET study by Dolan and Fletcher (1997) paired associates (*e.g.*, DOG...LABRADOR) were repeatedly encoded and then, following learning, changed (*e.g.*, DOG...BOXER). This change produced activation in left dorsolateral FC (DLFC) exceeding that occurring during the initial encoding of novel pairs. It is possible that the changed pairings would engender the requirement for greater selectivity without producing an increase in the overall amount of semantic material that was processed. If so, these findings are supportive for a role of left FC in selection.

Thompson-Schill and colleagues (1997) tested this possibility more thoroughly across a series of word and picture processing tasks. Higher selection demands were associated with increased left FC activity (ventrolateral and dorsolateral regions) across three semantic tasks (generation, classification, and comparison). While the purity with which they have isolated selection from retrieval and maintenance demands is not absolutely clear (discussed in Fletcher and Henson, 2001), the consistency of the left FC response across three different tasks argues strongly for the role of left FC in selection from among competing semantic alternatives. Furthermore, in a subsequent study using competition to engender higher selection demands, left posterior ventrolateral FC activity was greater when an item was processed according to criteria that had changed compared to those required on a previous presentation (Thompson-Schill *et al.*, 1999). This is highly consistent with the left FC response to changed paired associates (Dolan and Fletcher, 1997), a finding that was subsequently replicated using functional magnetic resonance imaging (fMRI) (Fletcher *et al.*, 2000).

Left FC Activation at Encoding Reflects Control of Semantic Retrieval

Wagner *et al.* (Wagner, 2001; Wagner *et al.*, 2001b) have also framed the role of left VLFC in terms of retrieval of material from semantic memory; however, they propose that its specific role lies in controlling retrieval irrespective of whether selection from among competing items is required. Such control processes would be called into play when the cue that provokes the recovery of semantic information does not strongly specify which item should be recovered. In contrast, when the cue has semantic overlap with the required response, it may be sufficient to facilitate retrieval without the need for the top-down control provided by left VLFC.

Wagner and colleagues (2001b) carried out an ingenious experiment to test this hypothesis. In an event-related fMRI study, the strength of relatedness between cue and targets was taken as an inverse measure of the degree to which control processes would be invoked. Subjects were required to judge which of two words was most closely associated with a cue. In low-control tasks, the correct response was associated strongly with the cue (*e.g.*, cue, CANDLE; target choice, FLAME or BALD). In the task designed to require a high degree of retrieval control, the correct response was only weakly related (choice: EXIST or HALO). In addition, they varied the number of possible targets (between two and four) from which to choose. Left VLFC activation was seen in the contrast of weak with strong cue–target relatedness and four items with two items (see Fig. 25.1). These investigators argued that this finding is compatible with a ventrolateral prefrontal cortex (VLPFC) role in control of retrieval given that there is no reason to suppose that selection demands would change across these tasks.

Left FC Activation at Encoding Reflects Organisation of Semantic Information

Shallice *et al.* (1994) suggested that left FC activation in verbal encoding tasks reflects the tendency to organise or group material (for example, according to semantic attributes), a view based, in part, upon neuropsychological observations (Incissa Della Rochetta and Milner, 1993; Gershberg and Shimamura, 1995). Fletcher and colleagues (1998a) tested this suggestion using a word encoding task in which the extent to which subjects were required to organise material (according to headings and subheadings) was varied. Left DLFC showed greater activity when organisational demands were increased. Moreover, when encoding occurred in association with a motor distracting task, this organisation-related left frontal activation was attenuated, and there was a simultaneous impairment in subjects' ability to carry out the task efficiently. This latter observation—a behavioural deficit (produced by distraction) associated with a neurophysiological deficit (attenuated left FC response)—provides strong grounds for an intimate link between left dorsolateral FC and organisational processes. Additionally, work by Wagner *et al.* (2001a) suggests that there may be a dissociation in function between ventrolateral and dorsolateral left frontal regions. They showed that simple maintenance of words was associated with left VLFC activation, but when those words had to be reordered according to a semantic dimension a more dorsal activation was seen. More recent support for the idea of a semantic organisational role comes from a study by Savage and colleagues (2001) who showed that left VLFC and DLFC (the latter with a focus at coordinates identical to those found by Fletcher *et al.*) were active in response to an increasing tendency to semantically cluster words in an encoding task.

Encoding Processes Identified Through Subsequent Retrieval Success

The majority of the studies described above identify encoding processes through manipulating task demands. Tasks that promote higher levels of subsequent retrieval success (deep encoding tasks) are presumed to activate brain systems that include regions specifically related to encoding. Two criticisms can be levelled at these studies. First, most used a blocked experimental design. In these instances, average brain activity measurements acquired in association with a block of one task performed repeatedly are compared to those associated with a block of

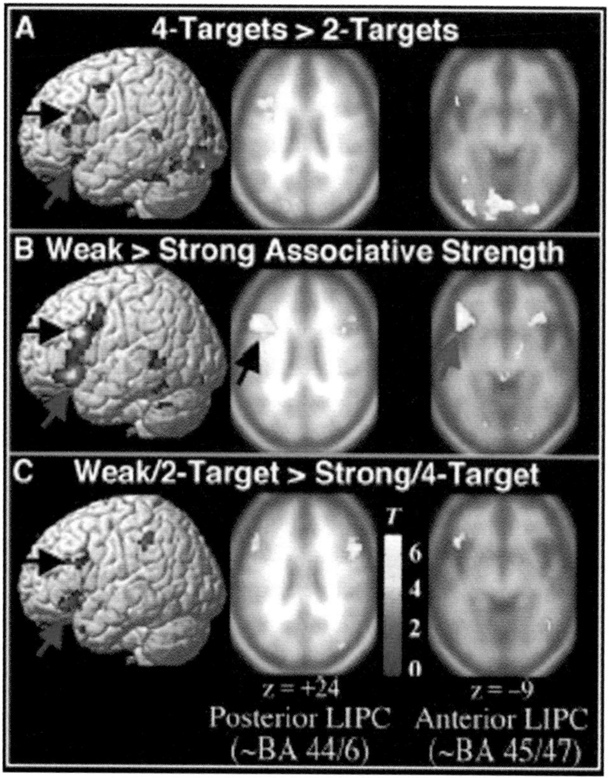

FIGURE 25.1
Main findings from Wagner *et al.* (2001b) exploring the effects of controlled retrieval. (A) Left VLPFC (more posterior dorsal region, black arrow; more anterior ventral region, red arrow) showed greater activation when subjects were required to match a probe word to a target word that is only weakly semantically associated with it. (B) Furthermore this region is activated, though to a lesser extent, when there is a greater choice of targets from which to select. (C) The relatively greater effect of the weak semantic association, as opposed to target number, is suggested by the fact that these regions are more active for weak association/low target numbers than for strong association/high target numbers. (From Wagner, A. D. *et al.*, *Neuron*, 31, 329–338, 2001. With permission.)

another task. The problem with this approach is that different tasks are not randomised but are performed predictably and repeatedly. Consequently, there may be dilution of key cognitive processes because not all items within a high encoding block will be successfully encoded and not all items in the low encoding block will remain unencoded. The predictability of task performance requirements within a block may encourage subjects to adopt optimising strategies that are only indirectly related to encoding. Second, this indirect approach to encoding often means that the two tasks will differ markedly in a number of ways that may or may not be directly related to the encoding process (*e.g.*, semantic versus non-semantic processing). If we wish to identify encoding processes in some pure form, this approach is therefore limited. Of course, this criticism is based upon our general uncertainty as to what precisely constitutes a pure encoding process.

Some studies have used blocked designs with a different aim: to identify brain regions where activity correlates with the learning process. While an event-related design is more suitable for this approach, it has nevertheless been used to good effect in a block-design experiment (Kopelman *et al.*, 1998) to show that left VLFC is more responsive to presentation of novel words (in the setting of an encoding task) and left DLFC more responsive in cases where learning actually occurred.

Event-related designs have been more frequently used to separate the haemodynamic responses associated with successfully encoded (subsequently remembered) items from those associated with unsuccessfully encoded (subsequently forgotten) items. Moreover, in such a design, because different tasks are carried out in a random and unpredictable order, the problems arising from the structure inherent in block designs are obviated. The exploration of successful versus unsuccessful encoding has been carried out with great success in event-related potential studies, deemed the D_m (difference due to subsequent memory) effect (Paller, *et al.*, 1987; Rugg,

1995). This approach offers the possibility of separating encoding processes from more general task demands.

The earliest studies showed that frontal activation at encoding was predictive of subsequent memory for verbal (Wagner *et al.*, 1998b) and visuospatial (Brewer *et al.*, 1998) material. The former study identified left ventrolateral, the latter right dorsolateral FC activation. Further studies have provided evidence for the sensitivity of left FC as a predictor of subsequent memory and of the relative strength of that subsequent memory (Henson *et al.*, 1999a; Kirchoff *et al.*, 2000; Buckner *et al.*, 2001).

Note that, in both of these studies, the D_m effect was seen within the setting of the same explicit task. Wagner and colleagues pointed to an overlap between brain regions (including left FC) that predict subsequent memory and those that subserve a semantic task compared to a non-semantic baseline (Wagner *et al.*, 1998b). This observation offers potentially important insights with respect to the cognitive nature of memory encoding, and they suggested that the overlap might be indicative that the cognitive mechanisms underlying encoding and those serving semantic deep processing are the same. Otten and colleagues explored this question further in an event-related fMRI experiment in which the D_m effect was examined subsequent to both a deep (semantic) and a shallow (alphabetical order) judgment (Otten *et al.*, 2001). A key finding was that left VLFC activity in both tasks predicts subsequent successful recognition (see Fig. 25.2). Moreover, the region showing a D_m effect is also one that shows a task effect (greater activity in the deep compared to the shallow task). Thus, their findings are compatible with those of Wagner *et al.* with respect to the overlap between a deep processing task and a successful encoding event. The question of how we are to interpret the observation that, within the setting of a shallow encoding task, left VLFC predicts subsequent memory is an interesting one. Otten and colleagues suggest that this effect occurs because there is an incidental semantic processing of items even when subjects are ostensibly carrying out the non-semantic task. This is a plausible suggestion but one that raises issues with regard to whether functional neuroimaging studies can ever offer an unambiguous understanding of the neuronal instantiation of encoding processes. It also highlights the ever-present possibility that, irrespective of overt task demands, subjects may engage in incidental processing of stimuli. If this is so, then it may be very difficult to design tasks that are pure enough to isolate a basic encoding system. Of course, this observation may provide grounds for optimism, too, as it suggests that a functional neuroimaging measure may provide an index of what the subject is actually doing during a task rather than what they have been instructed to do. The possibility of a neurophysiological indicator of an occult processing may prove useful, if it can be harnessed.

Thus, exploring the functional neuroanatomy of encoding is ultimately complex, in large part because our ideas of what constitutes an encoding process are imprecise. We may be clear as to what sorts of task conditions appear to promote encoding and we may observe when encoding has occurred through identifying items that are later remembered. However, it is unclear whether brain activations observed in association with encoding tasks are actually involved in some specific processes that we deem "encoding" or merely correlate with it in that they reflect tasks

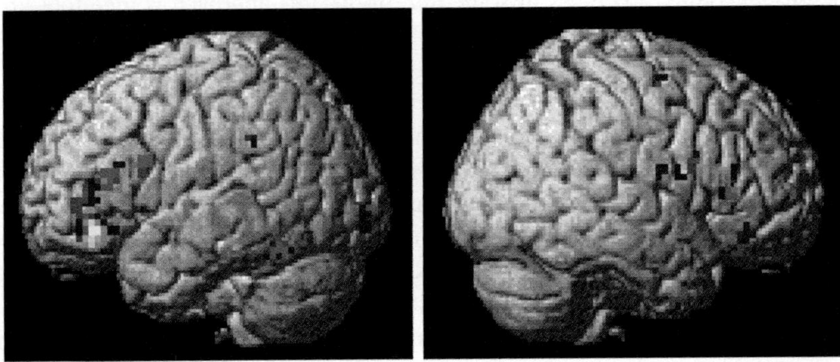

FIGURE 25.2
Subsequent memory effects in the setting of a deep (animacy judgement) encoding task. Left ventrolateral PFC activation is predictive of subsequent recognition memory. This region overlaps with a left VLPFC subsequent memory effect in a shallow encoding task. (From Otten, L. J. *et al.*, *Brain*, 124, 399–412, 2001. With permission.)

that promote encoding. Even sophisticated event-related studies that are sensitive to encoding success are limited. The challenge must lie in a more profound understanding of deep encoding processes and whether they are synonymous with or merely correlated with encoding processes. Ultimately, it seems that encoding processes may be more fruitfully described at a level other than that of regional activation such as changing inter-regional relationships or at the level of neurochemistry and synaptic plasticity.

Frontal Cortex and Encoding: A Synthesis of Evidence from Functional Neuroimaging

We now consider the broad array of findings from imaging studies of encoding with respect to two issues: (1) localisation of lateral FC activation with respect to the putative subprocesses, and (2) lateralisation of frontal activation.

Subregions and Subprocesses

The set of hypotheses outlined above has provided a useful heuristic with which to frame imaging studies and to develop imaging paradigms. The suggested processes are intimately related and, descriptively at least, hierarchically organised. At what point does retrieval merge into maintenance? How can we have selection without retrieval and maintenance? If we wish to increase selection demands, how do we do so without making greater demands on retrieval/maintenance? How might we increase demands to control semantic retrieval or to organise studied items without increasing the demand to select the semantic features that form the basis for an organisation scheme? In short, it may prove difficult to apply the standard imaging experimental design—in which groups of cognitive processes must be subtracted from each other to leave the processes of interest—to address this multilevel processing model. In any case, it seems most unlikely that any single experimental manipulation could perform this function satisfactorily. Moreover, as ever, we must consider closely the issue of whether our descriptive model of encoding has validity at a neurobiological level.

Leaving aside these caveats, there is compelling and consistent evidence that tasks requiring semantic processing of stimuli are associated with activation of various regions of left VLFC and, in some studies, left DLFC. Such processing optimises encoding (*i.e.*, it improves levels of subsequent retrieval), but for this to occur subjects need not be actively trying to remember the material. Almost invariably, semantic processing requirements encompass semantic retrieval, maintenance, and selection commonly associated with VLFC activation. It has also been suggested that the locus of semantic-related activation may lie in an anterior portion of VLFC, but this has not proved entirely consistent. Thus, while some evidence supports this viewpoint (Poldrack *et al.*, 1999), others localise it to a posterior region of VLFC, extending into DLFC (Thompson-Schill *et al.*, 1997, 1999). In addition to this localisation of the semantic processing requirement to VLFC, in the setting of both a semantic and a non-semantic task, a left VLFC region shows activity that is predictive of subsequent memory (Otten *et al.*, 2001). Moreover, within subjects there is overlap between the regions subserving semantic processing and those predicting subsequent memory, even when the task demands did not require semantic processing.

While imaging evidence therefore suggests that VLFC activation is strongly related (though in a way that is yet to be fully elucidated) to memory encoding, there are also some studies that show as strong association with DLFC activation. More dorsal activation is seen when the task demands are greater than simple semantic processing. Thus, the requirement to reorder or to organise is associated with DLFC activity (Fletcher *et al.*, 1998; Savage *et al.*, 2001; Wagner *et al.*, 2001a). Additionally, in tasks where stimuli were processed in conditions that contrasted with previous presentations of the same stimuli, dorsolateral activation was observed (Dolan and Fletcher, 1997; Thompson-Schill *et al.*, 1999). Further, the explicit manipulation of selection demands (Thompson-Schill *et al.*, 1997) produces dorsolateral activation in addition to ventrolateral FC activation.

Lateralisation of Frontal Activation at Encoding

The hemispheric encoding retrieval asymmetry (HERA) model of frontal contribution to episodic memory (Tulving *et al.*, 1994) has been highly influential. This theory was based on an early observation that many semantic and encoding tasks are associated with left FC activation and many retrieval tasks were associated with right FC activation. It has subsequently been suggested that lateralisation of activation reflects the material that has been used rather than the memory stage that was imaged. If this were so, we would expect to find that encoding of non-verbal material produces right-sided activation. Kelley and colleagues (1998) appeared to confirm that this was the case through their observation that encoding of words is associated with left (dorsolateral) FC activation, encoding of nameable objects with bilateral FC activation, and encoding of unknown faces with right FC activation. Wagner and colleagues (1998a) also demonstrated lateralisation of FC activation in an encoding task that reflected the nature of the encoded material. Furthermore, Grady and colleagues (1998) have convincingly shown that left VLFC activity is significantly greater with encoding of words compared to pictures. Nevertheless despite an apparent clarity in these observations it much be recognised that studies of encoding of verbal material have produced right as well as left FC activation (Thompson-Schill *et al.*, 1997; Poldrack *et al.*, 1999; Otten *et al.*, 2001).

BRAIN ACTIVATIONS ASSOCIATED WITH EPISODIC MEMORY RETRIEVAL

The question of whether or not an item or event has been retrieved is less problematic than whether it has been encoded. By definition, subjects are aware that a retrieved memory has come into consciousness. Retrieval may occur whether or not a subject was searching for an item, and there may be varying degrees of richness of retrieval as well as varying levels of confidence in that retrieval. The less problematic nature of retrieval is likely to account for the fact that there is considerably more functional neuroimaging data on retrieval than encoding. We have previously found it convenient to discuss retrieval-related neuroimaging studies in terms of two main groupings (Fletcher and Henson, 2001) and follow this approach here. In brief, we consider those studies that have manipulated the type of retrieval tasks and those that have manipulated the amount of material retrieved.

Studies Manipulating the Type of Retrieval Task

Intentional Versus Incidental Retrieval

The feeling of a memory simply coming to mind, in the absence of any particular aim to recall it, is a familiar one. This contrasts with the intentional retrieval of previously studied items that subjects find effortful and attention-demanding and which is often achieved through controlled and strategic memory searches. One of the earliest functional imaging studies of retrieval provided some clues as to the neurophysiological differences between these two phenomena. Squire *et al.* (1992) showed that, when subjects used word stems (*e.g.*, GAR…) as the basis for retrieving previously presented words (*e.g.*, GARAGE), activation in bilateral FC was greater than when they were instructed to complete stems merely with the first word that came to mind. The activation was located in right and left anterior FC (AFC) and in right DLFC. This finding was subsequently replicated with respect to the right AFC activation (Buckner *et al.*, 1995). Subsequently, Rugg *et al.* (1997) replicated and extended this result, showing that several regions of FC were more active during intentional than incidental recognition but that, in the case of right AFC, the response to intentional recognition occurred to a significantly greater extent when the words were more difficult to recognise (because they had been studied less efficiently at encoding). Taken together, these findings suggest that a number of frontal regions, most especially right AFC, may be related to an effortful search of the contents of memory (with greater activity when that search is rendered more difficult by poorer encoding).

Paired-Associate Cued Recall, Free Recall, Recognition Memory, and Source Memory

Memory retrieval may be tested in a number of ways. One common approach is to manipulate the degree to which subjects are prompted in their recall of an encoded event or stimulus. In tests of *recognition*, the prompt is most direct and complete, being a copy cue. For example subjects may be prompted with an entire word and required to indicate whether or not it was among those previously studied. By contrast, in tests of *free recall* subjects are completely unprompted. A variant of these two extremes is manipulation of the degree of prompting. For example, subjects may be presented with an associate (semantic or otherwise) of an item that was previously seen, or they may see some portion of the item and use this to recall the whole (*paired-associate cued recall*). In the case of words, for example, the first two or three letters of the word may be presented (*stem cued recall*) or perhaps only selected letters (*fragment cued recall*). A *source memory* task is distinct in many regards in so far as it is defined by the nature of the information that must be retrieved. A subject is not merely required to specify whether an item was previously presented but also the context (or source) of that memory. For example, a subjects may be required to specify whether an item occurred before or after a certain time point (temporal source memory) or specify which of several positions on a screen the item occupied at presentation (spatial source memory). To some extent, source memory tasks may be considered as another variation on the type of cueing that is presented, as the subject uses the retrieved item as a cue also. All of these manipulations, as we shall see, produce large effects on the magnitude and distribution of neurophysiological responses, effects that are explicable in terms of the influences that they have upon subjects' strategic approaches to a task.

The early study by Squire *et al.* (1992) of stem-cued recall produced predominantly right-sided FC activation. This finding was similar to that seen subsequently by Shallice *et al.* (1994) in a study of paired-associate cued recall. In the latter study, however, a focus of activation in right VLFC was observed in addition to that seen in DLFC (and, in contrast to Squire's study, no AFC activation was seen). Subsequently, Fletcher *et al.* (1998b) explored the effects of right FC activation of cued recall (paired-associate) compared to free recall and provided evidence for a ventrolateral–dorsolateral dissociation. In a free verbal recall task, subjects showed significantly greater activation of right DLFC, whereas cued retrieval produced significantly greater activation in right VLFC. These authors suggested that the two regions were performing qualitatively different functions in memory retrieval (VLFC in cue-specified retrieval of individual items, DLFC in the monitoring of item retrieval with respect to the overall list and the yet-to-be retrieved items). Further evidence for the role of DLFC (and AFC) in monitoring was provided by the observation that activity in this region was sensitive to the likelihood that retrieval errors may be committed during cued retrieval (Fletcher *et al.*, 1996). In a study comparing cued and free recall, however, Petrides *et al.* (1995) found the opposite pattern of response in ventrolateral FC. This may be explained by the fact that, in the latter study, items for the cued recall task were fewer and well practiced. Cabeza *et al.* (1997a) showed that neither VLFC nor DLFC appeared to differentiate between cued recall and recognition memory tasks, a finding at odds with the proposal that DLFC subserves monitoring processes required when retrieval is less specified or more demanding. However, because performance was carefully matched across the two tasks, it is feasible that monitoring requirements did not actually differ.

In a subsequent study, Cabeza and colleagues (1997b) identified greater DLFC response in a temporal source memory task (in which subjects had to decide which of two items had been presented more recently) compared to simple recognition. While this finding is consistent with a subsequent study of both temporal and spatial source retrieval (showing bilateral DLFC sensitivity to both; see Henson *et al.*, 1999b), it appears to be at odds with studies of Nyberg *et al.* (1995) and of Rugg *et al.* (1999). In both of these studies, comparisons were made between source and simple recognition memory. In the former, no FC regions showed greater activation in source memory (indeed, right VLFC activation was greater for the recognition memory task). In the latter, left AFC and VLFC were relatively more active in a spatial source judgment task. It is therefore difficult to equate the results of source memory tasks with the idea that DLFC subserves retrieval monitoring and that this monitoring is increased in such tasks compared to recognition. It should be remembered, however, that in the study by Rugg *et al.* study (1999) steps were taken to optimise source retrieval (by designing study tasks to optimise the encoding of source information). Such a manipulation may have had a critical effect on the degree to which monitoring became necessary at the retrieval stage.

In summary, the evidence from different types of verbal memory retrieval tasks is complex and rather inconclusive. FC regions are more active when subjects are engaged in intentional rather than incidental retrieval, suggesting that activation here does not reflect merely the effortless appearance of memories but rather the need to search within memory and evaluate products of that search. This view is supported by the observation that words that were subject to shallow encoding (and, hence, are more difficult to retrieve) provoke greater FC activity (in right AFC). The participation of separate FC regions in different aspects of intentional retrieval is suggested by the observation that free recall (requiring an internally guided memory search) preferentially activates right DLFC, whereas right VLFC is active in response to externally cued, paired-associate retrieval. This suggestion, while it is compatible with models of ventral–dorsal function devised on the basis of primate work (Petrides, 1998) and imaging studies of working memory (Petrides *et al.*, 1993a,b; Owen *et al.*, 1996), must be treated with caution in view of apparently contradictory data (Nyberg *et al.*, 1995; Rugg *et al.*, 1999). In the next section, we consider effects to determine the extent to which the memory search produces recollection.

The Amount and Type of Information Retrieved

The earliest studies attempting to dissociate the neuronal correlates of successful retrieval from the retrieval attempt were forced, by the temporal limitations of the PET technique, to use blocked experimental designs. In these instances experimenters compared blocks of predominantly successful memory retrieval (usually single words) with blocks in which words were mainly unstudied. There is a very real danger in these designs that subjects may quickly become aware that, in some blocks, words are old/studied and in others the words are new/unstudied. As a result, for unstudied items, subjects will realise that there is no need to engage in a retrieval attempt. Consequently, blocks may differ, not just according to retrieval success, but also according to retrieval attempt. These difficulties can be overcome in event-related designs, where it is possible to characterise differences between attempted and successful retrieval less ambiguously.

The majority of studies exploring the neuronal response to retrieval success have used word recognition paradigms; however, in the majority of memory retrieval studies, whether they have used recognition, cued recall, or free recall, the activated brain systems must include those associated with retrieval success as well as the retrieval attempt. An early study showed a dissociation between these two features by asking subjects to assess whether or not they had heard sentences before (Tulving *et al.*, 1994b). When blocks of old sentences were compared to blocks of new sentences, right DLFC and VLFC and bilateral AFC were activated. Rugg and colleagues (1996) showed that right DLFC and bilateral AFC were active when a block contained a higher proportion of words that subjects were able to recognise. The same group also showed right AFC activation in association with a memory task in which there was a higher proportion of studied words (Rugg *et al.*, 1998). In this latter study, an interaction between success and task type was observed (discussed below).

The frontal sensitivity to retrieval success is not clear cut, however. Kapur and colleagues (1995) showed that FC did not differentiate between blocks in which 85% of items were old and those in which only 15% were old (Kapur *et al.*, 1995). Rugg *et al.* (1996) made a similar observation showing that an 80:20 old/new ratio did not index measurably greater FC activity than a 20:80 ratio, but that both types of block produced significantly greater activation than a 0:100 ratio. The suggestion here was that blood flow changes occurring after each successful retrieval might be prolonged such that only a few such events within a block were sufficient to produce asymptote. This would make it difficult to unpick the effects of subtler manipulations of the proportion of old items using the blocked PET design. In other words, such designs may only be sensitive to old items (retrieval success) when a zero success baseline is used. Nyberg and colleagues (1995) showed that comparison of 100% studied word with 0% studied blocks was not associated with FC activation. It was suggested that the absence of FC activation in this study might reflect a tendency for subjects, in the conditions in which all items were new, to falsely identify some of the words as old. If true, this provides evidence that FC is sensitive to recognising or recalling items even when the memory is a false one. Studies addressing this question, by comparing true to illusory recognition indicate that this is indeed the case (Schacter *et al.*, 1996b, 1997; Cabeza *et al.*, 2001). Interestingly, Cabeza and colleagues showed a dissociation between patterns in DLFC and VLFC, with the former showing greater activity for old items and for illusory recognition and the latter for new items.

The majority of the experiments described above used blocked designs, leaving an ambiguity in interpretation of frontal responses to memory retrieval. The earliest event-related studies to address this issue found that FC did not differentiate between studied and unstudied words during a recognition test (Schacter *et al.*, 1997; Buckner *et al.*, 1998). Saykin *et al.* (1999) subsequently used an event-related design to show retrieval-related activation in right DLFC. Furthermore, Henson and colleagues (1999a) related the level of FC activity to both identifying previously studied words and the strength of this recollection. The pattern was a complex one, with both recollected (strongly remembered) and familiar (less strongly remembered) words generating FC activation, but the level of left AFC activity was greater for the former and the level of right DLFC was greater for the latter. In a further study, Henson and colleagues (2000) found broadly compatible results, showing that bilateral AFC and left DLFC were sensitive to recognised (versus new) items and that bilateral DLFC activity was greater when subjects were less confident about the veracity of their recognition (Henson *et al.*, 2000).

While certain frontal regions show sensitivity to retrieval success, over and above the attempt to retrieve material, a factor that must be taken into account is the confidence with which subjects recognise an item. Schacter and colleagues (1996a) showed that bilateral AFC activation occurred in association with cued retrieval of shallowly encoded but not deeply encoded words. While this may constitute evidence in favour of increased FC activation required in association with less confident retrieval, it also speaks against the suggestion we have developed linking FC to successful retrieval. Added complexity comes from the finding that right AFC activation can occur in association with recognition of deeply encoded words, but left DLFC and bilateral VLFC activation occurs with recognition of shallowly encoded words (Buckner *et al.*, 1998). With regard to both these studies, a manipulation of pre-scan encoding tasks is likely to have effects on the amount of success and, simultaneously, on the degree of confidence with which material is recalled. Because these studies show that FC activity is sensitive to both of these factors, a clear interpretation is difficult. Next, we consider the degree to which the type of task carried out has an influence upon the success achieved and the accompanying FC activations.

The Influence of Task Type on the FC Activations Engendered by Retrieval Success

The findings of Buckner and colleagues (1998), as well as those of Schacter and colleagues (1998), are apparently inconsistent with other retrieval data. They are, however, compatible with an observation by Rugg and colleagues (1998) that retrieval success in the setting of recognition memory produces differential FC activation to those accompanying cued retrieval tasks. In brief, while cued recall produces greater activation in bilateral AFC and left DLFC during cued recall, high success during the recognition task was associated with greater right AFC activity, while lower success in the cued retrieval task produced greater bilateral AFC activity. This set of observations suggests that, while successful recognition is associated with additional frontally mediated processes, it is failure in the cued recall tasks that requires further processing. One clear difference between a failure to recognise an item and a failure to generate a remembered word (in response to a word stem) is that, in the latter case, one is likely to continue to generate candidate responses in the hope that a remembered one may arise. This strategy is unhelpful in a recognition task, where there is little further that can be done to prompt retrieval. A key difference then in the response to recognition failure and to cued retrieval failure lies in a tendency, in the latter case, to switch between retrieval search and monitoring. Thus, a search that produces a candidate response that is deemed incorrect will invoke further search and monitoring (Fletcher and Henson, 2001). We interpret AFC activations that accompanied retrieval failure in cued recall (but not in recognition memory) as reflecting the control of repeated switching between search and retrieval processes.

Allen and colleagues (2000) carried out a further study that addressed this issue by exploring the effects of retrieval success across two types of cued recall tasks. They examined word stem cued and fragment cued retrieval in high- and low-success blocks. As with the experiments above, AFC (on the right) was activated for low success in the stem cued retrieval, and this effect was significantly greater than for low success in the fragment cued condition, in which fewer completions were possible. This pattern is compatible with the idea of a role for right AFC in switching between search and monitoring processes because such switching will occur in cases where more (incorrect) candidate responses are generated (in this case, for stem cued rather than fragment cued retrieval). This study also produced less consistent results in that left AFC activity was greater for successful than unsuccessful stem cued retrieval, and right DLFC activity was greater for successful than unsuccessful fragment cued retrieval.

One study that that has bearing on search/monitoring processing is an investigation into the *tip of the tongue* phenomenon (Maril *et al.*, 2001). This term refers to the commonly experienced phenomenon of knowing something but not being able to access it. Maril and colleagues elicited this in healthy volunteers and showed an association with activation in right AFC and VLFC. This activation was significantly greater than that associated with both correct responses and with "don't know" responses not accompanied by the tip of the tongue phenomenon. The implication is that these regions reflect processes associated with a continuing memory search and, particularly, with a search in which candidate responses may be produced but rejected.

Frontal Cortex and Retrieval: A Synthesis of Evidence from Functional Neuroimaging

We now consider the findings from imaging studies of episodic memory retrieval with respect to the same two issues covered at the end of the section on encoding: (1) localisation of lateral FC activation with respect to the putative subprocesses, and (2) lateralisation of frontal activation.

Subregions and Subprocesses

The patterns to emerge from episodic memory retrieval studies are much less clear than from encoding studies. A large number of inconsistencies may in part be explained by technical and design limitations (for discussion, see Fletcher and Henson, 2001); however, there are grounds for suggesting that existing imaging data may be usefully, albeit incompletely, explained in terms of a proposed model of memory retrieval (Burgess and Shallice, 1996). This model includes two stages of the retrieval process, the first of which lies in the identification and specification of search parameters and the second in the post-retrieval appraisal of the products of that memory search. An inclusion of a third component to this model (the additional control processes that must be required to integrate and adjust the components of the search–monitor–verify process) allows us to account for the retrieval imaging data more fully. In brief, the three main areas of lateral FC activation that have repeatedly been found across episodic memory retrieval studies may be usefully related to these three cognitive components of the retrieval process (Fletcher and Henson, 2001). More specifically, we suggest that VLFC activation tends to reflect the initial specification of the search process, DLFC reflects the post-retrieval monitoring/verification processes, and AFC activation reflects the higher order processes that are used in controlling the overall memory search with regard to its ongoing success and to changes that occur due to lack of success or task demands. It must be conceded that the experimental support for this tentative model is weak and inconsistent and that direct experimental testing is required.

Ventrolateral frontal cortex activity has been associated with cued paired-associate retrieval (Shallice *et al.*, 1994), and it has been observed that free recall produced a lesser activation in the same region (Fletcher *et al.*, 1998b). One clear difference between these two tasks was that, in the cued recall condition, the search spaced was repeatedly defined and redefined on the basis of experimentally provided cues. The particular sensitivity of VLFC to this task is therefore compatible with the model's prediction. Moreover, in an extreme case of memory searching, when something is on the tip of the tongue the increase in VLFC activity invites a similar explanation. An inconsistency of VLFC activity associated with recognition memory tasks is perhaps unsurprising because, in many instances, no real search is required; a copy cue is presented and defines precisely the response that is required. In other cases, the recognition task may be more demanding, with the copy cue providing the impetus for a search that becomes more far reaching, in which case VLFC activation may occur.

The role of DLFC in monitoring, selection, and manipulation of the products of episodic retrieval is supported by a general pattern of activation seen when a task demands that retrieved material is subject to further processing. Further processing is a necessity for retrieval of source material that consistently leads to DLFC activation (Cabeza *et al.*, 1997b; Henson *et al.*, 1999b; Rugg *et al.*, 1999). In addition, if each retrieved item must be incorporated into a predefined structure in order to guide further retrieval success (*i.e.*, to prevent repetition or omission), DLFC activation is seen. Note that, here, the idea is not simply that DLFC activation occurs when the task is simply more difficult for the subject but rather when there is a particular demand to assess and possibly further evaluate retrieved material. Thus, VLFC and AFC activation has been observed in the study of tip of the tongue phenomena (Maril *et al.*, 2001), which is highly demanding, whereas in a recognition task (in which demands were held constant) DLFC activity was sensitive to the trials in which subjects were not confident that their response was correct, a setting in which one would predict higher levels of evaluation of the retrieved material (Henson *et al.*, 2000).

The activation of AFC may reflect higher level controlling processes required under a number of circumstances. An early observation was that AFC activity is greater for intentional than incidental retrieval and that more demanding retrieval tasks (*e.g.*, when the preceding encoding task was a shallow rather than a deep one) tend to provoke greater activation here. These observations in themselves are suggestive that AFC may have such a controlling role but the picture is not an entirely consistent. One factor that must be taken into account is that a memory retrieval task will, in different circumstances and subjects, be comprised of many different processes and strategies. In dealing with blocks of stimuli, subjects are likely to evaluate each component stimulus not only in isolation but also with respect to the overall task design, expectancy, and changing strategies. Thus, subjects working with blocks where the number of targets have been manipulated but who remain unaware of this manipulation may interpret the fact that they are identifying a lot of items as "old" as evidence that their memory is faulty and that they should reevaluate the threshold for such an identification. The suggestion is that AFC may play a part in precisely this sort of evaluation and reappraisal. As a result, its activity may very from study to study in a way that is inconsistent with respect to task demands but may be perfectly consistent when the subject's covert behaviour is considered more closely. This is a speculative notion but it does provide an explanation for some of the FC activity patterns (*e.g.*, the task-by-success interaction observed by Rugg *et al.*, described above).

Lateralisation of Frontal Activation at Retrieval

According to the HERA model, retrieval of verbal (or verbalisable) material should be associated with right FC activation. As with the left-sided activation that is seen at encoding, this may be a reflection of material rather than a reflection of differential processes that occur at these stages. Relevant to this, Wagner and colleagues (1998a) showed that retrieval of verbal material was associated with left and retrieval of non-verbal material with bilateral VLFC. In addition, the lateralisation of retrieval-related FC activation is highly inconsistent (more so than in verbal encoding studies). In a review of encoding and retrieval studies (Fletcher and Henson, 2001) we observed that, out of 22 verbal encoding studies, 17 contained encoding-related contrasts that were associated with FC activation solely on the left side. Out of 25 verbal retrieval studies, only 11 showed a purely right-sided effect. This is a highly informal analysis, and the question is only likely to be settled by further work directly comparing encoding with retrieval and verbal with non-verbal material.

SUMMARY

Functional neuroimaging techniques have had a major impact on views regarding the contributions of FC to verbal memory encoding and retrieval; however, at present we must acknowledge that interpretation of localised activations is constrained by inadequate models of the frontal role in memory and, indeed, in cognition more generally. A valuable contribution of the functional neuroimaging techniques may lie in extending, refining, and testing theoretical models of frontal function rather than in the more widely used brain mapping process in which cognitive processes are localised to specific regions. This use of neuroimaging as a basis for exploring cognitive models may be approached in several ways. For example, imaging observations can provide evidence that tasks that are behaviourally identical in other ways have different neurophysiological correlates and, therefore, are likely to engage different cognitive processes. Conversely, imaging observations may point to neurophysiological overlap in seemingly diverse tasks and, by extrapolation, may show that common cognitive subprocesses underlie a variety of behaviourally diverse situations. In view of the likelihood that any given frontally mediated process is likely to occur across a number of task domains and contexts, this latter area of exploration, which forms the basis for the review in this chapter, may prove valuable.

References

Allan, K., Dolan, R. J., Fletcher, P. C., and Rugg, M. D. (2000). The role of right anterior prefrontal cortex in episodic memory retrieval. *NeuroImage*, **11**, 217–227.

Binder, J. R., Frost, J. A., Hammeke, T. A., Cox, R. W., Rao, S. M., and Prieto, T. (1997). Human brain language areas identified by functional magnetic resonance imaging. *J. Neurosci.*, **17**(1), 353–362.

Brewer, J. B., Zhao, Z., Desmond, J. E., Glover, G. H., and Gabrieli, J. D. (1998). Making memories: brain activity that predicts how well visual experience will be remembered [see comments]. *Science*, **281**, 1185–1187.

Buckner, R. L., Koutstaal, W., Schacter, D. L., Dale, A. M., Rotte, M., and Rosen, B. R. (1998). Functional-anatomic study of episodic retrieval. II. Selective averaging of event-related fMRI trials to test the retrieval success hypothesis. *NeuroImage*, **7**, 163–175.

Buckner, R. L., Raichle, M. E., and Petersen, S. E. (1995). Dissociation of human prefrontal cortical areas across different speech production tasks and gender groups. *J. Neurophysiol.*, **74**, 2163–2173.

Buckner, R. L., Wheeler, M. A., and Sheridan, M. (2001). Encoding processes during retrieval tasks. *J. Cogn. Neurosci.*, **13**(3), 406–415.

Burgess, P. W., and Shallice, T. (1996). Confabulation and the control of recollection. *Memory*, **4**(2), 359–412.

Cabeza, R., Kapur, S., Craik, F. I. M., Mcintosh, A. R., Houle, S., and Tulving, E. (1997a). Functional neuroanatomy of recall and recognition: a PET study of episodic memory. *J. Cogn. Neurosci.*, **9**, 254–265.

Cabeza, R., Mangels, J., Nyberg, L., Habib, R., Houle, S., Mcintosh, A. R., and Tulving, E. (1997b). Brain regions differentially involved in remembering what and when: a PET study. *Neuron*, **19**, 863–870.

Cabeza, R., Rao, S. M., Wagner, A. D., Mayer, A. R., and Schacter, D. L. (2001). Can medial temporal lobes distinguish true from false? An event-related functional MRI study of veridical and illusory recognition memory. *Proc. Natl. Acad. Sci. U.S.A.*, **98**(8), 4805–4810.

Craik, F. I. and Lockhart, R. S. (1972). Levels of processing: a framework for memory research. *J. Verbal Learn. Verbal Behav.*, **11**, 671–684.

Demb, J. B., Desmond, J. E., Wagner, A. D., Vaidya, C. J., Glover, G. H., and Gabrieli, J. D. (1995). Semantic encoding and retrieval in the left inferior prefrontal cortex: a functional MRI study of task difficulty and process-specificity. *J. Neurosci.*, **15**(9), 5870–5878.

Dolan, R. J. and Fletcher, P. C. (1997). Dissociating prefrontal and hippocampal function in episodic memory encoding. **388**, 582–585.

Fletcher, P. C. and Henson, R. N. A. (2001). Frontal lobes and human memory: insights from functional neuroimaging. *Brain*, **124**, 849–881.

Fletcher, P. C., Shallice, T., Frith, C. D., Frackowiak, R. S., and Dolan, R. J. (1996). Brain activity during memory retrieval: the influence of imagery and semantic cueing. *Brain*, **119**, 1587–1596.

Fletcher, P. C., Shallice, T., and Dolan, R. J. (1998a). The functional roles of prefrontal cortex in episodic memory. I. Encoding. *Brain*, **121**, 1239–1248.

Fletcher, P. C., Shallice, T., Frith, C. D., Frackowiak, R. S., and Dolan, R. J. (1998b). The functional roles of prefrontal cortex in episodic memory. II. Retrieval. *Brain*, **121**, 1249–1256.

Fletcher, P. C., Shallice, T., and Dolan, R. J. (2000). Sculpting the response space: an account of left prefrontal activation at encoding. *NeuroImage*, **12**(4), 404–417.

Frith, C. D., Friston, K. J., Liddle, P. F., and Frackowiak, R. S. J. (1991). Willed action and the prefrontal cortex in man: a study with PET. *Proc. Roy. Soc. London Ser. B*, **244**, 241–246.

Gabrieli, J. D., Poldrack, R. A., and Desmond, J. E. (1998). The role of left prefrontal cortex in language and memory. *Proc. Natl. Acad. Sci. U.S.A.*, **95**, 906–913.

Gershberg, F. B. and Shimamura, A. P. (1995). Impaired use of organisational strategies in free recall following frontal lobe damage. *Neuropsychologia*, **33**, 1305–1333.

Goldman-Rakic, P. S. (1998). The prefrontal landscape: implications of functional architecture for understanding human mentation and the central executive, in *The Prefrontal Cortex: Executive and Cognitive Functions*, Roberts, A., Robbins, T. W. and Weizkrantz, L., Eds., pp. 87–102. Oxford University Press, London.

Grady, C. L., Mcintosh, A. R., Rajah, M. N., and Craik, F. I. M. (1998). Neural correlates of the episodic encoding of pictures and words. *Proc. Natl. Acad. Sci. USA*, **95**, 2703–2708.

Henson, R. N. A., Rugg, M. D., Shallice, T., Josephs, O., and Dolan, R. J. (1999a). Recognition and familiarity in recognition memory: an event-related functional magnetic resonance imaging study. *J. Neurosci.*, **19**(10), 3962–3972.

Henson, R. N. A., Shallice, T., and Dolan, R. J. (1999b). Right prefrontal cortex and epsiodic memory retrieval: a functional MRI test of the monitoring hypothesis. *Brain*, **122**, 1367–1381.

Henson, R. N. A., Rugg, M. D., Shallice, T., and Dolan, R. J. (2000). Confidence in recognition memory for words: dissociating right prefrontal roles in episodic retrieval. *J. Cogn. Neurosci.*, **12**(6), 913–923.

Incissa Della Rochetta, A. and Milner, B. (1993). Strategic search and retrieval inhibition: the role of the frontal lobes. *Neuropsychologia*, **31**, 503–524.

Kapur, S., Craik, F. I., Tulving, E., Wilson, A. A., Houle, S., and Brown, G. M. (1994). Neuroanatomical correlates of encoding in episodic memory: levels of processing effect. *Proc. Natl. Acad. Sci. U.S.A.*, **91**, 2008–2011.

Kapur, S., Craik, F. I., Jones, C., Brown, G. M., Houle, S., and Tulving, E. (1995). Functional role of the prefrontal cortex in retrieval of memories: a PET study. *Neuroreport*, **6**, 1880–1884.

Kelley, W. M., Miezin, F. M., McDermott, K. B., Buckner, R. L., Raichle, M. E., Cohen, N. J., Ollinger, J. M., Akbudak, E., Conturo, T. E., Snyder, A. Z., and Petersen, S. E. (1998). Hemispheric spcialisation in human dorsal frontal cortex and medial temporal lobe for verbal and nonverbal memory encoding. *Neuron*, **20**, 927–938.

Kirchoff, B. A., Wagner, A. D., Maril, A., and Stern, C. E. (2000). Prefrontal-temporal circuitry for episodic encoding and subsequent memory. *J. Neurosci.*, **20**(16), 6173–6180.

Kopelman, M. D., Stevens, T. G., Foli, S., and Grasby, P. (1998). PET activation of the medial temporal lobe in learning. **121**(Pt. 5), 875–887.

Maril, A., Wagner, A. D., and Schacter, D. L. (2001). On the tip of the tongue: an event-related fMRI study of semantic retrieval failure and cognitive conflict. *Neuron*, **31**, 653–660.

Nyberg, L., Tulving, E., Habib, R., Nilsson, L. G., Kapur, S., Houle, S., Cabeza, R., and Mcintosh, A. R. (1995). Functional brain maps of retrieval mode and recovery of episodic information [see comments]. *Neuroreport*, **7**, 249–252.

Otten, L. J., Henson, R. N. A., and Rugg, M. D. (2001). Depth of processing effects on neural correlates of memory encoding: relationship between findings from across- and within-task comparisons. *Brain*, **124**, 399–412.

Owen, A. M., Evans, A. C., and Petrides M. (1996). Evidence for a two-stage reader of spatial working memory processing within the lateral frontal cortex model positron: a emision tomography study. *Cereb. Cortex*, **6**, 31–38.

Paller, K. A., Kutas, M., and Mayes, A. M. (1987). Neural correlates of encoding in an incidental learning paradigm. *Electroencephalography and Clin. Neurophysiol.*, **67**, 360–371.

Petersen, S. E., Fox, P. T., Posner, M. I., Mintun, M., and Raichle, M. E. (1988). Positron emission tomographic studies of the cortical anatomy of single-word processing. *Nature*, **331**, 585–589.

Petrides, M. (1998). Specialised systems for the processing of mnemonic information within the primate frontal cortex, in *The Prefrontal Cortex: Executive and Cognitive Functions*, Roberts, A., Robbins, T. W., and Weizkrantz, L., Eds., pp. 103–116. Oxford University Press, London.

Petrides, M., Alivisatos, B., Evans, A. C., and Meyer, E. (1993a). Dissociation of human mid-dorsolateral from posterior dorsolateral frontal cortex in memory processing. *Proc. Natl. Acad. Sci. U.S.A.*, **90**(3), 873–877.

Petrides, M., Alivisatos, B., Meyer, E., and Evans, A. C. (1993b). Functional activation of the human frontal cortex during the performance of verbal working memory tasks. *Proc. Natl. Acad. Sci. U.S.A.*, **90**, 878–882.

Petrides, M., Alivisatos, B., and Evans, A. C. (1995). Functional activation of the human ventrolateral frontal cortex during mnemonic retrieval of verbal information. *Proc. Natl. Acad. Sci. U.S.A.*, **92**, 5803–5807.

Poldrack, R. A., Wagner, A. D., Prull, M. W., Desmond, J. E., Glover, G. H., and Gabrieli, J. D. E. (1999). Functional specialisation for semantic and phonological processing in the left inferior prefrontal cortex. *NeuroImage*, **10**, 15–35.

Price, C. J., Moore, C. J., Humphreys, G. W., and Wise, R. S. J. (1997). Segregating semantic from phonological processes during reading. *J. Cogn. Neurosci.*, **9**, 727–733.

Raichle, M. E., Fiez, J. A., Videen, T. O., MacLeod, A. M., Pardo, J. V., Fox, P. T., and Petersen, S. E. (1994). Practice-related changes in human brain functional anatomy during nonmotor learning. *Cereb. Cortex*, **4**, 8–26.

Rugg, M. D., Fletcher, P. C., Frith, C. D., Frackowiak, R. S., and Dolan, R. J. (1996). Differential activation of the prefrontal cortex in successful and unsuccessful memory retrieval. *Brain*, **119**, 2073–2083.

Rugg, M. D., Fletcher, P. C., Frith, C. D., Frackowiak, R. S., and Dolan, R. J. (1997). Brain regions supporting intentional and incidental memory: a PET study. *Neuroreport*, **8**, 1283–1287.

Rugg, M. D., Fletcher, P. C., Allan, K., Frith, C. D., Frackowiak, R. S., and Dolan, R. J. (1998). Neural correlates of memory retrieval during recognition memory and cued recall. *NeuroImage*, **8**, 262–273.

Rugg, M. D., Fletcher, P. C., Chua, P. M.-L., and Dolan, R. J. (1999). The role of prefrontal cortex in recognition memory and memory for source: an fMRI study. *NeuroImage*, **10**(5), 520–529.

Rugg, M. D. (1995). ERP studies of memory, In: *Electrophysiology of Mind: Event-related Brain Potentials and Cognition*. Rugg, M. D. and Coles, G. H., Eds., pp. 132–170. Oxford University Press, Oxford.

Savage, C. R., Deckersback, T., Heckers, S., Wagner, A. D., Schacter, D. L., Alpert, N. M., Fischman, A. J., and Rauch, S. L. (2001). Prefrontal regions supporting spntaneous and directed application of verbal learning strategies. *Brain*, **124**(1), 219–231.

Saykin, A. J., Johnson, S. C., Flashman, L. A., McAllister, T. W., Sparling, M., and Darcey, T. M. (1999). Functional differentiation of medial temporal and frontal regions involved in processing novel and familiar words: an fMRI study. *Brain*, **122**, 1963–1971.

Schacter, D. L., Alpert, N. M., Savage, C. R., Rauch, S. L., and Albert, M. S. (1996a). Conscious recollection and the human hippocampal formation: evidence from positron emission tomography. *Proc. Natl. Acad. Sci. U.S.A.*, **93**, 321–325.

Schacter, D. L., Reiman, E., Curran, T., Yun, L. S., Bandy, D., McDermott, K. B., and Roediger, H. L.-R. (1996b). Neuroanatomical correlates of veridical and illusory recognition memory: evidence from positron emission tomography [see comments]. *Neuron*, **17**, 267–274.

Schacter, D. L., Buckner, R. L., Koutstaal, W., Dale, A. M., and Rosen, B. R. (1997). Late onset of anterior prefrontal activity during true and false recognition: an event-related fMRI study. *NeuroImage*, **6**, 259–269.

Shallice, T., Fletcher, P., Frith, C. D., Grasby, P., Frackowiak, R. S., and Dolan, R. J. (1994). Brain regions associated with acquisition and retrieval of verbal episodic memory. *Nature*, **368**, 633–635.

Squire, L. R., Ojemann, J. G., Miezin, F. M., Petersen, S. E., Videen, T. O., and Raichle, M. E. (1992). Activation of the hippocampus in normal humans: a functional anatomical study of memory. *Proc. Natl. Acad. Sci. U.S.A.*, **89**, 1837–1841.

Thompson-Schill, S. L., D'Esposito, M., Aguirre, G. K., and Farah, M. J. (1997). Role of left inferior prefrontal cortex in retrieval of semantic knowledge: a re-evaluation. *Proc. Natl. Acad. Sci. USA*, **94**, 14792–14797.

Thompson-Schill, S. L., D'Esposito, M., and Kan, I. P. (1999). Effects of repetition and competition on activity in left prefrontal cortex during word generation. *Neuron*, **23**, 513–522.

Tulving, E., Kapur, S., Craik, F. I., Moscovitch, M., and Houle, S. (1994a). Hemispheric encoding/retrieval asymmetry in episodic memory: positron emission tomography findings. *Proc. Natl. Acad. Sci. USA*, **91**(6), 2016–2020.

Tulving, E., Kapur, S., Markowitsch, H. J., Craik, F. I., Habib, R., and Houle, S. (1994b). Neuroanatomical correlates of retrieval in episodic memory: auditory sentence recognition [see comments]. *Proc. Natl. Acad. Sci. U.S.A.*, **91**, 2012–2015.

Vandenberghe, R., Price, C., Wise, R., Josephs, O., and Frackowiak, R. S. (1996). Functional anatomy of a common semantic system for words and pictures. *Nature*, **383**(6597), 254–256.

Wagner, A. D. (2001). Cognitive control and episodic memory: contributions from prefrontal cortex, in *Neuropsychology of Memory*, Squire, L. R. and Schacter, D. L., Eds., Guildford Press, New York.

Wagner, A. D., Poldrack, R. A., Eldridge, L. L., Desmond, J. E., Glover, G. H., and Gabrieli, J. D. E. (1998a). Material-specific lateralisation during episodic encoding and retrieval. *NeuroReport*, **9**(16), 3711–3717.

Wagner, A. D., Schacter, D. L., Rotte, M., Koutstaal, W., Maril, A., Dale, A. M., Rosen, B. R., and Buckner, R. L. (1998b). Building memories: remembering and forgetting of verbal experiences as predicted by brain activity. *Science*, **281**(5380), 1188–1191.

Wagner, A. D., Maril, A., Bjork, R. A., and Schacter, D. L. (2001a). Prefrontal contributions to executive control: fMRI evidence for functional distinctions within lateral prefrontal cortex. *NeuroImage*, **14**, 1337–1347.

Wagner, A. D., Pare-Blaegov, E. J., Clark, J., and Poldrack, R. A. (2001b). Recovering meaning: left prefrontal cortex guides controlled semantic retrieval. *Neuron*, **31**, 329–338.

Wiggs, C. L., Weisberg, J., and Martin, A. (1999). Neural correlates of semantic and episodic memory retrieval. *Neuropsychologia*, **37**, 103–118.

SECTION FIVE

LANGUAGE AND SEMANTICS

This section considers the functional neuroanatomy that underlies the comprehension and production of spoken and written words. This first chapter addresses three of the fundamental components of language: auditory speech comprehension, speech production, and semantic retrieval (see Fig. 26.1). This is followed by a more detailed consideration of the organisation of the semantic system in Chapter 27, the neural systems for reading in Chapter 28, and the nature of the neuronal abnormality in developmental dyslexia in Chapter 29. The section then concludes in Chapter 30 with a methodological review of the most efficient experimental designs and analysis for functional imaging studies of language.

CHAPTER

26

An Overview of Speech Comprehension and Production

SPEECH COMPREHENSION AND PRODUCTION

Words are learned by associating sounds and visual symbols with information in our external environment and inner world. The neural systems for speech comprehension and production therefore develop from cortical activity in sensory and motor areas. A recurrent theme in this chapter concerns the specificity of language processing: Are certain brain areas specific to language processing (*e.g.*, areas specialised for phonology), or does language emerge at the systems level from interactions among areas that each serve multiple (including non-linguistic) functions? For example, if brain areas are specialised for auditory speech comprehension, then we would expect to find responses in auditory areas that are primarily driven by speech input. Conversely, if auditory speech comprehension emerges at the systems level from interactions among areas responding to acoustic activity, motor control, and cognitive processing, then other complex auditory stimuli will evoke similar effects in auditory association cortex. In order to establish speech specificity, we therefore contrast auditory speech comprehension to complex environmental sound processing and speech production with other motor tasks (*e.g.*, tongue and finger movements). Similarly, at the level of word meaning, we ask: Does semantic retrieval activate the same neural system irrespective of the stimulus modality, or are the semantic retrieval areas specific for linguistic input? The hypothesised relationships between the sensory and motor components of speech processing are illustrated in Fig. 26.1.

Auditory Speech Comprehension

The comprehension of auditory speech includes the acoustic analysis of the auditory input, the recognition of speech sounds (phonemes), and access to the semantic system. Acoustically, the differentiation of speech sounds requires a continuous and rapid analysis of the distribution of sound frequencies (the spectral structure) and how these frequencies and their relative amplitudes change over time (the temporal structure). Lesion studies have suggested that the left auditory cortex is necessary for the perception of temporal information while the right auditory cortex is necessary for the perception of spectral information (Robin *et al.*, 1990). Nevertheless, because deficits specific to the discrimination of speech sounds (pure word deafness) are usually only reported after bilateral lesions restricted to the superior temporal lobes (Auerbach *et al.*, 1982; Buchman *et al.*, 1986), it is clear that either the left or the right superior temporal cortex can sustain the acoustic analysis of speech. In contrast, deficits in auditory speech recognition (the post-phonemic analysis stage) have traditionally been associated with lesions to the left posterior third of the superior temporal gyrus, where the memories for speech sounds were

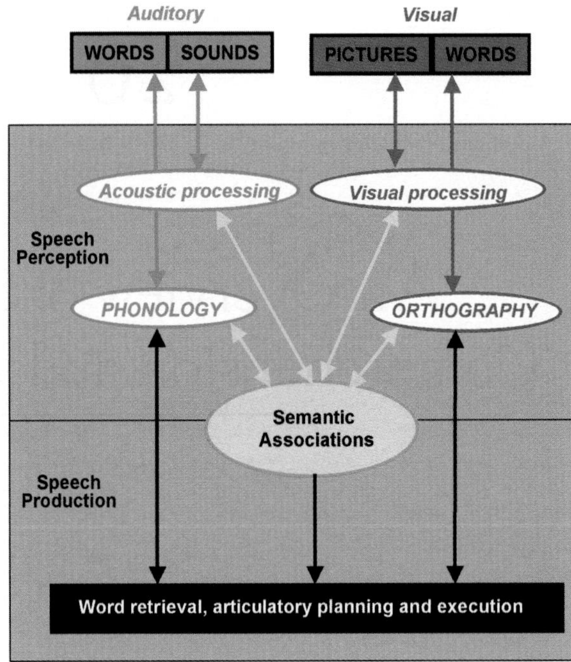

FIGURE 26.1
Building blocks for speech comprehension and production.

thought to be stored (Geschwind, 1965; Lichtheim, 1885; Wernicke, 1874). The relative importance of the left posterior superior temporal cortex has also been highlighted by findings that, in normal brains, the posterior third of the left superior temporal gyrus (especially the planum temporale) is larger than its homologue in the right hemisphere (Galaburda *et al.*, 1978).

In the last 15 years, functional imaging studies have sought to specify the anatomy of the different speech processes more precisely. These studies have compared cortical activation for auditory speech input to a range of nonlinguistic auditory stimuli that are matched to speech for various dimensions of the sound structure. On the basis of the lesion data discussed above, it might be expected that the left posterior superior temporal cortex, especially the planum temporale, would be differentially responsive to speech. In contrast, functional imaging studies have shown that: (1) the response of the left planum temporale is on the same order of magnitude for tones as it is for speech (Binder *et al.*, 2000), and (2) speech (relative to complex acoustic stimuli) activates the superior temporal sulci bilaterally, with peak activation lateral and ventral to Heschl's gyri (Binder *et al.*, 2000; Mummery *et al.*, 1999; Vouloumanos *et al.*, 2001). Vouloumanos *et al.* (2001) and Janke *et al.* (2002) have therefore concluded that the activations in superior temporal sulci demonstrate specialisation for speech processing. This conclusion, however, is based on two assumptions. The first is that the superior temporal activation did not reflect acoustic processes that were shared by speech and non-speech but enhanced during speech as a consequence of increased attention to the presence of familiar stimuli. Indeed, the mid-portions of the superior temporal sulci ($y = -10$ to -26 in Talairach and Tournoux space) are also activated by the perception of fine grained (millisecond) modulations in the amplitude and frequency structure of tones and noise (Belin *et al.*, 1998; Giraud *et al.*, 2000; Griffiths *et al.*, 1998; Hall *et al.*, 2002). The second assumption, with respect to specialisation for speech, is that the complex non-speech stimuli controlled for all levels of prelexical acoustic analysis. Vouloumanos *et al.* (2001) used "complex sine wave analogues" which controlled for the duration, pitch contour, amplitude envelope, relative formant amplitude, and intensity of speech but not the broader band formant information and parts of the harmonic spectrum. Likewise, spectral structure (*i.e.*, the pitch/frequency composition) was not controlled in the "signal correlated noise" used by Mummery *et al.* (1999). Therefore, although the extensive bilateral superior temporal activations may be analysing acoustic information that is necessary for speech

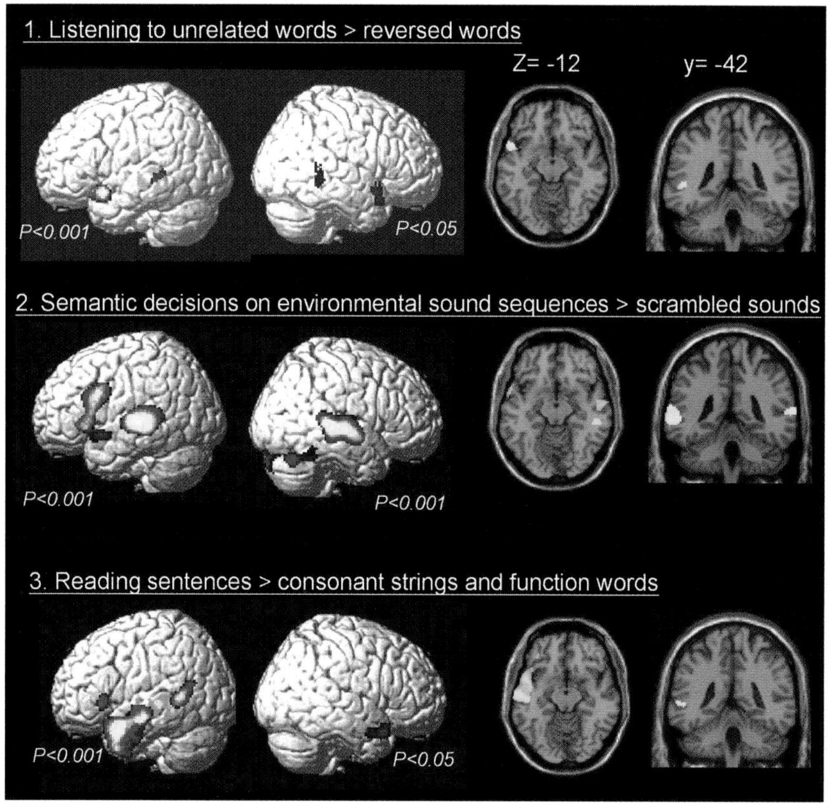

	1. Listen Words *(Price et al., '96)*	**2. Environmental sounds** (Thierry et al., '03)	**3. Written sentences** *(Vandenberghe et al.'01)*
Anterior STS			
Left:	-54, 16, -10 (3.8)	-58, 10, -10 (3.7)	-50, 8, -20 (7.0)
Right:	60, 14, -16 (2.3)	*ns*	56,12, -26 (2.9)
Posterior STS			
Left:	-50, -42, 0 (3.3)	-64, -36, 2 (5.6)	-58, -52, 6 (5.9)
Right:	46, -40, 0 (2.8)	52, -30, -4 (5.4)	*ns*

FIGURE 26.2
Speech perception areas.

recognition, these paradigms do not isolate the areas involved in speech recognition or determine whether the responses are specific to speech.

When the spectral structure is controlled by comparing speech to reversed speech, activation in the superior temporal sulci is greatly reduced (Binder *et al.*, 2000; Hickok *et al.*, 1997; Howard *et al.*, 1992; Price *et al.*, 1996). Figure 26.2 (row 1) shows the comparison of hearing words and reversed words reported in Price *et al.* (1996). Discrete regions of the left anterior and posterior superior temporal sulcus can be observed, with even smaller effects in the corresponding right hemisphere areas. Because reversed words control for amplitude modulations and the average spectral content of speech but not the temporal ordering of frequency and amplitude changes (the abrupt onsets and long delays in speech are reversed), the anterior and/or posterior activation differences between speech and reversed speech may reflect analysis of the temporal structure. Indeed, when speech was contrasted to rotated speech (Scott *et al.*, 2000), which controls for spectral and temporal processing but not speech recognition, activation was only observed in the left anterior superior temporal sulcus ($x = -54$, $y = +6$, $z = -16$), whereas the posterior superior temporal area (–64, –38, 0) responded to both speech and rotated speech. On the basis of these results, Scott *et al.* (2000) have associated the posterior area with analysis of the phonetic cues and features that are determined by the temporal ordering of events (in speech and rotated speech but not reversed speech) and the left anterior superior temporal area with intelligibility (word form recognition and beyond).

The question we come back to concerns the specificity of auditory responses for speech processing. Can the posterior and anterior speech areas also be activated by non-speech sounds? The answer to this question appears to be "yes." For example, a study by Griffiths *et al.* (1998) demonstrated that the anterior and posterior superior temporal areas observed for listening to words relative to reversed words (see Fig. 26.2) also respond during analysis of the time structure of "rippled noise" when the pitch variation corresponded to novel diatonic melodies that occur over seconds relative to milliseconds. The coordinates of these activations (Talairach and Tournoux, 1988; see Table 1 of Griffiths *et al.*, 1998) were (–54, +10, –18) in the left anterior temporal area, (–58, –42, –2) in the left posterior temporal area, (+58, +12, –26) in the right anterior temporal area, and (+72, –40, 6) in the right posterior temporal area. Despite the remarkable correspondence between these values and those shown for speech relative to reversed speech in Fig. 26.2, the stimuli of Griffith *et al.* (1998) were not speech like. Thus, the left anterior and posterior areas that Scott *et al.* have associated with intelligibility and phonemic feature analysis, respectively, are not speech specific.

A second line of evidence that the anterior and posterior speech areas are not speech specific comes from a recent study by Thierry *et al.* (2003) that observed increased activity in the left anterior and posterior "speech areas" when subjects listened to sequences of environmental sounds and decided if the sequence follows a logical order (*e.g.*, sounds of cork being pulled, popping noise, liquid pouring over ice cubes, someone sipping, someone sighing) relative to hearing scrambled sounds and responding to the beep at the end of the sequence (see Fig. 26.2, row 2). Although activation in the left anterior temporal area might be a consequence of the intelligibility of the familiar environmental sounds, activation in the left posterior temporal area is not consistent with analysis of the phonetic cues and features because there were no phonetic cues or features in the environmental sound stimuli. It is also worth noting that the activation profile for silently reading visually presented sentences overlaps with the areas observed for listening to speech, even though the reading conditions do not entail any auditory input. As can be seen in Fig. 26.2 (row 3), the peak coordinates for the anterior temporal activations that Vandenberghe *et al.* (2002) reported for reading sentences are within 2 mm of the activations reported by Griffiths *et al.* (1998) for the analysis of the long-term temporal structure. The posterior temporal activation for reading sentences also overlaps with those reported for auditory processing, but the peak coordinates (–58, –52, +6) lie posterior and dorsal to those observed for speech relative to reversed speech (–50, –42, 0).

Finally, the degree to which different stages of auditory speech comprehension are lateralised in left and right hemispheres remains to be understood. The rapid (millisecond) analysis of frequency and amplitude changes that is required to discriminate different phonemes has traditionally been associated with the left auditory cortex (Efron, 1963; Hammond, 1982; Lackner and Teuber, 1973). Functional imaging studies of temporal processing, in contrast, have consistently shown bilateral activation in auditory cortices (Belin *et al.*, 1998; Griffiths *et al.*, 1998; Hall *et al.*, 2002; Thivard *et al.*, 2000), with only a small left-hemisphere advantage for temporal analysis and a correspondingly small right-hemisphere advantage for spectral analysis (Zatorre and Belin, 2001). Likewise, speech recognition has been associated with left posterior temporal structures since the days of Wernicke (1874), but several functional imaging studies have shown homologous effects in the right hemisphere. For example, although Mummery *et al.* (1999) demonstrated left lateralised responses in the posterior superior temporal cortex, the data reported in Leff *et al.* (2002) suggest that the homologous area in the right hemisphere shows similar, but smaller effects in most normal subjects (see Fig. 1 in Leff *et al.*, 2002). Likewise, it might be the case that the right anterior temporal cortex is inconsistently or weakly activated for speech relative to rotated speech, but further studies are required to investigate this and to compare the inter-subject variability in left and right auditory cortex activation.

Summary of Auditory Speech Comprehension

In summary, auditory speech comprehension requires: (1) the continuous analysis of rapidly changing sound frequencies and their amplitudes, (2) recognition of phonetic cues and features, and (3) access to the semantic system. The lesion studies suggest that the early acoustic processing of speech is bilaterally distributed, but the auditory speech recognition stage is left lateralised. The functional imaging data have provided a more detailed picture: Acoustic processing of speech relative to tones and complex non-speech occurs in bilateral superior temporal sulci (STS) laterally and ventrally to the primary auditory cortex extending both anteriorly and posteriorly. Activation in a left anterior region indexes speech recognition, and activation in a left posterior region indexes phonetic analyses of the features (Scott *et al.*, 2000); however, none of these areas is specific for speech. Mid-portions of the superior temporal sulci (lateral and ventral to the primary auditory cortex) also respond during the analysis of time structure at the level of milliseconds (Belin *et al.*, 1998; Giraud *et al.*, 2000; Griffiths *et al.*, 1998; Hall *et al.*, 2002). The posterior and anterior portions of the superior temporal sulci also respond to environmental sound stimuli (Thierry *et al.*, 2003) and the melodic structure in noise (Griffiths *et al.*, 1998). Furthermore, the anterior area (associated with intelligibility) is also involved in visual sentence comprehension.

These results can be interpreted in two different ways. One possibility relates to the claim that any given cortical area can have different functions depending on which areas it is interacting with (see Friston and Price, 2001); thus, for instance, an area might have one role during auditory speech processing but another role during visual sentence processing. The other possibility is that a common function underlies all known responses; thus, it might be the case that the left anterior "intelligibility" area is involved in the long-term integration of auditory or visual information that is acquired over time. This would account for activation during the melodic (Griffiths *et al.*, 1998), environmental sound (Thierry *et al.*, 2003), auditory (Scott *et al.*, 2000), and written (Vandenberghe *et al.*, 2002) sentence conditions. It could also explain activation for single words relative to reversed words (see Fig. 26.2) if we assume that when auditory sounds become recognisable as speech, there is implicit/incidental processing in areas involved in the analysis of the long-term time structure of the auditory input. As a result, increased activation will be observed when speech is compared to non-speech, even when every attempt has been made to match spectral and temporal components in the speech and non-speech conditions. This is analogous to the well known modulations in early visual activity when the visual input is meaningful (Shulman *et al.*, 1997). With respect to the posterior area, it is more difficult to assign a single function that accounts for sensitivity to (1) phonetic structure, (2) melodies, and (3) environmental sounds. One possibility relates to the integration of acoustic sequences, and another possibility relates to the demands placed on linking fine-grained auditory information to higher order processing, but further studies are required.

SPEECH PRODUCTION

Cognitive models of speech production postulate a series of different processes that are required to generate even the simplest utterance. At a minimum, these are thought to include a conceptual representation of what needs to be articulated, lexical retrieval, procedures for combining and ordering the sounds, articulatory planning, and execution (Bock and Griffin, 2000). These processes should all be substantiated during picture naming; therefore, the following text considers the neural system for picture naming and compares this system to that observed during other speech production (*e.g.*, verbal fluency, propositional speech, colour naming) and motor execution (tongue and hand movements) tasks. As in the previous section on auditory speech comprehension, particular consideration is given to any components of the speech production system that might be speech specific.

Picture Naming

When overt picture naming is contrasted to silent viewing of abstract shapes that only control for some elements of the visual input, highly significant activation has been observed in a widely distributed left lateralised system; see Bookheimer *et al.* (1995) and Murtha *et al.* (1999) for remarkably consistent localisation of the areas. Activations during *overt* picture naming can be divided into two different groups depending on whether or not the areas are also activated during *silent* picture naming. The first group entails the left precentral, supplementary motor, anterior cingulate, and superior temporal areas which are *not* observed when silent picture naming is compared with viewing pictures of unfamiliar objects (Martin *et al.*, 1996; van Turennout *et al.*, 2000). These areas are therefore likely to be involved in the execution of the motor response and auditory processing of the spoken name. Indeed, Murphy *et al.* (1997) have demonstrated activation in these areas when subjects produce unarticulated vocalisation (*e.g.*, saying aloud "aah, aah, aah") (see Fig. 6 in Murphy *et al.*, 1997, and Figs. 5 and 6 in Wise *et al.*, 2001). The second group of areas entails bilateral temporal-occipital areas, left anterior insula, left thalamus, and mid- or right lateralised areas in the cerebellum. These areas are observed for both *silent* and *overt* picture naming relative to abstract patterns and non-objects. They are therefore the most likely candidates for conceptualisation, lexical retrieval, and articulatory planning.

Figure 26.3 shows the results of an experiment by Price *et al.*, (submitted) that attempted to tease apart the effects of object recognition from speech production. The stimuli were either pictures of objects and animals or visual noise patterns created by scrambling the object images. Half of the objects had a displaced feature and half of the scrambled images had a black circle superimposed in the centre of the stimulus (see top of Fig. 26.3 for examples). The task required either vocal or manual responses. When objects were presented, the vocal task was silent picture naming (move lips to articulate the name silently but without generating any sound to prevent

DESIGN

		Task: Vocal	Task: Manual
Stimuli	*Scrambled*	Say "OK"	Circle detection
	Objects (*Configuration change*)	Name	Object Decision (correct configuration?)

RESULTS

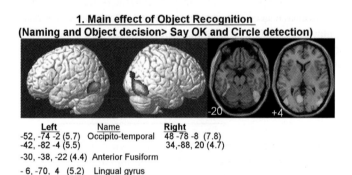

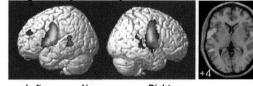

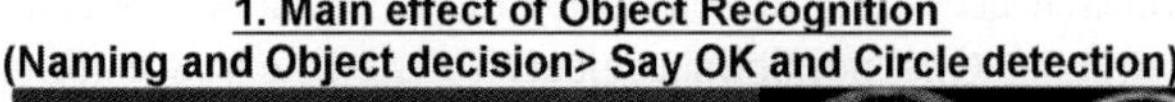

1. Main effect of Object Recognition
(Naming and Object decision> Say OK and Circle detection)

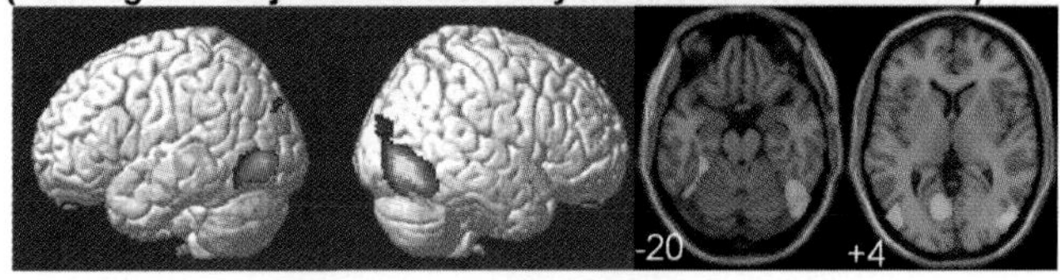

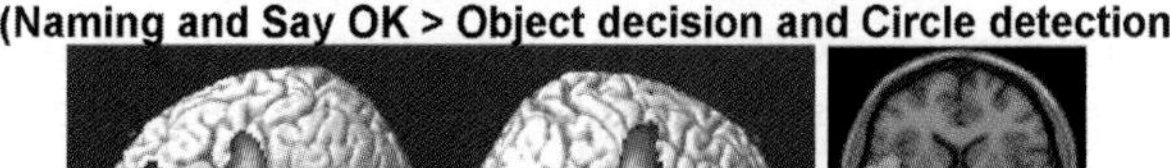

FIGURE 26.3
Object recognition and speech production areas.

auditory processing of the spoken response) and the manual task was object decision (key press response when the object had the correct configuration). When scrambled images were presented, the vocal task was silently articulating "OK" to the presentation of each picture, and the manual task was "circle decision" (key press response when a circle was present). From these four conditions, it was then possible to find: (1) the main effect of object recognition by comparing pictures of objects to scrambled images; (2) the main effect of articulation by comparing naming to object decision and saying "OK" to circle decision; and (3) the interaction of object naming and articulation (*i.e.*, increased activation for object naming only). As seen in many previous experiments (Bar *et al.*, 2001; Gerlach *et al.*, 1999; Martin *et al.*, 1996; Moore and Price, 1999; Vuilleumier *et al.*, 2002), the main effect of object recognition revealed bilateral occipito-temporal areas and the left lingual gyrus (see Fig. 26.3). In contrast, the main effect of articulation revealed bilateral precentral cortices, left anterior insula, bilateral posterior superior temporal regions, the precuneus, and a left middle/superior frontal area but no activation in the supplementary motor area, anterior cingulate, cerebellum, or thalami, suggesting that the latter areas were equally responsive for articulation and button presses. Interestingly, there was no interaction between object recognition and articulation (*i.e.*, no increased activation for object naming only), suggesting that picture naming involves the integration of object recognition and articulation areas.

The "articulation" areas illustrated in Fig. 26.3 can be subdivided further. Activation in bilateral sensorimotor cortices and the left anterior insula is consistently reported for all types of speech production tasks (Blank *et al.*, 2002; Murphy *et al.*, 1997; Warburton *et al.*, 1996). Critically, the loci of sensorimotor and insula activations reported in Fig. 26.3 ([–62, –4, 18], [62, –8, 16], [–46, 10, 2]) correspond almost exactly to those reported by Corfield *et al.* (1999) for simple tongue movements ([–62, –6, 22], [64, –4, 18], [–46, 6, 0]). Therefore, activation in these areas during speech production may be a reflection of the tongue movements required to speak but this is not consistent with speech specificity. Another plausible candidate for speech specific production is the posterior superior temporal cortex, or Wernicke's area. The same area is reported for verb and noun generation (Papathanassiou *et al.*, 2000; Warburton *et al.*, 1996; Wise *et al.*, 2001) relative to non-articulatory baseline conditions, but it is not observed for verb generation relative to auditory repetition or reading (Frith *et al.*, 1991; Petersen *et al.*, 1988). It is also very close to the posterior superior temporal areas associated with speech perception (see Fig. 26.2), but, as shown in Fig. 26.4, the speech production area is more dorsal and posterior to the speech perception area. These activations might represent two discrete areas, with the ventral area involved in auditory perception, the dorsal area involved in articulatory processing, and the small area of overlap resulting from the spatial smoothing used in the analysis procedure; however, this conclusion requires data from the same group of subjects. The alternative possibility is that one area is involved in both speech perception and speech production. Wise and colleagues (2001) have argued for a common posterior superior temporal area involved in speech perception and speech production with the role being to "transiently represent phonetic sequences, whether heard or internally generated and rehearsed." Certainly this explanation would be consistent with activation during speech perception, picture naming, and saying "OK" repeatedly, but any specificity for phonetic input can be excluded because the same area is also involved in the analysis of environmental sounds (Thierry *et al.*, 2003) and melodies (Griffiths *et al.*, 1998) (see Fig. 26.2). A related possibility is that the posterior superior temporal activation reflects transient representation of any acoustic sequences (*i.e.*, not specific to phonetic sequences). In contrast, it might be the case that the area is specialised for speech production, and speech production mechanisms are automatically activated during speech perception, the analysis of melodies, and environmental sound processing. Dissociating these different accounts will require further experimentation.

Finally, the experiment illustrated in Fig. 26.3 highlighted the left superior frontal cortex and precuneus during articulation. However, because these areas have not been reported for speech production during verbal fluency (Papathanassiou *et al.*, 2000; Warburton *et al.*, 1996), propositional speech (the natural expression of a concept; see (Blank *et al.*, 2002), or other picture naming paradigms (Bookheimer *et al.*, 1995; Martin *et al.*, 1996; Murtha *et al.*, 1999) they appear to be specific to the experiment illustrated in Fig. 26.3 and may be a consequence of deactivation for object and circle decisions.

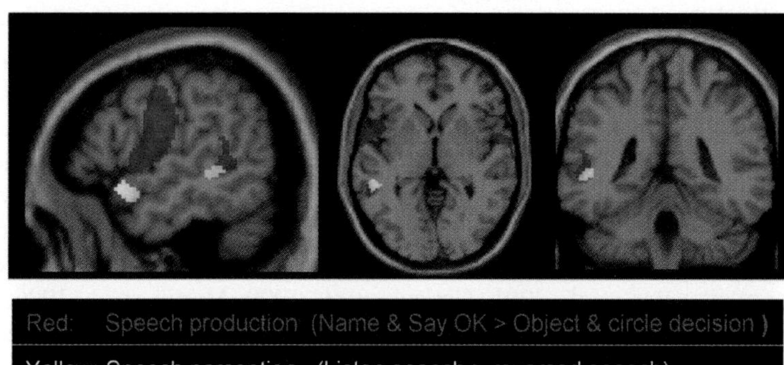

FIGURE 26.4
Speech production and perception.

Summary of Speech Production

In summary, at a cognitive level, speech production involves many putatively distinct stages. At a neuroanatomical level, picture naming studies have highlighted:

1. *Bilateral occipito-temporal areas*, which are involved in all paradigms involving object recognition irrespective of whether speech production is required (*e.g.*, during picture naming) or not (*e.g.*, during object decision); therefore, they are not speech specific.
2. *Left anterior fusiform*, which has been reported for picture naming (–30, –38, –22 in Fig. 26.3) and by Blank *et al.* (2002) for propositional speech production (–24, –38, –18). The same area (–31, –40, –18) has also been reported for reading and repeating words with high relative to low imageability (D'Esposito *et al.*, 1997; Wise *et al.*, 2000); therefore, it is likely to be involved at the conceptual stage of speech production.
3. *Posterior superior temporal cortex*, which is associated with picture naming and verbal fluency and appears to be involved in articulation rather than conceptualisation or lexical retrieval because it is activated when subjects continuously articulate "OK" irrespective of the input with no advantage for picture naming relative to saying "OK" (experiment illustrated in Fig. 26.3). Activation is also unlikely to be related to motor execution or monitoring the sound of the spoken response because it is also observed during silent word retrieval (Warburton *et al.*, 1996). It may have a potential role in procedures for combining and ordering the sounds/ articulatory planning (Levelt *et al.*, 1998; Wise *et al.*, 2001), but further experimentation is required.
4. *Auditory regions in the superior temporal cortices*, which are associated with hearing one's own voice. Activation in these areas is observed during unarticulated vocalisation but not when subjects are instructed to articulate silently (move lips without generating any sound).
5. *Bilateral sensorimotor cortices and the left anterior insula*, which are more active for speech than manual responses (see Fig. 26.3) but are not specific to speech because they also respond during the planning and execution of simple tongue movements.
6. *Anterior cingulate, supplementary motor area, bilateral cerebellum, and left thalamus*, which are not specific to speech because they are also observed for unarticulated vocal sounds (Murphy *et al.*, 1997) nor are they specific to vocal/facial movements because they are equally active for vocal and manual responses (for a discussion of activation during finger movements, see Sakai *et al.*, 2002); therefore, they are likely to be involved in planning both facial and manual motor execution.

Notably, this summary has not isolated any cortical areas that might be dedicated to word retrieval *per se*. For instance, the picture naming system segregated into areas involved in object recognition and articulation but there was no interaction to indicate areas involved in linking object recognition to later stages of speech production. Thus, it is possible that word retrieval may be instantiated by the anatomical connections between cortical areas involved in conceptual processing and articulation. Indeed, reports of direct anatomical connections between the inferior temporal cortex and the posterior superior temporal cortex (Di Virgilio and Clarke, 1997) may reflect the pathways from the anterior fusiform conceptualisation area (see above) to the beginnings of speech production in the posterior superior temporal cortex. Obviously, future experiments are required to test these hypotheses.

SEMANTIC RETRIEVAL

This section considers the neural systems required to retrieve conceptual information in order to make semantic decisions on words and pictures. Many different semantic retrieval tasks have been investigated with functional imaging, including living/non-living decisions, concrete/ abstract decisions, association decisions (*e.g.*, matching two items that are semantically associated with one another), verb generation (when a semantically related verb is retrieved in response to a noun), subordinate feature decisions (*e.g.*, does the animal have a long tail?), and complex monitoring tasks (press button if the words in a pair are pleasant or bigger than a chicken). Chapter 27 considers some of the differences between tasks and stimuli. Here, we focus on areas that are consistently activated regardless of task and stimulus modality (auditory words, visual words, and pictures).

Figure 26.5 illustrates the results of semantic decision tasks on heard words, written words, and pictures, relative to baseline conditions that control for perceptual processing. The tasks and stimuli varied in each experiment yet a remarkably similar pattern of activation is revealed. The activation pattern for heard words was derived from the combination of two experiments reported by Noppeney and Price (2002, 2003). In one experiment, subjects made semantic decisions (*e.g.*, is it red?) regarding food items (*e.g.*, cheese). In the other experiment, the stimuli referred to visual features ("black"), auditory features ("echo"), or abstract words (e.g., "prayer"), and subjects had to decide, for example, if the item was "dark," "loud," or "religious," respectively. For both experiments, the baseline conditions involved listening to reversed words and deciding if the word had been spoken by a male or female voice. Figure 26.5 (row 1) shows the main effect of words (in both experiments) relative to the baselines, thereby highlighting the common areas involved in auditory semantic retrieval.

The activation patterns for the written words and pictures (Figure 26.5, rows 2 and 3) were derived from a combination of the experiments reported by Vandenberghe *et al.* (1996) and Phillips *et al.* (2002). In the Vandenberghe *et al.* (1996) experiment, triads of written words referring to objects or animals were presented with a target word above and two response options below, and subjects had to decide which of the words below was most semantically related to the target word above. In the Phillips *et al.* (2002) experiment, single words referring to objects or fruit were presented, and subjects had to make either action decisions (*e.g.*, "would you twist this object?") or real-life size decisions (*e.g.*, "is the object bigger than a hammer?"). The baseline conditions for both experiments involved a perceptual decision on the same stimuli. As can be seen from Figure 26.5, a similar activation pattern is observed for each input modality (auditory words, visual words, pictures), despite the diversity of semantic content (objects, animals, features, abstract words) and tasks. The most significant effect is the extensive inferior frontal activation with several distinct subpeaks (*e.g.*, the ventral peak for the auditory and visual paradigms respectively were [–30, 34, –16] and [–30, 30, –14]). In addition, consistent activation is reported in left middle and inferior temporal regions (*e.g.*, [–54, –40, –14] and [–48, –60, –22] for auditory words; [–52, –42, –12] and [–42, –56, –20] for pictures), the left angular gyrus (*e.g.*, [–54, –72, 30] for auditory words; [–54, –70, 28] for pictures), and the right cerebellum (*e.g.*, [42, –72, –42] for auditory words; [42, –68, –50] for pictures), with weaker and less consistent effects in the left anterior fusiform (*e.g.*, [–32, –22, –34] for auditory words; [–38, –28, –20] for pictures) and left anterior temporal cortex (*e.g.*, [–66, –4, –22] for auditory words; [–58, –4, –20] for visual words).

Many functional imaging studies have focused on left inferior frontal activation during semantic retrieval (Binder *et al.*, 1997; Buckner *et al.*, 1995; Demb *et al.*, 1995; Fiez, 1997; Gabrieli *et al.*, 1996; Kapur *et al.*, 1994; Klein *et al.*, 1997; McCarthy *et al.*, 1993; Petersen *et al.*, 1988–1990; Poldrack *et al.*, 1999; Raichle *et al.*, 1994; Roskies *et al.*, 2001; Shaywitz *et al.*, 1995; Thompson-Schill *et al.*, 1997–1999; Wagner *et al.*, 2001). Critically, it is temporal, not frontal, lesions that typically result in semantic processing deficits. This has led to the hypothesis

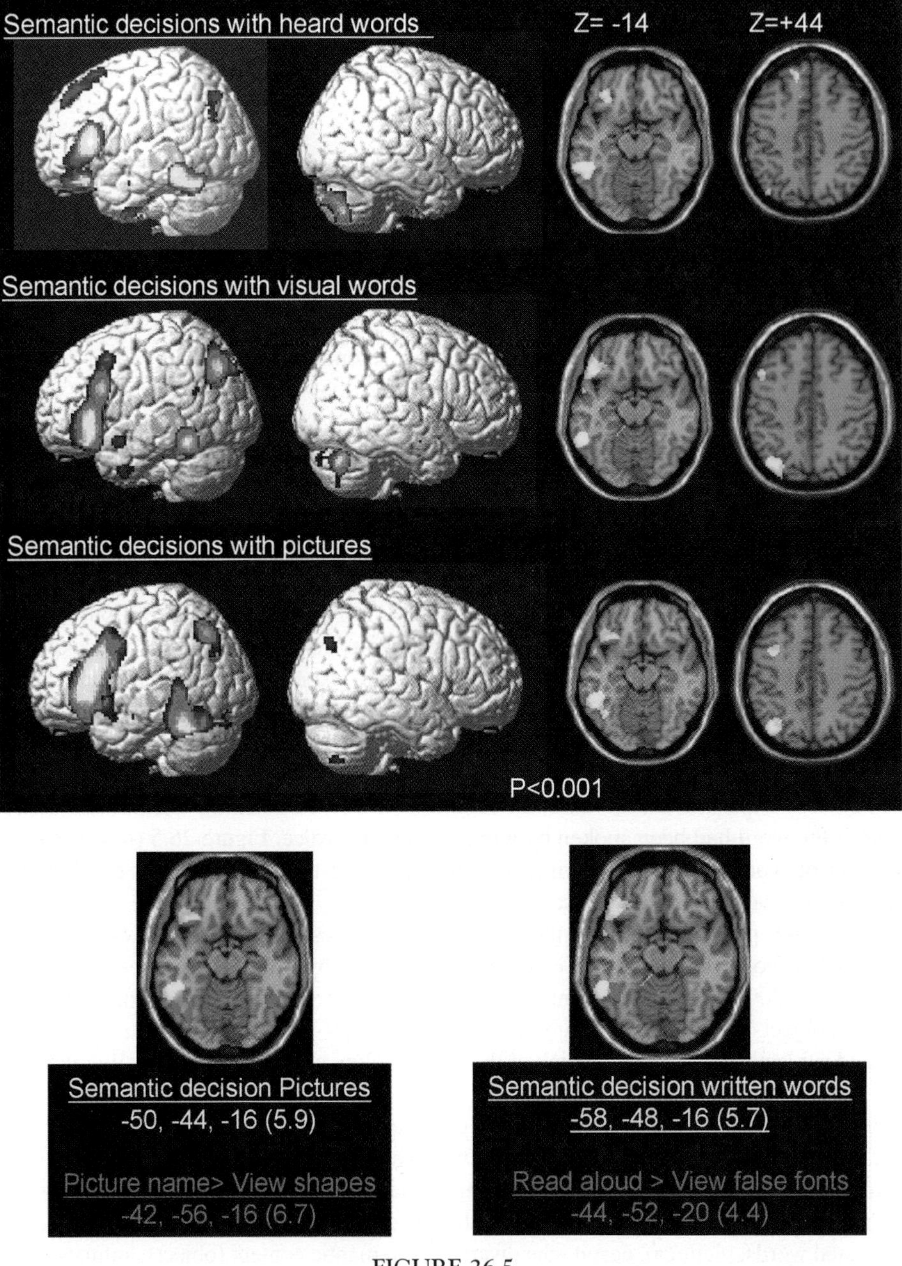

FIGURE 26.5
Semantic retrieval.

that frontal and temporal activation must reflect different underlying semantic functions. The temporal lobes are thought to be involved in the storage of semantic memories, while the left inferior frontal cortex is thought to play a more executive role (Fiez, 1997; Thompson-Schill *et al.*, 1997–1999; Wagner *et al.*, 2001). The distinction between frontal and temporal activations, however, is not clearly established. For instance, Wagner *et al.* (2001) and Noppeney and Price (2002) report similar effects of retrieval demand in frontal and temporal areas, suggesting that executive semantic processes are distributed throughout the semantic system rather than confined to the frontal lobe. Reexamination of the lesion data are consistent with this account because focal lesions in the temporal or parietal areas that activate during functional imaging studies of semantic retrieval do not result in semantic retrieval deficits (Price and Friston, 2002). Indeed, semantic deficits are usually only observed after extensive left temporoparietal (Alexander *et al.*, 1989) or bilateral anterior temporal lobe damage (Hodges *et al.*, 1992; Mummery *et al.*, 2000) .

It may therefore be the case that all the areas activated by the semantic retrieval paradigms summarised in the top three rows of Fig. 26.5 are involved in strategic elements of semantic retrieval rather than the conceptual representations themselves. Indeed, it is possible that the baseline tasks used to identify the semantic retrieval system removed any signal in areas that might be related to conceptual representations. This is illustrated in the lower part of Fig. 26.5, which compares the activation for picture naming and reading (see Chapter 28) to the activation related to semantic retrieval (upper part of Fig. 26.5). As can be seen, the semantic retrieval areas are lateral and anterior to the areas involved in picture naming and reading.

If the semantic retrieval areas illustrated in Fig. 26.5 do not reflect conceptual representations, then where might conceptual representations be? One theory is that the conceptual representations of objects are distributed in the sensory and motor cortices that perceive and respond to the presence of objects (Damasio, 1989). In this case semantic areas become synonymous with sensory and motor areas and the distinction between perception and semantics rests on whether activation in an area is driven by the sensory input or the mechanisms that enable the retrieval of learnt information in the absence of the stimulus; however, as illustrated in Fig. 26.6 there is no overlap between the sensory, motor, or semantic retrieval areas. One possibility is that the semantic retrieval areas represent the convergence of information from multiple modalities and correspond to high-level object representations, our amodal semantic system. However, according to Damasio (1989), the higher order convergence zones are not accumulators of all information described in earlier regions; rather, they serve to reactivate sensory and motor cortices during recall. Thus, the retrieval of sensory or motor information can only be achieved by recourse to unimodal cortices. Chapter 27 addresses this theory and considers whether the activation pattern during semantic retrieval depends on the type of information that is being abstracted (*e.g.*, activation in motor areas when the action semantics is being retrieved).

In summary, multiple studies of semantic retrieval have highlighted the importance of a distributed, modality-independent, left-lateralised neural network in frontal and extra-sylvian temporal and parietal areas. The frontal areas are thought to be involved in executive semantic functions, and conceptual knowledge is thought to be a property of the temporal lobes. As yet, however, there is no anatomical or cognitive model of semantic processing that explains all the data. The critical challenges that functional imaging methodology must overcome to advance our understanding of semantic retrieval are considered further in Chapter 27.

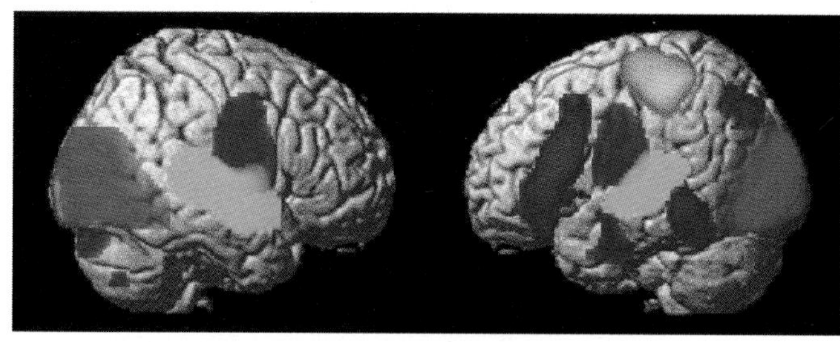

Color coding

Data from:

Visual input: False fonts > Auditory noise
Auditory input: Auditory noise > False fonts

Price et al. 2003

Vocal movements: Say "OK" > Tap finger
Finger movements: Tap finger > Say "OK"

Biggio et al. (in prep)

Semantic > Perceptual associations

Vandenberghe et al., 1996

FIGURE 26.6
Sensorimotor and semantic retrieval areas. (From Price *et al.*, submitted.)

CONCLUDING COMMENTS

The aim of this chapter was to provide an overview of the neural systems involved in single word speech comprehension and production. The conclusions are summarised in Figs. 26.7 and 26.8. Figure 26.7 compiles and integrates the data from Figs. 26.2, 26.3, and 26.5 to model the possible connections from speech perception and object recognition to speech production. Speech perception is localised to the superior temporal gyri and sulci with particular sensitivity to heard words in specific regions of the anterior and posterior superior temporal sulci. This contrasts with picture perception, which engages bilateral occipito-temporal cortices (see Fig. 26.3). The areas involved in conceptualisation and semantic processing may depend on the task, but the studies considered in this chapter highlighted the role of a left anterior fusiform area during picture naming, propositional speech, and visual and auditory word processing. In addition, semantic retrieval tasks engage a distributed, left-lateralised frontotemporal system that may be involved in cohering sensory and motor memories. No such system was observed for lexical retrieval. Therefore, it is proposed that the cognitive process (referred to as lexical retrieval) is implemented by the connections between conceptual and articulation areas. Finally, speech production activates bilateral sensorimotor cortices (a superior temporal area that lies dorsal to the speech perception areas) and other motor areas such as the supplementary motor area, anterior cingulate, cerebellum, and thalami that also respond during non-vocal tasks (and therefore are not shown in Fig. 26.3 or 26.7). On the basis of the evidence presented, only the dorsal superior temporal area could be considered specific to speech stimuli because, to the author's knowledge, it is not activated by manual or tongue movements. However, it is difficult to prove specificity on the basis of a lack of conflicting evidence.

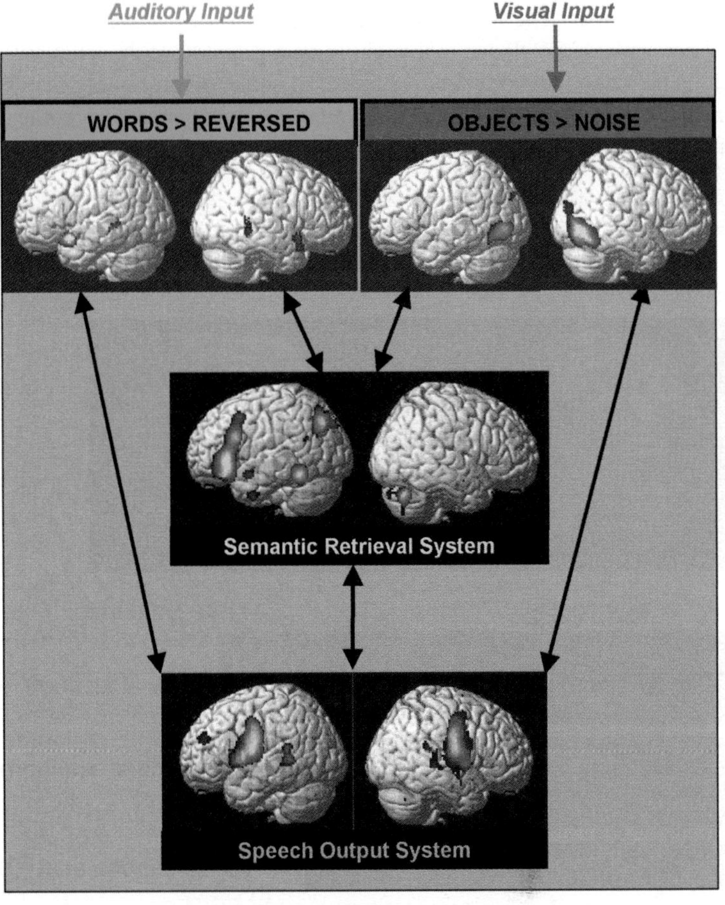

FIGURE 26.7
Neural systems underlying word processing.

Figure 26.8 compares the model presented in Fig. 26.7 with the 19th-century neurological model. The latter highlights Wernicke's area and Broca's area associated with speech comprehension and production, respectively (P. A. C. in Fig. 26.8 refers to the primary auditory cortex). The functional imaging data also highlight Wernicke's and Broca's areas but require two distinct modifications to the neurological model. The first relates to a possible subdivision within Wernicke's area, with the ventral portion (in yellow) activated during auditory speech perception and the dorsal region (in red) activated during speech production (see Fig. 26.4). The second relates to the role of the left anterior superior temporal sulcus (antSTS) in speech perception that was not predicted by the neurological model. As discussed in the section on auditory speech comprehension, this anterior STS area may have a role in integrating auditory and visual input, a function that would be particularly important during sentence processing (see Fig. 26.2 for activation during written sentence processing). Thus, this area may not be involved in auditory word repetition *per se* but may play a role in syntactic and semantic processing. In conclusion, the functional imaging data are remarkably consistent with the 19th-century neurological model that was based on postmortem studies. Nevertheless, functional imaging data provide increased spatial resolution that allows us to consider whether the speech areas correspond to those that are involved in non-linguistic sensory and motor functions. Furthermore, functional imaging studies can characterise individual variability that might provide important clues for how some patients recover their language abilities after lesions to the areas thought to be necessary for language.

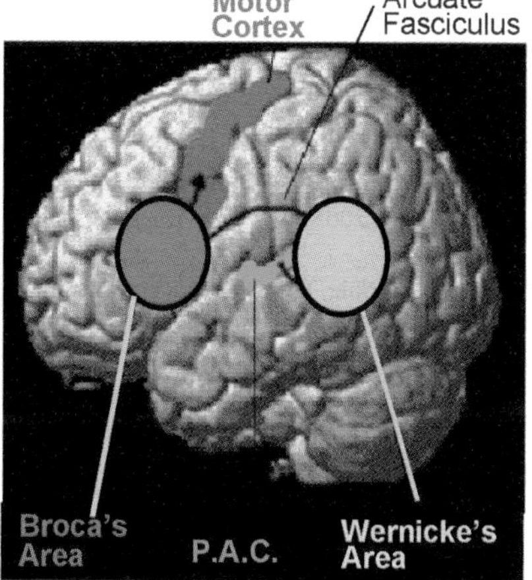

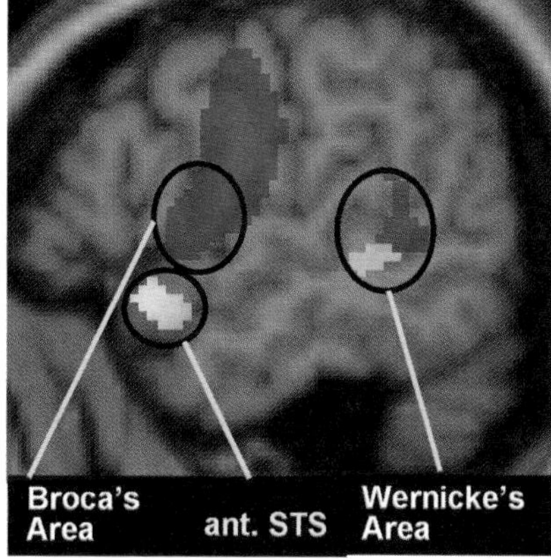

FIGURE 26.8
Changes to the neurological model.

References

Alexander, M. P., Hiltbrunner, B., and Fischer, R. S. (1989). Distributed anatomy of transcortical sensory aphasia. *Arch. Neurol.,* **46**(8), 885–892.

Auerbach, S. H., Allard, T., Naeser, M., Alexander, M. P., and Albert, M. L. (1982). Pure word deafness: analysis of a case with bilateral lesions and a defect at the prephonemic level. *Brain,* **105**(Pt. 2), 271–300.

Bar, M., Tootell, R. B., Schacter, D. L., Greve, D. N., Fischl, B., Mendola, J. D., Rosen, B. R., and Dale, A. M. (2001). Cortical mechanisms specific to explicit visual object recognition. *Neuron,* **29**, 529–535.

Belin, P., Zilbovicius, M., Crozier, S., Thivard, L., Fontaine, A., Masure, M. C., and Samson, Y. (1998). Lateralisation of speech and auditory temporal processing. *J. Cogn. Neurosci.,* **10**(4), 536–540.

Binder, J. R., Frost, J. A., Hammeke, T. A., Cox, R. W., Rao, S. M., and Prieto, T. (1997). Human brain language areas identified by functional magnetic resonance imaging. *J. Neurosci.,* **17**(1), 353–362.

Binder, J. R., Frost, J. A., Hammeke, T. A., Bellgowan, P. S., Springer, J. A., Kaufman, J. N., and Possing, E. T. (2000). Human temporal lobe activation by speech and nonspeech sounds. *Cereb. Cortex,* **10**, 512–528.

Blank, S. C., Scott, S. K., Murphy, K., Warburton, E., and Wise, R. J. (2002). Speech production: Wernicke, Broca and beyond. *Brain,* **125**(Pt. 8), 1829–1838.

Bock, K. and Griffin, Z. M. (2000). Producing words: how minds meet mouth, in *Aspects of Language Production,* Wheeldon, L. R., Ed., pp. 7–47. Psychology Press, Hove, U.K.

Bookheimer, S. Y., Zeffiro, T. A., Blaxton, T., Gaillard, W., and Theodore, W. (1995). Regional cerebral blood flow during object naming and word reading. *Hum. Brain Mapping,* **3**, 93–106.

Buchman, A. S., Garron, D. C., Trost-Cardamone, J. E., Wichter, M. D., and Schwartz, M. (1986). Word deafness: one hundred years later. *J. Neurol. Neurosurg. Psychiatry,* **49**(5), 489–499.

Buckner, R. L., Raichle, M. E., and Petersen, S. E. (1995). Dissociation of human prefrontal cortical areas across different speech production tasks and gender groups. *J. Neurophysiol.,* **74**(5), 2163–2173.

Corfield, D. R., Murphy, K., Josephs, O., Fink, G. R., Frackowiak, R. S., Guz, A., Adams, L., and Turner, R. (1999). Cortical and subcortical control of tongue movement in humans: a functional neuroimaging study using fMRI. *J. Appl. Physiol.,* **86**(5), 1468–1477.

Damasio, A. R. (1989). Time locked multiregional retroactivation: a systems level proposal for the neural substrates of recall and recognition. *Cognition,* **33**, 25–62.

Demb, J. B., Desmond, J. E., Wagner, A. D., Vaidya, C. J., Glover, G. H., and Gabrieli, J. D. E. (1995). Semantic encoding an retrieval in the left inferior prefrontal cortex: a functional MRI study of task difficulty and process specificity. *J. Neurosci.,* **15**, 5870–5878.

Di Virgilio, G. and Clarke, S. (1997). Direct interhemispheric visual input to human speech areas. *Hum. Brain Mapping,* **5**, 347–354.

Efron, R. (1963). Temporal perception, aphasia, and *deja vu. Brain,* **86**, 403–424.

Fiez, J. A. (1997). Phonology, semantics, and the role of the left inferior prefrontal cortex. *Hum. Brain Mapping,* **5**, 79–83.

Friston, K. J. and Price, C. J. (2001). Dynamic representations and generative models of brain function. *Brain Res. Bull.,* **54**(3), 275–285.

Frith, C. D., Friston, K. J., Liddle, P. F., and Frackowiak, R. S. (1991). A PET study of word finding. *Neuropsychologia,* **29**(12), 1137–1148.

Gabrieli, J. D., Desmond, J. E., Demb, J. B., Wagner, A. D., Stone, M. V., Vaidya, C. J., and Glover, G. H. (1996). Functional magnetic resonance imaging of semantic memory processes. *Psychol. Sci.,* **7**, 278–283.

Galaburda, A. M., Sanides, F., and Geschwind, N. (1978). Human brain: cytoarchitectonic left–right asymmetries in the temporal speech region. *Arch. Neurol.,* **35**(12), 812–817.

Gerlach, C., Law, I., Gade, A., and Paulson, O. B. (1999). Perceptual differentiation and category effects in normal object recognition: a PET study. *Brain,* **122**, 2159–2170.

Geschwind, N. (1965). Disconnection syndromes in animals and man. *Brain,* **88**, 237–294.

Giraud, A.-L., Lorenz, C., Ashburner, J., Wable, J., Johnsrude, I., Frackowiak, R., and Kleinschmidt, A. (2000). Representation of the temporal envelope of sounds in the human brain. *J. Neurophysiol.,* **84**, 1588–1598.

Griffiths, T. D., Buchel, C., Frackowiak, R. S., and Patterson, R. D. (1998). Analysis of temporal structure in sound by the human brain. *Nat. Neurosci.,* **1**(5), 422–427.

Hall, D. A., Johnsrude, I. S., Haggard, M. P., Palmer, A. R., Akeroyd, M. A., and Summerfield, A. Q. (2002). Spectral and temporal processing in human auditory cortex. *Cereb. Cortex,* **12**, 140–149.

Hammond, G. R. (1982). Hemispheric differences in temporal resolution. *Brain Cogn.,* **1**(1), 95–118.

Hickok, G., Love, T., Swinney, D., Wong, E. C., and Buxton, R. B. (1997). Functional MR imaging during auditory word perception: a single trial presentation paradigm. *Brain Language,* **58**, 197–201.

Hodges, J., Patternson, K., Oxbury, S., and Funnell, E. (1992). Semantic dementia: Progressive fluent – aphasia with temporal lobe atrophy. *Brain,* **115**, 1783–1806.

Howard, D., Patterson, K., Wise, R., Brown, W. D., Friston, K., Weiller, C., and Frackowiak, R. (1992). The cortical localisation of the lexicons: positron emission tomography evidence. *Brain,* **115**(Pt. 6), 1769–1782.

Jancke, L., Wustenberg, T., Scheich, H., and Heinze, H. J. (2002). Phonetic perception and the temporal cortex. *NeuroImage,* **15**(4), 733–746.

Kapur, S., Rose, R., Liddle, P. F., Zipursky, R. B., Brown, G. M., Stuss, D., Houle, S., and Tulving, E. (1994). The role of the left prefrontal cortex in verbal processing: semantic processing or willed action? *NeuroReport,* **5**(16), 2193–2196.

Klein, D., Olivier, A., Milner, B., Zatorre, R. J., Johnsrude, I., Meyer, E., and Evans, A. C. (1997). Obligatory role of the LIFG in synonym generation: evidence from PET and cortical stimulation. *NeuroReport,* **8**(15), 3275–3279.

Lackner, J. R. and Teuber, H. L. (1973). Alterations in auditory fusion thresholds after cerebral injury in man. *Neuropsychologia,* **11**(4), 409–415.

Leff, A., Crinion, J., Scott, S., Turkheimer, F., Howard, D., and Wise, R. (2002). A physiological change in the homotopic cortex following left posterior temporal lobe infarction. *Ann. Neurol.,* **51**(5), 553–558.

Levelt, W. J., Praamstra, P., Meyer, A. S., Helenius, P., and Salmelin, R. (1998). An MEG study of picture naming. *J. Cogn. Neurosci.,* **10**(5), 553–567.

Lichtheim, L. (1885). On aphasia. *Brain,* **7**, 433–484.

Martin, A., Wiggs, C., Ungerleider, L., and Haxby, J. (1996). Neural correlates of category-specific knowledge. *Nature,* **379**, 649–652.

McCarthy, G., Blamire, A. M., Rothman, D. L., Gruetter, R., and Shulman, R. G. (1993). Echo-planar magnetic resonance imaging studies of frontal cortex activation during word generation in humans. *Proc. Natl. Acad. Sci. USA,* **90**(11), 4952–4956.

Moore, C. J. and Price, C. J. (1999). Three distinct ventral occipitotemporal regions for reading and object naming. *NeuroImage,* **10**(2), 181–192.

Mummery, C. J., Ashburner, J., Scott, S. K., and Wise, R. J. (1999a). Functional neuroimaging of speech perception in six normal and two aphasic subjects. *J. Acoust. Soc. Am.,* **106**(1), 449–457.

Mummery, C. J., Patterson, K., Wise, R. J., Vandenbergh, R., Price, C. J., and Hodges, J. R. (1999b). Disrupted temporal lobe connections in semantic dementia. *Brain,* **122**, 61–73.

Mummery, C. J., Patterson, K., Price, C. J., Ashburner, J., Frackowiak, R. S. J., and Hodges, J. R. (2000). A voxel-based morphometry study of semantic dementia: relationship between temporal lobe atrophy and semantic memory. *Ann. Neurol.,* **47**(1), 36–45.

Murphy, K., Corfield, D. R., Guz, A., Fink, G. R., Wise, R. J., Harrison, J., and Adams, L. (1997). Cerebral areas associated with motor control of speech in humans. *J. Appl. Physiol.,* **83**(5), 1438–1447.

Murtha, S., Chertkow, H., Beauregard, M., and Evans, A. (1999). The neural substrate of picture naming. *J. Cogn. Neurosci.,* **11**(4), 399–423.

Nopenney, U. and Price, C. J. (2002). A PET study of stimulus and task-induced semantic processing. *NeuroImage,* **15**(4), 927–935.

Noppeney, U. and Price, C. J. (2003). Functional imaging of the semantic system: retrieval of sensory experienced and verbally learnt knowledge. *Brain Language,* **84**, 120–133.

Noppeney, U. and Price, C. J. (submitted). The neural areas that control. The retrieval and selection of semantics.

Papathanassiou, D., Etard, O., Mellet, E., Zago, L., Mazoyer, B., and Tzourio-Mazoyer, N. (2000). A common language network for comprehension and production: a contribution to the definition of language epicenters with PET. *NeuroImage,* **11**(4), 347–357.

Petersen, S. E., Fox, P. T., Posner, M. I., Mintun, M., and Raichle, M. E. (1988). Positron emission tomographic studies of the cortical anatomy of single-word processing. *Nature,* **331**(6157), 585–589.

Petersen, S. E., Fox, P. T., Posner, M. I., Mintun, M., and Raichle, M. E. (1989). Positron emission tomographic studies of the processing of single words. *J. Cogn. Neurosci.,* **1**(2), 153–170.

Petersen, S. E., Fox, P. T., Snyder, A. Z., and Raichle, M. E. (1990). Activation of extrastriate and frontal cortical areas by visual words and word-like stimuli. *Science,* **249**(4972), 1041–1044.

Phillips, J., Noppeney, U., Humphreys, G. W., and Price, C. J. (2002). Can segregation within the semantic system account for category-specific deficits? *Brain,* **125**, 2067–2080.

Poldrack, R. A., Wagner, A. D., Prull, M. W., Desmond, J. E., Glover, G. H., and Gabrieli, J. D. (1999). Functional specialisation for semantic and phonological processing in the left inferior prefrontal cortex. *NeuroImage,* **10**, 15–35.

Price, C. J. and Friston, K. J. (2002). Degeneracy and cognitive anatomy. *Trends Cogn. Sci.,* **6**(10), 416–421.

Price, C. J., Devin, J. T., Noppeney, U., McCrory, E., Mechelli, A., Biggio, N., Philips, J., Moore, C. J., and Friston, K. J., Reading: An acquired specialization of object naming, (in submission).

Price, C. J., Wise, R. J. S., Warburton, E. A., Moore, C. J., Howard, D., Patterson, K., Frackowiak, R. S. J., and Friston, K. J. (1996). Hearing and saying: the functional neuro-anatomy of auditory word processing. *Brain,* **119**(Pt. 3), 919–931.

Price, C. J., Winterburn, D., Giraud, A. L., Moore, C. J., and Noppeney, U. (2003). Cortical localisation of the visual and auditory word form areas: a reconsideration of the evidence. *Brain Language*, **86**, 272–288.

Raichle, M. E., Fiez, J. A., Videen, T. O., MacLeod, A. M., Pardo, J. V., Fox, P. T., and Petersen, S. E. (1994). Practice-related changes in human brain functional anatomy during nonmotor learning. *Cereb. Cortex,* **4**(1), 8–26.

Robin, D. A., Tranel, D., and Damasio, H. (1990). Auditory perception of temporal and spectral events in patients with focal left and right cerebral lesions. *Brain Language,* **39**(4), 539–555.

Roskies, A. L., Fiez, J. A., Balota, D. A., Raichle, M. A., and Petersen, S. E. (2001). Task-dependent modulation of regions in the left inferior frontal cortex during semantic processing. *J. Cogn. Neurosci.,* **13**(6), 829–843.

Sakai, K., Ramnani, N., and Passingham, R. E. (2002). Learning of sequences of finger movements and timing: frontal lobe and action-oriented representation. *J. Neurophysiol.,* **88**(4), 2035–2046.

Scott, S. K., Blank, C. C., Rosen, S., and Wise, R. J. (2000). Identification of a pathway for intelligible speech in the left temporal lobe. *Brain,* **123**(Pt. 12), 2400–2406.

Shaywitz, B. A., Pugh, K. R., Constable, R. T. *et al.* (1995). Localisation of semantic processing using functional magnetic resonance imaging. *Hum. Brain Mapping,* **2**, 149–158.

Shulman, G. L., Corbetta, M., Buckner, R. L., Raichle, M. E., Fiez, J. A., Miezin, F. M., and Petersen, S. E. (1997). Top-down modulation of early sensory cortex. *Cereb. Cortex,* **7**(3), 193–206.

Talairach, J. and Tournoux, P. (1988). *Co-planar Stereotaxic Atlas of the Human Brain.* Thieme, Stuttgart.

Thierry, G., Giraud, A.-L., and Price, C. J. (2003). Hemispheric dissociation in access to the human semantic system. *Neuron*, **38**, 499–506.

Thivard, L., Belin, P., Zilbovicius, M., Poline, J. B., and Samson, Y. (2000). A cortical region sensitive to auditory spectral motion. *NeuroReport,* **11**(13), 2969–2972.

Thompson-Schill, S. L., D'Esposito, M., Aguirre, G. K., and Farah, M. J. (1997). Role of left inferior prefrontal cortex in retrieval of semantic knowledge: a re-evaluation. *Proc. Natl. Acad. Sci. USA,* **94**, 14792–14797.

Thompson-Schill, S. L., Swick, D., Farah, M. J., D'Esposito, M., Kan, I. P., and Knight, R. T. (1998). Verb generation in patients with focal frontal lesions: a neuropsychological test of neuroimaging findings. *Proc. Natl. Acad. Sci. USA,* **95**(26), 15855–15860.

Thompson-Schill, S. L., D'Esposito, M., and Kan, I. P. (1999). Effects of repetition and competition on activity in the left prefrontal cortex during word generation. *Neuron,* **23**, 5113–5522.

Vandenberghe, R., Nobre, A. C., and Price, C. J. (2002). The response of left temporal cortex to sentences. *J. Cogn. Neurosci.,* **14**(4), 550–560.

Vandenberghe, R., Price, C. J., Wise, R., Josephs, O., and Frackowiak, R. S. J. (1996). Functional anatomy of a common semantic system for words and pictures. *Nature,* **383**, 254–256.

van Turennout, M., Ellmore, T., and Martin, A. (2000). Long lasting cortical plasticity in the object naming system. *Nat. Neurosci.,* **3**(12), 1329–1334.

Vouloumanos, A., Kiehl, K. A., Werker, J. F., and Liddle, P. F. (2001). Detection of sounds in the auditory stream: event-related fMRI evidence for differential activation to speech and nonspeech. *J. Cogn. Neurosci.,* **13**(7), 994–1005.

Vuilleumier, P., Henson, R. N., Driver, J., and Dolan, R. J. (2002). Multiple levels of visual object constancy revealed by event related fMRI of repetition priming. *Nat. Neurosci.,* **5**(5), 491–499.

Wagner, A. D., Pare-Blagoev, E. J., Clark, J., and Poldrack, R. A. (2001). Recovering meaning: left prefrontal cortex guides controlled semantic retrieval. *Neuron,* **31**(2), 329–338.

Warburton, E., Wise, R. J. S., Price, C. J., Weiller, C., Hadar, U., Ramsay, S., and Frackowiak, R. S. J. (1996). Noun and verb retrieval by normal subjects studies with PET. *Brain,* **119**(Pt. 1), 159–179.

Wernicke, C. (1874). *Der Aphasiche Symptomenkomplex.* Cohen and Weigert, Breslau, Poland.

Wise, R. J., Scott, S. K., Blank, S. C., Mummery, C. J., Murphy, K., and Warburton, E. A. (2001). Separate neural subsystems within 'Wernicke's area.' *Brain,* **124**(Pt. 1), 83–95.

Zatorre, R. J. and Belin, P. (2001). Spectral and temporal processing in human auditory cortex. *Cereb. Cortex,* **11**(10), 946–953.

C H A P T E R

27

The Feature-Based Model of Semantic Memory

This chapter discusses the contributions of functional imaging to our understanding of how conceptual knowledge is represented in the human brain. The first section outlines the feature-based account of semantic organisation. The second section describes the potential and pitfalls of functional imaging as a means to investigate the organisational principles of semantic memory. The third and fourth sections review functional imaging evidence for a role of a left posterior middle temporal area in action semantics and a left fusiform area in visual semantics. Finally, the fifth section revisits the feature-based account and concludes that specialisation of brain regions for different types of semantic knowledge can only be understood within particular task contexts.

THE FEATURE-BASED ACCOUNT OF SEMANTIC ORGANISATION

Since the seminal work of Warrington and Shallice (1984), double dissociations of semantic deficits for animate and inanimate items have been firmly established (for reviews, see Gainotti, 1995; Warrington and Shallice, 1984). Among the many cognitive models that have been offered to explain these category-specific deficits, the feature-based account has received particular attention. Within this framework (Allport, 1985; Gainotti, 1996; Martin *et al.*, 2000; Shallice, 1988; Warrington and Shallice, 1984), conceptual knowledge is thought to be represented in a large distributed network, indexing a range of semantic features (*e.g.*, visual, auditory, action, functional) that vary in their contributions to the meanings of concepts from different semantic categories. In particular, a distinction is drawn between sensory (*e.g.*, visual, auditory) and action (*e.g.*, hand action, body motion) features. While sensory features are important for distinguishing between living items, action semantics plays a critical role in the representations of inanimate items, especially tools. As a consequence, loss of sensory or action knowledge differentially disrupts the semantic representations of animate or inanimate objects, respectively. In this way, the feature-based account can explain category-specific semantic deficits for living and non-living items without assuming category-specificity as an underlying organisational principle of semantic memory. The feature-based model is thought to be implemented in the human brain in terms of input and output channels (Martin *et al.*, 2000). While sensory features are supposed to be subserved by brain regions close to or even overlapping with areas involved in modality-specific perception (*e.g.*, visual association areas), action semantics is hypothesised to be related to motor output regions as well as to brain areas involved in motion/action perception. Thus, the neural substrates underlying semantic features are related to or even identical with the regions that were engaged when the particular type of semantic knowledge was acquired during original sensorimotor experience. The first case proposes *semantic regions* that are selective for a particular type of semantic feature due to their afferent or efferent connections to *sensorimotor regions*. The second case assumes that sensorimotor regions themselves can sustain semantic representations or processes. The function of a sensorimotor region would then depend on the particular task context, which influences the strengths of the connections to other brain areas. For instance, visual association areas might be involved in perception when being activated via forward (bottom-up) connections from early visual areas and in semantic processes when being activated via backward (top-down) connections from semantic retrieval regions (Damasio, 1989; Price *et al.*, 2003).

Although the feature-based framework remains the dominant model for semantic organisation, it is not without criticism. For example, Caramazza and Shelton (1998) have argued that category-specific deficits do not correlate with the degree of impairment in sensory and motor knowledge. Instead, they suggest that conceptual knowledge is represented in segregated brain areas that have developed specialised neural mechanisms for processing objects from different semantic categories (*e.g.*, living items or artefacts) due to evolutionary pressures. Other models such as the conceptual structure account (Tyler and Moss, 2001) assume a unitary distributed conceptual system that is structured according to the correlations among semantic features (*i.e.*, the degree to which semantic features co-occur in the environment). Selective semantic deficits are explained by differences in the structure of concepts across categories. While living items are characterised by many features that are shared across categories, artefacts are defined by fewer and often more distinctive features.

POTENTIAL AND PITFALLS OF FUNCTIONAL NEUROIMAGING OF SEMANTIC ORGANISATION

Functional imaging experiments investigating the organisation of the semantic system have evolved along two lines of reasoning: The first approach compares brain activation elicited by stimuli from different object categories (*e.g.*, animals, tools) or feature categories (*e.g.*, colour, sound, taste) while keeping the task constant. The second approach holds the stimuli constant but changes the task instruction to focus the subject's attention selectively on different object features. For instance, subjects are required to make a semantic decision regarding the colour (*e.g.*, is it yellow?) or an associated action (*e.g.*, do you peel it?) of fruits. These specific task instructions thus differentially weight access to perceptual or action features.

Although these two approaches are founded on rational grounds, a clear interpretation of their activation results is impeded by several confounding factors and unresolved problems. Because the first approach compares brain activation evoked by stimuli from different categories, semantic as well as non-semantic properties of the stimuli might contribute to differences in brain response (Humphreys and Forde, 2001). Most notably, pictures of animate and inanimate objects differ in visual complexity and similarity; therefore, increased brain responses to picture naming of the animate category, for example, does not necessarily reflect a category-specific semantic organisation, but might instead arise at the levels of early visual processing, structural encoding, or object identification. Similar problems arise when using words as stimuli, as they place varying demands on phonological or orthographic processing. These examples demonstrate the importance of equating stimuli on their characteristic dimensions such as word frequency, familiarity, word length, structural complexity, and visual or auditory features. However, a perfect stimulus match often will not be achieved. Some confounds can be removed by looking for effects that are common to different stimulus (*i.e.*, picture or word) or input (heard or seen words) modalities using a conjunction analysis (Price and Friston, 1997). As activation that is observed irrespective of stimulus/input modality is less likely to be affected by pre-semantic processing differences, a conjunction can dissociate activations due to semantic factors from those reflecting irrelevant non-semantic processing.

Manipulating the task on the same stimuli avoids the problems of stimulus matching by comparing the brain responses to equivalent stimuli. In this case, the semantic task is designed to explicitly focus the subject's attention on different types of semantic features and thus differentially weigh their processing. Consequently, this approach is particularly susceptible to the effects of implicit processing. Implicit processing refers to the fact that many linguistic attributes are automatically processed by the human brain regardless of the explicit task demands (*e.g.*, the Stroop effect; see MacLeod, 1991). In imaging studies, task-irrelevant activation is illustrated by widespread activation in left-lateralised language areas for words compared to consonant letter strings during a feature detection task (Price *et al.*, 1996), which does not explicitly require the processing of words at a linguistic level. What does this imply for studies on the structure of the semantic system? Despite task-induced attentional shifts to specific semantic properties of an object, the entire semantic system might be activated in a highly connected way, and differential activation across types of semantic representations may thus be reduced or missed.

In addition, both stimulus and task changes are also confounded by general executive and specific strategic processes:

1. *Executive processes* include (effortful) retrieval, selection, and evaluation of semantic information; working memory; and response selection (Fiez, 1997; Gabrieli *et al.*, 1998; Noppeney and Price, 2002a; Roskies *et al.*, 2001; Thompson-Schill *et al.*, 1997, 1999b). Even subtle task differences that might not be sensitively reflected in reaction times can place differential demands on these various executive processes and cause profound differences in activation pattern. For instance, Perani *et al.* (1999a) report increased activation in a system comprised of the left dorso- and inferolateral prefrontal cortex, the superior and middle temporal, and the left occipital gyri for verbs relative to nouns, while no region was found more active for the reverse contrast. The activation pattern for verbs can easily be interpreted in terms of increased executive demands for verbs (in the context of longer reaction times) and therefore cannot be taken as evidence for an underlying segregation of verb/action and noun processing.
2. Confounds from specific strategies are illustrated in the study reported by Phillips *et al.* (2002b), which used the question "Is it bigger than a kiwi?" for retrieval of visual knowledge and "Do you peel it?" for retrieval of the action semantics. Only the visual question requires subjects to keep two objects in mind and make a size comparison, which might thus contribute to the activation differences.

These examples highlight the importance of a thorough task analysis to equate the cognitive processes involved across tasks accessing different types of semantics. As it will often be difficult to fully discard task-induced confounds, experimental designs are required that modulate the task variable by either changing the task instructions (*e.g.*, "Is it bigger than a kiwi?" vs. "Is it round?" for accessing visual knowledge) or introducing several different tasks (*e.g.*, semantic decision versus picture naming or semantic generation) that do not share the same confound. Only brain regions that show consistently greater activation for one type of semantics relative to all others can be uniquely associated with a specific type of semantic representation.

In conclusion, in order to distinguish differential activation patterns that reflect the underlying semantic organisation from spurious activation, differences due to confounds from non-semantic stimulus properties, or general/specific strategic processes, one needs to identify brain areas that respond specifically to one type of semantic representation irrespective of stimulus or input modality and instruction or task type. This requires either the integration of data from many studies or multifactorial designs that independently manipulate the factors of (1) semantic type, (2) stimulus or input modality, and (3) task instruction or task type.

Functional Imaging Studies Investigating the Feature-Based Model of Semantic Organisation

Most functional imaging studies have focused on category-specific effects and compared activations elicited by stimuli from different semantic categories, in particular tools and animals. Tools have mainly been associated with regions taking part in a visuomotor action network such as the left premotor cortex (Chao and Martin, 2000; Devlin *et al.*, 2002; Grabowski *et al.*, 1998; Grafton *et al.*, 1997; Martin *et al.*, 1996), the left posterior middle temporal (Cappa *et al.*, 1998; Chao *et al.*, 1999; Damasio *et al.*, 1996; Devlin *et al.*, 2002; Martin *et al.*, 1996; Moore and Price, 1999; Mummery *et al.*, 1996, 1998; Perani *et al.*, 1999b), and the supramarginal gyri

(Chao and Martin, 2000; Devlin *et al.*, 2002). In addition, some studies have reported enhanced left medial fusiform activation (Chao and Martin, 1999; Chao *et al.*, 2002) for tools relative to animals. Activations related to processing of animals have been even less consistent. While some studies have associated animals with visual association cortices—in particular, the lateral fusiform gyri (Chao and Martin, 1999; Chao *et al.*, 2002; Damasio *et al.*, 1996; Martin *et al.*, 1996; Perani *et al.*, 1995) and the superior temporal sulcus (Chao and Martin, 1999; Chao *et al.*, 2002)—others have linked them with the anterior temporal poles bilaterally (Devlin *et al.*, 2002; Moore and Price, 1999; Mummery *et al.*, 1996). Thus, studies contrasting different semantic categories have yielded inconsistent results (for a review, see Price and Friston, 2002). Moreover, category-specific effects can be accounted for by any cognitive model of semantic memory. In fact, they have been interpreted as evidence for the category-specific (Gerlach *et al.*, 2000; Spitzer *et al.*, 1998), the feature-based (Chao *et al.*, 1999; Grabowski *et al.*, 1998; Martin *et al.*, 1996, 2000; Perani *et al.*, 1995, 1999b; Phillips *et al.*, 2002b) and the conceptual structure (Devlin *et al.*, 2002; Tyler *et al.*, 2000) account. For instance, tool-specific activation in the left posterior middle temporal gyrus supports the category-specific framework but has also been attributed to implicit action retrieval within the feature-based framework. Conversely, the anterior temporal pole activation for animals can be interpreted as regional selectivity for animals or attributed to the greater demands that animals place on integration of semantic features during identification and semantic decision tasks (Devlin *et al.*, 2002) as suggested by the conceptual structure account.

This chapter focuses on functional imaging studies that investigated the feature-based model of semantic organisation and tested for anatomical segregation underlying different types of semantic features. For this, imaging studies:

1. Compared stimuli that referred to different semantic features (*e.g.*, colour versus hand action words) while holding the task constant (*e.g.*, repetition, semantic similarity judgments on triads of words) (Contreras, 2002; Noppeney *et al.*, 2002b).
2. Changed the task instructions to direct the subject's attention to different semantic aspects while holding the stimuli constant (*e.g.*, semantic decisions on tool stimuli with the task instructions "Do you twist the object?" versus "Is the object bigger than a kiwi?") (Martin *et al.*, 1995; Phillips *et al.*, 2002b).
3. Compared stimuli that referred to different semantic features (*e.g.*, colour relative to hand action words), where the task changed to explicitly direct the subject's attention to the semantic content of the stimulus (*e.g.*, semantic decision on colour words with the task instruction "Is it a dark colour?" vs. action words with the task instruction "Does the action involve a tool?") (Kellenbach *et al.*, 2001; Noppeney and Price, submitted; Noppeney *et al.*, 2002b).

While a range of different types of semantics such as auditory (Noppeney and Price, submitted; Noppeney *et al.*, 2002b), taste (Noppeney and Price, 2003a), functional-associative (Thompson-Schill and Gabrieli, 1999; Vandenberghe *et al.*, 1996), abstract (Kiehl *et al.*, 1999), and location (Cappa *et al.*, 1998; Mummery *et al.*, 1998; Noppeney and Price, 2003a) knowledge have been investigated, most studies have focused on action and visual semantics, which will be addressed in turn.

ACTION SEMANTICS AND THE LEFT POSTERIOR MIDDLE TEMPORAL GYRUS (LPMT)

The feature-based account (Martin *et al.*, 2000) proposes that the neural substrates underlying action representations are anatomically and functionally related to brain regions involved in motion perception (*i.e.*, MT/V5) and motor output (*i.e.*, premotor). In particular, the left posterior middle temporal gyrus (LPMT) has been associated with action semantics. As LPMT is anterior to motion area MT/V5, its role in action semantics might be engendered by its functional relation to action/motion perception mediated by afferents from area MT/V5. Consistent with this conjecture, LPMT is activated for observing grasping movements relative to static objects (Perani *et al.*, 2001; Rizzolatti *et al.*, 1996), hands (Grezes *et al.*, 1998, 1999) or random motion (Beauchamp *et al.*, 2002; Bonda *et al.*, 1996; Grezes *et al.*, 2001). While these activation differences might be due to specific motion characteristics of the stimuli at the perceptual level, LPMT activation was also increased for static pictures or sentences with implied motion/action relative to similar stimuli that did not imply motion (Kourtzi and Kanwisher, 2000; Ruby and Decety, 2001; Senior *et al.*, 2000). Most importantly, in semantic decision or generation tasks, LPMT is activated for retrieval of action (*e.g.*, "Do you twist this object?") relative to retrieval of visual semantics (*e.g.*, "Is the object bigger than a kiwi?"), when the stimuli were written words or pictures referring to real world objects (Martin *et al.*, 1995; Phillips *et al.*, 2002b). Similarly, LPMT activation is increased for semantic tasks on heard or seen words referring to action (*e.g.*, TWIST) relative to visual (*e.g.*, RED), auditory (*e.g.*, POP), motion (*e.g.*, RUN), or abstract (*e.g.*, IDEA) semantic features (Noppeney *et al.*, submitted). These effects were observed when the semantic task was held constant across conditions (*i.e.*, semantic similarity judgment on triads of words) as well as when the task instructions changed to direct the subject's attention to the specific semantic content of the stimulus (*e.g.*, "Does the hand action involve a tool?"). Taken together, these studies demonstrate that LPMT is more engaged in action semantics relative to a range of other semantic types regardless of whether action semantics is invoked by the task instruction or by the stimulus. Moreover, action selectivity in LPMT is observed irrespective of whether the stimuli are (1) written words or pictures or (2) heard or seen. Thus, the activations cannot be attributed to low-level stimulus characteristics. Instead, these results characterise LPMT as a multimodal semantic region associated with action semantics.

LPMT Is Selective for Action Semantics and for the Category of Tools

The feature-based theory predicates category-specific effects on anatomical segregation for different types of semantics. In particular, it links the category-specific effects of tools to effects specific to action semantics. In support of this hypothesis, many studies have consistently reported increased activation in LPMT for pictures or words depicting tools relative to animals or fruits during picture naming, semantic decision or generation tasks (Cappa *et al.*, 1998; Chao and Martin, 2000; Chao *et al.*, 1999, 2002; Devlin *et al.*, 2002; Martin *et al.*, 1996; Moore and Price, 1999; Mummery *et al.*, 1996, 1998; Phillips *et al.*, 2002a). These studies suggest that semantic category (*e.g.*, tools versus animals) and semantic type (*e.g.*, action versus visual) might modulate the neural response in overlapping LPMT regions and that LPMT action selectivity thus can account for category-specific effects of tools. Indeed, a recent study that independently manipulated stimulus category (*e.g.*, tools versus fruits; see Phillips *et al.*, 2002b) and task/type of semantics (*i.e.*, action vs. visual) in a 2×2 factorial design revealed that the tool and the action-selective effect influence LPMT in an additive fashion: Tools relative to fruits activated LPMT irrespective of whether the action or visual semantics is retrieved. Conversely, retrieval of action relative to visual knowledge activated LPMT regardless of whether tools or fruits are presented (see Fig. 27.1a). Thus, even when the stimuli were fruits, LPMT was more active when subjects made a semantic decision on an appropriate action (*e.g.*, "Can you peel it by hand") than on its real life size (*i.e.*, "Is it bigger than a lemon?"). This pattern of results was replicated in a follow-up study (Contreras, 2002), where subjects made semantic judgments on visual or action features that referred to animals or tools. Again, tools relative to animals and action relative to visual features increased LPMT activation in an additive fashion (see Fig. 27.1b). In conclusion, consistent with the feature-based account, tools that are more strongly linked to action semantics than animals or fruits activate an area that also responds to action retrieval. Moreover, both action semantics and tools increase LPMT responses independently.

The Distinction Between Hand Manipulations and Whole Body Movements

Actions can be classified as hand manipulations or whole body movements. A distinction between these two categories can be drawn at the perceptual and at the semantic level. At the perceptual level, hand manipulation movements are characterised by simple motion trajectories. For instance, the movement for using a saw is primarily a simple translation movement. By contrast, whole body movements are described by complex motion trajectories. Thus, humans can independently move different body parts that are connected by articulated joints. At the

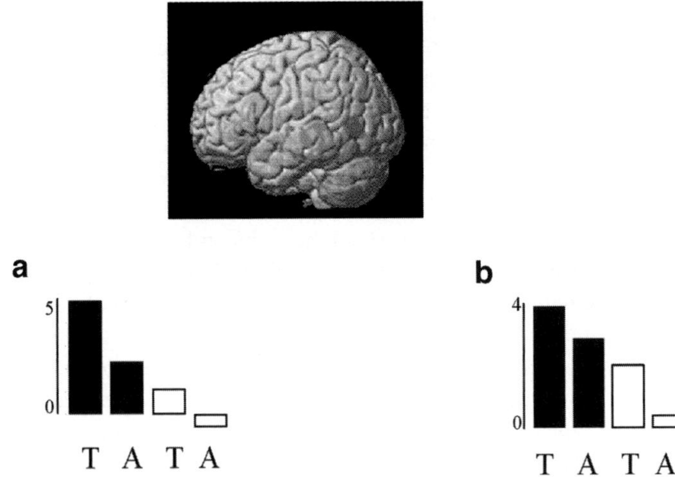

FIGURE 27.1
Additive effects of tool category and action retrieval in LPMT. Bottom: Top: Activation for action > visual semantics ($p < 0.05$, corrected) masked with action semantics : baseline ($p < 0.001$, uncorrected) is rendered on an averaged normalised brain. (a) Subjects were presented pictures or written words that referred to tools or fruits. In the activation conditions, they made a decision on action (*e.g.*, do you peel it by hand?) or visual (*e.g.*, is it bigger than a kiwi?) semantics. In the baseline condition, they made a decision on the screen size of the stimulus (Phillips *et al.*, 2002b). Left: Parameter estimates for semantic conditions averaged over pictures and words relative to baseline are shown at the peak coordinate of action > visual semantics (–56, –60, 0). T, tools; A, animals; black bars, action; white bars, visual. (b) In the activation conditions, subjects were presented with two written words referring to the properties of an object (*e.g.*, WEIGH and MEASURE) followed by three potential written object names (*e.g.*, SCALES, MIRROR, BED). The properties were visual, action, or functional attributes and the objects were household items or animals. Subjects decided which of the three objects was described by the two properties (Contreras, 2002). Parameter estimates for each semantic condition relative to baseline are shown at the peak coordinate of action : visual semantics (–62, –58, 2). T, tools; A, animals; black bars, action; white bars, visual.

semantic level, hand manipulations are more strongly associated with tools and utensils, while whole body movements are primarily linked with humans and animals. Based on these distinctions, the question arises whether LPMT responds more to hand manipulations than to whole body movements. At the perceptual level, this question has recently been addressed (Beauchamp *et al.*, 2002) by comparing the activations during observation of (1) natural simple tool movements (*e.g.*, sawing), (2) artificial simple tool movements (*e.g.*, a rotating saw), (3) natural complex human movements (*e.g.*, running), and (4) artificial simple human movements (*e.g.*, a rotating human). All types of tool and human movements activated area LPMT relative to moving gratings. Consistent with studies of category-specific effects, activation in LPMT was higher for moving tools than moving humans. Similarly, semantic decisions on words referring to whole body movements and hand manipulations increased LPMT activation relative to judgments on words referring to visual features (Contreras, 2002) or a non-semantic baseline. Consistent with the category-specific effect for tools, LPMT activation was higher for tool manipulations than for animal whole body movements. However, a direct comparison of hand manipulations and whole body movements (after accounting for the category effect of tools) has yielded inconclusive results with very small insignificant activation increases for hand manipulations relative to whole body movements at the perceptual and semantic level (Beauchamp *et al.*, 2002; Noppeney *et al.*, submitted). In summary, studies on action observation and semantic retrieval provide converging evidence that LPMT activation is commonly increased for hand manipulation as well as whole body movements. However, so far there is only weak evidence that hand manipulations relative to whole body movements enhance LPMT activation.

The Distinction Between Manipulation and Functional Knowledge: Knowing "How" and Knowing "What For"

Tools or objects can be characterised by the motion features of an associated hand action (*i.e.*, knowing "how" = manipulation knowledge) and by their function (*i.e.*, knowing "what for" or the context of usage = functional knowledge). Although a particular type of manipulation can sometimes be associated with a specific function (*e.g.*, a saw and a knife are associated with similar actions and have similar functions), the mapping between manipulation and functional properties is many to many. For instance, a piano and a record player subserve similar functions but are manipulated differently, while a piano and a typewriter fulfil different functions but are manipulated similarly. Recently, neuropsychological studies (Buxbaum *et al.*, 2000; Sirigu *et al.*, 1991) have reported patients who could match items on the basis of their function but not on the basis of how they are manipulated and vice versa. This double dissociation suggests that the neural substrates of function and manipulation knowledge may be anatomically segregated. Based on the putative relationship between LPMT and area MT/V5, one might hypothesise that LPMT responds to manipulation more than functional knowledge. Consistent with this notion, previous studies (Cappa *et al.*, 1998; Mummery *et al.*, 1998; Thompson-Schill *et al.*, 1999a) have not reported LPMT activation for retrieval of functional relative to visual semantics. A recent study (Kellenbach *et al.*, 2002) directly compared retrieving (1) an action associated with a manipulable object (*e.g.*, "Does using a saw involve a twisting or a turning movement?"), (2) a function of a manipulable object (*e.g.*, "Is a saw used to put a substance on another object?"), and (3) a function of a non-manipulable object (*e.g.*, a traffic light). While LPMT activation was significantly increased for manipulable relative to non-manipulable objects, it was only insignificantly enhanced when comparing retrieval of action with functional knowledge for manipulable objects. Thus, LPMT only showed an effect of stimulus (manipulable versus non-manipulable objects) but not task (action versus function retrieval) when manipulable objects are used as stimuli. Together with the series of previous null findings for functional knowledge (Cappa *et al.*, 1998; Mummery *et al.*, 1998; Thompson-Schill *et al.*, 1999a), these results suggest that LPMT activation is primarily driven by manipulation knowledge, which is automatically/implicitly invoked by manipulable objects irrespective of the specific task instructions.

The Influence of Sensory Experience

The *sensorimotor theory* hypothesises that semantic information is represented in a distributed neuronal network encoding semantic features (*e.g.*, visual, auditory, action), which are anatomically linked to the sensory (or motor) areas that are active when the features (*e.g.*, motion, colour) are experienced (Allport, 1985; Martin *et al.*, 2000; Warrington and McCarthy, 1987). Thus, the functional anatomy of semantic memory is predicated on the organisation of sensory systems. From this perspective, one might expect that sensory deprivation that leads to the restructuring of sensory systems will also modify the neural systems underlying semantic representations. In particular, one might hypothesise that visual deprivation, which enforces action experience via somatosensorimotor associations rather than visual motion perception, reduces the action-selective response in LPMT. Contrary to this conjecture, in both blind and sighted subjects, LPMT activation increased for semantic decisions on heard words referring to actions relative to words referring to visual, auditory, or motion features (Noppeney *et al.*, 2003b) (Fig. 27.2). This surprising resilience of LPMT action selectivity to visual deprivation suggests that the action-selective role of LPMT develops due to innately specified neurobiological mechanisms and not just experiential factors or it depends on its efferent connections to motor areas.

The Effects of Task-Context on Action-Selective LPMT Responses

The results reported so far have emphasised that LPMT responds selectively to action retrieval during focused semantic tasks. One might therefore be tempted to label LPMT as an "action semantic area;" however, this assertion might suggest that LPMT has a single function and that action selectivity occurs irrespective of the task context. In contrast, a recent study (Noppeney *et al.*, submitted) demonstrated that although LPMT is more active for action relative to visual, auditory, or motion features during focused semantic decision tasks, it responds equally to all semantic features when subjects silently repeat/read and think about the meaning of the words (see Fig. 27.3). The LPMT response to auditory and visual features during repetition is incompatible with an action-selective role for LPMT irrespective of the task context. Instead, this

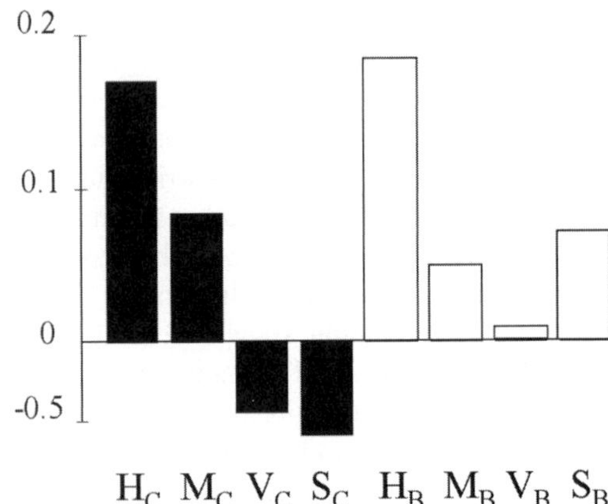

FIGURE 27.2
Resiliency of the action-selective LPMT response to visual deprivation. Blind and sighted subjects were presented with spoken words referring to hand actions (*e.g.*, TICKLE), body motions (*e.g.*, JUMPING), visual features (*e.g.*, BLUE), or auditory features (*e.g.*, POP) and made semantic decisions that explicitly focused their attention on the semantic content of each word (*e.g.*, JUMPING: Is it a quick movement?) (Noppeney *et al.*, 2003b). Parameter estimates for each semantic condition relative to baselines are shown at the peak coordinate of action > other semantic types (–54, –66, 3). Blind and sighted subjects show increased activation for hand actions relative to all other semantic types. H, hand action; M, body motion; V, visual; S, sound; black bars, sighted (C); white bars, blind (B).

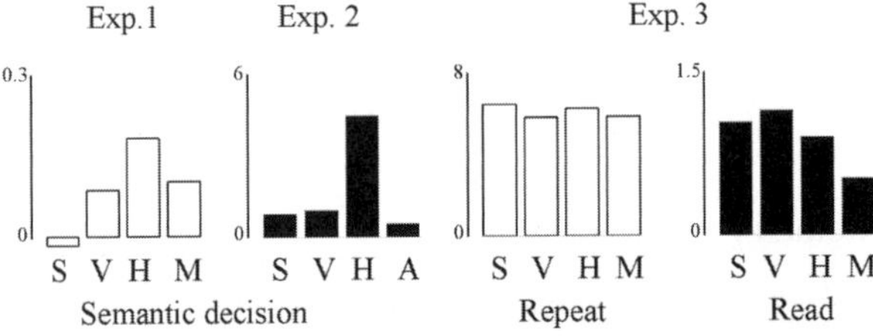

FIGURE 27.3
Task dependency of LPMT action selectivity. In all three experiments, subjects were presented with spoken or written words referring to hand actions, body motions, auditory features, visual features, or abstract concepts. In experiment 1, subjects engaged in decisions that explicitly focused their attention on the semantic content of each word. In experiment 2, they made semantic similarity judgments on triads of stimuli. In experiment 3, they thought about the meaning of words after reading or repeating (Noppeney *et al.*, submitted). Parameter estimates for each semantic activation relative to non-semantic baseline for semantic decision, repetition, and reading at the peak coordinate of hand action > other semantic types in experiments 1 and 2 (–57, –63, –3). S, sound; V, visual; H, hand action; M, body motion; A, abstract semantics; black bars, written words; white bars, spoken words.

activation pattern suggests that LPMT action selectivity may be better understood as an interaction between semantic type and task, which might be interpreted in two ways: From one perspective, LPMT performs the same process in both task contexts, and this is either enhanced for action or suppressed for non-action words during the semantic decision task. Alternatively, LPMT may perform different functions during repetition and semantic decision. For instance, during repetition LPMT might be involved in phonological processing, while during semantic decisions on action words it might subserve task-induced strategies such as action imagery, which are not required for retrieval of the other types of semantics. Irrespective of the precise function(s) the implication is that LPMT action selectivity depends on the task context.

Summary

Consistent with the feature-based account, retrieval of action semantics and action observation increase activation in LPMT that may be functionally and anatomically linked with area MT/V5. In particular, LPMT activation has been reported for tasks accessing action relative to visual, sound, and abstract semantics irrespective of whether the stimuli were words or pictures or were seen or heard. Moreover, LPMT also responds to tools that are more strongly linked with action/manipulation semantics than to other semantic categories such as animals or fruits. In fact, both action semantics and tools independently increase LPMT activation in an additive fashion. Some evidence has been provided for the notion that LPMT action selectivity is primarily engendered by its response to hand manipulations rather than whole body movements. The action-selective LPMT response in early blind subjects, who experienced actions primarily via sensorimotor associations, supports the emphasis on manipulation rather than visual associations. Together, these results might suggest that LPMT is specific to action retrieval; however, during repetition tasks, LPMT responds irrespective of the type of semantics. Here, the LPMT response to non-action words is incompatible with an action-selective role of LPMT irrespective of the task context. Instead, it suggests that LPMT action selectivity emerges only in a limited set of contexts.

VISUAL SEMANTICS AND THE FUSIFORM REGION

The feature-based account of semantic memory hypothesises an association between visual semantics and a left anterior fusiform region which is anterior and lateral to the fusiform area involved in colour perception (Lueck *et al.*, 1989). So far, only a few functional imaging studies on (1) retrieval of colour semantics and (2) visual imagery have provided evidence for this hypothesis. The initial evidence was provided by a study that compared generation of colour to generation of action words and reported increased activation in the bilateral fusiform when the stimuli were pictures and in the right fusiform when the stimuli were written words (Martin *et al.*, 1995). Further studies by the same group have also reported left fusiform/inferior temporal activation for colour generation relative to object naming (Chao and Martin, 1999; Wiggs *et al.*, 1999); however, as this comparison involved a task change (*i.e.*, semantic generation versus picture naming) and picture naming did not control for many cognitive processes involved in colour generation (*e.g.*, suppression of verbalising the name of the object, semantic search, working memory), activation was also enhanced in a widespread frontoparietal system rather than specifically in the fusiform area. Therefore, the fusiform/inferior temporal activation increase might be due to task-related processing differences rather than reflecting colour retrieval *per se*. Studies on visual imagery have also provided evidence for a role of the fusiform gyrus in visual semantics. Left anterior fusiform activation has been revealed when (1) comparing imagery of concrete words with listening to abstract words (D'Esposito *et al.*, 1997) and (2) correlating the effect of word imageability during listening, reading, and semantic decision (Wise *et al.*, 2000). By contrast, the right fusiform has been associated with colour imagery (Howard *et al.*, 1998). The degree of lateralisation and the exact locations of left anterior fusiform responses to visual semantics therefore show considerable variation.

Other studies have not observed activation specific to visual semantics, either in the fusiform area or elsewhere in the brain. For instance, left anterior fusiform activation was equal for retrieval of colour and verbally learned knowledge (Noppeney and Price, 2002b). Likewise, studies investigating visual semantics using real-life size judgments did not observe any significant activation difference (Phillips *et al.*, 2002b; Vandenberghe *et al.*, 1996) anywhere in the brain. To add to this inconsistency, several studies have associated retrieval of visual semantics with regions outside of the fusiform area. Thus, associating words on the basis of colour relative to location increased activation in the left anterior temporal gyrus (Mummery *et al.*, 1998), while retrieval of colour/size relative to sound features enhanced activation in the right inferior temporal gyrus (Kellenbach *et al.*, 2001). Furthermore, semantic decisions regarding luminance/form (*e.g.*, blue, light) and auditory features (*e.g.*, pop, noisy) relative to abstract concepts (*e.g.*, value, truth) increased activation in a left anterior temporal pole region but only during semantic decisions and not during auditory repetition (Noppeney and Price, 2002c). These effects have not been replicated in subsequent studies even when identical stimuli and focused semantic decisions were used, thus illustrating the confounding influence of (1) task-type, (2) specific instruction, and (3) possibly subject-specific strategies on the activation evoked by different types of semantic features. Taken collectively, it suggests that the anterior temporal pole activation does not reflect visual semantic retrieval but rather task-induced strategies that might vary across subjects.

Summary

Studies on visual semantics have primarily produced inconsistent results. While studies on visual imagery and some studies using semantic retrieval tasks have implicated the left/right anterior fusiform gyrus in visual semantics, others have reported null results (Noppeney and Price, 2003a; Phillips *et al.*, 2002b; Vandenberghe *et al.*, 1996) or activation specific to visual semantics elsewhere in the brain (Kellenbach *et al.*, 2001; Mummery *et al.*, 1998; Noppeney and Price, 2002c). One way to explain these divergent results is to appreciate the effects of implicit and task-induced semantic processing. For instance, as semantic knowledge about objects is strongly based on visual experience (at least in sighted subjects), one might hypothesise that brain areas related to visual semantics are implicitly activated even when stimuli or task direct the subject's attention to other types of semantics. As a consequence, differential activation between visual and non-visual semantic conditions might be reduced and thus missed in the analysis. Implicit processing might therefore explain the series of null results. Conversely, the inconsistent positive activation results might reflect strategic processes that depend on the task type, the specific task instructions and subject-specific strategies. Thus, further studies are required to ascertain whether visual semantic knowledge is segregated from other types of semantics, as predicted by the sensorimotor theory.

CONCLUSIONS AND FUTURE DIRECTIONS

Numerous studies have been designed to define the neural correlates of feature-based semantic representations. The only consistent finding that has emerged so far is an association of action retrieval with a left posterior middle temporal region (LPMT); however, an action-selective response in LPMT was only observed during focused semantic decision tasks, while LPMT responded equally to different semantic features during repetition tasks. This activation pattern is not compatible with an action-selective role of LPMT irrespective of the task context. Instead, it suggests that semantic specificity might be profoundly context sensitive and better understood as an interaction between semantic feature and task context.

Task by stimulus interactions of this sort can be understood from two perspectives. From a cognitive perspective, they demonstrate the fallacy of assigning brain regions with specific functions that are either stimulus bound or task bound. Instead, a brain region that shows a task by semantic type interaction might reflect a process that is involved irrespective of the semantic feature in one task but is suppressed/increased for one particular semantic feature in another task. Alternatively, a brain region might be involved in different processes during different tasks. For instance, it might take part in phonological processing during repetition and reflect specific retrieval strategies that are only relevant for one type of semantic feature during focused semantic decisions.

In terms of neural mechanisms, task by stimulus interactions are consistent with the well-established notion that functional specialisation emerges from changes in the interactions among brain areas that serve different functions (McIntosh, 2000; Mesulam, 1990). Accordingly, the functional role played by any neuronal system is defined by its interactions with other neuronal systems. Interactions can be via either forward connections (from lower to higher areas) or backward connections (from higher to lower areas) (Friston and Price, 2001). Backward connections may mediate the top-down effects of task. Thus, context-sensitive differential semantic activation might be mediated by task-dependent, top-down influences on responses to one semantic feature type. For instance, context-sensitive, action-selective activations in LPMT might be engendered by input from common semantic retrieval areas (*e.g.*, the left inferior frontal cortex) that selectively curtail or enhance responses to one particular semantic feature and is increased during focused semantic tasks.

What does this discussion imply for future studies investigating the organisational principles of semantic representations? First, semantic segregation needs to be considered within different task contexts. For this, multifactorial designs are required that enable (1) the dissociation of context-independent from context-sensitive effects, and (2) characterise interactions between semantic type and task context. We hypothesise that this approach will reveal that semantic-selective activation is profoundly sensitive to the context as defined by the task-type (*e.g.*, repetition, semantic decision) and the specific task instructions (*e.g.*, different instructions used for action retrieval). Investigating the retrieval of a particular semantic type in a series of task contexts and redefining semantic specificity as stimulus by task interactions might thus help us to explain the inconsistent results in the current literature; however, the context might not be entirely defined by the task instructions but might also depend on the individual subjects due to subject-specific strategies. To account for these subject-specific strategies, future studies are required that not only evaluate semantic activation that is consistent across subjects but also investigate intersubject variability.

Second, in terms of neural mechanisms, "context" is defined by the integration of activation in distributed brain regions. In order to study how a regionally semantic-selective response emerges from its interactions with other brain regions, we need to investigate semantic-selective responses within the framework of effective connectivity, which describes the influence that one area exerts over another. Effective connectivity studies will allow us to infer whether context-sensitive semantic selectivity is mediated by increased top-down modulation in a particular task context (*e.g.*, action selectivity in LPMT during focused semantic tasks). Moreover, they will enable us to formally address and test whether identical brain regions can sustain sensory functions when being activated via forward connections but semantic representational functions when being activated via backwards connections.

In conclusion, previous functional imaging studies on semantic organisation have focused on semantic-selective responses independent of the particular task context. This segregationist approach has primarily produced inconsistent results. Future studies might help us to resolve these inconsistencies by investigating how the semantic-selective response in a brain area is defined and modulated by a particular task context from a cognitive perspective and its interactions with other brain areas from the perspective of neuronal mechanisms.

References

Allport, D. A. (1985). Distributed memory, modular subsystems and dysphasia, in *Current Perspectives in Dysphasia*, Newman, S. K. and Epstein, R., Eds., pp. 32–60. Churchill Livingstone, Edinburgh.

Beauchamp, M. S., Lee, K. E., Haxby, J. V., and Martin, A. (2002). Parallel visual motion processing streams for manipulable objects and human movements. *Neuron,* **34**, 149–159.

Bonda, E., Petrides, M., Ostry, D., and Evans, A. 1996. Specific involvement of human parietal systems and the amygdala in the perception of biological motion. *J. Neurosci.,* **16**, 3737–3744.

Buxbaum, L., Veramonti, T., and Schwartz, M. (2000). Function and manipulation tool knowledge in apraxia: knowing 'what for' but not 'how.' *NeuroCase,* **6**, 83–97.

Cappa, S. F., Perani, D., Schnur, T., Tettamanti, M., and Fazio, F. (1998). The effects of semantic category and knowledge type on lexical-semantic access: a PET study. *Neuroimage,* **8**, 350–359.

Caramazza, A. and Shelton, J. R. (1998). Domain-specific knowledge systems in the brain the animate-inanimate distinction. *J. Cogn. Neurosci.,* **10**, 1–34.

Chao, L. L. and Martin, A. (1999). Cortical regions associated with perceiving, naming, and knowing about colors. *J. Cogn. Neurosci.,* **11**, 25–35.

Chao, L. L. and Martin, A. (2000). Representation of manipulable man-made objects in the dorsal stream. *NeuroImage,* **12**, 478–484.

Chao, L. L., Haxby, J. V., and Martin, A. (1999). Attribute-based neural substrates in temporal cortex for perceiving and knowing about objects. *Nat. Neurosci.,* **2**, 913–919.

Chao, L. L., Weisberg, J., and Martin, A. (2002). Experience-dependent modulation of category-related cortical activity. *Cereb. Cortex,* **12**, 545–551.

Contreras, V. (2002). Category-Specific Effects: Segregation of Semantic Knowledge and Degree of Feature Processing in the Brain, M.Sc. thesis. Welcome Department of Imaging Neuroscience, University College, London.

Damasio, A. R. (1989). Time-locked multiregional retroactivation: a systems-level proposal for the neural substrates of recall and recognition. *Cognition,* **33**, 25–62.

Damasio, H., Grabowski, T. J., Tranel, D., Hichwa, R. D., and Damasio, A. R. (1996). A neural basis for lexical retrieval [see comments]. *Nature,* **380**, 499–505 (published erratum in *Nature*, **381**(6595), 810, 1996).

D'Esposito, M., Detre, J. A., Aguirre, G. K., Stallcup, M., Alsop, D. C., Tippet, L. J., and Farah, M. J. (1997). A functional MRI study of mental image generation. *Neuropsychologia,* **35**, 725–730.

Devlin, J. T., Moore, C. J., Mummery, C. J., Gorno-Tempini, M. L., Phillips, J. A., Noppeney, U., Frackowiak, R. S., Friston, K. J., and Price, C. J. (2002). Anatomic constraints on cognitive theories of category specificity. *NeuroImage,* **15**, 675–685.

Fiez, J. A. (1997). Phonology, semantics, and the role of the left inferior prefrontal cortex. *Hum. Brain Mapping,* **5**, 79–83.

Friston, K. J. and Price, C. J. (2001). Generative models, brain function and neuroimaging. *Scand. J. Psychol.,* **42**, 167–177.

Gabrieli, J. D., Poldrack, R. A., and Desmond, J. E. (1998). The role of left prefrontal cortex in language and memory. *Proc. Natl. Acad. Sci. USA,* **95**, 906–913.

Gainotti, G., Silveri, M. C., Daniele, A., and Ginstolisi, L. (1995). Neuroanatomical correlates of category-specific semantic disorders: A critical survey. *Memory* **3**, 247–264.

Gainotti, G. and Silveri, M. C. (1996). Cognitive and anatomical locus of lesion in a patient with a category-specific semantic impairment for living beings. *Cogn. Neuropsychol.,* **13**, 357–389.

Gerlach, C., Law, I., Gade, A., and Paulson, O. B. (2000). Categorisation and category effects in normal object recognition: a PET study. *Neuropsychologia,* **38**, 1693–1703.

Grabowski, T. J., Damasio, H., and Damasio, A. R. (1998). Premotor and prefrontal correlates of category-related lexical retrieval. *NeuroImage,* **7**, 232–243.

Grafton, S. T., Fadiga, L., Arbib, M. A., and Rizzolatti, G. (1997). Premotor cortex activation during observation and naming of familiar tools. *NeuroImage,* **6**, 231–236.

Grezes, J., Costes, N., and Decety, J. (1998). Top-down effect of strategy on the perception of human biological motion: a PET investigation. *Cogn. Neuropsychol.,* **15**, 553–582.

Grezes, J., Costes, N., and Decety, J. (1999). The effects of learning and intention on the neural network involved in the perception of meaningless actions. *Brain,* **122**, 1875–1887.

Grezes, J., Fonlupt, P., Bertenthal, B., Delon-Martin, C., Segebarth, C., and Decety, J. (2001). Does perception of biological motion rely on specific brain regions? *NeuroImage,* **13**, 775–785.

Howard, R. J., ffytche, D. H., Barnes, J., McKeefry, D., Ha, Y., Woodruff, P. W., Bullmore, E. T., Simmons, A., Williams, S. C., David, A. S., and Brammer, M. (1998). The functional anatomy of imagining and perceiving colour. *NeuroReport,* **9**, 1019–1023.

Humphreys, G. W. and Forde, E. M. (2001). Hierarchies, similarity, and interactivity in object recognition: 'category-specific' neuropsychological deficits. *Behav. Brain Sci.,* **24**, 453–476.

Kellenbach, M. L., Brett, M., and Patterson, K. (2001). Large, colorful, or noisy? Attribute- and modality-specific activations during retrieval of perceptual attribute knowledge. *Cogn. Affect. Behav. Neurosci.,* **1**, 207–221.

Kellenbach, M., Brett, M., and Patterson, K. (2003). Action speak louder than functions: the importance of manipulability and action in tool representation. *J. Cogn. Neurosci.,* **15**(1), 30–46.

Kiehl, K. A., Liddle, P. F., Smith, A. M., Mendrek, A., Forster, B. B., and Hare, R. D. (1999). Neural pathways involved in the processing of concrete and abstract words. *Hum. Brain Mapping,* **7**, 225–233.

Kourtzi, Z. and Kanwisher, N. (2000). Activation in human MT/MST by static images with implied motion. *J. Cogn. Neurosci.,* **12**, 48–55.

Lueck, C. J., Zeki, S., Friston, K. J., Deiber, M. P., Cope, P., Cunningham, V. J., Lammertsma, A. A., Kennard, C., and Frackowiak, R. S. (1989). The colour centre in the cerebral cortex of man. *Nature,* **340**, 386–389.

MacLeod, C. M. (1991). Half a century of research on the Stroop effect: an integrative review. *Psychol. Bull.,* **109**, 163–203.

Martin, A., Haxby, J. V., Lalonde, F. M., Wiggs, C. L., and Ungerleider, L. G. (1995). Discrete cortical regions associated with knowledge of color and knowledge of action. *Science,* **270**, 102–105.

Martin, A., Wiggs, C. L., Ungerleider, L. G., and Haxby, J. V. (1996). Neural correlates of category-specific knowledge. *Nature,* **379**, 649–652.

Martin, A., Ungerleider, L. G., and Haxby, J. V. (2000). Category-specificity and the brain: the sensory/motor model of semantic representations of objects, in *The Cognitive Neurosciences*, Gazzaniga, M. S., Ed., pp. 1023–1037. MIT Press, Cambridge, MA.

McIntosh, A. R. (2000). Towards a network theory of cognition. *Neural Netw.,* **13**, 861–870.

Mesulam, M. M. (1990). Large-scale neurocognitive networks and distributed processing for attention, language, and memory. *Ann. Neurol.,* **28**, 597–613.

Moore, C. J. and Price, C. J. (1999). A functional neuroimaging study of the variables that generate category-specific object processing differences. *Brain,* **122**, 943–962.

Mummery, C. J., Patterson, K., Hodges, J. R., and Wise, R. J. (1996). Generating 'tiger' as an animal name or a word beginning with T: differences in brain activation. *Proc. Roy. Soc. London, Ser. B, Biol. Sci.,* **263**, 989–995 (published erratum in *Proc. Roy. Soc. London, Ser. B, Biol. Sci.,* **263**(1377), 1755–1756, 1996).

Mummery, C. J., Patterson, K., Hodges, J. R., and Price, C. J. (1998). Functional neuroanatomy of the semantic system: divisible by what? *J. Cogn. Neurosci.,* **10**, 766–777.

Noppeney, U. and Price, C. J. (2002a). A PET study of stimulus- and task-induced semantic processing. *NeuroImage,* **15**, 927–935.

Noppeney, U. and Price, C. J. (2002b). Retrieval of visual, auditory, and abstract semantics. *NeuroImage,* **15**, 917–926.

Noppeney, U. and Price, C. J. (2003a). Functional imaging of the semantic system: retrieval of sensory-experienced and verbally-learnt knowledge. *Brain Language*, **84**, 120–133.

Noppeney, U., Friston, K., and Price, C. (2003c). Effects of visual deprivation on the organisation of the semantic system. *Brain,* **126**(Pt. 7), 1620–1627.

Noppeney, U., Josephs, O., Kiebel, S., Winterburn, D., Friston, K., and Price, C. (2003b). Task-dependent selectivity for action in the left posterior middle temporal cortex, submitted.

Perani, D., Cappa, S. F., Bettinardi, V., Bressi, S., Gorno-Tempini, M., Matarrese, M., and Fazio, F. (1995). Different neural systems for the recognition of animals and man-made tools. *NeuroReport,* **6**, 1637–1641.

Perani, D., Cappa, S. F., Schnur, T., Tettamanti, M., Collina, S., Rosa, M. M., and Fazio, F. (1999a). The neural correlates of verb and noun processing. A PET study. *Brain* **122**, 2337–44.

Perani, D., Schnur, T., Tettamanti, M., Gorno-Tempini, M., Cappa, S. F., and Fazio, F. (1999b). Word and picture matching: a PET study of semantic category effects. *Neuropsychologia,* **37**, 293–306.

Perani, D., Fazio, F., Borghese, N. A., Tettamanti, M., Ferrari, S., Decety, J., and Gilardi, M. C. (2001). Different brain correlates for watching real and virtual hand actions. *NeuroImage,* **14**, 749–758.

Phillips, J. A., Humphreys, G. W., Noppeney, U., and Price, C. J. (2002a). The neural substrates of action retrieval: an examination of semantic and visual routes to action. *Vision and Cogn.,* **9**(4), 662–684.

Phillips, J. A., Noppeney, U., Humphreys, G. W., and Price, C. J. (2002b). Can segregation within the semantic system account for category-specific deficits? *Brain,* **125**, 2067–2080.

Price, C. J. and Friston, K. J. (1997). Cognitive conjunction: a new approach to brain activation experiments. *NeuroImage,* **5**, 261–270.

Price, C. and Friston, K. (2002). Functional imaging studies of category specificity, in *Category Specificity in Brain and Mind*, Forde, E. M. and Humphreys, G. W., Eds., pp. 427–447, Psychology Press.

Price, C. J., Wise, R. J., and Frackowiak, R. S. (1996). Demonstrating the implicit processing of visually presented words and pseudowords. *Cereb. Cortex,* **6**, 62–70.

Price, C. J., Noppeney, U., Phillips, J. A., and Devlin, J. T. (2003). How is the fusiform gyrus related to category-specificity? *Cogn. Neuropsychol.*, **20**, 561–576.

Rizzolatti, G., Fadiga, L., Matelli, M., Bettinardi, V., Paulesu, E., Perani, D., and Fazio, F. (1996). Localisation of grasp representations in humans by PET. 1. Observation versus execution. *Exp. Brain Res.,* **111**, 246–252.

Roskies, A. L., Fiez, J. A., Balota, D. A., Raichle, M. E., and Petersen, S. E. (2001). Task-dependent modulation of regions in the left inferior frontal cortex during semantic processing. *J. Cogn. Neurosci.,* **13**, 829–843.

Ruby, P. and Decety, J. (2001). Effect of subjective perspective taking during simulation of action: a PET investigation of agency. *Nat. Neurosci.,* **4**, 546–550.

Senior, C., Barnes, J., Giampietro, V., Simmons, A., Bullmore, E. T., Brammer, M., and David, A. S. (2000). The functional neuroanatomy of implicit-motion perception or representational momentum. *Curr. Biol.,* **10**, 16–22.

Shallice, T. (1988). *From Neuropsychology to Mental Structure*. Cambridge University Press, Cambridge, U.K.

Sirigu, A., Duhamel, J. R., and Poncet, M. (1991). The role of sensorimotor experience in object recognition: a case of multimodal agnosia. *Brain,* **114**, 2555–2573 (published erratum in *Brain*, **115**(Pt. 2), 645, 1992).

Spitzer, M., Kischka, U., Guckel, F., Bellemann, M. E., Kammer, T., Seyyedi, S., Weisbrod, M., Schwartz, A., and Brix, G. (1998). Functional magnetic resonance imaging of category-specific cortical activation: evidence for semantic maps. *Brain Res. Cogn. Brain Res.,* **6**, 309–319.

Thompson-Schill, S. L. and Gabrieli, J. D. (1999). Priming of visual and functional knowledge on a semantic classification task. *J. Exp. Psychol. Learn. Mem. Cogn.,* **25**, 41–53.

Thompson-Schill, S. L., D'Esposito, M., Aguirre, G. K., and Farah, M. J. (1997). Role of left inferior prefrontal cortex in retrieval of semantic knowledge: a reevaluation. *Proc. Natl. Acad. Sci. USA,* **94**, 14792–14797.

Thompson-Schill, S. L., Aguirre, G. K., D'Esposito, M., and Farah, M. J. (1999a). A neural basis for category and modality specificity of semantic knowledge. *Neuropsychologia,* **37**, 671–676.

Thompson-Schill, S. L., D'Esposito, M., and Kan, I. P. (1999b). Effects of repetition and competition on activity in left prefrontal cortex during word generation. *Neuron,* **23**, 513–522.

Tyler, L. K. and Moss, H. E. (2001). Towards a distributed account of conceptual knowledge. *Trends Cogn Sci.* **5**, 244–252.

Tyler, L. K., Moss, H. E., Durrant-Peatfield, M. R., and Levy, J. P. (2000). Conceptual structure and the structure of concepts: a distributed account of category-specific deficits. *Brain Language,* **75**, 195–231.

Vandenberghe, R., Price, C., Wise, R., Josephs, O., and Frackowiak, R. S. (1996). Functional anatomy of a common semantic system for words and pictures [see comments]. *Nature,* **383**, 254–256.

Warrington, E. K. and McCarthy, R. A. (1987). Categories of knowledge: further fractionations and an attempted integration. *Brain,* **110**, 1273–1296.

Warrington, E. K. and Shallice, T. (1984). Category specific semantic impairments. *Brain,* **107**, 829–854.

Wiggs, C. L., Weisberg, J., and Martin, A. (1999). Neural correlates of semantic and episodic memory retrieval. *Neuropsychologia,* **37**, 103–118.

Wise, R. J., Howard, D., Mummery, C. J., Fletcher, P., Leff, A., Buchel, C., and Scott, S. K. (2000). Noun imageability and the temporal lobes. *Neuropsychologia,* **38**, 985–994.

C H A P T E R

28

The Functional Anatomy of Reading

This chapter focuses exclusively on the neural systems that sustain reading. The first section considers the neuropsychological studies of acquired alexia that led to the 19th-century neurological model of reading and the 20th-century cognitive models of reading. The second section describes the neural systems for reading that have been revealed by functional imaging studies. In the next two sections, these findings are compared to the neural system for auditory word repetition and the picture naming system. The studies that have attempted to tease apart different reading routes are then considered, followed by a reconsideration of the neurological model of reading. We conclude that there may only be one route for reading which develops from an adaptation of the object naming system.

NEUROPSYCHOLOGICAL STUDIES OF ACQUIRED ALEXIA AND MODELS OF READING

The first neurological model of reading can be credited to Dejerine (1891), who contrasted two distinct types of alexia (the inability to read). In alexia *with* agraphia, the patient is unable to read or write; on the basis of a postmortem study, Dejerine associated this deficit to a lesion in the left angular gyrus and proposed that this was the site of visual images of speech—the so-called *word form area*. Patients suffering from alexia *without* agraphia show a more selective reading deficit because they do not lose the ability to write or speak; therefore, this syndrome is also referred to as *pure alexia*, and when patients are able to decode words by assembling the components letter by letter, the term *letter-by-letter readers* has been used. A case reported by Dejerine (1892) had sustained a left occipito-temporal lesion. Because the patient was able to write, knowledge of visual word forms appeared to be intact; therefore, the deficit was attributed to a disconnection between visual processing in the occipital cortex and word form recognition in the angular gyrus (for a full discussion of this and other disconnection syndromes, see Geschwind, 1965).

There have been many subsequent reports of patients with pure alexia, and a comprehensive review can be found in Damasio and Damasio (1983). The most consistent lesion results from occlusion of the left posterior cerebral artery with damage, including the medial occipital lobe (cuneus and lingual gyrus), the mesial temporal lobes (including the fusiform), the splenium of the corpus callosum, and the thalamus. Usually (but not always), this results in a right hemianopia which, in the context of corpus callosum damage, prevents visual input from the left visual field (right visual cortex) accessing the left angular gyrus. Pure alexia, therefore, results from damage to fibers connecting both visual fields to the language system (Damasio and Damasio, 1983; Geschwind, 1965).

The model of reading that emerged was based on a combination of Dejerine's reading studies and the early postmortem findings of Broca (1861) and Wernicke (1874) indicating speech production in the left posterior inferior frontal cortex (Broca's area) and speech comprehension in the left posterior superior temporal cortex (Wernicke's area). As illustrated in the upper part of Fig. 28.1, written word processing starts in occipital cortex with hypothetical links to speech output via the left angular gyrus, Wernicke's area, Broca's area, and the motor cortex. The functions associated with these five areas were, respectively, visual processing, visual word form images, auditory word form images, motor images, and articulation (see lower part of Fig. 28.1). To enable word comprehension, Lichtheim (1885) introduced the notion of a *concept centre* having connections to and from the auditory and motor images.

Understanding the nature of pure alexia is crucial for understanding the neural systems that sustain reading because if pure alexia only affects reading then this would suggest neuronal specialisation for reading; however, most studies of pure alexia that have examined visual processing in depth report concurrent deficits in non-reading domains. Deficits in colour naming and picture naming, for example, are frequently reported (Damasio and Damasio, 1983; De Renzi *et al.*, 1987; Geschwind, 1965). The inconsistent co-occurrence of letter, number, picture, and colour naming deficits has been explained in terms of the extent of the lesion. For example, Kurachi *et al.* (1979) claim that object naming disturbances depend on the extent of damage to

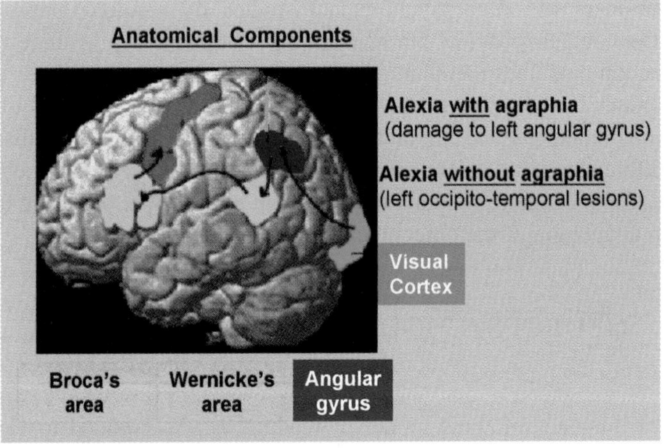

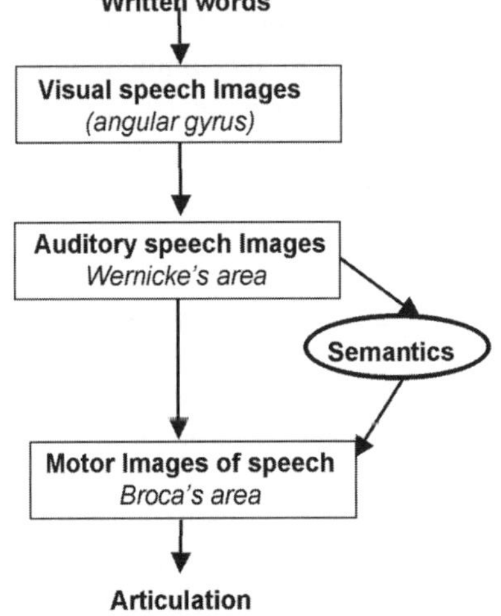

FIGURE 28.1
The 19th-century neurological model of reading.

the left cuneus, and Damasio and Damasio (1983) observed that colour anomia is always accompanied by damage to the lingual gyrus that extends into the left hippocampal region. Conversely, picture, colour, and letter naming can be spared while reading is impaired because reading is more complex and imposes greater demands on visual processing (Benson and Geshwind, 1969; Friedman and Alexander, 1984; Geschwind, 1965). In other words, according to the disconnection account of pure alexia, the reading problem is the most salient manifestation of a more general visual problem.

The most quoted exception to the nonspecificity of pure alexia and its anatomical basis is a study by Warrington and Shallice (1980). These authors dismissed the possibility that the reading impairment in pure alexia was due to visual or perceptual deficits because the patients they report showed no impairment with (1) complex picture interpretation, (2) recognition of pictures of objects in unconventional views, (3) selective attention, or (4) visual short-term memory; also, their patients were more impaired in regard to tachistoscopic presentation of words than pictures. Warrington and Shallice (1980) therefore localised the deficit in their patients to the function of a word form system that "parses (multiple and in parallel) letter strings into ordered familiar units and categorises these units visually" (p. 109). This explanation differs from the neurological model presented in Fig. 28.1 because it requires separate word form areas for reading and writing; however, the problem with this and all neuropsychological studies that claim to have found deficits that are specific to alphabetic stimuli is that there are no detailed task analyses of the visual processes is involved in reading or other visual tasks such as complex picture interpretation. Moreover, complex picture interpretation is a slow serial process, whereas whole word reading requires fast parallel letter identification; consequently, reading may be most affected by minor perceptual deficits.

Many other neuropsychological studies of reading have also challenged the 19th-century neurological model of reading presented in Fig. 28.1. For example, if the concept centre can only be accessed after conversion of visual word forms to auditory word forms, then we would not be able to distinguish the meaning of words that have the same sound (for example, *pain* and *pane*). Furthermore, the model does not account for two other forms of acquired dyslexia traditionally referred to as *surface dyslexia* and *phonological dyslexia*. Surface dyslexics typically have semantic deficits and particular difficulty reading words with exceptional spellings (for example, *choir* or *yacht*), although they can read meaningless words on the basis of spelling-to-sound rules (for example, *shoir* or *moof*). In contrast, phonological dyslexics have the opposite pattern of reading errors to surface dyslexics; that is, they are better at reading meaningful (*choir*) than meaningless (*shoir*) words. On the basis of this apparent "double dissociation," cognitive models of reading started to incorporate at least two routes to meaning (Coltheart *et al.*, 1993; Marshall and Newcombe, 1973).

Figure 28.2 illustrates two of the most popular formalisations of reading. The terminology has changed, with visual word forms referred to as *orthography* and auditory word forms referred to as *phonology*. These terms are more accurate because they incorporate both lexical (whole word) and sublexical (parts of words) processes. On the left of Fig. 28.2, a three-route model of reading is illustrated that shows the sublexical route, which allows unfamiliar non-words to be read; the lexical route, which allows familiar words to be read even in the absence of semantic knowledge; and the semantic route, which provides meaning to the words on the basis of orthography rather than phonology. Notably, meaningful words with regular spellings (for example, *ship*) can be read by all three routes (Coltheart *et al.*, 1993; Patterson and Shewell, 1987; Zorzi *et al.*, 1998). A contrasting formulation has been proposed on the basis of computational modelling (Seidenberg and McClelland, 1989). Here, the argument is that the same number of neuropsychological deficits and cognitive processes can emerge from changes in the availability of interactions in a system with far fewer components. More specifically, the so-called *triangular model* illustrated on the right of Fig. 28.2 is composed of three components: orthography, semantics, and phonology. Meaningless non-words can only be read via orthographic to phonological connections, meaningful words with irregular spellings require access to semantics, and meaningful words with regular spellings can be read by either route. Critically, however, neither of the models illustrated in Fig. 28.2 has physiological validity; there is no clear one-to-one mapping between reading deficit and lesion site, and the cognitive dissociations seen in patients are never all or none.

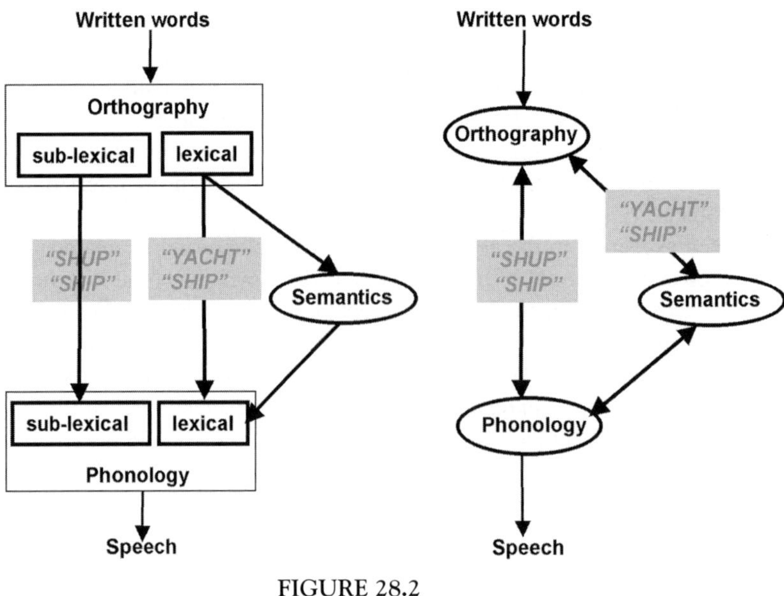

FIGURE 28.2
Multiple routes for reading.

THE NEURAL SYSTEMS FOR READING: EVIDENCE FROM FUNCTIONAL NEUROIMAGING

Functional imaging has allowed us to explore the neural systems for reading in neurologically normal subjects. Responses across the whole brain can be measured, rather than relying on the site of lesion as in neuropsychological studies of patients. Furthermore, by changing the relationship between the activation and baseline conditions, functional imaging experiments can segregate the subcomponents of the neural systems for reading and suggest hypotheses about the role of different areas (Fiez and Petersen, 1998; Petersen *et al.*, 1988–1990).

Figure 28.3 shows the neural systems for reading relative to resting with eyes closed (for a meta-analysis of other studies, see Turkeltaub *et al.*, 2002). The data come from two studies reported in Price and Friston (1997) and Price *et al.* (1996a), and the results of the new analysis are detailed using the conventional *x*, *y*, *z* coordinates of standard space (Talairach and Tournoux, 1988) with the corresponding *Z* score in brackets. The different colors used in Fig. 28.3 indicate the common and differential effects of three reading tasks that put increasing demands on speech production: reading silently without any mouth movements; mouthing, when the word is articulated overtly without producing any sound; and reading aloud, when the sound of the word is also generated. The red areas (and coordinates) in Fig. 28.3 indicate common activation for all three tasks relative to rest. Irrespective of the task, activation is observed in visual processing areas (bilateral occipito-temporal) and areas involved in speech output (sensorimotor and cerebellar regions, the supplementary motor cortex [SMA], left thalamus, and a dorsal region of the left posterior superior temporal cortex). The strong effects in articulation areas, even during silent reading, can be explained by the automaticity of reading in normal literate adults (MacLeod, 1991; Price *et al.*, 1996c). The green areas in Fig. 28.3 illustrate increased activation for "mouthing" relative to reading silently in bilateral anterior ingulae and sensomotor areas that are associated with articulation. Finally the blue areas in Fig. 28.3 illustrate increased activation for reading aloud than mouthing in bilateral superior temporal areas that have been associated with hearing the sound of the spoken response (Blank *et al.*, 2002; Price, 2000; Price *et al.*, 1996a,d; Wise *et al.*, 2001).

Taken together, the activations shown in Fig. 28.3 show a great deal of consistency with those hypothesised on the basis of the neurological model (Fig. 28.1), but there are some notable exceptions. First, no activation is observed in the left angular gyrus which would be predicted if this were a visual word form area. Second, activation does not extend anteriorly in the inferior

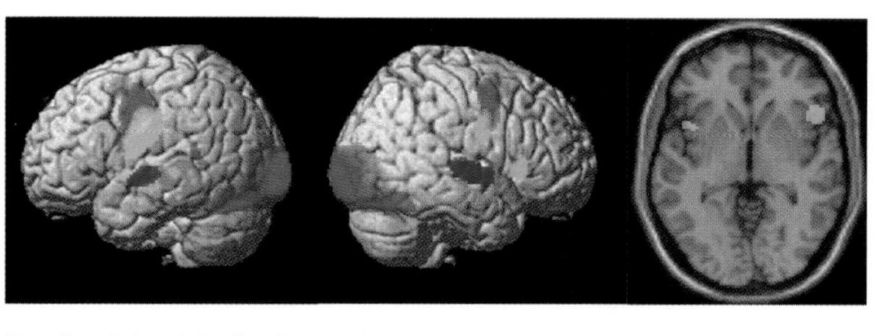

Reading (aloud & silent) > rest

Visual LH	Visual RH
-26, -98 0 (>8)	22, -98 –2 (>8)
-10, -96 2 (>8)	8, -84 4 (>8)
-16, -100 2 (>8)	
-32, -90 –16 (5.4)	0 –76 –12 (7.6)
-4, -96 2 (>8)	6, -92, -2 (>8)

Motor LH	Motor RH
-50, -8 44 (>8)	56, 4, 48 (>8)
-60, 2, 28 (6.3)	
-64, 4, 18 (5.3)	SMA
	4, 10, 54 (6.3)
	8, 4, 58 (5.7)

Cerbellum	
-30, -70, -20 (>8)	0 -72, -24 (>8)
	30, -62, -22 (>8)
	14, -70 –20 (.8)

left thalamus
-12, -20, 0 (4.8)

L. Superior temporal
-56, -44 14 (5.3)
-56, -50, 6 (5.2)

Mouthing – silent

Insula LH	Insula RH
-44, 12, 0 (4.5)	36 12, 2 (3.9)
-28, 6 0 (4.9)	
-28, 2, -2 (4.8)	
-32, 8 0 (4.8)	
-28, 4, -4 (4.7)	

Motor LH	Motor RH
-52, -12, 32 (6.3)	52, -2, 36 (5.1)
-58, -10, 24 (6.1)	62, -4, 20 (4.7)
-62, -12, 18 (5.6)	
-60, -2 16 (5.8)	
	Frontal RH
	52, 22 0 (5.2)

Aloud – Mouthing

L.superior temporal	R. superior temporal
-60, -8 –4 (5.2)	64, 2 –2 (5.0)
-64, -14, -2 (5.3)	70, - 4 –4 (5.7)
	72, –12 0 (5.9)
	72, -20 4 (5.4)
	48, -34, 8 (4.5)

FIGURE 28.3
Reading relative to resting with eyes closed.

frontal cortex, consistent with claims that the critical site for articulatory planning is in the left anterior insula (Dronkers, 1996; Wise *et al.*, 1999). Third, with the exception of the left posterior superior temporal cortex, activation is bilaterally distributed in both left and right hemispheres. To explain these inconsistencies, we need to segregate the reading system into the components that might underlie different reading functions (orthography, phonology, semantics) by contrasting reading activation to a variety of baseline tasks.

Figure 28.4 illustrates the activation for reading relative to viewing false fonts that control for early visual feature analysis without any orthographic input (letter processing). This has the effect of reducing the extensive occipito-temporal activation (seen when reading is contrasted to rest) to an area in the left mid-fusiform gyrus. As Fig. 28.4 illustrates, activation in this area is consistent across a range of reading tasks. The top row shows activation for passively viewing words relative to false fonts (using data previously reported in Price *et al.*, 1994). In addition to the left mid-fusiform, activation is observed in left posterior middle and superior temporal cortices, sensorimotor areas, and the cerebellum. The second row of Fig. 28.4 shows activation for words relative to false fonts when subjects are engaged in a visual feature detection task that was common to all stimuli (press a button if the stimulus has a visual feature that ascends above the rest of the letters/symbols). In this paradigm, the task is matched in the reading and baseline conditions, and activation pertains to the implicit processing of words while subjects are engaged in an irrelevant/incidental task (data for six subjects previously reported by Brunswick *et al.*,

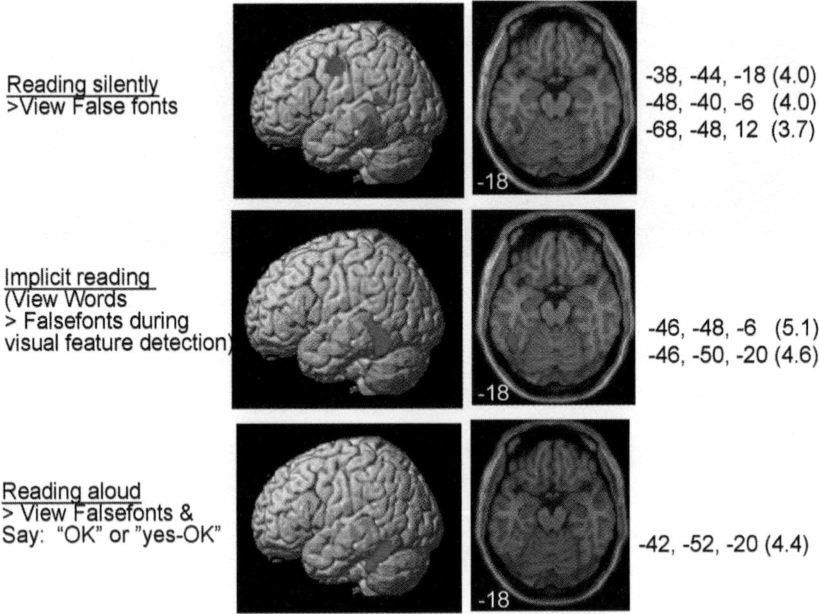

FIGURE 28.4
Reading relative to viewing false fonts.

1999, and for nine subjects previously reported by Price *et al.*, 1996c). Activation is observed in the left mid-fusiform and middle temporal cortex (as seen for silent reading without feature detection) but not in the left posterior superior temporal cortex or sensorimotor areas, suggesting that these speech production areas (see Chapter 26) were not implicitly activated during feature detection. Finally, the third row of Fig. 28.4 shows activation when reading aloud is compared to viewing false fonts and saying "OK," with the "OK" response included to control for articulation and hearing the sound of the spoken response (data for 8 subjects from Moore and Price, 1999, and for 10 subjects from McCrory, 2001). As in the silent reading and feature detection paradigms (rows 1 and 2 of Fig. 28.4), activation is observed in the left mid-fusiform and left middle temporal gyrus. The location of the mid-fusiform activation for each paradigm can be seen in the coordinates and *Z* scores (in brackets) given in the right-hand column of Fig. 28.4. In addition, it should be noted that the left superior temporal, sensorimotor, and cerebellar activations that are seen for reading silently relative to false fonts (row 1 of Fig. 28.4) are not observed when reading aloud is contrasted to saying "OK" to false fonts (row 3 of Fig. 28.4). This is because the "OK" response controls for speech output processing (see Chapter 26 for evidence).

In summary, the most consistent activation for the reading paradigms illustrated in Fig. 28.4 is located in the left mid-fusiform gyrus; however, a specific left mid-fusiform area is not associated with a particular cognitive process in the neurological model of reading (see Fig. 28.3) even though it is in the vicinity of the typical lesion site for pure alexia. Cohen and colleagues (Cohen *et al.*, 2000, 2002; Dehaene *et al.*, 2002) have therefore labelled the most posterior part of this area centred around the Talairach coordinates ($x = -43$, $y = -54$, $z = -12$) as the *visual word form area*. The problem with this assertion is that the posterior part of the left mid-fusiform is involved in many other tasks (Price and Devlin, 2003). For example, Fig. 28.5 illustrates the correspondence in the left mid-fusiform activation observed for: (1) reading relative to saying "OK" to false fonts (top row); (2) picture naming relative to saying "OK" to non-objects (second row); (3) colour naming relative to saying "OK" to the same stimuli (third row); and (4) auditory word repetition relative to saying "OK" to noise bursts (bottom row) (using data from McCrory, 2001; Moore and Price, 1999; Noppeney and Price, 2002; Price *et al.*, 1996c, 2003). Despite the different experiments and subjects, the peak locations of the activations are all less than 4 mm from the peak location of the reading area (see Fig. 28.4 or the coordinates specified by Cohen and colleagues above). Activation in the left mid-fusiform for all these diverse tasks can be interpreted in two ways. Either there is one function that underlies all the activations, in which

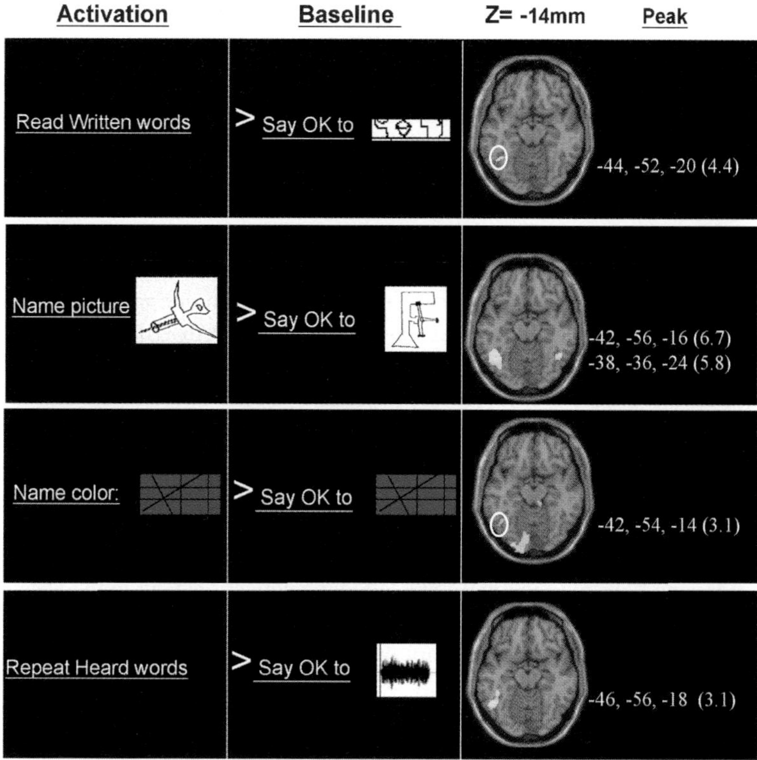

FIGURE 28.5
The left mid-fusiform.

case it is not specific to reading, or the left mid-fusiform area might be composed of multiple different regions, each with different functions and only one of the regions specialised for visual word forms. These possibilities are discussed in turn below.

If the posterior left mid-fusiform reading area has a single function that also underlies activation in non-reading tasks, what might this function be? Because the left mid-fusiform is within the visual processing stream, a role in visual processing/representations is the most likely possibility. Indeed, Martin and colleagues (Chao *et al.*, 1999, 2002; Martin and Chao, 2001) have reported increased activation for viewing pictures of animals relative to tools in a left posterior mid-fusiform area (peak: –40, –59, –10) that is only 5 mm away from the area (–43, –54, –12) that Cohen *et al.* refer to as the visual word form area. Furthermore, Martin and Chao (2001) have claimed that the category-sensitive fusiform activations are "driven by stored object information," with objects from the same category tending to share the same combination of features. An explanation in terms of visual form processing, however, is still not consistent with the response we observe for colour naming and auditory word repetition (see Fig. 28.4). In the colour naming paradigm, the visual form was identical in the activation and baseline conditions and the task did not rely on form information (although it is possible that increased attention to the stimulus during colour naming enhanced responses to the visual structure of the stimulus). In the auditory repetition task, posterior left mid-fusiform activation was observed even for heard words that did not have any clear visual associations (for example, *bleep*, *chime*, or *echo*) suggesting that activation is not specific to visual input or to visual associations. Another possibility is that the left posterior mid-fusiform acts as a "convergence zone" for the connections between visual and language domains (for a similar argument, see Tarkiainen *et al.*, 1999). In light of our observation (Phillips *et al.*, 2002; Price and Devlin, 2003) that the same area (–46, –56, –14) also responds during manipulation of unfamiliar objects that do not require linguistic processing, the convergence is likely to be a general one linking visual and motor areas. If we then propose that the left mid-fusiform has bidirectional links between visual and motor areas, then activation during auditory word processing can also be explained even when there is no visual processing involved in the task.

The alternative explanation is that the left posterior mid-fusiform area might be composed of multiple different regions, each with multiple different functions and only one of the regions being specialised for visual word forms. The precision with which activation is localised in functional magnetic resonance imaging (fMRI) and positron emission tomography (PET) is on the order of about 2 to 3 mm; therefore, at present, it is difficult to distinguish regions that were closer than 2 to 3 mm. Future studies are required to explore the possibility that there are fine-grained subdivisions within the left mid-fusiform; however, it should be noted that if specialisation for word form processing is at a microscopic level, no one-to-one correspondence would be observed between lesions and visual word form deficits. Lesions occur at a macroscopic level and a lesion to the left mid-fusiform area would impair all possible functions.

In summary, functional imaging studies have revealed a distributed set of areas for reading and highlighted an important role for a left mid-fusiform area that was not specified in the neurological model. We have considered the possibility that this fusiform area may serve as a visual word form area, an explanation that would also account for the absence of reading activation in the left angular gyrus where visual word form processing was expected on the basis of the neurological model; however, the data illustrated in Fig. 28.5 have demonstrated that the posterior part of the left mid-fusiform area is not dedicated to reading at the macroscopic (3-mm) level. It is therefore possible that the left mid-fusiform acts as a convergence zone linking visual and motor processing with bidirectional links, allowing activation even in the absence of visual processing. The next section explores specialisation for reading further by comparing the areas that are more active for reading than auditory word repetition.

READING COMPARED TO AUDITORY WORD REPETITION

According to the neurological model of reading (see Fig. 28.1), a comparison between reading and auditory word repetition should reveal the visual cortex and the left angular gyrus. In Price *et al.* (2003), we compared activation in four conditions: (1) reading, (2) auditory word repetition; (3) saying "OK" to false fonts; and (4) saying "OK" to auditory noise. Reading relative to auditory word repetition evoked highly significant effects throughout the whole of the occipital lobes ($p < 0.01$, corrected for multiple comparisons) but no effect ($p > 0.05$, uncorrected) in the left angular gyrus or any other area (see top of Fig. 28.6). These findings suggest that, as proposed by the neurological model, activation in Wernicke's area and Broca's area is common to reading and repeating (for further evidence, see Price *et al.*, 2003), and reading differs only by the input modality. However, the latter conclusion requires further investigation because it is based on a null effect and it assumes that the occipital activation relates only to visual processing.

The axial slice in the middle of Fig. 28.6 compares the extent of activation for reading relative to repeating (yellow) and reading relative to saying "OK" to false fonts (red) to segregate areas involved in early visual processing and later stages of word form processing. As can be seen, the posterior part of the left mid-fusiform area for words relative to false fonts lies within, or adjacent to, the visual processing areas. The graph at the bottom of Fig. 28.6 shows the relative effect sizes in the left posterior mid-fusiform for auditory word repetition (Rp), hearing noise bursts and saying "OK" (Ns), reading (Rd), and seeing false fonts and saying "OK" (Ff). A particularly interesting point to note here is that, although both reading and repeating activate this area relative to their corresponding baseline conditions (Ns and Ff), activation is greater for visual stimuli than auditory stimuli *irrespective of lexicality*. Thus, activation for viewing false font stimuli was significantly greater than that for listening to noise bursts ($Z = 5.4$; $p < 0.01$, corrected for multiple comparisons across the whole brain). Moreover, there was also an effect of lexicality (words > baseline) but no interaction between stimulus modality (visual or auditory) and lexicality (words or baseline). The activation difference between reading and auditory word repetition (Rd > Rp) is therefore not specific to visual word forms, as suggested by Dehaene *et al.* (2002). In conclusion, the posterior part of the left mid-fusiform area appears to be visually driven but modulated by the presence of meaningful stimuli.

If the only area to be more active for reading than auditory word repetition and false fonts is also activated during auditory word repetition (Rp > Ns in Fig. 28.6), which areas are specific to reading? The hypothesis we are pursuing is that, although there are no reading-specific areas,

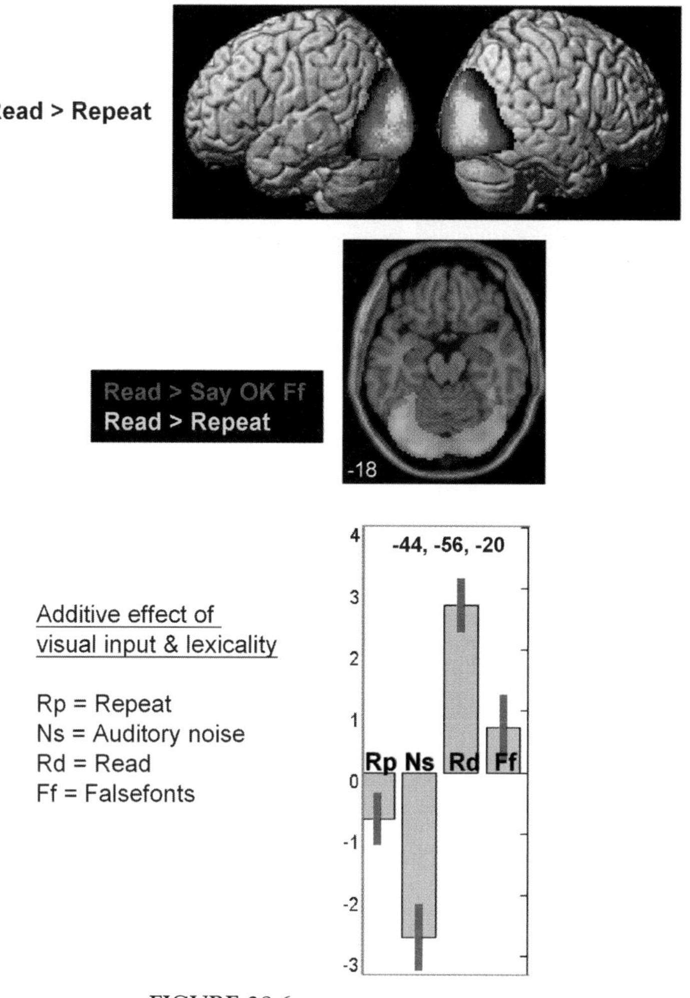

FIGURE 28.6
Reading relative to auditory word repetition.

specialisation for reading emerges at a systems level from changes in the interactions between areas that each serve multiple functions. In addition, it is possible that, although false fonts are not words, the visual system may implicitly treat them as words with potential meanings. Thus, the comparison of words to false fonts might hide reading areas in the visual cortex. In the next section, we therefore consider areas that are more active for reading than picture naming.

READING COMPARED TO PICTURE NAMING

As discussed previously, reports of patients with pure alexia suggest that neural systems might have become specialised for reading. It might therefore be expected that there would be at least some areas where there was increased activation for reading relative to equivalent tasks with pictures. Figure 28.7 illustrates the results of an analysis that compared object processing when the stimuli were presented as pictures or the written names of objects. The tasks were (1) semantic decisions; (2) perceptual decisions regarding the actual size of a stimulus on the screen (large or small?); and (3) naming pictures and words (using data collated from McCrory, 2001; Moore and Price, 1999; Phillips *et al.*, 2002). Irrespective of the task, written names increased activation relative to pictures in the left dorsal superior temporal area that is associated with speech production (see Chapter 26). Figure 28.7 (blue areas) also illustrates that, for reading relative to picture naming, written words also increased bilateral sensorimotor activation (blue

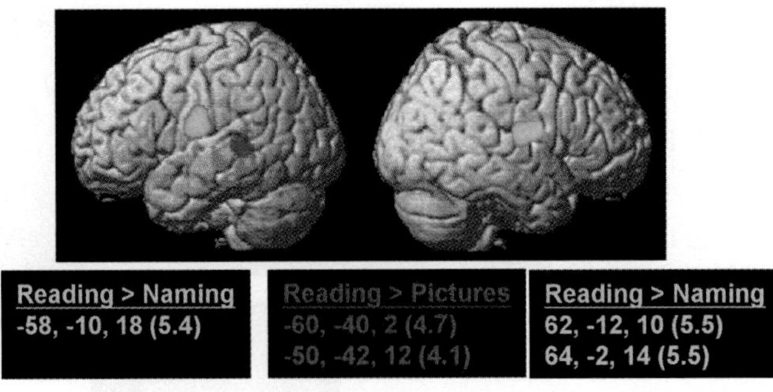

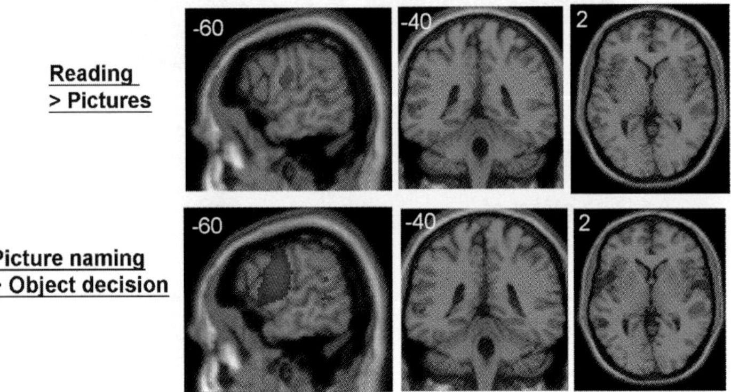

FIGURE 28.7
Reading relative to picture naming.

areas in Fig. 28.7), suggesting that the degree to which written word and picture processing differ depends on the task.

The advantage for written words in the left superior temporal and sensorimotor areas was highly significant but we still cannot claim that these areas are specific for reading. Activation in the same areas is also highly significant during picture naming and when subjects are instructed to say "OK" to visual noise displays (see Chapter 26). Increased activation for written names relative to picture naming therefore indicates a greater reliance on these speech production mechanisms, particularly when the word/name must be articulated. The bottom part of Fig. 28.7 illustrates the remarkably consistent correspondence between the areas activated for picture naming relative to object decisions (see also Fig. 26.3 from Chapter 26) and the areas more active for reading than picture naming. The conclusion is that these areas are not specific for reading.

DIFFERENT SPELLING-TO-SOUND ROUTES FOR READING?

If reading utilises the picture naming system, then how can we account for the different patterns of alexia discussed earlier (see Fig. 28.1)? Although reading object names activated the same areas as seen for picture naming, there may be alternative reading routes for other types of words which have less concrete meanings. The cognitive models illustrated in Fig. 28.2 suggest that reading routes are most likely to be distinguished for meaningless non-words and meaningful words. Several functional neuroimaging studies have contrasted activation for these different word types (Brunswick *et al.*, 1999; Fiebach *et al.*, 2002; Fiez *et al.*, 1999; Hagoort *et al.*, 1999; Herbster *et al.*, 1997; Mechelli *et al.*, 2003; Rumsey *et al.*, 1997; Tagamets *et al.*, 2000). The most consistent finding is that reading pseudo-words relative to words increases activity in the left posterior inferior temporal cortex, the left inferior frontal gyrus, and the left anterior insula, but there have been no replications across studies when reading words is contrasted to reading pseudo-words (for a review, see Mechelli *et al.*, 2003). Furthermore, increased activation for

Author	Date	Left temporal	Left frontal	Left insula
Price et al.	1996	-48, -62, -4	--------------	
Herbster et al.	1997	--------------	-44, 4, 16	
Rumsey et al.	1997	--------------	--------------	
Brunswick et al.	1999	-42, -54, -20	-48, 6, 26	
Hagoort et al.	1999	-34, -55, -11	-46, 17, -8	
Fiez et al.	1999	-43, -45, -8	-------------	-35, 15, 6
Xu et al.	2001	-46, -66 -10	-52, 10 12	
Fiebach et al.	2002	--------------	-47, 10,13	-37, 16, 0
Mechelli et al.	2003	-44, -64 -16	-48, 8 22	

Pseudowords > Words (Mechelli et al., 2003)

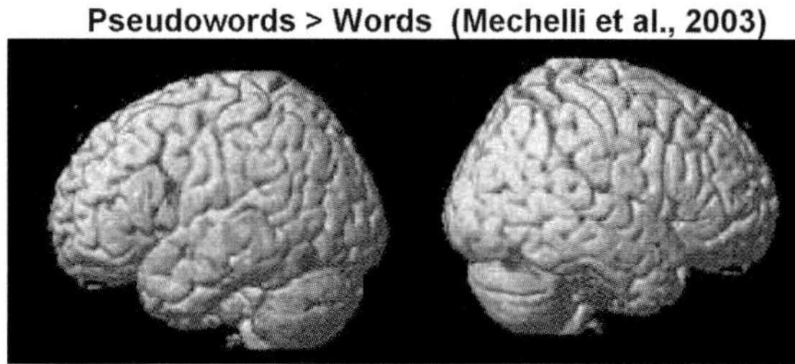

Reading > Rest (See Figure 3)

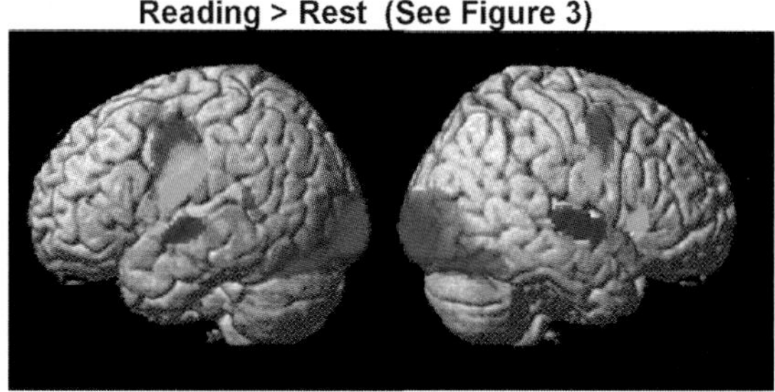

FIGURE 28.8
Pseudo-words relative to words ($p < 0.001$).

pseudo-words compared to words is still only a relative effect. In other words, activation in the temporal and frontal areas that are more active for pseudo-words is also observed for real word and picture processing. The top part of Fig. 28.8 shows the coordinates of the areas that most previous studies have found to be more activated by pseudo-words than real words. The middle row of Fig. 28.8 illustrates activation in these areas as depicted by Mechelli *et al.* (2003), and the bottom row of Fig. 28.8 illustrates the areas activated for real words relative to rest (from Fig. 28.3) to demonstrate that reading pseudo-words only enhances part of the distributed reading system.

With respect to the inconsistencies for real words relative to pseudo-words, the reported effects may reflect false positives due to the low statistical thresholds applied (no correction was made for the number of comparisons being made) or they may be due to confounds from non-lexical aspects of the stimuli (*e.g.*, differences in bigram frequency, visual input, or number of syllables). Alternatively, they may reflect true effects that are inconsistent across subjects (different subjects may use different reading strategies) or subtle effects that are not replicated across studies because of insufficient statistical power. Further experiments are required to pursue these possibilities. Meanwhile, we are reduced to the same conclusion: We have found no areas that are specific for reading.

An alternative, way to segregate different reading routes is to conduct functional imaging studies of patients with contrasting patterns of dyslexia (see Price *et al.*, in press). The results of a study of a surface dyslexic patient are summarised in Fig. 28.9. The patient (JH) had bilateral anterior temporal lobe atrophy that is characteristic of semantic dementia but she was able to

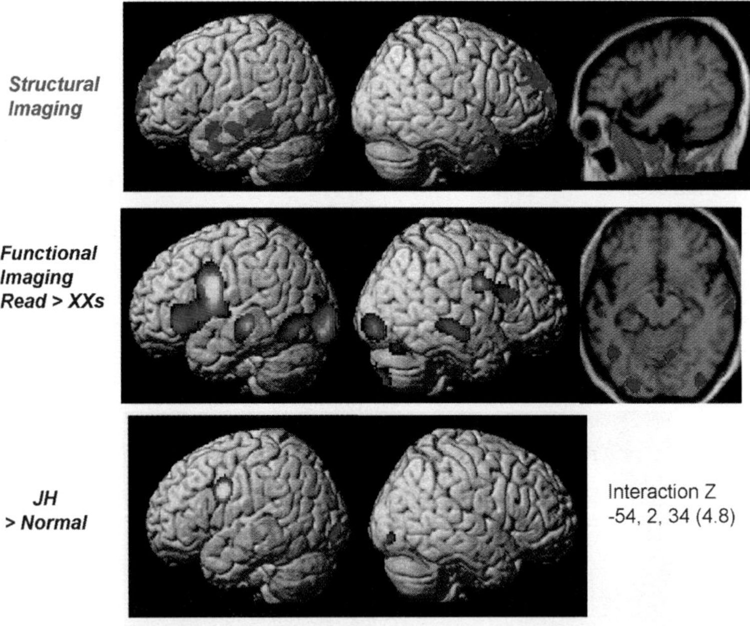

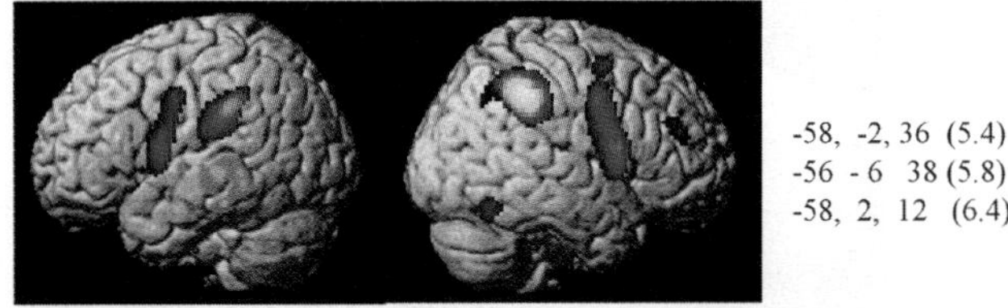

FIGURE 28.9
Phonological reading in a surface dyslexic (data from Price *et al.*, in press.) and phonological processing in normal subjects (data from Mummery *et al.*, 1998).

read high-frequency, three-letter words. Relative to viewing rows of XXXs and deciding if the letters were big or small, reading resulted in a distributed set of areas as reported in normal subjects (see Figs. 28.3 and 28.4). In addition, a left sensorimotor area was more active in JH relative to an age-matched control group. This area is close to the area that Mechelli *et al.* (2003) reported for pseudo-word relative to word reading (see Fig. 28.8), consistent with behavioural data that JH's reading was more reliant than normal on phonology than semantics. Moreover, in normal subjects, the left sensorimotor area where activation was enhanced in the surface dyslexic is more active for phonological decisions (judging the number of syllables) than semantic decisions (see lower part of Fig. 28.9). A preliminary investigation of surface dyslexia is therefore consistent with the conclusion that reading engages the same system as picture naming, but different components of the system can be modulated by word type and task.

A RECONSIDERATION OF THE NEUROLOGICAL MODEL OF READING

Taken together, the functional neuroimaging results are highly consistent with the neurological model illustrated in Fig. 28.1. The critical differences are that word form processing engages the left mid-fusiform gyrus, but there is no detectable activation in the left angular gyrus when the instructions are to pronounce written words, either aloud or silently. This is not to say that the left angular gyrus is not involved in reading. Fig. 28.10 demonstrates activation in the left angular gyrus when subjects are instructed to focus on the meaning of words rather than their

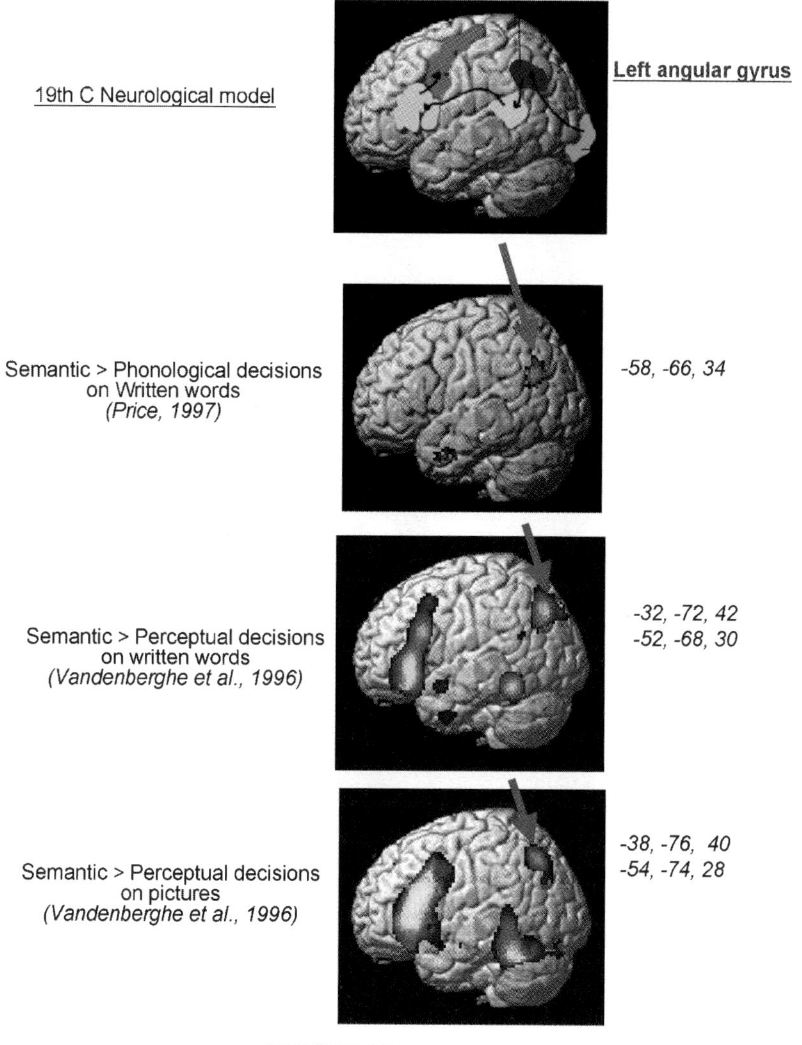

FIGURE 28.10
Role of the left angular gyrus.

sounds. The same area is also activated for semantic judgments on pictures of objects; therefore, it is not the case that the left angular gyrus is specific for the meaning of written words.

Figure 28.11 summarises the results of the studies reported in this chapter. The neural system for reading has been divided into four components: (1) the occipito-temporal areas that are activated for reading relative to rest; (2) the left mid-fusiform area that is activated for reading relative to false fonts; (3) the semantic retrieval areas as illustrated in Fig. 28.10; and (4) posterior superior temporal, insulae, and sensorimotor cortices that are activated by all speech production tasks, including saying "OK" repeatedly to meaningless stimuli (see Chapter 26). In cognitive terms, this model is most similar to the triangular model of reading (see Fig. 28.2); however, it contrasts to the dual route model of reading previously advocated (Price, 2000). This change of opinion results from a deeper appreciation of the system for picture naming. In Price (2000), I claimed that activation in the left posterior superior temporal area was not involved in picture naming, which proceeded via direct routes from the left posterior inferior temporal cortex to the left anterior insula. This was based on the assumption that the superior temporal activation seen when picture naming has been contrasted to low-level baselines (Bookheimer *et al.*, 1995; Murtha *et al.*, 1999) was a consequence of auditory processing of the spoken response. Consideration of new data that has segregated the components of picture naming system (see Fig. 26.3 in Chapter 26) and the distinction between two posterior superior temporal areas involved, respectively, in speech perception and speech production (see Fig. 26.4 in Chapter 26) has convinced me that picture naming also activates the same speech production system as

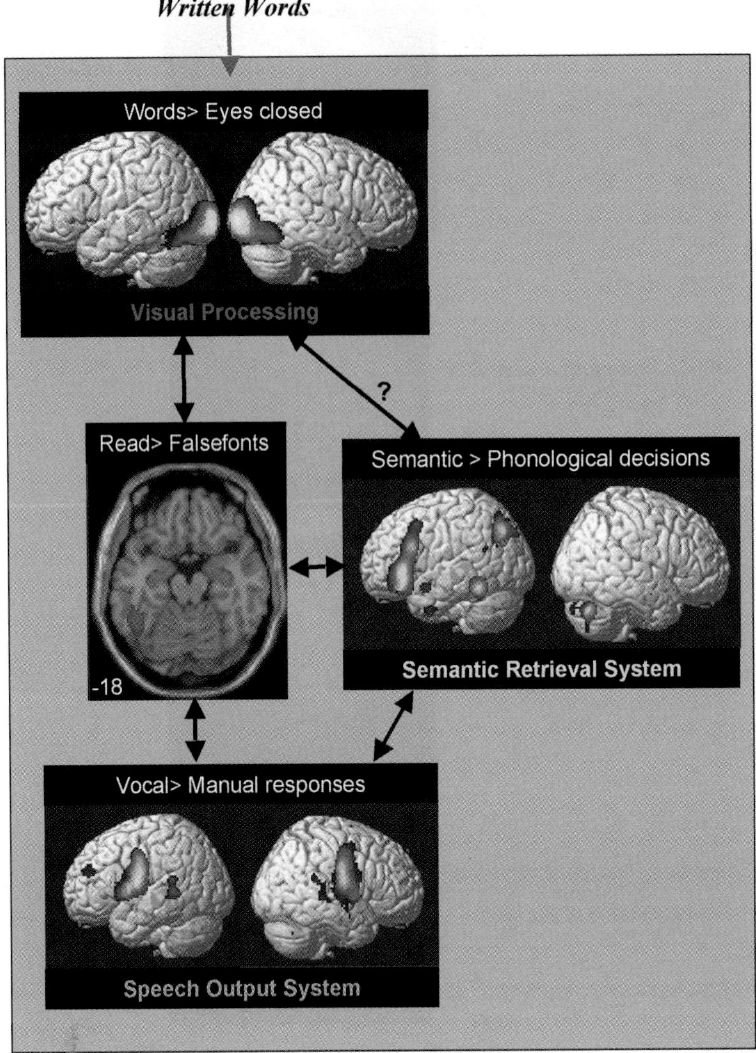

FIGURE 28.11
Proposed anatomical and cognitive model of reading.

reading. Within this system, picture naming elicits more occipito-temporal activation and words elicit more peri-Sylvian activation. Future studies are required to ascertain whether there are other neural systems for reading (for instance, in the right hemisphere).

References

Benson, D. F. and Geshwind, N. (1969). The alexias, in *Handbook of Clinical Neurology*, Vol. 4, Vinken, P. J. and Bruyn, G. W., Eds., pp. 112–140. Elsevier, Amsterdam.

Blank, S. C., Scott, S. K., Murphy, K., Warburton, E., and Wise, R. J. (2002). Speech production: Wernicke, Broca and beyond. *Brain*, **125**(Pt. 8), 1829–1838.

Bookheimer, S. Y., Zeffiro, T. A., Blaxton, T., Gaillard, W., and Theodore, W. (1995). Regional cerebral blood flow during object naming and word reading. *Hum. Brain Mapping*, **3**, 93–106.

Broca, P. (1861). Remarques sur le siège de la faculté du langage articulé; suivies d'une observation d'aphemie. *Bulletin de la Société Anatomique de Paris*, **6**, 330–357.

Brunswick, N., McCrory, E., Price, C. J., Frith, C. D., and Frith, U. (1999). Explicit and implicit processing of words and pseudowords by adult developmental dyslexics: a search for Wernicke's Wortschatz? *Brain*, **122**(Pt. 10), 1901–1917.

Chao, L., Haxby, J. V., and Martin, A. (1999). Attribute-based neural substrates in temporal cortex for perceiving and knowing about objects. *Nat. Neurosci.*, **2**(10), 913–919.

Chao, L., Weisberg, J., and Martin, A. (2002). Experience dependent modulation of category-related cortical activity. *Cereb. Cortex*, **12**, 545–551.

Cohen, L., Dehaene, S., Naccache, L., Lehericy, S., Dehaene-Lambertz, G., Henaff, M., and Michel, F. (2000). The visual word form area: spatial and temporal characterization of an initial stage of reading in normal subjects and posterior split-brain patients. *Brain*, **123**, 291–307.

Cohen, L., Lehericy, S., Chochon, F., Lemer, C., Rivard, S., and Dehaene, S. (2002). Language-specific tuning of visual cortex? Functional properties of the visual word form area. *Brain*, **125**, 1054–1069.

Coltheart, M., Curtis, B., Atkins, P., and Haller, M. (1993). Models of reading aloud: dual-route and parallel-distributed-processing approaches. *Psychol. Rev.*, **100**, 589–608.

Corfield, D. R., Murphy, K., Josephs, O., Fink, G. R., Frackowiak, R. S., Guz, A., Adams, L., and Turner, R. (1999). Cortical and subcortical control of tongue movement in humans: a functional neuroimaging study using fMRI. *J. Appl. Physiol.*, **86**(5), 1468–1477.

Damasio, A. and Damasio, H. (1983). The anatomic basis of pure alexia. *Neurology*, **33**, 1573–1583.

Dehaene, S., Le Clec, H., G., Poline, J. B., Bihan, D. L., and Cohen, L. (2002). The visual word form area: a prelexical representation of visual words in the left fusiform gyrus. *NeuroReport*, **13**(3), 321–325.

Dejerine, J. (1891). Sur un cas de cecite verbale avec agraphie, suivi d'autopsie. *Memoires Societe Biologique*, **3**, 197–201.

Dejerine, J. (1892). Contribution a l'etude anatomoclinique et clinique des differentes varietes de cecite verbal. *C.R. Hebdomadaire des Sceances et Memories de la Societe de Biologie*, **4**, 61–90.

De Renzi, E., Zambolin, A., and Crisi, G. (1987). The pattern of neuropsychological impairment associated with left posterior cerebral artery infarcts. *Brain*, **110**, 1099–1116.

Dronkers, N. F. (1996). A new brain region for coordinating speech articulation. *Nature*, **384**(6605), 159–161.

Fiebach, C. J., Friederici, A. D., Muller, K., and von Cramon, D. Y. (2002). fMRI evidence for dual routes to the mental lexicon in visual word recognition. *J. Cogn. Neurosci.*, **14**(1), 11–23.

Fiez, J. A. and Petersen, S. E. (1998). Neuro-imaging studies of word reading. *Proc. Natl. Acad. Sci. USA*, **95**, 914–921.

Fiez, J. A., Balota, D. A., Raichle, M. E., and Petersen, S. E. (1999). Effects of lexicality, frequency, and spelling-to-sound consistency on the functional anatomy of reading. *Neuron*, **24**(1), 205–218.

Friedman, R. B. and Alexander, M. P. (1984). Pictures, images and pure alexia; a case study. *Cogn. Neuropsychol.*, **1**, 9–23.

Geschwind, N. (1965). Disconnection syndromes in animals and man. *Brain*, **88**, 237–294.

Hagoort, P., Indefrey, P., Brown, C., Herzog, H., Steinmetz, H., and Seitz, R. J. (1999). The neural circuitry involved in the reading of German words and pseudowords: a PET study. *J. Cogn. Neurosci.*, **11**(4), 383–398.

Herbster, A. N., Mintun, M. A., Nebes, R. D., and Becker, J. T. (1997). Regional cerebral blood flow during word and nonword reading. *Hum. Brain Mapping*, **5**(2), 84–92.

Ishai, A., Ungerleider, L. G., Martin, A., Schouten, J. L., and Haxby, J. V. (1999). Distributed representation of objects in the human ventral visual pathway. *Proc. Natl. Acad. Sci. USA*, **96**, 9379–9384.

Kurachi, M., Yamaguchi, N., Inasaka, T., and Torii, H. (1979). Recovery from alexia without agraphia: report of an autopsy. *Cortex*, **15**, 297–312.

Lichtheim, L. (1885). On aphasia. *Brain*, **7**, 433–484.

MacLeod, C. M. (1991). Half a century of research on the Stoop effect: an integrative review. *Psychol. Bull.*, **109**, 163–203.

Marshall, J. C. and Newcombe, F. (1973). Patterns of paralexia: a psycholinguistic approach. *J. Psycholinguistic Res.*, **2**, 175–199.

Martin, A. and Chao, L. L. (2001). Semantic memory and the brain: structure and processes. *Curr. Opin. Neurobiol.*, **11**, 194–201.

Mechelli, A., Gorno-Tempini, M. L., and Price, C. J. (2003). Neuroimaging studies of word and pseudoword reading: consistencies, inconsistencies, and limitations. *J. Cogn. Neurosci.*, **15**, 260–271.

Moore, C. J. and Price, C. J. (1999). Three distinct ventral occipitotemporal regions for reading and object naming. *NeuroImage*, **10**(2), 181–192.

Mummery, C. J., Patterson, K., Hodges, J. R., and Price, C. J. (1998). Functional neuroanatomy of the semantic system: divisible by what? *J. Cogn. Neurosci.*, **10**(6), 766–777.

Murtha, S., Chertkow, H., Beauregard, M., and Evans, A. (1999). The neural substrate of picture naming. *J. Cogn. Neurosci.*, **11**(4), 399–423.

Noppeney, U. and Price, C. J. The neural areas that control the retreival and selection of semantics, submitted.

Noppeney, U. and Price, C. J. (2002). A PET study of stimulus and task-induced semantic processing. *NeuroImage*, **15**(4), 927–935.

Noppeney, U. and Price, C. J. (2003). *Brain and Language*, **84**, 120–133.

Patterson, K. and Shewell, C. (1987). Speak and spell: dissociations and word class effects, in *The Cognitive Neuropsychology of Language*, Coltheart, M., Sartori, G., and Job, R., Eds., pp. 273–294. Lawrence Erlbaum, London.

Petersen, S. E., Fox, P. T., Posner, M. I., Mintun, M., and Raichle, M. E. (1988). Positron emission tomographic studies of the cortical anatomy of single-word processing. *Nature*, **331**(6157), 585–589.

Petersen, S. E., Fox, P. T., Posner, M. I., Mintun, M., and Raichle, M. E. (1989). Positron emission tomographic studies of the processing of single words. *J. Cogn. Neurosci.*, **1**(2), 153–170.

Petersen, S. E., Fox, P. T., Snyder, A. Z., and Raichle, M. E. (1990). Activation of extrastriate and frontal cortical areas by visual words and word-like stimuli. *Science*, **249**(4972), 1041–1044.

Phillips, J. A., Humphreys, G. W., Noppeney, U., and Price, C. J. (2002). The neural substrates of action retrieval: an examination of semantic and visual routes to action. *Visual Cogn.*, **9**(4), 662–684.

Price, C. J. (2000). The anatomy of language: contributions from fuctional neuroimaging. *J. Anat.*, **197**, 335–359.

Price, C. J. and Devlin, J. T. (2003). The myth of the visual word form area. *NeuroImage*, **19**, 473–481.

Price, C. J., Devlin, J. T., Noppeney, U., McCrory, E., Mechelli, A., Biggio, N., Phillips, J., Moore, C. J., and Friston, K. J., Reading: An acquired specialization of object naming (in submission).

Price, C. J. and Friston, K. J. (1997). The temporal dynamics of reading: a PET study. *Proc. Roy. Soc. London Ser. B, Biol. Sci.*, **264**, 1785–1791.

Price, C. J., Gorno-Tempini, M.-L., Graham, K. S., Biggio, N., Mechelli, A., Patternson, K., and Noppeney, U. (2003). Normal and pathological reading: Converging data from lesion and imaging studies. *NeuroImage*, in press.

Price, C. J. *et al.* (2003). *Brain and Language*, **86**, 272–286.

Price, C. J., Wise, R. J., Watson, J. D., Patterson, K., Howard, D., and Frackowiak, R. S. (1994). Brain activity during reading: the effects of exposure duration and task. *Brain*, **117**(6), 1255–1269.

Price, C. J., Moore, C. J., and Frackowiak, R. S. J. (1996a). The effect of varying stimulus rate and duration on brain activity during reading. *NeuroImage*, **3**(1), 40–52.

Price, C. J., Moore, C. J., Humphreys, G. W., Frackowiak, R. S. J., and Friston, K. J. (1996b). The neural regions sustaining object recognition and naming. *Proc. Roy. Soc. London Ser. B, Biol. Sci.*, **263**(1376), 1501–1507.

Price, C. J., Wise, R. J. S., and Frackowiak, R. S. J. (1996c). Demonstrating the implicit processing of visually presented words and pseudowords. *Cereb. Cortex*, **6**(1), 62–70.

Price, C. J., Wise, R. J. S., Warburton, E. A., Moore, C. J., Howard, D., Patterson, K., Frackowiak, R. S. J., and Friston, K. J. (1996d). Hearing and saying: the functional neuro-anatomy of auditory word processing. *Brain*, **119**(Pt. 3), 919–931.

Price, C. J. Moore, C. J., Humphreys, G. W., and Wise, R. J. S. (1997) Segregating semantic from phonological processing. *J. Cogn. Neurosci.*, **9**(6), 727–733.

Price, C. J., Winterburn, D., Giraud, A. L., Moore, C. J., and Noppeney, U. (2003). Cortical localisation of the visual and auditory word form areas: a reconsideration of the evidence. *Brain Language*, **86**, 272–286.

Rumsey, J. M., Horwitz, B., Donahue, B. C., Nace, K., Maisog, J. M., and Andreason, P. (1997). Phonological and orthographic components of word recognition: a PET-rCBF study. *Brain*, **120**(5), 739–759.

Seidenberg, M. and McClelland, J. (1989). A distributed, developmental model of word recognition and naming. *Psychol. Rev.*, **96**, 523–568.

Tagamets, M. A., Novick, J. M., Chalmers, M. L., and Friedman, R. B. (2000). A parametric approach to orthographic processing in the brain: an fMRI study. *J. Cogn. Neurosci.*, **12**(2), 281–297.

Talairach, J. and Tournoux, P. (1988). *Co-planar Stereotaxic Atlas of the Human Brain*. Thieme, Stuttgart.

Tarkiainen, A., Helenius, P., Hansen, P.C., Cornelissen, P. L., and Salmelin, R. (1999). Dynamics of letter-string perception in the human occipito-temporal cortex. *Brain*, **122**, 2119–2131.

Thierry *et al.* (2003). *Neuron*, **38**, 499–506.

Turkeltaub, P. E., Eden, G. F., Jones, K. M., and Zeffiro, T. A. (2002). Meta-analysis of the functional neuroanatomy of single-word reading: method and validation. *NeuroImage*, **16**, 765–780.

Vandenberghe, R., Price, C. J., Wise, R., Josephs, O., and Frackowiak, R. S. J. (1996). Functional anatomy of a common semantic system for words and pictures. *Nature*, **383**, 254–256.

Warrington, E. K. and Shallice, T. (1980). Word form dyslexia. *Brain*, **103**, 99–112.

Wernicke, C. (1874). *Der Aphasiche Symptomenkomplex*. Cohen and Weigert, Breslau, Poland.

Wise, R. J., Greene, J., Buchel, C., and Scott, S. K. (1999). Brain regions involved in articulation. *Lancet*, **353**(9158), 1057–1061.

Wise, R. J., Scott, S. K., Blank, S. C., Mummery, C. J., Murphy, K., and Warburton, E. A. (2001). Separate neural subsystems within 'Wernicke's area'. *Brain*, **124**(Pt. 1), 83–95.

Xu, B., Grafman, J., Gaillard, W. D., Ishii, K., Vega-Bermudez, F., Pietrini, P., Reeves-Tyler, P., DiCamillo, P., and Theodore, W. (2001). Conjoint and extended neural networks for the computation of speech codes: the neural basis of selective impairment in reading words and pseudowords. *Cereb. Cortex*, **11**, 267–277.

Zorzi, M., Houghton, G., and Butterworth, B. (1998). Two routes or one in reading aloud: a connectionist dual-process model. *J. Exp. Psychol. Hum. Percept. Perform.*, **24**(4), 1131–1161.

CHAPTER

29

The Neurocognitive Basis of Developmental Dyslexia

INTRODUCTION

Developmental dyslexia is traditionally defined as a specific impairment in learning to read, despite normal intelligence and adequate reading instruction. This rather atheoretical definition has formed the basis of a diverse array of theories regarding the cause of dyslexia spanning psychological, biological, and educational domains; however, there is increasing agreement that the central difficulty in dyslexia relates to deficits in phonological processing—that is, deficits in processing the sounds of language (Pennington *et al.*, 1990; Snowling, 2000). The advent of neuroimaging techniques has provided the means to investigate the neural basis of phonological processing in dyslexia, with the majority of studies reporting reduced activation of the left temporo-parietal cortex. In addition, these techniques have facilitated the investigation of other putative deficits in dyslexia, in both visual and auditory processing. The evidence for neuro-functional impairments in each of these domains are reviewed in turn. The first section reviews early (1991–1996) functional imaging approaches to the study of developmental dyslexia; the next section considers, in detail, the results of more recent studies of reading and the phonological impairment in dyslexia; the third and fourth sections discuss studies of visual and auditory processing, respectively; and the last section summarises the caveats in the interpretation of abnormal activation and future directions for further studies.

THE EARLY STUDIES

In the context of well-documented behavioural evidence for a persistent impairment in phonological processing in dyslexia, imaging studies have aimed to identify the neural system underlying such a deficit. The first studies to evaluate phonological processing were undertaken early in the development of positron emission tomography (PET). In a PET study of glucose metabolism, Gross-Glenn *et al.* (1991) employed a task of serial reading of single words. Decreases in the normal asymmetries of frontal and occipital regions in the dyslexic group were reported: The control group showed greater leftward asymmetry in the lingual gyrus, but more rightward asymmetry in frontal regions. A separate study, also employing PET with glucose uptake as the dependent measure, reported significantly higher regional cerebral blood flow (rCBF) by dyslexic subjects in bilateral medial temporal lobes during a task of auditory syllable discrimination (Hagman *et al.*, 1992). Unfortunately these early studies were characterised by the absence of baseline conditions and limitations of statistical power necessary to reliably identify population differences.

Two other studies at this time implicated the left temporo-parietal region (Flowers *et al.*, 1991; Rumsey *et al.*, 1992). Flowers *et al.* (1991) carried out a xenon inhalation study of rCBF during an orthographic task, where subjects were required to identify correctly spelled words of four letters presented orally. Childhood reading impairment was related to excessive blood flow in a posterior temporo-parietal region. In the study by Rumsey *et al.* (1992)—the first to use PET and ^{15}O-labeled water in dyslexics—subjects listened to paired presentations of one-, two-, and three-syllable words. Their task was to make a button press response if the pair rhymed. The baseline task required the detection of a low tone among a series of distracters. The dyslexic group performed the task more poorly and showed significantly less activation in two left temporo-parietal regions activated by rhyme detection in controls. Limitations of spatial resolution did not allow Talairach coordinates to be reported, but the areas were believed to fall within left middle temporal and parietal regions that encompassed the angular gyrus. The authors explicitly argue for "a link between angular gyrus activity during phonologic processing and dyslexia," a position that they later develop. The region-of-interest method employed by this study somewhat limits the scope of these results. The possibility that differences existed in other areas, outside the chosen regions, cannot be excluded.

Rumsey and colleagues (1994) specifically investigated the role of the right hemisphere in dyslexia using a task of tonal memory using PET. Dyslexic and control subjects, matched on age, gender, handedness, educational level, and performance IQ, listened to paired sequences of tones (three or four notes long). Their task was to press a button if the sequences in a pair was identical. The baseline condition was rest, where subjects were instructed to lie still with their eyes closed. Behaviourally, the dyslexic group was found to be impaired, making significantly more errors. Relative to controls, they also failed to activate three right frontotemporal regions, for which Talairach coordinates were not made available; however, these regions are taken to reflect reduced activation in the right superior temporal gyrus, as well as right middle and inferior frontal gyri. These right hemisphere differences contrast with normal activation of left hemisphere regions and are interpreted in the context of a rapid temporal processing deficit.

Finally, Paulesu and colleagues (1996) contrasted neural activation in five dyslexic and five control participants during a rhyme judgment and a working memory task, with behavioural performance matched across groups. The dyslexic sample exhibited frontal activation (Broca's area) during rhyme judgment and activation of the posterior superior temporal gyrus (Wernicke's area) during a working memory task. The controls activated these areas and the insula during both tasks, leading the authors to suggest that dyslexia is a disconnection syndrome, with the insula playing the role of a bridge between these neighbouring regions; however, differences in insula activation have not been reported elsewhere. This discrepancy may reflect either the low numbers of participants in this study or the unusual inclusion of a working memory component to the scanning task.

Although insula dysfunction has not been replicated by other studies (see next section), it remains possible that a functional or anatomical disconnection exists in the dyslexic reader. That is, while the components of the language system in the dyslexic may be intact, they may be weakly interconnected within the language system as a whole. Horwitz *et al.* (1998) make a similar claim. The popularity of a functional disconnection hypothesis derives partly from the fact that it does not necessarily imply structural damage to a particular region. Instead, functional disruption may result from impaired input or output to a given region. To infer such a functional impairment, it would be important to show that the region in question can activate normally during other tasks, thereby demonstrating the absence of intrinsic damage.

READING AND PHONOLOGICAL PROCESSING

Over the past 20 years, a broad consensus has emerged in the field of dyslexia: that the core deficit is phonological in nature (Vellutino, 1979; Snowling, 2000); that is, impairments in learning to read have to do with oral language rather than visual perception. The phonological deficit refers to the processing or representation of the sound constituents of words and is indexed indirectly by a number of cognitive tasks. For example, tasks of phonological awareness require words to be segmented into smaller units (syllables or phonemes). Studies have shown that dyslexic children (Bowey *et al.*, 1992) and dyslexic adults (Bruck, 1992) are reliably impaired on these tasks.

Over recent years a number of functional imaging studies have specifically investigated phonological processing in dyslexia. Now that a pattern of findings is beginning to emerge across a number of studies, it is becoming increasingly necessary to consider their theoretical significance at the cognitive level. For example, we need to determine which regions, if any, index impaired phonological processing and which reflect compensatory activity. Likewise, we need to be open to the possibility that differences in neural activity may in fact be secondary or downstream of any phonological impairment.

In general, dyslexic participants have been reported to show a pattern of differential activation relative to normal readers that has clustered in three key left hemisphere regions: (1) a set of left frontal regions largely centred on the inferior frontal gyrus, (2) the angular gyrus, and adjacent regions including the supramarginal gyrus and the posterior aspect of the superior temporal gyrus (Wernicke's Area), and (3) the left posterior inferior temporal lobe (BA37), sometimes referred to as the occipito-temporal region. These are schematically represented in Fig. 29.1. The empirical evidence that implicates these regions in dyslexia and the theoretical conclusions that can be drawn regarding their significance will be discussed in turn. First, however, the six major studies that provide the body of evidence for this discussion are reviewed in detail.

Rumsey *et al.* (1997)

This study by Rumsey and colleagues assessed word and non-word reading in 17 dyslexic and 14 control male adults. The data provided by this group were used for correlational analyses in two later papers (Horwitz *et al.*, 1998; Rumsey *et al.*, 1999); these will be discussed following a discussion of the primary study. Rumsey and colleagues (1997) used whole brain analysis to measure rCBF with ^{15}O PET during two pronunciation tasks and two lexical decision tasks. In the first pronunciation task, participants were required to read aloud a series of pseudo-words constructed so that they did not resemble real words (*e.g.*, "chirl" and "phalbap"), while in the second pronunciation task participants were required to read aloud a series of irregular real words (*e.g.*, "choir" and "cocoa"). In the two lexical decision tasks, participants viewed pairs of items on either side of a monitor. In one condition, phonological decisions were made with participants being required to decide which of two pseudo-words sounded like a real word if pronounced correctly (*e.g.*, "bape" or "baik"). In the second condition, orthographic decisions were made with participants being required to choose the correctly spelled word from a real word and a pseudo-word distracter (*e.g.*, "hole" or "hoal"). Responses were made silently by pressing a button held in either the right or left hand. Visual fixation on a cross hair represented the baseline condition. The dyslexic sample all had a history of reading impairment identified in childhood, met DSM-IV criteria for developmental reading disorder, and had at least average intelligence and good spoken language. The control participants were matched on the basis of handedness, age, social class, and IQ.

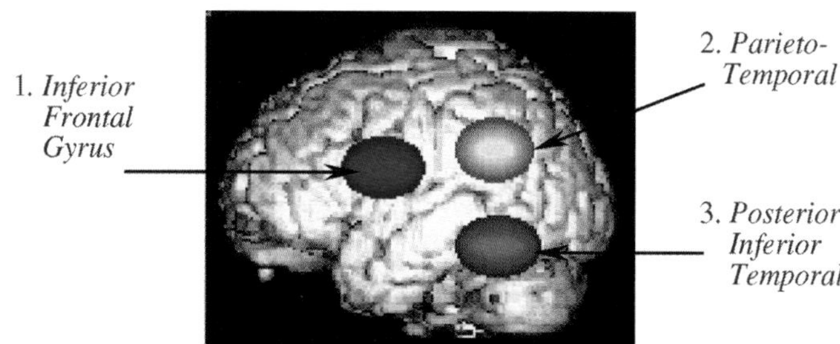

FIGURE 29.1

Three neural systems implicated in reading. (1) Left inferior frontal gyrus; (2) dorsal parieto-temporal region, incorporating the angular and supramarginal gyri and the superior temporal gyrus; and (3) posterior inferior temporal area (BA37), sometimes referred to as the occipito-temporal system and which incorporates fusiform and middle temporal gyri.

The dyslexic readers showed relatively less activation in a range of areas. Across both reading and lexical decision tasks, dyslexic participants showed reduced rCBF in mid- to posterior temporo-parietal cortex, including the angular/supramarginal region, the left superior temporal and middle temporal gyri, and in the left fusiform region. However, essentially normal activation was reported for the same tasks in the left inferior frontal regions. This, the authors suggest, is compatible with the hypothesis of bilateral involvement of posterior temporal and parietal cortices in dyslexia. This observed pattern of activation in the dyslexic participants was the same during both the word and pseudo-word conditions. On this basis, the authors suggest that a common impairment underlies the difficulty experienced by dyslexic participants in both kinds of reading task.

These same data provided the basis for two further papers (Horwitz *et al.*, 1998; Rumsey *et al.*, 1999) in which correlational analyses were reported. In the first, the authors aimed to establish the functional connectivity of the angular gyrus in both groups by evaluating inter-regional correlations of rCBF. A reference voxel was chosen on the basis of several previous studies of normal readers (BA39; [–44, –54, 24]). They report that, during pseudo-word reading, the control group displayed significant positive correlations between left angular gyral activity and several other left hemisphere areas, including inferior temporal gyrus (BA37), occipital gyrus (BA 19), lingual and fusiform gyri (BA18 and 20), superior temporal gyrus (BA 22), and left inferior frontal gyrus (BA 45). Non-significant or weaker correlations were observed when the reference voxel was placed in the right angular gyrus. A comparable but less significant pattern was observed for the exception word condition in the control group. When degree of correlation was statistically compared across groups, dyslexic readers failed to display strong functional relationships with several of these left hemisphere regions, including the inferior frontal cortex and middle and inferior temporal cortex (BA21/37), as well as superior temporal (BA38) and occipitotemporal cortices (BA19). This, it is argued, indicates a functional disconnection of the angular gyrus and these areas.

In a second paper (1999), again using the same set of data from Rumsey *et al.* (1997), the same authors provide further support for the role of the angular gyrus in dyslexia by establishing correlations between blood flow and reading ability as measured outside the scanner. These correlations, while uniformly positive for the control group, were reported to be uniformly negative for the dyslexic group. While greater rCBF in the angular gyrus was associated with better reading in the control group, in the dyslexic group it was associated with worse reading skill. On the basis of these results the authors again suggest a functional lesion in the angular gyrus in dyslexia.

As noted previously, disordered processing in the angular gyrus in these three papers is predicated on one dataset and drawn from one set of dyslexic participants (Rumsey *et al.*, 1997). A consideration of two methodological aspects of the original study leads to a somewhat different interpretation of the findings relating to the angular gyrus. First, the activation differences reported in the dyslexic participants were accompanied by highly significant deficits in task performance. Second, as the tasks were self-paced, the number of items viewed by each participant varied. This was reflected in a difference in the mean reaction times between the dyslexic and control subjects, again across all four tasks.

The consequence of widely differing levels of performance was, as the authors point out, a much more widespread and diffusely distributed spatial extent in the areas of activation and deactivation in the dyslexic sample. They suggest that while differences in spatial extent may be generalised to effects of difficulty level, localised differences appear to be more task related. In practice, however, it is extremely difficult to confidently partition activation differences arising from gross behavioural impairments from those attributable to differences in phonological processing. This is particularly the case given the degree of deficit displayed by the dyslexic sample, which led not only to more errors but also to a much slower rate of stimulus presentation. These factors substantially affect the putative cognitive processes that the measurements of blood flow are taken to reflect (Price *et al.*, 1996a; also see Price and Friston, 1999). The question arises whether a control group of non-dyslexic poor readers, making a comparable number of errors or carrying out the task at a similarly slow pace, would show a pattern of activation similar to that reported for the dyslexic group in this study.

With respect to presentation rate, previous studies of the normal population have shown that differences in rCBF can emerge as a result of different presentation rates in fixed rate designs

(Price *et al.*, 1996a). The self-paced nature of the study reported by Rumsey *et al.* (1997) and the behavioural differences that inevitably arose as a consequence may have contributed to the correlations observed between the rCBF measured in the angular gyrus and reading skill (Rumsey *et al.*, 1999). In order to address this concern, the authors calculated the correlation between rCBF and subject's mean reaction times to determine if there was a general correlation with the rate at which the task proceeded and rCBF. This correlation failed to reach significance for either group, leading the authors to conclude that the relationship between reading skill and rCBF were not an artefact of subject-induced differences in the rate of stimulus presentation; however, the failure to detect a correlation between rCBF and an approximate indication of presentation rate does not eliminate the concern that correlations in the angular gyrus, and reading skill are merely secondary to dyslexia. Mean reaction time represents a gross indication of exposure duration, which is likely to have varied across the course of the experiment. While some subjects may have presented with a consistent level of performance deviating little from a given pace, others may have shown considerable variability, responding sometimes more slowly and at other times quite rapidly. Both kinds of subjects may have had identical mean reaction times, yet this single measure would poorly characterise their very different experiences in the scanner.

Shaywitz *et al.* (1998)

The role of the left angular gyrus has also been given particular emphasis in a functional magnetic resonance imaging (fMRI) study by Shaywitz and colleagues (1998). In an effort to systematically vary the level of phonological processing, they presented a hierarchy of tasks to a group of 29 dyslexic readers and 32 control readers. These tasks were hypothesised to make progressively greater demands on phonological analysis. At the base of the hierarchy was a line orientation judgment task that required only visuospatial processing (*e.g.*, do \\\V and \\\V match?). In the second task, letter case judgment (*e.g.*, do bbBb and bbBb match?), the authors suggest that orthographic but not phonological processing is required because the consonant strings are phonotactically illegal; however, it is likely that some phonological processing was elicited given that the letters are readily nameable and highly familiar. Next, the letter rhyme task (*e.g.*, do T and V rhyme?) necessitated a phonological in addition to an orthographic component. A fourth task requiring a rhyme judgment of non-words increased the phonological component further (*e.g.*, do "lete" and "jete" rhyme?). In addition, the fifth and final task required subjects to decide whether two words (*e.g.*, "corn" and "rice") were in the same semantic category.

Behavioural performance of the dyslexic participants was significantly impaired on each of these tasks except for the initial line judgment task; yet, even for this baseline task, they were tending to make more errors (5.1% vs. 3.0% for the control participants). With regard to the functional imaging data, 17 regions of interest were identified in each hemisphere. Shaywitz *et al.* identified group differences in activation across tasks. Four regions were noted: the superior temporal gyrus (posterior STG, Wernicke's area), the angular gyrus (BA39), striate cortex (BA17), and inferior frontal gyrus (IFG, BA44/45). In addition marginally significant interactions were reported for the inferior lateral extrastriate cortex (ILES) and the anterior inferior frontal gyrus (BA46/47/11).

The posterior areas (Wernicke's area, angular gyrus, striate cortex, and ILES) demonstrated the same pattern of increasing activation across tasks in the control group. That is, an increase in activation going from the letter-case judgment to letter and non-word rhyme tasks. The dyslexic group failed to modulate activation in this way; levels of activation were lower, and the systematic increase across tasks observed in the control group was absent.

These data are taken by the authors to represent evidence of a "...functional disruption in an extensive system in posterior cortex encompassing both traditional visual and traditional language regions..." (Shaywitz *et al.*, 1998, p. 2639). Like Rumsey *et al.* (1992, 1997) particular attention is drawn to the abnormal activation of the angular gyrus within this system, which they state "...is considered pivotal in carrying out those cross-modal integrations necessary for reading" (Shaywitz *et al.*, 1998, p. 2639). The occurrence of neuroanatomic lesions to this region in acquired alexia is noted. Shaywitz *et al.* argue that, even though such a condition involves damage to an already existing system and dyslexia is a disorder that will produce cumulative effects over development, the important point is that disruption of the angular gyrus represents an abnormality within the same neuroanatomic system.

As in the Rumsey *et al.* (1997) study, however, the study by Shaywitz *et al.* was characterised by a confound in task performance across dyslexic and control groups. This was the case even for the case-judgment task which represented the baseline condition. When rCBF differences co-occur with significant impairments in task performance, then it becomes impossible to distinguish the causal relationship between these factors. Once again, the lower level of activation observed in the left angular gyrus in the dyslexic group might simply reflect reduced semantic processing related to their lower levels of accuracy across tasks.

Furthermore, the poorer performance even on the baseline task suggests that the control and dyslexic participants differed not only in reading skill, but also in cognitive abilities beyond those expected by such an impairment. Normal performance by dyslexic participants on tasks of physical matching of letters has been shown in the behavioural literature (Ellis, 1981). It is somewhat unsurprising, therefore, that this dyslexic group was characterised by a significantly lower full-scale IQ (FSIQ, 91) relative to their control group (FSIQ, 115). This discrepancy in overall cognitive ability renders the origin of any differences in task-specific rCBF changes uncertain. Unfortunately, we still have little idea how general cognitive ability influences neural processing in individual cognitive domains such as language.

Brunswick *et al.* (1999)

Brunswick *et al.* (1999) report two PET studies of reading. In the first, six control and six dyslexic participants, matched for age, IQ, and educational level, were asked to read aloud a series of words and non-words. An important consideration in the selection of these stimuli was that they would elicit as few errors as possible from both groups. Consequently, highly familiar short words were used (*e.g.*, "valley," "body," "carrot") in a straightforward reading task. Non-words were generated from these real words by maintaining the onset and coda while changing the internal consonants (*e.g.*, "vassey," "bofy," "cassot"). In addition, the design was a fixed pace to ensure identical presentation rates across all participants.

For the second study, another group of six dyslexic and six control participants, matched on the same criteria as in the first study, were recruited. Here, the authors aimed to reduce the possibility of differences in cognitive strategy (which the dyslexic participants might invoke during explicit reading) by making reading *incidental* to a feature detection task. Participants were required to decide whether an ascender (a letter going above the midline of the word) was present in a word, non-word, or false-font string, depending on the condition. This feature detection task was closely modelled on that of Price *et al.* (1996b), who demonstrated that the presence of words or pseudo-words in the visual field implicitly activates the neural system for reading even when the intention is not to read.

Behavioural performance did not differ between the dyslexic and control groups in either study. In the explicit study, word reading accuracy was comparable across groups; in the non-word reading condition, there was a tendency for the dyslexic participants to make a greater number of errors, although this did not reach significance (p = .06). Reaction times, however were not recorded. In the incidental reading task, in which reaction times were recorded, both speed of response and accuracy of detection did not differ significantly between the dyslexic and control participants.

Across both tasks, the dyslexic participants displayed significantly lower activation in the left inferior and middle temporal lobe (BA37; Talairach coordinates [–42, –60, –12] and [–42, –48, –6]) and in the left frontal operculum (–40, 4, 22). Lower activation was also observed bilaterally in the cerebellum. In the explicit reading condition only (where participants were required to read the words aloud), the dyslexic participants displayed significantly increased activation in a left premotor area 20 mm lateral to the area of reduced activation (BA6/44; [–64, 0, 26]). The authors suggest that the reduced activation in BA37 is consistent with a deficit in retrieving lexical phonology and represents an important locus of disordered phonological processing in dyslexic individuals. With regard to the increased activation observed in the left premotor region of Broca's area, also reported by Shaywitz *et al.* (1998), it is suggested that this increased activation reflects the enforced use of an effortful compensatory strategy involving articulatory routines. No differences were reported for the dyslexic group in the region of the angular gyrus during the explicit or incidental reading tasks.

In this study, therefore, task performance was largely matched across the dyslexic and control groups; however, while no differences in performance accuracy were reported during the explicit reading task, it is possible that control and dyslexic readers exhibited different reaction times during scanning, especially considering that such differences were found during the behavioural assessment battery. Without such reaction time data, it is impossible to discount the possibility that such a difference in performance contributed to the reported activation differences. To address this concern, the authors point out that the activation differences observed in BA37 during the task of incidental reading were independent of performance. Not only was reading not required for this task, but incidental task performance was matched across control and dyslexic groups, for both speed and accuracy of response during the scanning task.

With measures of general cognitive ability matched across groups, the consequence of uncontrolled factors appeared to be fewer with less widespread activation differences relative to previous studies. The absence of differences in the temporo-parietal region suggests that reduced activation here observed previously may have indexed poorer performance accuracy. Reduced activation in the posterior inferior temporal lobe (BA37) remained robust. The significance of differences in this region is discussed later in greater detail.

Paulesu *et al.* (2001)

Paulesu *et al.* (2001) adopted the identical explicit and incidental reading paradigms reported by Brunswick *et al.*(1999) using French and Italian orthographies. They then combined the data from the 12 English dyslexic subjects reported by Brunswick *et al.* (1999) with that obtained from 12 French dyslexics, 12 Italian dyslexics, and their corresponding control groups. Performance of the dyslexics and control subjects was matched within language. This cross linguistic comparison not only significantly increased the number of participants but is unique in identifying those regions that shows common differences in dyslexic readers across several different or thographies. As in Brunswick *et al.* (1999), significantly reduced activation in posterior and inferior temporal areas are reported, with peaks in the inferior, middle, and superior temporal gyri and the middle occipital gyrus. While variations in the degree of behavioural impairment point to differences specific to each orthography, the striking pattern of phonological deficit and of common neural differences, supports the existence of a culturally invariant neurocognitive basis of dyslexia.

Temple *et al.* (2001)

This fMRI study assessed the neural correlates of phonological processing in a group of 24 dyslexic children (8 to 12 years old) relative to a group of 15 control children matched in age and gender. Overall, the dyslexic children presented with a significantly lower FSIQ. In the experimental task, all children were required to judge whether a pair of visually presented letters rhymed, making their response using a hand-held response button. Stimulus pairs were presented in blocks of five and were preceded by the prompt “Rhyme?”. There were two baseline conditions. In the first, participants viewed two letters and pressed a button if the letters matched; in the second, they viewed two lines from a possible set of three (| / \) and pressed a button if they were the same. These were also presented in blocks of five and were preceded by the prompt “Same?”. Analysis of the behavioural performance indicated that the dyslexic children were significantly less accurate and slower in the rhyme letter condition than their peers. During both baseline conditions, where participants had to make visual decisions on letters or lines, dyslexic children were equally accurate but again slower than the control readers.

With regard to the fMRI results, the authors report that when the matching letter condition is used as the baseline for the rhyme letter condition, the normal reading children and the dyslexic children show activation in left hemisphere frontal regions; however, only the control children showed activation in the left temporo-parietal region. Activity in this region was not compared directly across groups; rather, a region-of-interest analysis was carried out on the basis of where the control children displayed significant activation during this contrast. The dyslexic children did not show significant difference in activity between the rhyme condition and the match letters baseline. In view of the fact that the control and dyslexic children were not matched in general ability, it was possible that any differences were due to differences in IQ between the two groups. To address this concern, the authors took subsets of 13 children from each group in order to create IQ-matched groups. A comparison of these groups produced similar results.

Like both Rumsey *et al.* (1997) and Shaywitz *et al.* (1998), Temple *et al.* drew particular attention to the reduced activation observed in the dyslexic children in the left temporo-parietal region centred on the angular gyrus and concluded that the impaired neural responses in this region reflect abnormal phonological processing in the dyslexic children; however, this conclusion is once again predicated on the assumption that differences in neural activation across the groups is not a function of differences in behavioural performance. In this study, the dyslexic children were both significantly slower and significantly less accurate in the rhyme letter condition than their peers. The authors address this concern directly: "Inevitably, the coupling of such behavioural and neural impairment raises the question of whether the altered neural response is the cause or the consequence of the phonological impairment. The discovery in this study that the altered neural response, especially the absence of temporo-parietal activation during phonological performance, *is present in childhood* favours the view that the neural response is causal rather than a compensatory response" (Temple *et al.*, 2001, p. 8; italics added). Unfortunately, this defence is groundless. While the authors accept that differences in behavioural performance might give rise to differences in neural activation, they point out that in their case this is unlikely because they observed such differences in a group of dyslexic *children*. There is every reason to suppose that children, like adults who perform poorly, will present with an altered pattern of neural responses.

A second concern with this study relates to the way in which the region of interest (ROI) was identified. If a region is selected on the basis that it is shown to be strongly activated in one group (here, the control group), then comparison with any other group statistically inflates the chances that increased activation in the first group will be found, thereby increasing the probability of a type I error. If a region is selected on an *a priori* basis, then both groups may or may not show significant activation of that area.

Shaywitz *et al.* (2002)

This recent fMRI study represents by far the most substantial investigation of phonological processing in dyslexic children. Of the 144 children scanned, 70 were dyslexic while 74 did not present with reading impairment. The children ranged in age between 7 and 18 years of age. The experimental tasks, designed to differentially tap the component processes of reading, largely mirrored those employed in their previous study with adults (reviewed above). The same baseline task, a judgment of line orientation, required the children to decide whether two groups of lines were the same (*e.g.*, do \\\V and \\\V match?). The authors chose to focus on two of the language-related tasks: the non-word rhyme task (*e.g.*, do "lete" and "jete" rhyme?) and a category judgment task (*e.g.*, are "corn" and "rice" in the same semantic category?). Word or symbol pairs were presented on a screen, and the participants were required to respond to the task with a button press, pressing one button for "yes" and another for "no."

As in the adult study, behavioural performance of the dyslexic participants was impaired relative to that of the control participants. For the non-word rhyme and the category judgment tasks, dyslexic children scored 59 and 75% correct, respectively, while the control children scored 79 and 91% correct, respectively. These levels of performance are not statistically compared in the paper nor are reaction times given. In addition, as in the adult study, the children constituting the dyslexic group were characterised by a significantly lower FSIQ than their peers. It would be of interest to establish whether this difference was confined to the verbal scales, or whether both verbal and performance scales were depressed.

With regard to the functional imaging data, a number of areas of reduced activation in the left hemisphere were reported in dyslexic readers. For the non-word rhyme task, dyslexic readers displayed significantly less activation in the inferior frontal gyrus, superior temporal sulcus, posterior aspect of the superior and middle temple gyri, and anterior aspect of the middle occipital gyrus. In the category judgment task, differences were confined to the angular gyrus, posterior aspect of the middle temporal gyrus, and anterior aspect of the occipital gyrus. Again, it is difficult to determine the extent to which disparities in the level of behavioural performance influenced these differential patterns of brain activation.

Two further analyses were reported. In the first, a correlation analysis was carried out between individual differences on measures of reading performance obtained outside the scanner and brain activation during the experimental tasks. Positive correlation (increased activation with greater reading skill) was found in the inferior aspect of the left occipitotemporal region (–42, –42, –5) during the non-word rhyme task and the category judgment task, with negative correlations in the right occipitotemporal region. In addition, bilateral parietotemporal activation (incorporating the angular gyrus) was positively correlated with reading ability but only during the category judgment task.

It is of interest that the precise region that correlated with reading ability during both tasks was the same region (–42, –48, –6) reported by Brunswick *et al.* (1999) as showing reduced activation during implicit and explicit reading in adult dyslexics. This suggests that even by childhood activation in the posterior inferior temporal area accurately indexes reading ability and, potentially, phonological processing. In contrast, the activity in the region around the angular gyrus only correlated with reading skill during the category judgment task. It may be of importance that only this task, and not the non-word rhyming task, entailed an explicit semantic component.

In the second analysis, age was correlated with degree of activation during the non-word rhyme and category judgment task. Here, the results were split according to group. On the non-word rhyme task, dyslexic participants showed a positive correlation between age and activation of bilateral inferior frontal gyri, as well as in a number of other areas. This correlation was not observed in controls, who instead showed a negative correlation with age and activation of the superior frontal sulcus and middle frontal gyri regions bilaterally. This pattern differed in the category judgment task, with control children showing a positive correlation between age and activation in the left inferior frontal gyrus and right precentral sulcus and the dyslexic children tending to show a correlation in the right inferior frontal gyrus.

Consistent Findings Across Studies

According to the functional imaging studies described above, the most consistent abnormalities in neural activation for reading developmental dyslexia are in the left posterior inferior temporal cortex (BA37), the left angular gyrus (BA39), and the left inferior frontal cortex. These areas are now discussed in turn. Significantly lower levels of activation in the posterior inferior temporal lobe were observed in dyslexic adults during word and non-word reading (Rumsey *et al.*, 1997; Brunswick *et al.*, 1999; Paulesu *et al.*, 2001) and lexical decision (Rumsey *et al.*, 1997). Shaywitz *et al.* (2002) report that activation in this region correlates significantly with standard measures of reading ability in children assessed prior to scanning. So poor readers, including dyslexics, were found to weakly activate this region relative to good readers when asked to carry out rhyme or category judgements. A magnetoencephalography (MEG) study by Salmelin *et al.* (1996) also provided evidence for disordered processing in the left inferior temporo-occipital region in Finnish dyslexic subjects during silent reading. This region becomes active as early as 180 ms after the presentation of a word and is therefore likely to represent very early stages in visual and/or phonological processing. Even up to 700 ms after stimulus onset, the activation of the left temporal lobe in the dyslexics was significantly less than that for the control subjects.

Converging evidence, therefore, strongly implicates the posterior inferior temporal region in the impaired phonological processing observed in dyslexic children and adults. There is increasing interest in the functional specialisation of this area, with some studies emphasising a role in retrieving phonology from semantics (Price and Friston, 1997; Usui *et al.*, 2003) and others postulating a role as the "visual word form area" (Cohen *et al.*, 2000; Pugh *et al.*, 2002). In view of the fact that dyslexic children, in addition to their reading impairment, are also poor in retrieving picture names (Badian *et al.*, 1990) one might predict reduced activation in BA37 during reading *and* picture naming. This would follow if both reading and naming impairments stem from a common deficit in phonological retrieval.

Evidence implicating the left angular gyrus (BA39) historically came from studies that demonstrated an inability to read (alexia) after left temporo-parietal lesions (Fig. 29.1, Region 1) particularly to the angular gyrus. It was Dejerine's proposal in 1891 that this region was critical for the reading process that marked the beginning of a substantial literature that was also to incorporate evidence implicating the supramarginal gyrus and the posterior area of the superior temporal gyrus. On the basis of this rather distinguished historical lineage, a natural expectation emerged that individuals with a *developmental* impairment in reading (developmental dyslexia) would also show abnormalities in the functioning of the angular gyrus. Several of the neuro-imaging studies discussed in this section have indeed reported a pattern of reduced activation in dyslexic participants in this precise region. The question arises, however, whether this pattern reflects impaired phonological processing or whether it is in fact a *consequence* of impaired phonological processing.

A careful consideration of methodological issues may be particularly relevant to understanding the pattern of reduced activation in the angular gyrus. Specifically, those studies that have reported such a pattern (Rumsey *et al.*, 1992, 1997; Shaywitz *et al.*, 1998; Temple *et al.*, 2001) were characterised by impaired behavioural performance by the dyslexic participants. How might this affect activation of the angular gyrus? Well, one possibility is that poorer performance will naturally lead to reduced semantic processing—words are unlikely to elicit the same level of semantic processing if they have not been successfully decoded. So, the abnormal activation in the angular gyrus, rather than representing the neuroanatomical locus of the dyslexics' phonological impairment, may in fact reflect their poorer reading accuracy. That is, the differences in activation may be secondary to online behavioural effects. Differences in the angular gyrus have not been reported when performance accuracy has been matched with that of the control group (Brunswick *et al.*, 1999; Paulesu *et al.*, 2001).

Such a conclusion would of course follow only if it was the case that the angular gyrus was implicated in semantic processing. A variety of functional imaging studies in the normal population have demonstrated precisely that. For example, this region has been shown to be more active when participants read words relative to reading non-words (Brunswick *et al.*, 1999), read the names of objects and famous people relative to letter strings (Gorno-Tempini *et al.*, 1998), and make semantic decisions on written words (*e.g.*, living or non-living?) relative to phonological decisions (*e.g.*, two syllables or not?) with the same stimuli (Price *et al.*, 1997). Crucially, it is also activated during semantic decisions with non-orthographic stimuli: with pictures (Vandenberghe *et al.*, 1996; Mummery *et al.*, 1998) and words presented orally (Binder *et al.*, 1997). As such, the angular gyrus appears to play a key role in processing semantic information across input modalities and not just in reading. The evidence, therefore, tends to suggest that the observed differences in activation of the angular gyrus may not index the phonological processing deficit in dyslexia, but the secondary impact of that deficit.

Finally, with respect to the left frontal/precentral regions, Shaywitz *et al.* (1998), Brunswick *et al.* (1999), and Temple *et al.* (2001) reported significantly greater activation in the dyslexics relative to the controls with activation increases during non-word rhyming correlating with the age of dyslexia (Shaywitz *et al.*, 2002). However, these effects appear to be task/study specific because increased left frontal activation was not observed during incidental reading when cognitive strategy was controlled (Brunswick *et al.*, 1999); therefore, Brunswick *et al.* (1999) and Shaywitz *et al.* (1998) have suggested that this left frontal activation may reflect an effortful compensatory strategy, involving sublexical assembly of articulatory routines. This would help the individual with dyslexia develop a more accurate representation of a given word sound if the phonological specification by posterior brain areas was inadequate or impaired. Alternatively, this increased activation may represent an excessive output of the developing reading system. For example, if dyslexic individuals were impaired in managing the phonological competition generated in posterior areas, then this would lead to excessive output to the IFG when they read an irregular orthography such as English. The competition between sublexical phonological alternatives, normally resolved by processing in posterior areas, must then be dealt with by this frontal region. The increased activation observed may directly reflect compensatory processes (for example, inhibitory processes) or it may reflect the increased output itself.

VISUAL PROCESSING AND THE MAGNOCELLULAR SYSTEM

The hypothesis that a core deficit in phonological processing characterises individuals with dyslexia is one that has gained much consensus and a great deal of empirical support (for a review, see Snowling and Nation, 1997); nevertheless, a variety of studies have shown additional visual and oculomotor abnormalities in some dyslexic subjects. These visual deficits have generally been interpreted in the context of an impaired transient or magnocellular system. Such a system is associated with high temporal resolution and sensitivity to low contrast and low spatial resolution. Poor contrast sensitivity (Lovegrove, 1993), temporal judgment (Eden *et al.*, 1995), and visual instability (Eden *et al.*, 1994), as well as higher coherence motion-detection thresholds (Cornelissen *et al.*, 1995), have all been taken as evidence of a dysfunction in the magnocellular system in dyslexic readers (Stein and Talcott, 1999). The magnocellular hypothesis, however, rests on a rather fragile empirical basis, and several studies have failed to replicate the findings cited above (see, for example, Walther-Muller, 1995; Johannes *et al.*, 1996). One possibility is that the group differences reported between dyslexics and controls in visual tasks are attributable to a minority of individuals within the dyslexic group who present with a range of sensory deficits (Rosens *et al.*, 2003). In view of the fact that dyslexia is often associated with other developmental disorders, including specific language impairment (SLI) and attention deficit disorder (ADHD), it is possible that those individuals showing sensory deficits are those with an additional disorder (Ramus, 2002). These co-morbid individuals may perform sensory tasks marginally more poorly as a result of strategic rather than perceptual deficits.

Even if some dyslexic individuals display visual processing deficits, it remains unclear whether these can be accounted for by the magnocellular theory. The magnocellular visual pathway is postulated to be most sensitive to stimuli at low spatial frequencies presented at low contrast and low luminance. A weakness in this system would be expected to be observable under those conditions. Yet, dyslexics are typically found to be poorer at all spatial frequencies or in tasks where frequencies are not entirely controlled (Skottun, 2000). Current evidence for an impairment in the magnocellular pathway in dyslexia therefore remains at best equivocal. Two fMRI studies have been carried out in order to investigate the neural basis of the postulated visual processing impairment in dyslexia.

Eden *et al.* (1996)

Eden *et al.* (1996) reported a remarkable failure of a group of six dyslexic volunteers to activate V5/MT while viewing low-contrast moving dots (M-stimulus). Such stimuli have reliably elicited activation of V5/MT in normal subjects (Cheng *et al.*, 1995) and are believed to activate the magnosystem preferentially. In the control task, participants were required to look at a stationary pattern (P-stimulus). A single subject analysis indicated that, while all of the control subjects showed bilateral activation of V5/MT when viewing the moving stimulus, only one dyslexic did so, and then only on the left side. In contrast, presentation of stationary patterns resulted in equivalent activation in both groups, which ruled out any interpretation in terms of a general visual deficit. The dyslexic group were also found to have a subtle impairment in detecting visual motion on a separate behavioural task. The authors interpret their results in the context of the magnocellular hypothesis and a general deficit in processing the temporal properties of stimuli. This, it is suggested, might account for both visual and phonological processing deficits.

Demb *et al.* (1998)

Demb *et al.* (1998) also investigated the magnocellular pathway in dyslexia using fMRI. Behaviourally, the dyslexic participants presented with poorer speed discrimination thresholds. Unlike the results of Eden *et al.* (1996), it was reported that the dyslexic group did activate V5/MT bilaterally when viewing moving versus stationary dot patterns under the low mean luminance conditions that weight the M pathway. However, when the groups were contrasted, the dyslexic responses were found to be significantly lower in MT+ (MT and adjacent motion-sensitive areas) and V1, as well as V2, V3, V3a, and V4v. Under conditions of high mean luminance, no difference emerged between dyslexic and control groups in V1 and these extrastriate areas. Given that low mean luminance emphasises M pathway inputs to cortex, the authors conclude that their results are consistent with a specific M pathway deficit in dyslexia.

In two further analyses, the authors evaluated the correlations between both performance on the psychophysical visual tasks and reading performance. With regard to motion discrimination performance, lower speed discrimination thresholds were correlated with stronger fMRI responses in V1 and MT+. These thresholds, however, were not correlated with brain activity in other cortical areas, including V2, V3, and V4v. With regard to reading performance, individual differences in reading rate were found to correlate with MT+ response ($r = 0.80$; $p < .005$) and more weakly with activity in V1 ($p < 0.05$). These results, therefore, indicate a three-way correlation between V1 and MT+ activity, speed discrimination thresholds, and reading speed. While only a correlation is suggested, the authors argue that it is difficult to imagine that a deficit in the M pathway "...would fail to have consequences for a complex visual behaviour like reading."

Discussion

While a cursory review of the evidence suggests a neuroanatomical basis for an impaired M pathway in dyslexia, closer inspection necessitates a more cautious conclusion. With regard to the finding by Eden *et al.* (1996) that dyslexic individuals failed to activate V5 during the perception of moving dots, it should be noted that neither Demb *et al.* (1998) nor Vanni *et al.* (1997) replicated this result. As indicated earlier, Demb *et al.* (1998) found that dyslexic subjects did show bilateral activation of V5 in a comparable task, albeit weaker than that shown by controls. Similarly Vanni *et al.* (1997) used MEG to measure neural activity in V5 while participants observed transient movement of high-contrast foveal stimuli, similar to that employed by Eden *et al.* (1996). While there was a slight trend for response delays in dyslexics, V5 was normally activated. Further research is needed to determine whether this inconsistency is due to the small number of individuals tested or to differences in the stimuli used. Disordered processing in V5 may occur in only a subset of dyslexic readers and may then only be a subtle effect.

The results of Demb *et al.* (1998) unlike those of Eden *et al.* (1996) paint a more complex picture: the dyslexic group showed lower levels of activation in several areas associated with visual processing (V1, V2, V3, V3a, and V4v), not just in V5 or MT. In the control, high-contrast condition, normal activation was demonstrated in these areas (V2, V3, V3a, and V4v); however, the crucial comparison (responses in MT+ during the high mean luminance control) was not made as a result of methodological limitations. Consequently, any claim of a selective impairment in this region during motion processing *specifically* cannot be substantiated. In general, it appears that the dyslexic group manifested differences across a range of visual processing areas, a finding that is not consistent with a specific impairment of the magnocellular pathway.

Furthermore, an inspection of the sample used by Demb *et al.* (1998) further weakens the conclusion that the magnocellular system is impaired in dyslexia. First, an unusually small number of dyslexic subjects were recruited ($n = 5$). Second, of these five, two were co-diagnosed with ADHD and were normally taking Ritalin. Third, dyslexic and control participants were only assumed to be matched for intelligence (this was not assessed); thus, the observed differences, rather than reflecting a primary cognitive deficit, may simply reflect domain general differences in IQ or differences in attentional processing. These factors are likely to substantially weaken the extent to which the pattern of results shown by these individuals are applicable to a dyslexic population as a whole. While future studies should be able to address these methodological limitations, one particular challenge will be to exclude the possibility that any differences in visual processing merely reflect a dyslexic's reduced exposure to print across development. If it is the case that dyslexic individuals experience significantly less exposure to print and therefore less "training" in the visual demands peculiar to the reading process, then they are likely to show differences in the neural activation of visual processing regions. As such, activation differences of this kind may represent a developmental and secondary consequence of dyslexia.

AUDITORY PROCESSING

It has been shown that some dyslexics perform less well on several auditory tasks that require the perception of brief or rapid speech and non-speech sounds (Tallal *et al.*, 1993). Like the deficit in visual processing, it is suggested that such auditory deficits are secondary to general magnocellular dysfunction; however, the degree to which dyslexic individuals manifest consistent deficits in non-linguistic domains, such as rapid temporal processing (as in visual processing), remains a matter of controversy (Mody *et al.*, 1997). As noted previously, it is likely that only a minority of dyslexic participants are impaired on these sensory tasks (Ramus *et al.*, 2003). The occurrence of other developmental disorders, such as SLI or ADHD, may characterise the impaired individuals (Heath *et al.*, 1999). An alternative hypothesis is that deficits observed on such tasks actually reflect non-sensory components of the task but relate to differences in short-term memory and the efficiency with which dyslexic individuals can employ verbal strategies (Marshall, 2001; McCrory, 2001).

The impetus to postulate a low-level cognitive impairment that attempts to explain the variety of deficits reported in the dyslexic literature is inevitably fraught with difficulty. Habib (2000), for example, argues that a deficit in temporal processing can account for the reported impairments shown by dyslexics on tasks across visual, auditory, and motor domains. The difficulty with such an approach is that we do not know whether any given dyslexic individual displays consistent deficits across these domains, as deficits reported in the literature almost invariably rely on group data. Not only do such all-encompassing theories need to account for why dyslexics appear impaired on a range of tasks, but they must also explain why they perform well on others. For example, recent cross-linguistic research has demonstrated that the severity of impairments in dyslexia interacts significantly with orthography. So, while Italian and English dyslexics present with common patterns of linguistic impairment and neural activation, only English dyslexics are functionally impaired in their everyday lives (Paulesu *et al.*, 2001). There is no suggestion that the temporal processing demands of these two alphabetic orthographies differ. In the same way, such an all-encompassing theory does not explain differential pattern impairments in naming and reading, if in both cases a common phonological representation is accessed (McCrory, 2001).

To date there have been three neuroimaging studies of auditory processing in developmental dyslexia. The first study, Rumsey *et al.* (1994), discussed in the first section, reported reduced right hemisphere activation for dyslexics during a tonal memory task (decide if two sequences are identical). Right hemisphere differences were also the primary finding in a more recent study involving auditory repetition (McCrory *et al.*, 2000), but Temple *et al.* (2001) found reduced activation only in left prefrontal cortex (see below for details).

McCrory *et al.* (2000)

Eight dyslexic subjects matched for age and general ability with a control group were scanned using PET during three conditions: repeating real words, repeating pseudo-words, and at rest. In both groups, speech repetition relative to rest elicited widespread bilateral activation in areas associated with auditory processing of speech, and there were no significant differences between words and pseudo-words. However, irrespective of word type, the dyslexic group was found to show less activation than the control group in the right superior temporal and right post-central gyri and also in the left cerebellum. Notably, the right anterior superior temporal cortex (BA22) was less activated in each of the eight dyslexic subjects, compared to each of the six control subjects. Interestingly, this deficit appeared to be specific to auditory repetition, as it was not detected in a previous study of reading that used the same sets of stimuli (Brunswick *et al.*, 1999); however, activation in this area does decrease when normal participants attend to the phonetic structure of speech. On this basis, it is suggested that the observed lower right hemisphere activation in the dyslexic group indicates compensatory processing; that is, dyslexic individuals engage in less processing of non-phonetic aspects of attended speech so that greater salience may be accorded to its phonological content.

Temple *et al.* (2000)

Temple *et al.* (2000) presented stimuli containing rapid and slow auditory transitions to dyslexic and control participants. The stimuli were non-linguistic in nature but designed to mimic the rapid temporal changes characteristic of speech syllables. Participants were required to perform an incidental task involving a pitch judgment in both conditions, pressing a button if the stimulus was judged to be high pitched. Temple and colleagues reported reduced activation in the dyslexic group relative to the control group in the left prefrontal cortex during the rapid stimuli condition. This region was located in the middle and superior frontal gyri, (BA46/10/9). In addition, the authors report that the left prefrontal response to the rapid stimuli was correlated with rapid auditory processing ability, as measured by auditory psychophysics performed outside the scanner. The authors also described a training program of a subset of these dyslexic participants. It was reported that these participants showed changes in brain responses to rapid stimuli before and after training, and some of these participants showed an improvement in rapid auditory processing and auditory language comprehension tests after training.

Like a number of previous studies, the tasks employed in this study elicited undesirable behavioural confounds. First, the dyslexic group performed worse on the incidental task (pitch discrimination) which is unfortunate because the purpose of this task was to match behavioural performance across the groups while the experimental stimuli are presented. Additionally, both groups were reported to perform this incidental task less accurately with the rapid vs. slow condition, indicating that both dyslexic and control groups found pitch detection more difficult in the rapid condition. So, the rapid and slow conditions differ not only on the factor of interest (speed of transition) but also on task difficulty, making it impossible to safely attribute any within-group differences on this task to acoustic processing as opposed to task difficulty.

Furthermore, the left prefrontal area (–36, 20, 32) reported to show reduced activation in the dyslexic group is in the same vicinity as the area showing reduced activation for dyslexics during phonological tasks ([–40, 14, 24], Rumsey *et al.*, 1997; [–40, 4, 22], Brunswick *et al.*, 1999) even when there was no acoustic input. It is therefore possible that the abnormality during temporal processing of sounds does not reflect the "rapid temporal processing deficit" but differences in a verbally mediated strategy that varied with task difficulty. For example, imagine that the control group employed the verbal strategy of labelling high-pitched stimuli "high" and low-pitched stimuli "low". Given the greater difficulty of the task with the rapid stimuli, then this strategy may have been more heavily employed in this condition. This would led to greater frontal activation (as reported). If the dyslexic subjects were not relying on a verbally mediated strategy, little frontal activation would be observed in the dyslexic group, and little difference would be observed between the rapid and slow conditions. Indeed, a study of rapid temporal processing in the normal population (Belin *et al.*, 1998) using precisely the same stimuli with PET found no differential sensitivity of this prefontal area to rapid non-speech analogues as compared to slow stimuli.

The training study reported by the authors is also characterised by a number of limitations. First, the training study reported involved only three participants. Second, all three participants were dyslexic; that is, no control group was utilised to evaluate whether any changes occurred as a consequence of repeated scanning as opposed to the impact of the training program. Third, only two out of the three subjects showed any difference on retest, precluding any possibility that general conclusions regarding the general dyslexic population might be drawn. Even if these concerns were met, caution should be exercised in inferring "plasticity" on the basis of such training studies. It is possible, or even likely, that participants may develop different strategies with practice. This has nothing to do with plasticity, rather with the fact that changing the nature of the subject's behaviour or experience will have a neural correlate. To call this "brain plasticity" is misleading, as it implies something much more substantial: a neuroanatomical reorganisation.

CONCLUSIONS AND FUTURE DIRECTIONS

It has been demonstrated that dyslexia, as a developmental disorder, presents an array of unique challenges to the neuroimaging researcher. On the one hand, the early emergence of phonological deficits (detectable even in 2 year olds; Scarborough, 1990), and their persistence across the life span (Pennington *et al.*, 1990) allows the neuroimaging researcher to investigate dyslexia in childhood and adulthood. On the other hand, these same developmental factors serve to complicate our understanding of the different patterns of neural activation observed in dyslexic readers.

In all of the studies reviewed in this chapter, there has been a tendency to interpret activation differences as reflections of the primary cognitive deficit in dyslexia. While such an interpretation is clearly attractive (allowing alternative theories to be falsified or supported), it can lead us to ignore a number of less glamorous but potentially more valid interpretations. These alternatives tend to be less appealing because they do not deliver the prized causal mechanisms. They are invaluable, however, in constructing the framework within which these mechanisms operate. An accurate neurocognitive picture of dyslexia can be obtained only when we consider all reasonable interpretations that may underlie our observed group differences. For example, group differences between dyslexic and non-impaired readers may reflect:

1. *Primary cognitive deficits.* In theory, these differences may manifest as significantly increased or decreased activation; in practice, however, cognitive deficits are almost always inferred on the basis of areas of decreased activation.
2. *Secondary consequences of the cognitive deficit.* The broad impact that dyslexia has on life experience (from number of books read to level of self-esteem) will inevitably have neurofunctional correlates. For example, dyslexics may experience reduced exposure to print across their life spans, leading to differences in visual processing. Alternatively, they may reflect differences in online processing; for example, dyslexic individuals may be less able to invoke verbal strategies to perform ostensibly non-verbal tasks (see section on rapid auditory processing above; McCrory, 2001).
3. *Compensatory processing.* This represents a response by the system to compensate for the impact of the cognitive deficit, such processing may either be online (and reflect quantitative differences in normal processing resources) or developmental in nature. This might be understood as a contrast between an increased utilisation of normal processing resources (*e.g.*, an increased reliance on articulatory information; Shaywitz *et al.*, 1998; Brunswick *et al.*, 1999) versus the actual modulation of the functionality of given areas (*e.g.*, the novel recruitment of right hemisphere regions; Shaywitz *et al.*, 2002).
4. *Online behavioural impairment.* A difficulty inherent in assessing language function in dyslexic individuals is that they are generally likely to perform less accurately and more slowly than non-impaired controls. Many studies reviewed in this chapter report dyslexic individuals who show precisely such impaired performance. One cannot ignore the fact that such differences in behavioural response confound the cause of neuronal abnormalities.
5. *Domain general differences.* As with behavioural performance, differences between participants in non-language domains (such as IQ) may significantly interact with neural activation in language areas. Unfortunately, a systematic investigation of how IQ interacts with language function remains an outstanding task for future research. In the meantime, it would seem advisable to pursue a cautionary approach (Rumsey *et al.*, 1997; Brunswick *et al.*, 1999; Temple *et al.*, 2001) by matching groups on IQ and indeed on any factors known to affect behavioural performance.

It is no accident that the majority of activation differences reviewed in this chapter have been taken to reflect primary or causal cognitive deficits. Such an approach gains impetus from the influence of cognitive neuropsychology. Within this framework, a cognitive deficit within a developed language system can be "acquired"—that is, the function of a specific component can be selectively compromised. As Bishop (1997) argues, the "dissociation" logic at the centre of this approach is not well suited to the developmental context. She points out that representations and relationships between components of a *developing* system change over time. As a result, cross-sectional psychological data at a particular point in development (as with neuroimaging data) can provide misleading indicators of the primary deficit. It is critical, therefore, that when activation differences are observed their significance is interpreted within a developmental context.

Toward an Integrated Neurocognitive Account

The consensus in the psychological literature is that a linguistic deficit (currently conceptualised in phonological terms) best explains the pattern of difficulties shown by dyslexic individuals.

The majority of neuroimaging studies to date have reflected this consensus, reporting differences in left posterior language regions in both dyslexic adults and children across different orthographies. Furthermore, these activation differences have been interpreted within a framework of phonological processing (Rumsey *et al.*, 1997; Shaywitz *et al.*, 1998; Brunswick *et al.*, 1999; Paulesu *et al.*, 2001; Temple *et al.*, 2001; Shaywitz *et al.*, 2002).

The need to provide a clear conceptualisation of what is meant by a deficit in phonological processing remains an outstanding task for future research. A common view is that the deficit reflects an impairment in phonological representation. For example, Snowling and Hulme (1989), Hulme and Snowling (1992), McDougall *et al.* (1994), and Swan and Goswami (1997a,b), among others, have suggested that it is the accuracy of the underlying phonological representations of words that is compromised. Similarly, Fowler (1991) has suggested that this poor specification at the representational level reflects a failure of the phonological forms to properly undergo a normal developmental progression from a holistic state to one of segmental organisation. Viewing the phonological deficit in this way follows naturally from a "box-and-arrows" conceptualisation of information processing. Yet, while such an approach can be useful within cognitive psychology, it has limited applicability when trying to account for the dynamic changes in blood flow captured by neuroimaging studies. A phonological representation is not located in a particular brain area; rather, phonological information is likely to reflect computational processes that interact across a number of brain regions.

Viewing the phonological deficit in this way, as an impairment in phonological processes, provides an explanatory model more fitted to contemporary computational modelling and neuroimaging data. One theory is that the phonological representations are in fact fully specified, but the functional access of the phonological code is compromised. In particular dyslexic individuals have difficulty resolving the competition at the phonological level when multiple phonological codes are activated. According to this phonological competition account (McCrory, 2001), dyslexics would experience greater difficulty with more irregular orthographies such as English, whose orthography generates a higher level of ambiguity and elicits the activation of multiple and competing sublexical codes. Likewise, naming pictures at a rapid pace might have little to do with a deficit in "rapid temporal processing" but might relate instead to a longer refractory period at the phonological level for dyslexic readers, so pictures are named normally at a slow pace but inaccurately when the pace of presentation is speeded (Wolff *et al.*, 1990) because dyslexic readers are unable to efficiently quell the competition from preceding items. In this way, representations are not viewed as static entities that are fully specified or not, but as dynamic states of informational representation that are affected by such factors as concurrent competition. On this basis, one would predict that dyslexic individuals would be able to spell or read a given word correctly in one situation but fail to do so in another.

At a neural level, the consistently reported pattern of reduced activation of the left inferior posterior temporal lobe (BA37) in dyslexic individuals may reflect a paucity of phonological inhibitory processes to manage such competition. Alternatively, it may represent a different role for semantic input in differentiating phonological competitors. Such hypotheses are consistent with the observation that skilled readers of English, who must contend with much higher levels of phonological ambiguity, show greater activation of this region during reading than do skilled Italian readers (Paulesu *et al.*, 2000). Viewing the phonological deficit within a dynamic context such as this arguably provides a richer explanatory framework within which activation differences may be interpreted.

Future studies now have the opportunity to investigate such hypotheses within a longitudinal framework. Such an approach is best placed to distinguish the developmental significance of the brain activation differences reported in the adult literature. Likewise, the use of cross-cultural comparisons will allow us to tease apart behavioural and environmental influences for the first time. Combined with improved neuroimaging techniques, these approaches provide a real opportunity to determine how differences in brain function relate to the aetiology of dyslexia at both the biological and cognitive levels.

References

Badian, N. A., McAnulty, G. B., Duffy, F. H., and Als, H. (1990). Prediction of dyslexia in kindergarten boys. *Ann. Dyslexia*, **40**, 152–169.

Belin, P., Zilbovicius, M., Crozier, S., Thivard, L., Fontaine, A., Masure, M. C., and Samson, Y. (1998). Lateralisation of speech and auditory temporal processing. *J. Cogn. Neurosci.*, **10**, 536–540.

Binder, J. R., Frost, J. A., Hammeke, T. A., Cox, R. W., Rao, S. M., and Prieto, T. (1997). Human brain language areas identified by functional magnetic resonance imaging. *J. Cogn. Neurosci.*, **17**, 353–362.

Bishop, D. V. M. (1997). Cognitive Neuropsychology and Developmental Disorders: Uncomfortable Bedfellows. *Quarterly J. Exp. Psychol.*, **50A**(4), 899–923.

Bowey, J. A., Cain, M. T., and Ryan, S. M. (1992). A reading level design of phonological skills underlying fourth grade children's word reading difficulties. *Child Develop.*, **63**, 999–1011.

Bruck, M. (1992). Persistence of dyslexics' phonological awareness deficits. *Develop. Psychol.*, **28**, 874–886.

Brunswick, N., McCrory, E., Price, C., Frith, C. D., and Frith, U. (1999). Explicit and implicit processing of words and pseudowords by adult developmental dyslexics: a search for Wernicke's Wortschatz? *Brain*, **122**, 1901–1917.

Cheng, K., Fujita, H., Kanno, I., Miura, S., and Tanaka, K. (1995). Human cortical fields activated by a wide-field visual motion: an H2 150 study. *J Neurophysiol.*, **74**, 413–427.

Cohen, L., Dehaene, S., Naccache, L., Lehericy, S., Dehaene-Lambertz, G., Henaff, M. A., and Michel, F. (2000). The visual word form area: spatial and temporal characterisation of an initial stage of reading in normal subjects and posterior split-brain patients. *Brain*, **123**, 291–307.

Cornelissen, P. L., Richardson, A., Mason, A., Fowler, S., and Stein, J. (1995). Contrast sensitivity and coherent motion detection measured at phototopic luminance levels in dyslexics and controls. *Vis. Res.*, **35**, 1483–1494.

Déjerine, J. (1891). Sur un cas de cecité verbale avec graphie, suivi d'autopsie. *Compte Rendu des Séances de la Société de Biologie*, **3**, 197–201.

Déjerine, J. (1892). Contribution à l'étude anatomo-pathologique et cliniques des differentes variétés de cécité verbale. *Compte Rendu Hebdomadaire des Séances et Memoires de la Société de Biologie*, **4**, 61–90.

Demb, J. B., Boynton, G. M., and Heeger, D. J. (1998). Functional magnetic resonance imaging of early visual pathways in dyslexia. *J. Neurosci.*, **18**, 6939–6951.

Demb, J. B., Poldrack, R. A., and Gabrieli, J. D. (1999). Functional neuroimaging of word processing in normal and dyslexic readers, in *Converging Methods for Understanding Reading and Dyslexia: Language, Speech, and Communication* Klein, R. M. and McMullen, P. A., Eds., pp. 245–304. MIT Press, Cambridge, MA.

Eden, G. F., Stein, J. F., Wood, H. M., and Wood, F. B. (1994). Differences in eye movements and reading problems in dyslexic and normal children. *Vision Res.*, **34**(10), 1345–1358.

Eden, G. F., Stein, J. F., Wood, M. H., and Wood, F. B. (1995). Verbal and visual problems in reading disability. *J Learning Disabilities*, **28**(5), 272–290.

Eden, G. F., VanMeter, J. W., Rumsey, J. M., Maisog, Woods, R. P., and Zeffiro, T. A. (1996). Abnormal processing of visual motion in dyslexia revealed by functional brain imaging. *Nature*, **382**, 66–69.

Ellis, N. (1981). Visual and name coding in dyslexic children. *Psychol. Res.*, **43**(2), 201–218.

Flowers, D. L., Wood, F. B., and Naylor, C. E. (1991). Regional cerebral blood flow correlates of language processes in reading disabilities. *Arch. Neurol.*, **48**, 637–643.

Fowler, A. (1991). How early phonological development might set the stage for phoneme awareness, in *Phonological Processes in Literacy: A Tribute to I. Y. Liberman*, Brady, S. and Shankweiler, D., Eds., pp. 97–117. Lawrence Erlbaum, Hillsdale, NJ.

Gorno-Tempini, M. L., Price C. J., Josephs O., Vandenberghe R., Cappa S. F., Kapur N., and Frackowiak R. S. (1998). The neural systems sustaining face and proper-name processing. *Brain*, **121**(11), 2103–2118.

Gross-Glenn, K., Duara, R., Loewenstein, D., Chang, J. Y., Yoshii F., Apicella A. M., Pascal, S., Boothe, T., Sevush, S. *et al.*, (1991). Positron emission tomographic studies during serial word reading by normal and dyslexic adults. *J. Clin. Exp. Neuropsychol.*, **13**, 531–544.

Habib, M. (2000). The neurological basis of developmental dyslexia: an overview and working hypothesis [review]. *Brain*, **123**(12), 2373–2399.

Hagman, M. D., Wood, F., Buchsbaum, M. S., Tallal, P., Flowers, L., and Katz, W. (1992). Cerebral brain metabolism in adult dyslexic subjects assessed with positron emission tomography during performance of an auditory task. *Arch. Neurol.*, **49**, 734–739.

Horwitz, B., Rumsey, J. M., and Donohue, B. C. (1998). Functional connectivity of the angular gyrus in normal reading and dyslexia. *Proc. Natl. Acad. Sci. USA*, **95**, 8939–8944.

Hulme, C. and Snowling, M. (1992). Deficits in output phonology: an explanation of reading failure? *Cogn. Neuropsychol.*, **9**, 47–72.

Johannes, S., Kaussmaul, C. L., Munte, R. F., and Mangun, G. R., (1996). Developmental dyslexia: passive visual stimulation provides no evidence for a magnocellular processing defect. *Neuropsychol.*, **34**, 1123–1127.

Lovegrove, W. (1993). Weakness in the transient visual system: a causal factor in dyslexia?, in *Temporal Information Processing in the Nervous System*, Vol. 682, Tallal, P., Galaburda, A., Llinas, R., and von Euler, C., Eds., pp. 57–69. Annals of the New York Academy of Sciences, New York.

Marshall, C. M., Snowling, M. J., and Bailey, P. J. (2001). The Effect of a Verbal-Labelling Strategy on Rapid Auditory Processing: Evidence from Normal and Dyslexic Readers, poster presentation at Essex University Conference: The Sensory Bases of Reading and Language Disorders, May.

McCrory, E. (2001). A Neurocognitive Investigation of Phonological Processing in Developmental Dyslexia, unpublished Ph.D. thesis, London University.

McCrory, E., Frith, U., Brunswick N., and Price, C. (2000). Abnormal functional activation during a simple word repetition task: a PET study of adult dyslexics. *J. Cogn. Neurosci.*, **12**(5),753–762.

McDougall, S., Hulme, C., Ellis, A. W., and Monk, A. (1994). Learning to read: the role of short-term memory and phonological skills. *J. Exp. Child Psychol.*, **58**, 112–123.

Mody, M., Studdert-Kennedy, M., and Brady, S. (1997). Speech perception deficits in poor readers: auditory processing or phonological coding? *J. Exp. Child Psychol.*, **64**, 199–231.

Mummery, C. J., Patterson, K., Hodges, J., and Price, C. J. (1998). Organisation of the semantic system: divisible by what? *J. Cogn. Neurosci.*, **10**, 766–777.

Paulesu, E., Frith, U., Snowling, M., Gallagher, A., Morton, J., Frackowiak, R. S., and Frith, C. D. (1996). Is developmental dyslexia a disconnection syndrome? Evidence from PET scanning. *Brain*, **119**, 143–157.

Paulesu, E., McCrory, E., Fazio, F., Menoncello, L., Brunswick, N., Cappa, S. F., Cotelli, M., Cossu, G., Corte, F., Lorusso, M., Pesenti, S., Gallagher, A., Perani, D., Price, C., Frith, C. D., and Frith, U. (2000). A cultural effect on brain function. *Nat. Neurosci.*, **3**(1), 91–96.

Paulesu, E., Demonet, J. F., Fazio, F., McCrory, E., Chanoine, V., Brunswick, N., Cappa, S. F., Cossu, G., Habib, M., Frith, C. D., and Frith, U. (2001). Dyslexia: cultural diversity and biological unity. *Science*, 291, 2165–2167.

Pennington, B. F., Van-Orden, G. C., Smith, S. D., Green, P. A., and Haith, M. M. (1990). Phonological processing skills and deficits in adult dyslexics. *Child Develop.*, **61**, 1753–1778.

Price, C. J. (1998). The functional anatomy of word comprehension and production. *Trends Cogn. Sci.*, **2**, 281–288.

Price, C. J. (2000). The anatomy of language: contributions from functional neuroimaging. *J. Anat.*, **197**, 335–359.

Price, C. J. and Friston, K. J. (1997). Cognitive conjuctions: a new approach to brain activation experiments. *NeuroImage*, **5**, 261–270.

Price, C. J. and Friston, K. J. (1999). Scanning patients with tasks they can perform. *Hum. Brain Mapping*, **8**, 102–108.

Price, C. J., Moore, C. J., and Frackowiak, R. S. (1996a). The effect of varying stimulus rate and duration on brain activity during reading. *NeuroImage*, **3**, 40–52.

Price, C. J., Wise, R. J., and Frackowiak, R. S. (1996b). Demonstrating the implicit processing of visually presented words and pseudowords. *Cereb. Cortex*, **6**, 62–70.

Price, C. J., Moore, C. J., Humphreys, G. W., and Wise, R. J. S. (1997). Segregating semantic from phonological processing. *J. Cogn. Neurosci.*, **9**, 727–723.

Ramus, F. (2001). Talk of two theories. *Nature*, **412**, 393–395.

Ramus, F., Rosen, S., Dakin, S. C., Day, B. L., Castellote, J. M., White, S., and Frith, U. (2003). Theories of developmental dyslexia: insights from a multiple case study of dyslexic adults. *Brain*, **126**(4), 841–865.

Rumsey, J. M., Andreason, P., Zametkin, A. J., Aquino, T., King, C., Hamburger, S. D., Pikus, A., Rapoport, J. L., and Cohen, R. (1992). Failure to activate the left temporal cortex in dyslexia: an oxygen 15 positron emission tomographic study. *Arch. Neurol.*, **49**, 527–534.

Rumsey, J. M., Andreason, P., Zametkin, A. J., King, A. C., Hamburger, S. D., Aquino, T., Hanahan, A. P., Pikus, A., and Cohen, R. M. (1994). Right frontotemporal activation by tonal memory in dyslexia: an $H_2{}^{15}O$ PET study. *Biol. Psychiatry*, **36**, 171–180.

Rumsey, J. M., Nace, K., Donohue, B., Wise, D., Maisog, M., and Andreason, P. (1997). A positron emission tomographic study of impaired word recognition and phonological processing in dyslexic men. *Arch. Neurol.*, **54**, 562–573.

Rumsey, J. M., Horwitz, B., Donohue, B. C., Nace, K. L., Maisog, J. M., and Andreason, P. (1999). A functional lesion in developmental dyslexia: left angular blood flow predicts severity. *Brain Language*, **70**, 187–204.

Salmelin, R., Service, E., Kiesila, P., Uutela, K., and Salonen, O. (1996). Impaired visual word processing in dyslexia revealed with magnetoencephalography. *Ann. Neurol.*, **40**(2), 157–162.

Scarborough, H. S. (1990). Very early language deficits in dyslexic children. *Child Develop.*, **61**, 1728–1743.

Shaywitz, S. E., Shaywitz, B. A., Pugh, K. R., Fulbright, R. K., Constable, R. T., Menci, W. B., Shankweiler, D. P., Liberman, A. M., Skudlarski, P., Fletcher, J. M., Katz, L., Marchione, K. E., Lacadie, C., Gatenby, C., and Gore, J. C. (1998). Functional disruption in the organisation of the brain for reading in dyslexia. *Proc. Natl. Acad. Sci. USA*, **95**, 2636–2641.

Shaywitz, S. E., Shaywitz, B. A., Pugh, K. R., Mencl, E., Fulbright, R. K., Skudlarski P., Constable, R. T., Marchione, K. E., Fletcher, Lyon G. R., and Gore, J. C. (2002) Disruption of posterior brain systems for reading in children with developmental dyslexia. *Soc. Biol. Psychiatry*, **52**, 101–110.

Skottun, B. (2000). The magnocellular deficit theory of dyslexia: the evidence from contrast sensitivity. *Vision Res.*, **40**, 111–127.

Snowling, M. (2000). *Dyslexia*. Blackwell, Oxford.

Snowling, M. and Hulme, C. (1989). A longitudinal case study of developmental phonological dyslexia. *Cogn. Neuropsychol.*, **6**, 379–403.

Snowling, M. and Nation, K. (1997). Language, phonology and learning to read, in *Dyslexia: Biology, Cognition and Intervention,* Hulme, C. and Snowling, M., Eds., pp. 153–166. Athanaeum Press, Gateshead, Tyne and Wear.

Spring, C. and Davis J. M. (1988). Relations of digit naming speed with three components of reading. *Appl. Psycholing.*, **9**, 315–334.

Stanovich, K. E. (1986). Matthew effects in reading: some consequences of individual differences in the acquisition of literacy. *Reading Res. Q.*, **21**, 360–364.

Stanovich, K. E. (1988). Research Colloquium, presented at Harvard University, Cambridge, MA.

Stanovich, K. E., Freeman, D. J., and Cunningham, A. E. (1983). The development of the relation between letter-naming speed and reading ability. *J. Psychonomic Soc.*, **21**, 199–202.

Stein, J. and Talcott, J. (1999). Impaired neuronal timing in developmental dyslexia: the magnocellular hypothesis. *Dyslexia*, **5**, 59–77.

Swan, D. and Goswami, U. (1997a). Picture naming deficits in developmental dyslexia: the phonological representation hypothesis. *Brain Language*, **56**, 334–353.

Swan, D. and Goswami, U. (1997b). Phonological awareness deficits in developmental dyslexia and the phonological representations hypothesis. *J. Exp. Child Psychol.*, **66**, 18–41.

Tallal, P., Miller, S., and Fitch, R. H. (1993). Neurobiological basis of speech: a case for the preeminence of temporal processing, in *Temporal Information Processing in the Nervous System*, Vol. 682, Tallal, P., Galaburda, A. M., Llinas, R. R., and von Euler, C., Eds., pp. 27–47. Annals of the New York Academy of Sciences, New York.

Temple, E., Poldrack, R. A., Protopapas, A., Nagarajan, S., Salz, T., Tallal, P., Merzenich, M. M., and Gabrieli, J. D. (2000). Disruption of the neural response to rapid acoustic stimuli in dyslexia: evidence from functional MRI. *Proc. Natl. Acad. Sci.*, **97**(25), 13907–13912.

Temple, E., Poldrack, R. A., Salidis, J., Deutsch, G. K., Tallal, P., Merzenich, M. M., and Gabrieli, J. D. (2001). Disrupted neural responses to phonological and orthographic processing in dyslexic children: an fMRI study. *NeuroReport*, **12**(2), 299–307.

Usui, K., Ikeda, A., Takayama, M., Matsuhashi, M., Yamamoto, J.-I., Satoh, T., Begum, T. *et al.* (2003) Conversion of semantic information into phonological representation: a function in left posterior basal temporal area. *Brain*, **126**, 632–641.

Vandenberghe, R., Price, C. J., Wise, R., Josephs, O., and Frackowiak R. S. J. (1996). Semantic system(s) for words and pictures: functional anatomy. *Nature*, **383**, 254–256.

Vanni, S., Uusitalo, M. A., Kiesila, P., and Hari, R. (1997). Visual motion activates V5 in dyslexics. *Neuroreport*, **8**(8), 1939–1943.

Walther-Muller, P. U. (1995). Is there a deficit of early vision in dyslexia? *Perception*, **24**, 919–936.

Wolff, P. H., Michel, G. F., and Ovrut, M. (1990). Rate variables and automatised naming in developmental dyslexia. *Brain Language*, **39**, 556–575.

CHAPTER

30

Detecting Language Activations with Functional Magnetic Resonance Imaging

INTRODUCTION

This chapter discusses a number of factors that affect sensitivity to language activations in functional magnetic resonance imaging (fMRI) measuring blood-oxygenation-level-dependent (BOLD) contrast. Here, sensitivity is referred to as the ability to detect experimentally induced activations, which is a function of (1) the size of the effect of interest, and (2) the efficiency of the design with which the haemodynamic responses are estimated. These, in turn depend on a number of issues related to data acquisition and analysis. The first requirement for detecting activations reliably throughout the brain is unbiased sampling of the haemodynamic response, which is considered in the first section. Once unbiased sampling is achieved, the ability to detect activations will depend on experimental design parameters such as stimulus rate, stimulus duration, stimulus size, epoch length, and stimulus ordering. These can affect sensitivity through BOLD saturation, neurophysiological, and efficiency-mediated effects, as discussed in the second section. The reasons why these effects may vary with imaging modality (*i.e.*, fMRI vs. positron emission tomography) are considered in the third section. Finally, the last section considers the relative sensitivity of event-related and epoch models in the context of blocked-design fMRI, using a single word reading paradigm.

RESPONSE SAMPLING

The first condition required to estimate activations reliably throughout the brain with fMRI is unbiased sampling of the haemodynamic response. FMRI acquires whole brain images by collating data from slices of the brain that have been sampled sequentially over time (rather than simultaneously, as in positron emission tomography). If the temporal relationship between data acquisition and stimulus presentation is fixed, different slices are acquired at fixed peristimulus times throughout the experiment. This may lead to a bias in the estimated activation, which depends on when the evoked BOLD response is sampled relative to the stimulus onset asynchrony (SOA). For instance, in both event-related and blocked-design fMRI, sampling the peak of the evoked haemodynamic response will lead to an overestimate of activation, whereas sampling any initial dip, the undershoot, or the troughs will lead to biased underestimates (see upper panels of Fig. 30.1). Biased sampling of peristimulus time was not originally considered to be a problem in blocked-design fMRI because of the implicit assumption that steady-state dynamics are attained within each block; however, when the SOA is relatively long, the evoked

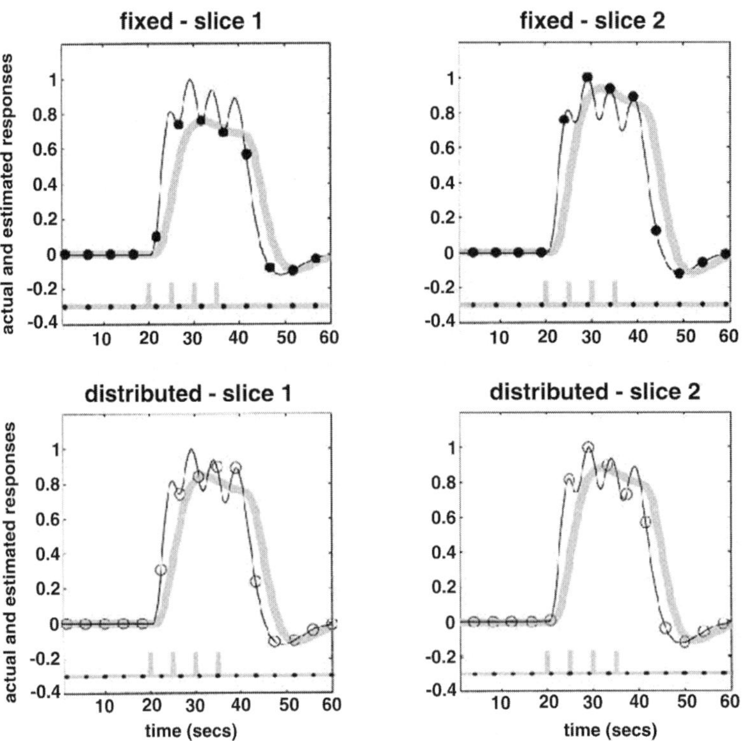

FIGURE 30.1
Differences between fixed (upper panels) and distributed (lower panels) sampling when a stimulus onset asynchrony (SOA) of 4 s is used in the context of blocked-design fMRI. In this simulation, the actual haemodynamic response (thin black line) is obtained by convolving an underlying stick function, which represents the stimulus onsets, with a synthetic haemodynamic response function. The thick grey line represents the estimated haemodynamic response. Upper panels: When acquisition and stimulus presentation are fixed, the estimated average activation is higher for slice 2 than slice 1 even though the actual haemodynamic response is the same. The bias is due to sampling the data slightly later in slice 2 than in slice 1 in each scan. Lower panels: When the sampling is distributed over the SOA, a less biased estimate is obtained. (From Price, C. J. *et al.*, *NeuroImage*, 10, 36–45, 1999. With permission.)

BOLD response may not conform to steady-state dynamics even in the context of blocked-design fMRI. It may also be the case that some language responses do not evoke a steady state because they are more transient or dynamically complex over peristimulus time than sensory or motor responses; however, in both event-related and blocked-design fMRI, an unbiased estimate of the response can be ensured by sampling the data in a distributed way over peristimulus time (see lower panels of Fig. 30.1).

Distributed sampling can be achieved in two ways. First, the presentation of the stimuli can be jittered by varying the SOA (Josephs and Henson, 1999; Josephs *et al.*, 1997). For example, the scan repetition time (*i.e.*, the time required to acquire one image) might be 2 s and the SOA might be 2 s ± 150 ms. Alternatively, distributed sampling can be achieved by using a scan repetition time and a SOA that are not integer multiples of each other.

The importance of distributed sampling, even in the context of blocked design fMRI, has been illustrated empirically. Price *et al.* (1999), using a word rhyming paradigm, showed that activation in Wernicke's area was only detected when data acquisition was distributed throughout the peristimulus time. This suggests that a steady-state BOLD signal did not develop even if stimuli were only 3 s apart, an observation that is consistent with the finding that neuronal responses in Wernicke's area express transient temporal profiles (Cannestra *et al.*, 2000). Veltman *et al.* (2002) made direct statistical comparisons between data acquired from one or multiple time points and found that nondistributed sampling led to biased estimates of activations in a number of prefrontal and temporal regions.

It should be noted that the risk of incorrect inference, due to biased estimates of activation, is greater in single-session experiments than in experiments in which independent sessions are pooled from the same subject or from different subjects. This is because variability in acquisition parameters (*e.g.*, different positioning in the scanner) will introduce some variability in the peristimulus time at which data are acquired. The mean response in a pooled analysis will therefore be a less biased estimate of the true response.

To summarise, when the temporal relationship between data acquisition and stimulus presentation is fixed, some slices are less sensitive to activations than others; however, by sampling the data in a distributed way over the SOA, one can ensure that all components of the BOLD signal are detected over scans. In practice, this can be achieved by using an SOA and a scan acquisition time that are not integer multiples of each other or, alternatively, by varying the SOA while keeping the scan acquisition time fixed.

THE EFFECTS OF EXPERIMENTAL DESIGN IN fMRI

Once unbiased sampling of the haemodynamic response is ensured, the sensitivity with which activations are detected will depend on the experimental design. This can be characterised in terms of the design parameters, which may affect the ability to detect significant activations in multiple ways. Below, the impact of design parameters on sensitivity through BOLD saturation effects is considered. Then a distinction is made between two further ways in which design parameters may affect the sensitivity to neuronal activations. These are referred to as neurophysiological and efficiency-mediated effects.

BOLD Saturation Effects

There is good evidence for nonlinearity in the BOLD response measured in fMRI (Miezin *et al.*, 2000; Miller *et al.*, 2001; Friston *et al.*, 1998; Pollmann *et al.*, 1998). This nonlinearity can be thought of as a "saturation" or "refractoriness" effect whereby the response to a run of events is smaller than would be predicted by the summation of responses to each event alone. This saturation is believed to arise in the mapping from cerebral blood flow to BOLD signal (Friston *et al.*, 2000; Huettel and McCarthy, 2000; Rees *et al.*, 1997), although it may also have a neuronal component.

Because the degree of saturation in the evoked BOLD response depends on prior activation history, nonlinearity is clearly a function of the design parameters used. In Mechelli *et al.* (2001), we explored the impact of saturation effects on BOLD responsiveness across a range of different design parameters by performing biophysical simulation studies based on a dynamical model of perfusion changes (Friston *et al.*, 2000). The model was derived by combining the balloon/Windkessel model of nonlinear coupling between regional cerebral blood flow (rCBF) and BOLD signals (Buxton *et al.*, 1998) and a linear model of how regional flow changes with synaptic activity. We were interested in the estimated average rCBF and BOLD responses per stimulus or event rather than the statistical efficiency with which these responses are detected. The results confirmed that the BOLD response to a stimulus is modulated by preceding stimuli to give a BOLD refractoriness (Fig. 30.2a). As a result, the average BOLD response per stimulus or event decreases with increasing epoch length (for as fixed SOA; Fig. 30.2b). Furthermore, the average BOLD response per stimulus or event decreases with a short SOA (for a fixed number of events; Fig. 30.2c). Finally, the BOLD response shows some highly nonlinear behaviour when stimulus amplitude is negative, as represented in Fig. 30.2d. This corresponds to a rectification-like effect (here, *rectification* refers to the selective attenuation of negative signal components) and indicates that fMRI can be asymmetric in its ability to detect deactivations relative to activations. In contrast, as stipulated by the model, the rCBF response per stimulus or event is not modulated by the design parameters used.

It is important to keep in mind that the results above are concerned with the rCBF and BOLD response estimates per stimulus and not with the statistical efficiency with which these responses are estimated. This means that, for example, the choice of a very short epoch length may be ideal in terms of minimising BOLD refractoriness but is not optimal in terms of design flexibility and statistical power (see below).

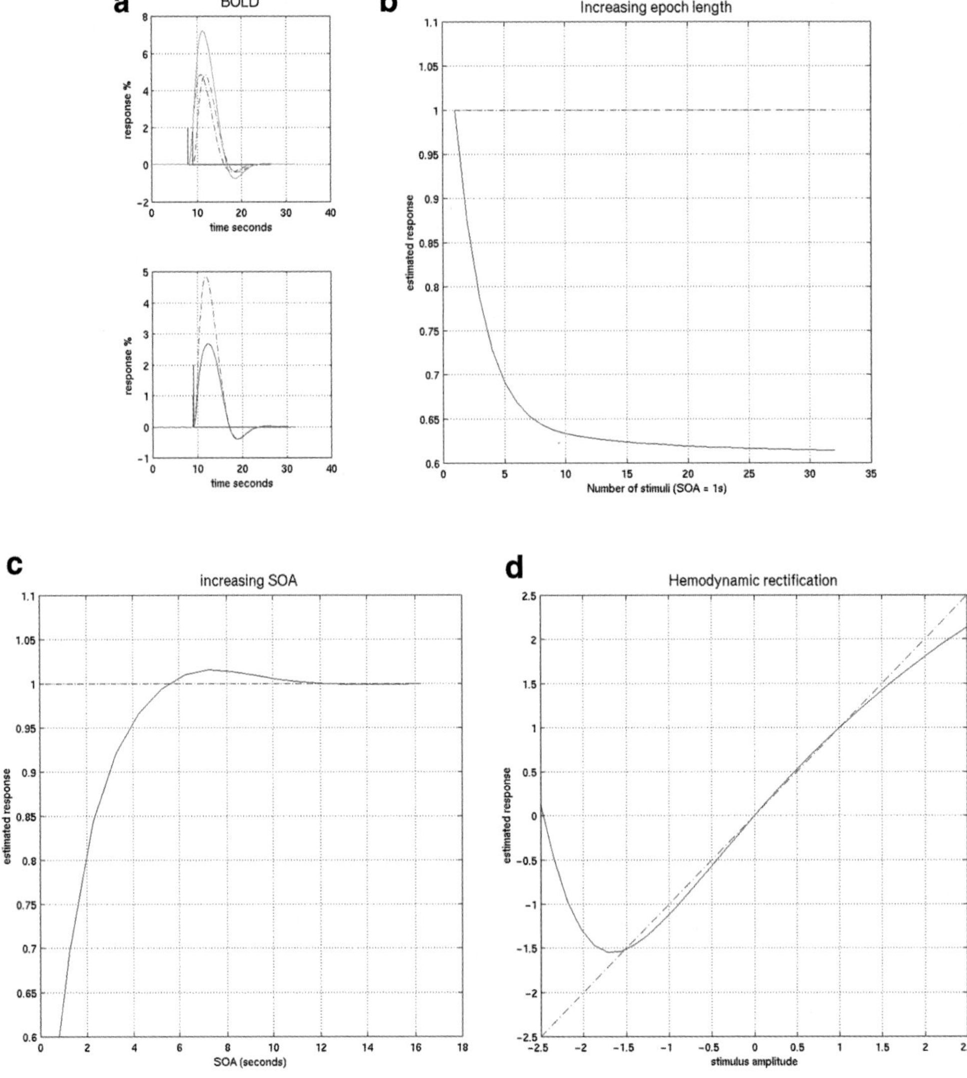

FIGURE 30.2
(a) Upper panel: simulated BOLD responses to a pair of words (bars) 1 s apart, presented together (light blue solid line) and separately (red and green broken lines). Lower panel: simulated BOLD responses to the second word when presented alone (red broken line as above) and when preceded by the first word (green solid line). The latter is obtained by subtracting the response to the first word from the response to both; the difference reflects the effect of the first word on the response to the second. It can be seen that the BOLD response to the second stimulus is markedly attenuated. (b) Effect of epoch length (for a fixed SOA) on simulated rCBF and BOLD responses per stimulus or event. The BOLD estimates (solid line) falls dramatically with increasing epoch length and then levels out at around 10 seconds; on the other hand, the rCBF estimates (broken line) are not affected by the epoch length. (c) Effect of epoch length (for a fixed number of events) on simulated rCBF and BOLD responses per stimulus or event as functions of the SOA. The estimated BOLD response increases dramatically with SOA until it reaches a maximum for an SOA of around 8 s. As the SOA increases further, the estimated BOLD response decreases slightly until it reaches a plateau for an SOA of around 12 s. On the contrary, the estimated rCBF response (broken line) is not modulated by the SOA. (d) Effect of stimulus amplitude on simulated rCBF (dotted line) and BOLD (solid line) responses. The simulated BOLD response increases when stimulus amplitude increases, but when stimulus amplitude decreases below 0 nonlinearities are expressed. On the other hand, the estimated rCBF response is linearly dependent on stimulus amplitude over positive and negative values.

Efficiency-Mediated Effects

Efficiency-mediated or "indirect" effects pertain to the efficiency with which haemodynamic responses are estimated. Efficiency of response estimation is a measure of how reliable the parameter estimates are and depends on the design variance (*i.e.*, it is a function of the contrast tested and the design matrix) and the error variance (the variance in the data not modelled by explanatory variables in the design matrix). The relative efficiency of different experimental designs is expressed as differences in standard error that can have substantial effects on the ensuing statistics. For instance, under the assumption that the error variance is independent of changes in the experimental design, blocked designs are more efficient than randomised designs (Friston *et al.*, 1999). This means that the standard error will be smaller for contrasts testing for activations in blocked than randomised designs. As a result, the T values will be higher in the blocked designs even if the amplitude of the haemodynamic responses and the parameter estimates are identical. In a design that includes both blocked and randomised components, this means it should be possible to show significant effects within the blocked but not the randomised component and yet no interaction between the effects and presentation mode. This was illustrated in Mechelli *et al.* (2003b), in which an event-related study of single word reading was presented which involved acquiring data using an experimental design that embodied both blocked and randomised trials. Significant effects were found in the blocked but not the randomised design in a number of occipital and frontal regions, yet the amplitude of the haemodynamic responses for the two presentation modes was the same. For instance, in the left superior occipital gyrus, the Z-score was 6.2 for blocked presentations but only 3.5 for randomised presentations, yet the parameter estimates for the two presentation models were identical. The disparity in statistical significance was a reflection of, and only of, smaller standard error (and therefore greater design efficiency) for blocked compared to randomised presentation (*i.e.*, 0.27 and 0.50, respectively).

As stated above, efficiency can be factorised into design variance and error variance. It should be noted that the design variance: (1) depends on the contrast and design matrix only, (2) can be computed *a priori*, and (3) is the same across the whole brain. In contrast, the error variance: (1) depends on cognitive/physiological effects (*e.g.*, the haemodynamic responses may be more variable in one context relative to another), (2) can only be estimated by performing a statistical analysis, and (3) is voxel-specific. This means that efficiency-mediated effects (*i.e.*, the relative efficiency for two or more experimental designs) can only be quantified *a priori* by assuming that the error variance is independent of changes in the experimental design. For this assumption to be met, the responses must conform to a linear convolution model that embodies two further assumptions: BOLD nonlinearities can be discounted and the form of the haemodynamic response function is the same for different experimental designs. When these assumptions are violated, differences in error variance may arise, thereby compounding the relative efficiency of the designs. In Mechelli *et al.* (2003b), we investigated whether the relative efficiency of blocked and randomised designs can be predicted under the assumptions adopted generally in the context of *a priori* estimation of efficiency. Differences in the error variance would indicate that both the error variance and the design must be considered when estimating efficiency. Alternatively, if differences in error variance are negligible, the relative efficiency can be predicted from the design alone. The results showed that it may not be correct to assume that the error variance (*i.e.*, the residual variance after evoked changes, modelled by the design matrix, have been discounted) is independent of changes in the experimental design. This makes *a priori* estimation of efficiency-mediated effects problematic, as the error variance must be taken into account but can only be estimated by performing a statistical analysis.

Neurophysiological Effects

Neurophysiological or "direct" effects pertain to the influence that one experimental parameter exerts on neuronal response. These are the effects of interest in most functional neuroimaging experiments, in which the neuronal correlates of sensorimotor and cognitive functions are investigated. As shown originally by a number of PET studies (see, for example, Price *et al.*, 1996, 1997, 1992), the neurophysiological effects of the experimental design parameters differ from region to region. For instance, during single word reading, bilateral occipital and left superior parietal areas activate throughout the time a word is presented, thereby showing a linear increase in activity with stimulus duration; in contrast, right hemisphere temporal and inferior parietal areas show a monotonic decrease in activity with increased duration (Price *et al.*, 1997). Investigating the neurophysiological effects of experimental design parameters not only identifies the optimum design parameters for maximising sensitivity in regions of interest but also enables the segregation of brain regions showing differential responses. In fMRI, examples

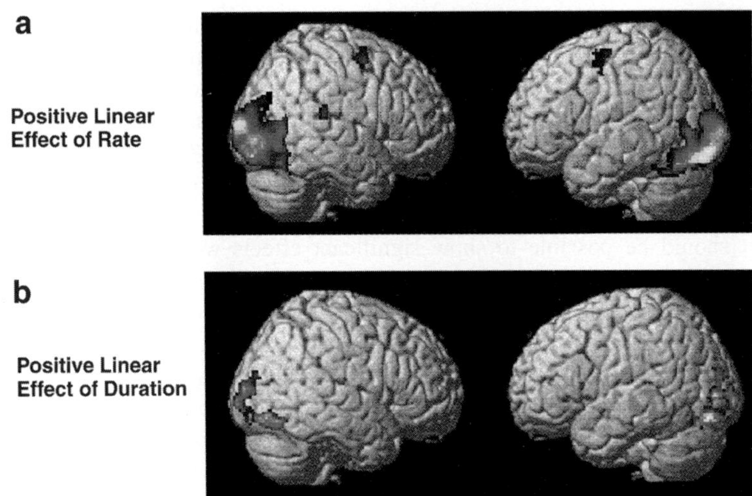

FIGURE 30.3
Examples of neurophysiological effects in the context of single word and pseudo-word reading ($p < 0.05$ corrected for multiple comparisons). (a) Regions showing positive linear effects of stimulus rate (from 20 to 60 words per minute). (Data from Mechelli *et al.*, 2000.) (b) Regions where activity increases with stimulus duration (200, 600, and 1000 ms). (Data from Mechelli *et al.*, 2003a.) Stimuli were presented in blocks of 21 s alternated to fixation, and the data were analysed using an epoch-related statistical model.

of neurophysiological effects of stimulus rate and duration during single word and pseudo-word reading are reported in Mechelli *et al.* (2000) and (2003a), respectively. For instance, positive linear effects of stimulus rate occur in regions associated with visual processing and response generation (Fig. 30.3a). In contrast, positive linear effects of stimulus duration occur in visual areas only (Fig. 30.3b). A question of interest is whether rate and duration effects reflect intrinsic properties of specific brain regions and, as a result, are expressed across a wide range of language tasks. Alternatively, rate and duration effects may be context specific and disappear when different language tasks, such as rhyming and lexical decision, are performed. To address this issue, a number of language tasks could be used that engage the same regions but rely on different cognitive processes.

Relation Between BOLD Saturation, Efficiency-Mediated, and Neurophysiological Effects

As discussed above, experimental design parameters may affect sensitivity in many ways as a consequence of BOLD saturation, efficiency-mediated, and neurophysiological effects. Critically, these effects are not independent but interact as represented in Fig. 30.4. The relationship between neurophysiological, BOLD saturation, and efficiency-mediated effects can be described as follows. First, neurophysiological effects may modulate the degree of saturation in the BOLD signal. This is illustrated in Mechelli *et al.* (2001), in which increased neuronal activation is shown to reduce the BOLD response per stimulus or event even when the rCBF estimates remain constant. Another example is given by haemodynamic rectification as discussed before. Here, BOLD saturation effects are proportional to the degree of neuronal deactivation (see Fig. 30.2d).

Second, neurophysiological effects may contribute to the error variance (*i.e.*, the residual variance after evoked changes modelled by the design matrix have been discounted), which in turn influences the efficiency with which parameters are estimated. For instance, neurophysiological effects that conform to the expected response, as modelled by the design matrix, will be associated with minimal error variance, and parameters will be estimated efficiently. In contrast, neurophysiological effects that deviate from the expected response will induce greater error variance, which may compromise design efficiency. An example is given in Mechelli *et al.* (2003b), in which greater error variance for randomised relative to blocked presentations was found in a number of frontal and occipital areas. We suggested that differential error variance

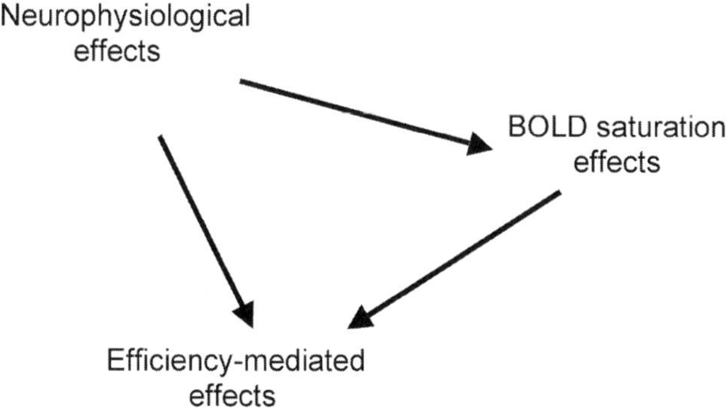

FIGURE 30.4
The relationship between BOLD saturation, neurophysiological, and efficiency-mediated effects. Arrows indicate the direction of the influence, with neurophysiological effects influencing BOLD saturation and efficiency-mediated effects, and BOLD saturation influencing efficiency-mediated effects.

resulted from neurophysiological effects (*i.e.*, differences in the shape and timing of the neuronal response due to different cognitive strategies for the two presentation modes).

Third, BOLD saturation effects may affect the efficiency with which effects are detected by contributing to the error variance. Specifically, the design efficiency will be reduced if strong BOLD nonlinearities occur that are not modelled by the design matrix. In contrast, design efficiency will be preserved if nonlinearities in the BOLD signal are negligible or modelled appropriately.

A critical consequence of these observations is that multiple effects of design parameters should be considered when constructing sensitive experimental designs. In practice, this may not be easy because, for example, the degree of BOLD saturation is likely to vary across different brain regions (Birn *et al.*, 2001; Miezin *et al.*, 2000). Furthermore, as discussed previously, it may be problematic to estimate the relative efficiency of two or more experimental designs prior to statistical analysis. The multiple effects of design parameters should also be considered when assessing functional imaging results. For instance, the contribution of efficiency-mediated effects to the statistics means that one should never compare statistics to make inferences about differential responses (*i.e.*, neurophysiological effects); rather, one should always make a statistical comparison of the data, generally testing for an interaction, in order to identify differential responses that are not confounded by efficiency-mediated effects. However, it may not be possible to assess whether saturation effects observed at the haemodynamic level are due to neurophysiological effects (*e.g.*, neuronal habituation) or BOLD nonlinearities. This is because neurophysiological effects and BOLD saturation can only be segregated by acquiring the BOLD signal in conjunction with more direct measures of neuronal activity, such as event-related potentials. Despite these difficulties, it is important to appreciate the distinction between BOLD saturation, efficiency-mediated, and neurophysiological effects when (1) constructing sensitive designs, and (2) assessing functional imaging results.

THE EFFECTS OF EXPERIMENTAL DESIGN IN PET AND FMRI

In the previous section, the ways in which experimental design parameters may affect sensitivity in fMRI were discussed. In this section, the differential ways that experimental design parameters can affect sensitivity in positron emission tomography (PET) and fMRI are considered. This is an important issue because the replication of results across imaging modalities identifies effects that are more likely to have a face validity (*i.e.*, true neurophysiological effects). The discrepancy between the effects of experimental design parameters in PET and fMRI has already been shown for auditory words. For instance, within the range of 10 to 90 words per minute (wpm), the rCBF in primary auditory cortex is proportional to auditory word presentation rate (Price *et al.*, 1992; Rees *et al.*, 1997), whereas the BOLD signal in the same region shows a saturable effect for high presentation rates (Rees *et al.*, 1997). On the other hand, rCBF in the left posterior superior temporal gyrus (Wernicke's area) increases in response to auditory words irrespective of their presentation rate (Price *et al.*, 1992), whereas the BOLD signal in the same region is proportional to presentation rate (Dhankhar *et al.*, 1997). The discrepancy between the dependence of PET and fMRI signals on stimulus rate may be due to: (1) PET and fMRI measuring different physiological parameters (rCBF and deoxyhemoglobin concentration) that do not share a common stimulus rate dependency, (2) differences in signal acquisition, and (3) differences in the nature of the baseline in PET and fMRI. These are now discussed in turn.

Physiological Parameters Measured in PET and fMRI

Understanding the nature of activity-dependent haemodynamic changes may help interpret the discrepancy between PET and fMRI responses when stimulus rate or other experimental design parameters vary. The presentation of a stimulus involves, in the first instance, neural activity in specific brain regions. This activity elicits (1) electrical signals in nerves to arterioles, and (2) the synthesis of nitric oxide. Nitric oxide is an informational, as opposed to energetic, substance that mediates vasodilatation by rapidly diffusing from the site of neural activity to sites of action in the microvessels (for a review, see Friston, 1995; Iadecola *et al.*, 1993). Both neurogenic and passive diffusion signals ensure muscle relaxation around vessels and mediate the coupling between neural activation and blood flow changes within a few hundred milliseconds. A modest increase in the cerebral metabolic rate of oxygen consumption is accompanied by a much larger increase in local blood flow. Because of this imbalance, the local deoxyhemoglobin concentration decreases during brain activation. The increase in blood flow is the basis for measuring activations with PET, whereas the decrease in local deoxyhemoglobin concentration is the basis for measuring responses with fMRI. When a second stimulus is presented, the coupling between neuronal dynamics and blood flow is believed to be unaffected by the occurrence of the first stimulus. In contrast, the coupling between neuronal activity and the BOLD signal depends on prior stimulation (Huettel and McCarthy, 2000; Rees *et al.*, 1997). Buxton and colleagues (1998) have proposed that the presentation of a stimulus inflates a venous "balloon." When this balloon is inflated, the rate at which diluted deoxyhemoglobin is expelled in response to the underlying neuronal activity is compromised and the BOLD signal is reduced. The response to the second stimulus will therefore be different in PET and fMRI because the physiological parameters they measure (rCBF and deoxyhemoglobin concentration) do not share a common dependency on the underlying neuronal activity. The reduced BOLD responsiveness to a second stimulus, or BOLD refractoriness, may account for the saturable effect of auditory stimulus rate detected in fMRI (Rees *et al.*, 1997) but not in PET (Price *et al.*, 1992; Rees *et al.*, 1997). This dependency of fMRI sensitivity on previous stimulation, and therefore on stimulus rate, makes the choice of the appropriate SOA a crucial factor in designing fMRI experiments.

Data Acquisition in PET and fMRI

If we ignore true differences in rate dependence between PET and fMRI due to nonlinearities inherent in the latter, then PET and fMRI should show the same rate dependence; however, this does not imply that a given dependency will be detected with equal sensitivity by PET and fMRI (*i.e.*, although the regression slopes of signal dependence on rate may be identical, the significance of T values may not be). Differences in sensitivity between PET and fMRI may reflect differences in the acquisition of the two datasets. In PET, haemodynamic responses are measured continuously and summed over a 60- to 90-s scan (an epoch of stimuli) at a given rate. Statistical inferences depend on the mean signal per epoch and the between-epoch variability and are not affected by the distribution of the haemodynamic responses within the epoch. On the other hand, fMRI data are acquired by sampling the haemodynamic response every 2 to 4 seconds. This means that data are sampled 20 to 40 times more often than in PET over the same time. In block designs, the statistical inference is therefore affected by the distribution of the haemodynamic responses within the presentation epoch. In short, fMRI inferences are based on within-epoch error variance, which is used to assess the variability in between-epoch estimates and their significance. In PET, inference is based directly on between-epoch error variance. If the within-epoch error is substantially smaller than between-epoch error, fMRI inferences may be, apparently, much more sensitive. This difference in sensitivity may have contributed to the proportional effect of stimulus rate detected in Wernicke's area using fMRI (Dhankhar *et al.*, 1997) but not in PET (Price *et al.*, 1992) during auditory word processing (but see discussion below).

The Nature of the Baseline in PET and fMRI

Finally, differences between PET and fMRI may be due to differences concerning the behavioural baseline. During PET data acquisition, each scan is clearly separated from the others, the inter-scan interval being 8 min or more. Subjects are therefore aware that stimuli will not occur while the resting scans are acquired. During fMRI data acquisition, however, resting time and stimulus presentation usually alternate without long intervals of rest. While the resting scans are acquired, subjects are therefore aware that stimuli may be presented at any time and their attention or expectation may enhance activity in stimulus processing areas, thereby reducing activation differences in fMRI relative to PET (Veltman *et al.*, 2000). If the experiment varies presentation rate and 0 wpm is included in the statistical regression, then the differential expectation in fMRI and PET baselines may introduce or exaggerate nonlinearities in rate effects in PET relative to fMRI. This is illustrated in a study by Rees *et al.* (1997) (Fig. 30.5).

Baseline differences may explain why, in Wernicke's area, the effect of increasing the rate of auditory word presentation was found to be (1) non-proportional to rCBF in the study by Price *et al.* (1992) when the baseline was rest with no expectation that any stimuli would be presented;

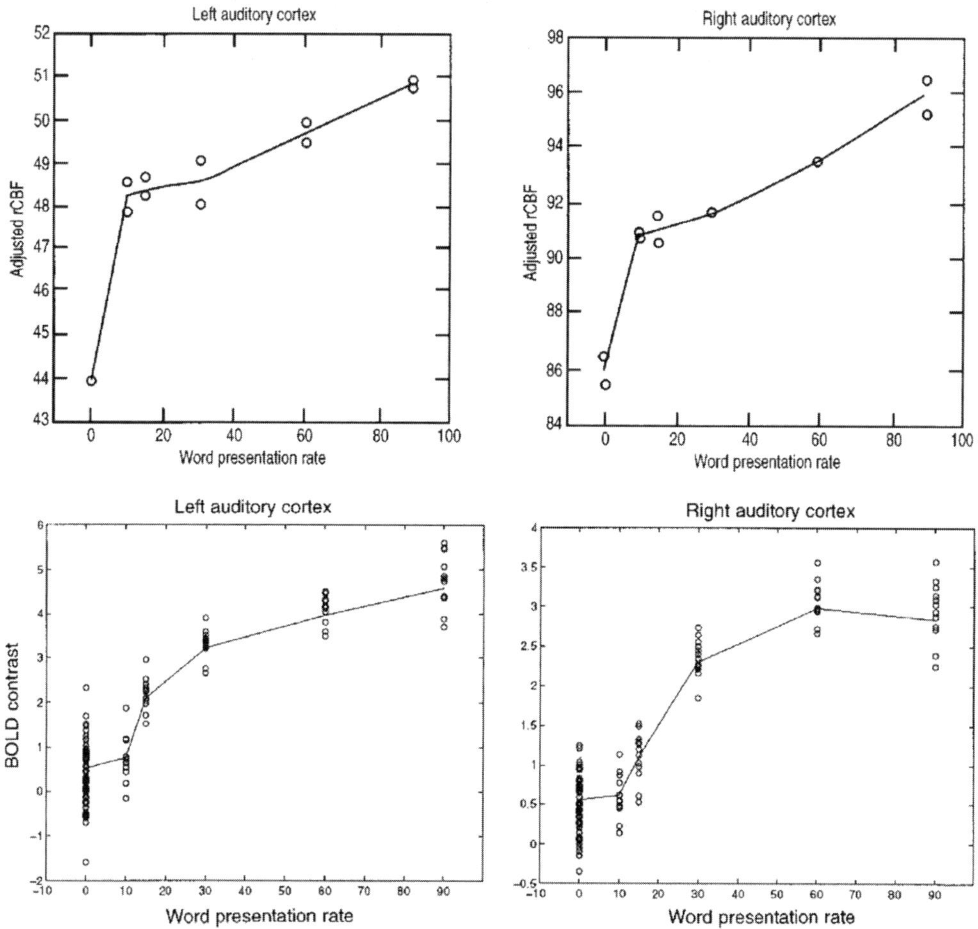

FIGURE 30.5
The effect of stimulus rate on rCBF (upper panels) and BOLD (lower panels) in the left and right auditory cortex during single auditory word processing (as reported by Rees *et al.*, 1997). It can be seen that the difference between PET and fMRI baselines introduced or exaggerated nonlinearities in rate effects in PET relative to fMRI if rest is treated as 0 wpm.

(2) proportional to rCBF in the study by Mummery *et al.* (1999) when subjects expected to hear words in the baseline (although none arrived); and (3) proportional to the BOLD response in the study by Dhankhar *et al.* (1997) when the baseline was rest in fMRI and subjects expected stimuli to be delivered within seconds.

In summary, (1) PET and fMRI measure different physiological parameters which may explain why the effect of stimulus rate in sensory cortex is nonlinear with BOLD and linear with rCBF; (2) different variance component estimations (within-epoch versus between-epoch) may explain why the effect of stimulus rate can be declared significant in BOLD and not in PET; and (3) differences in attentional set between PET and fMRI baselines may account for further discrepancies if rest is entered into the regression parametrically. It should be noted that these factors correspond to BOLD saturation, efficiency-mediated, and neurophysiological effects, as discussed in the previous section.

EPOCH VERSUS EVENT-RELATED ANALYSIS

While the first part of the chapter considered a number of issues related to data acquisition, the last section focuses on data analysis. As mentioned in the first section, a distinction is made in fMRI between event-related designs, in which stimuli of different types are intermixed, and blocked designs, in which stimuli of the same type are presented in blocks. Effects of interest in blocked designs are usually modelled with some form of boxcar regressor convolved with a synthetic haemodynamic response function (HRF). Implicit in this model is the assumption that steady-state synaptic activity and haemodynamics are attained within each block. In contrast, effects of interest in event-related designs are modelled by convolving each trial onset (*i.e.*, a stick function) with a synthetic HRF or temporal basis set. Here, the haemodynamic response to stimulus-induced neuronal transients is modelled without assuming constant within-block activity.

Epoch and Event-Related Models May Provide Differential Sensitivity

This section discusses the use of epoch and event-related analyses of data collected in blocked-design fMRI and notes that the two statistical models may provide differential sensitivity to experimentally induced effects. This is because the two types of models may differ with respect to the temporal shape of the predicted response in two fundamental ways. First, for relatively long SOAs (*e.g.*, 3 s or more), an epoch model will predict steady-state dynamics, whereas an event-related model will predict a periodic and dynamically modulated response, as represented in Fig. 30.6c. If the measured BOLD response to a train of stimuli is transient relative to the SOA, the response to any stimulus will have died away before the presentation of a subsequent stimulus. This will result in a periodic and dynamically modulated response as predicted by the event-related model, which would explain the data better than the epoch model. However, if the measured BOLD response has an unusual (unpredicted) shape, the epoch model is less likely to be out of phase and may explain the data better than the event-related model. It should be noted that the two types of models will differ, as represented in Fig. 30.6c, only when the SOA is long relative to the scan acquisition time.

Second, event-related and epoch models may differ with respect to the onset and offset of the predicted response to a train of stimuli. Fig. 30.6 illustrates differences in onset and offset latencies between epoch (red solid line) and event-related (blue broken line) models, when stimulus onset asynchrony (SOA) is 3 s. It can be seen that, although the two models assume the same amount of integrated synaptic activity, the event-related model expresses higher frequencies than the epoch model (Fig. 30.6a). Once the assumed synaptic activity is convolved with the HRF (Fig. 30.6b), the two models predict differential haemodynamic responses, with the epoch model reaching its peak later and returning to baseline sooner than the event-related model (Fig. 30.6c). This corresponds to differential response onsets and offsets for the event-related and the epoch model. When the epoch model is orthogonalised with respect to the event-related model (Fig. 30.6d), effects that are modelled by the event-related but not by the epoch model are identified. It appears that the event-related model explains changes in activity at the beginning

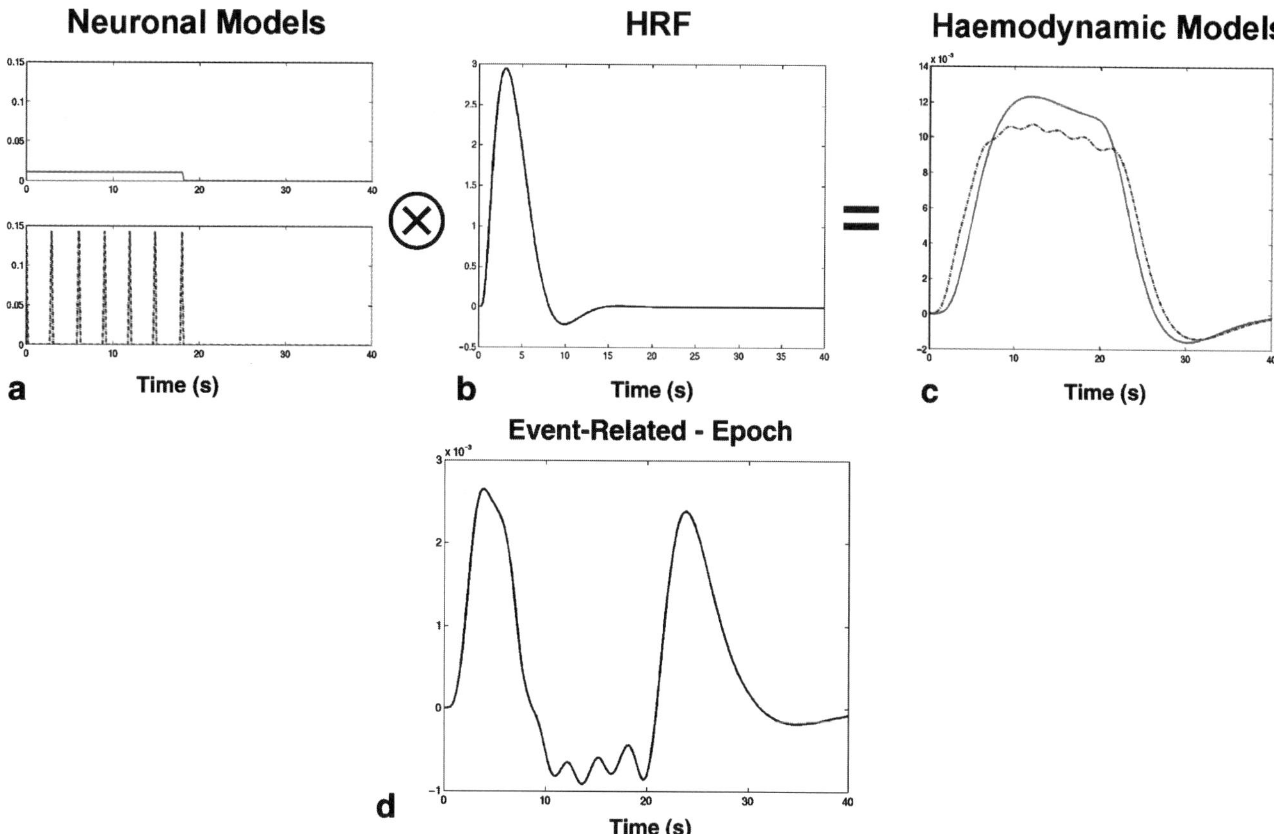

FIGURE 30.6
Difference in onset and offset latencies between epoch (red solid line) and event-related (blue broken line) models when the SOA is 3 seconds. (a) Neuronal models for epoch and event-related models. (b) The neuronal models are convolved with the HRF to predict the haemodynamic responses. (c) Differential haemodynamic responses predicted by the epoch and the event-related model. Although the areas under the curves are the same, the epoch model reaches its peak later and returns to baseline sooner than the event-related model. (d) When the epoch model is orthogonalised with respect to the event-related model, effects that are modelled by the event-related but not by the epoch model are identified. It can be seen that the event-related model explains changes in activity at the beginning and at the end of the block that are not accounted for by the epoch model.

and at the end of the block that are not accounted for by the epoch model.

In short, although both event-related and blocked models can be used to analyse data acquired using a blocked design paradigm, the two types of models may differ because: (1) the epoch model always predicts steady-state dynamics whereas an event-related model may predict a periodic and dynamically modulated response; and (2) the event-related model may reach its peak earlier and return to baseline later than the epoch model. It should be noted that the differences between event-related and epoch models are a function of stimulus rate. These differences would disappear in the limit of very fast presentation rates because the epoch and event-related regressors would be the same.

A critical question is which model one should use to best explain the data, thereby maximising the sensitivity with which statistical inferences are drawn. Mechelli *et al.* (2003c) explored the impact on sensitivity of differences in response onsets and offsets between event-related and epoch models. We presented data from a blocked-design fMRI study of single word reading alternated with fixation. Conventionally, such a design would be analysed using an epoch analysis with box-car regressors; however, a mixed model was used in which trials were modelled as both single events and epochs. This allowed us to estimate the variance in the BOLD signal that was explained by either the event-related or epoch regressors having discounted the effect of the other. The results showed that, in a number of critical language regions, the event-related model explained changes in activity for reading relative to fixation that were not accounted for by the epoch model (Fig. 30.7). In addition, the authors showed that the advantage of the event-related over epoch model was engendered by its early onset rather than its late

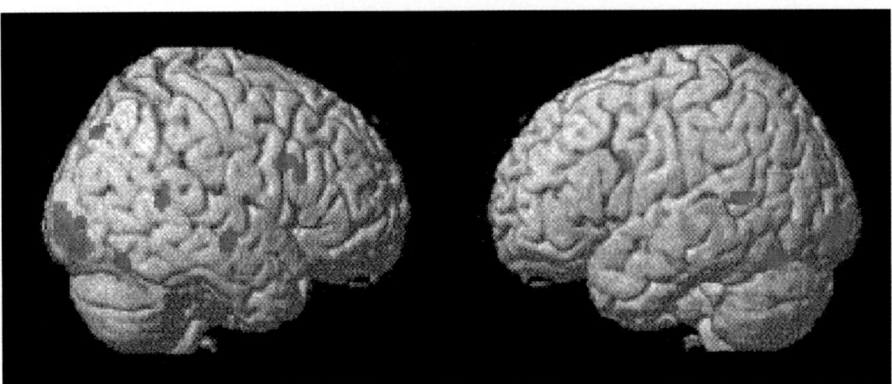

FIGURE 30.7
Regions that showed increased activity for reading relative to fixation that was explained by the event-related but not by the epoch model. These include critical language areas such as left mid-fusiform, posterior superior temporal, and inferior frontal cortex.

offset, relative to the epoch model.

It should be noted, however, that under other circumstances (*i.e.*, different cognitive paradigms), an epoch model may in fact provide greater sensitivity than an event-related model. For instance, neuronal activity may be sustained over time even if stimuli are presented intermittently. This would result in a steady-state haemodynamic response better explained by an epoch model than an event-related model.

Epoch and Event-Related Models May Address Different Effects

The choice between an epoch and an event-related model may also depend on the research hypothesis that motivates the study. It is important to bear in mind that an epoch analysis models the mean activity within each block for each experimental condition. In contrast, the parameters of an event-related model encode the average response per stimulus or event for each experimental condition. This has practical implications when experimental conditions are compared that involve different stimulus rates (*e.g.*, 20 and 60 wpm). Here, an epoch model contrast would compare the mean activity during blocks of 20 wpm to the mean activity during blocks of 60 wpm (as in PET). In contradistinction, an event-related contrast would compare the average response per stimulus for reading 20 wpm to the average response per stimulus for reading 60 wpm. As a result, the epoch model will indicate a significant effect of rate even when the response per stimulus or event is unaffected by rate, whereas the event-related model will not. In contrast, the event-related model will indicate a significant effect of rate if the evoked haemodynamic response per stimulus or event is modulated by presentation rate. Figure 30.8 illustrates the counterintuitive possibility that a positive effect of stimulus rate can be found using an epoch-related model, yet a negative effect of stimulus rate may be detected when an event-related model is applied to the same data. As can be seen, the expected haemodynamic response to a train of stimuli is modulated by stimulus rate in the event-related but not the epoch model. Clearly, here the two analyses address different types of effects, and the most appropriate model depends on the research question that motivates the study.

SUMMARY

In this chapter, some of the main factors that affect sensitivity to experimentally induced activations in fMRI studies have been reviewed. The first part of the chapter has considered a number of issues related to data acquisition. As discussed in the first section, multislice data acquisition may lead to an overestimate or underestimate of activation when only the peak or the undershoot is sampled. However, one can ensure distributed sampling of the haemodynamic responses by either (1) varying the SOA while keeping the scan acquisition time fixed, or (2)

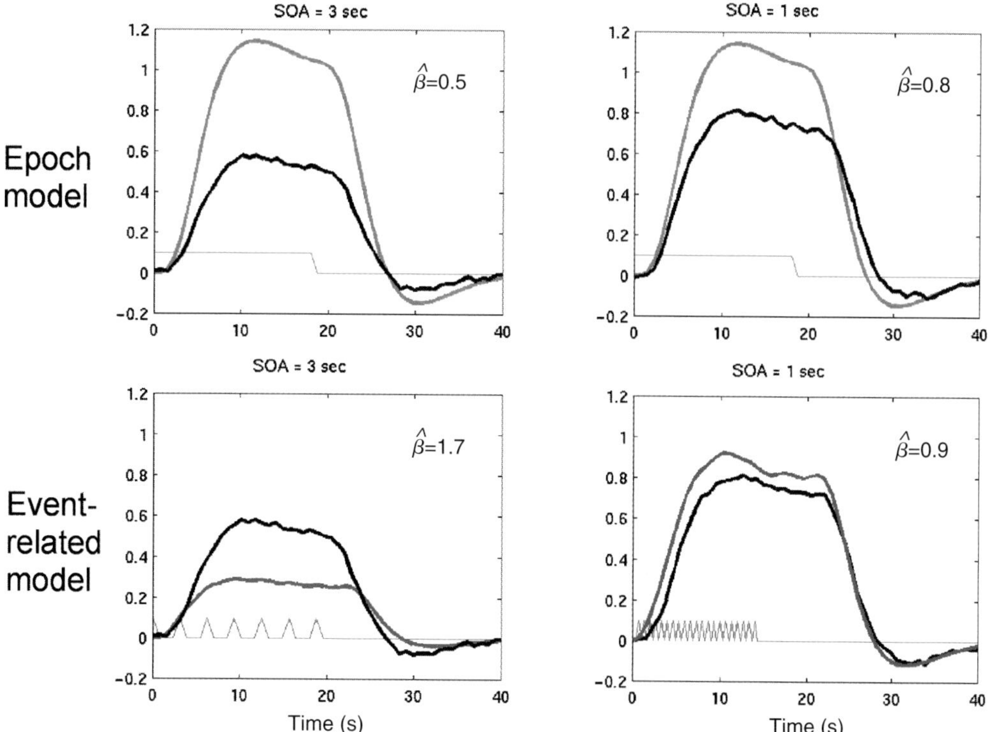

FIGURE 30.8
Simulated haemodynamic response (black line) to a train of stimuli when block length is 21 s and the SOA is either 3 s (left panels) or 1 s (right panels). Parameter estimates ($\hat{\beta}$) were obtained using an epoch model (red lines, upper panels) or an event-related model (blue lines, lower panels). The thin lines represent the underlying epoch and event-related neuronal models. In this simulation, the mean activity within the block increases as the number of stimuli increases or, equivalently, as the SOA decreases. As a result, when the epoch model was used, the parameter estimates increased with stimulus rate (*i.e.*, from 0.5 to 0.8) (upper right); however, the increase in activity is not proportional to the number of stimuli being presented. Hence, the average evoked haemodynamic response per stimulus or event decreases as the number of stimuli increases. This is why, when the event-related model was used, the parameter estimates decreased with stimulus rate (*i.e.*, from 1.7 to 0.9) (lower right).

using a scan repetition time and a SOA that are not integer multiples of each other. Once unbiased sampling of the haemodynamic response is achieved, the sensitivity with which effects are detected will depend on the experimental design. The next section considered the multiple ways in which experimental design parameters may affect the ability to detect language activations. BOLD saturation, neurophysiological, and efficiency-mediated effects should all be considered when constructing sensitive designs and interpreting functional imaging results. The reasons why these effects may vary with imaging modality (*i.e.*, fMRI versus positron emission tomography) were then considered, after which the discussion turned to issues in data analysis and addressed the relative sensitivity of event-related and epoch models in the context of blocked design fMRI. It was shown that an event-related analysis may provide greater sensitivity than an epoch analysis to experimentally induced effects, even in the context of blocked design fMRI. However, when experimental conditions are compared that involve different stimulus rates, the two approaches address different types of effects, and the most appropriate model depends on the research question that motivates the study.

References

Birn, R. M., Saad, Z., and Bandettini, P. A. (2001). Spatial heterogeneity of the nonlinear dynamics in the fMRI BOLD response. *NeuroImage*, **14**, 817–826.

Buxton, R. B., Wong, E. C., and Frank, L. R. (1998). Dynamics of blood flow and oxygenation changes during brain activation: the balloon model. *Magn. Res. Med.*, **39**, 855–864.

Cannestra, A. F., Bookheimer, S. Y., Pouratian, N., O'Farrell, A., Sicotte, N., Martin, N. A., Becker, D., Rubino, G., and Toga, A. W. (2000). Temporal and topographical characterisation of language cortices using intraoperative optical intrinsic signals. *NeuroImage*, **12**, 41–54.

Dhankhar, A., Wexler, B. E., Fulbright, R. K, Halwes, T., Blamire, A. M., and Shulman, R. G. (1997). Functional magnetic resonance imaging assessment of the human brain auditory cortex response to increasing word presentation rates. *J. Neurophysiol.*, **1**, 476–483.

Friston, K. J. (1995). Regulation of rCBF by diffusible signals: an analysis of constrains on diffusion and elimination. *Hum. Brain Mapping*, **3**, 56–65.

Friston, K. J., Josephs, O., Rees, G., and Turner, R. (1998). Nonlinear event-related responses in fMRI. *Magn. Res. Med.*, **39**, 41–52.

Friston, K. J., Zarahn, E., Josephs, O., Henson, R. N. A., and Dale, A. M. (1999). Stochastic designs in event-related fMRI. *NeuroImage*, **10**, 607–619.

Friston, K. J., Mechelli, A., Turner, R., and Price, C. J. (2000). Nonlinear responses in fMRI: the balloon model, Volterra kernels and other hemodynamics. *NeuroImage*, **12**, 466–477.

Huettel, S. A. and McCarthy, G. (2000). Evidence for a refractory period in the hemodynamic response to visual stimuli as measured by MRI. *NeuroImage*, **11**, 547–553.

Iadecola, C., Beitz, A. J., Renno, W., Xu, X., Mayer, B., and Zhang, F. (1993). Nitric oxide synthase-containing neural processes on large cerebral arteries and cerebral microvessels. *Brain Res.*, **606**, 148–155.

Josephs, O. and Henson, R. N. A. (1999). Event-related fMRI: modelling, inference and optimisation. *Philos. Trans. Roy. Soc. London*, **354**, 1215–1228.

Josephs, O., Turner, R., and Friston, K. J. (1997). Event-related fMRI. *Hum. Brain Mapping*, **5**, 243–248.

Mechelli, A., Friston, K. J., and Price, C. J. (2000). The effects of presentation rate during word and pseudoword reading: a comparison of PET and fMRI. *J. Cogn. Neurosci.*, **12**(Suppl. 2),145–156.

Mechelli, A., Price, C. J., and Friston, K. J. (2001). Nonlinear coupling between evoked rCBF and bold signals: a simulation study of hemodynamic responses. *NeuroImage*, **14**, 862–872.

Mechelli, A., Gorno-Tempini, M. L., and Price, C. J. (2003a) Neuroimaging studies of word and pseudoword reading: consistencies, inconsistencies and limitations. *J. Cogn. Neurosci.*, **15**, 260–271.

Mechelli, A., Price, C. J., Henson, R. N. A., and Friston K. J. (2003b). Estimating efficiency *a priori*: a comparison of blocked and randomised designs. *NeuroImage*, **18**, 798–805.

Mechelli, A., Henson, R. N. A., Price, C. J., and Friston, K. J. (2003c). Comparing event-related and epoch analysis in blocked design fMRI. *NeuroImage*, **18**, 806–810.

Miezin, F. M., Maccotta, L., Ollinger, J. M., Petersen, S. E., and Buckner, R. L. (2000). Characterizing the hemodynamic response: effects of presentation rate, sampling procedure, and possibility of ordering brain activity based on relative timing. *NeuroImage*, **11**, 735–759.

Miller, K. L., Luh, W.-M., Liu, T. T., Martinez, A., Obata, T., Wong, E. C., Frank, L. R., and Buxton, R. B. (2001). Nonlinear temporal dynamics of the cerebral blood flow response. *Hum. Brain Mapping*, **13**, 1–12.

Mummery, C. J., Ashburner, J., Scott, S. K., and Wise, R. J. S. (1999). Functional neuroimaging of speech perception in six normal and two aphasic subjects. *J. Acoust. Soc. Am.*, **106**, 449–457.

Pollmann, S., Wiggins, C. J., Norris, D. J., von Cramon, D. Y., and Schubert, T. (1998). Use of short intertrial intervals in single-trial experiments: a 3T fMRI study. *NeuroImage*, **8**, 327–339.

Price, C. J. and Friston, K. J. (1997). The temporal dynamics of reading: a PET study. *Proc. Roy. Soc. London Ser. B*, **264**, 1785–1791.

Price, C. J., Wise, R., Ramsay, S., Friston, K. J., Howard, D., Patterson, K., and Frackowiak, R. S. J. (1992). Regional response differences within the human auditory cortex when listening to words. *Neurosci. Lett.*, **146**, 179–182.

Price, C. J., Moore, C. J., and Frackowiak, R. S. J. (1996). The effect of varying stimulus rate and duration on brain activity during reading. *NeuroImage*, **3**, 40–52.

Price, C. J., Veltman, D., Ashburner, J., Josephs, O., and Friston, K. (1999). The critical relationship between the timing of stimulus presentation and data acquisition in fMRI. *NeuroImage*, **10**, 36–45.

Rees, G., Howseman, A., Josephs, O., Frith, C. D., Friston, K. J., Frackowiak, R. S. J., and Turner, R. (1997). Characterizing the relationship between BOLD contrast and regional cerebral blood flow measurements by varying the stimulus presentation rate. *NeuroImage*, **6**, 270–278.

Veltman, D. J., Friston, K. J., Sanders, G., and Price, C. J. (2000). Regionally specific sensitivity differences in fMRI and PET: where do they come from? *NeuroImage*, **11**, 575–588.

Veltman, D. J., Mechelli, A., Friston, K. J., and Price, C. J. (2002). The importance of distributed sampling in blocked fMRI designs. *NeuroImage*, **17**,1203–1206.

Vazquez, A. L. and Noll, D. C. (1998). Non-linear temporal aspects of the BOLD response in fMRI. *NeuroImage*, **7**, 108–118.

PART TWO

IMAGING NEUROSCIENCE—THEORY AND ANALYSIS

CHAPTER

31

Experimental Design and Statistical Parametric Mapping

INTRODUCTION

This chapter previews the ideas and procedures used in the analysis of brain imaging data. It serves to introduce the main themes covered, in depth, by the following chapters. The material presented in this chapter also provides a sufficient background to understand the principles of experimental design and data analysis referred to by the empirical chapters in the first part of this book. The following chapters on theory and analysis have been partitioned into four sections. The first three sections conform to the key stages of analysing imaging data sequences: computational neuroanatomy, modelling, and inference. These sections focus on identifying, and making inferences about, regionally specific effects in the brain. The final section addresses the integration and interactions among these regions through analyses of functional and effective connectivity.

Characterising a regionally specific effect rests on estimation and inference. Inferences in neuroimaging may be about differences expressed when comparing one group of subjects to another or, within subjects, changes over a sequence of observations. They may pertain to structural differences (e.g., in voxel-based morphometry; Ashburner and Friston, 2000) or neurophysiological indices of brain functions (e.g., fMRI). The principles of data analysis are very similar for all of these applications and constitute the subject of this and subsequent chapters. We will focus on the analysis of fMRI time series because this covers most of the issues that are likely to be encountered in other modalities. Generally, the analysis of structural images and PET scans is simpler because they do not have to deal with correlated errors from one scan to the next.

About This Chapter

A general issue in data analysis is the relationship between the neurobiological hypothesis one posits and the statistical models adopted to test that hypothesis. This chapter begins by reviewing the distinction between functional *specialisation* and *integration* and how these principles serve as the motivation for most analyses of neuroimaging data. We will address the design and analysis of neuroimaging studies from these distinct perspectives but note that they have to be combined for a full understanding of brain mapping results.

Statistical parametric mapping is generally used to identify functionally specialised brain responses and is the most prevalent approach to characterising functional anatomy and disease-related changes. The alternative perspective, namely, that provided by functional integration, requires a different set of (multivariate) approaches that examine the relationship among changes in activity in one brain area versus others. Statistical parametric mapping is a voxel-based approach that employs classical inference to make some comment about regionally specific responses to experimental factors. To assign an observed response to a particular brain structure, or cortical area, the data must conform to a known anatomical space. Before considering statistical modelling, this chapter deals briefly with how a time series of images is realigned and mapped into some standard anatomical space (e.g., a stereotactic space). The general ideas behind statistical parametric mapping are then described and illustrated with attention to the different sorts of inferences that can be made with different experimental designs.

fMRI is special, in the sense that the data lend themselves to a signal processing perspective. This can be exploited to ensure that both the design and analysis are as efficient as possible. Linear time-invariant models provide the bridge between inferential models employed by statistical mapping and conventional signal processing approaches. Temporal autocorrelations in noise processes represent another important issue specific to fMRI, and approaches to maximising efficiency in the context of serially correlated errors will be discussed. Nonlinear models of evoked haemodynamics are considered here because they can be used to indicate when the assumptions behind linear models are violated. fMRI can capture data very fast (in relation to other imaging techniques), affording the opportunity to measure event-related responses. The distinction between event and epoch-related designs will be discussed and considered in relation to efficiency and the constraints provided by nonlinear characterisations.

Before considering multivariate analyses we will close the discussion of inferences about regionally specific effects by looking at the distinction between fixed and random-effect analyses and how this relates to inferences about the subjects studied or the population from which these subjects came. The final section will deal with functional integration using models of effective connectivity and other multivariate approaches.

FUNCTIONAL SPECIALISATION AND INTEGRATION

The brain appears to adhere to two fundamental principles of functional organisation, *functional integration* and *functional specialisation,* where the integration within and among specialised areas is mediated by effective connectivity. The distinction relates to that between *localisationism* and *(dis)connectionism* that dominated thinking about cortical function in the 19th century. Since the early anatomical theories of Gall, the identification of a particular brain region with a specific function has become a central theme in neuroscience. However functional localisation per se was not easy to demonstrate: For example, a meeting that took place on August 4, 1881, addressed the difficulties of attributing function to a cortical area, given the dependence of cerebral activity on underlying connections (Phillips *et al.,* 1984). This meeting was entitled "Localisation of Function in the Cortex Cerebri" Goltz (1881), although accepting the results of electrical stimulation in dog and monkey cortex, considered that the excitation method was inconclusive, in that movements elicited might have originated in related pathways, or current could have spread to distant centers. In short, the excitation method could not be used to infer functional localisation because localisationism discounted interactions or functional integration among different brain areas. It was proposed that lesion studies could supplement excitation experiments. Ironically, it was observations on patients with brain lesions some years later (see Absher and Benson, 1993) that led to the concept of *disconnection syndromes* and the refutation of localisationism as a complete or sufficient explanation of cortical organisation. Functional localisation implies that a function can be localised in a cortical area, whereas specialisation suggests that a cortical area is specialised for some aspects of perceptual or motor processing, and that this specialisation is anatomically segregated within the cortex. The cortical infrastructure supporting a single function may then involve many specialised areas whose union is mediated by the functional integration among them. In this view functional specialisation is only meaningful in the context of functional integration and vice versa.

Functional Specialisation and Segregation

The functional role played by any component (e.g., cortical area, subarea, or neuronal population) of the brain is largely defined by its connections. Certain patterns of cortical projections are so common that they could amount to rules of cortical connectivity. "These rules revolve around one, apparently, overriding strategy that the cerebral cortex uses—that of functional segregation" (Zeki, 1990). Functional segregation demands that cells with common functional properties be grouped together. This architectural constraint necessitates both convergence and divergence of cortical connections. Extrinsic connections among cortical regions are not continuous but occur in patches or clusters. This patchiness has, in some instances, a clear relationship to functional segregation. For example, V2 has a distinctive cytochrome oxidase architecture, consisting of thick stripes, thin stripes, and interstripes. When recordings are made in V2, directionally selective (but not wavelength or color selective) cells are found exclusively in the thick stripes. Retrograde (i.e., backward) labeling of cells in V5 is limited to these thick stripes. All of the available physiological evidence suggests that V5 is a functionally homogeneous area that is specialised for visual motion. Evidence of this nature supports the notion that patchy connectivity is the anatomical infrastructure that mediates functional segregation and specialisation. If it is the case that neurons in a given cortical area share a common responsiveness (by virtue of their extrinsic connectivity) to some sensorimotor or cognitive attribute, then this functional segregation is also an anatomical one. Challenging a subject with the appropriate sensorimotor attribute or cognitive process should lead to activity changes in, and only in, the area of interest. This is the anatomical and physiological model on which the search for regionally specific effects is based.

The analysis of functional neuroimaging data involves many steps that can be broadly divided into (1) spatial processing, (2) estimating the parameters of a statistical model, and (3) making inferences about those parameter estimates with appropriate statistics (see Fig. 31.1). We will deal first with spatial transformations: In order to combine data from different scans from the same subject, or data from different subjects, they must conform to the same anatomical frame of reference. The spatial transformations and morphological operations required are dealt with in depth in Section 1 of Part II.

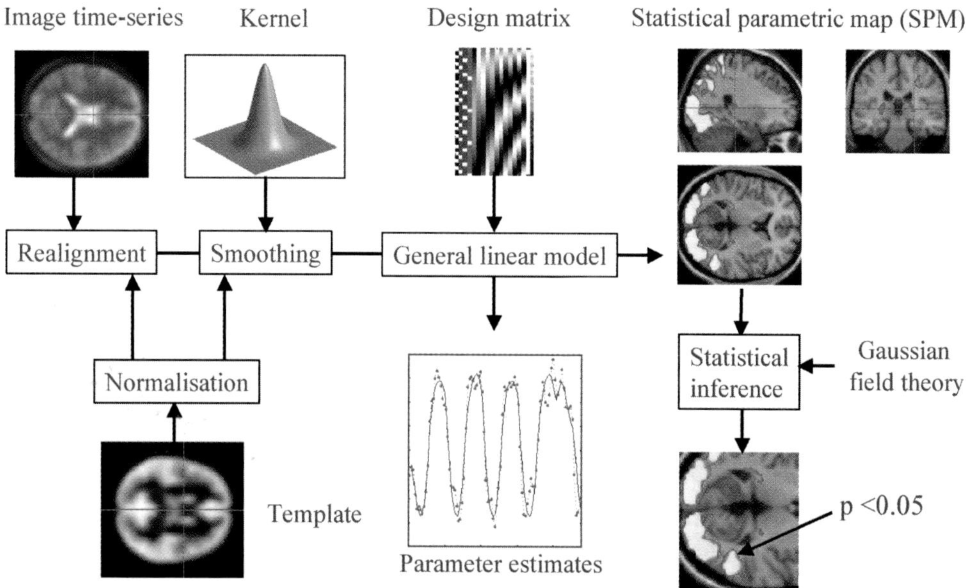

FIGURE 31.1
This schematic depicts the transformations that start with an imaging data sequence and end with a statistical parametric map (SPM). SPMs can be thought of as "X rays" of the significance of an effect. Voxel-based analyses require the data to be in the same anatomical space. This is effected by realigning the data (and removing movement-related signal components that persist after realignment). After realignment, the images are subject to nonlinear warping so that they match a template that already conforms to a standard anatomical space. After smoothing, the general linear model is employed to (1) estimate the parameters of the model and (2) derive the appropriate univariate test statistic at every voxel (see Fig. 31.4). The test statistics that ensue (usually T or F statistics) constitute the SPM. The final stage is to make statistical inferences on the basis of the SPM and random field theory (see Fig. 31.7) and characterise the responses observed using the fitted responses or parameter estimates.

SPATIAL REALIGNMENT AND NORMALISATION (SECTION 1, COMPUTATIONAL NEUROANATOMY)

The analysis of neuroimaging data generally starts with a series of spatial transformations. These transformations aim to reduce unwanted variance components in the voxel time series that are induced by movement or shape differences among a series of scans. Voxel-based analyses assume that the data from a particular voxel all derive from the same part of the brain. Violations of this assumption will introduce artifactual changes in the voxel values that may obscure changes, or differences, of interest. Even single-subject analyses proceed in a standard anatomical space, simply to enable reporting of regionally specific effects in a frame of reference that can be related to other studies.

The first step is to realign the data to "undo" the effects of subject movement during the scanning session. After realignment the data are then transformed using linear or nonlinear warps into a standard anatomical space. Finally, the data are usually spatially smoothed before entering the analysis proper.

Realignment (Chapter 32, Rigid Body Registration)

Changes in signal intensity over time, from any one voxel, can arise from head motion, and this represents a serious confound, particularly in fMRI studies. Despite restraints on head movement, cooperative subjects still show displacements of up to several millimeters. Realignment involves (1) estimating the six parameters of an affine "rigid-body" transformation that minimises the (sum of squared) differences between each successive scan and a reference scan (usually the first or the average of all scans in the time series) and (2) applying the transformation by resampling the data using trilinear, sinc, or spline interpolation. Estimation of the affine transformation is usually effected with a first-order approximation of the Taylor expansion of the effect of movement on signal intensity using the spatial derivatives of the images (see below). This allows for a simple iterative least-squares solution that corresponds to a Gauss-Newton search (Friston *et al.,* 1995a). For most imaging modalities this procedure is sufficient to realign scans to, in some instances, a hundred microns or so (Friston *et al.,* 1996a). However, in fMRI, even after perfect realignment, movement-related signals can still persist. This calls for a further step in which the data are *adjusted* for residual movement-related effects.

Adjusting for Movement-Related Effects in fMRI

In extreme cases as much as 90% of the variance in fMRI time series can be accounted for by the effects of movement *after* realignment (Friston *et al.,* 1996a). Causes of these movement-related components are due to movement effects that cannot be modeled using a *linear* affine model. These nonlinear effects include (1) subject movement between slice acquisition, (2) interpolation artifacts (Grootoonk *et al.,* 2000), (3) nonlinear distortion due to magnetic field inhomogeneities (Andersson *et al.,* 2001), and (4) spin-excitation history effects (Friston *et al.,* 1996a). The latter can be pronounced if the TR (repetition time) approaches T_1 making the current signal a function of movement history. These multiple effects render the movement-related signal (y) a nonlinear function of displacement (x) in the nth and previous scans $y_n = f(x_n, x_{n-1},\ldots)$. By assuming a sensible form for this function, its parameters can be estimated using the observed time series and the estimated movement parameters x from the realignment procedure. The estimated movement-related signal is then simply subtracted from the original data. This adjustment can be carried out as a preprocessing step or embodied in model estimation during the analysis proper. The form for $f(x)$, proposed by Friston *et al.* (1996a), was a nonlinear autoregression model that used polynomial expansions to second order. This model was motivated by spin-excitation history effects and allowed displacement in previous scans to explain the current movement-related signal. However, it is also a reasonable model for many other sources of movement-related confounds. Generally, for TRs of several seconds, interpolation artifacts supersede (Grootoonk *et al.,* 2000), and first-order terms, comprising an expansion of the current displacement in terms of periodic basis functions, are sufficient.

This subsection has considered *spatial* realignment. In multislice acquisition, different slices are acquired at slightly different times. This raises the possibility of *temporal* realignment to ensure that the data from any given volume were sampled at the same time. This is usually performed using sinc interpolation over time and only when (1) the temporal dynamics of evoked responses are important and (2) the TR is sufficiently small to permit interpolation. Generally timing effects of this sort are not considered problematic because they manifest as artifactual latency differences in evoked responses from region to region. Given that biophysical latency differences may be on the order of a few seconds, inferences about these differences are only made when comparing different trial types at the *same* voxel. Provided the effects of latency differences are modelled, this renders temporal realignment unnecessary in most instances.

Spatial Normalisation (Chapter 33, Spatial Normalisation Using Basis Functions)

After realigning the data, a mean image of the series, or some other coregistered (e.g., a T_1-weighted) image, is used to estimate some warping parameters that map it onto a template that already conforms to some standard anatomical space (e.g., Talairach and Tournoux 1988). This estimation can use a variety of models for the mapping, including (1) a 12-parameter affine transformation, where the parameters constitute a spatial transformation matrix; (2) low-frequency basis spatial functions (usually a discrete cosine set or polynomials), where the parameters are the coefficients of the basis functions employed; and (3) a vector field specifying the mapping for each control point (e.g., voxel). In the latter case, the parameters are vast in number and constitute a vector field that is bigger than the image itself. Estimation of the parameters of all of these models can be accommodated in a simple Bayesian framework, in which one is trying to find the deformation parameters θ that have the maximum posterior probability $p(\theta \mid y)$ given the data y, where $p(\theta \mid y)\, p(y) = p(y \mid \theta)\, p(\theta)$. Put simply, one wants to find the deformation that is most likely given the data. This deformation can be found by maximising the probability of getting the data, assuming the current estimate of the deformation is true, times the probability of that estimate being true. In practice, the deformation is updated iteratively using a Gauss-Newton scheme to maximise $p(\theta \mid y)$. This involves jointly minimising the likelihood and prior potentials and $H(y \mid \theta) = \ln p(y \mid \theta)$ and $H(\theta) = \ln p(\theta)$. The likelihood potential is generally taken to be the sum of squared differences between the template and deformed image and reflects the probability of actually getting that image if the transformation was correct. The prior potential can be used to incorporate prior information about the likelihood of a given warp. Priors can be determined empirically or motivated by constraints on the mappings. Priors play a more essential role as the number of parameters specifying the mapping increases and are central to high dimensional warping schemes (Ashburner *et al.,* 1997 and Chapter 34, High-Dimensional Image Warping).

In practice, most people use an affine or spatial basis function warps and iterative least squares to minimise the posterior potential. A nice extension of this approach is that the likelihood potential can be refined and taken as the difference between the index image and the best (linear) combination of templates (e.g., depicting gray, white, CSF, and skull tissue partitions). This models intensity differences that are unrelated to registration differences and allows different modalities to be coregistered (see Fig. 31.2).

A special consideration is the spatial normalisation of brains that have gross anatomical pathology. This pathology can be of two sorts: (1) quantitative changes in the amount of a particular tissue compartment (e.g., cortical atrophy) or (2) qualitative changes in anatomy involving the insertion or deletion of normal tissue compartments (e.g., ischemic tissue in stroke or cortical dysplasia). The former case is generally not problematic in the sense that changes in the amount of cortical tissue will not affect its optimum spatial location in reference to some template (and, even if it does, a disease-specific template is easily constructed). The second sort of pathology can introduce substantial "errors" in the normalisation unless special precautions are taken. These usually involve imposing constraints on the warping to ensure that the pathology does not bias the deformation of undamaged tissue. This involves "hard" constraints implicit in using a small number of basis functions or "soft" constraints implemented by increasing the role of priors in Bayesian estimation. An alternative strategy is to use another

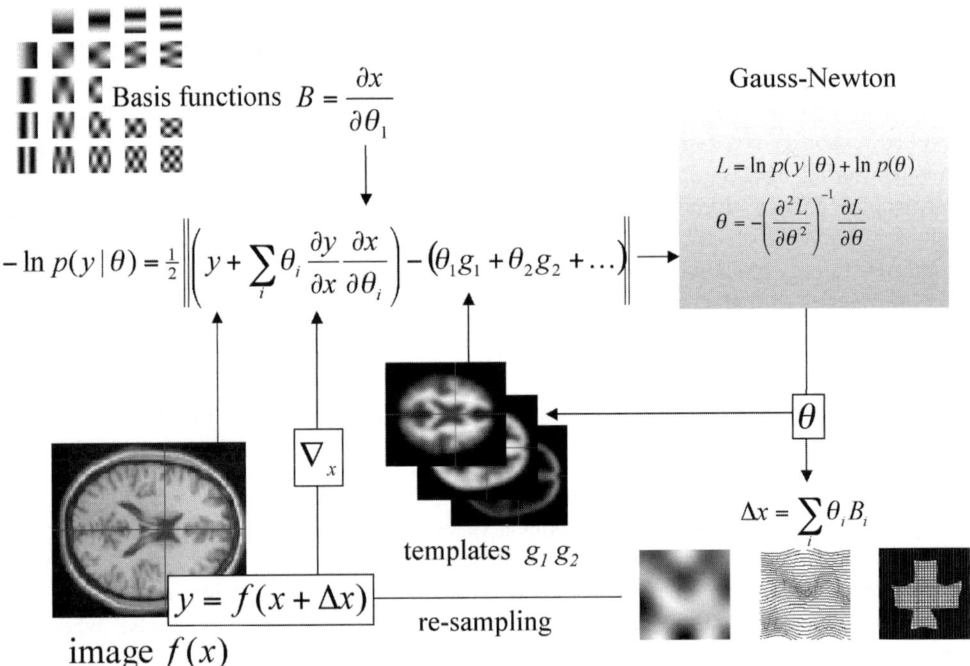

FIGURE 31.2
Schematic illustrating a Gauss-Newton scheme for maximizing the posterior probability $p(\theta \mid y)$ of the parameters required to spatially normalise an image. This scheme is iterative. At each step the conditional estimate of the parameters is obtained by jointly minimizing the likelihood and the prior potentials. The former is the difference between a resampled (i.e., warped) version y of the image f and the best linear combination of some templates g. These parameters are used to mix the templates and resample the image to progressively reduce both the spatial and intensity differences. After convergence, the resampled image can be considered normalised.

modality that is less sensitive to the pathology as the basis of the spatial normalisation procedure or to simply remove the damaged region from the estimation by masking it out.

Coregistration of Functional and Anatomical Data

It is sometimes useful to coregister functional and anatomical images. However, with echo-planar imaging, geometric distortions of T_2* images, relative to anatomical T_1-weighted data, are a particularly serious problem because of the very low frequency per point in the phase encoding direction. Typically for echo-planar fMRI magnetic field inhomogeneity, sufficient to cause dephasing of 2π through the slice, corresponds to an in-plane distortion of a voxel. "Unwarping" schemes have been proposed to correct for the distortion effects (Jezzard and Balaban, 1995). However, this distortion is not an issue if one spatially normalises the functional data.

Spatial Smoothing

The motivations for smoothing the data are fourfold:

1. By the matched filter theorem, the optimum smoothing kernel corresponds to the size of the effect that one anticipates. The spatial scale of haemodynamic responses is, according to high-resolution optical imaging experiments, about 2–5 mm. Despite the potentially high resolution afforded by fMRI, an equivalent smoothing is suggested for most applications.
2. By the central limit theorem, smoothing the data will render the errors more normal in their distribution and ensure the validity of inferences based on parametric tests.
3. When making inferences about regional effects using Gaussian random field theory (see below) the assumption is that the error terms are a reasonable lattice representation of an underlying and smooth Gaussian field. This necessitates that smoothness be substantially greater than voxel size. If the voxels are large, then they can be reduced by subsampling the data and smoothing (with the original point spread function) with little loss of intrinsic resolution.

4. In the context of intersubject averaging, it is often necessary to smooth more (e.g., 8 mm in fMRI or 16 mm in PET) to project the data onto a spatial scale where homologies in functional anatomy are expressed among subjects.

Summary

Spatial registration and normalisation can proceed at a number of spatial scales depending on how one parameterises variations in anatomy. We have focussed on the role of normalisation to remove unwanted differences to enable subsequent analysis of the data. However, it is important to note that the products of spatial normalisation are bifold; a spatially normalised image and a deformation field (see Fig. 31.3). This deformation field contains important information about anatomy, in relation to the template used in the normalisation procedure. The analysis of this information forms a key part of computational neuroanatomy. The tensor fields can be analysed directly (deformation-based morphometry) or used to create maps of specific anatomical attributes (e.g., compression, shears). These maps can then be analysed on a voxel-by-voxel basis (tensor-based morphometry). Finally, the normalised structural images can themselves be subject to statistical analysis after some suitable segmentation procedure (see Chapter 35, Image Segmentation). This is known as *voxel-based morphometry.* Voxel-based morphometry is the most commonly used voxel-based neuroanatomical procedure and can easily be extended to incorporate tensor-based approaches. See Chapter 36, Morphometry, for more details.

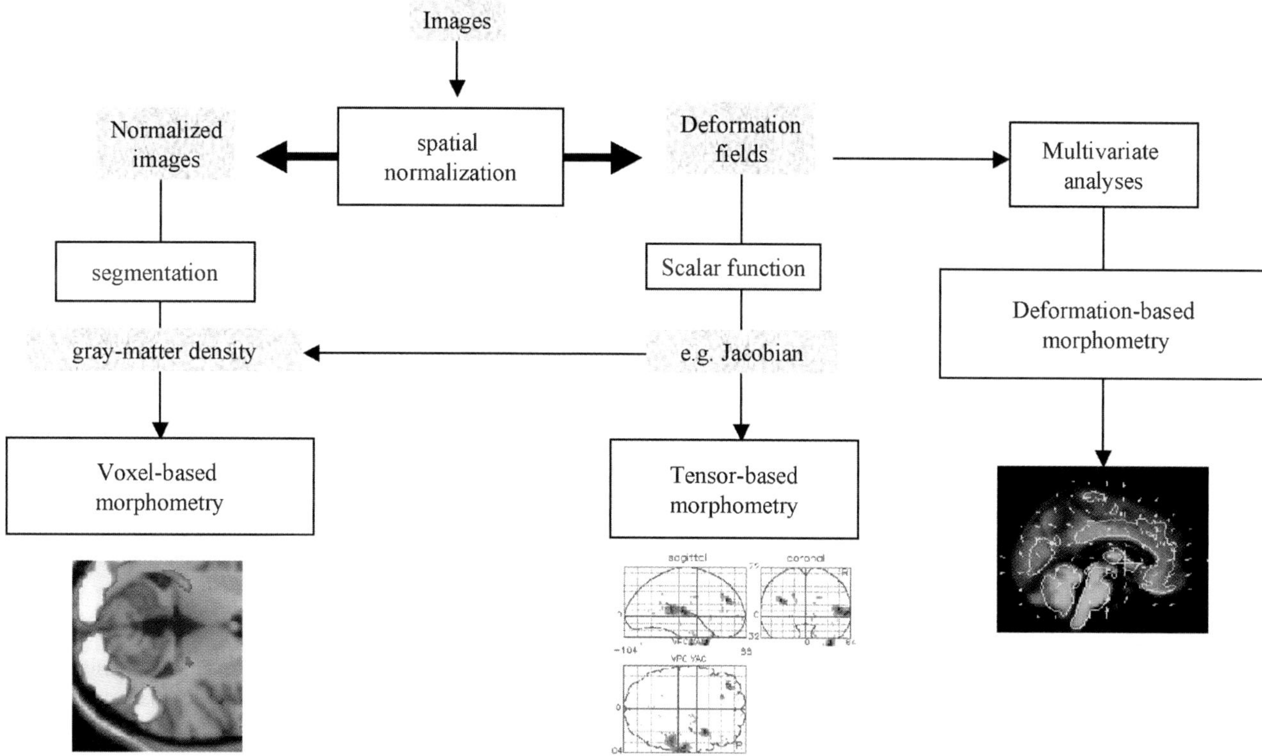

FIGURE 31.3
Schematic illustrating different procedures in computational anatomy. After spatial normalisation, one has access to the normalised image and the deformation field implementing the normalisation. The deformation or tensor field can be analysed directly (deformation-based morphometry) or can be used to derive maps of formal attributes (e.g., compression, dilatation, shear). These maps can then be subject to conventional voxel-based analyses (tensor-based morphometry). Alternatively, the normalised images can be processed (e.g., segmented) to reveal some interesting aspect of anatomy (e.g., the tissue composition) and analysed in a similar way (voxel-based morphometry). Techniques developed for tensor-based morphometry can be absorbed into voxel-based morphometry to prove a unified framework. For example, before statistical analysis, Jacobian, or voxel-compression, maps can be multiplied by gray-matter density maps. This endows volumetric changes, derived from the tensor, with tissue specificity, based on the segmentation.

STATISTICAL PARAMETRIC MAPPING (SECTIONS 2 AND 3, MODELLING AND INFERENCE)

Functional mapping studies are usually analysed with some form of statistical parametric mapping. Statistical parametric mapping entails the construction of spatially extended statistical processes to test hypotheses about regionally specific effects (Friston *et al.,* 1991). Statistical parametric maps (SPMs) are image processes with voxel values that are, under the null hypothesis, distributed according to a known probability density function, usually Student's T or F distributions. These are known colloquially as *T-maps* or *F-maps*. The success of statistical parametric mapping is due largely to the simplicity of the idea, namely, one analyses each and every voxel using any standard (univariate) statistical test. The resulting statistical parameters are assembled into an image—the SPM. SPMs are interpreted as spatially extended statistical processes by referring to the probabilistic behaviour of Gaussian fields (Adler, 1981; Worsley *et al.,* 1992, 1996; Friston *et al.,* 1994a). Gaussian random fields model both the univariate probabilistic characteristics of an SPM and any nonstationary spatial covariance structure. "Unlikely" excursions of the SPM are interpreted as regionally specific effects, attributable to the sensorimotor or cognitive process that has been manipulated experimentally.

Over the years statistical parametric mapping has come to refer to the conjoint use of the *general linear model* (GLM) and *Gaussian random field* (GRF) theory to analyze and make classical inferences about spatially extended data through SPMs. The GLM is used to estimate some parameters that could explain the spatially continuous data in exactly the same way as in conventional analyses of discrete data (see Chapter 37, The General Linear Model). GRF theory is used to resolve the multiple comparison problem that ensues when making inferences over a volume of the brain. GRF theory provides a method for correcting p values for the search volume of a SPM and plays the same role for *continuous* data (i.e., images) as the Bonferonni correction does for the number of discontinuous or *discrete* statistical tests (see Chapter 44, Introduction to Random Field Theory).

The approach was called SPM for three reasons: (1) to acknowledge significance probability mapping, the use of interpolated pseudo-maps of p values used to summarise the analysis of multichannel ERP studies; (2) for consistency with the nomenclature of parametric maps of physiological or physical parameters (e.g., regional cerebral blood flow rCBF or volume rCBV parametric maps); and (3) in reference to the *parametric* statistics that comprise the maps. Despite its simplicity there are some fairly subtle motivations for the approach that deserve mention. Usually, given a response or dependent variable comprising many thousands of voxels, one would use *multivariate* analyses as opposed to the *mass-univariate* approach that SPM represents. The problems with multivariate approaches are that (1) they do not support inferences about regionally specific effects, (2) they require more observations than the dimension of the response variable (i.e., number of voxels), and (3) even in the context of dimension reduction, they are less sensitive to focal effects than mass-univariate approaches. A heuristic argument for their relative lack of power is that multivariate approaches estimate the model's error covariances using lots of parameters (e.g., the covariance between the errors at all pairs of voxels). In general, the more parameters (and hyper-parameters) an estimation procedure has to deal with, the more variable the estimate of any one parameter becomes. This renders inferences about any single estimate less efficient.

Multivariate approaches consider voxels as different levels of an experimental or treatment factor and use classical analysis of variance, not at each voxel (c.f. SPM), but by considering the data sequences from all voxels together, as replications over voxels. The problem here is that regional changes in error variance, and spatial correlations in the data, induce profound nonsphericity[1] in the error terms. This nonsphericity would again require large numbers of

[1] *Sphericity* refers to the assumption of identically and independently distributed error terms (i.i.d.). Under i.i.d. the probability density function of the errors, from all observations, has spherical isocontours, hence, *sphericity.* Deviations from either of the i.i.d. criteria constitute nonsphericity. If the error terms are not identically distributed, then different observations have different error variances. Correlations among error terms reflect dependencies among the errors (e.g., serial correlation in fMRI time series) and constitute the second component of nonsphericity. In neuroimaging both spatial and temporal nonsphericity can be quite profound.

hyperparameters to be estimated for each voxel using conventional techniques. In SPM the nonsphericity is parameterised in a very parsimonious way with just two hyperparameters for each voxel. These are the error variance and smoothness estimators (see Section 3 and Fig. 31.2). This minimal parameterisation lends SPM a sensitivity that surpasses multivariate approaches. SPM can do this because GRF theory implicitly imposes constraints on the nonsphericity implied by the continuous and (spatially) extended nature of the data (see Chapter 45, Introduction to Random Field Theory). This is something that conventional multivariate and equivalent univariate approaches do not accommodate, to their cost.

Some analyses use statistical maps based on nonparametric tests that eschew distributional assumptions about the data (see Chapter 46, Nonparametric Permutation Tests for Functional Neuroimaging). These approaches are generally less powerful (i.e., less sensitive) than parametric approaches (see Aguirre *et al.,* 1998). However, they have an important role in evaluating the assumptions behind parametric approaches and may supercede in terms of sensitivity when these assumptions are violated (e.g., when degrees of freedom are very small and voxel sizes are large in relation to smoothness).

In Chapter 47, Classical and Bayesian Inference, we consider the Bayesian alternative to classical inference with SPMs. This rests on conditional inferences about an effect, given the data, as opposed to classical inferences about the data, given the effect is zero. Bayesian inferences about spatially extended effects use posterior probability maps (PPMs). Although less commonly used than SPMs, PPMs are potentially very useful, not least because they do not have to contend with the multiple comparisons problem induced by classical inference. In contradistinction to SPM, this means that inferences about a given regional response do not depend on inferences about responses elsewhere.

Next we consider parameter estimation in the context of the GLM. This is followed by an introduction to the role of GRF theory when making classical inferences about continuous data.

General Linear Model (Chapter 37)

Statistical analysis of imaging data corresponds to (1) modelling the data to partition observed neurophysiological responses into components of interest, confounds, and error and (2) making inferences about the interesting effects in relation to the error variance. This classical inference can be regarded as a direct comparison of the variance due to an interesting experimental manipulation with the error variance (c.f. the F statistic and other likelihood ratios). Alternatively, one can view the statistic as an estimate of the response, or difference of interest, divided by an estimate of its standard deviation. This is a useful way to think about the T statistic.

A brief review of the literature may give the impression that there are numerous ways to analyze PET and fMRI time series with a diversity of statistical and conceptual approaches. This is not the case. With very a few exceptions, every analysis is a variant of the general linear model. This includes (1) simple T tests on scans assigned to one condition or another, (2) correlation coefficients between observed responses and boxcar stimulus functions in fMRI, (3) inferences made using multiple linear regression, (4) evoked responses estimated using linear time-invariant models, and (5) selective averaging to estimate event-related responses in fMRI. Mathematically, they are all identical and can be implemented with the same equations and algorithms. The only thing that distinguishes among them is the design matrix encoding the experimental design. The use of the correlation coefficient deserves special mention because of its popularity in fMRI (Bandettini *et al.,* 1993). The significance of a correlation is identical to the significance of the equivalent T-statistic testing for a regression of the data on the stimulus function. The correlation coefficient approach is useful but the inference is effectively based on a limiting case of multiple linear regression that is obtained when there is only one regressor. In fMRI many regressors usually enter into a statistical model. Therefore, the T statistic provides a more versatile and generic way of assessing the significance of regional effects and is preferred over the correlation coefficient.

The general linear model is an equation $Y = X\beta + \varepsilon$ that expresses the observed response variable Y in terms of a linear combination of explanatory variables X plus a well-behaved error term (see Fig. 31.4; Friston *et al.,* 1995b). The general linear model is variously known as *analysis of covariance* or *multiple regression analysis* and subsumes simpler variants, like the T test for a difference in means, to more elaborate linear convolution models such as finite impulse response (FIR) models. Matrix X, which contains the explanatory variables (e.g., designed effects or confounds), is called the *design matrix*. Each column of the design matrix corresponds to some effect one has built into the experiment or that may confound the results. These are referred to as *explanatory variables, covariates,* or *regressors.* The example in Fig. 1 relates to a fMRI study of visual stimulation under four conditions. The effects on the response variable are modeled in terms of functions of the presence of these conditions (i.e., boxcars smoothed with a hemodynamic response function) and constitute the first four columns of the design matrix. A series of terms then follows that is designed to remove or model low-frequency variations in signal due to artifacts such as aliased biorhythms and other drift terms. The final column is whole brain activity. The relative contribution of each of these columns is assessed using standard least squares and inferences about these contributions are made using T or F statistics, depending on whether one is looking at a particular linear combination (e.g., a subtraction) or all of them together. The operational equations are depicted schematically in Fig. 31.4. In this scheme the general linear model has been extended (Worsley and Friston, 1995) to incorporate intrinsic nonsphericity, or correlations among the error terms, and to allow for some specified temporal filtering of the data with the matrix S. This generalisation brings with it the notion of *effective degrees of freedom,* which are less than the conventional degrees of freedom under i.i.d. assumptions (see footnote). They are smaller because the temporal correlations reduce the effective number of independent observations. The T and F statistics are constructed using Satterthwaite's approximation. This is the same approximation used in classical nonsphericity corrections such as the Geisser-Greenhouse correction. However, in the Worsley and Friston (1995) scheme, Satherthwaite's approximation is used to construct the statistics and appropriate degrees of freedom, not simply to provide a post hoc correction to the degrees of freedom.

A special case of temporal filtering deserves mention. This is when the filtering decorrelates (i.e., whitens) the error terms by using $S = \Sigma^{-1/2}$. This is the filtering scheme used in current implementations of software for SPM and renders the ordinary least-squares (OLS) parameter estimates maximum likelihood (ML) estimators. These are optimal in the sense that they are the minimum variance estimators of all unbiased estimators. The estimation of $S = \Sigma^{-1/2}$ uses expectation maximisation (EM) to provide restricted maximum likelihood (ReML) estimates of $\Sigma = \Sigma(\lambda)$ in terms of hyperparameters λ corresponding to variance components (see Chapter 39, Variance Components, and Chapter 47, Classical and Bayesian Inference, for an explanation of EM). In this case the effective degrees of freedom revert to the maximum that would be attained in the absence of temporal correlations or nonsphericity.

The equations summarised in Fig. 31.4 can be used to implement a vast range of statistical analyses. The issue is therefore not so much the mathematics but the formulation of a design matrix X appropriate to the study design and inferences that are sought. The design matrix can contain both covariates and indicator variables. Each column of X has an associated unknown parameter. Some of these parameters will be of interest (e.g., the effect of particular sensorimotor or cognitive condition or the regression coefficient of hemodynamic responses on reaction time). The remaining parameters will be of no interest and pertain to confounding effects (e.g., the effect of being a particular subject or the regression slope of voxel activity on global activity). Inferences about the parameter estimates are made using their estimated variance. This allows one to test the null hypothesis that all estimates are zero using the F statistic to give an SPM{F} or that some particular linear combination (e.g., a subtraction) of the estimates is zero using an SPM{T}. The T statistic is obtained by dividing a contrast or compound (specified by contrast weights) of the ensuing parameter estimates by the standard error of that compound. The latter is estimated using the variance of the residuals about the least-squares fit. An example of a contrast weight *vector* would be [–1 1 0 0 ...] to compare the difference in responses evoked by two conditions, modeled by the first two condition-specific regressors in the design matrix. Sometimes several contrasts of parameter estimates are jointly interesting, for example, when using polynomial (Büchel *et al.,* 1996) or basis function expansions of some experimental factor. In these instances, the SPM{F} is used and is specified with a *matrix* of contrast weights that can be thought of as a collection of "T contrasts" that one wants to test together. See Chapter 38,

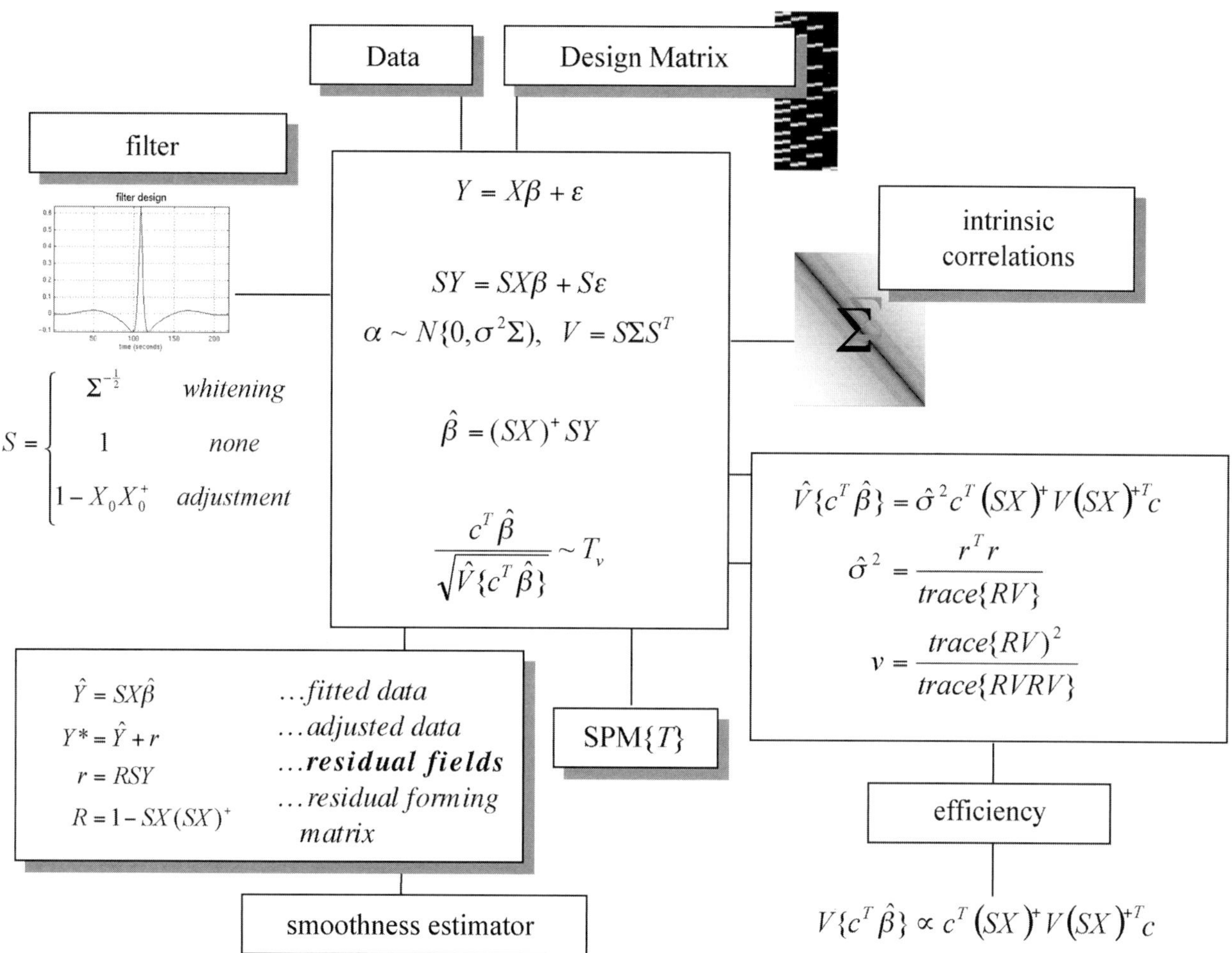

FIGURE 31.4
The general linear model. The general linear model is an equation expressing the response variable Y in terms of a linear combination of explanatory variables in a design matrix X and an error term with assumed or known autocorrelation Σ. In fMRI the data can be filtered with a convolution or residual forming matrix (or a combination) S, leading to a generalised linear model that includes (intrinsic) serial correlations and applied (extrinsic) filtering[2]. Different choices of S correspond to different estimation schemes as indicated on the upper left. The parameter estimates are obtained in a least-squares sense using the pseudoinverse (denoted by +) of the filtered design matrix. Generally an effect of interest is specified by a vector of contrast weights c that give a weighted sum or compound of parameter estimates referred to as a *contrast.* The T statistic is simply this contrast divided by its the estimated standard error (i.e., square root of its estimated variance). The ensuing T statistic is distributed with v degrees of freedom. The equations for estimating the variance of the contrast and the degrees of freedom associated with the error variance are provided in the right-hand panel. Efficiency is simply the inverse of the variance of the contrast. These expressions are useful when assessing the relative efficiency of experimental designs. The parameter estimates can either be examined directly or used to compute the fitted responses (see lower left panel). Adjusted data refers to data from which estimated confounds have been removed. The residuals r are obtained from applying the residual-forming matrix R to the data. These residual fields are used to estimate the smoothness of the component fields of the SPM used in random field theory (see Fig. 31.7).

Contrasts and Classical Inference, for a more detailed explanation. An "F contrast" might look like this:

$$\begin{bmatrix} -1 & 0 & 0 & 0 & \dots \\ 0 & 1 & 0 & 0 & \dots \end{bmatrix}$$

which would test for the significance of the first *or* second parameter estimates. The fact that the first weight is –1 as opposed to 1 has no effect on the test because the F statistic is based on sums of squares.

[2]Note that generalised linear models are much more extensive than linear models with nonspherical Gaussian errors and cover models with non-Gaussian errors. This means that the generalised linear models referred to in this book are the simplest generalisation of general linear models.

In most analyses, the design matrix contains indicator variables or parametric variables encoding the experimental manipulations. These are formally identical to classical analysis of covariance (AnCova) models. An important instance of the GLM, from the perspective of fMRI, is the linear time-invariant (LTI) model. Mathematically this is no different from any other GLM. However, it explicitly treats the data sequence as an ordered time series and enables a signal processing perspective that can be very useful (see Chapter 40, Analysis of fMRI Time Series).

LTI Systems and Temporal Basis Functions

In Friston *et al.* (1994b) the form of the hemodynamic impulse response function (HRF) was estimated using a least-squares deconvolution and a time-invariant model, where evoked neuronal responses are convolved with the HRF to give the measured hemodynamic response (see Boynton *et al.,* 1996). This simple linear framework is the cornerstone for making statistical inferences about activations in fMRI with the GLM. An impulse response function is the response to a single impulse, measured at a series of times after the input. It characterises the input–output behaviour of the system (i.e., voxel) and places important constraints on the sorts of inputs that will excite a response. The HRFs, estimated in Friston *et al.* (1994b) resembled a Poisson or Gamma function, peaking at about 5 sec. Our understanding of the biophysical and physiological mechanisms that underpin the HRF has grown considerably in the past few years (e.g., Buxton and Frank, 1997; Chapter 41, Hemodynamic Modelling). Figure 31.5 shows some simulations based on the hemodynamic model described in Friston *et al.* (2000a). Here, neuronal activity induces some autoregulated signal that causes transient increases in rCBF. The resulting flow inflates the venous balloon, increasing its volume (v) and diluting venous blood to decrease deoxyhemoglobin content (q). The BOLD signal is roughly proportional to the concentration of deoxyhemoglobin (q/v) and follows the rCBF response with about 1 sec of delay.

Knowing the forms that the HRF can take is important for several reasons, not least because it allows for better statistical models of the data to be designed. The HRF may vary from voxel to voxel and this has to be accommodated in the GLM. To allow for different HRFs in different brain regions, the notion of temporal basis functions, to model evoked responses in fMRI, was introduced (Friston *et al.,* 1995c) and applied to event-related responses by Josephs *et al.* (1997) (see also Lange and Zeger, 1997). The basic idea behind temporal basis functions is that the hemodynamic response induced by any given trial type can be expressed as the linear combination of several (basis) functions of peristimulus time. The convolution model for fMRI responses takes a stimulus function encoding the supposed neuronal responses and convolves it with an HRF to give a regressor that enters into the design matrix. When using basis functions, the stimulus function is convolved with all basis functions to give a series of regressors. The associated parameter estimates are the coefficients or weights that determine the mixture of basis functions that best models the HRF for the trial type and voxel in question. We find the most useful basis set to be a canonical HRF and its derivatives with respect to the key parameters that determine its form (e.g., latency and dispersion). The nice thing about this approach is that it can partition differences among evoked responses into differences in magnitude, latency, or dispersion that can be tested for using specific contrasts and the SPM{T} (Friston *et al.,* 1998b).

Temporal basis functions are important because they enable a graceful transition between conventional multilinear regression models with one stimulus function per condition and FIR models with a parameter for each time point following the onset of a condition or trial type. Figure 31.6 illustrates this graphically. In summary, temporal basis functions offer useful constraints on the form of the estimated response that retain (1) the flexibility of FIR models and (2) the efficiency of single regressor models. The advantage of using several temporal basis functions (as opposed to an assumed form for the HRF) is that one can model voxel-specific forms for hemodynamic responses and formal differences (e.g., onset latencies) among responses to different sorts of events. The advantages of using basis functions over FIR models are that (1) the parameters are estimated more efficiently and (2) stimuli can be presented at any point in the interstimulus interval. The latter is important because time-locking stimulus presentation and data acquisition give a biased sampling over peristimulus time and can lead to differential sensitivities, in multislice acquisition, over the brain.

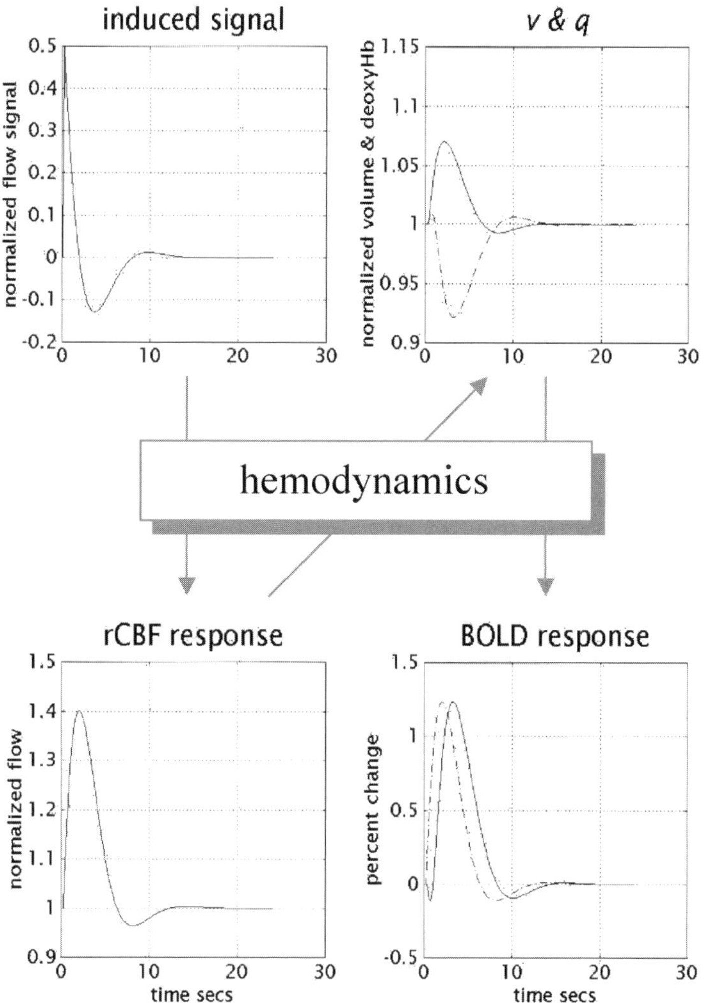

FIGURE 31.5
Hemodynamics elicited by an impulse of neuronal activity as predicted by a dynamical biophysical model (see Friston *et al.*, 2000a, for details). A burst of neuronal activity causes an increase in a flow-inducing signal that decays with first-order kinetics and is downregulated by local flow. This signal increases rCBF, which dilates the venous capillaries, increasing volume *(v)*. Concurrently, venous blood is expelled from the venous pool, decreasing deoxyhemoglobin content *(q)*. The resulting fall in deoxyhemoglobin concentration leads to a transient increases in the BOLD (blood oxygenation level dependent) signal and a subsequent undershoot.

Statistical Inference and the Theory of Random Fields (Chapters 44 and 45)

Classical inferences using SPMs can be of two sorts depending on whether one knows where to look in advance. With an anatomically constrained hypothesis about effects in a particular brain region, the uncorrected p value associated with the height or extent of that region in the SPM can be used to test the hypothesis. With an anatomically open hypothesis (i.e., a null hypothesis that there is no effect anywhere in a specified volume of the brain), a correction for multiple dependent comparisons is necessary. The theory of random fields provides a way of adjusting the p value that takes into account the fact that neighbouring voxels are not independent by virtue of continuity in the original data. Provided the data are sufficiently smooth, the GRF correction is less severe (i.e., is more sensitive) than a Bonferroni correction for the number of voxels. As noted above GRF theory deals with the multiple comparisons problem in the context of continuous, spatially extended statistical fields, in a way that is analogous to the Bonferroni procedure for families of discrete statistical tests. There are many ways to appreciate the difference between GRF and Bonferroni corrections. Perhaps the most intuitive is to consider the fundamental difference between a SPM and a collection of discrete T values. When declaring a connected volume or region of the SPM to be significant, we refer collectively to all voxels that

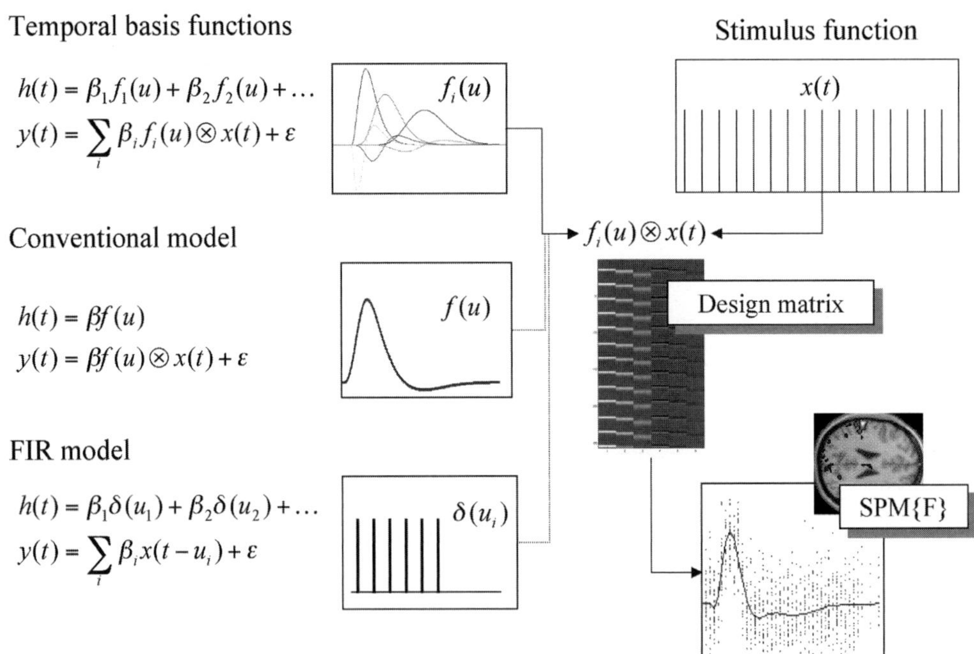

FIGURE 31.6
Temporal basis functions offer useful constraints on the form of the estimated response that retain (1) the flexibility of FIR models and (2) the efficiency of single regressor models. The specification of these constrained FIR models involves setting up stimulus functions *x(t)* that model expected neuronal changes [e.g., boxcars of epoch-related responses or spikes (delta functions) at the onset of specific events or trials]. These stimulus functions are then convolved with a set of basis functions $f(u)$ of peristimulus time u that model the HRF in some linear combination. The ensuing regressors are assembled into the design matrix. The basis functions can be as simple as a single canonical HRF (middle), through to a series of delayed delta functions (bottom). The latter case corresponds to a FIR model and the coefficients constitute estimates of the impulse response function at a finite number of discrete sampling times. Selective averaging in event-related fMRI (Dale and Buckner, 1997). is mathematically equivalent to this limiting case.

comprise that region. The false-positive rate is expressed in terms of connected (excursion) sets of voxels above some threshold, under the null hypothesis of no activation. This is not the expected number of false-positive voxels. One false-positive region may contain hundreds of voxels, if the SPM is very smooth. A Bonferroni correction would control the expected number of false-positive *voxels,* whereas GRF theory controls the expected number of false-positive *regions.* Because a false-positive region can contain many voxels the corrected threshold under a GRF correction is much lower, rendering it much more sensitive. In fact, the number of voxels in a region is somewhat irrelevant because it is a function of smoothness. The GRF correction discounts voxel size by expressing the search volume in terms of smoothness or resolution elements *(resels)* (see Fig. 31.7). This intuitive perspective is expressed formally in terms of differential topology using the *Euler characteristic* (Worsley *et al.,* 1992). At high thresholds the Euler characteristic corresponds to the number of regions exceeding the threshold.

There are only two assumptions underlying the use of the GRF correction: (1) The error fields (but not necessarily the data) are a reasonable lattice approximation to an underlying random field with a multivariate Gaussian distribution, and (2) these fields are continuous, with a differentiable and invertible autocorrelation function. A common misconception is that the autocorrelation function has to be Gaussian. It does not. The only way in which these assumptions can be violated is if (1) the data are not smoothed (with or without subsampling to preserve resolution), violating the reasonable lattice assumption, or (2) the statistical model is misspecified so that the errors are not normally distributed. Early formulations of the GRF correction were based on the assumption that the spatial correlation structure was wide-sense stationary. This assumption can now be relaxed due to a revision of the way in which the smoothness estimator enters the correction procedure (Kiebel *et al.,* 1999). In other words, the corrections retain their validity, even if the smoothness varies from voxel to voxel.

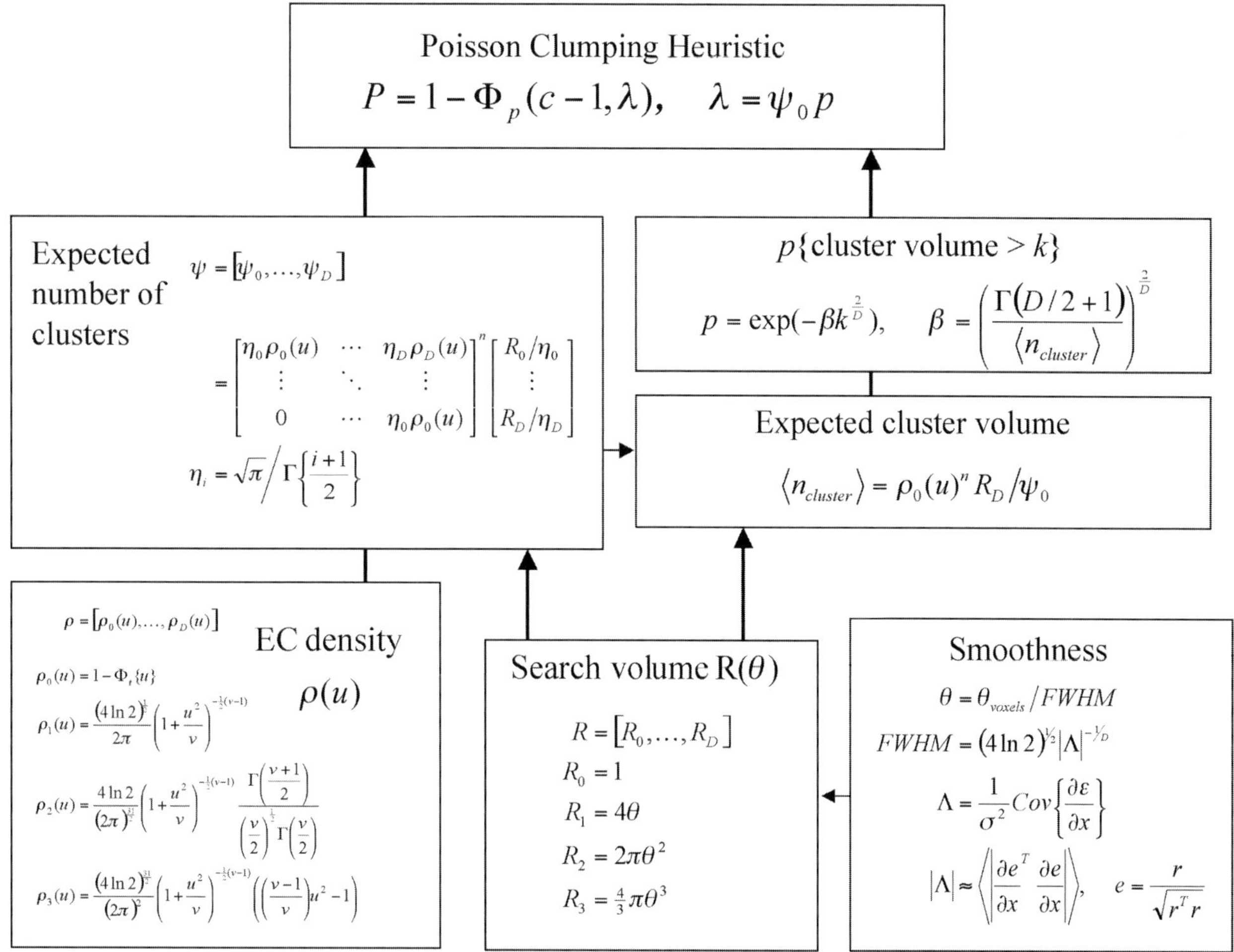

FIGURE 31.7
Schematic illustrating the use of random field theory in making inferences about SPMs. If one knows where to look exactly, then inference can be based on the value of the statistic at a specified location in the SPM, without correction. However, if one does not have an anatomical constraint *a priori,* then an adjustment for multiple dependent comparisons has to be made. These corrections are usually made using distributional approximations from GRF theory. This schematic deals with a general case of n SPM{T} whose voxels all survive a common threshold u (i.e., a conjunction of n component SPMs). The central probability, on which all voxel, cluster, or set-level inferences are made, is the probability P of getting c or more clusters with k or more resels (resolution elements) above this threshold. By assuming that clusters behave like a multidimensional Poisson point process (i.e., the Poisson clumping heuristic), P is simply determined. The distribution of c is Poisson with an expectation that corresponds to the product of the expected number of clusters, of any size, and the probability that any cluster will be bigger than k resels. The latter probability is shown using a form for a single Z-variate field constrained by the expected number of resels per cluster (<·> denotes expectation or average). The expected number of resels per cluster is simply the expected total number of resels divided by the expected number of clusters. The expected number of clusters is estimated with the Euler characteristic (EC) (effectively the number of blobs minus the number of holes). This estimate is, in turn, a function of the EC density for the statistic in question (with degrees of freedom v) and the resel counts. The EC density is the expected EC per unit of D-dimensional volume of the SPM where the D-dimensional volume of the search space is given by the corresponding element in the vector of resel counts. Resel counts can be thought of as a volume metric that has been normalised by the smoothness of the SPM component fields expressed in terms of the full width at half maximum (FWHM). This is estimated from the determinant of the variance-covariance matrix of the first spatial derivatives of e, the normalised residual fields r (from Fig. 31.4). In this example, equations for a sphere of radius θ are given, and Φ denotes the cumulative density function for the subscripted statistic in question.

Anatomically Closed Hypotheses

When making inferences about regional effects (e.g., activations) in SPMs, one often has some idea about where the activation should be. In this instance, a correction for the entire search volume is inappropriate. However, a problem remains in the sense that one would like to consider activations that are "near" the predicted location, even if they are not exactly coincident. One can adopt two approaches: (1) Prespecify a small search volume and make the appropriate GRF correction (Worsley *et al.,* 1996) or (2) use the uncorrected p value based on the spatial extent of the nearest cluster (Friston, 1997). This probability is based on getting the observed number of voxels, or more, in a given cluster (conditional on that cluster existing). Both of these procedures are based on distributional approximations from GRF theory.

Anatomically Open Hypotheses and Levels of Inference

To make inferences about regionally specific effects, the SPM is thresholded, using some height and spatial extent thresholds that are specified by the user. Corrected p values can then be derived that pertain to (1) the number of activated regions (i.e., number of clusters above the height and volume threshold), the *set-level inferences;* (2) the number of activated voxels (i.e., volume) comprising a particular region, the *cluster-level inferences;* and (3) the p value for each voxel within that cluster, the *voxel-level inferences.* These p values are corrected for the multiple dependent comparisons and are based on the probability of obtaining c, or more, clusters, with k, or more, voxels above a threshold u in an SPM of known or estimated smoothness. This probability has a reasonably simple form (see Fig. 31.7 for details).

Set level refers to the inference that the number of clusters comprising an observed activation profile is highly unlikely to have occurred by chance and is a statement about the activation profile, as characterised by its constituent regions. Cluster-level inferences are a special case of set-level inferences that occur when the number of clusters $c = 1$. Similarly, voxel-level inferences are special cases of cluster-level inferences that result when the cluster can be small (i.e., $k = 0$). Using a theoretical power analysis (Friston *et al.,* 1996b) of distributed activations, one observes that set-level inferences are generally more powerful than cluster-level inferences and that cluster-level inferences are generally more powerful than voxel-level inferences. The price paid for this increased sensitivity is reduced localising power. Voxel-level tests permit individual voxels to be identified as significant, whereas cluster- and set-level inferences only allow clusters or sets of clusters to be declared significant. Remember that these conclusions, about the relative power of different inference levels, are based on distributed activations. Focal activation may well be detected with greater sensitivity using voxel-level tests based on peak height. Typically, people use voxel-level inferences and a spatial extent threshold of zero. This reflects the fact that characterisations of functional anatomy are generally more useful when specified with a high degree of anatomical precision.

EXPERIMENTAL DESIGN

This section considers the different sorts of designs that can be employed in neuroimaging studies. Experimental designs can be classified as *single factor* or *multifactorial* designs; within this classification the levels of each factor can be *categorical* or *parametric.* We will start by discussing categorical and parametric designs and then deal with multifactorial designs.

Categorical Designs, Cognitive Subtraction, and Conjunctions

The tenet of cognitive subtraction is that the difference between two tasks can be formulated as a separable cognitive or sensorimotor component and that regionally specific differences in hemodynamic responses, evoked by the two tasks, identify the corresponding functionally specialised area. Early applications of subtraction range from the functional anatomy of word processing (Petersen *et al.,* 1989) to functional specialisation in extrastriate cortex (Lueck *et al.,* 1989). The latter studies involved presenting visual stimuli with and without some sensory attribute (e.g., color or motion). The areas highlighted by subtraction were identified with homologous areas in monkeys that showed selective electrophysiological responses to equivalent visual stimuli.

Cognitive conjunctions (Price and Friston, 1997) can be thought of as an extension of the subtraction technique, in the sense that they combine a series of subtractions. In subtraction one tests a *single* hypothesis pertaining to the activation in one task relative to another. In conjunction analyses *several* hypotheses are tested, asking whether all the activations, in a series of task pairs, are jointly significant. Consider the problem of identifying regionally specific activations due to a particular cognitive component (e.g., object recognition). If one can identify a series of task pairs whose differences have only that component in common, then the region that is activated, in all corresponding subtractions, can be associated with the common component. Conjunction analyses allow one to demonstrate the context-invariant nature of regional responses. One important application of conjunction analyses is in multisubject fMRI studies, where generic effects are identified as those that are conjointly significant in all the subjects studied (see below).

Parametric Designs

The premise behind parametric designs is that regional physiology will vary systematically with the degree of cognitive or sensorimotor processing or deficits thereof. Examples of this approach include the PET experiments of Grafton *et al.* (1992), which demonstrated significant correlations between hemodynamic responses and the performance of a visually guided motor tracking task. On the sensory side Price *et al.* (1992) demonstrated a remarkable linear relationship between perfusion in peri-auditory regions and frequency of aural word presentation. This correlation was not observed in Wernicke's area, where perfusion appeared to correlate, not with the discriminative attributes of the stimulus, but with the presence or absence of semantic content. These relationships or *neurometric functions* may be linear or nonlinear. Using polynomial regression, in the context of the GLM, one can identify nonlinear relationships between stimulus parameters (e.g., stimulus duration or presentation rate) and evoked responses. To do this one usually uses a SPM{F} (see Büchel *et al.,* 1996).

The example provided in Fig. 31.8 illustrates both categorical and parametric aspects of design and analysis. These data were obtained from a fMRI study of visual motion processing using radially moving dots. The stimuli were presented over a range of speeds using *isoluminant* and *isochromatic* stimuli. To identify areas involved in visual motion, a stationary dots condition was subtracted from the moving dots conditions (see the contrast weights on the upper right). To ensure significant motion-sensitive responses, using both color and luminance cues, a conjunction of the equivalent subtractions was assessed under both viewing contexts. Areas V5 and V3a are seen in the ensuing SPM{T}. The T values in this SPM are simply the minimum of the T values for each subtraction. Thresholding this SPM{T_{min}} ensures that all voxels survive the threshold u in each subtraction separately. This *conjunction* SPM has an equivalent interpretation; it represents the intersection of the excursion sets, defined by the threshold u, of each *component* SPM. This intersection is the essence of a conjunction. The expressions in Fig. 31.7 pertain to the general case of the minimum of n T values. The special case where n = 1 corresponds to a conventional SPM{T}.

The responses in left V5 are shown in the lower panel of Fig. 31.8 and speak to a compelling inverted "U" relationship between speed and evoked response that peaks at around 8 degrees per second. It is this sort of relationship that parametric designs try to characterise. Interestingly, the form of these speed-dependent responses was similar using both stimulus types, although luminance cues are seen to elicit a greater response. From the point of view of a factorial design there is a *main effect* of cue (isoluminant vs. isochromatic), a main (nonlinear) effect of speed, but no speed by cue *interaction.*

Clinical neuroscience studies can use parametric designs by looking for the neuronal correlates of clinical (e.g., symptom) ratings over subjects. In many cases multiple clinical scores are available for each subject and the statistical design can usually be seen as a multilinear regression. In situations where the clinical scores are correlated, principal component analysis or factor analysis is sometimes applied to generate a new, and smaller, set of explanatory variables that are orthogonal to each other. This has proved particularly useful in psychiatric studies where syndromes can be expressed over a number of different dimensions (e.g., the degree of psychomotor poverty, disorganisation and reality distortion in schizophrenia; see Liddle *et al.,* 1992). In this way, regionally specific correlates of various symptoms may point to their distinct pathogenesis in a way that transcends the syndrome itself. For example, psychomotor poverty may be associated with left dorsolateral prefrontal dysfunction irrespective of whether the patient is suffering from schizophrenia or depression.

Multifactorial Designs

Factorial designs are becoming more prevalent than single-factor designs because they enable inferences about interactions. At its simplest an interaction represents a change in a change. Interactions are associated with factorial designs where two or more factors are combined in the

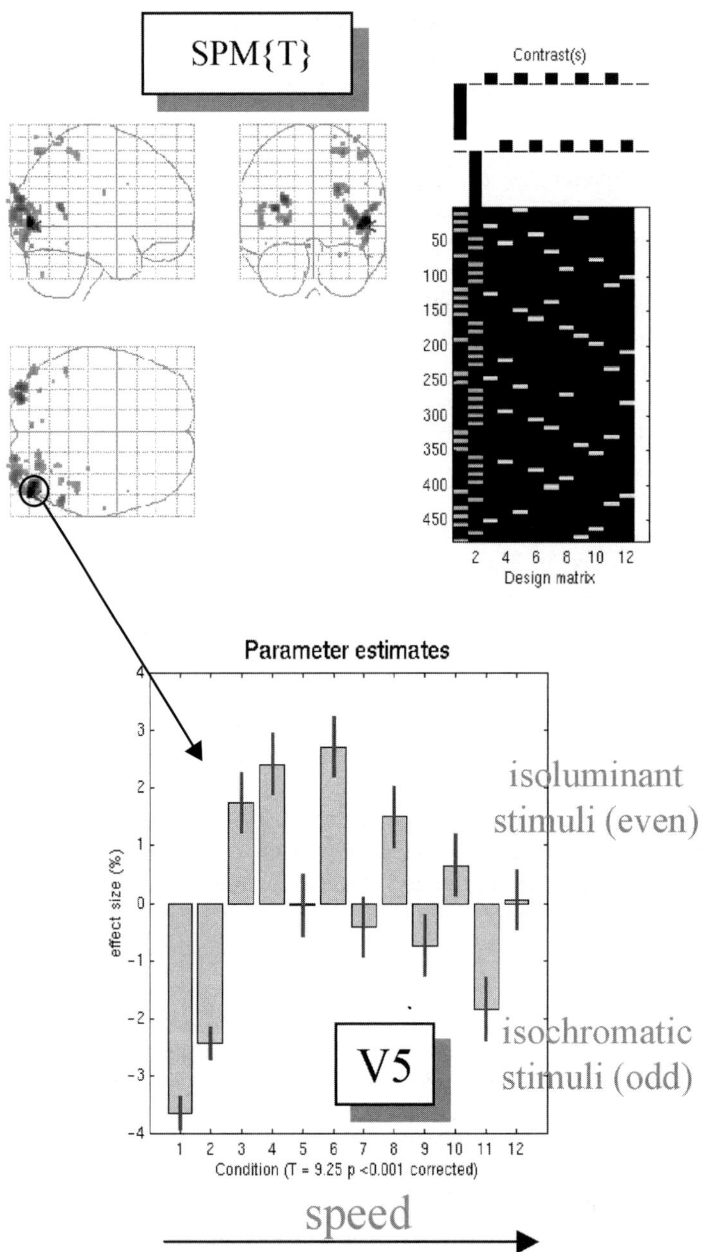

FIGURE 31.8
(Top right) Design matrix. This is an image representation of the design matrix. Contrasts: These are the vectors of contrast weights defining the linear compounds of parameters tested. The contrast weights are displayed over the column of the design matrix that corresponds to the effects in question. The design matrix here includes condition-specific effects (boxcars convolved with a hemodynamic response function). Odd columns correspond to stimuli shown under isochromatic conditions and even columns model responses to isoluminant stimuli. The first two columns are for stationary stimuli, and the remaining columns are for conditions of increasing speed. The final column is a constant term. (Top left) SPM{T}. This is a maximum intensity projection of the SPM{T} conforming to the standard anatomical space of Talairach and Tournoux (1988). The T values here are the minimum T values from both contrasts, thresholded at $p = 0.001$ uncorrected. The most significant conjunction is seen in left V5. (Lower panel) Plot of the condition-specific parameter estimates for this voxel. The T value was 9.25 ($p < 0.001$ corrected; see Fig. 7).

same experiment. The effect of one factor, on the effect of the other, is assessed by the interaction term. Factorial designs have a wide range of applications. An early application in neuroimaging examined physiological adaptation and plasticity during motor performance by assessing time by condition interactions (Friston *et al.,* 1992a). Psychopharmacological activation studies are further examples of factorial designs (Friston *et al.,* 1992b). In these studies cognitively evoked responses are assessed before and after being given a drug. The interaction term reflects the

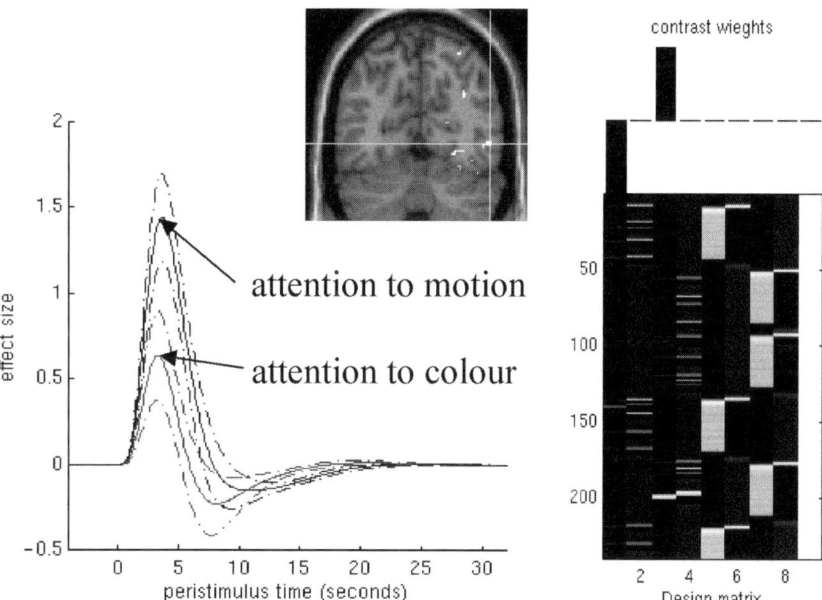

FIGURE 31.9
Results showing how to assess an interaction using an event-related design. Subjects viewed stationary monochromatic stimuli that occasionally changed color and moved at the same time. These compound events were presented under two levels of attentional set (attention to color and attention to motion). The event-related responses are modeled, in an attention-specific fashion, by the first four regressors (delta functions convolved with a hemodynamic response function and its derivative) in the design matrix on the right. The simple main effects of attention are modeled as similarly convolved boxcars. The interaction between attentional set and visually evoked responses is simply the difference in evoked responses under both levels of attention and is tested for with the appropriate contrast weights (upper right). Only the first 256 rows of the design matrix are shown. The most significant modulation of evoked responses, under attention to motion, was seen in left V5 (insert). The fitted responses and their standard errors are shown on the left as functions of peristimulus time.

pharmacological modulation of task-dependent activations. Factorial designs have an important role in the context of cognitive subtraction and additive factors logic by virtue of being able to test for interactions or context-sensitive activations (i.e., to demonstrate the fallacy of "pure insertion"; see Friston *et al.,* 1996c). These interaction effects can sometimes be interpreted as (1) the integration of the two or more (cognitive) processes or (2) the modulation of one (perceptual) process by another. See Fig. 31.9 for an example. From the point of view of clinical studies, interactions are central. The effect of a disease process on sensorimotor or cognitive activation is simply an interaction and involves replicating a subtraction experiment in subjects with and without the pathophysiology studied. Factorial designs can also embody parametric factors. If one of the factors has a number of parametric levels, the interaction can be expressed as a difference in regression slope of regional activity on the parameter, under both levels of the other (categorical) factor. An important example of factorial designs, which mix categorical and parameter factors, is those looking for *psychophysiological interactions.* Here the parametric factor is brain activity measured in a particular brain region. These designs have proven useful in looking at the interaction between bottom-up and top-down influences within processing hierarchies in the brain (Friston *et al.,* 1997). This issue will be addressed below and in Section 4, from the point of view of effective connectivity.

DESIGNING fMRI STUDIES (Chapter 40, Analysis of fMRI Time Series)

In this section we consider fMRI time series from a signal processing perspective with particular focus on optimal experimental design and efficiency. fMRI time series can be viewed as a linear admixture of signal and noise. The signal corresponds to neuronally mediated hemodynamic changes that can be modeled as a nonlinear convolution of some underlying neuronal process, responding to changes in experimental factors, by a HRF. Noise has many contributions that render it rather complicated in relation to other neurophysiological measurements. These include neuronal and non-neuronal sources. Neuronal noise refers to a neurogenic signal not modeled by the explanatory variables and has the same frequency structure as the signal itself. Non-neuronal components have both white (e.g., R. F. Johnson noise) and colored components (e.g., pulsatile motion of the brain caused by cardiac cycles and local modulation of the static magnetic field B_0 by respiratory movement). These effects are typically low frequency or wideband (e.g., aliased cardiac-locked pulsatile motion). The superposition of all components induces temporal correlations among the error terms (denoted by Σ in Fig. 31.4) that can effect sensitivity to experimental effects. Sensitivity depends on (1) the relative amounts of signal and noise and (2) the efficiency of the experimental design. Efficiency is simply a measure of how reliable the parameter estimates are and can be defined as the inverse of the variance of a contrast of parameter estimates (see Fig. 31.4). Two important considerations arise from this perspective on fMRI time series: The first pertains to optimal experimental design and the second to optimum deconvolution of the time series to obtain the most efficient parameter estimates.

Hemodynamic Response Function and Optimum Design

As noted above, an LTI model of neuronally mediated signals in fMRI suggests that only those experimentally induced signals that survive convolution with the HRF can be estimated with any efficiency. By convolution theorem the frequency structure of experimental variance should therefore be designed to match the transfer function of the HRF. The corresponding frequency profile of this transfer function is shown in Fig. 31.10, solid line). It is clear that frequencies around 0.03 Hz are optimal, corresponding to periodic designs with 32-sec periods (i.e., 16-sec epochs). Generally, the first objective of experimental design is to comply with the natural constraints imposed by the HRF and ensure that experimental variance occupies these intermediate frequencies.

Serial Correlations and Filtering

This is quite a complicated but important area. Conventional signal processing approaches dictate that whitening the data engenders the most efficient parameter estimation. This corresponds to filtering with a convolution matrix S (see Fig. 31.3) that is the inverse of the intrinsic convolution matrix K ($KK^T = \Sigma$). This *whitening strategy* renders the least-squares estimator in Fig. 31.4 equivalent to the ML or Gauss-Markov estimator. However, one generally does not know the form of the intrinsic correlations, which means they have to be estimated. This estimation usually proceeds using a restricted maximum likelihood (ReML) estimate of the serial correlations, among the residuals, that properly accommodates the effects of the residual-forming matrix and associated loss of degrees of freedom. However, using this estimate of the intrinsic nonsphericity to form a Gauss-Markov estimator at each voxel is not easy. First, the estimate of nonsphericity can itself be imprecise, leading to bias in the standard error (Friston *et al.,* 2000b). Second, ReML estimation requires a computationally prohibitive iterative procedure at every voxel. There are a number of approaches to these problems that aim to increase the efficiency of the estimation and reduce the computational burden. The approach adopted in current versions of our software is to use ReML estimates based on all voxels that respond to experimental manipulation. This affords very efficient hyperparameter estimates[3] and, furthermore, allows one to use the same matrices at each voxel when computing the parameter estimates.

Although we usually make $S = \Sigma^{-1/2} = K^{-1}$, using a first pass ReML estimate of the serial correlations, we will deal with the simpler and more general case where S can take any form. In this case the parameter estimates are *generalised* least-squares (GLS) estimators. The GLS estimator is unbiased and, luckily, is identical to the Gauss-Markov estimator if the regressors in the design matrix are periodic.[4] After GLS estimation, the ReML estimate of $V = S\Sigma S^T$ enters into the expressions for the standard error and degrees of freedom provided in Fig. 31.4.

[3] The efficiency scales with the number of voxels.

[4] More exactly, the GLS and ML estimators are the same if X lies within the space spanned by the eigenvectors of the Toeplitz autocorrelation matrix Σ.

$$y(t) = x(t) \otimes f(t)$$

by convolution theorem

$$g_y(\omega) = g_f(\omega) g_x(\omega)$$

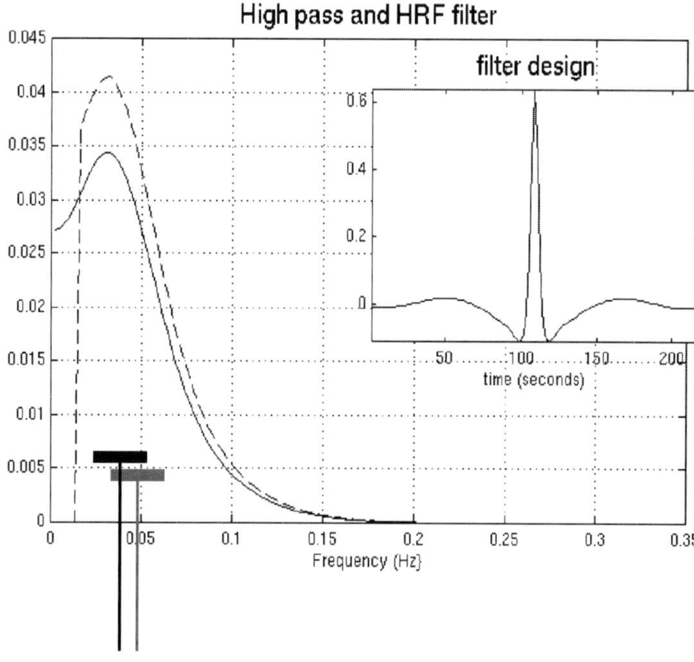

FIGURE 31.10
Modulation transfer function of a canonical HRF, with (broken line) and without (solid line) the application of a high-pass filter. This transfer function corresponds to the spectral density of a white noise process after convolution with the HRF and places constraints on the frequencies that survive convolution with the HRF. This follows from convolution theorem (summarised in the equations). The insert is the filter expressed in time, corresponding to the spectral density that is obtained after convolution with the HRF and high-pass filtering.

fMRI noise has been variously characterised as a $1/f$ process (Zarahn *et al.,* 1997) or an autoregressive process (Bullmore *et al.,* 1996) with white noise (Purdon and Weisskoff, 1998). Irrespective of the exact form these serial correlations take, treating low-frequency drifts as fixed effects can finesse the hyperparameterisation of serial correlations. Removing low frequencies from the time series allows the model to fit serial correlations over a more restricted frequency range or shorter time spans. Drift removal can be implemented by including drift terms in the design matrix or by including the implicit residual forming matrix in S to make it a high-pass filter. An example of a high-pass filter with a high-pass cutoff of 1/64 Hz is shown in the inset of Fig. 31.8. This filter's transfer function (the broken line in the main panel) illustrates the frequency structure of neurogenic signals after high-pass filtering.

Spatially Coherent Confounds and Global Normalisation

Implicit in the use of high-pass filtering is the removal of low-frequency components that can be regarded as confounds. Other important confounds are signal components that are artifactual or have no regional specificity. These are referred to as *global confounds* and have a number of causes. These can be divided into physiological (e.g., global perfusion changes in PET, mediated by changes in pCO_2) and nonphysiological (e.g., transmitter power calibration, B_1 coil profile and receiver gain in fMRI). The latter generally scale the signal before the MRI sampling process. Other nonphysiological effects may have a nonscaling effect (e.g., Nyquist ghosting, movement-related effects). In PET it is generally accepted that regional changes in rCBF, evoked neuronally, mix additively with global changes to give the measured signal. This calls for a global normalisation procedure in which the global estimator enters into the statistical model as a confound. In fMRI, instrumentation effects that scale the data motivate a global normalisation by proportional scaling, using the whole brain mean, before the data enter into the statistical model.

It is important to differentiate between global confounds and their estimators. By definition the global mean over intracranial voxels will subsume all regionally specific effects. This means that the global estimator may be partially collinear with effects of interest, especially if the evoked responses are substantial and widespread. In these situations global normalisation may induce apparent deactivations in regions *not* expressing a physiological response. These are not artifacts in the sense that they are real, relative to global changes, but they have little face validity in terms of the underlying neurophysiology. In instances where regionally specific effects bias the global estimator, some investigators prefer to omit global normalisation. Provided drift terms are removed from the time series, this is generally acceptable because most global effects have slow time constants. However, the issue of normalisation-induced deactivations is better circumnavigated with experimental designs that use well-controlled conditions, which elicit differential responses in restricted brain systems.

Nonlinear System Identification Approaches

So far we have only considered LTI models and first-order HRFs. Another signal processing perspective is provided by nonlinear system identification (Vazquez and Noll, 1998). This section considers nonlinear models as a prelude to the next subsection on event-related fMRI, where nonlinear interactions among evoked responses provide constraints for experimental design and analysis. We have described an approach to characterising evoked hemodynamic responses in fMRI based on nonlinear system identification, in particular the use of *Volterra series* (Friston *et al.,* 1998a). This approach enables one to estimate Volterra kernels that describe the relationship between stimulus presentation and the hemodynamic responses that ensue. Volterra series are essentially high-order extensions of linear convolution models. These kernels, therefore, represent a nonlinear characterisation of the HRF that can model the responses to stimuli in different contexts and interactions among stimuli. In fMRI, the kernel coefficients can be estimated by (1) using a second-order approximation to the Volterra series to formulate the problem in terms of a general linear model and (2) expanding the kernels in terms of temporal basis functions. This allows the use of the standard techniques described above to estimate the kernels and to make inferences about their significance on a voxel-specific basis using SPMs.

One important manifestation of the nonlinear effects, captured by the second-order kernels, is a modulation of stimulus-specific responses by preceding stimuli that are proximate in time. This means that responses at high stimulus presentation rates saturate and, in some instances, show an inverted U behaviour. This behaviour appears to be specific to BOLD effects (as distinct from evoked changes in cerebral blood flow) and may represent a *hemodynamic refractoriness.* This effect has important implications for event-related fMRI, in which one may want to present trials in quick succession.

The results of a typical nonlinear analysis are given in Fig. 31.11. The results in the right panel represent the average response, integrated over a 32-sec train of stimuli as a function of stimulus onset asynchrony (SOA) within that train. These responses are based on the kernel estimates (left-hand panels) using data from a voxel in the left posterior temporal region of a subject obtained during the presentation of single words at different rates. The solid line represents the estimated response and shows a clear maximum at just less than 1 sec. The dots are responses based on empirical data from the same experiment. The broken line shows the expected response in the absence of nonlinear effects (i.e., that predicted by setting the second-order kernel to zero). It is clear that nonlinearities become important at around 2 sec, leading to an actual diminution of the integrated response at sub-second SOAs. The implication of this sort

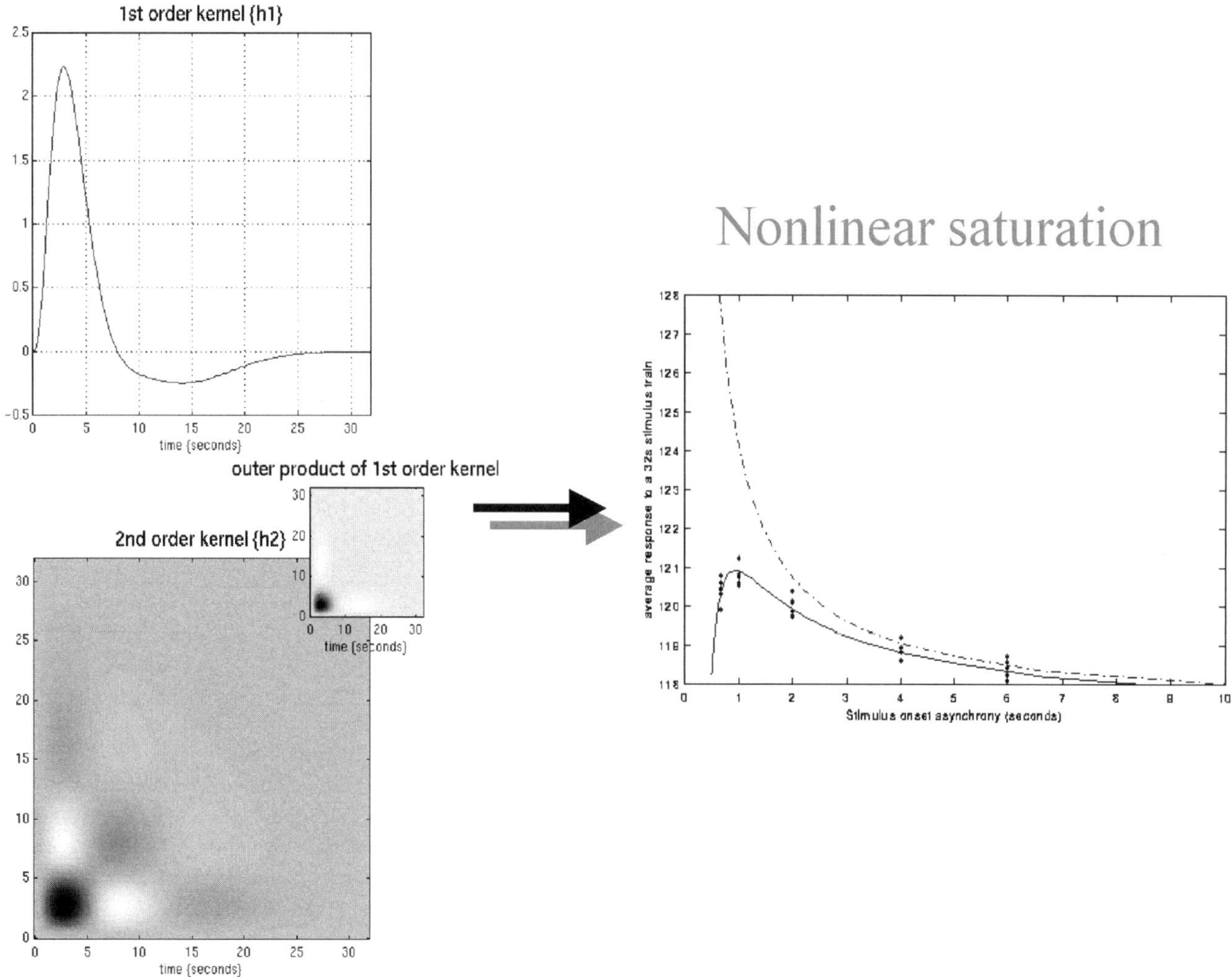

FIGURE 31.11
(Left). Volterra kernels from a voxel in the left superior temporal gyrus at –56, –28, and 12 mm. These kernel estimates were based on a single subject study of aural word presentation at different rates (from 0 to 90 words per minute) using a second-order approximation to a Volterra series expansion modelling the observed hemodynamic response to stimulus input (a delta function for each word). These kernels can be thought of as a characterisation of the second-order hemodynamic response function. The first-order kernel κ_1 (upper panel) represents the first-order component usually presented in linear analyses. The second-order kernel (lower panel) is presented in image format. The color scale is arbitrary; white is positive and black is negative. The insert on the right represents $\kappa_1\kappa_1^T$, the second-order kernel that would be predicted by a simple model that involved linear convolution with κ_1 followed by some static nonlinearity. (Right) Integrated responses over a 32-sec stimulus train as a function of SOA. Solid line: Estimates based on the nonlinear convolution model parameterised by the kernels on the left. Broken line: The responses expected in the absence of second-order effects (i.e., in a truly linear system). Dots: Empirical averages based on the presentation of actual stimulus trains.

of result is that (1) SOAs should not really fall much below 1 sec and (2) at short SOAs the assumptions of linearity are violated. Note that these data pertain to single word processing in auditory association cortex. More linear behaviours may be expressed in primary sensory cortex where the feasibility of using minimum SOAs as low as 500 ms has been demonstrated (Burock *et al.,* 1998). This lower bound on SOA is important because some effects are detected more efficiently with high presentation rates. We now consider this from the point of view of event-related designs.

Event and Epoch-Related Designs

A crucial distinction, in experimental designs for fMRI, is that between *epoch-* and *event-*related designs. In SPECT and PET only epoch-related responses can be assessed because of the relatively long half-life of the radiotracers used. However, in fMRI we have an opportunity to measure event-related responses that may be important in some cognitive and clinical contexts. An important issue in event-related fMRI is the choice of interstimulus interval or more precisely SOA. The SOA, or the distribution of SOAs, is a critical factor and is chosen, subject to psychological or psychophysical constraints, to maximise the efficiency of response estimation. The constraints on the SOA clearly depend on the nature of the experiment but are generally satisfied when the SOA is small and derives from a random distribution. Rapid presentation rates allow for the maintenance of a particular cognitive or attentional set, decrease the latitude that the subject has for engaging alternative strategies or incidental processing, and allows the integration of event-related paradigms using fMRI and electrophysiology. Random SOAs ensure that preparatory or anticipatory factors do not confound event-related responses and ensure a uniform context in which events are presented. These constraints speak to the well-documented advantages of event-related fMRI over conventional blocked designs (Buckner *et al.,* 1996; Clark *et al.,* 1998).

To compare the efficiency of different designs it is useful to have some common framework that encompasses all of them. The efficiency can then be examined in relation to the parameters of the designs. Designs can be *stochastic* or *deterministic* depending on whether there is a random element to their specification. In stochastic designs (Heid *et al.,* 1997) one needs to specify the probabilities of an event occurring at all times those events could actually occur. In deterministic designs the occurrence probability is unity and the design is completely specified by the times of stimulus presentation or trials. The distinction between stochastic and deterministic designs pertains to how a particular realisation or stimulus sequence is created. The efficiency afforded by a particular event sequence is a function of the event sequence itself, and not of the process generating the sequence (i.e., deterministic or stochastic). However, within stochastic designs, the design matrix X, and associated efficiency, are random variables and the *expected* or average efficiency over realisations of X is easily computed.

In the framework considered here (Friston *et al.,* 1999a) the occurrence probability p of any event occurring is specified at each time that it could occur (i.e., every SOA). Here p is a vector with an element for every SOA. This formulation engenders the distinction between *stationary* stochastic designs, where the occurrence probabilities are constant, and *nonstationary* stochastic designs, where they change over time. For deterministic designs the elements of p are 0 or 1, the presence of a 1 denoting the occurrence of an event. An example of p might be the boxcars used in conventional block designs. Stochastic designs correspond to a vector of identical values and are therefore stationary in nature. Stochastic designs with temporal modulation of occurrence probability have time-dependent probabilities varying between 0 and 1. With these probabilities the expected design matrices and expected efficiencies can be computed. A useful thing about this formulation is that by setting the mean of the probabilities p to a constant, one can compare different deterministic and stochastic designs given the same number of events. Some common examples are given in Fig. 31.12 (right panel) for an SOA of 1 sec and 32 expected events or trials over a 64-sec period (except for the first deterministic example with 4 events and an SOA of 16 sec). We can see that the least efficient is the sparse deterministic design (despite the fact that the SOA is roughly optimal for this class), whereas the most efficient is a block design. A slow modulation of occurrence probabilities gives high efficiency whilst retaining the advantages of stochastic designs and may represent a useful compromise between the high efficiency of block designs and the psychological benefits and latitude afforded by stochastic designs. However, it is important not to generalise these conclusions too far. An efficient design for one effect may not be optimum for another, even within the same experiment. This can be illustrated by comparing the efficiency with which evoked responses are detected and the efficiency of detecting the difference in evoked responses elicited by two sorts of trials, as discussed next.

Consider a stationary stochastic design with two trial types. Because the design is stationary the vector of occurrence probabilities for each trial type is specified by a single probability. Let us assume that the two trial types occur with the same probability $\mathbf{p}$. By varying $\mathbf{p}$ and SOA, one can find the most efficient design depending on whether one is looking for evoked responses per se or differences among evoked responses. These two situations are depicted in the left panels of Fig. 31.12. It is immediately apparent that, for both sorts of effects, very small SOAs are optimal. However, the optimal occurrence probabilities are not the same. More infrequent events (corresponding to a smaller $\mathbf{p} = 1/3$) are required to estimate efficiently the responses themselves.

$$X = SB$$

$$1/\text{Efficiency} \propto c^T \left\langle X^T X \right\rangle^{-1} c$$

$$\left\langle X^T X \right\rangle = \left\langle B^T S^T SB \right\rangle = p^T (S^T S - 1)p + diag(p)$$

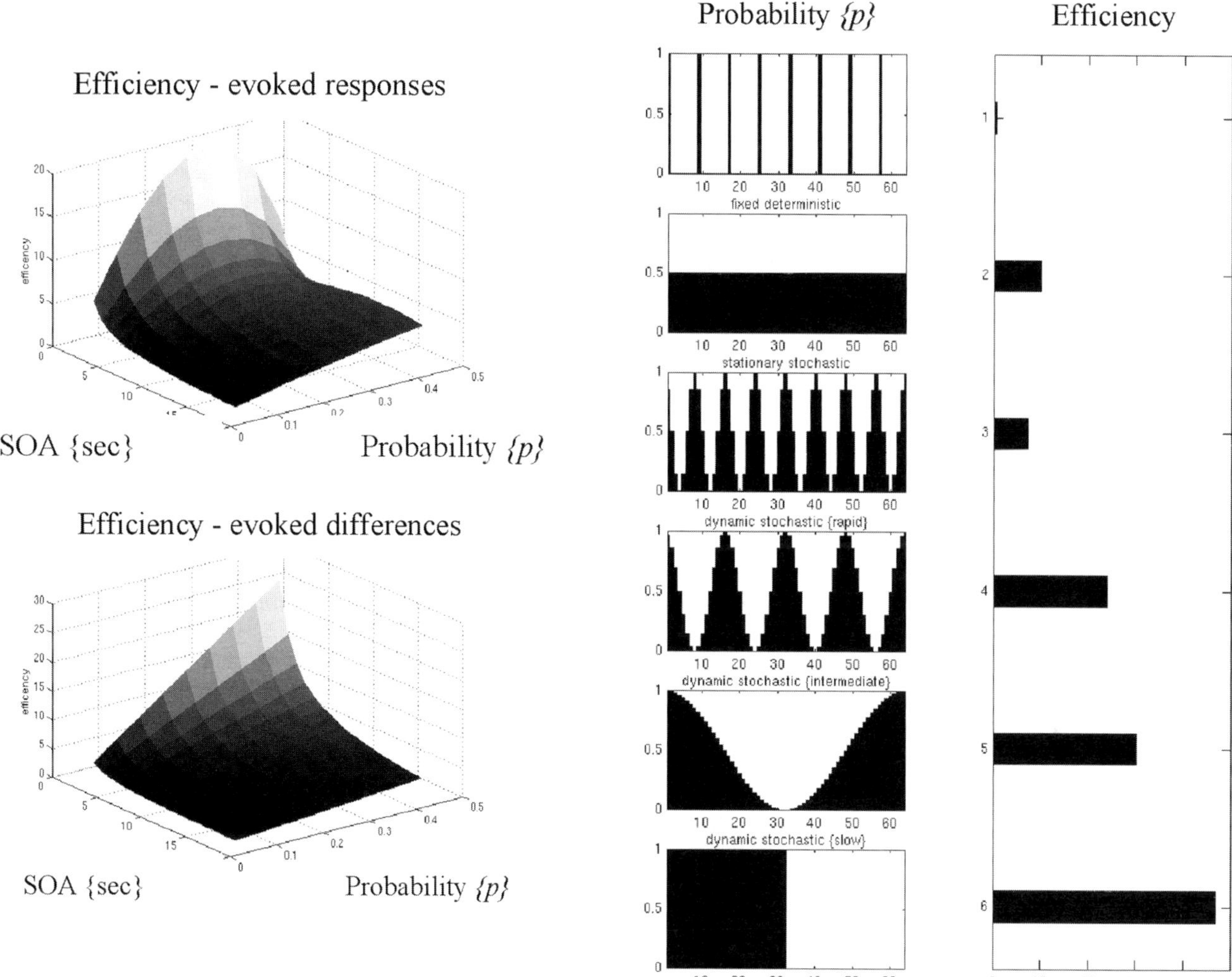

FIGURE 31.12
Efficiency as a function of occurrence probabilities p for a model X formed by postmultiplying S (a matrix containing n columns, modelling n possible event-related responses every SOA) by B, where B is a random binary vector that determines whether the nth response is included in X or not, where $\langle B \rangle = p$. (Right) A comparison of some common designs. A graphical representation of the occurrence probabilities p expressed as a function of time (seconds) is shown on the left and the corresponding efficiency is shown on the right. These results assume a minimum SOA of 1 sec, a time series of 64 sec, and a single trial-type. The expected number of events was 32 in all cases (apart from the first). (Left) Efficiency in a stationary stochastic design with two event types both presented with probability p every SOA. The upper graph is for a contrast testing for the response evoked by one trial type, and the lower graph is for a contrast testing for differential responses.

This is equivalent to treating the baseline or control condition as any other condition (i.e., by including null events, with equal probability, as further event types). Conversely, if we are only interested in making inferences about the differences, one of the events plays the role of a null event and the most efficient design ensues when one or the other event occurs (i.e., $\mathbf{p} = 1/2$). In short, the most efficient designs obtain when the events subtending the differences of interest occur with equal probability.

Another example of how the efficiency is sensitive to the effect of interest is apparent when we consider different parameterisations of the HRF. This issue is sometimes addressed through distinguishing between the efficiency of response *detection* and response *estimation.* However, the principles are identical and the distinction reduces to how many parameters one uses to model the HRF for each trail type (one basis function is used for detection and a number are required to estimate the shape of the HRF). Here the contrasts may be the same but the shape of the regressors will change depending on the temporal basis set employed. The conclusions above were based on a single canonical HRF. Had we used a more refined parameterisation of the HRF, say, using three-basis functions, the most efficient design to estimate one basis function coefficient would not be the most efficient for another. This is most easily seen from the signal processing perspective in which basis functions with high-frequency structures (e.g., temporal derivatives) require the experimental variance to contain high-frequency components. For these basis functions, a randomised stochastic design may be more efficient than a deterministic block design, simply because the former embodies higher frequencies. In the limiting case of FIR estimation the regressors become a series of stick functions (see Fig. 31.6), all of which have high frequencies. This parameterisation of the HRF calls for high frequencies in the experimental variance. However, the use of FIR models is contraindicated by model selection procedures (see Chapter 40, Analysis of fMRI Time Series) that suggest only two or three HRF parameters can be estimated with any efficiency. Results that are reported in terms of FIRs should be treated with caution because the inferences about evoked responses are seldom based on the FIR parameter estimates. This is precisely because they are estimated inefficiently and contain little useful information.

INFERENCES ABOUT SUBJECTS AND POPULATIONS

In this section we consider some issues that are generic to brain mapping studies that have repeated measures or replications over subjects. The critical issue is whether we want to make an inference about the effect in relation to the *within-subject variability* or with respect to the *between-subject variability.* For a given group of subjects, there is a fundamental distinction between saying that the response is significant relative to the precision[5] with which that response in measured and saying that it is significant in relation to the intersubject variability. This distinction relates directly to the difference between *fixed-* and *random-effect* analyses. The following example tries to make this clear. Consider what would happen if we scanned six subjects during the performance of a task and baseline. We then construct a statistical model, in which task-specific effects are modelled separately for each subject. Unknown to us, only one of the subjects activated a particular brain region. When we examine the contrast of parameter estimates, assessing the mean activation over all subjects, we see that it is greater than zero by virtue of this subject's activation. Furthermore, because that model fits the data extremely well (modelling no activation in five subjects and a substantial activation in the sixth) the error variance, on a scan-to-scan basis, is small and the T statistic is very significant. Can we then say that the group shows an activation? On the one hand, we can say, quite properly, that the mean group response embodies an activation but clearly this does not constitute an inference that the group's response is significant (i.e., that this sample of subjects shows a consistent activation). The problem here is that we are using the *scan-to-scan* error variance and this is not necessarily appropriate for an inference about group responses. To make the inference that the group showed a significant activation, we would have to assess the variability in activation effects from *subject to subject* (using the contrast of parameter estimates for each subject). This variability now constitutes the proper error variance. In this example the variance of these six measurements would be large relative to their mean and the corresponding T statistic would not be significant.

The distinction between the two approaches above relates to how one computes the appropriate error variance. The first represents a fixed-effect analysis and the second a random-effect analysis (or more exactly a mixed-effects analysis). In the former the error variance is estimated on a scan-to-scan basis, assuming that each scan represents an independent observation (ignoring serial correlations). Here the degrees of freedom are essentially the number of scans (minus the

[5] Precision is the inverse of the variance

rank of the design matrix). Conversely, in random-effect analyses, the appropriate error variance is based on the activation from subject to subject where the effect per se constitutes an independent observation and the degrees of freedom fall dramatically to the number of subjects. The term *random effect* indicates that we have accommodated the randomness of differential responses by comparing the mean activation to the variability in activations from subject to subject. Both analyses are perfectly valid but only in relation to the inferences that are being made: Inferences based on fixed-effects analyses are about the particular subject(s) studied. Random-effects analyses are usually more conservative but allow the inference to be generalised to the population from which the subjects were selected.

Random-Effects Analysis (Chapter 42)

The implementation of random-effect analyses in SPM is fairly straightforward and involves taking the contrasts of parameters estimated from a *first-level* (fixed-effect) analysis and entering them into a *second-level* (random-effect) analysis. This ensures that there is only one observation (i.e., contrast) per subject in the second-level analysis and that the error variance is computed using the subject-to-subject variability of estimates from the first level. The nature of the inference made is determined by the contrasts entered into the second level (see Fig. 31.13). The

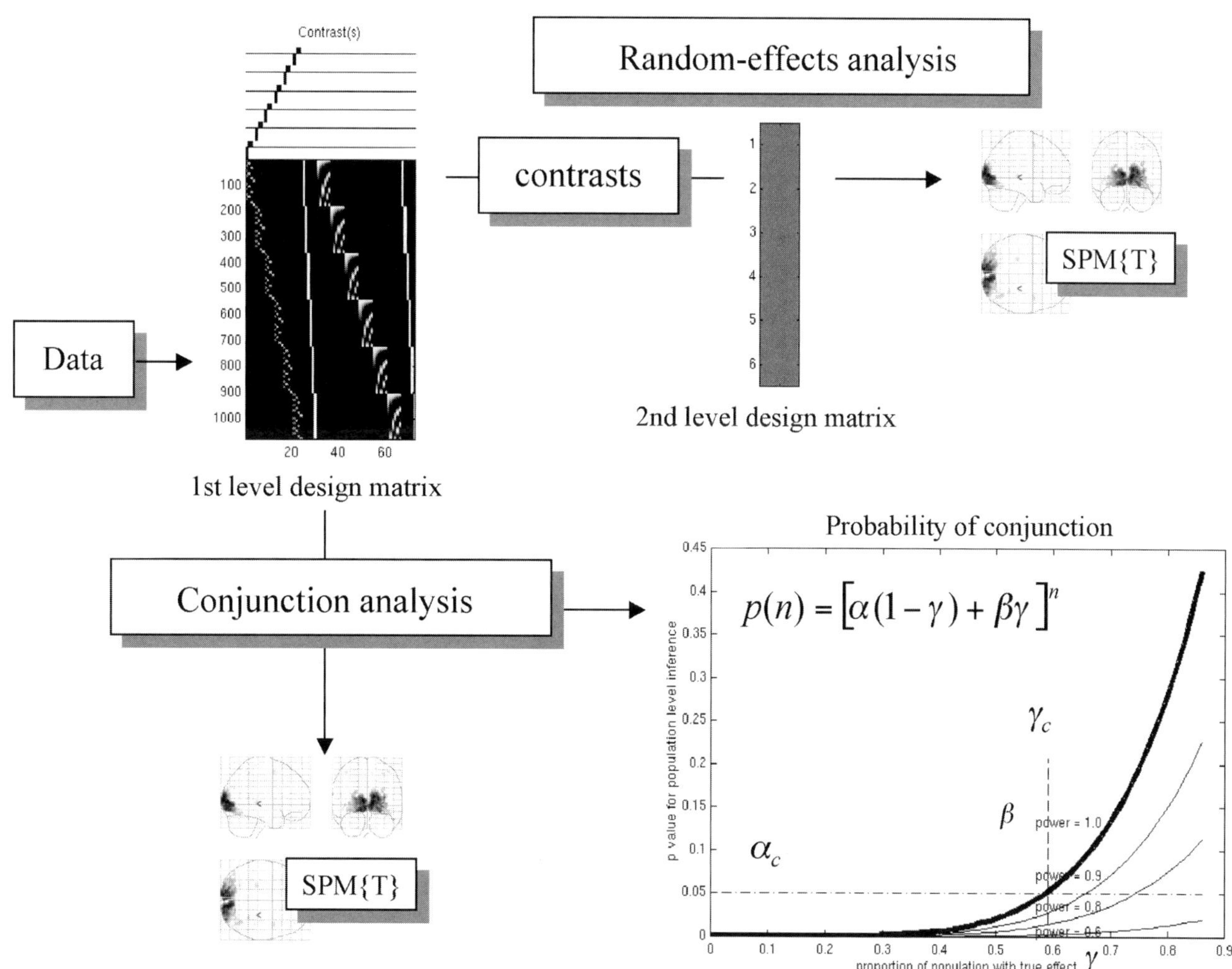

FIGURE 31.13
Schematic illustrating the implementation of random-effect and conjunction analyses for population inference. The lower right graph shows the probability $p(n)$ of obtaining a conjunction over n subjects, conditional on a certain proportion γ of the population expressing the effect, for a test with specificity of α = 0.05, at several sensitivities (β = 1, 0.9, 0.8, and 0.6). The broken lines denote the critical specificity for population inference α_c and the associated proportion of the population γ_c.

second-level design matrix simply tests the null hypothesis that the contrasts are zero (and is usually a column of ones, implementing a single sample T test).

The reason this multistage procedure emulates a full mixed-effects analysis, using a hierarchical observation model (see Chapter 43, Hierarchical Models), rests on the fact that the design matrices for each subject are the same (or sufficiently similar). In this special case, the estimator of the variance at the second level contains the right mixture of variance induced by observation error at the first level and between-subject error at the second. It is important to appreciate this because the efficiency of the design at the first level percolates to higher levels. It is therefore important to use efficient strategies at all levels in a hierarchical design.

Conjunction Analyses and Population Inferences

In some instances a fixed-effects analysis is more appropriate, particularly to facilitate the reporting of a series of single-case studies. Among these single cases it is natural to ask what are common features of functional anatomy (e.g., the location of V5) and what aspects are subject specific (e.g., the location of ocular dominance columns). One way to address commonalities is to use a conjunction analysis over subjects. It is important to understand the nature of the inference provided by conjunction analyses of this sort. Imagine that in 16 subjects the activation in V5, elicited by a motion stimulus, was greater than zero. The probability of this occurring by chance, in the same area, is extremely small and is the p value returned by a conjunction analysis using a threshold of $p = 0.5$ (T = 0) for each subject. This result constitutes evidence that V5 is involved in motion processing. However, note that this is not an assertion that each subject activated significantly. (We merely require the T value to be greater than zero for each subject.) In other words, a significant conjunction of activations is not synonymous with a conjunction of significant activations.

The motivations for conjunction analyses, in the context of multisubject studies, are twofold: (1) They provide an inference, in a fixed-effect analysis testing the null hypotheses of no activation in any of the subjects, that can be much more sensitive than testing for the average activation; and (2) they can be extended to make inferences about the population as described next.

If, for any given contrast, one can establish a conjunction of effects over n subjects using a test with a specificity of α and sensitivity β, the probability of this occurring by chance can be expressed as a function of γ, where γ is the proportion of the population that would have activated (see the equation in Fig. 31.13, lower right panel). This probability has an upper bound α_c corresponding to a critical proportion γ_c that is realised when (the generally unknown) sensitivity is one. In other words, under the null hypothesis that the proportion of the population evidencing this effect is less than or equal to γ_c, the probability of getting a conjunction over n subjects is equal to or less than α_c. In short, a conjunction allows one to say, with a specificity of α_c, that more than γ_c of the population shows the effect in question. Formally, we can view this analysis as a conservative $100\ (1 - \alpha_c)\%$ confidence region for the unknown parameter γ. These inferences can be construed as statements about how typical the effect is, without saying that it is necessarily present in every subject.

In practice, a conjunction analysis of a multisubject study comprises the following steps:

1. A design matrix is constructed in which the explanatory variables pertaining to each experimental condition are replicated for each subject. This subject-separable design matrix implicitly models subject by condition interactions (i.e., different condition-specific responses among sessions).
2. Contrasts are then specified that test for the effect of interest in each subject to give a series of SPM{T} that can be reported as a series of "single-case" studies in the usual way.
3. These SPM {T} are combined at a threshold u (corresponding to the specificity α in Fig. 31.13) to give a SPM{T_{min}} (i.e., conjunction SPM). The corrected p values associated with each voxel are computed as described in Fig. 31.7. These p values provide for inferences about effects that are common to the particular subjects studied. Because we have demonstrated regionally specific conjunctions, one can also proceed to make an inference about the population from which these subjects came using the confidence region approach described above (see Friston *et al.*, 1999b, for a fuller discussion).

FUNCTIONAL INTEGRATION (SECTION 4)

Functional and Effective Connectivity (Chapter 48, Functional Integration in the Brain)

Imaging neuroscience has firmly established functional specialisation as a principle of brain organisation in man. The integration of specialised areas has proven more difficult to assess. Functional integration is usually inferred on the basis of correlations among measurements of neuronal activity. Functional connectivity has been defined as statistical dependencies or correlations *among remote neurophysiological events.* However correlations can arise in a variety of ways. For example, in multiple-unit electrode recordings they can result from stimulus-locked transients evoked by a common input or reflect stimulus-induced oscillations mediated by synaptic connections (Gerstein and Perkel, 1969). Integration within a distributed system is usually better understood in terms of effective connectivity. Effective connectivity refers explicitly to *the influence that one neural system exerts over another,* either at a synaptic (i.e., synaptic efficacy) or population level. It has been proposed that "the [electrophysiological] notion of effective connectivity should be understood as the experiment- and time-dependent, simplest possible circuit diagram that would replicate the observed timing relationships between the recorded neurons" (Aertsen and Preißl, 1991). This speaks to two important points: (1) Effective connectivity is dynamic, i.e., activity and time dependent, and (2) it depends on a model of the interactions. The estimation procedures employed in functional neuroimaging can be classified as (1) those based on linear regression models (McIntosh and Gonzalez-Lima, 1994, Friston *et al.,* 1995d) or (2) those based on nonlinear dynamic models.

There is a necessary relationship between approaches to characterising functional integration and multivariate analyses because the latter are necessary to model interactions among brain regions. Multivariate approaches can be divided into those that are inferential in nature and those that are data led or exploratory. We will first consider multivariate approaches that are universally based on functional connectivity or covariance patterns (and are generally exploratory) and then turn to models of effective connectivity (which usually allow for some form of inference).

Eigenimage Analysis and Related Approaches (Chapter 49, Functional Connectivity)

Most analyses of covariances among brain regions are based on the singular value decomposition (SVD) of between-voxel covariances in a neuroimaging time series. Friston *et al.* (1993) introduced voxel-based principal component analysis (PCA) of neuroimaging time series to characterise distributed brain systems implicated in sensorimotor, perceptual, or cognitive processes. These distributed systems are identified with principal components or *eigenimages* that correspond to spatial modes of coherent brain activity. This approach represents one of the simplest multivariate characterisations of functional neuroimaging time series and falls into the class of exploratory analyses. Principal component or eigenimage analysis generally uses SVD to identify a set of orthogonal spatial modes that capture the greatest amount of variance expressed over time. As such, the ensuing modes embody the most prominent aspects of the variance-covariance structure of a given time series. Noting that covariance among brain regions is equivalent to functional connectivity renders eigenimage analysis particularly interesting because it was among the first ways of addressing functional integration (i.e., connectivity) with neuroimaging data. Subsequently, eigenimage analysis has been elaborated in a number of ways. Notable among these is canonical variate analysis (CVA) and multidimensional scaling (Friston *et al.,* 1996d,e). Canonical variate analysis was introduced in the context of MANCOVA (multiple analysis of covariance) and uses the generalised eigenvector solution to maximise the variance that can be explained by some explanatory variables relative to error. CVA can be thought of as an extension of eigenimage analysis that refers explicitly to some explanatory variables and allows for statistical inference.

In fMRI, eigenimage analysis (e.g., Sychra *et al.,* 1994) is generally used as an exploratory device to characterise coherent brain activity. These variance components may, or may not be, related to experimental design, and endogenous coherent dynamics have been observed in the motor system (Biswal *et al.,* 1995). Despite its exploratory power eigenimage analysis is fundamentally limited for two reasons. First, it offers only a linear decomposition of any set of neurophysiological measurements and, second, the particular set of eigenimages or spatial modes obtained is uniquely determined by constraints that are biologically implausible. These aspects of PCA confer inherent limitations on the interpretability and usefulness of eigenimage analysis of biological time series and have motivated the exploration of nonlinear PCA and neural network approaches (e.g., Mørch *et al.,* 1995).

Two other important approaches deserve mention here. The first is independent component analysis (ICA). ICA uses entropy maximisation to find, using iterative schemes, spatial modes or their dynamics that are approximately *independent.* This is a stronger requirement than *orthogonality* in PCA and involves removing high-order correlations among the modes (or dynamics). It was initially introduced as *spatial* ICA (McKeown *et al.,* 1998) in which the independence constraint was applied to the modes (with no constraints on their temporal expression). More recent approaches use, by analogy with magneto- and electrophysiological time-series analysis, *temporal* ICA, in which the dynamics are required to be independent. This requires an initial dimension reduction (usually using conventional eigenimage analysis). Finally, interest has been expressed in cluster analysis (Baumgartner *et al.,* 1997). Conceptually, this can be related to eigenimage analysis through multidimensional scaling and principal coordinate analysis. In cluster analysis voxels in a multidimensional scaling space are assigned belonging probabilities to a small number of clusters, thereby characterizing the temporal dynamics (in terms of the cluster centroids) and spatial modes (defined by the belonging probability for each cluster). These approaches eschew many of the unnatural constraints imposed by eigenimage analysis and can be a useful exploratory device.

Characterizing Nonlinear Coupling among Brain Areas (Chapters 50, Effective Connectivity)

Linear models of effective connectivity assume that the multiple inputs to a brain region are linearly separable. This assumption precludes activity-dependent connections that are expressed in one context and not in another. The resolution of this problem lies in adopting models that include interactions among inputs. These interactions or bilinear effects can be construed as a context- or activity-dependent modulation of the influence that one region exerts over another, where that context is instantiated by activity in further brain regions exerting modulatory effects. These nonlinearities can be introduced into structural equation modelling using so-called "moderator" variables that represent the interaction between two regions in causing activity in a third (Büchel and Friston, 1997). From the point of view of regression models, modulatory effects can be modeled with nonlinear input–output models and in particular the Volterra formulation described above. In this instance, the inputs are not stimuli but activities from other regions. Because the kernels are high order they embody interactions over time and among inputs and can be thought of as explicit measures of effective connectivity (see Fig. 31.14). An important thing about the Volterra formulation is that it has a high face validity and biological plausibility. The only thing it assumes is that the response of a region is some analytic nonlinear function of the inputs over the recent past. This function exists even for complicated dynamical systems with many unobservable state variables. Within these models, the influence of one region on another has two components: (1) the direct or *driving* influence of input from the first (e.g., hierarchically lower) region, irrespective of the activities elsewhere, and (2) an activity-dependent, *modulatory* component that represents an interaction with inputs from the remaining (e.g., hierarchically higher) regions. These are mediated by the first- and second-order kernels, respectively. The example provided in Fig. 31.15 addresses the modulation of visual cortical responses by attentional mechanisms (e.g., Treue and Maunsell, 1996) and the mediating role of activity-dependent changes in effective connectivity. The right panel in Fig. 31.15 shows a characterisation of this modulatory effect in terms of the increase in V5 responses to a simulated V2 input when posterior parietal activity is zero (broken line) and when it is high (solid line). The estimation of the Volterra kernels and statistical inference procedure is described in Friston and Büchel (2000).

The key thing about this example is that the most interesting thing is the change in effective connectivity from V2 to V5. Context-sensitive changes in effective connectivity transpire to be the most important aspect of functional integration and have two fundamental implications

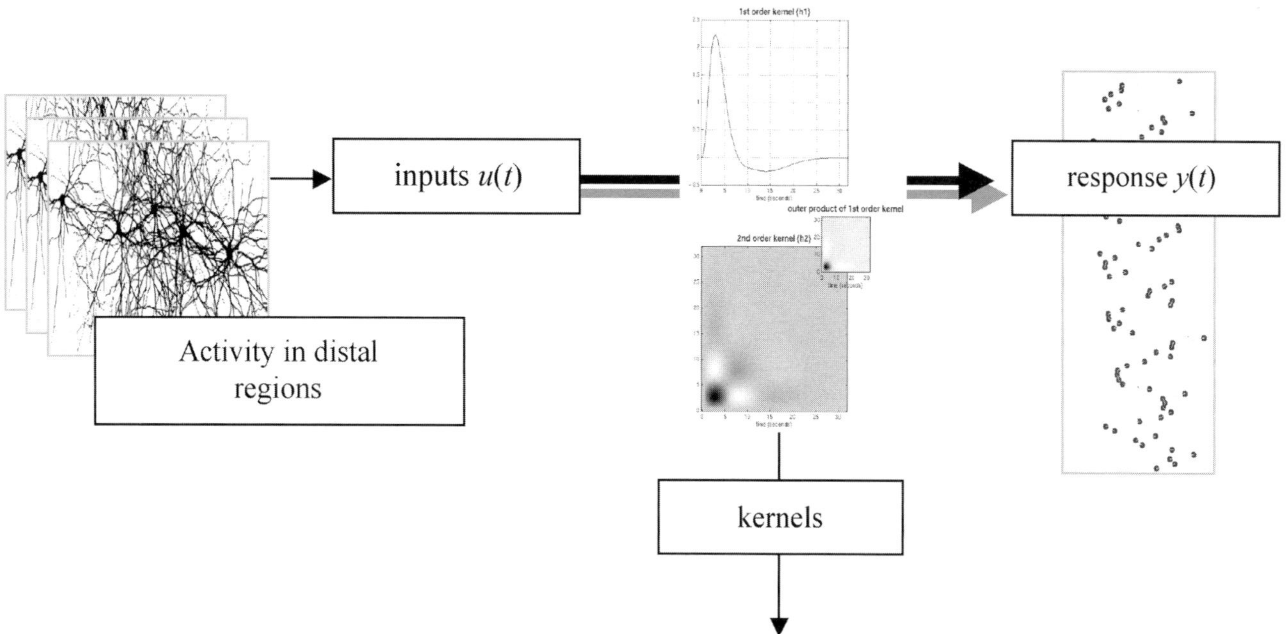

Volterra series a general nonlinear input-state-output characterization

$$y(t) = \kappa_0 + \sum_{i=1}^{\infty} \int_0^t \ldots \int_0^t \kappa_i(\sigma_1, \ldots \sigma_i) u(t-\sigma_1) \ldots u(t-\sigma_i) d\sigma_1 \ldots d\sigma_i$$

$$\kappa_i(\sigma_1) = \frac{\partial y(t)}{\partial u(t-\sigma_1)}, \qquad \kappa_2(\sigma_1, \sigma_2) = \frac{\partial^2 y(t)}{\partial u(t-\sigma_1) \partial u(t-\sigma_2)}, \qquad \ldots$$

FIGURE 31.14
Schematic depicting the causal relationship between the outputs and the recent history of the inputs to a nonlinear dynamical system, in this instance a brain region or voxel. This relationship can be expressed as a Volterra series, which expresses the response or output $y(t)$ as a nonlinear convolution of the inputs $u(t)$, critically without reference to any hidden state variables. This series is simply a functional Taylor expansion of $y(t)$ as a function of the inputs over the recent past. The term $\kappa_i(\sigma_1, \ldots, \sigma_i)$ represents the ith-order kernel. Volterra series have been described as "power series with memory" and are generally thought of as a high-order or "nonlinear" convolution of the inputs to provide an output. Volterra kernels are useful in characterizing the effective connectivity or influences that one neuronal system exerts over another because they represent the causal characteristics of the system in question. Neurobiologically they have a simple and compelling interpretation: *They are synonymous with effective connectivity.* It is evident that the first-order kernel embodies the response evoked by a change in input at $t - \sigma_1$. In other words it is a time-dependant measure of *driving* efficacy. Similarly the second-order kernel reflects the *modulatory* influence of the input at $t - \sigma_1$ on the evoked response at $t - \sigma_2$, and so on for higher orders.

for experimental design and analysis. First, experimental designs for analyses of effective connectivity are generally multifactorial. This is because one factor is needed to evoke responses and render the coupling among brain areas measurable and a second factor is required to induce changes in that coupling. The second implication is that models of effective connectivity should embrace changes in coupling. As will be seen in Section 4 these changes are usually modeled with *bilinear* terms or interactions. Bilinear terms appear in the simplest models of effective connectivity (e.g., psychophysiological interactions) through to nonlinear dynamic causal models (see Chapter 52, Dynamic Causal Modelling).

CONCLUSION

In this chapter we have reviewed the main components of image analysis and have touched briefly on ways of assessing functional integration in the brain. The key principles of functional specialisation and integration were used to motivate the various approaches considered. In the remaining chapters of this book we will revisit these procedures and disclose the details that underpin each component.

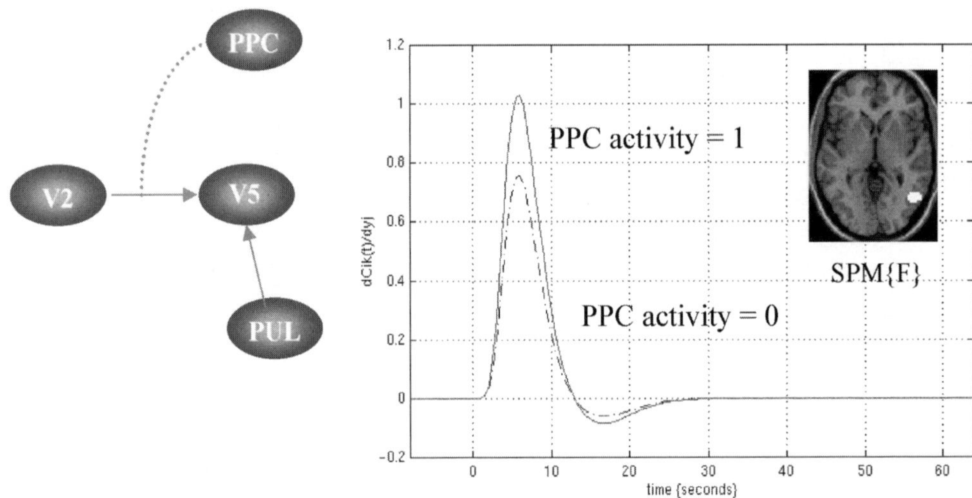

FIGURE 31.15
(Left) Brain regions and connections comprising an effective connectivity model formulated in terms of a Volterra series (see Fig. 31.14). (Right) Characterisation of the effects of V2 inputs on V5 and their modulation by posterior parietal cortex (PPC). The broken line represents estimates of V5 responses when PPC activity is zero, according to a second-order Volterra model of effective connectivity with inputs to V5 from V2, PPC, and the pulvinar (PUL). The solid curve represents the same response when PPC activity is one standard deviation of its variation over conditions. It is evident that V2 has an activating effect on V5 and that PPC increases the responsiveness of V5 to these inputs. In this study subjects were studied with fMRI under identical stimulus conditions (visual motion subtended by radially moving dots), whilst manipulating the attentional component of the task (detection of velocity changes). The insert shows all voxels in V5 that evidenced a modulatory effect ($p < 0.05$ uncorrected). These voxels were identified by thresholding a SPM{F} testing for the contribution of second-order kernels involving V2 and PPC while treating all other components as nuisance variables.

References

Absher, J. R., and Benson, D. F. (1993). Disconnection syndromes: an overview of Geschwind's contributions. *Neurology* **43,** 862–867.

Adler, R. J. (1981). In "The Geometry of Random Fields." Wiley, New York.

Aertsen, A., and Preißl, H. (1991). Dynamics of activity and connectivity in physiological neuronal Networks. In "Nonlinear Dynamics and Neuronal Networks," H. G. Schuster, ed., pp. 281–302. VCH Publishers, New York.

Aguirre, G. K., Zarahn, E., and D'Esposito, M. (1998). A critique of the use of the Kolmogorov-Smirnov (KS) statistic for the analysis of BOLD fMRI data. *Mag. Res. Med.* **39,** 500–505.

Andersson, J. L., Hutton, C., Ashburner, J., Turner, R., Friston, K. (2001). Modelling geometric deformations in EPI time series. *NeuroImage* **13,** 903–919.

Ashburner, J., and Friston, K. J. (1999). Nonlinear spatial normalisation using basis functions. *Hum Brain Mapping* **7,** 254–266.

Ashburner, J., and Friston, K. J. (2000). Voxel-based morphometry—the methods. *NeuroImage* **11,** 805–821.

Ashburner, J., Neelin, P., Collins, D. L., Evans, A., and Friston, K. (1997). Incorporating prior knowledge into image registration. *NeuroImage* **6,** 344–352.

Bandettini, P. A., Jesmanowicz, A., Wong, E. C., and Hyde, J. S. (1993). Processing strategies for time course data sets in functional MRI of the human brain. *Mag. Res. Med.* **30,** 161–173.

Baumgartner, R., Scarth, G., Teichtmeister, C., Somorjai, R., and Moser, E. (1997). Fuzzy clustering of gradient-echo functional MRI in the human visual cortex Part 1: reproducibility. *J. Mag. Res. Imaging* **7,** 1094–1101.

Biswal, B., Yetkin, F. Z., Haughton, V. M., and Hyde, J. S. (1995). Functional connectivity in the motor cortex of resting human brain using echo-planar MRI. *Mag. Res. Med.* **34,** 537–541.

Boynton, G. M., Engel, S. A., Glover, G. H., and Heeger, D. J. (1996). Linear systems analysis of functional magnetic resonance imaging in human V1. *J. Neurosci.* **16,** 4207–4221.

Büchel, C., and Friston, K. J. (1997). Modulation of connectivity in visual pathways by attention: cortical interactions evaluated with structural equation modelling and fMRI. *Cerebral Cortex* **7,** 768–778.

Büchel, C., Wise, R. J. S., Mummery, C. J., Poline, J.-B., and Friston, K. J. (1996). Nonlinear regression in parametric activation studies. *NeuroImage* **4,** 60–66.

Buckner, R., Bandettini, P., O'Craven, K., Savoy, R., Petersen, S., Raichle, M., and Rosen, B. (1996). Detection of cortical activation during averaged single trials of a cognitive task using functional magnetic resonance imaging. *Proc. Natl. Acad. Sci. USA* **93,** 14878–14883.

Bullmore, E. T., Brammer, M. J., Williams, S. C. R., Rabe-Hesketh, S., Janot, N., David, A., Mellers, J., Howard, R., and Sham, P. (1996). Statistical methods of estimation and inference for functional MR images. *Mag. Res. Med.* **35,** 261–277.

Burock, M. A., Buckner, R. L., Woldorff, M. G., Rosen, B. R., and Dale, A. M. (1998). Randomised event-related experimental designs allow for extremely rapid presentation rates using functional MRI. *NeuroReport* **9,** 3735–3739.

Buxton, R. B., and Frank, L. R. (1997). A model for the coupling between cerebral blood flow and oxygen metabolism during neural stimulation. *J. Cereb. Blood Flow Metab.* **17,** 64–72.

Clark, V. P., Maisog, J. M., and Haxby, J. V. (1998). fMRI study of face perception and memory using random stimulus sequences. *J. Neurophysiol.* **76,** 3257–3265.

Dale, A., and Buckner, R. (1997). Selective averaging of rapidly presented individual trials using fMRI. *Hum Brain Mapping* **5,** 329–340.

Friston, K. J. (1997). Testing for anatomical specified regional effects. *Hum. Brain Mapping* **5,** 133–136.

Friston, K. J., and Buchel, C. (2000). Attentional modulation of effective connectivity from V2 to V5/MT in humans. *Proc. Natl. Acad. Sci. USA* **97,** 7591–7596.

Friston, K. J., Frith, C. D., Liddle, P. F., and Frackowiak, R. S. J. (1991). Comparing functional (PET) images: the assessment of significant change. *J. Cereb. Blood Flow Metab.* **11,** 690–699.

Friston, K. J., Frith, C., Passingham, R. E., Liddle, P. F., and Frackowiak, R. S. J. (1992a) Motor practice and neurophysiological adaptation in the cerebellum: a positron tomography study. *Proc. Roy. Soc. London Series B* **248,** 223–228.

Friston, K. J., Grasby, P., Bench, C., Frith, C. D., Cowen, P. J., Little, P., Frackowiak, R. S. J., and Dolan, R. (1992b) Measuring the neuromodulatory effects of drugs in man with positron tomography. *Neurosci. Lett.* **141,** 106–110.

Friston, K. J., Frith, C., Liddle, P., and Frackowiak, R. S. J. (1993). Functional connectivity: the principal component analysis of large data sets. *J. Cereb. Blood Flow Metab.* **13,** 5–14.

Friston, K. J., Worsley, K. J., Frackowiak, R. S. J., Mazziotta, J. C., and Evans, A. C. (1994a) Assessing the significance of focal activations using their spatial extent. *Hum. Brain Mapping* **1,** 214–220.

Friston, K. J., Jezzard, P. J., and Turner, R. (1994b) Analysis of functional MRI time-series *Hum. Brain Mapping* **1,** 153–171.

Friston, K. J., Ashburner, J., Frith, C. D., Poline, J.-B., Heather, J. D., and Frackowiak, R. S. J. (1995a) Spatial registration and normalisation of images. *Hum. Brain Mapping* **2,** 165–189.

Friston, K. J., Holmes, A. P., Worsley, K. J., Poline, J. B., Frith, C. D., and Frackowiak, R. S. J. (1995b) Statistical parametric maps in functional imaging: a general linear approach *Hum. Brain Mapping* **2,** 189–210.

Friston, K. J., Frith, C. D., Turner, R., and Frackowiak, R. S. J. (1995c) Characterizing evoked hemodynamics with fMRI. *NeuroImage* **2,** 157–165.

Friston, K. J., Ungerleider, L. G., Jezzard, P., and Turner, R. (1995d) Characterizing modulatory interactions between V1 and V2 in human cortex with fMRI. *Hum. Brain Mapping* **2,** 211–224.

Friston, K. J., Williams, S., Howard, R., Frackowiak, R. S. J., and Turner, R. (1996a) Movement related effects in fMRI time series. *Mag. Res. Med.* **35,** 346–355.

Friston, K. J., Holmes, A., Poline, J.-B., Price, C. J., and Frith, C. D. (1996b) Detecting activations in PET and fMRI: levels of inference and power. *NeuroImage* **4,** 223–235.

Friston, K. J., Price, C. J., Fletcher, P., Moore, C., Frackowiak, R. S. J., and Dolan, R. J. (1996c) The trouble with cognitive subtraction. *NeuroImage* **4,** 97–104.

Friston, K. J., Poline, J.-B., Holmes, A. P., Frith, C. D., and Frackowiak, R. S. J. (1996d) A multivariate analysis of PET activation studies. *Hum. Brain Mapping* **4,** 140–151.

Friston, K. J., Frith, C. D., Fletcher, P., Liddle, P. F., and Frackowiak, R. S. J. (1996e) Functional topography: multidimensional scaling and functional connectivity in the brain. *Cerebral Cortex* **6,** 156–164.

Friston, K. J., Büchel, C., Fink, G. R., Morris, J., Rolls, E., and Dolan, R. J. (1997). Psychophysiological and modulatory interactions in neuroimaging. *NeuroImage* **6,** 218–229.

Friston, K. J., Josephs, O., Rees, G., and Turner, R. (1998a) Non-linear event-related responses in fMRI. *Mag. Res. Med.* **39,** 41–52.

Friston, K. J., Fletcher, P., Josephs, O., Holmes, A., Rugg, M. D., and Turner, R. (1998b) Event-related fMRI: characterizing differential responses. *NeuroImage* **7,** 30–40.

Friston, K. J., Zarahn, E., Josephs, O., Henson, R. N., Dale, A. M. (1999a) Stochastic designs in event-related fMRI. *NeuroImage* **10,** 607–619.

Friston, K. J., Holmes, A. P., Price, C. J., Buchel, C., Worsley, K. J. (1999b) Multisubject fMRI studies and conjunction analyses. *NeuroImage* **10,** 385–396.

Friston, K. J., Mechelli, A., Turner, R., Price, C. J. (2000a) Nonlinear responses in fMRI: the balloon model, Volterra kernels, and other hemodynamics. *NeuroImage* **12,** 466–477.

Friston, K. J., Josephs, O., Zarahn, E., Holmes, A. P., Rouquette, S., and Poline, J. (2000b) To smooth or not to smooth? Bias and efficiency in fMRI time-series analysis. *NeuroImage* **12,** 196–208.

Gerstein, G. L., and Perkel, D. H. (1969). Simultaneously recorded trains of action potentials: analysis and functional interpretation. *Science* **164,** 828–830.

Girard, P., and Bullier, J. (1989). Visual activity in area V2 during reversible inactivation of area 17 in the macaque monkey. *J. Neurophysiol.* **62,** 1287–1301.

Goltz, F. (1881). In "Transactions of the 7th International Medical Congress" (W. MacCormac, ed.), Vol. I, pp. 218–228. J. W. Kolkmann, London.

Grafton, S., Mazziotta, J., Presty, S., Friston, K. J., Frackowiak, R. S. J., and Phelps, M. (1992). Functional anatomy of human procedural learning determined with regional cerebral blood flow and PET. *J Neurosci.* **12,** 2542–2548.

Grootoonk, S., Hutton, C., Ashburner, J., Howseman, A. M., Josephs, O., Rees, G., Friston, K. J., Turner, R. (2000). Characterisation and correction of interpolation effects in the realignment of fMRI time series. *NeuroImage* **11,** 49–57.

Heid, O., Gönner, F., and Schroth, G. (1997). Stochastic functional MRI. *NeuroImage* **5,** S476.

Hirsch, J. A., and Gilbert, C. D. (1991). Synaptic physiology of horizontal connections in the cat's visual cortex. *J. Neurosci.* **11,** 1800–1809.

Jezzard, P., and Balaban, R. S. (1995). Correction for geometric distortion in echo-planar images from B0 field variations. *Mag. Res. Med.* **34,** 65–73.

Josephs, O., Turner, R., and Friston, K. J. (1997). Event-related fMRI *Hum. Brain Mapping* **5,** 243–248.

Kiebel, S. J., Poline, J. B., Friston, K. J., Holmes, A. P., Worsley, K. J. (1999). Robust smoothness estimation in statistical parametric maps using standardised residuals from the general linear model. *NeuroImage* **10,** 756–766.

Lange, N., and Zeger, S. L. (1997). Non-linear Fourier time series analysis for human brain mapping by functional magnetic resonance imaging (with discussion). *J. Roy. Stat. Soc. Ser C* **46,** 1–29.

Liddle, P. F., Friston, K. J., Frith, C. D., and Frackowiak, R. S. J. (1992). Cerebral blood-flow and mental processes in schizophrenia *J. Roy. Soc. Med.* **85,** 224–227.

Lueck, C. J., Zeki, S., Friston, K. J., Deiber, M. P., Cope, N. O., Cunningham, V. J., Lammertsma, A. A., Kennard, C., and Frackowiak, R. S. J. (1989). The color centre in the cerebral cortex of man. *Nature* **340,** 386–389.

McIntosh, A. R., and Gonzalez-Lima, F. (1994). Structural equation modelling and its application to network analysis in functional brain imaging. *Hum. Brain Mapping* **2,** 2–22.

McKeown, M., Jung, T.-P., Makeig, S., Brown, G., Kinderman, S., Lee, T.-W., and Sejnowski, T. (1998). Spatially independent activity patterns in functional MRI data during the Stroop color naming task. *Proc. Natl. Acad. Sci. USA* **95,** 803–810.

Mørch, N., Kjems, U., Hansen, L. K., Svarer, C., Law, I., Lautrup, B., and Strother, S. C. (1995). Visualisation of neural networks using saliency maps. In "IEEE International Conference on Neural Networks," Perth, Australia, pp. 2085–2090. IEEE, New York.

Petersen, S. E., Fox, P. T., Posner, M. I., Mintun, M., and Raichle, M. E. (1989). Positron emission tomographic studies of the processing of single words. *J. Cog. Neurosci.* **1,** 153–170.

Phillips, C. G., Zeki, S., and H. B., Barlow, H. B. (1984). Localisation of function in the cerebral cortex: past present and future. *Brain* **107,** 327–361.

Purdon, P. L., and Weisskoff, R. M. (1998). Effect of temporal autocorrelation due to physiological noise and stimulus paradigm on voxel-level false-positive rates in fMRI. *Hum. Brain Mapping* **6,** 239–495.

Price, C. J., and Friston, K. J. (1997). Cognitive conjunction: a new approach to brain activation experiments. *NeuroImage* **5,** 261–270.

Price, C. J., Wise, R. J. S., Ramsay, S., Friston, K. J., Howard, D., Patterson, K., and Frackowiak, R. S. J. (1992). Regional response differences within the human auditory cortex when listening to words. *Neurosci. Lett.* **146,** 179–182.

Sychra, J. J., Bandettini, P. A., Bhattacharya, N., and Lin, Q. (1994). Synthetic images by subspace transforms, I: principal component images and related filters. *Med. Physics* **21,** 193–201.

Talairach, P., and Tournoux, J. (1988). "A Stereotactic Coplanar Atlas of the Human Brain." Stuttgart Thieme.

Treue, S., and Maunsell, H. R. (1996). Attentional modulation of visual motion processing in cortical areas MT and MST. *Nature* **382,** 539–541.

Vazquez, A. L., and Noll, C. D. (1998). Nonlinear aspects of the BOLD response in functional MRI. *NeuroImage* **7,** 108–118.

Worsley, K. J., and Friston, K. J. (1995). Analysis of fMRI time-series revisited—again. *NeuroImage* **2,** 173–181.

Worsley, K. J., Evans, A. C., Marrett, S., and Neelin, P. (1992). A three-dimensional statistical analysis for rCBF activation studies in human brain. *J. Cereb. Blood Flow Metab.* **12,** 900–918.

Worsley, K. J., Marrett, S., Neelin, P., Vandal, A. C., Friston, K. J., and Evans, A. C. (1996). A unified statistical approach or determining significant signals in images of cerebral activation. *Hum. Brain Mapping* **4,** 58–73.

Zarahn, E., Aguirre, G. K., and D'Esposito, M. (1997). Empirical analyses of BOLD fMRI statistics: I Spatially unsmoothed data collected under null-hypothesis conditions. *NeuroImage* **5,** 179–197.

Zeki, S. (1990). The motion pathways of the visual cortex. In "Vision: Coding and Efficiency" (C. Blakemore, ed.), pp. 321–345. Cambridge University Press, UK.

SECTION ONE

COMPUTATIONAL NEUROANATOMY

CHAPTER

32

Rigid Body Registration

INTRODUCTION

Image registration is important in many aspects of functional image analysis. In imaging neuroscience, particularly for fMRI, the signal changes due to any hæmodynamic response can be small compared to apparent signal differences that can result from subject movement. Subject head movement in the scanner cannot be completely eliminated, so retrospective motion correction is performed as a preprocessing step. This is especially important for experiments where subjects may move in the scanner in a way that is correlated with the different conditions (Hajnal *et al.,* 1994). Even tiny systematic differences can result in a significant signal accumulating over numerous scans. Without suitable corrections, artifacts arising from subject movement correlated with the experimental paradigm may appear as activations. A second reason why motion correction is important is because it increases sensitivity. The t test is based on the signal change relative to the residual variance. The residual variance is computed from the sum of squared differences between the data and the linear model to which it is fitted. Movement artifacts add to this residual variance, and so reduce the sensitivity of the test to true activations.

For studies of a single subject, sites of activation can be accurately localised by superimposing them on a high-resolution structural image of the subject (typically a T_1-weighted MRI). This requires registration of the functional images with the structural image. As in the case of movement correction, this is normally performed by optimising a set of parameters describing a rigid body transformation, but the matching criterion needs to be more complex because the structural and functional images normally look very different. A further use for this registration is that a more precise spatial normalisation can be achieved by computing it from a more detailed structural image. If the functional and structural images are in register, then a warp computed from the structural image can be applied to the functional images.

Another application of rigid registration is within the field of morphometry and involves identifying shape changes within single subjects by subtracting coregistered images acquired at different times. The changes could arise for a number of different reasons, but most are related to pathology. Because the scans are of the same subject, the first step for this kind of analysis involves registering the images together by a rigid body transformation.

At its simplest, image registration involves estimating a mapping between a pair of images. One image is assumed to remain stationary (the reference image), whereas the other (the source image) is spatially transformed to match it. To transform the source to match the reference, it is necessary to determine a mapping from each voxel position in the reference to a corresponding position in the source. The source is then resampled at the new positions. The mapping can be thought of as a function of a set of estimated transformation parameters. A rigid body transformation in three dimensions is defined by six parameters: three translations and three rotations.

Two steps are involved in registering a pair of images together. There is the *registration* itself, whereby the set of parameters describing a transformation is estimated. Then there is the *transformation,* where one of the images is transformed according to the estimated parameters. Performing the registration normally involves iteratively transforming the source image many times, using different parameters, until some matching criterion is optimised.

First of all, this chapter will explain how images are transformed via the process of resampling. This chapter is about about rigid registration of images, so the next section describes the parameterisation of rigid body transformations as a subset of the more general affine transformations. The final two sections describe methods of rigid body registration, in both intra- and intermodality contexts. Intramodality registration implies registration of images acquired using the same modality and scanning sequence or contrast agent, whereas intermodality registration allows the registration of different modalities (e.g., T_1- to T_2-weighted MRI, or MRI to PET).

RESAMPLING IMAGES

An image transformation is usually implemented as a "pulling" operation (where pixel values are pulled from the original image into their new location) rather than a "pushing" one (where the pixels in the original image are pushed into their new location). This involves determining, for each voxel in the transformed image, the corresponding intensity in the original image. Usually, this requires sampling between the centers of voxels, so some form of interpolation is needed.

Simple Interpolation

The simplest approach is to take the value of the closest voxel to the desired sample point. This is referred to as *nearest neighbour* or *zero-order hold* resampling. This has the advantage of preserving the original voxel intensities, but the resulting image is degraded quite considerably, resulting in the resampled image having a "blocky" appearance.

Another approach is to use *trilinear interpolation (first-order hold)* to resample the data. This is slower than nearest neighbour, but the resulting images are less "blocky." However, trilinear interpolation has the effect of losing some high-frequency information from the image.

Figure 32.1 will now be used to illustrate bilinear interpolation (the two-dimensional version of trilinear interpolation). Assuming that there is a regular grid of pixels at coordinates x_a, y_a to x_p, y_p, having intensities v_a to v_p, and that the point to resample is at u. The values at points r and s are first determined (using linear interpolation) as follows:

$$v_r = \frac{(x_g - x_r)v_f + (x_r - x_f)v_g}{x_g - x_f}$$

$$v_s = \frac{(x_k - x_s)v_j + (x_s - x_j)v_k}{x_k - x_j}$$

Then v_u is determined by interpolating between v_r and v_s:

$$v_u = \frac{(y_u - y_s)v_r + (y_r - y_u)v_s}{y_r - y_s}$$

The extension of the approach to three dimensions is trivial.

Polynomial Interpolation

Rather than using only the eight nearest neighbours (in 3D) to estimate the value at a point, more neighbours can be used in order to fit a smooth function through the neighbouring voxels, and then read off the value of the function at the desired location. *Polynomial interpolation* is one such approach (zero- and first-order hold interpolations are simply low-order polynomial

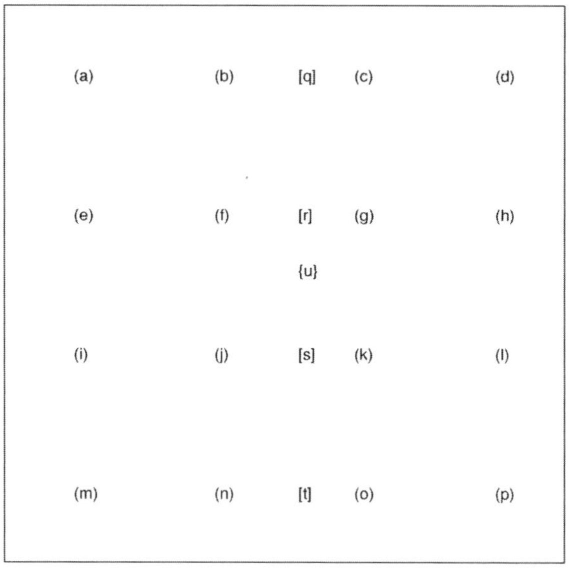

(a) (b) [q] (c) (d)

(e) (f) [r] (g) (h)

{u}

(i) (j) [s] (k) (l)

(m) (n) [t] (o) (p)

FIGURE 32.1
Illustration of image interpolation in two dimensions. Points a through to p represent the original regular grid of pixels. Point u is the point who's value is to be determined. Points q to t are used as intermediates in the computation.

interpolations). It is now illustrated how v_q can be determined from pixels a to d. The coefficients ($\mathbf{q}$) of a polynomial that runs through these points can be obtained by computing as follows:

$$\mathbf{q} = \begin{bmatrix} 1 & 0 & 0 & 0 \\ 1 & (x_b - x_a) & (x_b - x_a)^2 & (x_b - x_a)^3 \\ 1 & (x_c - x_a) & (x_c - x_a)^2 & (x_c - x_a)^3 \\ 1 & (x_d - x_a) & (x_d - x_a)^2 & (x_d - x_a)^3 \end{bmatrix}^{-1} \begin{bmatrix} v_a \\ v_b \\ v_c \\ v_d \end{bmatrix}$$

Then v_q can be determined from these coefficients by

$$v_q = [1 \; (x_q - x_a) \; (x_q - x_a)^2 \; (x_q - x_a)^3]\mathbf{q}$$

To determine v_u, a similar polynomial would be fitted through points q, r, s, and t. The Vandermonde matrices required for polynomial interpolation are very ill conditioned, especially for higher orders. A better way of doing polynomial interpolation involves using *Lagrange polynomials* (see Press *et al.*, 1992; Jain, 1989). Polynomial interpolation is a very crude approach, which has the disadvantage that discontinuities arise when moving from different sets of nearest neighbours.

Windowed Sinc Interpolation

The optimum method of applying rigid body transformations to images with minimal interpolation artifact is to do it in Fourier space. In real space, the interpolation method that gives results closest to a Fourier interpolation is *sinc interpolation.* This involves convolving the image with a sinc function centered on the point to be resampled. To perform a pure sinc interpolation, every voxel in the image should be used to sample a single point. This is not feasible due to speed considerations, so an approximation using a limited number of nearest neighbours is used. Because the sinc function extends to infinity, it is often truncated by modulating with a Hanning window (see Fig. 32.2). Because the function is separable, the implementation of sinc interpolation is similar to that for polynomial interpolation, in that it is performed sequentially in the three dimensions of the volume. For one dimension the windowed sinc function using the I nearest neighbours would be

$$\sum_{i=1}^{I} v_i \frac{\frac{\sin(\pi d_i)}{\pi d_i} \frac{1}{2}(1 + \cos(2\pi d_i/I))}{\sum_{j=1}^{I} \frac{\sin(\pi d_j)}{\pi d_j} \frac{1}{2}(1 + \cos(2\pi d_j/I))}$$

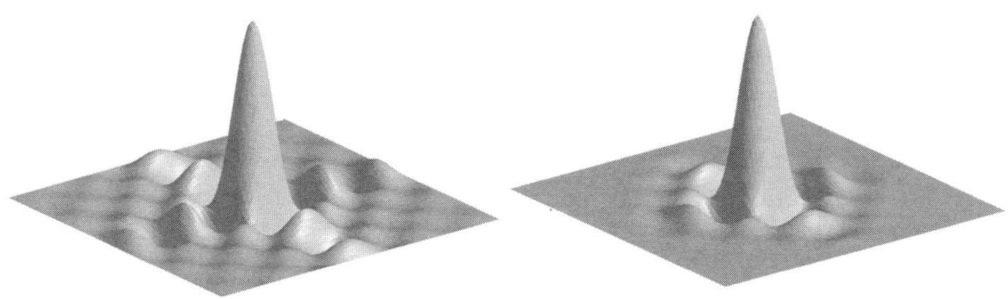

FIGURE 32.2
Sinc function in two dimensions, both with (right) and without (left) a Hanning window.

where d_i is the distance from the center of the ith voxel to the point to be sampled, and v_i is the value of the ith voxel.

Generalised Interpolation

The methods described so far are all classical interpolation methods that locally convolve the image with some form of interpolant.[1] Much more efficient resampling can be performed using *generalised interpolation* (Thévenaz *et al.*, 2000), where the images are first transformed into something else before applying the local convolution. Generalised interpolation methods model an image as a linear combination of basis functions with local support, typically *B-splines* or *o-Moms* (maximal-order interpolation of minimal support) basis functions (see Fig. 32.3). Before resampling begins, an image of basis function coefficients is produced, which involves a very fast deconvolution (Unser *et al.,* 1993a,b). Resampling at each new point then involves computing the appropriate linear combination of basis functions, which can be thought of as a local convolution of the basis function coefficients.

B-splines are a family of functions of varying degree. Interpolation using B-splines of degree 0 or 1 (first and second order) is identical to nearest neighbour[2] or linear interpolation, respectively. B-splines of degree n are given by:

$$\beta^n(x) = \sum_{j=0}^{n} \frac{(-1)^j (n+1)}{(n+1-j)!j!} \max\left(\frac{n+1}{2} + x - j, 0\right)^n$$

An nth degree B-spline has a local support of $n + 1$, which means that during the final resampling step, a linear combination of $n + 1$ basis functions is needed to compute an interpolated value. o-Moms are derived from B-splines, and consist of a linear combination of the B-spline and its derivatives. They produce the most accurate interpolation for the least local support, but lack some of the B-spline's advantages. Unlike the o-Moms functions, a B-spline of order n is $n - 1$ times continuously differentiable.

Fourier Methods

Higher order interpolation is slow when many neighbouring voxels are used, but there are faster ways of interpolating when doing rigid body transformations. Translations parallel to the axes are trivial, because these simply involve convolving with a translated delta function. For translations that are not whole numbers of pixels, the delta function is replaced by a sinc function centered at the translation distance. The use of fast Fourier transforms means that the convolution can be performed most rapidly as a multiplication in Fourier space. It is clear how translations can be performed in this way, but rotations are less obvious. One way that rotations can be effected involves replacing them by a series of shears (Eddy *et al.,* 1996) (see later section titled "shears"). A shear simply involves translating different rows or columns of an image by different amounts, so each shear can be performed as a series of one-dimensional convolutions.

[1] The polynomial interpolation can also be formulated this way by combining Eqs. (32.1) and (32.1) to eliminate the intermediate **q**.

[2] Except with a slightly different treatment exactly in the center of two voxels.

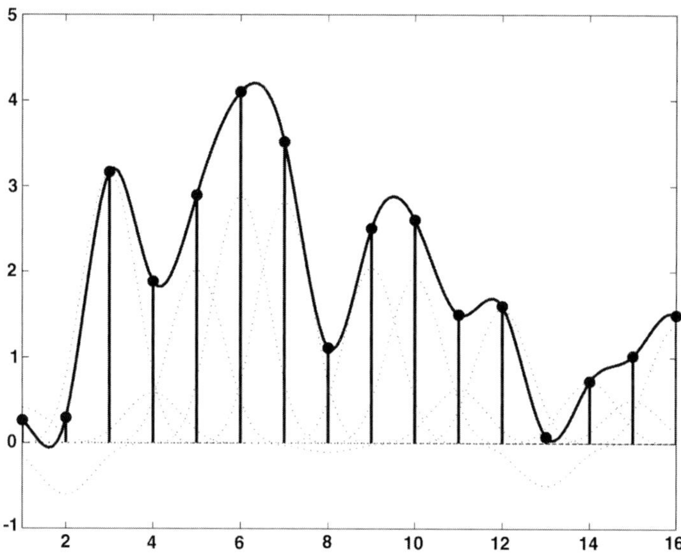

FIGURE 32.3
This figure illustrates a one-dimensional B-spline representation of an image, where the image is assumed to be composed of a linear combination of B-spline basis functions. The dotted lines are the individual basis functions, which sum to produce the interpolated function (solid line).

RIGID BODY TRANSFORMATIONS

Rigid body transformations consist of only rotations and translations, and leave given arrangements unchanged. They are a subset of the more general affine[3] transformations. For each point (x_1, x_2, x_3) in an image, an affine mapping can be defined into the coordinates of another space (y_1, y_2, y_3). This is expressed as

$$\begin{aligned} y_1 &= m_{11}x_1 + m_{12}x_2 + m_{13}x_3 + m_{14} \\ y_2 &= m_{21}x_1 + m_{22}x_2 + m_{23}x_3 + m_{24} \\ y_3 &= m_{31}x_1 + m_{32}x_2 + m_{33}x_3 + m_{34} \end{aligned}$$

which is often represented by a simple matrix multiplication ($\mathbf{y} = \mathbf{Mx}$):

$$\begin{bmatrix} y_1 \\ y_2 \\ y_3 \\ 1 \end{bmatrix} = \begin{bmatrix} m_{11} & m_{12} & m_{13} & m_{14} \\ m_{21} & m_{22} & m_{23} & m_{24} \\ m_{31} & m_{32} & m_{33} & m_{34} \\ 0 & 1 & 2 & 3 \end{bmatrix} \begin{bmatrix} x_1 \\ x_2 \\ x_3 \\ 1 \end{bmatrix}$$

The elegance of formulating these transformations in terms of matrices is that several of them can be combined, simply by multiplying the matrices together to form a single matrix. This means that repeated resampling of data can be avoided when reorienting an image. Inverse affine transformations are obtained by inverting the transformation matrix.

Translations

If a point $\mathbf{x}$ is to be translated by $\mathbf{q}$ units, then the transformation is simply

$$\mathbf{y} = \mathbf{x} + \mathbf{q}$$

In matrix terms, this can be considered as

$$\begin{bmatrix} y_1 \\ y_2 \\ y_3 \\ 1 \end{bmatrix} = \begin{bmatrix} 1 & 0 & 0 & q_1 \\ 0 & 1 & 0 & q_2 \\ 0 & 0 & 1 & q_3 \\ 0 & 0 & 0 & 1 \end{bmatrix} \begin{bmatrix} x_1 \\ x_2 \\ x_3 \\ 1 \end{bmatrix}$$

[3] *Affine* means that parallel lines remain parallel after the transformation.

Rotations

In two dimensions, a rotation is described by a single angle. Consider a point at coordinate (x_1, x_2) on a two-dimensional plane. A rotation of this point to new coordinates (y_1, y_2), by θ radians around the origin, can be generated by the following transformation:

$$\begin{aligned} y_1 &= \cos(\theta)x_1 + \sin(\theta)x_2 \\ y_2 &= -\sin(\theta)x_1 + \cos(\theta)x_2 \end{aligned}$$

This is another example of an affine transformation. For the three-dimensional case, an object can be rotated in three orthogonal planes. These planes of rotation are normally expressed as being around the axes. A rotation of q_1 radians about the first *(x)* axis is normally called *pitch,* and is performed by

$$\begin{bmatrix} y_1 \\ y_2 \\ y_3 \\ 1 \end{bmatrix} = \begin{bmatrix} 1 & 0 & 0 & 0 \\ 0 & \sin(q_1) & \sin(q_1) & 0 \\ 0 & -\sin(q_1) & \sin(q_1) & 0 \\ 0 & 0 & 0 & 1 \end{bmatrix} \begin{bmatrix} x_1 \\ x_3 \\ x_2 \\ 1 \end{bmatrix}$$

Similarly, rotations about the second *(y)* and third *(z)* axes (called *roll* and *yaw,* respectively) are carried out by the following matrices:

$$\begin{bmatrix} \sin(q_2) & 0 & \sin(q_1) & 0 \\ 0 & 1 & 0 & 0 \\ -\sin(q_2) & 0 & \sin(q_2) & 0 \\ 0 & 0 & 0 & 1 \end{bmatrix} \text{ and } \begin{bmatrix} \sin(q_3) & \sin(q_3) & 0 & 0 \\ -\sin(q_3) & \sin(q_3) & 0 & 0 \\ 0 & 0 & 1 & 0 \\ 0 & 0 & 0 & 1 \end{bmatrix}$$

Rotations are combined by multiplying these matrices together in the appropriate order. The order of the operations is important. For example, a rotation about the first axis of $\pi/2$ radians followed by an equivalent rotation about the second would produce a very different result than that obtained if the order of the operations were reversed.

Zooms

The affine transformations described so far will generate purely rigid body mappings. Zooms are needed to change the size of an image, or to work with images whose voxel sizes are not isotropic or that differ between images. These represent scalings along the orthogonal axes, and can be represented via

$$\begin{bmatrix} y_1 \\ y_2 \\ y_3 \\ 1 \end{bmatrix} = \begin{bmatrix} q_1 & 0 & 0 & 0 \\ 0 & q_2 & 0 & 0 \\ 0 & 0 & q_3 & 0 \\ 0 & 0 & 0 & 1 \end{bmatrix} \begin{bmatrix} x_1 \\ x_2 \\ x_3 \\ 1 \end{bmatrix}$$

A single zoom by a factor of -1 will flip an image (see later section on left- and right-handed coordinate systems). Two flips in different directions will merely rotate it by π radians (a rigid body transformation). In fact, any affine transformation with a negative determinant will render the image flipped.

Shears

Shearing by parameters q_1, q_2, and q_3 can be performed by the following matrix:

$$\begin{bmatrix} 1 & q_1 & q_2 & 0 \\ 0 & 1 & q_3 & 0 \\ 0 & 0 & 1 & 0 \\ 0 & 0 & 0 & 1 \end{bmatrix}$$

A shear by itself is not a rigid body transformation, but it is possible to combine shears in order to generate a rotation. In two dimensions, a matrix encoding a rotation of θ radians about the origin (see "Within-Modality Rigid Registration" section) can be constructed by multiplying together three matrices that effect shears (Eddy *et al.,* 1996):

$$\begin{bmatrix} \cos(\theta) & \sin(\theta) & 0 \\ -\sin(\theta) & \cos(\theta) & 0 \\ 0 & 0 & 1 \end{bmatrix} \equiv \begin{bmatrix} 1 & \tan(\theta/2) & 0 \\ 0 & 0 & 1 \\ 0 & 0 & 1 \end{bmatrix} \begin{bmatrix} 1 & 0 & 0 \\ \sin(\theta) & 1 & 0 \\ 0 & 0 & 1 \end{bmatrix} \begin{bmatrix} 1 & \tan(\theta/2) & 0 \\ 0 & 1 & 0 \\ 0 & 0 & 1 \end{bmatrix}$$

Rotations in three dimensions can be decomposed into four shears (Cox and Jesmanowicz, 1999). Because shears can be performed quickly as one-dimensional convolutions, then these decompositions are very useful for doing accurate and rapid rigid body transformations of images.

Parameterising a Rigid Body Transformation

When doing rigid registration of a pair of images, it is necessary to estimate six parameters that describe the rigid body transformation matrix. There are many ways of parameterising this transformation in terms of six parameters (**q**). One possible form is

$$\mathbf{M} = \mathbf{TR}$$

where

$$\mathbf{T} = \begin{bmatrix} 1 & 0 & 0 & q_1 \\ 0 & 1 & 0 & q_2 \\ 0 & 0 & 1 & q_3 \\ 0 & 0 & 0 & 1 \end{bmatrix}$$

and

$$\mathbf{R} = \begin{bmatrix} 1 & 0 & 0 & 0 \\ 0 & \cos(q_4) & \cos(q_4) & 0 \\ 0 & -\sin(q_4) & \cos(q_4) & 0 \\ 0 & 0 & 0 & 1 \end{bmatrix} \begin{bmatrix} \cos(q_5) & 0 & \sin(q_5) & 0 \\ 0 & 1 & 0 & 0 \\ -\sin(q_5) & 0 & \cos(q_5) & 0 \\ 0 & 0 & 0 & 1 \end{bmatrix} \begin{bmatrix} \cos(q_6) & \sin(q_6) & 0 & 0 \\ -\sin(q_6) & \cos(q_6) & 0 & 0 \\ 0 & 0 & 1 & 0 \\ 0 & 0 & 0 & 1 \end{bmatrix}$$

Sometimes it is desirable to extract transformation parameters from a matrix. Extracting these parameters **q** from **M** is relatively straightforward. Determining the translations is trivial, as they are simply contained in the fourth column of **M.** This just leaves the rotations:

$$\mathbf{R} = \begin{bmatrix} c_5c_6 & c_5s_6 & s_5 & 0 \\ -s_4s_5c_6 - c_4s_6 & -s_4s_5s_6 + c_4c_6 & s_4c_5 & 0 \\ -c_4s_5c_6 + s_4s_6 & -c_4s_5s_6 - s_4c_6 & c_4c_5 & 0 \\ 0 & 0 & 0 & 1 \end{bmatrix}$$

where s_4, s_5, and s_6 are the sines, and c_4, c_5, and c_6 are the cosines of parameters q_4, q_5, and q_6, respectively. Therefore, provided that c_5 is not zero:

$$\begin{aligned} q_5 &= \sin^{-1}(r_{13}) \\ q_4 &= \operatorname{atan2}(r_{23}/\cos(q_5), r_{33}/\cos(q_5)) \\ q_6 &= \operatorname{atan2}(r_{12}/\cos(q_5), r_{11}/\cos(q_5)) \end{aligned}$$

where atan2 is the four-quadrant inverse tangent.

Working with Volumes of Differing or Anisotropic Voxel Sizes

Voxel sizes need be considered during image registration. Often, the images (say, **f** and **g**) will have voxels that are anisotropic. The dimensions of the voxels are also likely to differ between images of different modalities. For simplicity, a Euclidean space is used, where measures of distance are expressed in millimeters. Rather than transforming the images into volumes with cubic voxels that are the same size in all images, one can simply define affine transformation matrices that map from voxel coordinates into this Euclidean space. For example, if image **f** is of size 128 × 128 × 43 and has voxels that are 2.1 mm × 2.1 mm × 2.45 mm, the following matrix can be defined:

$$\mathbf{M_f} = \begin{bmatrix} 2.1 & 0 & 0 & -135.45 \\ 0 & 2.1 & 0 & -135.45 \\ 0 & 0 & 2.45 & -53.9 \\ 0 & 0 & 0 & 1 \end{bmatrix}$$

This transformation matrix maps voxel coordinates to a Euclidean space whose axes are parallel to those of the image and distances are measured in millimeters, with the origin at the center of the image volume (i.e., $\mathbf{M_f}$ [64.5 64.5 22 1]^T = [0 0 0 1]^T. A similar matrix can be defined for **g** ($\mathbf{M_g}$). Because modern MR image formats such as DICOM generally contain information about image orientations in their headers, it is possible to extract this information to automatically compute values for $\mathbf{M_f}$ or $\mathbf{M_g}$. This makes it possible to easily register images that were originally acquired in completely different orientations.

The objective of a rigid body registration is to determine the affine transformation that maps the coordinates of image **g** to those of **f.** To accomplish this, a rigid body transformation matrix $\mathbf{M_r}$ is determined, such that $\mathbf{M_f}^{-1}\mathbf{M_r}^{-1}\mathbf{M_g}$ will map from voxels in **g** to those in **f.** The inverse of this matrix maps from **f** to **g.** Once $\mathbf{M_r}$ has been determined, $\mathbf{M_f}$ can be set to $\mathbf{M_r M_f}$. From there onward the mapping between the voxels of the two images can be achieved by $\mathbf{M_f}^{-1}\mathbf{M_g}$. Similarly, if another image (**h**) is also registered with **g** in the same manner, then not only is there a mapping from **h** to **g** (via $\mathbf{M_g}^{-1}\mathbf{M_h}$), but there is also one from **h** to **f,** which is simply $\mathbf{M_f}^{-1}\mathbf{M_h}$ (derived from $\mathbf{M_f}^{-1}\mathbf{M_g}\mathrm{M_g}^{-1}\mathbf{M_h}$).

Left- and Right-Handed Coordinate Systems

Positions in space can be represented in either a left- or right-handed coordinate system (see Fig. 32.4), where one system is a mirror image of the other. For example, the system used by the Talairach Atlas (Talairach and Tournoux, 1988) is right handed, because the first dimension (often referred to as the x direction) increases from left to right, the second dimension goes from posterior to anterior (back to front), and the third dimension increases from inferior to superior (bottom to top). The axes can be rotated by any angle, and they still retain their handedness. An affine transformation mapping between left- and right-handed coordinate systems has a negative determinant, whereas one that maps between coordinate systems of the same kind will have a positive determinant. Because the left and right sides of a brain have similar appearances, care must be taken when reorienting image volumes. Consistency of the coordinate systems can be achieved by performing any reorientations using affine transformations and by checking the determinants of the matrices.

Rotating Tensors

Diffusion tensor imaging (DTI) is becoming increasingly useful. These datasets are usually stored as six images containing a scalar field for each unique tensor element. It is worth noting that a rigid body transformation of a DTI dataset is not a simple matter of rigidly rotating the individual scalar fields.[4] Once these fields have been resampled, the tensor represented at every

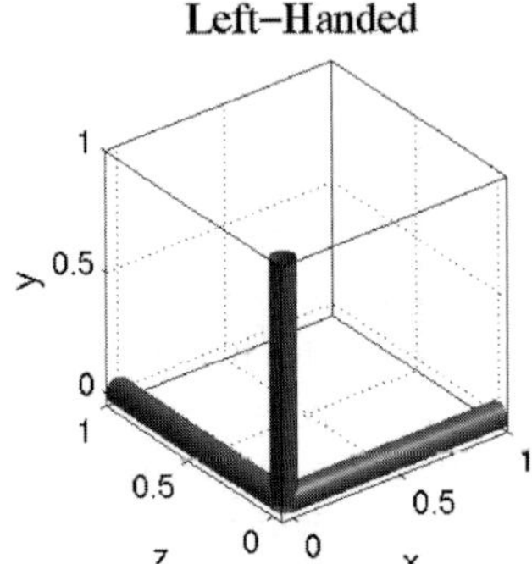

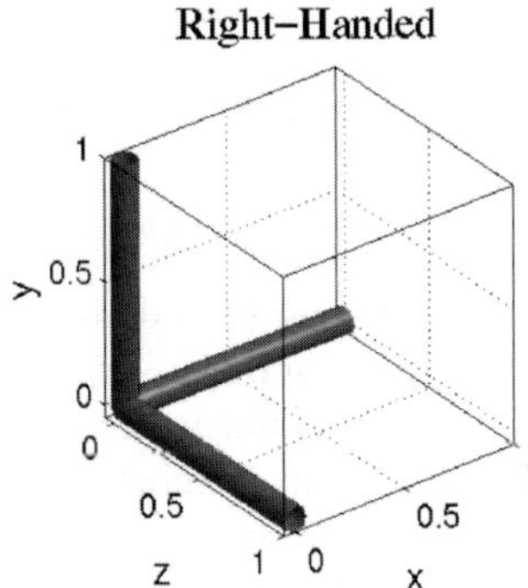

FIGURE 32.4
Left- and right-handed coordinate systems. The thumb corresponds to the x axis, the index finger to the y axis, and the second finger to the z axis.

[4] Some interpolation methods are unsuitable for resampling the raw scalar fields, because the introduction of sampling errors can cause the positive definite nature of the tensors to be lost.

voxel position needs to be rotated. A 3×3 tensor $\mathbf{T}$ can be rotated by a 3×3 matrix $\mathbf{R}$ by $\mathbf{T}' = \mathbf{R}\mathbf{T}\mathbf{R}^T$.

If DTI volumes are to be transformed using more complex warping models, then the local derivatives of the deformations (Jacobian matrices) need to be computed at each voxel. Suitable transformations can then be extracted from these derivatives, and applied to each element of the resampled tensor field (Alexander *et al.,* 1999, 2001).

WITHIN-MODALITY RIGID REGISTRATION

Whenever several images of the same subject have been acquired, it is extremely useful to have them all in register. Some of the simple benefits of this include allowing images to be averaged in order to increase the signal-to-noise ratio, or to subtract one image from another to emphasise differences between the images. Rigid[5] registration is normally used for retrospectively registering images of the same subject that have been collected at different times. Even if images were acquired during the same scanning session, the subject may have moved slightly between acquisitions.

The most common application of within-modality registration in functional imaging is to reduce motion artifacts by realigning the volumes in image time series. The objective of realignment is to determine the rigid body transformations that best map the series of functional images to the same space. This can be achieved by minimising the sum of squared differences between each of the images and a reference image, where the reference image could be one of the images in the series. For slightly better results, this procedure could be repeated, but instead of matching to one of the images from the series, the images would be registered to the mean of all of the realigned images. Because of the nonstationary variance in the images, a variance image could be computed at the same time as the mean, in order to provide better weighting for the registration. Voxels with a lot of variance should be given lower weighting, whereas those with less variance should be weighted more highly.

Within-modality image registration is also useful for looking at shape differences of brains. Morphometric studies sometimes involve looking at changes in brain shape over time, often to study the progression of a disease such as Alzheimer's or to monitor tumor growth or shrinkage. Differences between structural MR scans acquired at different times are identified by first coregistering the images and then looking at the difference between the registered images. Rigid registration can also be used as a preprocessing step before using nonlinear registration methods for identifying shape changes (Freeborough and Fox, 1998).

Image registration involves estimating a set of parameters describing a spatial transformation that "best" match the images together. The goodness of the match is based on a *cost function,* which is maximised or minimised using some *optimisation algorithm.* This section deals with registering images that have been collected using the same (or similar) modalities, allowing a relatively simple cost function to be used. In this case, the cost function is the mean squared difference between the images. A later section deals with the more complex task of registering images with different contrasts.

Optimisation

The objective of optimisation is to determine the values for a set of parameters for which some function of the parameters is minimised (or maximised). One of the simplest cases involves determining the optimum parameters for a model in order to minimise the sum of squared differences between a model and a set of real-world data (χ^2). Normally there are many parameters, and it is not possible to exhaustively search through the whole parameter space. The usual approach is to make an initial parameter estimate and begin iteratively searching from there. At each iteration, the model is evaluated using the current parameter estimates, and χ^2 computed. A judgment is then made about how the parameter estimates should be modified before continuing on to the next iteration. The optimisation is terminated when some convergence criterion is achieved (usually when χ^2 stops decreasing).

[5] Or affine registration if voxel sizes are not accurately known.

The image registration approach described here is essentially an optimisation. One image (the source image) is spatially transformed so that it matches another (the reference image), by minimising χ^2. The parameters that are optimised are those that describe the spatial transformation (although there are often other nuisance parameters required by the model, such as intensity scaling parameters). A good algorithm to use for rigid registration (Friston *et al.,* 1995; Woods *et al.,* 1998) is *Gauss-Newton* optimisation, which is illustrated here.

Suppose that $b_i(\mathbf{q})$ is the function describing the difference between the source and reference images at voxel i, when the vector of model parameters has values $\mathbf{q}$. For each voxel, a first approximation of Taylor's theorem can be used to estimate the value that this difference will take if the parameters $\mathbf{q}$ are decreased by $\mathbf{t}$:

$$b_i(\mathbf{q}-\mathbf{t}) \simeq b_i(\mathbf{q}) - t_1 \frac{\partial b_i(\mathbf{q})}{\partial q_1} - t_2 \frac{\partial b_i(\mathbf{q})}{\partial q_2}$$

This allows the construction of a set of simultaneous equations (of the form $\mathbf{At} \simeq \mathbf{b}$) for estimating the values that $\mathbf{t}$ should assume to in order to minimise $\Sigma_i b_i(\mathbf{q}-\mathbf{t})^2$:

$$\begin{bmatrix} \frac{\partial b_1(\mathbf{q})}{\partial q_1} & \frac{\partial b_1(\mathbf{q})}{\partial q_2} & \cdots \\ \frac{\partial b_2(\mathbf{q})}{\partial q_1} & \frac{\partial b_2(\mathbf{q})}{\partial q_2} & \cdots \\ \vdots & \vdots & \ddots \end{bmatrix} \begin{bmatrix} t_1 \\ t_2 \\ \vdots \end{bmatrix} \simeq \begin{bmatrix} b_1(\mathbf{q}) \\ b_2(\mathbf{q}) \\ \vdots \end{bmatrix}$$

From this, an iterative scheme can be derived for improving the parameter estimates. For iteration n, the parameters $\mathbf{q}$ are updated as

$$\mathbf{q}^{(n+1)} = \mathbf{q}^{(n)} - (\mathbf{A}^T\mathbf{A})^{-1}\mathbf{A}^T\mathbf{b} \tag{32.1}$$

where $\mathbf{A} = \begin{bmatrix} \frac{\partial b_1(\mathbf{q})}{\partial q_1} & \frac{\partial b_1(\mathbf{q})}{\partial q_2} & \cdots \\ \frac{\partial b_2(\mathbf{q})}{\partial q_1} & \frac{\partial b_2(\mathbf{q})}{\partial q_2} & \cdots \\ \vdots & \vdots & \ddots \end{bmatrix}$ and $\mathbf{b} = \begin{bmatrix} b_1(\mathbf{q}) \\ b_2(\mathbf{q}) \\ \vdots \end{bmatrix}$

This process is repeated until χ^2 can no longer be decreased—or for a fixed number of iterations. There is no guarantee that the best global solution will be reached, because the algorithm can get caught in a local minimum. To reduce this problem, the starting estimates for $\mathbf{q}$ should be set as close as possible to the optimum solution. The number of potential local minima can also be decreased by working with smooth images. This also has the effect of making the first-order Taylor approximation more accurate for larger displacements. Once the registration is close to the final solution, it can continue with less smooth images.

In practice, $\mathbf{A}^T\mathbf{A}$ and $\mathbf{A}^T\mathbf{b}$ from Eq. (32.1) are often computed "on the fly" for each iteration. By computing these matrices using only a few rows of $\mathbf{A}$ and $\mathbf{b}$ at a time, much less computer memory is required than is necessary for storing the whole of matrix $\mathbf{A}$. Also, the partial derivatives $\partial b_i(\mathbf{q})/\partial q_j$ can be rapidly computed from the gradients of the images using the chain rule (see Woods, 1999, for detailed information).

Note that element i of $\mathbf{A}^T\mathbf{b}$ is equal to $\frac{1}{2}\frac{\partial \chi^2}{\partial q_i}$, and that element i, j of $\mathbf{A}^T\mathbf{A}$ is approximately equal to $\frac{1}{2}\frac{\partial^2 \chi^2}{\partial q_i \partial q_j}$ (one-half of the Hessian matrix, often referred to as the curvature matrix; see Press *et al.,* 1992, Section 15.5, for a general description, or Woods, 1999, 2000, for more information related to image registration). Another way of thinking about the optimisation is that it fits a quadratic function to the error surface at each iteration. Successive parameter estimates are chosen such that they are at the minimum point of this quadratic (illustrated for a single parameter in Fig. 32.5).

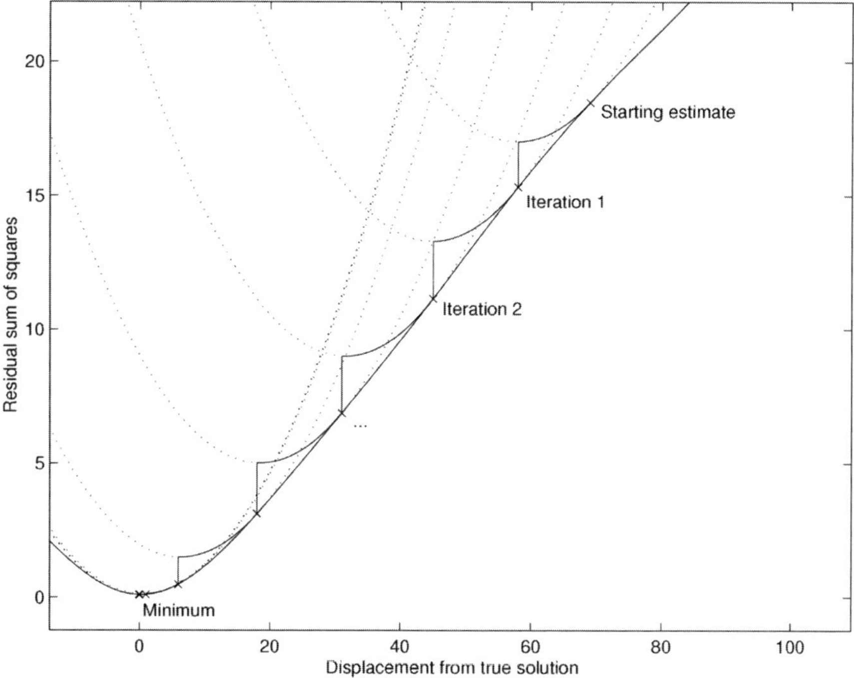

FIGURE 32.5
The optimisation can be thought of as fitting a series of quadratics to the error surface. Each parameter update is such that it falls at the minimum of the quadratic.

Implementation

This section is about estimating parameters that describe a rigid body transformation, but the principles can be extended to models that describe nonlinear warps. To register a source image **f** to a reference image **g,** a six-parameter rigid body transformation (parameterised by q_1 to q_6) would be used. To perform the registration, a number of points in the reference image (each denoted by $\mathbf{x}_i$) are compared with points in the source image (denoted by $\mathbf{Mx}_i$, where **M** is the rigid body transformation matrix constructed from the six parameters). The images may be scaled differently, so an additional intensity scaling parameter (q_7) may be included in the model. The parameters (**q**) are optimised by minimising the sum of squared differences[6] between the images according to the algorithm described in earlier sections and Eq. (32.1). The function that is minimised is

$$\sum_i [f(\mathbf{Mx}_i) - q_7 g(\mathbf{x}_i)]^2$$

where $\mathbf{M} = \mathbf{M_f}^{-1}\mathbf{M_r}^{-1}\mathbf{M_g}$, and $\mathbf{M_r}$ is constructed from parameters **q** (refer to section on working with volumes having differing voxel sizes). Vector **b** is generated for each iteration as

$$\mathbf{b} = \begin{bmatrix} f(\mathbf{Mx}_1) - q_7 g(\mathbf{x}_1) \\ f(\mathbf{Mx}_2) - q_7 g(\mathbf{x}_2) \\ \vdots \end{bmatrix}$$

Each column of matrix **A** is constructed by differentiating **b** with respect to parameters q_1 to q_7:

[6] Strictly speaking, it is the mean squared difference that is minimised, rather than the sum of squared differences. Inevitably, some values of $\mathbf{Mx}_i$ will lie outside the domain of **f,** so nothing is known about what the image intensity should be at these points. The computations are only performed for points where both $\mathbf{x}_i$ and $\mathbf{Mx}_i$ lie within the field of view of the images.

$$\mathbf{A} = \begin{bmatrix} \frac{\partial f(\mathbf{Mx}_1)}{\partial q_1} & \frac{\partial f(\mathbf{Mx}_1)}{\partial q_2} & \cdots & \frac{\partial f(\mathbf{Mx}_1)}{\partial q_6} & -g(\mathbf{x}_1) \\ \frac{\partial f(\mathbf{Mx}_2)}{\partial q_1} & \frac{\partial f(\mathbf{Mx}_2)}{\partial q_2} & \cdots & \frac{\partial f(\mathbf{Mx}_2)}{\partial q_6} & -g(\mathbf{x}_2) \\ \vdots & \vdots & \ddots & \vdots & \vdots \end{bmatrix}$$

Because nonsingular affine transformations are easily invertible, it is possible to make the registration more robust by also considering what happens with the inverse transformation. By swapping around the source and reference image, the registration problem also becomes one of minimising:

$$\sum_j [g(\mathbf{M}^{-1}\mathbf{y}_j) - q_7^{-1} f(\mathbf{y}_j)]^2$$

In theory, a more robust solution could be achieved by simultaneously including the inverse transformation to make the registration problem symmetric (Woods *et al.,* 1998). The cost function would then be

$$\lambda_1 \sum_i [f(Mx_i) - q_7 g(x_i)]^2 + \lambda_2 \sum_j [g(M^{-1}y_j) - q_7^{-1} f(y_j)]^2$$

Normally, the intensity scaling of the image pair will be similar, so equal values for the weighting factors (λ_1 and λ_2) can be used. Matrix **A** and vector **b** would then be formulated as follows:

$$\mathbf{A} = \begin{bmatrix} \lambda_1^{\frac{1}{2}} [f(\mathbf{Mx}_1) - q_7 g(\mathbf{x}_1)] \\ \lambda_1^{\frac{1}{2}} [f(\mathbf{Mx}_2) - q_7 g(\mathbf{x}_2)] \\ \vdots \\ \lambda_2^{\frac{1}{2}} [g(\mathbf{M}^{-1}\mathbf{y}_1) - q_7^{-1} f(\mathbf{y}_1)] \\ \lambda_2^{\frac{1}{2}} [g(\mathbf{M}^{-1}\mathbf{y}_2) - q_7^{-1} f(\mathbf{y}_2)] \end{bmatrix}$$

and

$$\mathbf{b} = \begin{bmatrix} \lambda_1^{\frac{1}{2}} [f(\mathbf{Mx}_1) - q_7 g(\mathbf{x}_1)] \\ \lambda_1^{\frac{1}{2}} [f(\mathbf{Mx}_2) - q_7 g(\mathbf{x}_2)] \\ \vdots \\ \lambda_2^{\frac{1}{2}} [g(\mathbf{M}^{-1}\mathbf{y}_1) - q_7^{-1} f(\mathbf{y}_1)] \\ \lambda_2^{\frac{1}{2}} [g(\mathbf{M}^{-1}\mathbf{y}_2) - q_7^{-1} f(\mathbf{y}_2)] \\ \vdots \end{bmatrix}$$

Residual Artifacts from PET and fMRI

Even after realignment, some motion-related artifacts may still remain in functional data. After retrospective realignment of PET images with large movements, the primary source of error is due to incorrect attenuation correction. In emission tomography methods, many photons are not detected because they are attenuated by the subject's head. Normally, a transmission scan (using a moving radioactive source external to the subject) is acquired before collecting the emission scans. The ratio of the number of detected photon pairs from the source, with and without a head in the field of view, produces a map of the proportion of photons that are absorbed along any line of response. If a subject moves between the transmission and emission scans, then the applied attenuation correction is incorrect because the emission scan is no longer aligned with the transmission scan. Methods exist for correcting these errors (Anderson *et al.,* 1995), but they are beyond the scope of this book.

In fMRI, there are many sources of motion-related artifacts. The most obvious ones are as follows:

- Interpolation error from the resampling algorithm used to transform the images can be one of the main sources of motion-related artifacts. When the image series is resampled, it is important to use a very accurate interpolation method.
- When MR images are reconstructed, the final images are usually the modulus of the initially complex data, resulting in any voxels that should be negative being rendered positive. This has implications when the images are resampled, because it leads to errors at the edge of the brain that cannot be corrected regardless of how good the interpolation method is. Possible ways to circumvent this problem are to work with complex data, or possibly to apply a low-pass filter to the complex data before taking the modulus.
- The sensitivity (slice selection) profile of each slice also plays a role in introducing artifacts (Noll *et al.,* 1997).
- fMRI images are spatially distorted, and the amount of distortion depends partly on the position of the subject's head within the magnetic field. Relatively large subject movements result in the brain images changing shape, and these shape changes cannot be corrected by a rigid body transformation (Jezzard and Clare, 1999; Anderson *et al.,* 2001).
- Each fMRI volume of a series is currently acquired a plane at a time over a period of a few seconds. Subject movement between acquiring the first and last plane of any volume is another reason why the images may not strictly obey the rules of rigid body motion.
- After a slice is magnetised, the excited tissue takes time to recover to its original state, and the amount of recovery that has taken place will influence the intensity of the tissue in the image. Out-of-plane movement will result in a slightly different part of the brain being excited during each repeat. This means that the spin excitation will vary in a way that is related to head motion, thus leading to more movement-related artifacts (Friston *et al.,* 1996).
- Nyquist ghost artifacts in MR images do not obey the same rigid body rules as the head, so a rigid rotation to align the head will not mean that the ghosts are aligned. The same also applies to other image artifacts such as those arising due to chemical shifts.
- The accuracy of the estimated registration parameters is normally in the region of tens of microns. This is dependent on many factors including the effects just mentioned. Even the signal changes elicited by the experiment can have a slight effect (a few microns) on the estimated parameters (Freire and Mangin, 2001).

These problems cannot be corrected by simple image realignment, so they may be sources of possible stimulus correlated motion artifacts. Systematic movement artifacts resulting in a signal change of only 1% or 2% can lead to highly significant false positives over an experiment with many scans. This is especially important for experiments where some conditions may cause slight head movements (such as motor tasks or speech), because these movements are likely to be highly correlated with the experimental design. In cases like these, it is difficult to separate true activations from stimulus correlated motion artifacts. Providing there are enough images in the series and the movements are small, some of these artifacts can be removed by using an ANCOVA model to remove any signal that is correlated with functions of the estimated movement parameters (Friston *et al.,* 1996). However, when the estimates of the movement parameters are related to the experimental design, it is likely that much of the true fMRI signal will also be lost. These are still unresolved problems.

BETWEEN-MODALITY RIGID REGISTRATION

The combination of multiple imaging modalities can provide enhanced information that is not readily apparent on inspection of individual image modalities. For studies of a single subject, sites of activation can be accurately localised by superimposing them on a high-resolution structural image of the subject (typically a T_1-weighted MRI). This requires registration of the functional images with the structural image. A further possible use for this registration is that a more precise spatial normalisation can be achieved by computing it from a more detailed structural image. If the functional and structural images are in register, then a warp computed from the structural image can be applied to the functional images. Normally a rigid body model is used for registering images of the same subject, but because fMRI images are usually severely distorted—particularly in the phase encode direction (Jezzard and Clare, 1999; Jezzard, 2000)—it is often preferable to do nonlinear registration (Studholme *et al.,* 2000; Kybic *et al.,* 2000). Rigid registration models require voxel sizes to be accurately known. This is a problem that is particularly apparent when registering images from different scanners.

Two images from the same subject acquired using the same modality or scanning sequences generally look similar, so it suffices to find the rigid body transformation parameters that minimise the sum of squared differences between them. However, for coregistration between modalities, there is nothing quite as obvious to minimise, because there is no linear relationship between the image intensities (see Fig. 32.6).

Older methods of registration involved the manual identification of homologous landmarks in the images. These landmarks are aligned together, thus bringing the images into registration. This is time consuming, requires a degree of experience, and can be rather subjective. One of the first widely used semiautomatic coregistration methods was that known as the *head-hat approach* (Pelizzari *et al.,* 1988). This method involved extracting brain surfaces of the two images and then matching the surfaces together. There are also a number of other between-modality registration methods that involve partitioning the images, finding common features between them, and then registering them together, but they are beyond the scope of this chapter.

The first intensity-based intermodal registration method was *AIR* (Woods *et al.,* 1993), which has been widely used for a number of years for registering PET and MR images. This method uses a variance of intensity ratios (VIR) cost function, and involves dividing the MR images into a number of partitions based on intensity. The registration is approximately based on minimising the variance of the corresponding PET voxel intensities for each partition. It makes a number of assumptions about how the PET intensity varies with the MRI intensity, which are generally valid within the brain, but do not work when nonbrain tissue is included. Because of this, the method has the disadvantage of requiring the MR images to be preprocessed, which normally involves editing to remove nonbrain tissue. For a review of a number of intermodality registration approaches up until the mid-1990s, see Zuk and Atkins (1996).

Information Theoretic Approaches

The most recent voxel-similarity measures to be used for intermodal (as well as intramodal; Holden *et al.,* 2000) registration have been based on *information theory.* These measures are based on joint probability distributions of intensities in the images, usually discretely represented in the form of 2D joint histograms. Once constructed, the joint histogram is normalised so that the bins integrate to unity.

The first information theoretic measure to be proposed was the entropy of the joint probability distribution (Studholme *et al.,* 1995), which should be minimised when the images are in register:

$$H(\mathbf{f},\mathbf{g}) = -\int_{-\infty}^{\infty}\int_{-\infty}^{\infty} P(\mathbf{f},\mathbf{g}) \log P(\mathbf{f},\mathbf{g}) \log P(\mathbf{f},\mathbf{g}) d\mathbf{f} d\mathbf{g}$$

The discrete representation of the probability distributions is from a joint histogram (that has been normalised to sum to unity), which can be considered an I by J matrix $\mathbf{P}$. The entropy is then computed from the histogram according to:

$$H(\mathbf{f},\mathbf{g}) = -\sum_{j=1}^{J}\sum_{i=1}^{I} p_{ij} \log p_{ij}$$

In practice, the entropy measure was found to produce poor registration results, but shortly afterward, a more robust measure of registration quality was introduced. This was based on *mutual information* (MI) (Collignon *et al.,* 1995; Wells III *et al.,* 1996), also known as *Shannon information,* which is given by

$$I(\mathbf{f},\mathbf{g}) = H(\mathbf{f}) + H(\mathbf{g}) - H(\mathbf{f},\mathbf{g})$$

where $H(\mathbf{f},\mathbf{g})$ is the joint entropy of the images, and $H(\mathbf{f})$ and $H(\mathbf{g})$ are their marginalised entropies given by

$$H(\mathbf{f}) = -\int_{-\infty}^{\infty} P(\mathbf{f}) \log P(\mathbf{f})\, d\mathbf{f}$$
$$H(\mathbf{g}) = -\int_{-\infty}^{\infty} P(\mathbf{g}) \log P(\mathbf{g})\, d\mathbf{g}$$

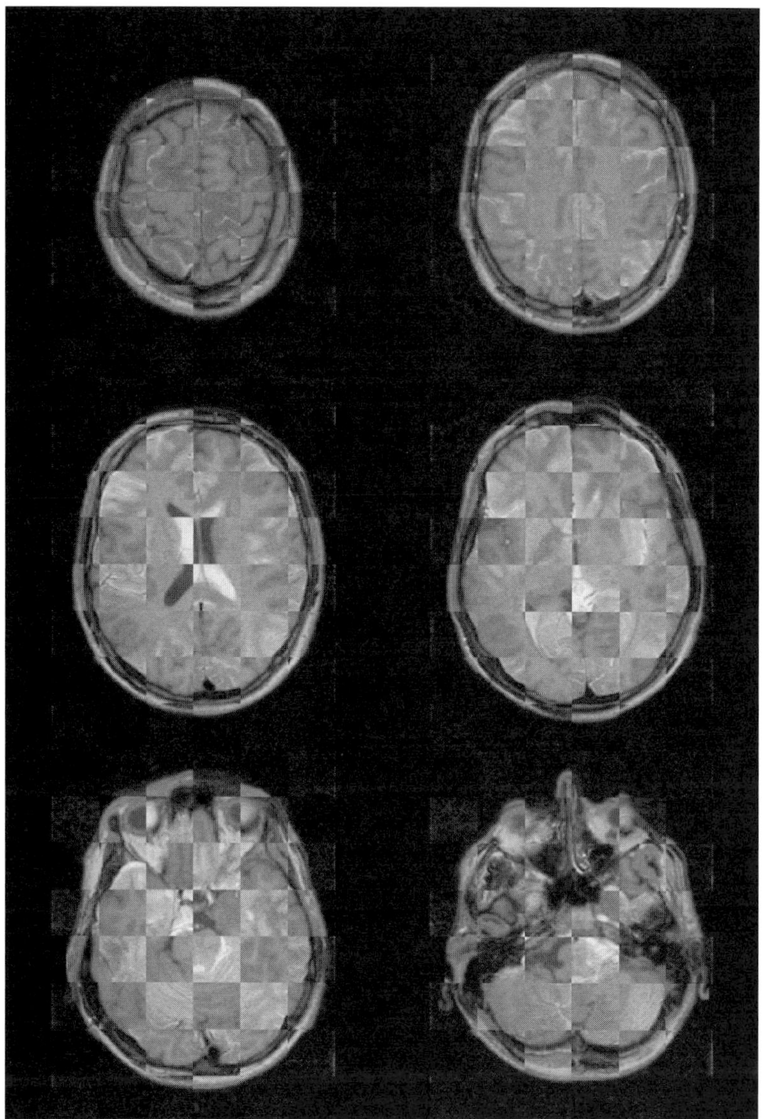

FIGURE 32.6
An example of T_1- and T_2-weighted MR images registered using mutual information. The two registered images are shown interleaved in a chequered pattern.

MI is a measure of dependence of one image on the other and can be considered to be the distance (Kullback-Leibler divergence) between the joint distribution [$P(\mathbf{f},\mathbf{g})$] and the distribution assuming complete independence [$P(\mathbf{f})P(\mathbf{g})$]. When the two distributions are identical, this distance (and the mutual information) is zero. After rearranging, the expression for MI becomes

$$I(\mathbf{f},\mathbf{g}) = KL\left[P(\mathbf{f},\mathbf{g})\,||\,P(\mathbf{f})P(\mathbf{g})\right] = \int_{-\infty}^{\infty}\int_{-\infty}^{\infty} P(\mathbf{f},\mathbf{g}) \log\left(\frac{P(\mathbf{f},\mathbf{g})}{P(\mathbf{f})P(\mathbf{g})}\right) d\mathbf{f}d\mathbf{g}$$

It is assumed that the MI between the images is maximised when they are in register (see Fig. 32.7). One problem though, is that MI is biased by the amount of overlap between the images (although it is still less influenced than the joint entropy). When there is less overlap, fewer samples are used to construct a joint histogram, meaning that it is more "spiky." This produces a slightly higher measure of MI. One overlap invariant information theoretic measure (Studholme *et al.,* 1999) that can be used for registration is

$$\tilde{I}(\mathbf{f},\mathbf{g}) = \frac{H(\mathbf{f}) + H(\mathbf{g})}{H(\mathbf{f},\mathbf{g})}$$

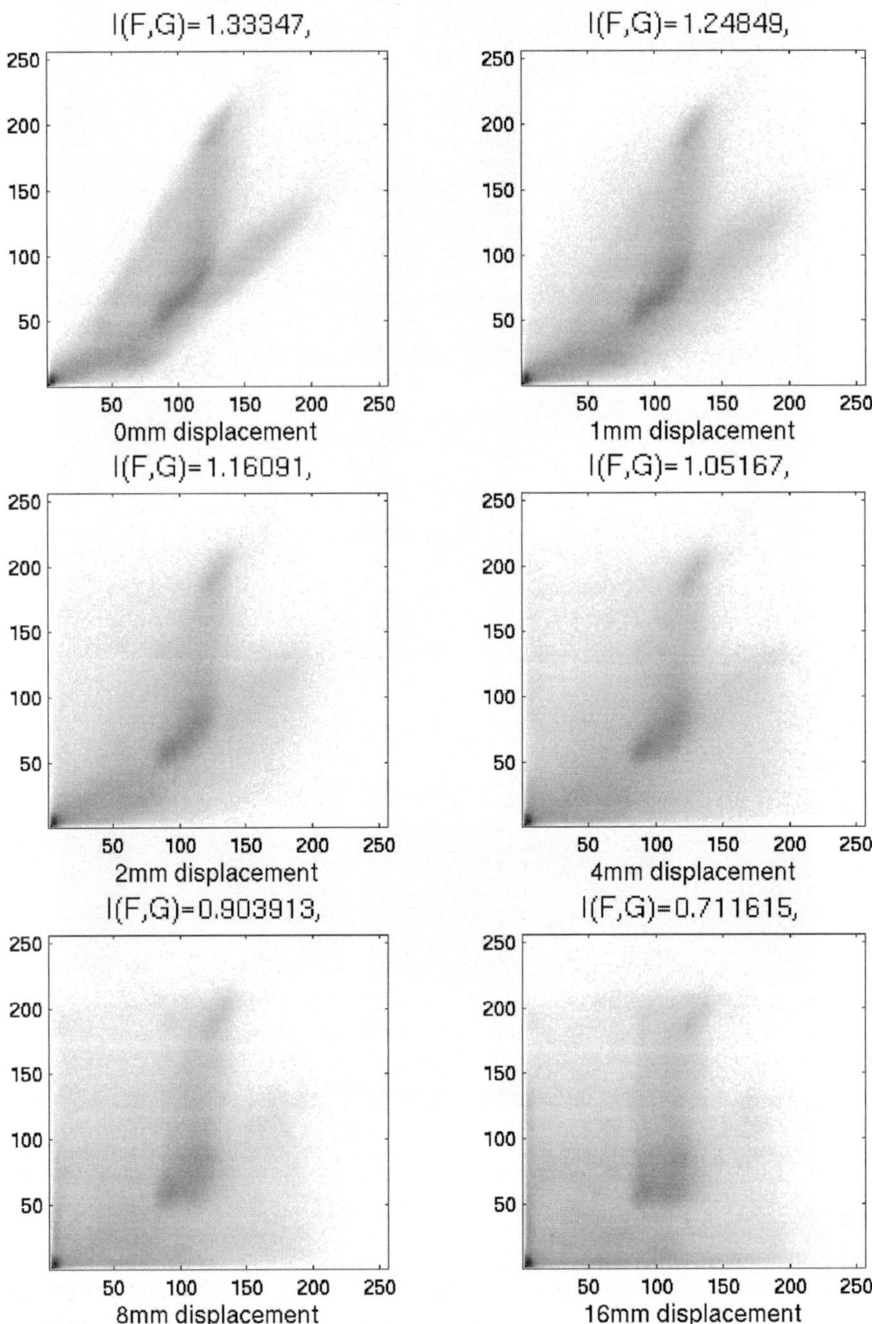

FIGURE 32.7
An illustration of how the joint histogram of an image pair changes as the images are displaced relative to each other. [Note that the pictures show $\log(1 + N)$, where N is the count in each histogram bin.] The MI of the images is also shown.

Another useful measure (Maes *et al.,* 1997) is

$$\tilde{I}(\mathbf{f},\mathbf{g}) = 2H(\mathbf{f},\mathbf{g}) - H(\mathbf{f}) - H(\mathbf{g})$$

and also the *entropy correlation coefficient* (Maes *et al.,* 1997; Press *et al.,* 1992, p. 634, for more information):

$$U(\mathbf{f},\mathbf{g}) = 2\,\frac{H(\mathbf{f}) + H(\mathbf{g}) - H(\mathbf{f},\mathbf{g})}{H(\mathbf{f}) + H(\mathbf{g})}$$

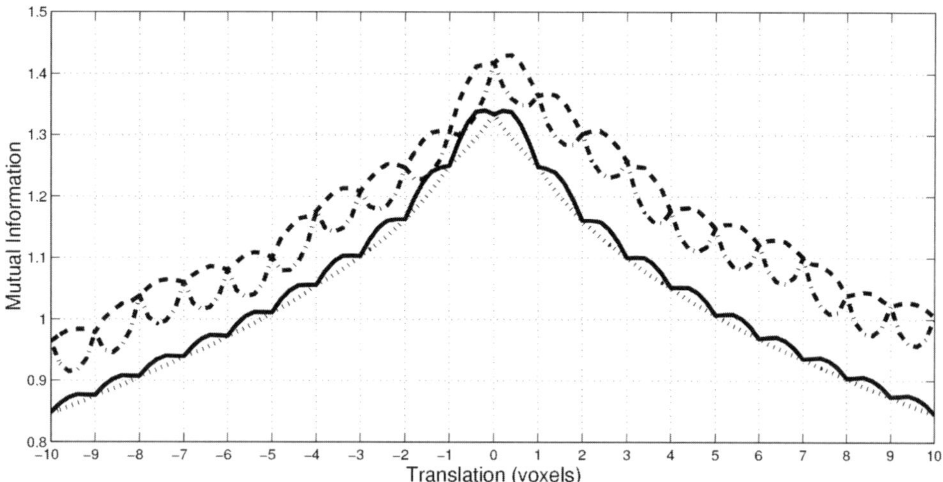

FIGURE 32.8
The mutual information cost function can be particularly susceptible to interpolation artifacts. This figure shows a plot of the MI between two images when they are translated with respect to each other. The dotted and dot-dashed lines show it computed using partial volume interpolation at high and lower sampling densities. The solid and dashed lines show MI computed by interpolating the images themselves.

Implementation Details

Generating a joint histogram involves scanning through the voxels of the reference image and finding the corresponding points of the source. The appropriate bin in the histogram is incremented by one for each of these point pairs. Pairs are ignored if the corresponding voxel is unavailable because it lies outside the image volume. The coordinate of the corresponding point rarely lies at an actual voxel center, meaning that interpolation is required.

Many developers use *partial volume interpolation* (Collignon *et al.,* 1995), rather than interpolating the images themselves, but this can make the MI cost function particularly susceptible to interpolation artifact (see Fig. 32.8). The MI tends to be higher when voxel centers are sampled, where one is added to a single histogram bin. MI is lower when sampling in the center of the eight neighbours, as an eighth is added to eight bins. These artifacts are especially prominent when fewer point pairs are used to generate the histograms.

A simpler alternative is to interpolate the images themselves, but this can lead to new intensity values in the histograms, which also cause interpolation artifacts. This artifact largely occurs because of aliasing after integer-represented images are rescaled so that they have values between zero and $I - 1$, where I is the number of bins in the histogram (see Fig. 32.9). If care is taken at this stage, then interpolation of the image intensities becomes less of a problem. Another method of reducing these artifacts is to not sample the reference image on a regular grid, by (for example) introducing a random jitter to the sampled points (Likar and Pernuš, 2001).

Histograms contain noise, especially if a relatively small number of points are sampled in order to generate them. The optimum binning to use is still not fully resolved, and is likely to vary from application to application, but most researchers use histograms ranging between about 16×16 and 256×256. Smoothing a histogram has a similar effect to using fewer bins. Another alternative is to use a continuous representation of the joint probability distribution, such as a Parzen window density estimate (Wells III *et al.,* 1996) or possibly even a Gaussian mixture model representation.

An earlier section introduced a method of optimisation based on the first and second derivatives of the cost function. Similar principles have been applied to minimising the VIR cost function (Woods *et al.,* 1993) and also to maximising MI (Thévenaz and Unser, 2000).[7]

[7] This paper uses Levenberg-Marquardt optimisation (Press *et al.,* 1992), which is a stabilised version of the Gauss-Newton method.

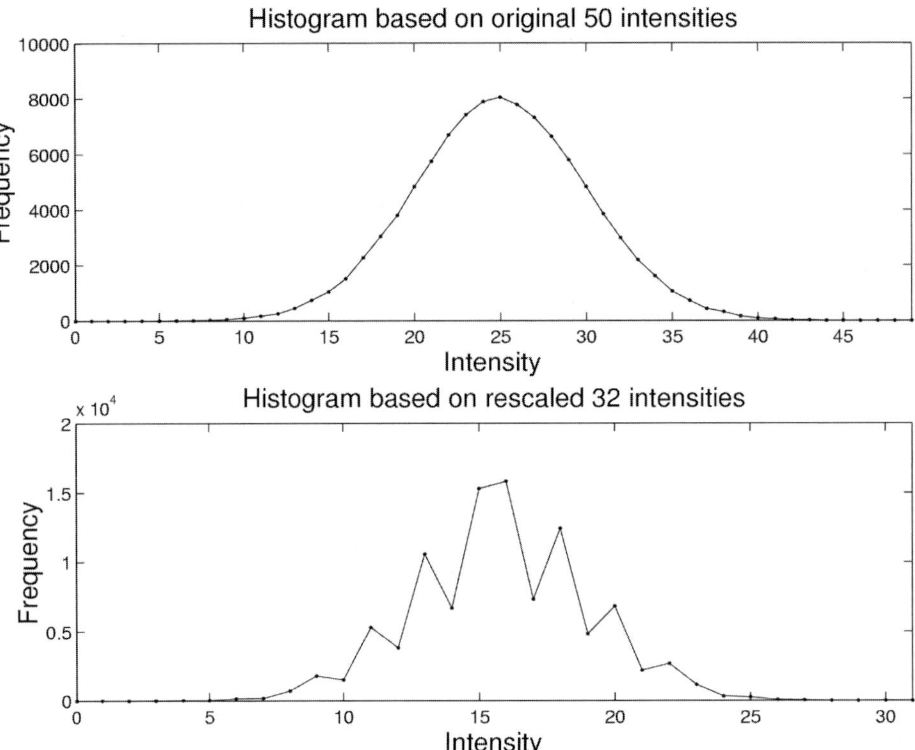

FIGURE 32.9
Rescaling an image can lead to aliasing artifacts in its histogram. (Top) Histogram based on original integer intensity values, simulated to have a Gaussian distribution. (Bottom) The histogram after the intensities are rescaled to between 0 and 63 shows aliasing artifacts.

However, the most widely adopted scheme for maximising MI is Powell's method (see Press *et al.,* 1992, p. 415), which involves a series of successive line searches. Failures occasionally arise if the voxel similarity measure does not vary smoothly with changes to the parameter estimates. This can happen because of interpolation artifacts or if insufficient data contribute to the joint histogram. Alternatively, the algorithm can get caught within a local optimum, so it is important to assign starting estimates that approximately register the images. The required accuracy of the starting estimates depends on the particular images, but an approximate figure for many brain images with a good field of view would be in the region of about 5 cm for translations and 15° for rotations.

References

Alexander, D. C., Gee, J. C., and Bajcsy, R. (1999). Strategies for data reorientation during nonrigid transformations of diffusion tensor images. *Lecture Notes Computer Sci.* **1679,** 463–472.

Alexander, D. C., Pierpaoli, C., Basser, P. J., and Gee, J. C. (2001). Spatial transformations of diffusion tensor magnetic resonance images. *IEEE Trans. Med. Imaging* **20**(11), 1131–1139.

Andersson, J. L. R., Vagnhammar, B. E., and Schneider, H. (1995). Accurate attenuation correction despite movement during PET imaging. *J. Nucl. Med.* **36**(4), 670–678.

Andersson, J. L. R., Hutton, C., Ashburner, J., Turner, R., and Friston, K. J. (2001). Modelling geometric deformations in EPI time series. *NeuroImage* **13**(5), 903–919.

Collignon, A., Maes, F., Delaere, D., Vandermeulen, D., Suetens, P., and Marchal, G. (1995). Automated multi-modality image registration based on information theory. In: "Proc. Information Processing in Medical Imaging" (Y. Bizais, C. Barillot, and R. Di Paola, eds.). Kluwer Academic Publishers, Dordrecht, The Netherlands.

Cox, R. W., and Jesmanowicz, A. (1999). Real-time 3D image registration for functional MRI. *Mag. Res. Med.* **42,** 1014–1018.

Eddy, W. F., Fitzgerald, M., and Noll, D. C. (1996). Improved image registration by using Fourier interpolation. *Mag. Res. Med.* **36,** 923–931.

Freeborough, P. A., and Fox, N. C. (1998). Modelling brain deformations in Alzheimer disease by fluid registration of serial MR images. *J. Computer Assisted Tomog.* **22**(5), 838–843.

Freire, L., and Mangin, J.-F. (2001). Motion correction algorithms of the brain mapping community create spurious functional activations. In: "Proc. Information Processing in Medical Imaging" (M. F. Insana and R. M. Leah, ed.). Springer-Verlag, Berlin, Heidelberg.

Friston, K. J., Ashburner, J., Frith, C. D., Poline, J.-B., Heather, J. D., and Frackowiak, R. S. J. (1995). Spatial registration and normalisation of images. *Hum. Brain Mapping* **2,** 165–189.

Friston, K. J., Williams, S., Howard, R., Frackowiak, R. S. J., and Turner, R. (1996). Movement-related effects in fMRI time-series. *Mag. Res. Med.* **35,** 346–355.

Hajnal, J. V., Mayers, R., Oatridge, A., Schwieso, J. E., Young, J. R., and Bydder, G. M. (1994). Artifacts due to stimulus correlated motion in functional imaging of the brain. *Mag. Res. Med.* **31,** 289–291.

Holden, M. H., Hill, D. L. G., Denton, E. R. E., Jarosz, J. M., Cox, T. C. S., Rohlfing, T., Goodey, J., and Hawkes, D. J. (2000). Voxel similarity measures for 3-D serial MR brain image registration. *IEEE Trans. Med. Imaging* **19**(2), 94–102.

Jain, A. K. (1989). "Fundamentals of Digital Image Processing" Prentice-Hall. Upper Saddle River, NJ.

Jezzard, P. (2000). "Handbook of Medical Imaging," chap. 26, pp. 425–438. Academic Press, San Diego.

Jezzard, P., and Clare, S. (1999). Source distortion in functional MRI data. *Hum. Brain Mapping* **8**(2), 80–85.

Kybic, J., Thévenaz, P., Nirkko, A., and Unser, M. (2000). Unwarping of unidirectionally distorted EPI images. *IEEE Trans. Med. Imaging* **19**(2), 80–93.

Likar, B., and Pernuš, F. (2001). A heirarchical approach to elastic registration based on mutual information. *Image Vis. Computing* **19,** 33–44.

Maes, F., Collignon, A., Vandermeulen, D., Marchal, G., and Seutens, P. (1997). Multimodality image registration by maximisation of mutual information. *IEEE Trans. Med. Imaging* **16,** 187–197.

Noll, D. C., Boada, F. E., and Eddy, W. F. (1997). A spectral approach to analyzing slice selection in planar imaging: optimisation for through-plane interpolation. *Mag. Res. Med.* **38,** 151–160.

Pelizzari, C. A., Chen, G. T. Y., Spelbring, D. R., Weichselbaum, R. R., and Chen, C. T. (1988). Accurate three-dimensional registration of CT, PET and MR images of the brain. *J. Computer Assisted Tomog.* **13,** 20–26.

Press, W. H., Teukolsky, S. A., Vetterling, W. T., and Flannery, B. P. (1992). "Numerical Recipes in C," 2nd ed. Cambridge University Press, Cambridge.

Studholme, C., Constable, R. T., and Duncan, J. S. (2000). Accurate alignment of functional EPI data to anatomical MRI using a physics-based distortion model. *IEEE Trans. Medical Imaging* **19**(11), 1115–1127.

Studholme, C., Hill, D. L. G., and Hawkes, D. J. (1995). Multiresolution voxel similarity measures for MR-PET coregistration. In: "Proc. Information Processing in Medical Imaging" (Y. Bizais, C. Barillot, and R. Di Paola, eds.). Kluwer Academic Publishers, Dordrecht, The Netherlands.

Studholme, C., Hill, D. L. G., and Hawkes, D. J. (1999). An overlap invariant entropy measure of 3D medical image alignment. *Patt. Recog.* **32,** 71–86.

Talairach, J., and Tournoux, P. (1988). "Coplanar Stereotaxic Atlas of the Human Brain." Thieme Medical, New York.

Thévenaz, P., Blu, T., and Unser, M. (2000). Interpolation revisited. *IEEE Trans. Med. Imaging* **19**(7), 739–758.

Thévenaz, P., and Unser, M. (2000). Optimisation of mutual information for multiresolution image registration. *IEEE Trans. Image Process.* **9**(12), 2083–2099.

Unser, M., Aldroubi, A., and Eden, M. (1993a). B-spline signal processing: part I—theory. *IEEE Trans. Signal Processing* **41**(2), 821–833.

Unser, M., Aldroubi, A., and Eden, M. (1993b). B-spline signal processing: part II—efficient design and applications. *IEEE Trans. Signal Processing* **41**(2), 834–848.

Wells III, W. M., Viola, P., Atsumi, H., Nakajima, S., and Kikinis, R. (1996). Multi-modal volume registration by maximisation of mutual information. *Med. Image Anal.* **1**(1), 35–51.

Woods, R. P. (1999). "Brain Warping," chap. 20, pp. 365–376. Academic Press, San Diego.

Woods, R. P. (2000). "Handbook of Medical Imaging," chap. 33, pp. 529–536. Academic Press, San Diego.

Woods, R. P., Mazziotta, J. C., and Cherry, S. R. (1993). MRI-PET registration with automated algorithm. *J. Computer Assisted Tomog.* **17,** 536–546.

Woods, R. P., Grafton, S. T., Holmes, C. J., Cherry, S. R., and Mazziotta, J. C. (1998). Automated image registration: I. general methods and intrasubject, intramodality validation. *J. Computer Assisted Tomog.* **22**(1), 139–152.

Zuk, T. D., and Atkins, M. S. (1996). A comparison of manual and automatic methods for registering scans of the head. *IEEE Trans. Med. Imaging* **15**(5), 732–744.

CHAPTER

33

Spatial Normalisation Using Basis Functions

INTRODUCTION

Sometimes it is desirable to warp images from a number of individuals into roughly the same standard space to allow signal averaging across subjects. This procedure is known as *spatial normalisation.* In functional imaging studies, spatial normalisation of the images is useful for determining what happens generically over individuals. A further advantage of using spatially normalised images is that activation sites can be reported according to their Euclidean coordinates within a standard space (Fox, 1995). The most commonly adopted coordinate system within the brain imaging community is that described by Talairach and Tournoux (1988), although new standards are now emerging that are based on digital atlases (Evans *et al.,* 1993, 1994; Mazziotta *et al.,* 1995).

Methods of registering images can be broadly divided into *label based* and *intensity based.* Label-based techniques identify homologous features (labels) in the source and reference images and find the transformations that best superpose them. The labels can be points, lines, or surfaces. Homologous features are often identified manually, but this process is time consuming and subjective. Another disadvantage of using points as landmarks is that there are very few readily identifiable discrete points in the brain. Lines and surfaces are more readily identified, and in many instances they can be extracted automatically (or at least semiautomatically). Once they are identified, the spatial transformation is effected by bringing the homologies together. If the labels are points, then the required transformations at each of those points is known. Between the points, the deforming behaviour is not known, so it is forced to be as "smooth" as possible. A number of methods are available for modelling this smoothness. The simplest models include fitting splines through the points in order to minimise *bending energy* (Bookstein, 1989, 1997a). More complex forms of interpolation, such as viscous fluid models, are often used when the labels are surfaces (Thompson and Toga, 1996; Davatzikos, 1996).

Intensity (nonlabel)-based approaches identify a spatial transformation that optimises some voxel-similarity measure between a source and reference image, where both are treated as unlabeled continuous processes. The matching criterion is usually based on minimising the sum of squared differences or maximising the correlation between the images. For this criterion to be successful, it requires the reference to appear like a warped version of the source image. In other words, there must be a correspondence in the gray levels of the different tissue types between the source and reference images. To warp together images of different modalities, a few intensity-based methods have been devised that involve optimising an information theoretic measure (Studholme *et al.,* 2000; Thévenaz and Unser, 2000). Intensity matching methods are usually very susceptible to poor starting estimates, so more recently a number of hybrid approaches have emerged that combine intensity-based methods with matching user-defined features (typically sulci).

A potentially enormous number of parameters are required to describe the nonlinear transformations that warp two images together (i.e., the problem is very high dimensional). However, much of the spatial variability can be captured using just a few parameters. Some research groups use only a 9- or 12-parameter affine transformation to approximately register images of different subjects, accounting for differences in position, orientation, and overall brain dimensions. Low spatial frequency global variability of head shape can be accommodated by describing deformations by a linear combination of low-frequency basis functions. One widely used basis function registration method is part of the AIR package (Woods *et al.,* 1998a,b), which uses polynomial basis functions to model shape variability. For example, a two-dimensional third-order polynomial basis function mapping can be defined as follows:

$$\begin{aligned} y_1 = {} & q_1 + q_2x_1 + q_3x_1^2 + q_4x_1^3 \\ & + q_5x_1 + q_6x_1x_2 + q_7x_1^2x_2 \\ & + q_8x_2^2 + q_9x_1x_2^2 \\ & + q_{10}x_2^3 \\ y_2 = {} & q_{11} + q_{12}x_1 + q_{13}x_1^2 + q_{14}x_1^3 \\ & + q_{15}x_2 + q_{16}x_1x_2 + q_{17}x_1^2x_2 \\ & + q_{18}x_2^2 + q_{19}x_1x_2^2 \\ & + q_{20}x_2^3 \end{aligned}$$

Other low-dimensional registration methods may employ a number of other forms of basis function to parameterise the warps. These include Fourier bases (Christensen, 1999), sine and cosine transform basis functions (Christensen, 1994; Ashburner and Friston, 1999), B-splines (Studholme *et al.,* 2000; Thévenaz and Unser, 2000), and piecewise affine or trilinear basis functions (see Glasbey and Mardia, 1998, for a review). The small number of parameters will not allow every feature to be matched exactly, but it will permit the global head shape to be modeled. The rationale for adopting a low-dimensional approach is that it allows rapid modelling of global brain shape.

The deformations required to transform images to the same space are not clearly defined. Unlike rigid-body transformations, where the constraints are explicit, those for warping are more arbitrary. Regularisation schemes are therefore necessary when attempting image registration with many parameters, thus ensuring that voxels remain close to their neighbours. Regularisation is often incorporated by some form of Bayesian scheme, using estimators such as the *maximum a posteriori* (MAP) estimate or the *minimum variance estimate* (MVE). Often, the prior probability distributions used by registration schemes are linear, and they include minimising the *membrane energy* of the deformation field (Amit *et al.,* 1991; Gee *et al.,* 1997), the *bending energy* (Bookstein, 1997a) or the *linear-elastic energy* (Miller *et al.,* 1993; Davatzikos, 1996). None of these linear penalties explicitly preserves the topology[1] of the warped images, although cost functions that incorporate this constraint have been devised (Edwards *et al.,* 1997; Ashburner and Friston, 1998). A number of methods involve repeated Gaussian smoothing of the estimated deformation fields (Collins *et al.,* 1995). These methods can be classed among the elastic registration methods because convolving a deformation field is a form of linear regularisation (Bro-Nielsen and Gramkow, 1996).

An alternative to using a Bayesian scheme incorporating some form of elastic prior could be to use a viscous fluid model (Christensen *et al.,* 1994, 1996; Bro-Nielsen and Gramkow, 1996; Thirion, 1995) to estimate the warps. In these models, finite difference methods are often used to solve the partial differential equations that model one image as it "flows" to the same shape as the other. The major advantage of these methods is that they are able to account for large deformations and also ensure that the topology of the warped image is preserved. Viscous fluid

[1] The word *topology* is used in the same sense as in "Topological Properties of Smooth Anatomical Maps" (Christensen *et al.,* 1995). If spatial transformations are not one to one and continuous, then the topological properties of different structures can change.

models are almost able to warp any image so that it looks like any other image, while still preserving the original topology. These methods can be classed as "plastic" because it is not the deformation fields themselves that are regularised, but rather the increments to the deformations at each iteration.

METHOD

This chapter describes the steps involved in registering images of different subjects into roughly the same coordinate system, where the coordinate system is defined by a template image (or series of images).

This section begins by introducing a modification to the optimisation method described in Chapter 32, such that more robust MAP parameter estimates can be obtained. It works by estimating the optimum coefficients for a set of bases, by minimising the sum of squared differences between the template and source image, while simultaneously minimising the deviation of the transformation from its expected value. To adopt the MAP approach, it is necessary to have estimates of the likelihood of obtaining the fit given the data, which requires prior knowledge of spatial variability and also knowledge of the variance associated with each observation. True Bayesian approaches assume that the variance associated with each voxel is already known, whereas the approach described here is a type of empirical Bayesian method, which attempts to estimate this variance from the residual errors (see Chapter 39). Because the registration is based on smooth images, correlations between neighbouring voxels are considered when estimating the variance. This makes the same approach suitable for the spatial normalisation of both high-quality MR images and low-resolution, noisy PET images.

The first step in registering images from different subjects involves determining the optimum 12-parameter affine transformation. Unlike Chapter 32—where the images to be matched together are from the same subject—zooms and shears are needed to register heads of different shapes and sizes. Prior knowledge of the variability of head sizes is included within a Bayesian framework in order to increase the robustness and accuracy of the method.

The next part describes nonlinear registration for correcting gross differences in head shapes that cannot be accounted for by the affine normalisation alone. The nonlinear warps are modeled by linear combinations of smooth discrete cosine transform basis functions. A fast algorithm is described that utilises Taylor's theorem and the separable nature of the basis functions, meaning that most of the nonlinear spatial variability between images can be automatically corrected within a few minutes. For speed and simplicity, a relatively small number of parameters (approximately 1000) are used to describe the nonlinear components of the registration. The MAP scheme requires some form of prior distribution for the basis function coefficients, so a number of different forms for this distribution are then presented.

The last part of this section describes a variety of possible models for intensity transforms. In addition to spatial transformations, it is sometimes desirable to also include intensity transforms in the registration model, because one image may not look exactly like a spatially transformed version of the other.

A MAP Solution

A Bayesian registration scheme is used in order to obtain a MAP estimate of the registration parameters. Given some prior knowledge of the variability of brain shapes and sizes that may be encountered, a MAP registration scheme is able to give a more accurate (although biased) estimate of the true shapes of the brains. This is illustrated by a very simple one-dimensional example in Fig. 33.1. The use of a MAP parameter estimate reduces any potential overfitting of the data, which may lead to unnecessary deformations that only reduce the residual variance by a tiny amount. It also makes the registration scheme more robust by reducing the search space of the algorithm and, therefore, the number of potential local minima.

Bayes' rule can be expressed as

$$p(\mathbf{q} \mid \mathbf{b}) \propto p(\mathbf{b} \mid \mathbf{q})p(\mathbf{q}) \tag{33.1}$$

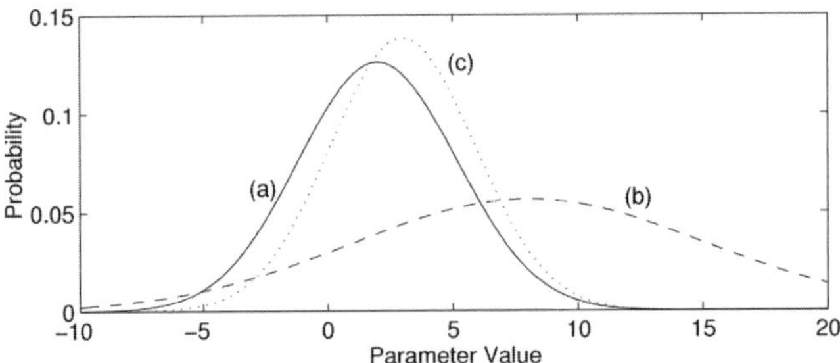

FIGURE 33.1
This figure illustrates a hypothetical example with one parameter, where the prior probability distribution is better described than the likelihood. The solid Gaussian curve (a) represents the prior probability distribution function (pdf), and the dashed curve (b) represents a maximum likelihood parameter estimate (from fitting to observed data) with its associated certainty. The true parameter is known to be drawn from distribution (a), but it can be estimated with the certainty described by distribution (b). Without the MAP scheme, a more precise estimate would probably be obtained for the true parameter by taking the most likely *a priori* value, rather than the value obtained from a maximum likelihood fit to the data. This would be analogous to cases where the number of parameters is reduced in a maximum likelihood registration model in order to achieve a better solution. The dotted line (c) shows the posterior pdf obtained using Bayesian statistics. The maximum value of (c) is the MAP estimate. It combines previously known information with that from the data to give a more accurate estimate.

where $p(\mathbf{q})$ is the prior probability of parameters $\mathbf{q}$, $p(\mathbf{b} \mid \mathbf{q})$ is the conditional probability that $\mathbf{b}$ is observed given $\mathbf{q}$, and $p(\mathbf{q} \mid \mathbf{b})$ is the posterior probability of $\mathbf{q}$, given that measurement $\mathbf{b}$ has been made. The *maximum a posteriori* (MAP) estimate for parameters $\mathbf{q}$ is the mode of $p(\mathbf{q} \mid \mathbf{b})$. The *maximum likelihood* (ML) estimate is a special case of the MAP estimate, in which $p(\mathbf{q})$ is uniform over all values of $\mathbf{q}$. For our purposes, $p(\mathbf{q})$ represents a known prior probability distribution from which the parameters are drawn, $p(\mathbf{b} \mid \mathbf{q})$ is the probability of obtaining the data $\mathbf{b}$ given the parameters (likelihood of $\mathbf{q}$), and $p(\mathbf{q} \mid \mathbf{b})$ is the function to be maximised. The optimisation can be simplified by assuming that all probability distributions can be approximated by multinormal (multidimensional and normal) distributions and can therefore be described by a mean vector and a covariance matrix.

A probability is related to its Gibbs form by $p(a) \propto e^{-H(a)}$. Therefore, the posterior probability is maximised when its Gibbs form is minimised. This is equivalent to minimising $H(\mathbf{b} \mid \mathbf{q}) + H(\mathbf{q})$ (the posterior potential). In this expression, $H(\mathbf{b} \mid \mathbf{q})$ (the likelihood potential) is related to the residual sum of squares. If the parameters are assumed to be drawn from a multinormal distribution described by a mean vector $\mathbf{q_0}$ and covariance matrix $\mathbf{C_0}$, then $H(\mathbf{q})$, the prior potential, is simply given by

$$H(\mathbf{q}) = (\mathbf{q} - \mathbf{q}_0)^T \mathbf{C}_0^{-1} (\mathbf{q} - \mathbf{q}_0)$$

Equation (32.1) in the preceding chapter gives the following maximum likelihood updating rule for the parameter estimation:

$$\mathbf{q}_{\mathrm{ML}}^{(n+1)} = \mathbf{q}^{(n)} - (\mathbf{A}^T\mathbf{A})^{-1} \mathbf{A}^T\mathbf{b} \tag{33.2}$$

Assuming equal variance for each observation (σ^2) and ignoring covariances among them, the formal covariance matrix of the fit on the assumption of normally distributed errors is given by $\sigma^2 (\mathbf{A}^T\mathbf{A})^{-1}$. When the distributions are normal, the MAP estimate is simply the average of the prior and likelihood estimates, weighted by the inverses of their respective covariance matrices:

$$\mathbf{q}^{(n+1)} = (\mathbf{C}_0^{-1} + \mathbf{A}^T\mathbf{A}/\sigma^2)^{-1} (\mathbf{C}_0^{-1}\mathbf{q}_0 + \mathbf{A}^T\mathbf{A}/\sigma^2\mathbf{q}_{\mathrm{ML}})^{(n+1)} \tag{33.3}$$

The MAP optimisation scheme is obtained by combining Eqs. (33.2) and (33.3):

$$\mathbf{q}^{(n+1)} = (\mathbf{C}_0^{-1} + \mathbf{A}^T\mathbf{A}/\sigma^2)^{-1} (\mathbf{C}_0^{-1}\mathbf{q}_0 + \mathbf{A}^T\mathbf{A}\mathbf{q}^{(n)}/\sigma^2 - \mathbf{A}^T\mathbf{b}/\sigma^2) \tag{33.4}$$

For the sake of the registration, it is assumed that the exact form for the prior probability distribution $[N(\mathbf{q_0}, \mathbf{C}_0)]$ is known. However, because the registration may need to be done on a wide range of different image modalities, with differing contrasts and signal-to-noise ratios, it is not possible to easily and automatically know what value to use for σ^2. In practice, σ^2 is assumed to be the same for all observations, and it is estimated from the sum of squared differences from the current iteration:

$$\sigma^2 = \sum_{i=1}^{I} b_i(\mathbf{q})^2/\nu$$

where ν refers to the degrees of freedom. If the sampling is sparse relative to the smoothness, then $\nu \simeq I - J$, where I is the number of sampled locations in the images and J is the number of estimated parameters.[2]

However, complications arise because the images are smooth, resulting in the observations not being independent and a reduction in the effective number of degrees of freedom. The degrees of freedom are corrected using the principles described by Friston *et al.* (1995b); although this approach is not strictly correct (Worsley and Friston, 1995), it gives an estimate that is close enough for these purposes. The effective degrees of freedom are estimated by assuming that the difference between **f** and **g** approximates a continuous, zero-mean, homogeneous, smoothed *Gaussian random field.* The approximate parameter of a Gaussian point spread function describing the smoothness in direction k (assuming that the axes of the Gaussian are aligned with the axes of the image coordinate system) can be obtained by (Poline *et al.*, 1995)

$$w_k = \sqrt{\frac{\sum_{i=1}^{I} b_i(\mathbf{q})^2}{2\sum_{i=1}^{I} (\nabla_k b_i(\mathbf{q}))^2}}$$

Multiplying w_k by $\sqrt{8 \log_e (2)}$ produces an estimate of the full-width at half-maximum (FWHM) of the Gaussian. If the images are sampled on a regular grid where the spacing in each direction is s_k, the number of effective degrees of freedom[3] becomes approximately:

$$\nu = (I - J) \prod_k \frac{s_k}{w_k(2\pi)^{1/2}}$$

This is essentially a scaling of $I - J$ by the number of resolution elements per voxel.

This approach has the advantage that when the parameter estimates are far from the solution, σ^2 is large, so the problem becomes more heavily regularised with more emphasis being placed on the prior information. For nonlinear warping, this is analogous to a coarse-to-fine registration scheme. The penalty against higher frequency warps is greater than that for those of low frequency (see later section). In the early iterations, the estimated σ^2 is higher, leading to a heavy penalty against all warps, but with more against those of higher frequency. The algorithm does not fit much of the high-frequency information until σ^2 has been reduced. In addition to a gradual reduction in σ^2 due to the decreasing residual squared difference, σ^2 is also reduced because the estimated smoothness is decreased, leading to more effective degrees of freedom. Both of these factors are influential in making the registration scheme more robust to local minima.

Affine Registration

Almost all between-subject coregistration or spatial normalisation methods for brain images begin by determining the optimal 9- or 12-parameter affine transformation that registers the images together. This step is normally performed automatically by minimising (or maximising) some mutual function of the images. The objective of affine registration is to fit the source image **f** to a template image **g,** using a 12-parameter affine transformation. The images may be scaled quite differently, so an additional intensity scaling parameter is included in the model.

Without constraints and with poor data, simple ML parameter optimisation (similar to that described in Chapter 32) can produce some extremely unlikely transformations. For example, when there are only a few slices in the image, it is not possible for the algorithms to determine an accurate zoom in the out-of-plane direction. Any estimate of this value is likely to have very

[2] Strictly speaking, the computation of the degrees of freedom should be more complicated than this, because this simple model does not account for the regularisation.

[3] Note that this only applies when $s_k < w_k (2\pi)^{1/2}$, otherwise $\nu = I - J$. Alternatively, to circumvent this problem, the degrees of freedom can be better estimated by $(I - J) \prod_k \text{erf}(2^{-3/2} s_k/w_k)$. This gives a similar result to the approximation by Friston *et al.* (1995b) for smooth images, but never allows the computed value to exceed $I - J$.

large errors. When a regularised approach is not used, it may be better to assign a fixed value for this difficult-to-determine parameter and simply fit for the remaining ones.

By incorporating prior information into the optimisation procedure, a smooth transition between fixed and fitted parameters can be achieved. When the error for a particular fitted parameter is known to be large, then that parameter will be based more on the prior information. To adopt this approach, the prior distribution of the parameters should be known. This can be derived from the zooms and shears determined by registering a large number of brain images to the template.

Nonlinear Registration

The nonlinear spatial normalisation approach described here assumes that the image has already been approximately registered with the template according to a 12-parameter affine registration. This section illustrates how the parameters describing global shape differences (not accounted for by affine registration) between an image and template can be determined.

The model for defining nonlinear warps uses deformations consisting of a linear combination of low-frequency periodic basis functions. The spatial transformation from coordinates $\mathbf{x}_i$ to coordinates $\mathbf{y}_i$ is

$$y_{1i} = x_{1i} + u_{1i} = x_{1i} + \sum_j q_{j1} d_j(\mathbf{x}_i)$$

$$y_{2i} = x_{2i} + u_{2i} = x_{1i} + \sum_j q_{j2} d_j(\mathbf{x}_i)$$

$$y_{3i} = x_{3i} + u_{3i} = x_{3i} + \sum_j q_{j3} d_j(\mathbf{x}_i)$$

where q_{jk} is the jth coefficient for dimension k, and $d_j(\mathbf{x})$ is the jth basis function at position $\mathbf{x}$.

The choice of basis functions depends on the distribution of warps likely to be required and also on how translations at borders should behave. If points at the borders over which the transform is computed are not required to move in any direction, then the basis functions should consist of the lowest frequencies of the three-dimensional discrete sine transform (DST). If there are to be no constraints at the borders, then a three-dimensional discrete cosine transform (DCT) is more appropriate. Both of these transforms use the same set of basis functions to represent warps in each of the directions. Alternatively, a mixture of DCT and DST basis functions can be used to constrain translations at the surfaces of the volume to be parallel to the surface only (*sliding* boundary conditions). By using a different combination of DCT and DST basis functions, the corners of the volume can be fixed and the remaining points on the surface can be free to move in all directions (*bending* boundary conditions) (Christensen, 1994). These various boundary conditions are illustrated in Fig. 33.2.

The basis functions used here are the lowest frequency components of the three- (or two)-dimensional DCT. In one dimension, the DCT of a function is generated by premultiplication with the matrix $\mathbf{D}^T$, where the elements of the $I \times M$ matrix $\mathbf{D}$ are defined as follows:

$$d_{i1} = \frac{1}{\sqrt{I}} \quad i = 1..I$$

$$d_{im} = \sqrt{\frac{2}{I}} \cos\left(\frac{\pi(2i-1)(m-1)}{2I}\right) \quad i = 1..I,\ m = 2..M$$

A set of low-frequency, two-dimensional DCT basis functions is shown in Fig. 33.3, and a schematic example of a two-dimensional deformation based on the DCT is shown in Fig. 33.4.

As for affine registration, the optimisation involves minimising the sum of squared differences between a source ($\mathbf{f}$) and template image ($\mathbf{g}$). The images may be scaled differently, so an additional parameter (w) is needed to accommodate this difference. The minimised function is then

$$\sum_i [f(\mathbf{y}_i) - wg(\mathbf{x}_i)]^2$$

The approach described in Chapter 32 is used to optimise the parameters $\mathbf{q}_1$, $\mathbf{q}_2$, $\mathbf{q}_3$, and w, and requires derivatives of the function $f(\mathbf{y}_i) - wg(\mathbf{x}_i)$ with respect to each parameter. These can be obtained using the chain rule:

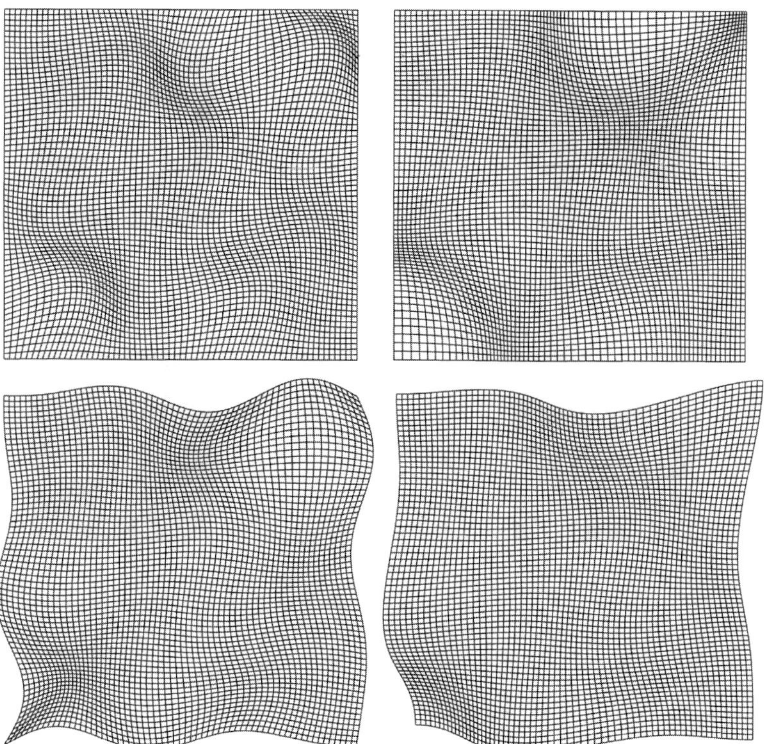

FIGURE 33.2
Different boundary conditions. (Above left) Fixed boundaries (generated purely from DST basis functions). (Above right) Sliding boundaries (from a mixture of DCT and DST basis functions). (Below left) Bending boundaries (from a different mixture of DCT and DST basis functions). (Below right) Free boundary conditions (purely from DCT basis functions).

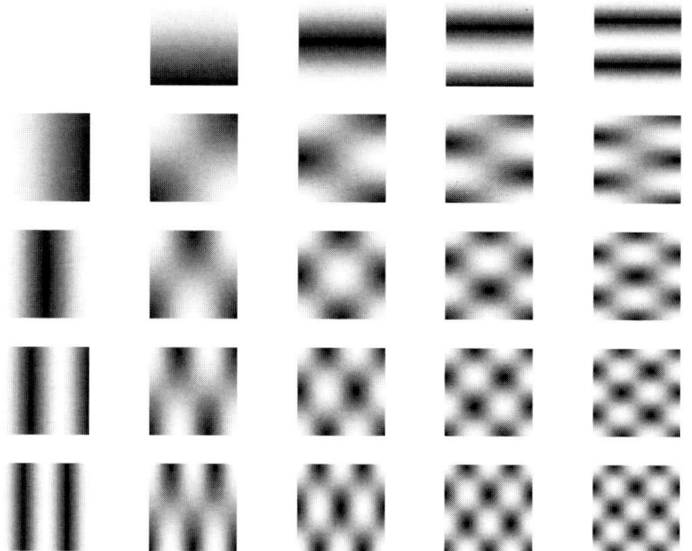

FIGURE 33.3
The lowest frequency basis functions of a two-dimensional DCT.

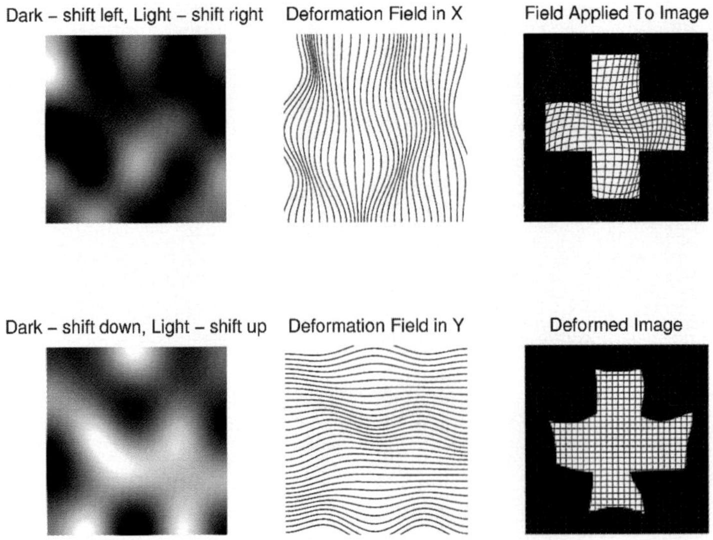

FIGURE 33.4
In two dimensions, a deformation field consists of two scalar fields: one for horizontal deformations, and the other for vertical deformations. The images on the left show deformations as a linear combination of basis images (see Fig. 33.3). The center column shows the same deformations in a more intuitive sense. The deformation is applied by overlaying it on a source image and resampling (right).

$$\frac{\partial f(\mathbf{y}_i)}{\partial q_{j1}} = \frac{\partial f(\mathbf{y}_i)}{\partial y_{1i}} \frac{\partial y_{1i}}{\partial q_{j1}} = \frac{\partial f(\mathbf{y}_i)}{\partial y_{1i}} d_j(\mathbf{x}_i)$$
$$\frac{\partial f(\mathbf{y}_i)}{\partial q_{j2}} = \frac{\partial f(\mathbf{y}_i)}{\partial y_{2i}} \frac{\partial y_{2i}}{\partial q_{j2}} = \frac{\partial f(\mathbf{y}_i)}{\partial y_{2i}} d_j(\mathbf{x}_i)$$
$$\frac{\partial f(\mathbf{y}_i)}{\partial q_{j3}} = \frac{\partial f(\mathbf{y}_i)}{\partial y_{3i}} \frac{\partial y_{3i}}{\partial q_{j3}} = \frac{\partial f(\mathbf{y}_i)}{\partial y_{3i}} d_j(\mathbf{x}_i)$$

The approach involves iteratively computing $\mathbf{A}^T\mathbf{A}$ and $\mathbf{A}^T\mathbf{b}$. However, because there are many parameters to optimise, these computations can be very time consuming. We now provide a description of a very efficient way to compute these matrices.

A *Fast Algorithm*

A fast algorithm for computing $\mathbf{A}^T\mathbf{A}$ and $\mathbf{A}^T\mathbf{b}$ is shown in Fig. 33.5. The remainder of this section explains the matrix terminology used and why it is so efficient.

For simplicity, the algorithm is only illustrated in two dimensions. Images **f** and **g** are considered to be $I \times J$ matrices **F** and **G,** respectively. Row i of **F** is denoted by $\mathbf{f}_{i,:}$, and column j by $\mathbf{f}_{:,j}$. The basis functions used by the algorithm are generated from a separable form from matrices $\mathbf{D}_1$ and $\mathbf{D}_2$, with dimensions $I \times M$ and $J \times N$, respectively. By treating the transform coefficients as $M \times N$ matrices $\mathbf{Q}_1$ and $\mathbf{Q}_2$, the deformation fields can be rapidly constructed by computing $\mathbf{D}_1\mathbf{Q}_1\mathbf{D}_2^T$ and $\mathbf{D}_1\mathbf{Q}_2\mathbf{D}_2^T$.

Between each iteration, image **F** is resampled according to the latest parameter estimates. The derivatives of **F** are also resampled to give ∇_1F and ∇_2F. The ith element of each of these matrices contains $f(\mathbf{y}_i)$, $\partial f(\mathbf{y}_i)/\partial y_i$, and $\partial f(\mathbf{y}_i)/\partial y_{2i}$, respectively.

The notation diag $(\nabla_1 \mathrm{f}_{:,j})\mathbf{D}_1$ simply means to multiply each element of row i of $\mathbf{D}_1$ by $\nabla_1\mathbf{f}_{i,j}$, and the symbol ⊗ refers to the *Kronecker tensor product.* If $\mathbf{D}_2$ is a matrix of order $J \times N$, and $\mathbf{D}_1$ is a second matrix, then

$$\mathbf{D}_2 \otimes \mathbf{D}_1 = \begin{bmatrix} d_{211}\mathbf{D}_1 & \dots & d_{21N}\mathbf{D}_1 \\ \vdots & \ddots & \vdots \\ d_{2J1}\mathbf{D}_1 & \dots & d_{2JN}\mathbf{D}_1 \end{bmatrix}$$

The advantage of the algorithm shown in Fig. 33.5 is that it utilises some of the useful properties of Kronecker tensor products. This is especially important when the algorithm is implemented in three dimensions. The limiting factor to the algorithm is no longer the time taken

$$\alpha = [0]$$

$$\beta = [0]$$

$$\begin{aligned}
&for \quad j = 1 \dots J\\
&\quad \mathbf{C} = \mathbf{d_2}_{j,:}{}^T \mathbf{d_2}_{j,:}\\
&\quad \mathbf{E_1} = diag(\nabla_1 \mathbf{f}_{:,j})\mathbf{D_1}\\
&\quad \mathbf{E_2} = diag(\nabla_2 \mathbf{f}_{:,j})\mathbf{D_1}\\
&\quad \alpha = \alpha + \begin{bmatrix} \mathbf{C} \otimes (\mathbf{E_1}^T\mathbf{E_1}) & \mathbf{C} \otimes (\mathbf{E_1}^T\mathbf{E_2}) & -\mathbf{d_2}_{j,:}{}^T \otimes (\mathbf{E_1}^T\mathbf{g}_{:,j}) \\ (\mathbf{C} \otimes (\mathbf{E_1}^T\mathbf{E_2}))^T & \mathbf{C} \otimes (\mathbf{E_2}^T\mathbf{E_2}) & -\mathbf{d_2}_{j,:}{}^T \otimes (\mathbf{E_2}^T\mathbf{g}_{:,j}) \\ (-\mathbf{d_2}_{j,:}{}^T \otimes (\mathbf{E_1}^T\mathbf{g}_{:,j}))^T & (-\mathbf{d_2}_{j,:}{}^T \otimes (\mathbf{E_1}^T\mathbf{g}_{:,j}))^T & \mathbf{g}_{:,j}{}^T\mathbf{g}_{:,j} \end{bmatrix}\\
&\quad \beta = \beta + \begin{bmatrix} \mathbf{d_2}_{j,:}{}^T \otimes (\mathbf{E_1}^T(\mathbf{f}_{:,j} - w\mathbf{g}_{:,j})) \\ \mathbf{d_2}_{j,:}{}^T \otimes (\mathbf{E_2}^T(\mathbf{f}_{:,j} - w\mathbf{g}_{:,j})) \\ \mathbf{g}_{:,j}{}^T(\mathbf{f}_{:,j} - w\mathbf{g}_{:,j}) \end{bmatrix}\\
&end
\end{aligned}$$

FIGURE 33.5
A two-dimensional illustration of the fast algorithm for computing $\mathbf{A}^T\mathbf{A}$ (α) and $\mathbf{A}^T\mathbf{b}$ (β).

to create the curvature matrix ($\mathbf{A}^T\mathbf{A}$), but is now the amount of memory required to store it and the time taken to invert it.

Linear Regularisation for Nonlinear Registration

Without regularisation in the nonlinear registration, it is possible to introduce unnecessary deformations that only reduce the residual sum of squares by a tiny amount (see Fig. 33.6). This could potentially make the algorithm very unstable. Regularisation is achieved by minimising the sum of squared difference between the template and the warped image, while simultaneously minimising some function of the deformation field. The principles are Bayesian and make use of the MAP scheme described earlier.

The first requirement for a MAP approach is to define some form of prior distribution for the parameters. For a simple linear[4] approach, the priors consist of an *a priori* estimate of the mean of the parameters (assumed to be zero) and also a covariance matrix describing the distribution of the parameters about this mean. Many forms are possible for these priors, each of which describes some form of "energy" term. If the true prior distribution of the parameters is known (somehow derived from a large number fo subjects), then $\mathbf{C}_0$ could be an empirically determined covariance matrix describing this distribution. This approach would have the advantage that the resulting deformations are more typically "brain like," and so increase the face validity of the approach.

The three distinct forms of linear regularisation that we describe next are based on *membrane energy, bending energy,* and *linear-elastic energy.* None of these schemes enforces a strict one-to-one mapping between the source and template images, but this makes little difference for the small deformations required here. Each of these models needs some form of elasticity constants (λ and sometimes μ). Values of these constants that are too large will provide too much regularisation and result in greatly underestimated deformations. If the values are too small, there will not be enough regularisation and the resulting deformations will overfit the data.

Membrane Energy

The simplest model used for linear regularisation is based on minimising the *membrane energy* of the deformation field $\mathbf{u}$ (Amit *et al.,* 1991; Gee *et al.,* 1997). By summing over i points in three dimensions, the membrane energy of $\mathbf{u}$ is given by

[4] Although the cost function associated with these priors is quadratic, the priors are linear in the sense that they minimise the sum of squares of a linear combination of the model parameters. This is analogous to solving a set of linear equations by minimising a quadratic cost function.

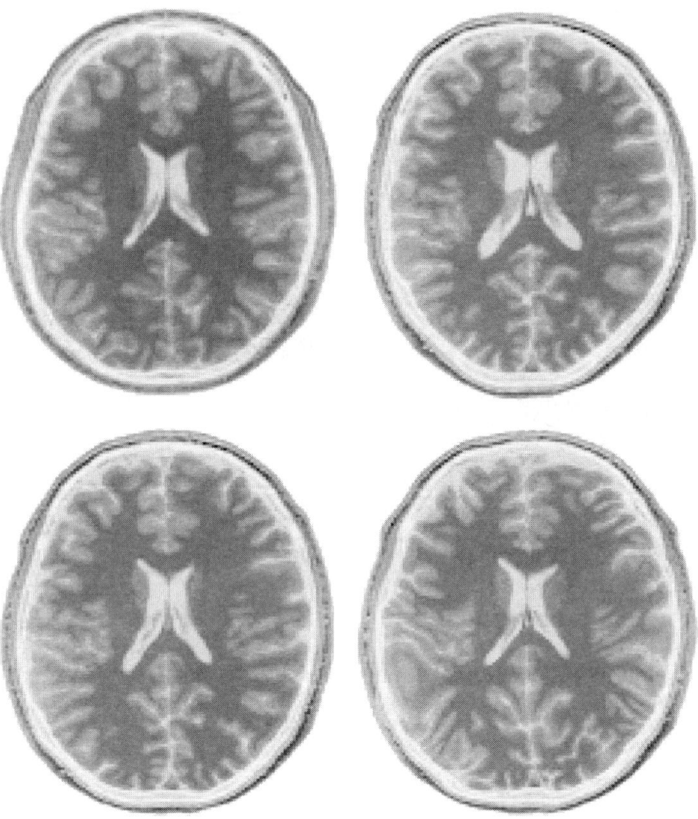

FIGURE 33.6
The image shown at top left is the template image. At top right is an image that has been registered with it using a 12-parameter affine registration. The image at bottom left is the same image registered using the 12-parameter affine registration, followed by a regularised global nonlinear registration. It should be clear that the shape of the image approaches that of the template much better after nonlinear registration. At bottom right is the image after the same affine transformation and nonlinear registration, but this time without using any regularisation. The mean squared difference between the image and template after the affine registration was 472.1. After the regularised nonlinear registration this was reduced to 302.7. Without regularisation, a mean squared difference of 287.3 is achieved, but this is at the expense of introducing a lot of unnecessary warping.

$$\sum_i \sum_{j=1}^{3} \sum_{k=1}^{3} \lambda \left(\frac{\partial u_{ji}}{\partial x_{ki}} \right)^2$$

where λ is simply a scaling constant. The membrane energy can be computed from the coefficients of the basis functions by $\mathbf{q}_1{}^T\, \mathbf{H}\mathbf{q}_1 + \mathbf{q}_2{}^T\, \mathbf{H}\mathbf{q}_2 + \mathbf{q}_3{}^T\, \mathbf{H}\mathbf{q}_3$, where $\mathbf{q}_1$, $\mathbf{q}_2$ and $\mathbf{q}_3$ refer to vectors containing the parameters describing translations in the three dimensions. The matrix $\mathbf{H}$ is defined by

$$\begin{aligned}\mathbf{H} = \lambda\, (\dot{\mathbf{D}}_3{}^T\dot{\mathbf{D}}_3) \otimes (\mathbf{D}_2{}^T\mathbf{D}_2) \otimes (\mathbf{D}_1{}^T\mathbf{D}_1)\\ + \lambda\, (\mathbf{D}_3{}^T\mathbf{D}_3) \otimes (\dot{\mathbf{D}}_2{}^T\dot{\mathbf{D}}_2) \otimes (\mathbf{D}_1{}^T\mathbf{D}_1)\\ + \lambda\, (\mathbf{D}_3{}^T\mathbf{D}_3) \otimes (\mathbf{D}_2{}^T\mathbf{D}_2) \otimes (\dot{\mathbf{D}}_1{}^T\dot{\mathbf{D}}_1)\end{aligned}$$

where the notation $\dot{\mathbf{D}}_1$ refers to the first derivatives of $\mathbf{D}_1$.

Assuming that the parameters consist of $[\mathbf{q}_1{}^T\mathbf{q}_2{}^T\mathbf{q}_3{}^T w]^T$, matrix $\mathbf{C}_0{}^{-1}$ from Eq. (33.4) can be constructed from $\mathbf{H}$ by

$$\mathbf{C}_0^{-1} = \begin{bmatrix} \mathbf{H} & \mathbf{0} & \mathbf{0} & \mathbf{0} \\ \mathbf{0} & \mathbf{H} & \mathbf{0} & \mathbf{0} \\ \mathbf{0} & \mathbf{0} & \mathbf{H} & \mathbf{0} \\ \mathbf{0} & \mathbf{0} & \mathbf{0} & \mathbf{0} \end{bmatrix}$$

$\mathbf{H}$ is all zeros, except for the diagonal. Elements on the diagonal represent the reciprocal of the *a priori* variance of each parameter. If all the DCT matrices are $I \times M$, then each diagonal element is given by

$$h_{j+M[k-1+M(l-1)]} = \lambda\pi^2 I^{-2} ((j-1)^2 + (k-1)^2 + (l-1)^2)$$
$$\text{over } j = 1\ldots M,\ k = 1\ldots M \text{ and } l = \ \ldots M$$

Bending Energy

Bookstein's thin plate splines (Bookstein, 1997a,b) minimise the *bending energy* of deformations. For a two-dimensional deformation, the bending energy is defined by

$$\lambda \sum_i \left[\left(\frac{\partial^2 u_{1i}}{\partial x_{1i}^2} \right)^2 + \left(\frac{\partial^2 u_{1i}}{\partial x_{2i}^2} \right)^2 + 2 \left(\frac{\partial^2 u_{1i}}{\partial x_{1i} \partial x_{2i}} \right)^2 \right] +$$
$$\lambda \sum_i \left[\left(\frac{\partial^2 u_{2i}}{\partial x_{1i}^2} \right)^2 + \left(\frac{\partial^2 u_{2i}}{\partial x_{2i}^2} \right)^2 + 2 \left(\frac{\partial^2 u_{2i}}{\partial x_{1i} \partial x_{2i}} \right)^2 \right] +$$

This can be computed by

$$\begin{aligned} &\lambda \mathbf{q}_1^T (\ddot{\mathbf{D}}_2 \otimes \mathbf{D}_1)^T (\ddot{\mathbf{D}}_2 \otimes \mathbf{D}_1)\mathbf{q}_1 + \lambda \mathbf{q}_1^T (\mathbf{D}_2 \otimes \ddot{\mathbf{D}}_1)^T (\mathbf{D}_2 \otimes \ddot{\mathbf{D}}_1)\mathbf{q}_1 \\ &+ 2\lambda \mathbf{q}_1^T (\dot{\mathbf{D}}_2 \otimes \dot{\mathbf{D}}_1)^T (\dot{\mathbf{D}}_2 \otimes \dot{\mathbf{D}}_1)\mathbf{q}_1 + \lambda \mathbf{q}_2^T (\ddot{\mathbf{D}}_2 \otimes \mathbf{D}_1)^T (\ddot{\mathbf{D}}_2 \otimes \mathbf{D}_1)\mathbf{q}_2 \\ &+ \lambda \mathbf{q}_2^T (\mathbf{D}_2 \otimes \ddot{\mathbf{D}}_1)^T (\mathbf{D}_2 \otimes \ddot{\mathbf{D}}_1)\mathbf{q}_2 + 2\lambda \mathbf{q}_2^T (\dot{\mathbf{D}}_2 \otimes \dot{\mathbf{D}}_1)^T (\dot{\mathbf{D}}_2 \otimes \dot{\mathbf{D}}_1)\mathbf{q}_2 \end{aligned}$$

where the notation $\dot{\mathbf{D}}_1$ and $\ddot{\mathbf{D}}_1$ refer to the column-wise first and second derivatives of $\mathbf{D}_1$. This is simplified to $\mathbf{q}_1^T\mathbf{H}\mathbf{q}_1 + \mathbf{q}_2^T\mathbf{H}\mathbf{q}_2$ where

$$\mathbf{H} = \lambda \left[(\ddot{\mathbf{D}}_2^T \ddot{\mathbf{D}}_2) \otimes (\mathbf{D}_1^T \mathbf{D}_1) + (\mathbf{D}_2^T \mathbf{D}_2) \otimes (\ddot{\mathbf{D}}_1^T \ddot{\mathbf{D}}_1) + 2 (\dot{\mathbf{D}}_2^T \dot{\mathbf{D}}_2) \otimes (\dot{\mathbf{D}}_1^T \dot{\mathbf{D}}_1) \right]$$

Matrix $\mathbf{C}_0^{-1}$ from Eq. (33.4) can be constructed from $\mathbf{H}$ as follows:

$$\mathbf{C}_0^{-1} = \begin{bmatrix} \mathbf{H} & \mathbf{0} & \mathbf{0} \\ \mathbf{0} & \mathbf{H} & \mathbf{0} \\ \mathbf{0} & \mathbf{0} & 0 \end{bmatrix}$$

with values on the diagonals of $\mathbf{H}$ given by

$$h_{j+(k-1)\times M} = \lambda \left(\left[\frac{\pi (j-1)}{I} \right]^4 + \left[\frac{\pi (k-1)}{I} \right]^4 + 2 \left[\frac{\pi (j-1)}{I} \right]^2 \left[\frac{\pi (k-1)}{I} \right]^2 \right)$$
$$\text{over } j = 1\ldots M \text{ and } k = 1\ldots M$$

Linear-Elastic Energy

The *linear-elastic energy* (Miller *et al.,* 1993) of a two-dimensional deformation field is

$$\sum_{j=1}^{2} \sum_{k=1}^{2} \sum_i \frac{\lambda}{2} \left(\frac{\partial u_{ji}}{\partial x_{ji}} \right) \left(\frac{\partial u_{ki}}{\partial x_{ki}} \right) + \frac{\mu}{4} \left(\frac{\partial u_{ji}}{\partial x_{ki}} + \frac{\partial u_{ki}}{\partial x_{ji}} \right)^2$$

where λ and μ are the *Lamé* elasticity constants. The elastic energy of the deformations can be computed by:

$$\begin{aligned} &(\mu + \lambda/2)\mathbf{q}_1^T(\mathbf{D}_2 \otimes \dot{\mathbf{D}}_1)^T (\mathbf{D}_2 \otimes \dot{\mathbf{D}}_1)\mathbf{q}_1 + (\mu + \lambda/2)\mathbf{q}_2^T(\dot{\mathbf{D}}_2 \otimes \mathbf{D}_1)^T (\dot{\mathbf{D}}_2 \otimes \mathbf{D}_1)\mathbf{q}_2 \\ &+ \mu/2\mathbf{q}_1^T(\dot{\mathbf{D}}_2 \otimes \mathbf{D}_1)^T (\dot{\mathbf{D}}_2 \otimes \mathbf{D}_1)\mathbf{q}_1 + \mu/2\mathbf{q}_2^T(\mathbf{D}_2 \otimes \dot{\mathbf{D}}_1)^T (\mathbf{D}_2 \otimes \dot{\mathbf{D}}_1)\mathbf{q}_2 \\ &+ \mu/2\mathbf{q}_1^T(\dot{\mathbf{D}}_2 \otimes \mathbf{D}_1)^T (\mathbf{D}_2 \otimes \dot{\mathbf{D}}_1)\mathbf{q}_2 + \mu/2\mathbf{q}_2^T(\mathbf{D}_2 \otimes \dot{\mathbf{D}}_1)^T (\dot{\mathbf{D}}_2 \otimes \mathbf{D}_1)\mathbf{q}_1 \\ &+ \lambda/2\mathbf{q}_1^T(\mathbf{D}_2 \otimes \dot{\mathbf{D}}_1)^T (\dot{\mathbf{D}}_2 \otimes \mathbf{D}_1)\mathbf{q}_2 + \lambda/2\mathbf{q}_2^T(\dot{\mathbf{D}}_2 \otimes \mathbf{D}_1)^T (\mathbf{D}_2 \otimes \dot{\mathbf{D}}_1)\mathbf{q}_1 \end{aligned}$$

A regularisation based on this model requires an inverse covariance matrix that is not a simple diagonal matrix. This matrix is constructed as follows:

$$\mathbf{C}_0^{-1} = \begin{bmatrix} \mathbf{H}_1 & \mathbf{H}_3 & \mathbf{0} \\ \mathbf{H}_3^T & \mathbf{H}_2 & \mathbf{0} \\ \mathbf{0} & \mathbf{0} & 0 \end{bmatrix}$$

where

$$\begin{aligned} \mathbf{H}_1 &= (\mu + \lambda/2)(\mathbf{D}_2^T \mathbf{D}_2) \otimes (\dot{\mathbf{D}}_1^T \dot{\mathbf{D}}_1) + \mu/2(\dot{\mathbf{D}}_2^T \dot{\mathbf{D}}_2) \otimes (\mathbf{D}_1^T \mathbf{D}_1) \\ \mathbf{H}_2 &= (\mu + \lambda/2)(\dot{\mathbf{D}}_2^T \dot{\mathbf{D}}_2) \otimes (\mathbf{D}_1^T \mathbf{D}_1) + \mu/2(\mathbf{D}_2^T \mathbf{D}_2) \otimes (\dot{\mathbf{D}}_1^T \dot{\mathbf{D}}_1) \\ \mathbf{H}_3 &= \lambda/2(\mathbf{D}_2^T \dot{\mathbf{D}}_2) \otimes (\dot{\mathbf{D}}_1^T \mathbf{D}_1) + \mu/2(\dot{\mathbf{D}}_2^T \mathbf{D}_2) \otimes (\mathbf{D}_1^T \dot{\mathbf{D}}_1) \end{aligned}$$

Templates and Intensity Transformations

Earlier sections modeled a single intensity scaling parameter (q_{13} and w), but more generally, the optimisation can be assumed to minimise two sets of parameters: those that describe spatial transformations ($\mathbf{q_s}$) and those for describing intensity transformations ($\mathbf{q_t}$). This means that the difference function can be expressed in the generic form:

$$b_i(\mathbf{q}) = f\,[\mathbf{s}(\mathbf{x}_i, \mathbf{q_s})] - t(\mathbf{x}_i, \mathbf{q_t})$$

where **f** is the source image, **s**() is a vector function describing the spatial transformations based on parameters $\mathbf{q_s}$, and $t()$ is a scalar function describing intensity transformations based on parameters $\mathbf{q_t}$; $\mathbf{x}_i$ represents the coordinates of the ith sampled point.

The previous subsections simply considered matching one image to a scaled version of another, in order to minimise the sum of squared differences between them. For this case, $t(\mathbf{x}_i, \mathbf{q_t})$ is simply equal to $q_{t1}g(\mathbf{x}_i)$, where q_{t1} is a simple scaling parameter and **g** is a template image. This is most effective when there is a linear relation between the image intensities. Typically, the template images used for spatial normalisation will be similar to those shown in the top row of Fig. 33.7. The simplest least-squares fitting method is not optimal when there is not a linear relationship between the images. Examples of nonlinear relationships are illustrated in Fig. 33.8, which shows histograms (scatterplots) of image intensities plotted against each other.

An important idea is that a given image can be matched not to one reference image, but to a series of images that all conform to the same space. The idea here is that (ignoring the spatial differences) any given image can be expressed as a linear combination of a set of reference images. For example, these reference images might include different modalities (PET, SPECT, ^{18}F-DOPA, ^{18}F-deoxy-glucose, T_1-weighted MRI, T^*_2-weighted MRI, etc.) or different anatomical tissues (gray matter, white matter, and CSF segmented from the same T_1-weighted MRI, etc.) or different anatomical regions (cortical gray matter, subcortical gray mater, cerebellum, etc.) or finally any combination of the above. Any given image, irrespective of its modality could be approximated with a function of these images. A simple example using two images would be

$$b_i(\mathbf{q}) = f\,[\mathbf{s}(\mathbf{x}_i, \mathbf{q_s})] - [q_{t1}g_1(\mathbf{x}_i) + q_{t2}g_2(\mathbf{x}_i)]$$

In Fig. 33.9, a plane of a T_1-weighted MRI is modeled by a linear combination of the five other template images shown in Fig. 33.7. Similar models were used to simulate T_2- and PD-weighted

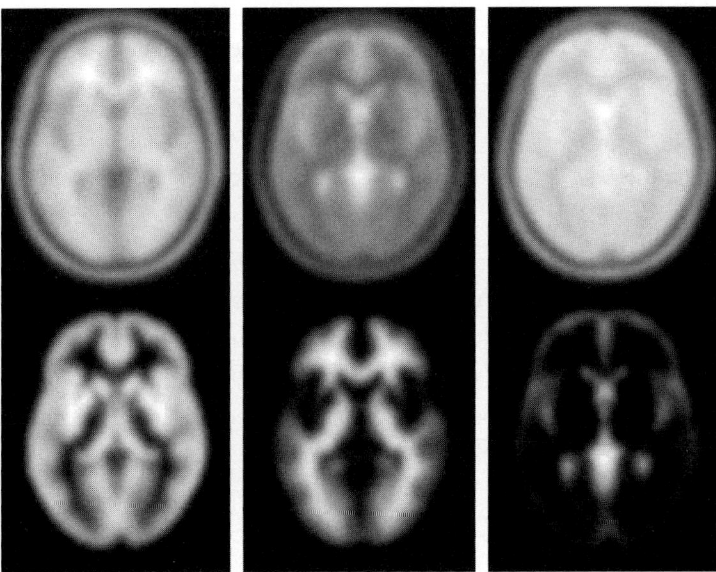

FIGURE 33.7
Example template images. (Top) T_1-weighted MRI, T_2-weighted MRI, and PD-weighted MRI. (Bottom) Gray matter probability distribution, white matter probability distribution, and CSF probability distribution. All data were generated at the McConnel Brain Imaging Center, Montréal Neurological Institute at McGill University, and are based on the averages of about 150 normal brains. The original images were reduced to 2-mm resolution and convolved with an 8-mm FWHM Gaussian kernel to be used as templates for spatial normalisation.

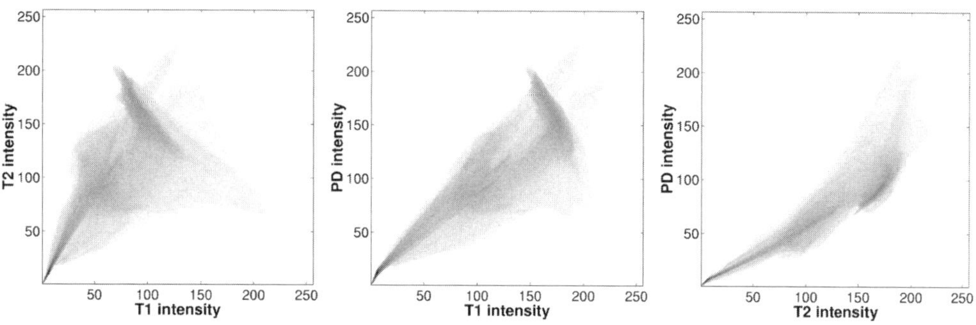

FIGURE 33.8
Two-dimensional histograms of template images [intensities shown as $\log(1 + n)$, where n is the value in each bin]. The histograms were based on the whole volumes of the template images shown in the top row of Fig. 33.7.

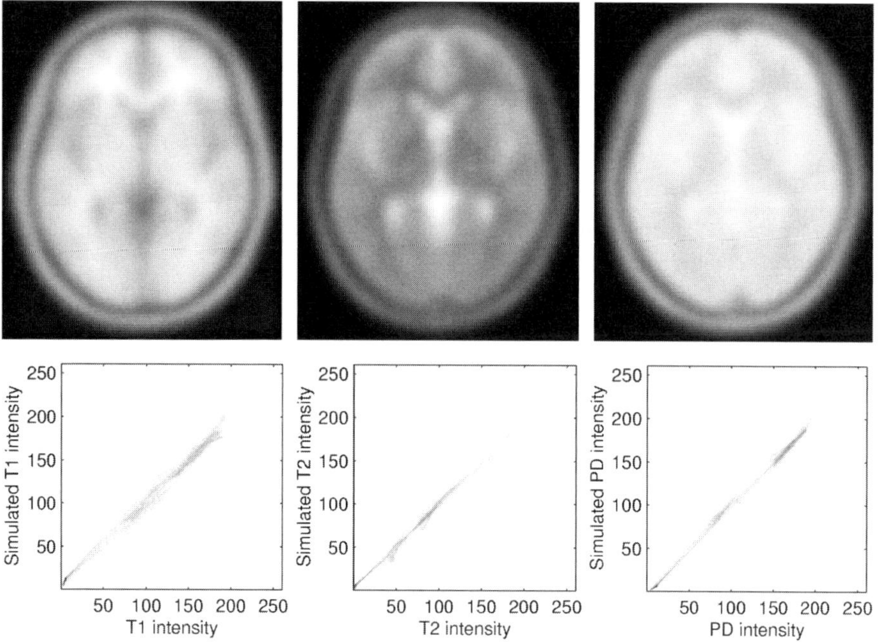

FIGURE 33.9
(Top) Simulated images of T_1-, T_2-, and PD-weighted images. (Bottom) Histograms of the real images versus the simulated images.

MR images. The linearity of the scatterplots (compared to those in Fig. 33.8) shows that MR images of a wide range of different contrasts can be modeled by a linear combination of a limited number of template images. Visual inspection shows that the simulated images are very similar to those shown in Fig. 33.7.

Alternatively, the intensities could vary spatially (for example, due to inhomogeneities in the MRI scanner). Linear variations in intensity over the field of view can be accounted for by optimising a function of the form:

$$b_i(\mathbf{q}) = f\,[\mathbf{s}(\mathbf{x}_i, \mathbf{q}_s)] - [q_{t1}g(\mathbf{x}_i) + q_{t2}x_{1i}g(\mathbf{x}_i) + q_{t3}x_{2i}g(\mathbf{x}_i) + q_{t4}x_{3i}g(\mathbf{x}_i)]$$

More complex variations could be included by modulating with other basis functions (such as the DCT basis function set described in an earlier section) (Friston *et al.*, 1995a). The examples shown so far have been linear in their parameters describing intensity transformations. A simple example of an intensity transformation that is nonlinear would be:

$$b_i(\mathbf{q}) = f\,[\mathbf{s}(\mathbf{x}_i, \mathbf{q}_s)] - q_{t1}g(\mathbf{x}_i)^{q_{t2}}$$

Collins *et al.* (1994) suggested that—rather than matching the image itself to the template—some function of the image should be matched to a template image transformed in the same way.

He found that the use of gradient magnitude transformations leads to more robust solutions, especially in cases of limited brain coverage or intensity inhomogeneity artifacts (in MR images). Other rotationally invariant moments also contain useful matching information (Shen and Davatzikos, 2002). The algorithms described here perform most efficiently with smooth images. Much of the high-frequency information in the images is lost in the smoothing step, but information about important image features may be retained in separate (smoothed) moment images. Simultaneous registrations using these extracted features may be a useful technique for preserving information, while still retaining the advantages of using smooth images in the registration.

Another idea for introducing more accuracy by making use of internal consistency would be to simultaneously spatially normalise coregistered images to corresponding templates. For example, by simultaneously matching a PET image to a PET template, at the same time as matching a structural MR image to a corresponding MR template, more accuracy could be obtained than by matching the images individually. A similar approach could be devised for simultaneously matching different tissue types from classified images together (Good *et al.*, 2001), although a more powerful approach is to incorporate tissue classification and registration into the same Bayesian model (Fischl *et al.*, 2002).

DISCUSSION

The criteria for "good" spatial transformations can be framed in terms of validity, reliability, and computational efficiency. The validity of a particular transformation device is not easy to define or measure and indeed varies with the application. For example, a rigid body transformation may be perfectly valid for realignment but not for spatial normalisation of an arbitrary brain into a standard stereotaxic space. Generally the sorts of validity that are important in spatial transformations can be divided into (1) *face validity,* established by demonstrating that the transformation does what it is supposed to, and (2) *construct validity,* assessed by comparison with other techniques or constructs. Face validity is a complex issue in functional mapping. At first glance, face validity might be equated with the coregistration of anatomical homologs in two images. This would be complete and appropriate if the biological question referred to structural differences or modes of variation. In other circumstances, however, this definition of face validity is not appropriate. For example, the purpose of spatial normalisation (either within or between subjects) in functional mapping studies is to maximise the sensitivity to neurophysiological change elicited by experimental manipulation of the sensorimotor or cognitive state. In this case a better definition of a valid normalisation is that which maximises condition-dependent effects with respect to error (and, if relevant, intersubject) effects. This will probably be effected when functional anatomy is congruent. This may or may not be the same as registering structural anatomy.

Because the deformations are only defined by a few hundred parameters, the nonlinear registration method described here does not have the potential precision of some other methods. High-frequency deformations cannot be modeled because the deformations are restricted to the lowest spatial frequencies of the basis functions. This means that the current approach is unsuitable for attempting exact matches between fine cortical structures (see Fig. 33.10 and 33.11).

The current method is relatively fast, taking on the order of 30 sec per iteration, depending on the number of basis functions used. The speed is partly a result of the small number of parameters involved and the simple optimisation algorithm that assumes an almost quadratic error surface. Because the images are first matched using a simple affine transformation, there is less "work" for the algorithm to do, and good registration can be achieved with only a few iterations (fewer than 20). The method does not rigorously enforce a one-to-one match between the brains being registered. However, by estimating only the lowest frequency deformations and by using appropriate regularisation, this constraint is rarely broken.

The approach in this chapter searches for a MAP estimate of the parameters defining the warps. However, optimisation problems for complex nonlinear models such as those used for image registration can easily get caught in local minima, so there is no guarantee that the

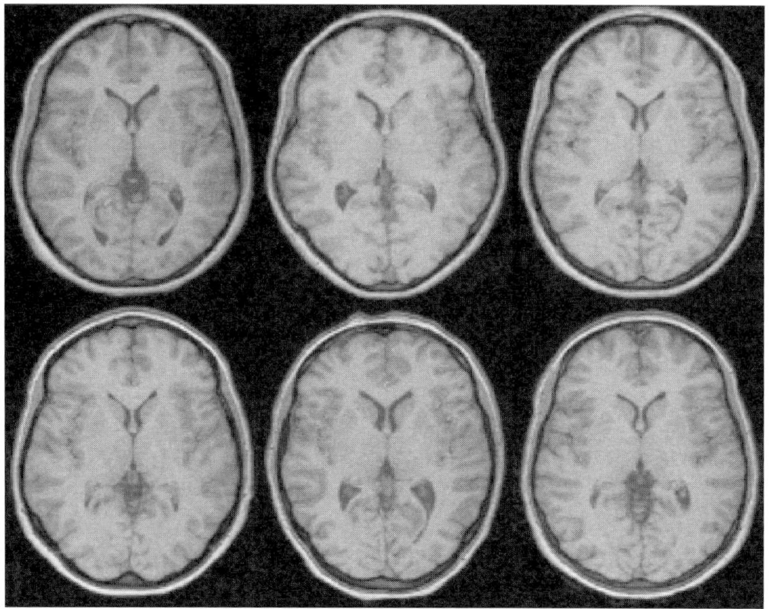

FIGURE 33.10
Images of six subjects registered using a 12-parameter affine registration (see also Fig. 33.11). The affine registration matches the positions and sizes of the images.

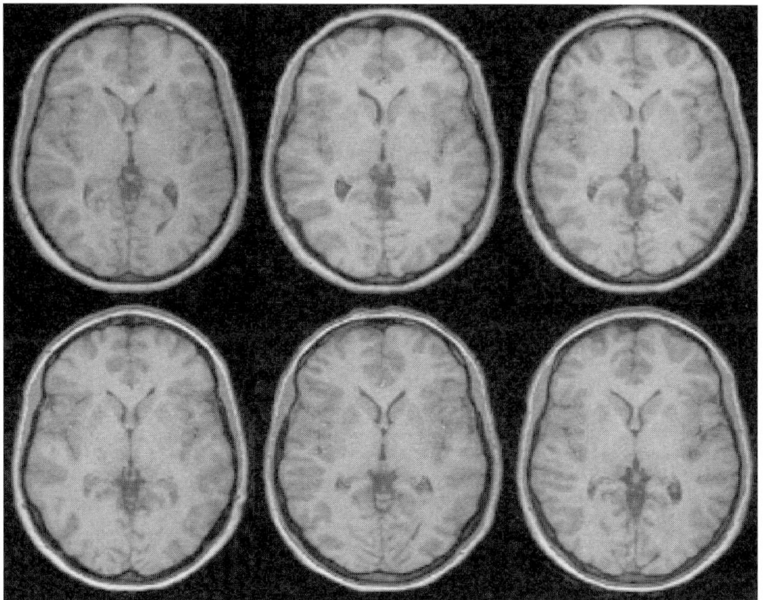

FIGURE 33.11
Six subjects' brains registered with both affine and basis function registration (see also Fig. 33.10). The basis function registration estimates the global shapes of the brains, but is not able to account for high spatial frequency warps.

estimate determined by the algorithm is globally optimum. Even if the best MAP estimate is achieved, there will be many other potential solutions that have similar probabilities of being correct. A further complication arises from the fact that there is no one-to-one match between the small structures (especially gyral and sulcal patterns) of any two brains. This means that it is not possible to obtain a single objective high-frequency match regardless of how good an algorithm is for determining the best MAP estimate. Because of these issues, registration using the *minimum variance estimate* (MVE) may be more appropriate. Rather than searching for the single most probable solution, the MVE is the average of all possible solutions, weighted by their individual posterior probabilities. Although useful approximations have been devised (Miller *et al.,* 1993; Christensen, 1994), this estimate is still difficult to achieve in practice because of the enormous amount of computing power required. The MVE is probably more appropriate than the MAP estimate for spatial normalisation, because it is (on average) closer to the "true" solution. However, if the errors associated with the parameter estimates and also the priors are normally distributed, then the MVE and the MAP estimate are identical. This is partially satisfied by smoothing the images before registering them.

When higher spatial frequency warps are to be fitted, more DCT coefficients are required to describe the deformations. Practical problems, however, occur when more than about the $8 \times 8 \times 8$ lowest frequency DCT components are used. One of these is the problem of storing and inverting the curvature matrix ($\mathbf{A}^T\mathbf{A}$). Even with deformations limited to $8 \times 8 \times 8$ coefficients, there are at least 1537 unknown parameters, requiring a curvature matrix of about 18 Mbytes (using double-precision floating-point arithmetic). High-dimensional registration methods that search for more parameters should be used when more precision is required in the deformations.

In practice, however, it may be meaningless to even attempt an exact match between brains beyond a certain resolution. There is no one-to-one relationship between the cortical structures of one brain and those of another, so any method that attempts to match brains exactly must be folding the brain to create sulci and gyri that do not really exist. Even if an exact match is possible, because the registration problem is not convex, the solutions obtained by high-dimensional warping techniques may not be truly optimum. High-dimensional registrations methods are often very good at registering gray matter with gray matter, for example, but there is no guarantee that the registered gray matter arises from homologous cortical features.

Also, structure and function are not always tightly linked. Even if structurally equivalent regions can be brought into exact register, it does not mean that the same is true for regions that perform the same or similar functions. For intersubject averaging, an assumption is made that functionally equivalent regions lie in approximately the same parts of the brain. This leads to the current rationale for smoothing images from multisubject functional imaging studies prior to performing statistical analyses. Constructive interference of the smeared activation signals then has the effect of producing a signal that is roughly in an average location. To account for substantial fine-scale warps in a spatial normalisation, it is necessary for some voxels to increase their volumes considerably and for others to shrink to an almost negligible size. The contribution of the shrunken regions to the smoothed images is tiny, and the sensitivity of the tests for detecting activations in these regions is reduced. This is another argument in favor of spatially normalising only on a global scale.

The constrained normalisation described here assumes that the template resembles a warped version of the image. Modifications are required in order to apply the method to diseased or lesioned brains. One possible approach is to assume different weights for different brain regions (Brett *et al.,* 2001). Lesioned areas can be assigned lower weights, so that they have much less influence on the final solution.

The registration scheme described in this chapter is constrained to describe warps with a few hundred parameters. More powerful and less expensive computers are rapidly evolving, so algorithms that are currently applicable will become increasingly redundant as it becomes feasible to attempt more precise registrations. Scanning hardware is also improving, leading to improvements in the quality and diversity of images that can be obtained. Currently, most registration algorithms only use the information from a single image from each subject. This is typically a T_1 MR image, which provides limited information that simply delineates gray and white matter. For example, further information that is not available in the more conventional sequences could be obtained from diffusion-weighted imaging. Knowledge of major white matter tracts should provide structural information more directly related to connectivity and implicit function, possibly leading to improved registration of functionally specialised areas.

References

Amit, Y., Grenander, U., and Piccioni, M. (1991). Structural image restoration through deformable templates. *J. Am. Statistical Assoc.* **86,** 376–387.

Ashburner, J., and Friston, K. J. (1998). High-dimensional nonlinear image registration. *NeuroImage* **7**(4), S737.

Ashburner, J., and Friston, K .J. (1999). Nonlinear spatial normalisation using basis functions. *Human Brain Mapping* **7**(4), 254–266.

Bookstein, F .L. (1989). Principal warps: Thin-plate splines and the decomposition of deformations. *IEEE Trans. Patt. Anal. Mach. Intell.* **11**(6), 567–585.

Bookstein, F .L. (1997a). Landmark methods for forms without landmarks: Morphometrics of group differences in outline shape. *Med. Image Anal.* **1**(3), 225–243.

Bookstein, F .L. (1997b). Quadratic variation of deformations. In: "Proc. Information Processing in Medical Imaging" (J. Duncan and G. Gindi, eds.). Springer-Verlag, Berlin.

Brett, M., Leff, A .P., Rorden, C., and Ashburner, J. (2001). Spatial normalisation of brain images with focal lesions using cost function masking. *NeuroImage* **14**(2), 486–500.

Bro-Nielsen, M., and Gramkow, C. (1996). Fast fluid registration of medical images. *Lect. Notes Computer Sci.* **1131,** 267–276.

Christensen, G .E. (1994). Deformable shape models for anatomy. Doctoral thesis, Washington University, Sever Institute of Technology.

Christensen, G. E. (1999). Consistent linear elastic transformations for image matching. In: "Proc. Information Processing in Medical Imaging" (A. K., *et al.,* eds.). Springer-Verlag, Berlin.

Christensen, G .E., Rabbitt, R. D., and Miller, M .I. (1994). 3D brain mapping using using a deformable neuroanatomy. *Phys. Med. Biol.* **39,** 609–618.

Christensen, G .E., Rabbitt, R .D., Miller, M .I., Joshi, S .C., Grenander, U., Coogan, T .A., and Van Essen, D .C. (1995). Topological properties of smooth anatomic maps. In: "Proc. Information Processing in Medical Imaging" (Y. Bizais, C. Barillot, and R. Di Paola, eds.). Kluwer Academic Publishers, Dordrecht, The Netherlands.

Christensen, G .E., Rabbitt, R .D., and Miller, M .I. (1996). Deformable templates using large deformation kinematics. *IEEE Trans. Image Proc.* **5,** 1435–1447.

Collins, D. L., Neelin, P., Peters, T .M., and Evans, A .C. (1994). Automatic 3D intersubject registration of MR volumetric data in standardised Talairach space. *J. Computer Assisted Tomog.* **18,** 192–205.

Collins, D .L., Evans, A .C., Holmes, C., and Peters, T .M. (1995). Automatic 3D segmentation of neuro-anatomical structures from MRI. In: "Proc. Information Processing in Medical Imaging" (Y. Bizais, C. Barillot, and R. Di Paola, eds.). Kluwer Academic Publishers, Dordrecht, The Netherlands.

Davatzikos, C. (1996). Spatial normalisation of 3D images using deformable models. *J. Computer Assisted Tomog.* **20**(4), 656–665.

Edwards, P .J., Hill, D .L. G., and Hawkes, D .J. (1997). Image guided interventions using a three component tissue deformation model. In: "Proc. Medical Image Understanding and Analysis."

Evans, A. C., Collins, D .L., Mills, S .R., Brown, E .D., Kelly, R .L., and Peters, T .M. (1993). 3D statistical neuro-anatomical models from 305 MRI volumes. In: "Proc. IEEE-Nuclear Science Symposium and Medical Imaging Conference."

Evans, A. C., Kamber, M., Collins, D .L., and Macdonald, D. (1994). An MRI-based probabilistic atlas of neuroanatomy. In: "Magnetic Resonance Scanning and Epilepsy," Vol. 24 (S. Shorvon, D. Fish, F. Andermann, G. M. Bydder, and S. H., eds.), Vol. 264 of *NATO ASI Series A, Life Sciences* pp. 263–274. Plenum Press, New York.

Fischl, B., Salat, D .H., Busa, E., Albert, M., Dieterich, M., Haselgrove, C., van der Kouwe, A., Killiany, R., Kennedy, D., Klaveness, S., Montillo, A., Makris, N., Rosen, B., and Dale, A. M. (2002). Whole brain segmentation: Automated labeling of neuroanatomical structures in the human brain. *Neuron* **33,** 341–355.

Fox, P .T. (1995). Spatial normalisation origins: Objectives, applications, and alternatives. *Hum. Brain Mapping* **3,** 161–164.

Friston, K. J., Ashburner, J., Frith, C .D., Poline, J.-B., Heather, J. D., and Frackowiak, R .S. J. (1995a). Spatial registration and normalisation of images. *Hum. Brain Mapping* **2,** 165–189.

Friston, K .J., Holmes, A .P., Poline, J.-B., Grasby, P .J., Williams, S .C .R., Frackowiak, R .S .J., and Turner, R. (1995b). Analysis of fMRI time series revisited. *NeuroImage* **2,** 45–53.

Gee, J .C., Haynor, D .R., Le Briquer, L., and Bajcsy, R. K. (1997). Advances in elastic matching theory and its implementation. In: "Proc. CVRMed-MRCAS'97" (P. Cinquin, R. Kikinis, and S. Lavallee, eds.). Springer-Verlag, Berlin.

Glasbey, C .A., and Mardia, K .V. (1998). A review of image warping methods. *J. Appl. Statistics* **25,** 155–171.

Good, C. D., Johnsrude, I .S., Ashburner, J., Henson, R .N .A., Friston, K. J., and Frackowiak, R .S .J. (2001). *NeuroImage* **14,** 21–36.

Mazziotta, J. C., Toga, A .W., Evans, A., Fox, P., and Lancaster, J. (1995). A probabilistic atlas of the human brain: Theory and rationale for its development. *NeuroImage* **2,** 89–101.

Miller, M .I., Christensen, G .E., Amit, Y., and Grenander, U. (1993). Mathematical textbook of deformable neuro-anatomies. *Proc. Natl. Acad. Sci. USA* **90,** 11944–11948.

Poline, J.-B., Friston, K .J., Worsley, K .J., and Frackowiak, R .S .J. (1995). Estimating smoothness in statistical parametric maps: Confidence intervals on p-values. *J. Computer Assisted Tomog.* **19**(5), 788–796.

Shen, D., and Davatzikos, C. (2002). HAMMER: Hierarchical attribute matching mechanism for elastic registration. *IEEE Trans. Med. Imaging* **21**(11), 1421–1439.

Studholme, C., Constable, R .T., and Duncan, J .S. (2000). Accurate alignment of functional EPI data to anatomical MRI using a physics-based distortion model. *IEEE Trans. Med. Imaging* **19**(11), 1115–1127.

Talairach, J., and Tournoux, P. (1988). "Coplanar Stereotaxic Atlas of the Human Brain." Thieme Medical, New York.

Thévenaz, P., and Unser, M. (2000). Optimisation of mutual information for multiresolution image registration. *IEEE Trans. Image Proc.* **9**(12), 2083–2099.

Thirion, J.-P. (1995). Fast non-rigid matching of 3D medical images. Tech. Rep. 2547, Institut National de Recherche en Informatique et en Automatique. Available from http://www.inria.fr/RRRT/RR-2547.html.

Thompson, P .M., and Toga, A .W. (1996). Visualisation and mapping of anatomic abnormalities using a probablistic brain atlas based on random fluid transformations. In: "Proc. Visualisation in Biomedical Computing."

Woods, R. P., Grafton, S .T ., Holmes, C .J., Cherry, S .R., and Mazziotta, J .C. (1998a). Automated image registration: I. General methods and intrasubject, intramodality validation. *J. Computer Assisted Tomog.* **22**(1), 139–152.

Woods, R. P., Grafton, S .T., Watson, J .D .G., Sicotte, N .L., and Mazziotta, J .C. (1998b). Automated image registration: II. Intersubject validation of linear and nonlinear models. *J. Computer Assisted Tomog.* **22**(1), 153–165.

Worsley, K .J., and Friston, K .J. (1995). Analysis of fMRI time-series revisited – again. *NeuroImage* **2,** 173–181.

C H A P T E R

34

High-Dimensional Image Warping

INTRODUCTION

Two brain images from the same subject can be coregistered using a six-parameter rigid body transformation, which simply describes the relative position and orientation of the images. However, for matching brain images of different subjects (or the brain of the same subject that may have changed shape over time; Freeborough and Fox, 1998), it is necessary to estimate a deformation field that also describes the relative shapes of the images. The previous chapter described a method of registering images of different subjects in order to match the overall shapes. However, many more parameters are required to describe the shape of a brain precisely, and estimating these can be very prone to error. This error can be reduced by ensuring that the deformation fields are internally consistent (Christensen, 1999). For example, suppose a deformation that matches brain **f** to brain **g** is estimated, and also a deformation that matches brain **g** to brain **f.** If one deformation field is not the inverse of the other, then at least one of them has to be wrong.

Often, the prior probability distributions used by Bayesian registration schemes are linear (see Chapter 33), and include minimising the *membrane energy* of the deformation field (Amit *et al.*, 1991; Gee *et al.*, 1997), the *bending energy* (Bookstein, 1997), or the *linear-elastic energy* (Miller *et al.*, 1993). None of these linear penalties is symmetric, and they do not explicitly preserve the topology[1] of the warped images.

An alternative to using a Bayesian scheme incorporating some form of elastic prior could be to use a viscous fluid model (Christensen *et al.*, 1994, 1996) to estimate the warps. In these models, finite difference methods are normally used to solve the partial differential equations that model one image as it "flows" to the same shape as the other. The major advantage of these methods is that they are able to account for large displacements and also ensure that the topology of the warped image is preserved, but they do have the disadvantage that they are computationally expensive. Viscous fluid models are almost able to warp any image so that it looks like any other image, while still preserving the original topology. In some respects these models may have too much freedom, in that extremely unlikely deformations are not penalised.

Viscous fluid models are one of many approaches that describe the spatial transformations in terms of a physical process. However, rather than obeying physical laws, the intensity-based registration model presented in this chapter utilises statistical rules. Unlikely deformations are

[1] The word *topology* is used in the same sense as in "Topological Properties of Smooth Anatomical Maps" (Christensen *et al.*, 1995). If spatial transformations are not one to one and continuous, then the topological properties of different structures can change.

penalised by incorporating prior information about the smoothness of the expected deformations using a *maximum a posteriori* (MAP) scheme. In addition, the topology of the deformed images is preserved by ensuring that the deformations are globally one to one.

The remainder of the chapter is divided into three main sections. The methods section describes the Bayesian principles behind the registration, which is essentially an optimisation procedure that simultaneously minimises a likelihood function (i.e., the sum of squared differences between the images), and a penalty function that relates to the prior probability of obtaining the deformations. A number of examples of registered images are provided in the next section. The final section discusses the validity of the method and includes a number of suggestions for future work.

METHODS

Registering one image volume to another involves estimating a vector field (deformation field) that maps from coordinates of one image to those of the other. In this work, one image (the template image) is considered to be fixed, and a mapping from this image to the second image (the source image) is estimated. The intensity of the ith voxel of the template is denoted by $g(\mathbf{x}_i)$, where $\mathbf{x}_i$ is a vector describing the coordinates of the voxel. The deformation field spanning the domain of the template is denoted by $\mathbf{y}_i$ [or $\mathbf{y}(\mathbf{x}_i)$] at each point, and the intensity of the source image at this mapped point is denoted by $f(\mathbf{y}_i)$. The source image is transformed to match the template by resampling it at the mapped coordinates.

This section begins by describing how the deformation fields are parameterised as piecewise affine transformations within a finite element mesh. The registration is achieved by matching the images while simultaneously trying to maximise the smoothness of the deformations. Bayesian statistics are used to incorporate this smoothness into the registration, and a method of optimisation is presented for finding the MAP estimate of the parameters. Suitable forms for the smoothness priors are presented. The first of these is the ideal form, which for practical reasons has only been developed for registration in two dimensions. The second form is an approximation to the ideal, and it has been developed for both two- and three-dimensional image registration.

Bayesian Framework

This approach to image registration estimates the required spatial transformation at every voxel and, therefore, requires many parameters. For example, to register two volumes of size $256 \times 256 \times 108$ voxels, we need 21,233,664 parameters. The number of parameters describing the transformations exceeds the number of voxels in the data. Because of this, it is essential that the effective degrees of freedom be reduced by imposing priors or constraints on the registration. As in the previous chapter, Bayesian statistics are used to incorporate a prior probability distribution into the warping model.

Bayes' theorem can be expressed as [see Eq. (33.1) in Chapter 33]

$$p(\mathbf{Y}|\mathbf{b}) \propto p(\mathbf{b}|\mathbf{Y})p(\mathbf{Y}) \tag{34.1}$$

where $p(\mathbf{Y})$ is the *a priori* probability of parameters $\mathbf{Y}$, $p(\mathbf{b}|\mathbf{Y})$ is the probability of observing data $\mathbf{b}$ given parameters $\mathbf{Y}$, and $p(\mathbf{Y}|\mathbf{b})$ is the *a posteriori* probability of $\mathbf{Y}$ given the data $\mathbf{b}$. Here, $\mathbf{Y}$ are the parameters describing the deformation, and $\mathbf{b}$ are the images to be matched. The estimate determined here is the MAP estimate, which is the value of $\mathbf{Y}$ that maximises $p(\mathbf{Y}|\mathbf{b})$. A probability is related to its Gibbs form by

$$p(\mathbf{Y}) \propto e^{-H(\mathbf{Y})} \tag{34.2}$$

Therefore, the MAP estimate is identical to the parameter estimate that minimises the Gibbs potential of the posterior distribution $[H(\mathbf{Y}|\mathbf{b})]$, where

$$H(\mathbf{Y}|\mathbf{b}) = H(\mathbf{b}|\mathbf{Y}) + H(\mathbf{Y}) + c \tag{34.3}$$

where c is a constant. The registration is therefore a nonlinear optimisation problem, whereby the cost function to be minimised is the sum of the likelihood potential $[H(\mathbf{b}|\mathbf{Y})]$ and the prior potential $[H(\mathbf{Y})]$. These potentials are now discussed in detail.

Likelihood Potentials

The registration matches a source image (**f**) to a template image (**g**). The current model assumes that one is simply a spatially transformed version of the other (i.e., there are no intensity variations between them), where the only intensity differences are due to uniform additive Gaussian noise. The Gibbs potential for this situation is given by

$$H(\mathbf{b}|\mathbf{Y}) = \frac{1}{2\sigma^2} \sum_{i=1}^{I} [f(\mathbf{y}_i) - \mathbf{g}(\mathbf{x}_i)]^2 \tag{34.4}$$

where $g(\mathbf{x}_i)$ is the ith pixel value of **g** and $f(\mathbf{y}_i)$ is the corresponding pixel value of **f.**

In this model, the variance (σ^2) is assumed to be the same for all voxels. A suitable value to use for each iteration is estimated by computing the residual sum of squared differences.[2] For the early iterations, σ^2 has a higher value, placing more weight on the priors, so the deformations are smoother. When close to the final solution, σ^2 has decreased, and the algorithm is able to compute more detailed deformations.

The potential is computed by sampling I discrete points within the template image, and equivalent points within the source image are sampled using trilinear interpolation. Gradients of the trilinearly interpolated source image are required for the registration, and these are computed using a finite difference method.

2D Prior Potentials

Consider the deformation fields that register two images **f** and **g.** The two fields that map from **f** to **g** and from **g** to **f** can be combined in order to map from **f** to **g** and then back to **f.** If the registrations are perfect, then the resulting deformation should be uniformly zero. Any deviations must be due to registration errors. To minimise these errors, there should be symmetry in the priors. In addition to considering the deforming forces that warp image **f** to match image **g,** the forces mediating the inverse of the deformation also need to be considered. To achieve this symmetry, the fundamental assumption is made that the probability of stretching a voxel by a factor of n is the same as the probability of shrinking n voxels by a factor of n^{-1}. For example, a deformation that stretches one voxel in the source image to fit two voxels in the template should incur the same penalty as the contraction of two voxels to fit one template voxel.

To compute these potentials in 2D, the pixels of the template image (**g**) are considered as being on a regular grid, with unit spacing between them. A triangular mesh connects the centers of each pixel (as shown in Fig. 34.1). Within each triangle, we assume a uniform affine mapping between the images. If the coordinates of the vertices of an undeformed triangle are (x_{11}, x_{21}), (x_{12}, x_{22}), and (x_{13}, x_{23}), and if they map to coordinates (y_{11}, y_{21}), (y_{12}, y_{22}), and (y_{13}, y_{23}), respectively, then the 3×3 affine mapping (**M**) can be obtained by

$$\mathbf{M} = \begin{bmatrix} m_{11} & m_{12} & m_{13} \\ m_{21} & m_{22} & m_{23} \\ 0 & 0 & 1 \end{bmatrix} = \begin{bmatrix} y_{11} & y_{12} & y_{13} \\ y_{21} & y_{22} & y_{23} \\ 1 & 1 & 1 \end{bmatrix} \begin{bmatrix} x_{11} & x_{12} & x_{13} \\ x_{21} & x_{22} & x_{23} \\ 1 & 1 & 1 \end{bmatrix} \tag{34.5}$$

The Jacobian matrix (**J**) of this affine mapping is simply obtained from matrix **M** by

$$\mathbf{J} = \begin{bmatrix} m_{11} & m_{12} \\ m_{21} & m_{22} \end{bmatrix} \tag{34.6}$$

The penalty for distorting each of these triangles is derived from its Jacobian matrix. By using singular value decomposition, **J** can be decomposed into two unitary matrices (**U** and **V**) and a diagonal matrix (**S**), such that $\mathbf{J} = \mathbf{USV}^T$. The unitary matrices simply represent rotations,[3] and are therefore not important to the penalty function. Diagonal matrix **S** contains the singular values, and these represent relative stretching in orthogonal directions. The determinant of **J** ($|\mathbf{J}|$) represents relative volume changes, and is simply the product of the singular values.

---

[2] Note that this is an empirical Bayesian approach because the variance component is derived from the data themselves, and that the variance estimate is just an approximation because the degrees of freedom are not properly computed.

[3] Complications arise when the determinant of **J** is negative. In such a case, either **U** or **V** will also incorporate a reflection by having a negative determinant. However, this should not cause problems since the registration prevents the determinant of **J** from becoming negative.

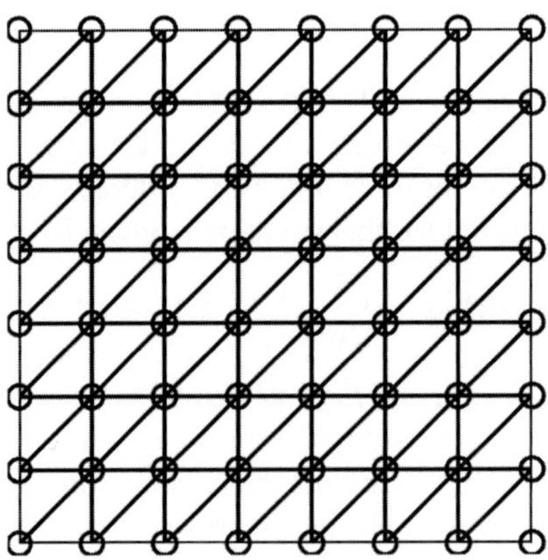

FIGURE 34.1
For the two-dimensional registration problem, the area of the template image (**g**) is divided into a triangular mesh where the nodes are centered on the pixels.

A suitable prior potential function should preserve a one-to-one mapping between **f** and **g** by constraining the determinants of the Jacobian matrices to be positive. The inverse of the mapping also needs to be considered in that the potential (per unit area) for **J** should be identical to that which would be obtained for $\mathbf{J}^{-1}$. A penalty such as $\log(|\mathbf{J}|)^2$ (or even $|\mathbf{J}| + |\mathbf{J}|^{-1} - 2$) would realise both of these criteria. However, relative lengths also need to be considered, and the length and volume changes should have similar distributions. A suitable form for this function is based on the logs of the diagonal elements of **S** being drawn from a normal distribution. The penalty per unit area is therefore $\lambda \log(s_{11})^2 + \lambda \log(s_{22})^2$, where λ is a "regularisation parameter."[4] If the logs of each diagonal element of **S** are normally distributed, then $\log |\mathbf{J}|$ is also normally distributed as $\log(|\mathbf{J}|) \equiv \log(s_{11}) + \log(s_{22})$ and both $\log(s_{11})$ and $\log(s_{22})$ are normally distributed. Each triangular patch has an area of 1/2 pixel, and it will have an area of $|\mathbf{J}|/2$ pixels when mapped to the space of image **f.** The total area affected by the penalty in both the template and source images is therefore $(1 + |\mathbf{J}|)/2$, so the penalty for each triangle becomes

$$h = \lambda(1 + |\mathbf{J}|)\,[\log(s_{11})^2 + \log(s_{22})^2]/2 \tag{34.7}$$

Examples of these penalties in terms of two-dimensional probability functions are illustrated in Fig. 34.2. The prior potential over the whole image is based on the sum of the potentials for each of the I triangles:

$$H(\mathbf{Y}) = \sum_{i=1}^{I} h_i \tag{34.8}$$

For simplicity, in the current description, the fact that the images have boundaries is ignored. In practice, the boundaries are fixed so that the deformation at the edges is always zero.

3D Prior Potentials

The preceding section described deformation fields consisting of a patchwork of triangles. The situation is more complex when working with three-dimensional deformations. For this case, the volume of the template image is divided into a mesh of tetrahedra, where the vertices of the tetrahedra are centered on the voxels. This is achieved by considering groups of eight voxels as little cubes. Each of these cubes is divided into five tetrahedra: one central one having 1/3 of the cube's volume, and four outer ones, each having 1/6 of the cube's volume (Guéziec and Hummel, 1995). There are two possible ways of dividing a cube into five tetrahedra. Alternating between the two conformations in a three-dimensional checkerboard pattern ensures that the whole template volume is uniformly covered (see Fig. 34.3). A deformation field is generated by

[4] Short of determining λ using a large number of "true" deformations, it is assigned some suitable value that facilitates rapid convergence to reasonable solutions.

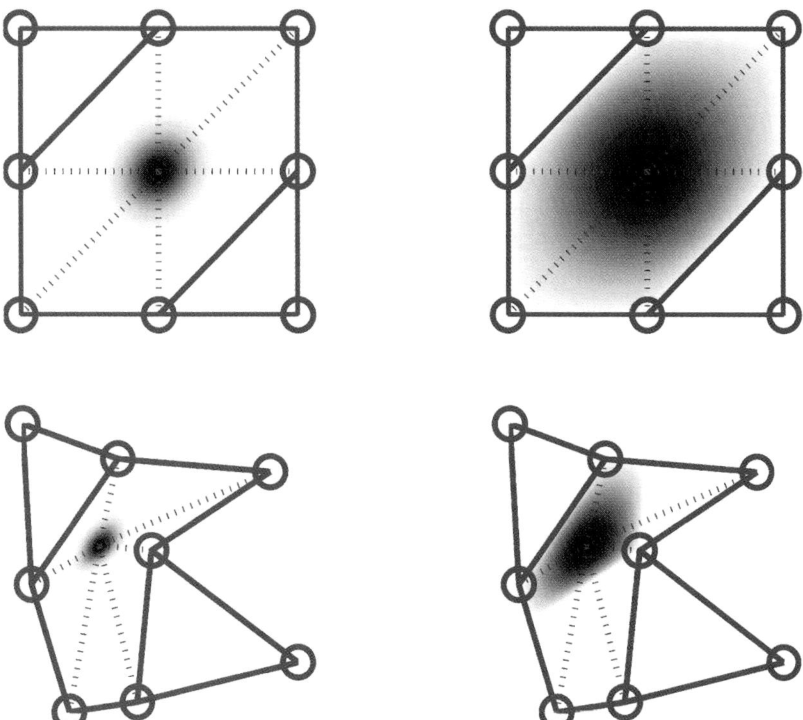

FIGURE 34.2
Probability density functions relating to the position of the center node, assuming that all other voxels remain at fixed locations on a regular grid. (Left) Using heavy regularisation $\lambda = 10$. (Right) Using light regularisation $\lambda = 1$. (Top) On a regular grid. (Bottom) On an irregular grid. The probabilities are defined as the exponent of the negative cost function [as in Eq. (34.2)], where the cost function is derived from the Jacobian matrices of the triangles that have the node as a vertex. The cost function is based on the sum of squares of the logs of the singular values. The dotted lines show the position of the node in the conformation with the lowest cost function.

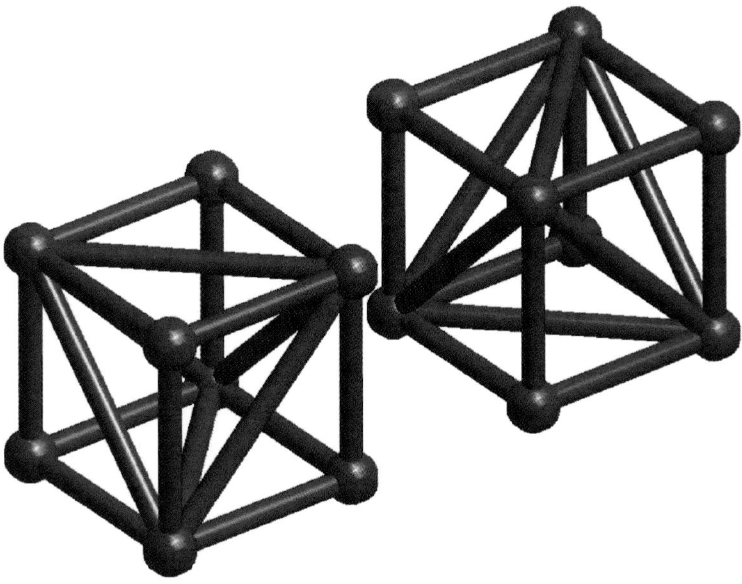

FIGURE 34.3
The volume of the template image is divided into a mesh of irregular tetrahedra, where the vertices of the tetrahedra are centered on the voxels. Groups of eight voxels are considered as little cubes. The volume of each cube is divided into five tetrahedra, in one of the two possible arrangements shown here. A face of a cube that is divided according to one arrangement opposes with the face of a cube that has been divided the other way. Because of this, it is necessary to arrange the two conformations in a three-dimensional checkerboard pattern.

treating the vertices of the tetrahedra as control points. These points are moved iteratively until the best match is achieved. The deformations are constrained to be locally one to one by ensuring that a tetrahedron never occupies any of the same volume as its neighbours. When a deformation is one to one, it is possible to compute its inverse (see later section titled "Inverting a Deformation Field").

The algorithm can use one of two possible boundary conditions. The simplest is when the vertices of tetrahedra that lie on the boundary remain fixed in their original positions (Dirichlet boundary condition). Providing that the initial starting estimate for the deformations is globally one to one, then the final deformation field will also satisfy this constraint (Christensen *et al.*, 1995). The other boundary condition involves allowing the vertices on the surface to move freely (analogous to the Neumann boundary condition). It is possible for the global one-to-one constraints to be broken in this case, as the volumes of non-neighbouring tetrahedra can now overlap. The examples shown later use the free boundary condition.

Within each tetrahedron, the deformation is considered to be a uniform affine transformation from which the Jacobian matrix is extracted in a way similar to that described in the previous section. A penalty is applied to each of the tetrahedra that constitute the volume covered. For each tetrahedron, it is the product of a penalty per unit volume and the total volume affected by the tetrahedron. The affected volume is the volume of the undeformed tetrahedron in the template image, plus the volume that the deformed tetrahedron occupies within the source image [$v(1 + |\mathbf{J}|)$, where v is the volume of the undeformed tetrahedron].

A good penalty against deforming each tetrahedron is based on the logs of the singular values of the Jacobian matrices at every point in the deformation being drawn from a normal distribution. The use of conventional methods for computing the SVD of a 3×3 matrix is currently too slow to be used within an image registration procedure.

Using the SVD regularisation, the penalty per unit volume is $\sum_{i=1}^{3} \log(s_{ii})^2$, where s_{ii} is the ith singular value of the Jacobian matrix. This function is equivalent to $\sum_{i=1}^{3} \log(s_{ii}^2)^2/4$. By using an approximation that $\log(x)^2 \simeq x + 1/x - 2$ for values of x very close to one, we now have the function $\sum_{i=1}^{3} (s_{ii}^2 + 1/s_{ii}^2 - 2)/4$. This function is relatively simple to evaluate, because the sum of squares of the singular values of a matrix is equivalent to the sum of squares of the individual matrix elements. This derives from the facts that the trace of a matrix is equal to the sum of its eigenvalues, and the eigenvalues of $\mathbf{J}^T\mathbf{J}$ are the squares of the singular values of $\mathbf{J}$. The trace of $\mathbf{J}^T\mathbf{J}$ is equivalent to the sum of squares of the individual elements of $\mathbf{J}$. Similarly, the sum of squares of the reciprocals of the singular values is identical to the sum of squares of the elements of the inverse matrix. The singular values of the matrix need not be calculated, and there is no longer a need to call the log function (which is relatively slow to compute). The penalty for each of the tetrahedra is now:

$$h = \lambda v(1 + |\mathbf{J}|) \operatorname{tr}(\mathbf{J}^T\mathbf{J} + (\mathbf{J}^{-1})^T\mathbf{J}^{-1} - 2\mathbf{I})/4 \tag{34.9}$$

where tr is the trace operation, $\mathbf{I}$ is a 3×3 identity matrix, v is the volume of the undeformed tetrahedron (either 1/6 or 1/3), and λ is a regularisation constant. The prior potential for the whole image is the sum of these penalty functions over all tetrahedra. Figure 34.4 shows a comparison of the potential based on the original $[\log(s_{ii})]^2$ cost function, and the potential based on $(s_{ii}^2 + s_{ii}^{-2} - 2)/4$.

The Optimisation Algorithm

The images are matched by estimating the set of parameters ($\mathbf{Y}$) that maximises their *a posteriori* probability. This involves beginning with a set of starting estimates and repeatedly making tiny adjustments such that the posterior potential is decreased. In each iteration, the positions of the control points (nodes) are updated *in situ,* by sequentially scanning through the template volume. During one iteration of the three-dimensional registration, the looping may work from inferior to superior (most slowly), posterior to anterior, and left to right (fastest). In the next iteration, the order of the updating is reversed (superior to inferior, anterior to posterior, and right to left). This alternating sequence is continued until there is no longer a significant reduction to the posterior potential, or for a fixed number of iterations.

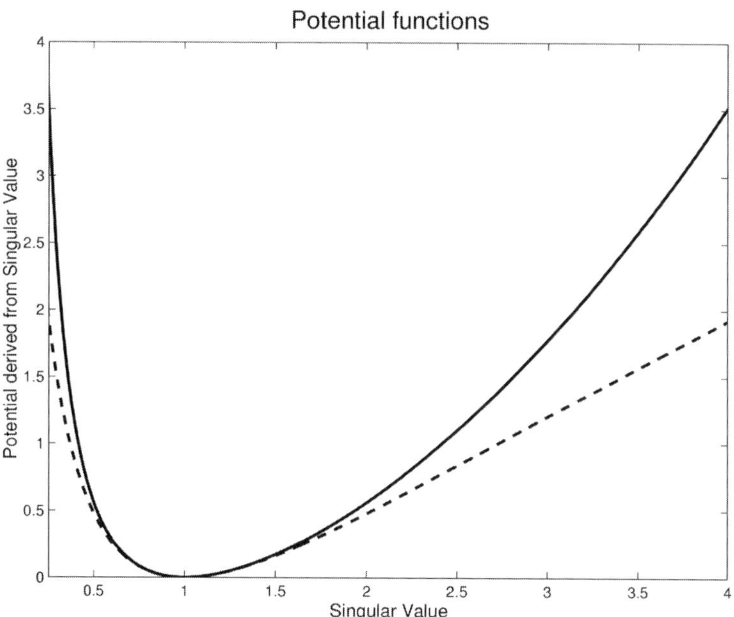

FIGURE 34.4
A comparison of the different cost functions. The dotted line shows the potential estimated from $\log(s_{ii})^2$, where s_{ii} is the ith singular value of a Jacobian matrix. The solid line shows the new potential, which is based on $(s_{ii}^2 + s_{ii}^{-2} - 2)/4$. For singular values very close to one, the potentials are almost identical.

Each iteration of the optimisation involves determining the rate of change of the posterior potential with respect to tiny changes in each element of **Y.** For the nth iteration, the estimates for the ith element of **Y** are modified according to:

$$\mathbf{y}_i^{(n+1)} = \mathbf{y}_i^{(n)} - \epsilon \frac{\partial H(\mathbf{Y}|\mathbf{b})}{\partial \mathbf{y}_i} = \mathbf{y}_i^{(n)} - \epsilon \left(\frac{\partial H(\mathbf{b}|\mathbf{Y})}{\partial \mathbf{y}_i} + \frac{\partial H(\mathbf{Y})}{\partial \mathbf{y}_i} \right) \quad (34.10)$$

where the value of ϵ is chosen to be suitably small (see below).

The term $\partial H(\mathbf{b}|\mathbf{Y})/\partial \mathbf{y}_i$ is the rate of change of likelihood potential with respect to changes in $\mathbf{y}_i$:

$$\frac{\partial H(\mathbf{b}|\mathbf{Y})}{\partial \mathbf{y}_i} = \frac{\partial [f(\mathbf{y}_i) - g(\mathbf{x}_i)]^2 /(2\sigma^2)}{\partial \mathbf{y}_i} = \frac{[f(\mathbf{y}_i) - g(\mathbf{x}_i)]}{\sigma_2} \frac{\partial f(\mathbf{y}_i)}{\partial \mathbf{y}_i} \quad (34.11)$$

where σ^2 is estimated as described earlier. In the updating, each node is moved along the direction that most rapidly decreases the *a posteriori* potential (a gradient descent method).

For the two-dimensional registration, $\partial H(\mathbf{Y})/\partial \mathbf{y}_i$ is dependent on changes to the Jacobian matrices of the six adjacent triangles shown in Fig. 34.5. Because the mathematics of computing these partial derivatives is algebraically dense, a C subroutine is provided in Fig. 34.6 that will compute the derivatives for a single triangular patch.

For the three-dimensional case, moving a node in the mesh influences the Jacobian matrices of the tetrahedra that have a vertex at that node, so the rate of change of the posterior potential is equal to the rate of change of the likelihood plus the rate of change of the prior potentials from these local tetrahedra. Approximately half of the nodes form a vertex in eight neighbouring tetrahedra, whereas the other half are vertices of 24 tetrahedra. The rate of change of the penalty function for each tetrahedron with respect to changes in position of one of the vertices is required. The Matlab 5.3 Symbolic Toolbox (The MathWorks, Natick, Massachusetts, USA) was used to derive expressions for analytically computing these derivatives, but these formulas are not given here. The ideas presented above assume that the voxel dimensions are isotropic and the same for both images. Modifications to the method that are required in order to account for the more general cases are trivial and are not shown here.

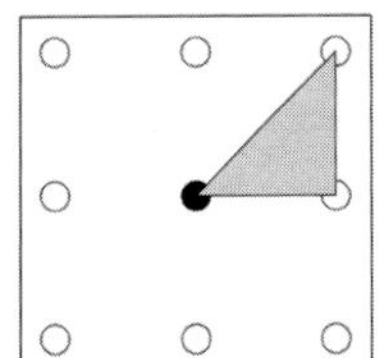
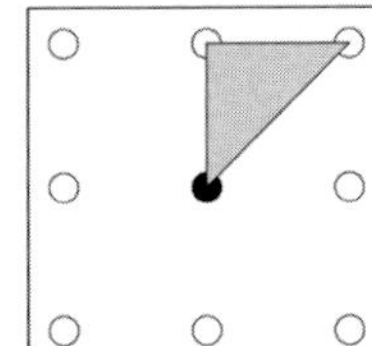
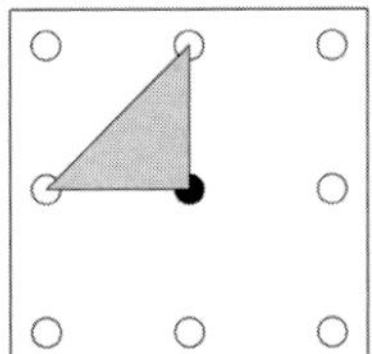
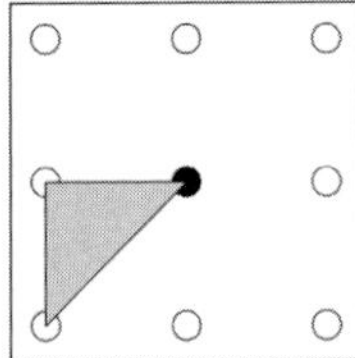
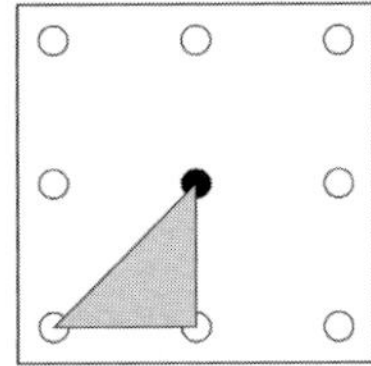
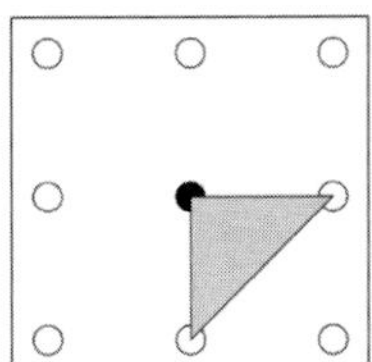

FIGURE 34.5
The six neighbouring triangles whose Jacobian matrices are influenced by translating the central point.

```
void dh_dy(double  *h, double *dh1, double *dh2, double lambda,
           double x11, double  x21, double  y11, double y21,
           double x12, double  x22, double  y12, double y22,
           double x13, double  x23, double  y13, double y23)
{
        double j11, j12, j21, j22, dj1, dj2;
        double w, w1, w2, dt, dt1, dt2, tm, tm1, tm2;
        double s1, s2, d1s1, d1s2, d2s1, d2s2;
        double dtx, t1, t2, t3, t4;
        dtx  =  x11*(x22-x23)+x12*(x23-x21)+x13*(x21-x22);
        j11  = (y11*(x22-x23)+y12*(x23-x21)+y13*(x21-x22))/dtx;
        j12  = (y11*(x13-x12)+y12*(x11-x13)+y13*(x12-x11))/dtx;
        j21  = (y21*(x22-x23)+y22*(x23-x21)+y23*(x21-x22))/dtx;
        j22  = (y21*(x13-x12)+y22*(x11-x13)+y23*(x12-x11))/dtx;
        dj1  = (x22-x23)/dtx; dj2 = (x13-x12)/dtx;
        w    = j11*j11+j12*j12+j21*j21+j22*j22;
        w1   = 2.0*(dj1*j11+dj2*j12); w2 = 2.0*(dj1*j21+dj2*j22);
        dt   = j22*j11-j12*j21;
        dt1  = j22*dj1-dj2*j21; dt2  = dj2*j11-j12*dj1;
        t1   = w+2.0*dt; t2    = w-2.0*dt; t3    = t1*t2;
        if (t3>1e-6){
                t3    = sqrt(t3); tm     = 2.0*t3;
                tm1   = (t2*(w1+2*dt1)+t1*(w1-2*dt1))/t3;
                tm2   = (t2*(w2+2*dt2)+t1*(w2-2*dt2))/t3;
        }
        else { tm = 0.0; tm1 = 1.0; tm2 = 1.0; }
        s1   = w *0.50 + tm *0.25; s2    = w *0.50 - tm *0.25;
        d1s1 = w1*0.50 + tm1*0.25; d1s2 = w1*0.50 - tm1*0.25;
        d2s1 = w2*0.50 + tm2*0.25; d2s2 = w2*0.50 - tm2*0.25;
        t1   = log(s1); t2     = log(s2);
        t3   = t1/s1;    t4    = t2/s2;
        dtx  = lambda*fabs(dtx)*0.5;
        t1   = 0.25*(t1*t1    + t2*t2  );
        t2   = 0.50*(t3*d1s1 + t4*d1s2);
        t3   = 0.50*(t3*d2s1 + t4*d2s2);
        *h   = dtx*t1*(dt+1);
        *dh1 = dtx*(t1*dt1 + t2*(dt+1));
        *dh2 = dtx*(t1*dt2 + t3*(dt+1));
}
```

FIGURE 34.6
C code for computing the rate of change of the prior potential (h) with respect to changes in y11 and y21. The arguments passed to the routine are the original coordinates at the vertices of the triangle. These are (x11,x21), (x12,x22), and (x13,x23), and they map to (y11,y21), (y12,y22), and (y13,y23), respectively. The values returned are h, dh1, and dh2, and these correspond to the potential of the deformation of the triangular patch, and the rate of change of the potential with respect to changes in y11 and y21. Note that the singular values of a 2×2 matrix **J** are $(\{w + [(w + 2d)(w - 2d)]^{1/2}\}/2)^{1/2}$ and $(\{w - [(w + 2d)(w - 2d)]^{1/2}\}/2)^{1/2}$, where $w = j^2_{11} + j^2_{12} + j^2_{21} + j^2_{22}$ and $d = j_{22}j_{11} - j_{12}j_{21}$.

If a node is moved too far, then the determinant of one or more of the Jacobian matrices associated with a neighbouring triangle or tetrahedron may become negative. This would mean a violation of the one-to-one constraint in the mapping (since neighbouring tetrahedra would occupy the same volume), so it is prevented by a bracketing procedure. The initial attempt moves the node by a small distance ϵ. If any of the determinants become negative, then the value of ϵ is halved and another attempt made to move the node the smaller distance from its original location. This continues for the node until the constraints are satisfied. A similar procedure is then repeated whereby the value of ϵ continues to be halved until the new potential is less than or equal to the previous value. By incorporating this procedure, the potential will never increase as a node is moved, therefore ensuring that the potential over the whole image will decrease with every iteration.

Inverting a Deformation Field

Occasionally it is desirable to compute the inverse of a deformation field. For example, if a deformation has been defined that warps brain A to match brain B, it may be useful to have the inverse of this deformation in order to warp brain B to match brain A. This section describes how to do this for three-dimensional transformations. The registration method estimates a deformation field that describes a mapping from points in the template volume to those in the source volume. Each point within the template maps to exactly one point within the source image, and every point within the source maps to a point in the template. For this reason, a unique inverse of the spatial transformation exists. To invert the deformation field, it is necessary to find the mapping from the voxels in the source image to their equivalent locations in the template.

The template volume is covered by a large number of contiguous tetrahedra. Within each tetrahedron, the mapping between the images is described by an affine transformation. Inverting the transformation involves sequentially scanning through all the deformed tetrahedra to find any voxels of the source image that lie inside. The vertices of each tetrahedron are projected onto the space of the source volume, and so form an irregular tetrahedron within that volume. All voxels within the source image (over which the deformation field is defined) should fall into one of these tetrahedra. Once the voxels within a tetrahedron are identified, the mapping to the template image is achieved simply by multiplying the coordinates of the voxels in the source image by the inverse of the affine matrix $\mathbf{M}$ for the tetrahedron (from an earlier section).

The first problem is to locate the voxels of the source image that lie within a tetrahedron, given the locations of the four vertices. This involves finding locations where the x, y, and z coordinates assume integer values within the tetrahedral volume. First of all, the vertices of the tetrahedron are sorted into increasing z coordinates. Planes where z takes an integer value are identified between the first and second, the second and third, and the third and fourth vertices. Between the first and second vertices, the cross-sectional shape of a tetrahedron (where it intersects a plane where z is an integer) is triangular. The corners of the triangle are at the locations where lines connecting the first vertex to each of the other three vertices intersect the plane. Similarly, between the third and fourth vertices, the cross section is again triangular, but this time the corners are at the intersects of the lines connecting the first, second, and third vertices to the fourth. Between the second and third vertex, the cross section is a quadrilateral, and this can be described by two triangles. The first can be constructed from the intersects of the lines connecting vertices one to four, two to four, and two to three. The other is from the intersects of the lines connecting vertices one to four, one to three, and two to three. The problem has now been reduced to the more trivial one of finding coordinates within the area of each triangle for which x and y are both integer values (see Fig. 34.7).

The procedure for finding points within a triangle is broken down into finding the ends of line segments in the triangle where y takes an integer value. To find the line segments, the corners of the triangle are sorted into increasing y coordinates. The triangle is divided into two smaller areas, separated by a line at the level of the second vertex. The method for identifying the ends of the line segments is similar to the one used for identifying the corners of the triangles. The voxels are then simply located by finding points on each of the lines where x is an integer.

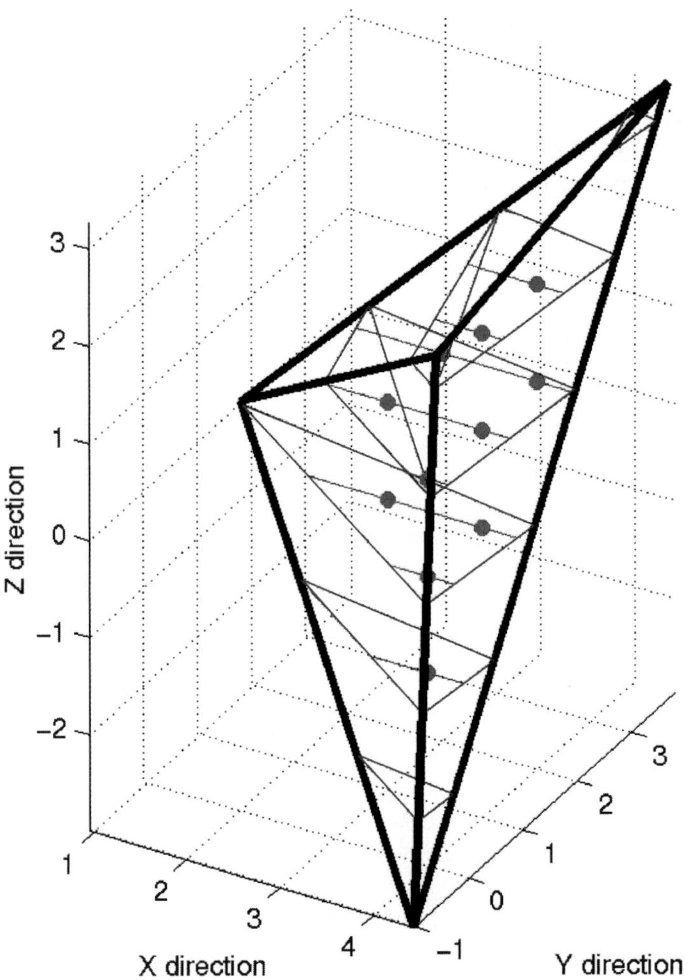

FIGURE 34.7
An illustration of how voxels are located within a tetrahedron.

EXAMPLES

A number of sets of examples are provided in this section. The first is based on simulated data and is designed to show the symmetric nature of the estimated warps. This is followed by examples of registering one brain to another, both in two and three dimensions. Finally, examples of several brains registered simultaneously are given, again in two and three dimensions.

Two-Dimensional Warping Using Simulated Data

Simulated data are used to demonstrate the reversibility of the deformation fields. Two images were constructed, one of them a circle, and the other a square. The circle was warped to match the square, and the square to match the circle. No noise was added to the images, so a constant variance was assumed for all iterations. The final results of the registration are shown in Fig. 34.8. To demonstrate the symmetry of the deformations, the two deformation fields were combined. These are shown in Fig. 34.9. If the deformations were perfectly symmetric, the combined deformations would be completely uniform. However, wrinkles can be seen that may be due to using finite approximations of continuous functions. Another contributing factor to the wrinkles may be because the likelihood potentials driving the registration are not symmetric.

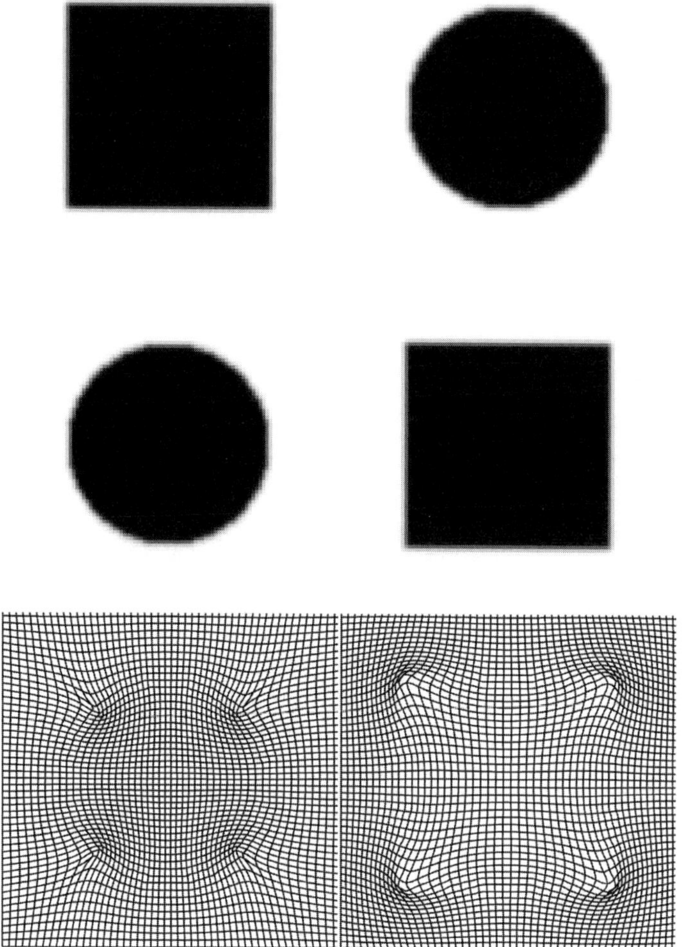

FIGURE 34.8
Demonstration using simulated data. (Above left) Original square. (Above right) Original circle. (Center left) Square deformed to match the circle. (Center right) Circle deformed to match the square. (Below left) Deformation field applied to the circle in order to warp it to match the square. The deformation field shows where data should be re-sampled from the original image in order to generate the warped version. (Below right) Deformation field required to deform the square to the circle.

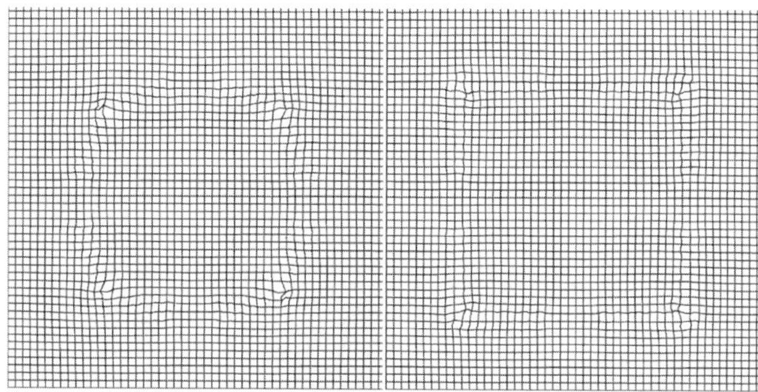

FIGURE 34.9
Demonstration of the reversibility of the deformations obtained by combining forward and reverse deformations. (Left) Deformation field that warps from the circle to the square and back to the circle. (Right) Deformation field that warps from the square to the circle and back to the square.

Registering Pairs of Images

Here are examples of registering pairs of images together, first in two dimensions, and then in three dimensions.

Two-Dimensional Example

Approximately corresponding slices through two MR images of different subjects were registered together using the current approach. To reduce the chance of the algorithm being caught in a local minimum, the first few iterations of the registration were carried out with the images smoothed using an 8-mm full-width at half-maximum Gaussian convolution kernel. Larger values for λ were also used for the early iterations in order to estimate the global head shape prior to estimating the more detailed deformations. The final results of the registration are shown in Fig. 34.10.

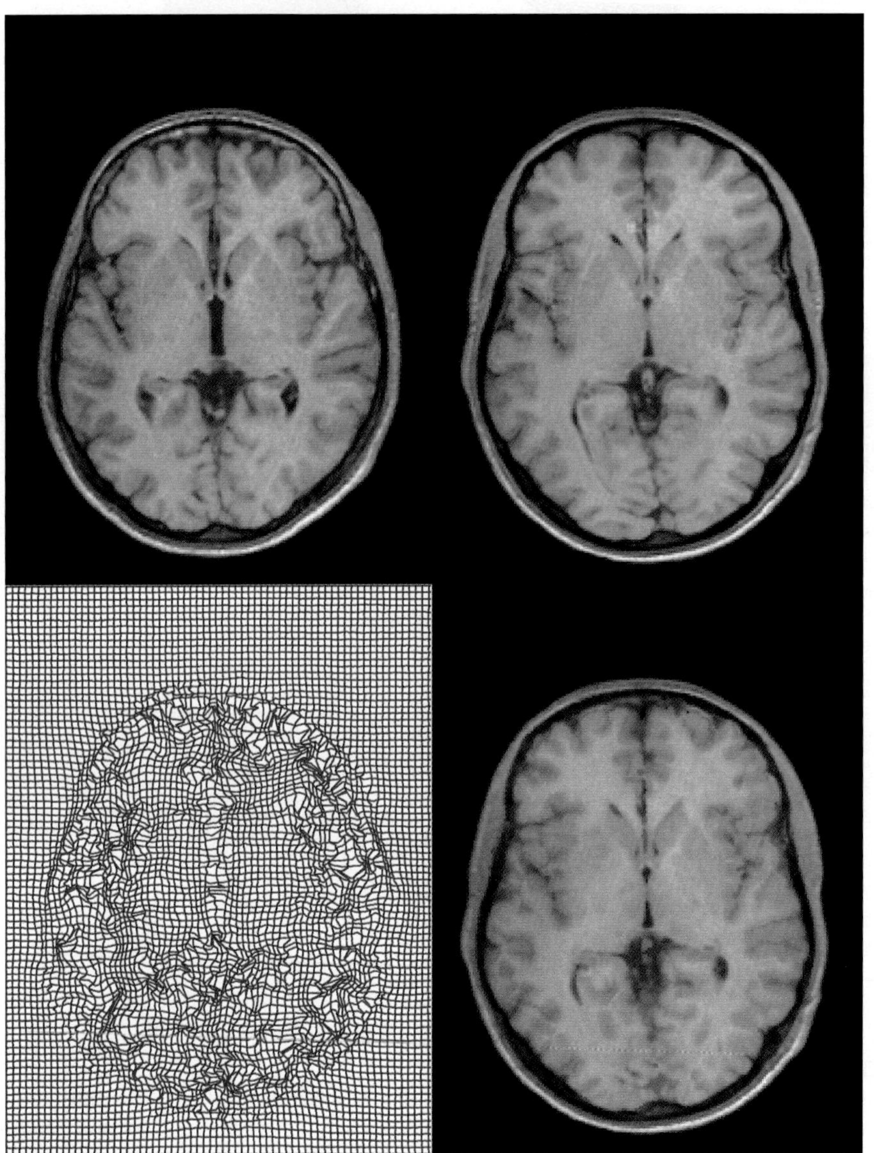

FIGURE 34.10
(Above left) The unwarped source image. (Above right) The template image. (Below left) The deformation field applied to the source image in order to warp it to match the template image. (Below right) The source image after warping to match the template.

Three-Dimensional Example

A pair of three-dimensional brain images were first registered using the global registration methods described in Chapter 33, which provide a good starting point for estimating the optimum high-dimensional deformation field. It took about 15.5 hours to estimate the 21,233,664 parameters on one of the processors of a SPARC Ultra 2 (Sun Microsystems, USA). Figure 34.11 shows the two registered brain images, and the corresponding deformation fields are shown in Fig. 34.12.

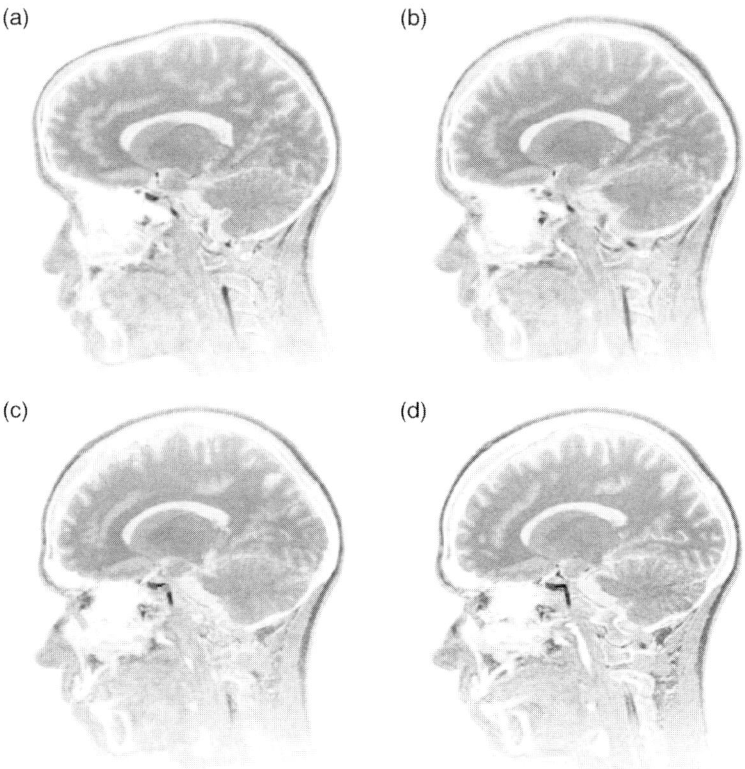

FIGURE 34.11
A sagittal plane from two images registered together. The template (reference) image is shown in (d). (a) shows the source image after affine registration to the template image. The source image after the basis function registration is shown in (b), and the final registration result is in (c). The deformation fields are shown in Fig. 34.12.

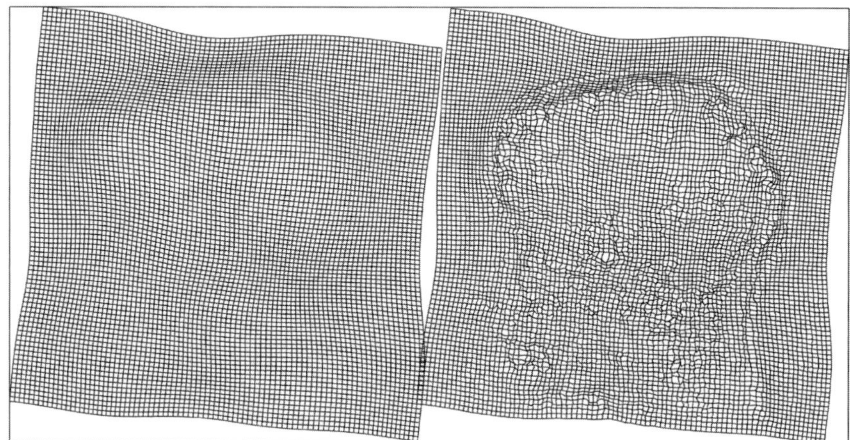

FIGURE 34.12
The deformation fields corresponding to the images in Fig. 34.11. Two components (vertical and horizontal translations) of the field after affine and basis function registration are shown on the left, whereas the final deformation field is shown on the right.

Registering to an Average

One of the themes of this chapter is about achieving internal consistency in the estimated warps. So far, only mappings between pairs of images have been discussed. When a number of images are to be registered to the same stereotaxic space, then there are more possible ways in which this can be achieved. The different routes that can be taken to achieve the same goal may not always produce consistent results (Le Briquer and Gee, 1997; Woods *et al.,* 1998; Christensen, 1999). To achieve more consistency in the warps, the images should all be registered to a template that is some form of average of all the individual images. A mapping between any pair of brains can then be obtained by combining the transformation from one of the brains to the template, with the inverse of the transformation that maps from the other brain to the template.

Two-Dimensional Example

An iterative procedure was used to generate such an average from a slice from the MR images of 29 subjects. The images were first registered to the same stereotaxic space using a 12-parameter affine registration, and the same slice extracted from all of the registered images. The first step involved averaging the intensities of the unwarped images to create an initial estimate for the template. Then an iteration of the registration procedure was used to bring each of the images slightly closer to the shape of the template. The warped brains were then averaged again, and this average was used as the template for the next round of the procedure. This was continued until the algorithm converged, and the Gibbs potential of the system was minimised. The template resulting from this procedure is shown in Fig. 34.13. A procedure similar to this may be a very useful and principled technique to generate templates and "canonical" references.

Three-Dimensional Example

A similar procedure was performed using the three-dimensional registration method, where an image that is the average of six normal subjects' brains was created. The image was an average not only of intensity, but also of shape. Again, the global registration methods described in Chapter 33 were first used. The procedure began by estimating the approximate deformations that map each of the images to a reference template, using the 12-parameter affine registration followed by the basis function approach (see Fig. 33.10 and 33.11). After the registration, each of the images were transformed according to the estimated parameters. The transformed images contained $121 \times 145 \times 121$ voxels, with a resolution of approximately $1.5 \times 1.5 \times 1.5$ mm. The first estimate of the new template was computed as the average of these images. The estimated 4×4 affine transformation matrices and basis function coefficients were used to generate starting parameters for estimating the high-dimensional deformation fields.

For each of the six images, 10 iterations of the current algorithm were used to bring the images slightly closer in to register with the template. The spatially transformed images were averaged again to obtain a new estimate for the template, after which the images were again registered to the template using a further 10 iterations. This process continued for a total of four times. A plane from each of the spatially transformed images is shown in Figure 34.14.

Visually, the registered images appear very similar. This is not always a good indication of the quality of the registration (but it does confirm that the optimisation algorithm has reduced the likelihood potentials). In theory, the wrong structures could be registered together, but distorted so that they look identical.

The brain surfaces of the original images were extracted using the procedures described in Chapter 35. This involved a segmentation of gray and white matter on which morphological operations were performed to remove the small amounts of remaining nonbrain tissue. The surfaces were then rendered. A number of points were selected that were near the surface of the template brain (the average of the spatially transformed images). By using the computed spatial transformations, these points were projected on to the closest corresponding location on the rendered brain surfaces. Figure 34.15 shows the rendered surfaces. Note that the large amount of cortical variability means that it is very difficult to objectively identify homologous locations on the surfaces of the different brains. The shapes of the internal brain structures are less variable, so the method is able to estimate transformations for these regions much more precisely.

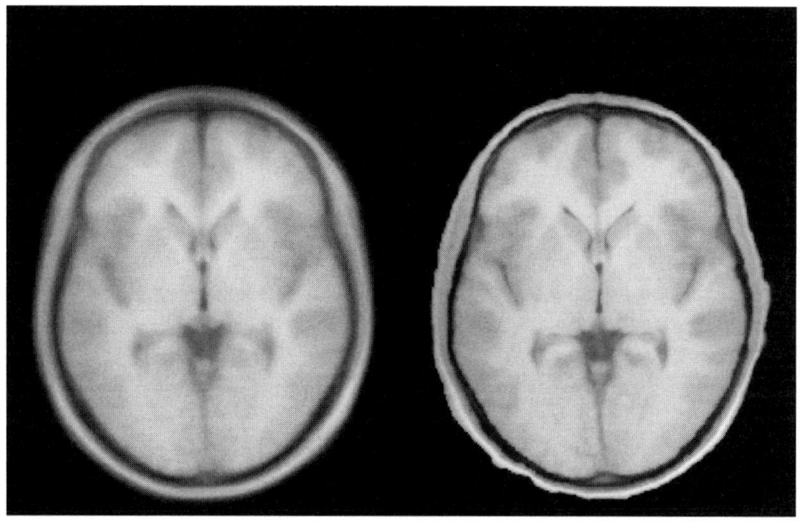

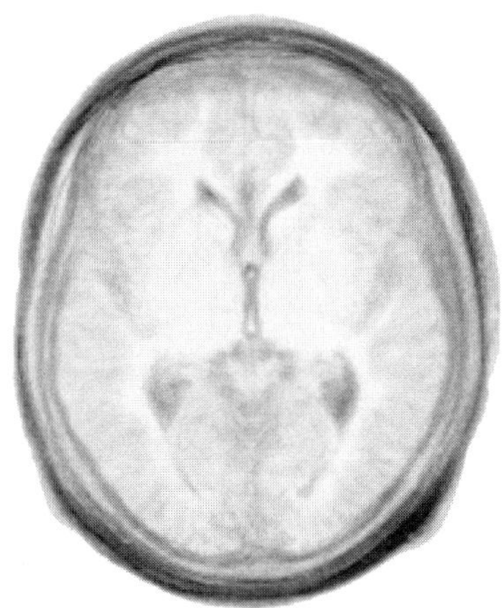

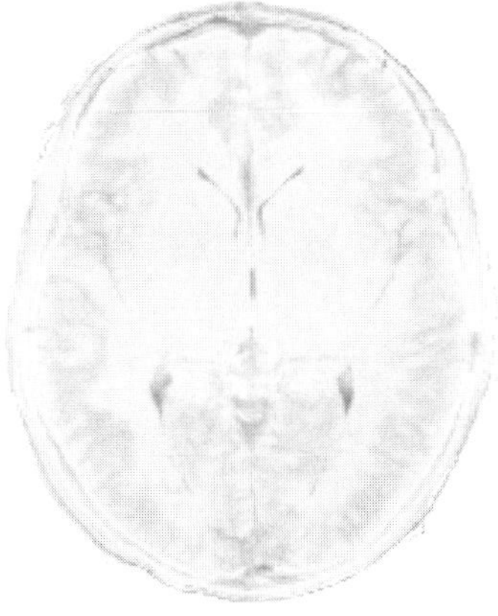

FIGURE 34.13
(Above left) The average of the MR images of 29 subjects registered together using a 12-parameter affine registration. (Above right) The average (both shape and intensity) of the same 29 MR images after registering together using the method described in the text. (Below left) The standard deviations of the affine registered MR images. (Below right) The standard deviations of the MR images after registration using the current method. The images of standard deviation are shown using the same intensity scaling.

Although the deformation fields contain a mapping from the average shaped template image to each of the individual images, it is still possible to compute the mapping between any image pair. This is done by combining a forward deformation that maps from the template image to the first image, with an inverse deformation (computed as described earlier) that maps from the second image to the template. Figure 34.16 shows five images that have been transformed in this way to match the same image.

DISCUSSION

Validation of warping methods is a complex area. The appropriateness of an evaluation depends on the particular application for which the deformations are to be used. For example, if the application was spatial normalisation of functional images of different subjects, then the most appropriate evaluation may be based on assessing the sensitivity of voxel-wise statistical tests. Because the warping procedure is based only on structural information, it is blind to the locations of functional activation. If the locations of activations can be brought into close correspondence

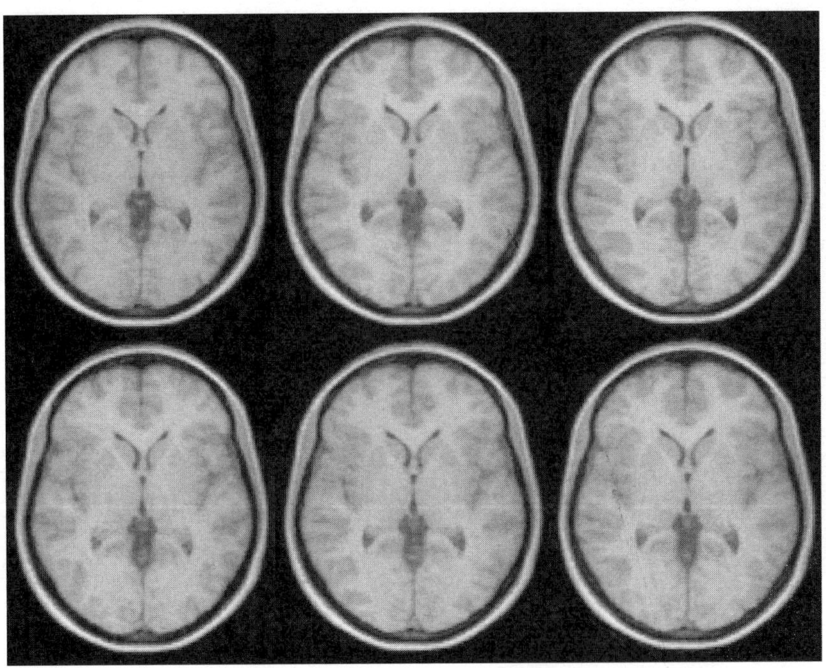

FIGURE 34.14
The images of the six brains after affine and basis function registration, followed by high-dimensional image registration using the methods described in this chapter (see also Fig. 33.10 and 33.11). The high-dimensional transformations are able to model high-frequency deformations that cannot be achieved using the basis function approach alone.

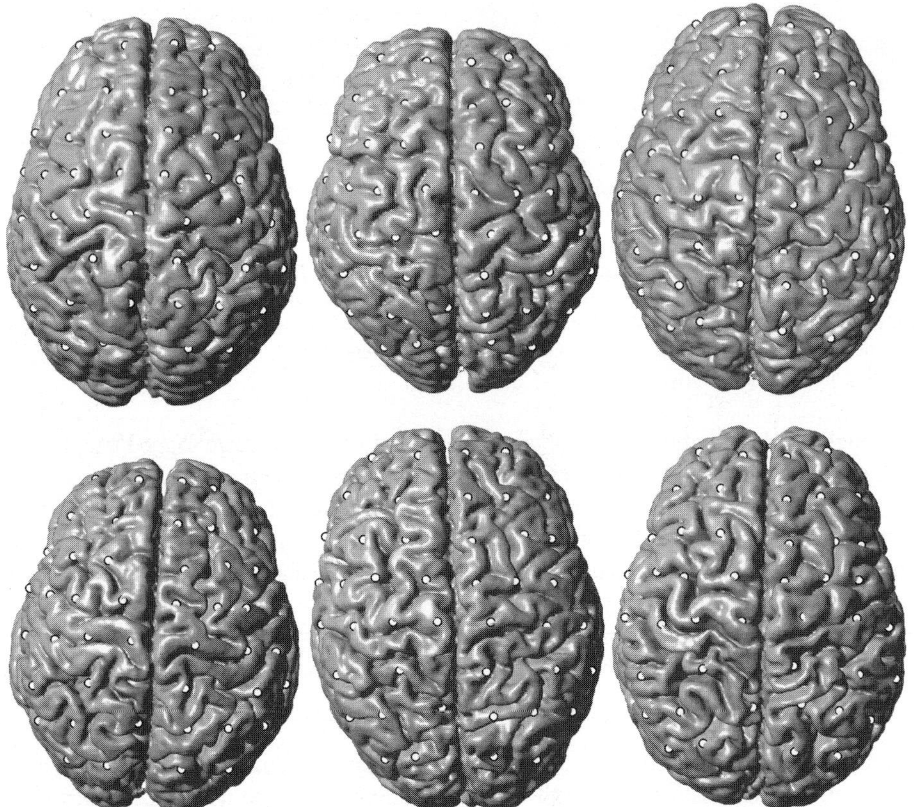

FIGURE 34.15
Rendered surfaces of the original six brains. The white markers correspond to equivalent locations on the brain surfaces as estimated by the registration algorithm.

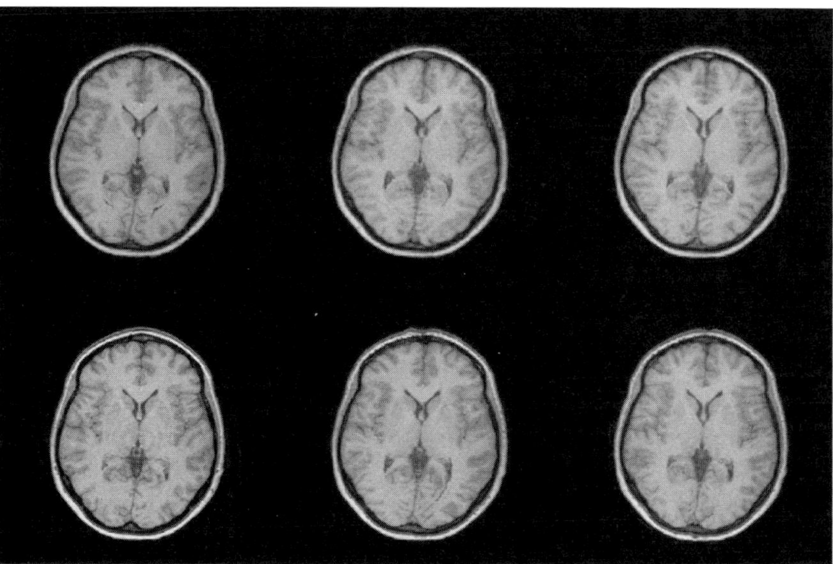

FIGURE 34.16
By combining the warps, it is possible to compute a mapping between any pair of images. In this example, the remaining images were all transformed to match the one shown at the lower left.

in different subjects, then it is safe to say that the spatial normalisation procedure is working well. The best measure of correspondence depends on how much the images are smoothed prior to performing the statistical tests. Different registration methods will perform differently depending on the amount of smoothing used. For example, the difference in performance of high- versus low-dimensional methods will be less when lots of smoothing is used. More discussion of this can be found in Chapter 33.

Another application may involve identifying shape differences among populations of subjects. In this case, the usefulness of the warping algorithm would be assessed by how well the deformation fields can be used to distinguish between the populations.

To know how well a new warping method works, it needs to be considered in relation to other available methods. There are also likely to be many hyperparameters to be tweaked for each of the models in order to obtain the best results. Optimum values for these hyperparameters are likely to depend on the types of images being registered. Rather than focusing on one of many possible evaluation strategies, this section considers the validity of the different components of the warping method described in the current chapter. The validity of the registration method is dependent on four main elements: the parameterisation of the deformations, the matching criteria, the priors describing the nature of the warps, and the algorithm for estimating the spatial transformations.

Parameterising the Deformations

The deformations are parameterised using regularly arranged piecewise affine transformations. The same principles described in this chapter can also be applied to more irregular arrangements of tetrahedra. Because much of an estimated deformation field is very smooth, whereas other regions are more complex, it may be advantageous in terms of speed to arrange the tetrahedra more efficiently. The layout of the triangles or tetrahedra described in this chapter is relatively simple, and it does have the advantage that no extra memory is required to store the original coordinates of vertices. It also means that some of the calculations required to determine the Jacobian matrices (part of a matrix inversion) can be precomputed and stored efficiently.

An alternative to using the linear mappings could be to use piecewise nonlinear mappings such as those described by Goshtasby (1987). However, such mappings would not fit easily into the current framework, because there would be no simple expression for the Gibbs potential for each of the patches of deformation field. This is because the Jacobian matrix is not constant within a patch, so computing the Gibbs potential would require a complicated integration procedure.

In terms of speed, this method does not compare favorably with some other high-dimensional intensity-based registration algorithms (Thirion, 1995), and this chapter has not concentrated on describing ways of making the algorithm more efficient. One way of achieving this would be to use an increasing density of nodes. For the early iterations, when estimating smoother deformations, fewer nodes are required to adequately define the deformations. The number of parameters describing the deformations is equal to three times the number of nodes, and a faster convergence should be achieved using fewer parameters. It is worth nothing that a coarse to fine scheme for the arrangement of the nodes is not necessary in terms of the validity of the method. A coarse to fine approach (in terms of using smoother images and deformations for the early iterations) can still be achieved even when the deformation field is described by an equally large number of nodes from start to finish.

The Matching Criterion

The matching criterion described here is fully automatic and produces reproducible and objective estimates of deformations that are not susceptible to bias from different investigators. It also means that relatively little user time is required to perform the registrations. However, this does have the disadvantage that human expertise and understanding (which are extremely difficult to encode into an algorithm) are not used by the registration. More accurate results may be possible if the method were semiautomatic, by also allowing user-identified features to be matched.

The current matching criterion involves minimising the sum of squared differences between source and template images. This same criterion is also used by many other intensity-based nonlinear registration methods and assumes that one image is just a spatially transformed version of the other, but with white Gaussian noise added. Note that this is not normally the case. After matching a pair of brain images, the residual difference is never purely uniform white noise, but tends to have a spatially varying magnitude. For example, the residual variance in background voxels is normally much lower than that in gray matter. An improved model would use a nonstationary variance map and possibly model covariance between neighbouring voxels, or even covariance between intensities in different regions (e.g., see Chapter 33).

The validity of the matching criterion depends partly on the validity of the template image. If the intensity values of the different tissues of the template image differ systematically from those of the corresponding tissues in the source image, then the validity of the matching will be impaired because the correlations introduced into the residuals are not accounted for by the model. Pathology is another case where the validity of the registration is compromised. This is because there is no longer a one-to-one correspondence between the features of the two images. An ideal template image should contain a "canonical" or average shaped brain. On average, registering a brain image to a canonical template requires smaller (and therefore less error prone) deformations than would be necessary for registering to an unusually shaped template.

Although the priors for the registration model are symmetric, the matching criterion is not. One effect of this is that the gradients of only one image are used to drive the registration, rather than the gradients of both. This is illustrated in Fig. 34.17. With a fully symmetric matching criterion, the evaluations in the "Two-Dimensional Warping Using Simulated Data" and "Registering Pairs of Images" sections would be expected to produce more consistent results. Note however, that the matching used in the "Registering to an Average" section can be considered as symmetric. When registering a pair of images together by matching them both to their average, the gradients of both images are considered equally. The result of this procedure would be two deformation fields that map "halfway." By combining the "halfway" deformations in the appropriate way (as shown in Fig. 34.16), a pair of deformation fields can be obtained that map between the images, and are both inverses of each other.

The Priors

Consider the transformations mapping between images **f** and **g.** By combining the transformation mapping from image **f** to image **g,** with the one that maps image **g** to image **f,** a third transformation can be obtained that maps from **f** to **g** and then back to **f.** Any nonuniformities in

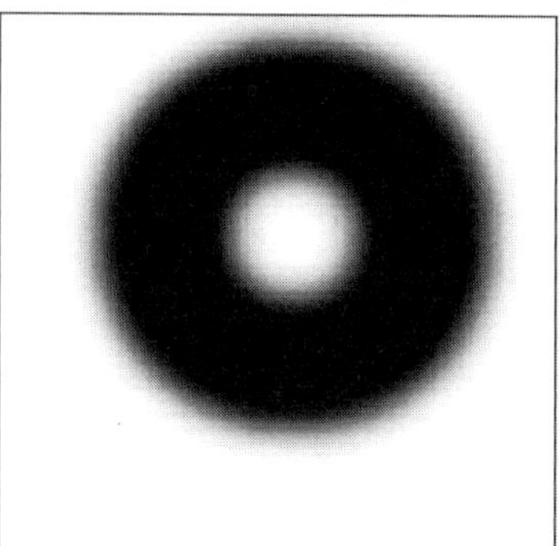

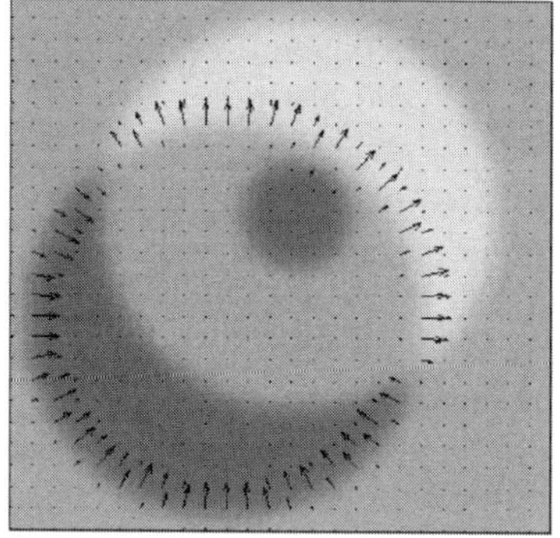

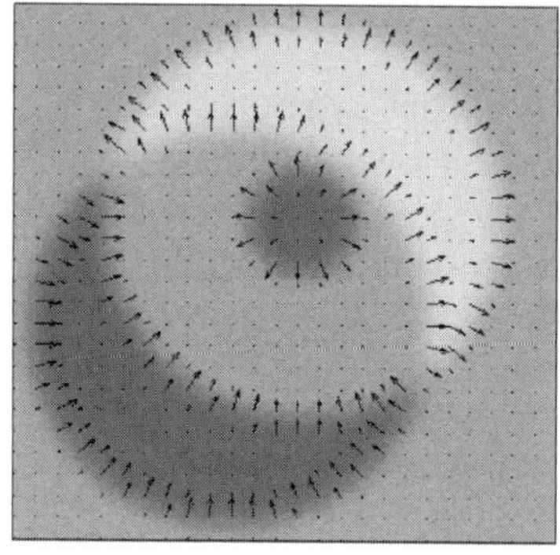

FIGURE 34.17
A comparison of a symmetric with an asymmetric likelihood potential. The arrows on the lower images show the directions in which the source image would be deformed. The template image contains a feature that is not found in the source image. If a registration is based only on gradients of the source image, then this feature is likely to have no effect on the final estimated spatial transformation. However, if the likelihood potential is symmetric, then this feature would drive a local expansion of the source image, until the likelihood potential is balanced by the prior potential.

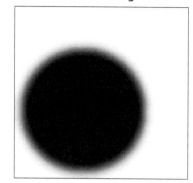

this resulting transformation represent errors in the registration process. The priors adopted in this chapter attempt to reduce any such inconsistencies in the deformation fields. The extreme case of an inconsistency between a forward and inverse transformation is when the one-to-one mapping between the images breaks down. Unlike many Bayesian registration methods that use linear priors (Amit *et al.,* 1991; Gee *et al.,* 1997; Miller *et al.,* 1993; Bookstein, 1997, 1989), the Bayesian scheme here uses a penalty function that approaches infinity if a singularity begins to appear in the deformation field. This is achieved by considering both the forward and inverse spatial transformations at the same time. For example, when the length of a structure is doubled in the forward transformation, it means that the length should be halved in the inverse transformation. Because of this, the penalty function used here is the same for both the forward and inverse of a given spatial transformation. The ideal form for this function should be based on the logs of the singular values of the Jacobian matrices having normal distributions, but the more rapidly computed function described earlier is a close enough approximation.

The penalty function is invariant to the relative orientations of the images. It does not penalise rotations or translations in isolation, only those relative to the position of neighbouring voxels. To reposition a region relative to its neighbours, it is necessary to introduce scaling and shearing into the affine transformations. It is this scaling and shearing that the model penalises, rather than the position and orientation itself (see Fig. 34.18).

Only the form of the prior potential has been stated, and little has been said about its magnitude relative to the likelihood potential. This is because it is not clear what the relative magnitudes of the two sets of potentials should be. The term λ relates to our belief in the amount of brain structural variability that is likely to be observed in the population. A relatively large

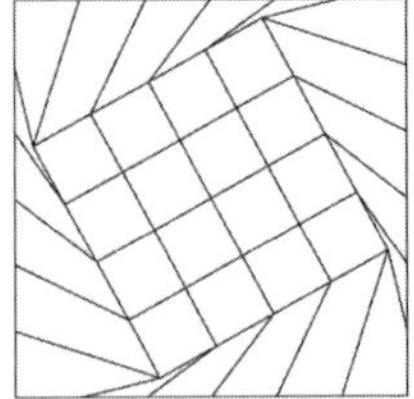
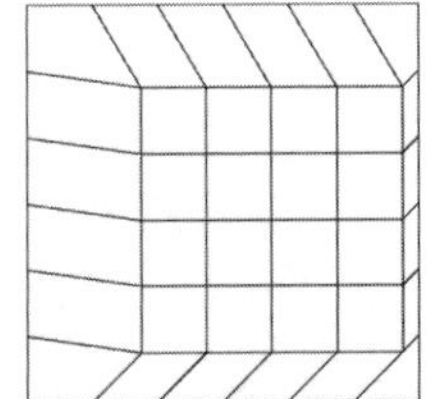

FIGURE 34.18
The objective of including the prior probability distribution in the registration model is to penalise shape changes of the source image. A rigid body rotation of a region of brain does nothing to the shape of that region. However, to rotate relative to the neighbouring regions, shears and zooms are necessary and these do change the shape of the image.

value for λ results in the deformations being more smooth, at the expense of a higher residual squared difference between the images, whereas a small value for λ will result in a lower residual squared difference, but fewer smooth deformations. The prior distributions described in this chapter are stationary (since λ is constant throughout). In reality, the true amount of brain structural variability is very likely to be different from region to region (Lester *et al.,* 1999), so a set of nonstationary priors should, in theory, produce more valid MAP estimates.

Much of the nonstationary variability will be higher in some directions than others. An alternative way of understanding the penalty function based on normally distributed logs of singular values is to consider the Hencky strain tensors of the deformations (see Chapter 36). The prior potential model described in this chapter is essentially minimising the sum of squares of the Hencky tensor elements. Anisotropic variability could be modeled by assuming different variances for each Hencky tensor element, thus allowing more stretching or contraction in some directions than others. Further material properties could be introduced by also modelling the covariance between the tensor elements. For example, by making all diagonal elements of the tensor correlated, then the deformations could be forced to be the same in all directions. Another covariance model could be used to force the deformations to be volume preserving (isochoric) by forcing the trace of the Hencky tensor to equal zero. Even more complex prior probability distributions could be devised that involve modelling covariance between the strain tensors of neighbouring (or even remote) triangles or tetrahedra. In theory, such models could be used to make whole regions stretch or contract uniformly.

Estimating the normal amount of structural variability is not straightforward. Registration methods could be used to do this by registering a large number of brain images to a canonical template. However, the estimates of structural variability will be heavily dependent on the priors used by the algorithm. A "chicken and egg" situation arises, whereby the priors are needed to estimate the optimum deformation fields, and the deformation fields are needed to estimate the correct priors. It may be possible to overcome this problem using an empirical Bayes method (see Chapter 39) to estimate the unknown hyperparameters (i.e., σ^2 and λ), which describe the relative importance of the different components of the objective function.

The Optimisation Algorithm

The method searches for the MAP solution, which is the single most probable realisation of all possible deformation fields. The steepest descent algorithm that is used does not guarantee that the globally optimum MAP solution will be achieved, but it does mean that a local optimum solution can be reached—eventually. Robust optimisation methods that almost always find the global optimum would take an extremely long time to run with a model that uses millions of parameters. These methods are simply not feasible for routine use on problems of this scale. However, if sulci and gyri can be easily labeled from the brain images, then robust methods can be applied in order to match the labeled features. Robust methods become more practical when the amount of information is reduced to a few key features. The robust match can then be used to bias the high-dimensional registration (Joshi *et al.,* 1995; Thompson and Toga, 1996; Davatzikos, 1996), therefore increasing the likelihood of obtaining the global optimum.

If the starting estimates are sufficiently close to the global optimum, then the algorithm is more likely to find the true MAP solution. Therefore, the choice of starting parameters can

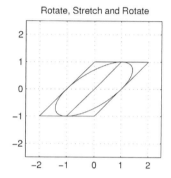

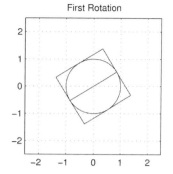

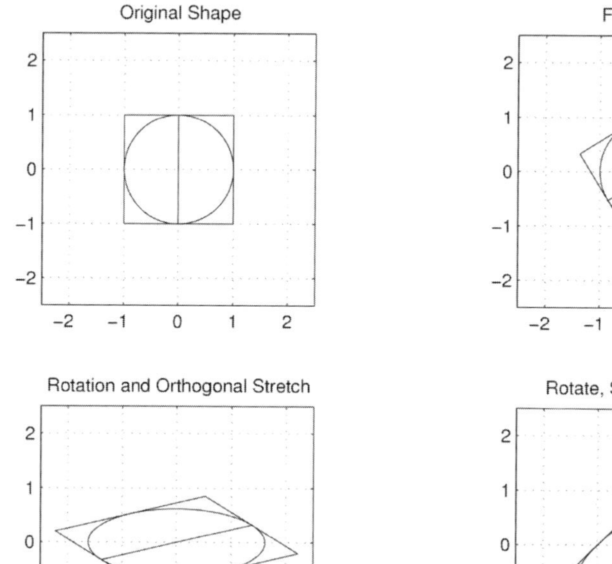

FIGURE 34.19
An affine transformation matrix that performs a shear must have singular values that are not equal to one. This figure shows a shear applied to a square and circle decomposed into the steps defined by singular value decomposition. The stretching that occurs between the upper right subfigure and that in the lower left is what would be penalised. Note that shearing does not change the area of the objects, so a penalty based only on the Jacobian determinants would have no effect on this type of distortion.

influence the validity of the final registration result. An error surface based only on the prior potential does not contain any local minima. However, there may be many local minima when the likelihood potential is added to this. Therefore, if the posterior potential is dominated by the likelihood potential, then it is much less likely that the algorithm will achieve the true MAP solution. If very high frequency deformations are to be estimated, then the starting parameters must be very close to the optimum solution.

One method of increasing the likelihood of achieving a good solution is to gradually reduce the value of λ relative to $1/\sigma^2$ over time. This has the effect of making the registration estimate the more global deformations before estimating more detailed warps. Most of the spatial variability is low frequency, so the algorithm can get reasonably close to a good solution using a relatively high value for lambda. This also reduces the number of local minima for the early iterations. The images should also be smoother for the earlier iterations in order to reduce the amount of confounding information and the number of local minima. A review of such approaches can be found in Lester and Arridge (1999).

A value for σ^2 is used that is based on the residual squared difference between the images after the previous iteration. The value of σ^2 is larger for the early iterations, so the posterior potential is based more on the priors. It decreases over time, thus decreasing the influence of the priors and allowing higher frequency deformations to be estimated. Similarly, for the example where images were registered to their average, the template image was smoothest at the beginning. Each time the template was recreated, it was slightly crisper than the previous version. High-frequency information that would confound the registration in the early iterations is gradually reintroduced to the template image as it is needed.

At first sight, it would appear that optimising the millions of parameters that describe a deformation field would be an impossible task. Note that these parameters are all related to each other since the regularisation tends to preserve the shape of the image and, hence, reduces the effective number of degrees of freedom that the model has to fit. The limiting case would be to set the regularisation parameter λ to infinity. Providing that the boundary conditions allowed it, this would theoretically reduce the dimensionality of the problem to a six-parameter rigid body transformation (although the current implementation would be unable to cope with a λ of infinity).

References

Amit, Y., Grenander, U., and Piccioni, M. (1991). Structural image restoration through deformable templates. *J. Am. Statistical Assoc.* **86,** 376–387.

Bookstein, F. L. (1989). Principal warps: Thin-plate splines and the decomposition of deformations. *IEEE Trans. Patt. Anal. Mach. Intell.* **11**(6), 567–585.

Bookstein, F. L. (1997). Landmark methods for forms without landmarks: Morphometrics of group differences in outline shape. *Med. Image Anal.* **1**(3), 225–243.

Christensen, G. E. (1999). Consistent linear elastic transformations for image matching. In: "Proc. Information Processing in Medical Imaging" (A. K. *et al.,* eds.). Springer-Verlag, Berlin.

Christensen, G. E., Rabbitt, R. D., and Miller, M. I. (1994). 3D brain mapping using using a deformable neuroanatomy. *Phy. Med. Biol.* **39,** 609–618.

Christensen, G. E., Rabbitt, R. D., and Miller, M. I. (1996). Deformable templates using large deformation kinematics. *IEEE Trans. Image Proc.* **5,** 1435–1447.

Christensen, G. E., Rabbitt, R. D., Miller, M. I., Joshi, S. C., Grenander, U., Coogan, T. A., and Van Essen, D. C. (1995). Topological properties of smooth anatomic maps. In: "Proc. Information Processing in Medical Imaging" (Y. Bizais, C. Barillot, and R. Di Paola, eds.). Kluwer Academic Publishers, Dordrecht, The Netherlands.

Davatzikos, C. (1996). Spatial normalisation of 3D images using deformable models. *J. Computer Assisted Tomog.* **20**(4), 656–665.

Freeborough, P. A., and Fox, N. C. (1998). Modelling brain deformations in Alzheimer disease by fluid registration of serial MR images. *J. Computer Assisted Tomog.* **22**(5), 838–843.

Gee, J. C., Haynor, D. R., Le Briquer, L., and Bajcsy, R. K. (1997). Advances in elastic matching theory and its implementation. In: "Proc. CVRMed-MRCAS'97" (P. Cinquin, R. Kikinis, and S. Lavallee, eds.). Springer-Verlag, Berlin.

Goshtasby, A. (1987). Piecewise cubic mapping functions for image registration. *Patt. Recog.* **20**(5), 525–533.

Guéziec, A., and Hummel, R. (1995). Exploiting triangulated surface extraction using tetrahedral decomposition. *IEEE Trans. Visualisation Computer Graphics* **1,** 328–342.

Joshi, S. C., Miller, M. I., Christensen, G. E., Banerjee, A., Coogan, T. A., and Grenander, U. (1995). Hierarchical brain mapping via a generalised Dirichlet solution for mapping brain manifolds. In: "Proc. SPIE Int. Symp. Optical Science, Engineering and Instrumentation." SPIE, Bellingham, WA.

Le Briquer, L., and Gee, J. C. (1997). Design of a statistical model of brain shape. In: "Proc. Information Processing in Medical Imaging" (J. Duncan and G. Gindi, eds.). Springer-Verlag, Berlin.

Lester, H., and Arridge, S. R. (1999). A survey of hierarchical non-linear medical image registration. *Patt. Recog.* **32,** 129–149.

Lester, H., Arridge, S. R., Jansons, K. M., Lemieux, L., Hajnal, J. V., and Oatridge, A. (1999). Non-linear registration with the variable viscosity fluid algorithm. In: "Proc. Information Processing in Medical Imaging" (A. K. *et al.,* eds.). Springer-Verlag, Berlin.

Miller, M. I., Christensen, G. E., Amit, Y., and Grenander, U. (1993). Mathematical textbook of deformable neuroanatomies. *Proc. Natl. Acad. Sci. USA* **90,** 11944–11948.

Thirion, J.-P. (1995). Fast non-rigid matching of 3D medical images. Tech. Rep. 2547, Institut National de Recherche en Informatique et en Automatique. Available from http://www.inria.fr/RRRT/RR-2547.html.

Thompson, P. M., and Toga, A. W. (1996). Visualisation and mapping of anatomic abnormalities using a probablistic brain atlas based on random fluid transformations. In: "Proc. Visualisation in Biomedical Computing."

Woods, R. P., Grafton, S. T., Holmes, C. J., Cherry, S. R., and Mazziotta, J. C. (1998). Automated image registration: I. General methods and intrasubject, intramodality validation. *J. Computer Assisted Tomog.* **22**(1), 139–152.

CHAPTER

35

Image Segmentation

INTRODUCTION

Healthy brain tissue can generally be classified into three broad tissue types on the basis of an MR image. These are gray matter (GM), white matter (WM), and cerebrospinal fluid (CSF). This classification can be performed manually on a good-quality T_1 image by simply selecting suitable image intensity ranges that encompass most of the voxel intensities of a particular tissue type. However, this manual selection of thresholds is highly subjective.

Some groups have used clustering algorithms to partition MR images into different tissue types, either using images acquired from a single MR sequence or by combining information from two or more registered images acquired using different scanning sequences or echo times (e.g., proton density and T_2 weighted). The approach described here is a version of the *mixture model* clustering algorithm (Hartigan, 1975), which has been extended to include spatial maps of prior belonging probabilities, and also a correction for image intensity nonuniformity that arises for many reasons in MR imaging. Because the tissue classification is based on voxel intensities, partitions derived without the correction can be confounded by these smooth intensity variations.

The model assumes that the MR image or images consist of a number of distinct tissue types (clusters) from which every voxel has been drawn. The intensities of voxels belonging to each of these clusters conform to a normal distribution, which can be described by a mean, a variance, and the number of voxels belonging to the distribution. For multispectral data (e.g., simultaneous segmentation of registered T_2 and PD images), multivariate normal distributions can be used. In addition, the model has approximate knowledge of the spatial distributions of these clusters, in the form of prior probability images.

Before using the current method for classifying an image, the image has to be in register with the prior probability images. The registration is normally achieved by least-squares matching with template images in the same stereotaxic space as the prior probability images. This can be done using nonlinear warping, but the examples provided in this chapter were done using affine registration (see Chapter 33).

One of the greatest problems faced by tissue classification techniques is nonuniformity of the image intensity. Many groups have developed methods for correcting intensity nonuniformities, and the scheme developed here shares common features. Two basic models describe image noise properties: multiplicative noise and additive noise. The multiplicative model describes images that have noise added before being modulated by the nonuniformity field (i.e., the standard deviation of the noise is multiplied by the modulating field), whereas the additive version models noise that is added after the modulation (standard deviation is constant). The current method uses a multiplicative noise model, which assumes that the errors originate from tissue variability rather than additive Gaussian noise from the scanner. Figure 35.2 illustrates the model used by the classification.

Nonuniformity correction methods all involve estimating a smooth function that modulates the image intensities. If the function is is not forced to be smooth, then it will begin to fit the higher frequency intensity variations due to different tissue types, rather than the low-frequency intensity nonuniformity artifact. Spline (Yan and Karp, 1995; Sled *et al.,* 1998) and polynomial (Van Leemput *et al.,* 1999a,b) basis functions are widely used for modelling the intensity variation. In these models, the higher frequency intensity variations are restricted by limiting the number of basis functions. In the current method, a Bayesian model is used, where it is assumed that the modulation field (**U**) has been drawn from a population for which the *a priori* probability distribution is known, thus allowing high-frequency variations of the modulation field to be penalised.

METHODS

The explanation of the tissue classification algorithm will be simplified by describing its application to a single two-dimensional image. A number of assumptions are made by the classification model. The first is that each of the $I \times J$ voxels of the image (**F**) has been drawn from a known number (K) of distinct tissue classes (clusters). The distribution of the voxel intensities within each class is normal (or multinormal for multispectral images) and initially unknown. The distribution of voxel intensities within cluster k is described by the number of voxels within the cluster (h_k), the mean for that cluster (v_k), and the variance around that mean (c_k).

Because the images are matched to a particular stereotaxic space, prior probabilities of the voxels belonging to the GM, WM, and CSF classes are known. This information is in the form of probability images provided by the Montréal Neurological Institute (Evans *et al.,* 1992, 1993, 1994) as part of the ICBM, NIH P-20 project (principal Investigator John Mazziotta), and derived from scans of 152 young healthy subjects. These probability images contain values in the range of zero to one, representing the prior probability of a voxel being either GM, WM, or CSF after an image has been normalised to the same space (see Figure 35.1). The probability of a voxel at coordinate i, j belonging to cluster k is denoted by b_{ijk}.[1]

The final assumption is that the intensity and noise associated with each voxel in the image has been modulated by multiplication with an unknown smooth scalar field.

Many unknown parameters need to be determined by the classification algorithm, and estimating any of these requires knowledge of the others. Estimating the parameters that describe a cluster (h_k, v_k, and c_k) relies on knowing which voxels belong to the cluster and also the form of the intensity modulating function. Estimating which voxels should be assigned to each cluster requires the cluster parameters to be defined and also the modulation field. In turn, estimating the modulation field needs the cluster parameters and the belonging probabilities.

The problem requires an iterative algorithm (see Fig. 35.3). It begins by assigning starting estimates for the various parameters. The starting estimate for the modulation field is typically uniformly one. Starting estimates for the belonging probabilities of the GM, WM, and CSF partitions are based on the prior probability images. Because there are no prior probability maps for background and nonbrain tissue clusters, they are estimated by subtracting the prior probabilities for GM, WM, and CSF from a map of all ones, and dividing the result equally between the remaining clusters.[2]

Each iteration of the algorithm involves estimating the cluster parameters from the nonuniformity corrected image, assigning belonging probabilities based on the cluster parameters, checking for convergence, and reestimating and applying the modulation function. With each

[1] Note that ij subscripts are used for voxels rather than the single subscripts used in the previous chapters. This is to facilitate the explanation of how the modulation field is estimated for 2D images as described in a later section.

[2] Where identical prior probability maps are used for more than one cluster, the affected cluster parameters need to be modified so that separate clusters can be characterised. This is typically done after the first iteration, by assigning different values for the means uniformly spaced between zero and the intensity of the WM cluster.

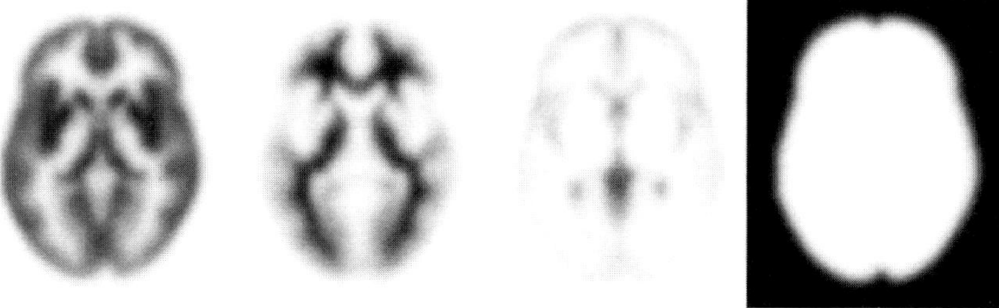

FIGURE 35.1
The *a priori* probability images of GM, WM, CSF, and nonbrain tissue. Values range between zero (white) and one (black).

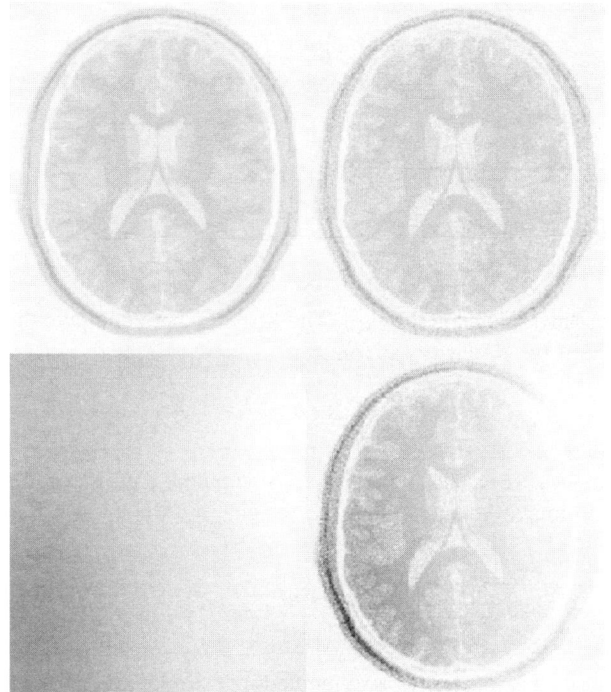

FIGURE 35.2
The MR images are modeled as a number of distinct clusters (top left), with different levels of Gaussian random noise added to each cluster (top right). The intensity modulation is assumed to be smoothly varying (bottom left) and is applied as a straightforward multiplication of the modulation field with the image (bottom right).

iteration, the parameters describing the distributions move toward a better fit and the belonging probabilities (**P**) change slightly to reflect the new distributions. This continues until a convergence criterion is satisfied. The parameters describing clusters with corresponding prior probability images tend to converge more rapidly than the others. This may be partly due to the better starting estimates. The final values for the belonging probabilities are in the range of 0 to 1, although most values tend to stabilise very close to one of the two extremes. The algorithm is in fact an *expectation maximisation* (EM) approach, where the *E-step* is the computation of the belonging probabilities, and the *M-step* is the computation of the cluster and nonuniformity correction parameters. The individual steps involved in each iteration are now described in more detail.

Estimating the Cluster Parameters

This stage requires the most recent estimate of the modulation function (**U,** where u_{ij} is the multiplicative correction at voxel i,j), and the current estimate of the probability of voxel i,j

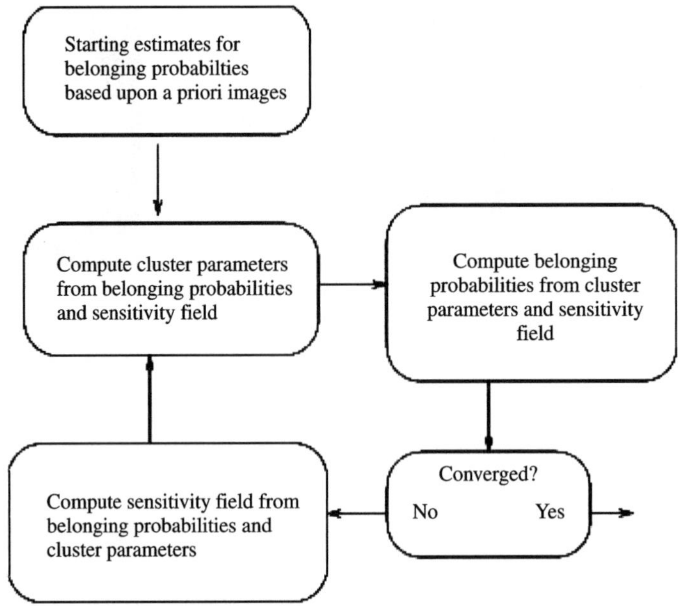

FIGURE 35.3
A flow diagram for the tissue classification.

belonging to class k, which is denoted by p_{ijk}. The first step is to compute the number of voxels (**h**) belonging to each of the K clusters as follows:

$$h_k = \sum_{i=1}^{I} \sum_{j=1}^{J} p_{ijk} \text{ over } k = 1..K$$

Mean voxel intensities for each cluster (**v**) are computed. This step effectively produces a weighted mean of the image voxels, where the weights are the current belonging probability estimates:

$$v_k = \frac{\sum_{i=1}^{I} \sum_{j=1}^{J} p_{ijk} f_{ij} u_{ij}}{h_k} \text{ over } k = 1..K$$

Then the variance of each cluster (**c**) is computed in a similar way to the mean:

$$c_k = \frac{\sum_{i=1}^{I} \sum_{j=1}^{J} p_{ijk} (f_{ij} u_{ij} - v_k)^2}{h_k} \text{ over } k = 1..K$$

Assigning Belonging Probabilities

The next step is to recalculate the belonging probabilities. This step uses the cluster parameters computed in the previous step, along with the prior probability images and the intensity-modulated input image. Bayes' rule is used to assign the probability of each voxel belonging to each cluster:

$$p_{ijk} = \frac{r_{ijk} s_{ijk}}{\sum_{l=1}^{K} r_{ijl} s_{ijl}} \text{ over } 1 = 1..I, j = 1..J, \text{ and } k = 1..K$$

where p_{ijk} is the *a posteriori* probability that voxel i,j belongs to cluster k given its intensity of f_{ij}; r_{ijk} is the likelihood of a voxel in cluster k having an intensity of f_{ik}; and s_{ijk} is the *a priori* probability of voxel i,j belonging in cluster k.

The likelihood function is obtained by evaluating the probability density functions for the clusters at each of the voxels:

$$r_{ijk} = \frac{u_{ij}}{(2\pi c_k)^{1/2}} \exp\left[\frac{-(f_{ij} u_{ij} - v_k)^2}{2c_k}\right] \text{ over } i = 1..I, j = 1..J, \text{ and } k = 1..K$$

The prior (s_{ijk}) is based on two factors: the number of voxels currently belonging to each cluster (h_k) and the prior probability images derived from a number of images (b_{ijk}). With no knowledge of the spatial prior probability distribution of the clusters or the intensity of a voxel, then the *a priori* probability of any voxel belonging to a particular cluster is proportional to the number of voxels currently included in that cluster. However, with the additional data from the prior probability images, a better estimate for the priors can be obtained:

$$s_{ijk} = \frac{h_k b_{ijk}}{\sum_{l=1}^{I}\sum_{m=1}^{J} b_{lmk}} \text{ over } i = 1..I,\ j = 1..J, \text{ and } k = 1..K$$

Convergence is ascertained by following the log-likelihood function:

$$\sum_{i=1}^{I}\sum_{j=1}^{J} \log\left(u_{ij}\sum_{k=1}^{K} r_{ijk}s_{ijk}\right)$$

The algorithm is terminated when the change in log-likelihood from the previous iteration becomes negligible.

Estimating the Modulation Function

To reduce the number of parameters describing an intensity modulation field, the field is modeled by a linear combination of low-frequency discrete cosine transform (DCT) basis functions (see Chapter 33) that were chosen because there are no constraints at the boundary. A two- or three-dimensional DCT is performed as a series of one-dimensional transforms, which are simply multiplications with the DCT matrix. The elements of a matrix (**D**) for computing the first M coefficients of the one-dimensional DCT of a vector of length I are given by:

$$d_{i1} = \frac{1}{\sqrt{I}} \quad i = 1..I$$

$$d_{im} = \sqrt{\frac{2}{I}} \cos\left[\frac{\pi(2i-1)(m-)}{2I}\right] \quad i = 1..I,\ m = 2..M \tag{35.1}$$

The matrix notation for computing the first $M \times N$ coefficients of the two-dimensional DCT of a modulation field $\mathbf{U}$ is $\mathbf{Q} = \mathbf{D}_1{}^T\mathbf{U}\mathbf{D}_2$, where the dimensions of the DCT matrices $\mathbf{D}_1$ and $\mathbf{D}_2$ are $I \times M$ and $J \times N$, respectively, and $\mathbf{U}$ is an $I \times J$ matrix. The approximate inverse DCT is computed by $\mathbf{U} \simeq \mathbf{D}_1\mathbf{Q}\mathbf{D}_2{}^T$. An alternative representation of the two-dimensional DCT is obtained by reshaping the $I \times J$ matrix $\mathbf{U}$ so that it is a vector ($\mathbf{u}$). Element $i + (j-1) \times I$ of the vector is then equal to element i,j of the matrix. The two-dimensional DCT can then be represented by $\mathbf{q} = \mathbf{D}^T\mathbf{u}$, where $\mathbf{D} = \mathbf{D}_2 \otimes \mathbf{D}_1$ (the Kronecker tensor product of $\mathbf{D}_2$ and $\mathbf{D}_1$), and $\mathbf{u} \simeq \mathbf{D}\mathbf{q}$.

The sensitivity correction field is computed by reestimating the coefficients ($\mathbf{q}$) of the DCT basis functions such that the product of the likelihood and a prior probability of the parameters are increased. This can be formulated as an iteration of a Gauss-newton optimisation algorithm (compare with Chapter 33):

$$\mathbf{q}^{(n+1)} = (\mathbf{C}_0^{-1} + \mathbf{A})^{-1}(\mathbf{C}_0^{-1}\mathbf{q}_0 + \mathbf{A}\mathbf{q}^{(n)} - \mathbf{b}) \tag{35.2}$$

where $\mathbf{q}_0$ and $\mathbf{C}_0$ are the means and covariance matrices describing the *a priori* probability distribution of the coefficients. Vector $\mathbf{b}$ contains the first derivatives of the log-likelihood cost function with respect to the basis function coefficients, and matrix $\mathbf{A}$ contains the second derivatives of the log-likelihood. These can be constructed efficiently using the properties of Kronecker tensor products (see Figure 33.5 in Chapter 33):

$$b_{l_1} = \sum_{j=1}^{J} d_{2jn_1} \sum_{i=1}^{I} d_{1im_1}\left[-u_{ij}^{-1} + f_{ij}\sum_{k=1}^{K}\frac{p_{ijk}(f_{ij}u_{ij} - v_k)}{c_k}\right]$$

$$A_{l_1l_2} = \sum_{j=1}^{J} d_{2jn_1}d_{2jn_2} \sum_{i=1}^{I} d_{1im_1}d_{1im_2}\left(u_{ij}^{-2} + f_{ij}^2\sum_{k=1}^{K}\frac{p_{ijk}}{c_k}\right)$$

where $l_1 = m_1 + M(n_1 - 1)$ and $l_2 = m_2 + M(n_2 - 1)$.

Once the coefficients have been reestimated, then the modulation field **U** can be computed from the estimated coefficients (**Q**) and the basis functions ($\mathbf{D}_1$ and $\mathbf{D}_2$).

$$u_{ij} = \sum_{n=1}^{N} \sum_{m=1}^{M} d_{2jn}\, q_{mn}\, d_{1im} \text{ over } i = 1..I, j = 1..J$$

Prior Probability Distribution

In Eq. (35.2), $\mathbf{q}_0$ and $\mathbf{C}_0$ represent a multinormal *a priori* probability distribution for the basis function coefficients. The mean of the prior probability distribution is such that it would generate a field that is uniformly one. For this, all elements of the mean vector are set to zero, apart from the first element that is set to $\sqrt{IJ}$.

The covariance matrix $\mathbf{C}_0$ is such that $(\mathbf{q} - \mathbf{q}_0)^T\mathbf{C}_0^{-1}(\mathbf{q} - \mathbf{q}_0)$ produces an "energy" term that penalises modulation fields that would be unlikely *a priori*. There are many possible forms for this penalty function (see Chapter 33). Some widely used simple penalty functions include the *membrane energy* and the *bending energy*, which (in three dimensions) have the forms $h = \sum_i \sum_{j=1}^{3} \lambda\left[\frac{\partial u(\mathbf{x}_i)}{\partial x_{ji}}\right]^2$ and $h = \sum_i \sum_{j=1}^{3} \sum_{k=1}^{3} \lambda\left[\frac{\partial^2 u(\mathbf{x}_i)}{\partial x_{ji}\partial x_{ki}}\right]^2$ respectively. In these formulas, $\frac{\partial u(\mathbf{x}_i)}{\partial x_{ji}}$ is the gradient of the modulating function at the ith voxel in the jth orthogonal direction, and λ is a user-assigned constant. However, for the purpose of modulating the images, a smoother cost function is used that is based on the squares of the third derivatives (third-order regularisation):

$$h = \sum_i \sum_{j=1}^{3} \sum_{k=1}^{3} \sum_{l=1}^{3} \lambda\left(\frac{\partial^3 u(\mathbf{x}_i)}{\partial x_{ji}\partial x_{ki}\partial x_{li}}\right)^2$$

This model was chosen because it produces slowly varying modulation fields that can represent the variety of nonuniformity effects that are likely to be encountered in MR images (see Fig. 35.4). In two dimensions it can be computed from

$$\begin{aligned}\mathbf{C}_0^{-1} = {} & \lambda\,(\dddot{\mathbf{D}}_2^T\dddot{\mathbf{D}}_2) \otimes (\mathbf{D}_1^T\mathbf{D}_1) + 3\lambda\,(\ddot{\mathbf{D}}_2^T\ddot{\mathbf{D}}_2) \otimes (\dot{\mathbf{D}}_1^T\dot{\mathbf{D}}_1) \\ & + 3\lambda\,(\dot{\mathbf{D}}_2^T\dot{\mathbf{D}}_2) \otimes (\ddot{\mathbf{D}}_1^T\ddot{\mathbf{D}}_1) + \lambda\,(\mathbf{D}_2^T\mathbf{D}_2) \otimes (\dddot{\mathbf{D}}_1^T\dddot{\mathbf{D}}_1)\end{aligned}$$

where the notation $\dot{\mathbf{D}}_1$, $\ddot{\mathbf{D}}_1$, and $\dddot{\mathbf{D}}_1$ refer to the first, second, and third derivatives [by differentiating Eq. (35.1) with respect to i] of $\mathbf{D}_1$, respectively, and λ is a user-specified hyperparameter.

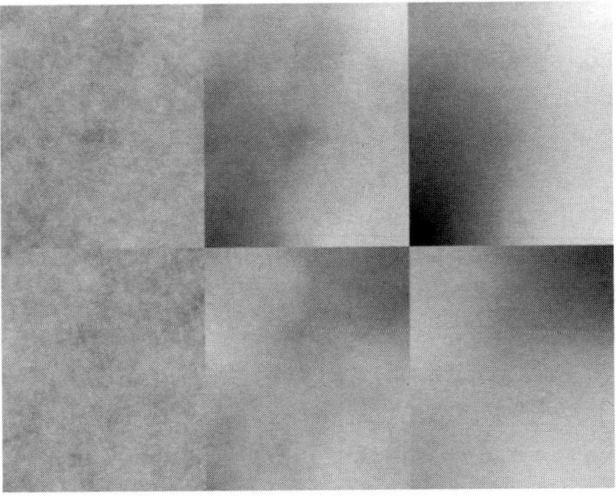

FIGURE 35.4
Randomly generated modulation fields generated using the membrane energy cost function (left), the bending energy cost function (center) and the squares of the third derivatives (right). These can be referred to as first-, second-, and third-order regularisation.

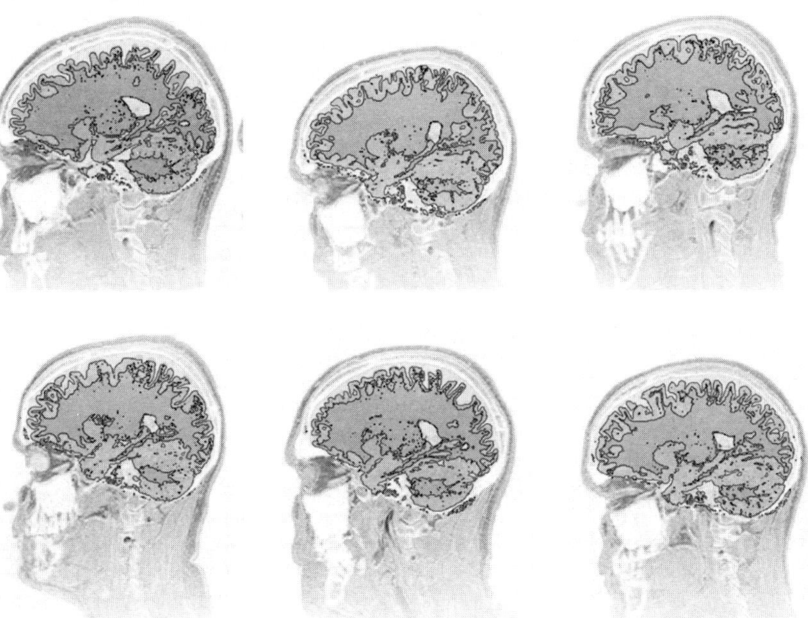

FIGURE 35.5
A single sagittal slice through six T_1-weighted images (2 Tesla scanner, with an MPRAGE sequence, 12° tip angle, 9.7-ms repeat time, 4-ms echo time, and 0.6-ms inversion time). Contours of extracted gray and white matter are shown superimposed on the images.

EXAMPLES

Figure 35.5 shows a single sagittal slice through six T_1-weighted images. The initial registration to the prior probability images was via the 12-parameter affine transformation described in Chapter 33. The images were automatically classified using the method described here, and contours of extracted gray and white matter are shown superimposed on the images.

Tissue classification methods are often evaluated using simulated images generated by the Brain Web simulator (Cocosco *et al.,* 1997; Kwan *et al.,* 1996; Collins *et al.,* 1998). It is then possible to compare the classified images with ground truth images of gray and white matter using the κ statistic (a measure of inter-rater agreement):

$$\kappa = \frac{p_o - p_e}{1 - p_e}$$

where p_o is the observed proportion of agreement, and p_e is the expected proportion of agreements by chance. If there are N observations in K categories, the observed proportional agreement is:

$$p_o = \sum_{k=1}^{K} f_{kk}/N$$

where f_{kk} is the number of agreements for the kth category. The expected proportion of agreements is given by

$$p_e = \sum_{k=1}^{K} r_k c_k/N^2$$

where r_k and c_k are the total number of voxels in the kth class for both the "true" and estimated partitions.

The classification of a single plane of the simulated T_1-weighted BrainWeb image with 100% nonuniformity is illustrated in Fig. 35.6. Note that no preprocessing to remove scalp or other nonbrain tissue was performed on the image. In theory, the tissue classification method should produce slightly better results if this nonbrain tissue is excluded from the computations. As the algorithm stands, a small amount of nonbrain tissue remains in the gray matter partition, which has arisen from voxels that lie close to gray matter and have similar intensities.

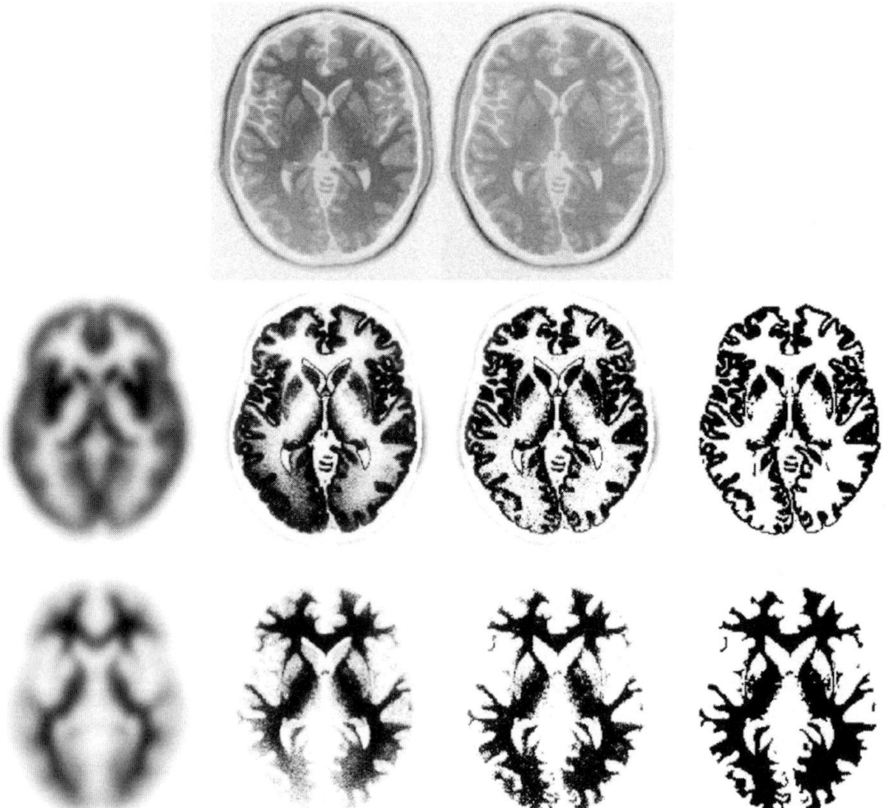

FIGURE 35.6
The classification of the simulated BrainWeb image. The top row shows the original simulated T_1-weighted MR image with 100% nonuniformity and the nonuniformity corrected version. From left to right, the middle row shows the *a priori* spatial distribution of gray matter used for the classification, gray matter extracted without nonuniformity correction, gray matter extracted with nonuniformity correction, and the "true" distribution of gray matter (from which the simulated images were derived). The bottom row is the same as the middle, except that it shows white matter rather than gray. Without nonuniformity correction, the intensity variation causes some of the white matter in posterior areas to be classified as gray. This was also very apparent in the cerebellum because of the intensity variation in the inferior-superior direction.

DISCUSSION

The current segmentation method is fairly robust and accurate for high quality T_1-weighted images, but is not beyond improvement. Currently, each voxel is assigned a probability of belonging to a particular tissue class based only on its intensity and information from the prior probability images. A great deal of other knowledge could be incorporated into the classification. For example, if all of a voxel's neighbours are gray matter, then there is a high probability that it is also gray matter. Other researchers have successfully used Markov random field models to include this information in a tissue classification model (Yan and Karp, 1995; Vandermeulen *et al.,* 1996; Van Leemput *et al.,* 1999b; Ruan *et al.,* 2000; Zhang *et al.,* 2001). Another very simple prior, that can be incorporated, is the relative intensity of the different tissue types (Fischl *et al.,* 2002). For example, when segmenting a T_1-weighted image, we know that the white matter should have a higher intensity than the gray matter, which in turn should be more intense than the CSF. When computing the means for each cluster, this prior information could sensibly be used to bias the estimates.

To function properly, the classification method requires good contrast between the different tissue types. However, many central gray matter structures have image intensities that are almost indistinguishable from that of white matter, so the tissue classification is not always very accurate in these regions. Another related problem is that of partial volume. Because the model assumes that all voxels contain only one tissue type, the voxels that contain a mixture of tissues

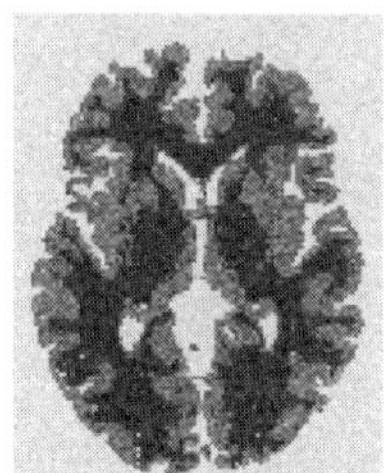

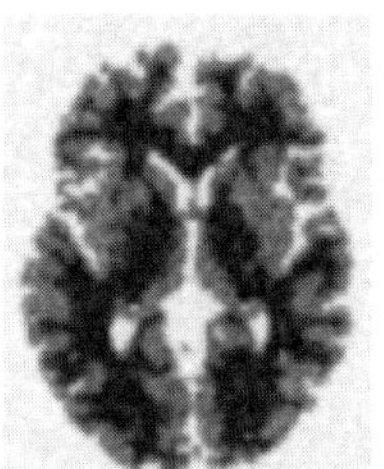

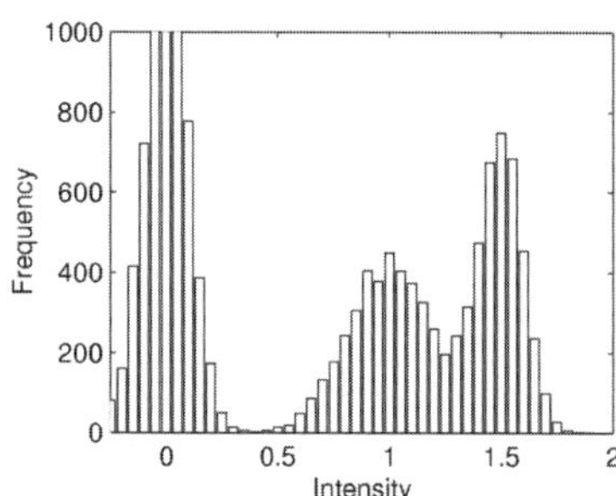

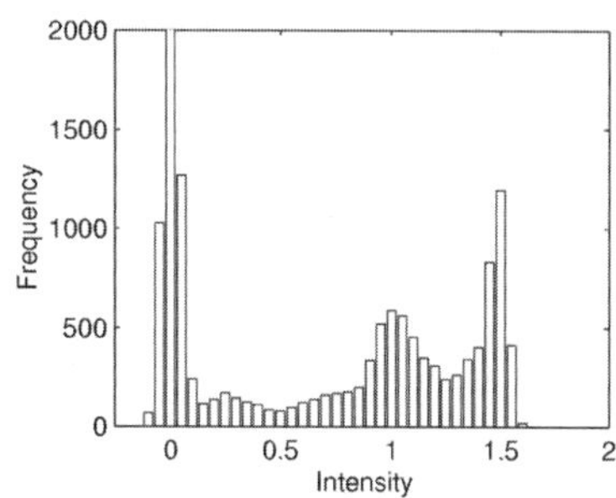

FIGURE 35.7
Simulated data showing the effects of partial volume on the intensity histograms. On the upper left is a simulated image consisting of three distinct clusters. The intensity histogram of this image is shown on the lower left and consists of three Gaussian distributions. The image at the top right is the simulated image after a small amount of smoothing. The corresponding intensity histogram no longer shows three distinct Gaussian distributions.

may not be modeled correctly. In particular, those voxels at the interface between white matter and ventricles will often appear as gray matter. This can be seen to a small extent in Fig. 35.5 and 35.6. Each voxel is assumed to be of only one tissue type, and not a combination of different tissues, so the model's assumptions are violated when voxels contain signal from more than one tissue type. This problem is greatest when the voxel dimensions are large, or if the images have been smoothed, and is illustrated using simulated data in Fig. 35.7. The effect of partial volume is that it causes the distributions of the intensities to deviate from normal. Some authors have developed more complex models than mixtures of Gaussians to describe the intensity distributions of the classes (Bullmore *et al.,* 1995). A more recent commonly adopted approach involves modelling separate classes of partial volume voxels (Laidlaw *et al.,* 1998; Ruan *et al.,* 2000; Shattuck *et al.,* 2001).

In order for the Bayesian classification to work properly, an image volume must be in register with a set of prior probability images used to instate the priors. Figure 35.8 shows the effects of misregistration on the accuracy of segmentation. This figure also gives an indication of how far a brain can deviate from the normal population of brains (that constitute the prior probability images) in order for it to be segmented adequately. Clearly, if the brain cannot be well registered with the probability images, then the segmentation will not be as accurate. This fact also has implications for severely abnormal brains, because they are more difficult to register with images that represent the prior probabilities of voxels belonging to different classes. Segmenting such abnormal brains can be a problem for the algorithm, because the prior probability images are based on normal healthy brains. The profile in Fig. 35.8 depends on the smoothness or resolution of the prior probability images. By not smoothing the prior probability images, the segmentation would be optimal for normal, young, and healthy brains. However, these images may need to be smoother in order to encompass more variability when patient data are to be processed.

As an example, consider a subject with very large ventricles. CSF may appear where the priors suggest that tissue should always be WM. These CSF voxels are forced to be misclassified as WM, and the intensities of these voxels are incorporated into the computation of the WM means and variances. This results in the WM being characterised by a very broad distribution, so the algorithm is unable to distinguish it from any other tissue. For young healthy subjects, the classification is normally good, but caution is required when the method is used for severely pathological brains.

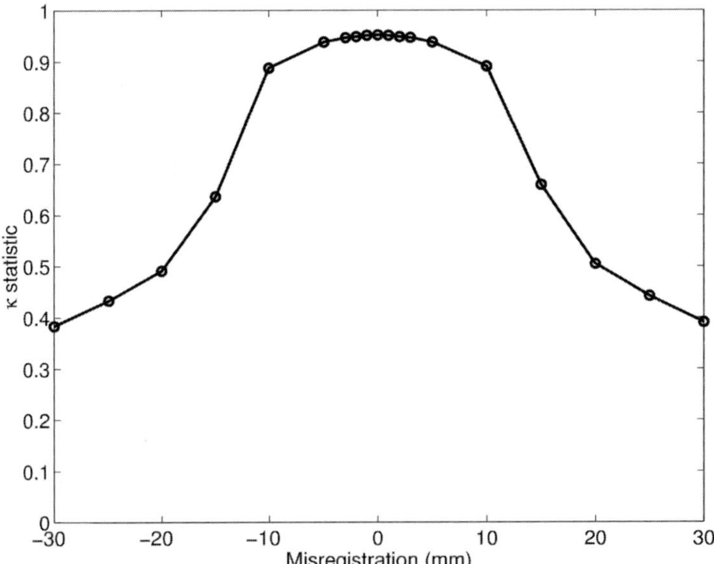

FIGURE 35.8
Segmentation accuracy with respect to misregistration with the prior probability images.

MR images are normally reconstructed by taking the modulus of complex images. Normally distributed complex values are not normally distributed when the magnitude is taken. Instead, they obey a Rician distribution. This means that any clusters representing the background are not well modeled by a single Gaussian, but it makes very little difference for most of the other clusters.

The segmentation is normally run on unprocessed brain images, where nonbrain tissue is not first removed. This results in a small amount of nonbrain tissue being classified as brain. However, by using morphological operations on the extracted GM and WM segments, it is possible to remove most of this extra tissue. The procedure begins by eroding the extracted WM image, so that any small specs of misclassified WM are removed. This is followed by conditionally dilating the eroded WM, such that dilation can only occur where GM and WM were present in the original extracted segments. Although some nonbrain structures (such as part of the sagittal sinus) may remain after this processing, most nonbrain tissue is removed. Figure 35.9 shows how the GM and WM partitions can be cleaned up using this procedure, and surface rendered images of brains automatically extracted this way are shown in Figure 34.15 in the previous chapter.

References

Bullmore, E., Brammer, M., Rouleau, G., Everitt, B., Simmons, A., Sharma, T., Frangou, S., Murray, R., and Dunn, G. (1995). Computerised brain tissue classification of magnetic resonance images: a new approach to the problem of partial volume artifact. *NeuroImage* **2,** 133–147.

Cocosco, C., Kollokian, V., Kwan, R.-S., and Evans, A. (1997). Brainweb: online interface to a 3D MRI simulated brain database. *NeuroImage* **5**(4), S425.

Collins, D., Zijdenbos, A., Kollokian, V., Sled, J., Kabani, N., Holmes, C., and Evans, A. (1998). Design and construction of a realistic digital brain phantom. *IEEE Trans. Med. Imaging* **17**(3), 463–468.

Evans, A. C., Collins, D. L., and Milner, B. (1992). An MRI-based stereotactic atlas from 250 young normal subjects. *Soc. Neurosci. Abstr.* **18,** 408.

Evans, A .C., Collins, D .L., and Mills, S .R., Brown, E .D., Kelly, R .L., and Peters, T .M (1993). 3D statistical neuroanatomical models from 305 MRI volumes. In "Proc. IEEE-Nuclear Science Symposium and Medical Imaging Conference. IEEE, New York.

Evans, A .C., Kamber, M., Collins, D. L., and Macdonald, D. (1994). An MRI-based probabilistic atlas of neuroanatomy. In "Magnetic Resonance Scanning and Epilepsy" (S. Shorvon, D. Fish, F. Andermann, G. M. Bydder, and S. H., eds.), Vol. 264 of *NATO ASI Series A, Life Sciences,* pp. 263–274. Plenum Press, New York.

Fischl, B., Salat, D. H., Busa, E., Albert, M., Dieterich, M., Haselgrove, C., van der Kouwe, A., Killiany, R., Kennedy, D., Klaveness, S., Montillo, A., Makris, N., Rosen, B., and Dale, A. M. (2002). Whole brain segmentation: automated labeling of neuroanatomical structures in the human brain. *Neuron* **33,** 341–355.

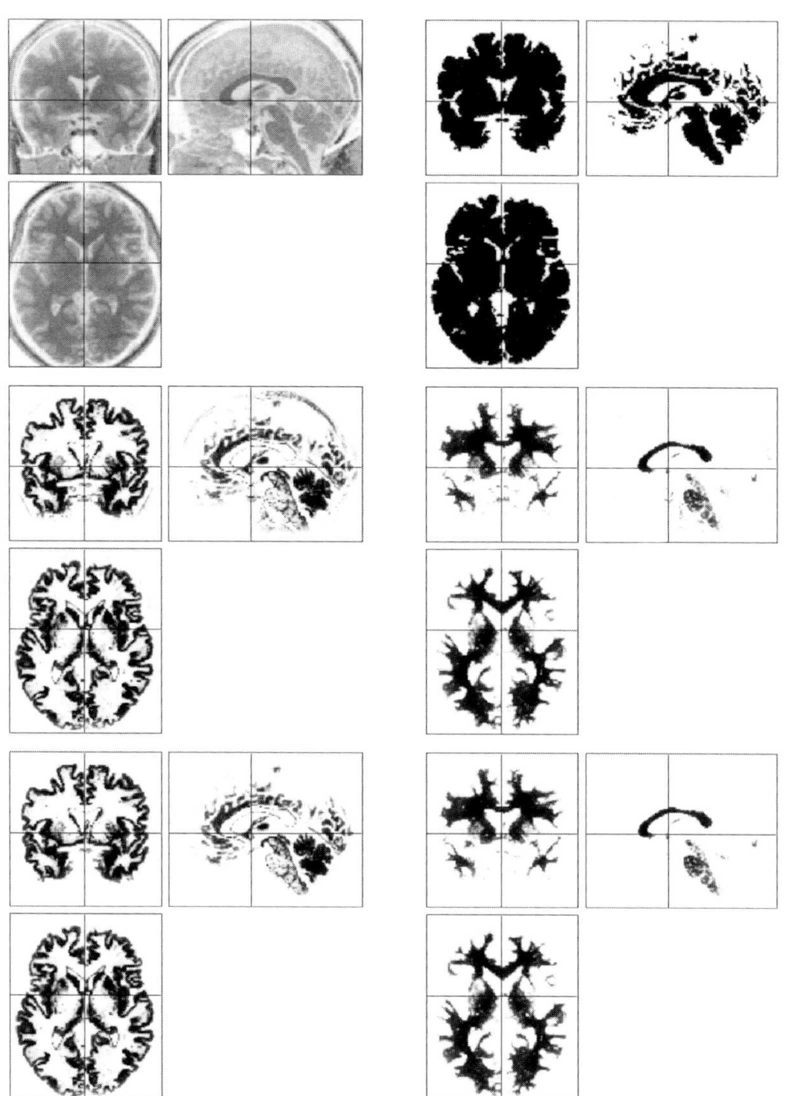

FIGURE 35.8
Example of automatically cleaned up segmented images. The top row shows the original T_1-weighted MR image, next to an automatically generated mask of brain derived from the initial gray and white matter partitions. The second row shows the initial extracted gray and white matter. The bottom row shows the gray and white matter partitions after cleaning up by multiplying with the brain mask.

Hartigan, J. A. (1975). "Clustering Algorithms," pp. 113–129. Wiley & Sons, New York.

Kwan, R. K.-S., Evans, A .C., and Pike, G .B. (1996). An extensible MRI simulator for post-processing evaluation. In: "Proc. Visualisation in Biomedical Computing."

Laidlaw, D. H., Fleischer, K .W., and Barr, A .H. (1998). Partial-volume bayesian classification of material mixtures in MR volume data using voxel histograms. *IEEE Trans. Med. Imaging* **17**(1), 74–86.

Ruan, S., Jaggi, C., Xue, J., Fadili, J., and Bloyet, D. (2000). Brain tissue classification of magnetic resonance images using partial volume modelling. *IEEE Trans. Med. Imaging* **19**(12), 1179–1187.

Shattuck, D .W., Sandor-Leahy, S .R., Schaper, K .A., Rottenberg, D .A., and Leahy, R .M. (2001). Magnetic resonance image tissue classification using a partial volume model. *NeuroImage* **13**(5), 856–876.

Sled, J. G., Zijdenbos, A .P., and Evans, A .C. (1998). A non-parametric method for automatic correction of intensity non-uniformity in MRI data. *IEEE Trans. Med. Imaging* **17**(1), 87–97.

Van Leemput, K., Maes, F., Vandermeulen, D., and Suetens, P. (1999a). Automated model-based bias field correction of MR images of the brain. *IEEE Trans. Med. Imaging* **18**(10), 885–896.

Van Leemput, K., Maes, F., Vandermeulen, D., and Suetens, P. (1999b). Automated model-based tissue classification of MR images of the brain. *IEEE Trans. Med. Imaging* **18**(10), 897–908.

Vandermeulen, D., Descombes, X., Suetens, P., and Marchal, G. (1996). Unsupervised regularised classification of multi-spectral MRI. In: "Proc. Visualisation in Biomedical Computing."

Yan, M. X. H., and Karp, J .S. (1995). An adaptive Bayesian approach to three-dimensional MR brain segmentation. In: "Proc. Information Processing in Medical Imaging" (Y. Bizais, C. Barillot, and R. Di Paola, eds.). Kluwer Academic Publishers, Dordrecht, The Netherlands.

Zhang, Y., Brady, M., and Smith, S. (2001). Segmentation of brain MR images through a hidden Markov random field model and the expectation-maximisation algorithm. *IEEE Trans. Med. Imaging* **20**(1), 45–57.

CHAPTER

36

Morphometry

INTRODUCTION

The morphometric methods described in this chapter relate to ways of statistically identifying and characterising structural differences among populations or for finding correlations between brain shape and, for example, disease severity. A large number of approaches for characterising differences in the shape and neuro-anatomical configuration of different brains have recently emerged due to improved resolution of anatomical human brain scans and the development of new sophisticated image processing techniques.

Studies of brain shape have been carried out by many researchers on a number of different populations, including patients with schizophrenia, autism, dyslexia, and Turner's syndrome. Often, the morphometric measurements used in these studies have been obtained from brain regions that can be clearly defined, resulting in a wealth of findings pertaining to these particular measurements. The measures are typically volumes of unambiguous structures such as the hippocampi or the ventricles. However, there are a number of morphometric features that may be more difficult to quantify by inspection, meaning that many observable structural differences may be overlooked. This chapter describes morphometric approaches that are not biased to one particular structure or tissue and give even-handed and comprehensive assessments of anatomical differences throughout the brain.

The approaches described here require the images of multiple subjects to be registered together by some form of spatial normalisation. The primary result of spatially normalising a series of images is that they all conform to the same stereotaxic space, enabling region-by-region comparisons to be performed. A second result is a series of deformation fields that describe the spatial transformations required to match the different shaped brains to the same template. Encoded within each deformation field is information about the individual image shapes, which can be further characterised using a number of statistical procedures.

The terms *deformation-based* and *tensor-based morphometry* will be used to denote methods of studying brain shape that are based on deformation fields. When comparing groups, deformation-based morphometry (DBM) uses deformation fields to identify differences in the relative positions of structures within subjects' brains. Tensor-based morphometry (TBM) refers to those methods that identify differences in the local shape of brain structures (see Fig. 36.1).

Characterisation using DBM can be global, pertaining to the entire field as a single observation, or can proceed on a voxel-by-voxel basis to make inferences about regionally specific positional differences. This simple approach to the analysis of deformation fields involves treating them as vector fields representing absolute displacements. However in this form, in addition to shape information, the vector fields also contain information on position and size that

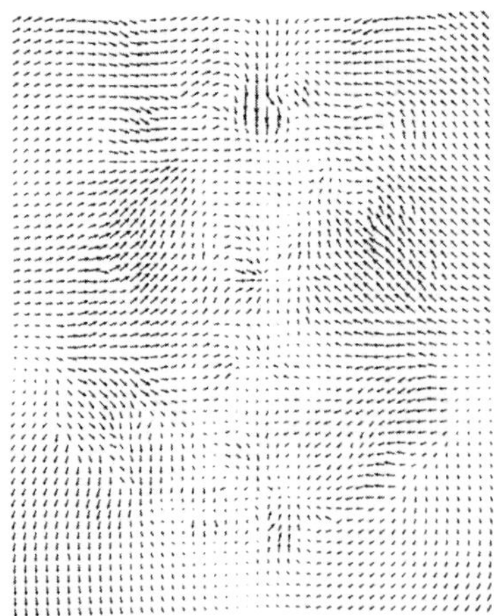

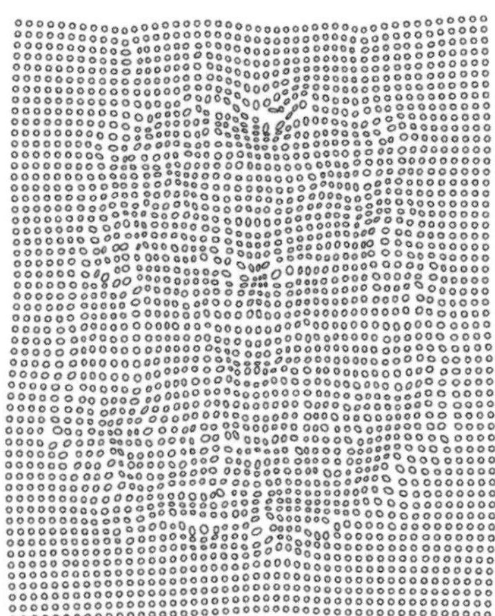

FIGURE 36.1
The term *deformation-based morphometry* will be used to describe methods of studying the positions of structures within the brain (left), whereas the term *tensor-based morphometry* will be used for methods that look at local shapes (right). Currently, the main application of tensor-based morphometry involves using the Jacobian determinants to examine the relative volumes of different structures. However, other features of the Jacobian matrices could be used, such as those representing elongation and contraction in different directions. The arrows in the panel on the left show absolute displacements after making a global correction for rotations and translations, whereas the ellipses on the right show how the same circles would be distorted in different parts of the brain.

is likely to confound an analysis. Much of the confounding information is first removed by global rotations, translations, and a zoom of the fields (Bookstein, 1997a).

When applied on a global scale, DBM simply identifies whether there are significant differences in overall shapes (based on a small number of parameters) among the brains of different populations. Generally, a single multivariate test is performed using parameters describing the deformations—often after parameter reduction with singular value decomposition. The Hotelling's T^2 statistic can be used for such simple comparisons between two groups of subjects (Bookstein, 1997a, 1999; Dryden and Mardia, 1998), but for more complex experimental designs, a multivariate analysis of covariance can be used to identify differences via the Wilk's λ statistic.

An alternative approach to DBM involves producing a statistical parametric map that locates any regions of significant positional differences among the groups of subjects. An example of this approach involves using a voxel-wise Hotelling's T^2 test on the vector field describing the displacements at each and every voxel (Thompson and Toga, 1999; Gaser *et al.,* 1999). The significance of any observed differences can be assessed by modelling the statistic field as a T^2 random field (Cao and Worsley, 1999). Note that this approach does not directly localise brain regions with different shapes, but rather identifies those brain structures that are in relatively different positions. The locations of the results will be highly dependent on how the positions and sizes of the brains are standardised.

If the objective is to localise structures whose shapes differ among groups, then some form of tensor-based morphometry is preferable for producing statistical parametric maps of regional shape differences. A deformation field that maps one image to another can be considered as a discrete vector field. By taking the gradients at each element of the field, a Jacobian matrix field is obtained, in which each element is a tensor describing the relative positions of neighbouring elements. Morphometric measures derived from such a tensor field can be used to locate regions with different shapes. The field obtained by taking the determinants at each point gives a map of structural volumes relative to those of a reference image (Freeborough and Fox, 1998; Gee and Bajcsy, 1999; Davatzikos, 2000; Chung *et al.,* 2001). Statistical parametric maps of these determinant fields can then be used to compare the anatomy of groups of subjects. A number of other measures derived from tensor fields have also been used by other researchers (Thompson and Toga, 1999; Thompson *et al.,* 2000).

Another form of morphometry involves examining the local composition of brain images. Gray and white matter voxels can be identified by image segmentation, before applying morphometric methods to study the spatial distribution of the tissue classes. These techniques will be referred to as *voxel-based morphometry* (VBM). Currently, the difficulty of computing very high resolution deformation fields (required for TBM at small scales) makes voxel-based morphometry a simple and pragmatic approach to addressing small-scale differences that is within the capabilities of most research units.

Morphometric methods have a number of different aims. They can be used for localising significant structural differences among populations, or for showing that overall brain structure is related to some effect of interest. When testing the overall brain structure, multivariate statistical methods are used to analyze groups of parameters for the whole brain (e.g., the deformation-based morphometry described in this chapter). The result of the forms of morphometry that localise structural differences would typically be a statistical parametric map (Friston *et al.,* 1995) of regional differences. Statistical parametric maps (SPMs) can be derived from univariate data where there is a single variable at each voxel (e.g., the voxel-based morphometry method described here), or from multivariate data, where there are several different variables at each voxel (e.g., tensor-based morphometry).

Another use for morphometric methods is for characterising essential differences or for producing some form of classification. Linear methods such as canonical correlation analysis or nonlinear classification methods can be used for these purposes. This chapter will be restricted to simple linear methods, which model data as multivariate normal distributions. Nonlinear classification methods can assume more complex distributions for the data, but they tend to be much more computationally expensive.

DEFORMATION-BASED MORPHOMETRY

Deformation-based morphometry (DBM) is a characterisation of the differences in the vector fields that describe global or gross differences in brain shape. These vector fields are the deformation fields used to effect nonlinear variants of spatial normalisation, when one of the images is a template that conforms to some standard anatomical space.

Spatially normalising a series of image volumes to match the same template will result in a series of deformation fields—one for each image. A deformation field can be considered as a continuous 3D vector field, containing a three-element vector at each point. After spatial normalisation, what each deformation field contains is a mapping from each voxel in the template image[1] to its corresponding voxel in the unwarped image. A simple representation of a deformation field is a series of three volumes of the same dimensions as the template image. The lattice location in one of these volumes corresponds to the same location in the template. The contents of a lattice location in the three volumes constitutes a vector that points to the coordinate of the equivalent structure in the unnormalised image. Therefore, the contents of voxel $\mathbf{x}$ in each of the deformation fields will be the coordinate of the same structure in each of the unwarped images. This allows statistical analysis methods to be used for comparing the positions of structures in different subject's images. The shape of an object is defined by the relative positions of its components, so in studying the relative positions of structures within a brain, we are actually finding out about the brain's shape.

In addition to encoding the shape of a subject's brain, a deformation field also encodes its pose and size. To make inferences about shape alone, these confounding components need to be removed.

Because deformation fields are multivariate, standard multivariate statistical techniques can be employed to estimate the nature of the differences and to make inferences about them. The end point of this form of DBM is a p value, derived via the Wilk's λ or Hotelling's T^2 statistic, pertaining to the significance of the effect and one or more canonical vectors, or deformations, that characterise their nature. These results can be obtained using multivariate analysis of

---

[1] Actually, it is a mapping from each voxel in a spatially normalised image to its voxel in the original unwarped image. We are assuming that the spatial normalisation is 100% accurate, such that each voxel in the template exactly matches the same voxel in the normalised image.

covariance (MANCOVA) and canonical correlation analysis (CCA) respectively. Before proceeding with the multivariate analyses, it is necessary for the information in the deformations to be compacted to just a few parameters. This is usually done by generating *eigenwarps* (principal modes of variation of the warps; Gee and Bajesy, 1999) using singular value decomposition.

Extracting Shape Information

Given a series of deformation fields, it is necessary to decompose each deformation into components relating to global position, orientation and size[2] (uninteresting components), and shape (the components of interest). Each field provides a mapping from points in the template to points in the source image, allowing well-known landmark methods (Bookstein, 1997b; Dryden and Mardia, 1998) to be used to extract the size and positional information. The extracted measures are such that the remaining shapes minimise the squared Procrustes distance between the template and images. Rather than basing the procedure on a few landmarks, all elements of the deformation field corresponding to voxels within the brain are considered. This involves first determining translations by computing centers of mass:

$$\bar{\mathbf{x}} = \frac{\sum_{i=1}^{I} \mathbf{x}_i w_i}{\sum_{i=1}^{I} w_i}$$

$$\bar{\mathbf{y}} = \frac{\sum_{i=1}^{I} \mathbf{y}_i w_i}{\sum_{i=1}^{I} w_i}$$

where $\mathbf{x}_i$ is the coordinate of the ith voxel of the template, $\mathbf{y}_i$ is the location that it maps to, and w_i is a weighting for that element. Nonbrain voxels are typically given zero weighting. The rotations are computed from the cross-covariance matrix (**C**) between the elements and deformed elements (after removing the effects of position):

$$c_{jk} \propto \sum_{i=1}^{I} w_i(x_{ij} - \bar{x}_j)\,(y_{ik} - \bar{y}_k)$$

The 3×3 matrix **C** is decomposed using singular value decomposition to give three matrices: **U, S,** and **V** (such that $\mathbf{C} = \mathbf{USV}^T$, where **U** and **V** are unitary, and **S** is a diagonal matrix). The rotation matrix (**R**) can then be reconstituted from these matrices by $\mathbf{R} = \mathbf{UV}^T$. If size effects are to be removed, then finally, moments around the centers are used to correct for relative size differences (z):

$$z = \sqrt{\frac{\sum_{j=1}^{3}\sum_{i=1}^{I} (x_{ij} - \bar{x}_j)^2 w_i}{\sum_{j=1}^{3}\sum_{i=1}^{I} (y_{ij} - \bar{y}_j)^2 w_i}}$$

Multivariate Analysis of Covariance

Following this, a data matrix is generated, where each row contains a corrected deformation field for one subject represented by a single vector. For multivariate analysis, it is necessary to have a representation of each deformation that is parameterised by far fewer variables than the number of subjects included in the study. Singular value decomposition can be used to compact this information, such that most of the variance of the nonlinear deformations can be represented by only a few parameters for each subject. MANCOVA is then used to make inferences about the effects of interest (i.e., provide p values).

A multivariate analysis of covariance (MANCOVA) assumes that there are several dependent variables for each observation, where an observation refers to a collection of data for a subject. These data can be represented by an $M \times I$ matrix **X,** where M is the number of subjects in the analysis, and I is the number of variables for each subject.

The columns of **X** are modeled by a linear combination of basis functions. Some of these basis functions represent effects that are not considered interesting in the study, but may still be significant. For example, linear age effects may confound a study of handedness. If a left-handed group is not perfectly age matched with a right-handed group, then findings that are actually due

[2] Although the total size of a brain is also often of interest.

to age could be attributed to handedness differences. In addition, the inclusion of confounding effects (such as age) in a model can result in a better fit to the data, possibly making the test more sensitive to the effects of interests.

Confounding effects are modeled by an $M \times K$ design matrix **G.** Each column of **G** can be a vector of covariates (e.g., the age of each subject), or alternatively can be arranged in blocks (e.g., there may be a column containing ones for left-handed subjects, and zeros for right-handed). In almost all cases, a column of ones is included in order to model a mean effect. First of all, any variance in the data that could be attributed to the confounds is removed by an orthogonalisation step:

$$\mathbf{X_a} = \mathbf{X} - \mathbf{G}(\mathbf{G}^T\mathbf{G})^{-1}\,\mathbf{G}^T\mathbf{X} \tag{36.1}$$

Similarly, the effects of interest are modeled by an $M \times J$ design matrix **Y.** The columns of **Y** can represent group memberships, where elements contain a one for subjects who are in a particular group, or a zero if they do not. Alternatively, the columns may contain covariates of interest such as disease severity for each subject. The columns in this design matrix are orthogonalised with respect to matrix **G:**

$$\mathbf{Y_a} = \mathbf{Y} - \mathbf{G}(\mathbf{G}^T\mathbf{G})^{-1}\,\mathbf{G}^T\mathbf{Y} \tag{36.2}$$

A MANCOVA involves assessing how the predictability of the observations changes when the effects of interest are discounted. This is based on the distributions of the residuals, which are assumed to be multinormal. The statistic is related to the determinants of the covariance matrices describing these distributions. In practice, the residual sum of squares and products (SSP) matrix (**W**) is compared to the SSP matrix of the fitted effects (**B**). These matrices are obtained as follows:

$$\mathbf{T} = \mathbf{Y_a}\,(\mathbf{Y_a}^T\mathbf{Y_a})^{-1}\mathbf{Y_a}^T\mathbf{X_a}$$
$$\mathbf{B} = \mathbf{T}^T\mathbf{T}$$
$$\mathbf{W} = (\mathbf{X_a} - \mathbf{T})^T\,(\mathbf{X_a} - \mathbf{T})$$

The statistic is called *Wilk's lambda* (Λ) and is based on the ratios of the determinants:

$$\Lambda = \frac{|\mathbf{W}|}{|\mathbf{B} + \mathbf{W}|}$$

The Wilk's lambda statistic can range between zero and one, where a value of one suggests no relationship between the effects of interest and the data, and a value of zero indicates a perfect relationship. This statistic is transformed to a χ^2 statistic (with IJ degrees of freedom under the null hypothesis) using the approximation of Bartlett[3]:

$$\chi^2 \approx -(M - K - (I + J + 1)/2)log_e(\Lambda)$$

Finally, the cumulative χ^2 distribution function is used to make inferences about whether the null hypothesis (that there is no difference between the distributions) can be rejected.

This multivariate approach fails when the number of variables approaches the number of subjects [$M - K - (I + J + 1)/2$ approaches zero, or becomes negative]. In many situations, it is necessary to regularise the problem by reducing the number of variables with respect to the number of subjects. One way of doing this involves using singular value decomposition to decompose the original data matrix **X** into unitary matrices **U** and **V,** and diagonal matrix **S,** such that $\mathbf{X} = \mathbf{USV}^T$. The diagonal elements of **S** are arranged in decreasing importance, so it is possible to reconstruct an approximation of **X** using only the first L diagonal elements of **S** and the first L columns of **U** and **V,** such that $\mathbf{X} \simeq \mathbf{U^*S^*V^{*T}}$. The MANCOVA would be performed using $\mathbf{U^*}$ (the first L columns of **U**).

Canonical Correlation Analysis

To characterise differences among groups of subjects, one usually uses CCA, which is a device that finds the linear combination of dependent variables (in this case the deformations) that is

[3] This is true provided the matrices do not contain any redundant columns; otherwise matrix pseudo-inverses are required in the computations, and the numbers of columns replaced by the matrix ranks.

maximally correlated with the explanatory variables (e.g., male vs. female). In a simple case of one categorical explanatory variable (e.g., sex) this will be the deformation field that best discriminates between the groups. Note that this is not the same as simply subtracting the deformation fields of two groups. This is because (1) the MANCOVA includes the effects of confounds that are removed and (2) some aspects of the deformations may be less reliable than others. (CCA gives deformations that explicitly discount error in relation to predicted differences.) The canonical deformations can either be displayed directly as deformation fields or can be applied to some image to "caricature" the effect detected.

Canonical correlation analysis is used to measure the strength of association between two sets of variables. In this case, the variables are $\mathbf{X_a}$ and $\mathbf{Y_a}$, which are the data and design matrix from the preceding section after having been orthogonalised with respect to a set of confounding effects. The first canonical variate pair is the linear combination of columns of $\mathbf{X_a}$ and the linear combination of columns of $\mathbf{Y_a}$ that has the maximum correlation. The second canonical variate pair consists of linear combinations that maximise the correlation subject to the constraint that they are orthogonal to the first pair of canonical variables. Similarly, all subsequent pairs maximise the correlations and are orthogonal to all previous pairs.

The weights used to determine the linear combinations are derived from the unitary matrices (**U** and **V**) obtained by singular value decomposition:

$$\mathbf{USV}^T = (\mathbf{X_a}^T\mathbf{X_a})^{-\frac{1}{2}} (\mathbf{X_a}^T\mathbf{Y_a}) (\mathbf{Y_a}^T\mathbf{Y_a})^{-\frac{1}{2}}$$

Then the weights (**A** and **B**) are derived by:

$$\mathbf{A} = (\mathbf{X_a}^T\mathbf{X_a})^{-\frac{1}{2}} \mathbf{U} \text{ and } \mathbf{B} = (\mathbf{Y_a}^T\mathbf{Y_a})^{-\frac{1}{2}} \mathbf{V}$$

The canonical variate pairs are obtained from the columns of $\mathbf{X_a}$A and $\mathbf{Y_a}$B.

When the number of variables approaches the number of observations, the problem needs to be regularised. This can be done by computing the canonical variates from data that have been compacted using singular value decomposition as in the preceding section. If **X** has been decomposed such that it can be approximated by $\mathbf{X} \simeq \mathbf{U^*S^*V^{*T}}$, and canonical correlation analysis performed on **U*** and **Y** to give weight matrices **A*** and **B***, then the weights to be applied to the original data (**X**) can be reconstructed by $\mathbf{V^*S^{*-1}A^*}$.

Figure 36.2 shows CCA as it would be used to graphically describe the differential features of three groups. However, it can also be used to aid classification. Once derived, the same weighting matrix (**A**) can be applied to new datasets that were not involved in its derivation. If there are only two groups involved in a study, then CCA can be used directly to assign group

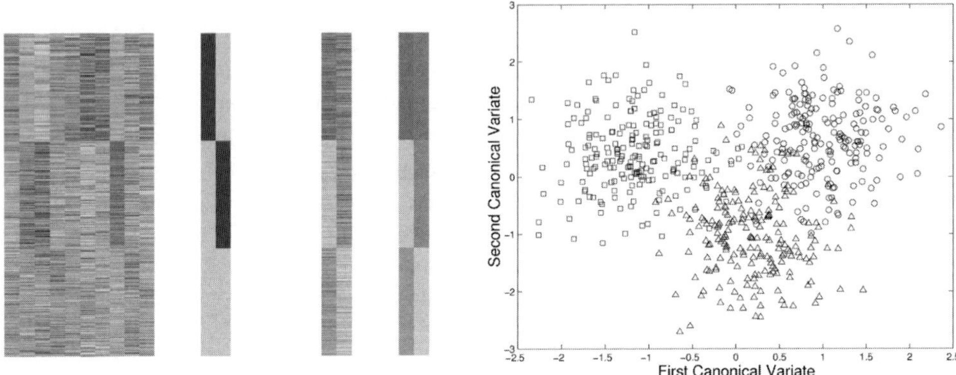

FIGURE 36.2
This figure illustrates canonical correlation analysis using simulated data. The two matrices on the left are a 600 × 10 data matrix ($\mathbf{X_a}$) and a 600 × 2 design matrix ($\mathbf{Y_a}$) after centering by orthogonalising with respect to a column of ones as described in Eqs. (36.1) and (36.2). The design matrix represents a partitioning of the data into three groups. The canonical variates for $\mathbf{X_a}$ and $\mathbf{Y_a}$ are shown in the third and fourth matrices ($\mathbf{X_a}$A and $\mathbf{Y_a}$B). The left-hand columns of these two matrices contain the first canonical variate pair, whereas the second pair are in the right-hand columns. The graph on the right shows the two columns of $\mathbf{X_a}$A plotted against each other, where the different symbols used represent memberships of the three different groups.

memberships to new observations.[4] With more groups, CCA serves as a graphical aid for assigning new observations to the groups.

TENSOR-BASED MORPHOMETRY

There is a near infinite number of ways in which the shapes of brains can differ among populations of subjects. Many thousands or millions of parameters are required to precisely describe the shape of a brain at the resolution of a typical structural MR image. Given, say, 10 schizophrenic and 10 control brain images, there are lots of ways of inventing a measure that would differentiate between the groups. In most cases though, this measure will not provide any distinguishing power in a comparison between further groups of schizophrenics and controls. In other words, the measure would be specific to the subjects included in the study, and not generalisable to the populations as a whole. It is therefore not feasible to use methods that try to detect *any* difference. One has to be specific about the types of differences that are searched for.

The multivariate methods described in the preceding section require that the deformations are parameterised by only a few eigenwarps, on which the statistical tests are performed. This only allows inferences about those eigenwarps included in the analyses, so much of the information in the deformation fields is lost.

A more useful analysis involves identifying focal differences in the form of a statistical parametric map. SPMs of univariate statistical measures often allow relatively simple questions to be addressed, such as where there is significantly more of a particular measure that happens to correlate with a particular effect of interest. Standard parametric statistical procedures (t tests and F tests) can be used to test the hypotheses within the framework of the general linear model (GLM; see Chapter 37), whereby a vector of observations is modeled by a linear combination of user-specified regressors (Friston *et al.,* 1995). The GLM is a flexible framework that allows many different tests to be applied, ranging from group comparisons and identification of differences that are related to specified covariates such as disease severity or age, to complex interactions between different effects of interest.

Performing comparisons at each voxel results in many statistical tests being done. Without any correction, the number of false-positive results would be proportional to the number of independent tests. A Bonferroni correction would be applied if the tests were independent, but this is not normally the case because of the inherent spatial smoothness of the data. In practice, the effective number of independent statistical tests is determined using Gaussian random field (GRF) theory (Friston *et al.,* 1996; Worsley *et al.,* 1996) (see Chapters 44 and 45). By using GRF theory, a correction for multiple dependent comparisons can be made to produce the appropriate rate of false-positive results.

SPMs can also be obtained from the results of voxel-wise multivariate tests. Instead of one variable per voxel of a subject, multivariate tests could effectively involve two or more variables. Following the voxel-wise multivariate tests, similar corrections based on GRF theory can be applied as in the univariate case. GRF theory has not yet been extended for Wilk's Λ fields, so approximations would need to be made that involve transforming the resulting Wilk's Λ fields to random fields of other statistics, such as χ^2 or F fields. Subsequent processing would then need to assume that the transformed fields have the same properties as true χ^2 or F fields. Another useful multivariate measure is Hotelling's T^2 statistic, for which GRF theory has recently been extended (Cao and Worsley, 1999).

The objective of TBM is to localise regions of shape differences among groups of brains, based on deformation fields that map points in a template (x_1, x_2, x_3) to equivalent points in individual source images (y_1, y_2, y_3). In principle, the Jacobian matrices of the deformations (a second-order tensor field relating to the spatial derivatives of the transformation) should be more reliable indicators of local brain shape than absolute deformations. Absolute deformations represent positions of brain structures, rather than local shape, and need to be quantified relative to some arbitrary reference position.

---

[4] Providing that the signs of the canonical variates are adjusted accordingly.

A Jacobian matrix contains information about the local stretching, shearing, and rotation involved in the deformation, and is defined at each point by

$$\mathbf{J} = \begin{bmatrix} \partial y_1/\partial x_1 & \partial y_1/\partial x_2 & \partial y_1/\partial x_3 \\ \partial y_2/\partial x_1 & \partial y_2/\partial x_2 & \partial y_2/\partial x_3 \\ \partial y_3/\partial x_1 & \partial y_3/\partial x_2 & \partial y_3/\partial x_3 \end{bmatrix}$$

A simple form of TBM involves comparing relative volumes of different brain structures, where the volumes are derived from Jacobian determinants at each point (see Figs. 36.3 and 36.4). Simple univariate statistics (t or F tests) can then be used to make inferences about regional volume differences among populations. This type of morphometry is useful for studies that have specific questions about whether growth or volume loss has occurred.

When many subjects are included in a study, a potentially more powerful form of TBM can be attained using multivariate statistics on other measures derived from the Jacobian matrices. This use of multivariate statistics not only tests for volumetric differences, but indicates whether there are any differences among lengths, areas, and the amount of shear. It may therefore be useful when there is no clear hypothesis about the nature of the differences, as may be the case when studying the effects of maturation on the human brain. This form of morphometry should be able to identify shape differences even when volumes are the same.

Because a Jacobian matrix encodes both local shape (zooms and shears) and orientation, it is necessary to remove the latter before making inferences. According to the polar decomposition theorem (Ogden, 1984), a nonsingular Jacobian matrix can be decomposed into a rotation matrix (**R**) and a symmetric positive definite matrix (**U** or **V**), such that $\mathbf{J} = \mathbf{RU} = \mathbf{VR}$. Matrices **U** and **V** (called the *right* and *left stretch* tensors, respectively) are derived by $\mathbf{U} = (\mathbf{J}^T \mathbf{J})^{1/2}$ and $\mathbf{V} =$

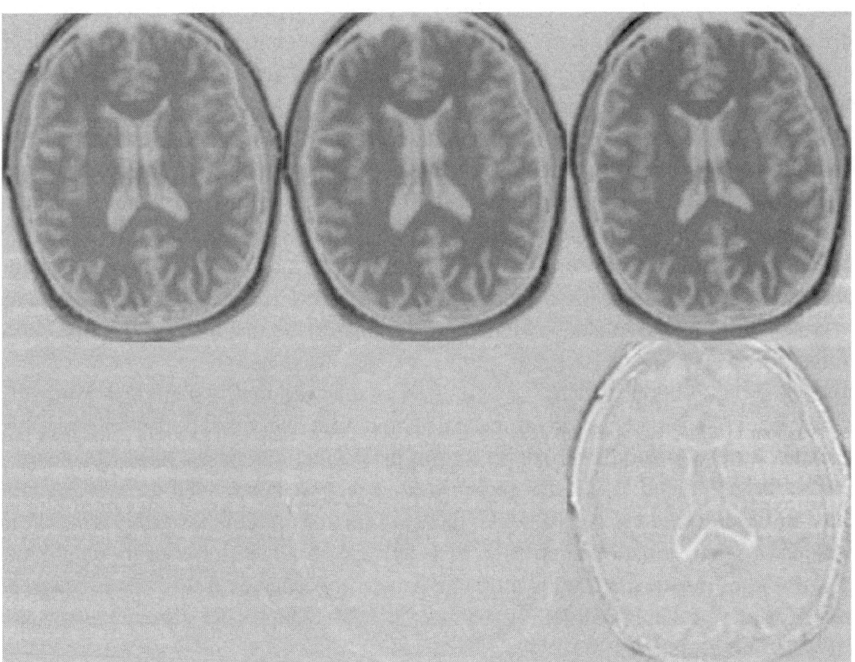

FIGURE 36.3
This figure illustrates warping together a pair of serial scans of the same Alzheimer's subject, using the three dimensional method presented in Chapter 34. The data were provided by the Dementia Research Group, National Hospital for Neurology and Neurosurgery, London. From left to right, the top row shows a slice from the late scan (used as the template), the early scan after rigid body registration followed by warping, and the early scan after rigid registration only. The bottom row shows the difference between the late and early scan, with and without warping. All images are displayed with the same intensity scaling. With only rigid registration, the difference between the early and late scan exhibits a difference at the edges of the ventricles (among other regions). This difference is greatly reduced by including warping in the spatial transformation. The informative contained in the difference image is transferred to the deformation fields. One informative feature of the deformation fields is the Jacobian determinants, which reflect volume changes. These are shown in Fig. 36.4.

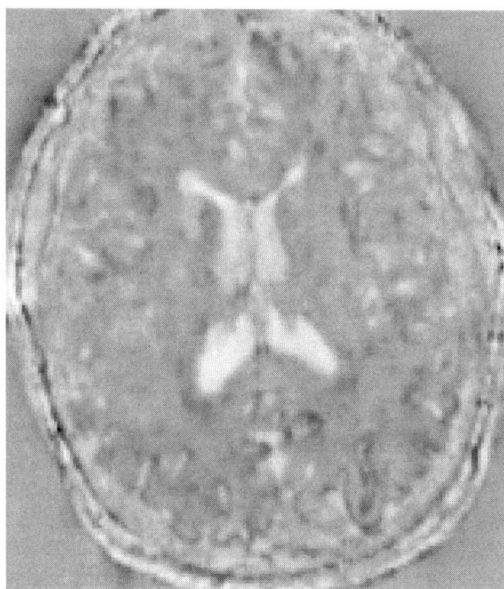

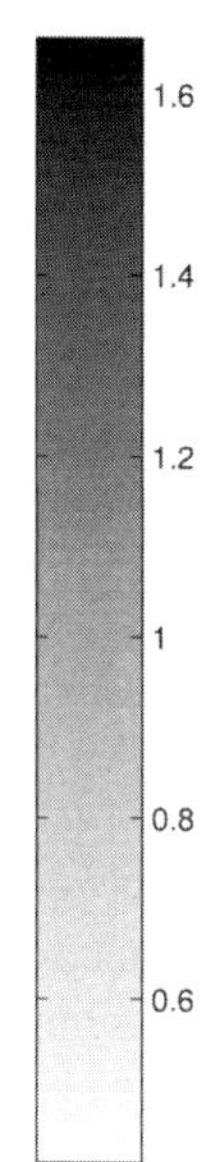

FIGURE 36.4
This figure illustrates the volume changes estimated by warping together the images shown in Fig. 36.3. The relative volumes are the Jacobian determinants of the deformation field. Smaller determinants are obtained when a region of the template maps to a smaller region in the source image. In this example, they represent regions that have expanded between the early and late scans. Regions where there are no measurable volume changes have Jacobian determinants with a value of one.

$(\mathbf{JJ}^T)^{1/2}$. Matrix **R** is then given by $\mathbf{R} = \mathbf{JU}^{-1}$ or $\mathbf{R} = \mathbf{V}^{-1}\mathbf{J}$. For a purely rigid body transformation, $\mathbf{U} = \mathbf{V} = \mathbf{I}$ (the identity matrix). Similarly, if $\mathbf{R} = \mathbf{I}$, then the deformation can be considered as *pure strain.* Deviations of **U** or **V** away from **I**, indicate a shape change, which can be represented by a strain tensor **E.** Depending on the reference coordinate system, the strain tensor is referred to as either a *Lagrangean* or an *Eulerian* strain tensor. When the strain tensor is derived from **U,** it is referred to as a Lagrangean strain tensor, whereas when it is derived from **V,** it is Eulerian. Spatial normalisation of a series of source images involves determining a mapping from each point in the template image to corresponding points in the source images. To compare image shapes, it is necessary to derive measures of shape within the coordinate system of the template image, rather than within the different coordinate systems of the individual source images. Therefore, the Lagrangean framework should be used.

For any deformation, there is a whole continuum of ways of defining strain tensors, based on a parameter m. When m is nonzero, the family of Lagrangean strain tensors **E** is given by $\mathbf{E}^{(m)} = m^{-1}(\mathbf{U}^m - \mathbf{I})$. For the special case when m is zero, the strain tensor is given by $\mathbf{E}^{(0)} = \ln(\mathbf{U})$, where the ln refers to a matrix logarithm. When m assumes values of –2, 0, 1 or 2, then the tensors are called the *Almansi, Hencky, Biot,* or *Green* strain tensors, respectively. For deformations derived using the methods in Chapter 34,[5] the Hencky tensor may be the most appropriate measure of local shape, providing the priors exert enough influence on the resulting deformation fields. One advantage of basing measures on the Hencky tensor is that it allows relative changes in length, volume, and area to be modeled using similar log-normal distributions. This would not be possible if the measures were modeled by normal distributions, because if a variable l is normally distributed, then l^3 is not. Also, it would not make sense to assume distributions that allow negative lengths or volumes if these are explicitly prohibited by the warping algorithm.

In three dimensions, a strain tensor has six unique elements (because it is a symmetric 3×3 matrix). Within a TBM framework, multivariate statistics would be applied to these elements in order to localise volume, area, and length differences, whereas DBM would involve performing a single, global multivariate test to compare the shapes. In principle, the difference between these

[5] Note that the sum of squares of the Hencky tensor elements is equivalent to the sum of squares of the logs of the singular values of **J,** meaning that the priors described in Chapter 34 are effectively minimising the squares of the Hencky tensor.

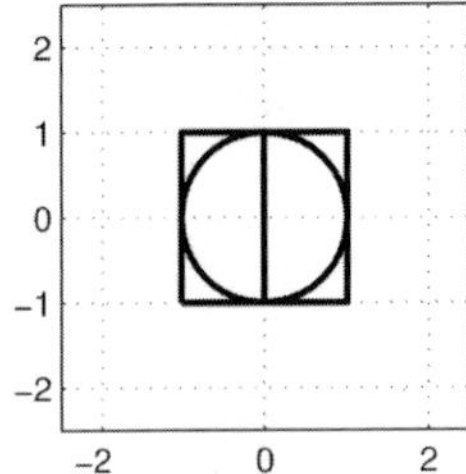

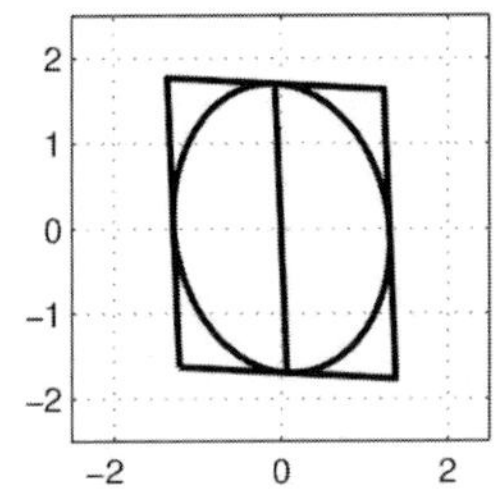

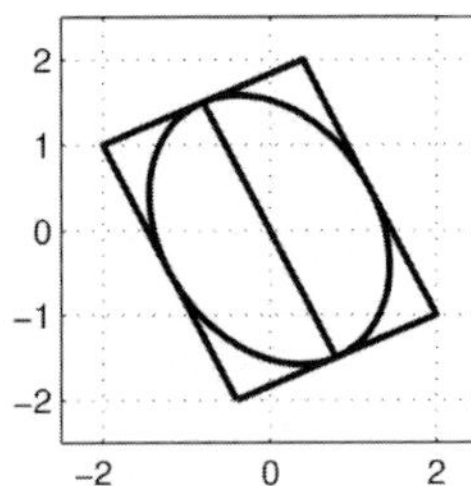

FIGURE 36.5
This figure illustrates polar decomposition, whereby the regular shape in the left-hand panel is transformed via shears and zooms to give the shape in the center, before being rotated to give the right-hand shape.

approaches need not be quite so distinct. Rather than basing the tests either on information at each voxel or on information from the whole brain, it is easy to see that forms of morphometry could be devised that are based on regional analyses. For example, DBM could be done region by region (after factoring out positional information), or multivariate TBM could be applied such that the tests include information from strain tensors in regions of neighbouring lattice locations. Both of these approaches should produce similar results. The regions could be based on predefined structures on the template image. Alternatively, they could involve some weighted combination of information from the neighbourhood of each voxel, with weights based on a function such as a Gaussian kernel or some other windowing function.

VOXEL-BASED MORPHOMETRY

A number of studies have already demonstrated structural brain differences among different patient populations using the technique of voxel-based morphometry (Wright *et al.,* 1995, 1999; Ashburner and Friston, 2000) or a related method that involves parceling the images into different regions (Goldszal *et al.,* 1998; Davatzikos, 2000).

VBM is another technique for producing SPMs of volumetric differences. Structural MR images of brains can differ among subjects in many ways. A useful measure of structural difference among populations is derived from a comparison of the local composition of different brain tissue types (gray matter, white matter, etc.). VBM has been designed to be sensitive to these differences, while discounting positional and other large scale volumetric differences in gross anatomy. The technique involves spatially normalising all subjects' MR images to the same stereotaxic space, extracting the gray matter from the normalised images, smoothing, and finally performing a statistical analysis to localise, and make inferences about, group differences. The output from the method is an SPM showing regions where gray matter concentration differs significantly among the groups.

VBM was originally devised to detect cortical thinning in a way that was not confounded by volume changes of the sort that are characterised by classical volumetric analyses of large brain structures (e.g., the temporal lobe). It does this by removing positional and volume difference (down to a specified spatial scale) through spatial normalisation. Differences in gray matter density are then detected by comparing the local intensities of gray matter maps after smoothing. Since its inception (Wright *et al.,* 1995) VBM has become an established tool in morphometry, being used to detect cortical atrophy and differences in slender white matter tracts. The classical perspective on VBM partitions volume changes into two spatial scales: (1) macroscopic volume or shape differences that can be modeled in the spatial normalisation procedure and (2) mesoscopic volume differences that cannot. The latter persist after normalisation and are detected after spatial smoothing of gray matter maps (i.e., partitions or segments)—smoothing transforms these volume differences into image intensity differences through the partial volume effect.

More recently, this perspective has changed with the incorporation of an additional step, introduced to compensate for the effect of spatial normalisation. When warping a series of images to match a template, it is inevitable that volumetric differences will be introduced into the warped images. For example, if one subject's temporal lobe has half the volume of that of the template, then its volume will be doubled during spatial normalisation. This will also result in a doubling of the voxels labeled gray matter. To remove this confound, the spatially normalised gray matter (or other tissue class) is adjusted by multiplying by its relative volume before and after warping. If warping results in a region doubling its volume, then the correction will halve the intensity of the tissue label. This whole procedure has the effect of preserving the total amount of gray matter signal in the normalised partitions (Goldszal *et al.*, 1998; Davatzikos *et al.*, 2001).[6] Classical VBM assumed that the warps were so smooth that these volume changes could be ignored. However, advances in normalisation techniques now allow for high-resolution warps.

If brain images from different subjects can be matched together exactly,[7] then a complete analysis of the volumetric differences could proceed using only the derived warps. Expansions and contractions occur when an image from one subject is warped to match that of another. These volume changes (hence also the relative volumes of structures) are encoded by the warps. One form of tensor-based morphometry involves analyzing these relative volumes (more formally, the Jacobian determinants of the deformation field) in order to identify regions of systematic volumetric difference. The adjustment step mentioned above can be considered from the perspective of TBM, in which volumetric changes derived from the warps are endowed with tissue specificity. By multiplying the relative volumes by the tissue class of interest, volumetric information about other tissue classes is discounted (i.e., there will be no changes attributed to gray matter in purely white matter regions). In other words, the product of gray matter and volume change has two equivalent interpretations: (1) In VBM it represents the proportion of the voxel that is gray matter, having adjusted for the confounding effects of warping the brains, and (2) it represents the proportion of volume change attributable to gray matter.

By including the multiplication step, a continuum is introduced between the methods of VBM and TBM. At the extreme where little or no warping is used, most of the information pertaining to volumetric differences will be derived from systematic differences in the spatial distribution of the tissue under study. At the other extreme, where registration between images is exact, all volumetric information will be encoded by the warps (because the normalised partitions will be identical). The product remains sensitive to differences at either extreme and can be regarded as an integration of classical VBM and TBM.

This dual perspective is illustrated in Fig. 36.6, using brain images of a subject suffering from Alzheimers disease. This example illustrates progressive volumetric changes of CSF, particularly in the ventricles. The first column of the figure shows how the later of the two images was processed by classifying the CSF (see Chapter 35) and smoothing it using an isotropic 12-mm FWHM Gaussian kernel. The column in the center shows the processing of the earlier image, which was first rigidly registered (see Chapter 32) with the late image and then the CSF was classified and smoothed. The difference between the smoothed CSF of the two images can be considered as analogous to VBM, where the spatial normalisation is restricted to a rigid body registration.

The third column shows processing that is analogous to the augmented approach. After rigid registration, the early image is precisely warped to match the late one. The warping method (see Chapter 34) attempts to estimate exact displacements at every voxel, so it is able to model the relative shapes of the pair of brains. The warped image is then classified, producing an image of CSF that is very similar to the CSF of the late image. A subtraction of these images would probably not show any meaningful differences. If the segmentation and warping were perfect, then the late CSF image would be identical to the warped early CSF image. To localise CSF volume differences, the volume changes resulting from the warping must also enter into the comparison. To do this, the warped CSF is simply multiplied by the relative volumes estimated from the warps. This means that the procedure preserves the amount of CSF from the original image, while also achieving a good registration. The figure shows an image of relative volumes, where lighter areas indicate a smaller volume in the early image. Following this multiplication, the data are smoothed. The difference between this image and the processed late image shows a

---

[6] Note that a uniformly smaller brain will have uniformly lower gray matter intensities after the correction. Any detected differences are therefore less regionally specific, unless some kind of "global" measures are modeled as confounding effects during the statistical analyses. These could pertain to the total amount of gray matter in each brain or, more usefully in many cases, the intracranial volume of each subject.

[7] Registered so that corresponding brain structures are matched, rather than solving the simpler problem of matching gray matter with gray matter, white with white, and CSF with CSF.

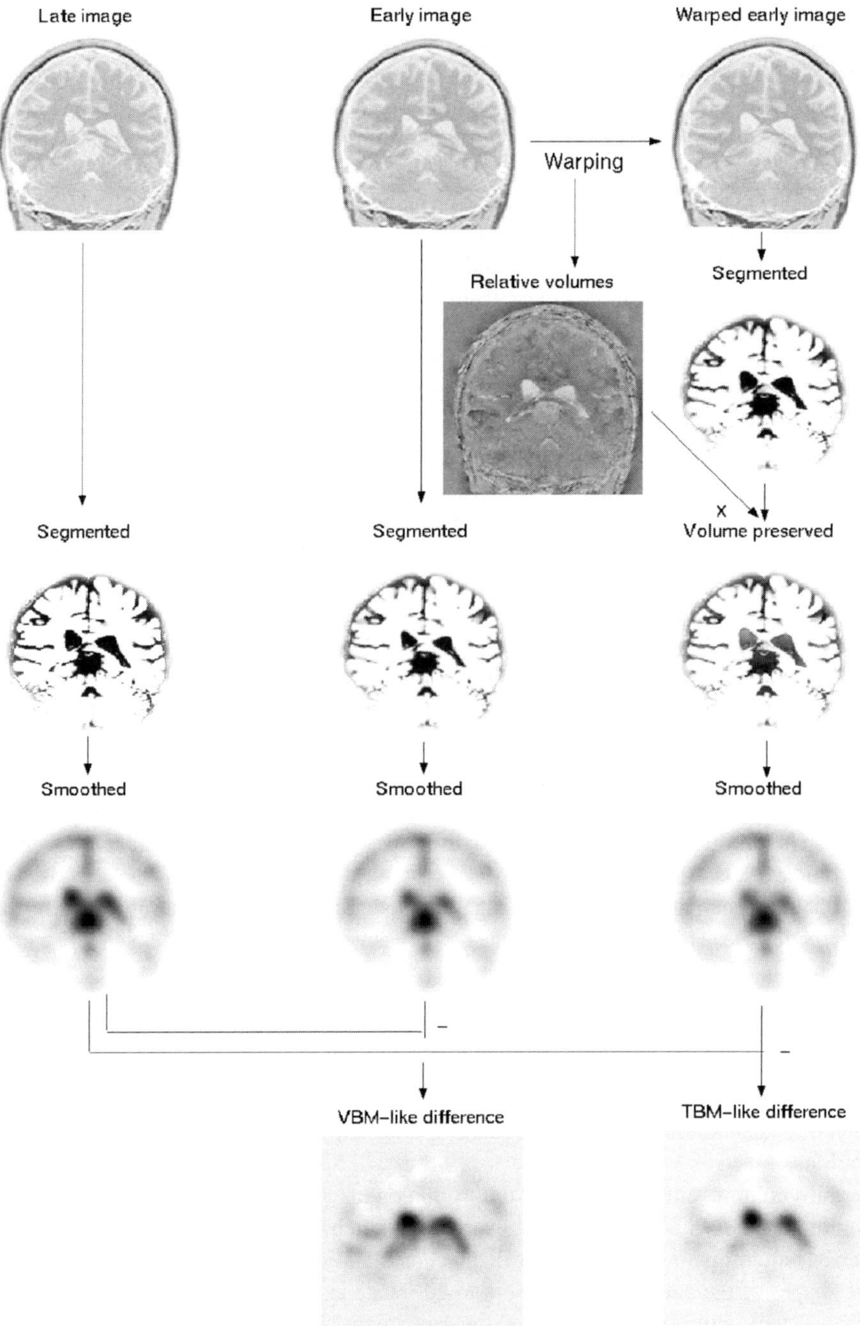

FIGURE 36.6
An illustration of the continuum between VBM and TBM. The center column illustrates a VBM processing stream, whereas the column on the right illustrates a TBM-like stream. The data were obtained from the Dementia Research Group, Queen Square, London.

picture of volumetric differences based on the warps (c.f., TBM). As can be seen from the bottom row of Fig. 36.6, the pattern of CSF volume differences estimated using the two methods is very similar.

Method

The steps involved in VBM are as follows:

- The procedure begins by spatially normalising all subjects' data to the same stereotaxic space, which is achieved by registering each image to the same template. The methods described in

Chapter 33 can be used to do this, although more precise methods can also be used. It is important that the quality of the registration be high and that the choice of template image does not bias the final solution. An ideal template consists of the average of a large number of MR images that have been registered to within the accuracy of the spatial normalisation technique. The spatially normalised images should have a relatively high resolution (1- or 1.5-mm isotropic voxels), so that the following gray matter extraction method is not excessively confounded by partial volume effects, where voxels contain a mixture of different tissue types.

The basis function approach of Chapter 33 is far from perfect,[8] but, with the right data, it gives a good "global" match between brain images. Because of this, there are cases when structural differences, not directly related to gray matter volumes, can be identified as significant. One obvious example is when one population has larger ventricles. Because the spatial normalisation method (Ashburner and Friston, 1999) cannot achieve an exact match, it has to change the volume of surrounding tissue when it attempts to make the ventricles of the individual subjects the same size. For example, if the ventricles are enlarged during spatial normalisation, then gray matter near to them also also needs to be enlarged. It is then possible for structural differences pertaining to ventricular volume to show up in a VBM study of gray matter volume. A way of circumventing this would be to base the spatial normalisation on only the segmented gray matter. If all data entering the statistical analysis were only derived from gray matter, then any significant differences must be due to gray matter.

- The spatially normalised images are then typically partitioned into different tissue classes using the segmentation technique described in Chapter 35. Note that if the segmentation step does not require prior probability maps of different tissue classes to be overlayed, then it should probably be performed first, in order to reduce the partial volume effects incurred by resampling the data. A further possible step after segmentation would be the binarisation of the resulting tissue class images. Many tissue classification methods produce images where each voxel is the *a posteriori* probability that that voxel should be assigned to a particular tissue type according to the model. These probabilities are values between zero and one. Binarisation would involve assigning each voxel to its most likely tissue class.
- Nonlinear spatial normalisation results in the volumes of certain brain regions increasing, whereas others decrease (Goldszal *et al.,* 1998; Davatzikos *et al.,* 2001). This has implications for the interpretation of what VBM actually tests. The objective of VBM is to identify regional differences in the amount of a particular tissue (gray or white matter). To preserve the actual amounts of gray matter within each structure, a further processing step can be incorporated that multiplies the partitioned images by the relative voxel volumes. These relative volumes are simply the Jacobian determinants of the deformation field (see above). Without this adjustment, VBM can be thought of as comparing the *relative concentration* of gray matter (i.e., the proportion of gray matter to other tissue types within a region). With the adjustment, VBM compares the *absolute amount* of gray matter in different regions.
- The gray matter images are now smoothed by convolving with an isotropic Gaussian kernel. This makes the subsequent voxel-by-voxel analysis comparable to a region of interest approach, because each voxel in the smoothed images contains the average amount of gray matter from around the voxel (where the region around the voxel is defined by the form of the smoothing kernel). This is often referred to as *gray matter density,* but should not be confused with cell packing density measured cytoarchitectonically. By the central limit theorem, smoothing also has the effect of rendering the data more normally distributed, thus increasing the validity of parametric statistical tests. Whenever possible, the size of the smoothing kernel should be comparable to the size of the expected regional differences between the groups of brains. The smoothing step also helps to compensate for the inexact nature of the spatial normalisation.

---

[8] Brain warping methods are still in their infancy. Most warping methods involve making MAP-like estimates of deformations, making use of suboptimal guesses for the likelihood and prior probability distributions. A single high-dimensional MAP estimate is not that useful when there are many other possible solutions with similar posterior probability, and estimating expectations over all MAP estimates is not feasible given the high dimensionality of the parameter space.

- Following the preprocessing, which involves spatial normalisation, tissue classification, and spatial smoothing, the final step in a VBM analysis is to perform voxel-wise statistical tests. The results of these tests are a SPM (Friston *et al.,* 1995) showing significant regional differences among the populations included in the study. Corrections for multiple dependent comparisons are then made using the theory of Gaussian random fields (Friston *et al.,* 1996; Worsley *et al.,* 1996, 1999).

  Statistical analysis using the GLM is used to identify regions of gray matter concentration that are significantly related to the particular effects under study (Friston *et al.,* 1995). The GLM is a flexible framework that allows many different tests to be applied, ranging from group comparisons and identification of regions of gray matter concentration that are related to specified covariates such as disease severity or age, to complex interactions between different effects of interest. Standard parametric statistical procedures (t tests and F tests) are used to test the hypotheses, so they are valid, providing the residuals, after fitting the model, are independent and normally distributed. If the statistical model is appropriate, there is no reason why the residuals should not be independent, but there are reasons why they may not be normally distributed. The original segmented images contain values between zero and one, where most of the values are very close to either of the extremes. Only by smoothing the segmented images does the behaviour of the residuals become more normally distributed.

  Following application of the GLM, the significance of any differences is ascertained using GRF theory (Friston *et al.,* 1996; Worsley *et al.,* 1996). A voxel-wise SPM comprises the result of many statistical tests, so it is necessary to correct for multiple dependent comparisons.

  Classical statistical tests cannot be used to prove a hypothesis, only to reject a null hypothesis. Any significant differences that are detected could be explained by a number of different causes, which are not disambiguated by the statistical inference. In other words, these tests are not concerned with accepting a specific hypothesis about the cause of a difference, but involve rejecting a null hypothesis with a given certainty. When the null hypothesis has been rejected, it does not impute a particular explanation for the difference if there are many potential causes that could explain it. The preprocessing employed by VBM manipulates the data so that the ensuing tests are more sensitive to some causes than others. In particular, VBM has been devised to be sensitive to systematic differences in the volumes of gray matter structures, but significant results can also arise for other reasons. Attribution of what may be the cause of any detected difference generally requires a careful characterisation of the parameter estimates after the inference has been made.

  An objection to VBM is that it is sensitive to systematic shape differences attributable to misregistration from the spatial normalisation step (Bookstein, 2001). This is one of a large number of potential systematic differences that can arise (Ashburner and Friston, 2001). For example, a particular subject group may move more in the scanner, so the resulting images contain motion artifact. This motion may interact with the segmentation to produce systematic classification differences. Another group may have systematic differences in the relative intensity of gray matter voxels compared to white matter or may have to be positioned differently in the scanner. All of these reasons, plus others, may produce differences that are detectable by VBM. They are all real differences among the data, but may not necessarily be due to reductions in gray matter density.

DISCUSSION

The morphometric methods developed here all attempt to automatically identify neuro-anatomical differences, either from features of spatially normalised images or from deformation fields that encode information about image shapes. Rather than focusing on particular structures, one important aspect of these methods is that the entire brain can be examined in a balanced way.

The different forms of morphometry have their own advantages and disadvantages, and the optimum approach may depend on the types of structural difference expected among the data. Where there are global patterns of difference, then the global approaches (that do not produce a SPM) may be more powerful, because they can model covariances between shapes of different structures. In contrast, the SPM approaches may be preferable where discrete focal differences are expected. The main disadvantages of global testing methods (as opposed to SPM methods) is that there are generally far more variables for each brain than there are brains in a study. This implies that covariances between all variables cannot be computed, so some form of dimensionality reduction (or regularisation) is required, leading to inevitable data loss.

A related issue is about how to normalise morphometric measures in order to produce the most useful results. This is particularly true for voxel-wise approaches, because relationships between other, more global, factors are not modeled. For example, consider a group of subjects with smaller hippocampi, but also smaller brains. Should the reduced hippocampi be considered significantly different if they correlate with a smaller brain? This size difference could also relate to lengths or volumes of temporal lobe or to a whole number of other measurements. Consider another example. If the right temporal lobe is relatively larger than the left temporal lobe for a particular group of subjects, then should these differences be localised in the left or right lobes? These are arguments for using global multivariate approaches.

Another challenge concerns visualising and communicating the results of morphometric tests. Three-dimensional volumes are quite difficult to visualise, especially within the limited space of most journals. However, the results of morphometric tests are often vector or tensor fields. These are quite difficult to visualise in two dimensions, but in three dimensions the challenge becomes much worse. The more useful results of global morphometric methods are the canonical variates that characterise the differences, and these are often some form of three-dimensional vector or tensor field. In comparison, differences localised by voxel-wise methods can be relatively easily presented as a SPM. Although the reasons may appear trivial, voxel-wise approaches will probably come to dominate because their results can be explained and presented much more easily.

When parametric statistical methods are used, statistical designs such as comparisons between single subjects and whole groups may not be as reliable as more balanced designs involving comparisons between groups of several subjects. It may be necessary to resort to nonparametric methods (Holmes *et al.,* 1996; Bullmore *et al.,* 1999) for such cases. The alternative may involve developing suitable transforms for the data that render them better behaved.

Other factors also influence the validity and sensitivity of the different morphometric approaches. In particular, the warping method used to register the images to the same stereotaxic space has a significant influence on the results. For DBM and TBM, the statistical tests are based entirely on the deformation fields produced by the warping methods. The warping methods described in this book are all nonlinear optimisation procedures and, therefore, can be susceptible to reaching local minima and, hence, nonoptimal solutions. These local minima have negative consequences for subsequent statistical tests, because the estimated shapes do not reflect the true shapes of anatomical structures. Other problems occur when warping brains containing severe pathologies. For example, if a brain contains features that are not present in the template image, then an accurate match cannot be achieved. The effects of this mismatch may also propagate to other brain regions because of the inherent smoothness of the deformation fields. Much more work is necessary in order to develop warping methods that can model the various forms of severe pathology that may be encountered.

References

Ashburner, J., and Friston, K. J. (1999). Nonlinear spatial normalisation using basis functions. *Hum. Brain Mapping* **7**(4), 254–266.

Ashburner, J., and Friston, K. J. (2000). Voxel-based morphometry—the methods. *NeuroImage* **11,** 805–821.

Ashburner, J., and Friston, K. J. (2001). Why voxel-based morphometry should be used. *NeuroImage* **14**(6), 1238–1243.

Bookstein, F. L. (1997a). Landmark methods for forms without landmarks: morphometrics of group differences in outline shape. *Med. Image Anal.* **1**(3), 225–243.

Bookstein, F. L. (1997b). Quadratic variation of deformations. In: "Proc. Information Processing in Medical Imaging" (J. Duncan and G. Gindi, eds.). Springer-Verlag, Berlin.

Bookstein, F. L. (1999). "Brain Warping," chap. 10, pp. 157–182. Academic Press, San Diego.

Bookstein, F. L. (2001). Voxel-based morphometry should not be used with imperfectly registered images. *NeuroImage* **14**(6), 1454–1462.

Bullmore, E., Suckling, J., Overmeyer, S., Rabe-Hesketh, S., Taylor, E., and Brammer, M. (1999). Global, voxel, and cluster tests, by theory and permutation, for a difference between two groups of structural MR images of the brain. *IEEE Trans. Med. Imaging* **18**(1), 32–42.

Cao, J., and Worsley, K. J. (1999). The geometry of the Hotelling's T^2 random field with applications to the detection of shape changes. *Ann. Statistics* **27**(3), 925–942.

Chung, M. K., Worsley, K. J., Paus, T., Cherif, C., Collins, D. L., Giedd, J. N., Rapoport, J. L., and Evans, A. C. (2001). A unified statistical approach to deformation-based morphometry. *NeuroImage* **14**(3), 595–606.

Davatzikos, C. (2000). "Handbook of Medical Imaging." chap. 16, pp. 249–260. Academic Press, San Diego.

Davatzikos, C., Genc, A., Xu, D., and Resnick, S. M. (2001). Voxel-based morphometry using the ravens maps: methods and validation using simulated longitudinal atrophy. *NeuroImage* **14**(6), 1361–1369.

Dryden, I. L., and Mardia, K. (1998). "Statistical Shape Analysis." John Wiley and Sons, New York.

Freeborough, P. A., and Fox, N. C. (1998). Modelling brain deformations in alzheimer disease by fluid registration of serial MR images. *J. Computer Assisted Tomog.* **22**(5), 838–843.

Friston, K. J., Holmes, A. P., Worsley, K. J., Poline, J.-B., Frith, C. D., and Frackowiak, R. S. J. (1995). Statistical parametric maps in functional imaging: a general linear approach. *Hum. Brain Mapping* **2,** 189–210.

Friston, K. J., Holmes, A. P., Poline, J.-B., Price, C. J., and Frith, C. D. (1996). Detecting activations in PET and fMRI: levels of inference and power. *NeuroImage* **4,** 223–235.

Gaser, C., Volz, H.-P., Kiebel, S., Riehemann, S., and Sauer, H. (1999). Detecting structural changes in whole brain based on nonlinear deformations—application to schizophrenia research. *NeuroImage* **10,** 107–113.

Gee, J. C., and Bajcsy, R. K. (1999). "Brain Warping," chap. 11, pp. 183–198. Academic Press, San Diego.

Goldszal, A. F., Davatzikos, C., Pham, D. L., Yan, M. X. H. , Bryan, R. N., and Resnick, S. M. (1998). An image-processing system for qualitative and quantitative volumetric analysis of brain images. *J. Computer Assisted Tomog.* **22**(5), 827–837.

Holmes, A. P., Blair, R. C., J, D. G. W., and Ford, I. (1996). Non-parametric analysis of statistic images from functional mapping experiments. *J. Cereb. Blood Flow Metab.* **16,** 7–22.

Ogden, R. W. (1984). "Non-Linear Elastic Deformations." Dover, New York.

Thompson, P. M., and Toga, A. W. (1999). "Brain Warping," chap. 18, pp. 311–336. Academic Press, San Diego.

Thompson, P. M., Giedd, J. N., Woods, R. P., MacDonald, D., Evans, A. C., and Toga, A. W. (2000). Growth patterns in the developing brain detected by using continuum mechanical tensor maps. *Nature* **404,** 190–193.

Worsley, K. J., Marrett, S., Neelin, P., Vandal, A. C. Friston, K. J., and Evans, A. C. (1996). A unified statistical approach for determining significant voxels in images of cerebral activation. *Hum. Brain Mapping* **4,** 58–73.

Worsley, K. J., Andermann, M., Koulis, T., MacDonald, D., and Evans, A. C. (1999). Detecting changes in non-isotropic images. *Hum. Brain Mapping* **8**(2), 98–101.

Wright, I. C., McGuire, P. K., Poline, J.-B., Travere, J. M., Murray, R. M., Frith, C. D., Frackowiak, R. S. J., and Friston, K. J. (1995). A voxel-based method for the statistical analysis of gray and white matter density applied to schizophrenia. *NeuroImage* **2,** 244–252.

Wright, I. C., Ellison, Z. R., Sharma, T., Friston, K. J., Murray, R. M., and Mcguire, P. K. (1999). Mapping of gray matter changes in schizophrenia. *Schizophrenia Res.* **35,** 1–14.

SECTION TWO

MODELLING

CHAPTER

37

The General Linear Model

INTRODUCTION

In the absence of prior anatomical hypotheses regarding the physical location of a particular function, the statistical analysis of functional mapping experiments must proceed by assessing the acquired data for evidence of an experimentally induced effect at every intracerebral voxel individually and simultaneously.

After reconstruction, realignment, spatial normalisation, and (possibly) smoothing, the data are ready for statistical analysis. This involves two steps: First, statistics indicating evidence against a null hypothesis of no effect at each voxel are computed. An image of these statistics is then produced. Second, this statistical image must be assessed, reliably locating voxels where an effect is exhibited while limiting the possibility of false positives. In this chapter we address the former topic, the formation of an appropriate statistical image.

Current methods for assessing the data at each voxel are predominantly parametric: Specific forms of probability distribution are assumed for the data, and hypotheses specified in terms of models assumed for the (unknown) parameters of these distributions. The parameters are estimated and a statistic reflecting evidence against the null hypothesis formed. Statistics with a known null distribution are used such that the probability of obtaining a statistic, given that the null hypothesis is true, can be computed. This is hypothesis testing in the classical parametric sense. The majority of the statistical models used are special cases of the general linear model.

SPM has become an acronym in common use for the theoretical framework of voxel-based analysis of functional imaging data, for the software package implementing this procedure, and for the statistical image (statistical parametric map). Here we use SPM to refer to (1) the software package in its current version SPM99 and (2) the conceptual and theoretical framework.

In what follows, we first go through the equations for the general linear model with a spherical error distribution (i.e., we assume an independently and identically distributed error). This theoretical part is presented without any reference to PET or fMRI data and is orientated toward a description as found in a classical statistics textbook. In the third section, we turn to the data in question and illustrate the use of the general linear model on some PET data examples. In the fourth and final section, we introduce the linear model used for fMRI data. This model is a linear model with a normally distributed and nonspherical error.

THE GENERAL LINEAR MODEL

Before turning to the specifics of PET and fMRI, we consider the general linear model, which requires some basic matrix algebra and statistical concepts. These will be used to develop an understanding of classical hypothesis testing. Healy (1986) presents a brief summary of matrix methods relevant to statistics. Newcomers to statistical methods are directed toward Mould's excellent text "Introductory Medical Statistics" (1989), while the more mathematically experienced will find Chatfield's "Statistics for Technology" (1983) useful. Draper and Smith (1981) give a good exposition of matrix methods for the general linear model and go on to describe regression analysis in general. The definitive tome for practical statistical experimental design is Winer *et al.* (1991). An excellent book about experimental design has been written by Yandell (1997). A rather advanced, but very useful, text on linear models is that of Christensen (1996).

The General Linear Model: Introduction

Suppose we are to conduct an experiment during which we will measure a *response variable* (such as rCBF at a particular voxel) Y_j, where $j = 1, \ldots, J$ indexes the observation. The variable Y_j is random and conventionally denoted by a capital letter.[1] Suppose also that for each observation we have a set of L ($L < J$) *explanatory* variables (each measured without error) denoted by x_{jl}, where $l = 1, \ldots, L$ indexes the explanatory variables. The explanatory variables may be continuous (or sometimes discrete) *covariates,* functions of covariates, or they may be *dummy* variables indicating the *levels* of an experimental *factor.*

A *general linear model* explains the response variable Y_j in terms of a linear combination of the explanatory variables plus an error term:

$$Y_j = x_{j1}\beta_1 + \ldots + x_{jl}\beta_l + \ldots + x_{jL}\beta_L + \epsilon_j \tag{37.1}$$

Here the β_l are (unknown) parameters, corresponding to each of the L explanatory variables x_{jl}. The errors ϵ_j are independent and identically distributed normal random variables with zero mean and variance σ^2, written $\epsilon_j \overset{iid}{\sim} \mathcal{N}(0, \sigma^2)$. Linear models with other error distributions are *generalised linear models,* for which the acronym GLM is usually reserved.

Examples: Dummy Variables

Many classical parametric statistical procedures are special cases of the general linear model. We will illustrate this point by going through the equations for two well-known models.

Linear regression A simple example is linear regression, where only one continuous explanatory variable x_j is measured (without error) for each observation $j = 1, \ldots, J$. The model is usually written

$$Y_j = \mu + x_j\beta + \epsilon_j \tag{37.2}$$

where the unknown parameters are μ, a *constant term* in the model, the regression slope β, and $\epsilon_j \overset{iid}{\sim} \mathcal{N}(0, \sigma^2)$. This can be rewritten as a general linear model by the use of a dummy variable taking the value $x_{j1} = 1$ for all j:

$$Y_j = x_{j1}\mu + x_{j2}\beta_2 + \epsilon_j \tag{37.3}$$

which is of the form of Eq. (37.1) on replacing β_1 with μ.

Two-sample* t *test Similarly the two-sample t test is a special case of a general linear model: Suppose Y_{1j} and Y_{2j} are two independent groups of random variables: The two-sample t test assumes $Y_{qj} \overset{iid}{\sim} \mathcal{N}(\mu, \sigma^2)$, for $q = 1,2$, and assesses the null hypothesis $\mathcal{H}: \mu_1 = \mu_2$. The index j indexes the data points in both groups. The standard statistical way of writing the model is

[1] We talk of *random variables,* and of observations prior to their measurement, because classical (frequentist) statistics is concerned with what could have occurred in an experiment. Once the observations have been made, they are known, the residuals are known, and there is no randomness.

$$Y_{qj} = \mu_q + \epsilon_{qj} \tag{37.4}$$

The q subscript on the μ_q indicates that there are two *levels* to the group *effect,* μ_1 and μ_2. Here, $\epsilon_j \overset{iid}{\sim} \mathcal{N}(0, \sigma^2)$. This can be rewritten using two dummy variables x_{qj1} and x_{qj2} as follows:

$$Y_{qj} = x_{qj1}\mu_1 + x_{qj2}\mu_1 + \epsilon_{qj} \tag{37.5}$$

which is of the form of Eq. (37.1) after reindexing for qj. Here the dummy variables indicate group membership, where x_{qj1} indicates whether observation Y_{qj} is from the first group, in which case it has the value 1 when $q = 1$, and 0 when $q = 2$. Similarly, $x_{qj2} = \begin{cases} 0 & \text{if } q = 1 \\ 1 & \text{if } q = 2 \end{cases}$.

Matrix Formulation

In the following few subsections, we use the general linear model in its matrix formulation and derive a least-squares parameter estimation. After this, we describe how one can make inferences based on a contrast of the parameters. This theoretical treatment of the model is useful to derive a set of equations that can be used for the analysis of any data set that can be formulated in terms of the general linear model.

The general linear model can be succinctly expressed using matrix notation. Consider writing Eq. (37.1) in full, for each observation j, giving a set of simultaneous equations:

$$\begin{aligned} Y_1 &= x_{11}\beta_1 + \ldots + x_{1l}\beta_l + \ldots + x_{1L}\beta_L + \epsilon_1 \\ \vdots &= \vdots \\ Y_j &= x_{j1}\beta_1 + \ldots + x_{jl}\beta_l + \ldots + x_{jL}\beta_L + \epsilon_j \\ \vdots &= \vdots \\ Y_J &= x_{J1}\beta_1 + \ldots + x_{Jl}\beta_l + \ldots + x_{JL}\beta_L + \epsilon_J \end{aligned}$$

This has an equivalent matrix form:

$$\begin{pmatrix} Y_1 \\ \vdots \\ Y_j \\ \vdots \\ Y_J \end{pmatrix} = \begin{pmatrix} x_{11} & \ldots & x_{1l} & \ldots & x_{1L} \\ \vdots & \ddots & \vdots & \ddots & \vdots \\ x_{j1} & \ldots & x_{jl} & \ldots & x_{jL} \\ \vdots & \ddots & \vdots & \ddots & \vdots \\ x_{J1} & \ldots & x_{Jl} & \ldots & x_{JL} \end{pmatrix} \begin{pmatrix} \beta_1 \\ \vdots \\ \beta_l \\ \vdots \\ \beta_L \end{pmatrix} + \begin{pmatrix} \epsilon_1 \\ \vdots \\ \epsilon_j \\ \vdots \\ \epsilon_J \end{pmatrix}$$

which can be written in matrix notation as

$$Y = X\beta + \epsilon \tag{37.6}$$

where Y is the column vector of observations, ϵ the column vector of error terms, and β the column vector of parameters; $\beta = [\beta_1, \ldots, \beta_l, \ldots, \beta_L]^T$. The $J \times L$ matrix X, with jlth element x_{jl} is the *design matrix.* This has one row per observation, and one column (explanatory variable) per model parameter. The important point about the design matrix is that it is a near complete description of our model with the remainder of the model being in the error term. The design matrix is where the experimental knowledge about the expected signal is quantified.

Parameter Estimation

Once an experiment has been completed, we have observations of the random variables Y_j, which we denote by y_j. Usually, the simultaneous equations implied by the general linear model (with $\epsilon = 0$) cannot be solved, because the number of parameters L is typically chosen to be less than the number of observations J. Therefore, some method of estimating parameters that "best fit" the data is required. This is achieved by the method of *ordinary least squares.*

Denote a set of parameter estimates by $\tilde{\beta} = [\tilde{\beta}_1,\ldots,\tilde{\beta}_L]^T$. These parameters lead to *fitted values* $\tilde{Y} = [\tilde{Y}_1,\ldots,\tilde{Y}_J]^T = X\tilde{\beta}$, giving residual errors $e = [e_1,\ldots,e_J]^T = Y - \tilde{Y} = Y - X\tilde{\beta}$. The *residual sum of squares* $S = \sum_{j=1}^{J} e_j^2 = e^Te$ is the sum of the square differences between the actual and fitted values and thus measures the fit of the model with these parameter estimates.[2] The *least-squares* estimates are the parameter estimates that minimise the residual sum of squares. In full,

[2] e^Te is the L_2 norm of e—geometrically equivalent to the distance between the model and data.

$$S = \sum_{j=1}^{J}(Y_j - x_j\tilde{\beta}_1 - \ldots - x_{jL}\tilde{\beta}_L)^2$$

This is minimised when

$$\frac{\partial s}{\partial \tilde{\beta}_l} = 2\sum_{j=1}^{J}(-x_{jl})(Y_j - x_{j1}\tilde{\beta}_1 - \ldots - x_{jL}\tilde{\beta}_L) = 0$$

This equation is the lth row of $X^TY = (X^TX)\tilde{\beta}$. Thus, the least-squares estimates, denoted by $\tilde{\beta}$, satisfy the *normal equations:*

$$X^TY = (X^TX)\hat{\beta} \tag{37.7}$$

For the general linear model, the least squares estimates are the *maximum likelihood estimates* and are the *best linear unbiased estimates.*[3] That is, of all linear parameter estimates consisting of linear combinations of the observed data whose expectation is the true value of the parameters, the least-squares estimates have the minimum variance.

If (X^TX) is invertible, which it is if and only if the design matrix X is of full rank, then the least squares estimates are

$$\hat{\beta} = (X^TX)^{-1}X^TY \tag{37.8}$$

Overdetermined Models

If X has linearly dependent columns, it is *rank deficient,* (X^TX) is singular, and has no inverse. In this case the model is overparameterised: There are infinitely many parameter sets describing the same model. Correspondingly, there are infinitely many least-squares estimates $\hat{\beta}$ satisfying the normal equations. We will illustrate the overdetermined case by an example and discuss the solution that is adopted in SPM.

One-Way ANOVA Example

A simple example of such a model is the classic Q group one-way analysis of variance (ANOVA) model. Generally, an ANOVA determines the variability in the measured response that can be attributed to the effects of factor levels. The remaining unexplained variation is used to assess the significance of the effects (Yandell, 1997, p. 4 and pp. 202ff). The model for a one-way ANOVA is given by

$$Y_{qj} = \mu + \alpha_q + \epsilon_{qj} \tag{37.9}$$

where Y_{qj} is the jth observation in group $q = 1,\ldots,Q$. This model clearly does not uniquely specify the parameters: For any given μ and α_q, the parameters $\mu' = \mu + d$ and $\alpha'_q = \alpha_q - d$ give an equivalent model for any constant d. That is, the model is indeterminate up to the level of an additive constant between the constant term μ and the group effects α_q. Similarly for any set of least-squares estimates $\hat{\mu}$, $\hat{\alpha}_q$. Here there is one degree of indeterminacy in the model, resulting in the design matrix having rank Q, which is one less than the number of parameters (the number of columns of X). If the data vector Y has observations arranged by group, then for three groups ($Q = 3$), the design matrix and parameter vectors are

$$X = \begin{bmatrix} 1 & 1 & 0 & 0 \\ \vdots & \vdots & \vdots & \vdots \\ 1 & 1 & 0 & 0 \\ 1 & 0 & 1 & 0 \\ \vdots & \vdots & \vdots & \vdots \\ 1 & 0 & 1 & 0 \\ 1 & 0 & 0 & 1 \\ \vdots & \vdots & \vdots & \vdots \\ 1 & 0 & 0 & 1 \end{bmatrix} \quad \beta = \begin{bmatrix} \mu \\ \alpha_1 \\ \alpha_2 \\ \alpha_3 \end{bmatrix}$$

[3] Gauss-Markov theorem.

Clearly this matrix is rank deficient: The first column is the sum of the others. Therefore, in this model, one cannot test for the effect of one or more groups. However, note that the addition of the constant μ does not affect the relative differences between pairs of group effects. Therefore, *differences* in group effects are uniquely estimated regardless of the particular set of parameter estimates used. In other words, even if the model is overparameterised, there are still useful linear combinations of parameters (i.e., differences between pairs of group effects). This important concept will emerge in many designs, especially for PET and multisubject data. It will be treated more thoroughly in the "Estimable Functions and Contrasts" section.

Pseudoinverse Constraint

In the overdetermined case, a set of least-squares estimates may be found by imposing constraints on the estimates, or by inverting $(X^T X)$ using a pseudoinverse technique which essentially implies a constraint. In either case it is important to remember that the actual estimates obtained depend on the particular constraint or pseudoinverse method chosen. This has implications for inference: It is only meaningful to consider functions of the parameters that are uninfluenced by the particular constraint chosen.

Some obvious constraints are based on removing columns from the design matrix. In the one-way ANOVA example, one can remove the constant term to construct a design matrix which has linearly independent columns. For more complex designs, the form of the design matrix can change a lot such that it becomes difficult to visually recognise the original model. Therefore, in SPM, the overall principle is that each experimentally induced effect is represented by one or more regressors. This excludes the removal of columns as an option to deal with overdetermined models.

Alternatively a pseudoinverse method can be used. Let $(X^TX)^-$ denote the pseudoinverse of (X^TX). Then we can use $(X^T X)^-$ in place of $(X^TX)^{-1}$ in Eq. (37.8). A set of least-squares estimates is given by $\hat{\beta} = (X^TX)^- X^T Y = X^- Y$. The pseudoinverse function implemented in MATLAB gives the Moore-Penrose pseudoinverse.[4] This results in the least-squares parameter estimates with the minimum sum of squares (minimum L_2 norm $||\hat{\beta}||_2$). For example, for the one-way ANOVA model, this can be shown to give parameter estimates $\hat{\mu} = \sum_{j=1}^{Q} (\bar{Y}_{q\bullet})/(1 + Q)$ and $\hat{\alpha}_q = \bar{Y}_{q\bullet} - \hat{\mu}$. By $\bar{Y}_{q\bullet}$ we denote the average of Y over the observation index j, i.e., the average of the data in group q.

Using the pseudoinverse for parameter estimation in overdetermined models is the solution adopted in SPM. As mentioned above, this still does not allow us to test for those linear combinations of effects for which an infinite number of parameter estimates exists. (This topic is covered in great detail in Chapter 8.) Note that the pseudoinverse constraint leaves us with all columns of X.

Geometrical Perspective

For some, a geometrical perspective provides an intuitive feel for the procedure. (This section can be omitted without loss of continuity.)

The vector of observed values Y defines a single point in $\Re^J$, J-dimensional Euclidean space. $X\tilde{\beta}$ is a linear combination of the columns of the design matrix X. The columns of X are J vectors, so $X\tilde{\beta}$ for a given $\tilde{\beta}$ defines a point in $\Re^J$. This point lies in the subspace of $\Re^J$ spanned by the columns of the design matrix, the X space. The dimension of this subspace is rank(X). Recall that the space spanned by the columns of X is the set of points Xc for all $c \in \Re^L$. The residual sum of squares for parameter estimates $\tilde{\beta}$ is the distance from $X\tilde{\beta}$ to Y. Thus, the least-squares estimates $\hat{\beta}$ correspond to the point in the space spanned by the columns of X that is nearest to the data Y. The perpendicular from Y to the X space meets the X space at $\hat{Y} = X\hat{\beta}$. It is now clear why there are no unique least-squares estimates if X is rank deficient; for then any point in the X space can be obtained by infinitely many linear combinations of the columns of X, i.e., the solution exists on a hyperplane and is not a point.

If X is of full rank, then define the projection matrix as $P_X = X\,(X^T X)^{-1}\,X^T$. Then $\hat{Y} = P_X Y$, and geometrically P_X is a projection onto the X space. Similarly, the residual forming matrix is

[4] If X is of full rank, then $(X^TX)^-$ is an inefficient way of computing $(X^TX)^{-1}$.

$R = (I_J - P_X)$, where I_J is the identity matrix of rank J. Thus $RY = e$, and R is a projection matrix onto the space orthogonal to the X space.

As a concrete example, consider a linear regression with only three observations. The observed data $y = [y_1, y_2, y_3]^T$ defines a point in three-dimensional Euclidean space ($\Re^3$). The model of Eq. (37.2) leads to a design matrix

$$X = \begin{bmatrix} 1 & x_1 \\ 1 & x_2 \\ 1 & x_3 \end{bmatrix}$$

Provided the x_j's are not all the same, the columns of X span a two-dimensional subspace of $\Re^3$, a plane (Fig. 37.1).

Inference

Here, we derive the t and F statistics, which are used to test for a linear combination of effects. We will also return to the issue of overdetermined models and determine which linear combinations (contrasts) we can test.

Residual Sum of Squares

The residual variance σ^2 is estimated by the residual sum of squares divided by the appropriate degrees of freedom:

$$\hat{\sigma}^2 = \frac{e^T e}{J-p} \sim \sigma^2 \frac{\chi^2_{J-P}}{J-p}$$

where p = rank (X). See also the Appendix for a derivation of this result.

Linear Combinations of the Parameter Estimates

It is not too difficult to show that the parameter estimates are normally distributed: If X is full rank then $\hat{\beta} \sim \mathcal{N}(\beta, \sigma^2(X^T X)^{-1})$. From this it follows that for a column vector c containing L weights, then

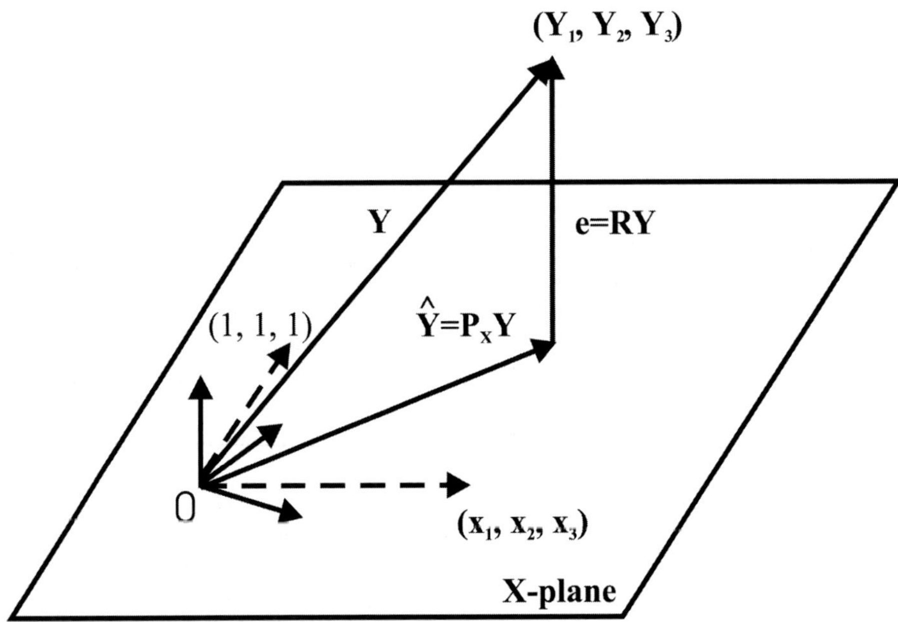

FIGURE 37.1
Geometrical perspective on linear regression: The three-dimensional data Y lies in a three-dimensional space. In this observation space, the (two-column) design matrix spans a subspace. Note that the axes of the design space are not aligned with the axes of the observation space. The least-squares estimate is the point in the space spanned by the design matrix that has minimal distance to the data point.

$$c^T\hat{\beta} \sim \mathcal{N}(c^T\beta, \sigma^2 c^T(X^TX)^{-1}c) \tag{37.10}$$

Furthermore, $\hat{\beta}$ and $\hat{\sigma}^2$ are independent (Fisher's law). Thus, prespecified hypotheses concerning linear compounds of the model parameters $c^T\beta$ can be assessed using

$$\frac{c^T\hat{\beta} - c^T\beta}{\sqrt{\hat{\sigma}^2 c^T(X^TX)^{-1}c}} \sim t_{J-p} \tag{37.11}$$

where t_{J-p} is a Student's t distribution with $J-p$ degrees of freedom. For example, the hypothesis $\mathcal{H}: c^T\beta = d$ can be assessed by computing

$$T = \frac{c^T\hat{\beta} - d}{\sqrt{\hat{\sigma}^2 c^T(X^TX)^{-1}c}} \tag{37.12}$$

and computing a p value by comparing T with a t distribution having $J-p$ degrees of freedom. In SPM, all tested null hypotheses are of the form $c^T\beta = 0$. Also note that in SPM tests based on this t value are always one sided.

Example: Two-Sample* t *Test For example, consider the two-sample t test. The model of Eq. (37.4) leads to a design matrix X with two columns of dummy variables indicating group membership and parameter vector $\beta = [\mu_1, \mu_2]^T$. Thus, the null hypothesis $\mathcal{H}: \mu_1 = \mu_2$ is equivalent to $\mathcal{H}: c^T\beta = 0$ with $c = [1, -1]^T$.

The first column of the design matrix contains n_1 1's and n_2 0's, indicating the measurements from group one, while the second column contains n_1 0's and n_2 1's for group two. Thus,

$$(X^TX) = \begin{pmatrix} n_1 & 0 \\ 0 & n_2 \end{pmatrix}, (X^TX)^{-1} = \begin{pmatrix} 1/n_1 & 0 \\ 0 & 1/n_2 \end{pmatrix}$$

and

$$c^T(X^TX)^{-1}c = 1/n_1 + 1/n_2$$

giving the t statistic [by Eq. (37.11)]

$$T = \frac{\hat{\mu}_1 - \hat{\mu}_2}{\sqrt{\hat{\sigma}^2(1/n_1 + 1/n_2)}}$$

which is the standard formula for the two-sample t statistic, with a Student's t distribution of $n_1 + n_2 - 2$ degrees of freedom under the null hypothesis.

Estimable Functions and Contrasts

Recall from an earlier section that if the model is overparameterised (i.e., X is rank deficient), then there are infinitely many parameter sets describing the same model. Constraints or the use of a pseudoinverse technique pull out only one set of parameters from infinitely many. Therefore, when examining linear compounds $c^T\beta$ of the parameters it is imperative to consider only compounds that are invariant over the space of possible parameters. Such linear compounds are called *contrasts*. In the following, we will characterise contrasts as linear combinations having two properties, which can be used to determine whether a linear compound is a proper contrast or not.

In detail (Scheffé, 1959), a linear function $c^T\beta$ of the parameters is *estimable* if there is a linear unbiased estimate c'^TY for some constant vector of weights c'. That is $c^T\beta = E(c'^TY)$. [$E(Y)$ is the expectation of the random variable Y.] The natural estimate $c^T\hat{\beta}$ is unique for an estimable function whatever solution, $\hat{\beta}$, of the normal equations is chosen (Gauss-Markov theorem). Further, $c^T\beta = E(c'^TY) = c'^TX\beta \Rightarrow c^T = c'^TX$, so c is a linear combination of the rows of X.

A *contrast* is an estimable function with the additional property $c^T\hat{\beta} = c'^T\hat{Y} = c'^TY$. Now $c'^T\hat{Y} = c'^TY \Leftrightarrow c'^TP_XY = c'^TY \Leftrightarrow c' = P_Xc'$ (since P_X is symmetric), so c' is in the X space. In summary, a contrast is an estimable function whose c' vector is a linear combination of the columns of X.[5]

[5] In statistical parametric mapping, one usually refers to the vector c as the *vector of contrast weights*. Informally, we will also refer to c as the *contrast*, a slight misuse of the term.

One can test whether c is a contrast vector by combining the two properties (1) $c^T = c'^T X$ and (2) $c' = P_X c'$ for some vector c'. Combining (1) and (2), it follows that $c^T = c'^T P_X X$. Because of (1), $c^T = c^T(X^TX)^- X^TX$. In other words, c is a contrast if it is unchanged by postmultiplication with $(X^TX)^- X^TX$. This test is used in SPM for user-specified contrasts.[6]

For a contrast it can be shown that $c^T\hat{\beta} \sim \mathcal{N}(c^T\beta, \sigma^2 c'^T c')$. Using a pseudoinverse technique, $P_X = X(X^TX)^- X^T$, so $c' = P_X c' \Rightarrow c'^T c' = c'^T X\,(X^TX)^- X^T c' = c^T(X^TX)^- c$ since $c = c'^T X$ for an estimable function.

This shows that the distributional results given above for unique designs [Eqs. (37.10) and (37.11)] apply for contrasts of the parameters of nonunique designs, where $(X^TX)^{-1}$ is replaced by a pseudoinverse.

It remains to characterise which linear compounds of the parameters are contrasts. For most designs, contrasts have weights that sum to zero over the levels of each factor. For example, for the one-way ANOVA with parameter vector $\beta = [\mu, \alpha_1, \ldots, \alpha_Q]^T$, the linear compound $c^T\beta$ with weights vector $c = [c_0, c_1, \ldots, c_Q]^T$ is a contrast if $c_0 = 0$ and $\sum_{q=1}^{Q} c_q = 0$.

Extra Sum-of-Squares Principle and F Contrasts

The *extra sum-of-squares* principle provides a method for assessing general linear hypotheses and for comparing models in a hierarchy, where inference is based on an F statistic. Here, we will describe the classical F test based on the assumption of an independent identically distributed error. In SPM, both statistics, the t and the F statistic, are used for making inferences.

We first describe the classical F test as found in nearly all introductory statistical texts. After that we will point at two critical limitations of this description and derive a more general and better suited implementation of the F test for typical models in neuroimaging.

Suppose we have a model with parameter vector β that can be partitioned into two, $\beta = [\beta_1^T \vdots \beta_2^T] \vdots$, and suppose we wish to test $\mathcal{H}: \beta_1 = 0$. The corresponding partitioning of the design matrix X is $X = [X_1 \vdots X_2]$, and the *full model* is

$$Y = [X_1 \vdots X_2]\begin{bmatrix}\beta_1 \\ \ldots \\ \beta_2\end{bmatrix} + \epsilon$$

which when $\mathcal{H}$ is true reduces to the *reduced model:* $Y = X_2\beta_2 + \epsilon$. Denote the residual sum of squares for the full and reduced models by $S(\beta)$ and $S(\beta_2)$, respectively. The *extra sum of squares* due to β_1 after β_2 is then defined as $S(\beta_1|\beta_2) = S(\beta_2) - S(\beta)$. Under $\mathcal{H}$, $S(\beta_1|\beta_2) \sim \sigma^2\chi_p^2$ independent of $S(\beta)$, where the degrees of freedom are $p = \text{rank}(X) - \text{rank}(X_2)$. [If $\mathcal{H}$ is not true, then $S(\beta_1|\beta_2)$ has a noncentral chi-squared distribution, still independent of $S(\beta)$.] Therefore, the following F statistic expresses evidence against $\mathcal{H}$:

$$F = \frac{\dfrac{S(\beta_2) - S(\beta)}{p - p_2}}{\dfrac{S(\beta)}{J - p}} \sim F_{p-p2, J-p} \tag{37.13}$$

where $p = \text{rank}(X)$ and $p_2 = \text{rank}(X_2)$. The larger F gets the more unlikely it is that F was sampled under the null hypothesis H. Significance can then be assessed by comparing this statistic with the appropriate F distribution. Draper and Smith (1981) give derivations.

This formulation of the F statistic has two limitations. The first is that two (nested) models, the full and the reduced model, have to be fitted subsequently to the data. In practice, this is implemented by a two-pass procedure on a, typically, large dataset. The second limitation is that a partitioning of the design matrix into two blocks of regressors is not the only way one can partition the design matrix space. Essentially, one can partition X into two sets of linear combinations of the regressors. As an example, one might be interested in the difference between two effects. If each of these two effects is modeled by one regressor, a simple partitioning is not possible and one cannot use Eq. (37.13) to test for the difference. Rather, one has to reparameterise the model such that the differential effect is explicitly modeled by a single regressor. As we will show in the following, this reparameterisation is unnecessary.

[6] The actual implementation of this test is based on a more efficient algorithm using a singular value decomposition.

The key to implementing an F test that avoids these two limitations is the notion of contrast matrices. A contrast matrix is a generalisation of a contrast vector. Each column of a contrast matrix consists of one contrast vector. Importantly, the contrast matrix controls the partitioning of the design matrix X.

A (user-specified) contrast matrix c is used to determine a subspace of the design matrix, i.e., $X_c = Xc$. The orthogonal contrast to c is given by $c_0 = I_p - cc^-$. Then, let $X_0 = Xc_0$ be the design matrix of the reduced model. We wish to compute what effects X_c explain, *after* first fitting the reduced model X_0. The important point to note is that although c and c_0 are orthogonal to each other, X_c and X_0 are possibly not, because the relevant regressors in the design matrix X can be correlated. If the partitions X_0 and X_c are not orthogonal, the temporal sequence of the subsequent fitting procedure attributes their shared variance to X_0. However, the subsequent fitting of two models is unnecessary, because one can construct a projection matrix from the data to the subspace of X_c, which is orthogonal to X_0. We denote this subspace by X_a.

The projection matrix M due to X_a can be derived from the residual forming matrix of the reduced model X_0. This matrix is given by $R_0 = I_J - X_0X_0^-$. The projection matrix is then $M = R_0 - R$, where R is the residual forming matrix of the full model, i.e., $R = I_J - XX^-$.

The F statistic can then be written as

$$F = \frac{(MY)^T MY}{(RY)^T RY} \frac{J-p}{p_1} = \frac{Y^T MY}{Y^T RY} \frac{J-p}{p_1} \sim F_{p_1, J-p} \tag{37.14}$$

where p_1 is the rank of X_a. Since M is a projector onto a subspace within X, we can also write

$$F = \frac{\hat{\beta}^T X^T M X \hat{\beta}}{Y^T RY} \frac{J-p}{p_1} = \sim F_{p_1, J-p} \tag{37.15}$$

This equation means that we can conveniently compute an F statistic for any user-specified contrast without any reparameterisation. In SPM, all F statistics are based on the full model so that Y^TRY need only be estimated once and then stored for subsequent use.

In summary, the formulation of the F statistic in Eq. (37.15) is a powerful tool, because by using a contrast matrix c we can test for a subspace spanned by contrasts of the design matrix X. Importantly, we do not need to reparameterise the model and estimate an additional parameter set, but use estimated parameters of the full model. More about F contrasts and their applications can be found in chapter 8.

Example: one-way ANOVA For example, consider a one-way ANOVA [Eq. (37.9)], where we wish to assess the omnibus null hypothesis that all the groups are identical: $\mathcal{H}: \alpha_1 = \alpha_2 = \ldots = \alpha_Q$. Under $\mathcal{H}$ the model reduces to $Y_{qj} = \mu + \epsilon_{qj}$. Since the ANOVA model contains a constant term, μ, $\mathcal{H}$ is equivalent to $\mathcal{H}: \alpha_1 = \alpha_2 = \ldots = \alpha_Q = 0$. Thus, let $\beta_1 = (\alpha_1,\ldots,\alpha_Q)^T$, and $\beta_2 = \mu$. Equation (37.13) then gives an F statistic that is precisely the standard F statistic for a one-way ANOVA.

Alternatively, we can apply Eq. (37.15). The contrast matrix c is a diagonal $Q + 1$ matrix with Q ones on the upper main diagonal and a zero in the Q + 1st element on the main diagonal (Fig. 37.2). This contrast matrix tests whether there was an effect due to any group after taking into account a constant term across groups. Application of Eq. (37.15) results in the same F value as compared to Eq. (37.13), but without the need to explicitly fit two models.

Adjusted and Fitted Data

Adjusted data can be used to illustrate the nature of an effect, some effects having been removed from the raw data Y. For example, when looking at the difference between two groups (two-sample t test), the effect that is of no interest is the mean over the two groups. Removing this overall mean allows one to have a better chance of visually assessing the difference which is otherwise *hidden away*, because its amplitude is typically only a small fraction of the mean amplitude. This principle of removing effects of no interest to better visually assess the overall effects of interest can be applied to any kind of design.

The question to answer is which effects are of interest and which are not. The partitioning of the design matrix into these two parts is based on the same principles as the F test developed in

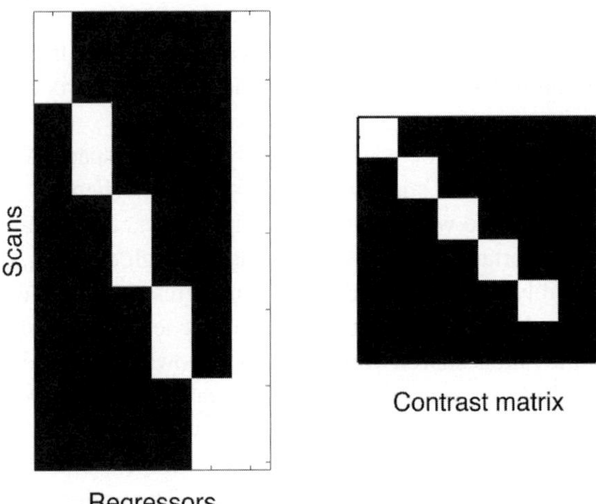

FIGURE 37.2
Example of ANOVA design and contrast matrix. Both matrices are displayed as images, where 0's are coded by black and 1's by white. (Left) Design matrix, where five groups are modeled by their mean and overall mean. The model is overdetermined by one degree of freedom. (Right) F-contrast matrix which tests for any group-specific deviation from the overall mean.

the preceding subsection. We can use an F contrast for the partitioning, which is equivalent to the specification of a full and reduced model. In this context, adjusted data are the residuals of the reduced model, i.e., components that can be explained by the reduced model have been removed from the data. In other words, to compute adjusted data, the user needs to tell SPM which part of the design matrix is of no interest (the reduced model). SPM then takes the part of the design matrix that is orthogonal to the reduced model as the effects of interest. This process will be illustrated below by an example. Note that the partitioning of the design matrix follows the same logic as the F test: First, any effect due to the reduced model is removed and only the remaining effects are taken to be of interest. An important point is that any overlap (correlation) between the reduced model and our *partition of interest* is explained by the reduced model. In the context of adjusted data this means that the adjusted data will not contain that component of the effects that can be explained by the reduced model.

Operationally, we compute the adjusted data using the same procedure that is used to calculate the F statistic. A user-specified contrast matrix c induces a partitioning of the design matrix X. The reduced model is given by $X_0 = Xc_0$ and its residual forming matrix $R_0 = I_J - X_0X_0^-$. The adjusted data can then be computed by $\tilde{Y} = R_0Y$. Note that this projection technique makes a reparameterisation redundant.

An alternative way of computing the adjusted data $\tilde{Y}$ is to compute the data explained by the design matrix partition orthogonal to X_0 and add the residuals of the full model, i.e., $\tilde{Y} = Y_f + e$. The residuals are given by $e = RY$, where R is the residual forming matrix of the full model, and $Y_f = MY$, where Y_f is referred to as *fitted data*. The projection matrix M is computed by $M = R_0 - R$. In other words, the fitted data are equivalent to the adjusted data minus the estimated error, i.e., $Y_f = \tilde{Y} - e$.

In SPM, both adjusted and fitted data can be plotted for any voxel. For these plots, SPM requires the specification of an F contrast, which encodes the partitioning of the design matrix into effects of interest and no interest.

Example

As an example, we look at a one-way ANOVA with four groups. The design matrix consists of four columns which indicate group membership. Each group has 12 measurements so that we have 48 measurements total. In our example, we are interested in the average of two differences. The first difference is between group 1 and 2 and the second difference between group 2 and 3. If we want to test this difference with a t statistic, the contrast vector will be $c = [-1, 1, -1, 1]^T$. In Fig. 37.3 (left), we show what the actual data look like. It is easy to see that there is a

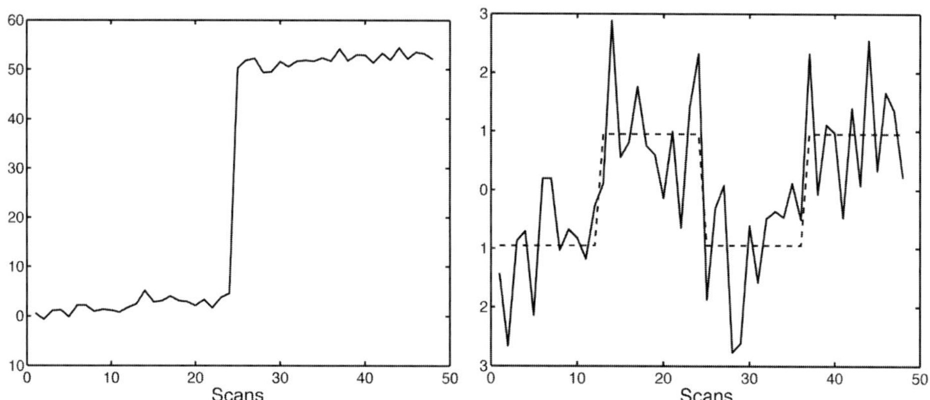

FIGURE 37.3
Adjusted and fitted data. (Left) Plot of raw data. (Right) Solid line: adjusted data; dashed line: fitted data.

difference between the average of the first two groups compared to the average of the last two groups. (This difference could be tested by using the contrast vector $c = [-1, -1, 1, 1]^T$.) However, by visual inspection, it is hard to tell whether there is a difference between the average of group 1 and 3 compared to the average of group 2 and 4. This is a situation where a plot of adjusted and fitted data is helpful. First, we have to specify a reduced model. One way of doing this is to specify a contrast vector or matrix that defines our effect of interest. In our example, the difference is represented by the contrast vector $c = [-1, 1, -1, 1]^T$. The contrast matrix c_0 is given by $c_0 = I_4 - cc^-$. With c_0, we can compute X_0, R_0, and M, all of which are needed to compute the adjusted and fitted data. In Fig. 37.3 (right), we show the fitted and adjusted data. In this plot, it is obvious that there actually is a difference between group 1 and 2 and between group 3 and 4. This example illustrates that plots of fitted and adjusted data are helpful, when the effect of interest is masked by a comparably large effect of no interest. This is very often the case in neuroimaging, where typically the effect of interest is very small compared to large confounding effects.

Note that a plot of adjusted or fitted data can never substitute for a test of significance. However, for illustration purposes, a plot of the adjusted/fitted data is the closest one can get to the effect that one wishes to test.

Design Matrix Images

SPM uses grayscale images of the design matrix to represent linear models. An example for a single subject PET activation study with four scans under each of three conditions is shown in Fig. 37.4. The first three columns contain indicator variables (consisting of zeros and ones) indicating the condition. The last column contains the (mean corrected) global cerebral blood flow (gCBF) values (see below).

In the grayscale design matrix images, –1 is black, 0 midgray, and +1 white. Columns containing covariates are scaled by subtracting the mean (zero for centered covariates). For display purposes regressors are divided by their absolute maximum, giving values in [–1, 1]. Design matrix blocks containing factor by covariate interactions are scaled such that the covariate values lie in [0,1], thus preserving representation of the padding zeros as midgray.

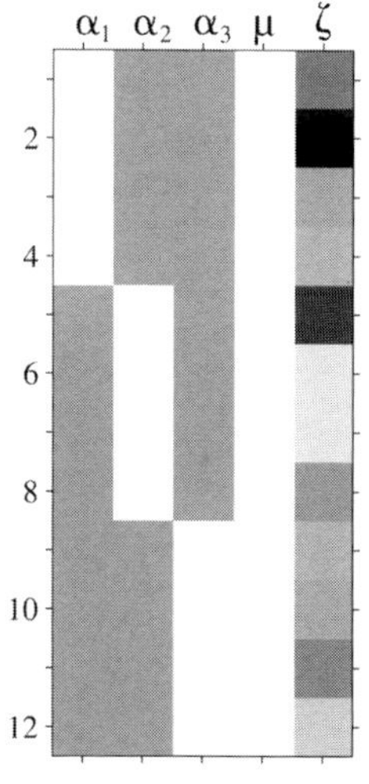

FIGURE 37.4
Single-subject activation experiment, ANCOVA design. Illustrations for a three-condition experiment with four scans in each of three conditions, ANCOVA design. Design matrix image, with columns labeled by their respective parameters. The scans are ordered by condition.

PET AND BASIC MODELS

With the details of the general linear model covered, we turn our attention to some actual models used in functional brain mapping, discuss the practicalities of their application, and introduce some terminology used in SPM. Because the approach is mass univariate, we must consider a model for each and every voxel. Bear in mind that in the mass univariate approach, the same model is used at every voxel simultaneously, with different parameters for each voxel. We concentrate on PET data, with its mature family of standard statistical experimental designs. Models of fMRI data will be presented in the next section.

Although most PET functional mapping experiments are on multiple subjects, many of the key concepts are readily demonstrated using single-subject data.

Heteroscedacity

Heteroscedacity in the context of neuroimaging means that the error variance is allowed to vary between voxels. In PET data, there is substantial evidence against an assumption of constant variance (homoscedasticity) at all points of the brain. This fact is perhaps to be expected, considering the different constituents and activities of gray and white matter. This is unfortunate, because the small sample sizes leave few degrees of freedom for variance estimation. If homoscedasticity could be assumed, variance estimates could legitimately be pooled across all voxels. Provided the image is much greater in extent than its smoothness, this gives an estimate with sufficiently high (effective) degrees of freedom such that its variability is negligible. (Since the images are smooth, neighbouring voxels are correlated and hence the variance estimates at neighbouring voxels are correlated.) The t statistics based on such a variance estimate are approximately normally distributed, the approximation failing only in the extreme tails of the distribution.

Global Normalisation

In neuroimaging, one can differentiate between regional and global activity. By regional activity one typically means the activity measured in a single voxel or a small volume of voxels. Global activity refers to a global measure of brain activity. These two informal descriptions of regional and global activity reflect the fact that there may be a number of different definitions. However, the reason why the concept of global activity is important is that there are effects in a single voxel that are caused by global effects. These are usually difficult to model. Typically, we use simple models for global effects. Modelling global effects enhances the sensitivity and accuracy of the subsequent inference step about experimentally induced effects.

As an example, consider a simple single-subject PET experiment. The subject is scanned repeatedly under both *baseline* (control) and *activation* (experimental) conditions. Inspection of regional activity, used as a measure of regional cerebral blood flow (rCBF), alone at a single voxel may not indicate an experimentally induced effect. However, the additional consideration of global activity, the global cerebral blood flow (gCBF), for the respective scans may clearly differentiate between the two conditions (Fig. 37.5).

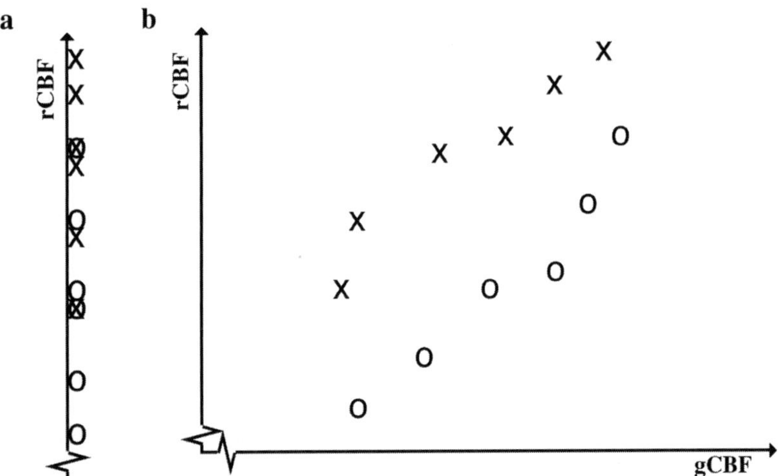

FIGURE 37.5
Single-subject PET experiment, illustrative plots of rCBF at a single voxel: (a) Dot-plots of rCBF. (b) Plot of rCBF vs. gCBF. Both plots indexed by condition: ○ for baseline, × for active.

In SPM, the precise definition of global activity is user dependent. The *default* definition is that global activity is the global average of image intensities of intracerebral tissue. If Y_j^k is the image intensity at voxel $k = 1,\ldots,K$ of scan j, then denote the estimated global activity by $g_j = \bar{Y}_j^{\bullet} = \sum_{k=1}^{K} Y_j^k/K$.

Having estimated the global activity for each scan, a decision must be made about what model of global activity should be used. In SPM, there are basically two alternatives or various mixtures between them. The first is *proportional scaling* and the second is an ANCOVA approach.

Proportional Scaling

One way to account for global changes is to adjust the data by scaling each scan by its estimated global activity. This approach is based on the assumption that the measurement process introduces a (global) scaling of the image intensities at each voxel, a gain factor. This has the advantage of converting the raw data into a physiological range to give parameters in interpretable scale. The mean global value is usually chosen to be the canonical normal gCBF of 50 mL/min/dL. The scaling factor is thus $\frac{50}{g.}$. We shall assume that the count rate recorded in the scanner (counts data) has been scaled into a physiologically meaningful scale. The normalised data are $Y_j'^k = (50/g_j)Y_j^k$. The model is then

$$Y_j^k = \frac{g_j}{50}(X\beta^k)_j + \epsilon_j'^k \tag{37.16}$$

where $\epsilon'^k \sim \mathcal{N}(0, \sigma_k^2 \times \text{diag}\,[(g_j/50)^2])$. The diag() operator transforms a column vector to a diagonal matrix with the vector on its main diagonal and zero elsewhere. This is a weighted regression; i.e., the shape of the error covariance matrix is no longer I_J, but a function of the estimated global activity. Also note that the jth row of X is weighted by $g_j/50$.

The adjustment of data, from Y to Y', is illustrated in Fig. 37.6a.

ANCOVA *Approach*

Another approach is to include the mean corrected global activity vector g as an additional regressor into the model. In this case the model of Eq. (37.6) becomes

$$Y_j^k = (X\beta)j + \zeta^k(g_j - \bar{g}_{\bullet}) + \epsilon_j^k \tag{37.17}$$

where $\epsilon^k \sim \mathcal{N}(0, \sigma^2_k I_J)$ and ζ^k is the slope parameter for the global activity vector. In this model, the data are explained as the sum of experimentally induced regional activity and some global activity which varies over scans. Note that the model of Eq. (37.17) can be considerably extended by allowing for different slopes between replications, conditions, subjects and groups.

Proportional Scaling versus ANCOVA

Clearly a decision has to be made about which global normalisation approach should be used for a given dataset. One cannot apply both, because proportional scaling will normalise the global mean activity such that the mean corrected g in the ANCOVA approach will consists of a zero vector. The proportional scaling approach is most appropriate for any dataset for which there is a gain (multiplicative) factor that varies over scans. This is a useful assumption for fMRI data (see next section). In contrast to this, an ANCOVA approach is appropriate if the gain factor does not change over scans. This is the case for PET scans acquired on modern scanners using protocols which control for the administered dose rate. This means that a change in estimated global activity reflects a change in a subject's global activity and not a change in a global (machine-specific) gain factor. Moreover, the ANCOVA approach assumes that regional experimentally induced effects are independent of changes in global activity. Note that the ANCOVA approach should not be used for PET data, where the administered dose is not controlled and varies over scans. In this case, the true underlying gCBF might be constant over scans, but the global gain factor varies. Similarly, for SPECT scans, it is known that the global gain factor can vary over scans, so that it is recommended to prefer proportional scaling over the ANCOVA approach for SPECT data.

Special considerations apply if there are condition-dependent changes in global activity.

Implicit in allowing for changes in gCBF (either by proportional scaling or ANCOVA), when assessing condition-specific changes in rCBF, is the assumption that gCBF represents the

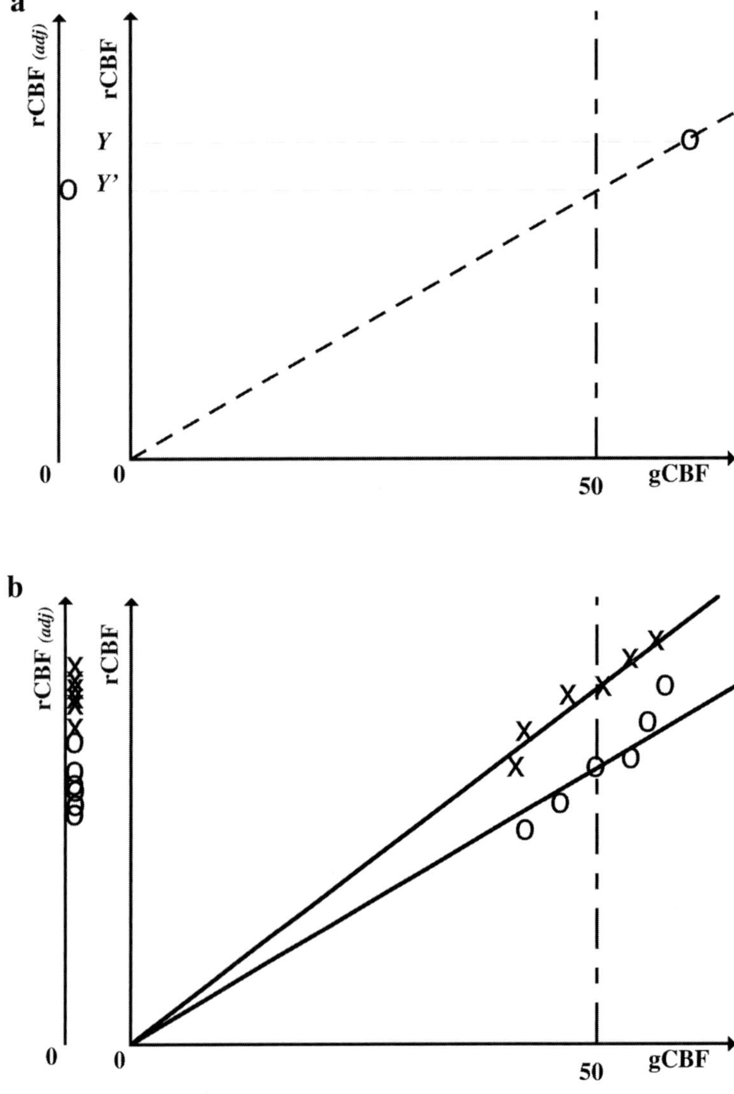

FIGURE 37.6
(a) Adjustment by proportional scaling. (b) Simple single-subject activation as a *t* test on adjusted rCBF: weighted proportional regression.

underlying background flow above which regional differences are assessed. That is, gCBF is independent of condition. Clearly, since gCBF is calculated as the mean intracerebral rCBF, an increase of rCBF in a particular brain region must cause an increase of gCBF unless there is a corresponding decrease of rCBF elsewhere in the brain. Similar problems can arise when comparing a group of subjects with a group of patients with brain atrophy, or when comparing pre- and postoperative rCBF.

If gCBF actually varies considerably between conditions, as in pharmacological activation studies, then testing for an activation after allowing for global changes involves extrapolating the relationship between regional and global flow outside the range of the data. This extrapolation might not be valid, as illustrated in Fig. 37.7a.

If gCBF is increased by a large activation that is not associated with a corresponding deactivation, then comparison at a common gCBF will make nonactivated regions (whose rCBF remained constant) appear falsely deactivated, and the magnitude of the activation will be similarly decreased. (Figure 37.7b illustrates the scenario for a simple single-subject activation experiment using ANCOVA.) In such circumstances a better measure of the underlying background flow should be sought, for instance, by examining the flow in brain regions known to be unaffected by the stimulus.

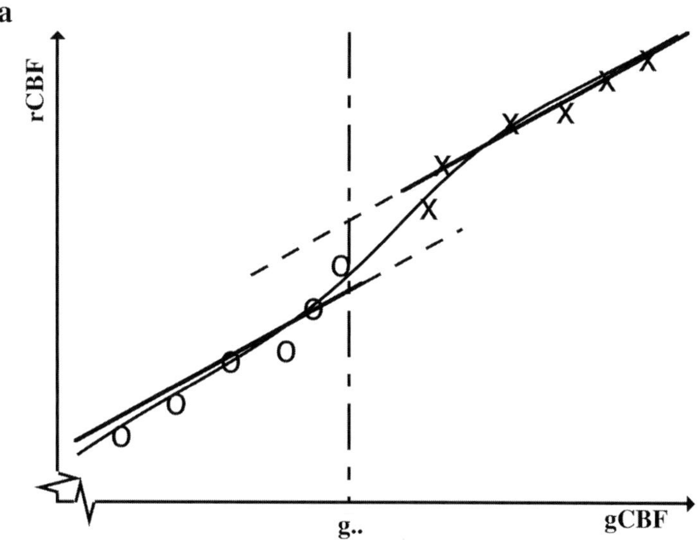

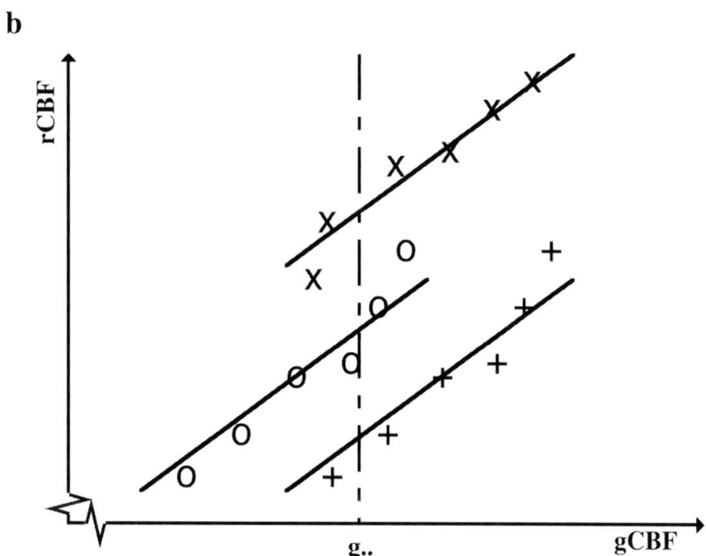

FIGURE 37.7
Single-subject data, illustrative ANCOVA plots of rCBF vs. rCBF at a single voxel showing potential problems with global changes: (a) Large change in gCBF between conditions. The apparent activation relies on linear extrapolation of the baseline and active condition regressions (assumed to have the same slope) beyond the range of the data. The actual relationship between regional and global for no activation may be given by the curve, in which case there is no activation effect. (b) Large activation inducing increase in gCBF measured as brain mean rCBF. Symbol • denotes rest, × denotes active condition values if this is a truly activated voxel (in which case the activation is underestimated), while + denotes active condition values where this voxel is not activated (in which case an apparent deactivation is seen).

Grand Mean Scaling

Grand mean scaling multiplies all scans by some factor such that the resulting estimated mean global activity is a user-specified constant over scans.[7] Note that this common factor has no effect on the inference, because in the t and F statistic [Eqs. (37.12) and (37.14)] such a factor cancels. It will also not change relative interpretations of the fitted or adjusted data. The default behaviour of SPM with respect to PET and fMRI data is described in §3 and §4.

[7] Clearly grand mean scaling is redundant when followed by proportional scaling.

Mixtures of Scaling and ANCOVA

For PET and SPECT data, the user can choose from a wide range of global normalisation models that lie between proportional scaling and an ANCOVA approach. An intermediate approach is possible by scaling groups of scans. These groups can be scaling by replication, condition, subject, and group grand mean. This can be then applied together with an ANCOVA approach that estimates different slopes for such a grouping. For example, one can apply proportional scaling by the grand mean within-subject and combine this with a within-subject ANCOVA approach.

PET Models

In the following subsections, the flexibility of the general linear model is demonstrated using models for various PET functional mapping experiments. For generality, ANCOVA style models are used, with gCBF included as a confounding covariate. The corresponding ANCOVA models for data adjusted by proportional scaling can be obtained by omitting the global terms. Voxel-level models are presented in the usual statistical notation, alongside the SPM description and design matrix images. The form of contrasts for each design are indicated, and some practicalities of the SPM interface are discussed.

Single-Subject Models

Single-subject activation design The simplest experimental paradigm is the single-subject activation experiment. Suppose we have Q conditions, with M_q scans under condition q. Let Y_{qj}^k denote the rCBF at voxel k in scan $j = 1,\ldots,M_q$ under condition $q = 1,\ldots,Q$. The model is

$$Y_{qj}^k = \alpha_q^k + \mu^k + \zeta^k(g_{qj} - \bar{g}_{\bullet\bullet}) + \epsilon_{qj}^k \tag{37.18}$$

There are $Q + 2$ parameters for the model at each voxel: the Q condition effects, the constant term μ^k, and the global regression effect, giving parameter vector $\beta^k = (\alpha_1^k,\ldots,\alpha_Q^k, \mu^k, \zeta^k)^T$ at each voxel. In this model, replications of the same condition are modeled with a single effect. The model is overparameterised, having only $Q + 1$ degrees of freedom, leaving $N - Q - 1$ residual degrees of freedom, where $N = \Sigma M_q$ is the total number of scans.

Contrasts are linear compounds $c^T \beta^k$ for which the weights sum to zero over the condition effects, and give zero weight to the constant term, i.e., $\sum_{q=1}^{Q} c_q = 0$ (Fig. 37.8). Therefore, linear compounds that test for a simple group effect or for an average effect over groups cannot be contrasts. However, one can test for differences between groups. For example, to test the null hypothesis $\mathcal{H}^k : \alpha_1^k = (\alpha_2^k + \alpha_3^k)/2$ against the one-sided alternative $\bar{\mathcal{H}}^k : \alpha_1^k > (\alpha_2^k + \alpha_3^k)/2$, the appropriate contrast weights would be $c = [1, -\frac{1}{2}, -\frac{1}{2}, 0,\ldots, 0]^T$. In words, one tests for a (positive) difference between the effect of group 1 compared to the average of groups 2 and 3. Large positive values of the t statistic express evidence against the null hypothesis, in favor of the alternative hypothesis.

Single-subject parametric design Consider the single-subject parametric experiment in which a single covariate of interest, or "score," is measured. For instance, the covariate may be a physiological variable, a task difficulty rating, or a performance score. We want to find regions where the rCBF values are highly correlated with the covariate, taking into account the effect of global changes. Figure 37.9a depicts the situation. If Y_j^k is the rCBF at voxel k of scan $j = 1,\ldots, J$ and s_j is the independent covariate, then a simple ANCOVA style model is a multiple regression with two covariates:

$$Y_j^k = \varrho^k(s_j - \bar{s}_\bullet) + \mu^k + \zeta^k(g_j - \bar{g}_\bullet) + \epsilon_{qj}^k \tag{37.19}$$

Here, ϱ^k is the slope of the regression plane in the direction of increasing score, fitted separately for each voxel.

There are three model parameters, leaving $J - 3$ residual degrees of freedom. The design matrix (Fig. 37.9b) has three columns, a column containing the (centered) score covariate, a column of dummy 1's corresponding to μ^k, and a column containing the (centered) global values.

In SPM this is a *single-subject, covariates only* design. The design is uniquely specified, so any linear combination of the three parameters is a contrast. The null hypothesis of no score

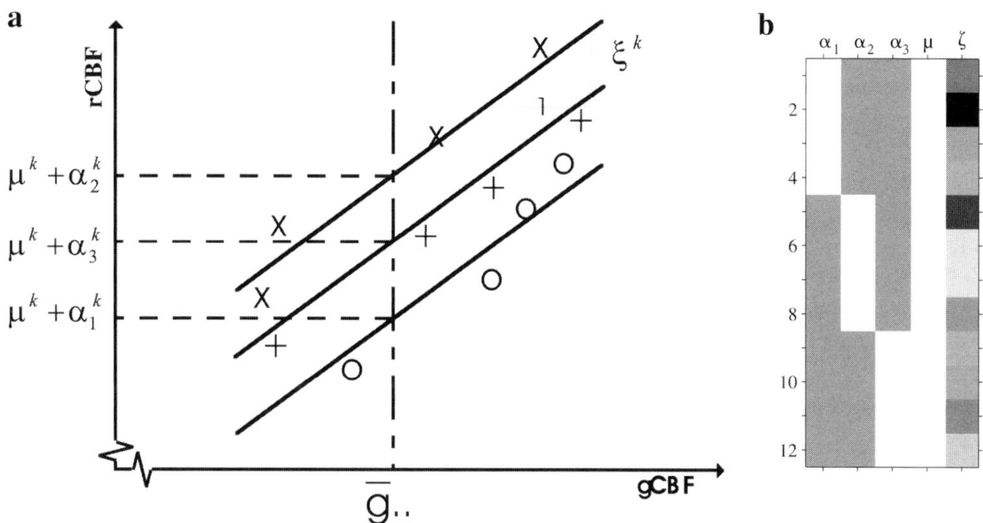

FIGURE 37.8
Single-subject study, ANCOVA design. Illustration of a three-condition experiment with four scans in each of three conditions, ANCOVA design. (a) Illustrative plot of rCBF vs. gCBF. (b) Design matrix image with columns labeled by their respective parameters. The scans are ordered by condition.

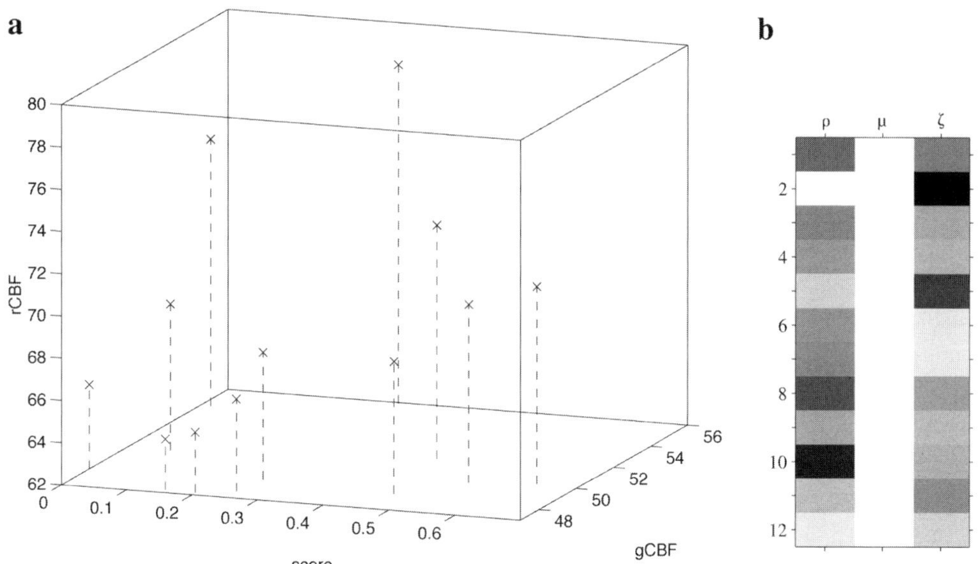

FIGURE 37.9
Single-subject parametric experiment: (a) Plot of rCBF vs. score and gCBF. (b) Design matrix image for Eq. (37.19), illustrated for a 12-scan experiment. Scans are ordered in the order of acquisition.

effect at voxel k, $\mathcal{H}^k : \varrho^k = 0$, can be assessed against the one-sided alternative hypotheses $\mathcal{H}^k : \varrho^k > 0$ (rCBF increasing with score) with contrast weight for the effect of interest $c_1 = +1$, and against $\overline{\mathcal{H}}^k : \varrho^k < 0$ (rCBF decreasing as score increases) with contrast weight $c_1 = -1$.

This simple model assumes a linear relationship between rCBF and the covariate (and other explanatory variables). More general relationships can be modeled by including other functions of the covariate. These functions are essentially new explanatory variables, which if linearly combined still fit in the framework of the general linear model. For instance, if an exponential relationship is expected, the logarithm of s_j, i.e., $\ln(s_j)$, would be used in place of s_j. Fitting powers of covariates as additional explanatory variables leads to *polynomial regression.* More generally, a set of *basis functions* can be used to expand the covariate to allow flexible modelling. This theme will be developed later in this chapter (for fMRI) and in other chapters.

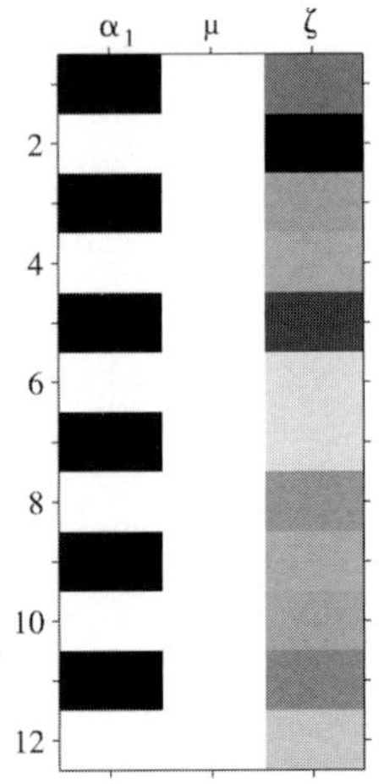

FIGURE 37.10
Example design matrix image for a single-subject activation study, with six scans in each of two conditions, formulated as a parametric design. The 12 scans are ordered alternating between baseline and activation conditions, as might have been the order of acquisition.

Simple single-subject activation revisited As discussed in the general linear model section, it is often possible to reparameterise the same model in many ways. As an example, consider a two-condition ($Q = 2$) single-subject experiment, discussed above. The model of Eq. (37.18) is

$$Y^k_{qj} = \alpha^k_q + \mu\mathrm{k} + \zeta^k\,(g_{qj} - \bar{g}_{\bullet\bullet}) + \epsilon^k_{qj}$$

The model is overdetermined, so consider a sum-to-zero constraint on the condition effects. For two conditions this implies $\alpha^k_1 = -\alpha^k_2$. Substituting for α^k_2 the resulting design matrix has a column containing +1's and −1's indicating the condition $q = 1$ or $q = 2$, respectively, a column of 1's for the overall mean, and a column containing the (centered) gCBF (Fig. 37.10). The corresponding parameter vector is $\beta^k = [\alpha^k_1, \mu^k, \zeta^k]^T$. Clearly this is the same design matrix as that for a parametric design with (noncentered) "score" covariate indicating the condition as active or baseline with +1 or −1, respectively. The hypothesis of no activation at voxel k, $\mathcal{H}^k$: $\alpha^k_1 = 0$ can be tested against the one-sided alternatives $\bar{\mathcal{H}}^k : \alpha^k_1 > 0$ (activation) and $\bar{\mathcal{H}}^k : \alpha^k_1 < 0$ with contrast weights for the effects of interest $c_1 = 1$ and $c_1 = -1$, respectively. This example illustrates how the SPM interface may be used to enter "hand-built" blocks of design matrix as noncentered covariates.

Single subject: conditions and covariates Frequently, other confounding covariates in addition to gCBF can be added into the model. For example, a linear time component could be modeled simply by entering the scan number as covariate. In SPM these appear in the design matrix as additional covariate columns adjacent to the global flow column.

Factor by covariate interactions A more interesting experimental scenario occurs when a parametric design is repeated under multiple conditions in the same subject(s). A specific example would be a PET language experiment in which, during each of 12 scans, lists of words are presented. Two types of word lists (the two conditions) are presented at each of six rates (the parametric component). Interest may lie in locating regions where there is a difference in rCBF between conditions (accounting for changes in presentation rate), the *main* effect of condition; locating regions where rCBF increases with rate (accounting for condition), the main effect of rate; and possibly assessing evidence for condition-specific responses in rCBF to changes in rate, an interaction effect.[8] Let Y^k_{qrj} denote the rCBF at voxel k for the jth measurement under rate $r = 1,\ldots, R$ and condition $q = 1,\ldots, Q$, with s_{qr} the rate covariate (some function of the rates). A suitable model is

$$Y^k_{qrj} = \alpha^k_q + \varrho^k_q\,(s_{qr} - \bar{s}_{\bullet\bullet}) + \mu^k + \zeta^k(g_{qrj} - \bar{g}_{\bullet\bullet\bullet}) + \epsilon^k_{qrj} \qquad (37.20)$$

Note the q subscript on the parameter ϱ^k_q, indicating different slopes for each condition. Ignoring for the moment the global flow, the model describes two simple regressions with common error variance (Fig. 37.11a). The SPM interface describes such factor by covariate interactions as *factor-specific covariate fits*. The interaction between condition and covariate effects is manifested as different regression slopes for each condition. There are $2Q + 2$ parameters for the model at each voxel, $\beta^k = [\alpha^k_1,\ldots, \alpha^k_Q, \varrho^k_1,\ldots, \varrho^k_Q, \mu^k, \zeta^k]^T$, with $2Q + 1$ degrees of freedom. A design matrix image for the two-condition example is shown in Fig. 37.11b. The factor by covariate interaction takes up the third and fourth columns, corresponding to the parameters ϱ^k_1 and ϱ^k_2, the covariate being split between the columns according to condition, the remaining cells filled with zeros.

Only the constant term and global slope are designated confounding, giving $2Q$ effects of interest to specify contrast weights for, $\beta^k_1 = [\alpha^k_1,\ldots, \alpha^k_Q, \varrho^k_1,\ldots, \varrho^k_Q]^T$. As with the activation study model, contrasts have weights which sum to zero over the condition effects. For the two-condition word presentation example, contrast weights $c_1 = [0, 0, 1, 0]^T$ for the effects of interest express evidence against the null hypothesis that there is no covariate effect in condition 1, with large values indicating evidence of a positive covariate effect. Weights $c_1 = [0, 0, \frac{1}{2}, \frac{1}{2}]^T$ address the hypothesis that there is no average covariate effect across conditions, against the one-sided alternative that the average covariate effect is positive. Weights $c_1 = [0, 0, -1, +1]^T$ address the

[8] Two experimental factors *interact* if the level of one affects the expression of the other.

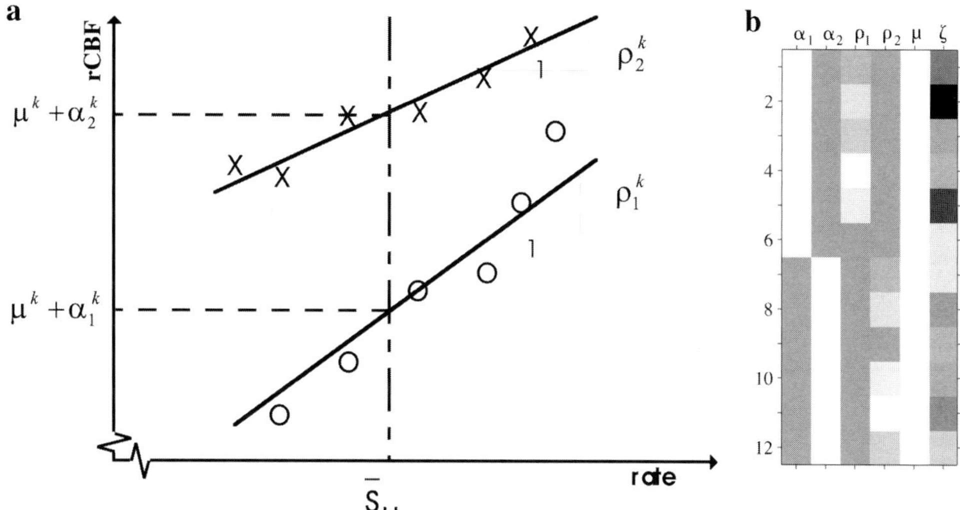

FIGURE 37.11
Single-subject experiment with conditions, covariate, and condition by covariate interaction. (a) Illustrative plot of rCBF vs. rate. (b) Design matrix image for Eq. (37.20). Both illustrated for the two-condition 12-scan experiment described in the text. The scans have been ordered by condition.

hypothesis that there is no condition by covariate interaction, that is, that the regression slopes are the same, against the alternative that the condition 2 regression is steeper.

Conceptually, contrast weights $c_1 = [-1, +1, 0, 0]^T$ and $c_1 = [+1, -1, 0, 0]^T$ for the effects of interest assess the hypothesis of no condition effect against appropriate one-sided alternatives. However, the comparison of main effects is confounded in the presence of an interaction: In the above model, both gCBF and the rate covariate were centered, so the condition effects α_q^k are the relative heights of the respective regression lines (relative to μ^k) at the mean gCBF and mean rate covariate. Clearly if there is an interaction, then differences in the condition effects (the separation of the two regression lines) depend on where you look at them. Were the rate covariate not centered, the comparison would be at mean gCBF and zero rate, possibly yielding a different result.

Thus the main effects of condition in such a design must be interpreted with caution. If there is little evidence for a condition-dependent covariate effect then there is no problem. Otherwise, the relationship between rCBF and other design factors should be examined graphically to assess whether the perceived condition effect is sensitive to the level of the covariate.

Multisubject Designs

Frequently, experimentally induced changes of rCBF are subtle, such that analyses must be pooled across subjects to find statistically significant evidence of an experimentally induced effect. In this chapter, we will discuss some fixed-effects models. Random or mixed effects models are covered in Chapter 12.

The single-subject designs presented above must be extended to account for subject-to-subject differences. The simplest type of subject effect is an additive effect, otherwise referred to as a *block effect.* This implies that all subjects respond in the same way, save for an overall shift in rCBF (at each voxel). We extend our notation by adding subscript i for subjects, so Y_{iqj}^k is the rCBF at voxel k of scan j under condition q on subject $i = 1,\ldots, N$.

Multisubject activation (replications) For instance, the single-subject activation model of Eq. (37.18) is extended by adding subject effects γ_i^k giving the model:

$$Y_{iqj}^k = \alpha_q^k + \gamma_i^k + \zeta^k(g_{iqj} - \bar{g}_{\ldots}) + \epsilon_{iqj}^k \tag{37.21}$$

A schematic plot of rCBF vs. gCBF for this model is shown in Fig. 37.12a. In SPM terminology, this is a *multisubject, replication of conditions* design. The parameter vector at voxel k is $\beta^k = [\alpha_1^k \ldots, \alpha_Q^k, \gamma_1^k, \ldots, \gamma_N^k, \zeta^k]^T$. The design matrix (Fig. 37.12b) has N columns of dummy variables

a

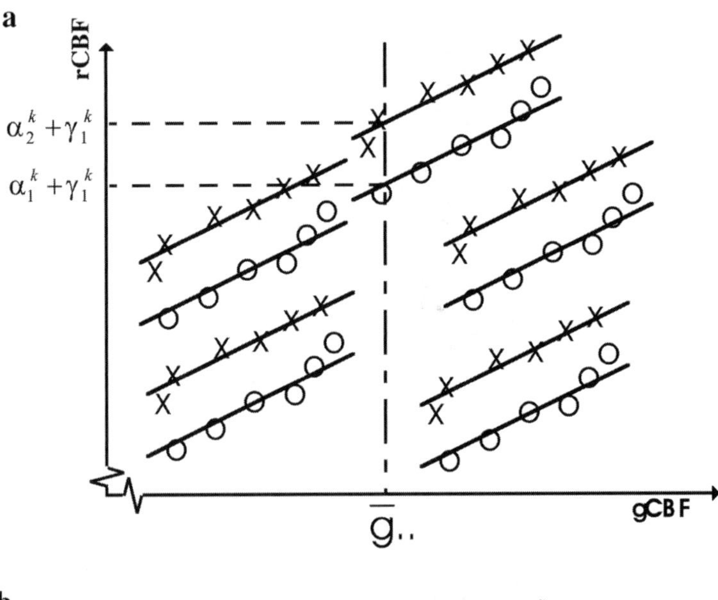

b

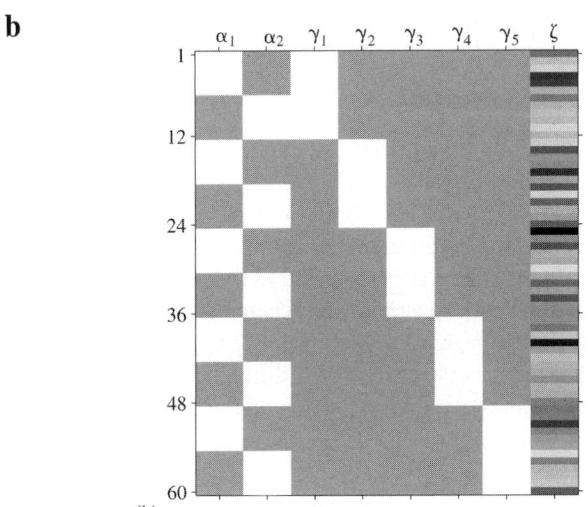

FIGURE 37.12
Multisubject activation experiment, replication of conditions of model Eq. (37.21). Illustrations for a five-subject study, with six replications of each of two conditions per subject: (a) Illustrative plot of rCBF vs. gCBF. (b) Design matrix image. The first two columns correspond to the condition effects, the next five to the subject effects, the last to the gCBF regression parameter. The design matrix corresponds to scans ordered by subject and by condition within subjects.

corresponding to the subject effects. (Similarly a multisubject parametric design could be derived from the single-subject case by including appropriate additive subject effects.)

Again, the model is overparameterised, though this time we have omitted the explicit constant term from the confounds, since the subject effects can model an overall level. Adding a constant to each of the condition effects and subtracting it from each of the subject effects gives the same model. Bearing this in mind, it is clear that contrasts must have weights that sum to zero over both the subject effects and the condition effects.

Condition by replication interactions The above model assumes that, accounting for global and subject effects, replications of the same condition give the same expected response. There are many reasons why this assumption may be inappropriate, such as learning effects or more generally effects that change as a function of time. For example, some time effects can be modeled by including appropriate functions of the scan number as confounding covariates. With multisubject designs we have sufficient degrees of freedom available to enable the consideration of replication by condition interactions. Such interactions imply that the expected response to each condition is different between replications (having accounted for other effects in the

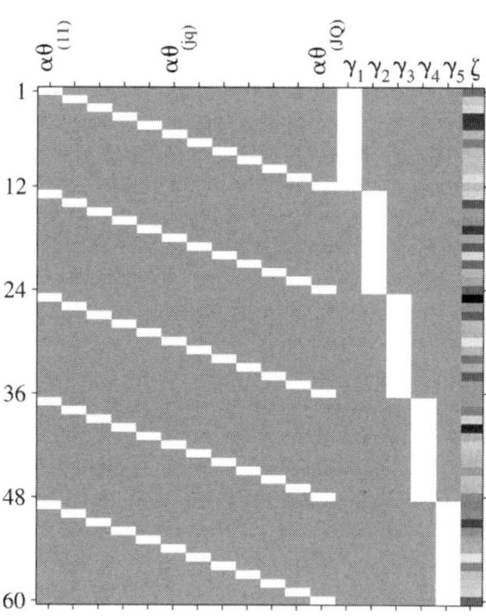

FIGURE 37.13
Multisubject activation experiment, "classic" SPM design, where each replication of each experimental condition is considered as a separate condition [Eq. (37.22)]. Illustrative design matrix image for five subjects, each having 12 scans, the scans having been ordered by subject and by condition and replication within subject. The columns are labeled with the corresponding parameter. The first 12 columns correspond to the "condition" effects, the next five to the subject effects, the last to the gCBF regression parameter.

model). Usually in statistical models, interaction terms are added to a model containing main effects. However, such a model is so overparameterised that the main effects may be omitted, leaving just the interaction terms. The model is

$$Y_{iqj}^{k} = \alpha\vartheta_{(qj)}^{k} + \gamma_{i}^{k} + \zeta^{k}(g_{iqj} - \bar{g}_{\bullet\bullet\bullet}) + \epsilon_{iqj}^{k} \tag{37.22}$$

where $\alpha\vartheta_{(qj)}^{k}$ is the interaction effect for replication j of condition q, the condition-by-replication effect. As with the previous model, this model is overparameterised (by one degree of freedom), and contrasts must have weights which sum to zero over the condition-by-replication effects. There are as many of these condition-by-replication terms as there are scans per subject. (An identical model is arrived at by considering each replication of each experimental condition as a separate condition.) If the scans are reordered such that the jth scan corresponds to the same replication of the same condition in each subject, then the condition-by-replication corresponds to the scan number. An example design matrix for five subjects scanned 12 times is shown in Fig. 37.13a, where the scans have been recorded. In SPM this is termed a *multisubject, conditions only* design.

This is the "classic" SPM ANCOVA described by Friston *et al.* (1990), and implemented in the original SPM software.[9] It offers great latitude for specification of contrasts. Appropriate contrasts can be used to assess main effects, specific forms of interaction, and even parametric effects. For instance, consider the verbal fluency dataset described by Friston *et al.* (1995)[10]: Five subjects were scanned 12 times, 6 times under each of two conditions, word shadowing (condition A) and intrinsic word generation (condition B). The scans were reordered to ABABABABABAB for all subjects. Then a contrast with weights (for the condition-by-replication effects) of $c_1 = [-1, 1, -1, 1, -1, 1, -1, 1, -1, 1, -1, 1]^T$ assesses the hypothesis of no main effect of word generation (against the one-sided alternative of activation). A contrast with weights of $c_1 = [5\frac{1}{2}, 4\frac{1}{2}, 3\frac{1}{2}, 2\frac{1}{2}, 1\frac{1}{2}, \frac{1}{2}, -\frac{1}{2}, -1\frac{1}{2}, -2\frac{1}{2}, -3\frac{1}{2}, -4\frac{1}{2}, -5\frac{1}{2}]^T$ is sensitive to linear decreases in rCBF over time, independent of condition, and accounting for subject effects and changes in gCBF. A contrast with weights of $c_1 = [1, -1, 1, -1, 1, -1, -1, 1, -1, 1, -1, 1]^T$ assesses the interaction of time and condition, subtracting the activation in the first half of the experiment from that in the latter half.

---

[9] The original SPM software is now fondly remembered as SPM *classic*.

[10] This dataset is available via http://www.fil.ion.ucl.ac.uk/spm/data/.

Interactions with subject Although it is usually reasonable to use ANCOVA style models to account for global flow, with regression parameters constant across conditions, the multisubject models considered thus far assume additionally that this regression parameter is constant across subjects. It is quite possible that rCBF at the same location for different subjects will respond differentially to changes in gCBF—a subject by gCBF covariate interaction. The gCBF regression parameter can be allowed to vary from subject to subject. Extending the multisubject activation (replication) model of Eq. (37.21) in this way gives

$$Y_{iqj}^k = \alpha_q^k + \gamma_i^k + \zeta_i^k(g_{iqj} - \bar{g}_{\bullet\bullet\bullet}) + \epsilon_{iqj}^k \tag{37.23}$$

Note the i subscript on the global slope term ζ_i^k, indicating a separate parameter for each subject. A schematic plot of rCBF vs. gCBF for this model and an example design matrix image are shown in Fig. 37.14. In the terminology of the SPM interface, this is an *ANCOVA by subject.* The additional parameters are of no interest, and contrasts are as before.

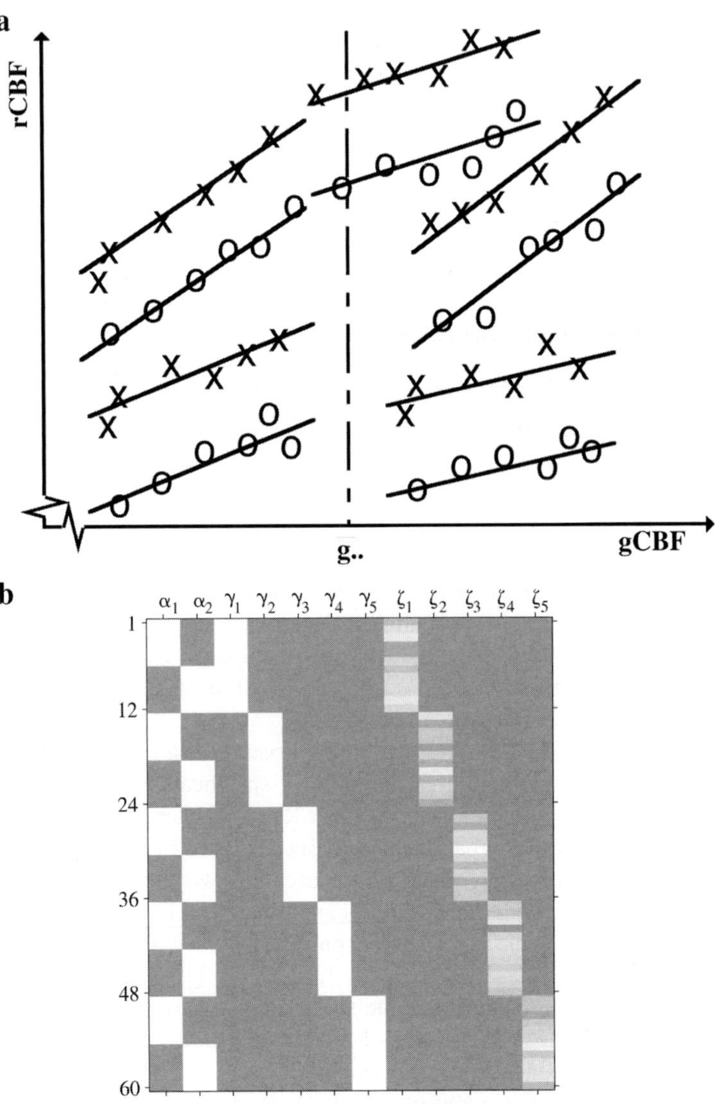

FIGURE 37.14
Multisubject activation experiment, replication of conditions, ANCOVA by subject for model of Eq. (37.23). Illustrations for a five-subject study, with six replications of each of two conditions per subject: (a) Illustrative plot of rCBF vs. gCBF. (b) Design matrix image. The first two columns correspond to the condition effects, the next five to the subject effects, the last five the gCBF regression parameters for each subject. The design matrix corresponds to scans ordered by subject and by condition within subjects.

Similarly, the SPM interface allows subject by covariate interactions, termed *subject-specific fits*. Subject by condition interactions can be entered by using *multisubject, conditions × subject interaction and covariates*.

Multistudy Designs

The last class of SPM models for PET we consider are the *multistudy models*. In these models, subjects are grouped into two or more *studies*. The multistudy designs fit separate condition effects for each study. In statistical terms this is a *split plot* design. As an example consider two multisubject activation studies, the first with five subjects scanned 12 times under two conditions (as described above), the second with three subjects scanned 6 times under three conditions. An example design matrix image for a model containing study-specific condition effects, subject effects, and study-specific global regression (termed *ANCOVA by group* in SPM) is shown in Fig. 37.15. The first two columns of the design matrix correspond to the condition effects for the first study, the next two to the condition effects for the second study, the next eight to the subject effects, and the last to the gCBF regression parameter. (The corresponding scans are assumed to be ordered by study, by subject within study, and by condition within subject.)

Contrasts for multistudy designs in SPM have weights that, when considered for each of the studies individually, would define a contrast for the study. Thus, contrasts must have weights which sum to zero over the condition effects within each study. Three types of useful comparison remain. The first is a comparison of condition effects within a single study, carried out in the context of a multistudy design; the contrast weights appropriate for the condition effects of the study of interest are entered, padded with zeros for the other study, e.g., $c_1 = [1, -1, 0, 0, 0]^T$ for the first study in our example. This may have additional power when compared to an analysis of this study in isolation, since the second study observations change the variance estimates. The second is an average effect across studies; contrasts for a particular effect in each of the studies are concatenated, the combined contrast assessing a mean effect across studies. For example, if the second study in our example has the same conditions as the first, plus an additional condition, then such a contrast would have weights for the effects of interest $c_1 = [-1, 1, -1, 1, 0]^T$. Last, differences of contrasts across studies can be assessed, such as differences in activation. The contrast weights for the appropriate main effect in each study are concatenated, with some studies' contrasts negated. In our example, $c_1 = [-1, 1, 1, -1, 0]^T$ would be appropriate for locating regions where the first study activated more than the second, or where the second deactivated more than the first.

Assumption of model fit in this case includes the assumption that the error terms have equal variance (at each voxel) across studies. For very different study populations, or studies from different scanners or protocols (possibly showing large differences in the measured global

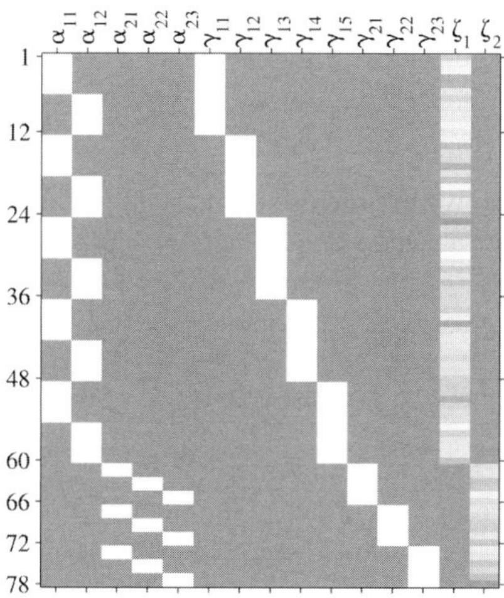

FIGURE 37.15
Design matrix image for the example multistudy activation experiment described in the text.

activity between studies), this assumption may not be tenable and the different variances should be modeled (Chapter 9).

Basic Models

In this section, we will discuss some of the models that are referred to in SPM as *basic models*. Typically, basic models are used for analyses at the second level to implement mixed effects models (Chapter 12). For example, basic models include the one-sample *t* test, the two-sample *t* test, the paired *t* test and a one-way ANCOVA, all of which are described in the following. For clarity, we drop the voxel superscript *k*.

One-Sample t Test

The one-sample *t* test can be used to test the null hypothesis that the mean of J scans equals zero. This is the simplest model available in SPM and the design matrix consists of just a constant regressor. The model is

$$Y = x_1\beta_1 + \epsilon \tag{37.24}$$

where x_1 is a constant vector of ones and $\epsilon \sim N(0, \sigma^2 I_J)$. The null hypothesis is $\mathcal{H}: \beta_1 = 0$ and the alternative hypothesis is $\overline{\mathcal{H}}: \beta_1 > 0$. The t value is computed using Eq. (37.12) as

$$T = \frac{\hat{\beta}_1}{\sqrt{\hat{\sigma}^2/J}} \sim t_{J-1} \tag{37.25}$$

where $\hat{\sigma}^2 = Y^T RY/(J-1)$, where R is the residual forming matrix (see above). In other words, $Y^T RY$ is the sum of squares of the residuals. This could also be expressed as $Y^T RY = \sum_{j=1}^{J} (Y_j - \hat{Y}_j)^2$, where $\hat{Y}_j = (x_1\hat{\beta}_1)_j = \hat{\beta}_1$.

Two-Sample t Test

The two-sample *t* test allows one to test the null hypothesis that the means of two groups are equal. The resulting SPM design matrix consists of three columns; the first two encode the group membership of each scan and the third models a common constant across scans of both groups. This model is overdetermined by one degree of freedom, i.e., the sum of the first two regressors equals the third regressor. Notice the difference in parameterisation compared to the earlier two-sample *t* test example. As it turns out, the resulting *t* value is nevertheless the same for a differential contrast. Let the number of scans in the first and second group be J_1 and J_2, where $J = J_1 + J_2$. The three regressors consists of ones and zeros, where the first regressor consists of J_1 ones, followed by J_2 zeros. The second regressor consists of J_1 zeros, followed by J_2 ones. The third regressor contains ones only.

Let the contrast vector be $c = [-1, 1, 0]^T$, i.e., the alternative hypothesis is $\overline{\mathcal{H}}: \beta_1 < \beta_2$. Then

$$(X^T X) = \begin{pmatrix} J_1 & 0 & J_1 \\ 0 & J_2 & J_2 \\ J_1 & J_2 & J \end{pmatrix}$$

This matrix is rank deficient so we use the pseudo-inverse $(X^T X)^-$ to compute the t statistic. We sandwich $(X^T X)^-$ with the contrast and get $c^T(X^T X)^- c = 1/J_1 + 1/J_2$. The t statistic is then given by

$$T = \frac{\hat{\beta}_2 - \hat{\beta}_1}{\sqrt{\hat{\sigma}^2/(1/J_1 + 1/J_2)}} \sim t_{J-2} \tag{37.26}$$

and $\hat{\sigma}^2 = Y^T \mathrm{RY}/(J-2)$. Note that one assumption for the two-sample *t* test is that $J_1 = J_2$, i.e., the number of scans in both groups is the same. However, it turns out that the two-sample *t* test is rather robust against a violation of this assumption. Another assumption which we implicitly made in Eq. (37.26) is that we have equal variance in both groups. This assumption may not be tenable (e.g., when comparing normal subjects with patients) and we potentially have to take this nonsphericity into account (Chapter 9).

Paired t Test

The model underlying the paired t test is an extension to the model underlying the two-sample t test. It is assumed that the scans come in pairs, i.e., one scan of each pair is in the first group and the other is in the second group. The extension is that the means over pairs are not assumed to be equal, i.e., the mean of each pair has to be modeled separately. For instance, let the number of pairs be $N_{\text{pairs}} = 5$, i.e., the number of scans is $J = 10$. The design matrix consists of seven regressors. The first two model the deviation from the pair-wise mean within group and the last five model the pair-specific means. The model has degrees of freedom one less than the number of regressors.

Let the contrast vector be $c = [-1, 1, 0, 0, 0, 0, 0]^T$, i.e., the alternative hypothesis is $\overline{\mathcal{H}} : \beta_1 < \beta_2$. This leads to

$$T = \frac{\hat{\beta}_2 - \hat{\beta}_1}{\sqrt{\hat{\sigma}^2/(1/J_1 + 1/J_2)}} \sim t_{J-J/2-1} \tag{37.27}$$

The difference to the two-sample t test lies in the degrees of freedom $J - J/2 - 1$. The two-sample t test and the paired t test are an example of compromising when selecting a model. The paired t test can be a more appropriate model for a given dataset, but more effects are modelled, i.e., there are fewer error degrees of freedom. This might come at the price of a decrease in sensitivity so that the two-sample t test can be less appropriate, but more sensitive. This compromise is increasingly harder to make with a smaller number of scans J.

One-Way ANCOVA

A one-way ANCOVA allows one to model group effects, i.e., the mean of each of Q groups. This model includes the one-sample and two-sample t tests, i.e., the cases, when $1 \leq Q \leq 2$.

In our example, let the number of groups be $Q = 3$, where there are five scans within each group, i.e., $J_q = 5$ for $q = 1,\ldots,Q$. A range of different contrasts is available. For instance, we could test the null hypothesis that the group means are all equal using the F contrast as described earlier. Here, we wish to test the null hypothesis, whether the mean of the first two groups is equal to the mean of the third group, i.e., $\mathcal{H}: (\beta_1 + \beta_2)/2 - \beta_3 = 0$. Our alternative hypothesis is $\overline{\mathcal{H}} : (\beta_1 + \beta_2)/2 < \beta_3$. This can be tested based on a t statistic, where we use the contrast $c = [-1/2, -1/2, 1, 0]^T$. The resulting t statistic and its distribution are

$$T = \frac{(\hat{\beta}_1 - \hat{\beta}_2)/2 - \hat{\beta}_3}{\sqrt{\hat{\sigma}^2/(1/J_1 + 1/J_2 + 1/J_3)}} \sim t_{J-Q} \tag{37.28}$$

fMRI MODELS

In this section, we describe the analysis of fMRI data. For PET, we showed that we can use the general linear model to analyze the data. The models used to interpret fMRI data are modified due to differences in the character of fMRI data compared to PET. These differences include (1) serial temporal correlations, (2) fast event-related designs, and (3) the large number of observations. A linear model can still be used, but the normally distributed error term is nonspherical.[11]

Historically, SPM was developed for and applied to PET data and therefore it is not a surprise that SPM for fMRI data was initially based on the understanding that SPM would just need some extensions to cope with the new kind of data. In this section, we therefore not only describe these extensions, but also describe the model from scratch. This has the benefits (1) that the modelling issues in fMRI analysis are described without the need to refer to PET issues and (2) that one can skip most of the PET section if trying to learn about fMRI analysis.

The topics of this section are a linear time-series model for fMRI data, temporal serial correlations and their estimation, temporal filtering, parameter estimation, and inference.

[11] *Nonsphericity* refers to the deviation of the error covariance matrix from a diagonal shape or a shape that can be transformed into a diagonal shape. See also Chapter 9.

Linear Time-Series Model

One of the mainstays of SPM is that we use the same temporal model at each voxel, i.e., we use a mass-univariate model and perform the same analysis at each voxel. Therefore, we can describe the complete temporal model for fMRI data by looking at how the data from a single voxel (a time series) is modeled. A time series consists of the sequential measures of fMRI signal intensities over the period of the experiment. Usually, fMRI data are acquired for the whole brain with a sample time of roughly 2–4 sec using an echo planar imaging (EPI) sequence. This means that a time series at a single voxel is acquired with a sample time of 2–4 sec.

Multisubject data are acquired in sessions, there being one or more sessions for each subject.[12] Here, we only talk about a model for one of these sessions, i.e., a single-subject analysis. Multisubject studies are based on multiple single-subject models and are described in Chapter 12.

The process we are going to describe in the following is at the heart of SPM. We take as an input a single time series and transform it to a single statistical value. This statistic can then be used to derive a p value. This is done simultaneously at all voxels so that a SPM is formed with one statistic at each voxel.

Suppose we have a time series of N observations $Y_1,\ldots,Y_s,\ldots,Y_N$, acquired at one voxel at times t_s, where $s = 1,\ldots,N$ is the *scan number.* The approach is to model at each voxel the observed time series as a linear combination of explanatory functions, plus an error term:

$$Y_s = \beta_1 f^1(t_s) + \ldots + \beta_l f^l(t_s) + \ldots + \beta_L f^L(t_s) + \epsilon_s \tag{37.29}$$

Here the L functions $f^1(.),\ldots,f^L(.)$ are a suitable set of *regressors,* designed such that linear combinations of them span the space of possible fMRI responses for this experiment, up to the level of error. Consider writing out the above Eq. (37.29) for all time points t_s, to give a set of equations as follows:

$$\begin{aligned}
Y_1 &= \beta_1 f^1(t_s) + \ldots + \beta_l f^l(t_1) + \ldots + f^L(t_1)\beta_L + \epsilon_1 \\
\vdots &= \vdots \\
Y_s &= \beta_1 f^1(t_s) + \ldots + \beta_l f^l(t_s) + \ldots + f^L(t_s)\beta_L + \epsilon_s \\
\vdots &= \vdots \\
Y_N &= \beta_1 f^1(t_N) + \ldots + \beta_l f^l(t_N) + \ldots + f^L(t_N)\beta_L + \epsilon_N
\end{aligned}$$

which in matrix form is

$$\begin{pmatrix} Y_1 \\ \vdots \\ Y_s \\ \vdots \\ Y_N \end{pmatrix} = \begin{pmatrix} f^1(t_1) & \ldots & f^l(t_1) & \ldots & f^L(t_1) \\ \vdots & \ddots & \vdots & \ddots & \vdots \\ f^1(t_s) & \ldots & f^l(t_s) & \ldots & f^L(t_s) \\ \vdots & \ddots & \vdots & \ddots & \vdots \\ f^1(t_N) & \ldots & f^l(t_N) & \ldots & f^L(t_N) \end{pmatrix} \begin{pmatrix} \beta_1 \\ \vdots \\ \beta_l \\ \vdots \\ \beta_L \end{pmatrix} + \begin{pmatrix} \epsilon_1 \\ \vdots \\ \epsilon_s \\ \vdots \\ \epsilon_N \end{pmatrix} \tag{37.30}$$

or in matrix notation

$$Y = X\beta + \epsilon \tag{37.31}$$

Here each column of the design matrix X contains the values of one of the continuous regressors evaluated at each time point t_s of the fMRI time series. That is, the columns of the design matrix are the discretised regressors.

The regressors must be chosen to span the space of all possible fMRI responses for the experiment in question, such that the error vector ϵ is normally distributed with zero mean. As will be discussed later, ϵ is not assumed to be spherically distributed. Rather, we will consider other forms for the covariance matrix of ϵ. This leads us out of the realm of the general linear model to the much broader class, the generalised linear model (GLM). However, because we are modelling the data with a normally distributed error term and do not consider other error distributions or so-called *link functions,* we look at a rather constrained class of GLMs.

---

[12] The term *session* will be defined later.

Proportional and Grand Mean Scaling

Before we proceed to the description of how the regressors in the design matrix are generated, we want to mention the issue of global normalisation. fMRI data are known to be subject to various processes that cause globally distributed confounding effects (e.g., Andersson et al., 2001). A rather simple global confounding source is the scanner gain. This volume-wise gain is a factor that scales the whole image and is known to vary slowly during a session. A simple way to remove the effect of such a varying gain is to estimate this gain per image and multiply all image intensities by this gain estimate. This method is known as *proportional scaling.*

If one does not use proportional scaling, SPM performs by default a session-specific scaling. This type of scaling divides each volume by a session-specific gain. This is known in SPM as *grand mean scaling.* Session-specific grand mean scaling is highly recommended, because the session-specific gains can strongly vary between sessions, masking any activations.

To estimate the gain factors, SPM uses a rough estimate of the volume-wise intracerebral mean intensity. Note that both kinds of scaling also scale the mean global activity (either of a volume or of a session) to 100. The data and a signal change can then be conveniently interpreted as percent with respect to the estimated global intracerebral mean.

Generation of Regressors

In the following, we will describe how the regressors in Eq. (37.30) are generated and what the underlying model of the BOLD response is. This process consists of several stages. Although these are mostly hidden from the user, it can be helpful to know about intermediate processing steps and their temporal sequence.

The overall aim of regressor generation is to come up with a design matrix that models the expected fMRI response at any voxel as a linear combination of its columns. Basically, SPM needs to know two things to construct the design matrix. The first is the timings of the experiment and the second is the expected shape of the BOLD response due to stimulus presentation. Given this information, SPM computes the design matrix. In the following, we will go through the stages of this process.

Timing

We describe how a design matrix for one session of functional data is generated. Let the number of scans in a session be N_{scans}. Furthermore, it is important that the data be ordered according to acquisition order.

In SPM a session starts at session time zero. This time point is given when the first slice of the first scan was started to be acquired by the scanner. Session time can be measured both in scans or in seconds. In both cases the session starts at time zero regardless of the units. The duration of a session is the number of scans multiplied by the volume repetition time (RT), which is the time spent from the beginning of the acquisition of one scan to the beginning of the acquisition of the next scan. We assume that RT stays constant throughout a session. The RT and the number of scans of a given session completely define the start and the end of a session. Moreover, because we assume that RT stays constant throughout the experiment, one also knows the onset of each scan.

The design of the experiment is described as a series of trials or events, where each trial is associated with a trial type. Let N^m_{trials} be the number of trials of trial type m and N_{types} the number of trial types. For each trial j of trial type m, one needs to specify its onset and duration. Note that we do not need to make a distinction between event-related or blocked designs so that a trial can be either a short event or an epoch. Let the onset vector of trial type m be O^m so that O^m_j is the onset of trial j of trial type m. For example, the onset of a trial that started at the beginning of scan 4 is at session time 3 (in scans) or at session time $3 \cdot \text{RT}$ (in seconds). Let vector D^m contain the user-specified stimulus durations of each trial for trial type m.

Given all onsets O^m and durations D^m, SPM generates an internal representation of the session and the experiment. This representation consists of the discretised stimulus function S^m for each trial type m. All time bins of a session are covered such that the vectors S^m represent a contiguous series of time bins. These time bins typically do not cover a time period of length RT, but a fraction of it to provide a well-sampled discretised version of the stimulus functions S^m, i.e., they are oversampled.

The occurrence of a stimulus is binarily represented in the stimulus functions. The elements of the stimulus function can also contain other values. An important application of this lies in the concept of *parametric modulation.*

Note that the degree of discretisation of the stimulus functions is controlled by the user. Time bin size is specified in number of time bins per RT.[13]

For example, assume the RT is 3.2 sec. Then each time bin given the default of 16 bins/RT covers 200 msec. The length of the vector S^m is $16N_{\text{scans}}$. Note that choosing a smaller time bin size does not necessarily provide a higher temporal precision for the resulting regressors in the design matrix. This is because the expected BOLD response is located in a rather low frequency band. Therefore, responses to trials being only a few milliseconds apart from each other are virtually indistinguishable.

High-Resolution Basis Functions

After the generation of the stimulus functions, we need to describe the shape of the expected response. This is done using temporal basis functions. During the development of SPM during the last few years, some effort has gone into designing sets of basis functions that appropriately model the expected blood oxygen level dependent (BOLD) response. The underlying model is that the BOLD response for a given trial type m is generated by feeding the stimulus function through a linear finite impulse response (FIR) system, whose output is the observed data Y. This is expressed by the model

$$Y = d\left(\sum_{m=1}^{N_{types}} h^m \otimes S^m\right) + \epsilon \tag{37.32}$$

where h^m is the impulse response function for trial type m. The $\otimes$ operator denotes the convolution of two vectors (Bracewell, 1986), and $d(\cdot)$ denotes the down-sampling operation which is needed to sample the convolved stimulus functions at each sampled time point. In other words, the observed data Y are modeled by summing the output of N_{types} different linear systems. Additionally, we add some measurement noise ϵ. The input to the mth linear system is the stimulus function of trial type m.

The impulse response functions h^m are not known, but we assume that they can be modeled as linear combinations of some basis functions b_i:

$$Y = \sum_{m=1}^{N_{types}} \sum_{i=1}^{N_{bf}} d(b_i \beta_i^m \otimes S^m) + \epsilon \tag{37.33}$$

where β_i^m is the ith coefficient for trial type m and N_{bf} is the number of basis functions b_i. We can move the coefficients so that we get

$$Y = d([(b \otimes S^1)\beta^1 + \ldots + (b \otimes S^{N_{types}})\beta^{N_{types}}]) + \epsilon \tag{37.34}$$

where

$$b = [b_1,\ldots,b_{N_{bf}}] \text{ and } \beta^m = [\beta_1^{mT},\ldots,\beta_{N_{bf}}^{mT}]^T$$

Note that we define the convolution to operate on the columns of matrix b. If we let

$$X = d[(b \otimes S^1):\ldots:(b \otimes S^{N_{types}})] \text{ and } \beta = [\beta^{1^T},\ldots,\beta^{N_{types}T}]^T$$

we see that Eq. (37.34) is a linear model like Eq. (37.31). The columns of the design matrix X are given by the discretely sampled convolution of each of the N_{types} stimulus functions with each of the N_{bf} basis functions. Note that although we assumed different impulse response functions for each trial type m, our parameterisation leads to the same basis functions b_i for each trial type, but different parameter vectors $\beta_1^m,\ldots, \beta_{N_{bf}}^m$.

In summary, when we choose a specific basis function set b_i, we express our belief that a linear combination of the convolved basis functions is able to model an experimentally induced effect. The question remains of which basis function set is appropriate for fMRI data. In SPM, the default choice is a parameterised model of the expected impulse response function. This

[13] The effective time bin size is accessible in SPM as variable fMRI_T. Its default value is 16.

function is a superposition of two gamma functions. To form an appropriate basis function set, one usually complements this function with its first partial derivatives with respect to some generating parameters. In SPM, the default choice is to add partial derivatives with respect to two generating parameters, the onset and dispersion. This gives a basis function set with three basis functions: b_1 is the expected response function, b_2 its partial derivative with respect to onset (time) and b_3 its partial derivative with respect to dispersion. In SPM, this set is usually referred to as the *hemodynamic response function (HRF) with derivatives*. In practice, this set can model a BOLD response that (1) can be slightly shifted in time with respect to the expected delay or (2) has a different width than the HRF model b_1. This issue is dealt within more detail in Chapter 10.

Parametric Modulation

When we first introduced the stimulus functions S^m they were described as vectors consisting of ones and zeros. However, one can also assign numbers other than 1 to the S^m. More interestingly, one can assign different values to different individual trials. As one can see from Eq. (37.34), after convolution of the S^m with the basis functions b_i, different weights in S^m essentially control the relative height of the expected response of all trials. This weighting allows models where one can parametrically modulate the relative response height over trials. There is a wide range of applications for parametric modulations. For instance, one can weight events by a linear function of time, which models a linear change in the individual responses over time. Another application is the weighting of S^m with some external measure that was acquired trial-wise, e.g., reaction times. Such a modulated regressor would allow one to test for a linear dependence between reaction times and height of response while taking into account all other modeled effects. Higher order modulations can be modeled by polynomial expansions of the modulation, which give us multiple parametrically modulated regressors per trial type.

Low-Resolution Basis Functions

In Eq. (37.34), a down-sampling operator d was applied to sample the high-resolution (continuous) regressors to the low-resolution space of the data Y. Here, one has to be aware of a slight limitation of the SPM model for event-related data that arises due to the use of the same temporal model at each voxel.

fMRI data are typically acquired slice-wise so that a small amount of time elapses from the acquisition of one slice to the next. Given standard EPI sequences, acquisition of one slice takes roughly 100 msec. Therefore, an optimal sampling of the high-resolution basis functions does not exist, because any chosen sampling will only be optimal for one slice, but not for all others. The largest timing error is given for a slice that lies in acquisition order $\lfloor N_{\text{slices}}/2 \rfloor$ slices away from the slice for which the temporal model is exact.[14] This sampling issue is only relevant for event-related designs, where one typically uses short stimulus durations that elicit BOLD responses lasting only some seconds. For these transient responses, an appropriate temporal model is critical. Any difference in expected and actual onset may decrease the sensitivity of the analysis if one uses a naive HRF model (e.g., only the HRF model without its derivatives). For blocked designs, timing errors are small compared to epoch length so that the potential loss in sensitivity is negligible.

In SPM, there are two ways to solve this timing issue and take the different slice acquisition times into account. The first is to choose one time point within volume acquisition time and temporally interpolate all slices at this time. This is called *slice timing correction*. However, note that this interpolation requires rather short RT (<3 sec), because the sampling should be dense enough in relation to the width of the BOLD response to capture its interesting peak. The second option is to model latency differences with the temporal derivative of the HRF set. As discussed above, the temporal derivative can model a temporal shift of the expected BOLD response. This temporal shift can not only capture onset timing differences due to different slice times, but also differences due to, for example, a different vascular response onset. However, due to the linear nature of the model, the temporal derivative can only model small shifts (forward or backward in time). With the HRF basis functions set, the temporal derivative can accommodate a shift

[14] $\lfloor x \rfloor$ denotes the nearest integer less or equal to x.

backward or forward of slightly more than 1 sec. The slice timing interpolation is recommended if one looks for voxel-specific timing differences between conditions. Independently of this, we recommend the use of the temporal derivative as part of the model to capture any potential latency differences.

One also needs to specify at what time bin, in scan time, SPM samples the regressors to generate the design matrix. The SPM default is 1, i.e., the first time bin after the start of a scan.[15]

Finally, the down-sampled basis functions are mean corrected and entered column-wise into the design matrix X [Eq. (37.30)]. A baseline is modeled by adding a constant regressor to the design matrix.

Additional Regressors

It is possible to use additional regressors in the model without going through the process described above. For instance, consider the case for which an additional physiological measurement was acquired during the session at a high temporal resolution. These measurements can be added to the design matrix after suitable down-sampling. Another important example for user-specified regressors is the modelling of movement correlated effects. These can be taken into account to a first order by adding the estimated movement parameters as regressors (see Chapter 2). Note that all user-specified regressors are automatically mean corrected by SPM.

Serial Correlations

fMRI data exhibit short-range serial temporal correlations. By this we mean that the error ϵ_s at a given scan s is correlated with its temporal neighbours. This has to be modeled, because correlations play an important role when assessing the significance of a test statistic. Ignoring correlations leads to an inappropriate estimate of the error covariance matrix, which is propagated to the estimated parameter covariance matrix. In other words, when forming a t or F statistic, we have a biased estimate of the variability of a contrast. Additionally, when using ordinary least-squares estimates, the null statistic, which is used when computing p values, is also dependent on the error covariance matrix. This dependency occurs when estimating the effective degrees of freedom of a null distribution.[16] With serial correlations present and modeled, the effective degrees of freedom are lower than in the independent case. The overall picture is that ignoring serial correlations leads generally to too lenient and therefore invalid tests. To derive correct tests we have to appropriately estimate the error covariance matrix by assuming some kind of nonsphericity (Chapter 9). Then, we use this estimate in the computation of the statistic and the effective degrees of freedom.

Note that we are only concerned about the serial correlations of the error component ϵ of the time series of Eq. (37.31). The correlations induced by the experimental design should be modeled by the design matrix X.

Serial correlations in fMRI data are caused by various sources including cardiac, respiratory, and vasomotor sources (Mitra et al., 1997).

Two issues need to be resolved. The first is how to estimate the error covariance matrix and the second is how to incorporate this estimate into our modelling framework and derive a valid statistical test. In what follows we describe the statistics that are based on ordinary least-squares (OLS) parameter estimates.

One model that seems to capture the observed form of serial correlations in fMRI data is the autoregressive (order 1) plus white noise model (AR(1)+wn) (Purdon and Weisskoff, 1998).[17] This model accounts for short-range correlations. Note that the order of the model (one) means that the form and amount of correlations can be modeled by one (AR) coefficient. The model order does not refer to the range of the serial correlations in time. We only need to model short-range correlations, because we also apply a high-pass filter to the data. The high-pass filter removes any low-frequency components and thus long-range correlations from the data.

[15] This sampling point is accessible in SPM as variable $fMRI_T0$ and lies between 1 and $fMRI_T$, the number of time bins.

[16] *Effective degrees of freedom* refers to the degrees of freedom of an approximation to the underlying null distribution (Worsley and Friston, 1995).

[17] The AR(1)+wn is also known as the autoregressive moving-average model of order (1,1) (ARMA(1,1)).

We refer the interested reader to the Appendix for a mathematical description of the AR(1)+wn model.

Estimation of the Error Covariance Matrix

Having decided that the AR(1)+wn is an appropriate model for the fMRI error covariance matrix, we need to estimate its three hyperparameters at each voxel. The hyperparameterised model gives an autocovariance matrix at each voxel [Eq. (37.45)], which we want to estimate. In SPM, an additional assumption is made to estimate this matrix more efficiently, which is described in the following.

Mathematically, the error covariance matrix can be partitioned into two components. The first component is the correlation matrix and the second component is the variance. The assumption made by SPM is that the correlation matrix is the same at all voxels of interest (see Chapter 9 for further details). The variance is assumed to be different between voxels. In other words, SPM assumes that the pattern of serial correlations is the same over all interesting voxels, but its amplitude is different at each voxel. This assumption seems to be quite a sensible one, because we observed that the serial correlations over voxels within tissue types are very similar. The estimate of the serial correlations is therefore extremely precise because of the large number of voxels involved in the estimation. Therefore, the correlation matrix at each voxel can be assumed to be known.

In the following, we describe the model and estimation of the error covariance matrix. Let us start with the linear model for voxel k:

$$Y^k = X\beta^k + \epsilon^k \tag{37.35}$$

where Y^k is an $N \times 1$ observed time-series vector at voxel k, X is an $N \times L$ design matrix, β^k is the parameter vector, and ϵ^k is the error at voxel k. The error ϵ^k is normally distributed with $\epsilon \sim N(0, \sigma^{k^2} V)$. The critical difference to Eq. (37.6) is the distribution of the error term where the identity matrix I is replaced by the correlation matrix V. Note that V does not depend on the voxel position k, i.e., we make the above-mentioned assumption that the correlation matrix V is the same for all voxels $k = 1,\ldots,K$. However, the variance σ^{k^2} is assumed to be different for each voxel.

How can the correlation matrix V be estimated over all voxels? Since we made the assumption that V is the same at each voxel, we can either estimate V at each voxel and then pool our estimate, or we can pool data from all voxels and then estimate V on this pooled data. We use the second method, because it is computationally much more efficient. The pooled data are given by summing the sampled covariance matrix of all interesting voxels k, i.e., $V_Y = \Sigma_k Y^k Y^k T$. Note that the pooled V_Y is a mixture of two components, the experimentally induced variance and the error variance component:

$$V_Y = \sum_k X\beta^k \beta^{k^T} X^T + \epsilon^k \epsilon^{k^T} \tag{37.36}$$

One way of estimating the error covariance matrix $\text{cov}(\epsilon^k) = \sigma^{k^2} V$ is to use the restricted maximum likelihood (ReML) method (Harville, 1977; Friston *et al.*, 2002). ReML takes the space spanned by the design matrix into account and is an unbiased estimator of the hyperparameters. ReML works with linear covariance constraints, i.e., the estimated covariance matrix is modeled as a linear combination of some covariance constraints. The concept of covariance constraints is a very general concept that can be used to model all kinds of nonsphericity (see Chapter 9). The model described in the Appendix, Eq. (37.44), is nonlinear in the hyperparameters so ReML cannot be used directly. But if we linearise the covariance constraints

$$V = \sum_l \lambda_l Q_l \tag{37.37}$$

where Q_l are $N \times N$ constraint matrices and the λ_l are the hyperparameters, ReML can be applied. We are interested in specifying the Q_l such that they form an appropriate model for serial correlations of fMRI data when using standard EPI sequences. The default model in SPM is to use two constraints, Q_1 and Q_2. These are $Q_1 = I_N$ and

$$Q_{2_{ij}} = \begin{cases} e^{-|i-j|} & : \; i \neq j \\ 0 & : \; i = j \end{cases} \tag{37.38}$$

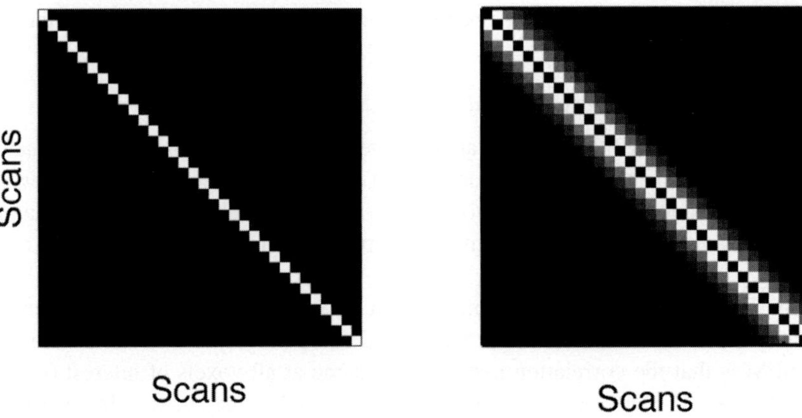

FIGURE 37.16
Graphical illustration of the two covariance constraints used for estimating the error correlation matrix. (Left) Constraint Q_1 imposes a stationary variance onto the estimate. (Right) Constraint Q_2 implements the AR(1) model part with an autoregressive coefficient of $1/e$.

Figure 37.16 shows the shape of Q_1 and Q_2.

A voxel-wide estimate of V is then derived by rescaling V such that V is a correlation matrix.

This method of estimating the covariance matrix at each voxel uses the two voxel-wide (global) hyperparameters λ_1 and λ_2. A third voxel-wise (local) hyperparameter (the *variance* σ^2) is estimated at each voxel using the usual estimator (Worsley and Friston, 1995):

$$\sigma^{k^2} = \frac{Y^{k^T} R Y^k}{\text{trace}(RV)} \tag{37.39}$$

where R is the residual forming matrix. This completes the estimation of the serial correlations at each voxel k. Before we can use these estimates to derive statistical tests, we still need to describe the high-pass filter and what role it plays in modelling fMRI data.

Temporal Filtering

The concept of filtering is based on the observation that certain frequency bands in the data contain more noise than others. In an ideal world, our experimentally induced effects would live in one frequency band and all of the noise in another. Applying a filter that removes the noise frequency range from the data would then give us increased sensitivity. However, the data are a mixture of activation and noise that can share some frequency bands. One of the experimenter's tasks is therefore to make sure that the interesting effects do not lie in a frequency range that is especially exposed to noise processes. In fMRI, the low frequencies (say, less than half a cycle per minute, i.e., 1/120 Hz) are known to contain scanner drifts and possibly cardiac/respiratory artifacts. Any activations that lie within this frequency range are virtually undistinguishable from these noise processes. This is why (1) fMRI data should be high-pass filtered to remove noise and (2) the experimenter should take care to construct a design that puts the interesting contrasts into higher frequencies than 1/120 Hz. This issue is especially important for event-related designs and is dealt with in Chapter 10. Here, we describe how the high-pass filter is implemented.

The *high-pass filter* is implemented using a set of discrete cosine transform (DCT) basis functions. These are part of the design matrix. To the user of SPM, they are *invisible* in the sense that the DCT regressors are never plotted. This is simply to save space on the display. In practice, the parameters of the DCT part of the design matrix are not estimated, but the residual forming matrix of the DCT regressors are applied to the data. Only after this step, the other (visible) part of the design matrix is fitted to the resulting residuals. This procedure is equivalent to estimating all model parameters simultaneously, where all tests of hypotheses automatically take low-frequency noise components into account.

Mathematically, for time points $t = 1,\ldots,N$, the discrete cosine set functions are $f_r(t) = \sqrt{2/N}\,[\cos(r\pi\frac{t}{N})]$. See Fig. 37.17 for an example. The integer index r ranges from 1 (giving half

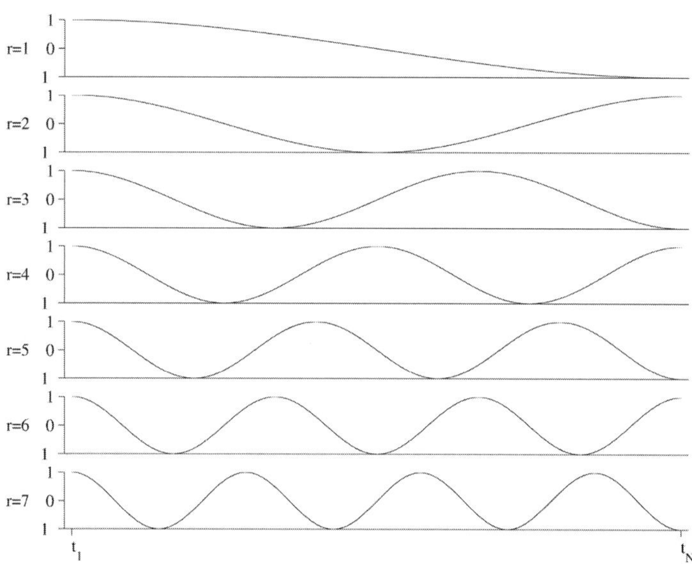

FIGURE 37.17
A discrete cosine transform set.

a cosine cycle over the N time points) to a user-specified maximum R. Note that SPM asks for a high-pass cutoff d_{cut} in seconds; R is then chosen as $R = \lfloor 2N\ RT/d_{cut} + 1 \rfloor$.

To summarise, the following picture emerges. The regressors in the design matrix X must account for all components in the fMRI time series up to the level of residual noise. The high-pass filter is part of the design matrix and removes unwanted low-frequency components from the data. The estimation of the error covariance matrix is based on a model similar to the AR(1)+wn model and uses the ReML method for estimation of the hyperparameters. In the next section, we describe how the model parameter estimates are used to form a t or F statistic at each voxel.

Parameter Estimates and Distributional Results

In this section, we describe the equations that lead to a t or F statistic. These statistics can be used to make inferences about the data by computing a p value at each voxel. For clarity, we drop the voxel index superscript k.

Ordinary least-squares parameter estimates $\hat{\beta}$ are given by

$$\hat{\beta} = (X^T X)^- X^T Y = X^- Y \tag{37.40}$$

As described above, we estimate the error correlation matrix V using the ReML method. The error covariance matrix is then given by $\hat{\sigma}^2 V$ [Eq. (37.39)]. The covariance matrix of the parameter estimate is

$$Var(\hat{\beta}) = \sigma^2 X^- V X^{-T} \tag{37.41}$$

A t statistic can then be formed by dividing a contrast of the estimated parameters $c^T\hat{\beta}$ by its estimated standard deviation:

$$T = \frac{c^T\hat{\beta}}{\sqrt{\hat{\sigma}^2 c^T X^- V X^{-T} c}} \tag{37.42}$$

where σ^2 is estimated using Eq. (37.39).

The key difference to the spherical case, i.e., when the error is i.i.d., is that the correlation matrix V enters into the denominator of the t value. This gives us a more accurate t statistic. However, because of V the denominator of Eq. (37.42) is not the square root of a χ^2 distribution. (The denominator would be exactly χ^2 distributed, when V describes a spherical distribution.) This means that Eq. (37.42) is not t distributed and we cannot simply make inferences by comparing with a t null distribution with trace (RV) degrees of freedom.

Instead, one approximates the denominator with a χ^2 distribution [Eq. (37.42)]. Consequently, T is then approximated by a t distribution. The approximation proposed by Worsley and Friston (1995) is the Satterthwaite approximation (see also Yandell, 1997), which is based on fitting the first two moments of the denominator distribution with a χ^2 distribution. The degrees of freedom of the approximating χ^2 distribution are called the *effective* degrees of freedom and are given by

$$v = \frac{2E(\hat{\sigma}^2)^2}{\text{var}(\hat{\sigma}^2)} = \frac{\text{trace}(RV)^2}{\text{trace}(RV\,RV)} \tag{37.43}$$

See the Appendix for a derivation of this Satterthwaite approximation.

Similarly, the null distribution of an F statistic in the presence of serial correlations can be approximated. In this case, both the numerator and denominator of the F value are approximated by a χ^2 distribution.

Summary

After reconstruction, realignment, spatial normalisation, and smoothing, functional imaging data are ready for statistical analysis. This involves two steps: First, statistics indicating evidence against a null hypothesis of no effect at each voxel are computed. An image of these statistics is then produced. Second, this statistical image must be assessed, reliably locating voxels where an effect is exhibited while limiting the possibility of false positives. These two steps are referred to as (1) modelling and (2) inference and they are covered separately in this book.

As models are designed with inference in mind, it is often difficult to separate the two issues. However, the inference section, Section 3 in Part II of this book, is largely concerned with the multiple comparison, that is, how to correctly make inferences from large volumes of statistic images. A distinction can be made between such *image-level* inference and statistical inference at a single voxel. This second sort of inference has been covered in this chapter and will be dealt with further in the remainder of Section 2.

We have shown how the general linear model, the workhorse of functional imaging analysis, provides a single framework for many statistical tests and models, giving great flexibility for experimental design and analysis. The use of such models will be further highlighted in the following chapters, especially Chapters 8 and 9. Additionally, to incorporate nonspherical error distributions, SPM uses covariance constraints and the ReML estimator. This is described further in Chapter 9.

In Chapters 10 and 11 we focus on modelling issues specific to fMRI and in Chapters 12 and 13 consider making inferences from multiple subject fMRI and PET studies. In Chapter 13 we take up recent developments in the field which make used of hierarchical models. This introduction to the area paves the way for further development in Section 2, in particular Chapter 17.

APPENDIX

Autoregressive Model of Order 1 Plus White Noise

Mathematically, the AR(1)+wn model at voxel k can be written in state-space form:

$$\begin{aligned} \epsilon(s) &= z(s) + \delta_\epsilon(s) \\ z(s) &= az(s-1) + \delta_z(s) \end{aligned} \tag{37.44}$$

where $\delta_\epsilon(s) \sim N(0, \sigma_\epsilon^2)$, $\delta_z(s) \sim N(0, \sigma_z^2)$, and a is the AR(1) coefficient. This model describes the error component $\epsilon(s)$ at time point s and at voxel k as the sum of an autoregressive component $z(s)$ plus white noise $\delta_\epsilon(s)$. We have three variance parameters at each voxel k, the variances of the two error components δ_ϵ and δ_z and the autoregressive coefficient a. The resulting error covariance matrix is then given by

$$E(\epsilon\epsilon^T) = \sigma_z^2(I_N - A)^{-1}(I_N - A)^{-T} + \sigma_\epsilon^2 \tag{37.45}$$

where A is a matrix with all elements of the first lower off-diagonal set to a and zero elsewhere, and I_N is the identity matrix of dimension N.

Satterthwaite Approximation

The unbiased estimator for σ^2 is given by dividing the sum of the squared residuals by its expectation (Worsley and Friston, 1995). Let e be the residuals $e = RY$, where R is the residual forming matrix:

$$\begin{aligned} E(e^Te) &= E[\text{trace}(ee^T)] \\ &= \text{E}[\text{trace}(RYY^T R^T)] \\ &= \text{trace}(R\sigma^2 V R^T) \\ &= \sigma^2 \,\text{trace}(RV) \end{aligned}$$

An unbiased estimator of σ^2 is given by $\hat{\sigma}^2 = \frac{e^T\text{e}}{\text{trace}(RV)}$. If V is a diagonal matrix with identical nonzero elements, trace(RV) = trace$(R) = J - p$, where J is the number of observations and p the number of parameters.

In what follows, we derive the Satterthwaite approximation to a χ^2 distribution given a nonspherical error covariance matrix.

We approximate the distribution of the squared denominator of the t value [Eq. (37.42)] $d = \hat{\sigma}^2 c^T(X^TX)^- X^TV\,\text{X}(X^TX)^- c$ with a scaled χ^2 variate, i.e.,

$$d \sim p(ay) \tag{37.46}$$

where $p(y) \sim \chi^2(\nu)$. We want to estimate the effective degrees of freedom ν. Note that, for a $\chi^2(\nu)$ distribution, $E(y) = \nu$ and var$(y) = 2\nu$. The approximation is made by matching the first two moments of d to the first two moments of ay:

$$E(d) = a\nu \tag{37.47}$$

$$var(d) = a^2 2\nu \tag{37.48}$$

If the correlation matrix V [Eq. (37.42)] is assumed to be known, it follows that

$$\nu = \frac{2E(\hat{\sigma}^2)^2}{\text{var}(\hat{\sigma}^2)} \tag{37.49}$$

With $E(\hat{\sigma}^2) = \sigma^2$ and

$$\begin{aligned} E(e^Tee^Te) &= E(2\text{trace}[(e_ie_i^T)^2] + \text{trace}(e_ie_i^T)^2) \\ &= \sigma^4[2\text{trace}(RV\,RV) + \text{trace}\,(RV)^2] \end{aligned}$$

we have

$$\begin{aligned} var(\hat{\sigma}^2) &= E(\hat{\sigma}^4) - E(\hat{\sigma}^2)^2 \\ &= \frac{\sigma^4[2\text{trace}(RV\,RV) + \text{trace}\,(RV)^2]}{\text{trace}\,(RV)^2} - \sigma^4 \\ &= \frac{2\sigma^4\text{trace}(RV\,RV)}{\text{trace}\,(RV)^2} \end{aligned}$$

Using Eq. (37.49), we get

$$\nu = \frac{\text{trace}(RV)^2}{\text{trace}\,(RV\,RV)} \tag{37.50}$$

References

Andersson, J. L., Huttton, C., Ashburner, J., Turner, R., and Friston, K. (2001). Modelling geometric deformations in EPI time series. *NeuroImage* **13,** 903–919.

Bracewell, R. (1986). "The Fourier Transform and Its Applications," 2nd ed. McGraw-Hill, New York.

Chatfield, C. (1983). "Statistics for Technology." Chapman & Hall, London.

Christensen, R. (1996). "Plane Answers to Complex Questions: The Theory of Linear Models." Springer-Verlag, Berlin.

Draper, N., and Smith, H. (1981). "Applied Regression Analysis," 2nd ed. John Wiley & Sons, New York.

Friston, K., Frith, C., Liddle, P., Dolan, R., Lammertsma, A., and Frackowiak, R. (1990). The relationship between global and local changes in PET scans. *J. Cereb. Blood Flow Metab.* **10,** 458–466.

Friston, K., Holmes, A., Worsley, K., Poline, J., Frith, C., and Frackowiak, R. (1995). Statistical parametric maps in functional imaging: A general linear approach. *Hum. Brain Mapping* **2,** 189–210.

Friston, K. J., Penny, W. D., Phillips, C., Kiebel, S. J., Hinton, G., and Ashburner, J. (2002). Classical and Bayesian inference in neuroimaging: Theory. *NeuroImage* **16,** 465–483.

Harville, D. A. (1977). Maximum likelihood approaches to variance component estimation and to related problems. *J. Am. Statistics Assoc.* **72,** 320–338.

Healy, M. (1986). "Matrices for Statistics." Oxford University Press, Oxford, UK.

Mitra, P., Ogawa, S., Hu, X., and Ugurbil, K. (1997). The nature of spatiotemporal changes in cerebral hemodynamics as manifested in functional magnetic resonance imaging. *Magn. Res. Imaging Med.* **37,** 511–518.

Mould, R. (1989). "Introductory Medical Statistics," 2nd ed. Institute of Physics Publishing, London.

Purdon, P., and Weisskoff, R. (1998). Effect of temporal autocorrelation due to physiological noise and stimulus paradigm on voxel-level false-positive rates in fMRI. *Hum. Brain Mapping* **6,** 239–249.

Scheffé, H. (1959). "The Analysis of Variance." Wiley, New York.

Winer, B., Brown, D., and Michels, K. (1991). "Statistical Principles in Experimental Design," 3rd ed. McGraw-Hill, New York.

Worsley, K., and Friston, K. (1995). Analysis of fMRI time-series revisited—again. *NeuroImage* **2,** 173–181.

Yandell, B. S. (1997). "Practical Data Analysis for Designed Experiments." Chapman & Hall, London.

CHAPTER

38

Contrasts and Classical Inference

INTRODUCTION

The general linear model (GLM) characterises postulated relationships between our experimental manipulations and the observed data. These relations may consist of multiple effects all of which are contained within a specified design matrix. To test for a specific effect we use a *contrast,* which allows us to focus on a particular characteristic of the data. The application of many different contrast vectors to the same design matrix allows us to test for multiple effects without having to refit the model. This is important in functional imaging because model fitting is computationally demanding.

There are often several ways to mathematically model an experimental paradigm. For example, in a functional imaging experiment the baseline condition can be modeled explicitly or not at all. This sort of issue generalises to more complex designs. Contrast specification and the interpretation of results are entirely dependent on the model specification, which in turn depends on the design of the experiment. The most important step is clearly the specification of the experimental paradigm since if a design is clearly thought through, the questions asked of the data are generally easily specified.

In general, it is not very useful to know simply that a specific brain area was more active during one condition than another. We wish to know whether this difference is statistically significant. The definition of contrasts is therefore intimately related to statistical tests. We will therefore review the aspects of hypothesis testing that relate directly to the specification of contrasts.

This chapter is organised as follows. We first review the basics beginning with some general comments about specification of contrasts and design matrices. We then review the raw material for the construction of contrasts, namely, the parameters of the linear model. Next we describe some rules for constructing contrasts based on the t test. We also discuss F contrasts and the important issue of correlation between regressors.

SOME GENERAL REMARKS

Thinking about which contrasts will be used should start before acquiring the data. Indeed, most of the problems concerning contrast specification come from poor design specification. Poor designs may be unclear about what the objective is or may try to answer too many questions in a single model. This often leads to a compromise in which it becomes difficult to provide clear answers to the questions of interest. This may seem obvious but still seems to be one of the main source of problems in functional imaging data analysis.

This previous remark does not completely preclude the use of a complex paradigm, in the sense that many conditions can and often should be included in the design. The process of recruiting subjects and acquiring the data is long and costly and therefore it is only natural that one would like to answer as many questions as possible with the same data. However, this requires careful thinking about which contrasts will then be specified and whether they actually answer the question of interest.

Complex designs may also lead to testing many hypotheses at each voxel. The fact that this will increase the risk of false positives is an issue that is overlooked more often than not. Indeed, it is somewhat surprising that the problem of multiple comparisons across voxels has received a large amount of attention during the last 10 years, while the problem of multiple comparisons across contrasts has not yet been addressed in the brain imaging literature. If there is no correction for the number of contrasts tested, results should be considered as exploratory (with an uncontrolled risk of error). Alternatively, Bonferroni correction can be applied to set a conservative bound on the risk of error.

One of the difficulties in brain imaging is that the form of the signal of interest is not precisely known because the hemodynamic response varies across subjects and brain regions. We therefore face a double task: estimation (What has happened?) and detection (Has anything happened?).

CONSTRUCTING MODELS

What Should Be Included in the Model?

Again, it is generally a good idea to think about how the experiment is going to be modeled and which comparison we wish to make *before* acquiring the data. We first review some of the questions often asked at the modelling step that have an impact on how the comparisons between conditions are going to be performed.

For a given experiment, different model parameterisations are usually possible and some of them may allow for an easier specification of contrasts. The specified model represents the *a priori* ideas about how the experimental paradigm influences the measured signal. The less prior information there is about the form of the induced signal, the larger the number of regressors required by the model, such that the combination of regressors can account for the possible signal variation.

To make this point clear, we take the example of an fMRI experiment investigating signal variation in the motor cortex when a subject is asked to press a device with four different forces (the "press" condition) interleaved with some "rest" periods.

The first question to be answered is whether the rest period should be modeled or not. In general, there is no difference whether the rest period is explicitly modeled or not; the only difference may arise because of edge effects during the convolution with the expected hemodynamic response function (for fMRI data). However, it has to be understood that the information contained in the data corresponds effectively to the difference between the conditions and the rest period. Therefore it is generally advisable not to model implicit conditions. One may think instead in terms of modelling the difference between two conditions. However, when the number of conditions is greater than 2, it is often easier to model each condition separately and accept that there will be redundancy in the model and that only some comparisons will be valid (see the section on estimability below).

The second question that may arise is how to model the "press" condition. Here the prior information on neural activity and its metabolic consequence is essential. One may have very specific prior assumptions, for example, that the response should be linear with the force developed by the subject. In this case, one regressor representing this linear increase should be included in the model with, for instance, a value of one for the smallest force and a value of four for the greatest. In this design, we might then ask what value should this covariate take during the "rest" periods? If zeros are assumed during this period, there is an explicit hypothesis in the model that the difference between the rest and the first force level is the same as the difference between the first and the second force level (or second and third, etc.). To relax this hypothesis, the difference between the "press" conditions and the rest period must be modeled explicitly.

Modelling the Baseline

Generally the constant offset of the signal has to be modeled (as a column of ones) since the measured signal has an offset (it is not on average zero even without stimuli or task). Figure 38.1 shows this simple design, referred to as *model 1,* which has three regressors.[1] This is a *linear parametric* model. Some questions that can then be put to the design would be as follows:

1. Is there a positive linear increase? (testing if the parameter associated with the first regressor is significantly greater than zero).
2. Is there a difference between the rest and the first force level that is not the same as the one between other force levels? In other words, is there an additive offset for the "press" condition not accounted for by the linear increase? This would be tested using the second coefficient.
3. Is the average value of the signal during the rest period different from zero (positive or negative)?

Note that in this first example the model could be reparameterised, for instance by removing the mean of the first and second regressors to model only the difference around the mean (in fact, this is done automatically in SPM). In that case, the first and second questions would still be valid and the corresponding parameters unchanged, but the interpretation of the third parameter would differ. It would take the value of the average of the measured data, therefore including a potential increase due to the first condition. On the other hand, if there is no information on whether the "press" condition might involve some negative response or not (this corresponds to the case where the only *a priori* information is the difference between the levels of force), then it is more reasonable to remove the mean.

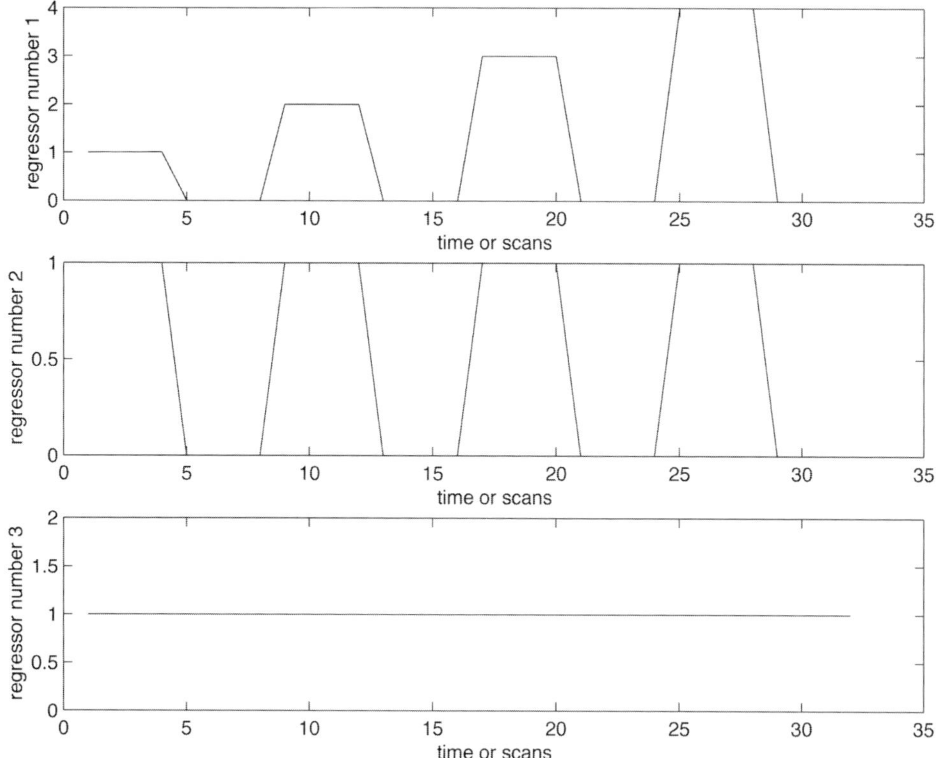

FIGURE 38.1
Simple linear increase design showing the three regressors constituting the design matrix for the experiment described in the text. The regressors, from top to bottom, model (1) the effects of a linear increase in force, (2) the effect of force itself, and (3) the baseline response.

---

[1] Whilst it is usual to convolve regressors with an assumed hemodynamic response function, as described in Chapter 37, we have skipped this step so as to focus more keenly on design issues.

The above points are clarified by the following example. Suppose that the data y come from model 1. We use parameters values [10 5 100] for the three regressors, respectively. Analysis with a model in which the first two covariates have been mean centered leads to an estimation of [10 5 115] in the absence of noise. Clearly, the parameter estimates corresponding to the first two conditions of interest (now centered) are unchanged, but the parameter modelling the mean is changed (from 100 to 115). The reason is that it now includes the average of regressors one and two weighted by their respective parameter estimates.

Extending Our First Model

The hypothesis that the response increases linearly is a rather strong one. There are basically two ways to relax this assumption.

First, the linear increase modeled in the first covariate can be developed in a Taylor-like expansion, such that not only linear increases but also quadratic or cubic increases can be modeled. This solution leads to the inclusion of a new regressor that is simply constructed by the square of values of the linear increase regressor. This new model, model 2, is shown in Fig. 38.2. This is a *quadratic-parametric model,* a type of parameteric modulation that is described further in Chapters 37 and 40.

The second solution is to have a nonparametric form, leaving the model completely free to capture any differences between the four force levels. This is achieved by representing each force level as a separate covariate. This example, model 3, is shown in Fig. 38.3. This is a *nonparameteric model.* Clearly, modelling the difference between each level and the rest period renders the modelling of the average "press" versus rest condition redundant, since the average can be formed from the sum of the different force levels.

Note that what we want to model can be seen as two independent components; the differences between levels 1 and 2, levels 2 and 3, and levels 3 and 4 for one part, and the average activation over all levels of force (the main effect of force) for the other part. Note that the difference between levels 1 and 4 can be created with (1–2)+(2–3)+(3–4). Modelling differences between

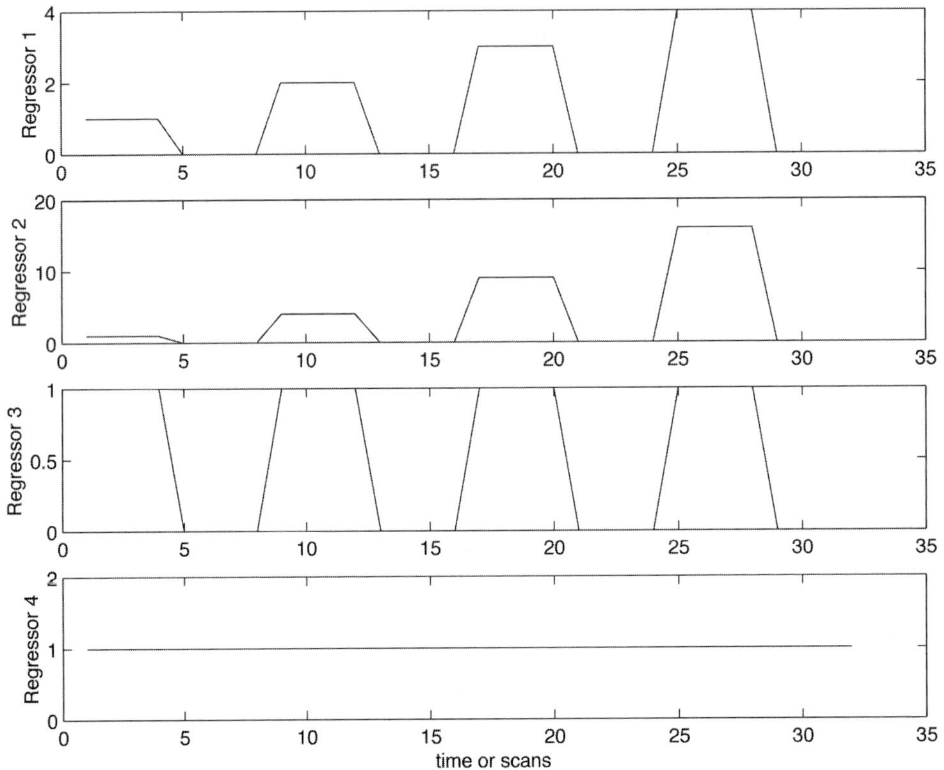

FIGURE 38.2
Linear and quadratic increase covariates. Note the scale of the second covariate.

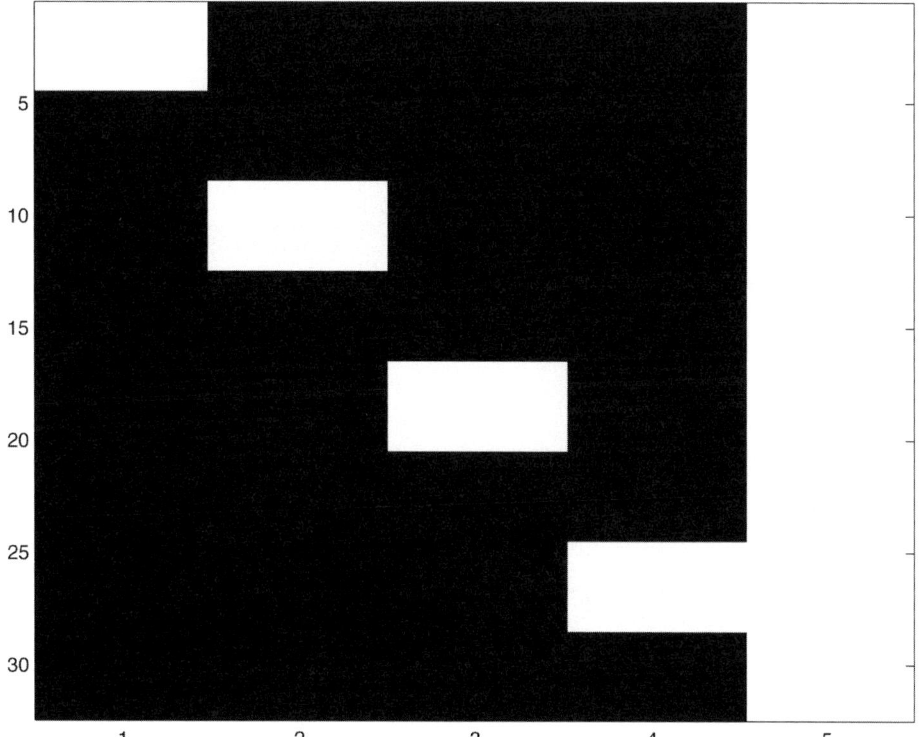

FIGURE 38.3
Different force levels are modeled using separate covariates. Black is 0 and white is 1 on this panel.

levels is similar to modelling interactions in factorial designs (see Chapter 37). We therefore have the choice here to model the difference of each level with the rest condition, or the main effect and the interaction. The questions that can be put to these two designs are exactly the same, they are just "rephrased." The two versions of this model, models 3 and 4, are shown in Figs. 38.3 (difference of each level with rest) and 38.4 (main effect and interactions).

The choice between parametric and nonparametric models often depends on the number of parameters that need to be modeled. If this number is large, then parametric models might be preferred. A limited number of parameters (compared to the number of data points) with little prior information would generally lead to nonparametric models.

In each case, we may be unsure about how to test the effect of the force levels and which effects to test. Before answering these question more formally in the next sections, we briefly describe the issues involved. For the parametric models, we might be interested in the following questions:

- Is there a linear increase or decrease in activation with force level (modeled by the first covariate)?
- Is there a quadratic increase or decrease in *addition* to the linear variation (modeled by the second covariate)?
- Is there anything that is either linear or quadratic in the response to the different levels of force (the joint use of the first and second covariate)?

Should we in this instance center the quadratic covariate or not? The first answer to this is that it generally makes no difference. In general, only variations around the averaged signal over time are easily interpretable. Not centering this covariate would only make a difference if one were interested in the "mean" parameter. Likewise, the quadratic increase shown in Fig. 38.2 can be decomposed into a linear increase and a "pure" quadratic increase (one decorrelated from a linear trend). Removing the component that can be explained by the linear increase from the quadratic increase makes the "linear increase" regressor parameter easier to interpret. But one has to be careful not to overinterpret a significant linear increase since even a signal equal to the

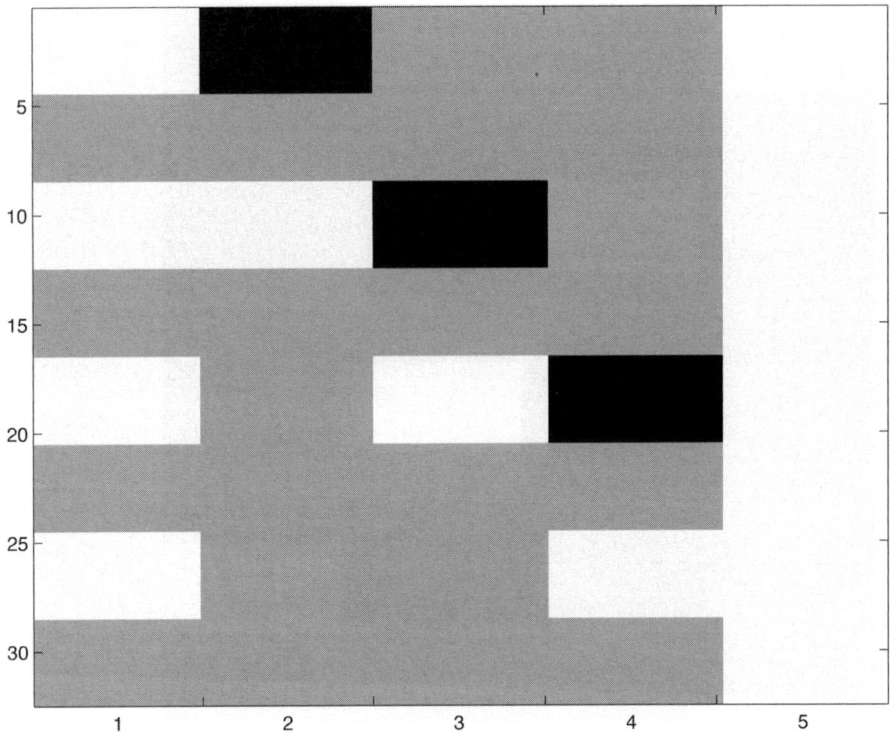

FIGURE 38.4
The main effect of force is modeled with the first regressor and the interactions are modeled with regressors 2 to 4.

second regressor in Fig. 38.2 may have a significant linear component.[2]

For the nonparametric models, interesting questions might be

- Is there an overall difference between force levels and the rest condition (average difference between force levels and rest)? This would involve the average of the first four regressors in model 3 and the first regressor in model 4.
- Are there differences between force conditions? This is resolved by looking conjointly at all differences in force levels versus rest in model 3 and at regressors 2 to 4 in model 4.
- Would it be possible to test for a linear increase of the signal as a function of the force level? Because any difference between condition levels has been modeled, it would not be easy to test for a *specific* linear increase. However, one can inspect the shape of the increase post hoc by displaying the parameter estimates.

The reparameterisation question is often framed in the following form. Should conditions A and B be modeled separately, or should the common part of A and B (A+B) be modeled as well as the difference (A–B)? Note that if there is no third condition (or implicit condition as a null event or baseline) only (A–B) can be estimated from the data.

Another example often considered is the case where the data acquired during a period of time correspond to several factors in an experiment. For instance, consider an experiment comprising two factors, for instance, a modality factor where stimuli are presented either auditorily or visually, and a word factor where stimuli are either names, verbs, or nonwords. Rather than trying to model the factors (and possibly their interaction), it is often easier to model each level of the factor (here 2 by 3, yielding six conditions). If there is no further implicit or explicit rest (or baseline) then the questions of interest can be framed in terms of differences between these conditions. We return to this example in a later section.

[2] Because there is a common part to these two regressors, it is really a matter of interpretation whether this common part should be attributed to one or the other component. See the later section on correlation and Andrade *et al.* (1999) for further discussion of this matter.

CONSTRUCTING AND TESTING CONTRASTS

Parameter Estimation

We now turn to the issue of parameter estimation. As thoroughly reviewed in Chapter 37, the model considered is

$$Y = X\beta + \epsilon \tag{38.1}$$

simply expressing that the data Y (here Y is any time series of length n at a given location in the brain; see Appendix A for notation) can be approximated with a linear combination of time series in X. The matrix X of dimension (n, p), therefore, contains all effects that may have an influence on the acquired signal. The quantity ϵ is additive noise and has a normal distribution with zero mean and covariance $\sigma^2\Sigma_i$. The parameters β can then be estimated using least squares.

The most important thing to realise about model of Eq. (38.1) is that it states that the expectation of the data Y is equal to $X\beta$. If this is not the case, then the model is not appropriate and statistical results are likely to be invalid. This will occur if X does not contain all effects influencing the data or contains too many regressors not related to the data.

A second important remark is that least-squares estimation is a "good" estimation only under the assumption of normally distributed noise. This means that if there are outliers, the estimate $\hat{\beta}$ may be biased. The noise in functional imaging, however, seems close to normal and many aspects of the data processing stream, e.g., spatial smoothing, have "normalising" properties.[3] The true parameters β are estimated from the data using

$$\hat{\beta} = (X^TX)^- X^TY \tag{38.2}$$

where X^- denotes the Moore-Penrose pseudo-inverse of X. The fitted data $\hat{Y}$ are defined as

$$\hat{Y} = X\hat{\beta} \tag{38.3}$$

and represent what is predicted by the model. The estimated noise is

$$Y - \hat{Y} = RY = r \tag{38.4}$$

where

$$R = I_n - XX^- \tag{38.5}$$

The noise variance is estimated with

$$\hat{\sigma}^2 = Y^T RY/\mathrm{tr}[R\Sigma_i] \tag{38.6}$$

Looking at formula (38.2) we realise the following:

- Parameters are dependent on the scaling chosen for the regressors in X. This scaling will not be important when the parameter estimate is compared to its standard deviation, but is important if regressors are entered "by hand" and then compared to each other in the same design. When entered through the dedicated interface in SPM, the regressors are appropriately scaled to yield sensible comparisons.
- Not all parameters may be estimable. This is the subject of the following subsection.

Estimability

One can appreciate that not all parameters may be estimable by taking the rather unlikely model that contains the same regressor twice, say, x_1 and $x_2 = x_1$ having corresponding parameters β_1 and β_2. Clearly, there is no information in the data on which to base the choice of $\hat{\beta}_1$ compared to $\hat{\beta}_2$. In this specific case, any solution of the form $\hat{\beta}_1 + \hat{\beta}_2$ = constant will provide the same fitted data, the same residuals, but an infinity of possible $\hat{\beta}_1$ and $\hat{\beta}_2$.

To generalise this argument, we consider linear functions of the parameter estimates

$$\lambda_1\hat{\beta}_1 + \lambda_2\hat{\beta}_2 + \ldots = \lambda^T\hat{\beta} \tag{38.7}$$

[3] If the original noise properties are well known, the most efficient way to analyze the data is to use the maximum likelihood procedure that would whiten the noise.

The constants λ_i are the coefficients of a function that "contrasts" the parameter estimates. The vector $\lambda^T = [\lambda_1\lambda_2\ldots\lambda_p]$, where p is the number of parameters in X, is referred to as the *contrast vector.* The word *contrast* is used for the result of the operation $\lambda^T\hat{\beta}$. A contrast is therefore a random variable, since $\hat{\beta}$ is estimated from noisy data.

This situation generalises each time a regressor can be constructed with a linear combination of the others. The matrix X is said to be rank deficient or degenerate if some of the parameter estimates are not unique and therefore do not convey any meaning by themselves. At first sight, this situation seems unlikely. However, especially for PET data, most design models are degenerate. This is because of the joint modelling of a constant term for the mean and of all the differences between any condition and the remaining scans.

A contrast is estimable if and only if the contrast vector can be written as a linear combination of the rows of X. This is because we get the information about a contrast through combinations of the rows of Y. If no combination of rows of X is equal to λ^T, then the contrast is not estimable.[4]

In more technical terms, the contrast λ has to lie within the space of X^T, denoted by $\lambda \subset C(X^T)$, or, equivalently, that λ is unchanged when projected orthogonally onto the rows of X (i.e., that $P_{X^T}\lambda = \lambda$ with P_{XT} being the "projector" onto X^T (see Appendix C).

The SPM interface ensures that any specified contrast is estimable, hence offering protection against contrasts that would not make sense in degenerate designs. A further possible difficulty is that a contrast may be estimable but may be misinterpreted. One of the goals of this chapter is to improve the interpretation of contrasts.

Constructing and Testing t Contrasts

If it is clear what the parameter estimates represent, then specification of contrasts is simple, especially in the case of t contrasts. These contrasts are of the form described above, i.e., univariate linear combinations of parameter estimates. For instance, for model 1 we can ask if there is a linear increase by testing β_1 using the combination $1\beta_1 + 0\beta_2 + 0\beta_3$, that is, with the contrast vector $\lambda^T = [1\ 0\ 0]$. A linear decrease can be tested with $\lambda^T = [-1\ 0\ 0]$.

To test for the additive offset of the "press" condition, not accounted for by the linear increase, we use $\lambda^T = [0\ 1\ 0]$. Note here that the linear increase is starting with a value of one for the first force level, up to 4 for the fourth level (see Fig. 38.1).

When testing for the second regressor, *we are effectively removing that part of the signal that can be accounted for by the first regressor.* This means that the second regressor is not giving the average value of the difference between the "press" conditions and the rest condition. To obtain this, we would have to construct a reparameterisation of model 1 and replace the first regressor so that it models *only* difference of "force levels" around an average difference between "press" and rest. This is achieved by orthogonalising the first regressor with respect to the second. This new model, model 5, is shown in Fig. 38.5. The parameter estimates of this new model are [10 30 100] as compared to [10 5 100] for model 1. This issue is detailed in Andrade *et al.* (1999), and the same effect can be seen in F tests (see later section). In other words, one should have clearly in mind not only what *is* but also what *is not* tested by the constructed statistics.

Another solution (useful in neuroimaging where estimating the parameters can be time consuming) is to work out the equivalent contrast (see later section).

The contrast vector $\lambda^T = [1\ 1\ 0]$ is valid but difficult to interpret. For example, the individual effects may be strong but because they can have different signs the overall effect may be weak.

For model 3 the average amplitude of the "press" condition compared to rest would be tested with $\lambda^T = [1\ 1\ 1\ 1\ 0]$. For model 4 the same effect can be tested with $\lambda^T = [1\ 0\ 0\ 0\ 0]$. The two contrasts give exactly the same t maps. Note that in both cases, it is the average over levels that is tested, and this could be significant just because of the impact of one level.

An interesting question is whether we can easily test the linearity of the response to the four levels in those models. For model 3 the intuitive contrast to enter would be $\lambda^T = [1\ 2\ 3\ 4\ 0]$. This

[4] Strictly, as we have described in Chapter 37, all contrasts are estimable by definition. If a linear combination of parameter estimates is not estimable then that linear combination is not a contrast. In this chapter, however, we often use the expression *estimable contrast* for purposes of emphasis and because this term is used in the neuroimaging community.

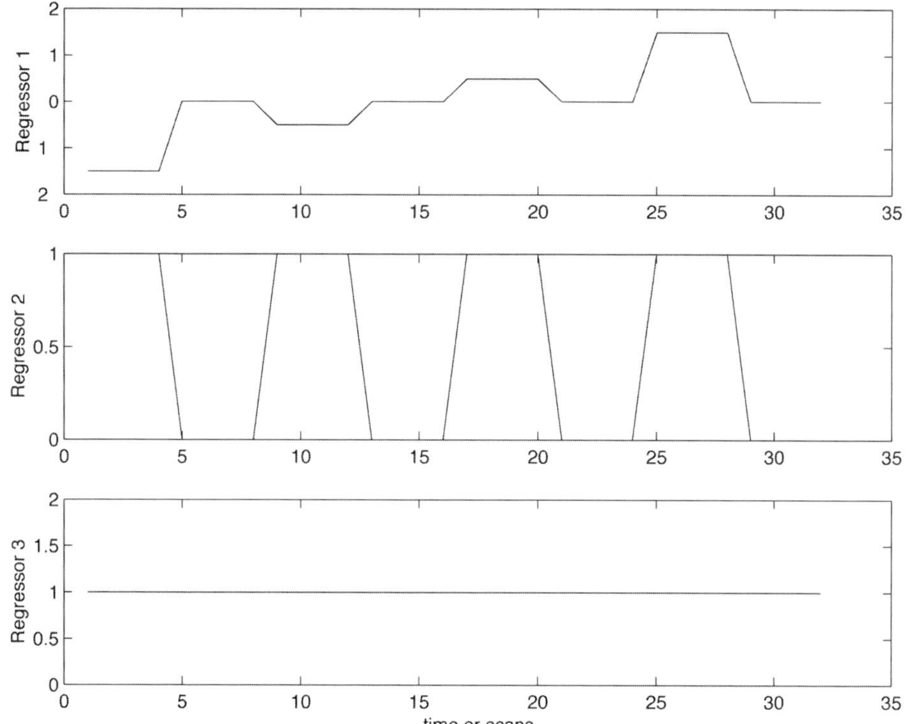

FIGURE 38.5
This is the same as model 1 but the main effect of force has been removed from the first regressor. This changes the interpretation of the second regressor.

would indeed test for a linear increase of the force level, but in a very unspecific manner, in the sense that the test might be significant in a situation where only the fourth condition has a greater signal than in the rest condition. This is because we are testing for the weighted sum of the related parameters. The test is therefore valid, but certainly does not ensure that the signal has a linear change with force levels. In other words, the model is flexible and we are testing a very restricted hypothesis, such that the shape of the predicted signal may be far away from the shape of the tested component.

Computing *t* Statistics

Whatever contrast is used, the contrast *t* statistics are produced using (Friston *et al.,* 1995; Worsley and Friston, 1995)

$$t_{df} = \lambda^T\hat{\beta}/SD(\lambda^T\hat{\beta}) \tag{38.8}$$

where SD(z) denotes the standard deviation of z and is computed from the variance

$$\text{var}[\lambda^T\hat{\beta}] = \hat{\sigma}^2\lambda^T(X^TX)^- X^T\Sigma_i X(X^TX)^-\lambda \tag{38.9}$$

For Gaussian errors t_{df} follows approximately a Student distribution with degrees of freedom given by $df = \text{tr}[R\Sigma_i]^2/\text{tr}[R\Sigma_i R\Sigma_i]$. At the voxel level, the value t_{df} is tested against the likeliness of this value under the null hypothesis.

The important point here is that the standard deviation of the contrast of parameter estimates depends on the matrix X. More specifically, when regressors are correlated, the variance of the corresponding parameter estimates increases. In other words, the stability of the estimation for one component is greater when other components included in the model are decorrelated. The dependence of the covariance of the estimated effects and the correlation within the model can be used, for instance, to optimise event-related designs.

The test of t_{df} is one tailed when testing for positivity only or negativity only and two tailed when jointly testing for positive or negative effects (see next section).

CONSTRUCTING AND TESTING F CONTRASTS

In this section, we will consider an experiment with two event-related conditions using the simple case of right and left motor responses. In this experiment, the subject is asked to press a button with the right or left hand depending on a visual instruction (involving some attention). The events arrive pseudo-randomly but with a long interstimulus interval. We are interested in finding the brain regions that respond more to the right than to the left motor movement.

Our first model supposes that the shape of the hemodynamic response function (HRF) can be modeled by a *canonical HRF* (see Chapter 40 for details). This model is shown in Fig. 38.6. To find the brain regions responding more to the left than to the right motor responses we can use $\lambda^T = [1\ -1\ 0]$. Application of this contrast produces the SPM t map shown in Fig. 38.7. This clearly shows activation of contralateral motor cortex plus other expected regions such as ipsilateral cerebellum.

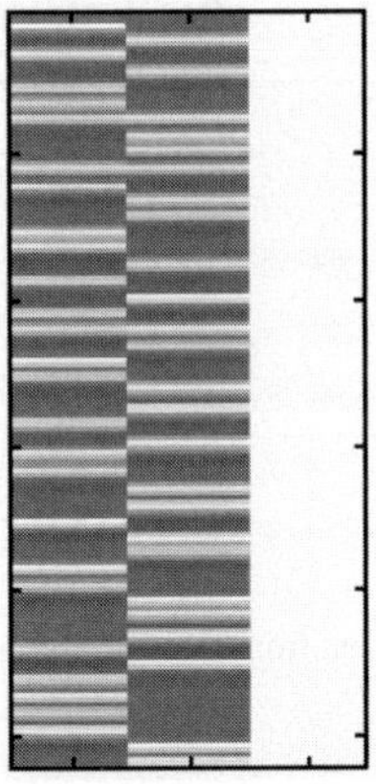

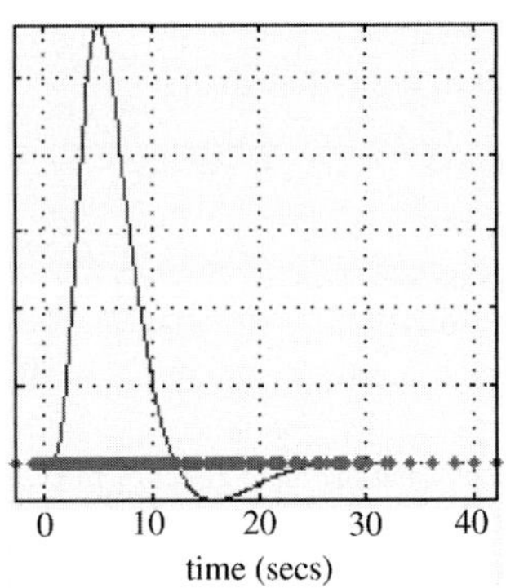

FIGURE 38.6
The left panel shows the design matrix for analyzing two event-related conditions (left or right motor responses) versus an implicit baseline in the case where the shape of the HRF is assumed known up to a scaling factor. This canonical HRF is shown on the right panel. This HRF has been convolved with the series of Dirac functions, which occur at event onset times, to form the two leftmost regressors in the design matrix on the left.

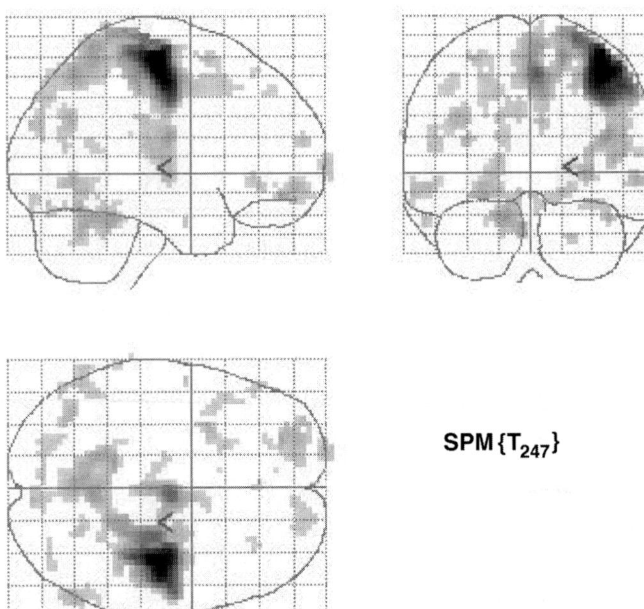

FIGURE 38.7
SPM t image corresponding to the overall difference between the left and right responses. This map was produced using the [1 – 1 0] contrast on the design matrix shown in Fig. 38.6.

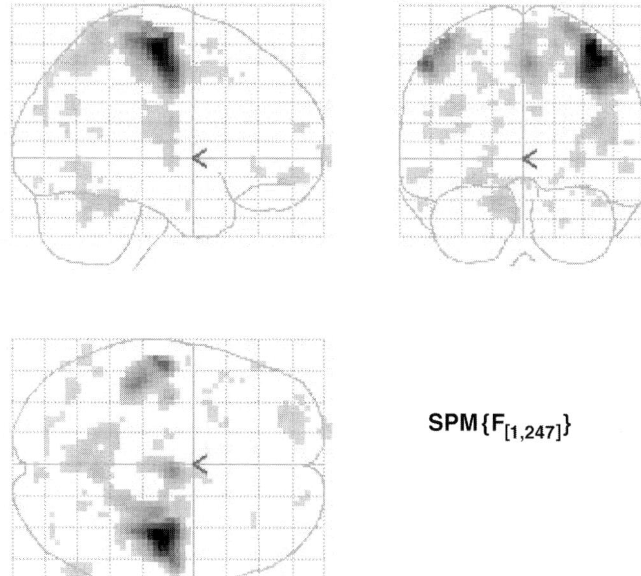

FIGURE 38.8
SPM F image corresponding to the overall difference (positive or negative) from the left and right responses. This map was produced using the F contrast [1 0 0; 0 1 0] on the design matrix shown in Fig. 38.6.

Because there is an implicit baseline, the parameters are also interpretable on their own and, when tested (SPM t maps not shown), they show responses not only for the motor regions but also the expected visual regions.[5] Instead of having the two regressors being one for the left response and one for the right response, an equivalent model would have two regressors, the first modelling the response common to right and left and the second modelling the difference between these responses.

The fact that the HRF varies across brain regions and subjects can be accommodated as follows. A simple extension of the model of Fig. 38.6 is presented later in Fig. 38.9, for which each response is modeled with three basis functions. These functions are able to model small variations in the delay and dispersion of the HRF, as described in Chapter 40. They are mean centered, so the mean parameter will represent the overall average of the data.

For this new model, how do we test for the effects of, for instance, the right motor response? The most reasonable approach in the first instance is to test for all regressors modelling this response. This does not mean the sum (or average) of the parameter estimates since the sign of those parameter estimates is not interpretable, but rather the (weighted) sum of squares of those parameter estimates. The appropriate F contrast is shown in Fig. 38.10.

One interpretation of the F contrast is of the specification of a series of one-dimensional contrasts, each of them testing against the null hypothesis that the parameter is zero. Because parameters are tested against zero, one would have to reconstruct the fitted data and check the positive or negative aspects of the response.

To test for the *overall* difference between right and the left responses we use the contrast shown in Fig. 38.11. Note that multiplying the F contrast coefficients by –1 does not change the value of the test. To see if the tested difference is "positive" or "negative" (if this makes sense since the modeled difference could be partly positive and partly negative) one has to look at the fitted signal corresponding to the extra sum of squares tested. The F-test image corresponding to this contrast is shown in Fig. 38.12. This image is very similar to the corresponding image for the simpler model (Fig. 38.8). Finally, Fig. 38.13 shows that the more complex model provides a better fit to the data.

[5] Interestingly, there is some ipsilateral activation in the motor cortex such that the "left–right" contrast is slightly less significant in the motor regions than the "left" [1 0 0] contrast.

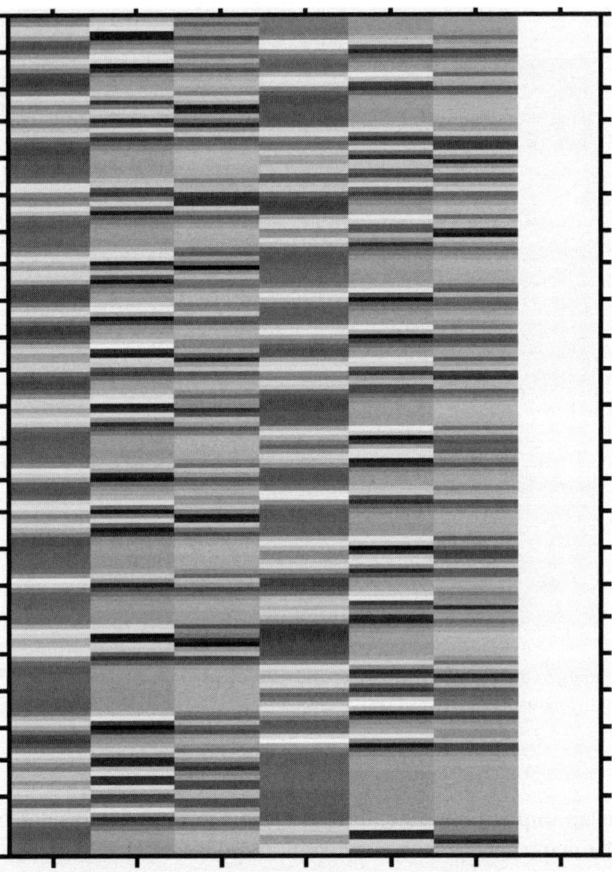

FIGURE 38.9
This is the same model as in Fig. 38.6, but we use three regressors to model each condition. The first three columns model the first condition (left motor response) while columns 4 to 6 model the second condition (right motor response). The three basis functions are the canonical HRF and its derivatives with respect to time and dispersion.

To conclude this section, we give a few more examples using the design described earlier. We suppose a 2 by 3 factorial design consisting of words presented either visually (V) or aurally (A) and belonging to three different categories (C1, C2, C3). The way the design is constructed is to model all six event types in the following order in the design matrix; V-C1 (presented visually and in category one), V-C2, V-C3, A-C1, A-C2, A-C3. We can then test for the interaction between the modality and category factors. We suppose that the experiment is a rapid event-related design with no implicit baseline, such that only comparisons between different kinds of events are meaningful (and not events in themselves). In a first example the events are modeled using only one basis function. A test for the main effect of modality would be the one presented in Fig. 38.14a. Figure 38.14b shows the test for the main effect of category. Note that because there is no implicit baseline here, the main effects of factors are differences between the levels. Finally, the interaction term would be tested for as in Fig. 38.14c.

The number of rows in an interaction contrast (without implicit baseline) is given by

$$N_{rows} = \prod_{i=1}^{N} (l_i - 1) \tag{38.10}$$

where N is the number of factors and l_i the number of levels of factor i.

Interpretations of F Contrasts

There are two equivalent ways of thinking about F contrasts. For example, we can think about the F contrast in Fig. 38.10 as fitting a reduced model that does not contain the "right motor response" regressors. This reduced model would have a design matrix X_0 with zero entries where

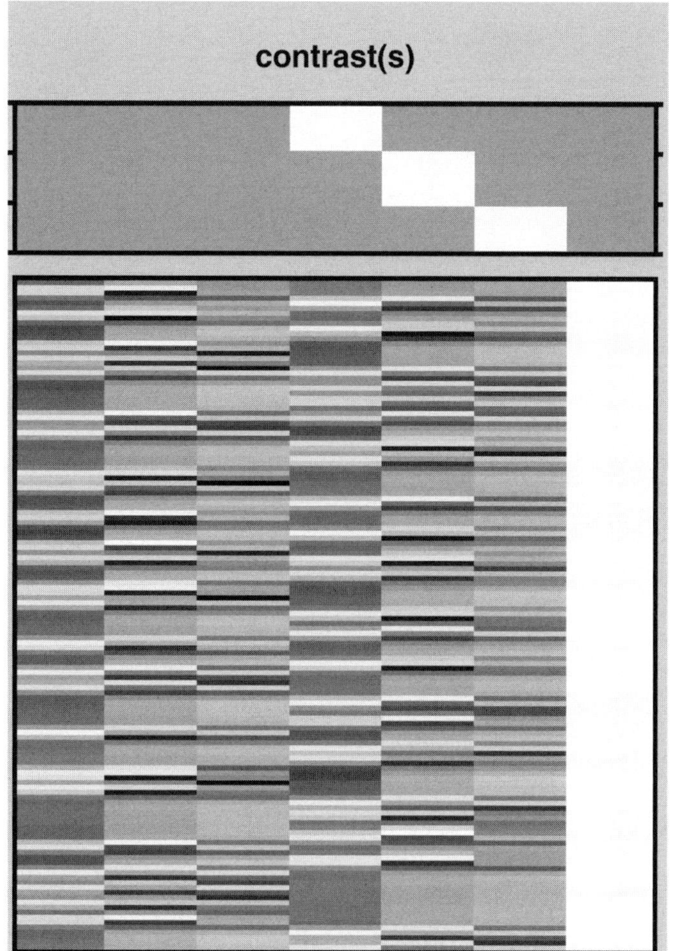

FIGURE 38.10
This figure shows a simple F contrast testing for the regressors modelling the right motor response. This corresponds to constructing the reduced model that does not contain the regressors that are "marked" with the F contrast.

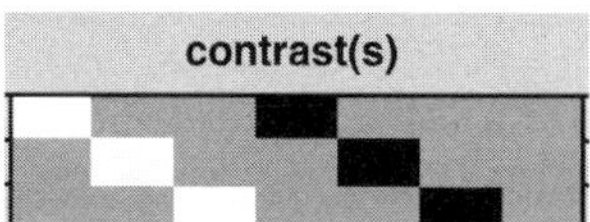

FIGURE 38.11
This figure shows the F contrast used to test the overall difference (across basis functions) between the left and right responses.

the "right motor response" regressors were in the "full" design matrix X. The test then looks at the variance of the residuals (see earlier section) as compared to that of the full model X. The F test simply computes the extra sum of squares that can be accounted for by the inclusion in the model of the three "right-hand" regressors. Following any statistical textbook (e.g., Christensen, 1996) and the work of Friston *et al.* (1995) and Worsley and Friston (1995), this is expressed by testing the following quantity:

$$F_{df_1,df_2} = \frac{[Y^T(I - P_{X_0})Y - Y^T(I - P_X)Y]/\nu_1}{Y^T(I - P_X)Y/\nu_2} \tag{38.11}$$

with

$$\begin{aligned} \nu_1 &= \mathrm{tr}[(R_0 - R)\Sigma_i] \\ \nu_2 &= \mathrm{tr}\,(R\Sigma_i) \end{aligned} \tag{38.12}$$

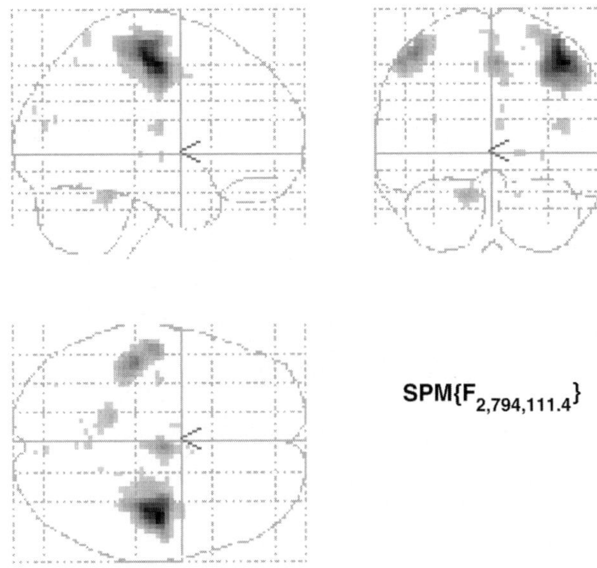

FIGURE 38.12
SPM F image corresponding to the overall difference between the left and right responses. This map was produced using the F contrast in Fig. 38.11 applied to the design matrix in Fig. 38.9.

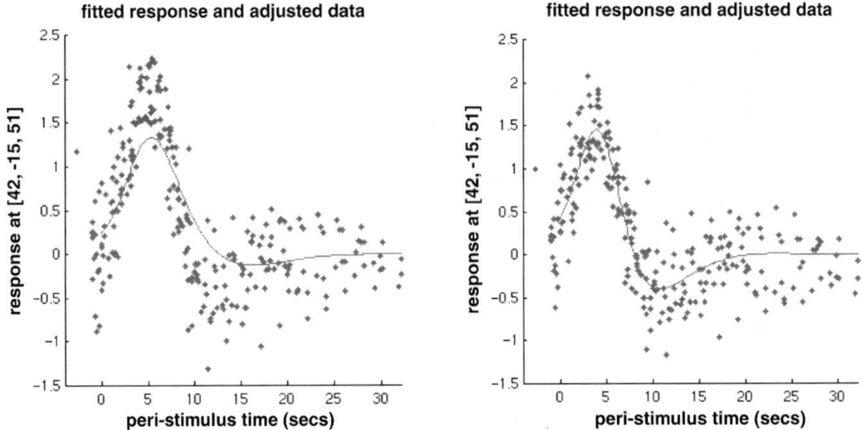

FIGURE 38.13
These plots show the hemodynamic response at a single voxel (the maxima of the SPM-F map in Fig. 38.12). The left plot shows the HRF as estimated using the simple model in Fig. 38.6 and demonstrates a certain lack of fit. This lack of fit is corrected (right panel) by using the more flexible model of Fig. 38.9.

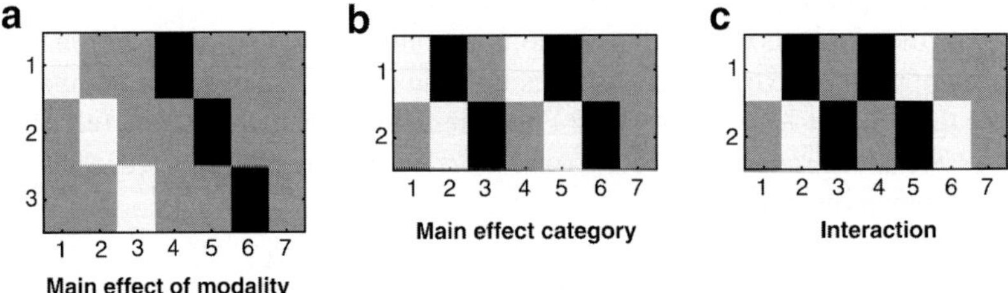

FIGURE 38.14
F contrasts testing, respectively, for (a) the main effect of modality (b) the main effect of category and (c) the interaction modality × category.

and

$$df_1 = \mathrm{tr}\,[(R_0 - R)\Sigma_i(R_0 - R)\Sigma_i]/\mathrm{tr}[(R_0 - R)\Sigma_i]^2 \tag{38.13}$$

$$df_2 = \mathrm{tr}(R\Sigma_i R\Sigma_i)/\mathrm{tr}(R\Sigma_i)^2 \tag{38.14}$$

where R_0 is the projector onto the residual space of X_0, and P_X is the orthogonal projector onto X (see Appendix C for a definition of a *projector.*) We also have[6]

$$F_{df_1,df_2} \sim F(df_1,df_2) \tag{38.15}$$

Such a test can be implemented by specifying the columns of the design matrix that should be kept for the reduced model.

The second interpretation of the F test is of the specification of a series of one-dimensional contrasts, each of them testing against the null hypothesis that the parameter is zero. Note that in this case, parameters are tested against zero and, therefore, to interpret this test one would have to reconstruct the fitted data and check the positive or negative aspects of the response.

We now formally show how the two interpretations of the F test are linked. The model in Eq. (38.1), $Y = X\beta + \epsilon$, is restricted by the test $c^T\beta = 0$ where c is now a *contrast matrix.* If c yields an estimable function, then we can define a matrix H such that $c = H^TX$. Therefore, $H^TX\beta = 0$ which, together with Eq. (38.1), is equivalent to $Y \subset C(X)$ and $Y \subset C(H^\perp)$, the space orthogonal to H. It can be shown that the reduced model corresponding to this test can be chosen to be $X_0 = P_X - P_H$. This is a valid choice if and only if the space spanned by X_0 is the space defined by $C(H)^\perp \cap C(X)$ and it is easy to show that it is indeed the case.

If $C(H) \subset C(X)$, the numerator of Eq. (38.11) can be rewritten as

$$Y^T(R_0 - R)Y = Y^T(X_0 - R)Y = Y^T(P_X - X_0)Y = Y^T(P_H)Y \tag{38.16}$$

We choose H such that it satisfies the condition above with $H = (X^T)^- c$, which yields

$$\begin{aligned} Y^T(P_H)Y &= Y^TX(X^TX)^-X^TH(H^TH)^-H^TX(X^TX)^-X^TY \\ &= \hat{\beta}^Tc(H^TH)^-c^T\hat{\beta} \end{aligned} \tag{38.17}$$

The above rewriting of the F test is important for several reasons. First it makes the specification and computation of F tests feasible in the context of large datasets. Specifying a reduced model and computing the extra sum of squares using Eq. (38.11) would be too computationally demanding. Second, it helps to make the link between a *t* test and the test of a reduced model and therefore helps to recall that what is tested is only the "extra" variability that cannot be explained by the reduced model. Third, it makes the test of complex interactions using F tests more intuitive.

The F contrast that looks at the total contribution of all the "right regressors" is, however, quite a nonspecific test. One may have a specific hypothesis about the magnitude or the delay of the response and would like to test specifically for this. In the first instance, it might be thought that a reasonable test would be to use a *t* test with contrast [0 0 0 1 0 0 0 0], testing for a positive parameter on the regressor modelling the standard HRF. This is perfectly valid, but it has to be remembered that what is tested here is the amount of adequacy of the BOLD response with this regressor, not the magnitude of the response. This means, for instance, that if the response has the shape of the one supposed by the standard model but is significantly delayed, the test might produce poor results even if the delay is appropriately taken into account by the other regressors. This might be quite important when comparing the magnitude of responses between two conditions: If this magnitude is the same but the delays are different across conditions, the test comparing simply the standard response regressors might be misinterpreted. A difference of delay might appear as a difference of magnitude *even if the basis function is decorrelated or orthogonal.* A related problem, the estimation of the delay of the HRF, has been considered in an earlier chapter.

[6] This is an approximate result with good properties when the number of points is not too small or if Σ_i is close to the identity matrix.

Note that the simplest F contrasts are unidimensional, in which case the F statistic is simply the square of the corresponding t statistic. To visually differentiate between unidimensional F contrasts and t contrasts in the SPM interface, the former are displayed in terms of images and the latter as bars.

An important remark is that, generally speaking, if we are confident about the shape of the expected response, F tests are often less sensitive than t tests. The reason is that the greater the flexibility of the tested space, the greater the possibility of finding a signal that can have an important part of its variability explained by the model, and there is an implicit correction for this in the numerator of Eq. (38.11).

CORRELATION BETWEEN REGRESSORS AND OTHER ISSUES

Correlation between model regressors makes the tests more difficult to interpret. Unfortunately, such correlation is often imposed by the brain's dynamics, experimental design, or external measurements. The risks of misinterpretation have been extensively discussed (Andrade *et al.*, 1999; Sen and Srivistava, 1990). To summarise, one could miss activations when testing for a given contrast of parameters if there is significant correlation with the rest of the design. An important example of this situation is when the response to a stimulus is highly correlated with a motor response.

If one believes that a region's activity will not be influenced by the motor response, then it is advisable to test this specific region by first removing from the motor response regressor all that can be explained by the stimulus. This is of course a "dangerous" action since if, in fact, the motor response does influence the signal in this region, then the test result will be overly significant. That is, experimental variance will be wrongly attributed to the stimulus.

Moving the Variance across Correlated Regressors

If one decides that a regressor, or indeed several regressors or combination of those, should be orthogonalised with respect to some part of the design matrix before performing a test, it is not necessary to reparameterise and fit the model again. Once the model has been fitted, all information needed to test some effects can be found in the fitted parameter estimates. For instance, instead of testing the additional variance explained by a regressor, one may wish to test for all the variance that can be explained by this regressor. Using the definitions given earlier, if c is the contrast testing for the extra sum of squares, it is easy to show that the contrast matrix

$$c_{\text{Full\_space}} = X^T X c \qquad (38.18)$$

tests for all the variance explained by the subspace of X defined by Xc since we then have $H = Xc$.

Contrasts and Reparameterised Models

The above principle can be generalised as follows. If the design matrix contains three subspaces, say (S_1, S_2, S_3), one may wish to test for what is in S_1, having removed what could be explained by S_2 (but not by S_3). Other examples are conjunction analyses in which a series of contrasts can be modified such that the effects they test are orthogonal. This involves orthogonalising the subsequent subspaces tested. Therefore, results may differ depending on the order in which these contrasts are entered.

The principle to compute the contrast testing for various subspaces from parameterised versions of the model is simple. If X and X_p are two differently parameterised versions of the same model, then we can define a matrix T such that $X_p = XT$. If c_p is a test expressed in X_p while the data have been fitted using X, the equivalent of c_p using the parameter estimates of X is

$$c = c_p (T^T X^T X T)^{-} T^T X^T X \qquad (38.19)$$

One should be careful using this sort of transformation; for instance; one should not put a variance of "no interest" in the space tested. Such transformations are often very useful, however, because the models do not require refitting. See Andrade *et al.* (1999) for further examples.

Estimation-Detection Dilemma

A crucial point when analyzing functional imaging data (PET and fMRI alike) is that in general the model is not well known. The larger the model, the better in general would be the estimation of the signal, as long as the model is not starting to capture noise components. This often leads to less specific questions and to less sensitive tests compared to situations where the difference is known with better precision. There are two extreme choices:

- The use of a simple model with the danger of not having modeled some effects properly, a situation that may lead to biased results
- The use of a very flexible model with less sensitive tests and difficulties in the interpretation of the results

In other words, it is difficult to estimate the signal and at the same time test for this signal. A possible strategy would consist of using part of the data in an estimation phase that is separate from a testing phase. This will, however, involve "losing" some data. For an instance of such a strategy, see Kherif *et al.* (2002).

FIR and Random Effects Analyses

A typical example of a flexible model is finite impulse response (FIR) modelling of event-related fMRI data, as described in Chapter 40. The model in this case is as flexible as possible since the hemodynamic response function is allowed to take any shape. A classic difficulty with this approach, however, is how to implement a random-effects analysis (see Chapter 42). The difficulty arises because, usually, one takes a single contrast image per subject up to the second level. With an FIR characterisation, however, one has multiple parameter estimates per subject and one must therefore take into account the covariance structure between parameters. While this was prohibited in SPM99 it is now possible in SPM2, by making use of the nonsphericity options as alluded to in Chapters 39, 42, and 47.

CONCLUSION

In a functional imaging experiment it is often the case that one is interested in many sorts of effects, e.g., the main effects of various conditions and the possible interactions between them. To investigate each of these effects, one could fit several different GLMs and test hypotheses by looking at individual parameter estimates. Because functional imaging datasets are so large, however, this approach is impractical. A more expedient approach is to fit larger models and test for specific effects using specific contrasts.

In this chapter we have shown how specification of the design matrix is intimately related to the specification of contrasts. For example, it is often the case that main effects and interactions can be set up using parametric or nonparametric designs. These different designs lead to the use of different contrasts. Parametric approaches are favored for factorial designs with many levels per factor. For contrasts to be interpretable they must be estimable and we have described the conditions for estimability.

In fMRI one can model hemodynamic responses using the canonical HRF. This allows one to test for activations using t contrasts. To account for the variability in hemodynamic response across subjects and brain regions, one can model the HRF using the canonical HRF plus its derivatives with respect to time and dispersion. Inferences about differences in activation can then be made using F contrasts. We have shown that there are two equivalent ways of interpreting F contrasts, one employing the extra sum-of-squares principle to compare the model and a reduced model and one specifying a series of one-dimensional contrasts. Designs with correlation between regressors are less efficient and correlation can be removed by orthogonalising one effect with respect to other effects. Finally, we have shown how such orthogonalisation can be applied retrospectively, i.e., without having to refit the models.

APPENDIX A NOTATION

Y	= Data	$(n, 1)$ time series, where n is the number of time points or scans.
c or λ	= Contrast	Weights of the parameter estimates used to form the (numerator) of the statistics
X	= Design matrix or design model	The (n, p) matrix of regressors
β	= Model parameters	True (unobservable) coefficients such that the weighted sum of the regressors is the expectation of our data (if X is correct)
$\hat{\beta}$	= Parameter estimates	Computed estimation of the β using the data $Y : \hat{\beta} = (X^TX)^- X^TY$
R	= Residual forming matrix	Given a model X, the residual forming matrix $R = I_n - X X^-$ transforms the data Y into the residuals $r = RY$
$\sigma^2\Sigma_i$	= scan (time) covariance	(n, n) matrix that describes the (noise) covariance between scans

APPENDIX B SUBSPACES

Let us consider a set of p vectors x_i of dimension $(n, 1)$ (with $p < n$), such as regressors in fMRI. The space spanned by this set of vectors is formed of all possible vectors (say, u) that can be expressed as a linear combination of the $x_i : u = \alpha_1 x_1 + \alpha_2 x_2 + \ldots \alpha_p x_p$. If the matrix X is formed with the x_i: $X = [x_1 x_2 \ldots x_p]$,we note this space as $C(X)$.

Not all the x_i may be necessary to form $C(X)$. The minimal number needed is called the *rank* of the matrix X. If only a subset of the x_i are selected, say that they form the smaller matrix X_0, the space spanned by X_0, $C(X_0)$ is called a subspace of X. A contrast defines two subspaces of the design matrix X: one that is tested and one of "no interest," corresponding to the reduced model.

APPENDIX C ORTHOGONAL PROJECTION

The orthogonal projection of a vector x onto the space of a matrix A is the vector (for instance, a time series) that is the closest to what can be predicted by linear combinations of the columns of A. The closest here is in the sense of a minimal sum of square errors. The projector onto A, denoted P_A, is unique and can be computed with $P_A = AA^-$, with A^- denoting the Moore-Penrose pseudo-inverse[7] of A. For instance, in the "Parameter Estimation" section, the fitted data $\hat{Y}$ can be computed with

$$\hat{Y} = P_X Y = XX^- Y = X(X^TX)^- XY = X\hat{\beta} \tag{38.20}$$

Most of the operations needed when working with linear models only involve computations in the parameter space, as is shown in Eq. (38.17). For a further gain, if the design is degenerate, one can work in an orthonormal basis of the space of X. This is how the SPM code is implemented.

References

Andrade, A., Paradis, A.-L., Rouquette, S., and Poline, J.-B. (1999). Ambiguous results in functional neuroimaging data analysis due to covariate correlation. *NeuroImage* **10,** 483–486.

Christensen, R. (1996). "Plane Answers to Complex Questions: The Theory of Linear Models." Springer, Berlin.

Friston, K. J., Holmes, A. P., Worsley, K. J., Poline, J.-B., Frith, C. D., and Frackowiak, R. S. J. (1995). Statistical parametric maps in functional imaging: a general linear approach. *Hum. Brain Mapping* **2,** 189–210.

[7] Any generalised inverse could be used.

Kherif, F., Poline, J.-B., Flandin, F., Benali, H., Dehaene, S., and Worsley, K. J. Multivariate model specification for fMRI data. *NeuroImage,* 2002.

Sen, A., and Srivastava, M. (1990). "Regression Analysis – Theory, Methods, and Applications." Springer-Verlag, Berlin.

Worsley, K. J., and Friston, K. J. (1995). Analysis of fMRI time-series revisited—again. *NeuroImage* **2,** 173–181.

CHAPTER

39

Variance Components

INTRODUCTION

The validity of F statistics for classical inference on imaging data depends on the sphericity assumption. This assumption states that the difference between two measurement sets (e.g., those for two levels of a particular variable) has equal variance for all pairs of such sets. In practice, this assumption can be violated in several ways, for example, by differences in variance induced by different experimental conditions and/or by serial correlations within imaging time series.

A considerable literature exists in applied statistics that describes and compares various techniques for dealing with sphericity violation in the context of repeated measurements (see, e.g., Keselman *et al.,* 2001). The analysis techniques exploited by the Statistical Parametrical Mapping (SPM) package also employ a range of strategies for dealing with the variance structure of imaging data. These are dealt with in this chapter and related to classical schemes.

Deductions about what is significant in imaging data depend on a detailed model of what might arise by chance. If you do not know about the structure of random fluctuations in your signal, you will not know what features you should find "surprising." A key component of this structure is the covariance of the data, that is, the extent to which different sets of observations within your experiment are dependent on one another. If this structure is wrongly identified, it can lead to incorrect estimates of the variability of the parameters estimated from the data. This, in turn, can lead to false inferences.

Classical inference requires the expected likelihood distribution of a test statistic under the null hypothesis. Both the statistic and its distribution depend on hyperparameters controlling different components of the error covariance (this can be just the variance, σ^2, in simple models). Estimates of variance components are used to compute statistics and variability in these estimates to determine the statistic's degrees of freedom. Sensitivity depends, in part, on precise estimates of the hyperparameters (i.e., high degrees of freedom).

In the early years of functional neuroimaging, debate arouse around whether one could "pool" (error variance) hyperparameter estimates over voxels. The motivation for this was an enormous increase in the precision of the hyperparameter estimates that rendered the ensuing T statistics normally distributed with very high degrees of freedom (see Chapter 7). The disadvantage was that pooling rested on the assumption that the error variance was the same at all voxels. Although this assumption was highly implausible, the small number of observations in PET renders the voxel-specific hyperparameter estimates highly variable and it was not easy to show significant regional differences in error variance. With the advent of fMRI and more precise hyperparameter estimation, this regional heteroscedasticity was established and conventional pooling was precluded. Consequently, most analyses of neuroimaging data now use voxel-specific hyperparameter estimation. This is quite simple to implement, provided there is only one hyperparameter, because its ReML estimate (see Section 4 of Part II and Chapter 47) can be obtained noniteratively and simultaneously through the sum of squared residuals at each voxel. However, in an increasing number of situations, the errors have a number of variance components (e.g., serial correlations in fMRI or inhomogeneity of variance in hierarchical models). The ensuing nonsphericity presents a potential problem for mass univariate tests of the sort implemented by SPM.

Currently, several approaches to this problem are being taken. First, departures from a simple distribution of the errors can be modelled using tricks borrowed from the classical statistical literature. This correction procedure is somewhat crude, but can protect to some extent against the tendency toward liberal conclusions. Second, a correlation structure can be imposed on the data by smoothing. This runs the risk of masking interesting features of the signal, but can coerce the noise into better behaviour. Finally, the kinds of tests performed can be restricted. For example, tests comparing several measures from each of several subjects from a larger population can be "forbidden" since they rely more heavily on unjustifiable assumptions about the noise structure.

In this chapter we describe how this problem has been addressed in various versions of SPM. We first point to a mathematical equivalence between the classical statistical literature and SPM99 in their treatment of violations of assumptions about covariance structure. Classically, the assumed structure is the most liberal and allows a model to be estimated without mathematical iteration. In SPM99, as described in Worsley and Friston (1995), a temporal smoothing stage before the main analysis "swamps" any intrinsic autocorrelation with an imposed temporal covariance structure. Although this structure does not correspond to the assumptions underlying the classical analysis, the same approach is used to take account of this known violation. Although it would be possible to estimate and correct directly for the intrinsic covariation structure rather than trying to swamp it, an error in this estimation has been shown to be very costly in terms of the accuracy of the subsequent inference (Friston *et al.,* 2000).

Defining sphericity as a quantitative measure of the departure from basic assumptions about the null distribution, we will show how SPM99 compensates only for sphericity violations associated with serial correlations. It employs a correction to the degrees of freedom that is mathematically identical to that employed by the Greenhouse-Geisser univariate F test. This correction is applied after a filtering stage that swamps the intrinsic autocorrelation with an imposed structure. It is the known nonsphericity of this imposed structure that is then used to approximate the degrees of freedom.

In the second part of the chapter, we broadly describe a new approach to the problem. Instead of assuming an arbitrarily restricted covariance structure, we show how new iterative techniques can be used to simultaneously estimate the actual nature of the errors alongside the estimation of the model. While traditional multivariate techniques also have estimated covariances, here we allow the experimenter to "build in" knowledge or assumptions about the data, reducing the number of parameters that must be estimated and restricting the solutions to plausible forms. These techniques are implemented in new versions of SPM. We describe briefly the types of previously "forbidden" models that can be estimated using the new techniques.

More recent approaches that we have developed use a parametric empirical Bayesian (PEB) technique to estimate whichever variance components are of interest. This is equivalent to an iterative restricted maximum likelihood (ReML) approach. In functional magnetic resonance imaging (fMRI) time series, for example, these variance components model the white noise component as well as the covariance induced by, for example, an AR(1) component. In a mixed-effects analysis, the components correspond to the within-subject variance (possibly different for each subject) and the between-subject variance. More generally, when the population of subjects consists of different groups, we may have different residual variance in each group. PEB partitions the overall degrees of freedom (e.g., total number of fMRI scans) in such a way as to ensure that the variance estimates are unbiased. This takes place using a version of an expectation maximisation (EM) procedure in which the model coefficients and variance estimates are reestimated iteratively.

Finally, we will provide a mathematical justification for the pooling of covariance estimates underlying this approach.

MATHEMATICAL EQUIVALENCES

Assumptions Underlying Repeated-Measures ANOVA

Inference in imaging, under the approach of SPM, proceeds by the construction of an F test based on the null distribution. Our inferences are vulnerable to violations of assumptions about the variance structure of the data in just the same way as, for example, in the behavioural sciences:

> *Specifically, the conventional univariate method of analysis assumes that the data have been obtained from populations that have the well-known normal (multivariate) form, that the degree of variability (covariance) among the levels of the variable conforms to a spherical pattern, and that the data conform to independence assumptions. Since the data obtained in many areas of psychological inquiry are not likely to conform to these requirements ... researchers using the conventional procedure will erroneously claim treatment effects when none are present, thus filling their literatures with false positive claims* (Keselman *et al.*, 2001)

It could be argued that limits on the computational power available to researchers have led to a concentration on the limits of models that can be estimated without recourse to iterative algorithms. On this account, sphericity and its associated literature can be considered a historically specific issue. Nevertheless, although the development of methods such as those described in Worsley and Friston (1995) and implemented in SPM99 do not explicitly refer to the repeated measures designs, they are in fact mathematically identical, as we will now show.

The assumptions required for both sorts of analysis can be most easily defined by considering the variance-covariance matrix of the observations. Consider a population variance-covariance matrix for a measurement x under k treatments with n subjects. The measurements on each subject can be viewed as a k-element vector with associated covariance matrix

$$\Sigma_x = \begin{bmatrix} \sigma_{11} & \sigma_{11} & \cdots & \sigma_{1k} \\ \sigma_{21} & \sigma_{22} & \cdots & \sigma_{2k} \\ \vdots & & & \vdots \\ \sigma_{k1} & \sigma_{k2} & \cdots & \sigma_{kk} \end{bmatrix} \tag{39.1}$$

This matrix can be estimated on the basis of the data by the sample variance-covariance matrix

$$\hat{\Sigma}_x = \Sigma_x = \begin{bmatrix} s_{11} & s_{12} & \cdots & s_{1k} \\ s_{21} & s_{22} & \cdots & s_{2k} \\ \vdots & & & \vdots \\ s_{k1} & s_{k2} & \cdots & s_{kk} \end{bmatrix} \tag{39.2}$$

What is the most liberal criterion that we can apply to this matrix without violating the assumptions underlying repeated-measures ANOVA? By definition, the following equivalent properties are obeyed by the variance covariance matrix if the covariance structure is *spherical:*

$$\begin{aligned} &\forall j \neq j' \\ \sigma_{jj} + \sigma_{j'j'} - 2\sigma_{jj'} &= 2\lambda \\ \sigma^2_{X_j - X_{j'}} &= 2\lambda \\ \bar{\sigma}_{jj} - \bar{\sigma}_{jj'} &= \lambda \end{aligned} \tag{39.3}$$

In words, the statements in Eq. (39.3) say that for any pair of levels, the sum of their variances minus twice their covariance is equal to a constant. Equivalently, the variance of the difference between a pair of levels is the same for all pairs. Intuitively, it is clear that this assumption is violated, for example, in the case of temporal autocorrelation. In such a case, by definition, pairs of nearby levels (in this case time points) are more highly correlated than those separated by longer times. Another example might be an analysis that took three activations from each of a group member of two groups of subjects. Consider, for example, activation while reading, while writing, and while doing arithmetic. Assume we wanted to test whether the populations from which the two groups were drawn were significantly different, but we wanted to consider the three types of task together. This would involve an F test, but it would assume that the covariation between the reading and writing activations was the same as that between the writing and arithmetic. This may or may not be true. If it were not, sphericity would be violated, and the test would be overly liberal.

To illuminate the derivation of the term *sphericity,* we state without proof an equivalent condition to that in Eq. (39.3). This condition is that there can be found an orthonormal projection matrix M^* that can be used to transform the variables X of the original distribution to a new set of variables Y. This new set of variables has a covariance matrix Σ_Y that is *spherical* (i.e., is a scalar multiple of the identity matrix). This relation is exploited in the next section.

$$M^*M^{*\prime} = I$$

$$M^*\Sigma_x M^{*\prime} = \Sigma_y = \lambda I = \begin{bmatrix} \lambda & 0 & \dots & 0 \\ 0 & \lambda & \dots & 0 \\ \vdots & & & \vdots \\ 0 & 0 & \dots & \lambda \end{bmatrix} \tag{39.4}$$

$$\lambda = \frac{\sigma_{jj} + \sigma_{jj'} - 2\sigma_{jj'}}{2}$$

It is worth mentioning for completeness that while the sphericity condition is necessary it is not necessarily that intuitive nor is it clear by inspection whether a dataset conforms. Historically, therefore, a more restricted sufficient condition has been adopted, namely, *compound symmetry.* A matrix has compound symmetry if it has the following form:

$$\Sigma_x = \begin{bmatrix} \sigma^2 & \rho\sigma^2 & \dots & \rho\sigma^2 \\ \rho\sigma^2 & \sigma^2 & \dots & \rho\sigma^2 \\ \vdots & & & \vdots \\ \rho\sigma^2 & \rho\sigma^2 & \dots & \sigma^2 \end{bmatrix} \tag{39.5}$$

To describe the relation in Eq. (39.5) in words, all within-group variances are assumed equal, and separately all covariances are assumed equal and this can be assessed directly from the data. Statistical approaches do exist to assess whether a dataset deviates from sphericity such as Mauchly's test (see, e.g., Winer *et al.,* 1991), but these have very low power.

A Measure of Departure from Sphericity

Using the notation of the variance-covariance matrix from Eq. (39.1), we can define a measure of departure from sphericity after Box (1954):

$$\varepsilon = \frac{k^2(\bar{\sigma}_{jj} - \bar{\sigma}_{..})^2}{(k-1)\sum\sum(\sigma_{jj'} - \sigma_{j.} - \sigma_{.j} + \sigma_{..})} \tag{39.6}$$

where σ_{jj} = mean for diagonal entries, $\sigma_{..}$ = mean for all entries, $\sigma_{j.}$ = mean for row j, $\sigma_{.j}$ = and mean for column j. We can rephrase Eq. (39.6) in terms of λ_j, the characteristic roots of the transformed matrix Σ_y from Eq. (39.4):

$$\varepsilon = \frac{(\Sigma\lambda_i)^2}{(k-1)\sum\sum\lambda_i^2} \tag{39.7}$$

We now informally derive upper and lower bounds for our new measure. If Σ_y is spherical, i.e., of the form λI, then the roots are equal and because Σ_y is of size $(k-1) \times (k-1)$ then

$$\varepsilon = \frac{(\Sigma\lambda)^2}{(k-1)\sum\lambda^2} = \frac{((k-1)\lambda)^2}{(k-1)(k-1)\lambda^2} = 1 \tag{39.8}$$

At the opposite extreme, it can be shown that for a maximum departure from sphericity,

$$\Sigma_x = \begin{bmatrix} c & c & \dots & c \\ c & c & & c \\ \vdots & \vdots & & \vdots \\ c & c & \dots & c \end{bmatrix} \tag{39.9}$$

for some constant c. Then the first characteristic root $\lambda_1 = (k-1)c$ and the rest are zeros. From this we see that

$$\varepsilon = \frac{(\Sigma\lambda_i)^2}{(k-1)\Sigma\lambda_i^2} = \frac{\lambda_i^2}{(k-1)\Sigma\lambda_i^2} = \frac{1}{(k-1)} \tag{39.10}$$

Thus we have the following bounds:

$$\frac{1}{(k-1)} \leq \varepsilon \leq 1 \tag{39.11}$$

We have seen that the measure ε can be well defined using basic matrix algebra and that it expresses the degree to which the standard assumptions underlying the distribution are violated. In the following section, we employ this measure to systematically protect ourselves against falsely positive inferences by correcting the parameters of the F distribution.

Correcting Degrees of Freedom Using ε: The Satterthwaite Approximation

Box's motivation for using this measure for the departure from sphericity was designed to harness an approximation due to Satterthwaite. This deals with the fact that the actual distribution of the variance estimator is not χ^2 if the data are not spherical, and thus the F statistic used for hypothesis testing is inaccurate. The solution adopted is to approximate the true distribution with a moment matched scaled χ^2 distribution matching the first and second moments. Using this approximation in the context of repeated-measures ANOVA with k measures and n subjects, the overall F statistic will be distributed as $F[(k-1)\varepsilon, (n-1)(k-1)\varepsilon]$. To understand the elegance of this approach, note that, as shown above, when the sphericity assumptions underlying the model are met, $\varepsilon = 1$ and the F distribution is then just $F[(k-1), (n-1)(k-1)]$, the standard degrees of freedom for this model. The correction "vanishes" when it is not needed.

Finally, we note that this approximation has been adopted for neuroimaging data in SPM. Consider the expression for the effective degrees of freedom from Worsley and Friston (1995) that is applied in SPM99. There

$$\nu = \frac{\text{trace}(RV)^2}{\text{trace}(RVRV)} \tag{39.12}$$

Compare Eq. (39.7) and also see Chapter 47 for a derivation. If we remember that the conventional degrees of freedom for the t statistic is $k-1$ and consider as a correction for the degrees of freedom, then

$$\nu = (k-1)\varepsilon = (k-1)\frac{(\Sigma\lambda_i)^2}{(k-1)\Sigma\lambda_i^2} = \frac{(\Sigma\lambda_i)^2}{\Sigma\lambda_i^2} = \frac{\text{trace}(RV)^2}{\text{trace}(RVRV)} \tag{39.13}$$

Thus SPM applies the Satterthwaite approximation to correct the F statistic, implicitly using a measure of sphericity violation. In the next section, we will see that this approach is similar to that employed in conventional statistical packages.

Which Covariance Matrix Should Be Used for Estimation of Corrected Degrees of Freedom?

Returning to the classical approach, in practice of course we do not know Σ_x and so it will be estimated by S_x, the sample covariance matrix of Eq. (39.2). From this we can generate an $\hat{\varepsilon}$ by substituting $s_{jj'}$ for the $\sigma_{jj'}$ in Eq. (39.6). This correction that uses the sample covariance is often referred to as '*Greenhouse-Geisser correction*' e.g., Winer *et al.*, 1991). An extensive literature treats the further steps in harnessing this correction and some variants on it in practice. For example, correction can be made more conservative by taking the lower bound on $\hat{\varepsilon}$ as derived in Eq. (39.10). This highly conservative test is—confusingly—also referred to as the *Greenhouse-Geisser conservative correction.*

The important point to note, however, is that the construction of the F statistic is predicated on a model covariance structure that satisfies the assumptions of sphericity as outlined above, but the degrees of freedom are adjusted based on the *sample* covariance structure. This contrasts

TABLE 39.1 Possible Combinations of Approaches

	Classical approach Greenhouse-Geisser	SPM99	SPM 2
Choice of model	Assume sphericity	Assume i.i.d. or AR(1)	Use ReML to estimate covariance structure parameterised with a basis set
Corrected degrees of freedom based on covariance structure of ...	Actual data	Model	Model
Estimation of degrees of freedom is voxel-wise or for whole brain		Whole brain	Whole brain

with the approach taken in, for example, SPM99, which assumed either i.i.d. errors (a covariance matrix that is a scalar multiple of the identity matrix) or a simple autocorrelation structure, but corrected the degrees of freedom only on the basis of the *modelled* covariance structure. In the i.i.d. case, no correction was made regardless of what the data looked like. In the autocorrelation case, an appropriate correction was made, but it ignored the sample covariance matrix and assumed that the data structure was as modelled. These strategic differences are summarised in Table 39.1.

Estimating Covariance Components

In SPM2, a refinement is made in that the covariance structure can be estimated from the data. This is accomplished by defining a basis set for the covariance matrix and then using an iterative restricted maximum likelihood (ReML) algorithm to estimate parameters controlling these bases. In this way a wide range of sphericity violations can be modelled explicitly. Examples include temporal autocorrelation and more subtle effects of correlations induced by taking several measures on each of several subjects. In all cases, however, the modelled covariance structure is used to calculate the appropriate degrees of freedom using the moment-matching procedure described in Chapter 37. We do not discuss estimation in detail because this topic is covered in Chapters 43 and 47. We simply state the form of the parameterisation of the variance components and give illustrations of their typical form. We model the covariance matrix as follows:

$$\Sigma_x = \sum \lambda_j Q_j \tag{39.14}$$

where λ_j are some hyperparameters and Q_j represent some basis set for the covariance matrices. The Q_j term embodies the form of the covariance components at any level and could model different variances for different blocks of data or different forms of correlations within blocks. Estimation takes place using a ReML procedure in which the model coefficients and variance estimates are reestimated iteratively.

As will be discussed in the final section, what we in fact estimate is an intercorrelation matrix or normalised covariance for many voxels at once. This can be multiplied by a scalar variance estimate calculated for each voxel separately. Because this scalar does not affect the correlation structure, the corrected degrees of freedom are the same for all voxels.

Schematic Form of Covariance Constraints

These can be thought of as "design matrices" for the second-order behaviour of the response variable. They form a basis set for estimating the error covariance, with the hyperparameters scaling the contribution of each constraint. Figure 39.1 illustrates two possible applications of this technique. One for first-level analysis and one for random effects.

Three independent choices need to be made when dealing with data that may not be distributed according to one's model. We can consider the issues described above separately and

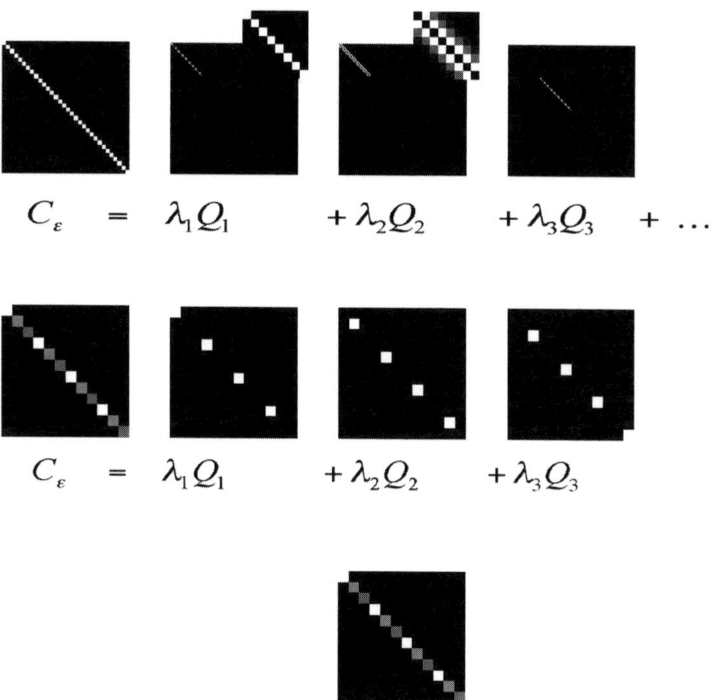

FIGURE 39.1
(Top row) Here we imagine that we have a number of observations over time and a number of subjects. We decide to model the autocorrelation structure by a sum of a simple autocorrelation AR(1) component and a white noise component. A separately scaled combination of these two can approximate a wide range of actual structures, since the white noise component affects the "peakiness" of the overall autocorrelation. For this purpose, we generate two bases for each subject, and here we illustrate the first three. The first is an identity matrix (no correlation) restricted to the observations from the first subject, the second is the same but blurred in time and with the diagonal removed. The third illustrated component is the white noise for the second subject and so on. (Bottom row) In this case we imagine that we have three measures for each of several subjects. For example, as suggested above, consider a second-level analysis in which we have a scan while reading, while writing and while doing arithmetic for several members of a population. We would like to make an inference about the population from which the subjects are drawn. We want to estimate what the covariation structure of the three measures is, but we assume that this structure is the same for each of the individuals. Here we generate three bases in total, one for all the reading scores, one for all the writing, and one for all the arithmetic. We then iteratively estimate the hyperparameters controlling each basis, and hence the covariance structure.

could in principle choose any combination of them for an analysis strategy. Table 39.1 illustrates the actual combination used in the approaches described in this chapter.

POOLING

So far we have discussed the variance structure of our data drawing from a univariate or mass univariate approach. In this section we ask whether we can harness the fact that our voxels come from the same brain. First, we motivate the question by demonstrating that sphericity estimation derives a noisy measure and that it might, therefore, be beneficial to pool over voxels. We will next show that under certain assumptions this strategy can be justified and then illustrate an implementation.

Simulating Noise in Sphericity Measures

To assess the practicality of voxel-wise estimation of the covariance structure we simulated 10,000 voxels drawn from a known population with eight measures of three levels of a repeated measure. For each voxel we estimated the variance-covariance matrix using a ReML procedure with a basis set corresponding to the true distribution. We then calculated the ε correction factor and plotted a histogram for the distribution of this over the 10,000 voxels (see Fig. 39.2). Note

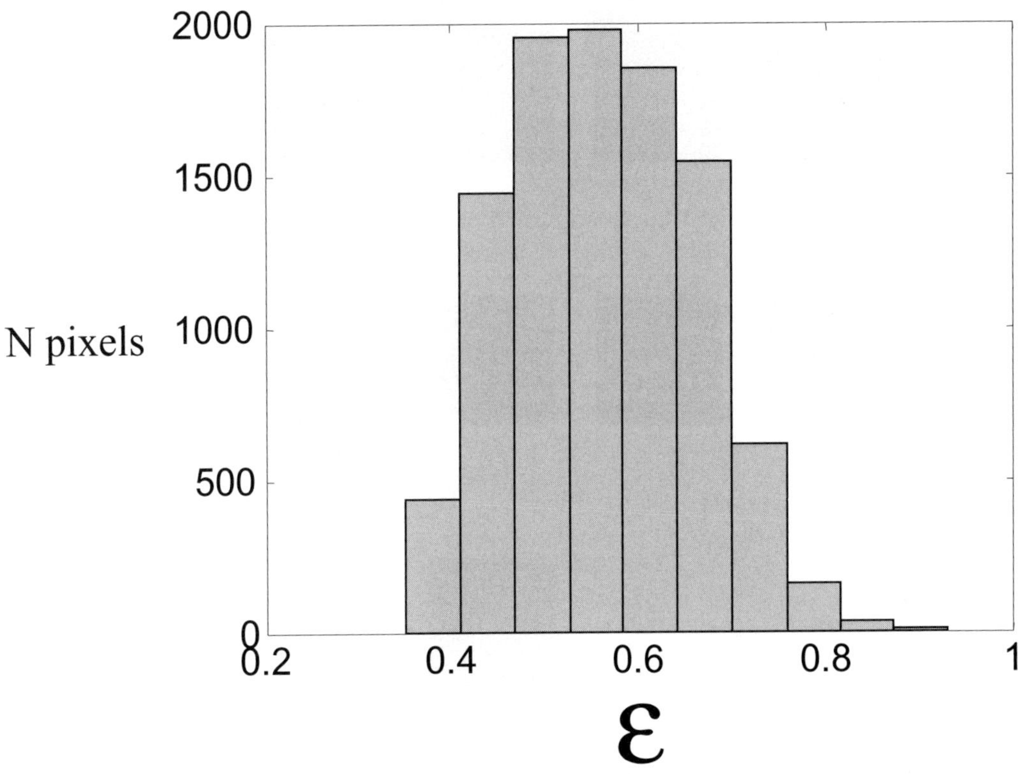

FIGURE 39.2
Histogram illustrating voxel-wise sphericity measure, ϵ, for 10,000 simulated voxels drawn from a known population with eight measures of three levels of a repeated measure. Average of the illustrated voxel-wise estimates is 0.56. The voxel-wide estimate was 0.65, and the ϵ for the generating distribution was indeed 0.65.

the wide distribution even for a uniform underlying variance structure, emphasising the utility of pooling the estimate over many voxels or even the whole brain to generate an intercorrelation matrix. The voxel-wide estimate was 0.65, which is higher (more spherical) than the average of the voxel-wise estimates illustrated above, which is 0.56. In this case the ε for the generating distribution was indeed 0.65.

Degrees of Freedom Reprised

As this simulation shows, to make the estimate of effective degrees of freedom valid, we require very precise estimates of nonsphericity. However, as mentioned at the start of this chapter, "pooling" is problematic because the true error variance may change from voxel to voxel. We now expand on the form described in Eq. (39.14) to describe in detail the strategy used by current fMRI analysis packages such as SPM and *multistat* (Worsley *et al.*, 2002). As stated, we hyperparameterise the error covariance in terms of a single hyperparameter that is voxel specific and a series of voxel-independent hyperparameters, which can be estimated with high precision over a large number of voxels. For the *i*th voxel, we are then assuming $\varepsilon_i \sim N\{0, \sigma_i^2 (\lambda_1 Q_1 +, \ldots, \lambda_n Q_n)\}$. This allows one to use the reduced single-hyperparameter model and the effective degrees of freedom as in Eq. (39.1) while still allowing error variance to vary from voxel to voxel. Here the pooling is over "similar" voxels (e.g., those that activate are spatially close), which are assumed to express various error variance components in the same proportion but not in the same amounts. In summary, we factorise the error covariance into voxel-specific variance and temporal covariance that is the same for all voxels in the subset. This effectively factorises the spatiotemporal covariance into nonstationary spatial covariance and stationary temporal nonsphericity. This enables pooling for, and only for, estimates of temporal covariances.

The problem is that estimating multiple hyperparameters (1) usually requires an iterative procedure that is computationally prohibitive for massive numbers of voxels and (2) gives imprecise estimates that render the inference less sensitive. The solution most commonly adopted is to retain the simplicity of the conventional single hyperparameter approach and use a generalised linear model with known nonsphericity (Worsley and Friston, 1995). In this approach the different variance components are estimated *a priori* and combined to give the nonsphericity structure in terms of a single error covariance matrix V. This reduces a problem with multiple variance components i.e., $\varepsilon \sim N\{0, \lambda_1 Q_1 +, \ldots, \lambda_n Q_n\}$ into a single component model $\varepsilon \sim N\{0, \sigma^2 V\}$ with a single hyperparameter σ^2. Inference can then proceed using OLS and the appropriate adjustments for the nonsphericity. As described in the previous section, the hyperparameter is estimated using the sum of squared residuals, and the Satterthwaite approximation is used to give the effective degrees of freedom.

The effective degrees of freedom can be thought of as adjusted for known nonsphericity. Here $V \propto \hat{\lambda}_1 Q_1 +, \ldots, \hat{\lambda}_n Q_n$ where the constant of proportionality is arbitrarily chosen to render $tr\{V\}$ equal to its size, cf. a correlation matrix. As stated above, the Satterthwaite approximation is exactly the same as that employed in the Greenhouse-Geisser (GG) correlation for nonsphericity in commercial packages. However, a fundamental distinction exists between the SPM adjustment and the GG correction. This is because the nonsphericity V enters as a known constant (or as an estimate with very high precision). In contradistinction, the nonsphericity in GG uses the sample covariance matrix or multiple hyperparameter estimates, usually ReML, based on the data themselves to give $\hat{V} \propto \hat{\boldsymbol{\lambda}}_1 Q_1 +, \ldots, \hat{\lambda}_n Q_n$. This gives corrected degrees of freedom that are generally too high, leading to mildly capricious inferences.[1] Compare the following with (39.12):

$$\nu_{GG} = tr\{R\}\varepsilon_{GG} = \frac{tr\{R\hat{V}\}^2}{tr\{R\hat{V}R\hat{V}\}} \tag{39.15}$$

The reason the degrees of freedom are too high is that GG fails to take into account the variability in the ReML hyperparameter estimates and ensuing variability in $\hat{V}$. There are simple solutions to this that involve abandoning the single variance component model and forming statistics using multiple hyperparameters directly (Kiebel *et al.*, 2003).

The critical difference between conventional GG corrections and the SPM adjustment lies in the fact that SPM is a mass univariate approach that can pool nonsphericity estimates $\hat{V}$ over subsets of voxels to give a highly precise estimate V. Conventional univariate packages cannot do this because there is only one data sequence.

Separable Errors

The final issue addressed in this chapter is how relative values of the voxel-independent hyperparameters are estimated and how precise these estimates are. There are many situations in which the hyperparameters of mass univariate observations factorise. In the present context we can regard fMRI time series as having both spatial and temporal correlations among the errors that factorise in a Kronecker tensor product. Consider the data matrix $Y = [y_i, \text{k}, y_n]$ with one column, over time, for each of n voxels. The spatiotemporal correlations can be expressed as the error covariance matrix in a vectored GLM:

$$Y = X\beta + \varepsilon$$

$$vec\{Y\} = \begin{bmatrix} y_i \\ \vdots \\ y_n \end{bmatrix} = \begin{bmatrix} X & & 0 \\ & \ddots & \vdots \\ 0 & \ldots & X \end{bmatrix} \begin{bmatrix} \beta_i \\ \vdots \\ \beta_n \end{bmatrix} + \begin{bmatrix} \varepsilon_i \\ \vdots \\ \varepsilon_n \end{bmatrix} \tag{39.16}$$

$$\text{cov}\ \{vec\{\varepsilon\}\ \} = \Sigma \otimes V = \begin{bmatrix} \Sigma_1 V & & \Sigma_{1n} V \\ & \ddots & \vdots \\ \Sigma_{n1} V & \ldots & \Sigma_n V \end{bmatrix}$$

Note that Eq. (39.16) assumes a separable form for the errors. This is the key assumption underlying the pooling procedure. Here V embodies the temporal nonsphericity and Σ the spatial nonsphericity. Notice that the elements of Σ are voxel specific, whereas the elements of V are the same for all voxels. We could now enter the vectored data directly into a ReML scheme to

[1] This is only a problem if the variance components interact (e.g., as with serial correlations in fMRI).

estimate the spatial and temporal hyperparameters. However, we can capitalise on the assumed separable form of the nonsphericity over time and space by estimating only the hyperparameters of V and then use the usual estimator (Worsley and Friston, 1995) to compute a single hyperparameter $\hat{\Sigma}_i$ for each voxel according to Eq. (39.16).

The hyperparameters of V can be estimated with the algorithm presented in Friston *et al.* (2002, Appendix 1). This uses a Fisher scoring scheme to maximise the log likelihood $\ln p(Y \mid \lambda, \Sigma)$ (i.e., the ReML objective function) to find the ReML estimates. In the current context this scheme is

$$\begin{aligned} \lambda &\leftarrow \lambda + W^{-1}g \\ g_i &= \frac{\partial \ln p\,(Y \mid \lambda, \Sigma)}{\partial \lambda_i} = \frac{n}{2}\, tr\{PQ_i\} + \frac{1}{2}\, tr\{P^T Q_i P Y \Sigma^{-1} Y^T\} \\ W_{ij} &= E\left\{-\frac{\partial^2 \ln p\,(Y \mid \lambda, \Sigma)}{\partial \lambda_{ij}^2}\right\} = \frac{n}{2}\, tr\{PQ_i PQ_j\} \\ P &= V^{-1} - V^{-1}X\,(X^T V^{-1} X)^{-1} X^T V^{-1} \\ V &= \lambda_1 Q_1 +, \ldots, \lambda_n Q_n \end{aligned} \tag{39.17}$$

where $E\{\,\}$ is the expectation operator. Notice that the Kronecker tensor products and vectorised forms disappear. Critically W, the precision of the hyperparameter estimates, increases linearly with the number of voxels. With sufficient voxels this allows us to enter the resulting estimates, through V, into Eq. (39.16) as known variables, because they are so precise. The nice thing about Eq. (39.17) is that the data enter only as $Y\Sigma^{-1}Y^T$ whose size is determined by the number of scans as opposed to the massive number of voxels. The term $Y\Sigma^{-1}Y^T$ is effectively the sample temporal covariance matrix, sampling over voxels (after spatial whitening), and can be assembled voxel by voxel in a memory efficient fashion. Equation (39.17) assumes that we know the spatial covariances. In practice, $Y\Sigma^{-1}Y^T$ is approximated by selecting voxels that are spatially dispersed (so that $\Sigma_{ij} = 0$) and scaling the data by a ReML estimate of Σ_i^{-1} that is obtained noniteratively assuming temporal sphericity.

CONCLUSIONS

We have shown that classical and recent approaches do not explicitly estimate the covariance structure of the noise in their data but instead assumed it has a tractable form, and then corrects for any deviations from the assumptions by an approximation. This approximation can be based on the actual data or on a defined structure that is imposed on the data. More modern approaches explicitly model the types of covariation that the experimenter expects to find in the data. This estimation can be noisy and, therefore, is best conducted over pooled collections of voxels.

The use of this technique allows the experimenter to perform types of analysis that were previously "forbidden" under the less sophisticated schemes. These are of real interest to many researchers and include better estimation of the autocorrelation structure for fMRI data and the ability to take more than one scan per subject to the second level and thus conduct F tests to draw conclusions about populations. In event-related studies where the exact form of the haemodynamic response can be critical, more than one aspect of this response can be analysed in a random-effects context. For example, a canonical form and a measure of latency or spread in time can jointly express a wide range of real responses. Alternatively, a more general basis set (e.g., Fourier or finite impulse response) can be used allowing for non-spherity among the different components of the set.

References

Box, G. E. P. (1954). Some theorems on quadratic forms applied in the study of analysis of variance problems. *Ann. Math. Statistics* **25,** 290–302.

Friston, K. J., Josephs, O., Zarahn, E., Holmes, A. P., Rouquette, S., and Poline J. (2000). To smooth or not to smooth? Bias and efficiency in fMRI time-series analysis. *NeuroImage* **12**(2), 196–208.

Friston, K. J., Glaser, D. E., Henson, R. N., Kiebel, S., Phillips, C., and Ashburner, J. (2002) Classical and Bayesian inference in neuroimaging: applications. *NeuroImage* **6**(2), 484–512.

Keselman, H. J., Algina, J., and Kowalchuk, R. K. (2001). The analysis of repeated measures designs: a review. *Br. J. Math. Stat. Psychol.* **54**(Pt 1), 1–20.

Kiebel, S. J., Glaser, D. E., and Friston, K.J. (2003) A heuristic for the degrees of freedom of statistics based on multiple hyperparameters.

Winer, B. J. *et al.* (1991). "Statistical Principles in Experimental Design." McGraw-Hill, New York.

Worsley, K. J., and Friston, K. J. (1995). Analysis of fMRI time-series revisited—again. *NeuroImage* **2,** 173—181.

Worsley, K. J., Liao, C. H., Aston, J., Petro, V., Duncan, G. H., Morales, F., and Evans, A. C. (2002). A general statistical analysis for fMRI data. *NeuroImage*, **15**, 1–15.

CHAPTER

40

Analysis of fMRI Time Series

Linear Time-Invariant Models, Event-Related fMRI, and Optimal Experimental Design

INTRODUCTION

This chapter discusses issues specific to the analysis of fMRI data. It extends the generalised linear model (GLM) introduced in Chapter 37 to linear time-invariant (LTI) systems, in which the blood oxygenation level dependent (BOLD) signal is modelled by neuronal causes that are expressed via a haemodynamic response function (HRF). The first section introduces the concepts of temporal basis functions, temporal filtering of fMRI data, and models of temporal autocorrelation. The second section describes the application of these ideas to event-related models, including issues relating to the temporal resolution of fMRI. The third section concerns the efficiency of fMRI experimental designs, as a function of the interstimulus interval and ordering of stimulus types. The final section illustrates some of the concepts introduced in the preceding sections with an example dataset from a single-subject event-related fMRI experiment.

fMRI TIME SERIES

Unlike PET scans, it is important to order fMRI scans as a function of time, i.e., treat them as a time series. This is because the BOLD signal will tend to be correlated across successive scans, meaning that they can no longer be treated as independent samples. The main reason for this correlation is the fast acquisition time (T_R) for fMRI (typically 2–4 sec compared to 8–12 minutes for PET) relative to the duration of the BOLD response (at least 30 sec). Treating fMRI data as time series also allows us to view statistical analyses in signal processing terms.

The GLM can be expressed as a function of time [Friston *et al.*, 1994; see Eq. (37.1) in Chapter 37]:

$$y(t) = x_c(t)\,\beta_c + \varepsilon(t) \qquad \varepsilon(t) \sim N(0,\sigma^2\Sigma) \tag{40.1}$$

where the data $y(t)$ comprise the fMRI time series (with each time point representing one scan), the explanatory variables, $x_c(t)$, $c = 1..N_c$ are now functions of time, β_c are the N_c (time-invariant) parameters, and Σ is the noise autocorrelation (see "Temporal Autocorrelation" section below). Though $y(t)$ and $x_c(t)$ are discrete (sampled) time series (normally represented by the vector **y** and design matrix **X**, respectively), we initially treat the data and model in terms of continuous time.

Stimulus, Neural and Haemodynamic Models, and Linear Time Invariance

An explanatory variable $x(t)$ represents the predicted BOLD response arising from a neural cause $u(t)$. These neural causes (e.g., the local field potentials of an ensemble of neurons) normally follow a sequence of experimental stimulation, $s(t)$. In SPM99, a distinction is made between neural activity that is impulsive (an *event*) and that which is sustained for several seconds after stimulation (an *epoch*). Both can be specified in terms of their onsets, but differ in the form of the neural model. For $i = 1.. N_i$ experimental conditions, each consisting of $j = 1, \ldots, N_j$ onset times o_{ij}, the stimulus model is as follows:

$$s_i(t) = \Sigma_{j=1\ldots Nj}\, \alpha_{ij}\, \delta(t{-}o_{ij}) \tag{40.2}$$

where α_{ij} is a scaling factor and $\delta(t)$ is the (Dirac) delta function. The vector $\boldsymbol{\alpha}_\mathbf{i}$ over the N_j replications of the ith condition corresponds to a *parametric modulation* of that condition (e.g., by behavioural data associated with each stimulus; see later "Parametric Model" section for an example).[1] Below we assume α_{ij} is fixed at 1.

For events, the neural activity $u_i(t)$ is equated with $s_i(t)$. For epochs, the neural activity, $r(\tau)$, is modelled by $b = 1\ldots N_b$ temporal *basis functions*, $g_b(\tau)$:

$$r(\tau) = \Sigma_{b=1\ldots Nb}\, \beta_b\, g_b(\tau) \tag{40.3}$$

where τ indexes a finite peristimulus time (PST) over the epoch duration T_E (and the β_b are parameters to be estimated). Some example epoch response functions are shown in Fig. 40.1A. The simplest is a single "boxcar" or "tophat" function that assumes a constant level of neural activity during the epoch. This can be supplemented by a mean-corrected exponential decay (e.g., of form $\exp[-\tau/(4T_E)]$) to capture adaptation effects within an epoch. Other examples include a half-sine, $\sin(\pi\tau/T_E)$ and a discrete cosine transform (DCT) set, $g_b(\tau) = \cos[(b - 1)\pi\tau/T_E]$. The latter can capture any shape of neural response up to frequency limit $(N_b - 1)/2T_E$. The neural activity, from Eqs. (40.2) and (40.3) then becomes

$$u_i(\tau) = s_i(\tau) \otimes r(\tau) = \Sigma_{j=1\ldots Nj}\, \Sigma_{b=1\ldots Nb}\, \beta_b g_b(t{-}o_{ij})$$

If we assume that the BOLD signal is the output of a LTI system (Boynton *et al.,* 1996), that is, that the form of the response is independent of time, and the responses to successive stimuli superpose in a linear fashion, then we can express $x_i(t)$ as the convolution of the neural activity with a HRF, $h(\tau)$:

$$x_i(t) = u_i(t) \otimes h(\tau) \tag{40.4}$$

where τ now indexes a finite period, T_H, over which the BOLD response lasts (a *finite impulse response*). The HRF $h(\tau)$ is equivalent to the first-order Volterra kernel (see Chapter 41).[2] Figure 40.1B shows the BOLD signal predicted from convolution of an epoch, modelled by boxcar and exponential decay response functions, with a "canonical" form for the HRF. Also shown in Fig. 40.1C is the BOLD signal predicted for a series of rapid events (delta functions); note the near-equivalent BOLD signal obtained[3] (provided the interevent interval is a few seconds or less).

In other situations, we may not want to assume a fixed form for the HRF. Instead, we can allow for variability in its form by another expansion in terms of temporal basis functions, $f_k(\tau)$:

$$h(\tau) = \Sigma_{k=1\ldots Nk}\, \beta_k\, f_k(\tau) \tag{40.5}$$

(see later "Temporal Basis Functions" section for some examples). For a sequence of events, the GLM then becomes [from ([40.1), (40.2) and (40.4)]

$$y(t) = \Sigma_{i=1\ldots Ni}\, \Sigma_{j=1\ldots Nj}\, \Sigma_{k=1\ldots Nk}\, \beta_{ijk}\, f_k(t - o_{ij}) + \varepsilon(t)$$

where β_{ijk} are the parameters to be estimated.

---

[1] A polynomial expansion of α_{ij} can be used to test for higher order (nonlinear) dependencies of neural activity on the parametric factor.

[2] It is also possible to model nonlinearities in the mapping from stimulus to neural activity in terms of a Volterra expansion (Josephs & Henson, 1999). However, because we normally only know the stimulus function (input) and the BOLD signal (output), we cannot attribute nonlinearities uniquely to the stimulus-to-neural or neural-to-BOLD (or blood flow-to-BOLD) mappings.

[3] Bar a small shift in latency (Mechelli *et al.,* in 2000b).

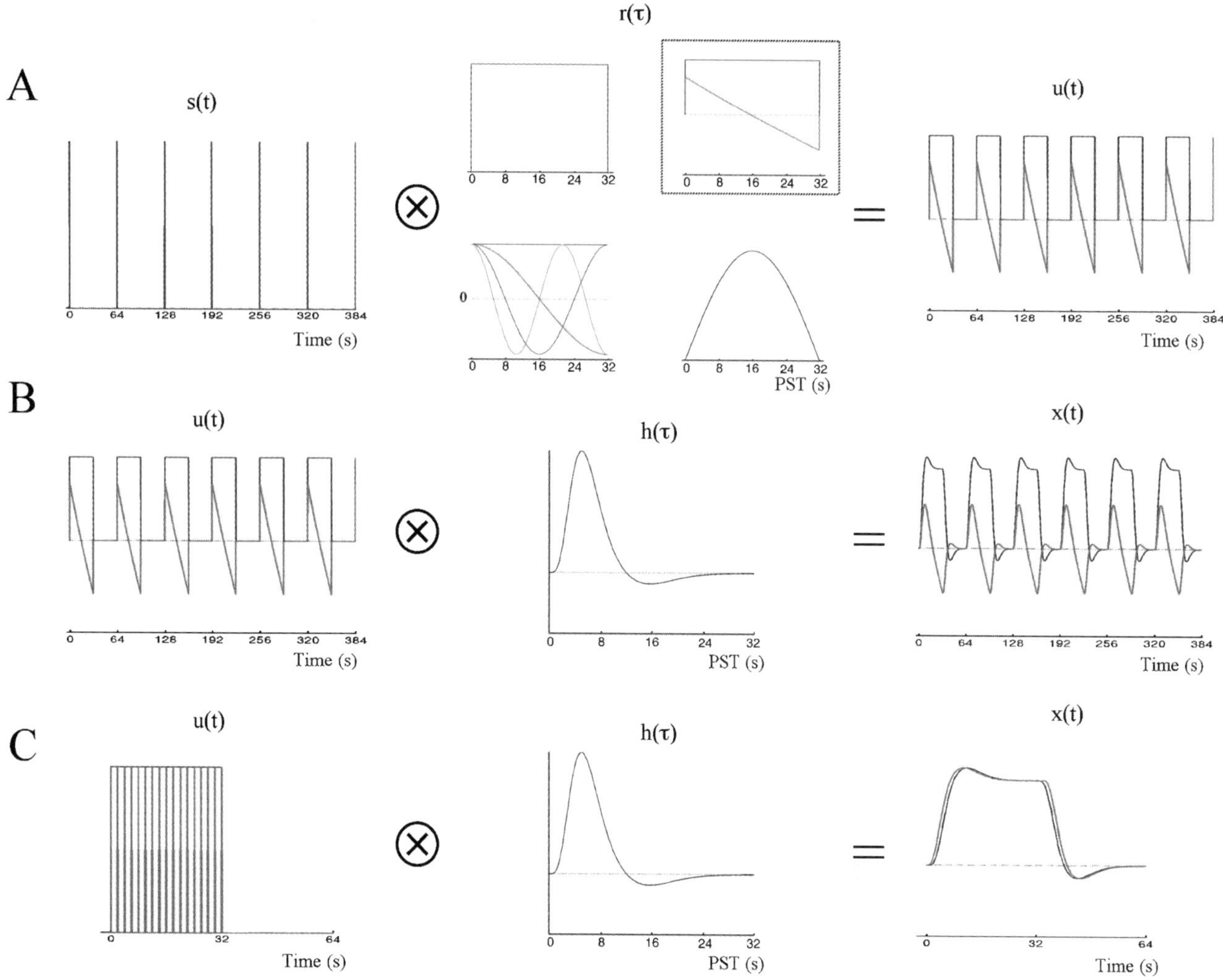

FIGURE 40.1
Stimulus, neural, and haemodynamic models. (A) Stimulus model, $s(t)$, for squarewave stimulation (32 sec on, 32 sec off) convolved with one of several possible epoch response function sets, $r(\tau)$, offered by SPM99 (clockwise: boxcar, boxcar plus exponential decay, half-sine, and DCT; boxcar plus exponential decay chosen here) to produce the predicted neural signal $u(t)$. (B) Neural signal convolved with a canonical HRF, $h(\tau)$, to produce the predicted BOLD signal, $x(t)$. (C) An alternative model of squarewave stimulation in terms of delta functions every 2 sec (green) predicts a BOLD response similar to a boxcar epoch response (blue) after scaling.

In practice, the above models are simulated in discrete time. Nonetheless, given that significant information may exist in the predicted signal at frequencies above that associated with typical T_R's, the simulations are performed in a time space with multiple ($T > 1$) time points per scan (i.e., with resolution, $dt = T_R/T$ sec). This means, for example, that events do not need to be synchronised with scans (their onsets can be specified in fractions of scans). The high-resolution time space also ensures that a sequence of delta functions (every dt sec) becomes an adequate discrete-time approximation to a continuous boxcar function. To create the explanatory vectors, $\mathbf{x}_c$, in units of scans, the predicted BOLD signal is down-sampled every T_R (at a specified time point T_0; Fig. 40.2). In the general case, the number of columns in the design matrix will be $N_c = N_i N_j N_k N_b$.

High-Pass Filtering

We can also view the frequency components of our time series $y(t)$ via the Fourier transform. A schematic of the power spectrum (the modulus of the complex Fourier components), typical of a subject at rest in the scanner, is shown in Fig. 40.3A. This "noise" spectrum is dominated by low frequencies and has been characterised by a $1/f$ form when expressed in amplitude (Zarahn

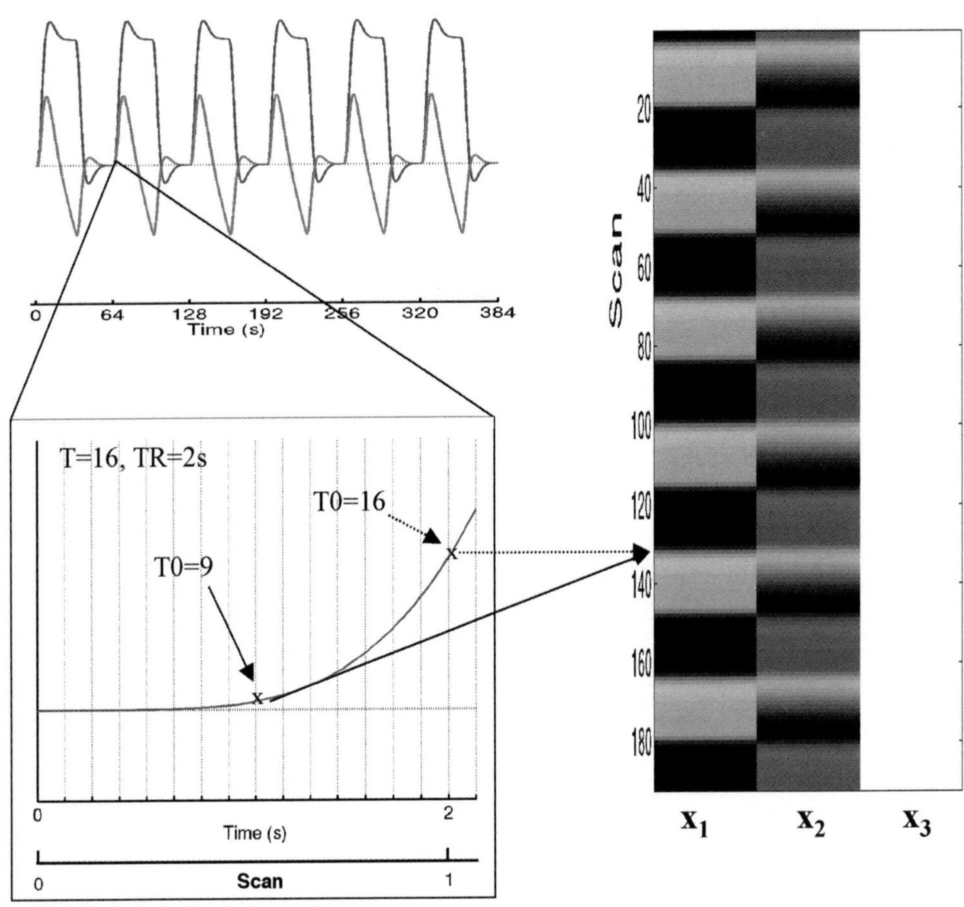

FIGURE 40.2
Creation of regressors for design matrix. Predicted BOLD signal $x(t)$ from Fig. 40.1B, simulated every $dt = T_R/T$ sec, is down-sampled every T_R at time point T_0 to create the columns $\mathbf{x}_1$ (boxcar) and $\mathbf{x}_2$ (exponential decay) of the design matrix (together with the mean or constant term $\mathbf{x}_3$). Two possible sample points are shown: at the middle and end of a 2-sec scan.

et al., 1997b). The noise arises from physical sources, sometimes referred to as *scanner drift* (e.g., slowly varying changes in ambient temperature), from physiological sources (e.g., biorhythms, such as ~1-Hz respiratory or ~0.25-Hz cardiac cycles, that are aliased by the slower sampling rate), and from residual movement effects and their interaction with the static magnetic field (Turner *et al.,* 1998). When the subject is performing a task, signal components are added that we wish to distinguish from this noise. Figure 40.3B, for example, shows the approximate signal spectrum imposed by an (infinite) square-wave stimulation of 32 sec on/32 sec off. When averaging over all frequencies, this signal might be difficult to detect against the background noise. However, by filtering the data with an appropriate high-pass filter (Fig. 40.3C), we can remove most of the noise. Ideally, the remaining noise spectrum would be flat (i.e., white noise, with equal power at all frequencies, though see next section).

The choice of the high-pass cutoff would ideally maximise the signal-to-noise ratio (SNR). However, we cannot distinguish signal from noise on the basis of the power spectrum of the data alone. One choice of cutoff is to minimise the loss of signal, the frequency components of which are inherent in the design matrix **X**. SPM99 offers such a cutoff by default (based on twice the maximum interval between the most frequently occurring condition). However, if this cutoff period is too great, the gain in signal passed can be outweighed by the extra noise passed. Thus, some loss of signal may be necessary to minimise noise.[4] Experimental designs should therefore

[4] In our experience, the $1/f$ noise becomes appreciable at frequencies below approximately 1/120 Hz, though this figure may vary considerably across scanners and subjects.

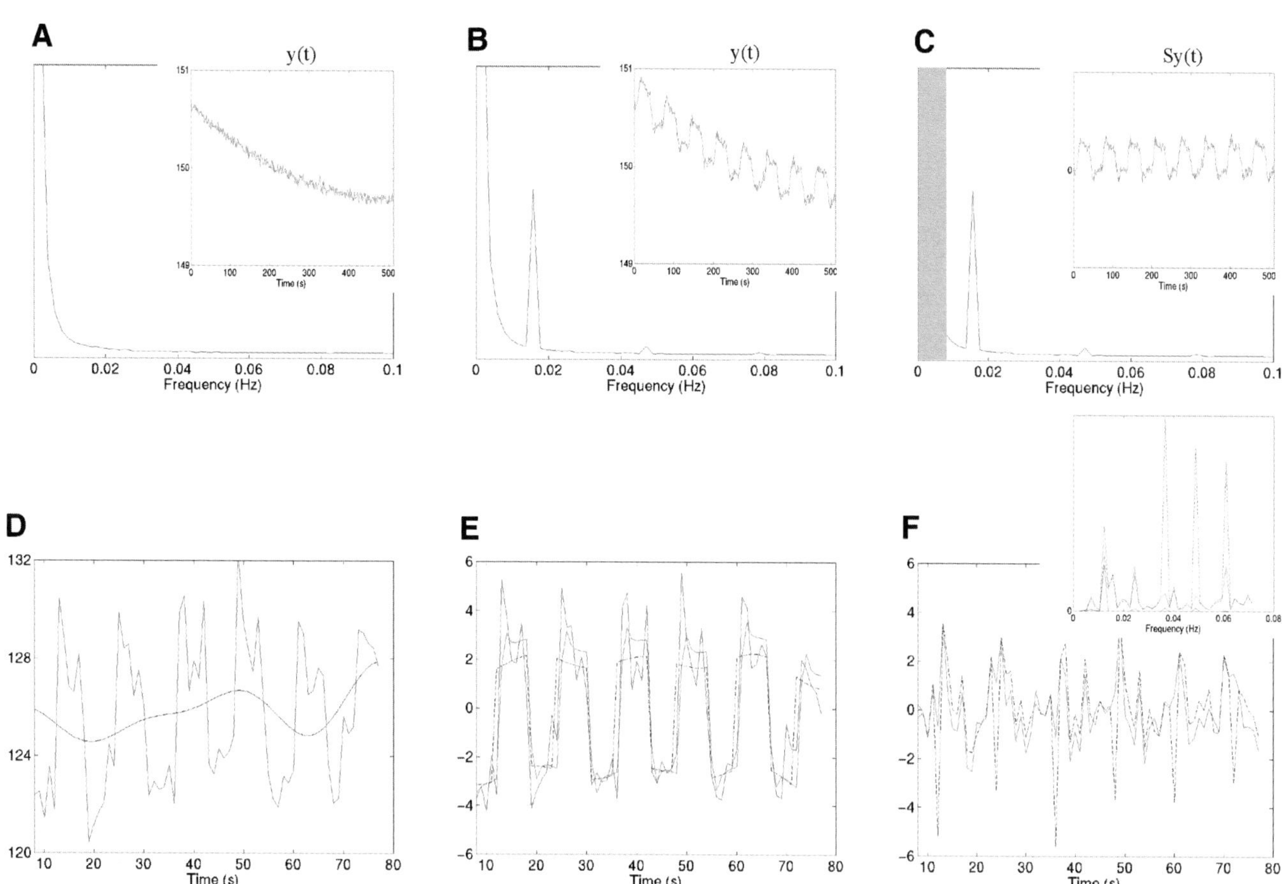

FIGURE 40.3
Power spectra, high-pass filtering, and HRF convolution. Schematic power spectrum and time series (inset) for (A) subject at rest, (B) after squarewave stimulation at 32 sec on, 32 sec off. (C) After high-pass filtering with a 128-sec cutoff. (D) Real data (blue) and low-frequency drift (black) fitted by DCT high-pass filter matrix **S** (with 168-sec cutoff) derived from the global maximum in a 42-sec-on, 42-sec-off auditory blocked design (T_R = 7 sec). (E) Fits of a boxcar epoch model with (red) and without (black) convolution by a canonical HRF, together with the data, after application of the high-pass filter. (F) Residuals after fits of models with and without HRF convolution. Note the large systematic errors for model without HRF convolution (black) at onset of each block, corresponding to (nonwhite) harmonics of the stimulation frequency in the residual power spectrum (inset).

not embody significant power at low frequencies (i.e., conditions to be contrasted should not live too far apart in time; see late "Efficiency and Optimisation of Experimental Design" section).

In the time domain, a high-pass filter can be implemented by a DCT with harmonic periods up to the cutoff. These basis functions can be made explicit as confounds in the design matrix, or they can be viewed as part of a temporal smoothing matrix, **S** (together with any low-pass filtering; see next section).[5] This matrix is applied to both data and model:

$$\mathbf{Sy} = \mathbf{SX}\beta + \mathbf{S}\boldsymbol{\varepsilon} \qquad \boldsymbol{\varepsilon} \sim N(0,\sigma^2\mathbf{V}) \qquad \mathbf{V} = \mathbf{S}\Sigma\mathbf{S}^{\mathrm{T}}$$

(treating the time series as vectors), with the classical correction for the degrees of freedom lost in the filtering inherent in the equation for the effective degrees of freedom (Chapter 39):

$$\nu = \mathrm{trace}\{\mathbf{RV}\}^2/\mathrm{trace}\{\mathbf{RVRV}\} \qquad \mathbf{R} = \mathbf{I} - \mathbf{SX}(\mathbf{SX})^+ \tag{40.6}$$

The effect of applying a high-pass filter to real data (taken from a 42-sec epoch experiment; http://www.fil.ion.ucl.ac.uk/spm/data#fMRI_MoAEpilot) is illustrated in Fig. 40.3D. Figure 40.3E shows the fitted responses after the filter **S** is applied to two boxcar models, one with and one without convolution with the HRF. The importance of convolving the neural model with an HRF is evident in the residuals (Fig. 40.3F). Had the explanatory variables been directly equated with the stimulus function, significant temporal structure would remain in the residuals (e.g., as

[5] Though the matrix form expediates mathematical analysis, in practice high-pass filtering is implemented by the computationally efficient subtraction of $RR^{T}y$, where **R** is the residual-forming matrix associated with the DCT.

negative deviations at the start of each block, that is, at higher frequency harmonics of the boxcar function).

Temporal Autocorrelation

There are various reasons why the noise component may not be white even after high-pass filtering. These include unmodelled neuronal noise sources that have their own haemodynamic correlates. Because these components live in the same frequency range as the effects of interest, they cannot be removed by the high-pass filter. These noise sources induce temporal correlation between the residual errors, $\varepsilon(t)$. Such autocorrelation is a special case of nonsphericity, which is treated more generally in Chapter 39. Here, we briefly review the various solutions to the specific problem of temporal autocorrelation in fMRI time series.

One solution proposed by Worsley and Friston (1995) is to apply a temporal smoothing. This is equivalent to adding a low-pass filter component to **S** (such that **S**, together with the high-pass filter, becomes a *bandpass* filter). If the time constants of the smoothing kernel are sufficiently large, the temporal autocorrelation induced by the smoothing can be assumed to swamp any intrinsic autocorrelation, Σ, such that

$$\mathbf{V} = \mathbf{S}\Sigma\mathbf{S}^{\mathrm{T}} \sim \mathbf{S}\mathbf{S}^{\mathrm{T}}$$

and thus the effective degrees of freedom can be calculated, using Eq. (40.6), solely via the known smoothing matrix. Low-pass filters derived from a Gaussian smoothing kernel with a full-width at half-maximum (FWHM) of 4–6 sec, or derived from a typical HRF, have been suggested (Friston *et al.,* 2000b).

An alternative solution is to estimate the intrinsic autocorrelation directly, which can be used to create a filter to "prewhiten" the data before fitting the GLM. In other words, the smoothing matrix is set to $\mathbf{S} = \mathbf{K}^{-1}$, where $\mathbf{K}\mathbf{K}^{\mathrm{T}}$ is the estimated autocorrelation matrix. If the estimation is exact, then

$$\mathbf{V} = \mathbf{K}^{-1}\Sigma(\mathbf{K}^{-1})^{\mathrm{T}} = \mathbf{K}^{-1}\mathbf{K}\mathbf{K}^{\mathrm{T}}(\mathbf{K}^{-1})^{\mathrm{T}} = \mathbf{I}$$

Two methods for estimating the autocorrelation are an autoregressive (AR) model (Bullmore *et al.,* 1996) and a $1/f$ model (Zarahn *et al.,* 1997b). An AR(p) is a pth-order autoregressive model, having the following time-domain form:

$$z(t) = a_1 z(t\text{-}1) + a_2 z(t\text{-}2)\ldots + a_p z(t\text{-}p) + w \Rightarrow \mathbf{z} = \mathbf{A}\mathbf{z} + \mathbf{w} \quad \mathbf{w} \sim N(0,\sigma^2\mathbf{I})$$

where **A** is a $(p + 1) \times (p + 1)$ lower triangular matrix of regression coefficients, a_i, that can be estimated by ordinary least squares. Several authors (e.g., Bullmore *et al.,* 1996; Kruggel and von Cramon, 1999b) use an AR(1) model, in which the autocorrelation (a_1) and noise (σ^2) parameters are estimated from the residuals ($\mathbf{z} = \varepsilon$) after fitting the GLM. These estimates are then used to create the filter $\mathbf{S} = (\mathbf{I} - \mathbf{A})^{-1}$ that is applied to the data before refitting the GLM (a procedure that can be iterated until the residuals are white).

The $1/f$ model is a linear model with the following frequency-domain form:

$$g(f) = b_1/f + b_2 \qquad p(f) = g(f)^2$$

where $p(f)$ is the power spectrum, the parameters of which, b_i, can be estimated from the Fourier-transformed data.

The advantage of these methods is that they produce the most efficient estimation of the GLM parameters under Gaussian assumptions (corresponding to Gauss-Markov or "minimum variance estimators"). Temporal smoothing is generally less efficient because it removes high-frequency components, which may contain signal. The disadvantage of the temporal autocorrelation models is that they can produce biased parameter estimates if the autocorrelation is not estimated accurately (i.e., do not necessarily produce "minimum bias estimators").

Friston *et al.* (2000b) argued that the AR(1) and $1/f$ models are not sufficient to estimate the typical autocorrelation in fMRI data. This is illustrated in Fig. 40.4A, which shows the power spectra and *autocorrelation functions*[6] for the residuals of an event-related dataset (as given in

[6] An autocorrelation function plots the correlation, $r(t)$, as a function of "lag", $t = 0..n - 1$, and is simply the Fourier transform of the power spectrum, $p(f)$, where $f = 2\pi i$, for $i = 1..n - 1$.

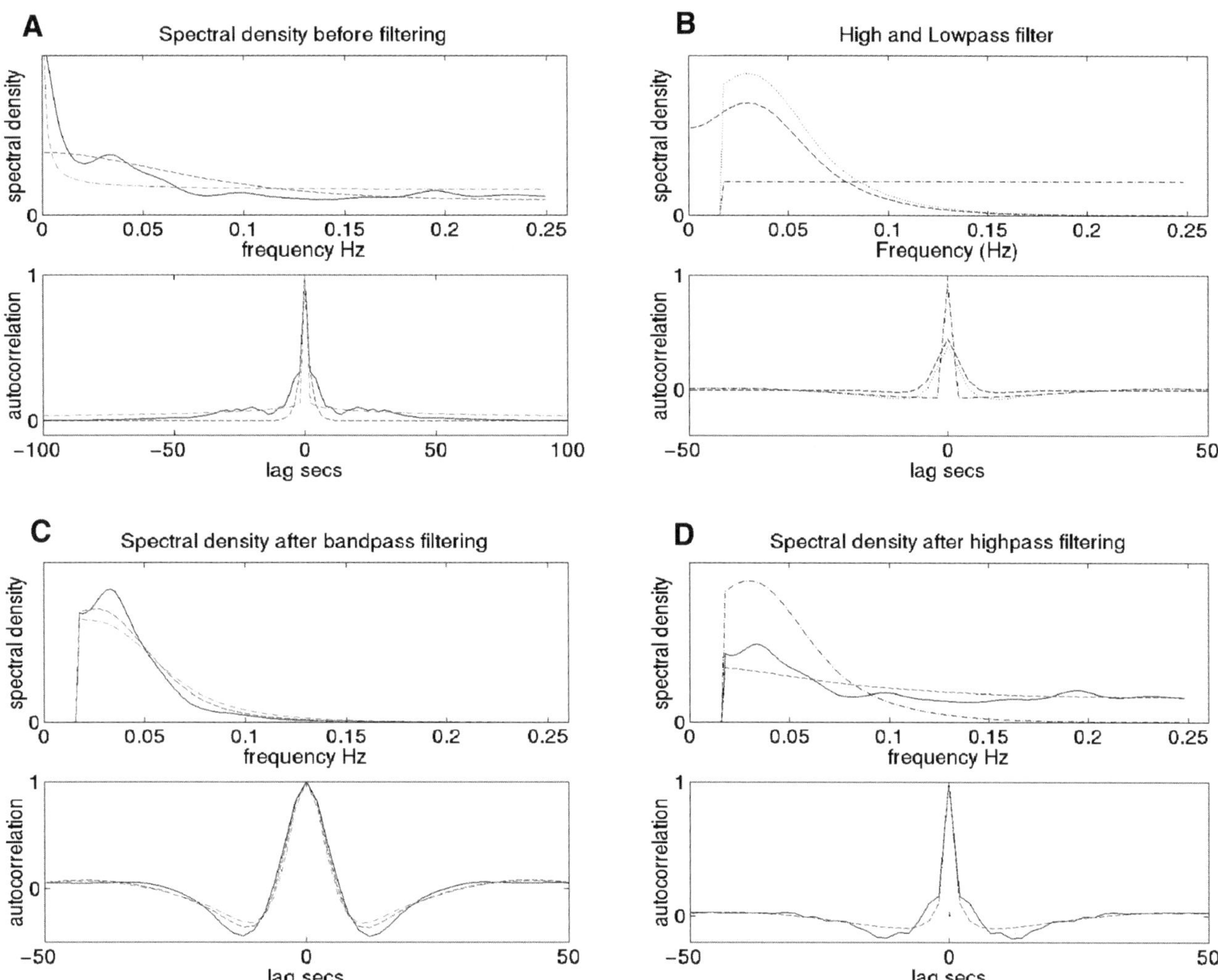

FIGURE 40.4

Models of fMRI temporal autocorrelation. Power spectra and autocorrelation functions for (A) data (solid black), derived from an AR(16) estimation of the mean, globally normalised residuals from one slice ($z = 0$) of an event-related dataset (described in the "Worked Example" section), together with fits of an AR(1) model (dashed blue) and $1/f$ amplitude model (dashed red); (B) high- (dot-dash) and low- (dotted) pass filters, comprising a bandpass filter (dashed); (C) data and both models after bandpass filtering [note that bandpass filter characteristics in (B) would also provide a reasonable approximation to residual autocorrelation]; (D) data (solid black) and ReML fit of AR(1)+white noise model (dashed blue) after high-pass filtering (also shown is the bandpass filter power spectrum, demonstrating the high-frequency information that would be lost by low-pass smoothing).

the later "Worked Example" section). We can see that the AR(1) model underpredicts the intermediate-range correlations, whereas the $1/f$ model overpredicts the long-range correlations. Such a mismatch between the assumed ($\mathbf{KK}'$) and intrinsic (Σ) autocorrelation will bias the statistics resulting from prewhitening the data.[7] This mismatch can be ameliorated by combining bandpass filtering (Fig. 40.4B) with modelling of the autocorrelation, in which case both models provide a reasonable fit (Fig. 40.4C). Indeed, high-pass filtering alone, with an appropriate cutoff, is normally sufficient to allow either model to fit the remaining autocorrelation (Friston *e*t al., 2000b).

SPM99 offers both an AR(1) model and low-pass smoothing as options (in conjunction with high-pass filtering). The AR(1) model parameters are estimated from the data covariance, rather than the residuals. This removes the potential bias resulting from correlation in the residuals induced by removing modelled effects (Friston *et al.,* 2002),[8] although it introduces potential

[7] More complex models of the temporal autocorrelation have since been shown to minimise bias, such as Tukey tapers (Woolrich *et al.,* 2001) and autoregessive moving average (ARMA) models, a special case of the latter being an AR(1)+white noise model (Burock & Dale, 2000).

[8] Note, however, that there are ways of reducing this bias (Worsely *et al.,* 2002).

bias resulting from signal and drifts in the data. The latter is ameliorated by pooling over voxels in the estimation of the AR(1) parameters, since only a minority of voxels typically contain signal. Another potential problem arises, however, if the temporal autocorrelation varies over voxels (Zarahn *et al.,* 1997b). For example, it has been argued to be higher in grey than white matter (Woolrich *et al.,* 2001). This can be accommodated by estimating voxel-specific AR(p) parameters (possibly together with some spatial regularisation; Worsley *et al.,* 2002), although this means that different voxels can have different effective degrees of freedom, which in strict terms violates the assumptions behind Gaussian field theory (Chapters 44 and 45). Such spatial variation is less of a problem for the temporal smoothing approach, which homogenises the autocorrelation across voxels.

A final problem with the above methods is that the model parameters and autocorrelation parameters are estimated separately, which requires multiple passes through the data and makes it difficult to properly accommodate the associated degrees of freedom. Iterative estimation schemes, such as restricted maximum likelihood (ReML), allow simultaneous estimation of model parameters and autocorrelation hyperparameters, together with proper partitioning of the effective degrees of freedom (see Chapter 39 for more details). This method can be used with any temporal autocorrelation model. Friston *et al.* (2002) chose an AR(1)+white noise model:

$$\mathbf{y} = \mathbf{X}\boldsymbol{\beta} + \mathbf{z}_1 + \mathbf{z}_2 \qquad \mathbf{z}_1 = \mathbf{A}\mathbf{z}_1 + \mathbf{w} \qquad \mathbf{w} = N(0,\sigma_1^2\mathbf{I}) \qquad \mathbf{z}_2 = N(0,\sigma_2^2\mathbf{I})$$

for which the autocorrelation coefficient a_1 was fixed to exp(−1), leaving two hyperparameters (σ_1^2 and σ_2^2). The additional white noise component ($\mathbf{z}_2$) contributes to the zero-lag autocorrelation, which in turn allows the AR(1) model to capture better the shape of the autocorrelation for longer lags. Note that this approach still requires a high-pass filter to provide accurate fits (Fig. 40.4D), although a subtle difference from the above residual-based approaches is that the high-pass filter is also treated as part of the complete model to be estimated, rather than as a prewhitening filter.

Such iterative schemes are computationally expensive when performed at every voxel. One possible solution is to assume that the ratio of hyperparameters is stationary over voxels, which allows the data to be pooled over voxels in order to estimate this ratio. Spatial variability in the absolute autocorrelation can be accommodated by subsequently estimating a single voxel-specific scaling factor (see Friston *et al.,* 2002, and Chapter 39 for further details). This scaling factor can be estimated in one step (because no iteration is required for ReML to estimate a single hyperparameter). This ReML solution to modelling the autocorrelation therefore shares the efficiency of prewhitening approaches, though with less potential bias; allows proper adjustment of the degrees of freedom; and makes some allowance for spatial variability in the temporal autocorrelation. This obviates the need for temporal smoothing, a consequence particularly important for event-related designs (below), in which appreciable signal can exist at high frequencies that would be lost by low-pass smoothing (see Fig. 40.4D). This approach has been implemented in SPM2.

EVENT-RELATED fMRI

Event-related fMRI (efMRI) is simply the use of fMRI to detect responses to individual trials, in a manner analogous to the time-locked event-related potentials (ERPs) recorded with EEG. The neural activity associated with each trial is normally (though not necessarily) modelled as a delta function—an "event"—at the trial onset.

Advantages of efMRI

The advent of event-related methods offers several advantages for experimental design. Foremost is the ability to intermix trials of different types (conditions), rather than blocking them in the manner required for PET and initially adopted for fMRI (cf. Figs. 40.5A and B). The counterbalancing or randomising of different trial types, as is standard in behavioural or electrophysiological studies, ensures that the average response to a trial type is not biased by a specific context or history of preceding trial types. This is important because the unbalanced

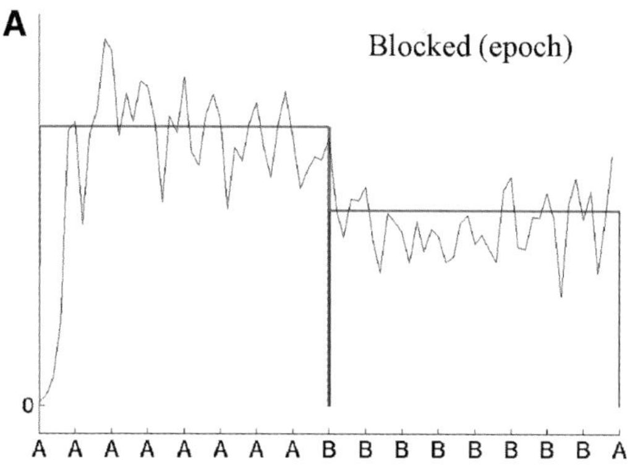

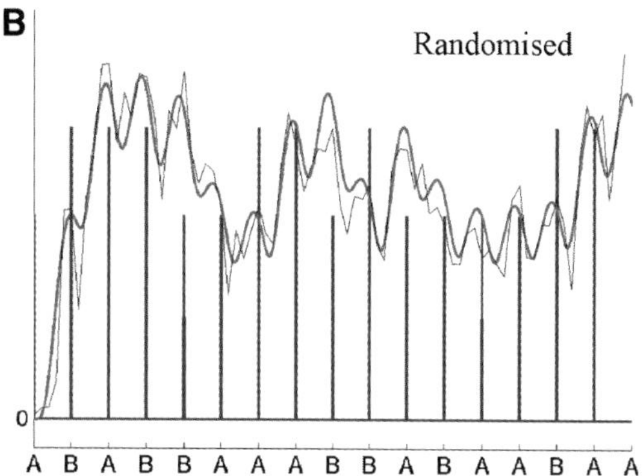

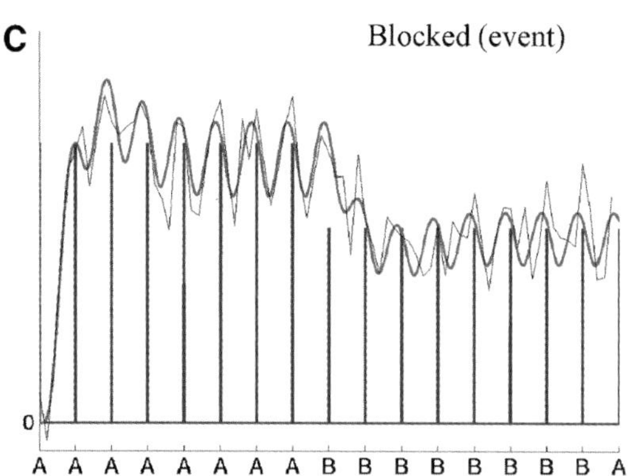

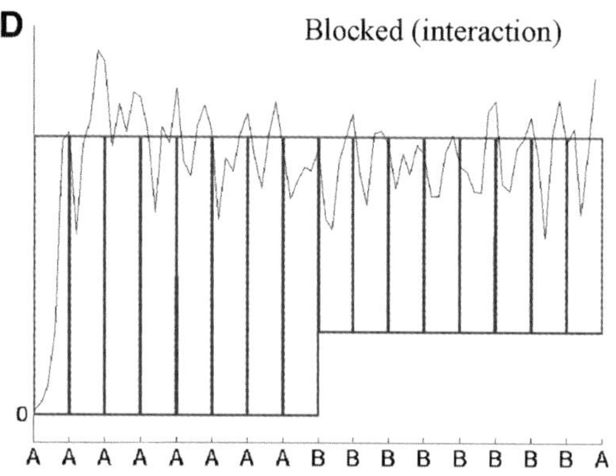

FIGURE 40.5
Blocked and randomised designs. Simulated data (black), neural model (blue), and schematic fitted response (red) for two event types (A and B) presented with SOA = 5 sec for (A) blocked design and boxcar epoch model; (B) randomised design and event-related model; (C) blocked design and event-related model; and (D) blocked design and response from a boxcar epoch model; neural model illustrates that equivalent response to A and B blocks does not distinguish item (event-related) effects from state (epoch-related) effects.

blocking of trial types might, for example, induce differences in the cognitive "set" or strategies adopted by subjects. This means that any difference in the mean activity during different blocks might reflect such "state" effects, rather than "item" effects specific to individual trials (e.g., Rugg and Henson, 2002). Johnson *et al.* (1997), for example, provided direct evidence that the presentation format—intermixed or blocked—can effect the ERP associated with a trial-based memory effect.[9]

A second advantage of event-related methods is that they allow categorisation of trial types according to the subject's behaviour. This might include separate modelling of trials with correct and incorrect task performance, or parametric modelling of trial-by-trial reaction times (modulations that are only possible indirectly when analysed at a block level). An appealing example of this facility occurs in *subsequent memory* experiments. In such experiments, subjects perform a simple "study" task on a series of items, followed by a surprise memory test. The latter allows the items in the study task to be categorised according to whether they were later remembered (a categorisation the researcher has little objective control over). Brain regions can then be isolated whose activity "predicts" subsequent memory (e.g., Henson *et al.,* 1999).

A third advantage reflects the identification of events whose occurrence can only be indicated by the subject. An example of such an event is the spontaneous transition between the perception of ambiguous visual objects, as in the face-vase illusion (Kleinschmidt *et al.,* 1998), or between 2D and 3D perception of 2D stereograms (Portas *et al.,* 2000), that is, situations in which the objective stimulation is constant. A fourth advantage is that event-related methods allow some

[9] Note that there are also disadvantages associated with randomised designs. Foremost, such designs are generally less efficient for detecting effects than blocked designs (with short SOAs and reasonable block lengths; see later "Efficiency and Optimisation of Experimental Design" section). In addition, some psychological manipulations, such as changes in selective attention or task, may exert stronger effects when blocked.

experimental designs that cannot be easily blocked. One example is an "oddball" design, in which the stimulus of interest is one that deviates from the prevailing context and, therefore, cannot be blocked by definition (Strange *et al.,* 2000).

A final advantage is that event-related methods potentially allow more accurate models of the data. Even when trial types are blocked, for example, modelling the BOLD response to each trial within a block may capture additional variability that is not captured by a simple boxcar neuronal model, particularly for intertrial intervals of more than a few seconds (Price *et al.,* 1999; Figs. 40.5A and C). Furthermore, it is possible distinguish between state effects and item effects. Chawla *et al.* (1999), for example, investigated the interaction between selective attention (a state effect) and transient stimulus changes (an item effect) in a *mixed epoch/event* design. Subjects viewed a visual stimulus that occasionally changed in either colour or motion. In some blocks, they were required to detect the colour changes; in other blocks they detected the motion changes. By varying the interval between changes within a block, Chawla *et al.* were able to reduce the correlation between the corresponding epoch- and event-related regressors. Tests of the epoch-related effect showed that attending toward a specific visual attribute (e.g., colour) increased the baseline activity in regions selective for that attribute (e.g., V4). Tests of the event-related effect showed that the impulse response to the same objective change in visual attribute was augmented when subjects were attending to that attribute. These combined effects of selective attention—raising endogenous baseline activity and increasing the gain of the exogenous response—could not be distinguished in blocked designs (Fig. 40.5D).

BOLD Impulse Response

A typical BOLD response to an impulse stimulation (event) is shown in Fig. 40.6A. The response peaks approximately 5 sec after stimulation, and is followed by an undershoot that lasts approximately 30 sec (at high magnetic fields, an initial undershoot can sometimes be observed; Malonek and Ginvald, 1996). Early event-related studies therefore used a long interstimulus interval (or more generally, stimulus onset synchrony, SOA, when the stimuli are not treated as delta functions) to allow the response to return to baseline between stimulations. However, although the responses to successive events will overlap at shorter SOAs, this overlap can be explicitly modelled (via an HRF). This modelling is simplified if successive responses can be assumed to add in a linear fashion, as discussed earlier. Short SOAs of a few seconds are desirable because they are comparable to those typically used in behavioural and electrophysiological studies, and because they are generally more efficient from the statistical perspective (see later "Efficiency and Optimisation of Experimental Design" section).

There is good evidence for nonlinearity in the BOLD impulse response as a function of SOA (Friston *et al.,* 1998a; Miezin *et al.,* 2000; Pollman *et al.,* 1997).[10] This nonlinearity is typically a "saturation" whereby the response to a run of events is smaller than would be predicted by the summation of responses to each event alone. This saturation is believed to arise in the mapping from blood flow to BOLD signal (Friston *et al.,* 2000a), although it may also have a neural locus, particularly for very short SOAs. (For biophysical models that such incorporate nonlinearities, see Chapter 41.) It has been found for SOAs below approximately 8 sec that the degree of saturation increases as the SOA decreases. For typical SOAs of 2–4 sec, however, the magnitude of the saturation is small (typically less than 20%; Miezin *et al.,* 2000).

Note that the dominant effect of increasing the duration of neural activity (up to 2–4 sec) in a linear-convolution model [Eq. (40.4)] is to increase the peak amplitude of the BOLD response (Fig. 40.6B). In other words, the BOLD response integrates neural activity over a few seconds. This is convenient because it means that neural activity can be reasonably modelled as a delta function (i.e., even though the amplitude of the response may vary nonlinearly with stimulus duration as noted in Vasquez and Noll, 1998, the shape of the response does not necessarily change dramatically). The corollary, however, is that a difference in the amplitude of the BOLD impulse response (as conventionally tested) does not imply a difference in the mean level of

[10] nonlinearities in the amplitude of the BOLD response are also found as a function of stimulus duration or stimulus magnitude (Vasquez and Noll, 1998). Nonlinearities also appear to vary considerably across different brain regions (Huettel and McCarthy, 2001; Birn *et al.,* 2001).

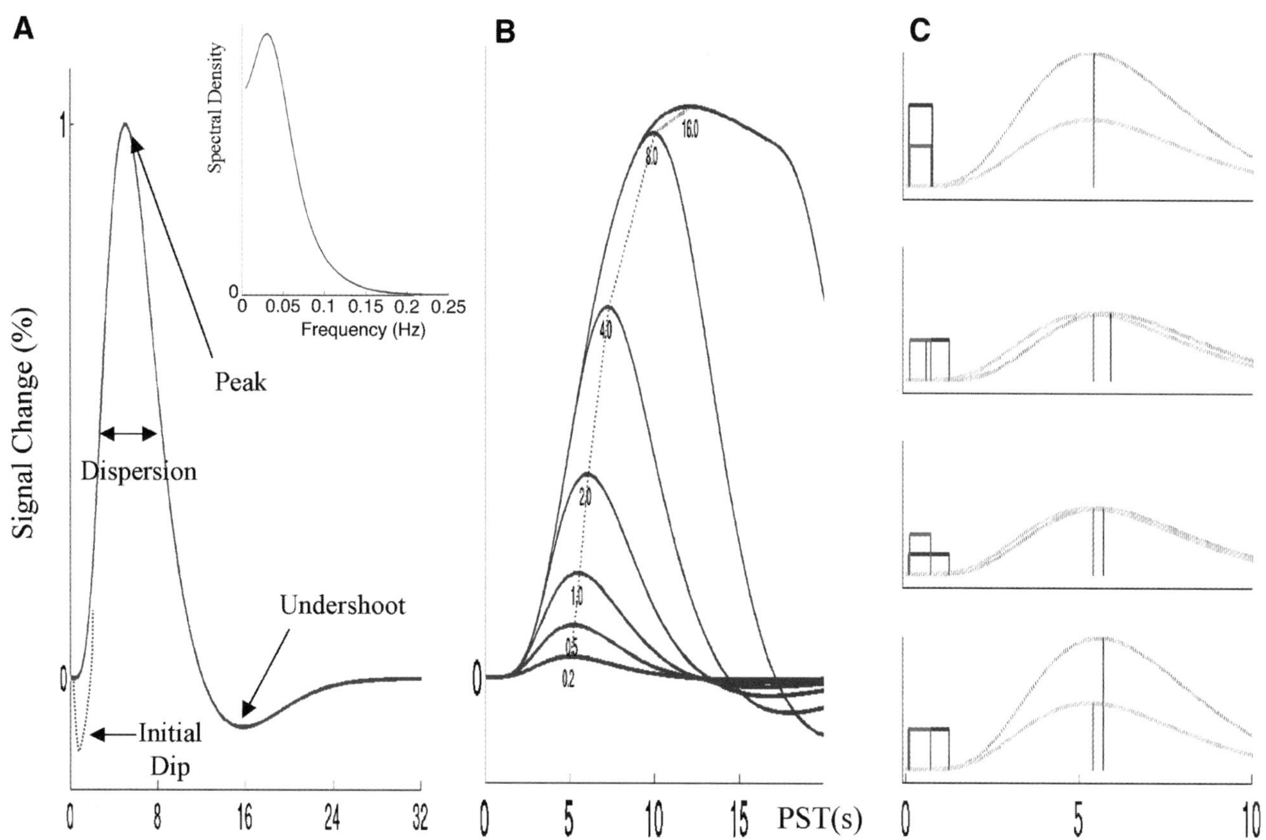

FIGURE 40.6
The BOLD response. (A) Typical (canonical) impulse response (power spectrum inset). (B) BOLD signal predicted from linear convolution by canonical impulse response of squarewave neural activity of increasing 200-ms to 16-sec durations. (C) BOLD signal predicted for two event types (red and blue) with squarewave neural activities of different (top to bottom) magnitude, onset, duration with same integrated activity, and duration with same mean activity. Vertical lines show peak of resulting BOLD response.

neural activity: The difference could reflect different durations of neural activity at same mean level. One way to tease these apart is to test for subtle differences in the peak latency of the BOLD impulse response (see later "Timing Issues: Theoretical" section), which will differ in the latter case but not former case (Fig. 40.5C).

The general shape of the BOLD impulse response appears similar across early sensory regions, such as V1 (Boynton *et al.,* 1996), A1 (Josephs *et al.,* 1997), and S1 (Zarahn *et al.,* 1997a). However, the precise shape has been shown to vary across the brain, particularly in higher cortical regions (Schacter *et al.,* 1997), presumably due mainly to variations in the vasculature of different regions (Lee *et al.,* 1995). Moreover, the BOLD response appears to vary considerably across people (Aguirre *et al.,* 1998).[11] These types of variability can be accommodated by expanding the HRF in terms of temporal basis functions of Eq. (40.5).

Temporal Basis Functions

Several temporal basis sets are offered in SPM. The most general are the finite impulse response (FIR) and Fourier basis sets, which make minimal assumptions about the shape of the response. The FIR set consists of N_k contiguous boxcar functions of PST, each of duration T_H/N_k sec (Fig. 40.7A), where T_H is the maximum duration of the HRF. The Fourier set (Fig. 40.7B) consists of N_s sine and N_s cosine functions of harmonic periods T_H, $T_H/2$ … T_H/N_s (i.e., $N_k = 2N_s$

[11] One possible solution is to use subject-specific HRFs derived from a reference region known to respond to a simple task (e.g., from central sulcus during a simple manual task performed during a pilot scan on each subject; Aguirre *et al.,* 1998). However, while this allows for intersubject variability, it does not allow for interregional variability within subjects (or potential error in estimation of the reference response).

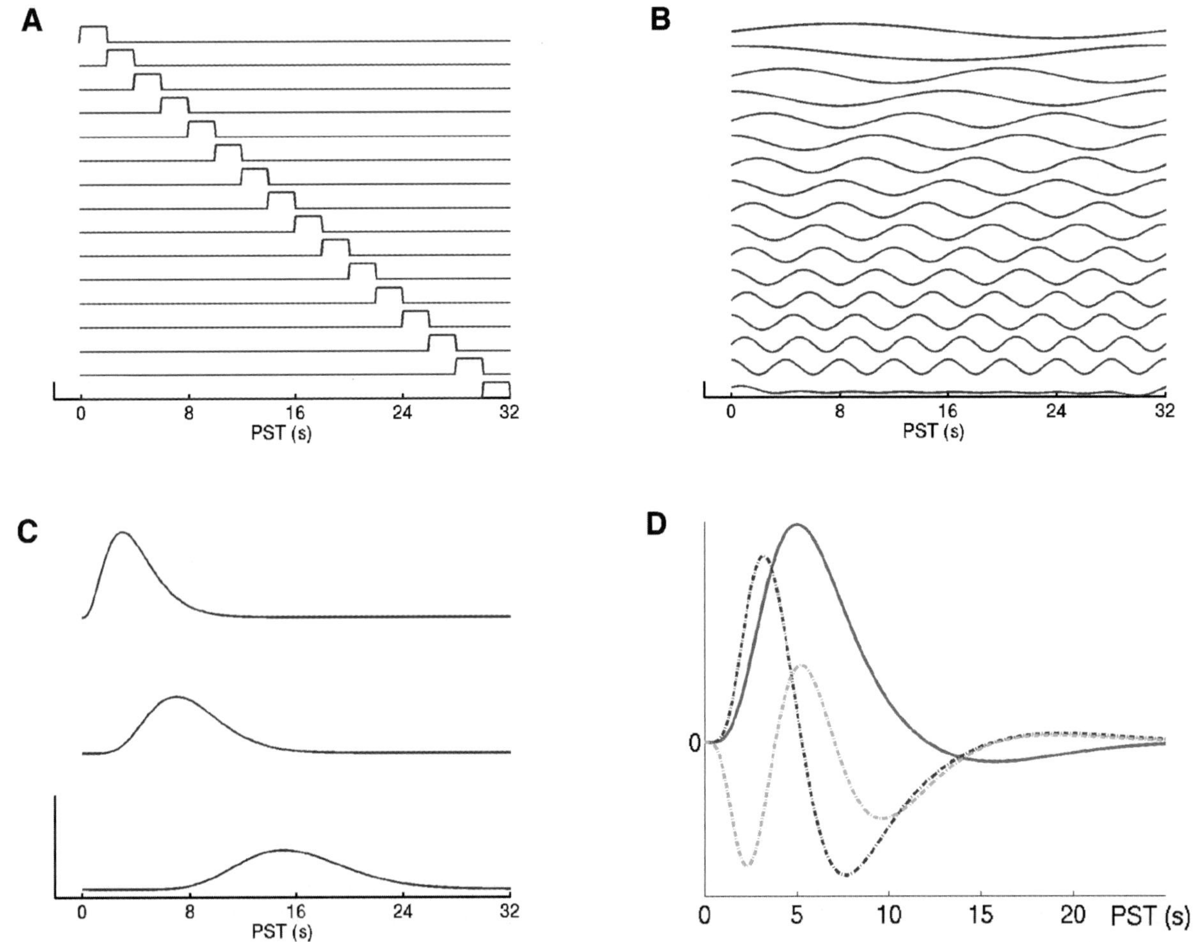

FIGURE 40.7
Temporal basis functions offered by SPM, $T_H = 32$ sec: (A) FIR basis set, $N_k = 16$; (B) Fourier basis set, $N_s = 8$; (C) Gamma functions, $N_k = 3$. (D) Canonical HRF (red) and its temporal (blue) and dispersion (green) derivatives. The temporal derivative is approximated by the orthogonalised finite difference between canonical HRFs with peak delay of 7 sec versus 6 sec; the dispersion derivative is approximated by the orthogonalised finite difference between canonical HRFs with peak dispersions of 1 versus 1.01.

+ 1 basis functions, where the last is the mean of the basis functions over T_H).[12] Linear combinations of the orthonormal FIR or Fourier basis functions can capture any shape of response up to a specified timescale (T_H/N_k in the case of the FIR) or frequency (N_s/T_H in the case of the Fourier set).[13]

In practice, there is little to choose between the FIR and Fourier sets: The Fourier set may be better suited when the PST sampling is nonuniform, whereas the parameter estimates for the FIR functions have a more direct interpretation in terms of "averaged" PST signal (effecting a linear "deconvolution"). Indeed, in the special case when $T_H/N_k = T_R$, the FIR functions are delta functions:

$$h(\tau) = \Sigma_{k=1\ldots Nk}\, \delta(\tau\text{-}k\text{-}1)$$

over the N_k poststimulus scans, and the design matrix for events onsetting at scan o_{ij} is as follows:

$$x_{tc} = \Sigma_{i=1\ldots Ni}\, \Sigma_{j=1\ldots Nj}\, \Sigma_{k=1\ldots Nk}\, \delta(t - (o_{ij} + k - 1))$$

where t indexes scans and c indexes the column for the kth basis function of the jth event of the ith type (Ollinger *et al.*, 2001; see Fig. 40.16A, later in this chapter, for an example). For the

[12] Since the HRF is assumed to be bounded at zero for $\tau <= 0$ and $\tau > T_H$, the Fourier basis functions can also be windowed (e.g., by a Hanning window) within this range.

[13] In practice, there is little point in making T_H/N_k smaller than the effective PST sampling interval, T_s, or specifying N_s/T_H higher than the Nyquist limit $1/(2T_s)$.

special case of nonoverlapping responses (i.e., that $o_{ij} + k \neq o_{uv} + w$ for all $i \neq u, j \neq v$ and $k \neq w$), the estimates β_{ik} of the FIR parameters are equivalent to the simple trial-averaged data:

$$\beta_{ik} = \Sigma_{j=1...Nj}\, y(o_{ij} + k - 1)/N_j$$

This estimation also approximates the HRF when the event types are fully counterbalanced (such that the number of occasions when $o_{ij} + k = o_{uv} + w$ is constant for all $i \neq u, j \neq v$ and $k \neq w$, which is approached when events are randomised and N_j is large[14]), a procedure that has been called *selective averaging* (Dale and Buckner, 1997). It is equivalent to noting that the covariance matrix $\mathbf{X}^T\mathbf{X}$ (sometimes called the *overlap correction matrix*; Dale, 1999) approaches the identity matrix (after mean correction), such that the ordinary least-squares estimates become

$$\beta = (\mathbf{X}^T\mathbf{X})^{-1}\mathbf{X}^T\mathbf{y} \cong \mathbf{X}^T\mathbf{y}$$

Note that such counterbalancing is not required by the full pseudo-inverse estimation used by SPM (though there may still be important psychological reasons for counterbalancing).

More parsimonious basis sets can be chosen that make various assumptions about the shape of the HRF.[15] One popular choice is the gamma function:

$$f(\tau) = ((\tau - o)/d)^{(p-1)}\, e^{-(\tau - o)/d}/(d(p-1)!) \tag{40.7}$$

where o is the onset delay, d is the time scaling, and p is an integer phase delay (the peak delay is given by pd, and the dispersion by pd^2). The gamma function has been shown to provide a reasonably good fit to the impulse response (Boynton *et al.,* 1996), although it lacks an undershoot (Fransson *et al.,* 1999; Glover, 1999). The first T_H sec of a set of N_k gamma functions of increasing dispersions can be obtained by incrementing $p = 2..N_k + 1$ (Fig. 40.7C), which can be orthogonalised with respect to one another (as in SPM). This set is more parsimonious in that fewer functions are required to capture the typical range of impulse responses than are required by the Fourier or FIR sets, reducing the degrees of freedom used in the design matrix and allowing more powerful statistical tests.

An even more parsimonious basis set, suggested by Friston *et al.* (1998b), is based on a *canonical HRF* and its partial derivatives (Fig. 40.7D). The canonical HRF is a "typical" BOLD impulse response characterised by two gamma functions, one modelling the peak and one modelling the undershoot. The canonical HRF is parameterised by an onset delay of 0 sec, peak delay of 6 sec, peak dispersion of 1, undershoot delay of 16 sec, undershoot dispersion of 1 and a peak-to-undershoot amplitude ratio of 6; these values were derived from a principal component analysis of the data reported in Friston *et al.* (1998a). To allow for variations about the canonical form, the partial derivatives of the canonical HRF with respect to, for example, its peak delay and dispersion parameters can be added as further basis functions. By a first-order multivariate Taylor expansion [cf. Eq. (40.8) below], the temporal derivative can capture differences in the latency of the peak response, while the dispersion derivative can capture differences in the duration of the peak response.[16]

Statistical Tests of Event-Related Responses and Choosing a Basis Set

Inferences using multiple basis functions are generally made with F contrasts (Chapter 8). An example F contrast that tests for any difference in the event-related response across trial types modelled by a canonical HRF basis set is shown later in Fig. 40.15C. Further assumptions about the shape of the response (or nature of differences between responses) can also be entered at the contrast level (Burock and Dale, 2000; Henson *et al.,* 2001a). One might restrict differential contrasts to a limited set of FIR time bins for example. In the extreme case, setting the contrast

---

[14] In strict terms, this also means an equal number of occasions (scans) when event types co-occur (i.e., are coincident), which is not normally the case.

[15] Unlike the Fourier or FIR sets, this set is not strictly a "basis" set in that it does not span the space of possible responses within the response window T_H, but we maintain the term here for convenience.

[16] A similar logic can be used to capture different latencies of epoch-related responses, namely, by adding the temporal derivatives of the HRF-convolved epoch response functions. Note that variations in the HRF can also be accommodated by nonlinear, iterative fitting techniques. (See Hinrichs *et al.,* 2000, for a combination of nonlinear estimation of HRF shape together with linear deconvolution of responses.)

weights for an FIR set to match an assumed HRF shape (e.g., Fig. 40.16B inset) will produce a parameter estimate for the contrast proportional to that obtained by using that HRF as a single basis function (assuming that FIR time bins have been sampled uniformly at each effective sampling interval).

However, when the real response resembles an assumed HRF, tests on a model using that HRF as a single basis function are more powerful (Ollinger *et al.,* 2001). In such cases, *t* tests on the parameter estimate for a canonical HRF, for example, can be interpreted in terms of the "amplitude" of the response. However, when the real response differs appreciably from the assumed form, tests on the HRF parameter estimates are biased (and an unmodelled structure will exist in the residuals). In such cases, a canonical HRF parameter estimate can no longer necessarily be interpreted in terms of amplitude (see Chapter 38). The addition of partial derivatives of the HRF (see above) can ameliorate this problem: The inclusion of a temporal derivative, for example, can reduce the residual error by capturing systematic delays relative to the assumed HRF.[17] Nonetheless, for responses that differ by more than 1 sec in their peak latency (i.e., when the first-order Taylor approximation fails), different canonical HRF parameters will be estimated even when the responses have identical peak amplitudes.

An important empirical question then becomes: How much variability exists around the canonical form? Henson *et al.* (2001b) addressed this question in a dataset involving rapid motor responses to brief presentations of faces across 12 subjects (the superset of the data in the "Worked Example" section). By modelling the event-related response with a canonical HRF, its partial derivatives, *and* an FIR basis set, the authors assessed the contribution of the different basis functions by a series of F contrasts. Significant variability was captured by both the temporal derivative and dispersion derivative, confirming that different regions exhibited different shaped responses. Little additional variability was captured by the FIR basis set, however, suggesting that the canonical HRF and its two partial derivatives were sufficient to capture the majority of experimental variability (at least in regions that were activated in this task).

This sufficiency may be specific to this dataset and may reflect the fact that neural activity was reasonably well modelled by a delta function. It is unlikely to hold for more complex experimental trials, such as working memory trials where information must be maintained for several seconds (e.g., Ollinger *et al.,* 2001). Nonetheless, such trials may be better accommodated by more complex neural models, expanding $u(t)$ in terms of multiple events/epochs [cf. Eq. (40.3)], while still assuming a fixed form for the HRF. This allows more direct inferences about stimulus, response, and delay components of a trial for example (Zarahn, 2000). More generally, the question of which basis set to use becomes a problem of model selection (Chapter 37).

A problem arises when one wishes to use multiple basis functions to make inferences in second-level analyses (e.g., in random-effects analyses over subjects; see Chapter 42). Subject-specific *beta images* created after fitting an FIR model in a first-level analysis could, for example, enter into a second-level model as a peristimulus time factor (differential F contrasts on which would correspond to a condition-by-time interaction in a conventional repeated-measures ANOVA). However, the parameter estimates are unlikely to be independent or identically distributed over subjects, violating the sphericity assumption of univariate tests (Chapter 39).[18] One solution is to use multivariate tests (Henson *et al.,* 2000a), although these are generally less powerful (by virtue of making minimal assumptions about the data covariance). The use of ReML or *parametric empirical Bayes* methods to estimate the hyperparameters governing constraints placed on the covariance matrix (Friston *et al.,* 2002; Chapter 39) resolves this problem.

[17] Note that the inclusion of the partial derivatives of an HRF does not necessarily affect the parameter estimate for the HRF itself, since the basis functions are orthogonal (unless correlations between the regressors arise owing to undersampling by the T_R or by temporal correlations between the onsets of events of different types). In other words, their inclusion does not necessarily affect second-level *t* tests on the HRF parameter estimates alone. Note also that *t* tests on the partial derivatives are not meaningful in the absence of information about the HRF parameter estimate: The derivative estimates depend on the size (and sign) of the HRF estimate and are unlikely to reflect plausible impulse responses (versus baseline) in the absence of a significant HRF parameter estimate (Henson *et al.*, 2002a).

[18] This is one reason why researchers have tended to stick with *t* tests on (contrasts of) the parameter estimate for a single canonical HRF at the second level, at the expense of generality (potentially missing responses with a noncanonical form).

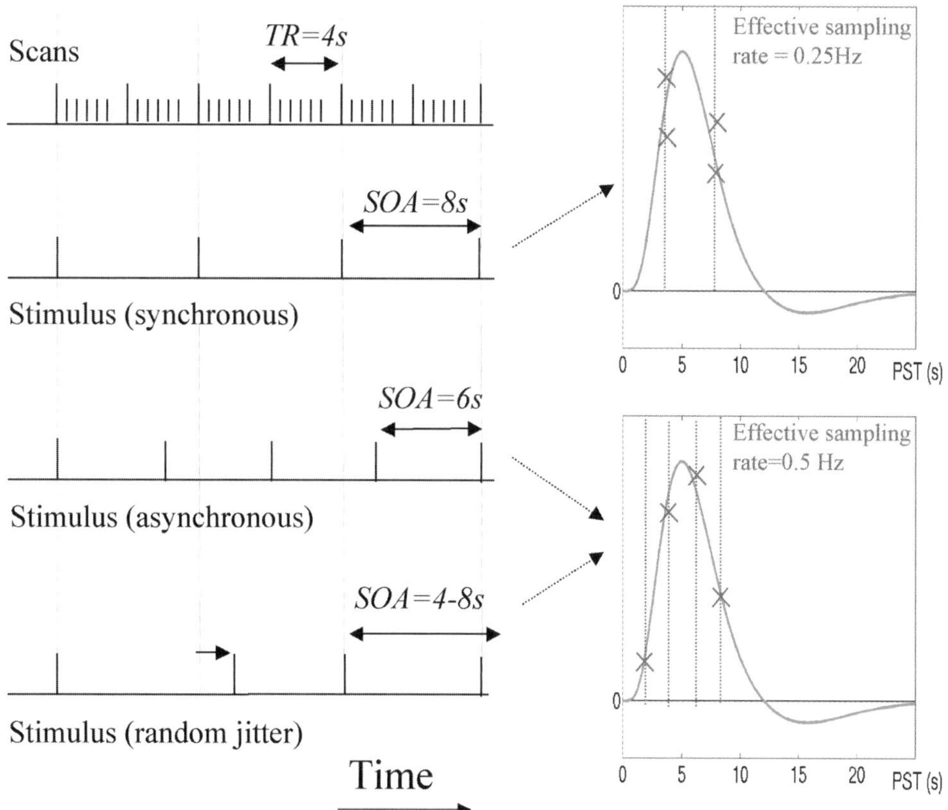

FIGURE 40.8
Effective sampling rate. Schematic (left) of stimulus event onsets relative to scan onsets (tall vertical lines represent first slice per scan; shorter lines represent subsequent slices) and resulting peristimulus sampling points (right).

Timing Issues: Practical

Both practical and theoretical issues surround the timing of BOLD responses. Two practical issues concern the effective sampling rate of the response and the different acquisition times for different slices (using EPI).

It is possible to sample the impulse response at poststimulus intervals, T_s, shorter than the interscan interval T_R by jittering event onsets with respect to scan onsets (Josephs *et al.,* 1997). Jittering can be effected by ensuring that the SOA is not a simple multiple of the T_R, or by adding a random trial-by-trial delay in stimulus onsets relative to scan onsets (Fig. 40.8). In both cases, different PSTs are sampled over trials, with the main difference between the two methods being whether the SOA is fixed or random. For example, an effective PST sampling of 0.5 Hz can be achieved with an SOA of 6 sec and a T_R of 4 sec; or by adding a delay of 0 or 2 sec randomly to each trial (producing SOAs of 4–8 sec, with a mean of 6 sec). While effective sampling rates higher than the T_R does not necessarily affect response detection for typical T_R's of 2–4 sec (since there is little power in the canonical response above 0.2 Hz; see Fig. 40.6A), higher sampling rates are important for quantifying the response shape, such as its latency (Miezin *et al.,* 2000).

Jittering event onsets with respect to scan onsets do not help the second practical issue concerning different slice acquisition times. This *slice-timing* problem (Henson *et al.,* 1999a) refers to the fact that, with a descending EPI sequence, for example, the bottom slice is acquired T_R sec later than the top slice. If a single basis function (such as a canonical HRF) were used to model the response, and onset times were specified relative to the start of each scan, the data in the bottom slice would be systematically delayed by T_R sec relative to the model.[19] This would

[19] One solution would be to allow different event onsets for different slices. SPM however assumes the same model (i.e., onsets) for all voxels (i.e., slices) in order to equate the degrees of freedom (e.g., residual autocorrelation) across voxels required for GFT (Chapters 44 and 45). Moreover, slice-timing information is lost as soon as images are resliced relative to a different orientation (e.g., during spatial normalisation).

produce poor and biased parameter estimates for later slices and would mean that different sensitivities would apply to different slices.[20] There are two main solutions to this problem: to interpolate the data in each slice as if the slices were acquired simultaneously or to use a basis set that allows for different response onset latencies.

Temporal interpolation of the data (using a full sinc interpolation) is possible during preprocessing of images in SPM99. For sequential acquisition schemes, temporal interpolation is generally better when performed after spatial realignment, since the timing error for a voxel resliced to nearby slices will be small relative to the potential error for a voxel that represents different brain regions owing to interscan movement. (This may not be true for interleaved acquisition schemes, for which temporal interpolation might be better before spatial realignment.) The data are interpolated by an amount proportional to their sampling time relative to a reference slice (whose data are unchanged). The event onsets can then be synchronised with the acquisition of the reference slice. In SPM, this is equivalent to maintaining event onsets relative to scan onsets, but setting the time point T_0 in the simulated time space of T time bins, from which the regressors are sampled, to

$$T_0 = \text{round}\{nT/N_s\}$$

where the reference slice is the nth slice acquired of the N_s slices per scan.

A problem with slice-timing correction is that the interpolation will alias frequencies above the Nyquist limit $1/(2T_R)$. Ironically, this means that the interpolation accuracy decreases as the slice-timing problem (i.e., T_R) increases. For short T_R's > 2–3 sec, the interpolation error is likely to be small. For longer T_R's, the severity of the interpolation error depends on whether appreciable signal power exists above the Nyquist limit (which is more likely for rapid, randomised event-related designs; see below).

An alternative solution to the slice-timing problem is to include additional basis functions that can accommodate timing errors. The Fourier basis set, for example, does not have a slice-timing problem (i.e., it is phase-invariant). For more constrained sets, the addition of the temporal derivatives of the functions may be sufficient. The parameter estimates for the derivatives will vary across slices, to capture shifts in the data relative to the model, while those for the response functions can remain constant (up to a first-order Taylor approximation). The temporal derivative of the canonical HRF, for example (Fig. 40.7D), can accommodate slice-timing differences of approximately ±1 s (i.e., T_R's of 2 sec, when the model is synchronised to the middle slice in time). A problem with this approach is that slice-timing differences are confounded with latency differences in the real response. This means that response latencies cannot be compared across different slices (see below).

Timing Issues: Theoretical

Assuming that the data are synchronised with the event onsets, there may be theoretical reasons for investigating aspects of the BOLD response latency, as well as its amplitude. For example, BOLD responses arising from blood vessels (e.g., veins) tend to have longer latencies than those from parenchyma (Saad *et al.*, 2001). Though absolute differences in response latency across brain regions are unlikely to be informative regarding underlying neural activity, since they may simply reflect differences in vasculature,[21] differences in the relative response latencies in different conditions may inform theories about the separate stages of underlying neural processes. Latency estimates may also correlate better with some behavioural measures, such as reaction times (Kruggel *et al.*, 2000).

For periodic responses, latency can be estimated easily using Fourier (Rajapakse *et al.*, 1998) or Hilbert (Saad *et al.*, 2001) transforms. For nonperiodic responses, the simplest approach is to construct a measure of latency from the trial-averaged response, such as the linear intercept to the ascending region of the peak response (using a very short T_R; Menon *et al.*, 1998), or the peak of a spline interpolation through the data (Huettel and McCarthy, 2001). Other approaches

[20] This is less of a problem for low-frequency responses, such as those induced by epochs of tens of seconds.

[21] Miezin *et al.* (2000), for example, showed that the peak response in motor cortex preceded that in visual cortex for events in which the motor response succeeded visual stimulation.

estimate the latency directly from a parameterised HRF, using either linear or nonlinear (iterative) fitting techniques.

A linear method for estimating latency within the GLM was proposed by Friston *et al.* (1998b). Using a first-order Taylor expansion of the response, these authors showed how the standard error of a fitted response can be estimated from the temporal derivative of an HRF. This approach was extended by Henson *et al.* (2002a) in order to estimate response latency directly. If the real response, $r(\tau)$, is a scaled (by α) version of an assumed HRF, $h(\tau)$, but shifted by a small amount $d\tau$, then

$$r(\tau) = \alpha\, h(\tau + \mathrm{d}\tau) \cong \alpha\, h(\tau) + \alpha\, h'(\tau)\, d\tau \tag{40.8}$$

where $h'(\tau)$ is the first derivative of $h(\tau)$ with respect to τ. If $h(\tau)$ and $h'(\tau)$ are used as two basis functions in the GLM to estimate the parameters β_1 and β_2 respectively, then

$$\beta_1 = \alpha \qquad \beta_2 = \alpha \mathrm{d}\tau \qquad \Rightarrow \qquad \mathrm{d}\tau = \beta_2/\beta_1$$

In other words, the latency shift can be estimated by the ratio of the derivative to HRF parameter estimates (a similar logic can be used for other parameters of the HRF, such as its dispersion). The first-order approximation holds when $d\tau$ is small relative to the time constants of the response (see Liao et al., 2002, for a more general treatment, using the first and second derivatives of a parameter representing the scaling of τ). When using SPM's canonical HRF and temporal derivative, for example, the approximation is reasonable for latency of shifts of $\pm$ 1 sec relative to the canonical HRF. Whole brain SPMs of differences in response latencies can be constructed simply by comparing the ratios (e.g., over subjects) of the temporal derivative to canonical HRF parameter estimates at every voxel (Fig. 40.9A).[22]

Other methods use nonlinear (iterative) fitting techniques. These approaches are more powerful (e.g., they can capture any size latency shift), but computationally expensive and, hence, often restricted to regions of interest. Various parameterisations of the HRF have been used, such as a Gaussian function parameterised by amplitude, onset latency and dispersion (Kruggel and von Cramon, 1999a) or a gamma function parameterised by amplitude, onset latency, and peak latency (Miezin *et al.,* 2000). Henson and Rugg (2001) used SPM's canonical HRF with the amplitude, onset latency, and peak latency parameters free to vary.[23] The latter was applied to a rapid event-related experiment in which an FIR basis set was used to first estimate the mean event-related response to first and second presentations of faces in a fusiform "face area." A subsequent nonlinear fit of the canonical HRF to these deconvolved data revealed significant differences (over subjects) in the amplitude and peak latency parameters, but not in the onset latency parameter (Fig. 40.9B). The most parsimonious explanation for this pattern is that repetition of a face decreased the duration of underlying neural activity (assuming a linear convolution model; see Fig. 40.6C).

A problem with unconstrained iterative fitting techniques is that the parameter estimates may not be optimal (because of local minima in the search space). Parameters that have correlated effects compound this problem; for example, situations can arise in noisy data where the estimates of onset and peak latency take implausibly large values of opposite sign. One solution is to put priors on the likely parameter distributions in a Bayesian estimation scheme (Chapter 41) to "regularise" the solutions (see Gossl *et al.,* 2001, for an example).

EFFICIENCY AND OPTIMISATION OF EXPERIMENTAL DESIGN

This section is concerned with optimising experimental designs in order to detect particular effects. The aim is to minimise the standard error of a contrast, $\mathbf{c}^T\beta$ (i.e., the denominator of a t

[22] To allow for voxels in which the approximation breaks down (e.g., for canonical HRF parameter estimates close to zero), Henson *et al.* (2002a) applied a sigmoidal squashing function to constrain the ratio estimates.

[23] The advantage of a Gaussian HRF is that its onset delay and dispersion are independent, unlike a gamma HRF [Eq. (40.7)]. A problem, however, is that a Gaussian HRF is not bounded for $\tau < 0$ and does not allow for the asymmetry typically found in the BOLD response. A problem with both a Gaussian HRF and a single gamma HRF is that they do not allow for a postpeak undershoot. A problem with the double (canonical) gamma HRF used by Henson and Rugg (2001) is that the onset latency and peak latency are correlated.

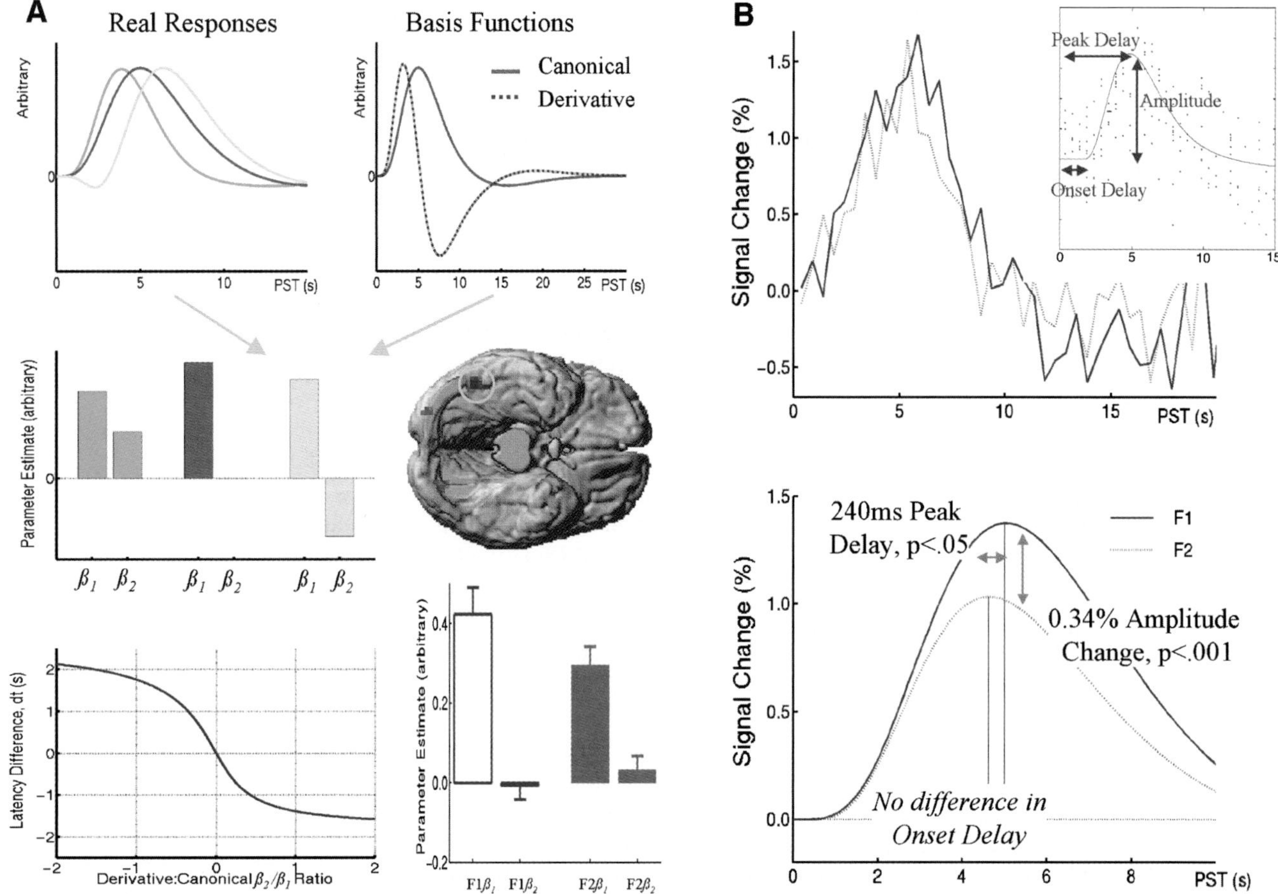

FIGURE 40.9
Estimating BOLD impulse response latency. (A) Top left: The canonical HRF (red) together with HRFs shifted 1 sec earlier (green) or later (yellow) in time. Top right: The canonical HRF and its temporal derivative. Middle left: Parameter estimates for canonical (β_1) and derivative (β_2) associated with fit to HRFs above. Middle right: Right fusiform region showing differential latency when tested across subjects (Henson *et al.,* 2002a; the superset of data in the "Worked Example" section). Bottom left: Relationship between the latency difference relative to the canonical HRF (*dt*) and the ratio of derivative-to-canonical parameter estimates (β_2/β_1). Bottom right: Canonical and derivative parameter estimates from right fusiform region above for first (F1) and second (F2) presentations of famous faces. (B) Event-related data (top) sampled every 0.5 sec from maximum of right fusiform region (+48, −54, −24) in (A) for F1 (solid) and F2 (dotted), fitted by HRF parameterised by peak amplitude, peak delay, and onset delay (inset) using Nelder-Mead iterative search, to give fitted responses (bottom) in which amplitude and peak latency, but not onset latency, differ significantly following repetition (using nonparametric tests across subjects; Henson and Rugg, 2001).

statistic; see Chapter 38), given a contrast matrix **c** and parameter estimates $\boldsymbol{\beta}$, whose variance is (Friston et al., 2000b) as follows:

$$\mathrm{var}\{\mathbf{c}^{\mathrm{T}}\beta\} = \sigma^2 \mathbf{c}^{\mathrm{T}} (\mathbf{SX})^{+}\mathbf{SVS}^{\mathrm{T}}(\mathbf{SX})^{+\mathrm{T}} \mathbf{c} \tag{40.9}$$

We want to minimise Eq. (40.9) with respect to the design matrix **X**, assuming that the filter matrix **S**, noise autocorrelation matrix **V**, and noise variance σ^2 are constant (although the autocorrelation and noise may in fact depend on the design; see below). If we incorporate **S** into **X**, and assume **V** = **I**, then this is equivalent to maximising the *efficiency, e,* of a contrast, defined as follows:

$$e(\mathbf{c},\mathbf{X}) = (\sigma^2 \mathbf{c}^{\mathrm{T}} (\mathbf{X}^{\mathrm{T}}\mathbf{X})^{-1} \mathbf{c})^{-1} \tag{40.10}$$

This equation can be split into the *noise variance*, σ^2, and the *estimator variance*, $\mathbf{X}^T\mathbf{X}$ (Mechelli *et al.,* in press-a).[24] If we are interested in multiple contrasts, expressed in a matrix **C**, and we assume σ^2 is constant, then the efficiency of a design can be defined (Dale, 1999) as follows:

$$e(\mathbf{X}) \propto \mathrm{trace}\{\mathbf{C}^{\mathrm{T}}(\mathbf{X}^{\mathrm{T}}\mathbf{X})^{-1}\mathbf{C}\}^{-1} \tag{40.11}$$

[24] Note that this measure of efficiency is not invariant to the scaling of the contrast vectors **c**, which should therefore be normalised.

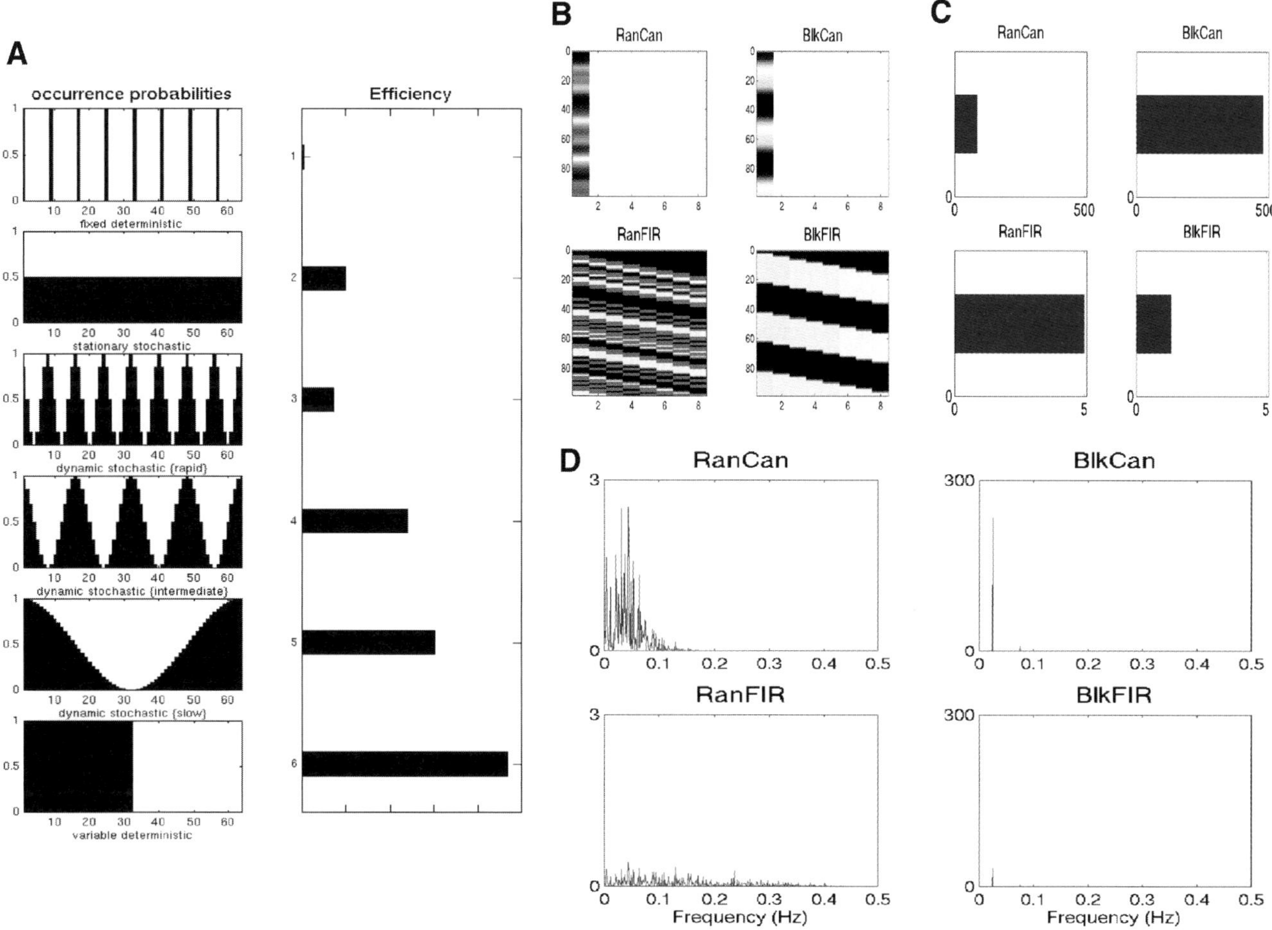

FIGURE 40.10

Efficiency for a single event type. (A) Probability of event each SOA_{min} (left column) and efficiency (right column, increasing left to right) for a deterministic design with SOA = 8 sec (first row), a stationary stochastic (randomised) design with $p = 0.5$ (second row), and dynamic stochastic designs with modulations of $p(t)$ by different sinusoidal frequencies (third to fifth rows), and in a blocked manner every 32 sec (sixth row). (B) Design matrices for randomised (Ran) and blocked (Blk) designs modelled with an FIR basis set (FIR, bin size = 4 sec) or canonical response function (Can), mean $p = 0.5$, $SOA_{min} = 2$ sec, $T_R = 1$ sec, block length = 20 sec. (C) Efficiencies for the four models (note change of scale between Can and FIR models). (D) Power spectra for the four models (note change of scale between Ran and Blk models).

Single-Event-Type Designs

For a single event type, the space of possible experimental designs can be captured by two parameters: the minimal SOA (SOA_m) and the probability, p, of an event occurring at every SOA_m (Friston *et al.,* 1999). In "deterministic" designs, $p = 1$ for every fixed multiple of SOA_m, and $p = 0$ otherwise (i.e., a series of events with fixed SOA; Fig. 40.10A). In "stochastic" designs, $0 < p < 1$, producing a range of SOAs. For "stationary" stochastic designs, p is constant, giving an exponential distribution of SOAs; for "dynamic" stochastic designs, p is itself a function of time. The temporal modulation of $p(t)$ in dynamic stochastic designs might be sinusoidal, for example, or a squarewave, corresponding to a blocked design. Also shown in Fig. 40.10A is the efficiency of each design (to detect a basic impulse response, i.e., $\mathbf{C} = [1]$, assuming a canonical HRF). For short SOA_m, the blocked design is most efficient, and the deterministic design least efficient. For stochastic designs, efficiency is generally maximal when the SOA_m is minimal and the (mean) $p = 0.5$ (Friston *et al.,* 1999).

Efficiency can also be considered in signal processing terms (Josephs & Henson, 1999). In the frequency domain, the HRF can be viewed as a filter. The most efficient contrast is one that passes maximum *neural signal* power at the dominant frequency of the HRF. Because the dominant frequency of a canonical HRF is approximately 30 sec (Fig. 40.6A), a blocked design with minimal SOA_m (large power) and a cycling frequency close to this figure (e.g., 15 sec on; 15 sec off) is very efficient. (Indeed, the most efficient design in this case would be a continuous sinusoidal modulation of neural activity with a period of 30 sec, corresponding to a delta function at 0.033 Hz in the power spectrum). The effect of bandpass filtering can also be viewed in these terms. Since the HRF and **S** matrix convolutions are commutative, a single equivalent filter can be calculated (the *effective HRF*; Josephs & Henson, 1999). Blocked designs with long cycling periods are undesirable since the majority of the induced variance is not passed by the high-pass filter (i.e., will be indistinguishable from low-frequency noise). Deterministic single-event designs with a short SOA_m will induce high-frequency neural variance that is not passed by the HRF (or low-pass filter). Stochastic designs, however, induce variance over a range of frequencies, so can be reasonably efficient with a short SOA_m.

A distinction has been made between *detection power* and *estimation efficiency* (Liu *et al.*, 2001; Birn *et al.*, 2002). The former refers to the ability to detect a significant response; the latter refers to the ability to estimate the shape of the response. The above examples, which assume a canonical HRF, relate to detection power. The concept of estimation efficiency can be illustrated simply by considering a more general basis set, such as an FIR. Multiple parameters now need to be estimated (**X** has multiple columns; Fig. 40.10B), and efficiency is maximal [Eq. (40.11)] when the covariance between the columns of **X** is minimal. In this case (with contrast **C** = **I**), blocked designs are less efficient than randomised designs (Fig. 40.10C), since the FIR regressors are highly correlated in blocked designs. This is the opposite of the situation with a single canonical HRF, for which blocked designs are more efficient than randomised designs. An alternative perspective is that the FIR basis functions have more high-frequency components and, therefore, "pass" more signal at the higher frequencies that arise from randomised designs (Fig. 40.10D).

Thus the different considerations of detecting a response versus characterising the form of that response require different types of experimental design. Hagberg *et al.* (2001) considered a range of possible SOA distributions (bimodal in the case of blocked designs; exponential in the case of fully randomised designs) and showed that "long-tail" distributions combine reasonable detection power and estimation efficiency (although uniform distributions, such as those based on a Latin Square, did as well on empirical data).

Multiple-Event-Type Designs

For multiple event types, the space of possible designs can be characterised by SOA_m and a *transition matrix* (Josephs & Henson, 1999). For N_i different event types, an N_i^m by N_i transition matrix captures the probability of an event being of each type, given the history of the last $1..m$ event types. Some examples are shown in Fig. 40.11. A fully randomised design with two event types (A and B) has a simple first-order transition matrix in which each probability is 0.5. The efficiencies (detection power) of two contrasts—[1 1], the main effect of A and B (versus baseline), and [1 −1], the differential effect—are shown as a function of SOA_m in Fig. 40.12A. The optimal SOA for the main effect under these conditions (for a finite sequence) is approximately 20 sec. The efficiency of the main effect decreases for shorter SOAs, whereas the efficiency of the differential effect increases. The optimal SOA thus depends on the specific contrast of interest.[25] Both patterns arise because of the increased summation of successive responses at shorter SOAs, producing greater overall signal power. In the case of the main effect, however, this power is moved to low frequencies that are not passed by the effective HRF (the signal simply becomes a "raised baseline" that is removed by the high-pass filter; Fig. 40.13A). For the differential effect, the extra power is maintained at higher frequencies because of the random modulation of the event types (i.e., greater experimentally induced variability about the mean signal over time; Fig. 40.13B).

Various experimental constraints on multiple-event-type designs can also be considered. In some situations, the order of event types might be fixed, and the design question relates to the optimal SOA. For an alternating A − B design (where A and B might reflect transitions

[25] The main effect, which does not distinguish A and B is, of course, equivalent to a deterministic design, whereas the differential effect is equivalent to a stochastic design (from the perspective of any one event type).

Design	Transition Matrix			Example Sequence
		A	B	
A. Randomised	A	0.5	0.5	ABBBAABABABAAAAB....
	B	0.5	0.5	
B. Alternating	A	0	1	ABABABABABABABAB....
	B	1	0	
C. Permuted	AA	0	1	ABBABAABBABABA....
	AB	0.5	0.5	
	BA	0.5	0.5	
	BB	1	0	
D. "Null events"	A	0.33	0.33	ABB--B-A---AABA--B....
	B	0.33	0.33	

FIGURE 40.11
Example transition matrices.

between two perceptual states, for example), the optimal SOA for a differential effect is 10 sec (Fig. 40.12B, i.e., half of that for the main effect).[26] In other situations, experimental constraints may limit the SOA, to at least 10 sec, say, and the design question relates to the optimal stimulus ordering. An alternating design is more efficient than a randomised design for such intermediate SOAs (since randomisation induces more low-frequency power that is lost to the high-pass filter; cf. Figs. 40.13B and C). However, an alternating design may not be advisable for psychological reasons (subjects' behaviour might be influenced by the predictable pattern). A permuted design (with second-order transition matrix shown in Fig. 40.11C) may be a more suitable choice (Fig. 40.12B). Such a design is random (counterbalanced) to first order, although fully deterministic to second order.

A further design concept concerns "null events" (or "fixation trials"). These are not real events, in that they do not differ from the interevent baseline and are not detectable by subjects (and hence are not modelled in the design matrix), but were introduced by Dale and Buckner (1997) to allow selective averaging (see "Temporal Basis Functions" section). In fact, they are simply a convenient means of creating a stochastic design by shuffling (permuting) a certain proportion of null events among the events of interest (and correspond to transition matrices whose columns do not sum to one; Fig. 40.11D). From the perspective of multiple-event-type designs, the reason for null events is to buy efficiency to both the main effect and differential effect at short SOA_m (at a slight cost to the efficiency for the differential effect; Fig. 40.12C). In other words, they provide better estimation efficiency in order to characterise the shape of the response at short SOA_m (by effectively producing an exponential distribution of SOAs).

The efficiencies shown in Fig. 40.12 are unlikely to map simply (e.g., linearly) onto the size of the t statistic. Nonetheless, if the noise variance [Eq. (40.9)] is independent of experimental design, the relationship should at least be monotonic (i.e., provide a rank ordering of the statistical power of different designs). Mechelli *et al.* (2003a) showed that the noise variance differed significantly between a blocked and a randomised design (both modelled with events, cf. Figs. 40.5B and 5C). This suggests that the stimulus ordering did affect unmodelled psychological or physiological effects in this dataset, contributing to the residual error (noise). When the data were high-pass filtered, however, the noise variance no longer differed significantly between the two designs. In this case, the statistical results were in agreement with the relative efficiencies predicted from the estimation variances.

Finally, note that the predictions in Fig. 40.12 are based on the LTI model; nonlinearities ensure that the efficiency of the differential effect does not increase indefinitely as the SOA tends

[26] This is the extreme case of a blocked design, with the alternation of longer runs of A and B becoming more efficient as the SOA decreases (Fig. 40.12D; i.e., the reason for blocking diminishes as the SOA increases).

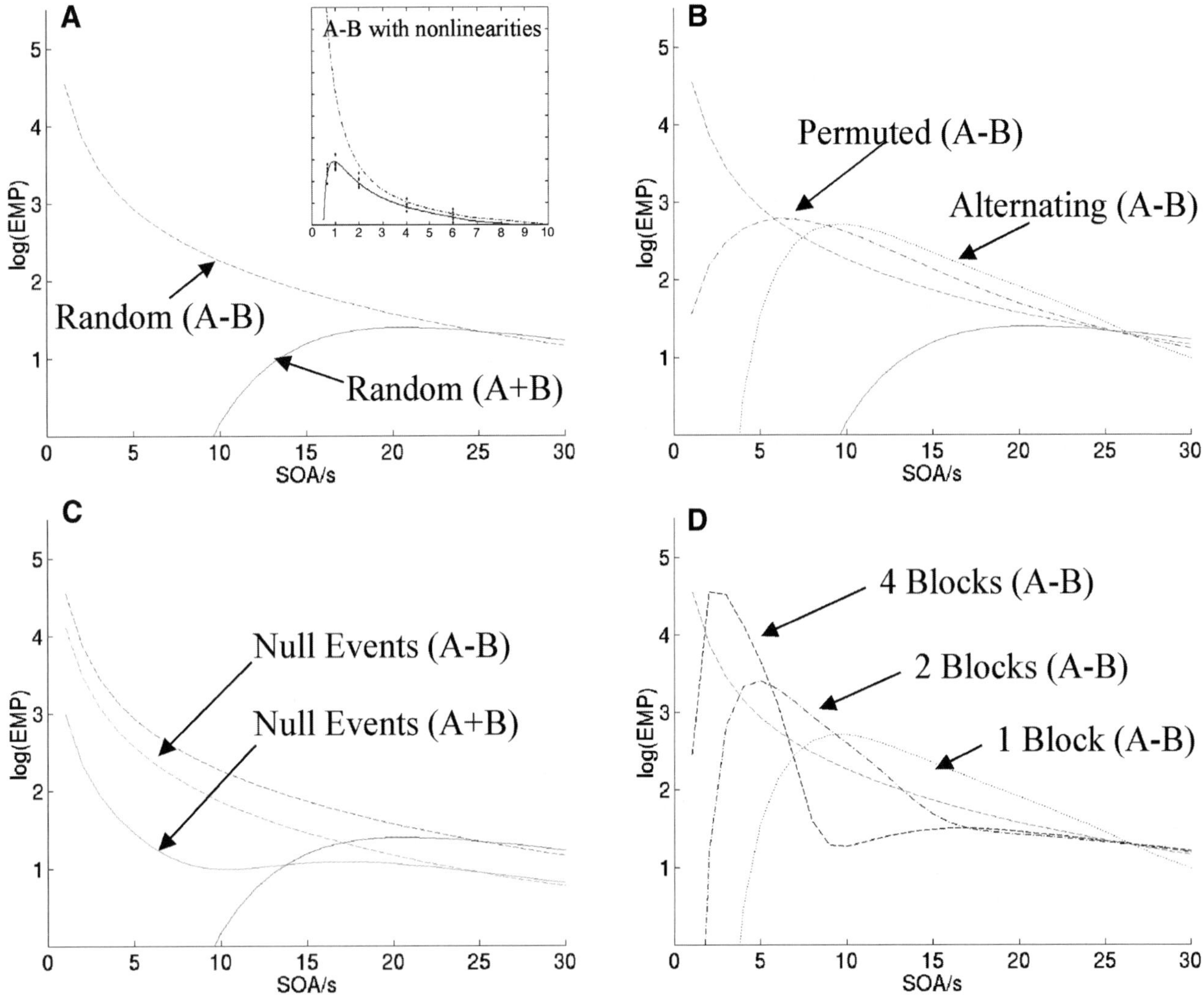

FIGURE 40.12
Efficiency for two event types. Efficiency is expressed in terms of *estimated measurable power* (EMP) passed by an effective HRF, characterised by a canonical HRF, high-pass filter with cutoff period of 60 sec and low-pass smoothing by a Gaussian 4-sec FWHM, as a function of SOA_{min} for main (solid) effect ([1 1] contrast) and differential (dashed) effect ([1 −1] contrast). (A) Randomised design. Inset is the efficiency for the differential effect with nonlinear saturation (solid) predicted from a second-order Volterra expansion (Friston *et al.,* 1998a). (B) Alternating (black) and permuted (blue) designs. (C) With (green) and without (red) null events. (D) Blocked designs with runs of one (dotted), two (dot-dash), or four (dashed) stimuli, for example, ABABABAB…, AABBAABB… and AAAABBBB, respectively.

to zero. In fact, the inclusion of nonlinearities in the form of the second-order Volterra kernel derived from one dataset (Friston *et al.,* 1998a; Chapter 41) suggests that efficiency continues to increase down to SOAs of 1 sec (after which it reverses), despite the presence of nonlinearities for SOAs below approximately 8 sec (Fig. 40.12A, inset). Nonetheless, differential responses have been detected with SOAs as short as 0.5 sec (Burock *et al.,* 1998).

WORKED EXAMPLE

In this section, some of the above ideas are illustrated in a single-session event-related fMRI dataset derived from one of the 12 subjects reported in Henson *et al.* (2002b), and freely available from the SPM website (http://www.fil.ion.ucl.ac.uk/spm/data/#SPM00AdvEFMRI). Events were 500-msec presentations of faces, to which the subject made a famous/nonfamous decision with the index and middle fingers of their right hand. One-half of the faces were

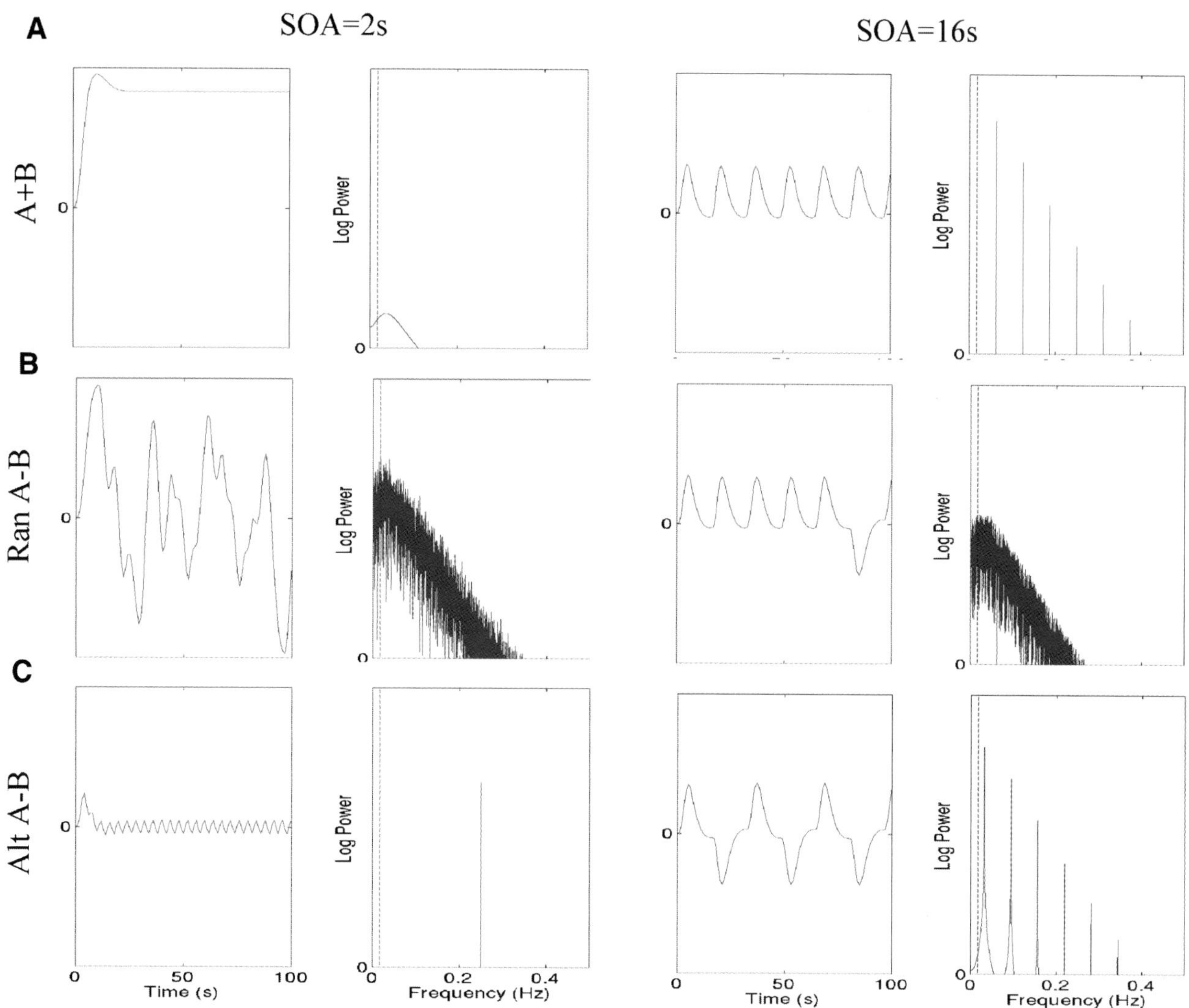

FIGURE 40.13
Frequency perspective on efficiency for two event types. Time series and power spectra, after canonical HRF convolution, with SOAs of 2 sec (left) and 16 sec (right), for (A) main effect, (B) differential effect in randomised design, and (C) differential effect in an alternating design. The high-pass filter is indicated as black dotted line in power spectra.

famous, one-half were novel (unfamiliar), and each face was presented twice during the session, producing a 2 × 2 factorial design consisting of first and second presentations of novel and famous faces (conditions N1, N2, F1, and F2, respectively, each containing $N_j = 26$ events). To these 104 events, 52 null events were added and the whole sequence permuted. This meant that the order of novel/famous faces was pseudo-randomised (given the finite sequence), though the order of first and second presentations, while intermixed, was constrained by the fact that second presentations were necessarily later than first presentations on average. SOA_{min} was 4.5 sec, but varied near exponentially over multiples of SOA_{min} owing to the null events. The time series comprised 351 images acquired continuously with a T_R of 2 sec. The images were realigned spatially, slice-time corrected to the middle slice, normalised with a bilinear interpolation to 3- × 3- × 3-mm voxels (Chapter 33), and smoothed with an isotropic Gaussian FWHM of 8 mm. The ratio of SOA_{min} to T_R ensured an effective peristimulus sampling rate of 2 Hz.

Analyses were performed with SPM99. Events were modelled with $N_k = 3$ basis functions consisting of the canonical HRF, its temporal derivative, and its dispersion derivative. The resolution of the simulated BOLD signal was set to 83 msec ($T = 24$), and the event onsets were synchronised with the middle slice ($T_0 = 12$). Also included in each model were six user-specified regressors derived from the rigid body realignment parameters (three translations and

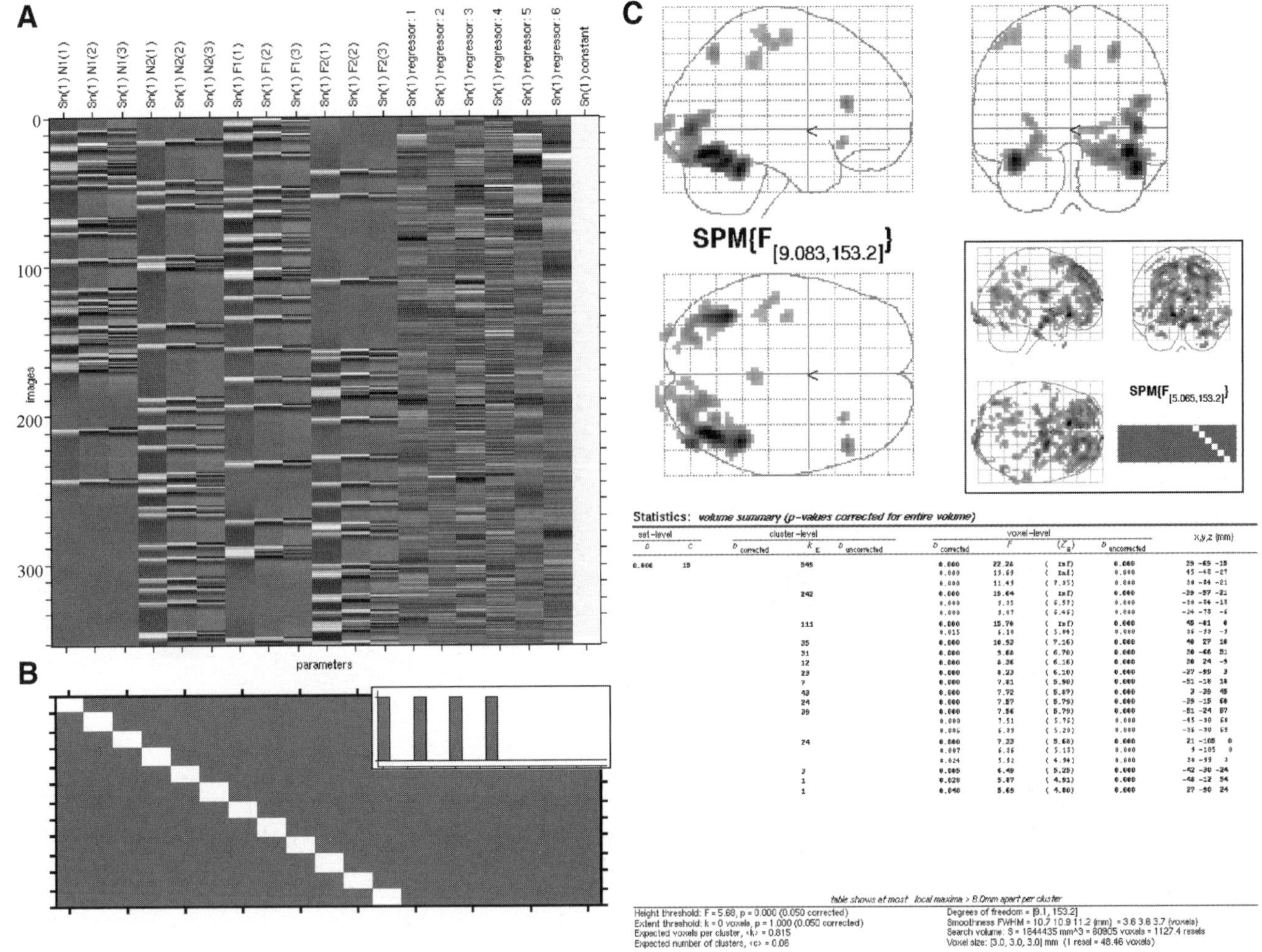

FIGURE 40.14
Categorical model: effects of interest. (A) Design matrix. (B) F contrast for effects of interest (inset is T contrast that tests for positive mean parameter estimate for canonical HRF). (C) SPM{F} MIP for effects-of-interest F contrast, thresholded at $p < .05$ whole brain corrected, together with SPM tabulated output (inset is SPM{F} for contrast on movement parameters, also at $p < .05$ corrected).

three rotations) to model residual (linear) movement effects.[27] A high-pass filter with a 120-sec cutoff was applied to both model and data, together with an AR(1) model for the residual temporal autocorrelation, as discussed earlier. No global scaling was used. Two different models are considered below: a *categorical* one and a *parametric* one. In the categorical model, each event type is modelled separately (N_i = 4). In the parametric model, a single event type representing all faces is modulated by their familiarity and the "lag" since their last presentation.

Categorical Model

The design matrix for the categorical model is shown in Fig. 40.14A. A (modified) effects-of-interest F contrast, corresponding to a reduced F test on the first 12 columns of the design matrix (i.e., removing linear movement effects), is shown in Fig. 40.14B and the resulting SPM{F} in Fig. 40.14C. The associated degrees of freedom [9,153] derive from the autocorrelation

[27] One might also include the temporal derivatives of the realignment parameters, and higher order interactions between them, in a Volterra approximation to residual movement effects, regardless of their cause. Note also that the rare events for which the fame decision was erroneous could be modelled as a separate event type (since they may involve physiological changes that are not typical of face recognition). This was performed in the demonstration on the website, but is ignored here for simplicity.

estimated from the AR(1) model.[28] Several regions, most notably in bilateral posterior inferior temporal, lateral occipital, left motor and right prefrontal cortices, show some form of reliable response to the events (versus baseline). Note that these responses could be activations (positive amplitude) or deactivations (negative amplitude), and may differ across the event types. A T contrast like that shown in the inset in Fig. 40.14B would test a more constrained hypothesis, namely, that the response is positive when averaged across all event types, and is a more powerful test for such responses (producing many more significant voxels in this dataset). Also inset in Fig. 40.14C is the SPM{F} from an F contrast on the realignment parameters, in which movement effects can be seen at the edge of the brain.

The parameter estimates (plotting the modified effects-of-interest contrast) and best fitting event-related responses for a right fusiform region (close to what has been called the *fusiform face area*; Kanwisher *et al.,* 1997) are shown in Figs. 40.15A and B. First presentations of famous faces produced the greatest response. Furthermore, responses in this region appear to be slightly earlier and narrower than the canonical response, as indicated by the positive parameter estimates for the temporal and dispersion derivatives.[29]

There are three obvious further effects of interest: the main effects of familiarity and repetition, and their interaction. The results from an F contrast for the repetition effect are shown in Fig. 40.15C, after inclusive masking with the effects-of-interest F contrast in Fig. 40.14C. This mask restricts analysis to regions that are generally responsive to faces (without needing a separate face localiser scan; cf. Kanwisher *et al.,* 1997) and could be used for a small-volume correction (Chapter 44). Note that this masking is facilitated by the inclusion of null events; otherwise the main effect of faces versus baseline could not be estimated efficiently "Multiple Event-Type Designs" section. Note also that the efficiency of the repetition effect is approximately 85% of that for the familiarity and interaction effects when we use Eq. (40.11) for the corresponding F contrasts. This reflects the unbalanced order of first and second presentations, meaning that more low-frequency signal power is lost to the high-pass filter. Incidentally, the inclusion of the movement parameters reduced the efficiency of these contrasts to only 97%.

The contrast of parameter estimates and fitted responses for the single right posterior occipitotemporal region identified by the repetition contrast are shown in Fig. 40.15D. Differential effects were seen on all three basis functions and represent decreased responses to repeated faces.[30]

Figure 40.16A shows the design matrix using a more general FIR basis set of $N_k = 16$, 2-sec time bins. The effects-of-interest contrast (Fig. 40.16B) reveals a subset of the regions identified with the canonical basis set (cf. Fig. 40.16C and Fig. 14C). The absence of additional regions using the FIR model suggests that no region exhibited a reliable event-related response with a noncanonical form (though this may reflect lack of power). Figure 40.16D shows the parameter estimates from the right fusiform region, which clearly demonstrate canonical-like impulse responses for the four event types. No right occipitotemporal region was identified by an F contrast testing for the repetition effect (Fig. 40.16C, inset) when using the FIR basis set. This reflects the reduced power of this unconstrained contrast. Note that constraints can be imposed on the contrasts, as illustrated by the T-contrast inset in Fig. 40.16B, which corresponds to a canonical HRF.

Parametric Model

In this model, a single event type was defined (collapsing the onsets for the four event types above), which was modulated by three parametric modulations. The first modelled how the response varied according to the recency with which a face had been seen (a suggestion made by Karl Friston, offering a continuous perspective on "repetition"). This was achieved by an exponential parametric modulation of the form:

---

[28] Applying a low-pass HRF smoothing instead resulted in degrees of freedom [10,106] and fewer significant voxels, while using a ReML estimation of an AR(1)+white noise model resulted in degrees of freedom [11,238] and a greater number of significant voxels.

[29] Indeed, several occipitotemporal regions were identified by an F contrast on the temporal derivative alone, demonstrating the importance of allowing for variability about the canonical form (reducing the residual error).

[30] Note that the difference in the temporal derivative parameter estimates does not imply a difference in latency, given the concurrent difference in canonical parameter estimates (Henson *et al.,* 2002a).

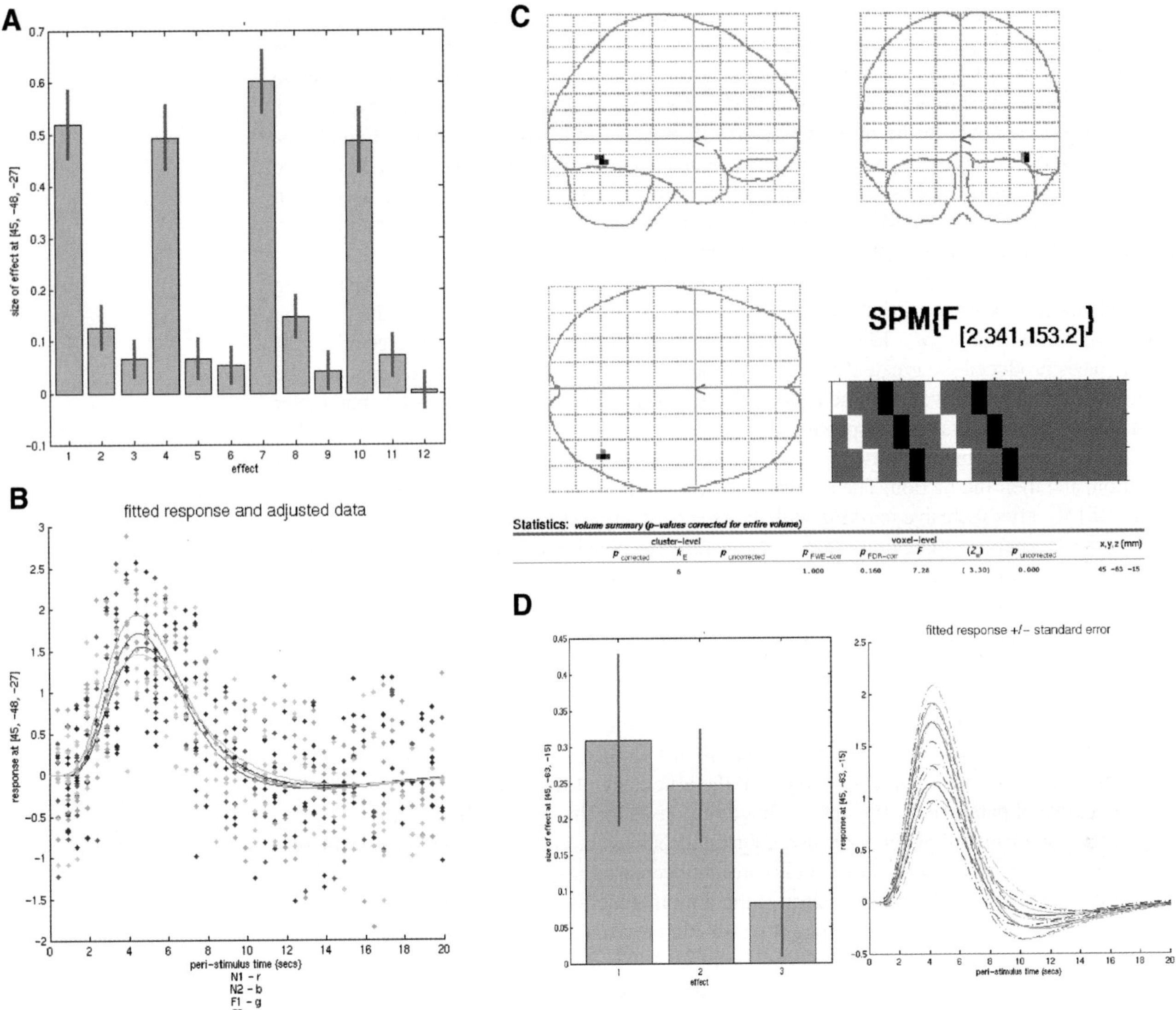

FIGURE 40.15
Categorical model: repetition effect. (A) Parameter estimates (scale arbitrary) from local maximum in right fusiform (+45, −48, −27), ordered by condition—N1, N2, F1, F2—and within each condition by basis function—canonical HRF, temporal derivative, and dispersion derivative. (B) Fitted event-related responses (solid) and adjusted data (dots) in terms of percentage signal change (relative to grand mean over space and time) against PST for N1 (red), N2 (blue), F1 (green), and F2 (cyan). (C). SPM{F} MIP for repetition effect contrast (inset), thresholded at $p < .001$ uncorrected, after inclusive masking with effects of interest (Fig. 40.12) at $p < .05$ corrected. (D) Contrast of parameter estimates for repetition effect (difference between first and second presentations) in right occipitotemporal region (+45 −63 −15) for canonical HRF, temporal derivative and dispersion derivative, together with fitted responses (solid) ±1 standard error (dashed).

$$\alpha_j = e^{-Lj/50}$$

where L_j is the "lag" for the jth face presentation, defined as the number of stimuli between that presentation and the previous presentation of that face.[31] Thus, as lag increases, the modulation decreases. For first presentations, $L_j = \infty$ and the modulation is zero[32] (though it becomes negative after mean correction).

The second parametric modulation had a binary value of 1 or −1, indicating whether the face was famous or novel; the third modulation was the interaction between face familiarity and lag

[31] The choice of an exponential function (rather than, say, a polynomial expansion) was based simply on the observation that many biological processes have exponential time dependency. The half-life of the function (50) was somewhat arbitrary; ideally it would be derived empirically from a separate dataset.

[32] This was for both famous and novel faces, though face familiarity could also be modelled this way by setting $L_j = \infty$ for N1, and $L_j = M$ for F1, where M is a large number (or some subjective recency rating).

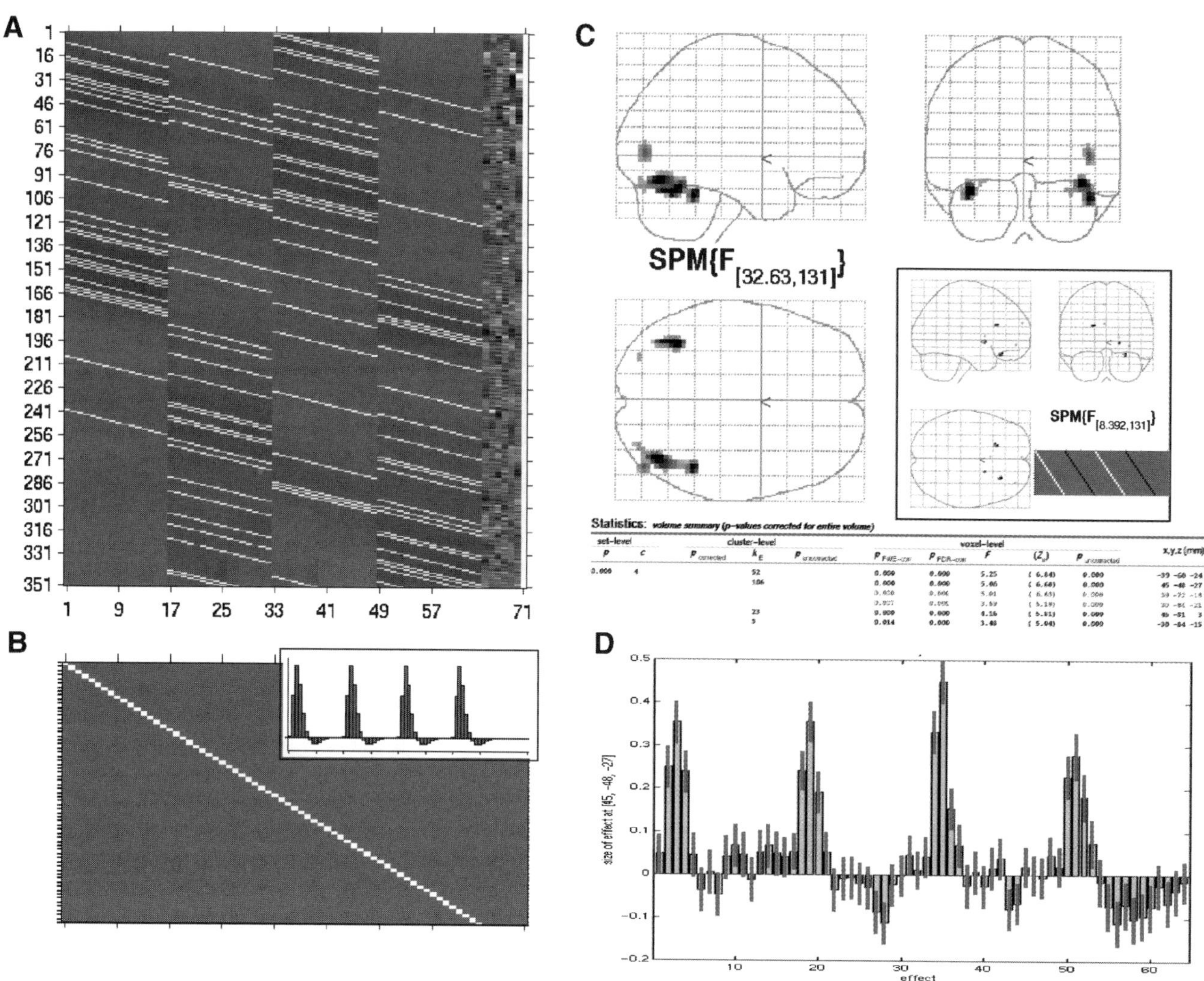

FIGURE 40.16
Categorical model: FIR basis set. (A) Design matrix. (B) Effects of interest F contrast (canonical HRF weighted T contrast inset). (C) SPM{F} MIP for effects of interest, thresholded at $p < .05$ whole brain corrected, together with SPM tabulated output. (Inset is SPM{F} for unconstrained repetition effect F contrast, thresholded at $p < .005$ uncorrected.) (D) Parameter estimates for effects of interest from right fusiform region (+45, −48, −27), as in Fig. 40.15A, ordered by conditions—N1, N2, F1, F2—and within each condition by the 16 basis functions (i.e., mean response every 2 sec from 0–32 sec PST).

(i.e., the product of the first and second modulations, after mean correction). Each modulation was applied to the three temporal basis functions, producing the design matrix in Fig. 40.17A. The F contrast for the main effect of faces versus baseline (upper contrast in Fig. 40.17B) identified regions similar to those identified by the effects-of-interest contrast in the categorical model presented above (since the models span similar spaces). As expected, the F contrast for the lag effect (lower contrast in Fig. 40.17B), after masking with the main effect, revealed the same right occipitotemporal region (Fig. 40.17C) that showed a main effect of repetition in the categorical model. The best fitting event-related parametric response in Fig. 40.17D shows that the response increases with lag, suggesting that the repetition-related decrease observed in the categorical model may be transient (consistent with the similar lag effect found when a parametric modulation was applied to second presentations only; Henson *et al.*, 2000b).

Acknowledgments

This work is funded by Wellcome Trust Fellowship 060924. The author would like to thank John Ashburner, Karl Friston, Dan Glaser and Will Penny for their comments.

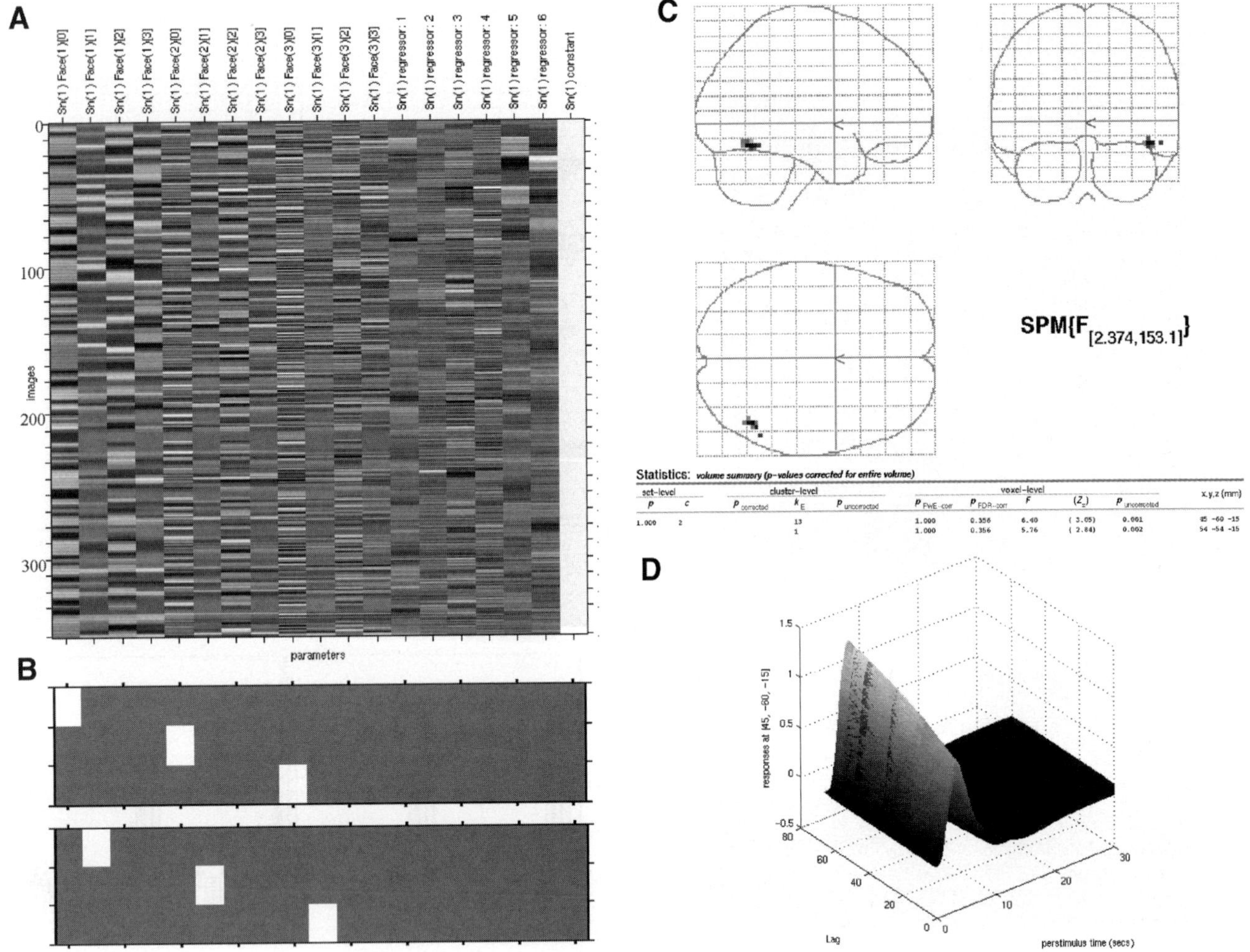

FIGURE 40.17
Parametric model: (A) Design matrix with columns ordered by basis function—canonical HRF, temporal derivative, dispersion derivative—and within each basis function by parametric effect—main effect, lag, familiarity, lag-x-familiarity. (B) F contrasts for main effect (top) and lag effect (bottom). (C) SPM{F} MIP for lag effect, together with SPM tabulated output, thresholded at $p < .005$ uncorrected, after inclusive masking with main effect at $p < .05$ corrected. (D) Parametric plot of fitted response from right occipitotemporal region (+45 −60 −15), close to that in Fig. 40.15C, in terms of percentage signal change versus PST and Lag (infinite lag values for first presentations not shown).

References

Aguirre, G. K., Zarahn, E., and D'Esposito, M. (1998. The variability of human, BOLD hemodynamic responses. *NeuroImage* **8,** 360–369.

Birn, R. M., Saad, Z. S., and Bandettini, P. A. (2001). Spatial heterogeneity of the nonlinear dynamics in the fMRI bold response. *NeuroImage* **14,** 817–826.

Birn, R. M., Cox, R. W., and Bandettini, P. A. (2002). Detection versus estimation in event-related fMRI: choosing the optimal stimulus timing. *NeuroImage,* **15,** 252–264.

Boynton, G. M., Engel, S. A., Glover, G. H., and Heeger, D. J. (1996). Linear systems analysis of functional magnetic resonance imaging in human V1. *J. Neurosci.* **16,** 4207–4221.

Bullmore, E. T., Brammer, M. J., Williams, S. C. R., Rabe-Hesketh, S., Janot, N., David, A., Mellers, J., Howard, R., and Sham, P. (1996). Statistical methods of estimation and inference for functional MR images. *Mag. Res. Med.* **35,** 261–277.

Burock, M. A., and Dale, A. M. (2000). Estimation and detection of event-related fMRI signals with temporally correlated noise: a statistically efficient and unbiased approach. *Hum. Brain Mapping* **11,** 249–260.

Burock, M. A., Buckner, R. L., Woldorff, M. G., Rosen, B. R., and Dale, A. M. (1998). Randomised event-related experimental designs allow for extremely rapid presentation rates using functional MRI. *NeuroReport* **9,** 3735–3739.

Chawla, D., Rees, G., and Friston, K. J. (1999). The physiological basis of attentional modulation in extrastriate visual areas. *Nat. Neurosci.* **2,** 671–676.

Dale, A. M. (1999). Optimal experimental design for event-related fMRI. *Hum. Brain Mapping* **8,** 109–114.

Dale, A., and Buckner, R. (1997). Selective averaging of rapidly presented individual trials using fMRI. *Hum. Brain Mapping* **5,** 329–340.

Fransson, P., Kruger, G., Merboldt, K. D., and Frahm, J. (1999). MRI of functional deactivation: temporal and spatial characteristics of oxygenation-sensitive responses in human visual cortex. *NeuroImage* **9,** 611–618.

Friston, K. J., Jezzard, P. J., and Turner, R. (1994). Analysis of functional MRI time-series. *Hum. Brain Mapping* **1,** 153–171.

Friston, K. J., Josephs, O., Rees, G., and Turner, R. (1998a). Non-linear event-related responses in fMRI. *Mag. Res. Med.* **39,** 41–52.

Friston, K. J., Fletcher, P., Josephs, O., Holmes, A., Rugg, M. D., and Turner, R. (1998b). Event-related fMRI: characterising differential responses. *NeuroImage* **7,** 30–40.

Friston, K. J., , Zarahn, E., Josephs, O., Henson, R. N., and Dale, A. M. (1999). Stochastic designs in event-related fMRI. *NeuroImage* **10,** 607–619.

Friston, K. J., Mechelli, A., Turner, R., and Price, C. J.(2000a). Nonlinear responses in fMRI: the balloon model, Volterra kernels, and other hemodynamics. *NeuroImage.* **12,** 466–477.

Friston, K. J., , Josephs, O., Zarahn, E., Holmes, A. P., Rouquette, S., and Poline, J. (2000b). To smooth or not to smooth? Bias and efficiency in fMRI time-series analysis. *NeuroImage.* **12,** 196–208.

Friston, K. J., Glaser, D. E., Henson, R. N. A., Kiebel, S., Phillips, C., and Ashburner, J. (2002). Classical and Bayesian inference in neuroimaging: applications. *NeuroImage* **16,** 484–512.

Glover, G. H. (1999). Deconvolution of impulse response in event-related BOLD fMRI. *NeuroImage* **9,** 416–429.

Gossl, C., Fahrmeir, L., and Auer, D. P. (2001). Bayesian modelling of the hemodynamic response function in BOLD fMRI. *NeuroImage* **14,** 140–148.

Hagberg, G. E., Zito, G., Patria, F., and Sanes, J. N. (2001). Improved detection of event-related functional MRI signals using probability functions. *NeuroImage* **14,** 1193–1205.

Henson, R. N. A., and Rugg, M. D. (2001). Effects of stimulus repetition on latency of the BOLD impulse response. *NeuroImage* **13,** 683.

Henson, R. N. A., Buechel, C., Josephs, O., and Friston, K. (1999a). The slice-timing problem in event-related fMRI. *NeuroImage* **9,** 125.

Henson, R. N. A., Rugg, M. D., Shallice, T., Josephs, O., and Dolan, R. (1999b). Recollection and familiarity in recognition memory: an event-related fMRI study. *J. Neurosci.* **19,** 3962–3972.

Henson, R., Andersson, J., and Friston, K. (2000a). Multivariate SPM: application to basis function characterisations of event-related fMRI responses. *NeuroImage* **11,** 468.

Henson, R., Shallice, T., and Dolan, R. (2000b). Neuroimaging evidence for dissociable forms of repetition priming. *Science,* **287,** 1269–1272.

Henson, R. N. A., Rugg, M. D., and Friston, K. J. (2001). The choice of basis functions in event-related fMRI. *NeuroImage* **13,** 149.

Henson, R. N. A., Price, C., Rugg, M. D., Turner, R., and Friston, K. (2002a). Detecting latency differences in event-related BOLD responses: application to words versus nonwords, and initial versus repeated face presentations. *NeuroImage,* **15,** 83–97.

Henson, R. N. A, Shallice, T., Gorno-Tempini, M.-L., and Dolan, R. J (2002b). Face repetition effects in implicit and explicit memory tests as measured by fMRI. *Cerebral Cortex* **12,** 178–186.

Hinrichs, H., Scholz, M., Tempelmann, C., Woldorff, M. G., Dale, A. M., and Heinze, H. J. (2000). Deconvolution of event-related fMRI responses in fast-rate experimental designs: tracking amplitude variations. *J. Cogn. Neurosci.* **12,** 76–89.

Huettel, S. A., and McCarthy, G. (2001). Regional differences in the refractory period of the hemodynamic response: an event-related fMRI study. *NeuroImage* **14,** 967–976.

Johnson, M. K., Nolde, S. F., Mather, M., Kounios, J., Schacter, D. L., and Curran, T. (1997). Test format can affect the similarity of brain activity associated with true and false recognition memory. *Psychol. Sci.* **8,** 250–257.

Josephs, O., and Henson, R. N. A. (1999). Event-related fMRI: modelling, inference and optimisation. *Phil. Trans. Roy. Soc. London,* **354,** 1215–1228.

Josephs, O., Turner, R., and Friston, K. J. (1997). Event-related fMRI *Hum. Brain Mapping* **5,** 243–248.

Kanwisher, N., McDermott, J., and Chun, M. M. (1997). The fusiform face area: a module in human extrastriate cortex specialised for face perception. *J. Neurosci.* **17,** 4302–4311.

Kleinschmidt, A., Buchel, C., Zeki, S., and Frackowiak, R. S. (1998). Human brain activity during spontaneously reversing perception of ambiguous figures. *Proc. Roy. Soc. Lond. B Biol. Sci.* **265**, 2427–33

Kruggel, F., and von Cramon, D. Y. (1999a). Modelling the hemodynamic response in single-trial functional MRI experiments. *Mag. Res. Med.* **42,** 787–797.

Kruggel, F., and von Cramon, D. Y. (1999b). Temporal properties of the hemodynamic response in functional MRI. *Hum. Brain Mapping* **8,** 259–271.

Kruggel, F., Zysset, S., and von Cramon, D. Y. (2000). Nonlinear regression of functional MRI data: an item recognition task study. *NeuroImage* **12,** 173–183.

Lee, A. T., Glover, G. H., and Meyer, C. H. (1995. Discrimination of large venous vessels in time-course spiral blood-oxygenation-level-dependent magnetic-resonance functional imaging. *Mag. Res. Med.* **33,** 745–754.

Liao, C. H., Worsley, K. J., Poline, J.-B., Duncan, G. H., and Evans, A. C. (2002). Estimating the delay of the hemodynamic response in fMRI data. *NeuroImage* **16,** 593–606.

Liu, T. T., Frank, L. R., Wong, E. C., and Buxton, R. B. (2001). Detection power, estimation efficiency, and predictability in event-related fMRI. *NeuroImage* **13,** 759–773.

Malonek, D., and Grinvald, A. (1996). Interactions between electrical activity and cortical microcirculation revealed by imaging spectroscopy: implications for functional brain mapping. *Science* **272,** 551–554.

Mechelli, A., Price, C. J., Henson, R. N. A., and Friston, K. J. (in press-a). The effect of high-pass filtering on the efficiency of response estimation: a comparison between blocked and randomised designs. *NeuroImage*, **18**, 798–805.

Mechelli, A., Henson, R. N. A., Price, C. J., and Friston, K. J. (in press-b). Comparing event-related and epoch analysis in blocked design fMRI. *NeuroImage*, **18**, 806–810.

Menon, R. S., Luknowsky, D. C., and Gati, J. S. (1998). Mental chronometry using latency-resolved functional MRI. *Proc. Natl. Acad. Sci. USA* **95,** 10902–10907.

Miezin, F. M., Maccotta, L., Ollinger, J. M., Petersen, S. E., and Buckner, R. L. (2000). Characterising the hemodynamic response: effects of presentation rate, sampling procedure, and the possibility of ordering brain activity based on relative timing. *NeuroImage* **11,** 735–759.

Ollinger, J. M., Shulman, G. L., and Corbetta, M. (2001). Separating processes within a trial in event-related functional MRI. *NeuroImage* **13,** 210–217.

Pollmann, S., Wiggins, C. J., Norris, D. G., von Cramon, D. Y., and Schubert, T. (1998). Use of short intertrial intervals in single-trial experiments: a 3T fMRI-study. *NeuroImage* **8,** 327–339.

Portas, C. M., Strange, B. A., Friston, K. J., Dolan, R. J., and Frith, C. D. (2000). How does the brain sustain a visual percept? *Proc. Roy. Soc. Lond. B Biol. Sci.* **267,** 845–850.

Price, C. J., Veltman, D. J., Ashburner, J., Josephs, O., and Friston, K. J. (1999). The critical relationship between the timing of stimulus presentation and data acquisition in blocked designs with fMRI. *NeuroImage* **10,** 36–44.

Rajapakse, J. C., Kruggel, F., Maisog, J. M., and von Cramon, D. Y. (1998). Modelling hemodynamic response for analysis of functional MRI time-series. *Hum. Brain Mapping* **6,** 283–300.

Rugg, M. D., and Henson, R. N. A. (2002). Episodic memory retrieval: an (event-related) functional neuroimaging perspective. In *The Cognitive Neuroscience of Memory Encoding and Retrieval* Parker, A. E., Wilding, E. L., and Bussey, T., Eds.). Psychology Press, Hove.

Saad, Z. S., Ropella, K. M., Cox, R. W., and DeYoe, E. A. (2001). Analysis and use of FMRI response delays. *Hum. Brain Mapping* **13,** 74–93.

Schacter, D. L., Buckner, R. L., Koutstaal, W., Dale, A. M., and Rosen, B. R. (1997. Late onset of anterior prefrontal activity during true and false recognition: an event-related fMRI study. *NeuroImage* **6,** 259–269.

Strange, B. A., Henson, R. N., Friston, K. J., and Dolan, R. J. (2000. Brain mechanisms for detecting perceptual, semantic, and emotional deviance. *NeuroImage* **12,** 425–433.

Turner, R., Howseman, A., Rees, G. E., Josephs, O., and Friston, K. (1998). Functional magnetic resonance imaging of the human brain: data acquisition and analysis. *Exp. Brain Res.* **123,** 5–12.

Vazquez, A. L., and Noll, C. D. (1998). Nonlinear aspects of the BOLD response in functional MRI. *NeuroImage* **7,** 108–118.

Woolrich, M. W., Ripley, B. D., Brady, M., and Smith, S. M. (2001). Temporal autocorrelation in univariate linear modelling of FMRI data. *NeuroImage* **14,** 1370–1386.

Worsley, K. J., and Friston, K. J. (1995), Analysis of fMRI time-series revisited—again. *NeuroImage* **2,** 173–181.

Worsley, K. J., Liao, C. H., Aston, J., Petre, V., Duncan, G. H., Morales, F., and Evans, A. C. (2002). A general statistical analysis for fMRI data. *NeuroImage,* **15,** 1–15.

Zarahn, E. (2000). Testing for neural responses during temporal components of trials with BOLD fMRI. *NeuroImage* **11,** 783–796.

Zarahn, E., Aguirre, G., and D'Esposito, M. (1997). A trial-based experimental design for fMRI. *NeuroImage* **6,** 122–138.

Zarahn, E., Aguirre, G. K., and D'Esposito, M. (1997). Empirical analyses of BOLD fMRI statistics: I Spatially unsmoothed data collected under null-hypothesis conditions. *NeuroImage* **5,** 179–197.

CHAPTER

41

Haemodynamic Modelling

INTRODUCTION

There is a growing appreciation of the importance of nonlinearities in evoked responses in fMRI, particularly with the advent of event-related fMRI. These nonlinearities are commonly expressed as interactions among stimuli that can lead to the suppression and increased latency of responses to a stimulus that is incurred by a preceding stimulus. We have presented previously a model-free characterisation of these effects using generic techniques from nonlinear system identification, namely, a Volterra series formulation. At the same time Buxton *et al.* (1998) described a plausible and compelling dynamic model of haemodynamic signal transduction in fMRI. Subsequent work by Mandeville *et al.* (1999) provided important theoretical and empirical constraints on the form of the dynamic relationship between blood flow and volume that underpins the evolution of the fMRI signal. In this chapter we combine these system identification and model-based approaches and ask whether the balloon model is sufficient to account for the nonlinear behaviours observed in real time series. We conclude that it can and, furthermore, that the model parameters that ensue are biologically plausible. This conclusion is based on the observation that the balloon model can produce Volterra kernels that emulate empirical kernels.

To enable this evaluation, we have had to embed the balloon model in a haemodynamic input–state–output model that included the dynamics of perfusion changes that are contingent on underlying synaptic activation. This chapter (1) presents the full haemodynamic model, (2) describes how its associated Volterra kernels can be derived, and (3) addresses the model's validity in relation to empirical nonlinear characterisations of evoked responses in fMRI and other neurophysiological constraints.

BACKGROUND

This chapter is about modelling the relationship between neural activity and the BOLD (blood-oxygenation-level-dependent) fMRI signal. Before describing a comprehensive model that can account for the most important types of nonlinearity empirically observed from fMRI studies, it is worth briefly putting this work into context. Essentially, three things need to be modelled in order to understand the neural-BOLD relationship. We must be clear about which aspects of neural activity are of interest to us and also about which give rise to the signals we measure. We should clarify the nature and properties of the mechanisms relating this activity, through metabolic demand, to the blood supply to the tissue containing the neurons. Finally, we need a model of how these changes in blood supply affect the signal measured in the scanner.

That there is a connection between blood supply and brain activity has been established for more than 100 years. In their seminal paper, Roy and Sherrington (1890) concluded that functional activity increased blood flow and inferred that a coupling was present that generated increased blood flow in response to increased metabolic demand. Interestingly, their observation of the consequences of metabolic demand came before the demonstration of the increase in demand itself. It was more than 70 years later that the regional measurement of the metabolic changes was convincingly achieved using an autoradiographic technique. This used a substitute for glucose, called *deoxyglucose* (2DG) radioactively labelled with ^{14}C. 2DG enters the cells by same mechanism as glucose but is not metabolised and thus accumulates inside the cells at a rate that is dependent on their metabolic activity. By examining the density of labelled 2DG in brain slices, Kennedy and colleagues (1976) obtained functional maps of the activity during the period in which 2DG was injected. This activity period was generally around 45 min, which limited the time resolution of the technique. In addition, only one measurement per subject could be made since the technique involves the sacrifice of the animal (further developments allowed the injection of two tracers, but this was still very restrictive). However, the spatial resolution could be microscopic since the label is contained in the cells themselves rather than being limited to the blood vessels surrounding them. Through theoretical modelling of the enzyme kinetics for the uptake of 2DG and practical experiments, the relationships between neural function and glucose metabolism have been established and underpin the development of *metabolic encephalography.*

Positron emission tomography (PET) measures an intermediate stage in the chain linking neural activity via metabolism to the BOLD signal. By using a tracer such as ^{15}O-labeled water, one can measure changes in regional cerebral blood flow (rCBF) that accompany changes in neural activity. This was originally thought of as an autoradiographic technique, but has many advantages over 2DG and is clearly much less invasive, making it suitable for human studies. Also, substantially shorter times are required for measurements, typically well below a minute. As suggested above, the elucidation of the mechanisms underlying the coupling of neural activity and blood flow lags behind the exploitation of the phenomenon. There are several candidate signals including the diffusible second messengers such as nitric oxide or intravascular responses to changes in blood oxygenation level caused by changes in oxygen consumption, and this remains an active area of research independent of its consequences for models of functional brain imaging.

In the treatment below, we follow evidence from Miller *et al.* (2000), among others, and assume that blood flow and neural activity are linearly related over normal ranges. However, there are ongoing arguments about the nature of the linkage between neural activity, the rate of metabolism of oxygen, and cerebral blood flow. Some PET studies have suggested that while an increase in neural activity produces a proportionate increase in glucose metabolism and cerebral blood flow, oxygen consumption does not increase proportionately (Fox and Raichle, 1986). This decoupling between blood flow and oxidative metabolism is known as the *anaerobic brain hypothesis* by analogy with muscle physiology. Arguing against this position, other groups have adopted an even more radical interpretation. They suggest that immediately following neural stimulation, transient decoupling occurs between neural activity and blood flow (Vanzetta and Grinvald, 1999). By this argument, there is an immediate increase in oxidative metabolism, which produces a transient localised increase in deoxyhemoglobin. Only later do the mechanisms regulating blood flow kick in, causing the observed increase in rCBF and hence blood volume. Evidence for this position comes from optical imaging studies and depends on modelling the absorption and light-scattering properties of cortical tissue and the relevant chromophores, principally (de)oxyhemoglobin. Other groups have questioned these aspects of the work, and the issue remains controversial (Lindauer *et al.*, 2001). One possible consequence of this position is that better spatial resolution would be obtained by focusing on this early phase of the haemodynamic response.

As this chapter demonstrates, the situation is even more complicated with regard to fMRI using a BOLD contrast. The technique uses the amount of oxygen in the blood as a marker for neural activity, exploiting the fact that deoxyhemoglobin is less diamagnetic than oxyhemoglobin. The term *blood oxygenation level* refers to the *proportion* of oxygenated blood, but the signal depends on the total amount of deoxyhemoglobin and so the total volume of blood is a factor. Another factor is the change in the amount of oxygen leaving the blood to enter the tissue and meet changes in metabolic demand. Because the blood that flows into the capillary bed is fully oxygenated, changes in blood flow also change blood oxygenation level. Finally, the elasticity of the vascular tissue of the veins and venules means that an increase in blood flow causes an increase in blood volume. All of these factors are modelled and discussed in the body of the chapter. Of course, even more factors can be considered; for example, Zheng *et al.* (2002) have extended the treatment described here to include, among others, the dynamics of oxygen buffered in the tissue.

Notwithstanding these complications, it is a standard assumption that "the fMRI signal is approximately proportional to a measure of local neural activity" (reviewed in Heeger & Ress, 2002), and this linear model is still used in many studies, particularly where interstimulus intervals are more than a second or two. Empirical evidence against this hypothesis is outlined below, but note that there are now theoretical objections too. In particular, the models that have been developed to account for observed nonlinearities embody our best knowledge about the physiological mechanisms at work in the regulation of blood volume and oxygenation. Because they generate nonlinearities in BOLD response given reasonable choices for the parameters (discussed below), one might consider the genie to have been let out of the bottle.

The last link in the chain concerns the relation between a complete description of the relevant aspects of blood supply and the physics underlying the BOLD signal. Although this is not the principal focus of this chapter, a couple of simple points are worth emphasising. First, differently sized blood vessels will give different changes in BOLD signal for the same changes in blood flow, volume, and oxygenation. This is because of differences in the inhomogeneity of the magnetic fields in their vicinity. Secondly, and for partially related reasons, heuristic equations as employed in this and other models are dependent on the strength of the magnet. In particular, the equation used here may be relevant only for 1.5-T scanners, although other versions for different field strengths have been developed.

Finally a word about "neural activity." So far in the discussion we have deliberately not specified what type of neural activity we are considering. Here again, theoretical and practical issues arise. First it is worth remembering that different electrophysiological measures can emphasise different elements of neural firing (also see below). In particular, recording of multiple single units with an intracortical microelectrode can tend to sample action potentials from large pyramidal output neurons. Such studies are frequently referred to when characterising the response properties of a primate cortical area. However, consideration of the metabolic demands of various cellular processes suggests that spiking is not the major drain on the resources of a cell but rather that synaptic transmission and conductances of postsynaptic potentials as well as cytoskeletal turnover are the dominating forces. Of course, such processes are just as important, whether in interneurons and whether excitatory or inhibitory. An example of the difference between these two views of the cortex might be feedforward versus feedback activity in low-level visual cortex. Indeed BOLD fMRI experiments in humans have shown good agreement with studies of spiking in V1 in response to modulating the contrast of a visual stimulus, but attentional (top-down) modulation effects in V1 have proved elusive in monkey electrophysiological studies but robust with BOLD studies in humans. Aside from their neurobiological significance, such discrepancies must be born in mind when defining the neural activity to which the BOLD signal might be responding linearly.

A further subtlety relates to the modelled time course of the neural activity. Even in everyday analysis of functional imaging data, it is natural to separate the model of the response into neural and haemodynamic components. However, a typical set of spikes or block functions often used to model the neural activity will fail to capture adaptation and response transients, which are well known from the neurophysiological literature. (Note that a recent set of studies has deliberately exploited these effects; Grill-Spector and Malach, 2001). In the worst case, an elaborate model designed to capture nonlinearities in the BOLD response may inadvertently pick up such components of the neural response, and in any case careful stimulus design and modelling of neural responses is called for.

Recent studies using simultaneous fMRI and intracortical electrical recording in monkey have empirically validated many of the theoretical points considered above (Logothetis *et al.*, 2001). In particular, the closeness of the BOLD signal to LFP and MUA rather than spiking activity have been emphasised. These studies also demonstrated that the linear assumption can predict up to 90% of the variance in BOLD responses in some cortical regions. However, there was considerable variability in the accuracy of prediction, with nearby sites sometimes being substantially worse. Overall, substantial nonlinearities were observed between stimulus contrast, blood flow, and BOLD signals.

Having surveyed the general issues surrounding the coupling of neural activity and the BOLD signal, we now proceed to outline a specific and detailed model. This should be considered as a partial instantiation of current knowledge, and further extensions of this model have been proposed that incorporate new data. Mechelli (Chapter 30) also presents further empirical verification of the parameter regime proposed here. What follows is largely a reprise of Friston *et al.* (2000) and contains some advanced mathematical material

NONLINEAR EVOKED RESPONSES

We now focus on the nonlinear aspects of evoked responses in functional neuroimaging and present a dynamic approach to modelling and characterising event-related signals in fMRI. We aim to (1) show that the balloon/windkessel model (Buxton and Frank, 1997; Buxton *et al.,* 1998; Mandeville *et al.,* 1999) is sufficient to account for nonlinearities in event-related responses that are seen empirically and (2) describe a nonlinear dynamic model that couples changes in synaptic activity to fMRI signals. This haemodynamic model obtains by combining the balloon/windkessel model (henceforth, balloon model) with a model of how synaptic activity causes changes in regional flow.

In Friston *et al.* (1994) we presented a linear model of haemodynamic responses in fMRI time series, wherein underlying neuronal activity (inferred on the basis of changing stimulus or task conditions) is convolved or smoothed with a *haemodynamic response function*. In Friston *et al.* (1998) we extended this model to cover nonlinear responses using a Volterra series expansion. At the same time, Buxton and colleagues (1998) developed a mechanistically compelling model of how evoked changes in blood flow were transformed into a BOLD signal. A component of the balloon model, namely, the relationship between blood flow and volume, was then elaborated in the context of standard windkessel theory by Mandeville *et al.* (1999). The Volterra approach, in contradistinction to other nonlinear characterisations of haemodynamic responses (cf. Vazquez and Noll, 1996), is model independent in the sense that Volterra series can model the behaviour of any nonlinear time-invariant dynamic system.[1] The principal aim of this work was to see if the theoretically motivated balloon model would be sufficient to explain the nonlinearities embodied in a purely empirical Volterra characterisation.

Volterra Series

Volterra series express the output of a system, in this case the BOLD signal from a particular voxel, as a function of some input, here the assumed synaptic activity that is changed experimentally. This series is a function of the input over its recent history and is expressed in terms of generalised convolution kernels. Volterra series are often referred to as nonlinear convolutions or polynomial expansions with memory. They are simply Taylor expansions extended to cover dynamic input–state–output systems by considering the effect of the input now and at all times in the recent past. The zeroth-order kernel is simply a constant about which the response varies. The first-order kernel represents the weighting applied to a sum of inputs over the recent past (cf. the haemodynamic response function) and can be thought of as the change in output for a change in the input at each time point. Similarly, the second-order coefficients represent interactions that are simply the effect of the input at one point in time on its contribution at another. The second-order kernel comprises coefficients that are applied to interactions among (i.e., products of) inputs, at different times in the past, to predict the response.

[1] In principle, the Volterra series can represent any dynamic input–state–output system and in this sense a characterisation in terms of Volterra kernels is model independent. However, by using basis functions to constrain the solution space, constraints are imposed on the form of the kernels and, implicitly, the underlying dynamic system (i.e., state-space representation). The characterisation is therefore only assumption free to the extent the basis set is sufficiently comprehensive.

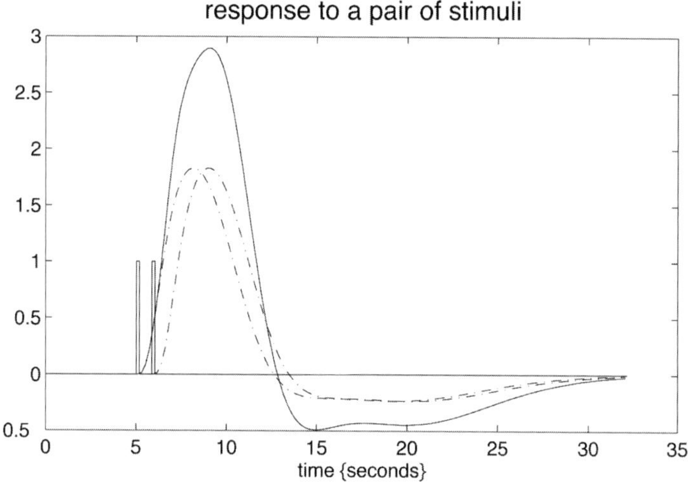

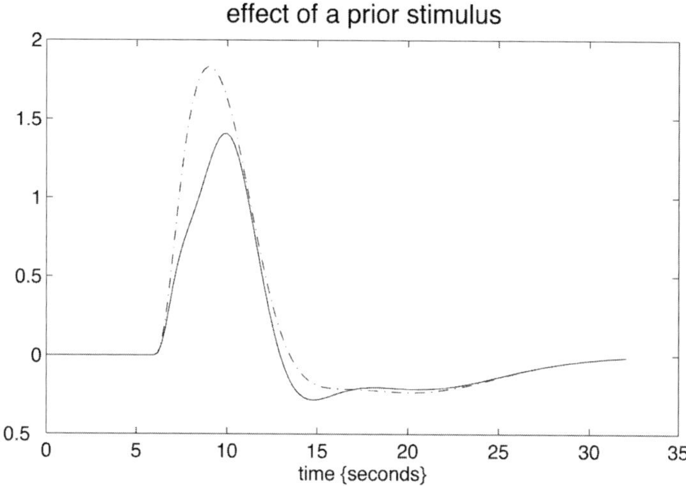

FIGURE 41.1
(Top) Simulated responses to a pair of words (bars) 1 sec apart, presented together (solid line) and separately (broken lines) based on the kernels shown in Fig. 41.4. (Lower) The response to the second word when presented alone (broken line as above) and when preceded by the first (solid line). The latter is obtained by subtracting the response to the first word from the response to both. The difference reflects the effect of the first word on the response to the second.

In short, the output can be considered a nonlinear convolution of the input where nonlinear behaviours are captured by high-order kernels. For example, the presence of a stimulus can be shown to attenuate the magnitude of, and induce a longer latency in, the response to a second stimulus that occurs within a second or so. The example shown in Fig. 41.1 comes from a previous analysis (Friston *et al.,* 1998) and shows how a preceding stimulus can modify the response to a subsequent stimulus. This sort of effect led to the notion of *haemodynamic refractoriness* and is an important example of nonlinearity in fMRI time series.

The important thing about Volterra series is that they do not refer to the hidden state variables that mediate between the input and output (e.g., blood flow, venous volume, oxygenation, the dynamics of endothelium-derived relaxing factor, kinetics of cerebral metabolism). This renders them very powerful because they provide for a complete specification of the dynamic behaviour of a system without ever having to measure the state variables or make any assumptions about how these variables interact to produce a response. On the other hand, the Volterra formulation is impoverished because it yields no mechanistic insight into how the response is mediated. The alternative is to posit some model of interacting state variables and establish the validity of that model in relation to observed input–output behaviours and the dynamics of the state variables themselves. This involves specifying a series of differential equations that express the change in one state variable as a function of the others and the input. Once these equations are specified, the equivalent Volterra representation can be derived analytically (see the Appendix for details). The balloon model is a comprehensive example of such a model.

Balloon Model

The balloon model (Buxton and Frank, 1997; Buxton *et al.,* 1998) is an input–state–output model with two state variables: volume (v) and deoxyhemoglobin content (q). The input to the system is blood flow (f_{in}) and the output is the BOLD signal (y). The BOLD signal is partitioned into extravascular and intravascular components, weighted by their respective volumes. These signal components depend on the deoxyhemoglobin content and render the signal a nonlinear function of v and q. The effect of flow on v and q (see below) determines the output, and it is these effects that are the essence of the balloon model: Increases in flow effectively inflate a venous "balloon" such that deoxygenated blood is diluted and expelled at a greater rate. The clearance of deoxyhemoglobin reduces intravoxel dephasing and engenders an increase in signal. Before the balloon has inflated sufficiently, the expulsion and dilution may be insufficient to counteract the increased delivery of deoxygenated blood to the venous compartment and an "early dip" in signal may be expressed. After the flow has peaked, and the balloon has relaxed again, reduced clearance and dilution contribute to the poststimulus undershoot commonly observed. This is a simple and plausible model that is predicated on a minimal set of assumptions and relates closely to the windkessel formulation of Mandeville *et al.* (1999). Furthermore, the predictions of the balloon model concur with the steady-state models of Hoge and colleagues, and their elegant studies of the relationship between blood flow and oxygen consumption in human visual cortex (e.g., Hoge *et al.,* 1999).

The balloon model is inherently nonlinear and may account for the sorts of nonlinear interactions revealed by the Volterra formulation. One simple test of this hypothesis is to see if the Volterra kernels associated with the balloon model compare with those derived empirically. The Volterra kernels estimated in Friston *et al.* (1998) clearly did not use flow as input because flow is not measurable with BOLD fMRI. The input comprised a stimulus function as an index of synaptic activity. To evaluate the balloon model in terms of these Volterra kernels, it has to be extended to accommodate the dynamics of how flow is coupled to synaptic activity encoded in the stimulus function. This chapter presents one such extension.

In summary, the balloon model deals with the link between flow and BOLD signal. By extending the model to cover the dynamic coupling of synaptic activity and flow, a complete model that relates experimentally induced changes in neuronal activity to BOLD signal is obtained. The input–output behaviour of this model can be compared to the real brain in terms of respective Volterra kernels.

The remainder of this chapter is divided into three sections. In the next section we present a haemodynamic model of the coupling between synaptic activity and BOLD response that builds on the balloon model. The second section presents an empirical evaluation of this model by comparing its Volterra kernels with those obtained using real fMRI data. This is not a trivial exercise because (1) there is no guarantee that the balloon model could produce the complicated forms of the kernels seen empirically and, (2) even if it could, the parameters needed to do so may be biologically implausible. This section provides estimates of these parameters, which allow some comment on the face validity of the model in relation to known physiology. The final section presents a discussion of the results in relation to known biophysics and neurophysiology.

This chapter is concerned with the validation and evaluation of the balloon model, in relation to the Volterra characterisations, and the haemodynamic model presented below in relation to real hemodynamics. Subsequent chapters will use the model to address some important issues related to Bayesian estimation of the parameters and the construction of dynamic causal models of brain responses (Chapters 47 and 53).

HAEMODYNAMIC MODEL

In this section we describe a haemodynamic model that mediates between synaptic activity and measured BOLD responses. This model essentially combines the balloon model and a simple

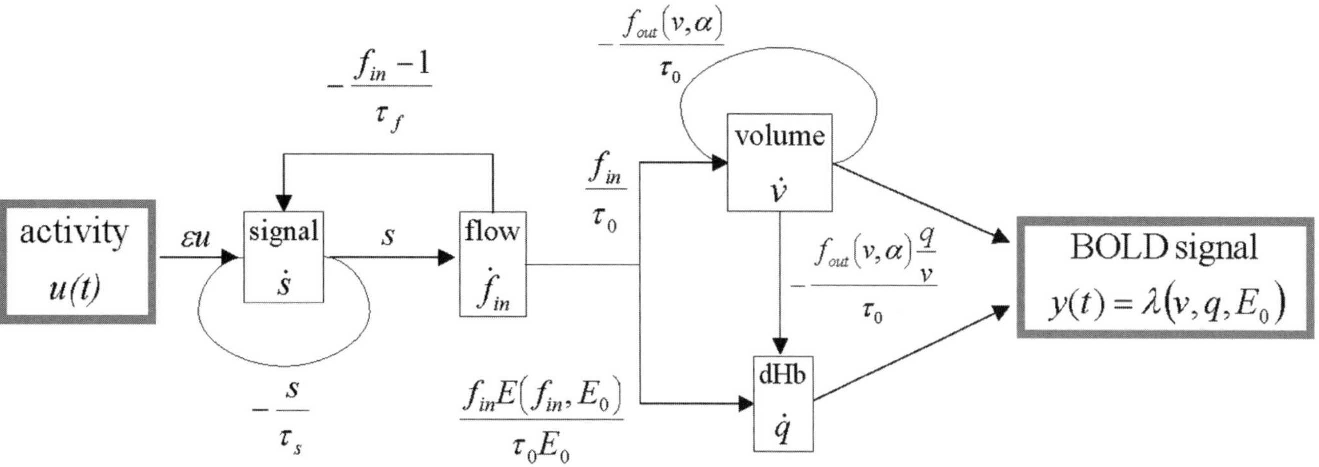

FIGURE 41.2
Schematic illustrating the organisation of the haemodynamic model. This is a fully nonlinear single input $u(t)$, single output $y(t)$ state model with four state variables s, f, v and q. The form and motivation for the changes in each state variable, as functions of the others, is described in the main text.

linear dynamic model of changes in rCBF caused by neuronal activity. The model architecture is summarised in Fig. 41.2. To motivate the model components more clearly, we will start at the output and work toward the input.

Balloon Component

This component links rCBF and the BOLD signal as described in Buxton *et al.* (1998). All variables are expressed in normalised form, relative to resting values. The BOLD signal $y(t) = \lambda(v,q,E_0)$ is taken to be a static nonlinear function of normalised venous volume (v), normalised total deoxyhemoglobin voxel content (q), and resting net oxygen extraction fraction by the capillary bed (E_0) :

$$\begin{aligned} y(t) &= \lambda(v, q, E_0) = V_0(k_1(1-q) + k_2(1-q/v) + k_3(1-v)) \\ k_1 &= 7E_0 \\ k_2 &= 2 \\ k_3 &= 2E_0 - 0.2 \end{aligned} \tag{41.1}$$

where V_0 is resting blood volume fraction. This signal comprises a volume-weighted sum of extravascular and intravascular signals that are functions of volume and deoxyhemoglobin content. The latter are the state variables whose dynamics need specifying. The rate of change of volume is simply

$$\tau_0 \dot{v} = f_{in} - f_{out}(v) \tag{41.2}$$

Mandeville *et al.* (1999) provide an excellent discussion of this equation in relation to windkessel theory. Eq. (41.2) says that volume changes reflect the difference between inflow f_{in} and outflow f_{out} from the venous compartment with a time constant τ_0. This constant represents the mean transit time (i.e., the average time it takes to traverse the venous compartment or for that compartment to be replenished) and is V_0/F_0 where F_0 is resting flow. The physiology of the relationship between flow and volume is determined by the evolution of the transit time. Mandeville *et al.* (1999) reformulated the temporal evolution of transit time into a description of the dynamics of resistance and capacitance of the balloon using windkessel theory (*windkessel* means "leather bag"). This enabled them to posit a form for the temporal evolution of a downstream elastic response to arteriolar vasomotor changes and estimate mean transit times using measurements of volume and flow, in rats, using fMRI and laser Doppler flowmetry. We compare these estimates to our empirical estimates in the next section.

Note that outflow is a function of volume. This function models the balloon-like capacity of the venous compartment to expel blood at a greater rate when distended. We model it with a single parameter based on the windkessel model:

$$f_{\text{out}}(v) = v^{1/\alpha} \tag{41.3}$$

where $1/\alpha = \gamma + \beta$ [cf. Eq. (6) in Mandeville *et al.,* 1999], $\gamma = 2$ represents laminar flow, and $\beta > 1$ models diminished volume reserve at high pressures and can be thought of as the ratio of the balloon's capacitance to its compliance. At steady state, empirical results from PET suggest $\alpha \approx 0.38$ (Grubb *et al.,* 1974). However, when flow and volume are changing dynamically, this value is smaller. Mandeville *et al.* (1999) were the first to measure the dynamic flow-volume relationship and estimated $\alpha \approx 0.18$, after 6 sec of stimulation, with a projected asymptotic steady-state value of 0.36.

The change in deoxyhemoglobin $\dot{q}$ reflects the delivery of deoxyhemoglobin into the venous compartment minus that expelled (outflow times concentration):

$$\tau_0 \dot{q} = f_{in} \frac{E(f_{in}, E_0)}{E_0} - f_{out}(v) q/v \tag{41.4}$$

where $E(f_{in}, E_0)$ is the fraction of oxygen extracted from the inflowing blood. This is assumed to depend on oxygen delivery and is consequently flow dependent. A reasonable approximation for a wide range of transport conditions is (Buxton *et al.,* 1998) as follows:

$$E(f_{in}, E_0) = 1 - (1 - E_0)^{1/f_{in}} \tag{41.5}$$

The second term in Eq. (41.4) represents an important nonlinearity: The effect of flow on signal is largely determined by the inflation of the balloon, resulting in an increase of $f_{\text{out}}(v)$ and clearance of deoxyhemoglobin. This effect depends on the concentration of deoxyhemoglobin such that the clearance attained by the outflow will be severely attenuated when the concentration is low (e.g., during the peak response to a prior stimulus). The implications of this will be illustrated in the next section.

This concludes the balloon model component, where there are only three unknown parameters that determine the dynamics: E_0, τ_0 and α, namely, resting oxygen extraction fraction (E_0), mean transit time (τ_0), and a stiffness exponent (α) specifying the flow-volume relationship of the venous balloon. The only thing required, to specify the BOLD response, is inflow.

rCBF Component

It is generally accepted that, over normal ranges, blood flow and synaptic activity are linearly related. A recent empirical verification of this assumption can be found in Miller *et al.* (2000) who used MRI perfusion imaging to address this issue in visual and motor cortices. After modelling neuronal adaptation, they were able to conclude that "Both rCBF responses are consistent with a linear transformation of a simple nonlinear neural response model." Furthermore, our own work using PET and fMRI replications of the same experiments suggests that the observed nonlinearities enter into the translation of rCBF into a BOLD response, as opposed to a nonlinear relationship between synaptic activity and rCBF, in the auditory cortices (see Friston *et al.,* 1998). Under the constraint that the dynamic system linking synaptic activity and rCBF is linear we have chosen the most parsimonious model:

$$\dot{f}_{in} = s \tag{41.6}$$

where s is some flow-inducing signal defined, operationally, in units corresponding to the rate of change of normalised flow (i.e., sec^{-1}). Although it may seem more natural to express the effect of this signal directly on vascular resistance (r), for example, $\dot{r} = -s$ Eq. (41.6) has the more plausible form. This is because the effect of signal (s) is much smaller when r is small. (When the arterioles are fully dilated, signals such as endothelium-derived relaxing factor or nitric oxide will cause relatively small decrements in resistance.) This can be seen by noting that Eq. (41.6) is equivalent to $\dot{r} = -r^2 s$, where $f_{in} = 1/r$.

The signal is assumed to subsume many neurogenic and diffusive signal subcomponents and is generated by neuronal activity $u(t)$:

$$\dot{s} = \varepsilon u(t) - s/\tau_s - (f_{in} - 1)/\tau_f \tag{41.7}$$

where ε, τ_s and τ_f are the three unknown parameters that determine the dynamics of this component of the haemodynamic model. They represent the efficacy with which neuronal activity causes an increase in signal, the time constant for signal decay or elimination, and the time constant for autoregulatory feedback from blood flow. The existence of this feedback term can be inferred from (1) poststimulus undershoots in rCBF (e.g., Irikura *et al.*, 1994) and (2) the well-characterised vasomotor signal in optical imaging (Mayhew *et al.*, 1998). The critical aspect of the latter oscillatory (~0.1 Hz) component of intrinsic signals is that it shows variable phase relationships from region to region, supporting strongly the notion of local closed-loop feedback mechanisms as modelled in Eqs. (41.6) and (41.7).

Each of the two components of the haemodynamic model above has three unknown components (see also Fig. 41.2 for a schematic summary). Figure 41.3 illustrates the behaviour of the haemodynamic model for typical values of the six parameters ($\varepsilon = 0.5$, $\tau_s = 0.8$, $\tau_f = 0.4$, $\tau_0 = 1$, $\alpha = 0.2$, $E_0 = 0.8$ and assuming $V_0 = 0.02$ here and throughout). We have used a very high value for oxygen extraction to accentuate the early dip (see discussion). Following a short-lived neuronal transient, a substantial amount of signal is created and starts to decay immediately. This signal induces an increase in flow that itself augments signal decay, to the extent the signal is suppressed below resting levels (see the upper left panel in Fig. 41.3). This behaviour is homologous to a very dampened oscillator. Increases in flow (lower left panel) dilate the venous balloon, which responds by ejecting deoxyhemoglobin. In the first few hundred milliseconds, the net deoxyhemoglobin (q) increases with an accelerating inflow-dependent delivery. It is then cleared by volume-dependent outflow expressing a negative peak a second or so after the positive volume (v) peak (the broken and solid lines in the upper right panel correspond to q and v, respectively). This results in an early dip in the BOLD signal followed by a pronounced positive peak at about 4 sec (lower right panel) that reflects the combined effects of reduced net deoxyhemoglobin, increased venous volume, and consequent dilution of deoxyhemoglobin. Note that the rise and peak in volume (solid line in the upper right panel) lags flow by about a second. This is very similar to the predictions of the windkessel formulation and the empirical results presented in Mandeville *et al.* (1999) (see their Fig. 41.2). After about 8 sec the inflow experiences a rebound due to its suppression of the perfusion signal. The reduced venous volume and ensuing outflow permit a reaccumulation of deoxyhemoglobin and a consequent undershoot in the BOLD signal.

The rCBF component of the haemodynamic model is a linear dynamic system and as such has only zeroth- and first-order kernels. This means it *cannot* account for the haemodynamic refractoriness and nonlinearities observed in BOLD responses. Although the rCBF component may facilitate the balloon component's capacity to model nonlinearities (by providing appropriate input), the rCBF component alone cannot generate second-order kernels. The question addressed in this chapter is whether the balloon component can produce second-order kernels that are realistic and do so with physiologically plausible parameters.

MODEL PARAMETER ESTIMATION

In this section we describe the data used to estimate Volterra kernels. The six unknown parameters of the haemodynamic model that best reproduce these empirical kernels are then identified. By minimising the difference between the model kernels and the empirical kernels, the optimal parameters for any voxel can be determined. The critical questions this section addresses are as follows: (1) Can the haemodynamic model account for the form of empirical kernels up to second order? and (2) Are the model parameters required to do this physiologically plausible?

Empirical Analyses

The data and Volterra kernel estimation are described in detail in Friston *et al.* (1998). In brief we obtained fMRI time series from a single subject at 2 T using a Magnetom VISION (by Siemens, Erlangen) whole body MRI system, equipped with a head volume coil. Contiguous

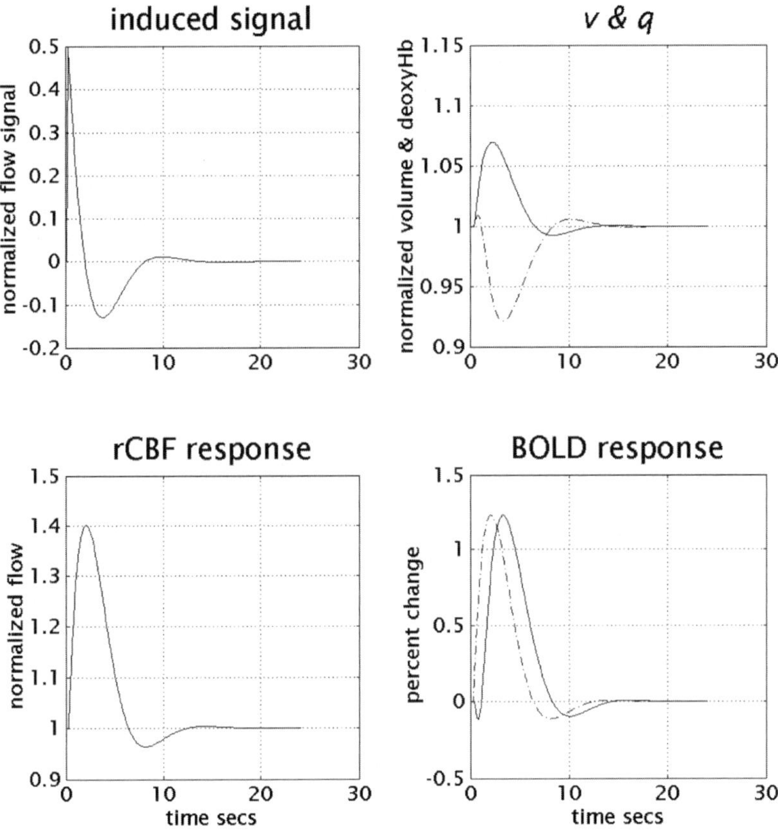

FIGURE 41.3
Dynamics of the haemodynamic model. (Upper left) The time-dependent changes in the neuronally induced perfusion signal that causes an increase in blood flow. (Lower left) The resulting changes in normalised blood flow (f). (Upper right) The concomitant changes in normalised venous volume (v) (solid line) and normalised deoxyhemoglobin content (q) (broken line). (Lower right) The percent change in BOLD signal that is contingent on v and q. The broken line is inflow normalised to the same maximum as the BOLD signal. This highlights the fact that BOLD signal lags the rCBF signal by about a second.

multislice T_2*-weighted fMRI images were obtained with a gradient echoplanar sequence using an axial slice orientation (TE = 40 ms, TR = 1.7 sec, $64 \times 64 \times 16$ voxels). After discarding initial scans (to allow for magnetic saturation effects), each time series comprised 1200 volume images with 3-mm isotropic voxels. The subject listened to monosyllabic or bisyllabic concrete nouns (i.e., *dog, mountain, gate*) presented at five different rates (10, 15, 30, 60, and 90 words per minute) for epochs of 34 sec, intercalated with periods of rest. The five presentation rates were successively repeated according to a Latin square design.

The data were processed within SPM (Wellcome Department of Cognitive Neurology, http://www.fil.ion.ucl.ac.uk/spm). The time series were realigned, corrected for movement-related effects, and spatially normalised into the standard space of Talairach and Tournoux (1988). The data were smoothed spatially with a 5-mm isotropic Gaussian kernel. Volterra kernels were estimated by expanding the kernels in terms of temporal basis functions and estimating the kernel coefficients up to second order using a generalised linear model (Worsley and Friston, 1995). The basis set comprised three gamma varieties of increasing dispersion and their temporal derivatives (as described in Friston *et al.,* 1998).

The stimulus function $u(t)$, the supposed neuronal activity, was simply the word presentation rate at which the scan was acquired. We selected voxels that showed a robust response to stimulation from two superior temporal regions in both hemispheres (see Fig. 41.4). These were the 128 voxels showing the most significant response when testing for the null hypothesis that the first- and second-order kernels were jointly zero. Selecting these voxels ensured that the kernel estimates had minimal variance.

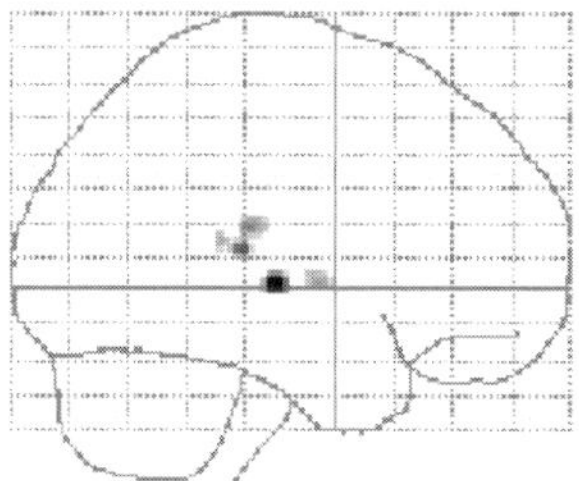
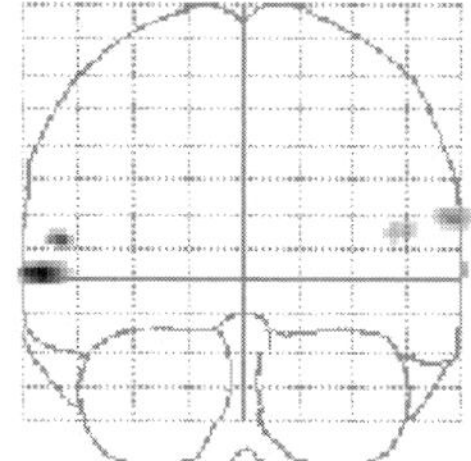
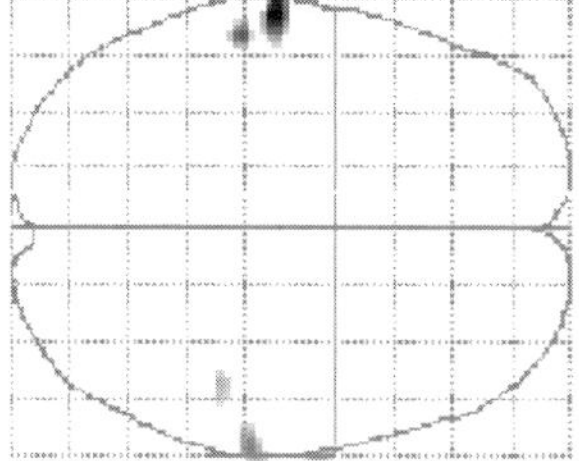

FIGURE 41.4
Voxels used to estimate the parameters of the haemodynamic model shown in Fig. 41.2. This is an SPM{F} testing for the significance of the first- and second-order kernel coefficients in the empirical analysis and represents a maximum intensity projection of a statistical process of the F ratio, following a multiple regression analysis at each voxel. This regression analysis estimated the kernel coefficients after expanding them in terms of a small number of temporal basis functions (see Friston *et al.*, 1998, for details). The format is standard and provides three orthogonal projections in the standard space conforming to that described in Talairach and Tournoux (1988). The gray scale is arbitrary and the SPM{F} has been thresholded to show the 128 most significant voxels.

Estimating the Model Parameters

For each voxel we identified the six parameters of the haemodynamic model of the previous section whose kernels corresponded, in a least-squares sense, to the empirical kernels for that voxel. To do this, we used nonlinear function minimisation as implemented in MATLAB5 (MathWorks Inc., Massachusetts). The model's kernels were computed, for a given parameter vector, as described in the Appendix and entered, with the corresponding empirical estimates, into the objective function that was minimised.

Results

The model-based and empirical kernels for the first voxel are shown in Fig. 41.5. Remarkable agreement is seen in terms of both the first- and second-order kernels. This is important because it suggests that the nonlinearities inherent in the balloon component of the haemodynamic model are sufficient to account for the nonlinear responses observed in real time series. The first-order kernel corresponds to the conventional (first-order) haemodynamic response function and shows the characteristic peak at about 4 sec and the poststimulus undershoot. The empirical undershoot appears more protracted than the model's prediction, suggesting that the model is not perfect in every respect. The second-order kernel has a pronounced negativity on the upper left, flanked by two smaller positivities. This negativity accounts for the refractoriness seen when two stimuli are temporally proximate, where this proximity is defined by the radius of the negative region. From the perspective of the balloon model, the second stimulus is compromised, in terms of elaborating a BOLD signal, because of the venous pooling, and consequent dilution of deoxyhemoglobin, incurred by the first stimulus. This means that less deoxyhemoglobin can be cleared for a given increase in flow. More interesting are the positive regions, which suggest that stimuli separated by about 8 sec should show superadditive effects. This can be attributed to the fact that, during the flow undershoot following the first stimulus, deoxyhemoglobin concentration is greater than normal (see the upper right panel in Fig. 41.3), thereby facilitating clearance of deoxyhemoglobin following the second stimulus.

Figure 41.6 shows the various functions implied by the haemodynamic model parameters averaged over all voxels. These include outflow as a function of venous volume $f_{out}(v,\alpha)$ and

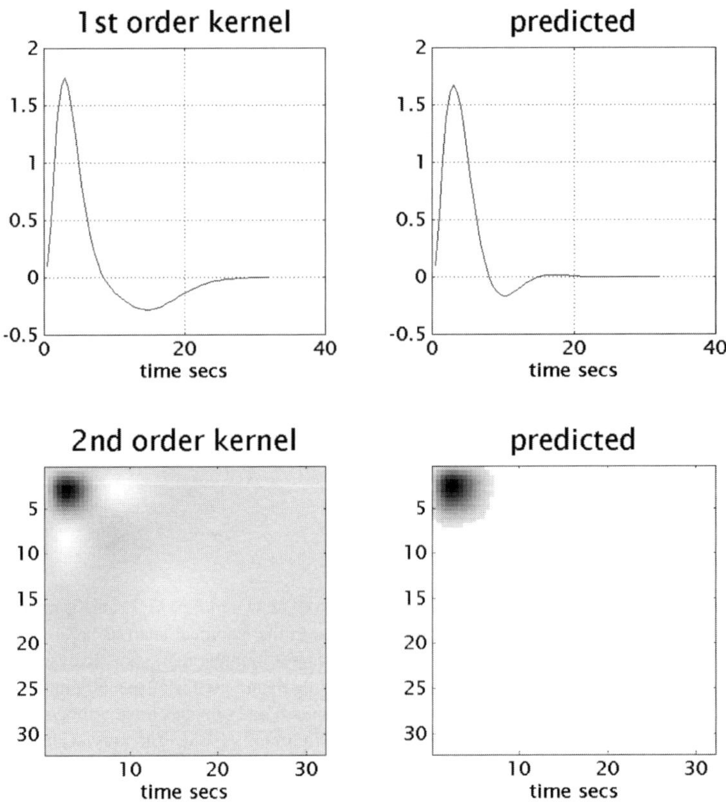

FIGURE 41.5
The first- and second-order Volterra kernels based on parameter estimates from a voxel in the left superior temporal gyrus at −56, −28, and 12 mm. These kernels can be thought of as a second-order haemodynamic response function. The first-order kernels (upper panels) represent the first-order component usually presented in linear analyses. The second-order kernels (lower panels) are presented in image format. The color scale is arbitrary; white is positive and black is negative. The left-hand panels are kernels based on parameter estimates from the analysis described in Fig. 41.4. The right-hand panels are the kernels associated with the haemodynamic model using parameter estimates that best match the empirical kernels.

oxygen extraction fraction as a function of inflow. The solid line in the upper right panel is extraction per se $E(f_{in}, E_0)$ and the broken line is the net normalised delivery of deoxyhemoglobin to the venous compartment $f_{in}E(f_{in}, E_0)/E_0$. Note that although the fraction of oxygen extracted decreases with flow, the net delivery of deoxygenated hemoglobin increases with flow. In other words, inflow increases per se actually reduce signal. It is only the secondary effects of inflow on dilution and volume-dependent outflow that cause an increase in BOLD signal. The lower panel depicts the nonlinear function of volume and deoxyhemoglobin that represents BOLD signal $y(t) = \lambda(v,q,E_0)$. Here one observes that positive BOLD signals are expressed only when deoxyhemoglobin is low. The effect of volume is much less marked and tends to affect signal predominantly through dilution. This is consistent with the fact that $k_2 > k_3$ [see Eq. (41.1)] for the value of E_0 estimated for these data.

The distributions of the parameters over voxels are shown in Fig. 41.7 with their mean in brackets at the top of each panel. Note that the data from which these estimates came were not independent. However, given they came from four different brain regions they are remarkably consistent. In the next section, we discuss each of these parameters and the effect it exerts on the BOLD response.

DISCUSSION

The main point to be made here is that the balloon model, suitably extended to incorporate the dynamics of rCBF induction by synaptic activity, is sufficient to reproduce the same form of Volterra kernels seen empirically. As such, the balloon model is sufficient to account for the more

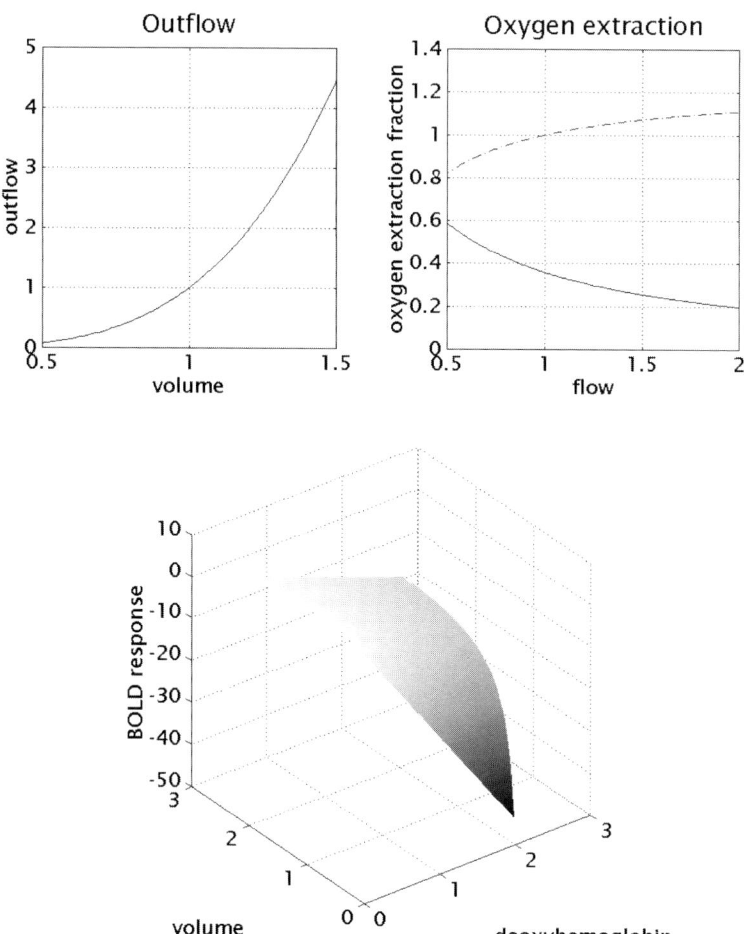

FIGURE 41.6
Functions implied by the mean haemodynamic model parameters over the voxels shown in Fig. 41.4. (Upper left) Outflow as a function of venous volume $f_{out}(v, a)$. (Upper right) Oxygen extraction as a function of inflow. The solid line is extraction per se $E(f_{in}, E_0)$ and the broken line is the net normalised delivery of deoxyhemoglobin to the venous compartment $f_{in}E(f_{in}, E_0)/E_0$. (Lower) This is a plot of the nonlinear function of volume and deoxyhemoglobin that represents BOLD signal $y(t) = l\ (v, q, E_0)$.

important nonlinearities observed in evoked fMRI responses. The remainder of this section deals with the validity of the haemodynamic model in terms of the plausibility of the parameter estimates from the previous section. The role of each parameter in shaping the haemodynamic response is illustrated in the associated panel in Fig. 41.8 and is discussed in the following subsections.

Neuronal Efficacy (ε)

Neuronal efficacy represents the increase in perfusion signal elicited by neuronal activity, expressed in terms of event density (i.e., number of evoked transients per second). From a biophysical perspective, it is not exceedingly interesting because it reflects both the potency of the stimulus in eliciting a neuronal response and the efficacy of the ensuing synaptic activity to induce the signal. It is interesting to note, however, that one word per second invokes an increase in normalised rCBF of unity (i.e., in the absence of regulatory effects, a doubling of blood flow over a second). As might be expected changes in this parameter simply modulate the evoked haemodynamic responses (see the first panel in Fig. 41.8).

Signal Decay (τ_s)

This parameter reflects signal decay or elimination. Transduction of neuronal activity into perfusion changes, over a few 100 microns, has a substantial neurogenic component (that may

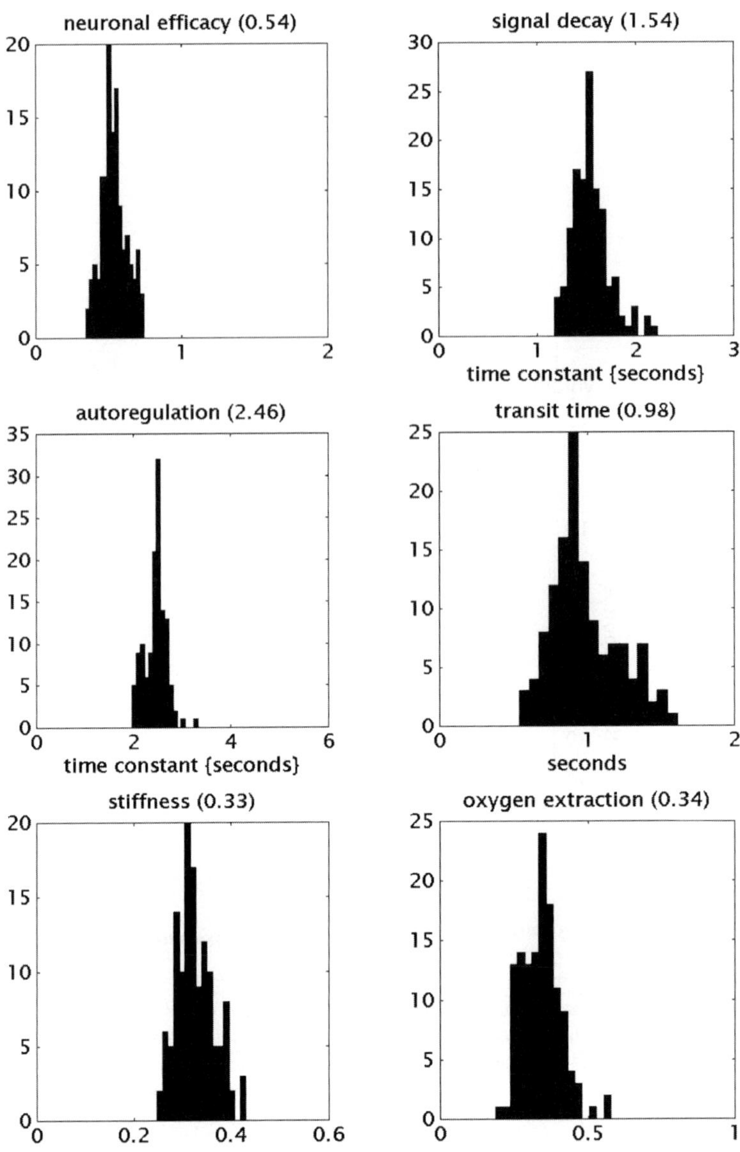

FIGURE 41.7
Histograms of the distribution of the six free parameters of the haemodynamic model estimated over the voxels shown in Fig. 41.3. The number in brackets at the top of each histogram is the mean value for the parameters in question: neuronal efficacy is ε, signal decay is τ_s, autoregulation is τ_f, transit time is τ_0, stiffness is α, and oxygen extraction is E_0.

be augmented by electrical conduction up the vascular endothelium). However, at spatial scales of several millimeters it is likely that rapidly diffusing spatial signals mediate increases in rCBF through relaxation of arteriolar smooth muscle. There are a number of candidates for this signal, nitric oxide (NO) being the primary one. It has been shown that the rate of elimination is critical in determining the effective time constants of haemodynamic transduction (Friston, 1995). Our decay parameter had a mean of about 1.54 sec giving a half-life $t_{1/2} = \tau_s \ln 2 = 1067$ ms. The half-life of NO is between 100 and 1000 ms (Paulson and Newman, 1987), whereas that of K^+ is about 5 sec. Our results are therefore consistent with spatial signalling with NO. Remember that the model signal subsumes all actual signalling mechanisms employed in the real brain. Increases in this parameter dampen the rCBF response to any input and will also suppress the undershoot (see next subsection) because the feedback mechanisms, which are largely responsible for the undershoot, are selectively suppressed (relative to just reducing neuronal efficacy during signal induction).

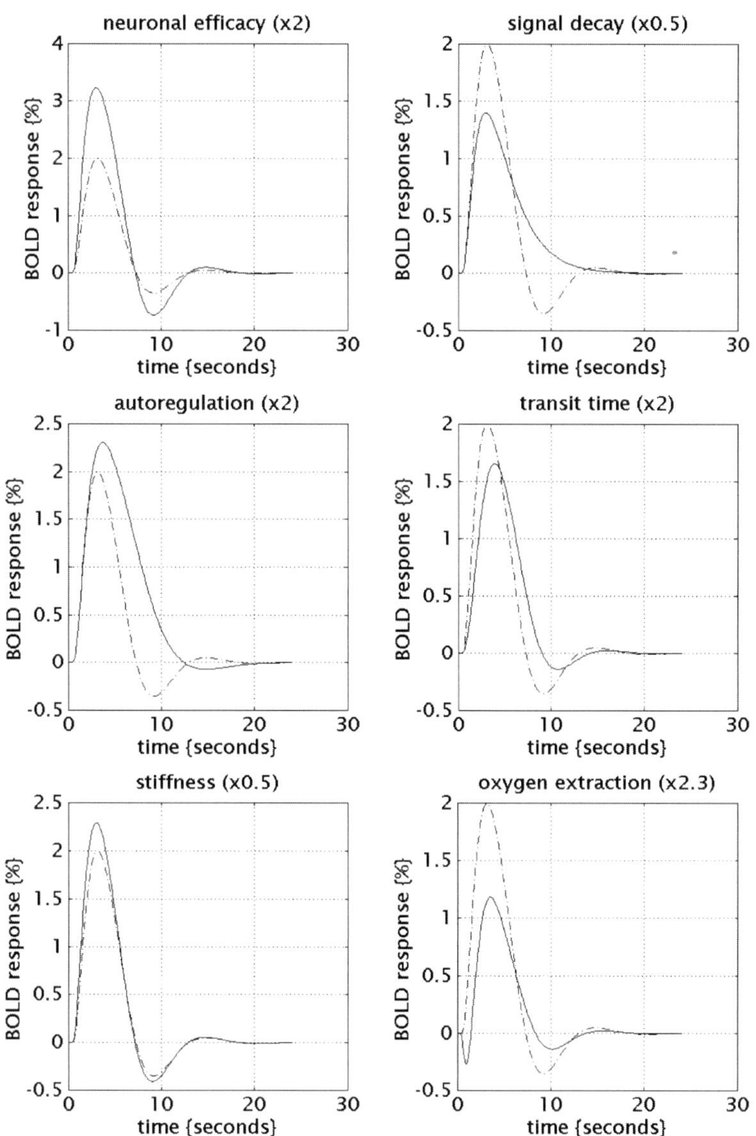

FIGURE 41.8
The effects of changing the model parameters on the evoked BOLD response. The number in brackets at the top of each graph is the factor applied to the parameter in question. Solid lines correspond to the response after changing the parameter and broken lines represent the response for the original parameter values (the mean values given in Fig. 41.7): neuronal efficacy is ε, signal decay is τ_s, autoregulation is τ_f, transit time is τ_0, stiffness is α, and oxygen extraction is E_0.

Autoregulation (τ_f)

This parameter is the time constant of the feedback autoregulatory mechanism whose physiological nature remains unspecified (but see Irikura *et al.,* 1994). The coupled differential equations [Eqs. (41.6) and (41.7)] represent a damped oscillator with a resonance frequency of $\omega = 1/(2\pi \quad \tau_f) \approx 0.101$ per second. This is exactly the frequency of the vasomotor signal that typically has a period of about 10 sec. This is a pleasing result that emerges spontaneously from the parameter estimation. The nature of these oscillations can be revealed by increasing the signal decay time constant (i.e., reducing the dampening) and presenting the model with low-level random neuronal input (uncorrelated Gaussian noise with a standard deviation of 1/64) as shown in Fig. 41.9. The characteristic oscillatory dynamics are readily expressed. The effect of increasing the feedback time constant is to decrease the resonance frequency and render the BOLD (and rCBF) response more enduring with a reduction or elimination of the undershoot. The third panel in Fig. 41.8 shows the effect of doubling τ_f.

Transit Time (τ_0)

This is an important parameter that determines the dynamics of the signal. It is effectively resting venous volume divided by resting flow, and in our data is estimated at 0.98 sec. The transit time through the rat brain is roughly 1.4 sec at rest and, according to the asymptotic projections for rCBF and volume, falls to 0.73 sec during stimulation (Mandeville *et al.*, 1999). In other words, it takes about a second for a blood cell to traverse the venous compartment. The effect of increasing mean transit time is to slow down the dynamics of the BOLD signal with respect to the flow changes. The shape of the response remains the same, but it is expressed more slowly. In the fourth panel of Fig. 41.8, a doubling of the mean transit time is seen to retard the peak BOLD response by about 1 sec and the undershoot by about 2 sec.

Stiffness Parameter (α)

Under steady-state conditions this would be about 0.38. The mean over voxels considered above was about 0.33. This discrepancy, in relation to steady-state levels, is anticipated by the windkessel formulation and is attributable to the fact that volume and flow are in a state of continuous flux during the evoked responses. Recall from Eq. (41.3) that $1/\alpha = \gamma + \beta = 3.03$ in our data. Under the assumption of laminar flow ($\gamma = 2$), $\beta \approx 1$, which is less than that found by Mandeville *et al.* (1999) for rats during forepaw stimulation but is certainly in a plausible range. Increasing this parameter increases the degree of nonlinearity in the flow-volume behaviour of the venous balloon that underpins the nonlinear behaviours for which we are trying to account. However, its direct effect on evoked responses to single stimuli is not very marked. The fifth panel of Fig. 41.8 shows the effects when α is decreased by 50%.

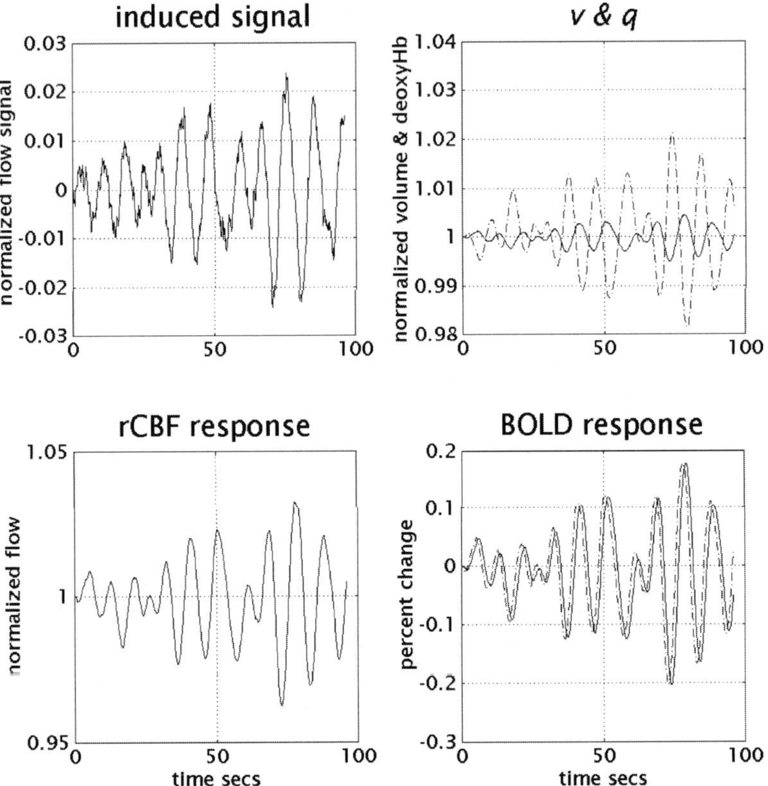

FIGURE 41.9
Simulated response to a noisy neuronal input (standard deviation 1/64 and mean of 0) for a model with decreased signal decay (i.e., less dampening). The model parameters were the same as those used in the Fig. 41.3 with the exception of τ_s, which was increased by a factor of 4. The characteristic 0.1-Hz oscillations are very similar to the oscillatory vasomotor signal seen in optical imaging experiments.

Resting Oxygen Extraction (E_0)

This is about 34% and the range observed in our data fits exactly with known values for resting oxygen extraction fraction (between 20% and 55%). Oxygen extraction fraction is a potentially important factor in determining the nature of evoked fMRI responses because it may be sensitive to the nature of the baseline that defines the resting state. Increases in this parameter can have quite profound effects on the shape of the response that bias it toward an early dip. In the example shown (last panel in Fig. 41.8), the resting extraction has been increased to 78%. This is a potentially important observation that may explain why the initial dip has been difficult to observe in all studies. According to the results presented in Fig. 41.8, the initial dip is very sensitive to resting oxygen extraction fraction, which should be high before the dip is expressed. Extraction fraction will be high in regions with very low blood flow or in tissue with endogenously high extraction. It may be that cytochrome oxidase rich cortex, like the visual cortices, may have a higher fraction and be more likely to evidence early dips.

In summary, the parameters of the haemodynamic model that best reproduce empirically derived Volterra kernels are all biologically plausible and lend the model a construct validity (in relation to the Volterra formulation) and face validity (in relation to other physiological characterisations of the cerebral haemodynamic reviewed in this section). In this extended haemodynamic model, nonlinearities inherent in the balloon model have been related directly to nonlinearities in responses. Their role in mediating the poststimulus undershoot is emphasised less here because the rCBF component can model undershoots.

The conclusions above are based only on data from the auditory cortex and from one subject. There is no guarantee that they will generalise. When submitted in paper form, one of our reviewers thought that it was more important for its conceptual motivation of modelling than for the specific findings. This is a very valid point. We anticipate that the framework presented here will be refined or changed when applied to other data, or the assumptions on which it is based are confirmed or refuted.

CONCLUSION

In conclusion, we have developed an input–state–output model of the haemodynamic response to changes in synaptic activity that combines the balloon model of flow to BOLD signal coupling and a dynamic model of the transduction of neuronal activity into perfusion changes. This model has been characterised in terms of its Volterra kernels and easily reproduces empirical kernels with parameters that are biologically plausible. This means that the nonlinearities inherent in the balloon model are sufficient to account for haemodynamic refractoriness and other nonlinear aspects of evoked responses in fMRI.

APPENDIX

Volterra kernels represent a generic and important characterisation of the invariant aspects of a nonlinear system (see Bendat, 1990). This appendix describes the nature of these kernels and how they are obtained given the differential equations describing the evolution of the state variables. Consider the following single input–single output (SISO) system:

$$\begin{aligned}\dot{X}(t) &= f(X, u(t)) \\ y(t) &= \lambda(X(t))\end{aligned} \tag{41.8}$$

where, for the haemodynamic model, $X = \{x_1, x_2, x_3, x_4\}^T = \{s, f_{in}, v, q\}^T$ with

$$\begin{aligned}
\dot{x}_1 &= f_1(X, u(t)) = \varepsilon u(t) - \frac{x_1}{\tau_s} - \frac{x_2 - 1}{\tau_f} \\
\dot{x}_2 &= f_2(X, u(t)) = x_1 \\
\dot{x}_3 &= f_3(X, u(t)) = \frac{1}{\tau_0}\,(x_2 - f_{out}\,(x_3, \alpha)) \\
\dot{x}_4 &= f_4(X, u(t)) = \frac{1}{\tau_0}\left(x_2\,\frac{E(x_2, E_0)}{E_0} - f_{out}\,(x_3, \alpha)\frac{x_4}{x_3}\right)
\end{aligned}$$

and $y(t) = \lambda(X(t)) = V_0(k_1(1 - x_4) + k_2(1 - x_4/x_3) + k_3(1 - x_3))$

The Volterra series expresses the output $y(t)$ as a nonlinear convolution of the neuronal inputs $u(t)$, critically without reference to the state variables $X(t)$. This series can be considered a nonlinear convolution that obtains from a functional Taylor expansion of $y(t)$ about $X(0) = X_0 = [0, 1, 1, 1]^T$ and $u(t) = 0$:

$$y(t) = \kappa_0(t) + \sum_{i=1}^{\infty} \int_0^t \ldots \int_0^t \kappa_i(t, \sigma_1, \ldots \sigma_i) u(\sigma_1) \ldots u(\sigma_i) d\sigma_1 \ldots d\sigma_i$$
$$\kappa_i(t, \sigma_1, \ldots \sigma_i) = \frac{\partial^i y(t)}{\partial u(\sigma_1) \ldots u(\sigma_i)} \tag{41.9}$$

where κ_i is the ith, generally time-dependent, kernel. The Taylor expansion of $\dot{X}(t)$ about X_0 and $u(t) = 0$:

$$\dot{X}(t) \approx f(X_0,0) + \frac{\partial f(X_0,0)}{\partial X}(X - X_0) + \frac{\partial^2 f(X_0,0)}{\partial X \partial u}(X - X_0)u + \frac{\partial f(X_0,0)}{\partial u}u$$

has a bilinear form following a change of variables [equivalent to adding an extra state variable $x_0(t) = 1$]:

$$\dot{X}'(t) \approx AX' + BX'u$$
$$X' = \begin{bmatrix} 1 \\ X \end{bmatrix}$$
$$A = \begin{bmatrix} 0 & 0 \\ \left(f(X_0,0) - \frac{\partial f(X_0,0)}{\partial X} X_0\right) & \frac{\partial f(X_0,0)}{\partial X} \end{bmatrix} \tag{41.10}$$
$$B = \begin{bmatrix} 0 & 0 \\ \left(\frac{\partial f(X_0,0)}{\partial u} - \frac{\partial^2 f(X_0,0)}{\partial X \partial u} X_0\right) & \frac{\partial^2 f(X_0,0)}{\partial X \partial u} \end{bmatrix}$$

This formulation is important because the Volterra kernels of bilinear systems have closed-form expressions. The existence of these closed-form expressions is due to the fact that the iterated integrals associated with the system's generating series can be expressed in terms of the generalised convolution integrals, of which the Volterra series is comprised (Fliess *et al.*, 1983). Here we take a more heuristic approach and consider the solution to Eq. (41.9) and its derivatives with respect to the inputs $u(t)$:

$$X'(\Delta t) \approx e^{\Delta t(A+Bu(0))} X'(0) \Rightarrow X'(T\Delta t) \approx \prod_{j=T-1}^{0} e^{\Delta t(A+Bu(j\Delta t))} X'(0), \quad \Delta t \to 0$$

$$\frac{\partial^i X'(T\Delta t)}{\partial u(\tau_1 \Delta t) \ldots u(\tau_i \Delta t)} = \prod_{j=T-1}^{\tau_i+1} e^{\Delta t(A+Bu(j\Delta t))} B \prod_{j=\tau_i}^{\tau_{i-1}+1} e^{\Delta t(A+Bu(j\Delta t))} \ldots B \prod_{j=\tau_1}^{0} e^{\Delta t(A+Bu(j\Delta t))} X'(0),$$

The kernels associated with the state variables X' are these derivatives evaluated at $u(t) = 0$

$$\chi_i(t, \sigma_1, \ldots \sigma_i) = \frac{\partial^i X'(t)}{\partial u(\sigma_1) \ldots u(\sigma_i)} = e^{(t-\sigma_i)A} B e^{(\sigma_i - \sigma_{i-1})A} \ldots B e^{\sigma_1 A} X'(0)$$

i.e.

$$\chi_0(t) = e^{tA} X'(0)$$
$$\chi_1(t, \sigma_1) = e^{(t-\sigma_1)A} B e^{\sigma_1 A} X'(0)$$
$$\chi_2(t, \sigma_1, \sigma_2) = e^{(t-\sigma_2)A} B e^{(\sigma_2 - \sigma_1)A} B e^{\sigma_1 A} X'(0)$$
$$\chi_2(t, \sigma_1, \sigma_2, \sigma_3) = \ldots$$

The kernels associated with the output $y(t)$ follow from the chain rule:

$$\kappa_0(t) = \lambda(\chi_0(t)$$
$$\kappa_1(t, \sigma_1) = \frac{\partial \lambda(\chi_0(t))}{\partial X} \chi_1(t, \sigma_1)$$
$$\kappa_2(t, \sigma_1, \sigma_2) = \frac{\partial \lambda(\chi_0(t))}{\partial X} \chi_2(t, \sigma_1, \sigma_2) + \chi_1(t, \sigma_1)^T \frac{\partial^2 \lambda(\chi_0(t))}{\partial X'^2} \chi_1(t, \sigma_2)$$
$$\kappa_2(t, \sigma_1, \sigma_2, \sigma_3) = \ldots$$

If the system is fully nonlinear, as in this case, then the kernels can be considered local approximations. In other words, the kernels are valid for inputs (i.e., neuronal activations) of a reasonable magnitude.

References

Bendat, J. S. (1990). *Nonlinear System Analysis and Identification from Random Data.* John Wiley and Sons, New York.

Buxton, R. B., and Frank, L. R. (1997). A model for the coupling between cerebral blood flow and oxygen metabolism during neural stimulation. *J. Cereb. Blood Flow Metab.* **17,** 64–72.

Buxton, R. B., Wong, E. C., and Frank, L. R. (1998). Dynamics of blood flow and oxygenation changes during brain activation: The balloon model. *MRM* **39,** 855–864.

Fliess, M., Lamnabhi, M., and Lamnabhi-Lagarrigue, F. (1983). An algebraic approach to nonlinear functional expansions. *IEEE Trans. Circuits Syst.* **30,** 554–570.

Fox, P. T., and Raichle, M. E. (1986). Focal physiological uncoupling of cerebral blood flow and oxidative metabolism during somatosensory stimulation in human subjects. *Proc. Natl. Acad. Sci. USA* **83**(4), 1140–1144.

Friston, K. J. (1995). Regulation of rCBF by diffusible signals: an analysis of constraints on diffusion and elimination *Hum. Brain Mapping* **3,** 56–65.

Friston, K. J., Jezzard, P., and Turner, R. (1994). Analysis of functional MRI time series. *Hum. Brain Mapping* **1,**153–171.

Friston, K. J., Josephs, O., Rees, G., and Turner, R. (1998). Nonlinear event-related responses in fMRI. *MRM* **39,** 41–52.

Friston, K. J., Mechelli, A., Turner, R., and Price, C. J. (2000). Nonlinear responses in fMRI: the balloon model, Volterra kernels, and other haemodynamic. *NeuroImage* **12**(4), 466–477.

Grill-Spector, K., and Malach, R. (2001). fMR-adaptation: a tool for studying the functional properties of human cortical neurons. *Acta Psychol. (Amst.)* **107**(1–3), 293–321..

Grubb, R. L., Rachael, M. E., Euchring, J. O., and Ter-Pogossian, M. M. (1974). The effects of changes in PCO_2 on cerebral blood volume, blood flow and vascular mean transit time. *Stroke* **5,** 630–639.

Heeger, D. J., and Ress, D. (2002). What does fMRI tell us about neuronal activity? *Nat. Rev. Neurosci.* **3**(2), 142–151.

Hoge, R. D., Atkinson, J., Gill, B., Crelier, G. R., Marrett, S., and Pike, G. B. (1999). Linear coupling between cerebral blood flow and oxygen consumption in activated human cortex. *Proc. Natl. Acad. Sci. USA* **96,** 9403–9408.

Irikura, K., Maynard, K. I., and Moskowitz, M. A. (1994). Importance of nitric oxide synthase inhibition to the attenuated vascular responses induced by topical l-nitro-arginine during vibrissal stimulation. *J. Cereb. Blood Flow Metab.* **14,** 45–48.

Kennedy, C., Des Rosiers, M. H., Sakurada, O., Shinohara, M., Reivich, M., Jehle, J. W., and Sokoloff, L. (1976). Metabolic mapping of the primary visual system of the monkey by means of the autoradiographic [14C]deoxyglucose technique. *Proc. Natl. Acad. Sci. USA* **73**(11), 4230–4234.

Lindauer, U., Royl, G., Leithner, C., Kuhl, M., Gold, L., Gethmann, J., Kohl-Bareis, M., Villringer, A., and Dirnagl, U. (2001). No evidence for early decrease in blood oxygenation in rat whisker cortex in response to functional activation. *NeuroImage* **13**(6 Pt 1) , 988–1001.

Logothetis, N. K., Pauls, J., Augath, M., Trinath, T., and Oeltermann, A. (2001). Neurophysiological investigation of the basis of the fMRI signal. *Nature* **412**(6843), 150–157.

Mandeville, J. B., Marota, J. J., Ayata, C., Zararchuk, G., Moskowitz, M. A., Rosen, B., and Weisskoff, R. M. (1999). Evidence of a cerebrovascular postarteriole windkessel with delayed compliance. *J. Cereb. Blood Flow Metab.* **19,** 679–689.

Mayhew, J., Hu, D., Zheng, Y., Askew, S., Hou, Y., Berwick, J., Coffey, P. J., and Brown, N. (1998). An evaluation of linear models analysis techniques for processing images of microcirculation activity *NeuroImage* **7,** 49–71.

Miller, K. L., Luh, W. M., Liu, T. T., Martinez, A., Obata, T., Wong, E. C., Frank, L. R., and Buxton, R. B. (2000). Characterising the dynamic perfusion response to stimuli of short duration. *Proc. ISRM* **8,** 580.

Paulson, O. B., and Newman, E. A. (1987). Does the release of potassium from astrocyte endfeet regulate cerebral blood? *Science* **237,** 896–898.

Roy, C. S. and Sherrington, C. S. (1890). On the regulation of the blood supply of the brain. *J. Physiol. Lond.* **11,** 85–108.

Talairach, J., and Tournoux, P. (1988). *A Co-Planar Stereotaxic Atlas of a Human Brain.* Thieme, Stuttgart.

Vanzetta, I., and Grinvald, A. (1999). Increased cortical oxidative metabolism due to sensory stimulation: implications for functional brain imaging. *Science* **286**(5444), 1555–1558.

Vazquez, A. L., and Noll, D. C. (1996). Non-linear temporal aspects of the BOLD response in fMRI. *Proc. Int. Soc. Mag. Res. Med.* **3**, S1765.

Worsley, K. J., and Friston, K. J. (1995). Analysis of fMRI time series revisited—again *NeuroImage* **2,**173–181.

Zheng, Y., Martindale, J., Johnston, D., Jones, M., Berwick, J., and Mayhew, J. (2002). A model of the hemodynamic response and oxygen delivery to brain. *NeuroImage* **16**(3 Pt 1), 617–637.

CHAPTER

42

Random-Effects Analysis

INTRODUCTION

In this chapter we are concerned with making statistical inferences from functional imaging studies involving many subjects. One can envisage two main reasons for studying multiple subjects. The first is that one may be interested in individual differences, as in many areas of psychology. The second, which is the one that concerns us here, is that one is interested in what is common to the subjects. In other words, we are interested in the stereotypical effect in the population from which the subjects are drawn.

As every experimentalist knows, a subject's response will vary from trial to trial. Further, this response will vary from subject to subject. These two sources of variability, within-subject (also called between-scan) and between-subject variability, must both be taken into account when making inferences about the population.

In statistical terminology, if we wish to take the variability of an effect into account we must consider the effect as a *random effect.* In a 12-subject PET study, for example, we can view those 12 subjects as being randomly drawn from the population at large. The subject variable is then a random effect and, in this way, we are able to take the sampling variability into account and make inferences about the population from which the subjects were drawn. Conversely, if we view the subject variable as a *fixed effect,* then our inferences will relate only to those 12 subjects chosen.

The majority of early studies in neuroimaging combined data from multiple subjects using a fixed-effects (FFX) approach. This methodology only takes into account the within-subject variability. It is used to report results as case studies. It is not possible to make formal inferences about population effects using FFX. Random-effects (RFX) analysis, however, takes into account both sources of variation and makes it possible to make formal inferences about the population from which the subjects are drawn.

In this chapter we describe FFX and RFX analyses of a multiple-subject PET study. In the next section, we show how the analyses are implemented and then describe the underlying mathematical models. In neuroimaging, RFX is implemented using the computationally efficient *summary statistic* approach. We also show that this is mathematically equivalent to the more computationally demanding maximum likelihood procedure.

ANALYSIS OF MULTISUBJECT DATA

Throughout this chapter we illustrate the different analysis methods using data from a PET study of verbal fluency. These data come from five subjects and were recorded under two alternating conditions. Subjects were asked to either repeat a heard letter or to respond with a word that began with that letter. These tasks are referred to as *word shadowing* and *word generation* and were performed in alternation over 12 scans and the order randomised over subjects. Both conditions were identically paced with one word being generated every 2 sec. PET images were realigned, normalised, and smoothed with a 16-mm isotropic Gaussian kernel.[1]

Fixed-Effects Analysis

Analysis of multiple-subject data takes place within the machinery of the general linear model (GLM) as described in earlier chapters. However, instead of having data from a single subject at each voxel we now have data from multiple subjects. This is entered into a GLM by concatenating data from all subjects into the single column vector Y. Commensurate with this augmented data vector is an augmented multisubject design matrix,[2] X, which is shown in Fig. 42.1. Columns 1 and 2 indicate scans taken during the word shadowing and word generation conditions, respectively. Columns 3 to 10 indicate these conditions for the other subjects. The time variables in columns 11 to 15 are used to probe habituation effects. These variables are not of interest to us in this chapter but we include them to improve the fit of the model. The GLM can be written as

$$Y = X\beta + E \tag{42.1}$$

where the β are regression coefficients and E is a vector of errors. The effects of interest can then be examined using an augmented contrast vector, c. For example, for the verbal fluency data the contrast vector

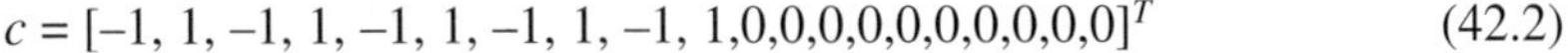

$$c = [-1, 1, -1, 1, -1, 1, -1, 1, -1, 1, 0, 0, 0, 0, 0, 0, 0, 0, 0, 0]^T \tag{42.2}$$

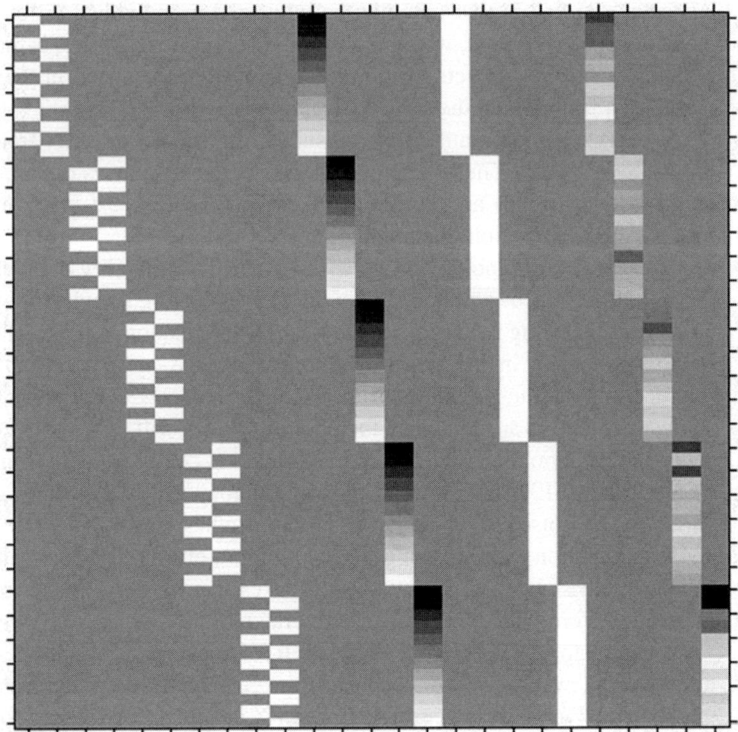

FIGURE 42.1
Design matrix for five-subject FFX analysis of PET data. There are 60 rows, 12 for each subject. The first 10 columns contain indicator variables showing which condition (word shadowing or word generation) relates to which scan. Columns 11 to 15 contain time variables, columns 16 to 20 subject-specific offsets, and the last 5 columns the global effect at each scan.

[1] This dataset and full details of the preprocessing are available from http://www.fil.ion.ucl.ac.uk/spm/data.

[2] This design was created using the "multisubject: condition by subject interaction and covariates" option in SPM99.

would be used to examine the differential effect of word generation versus word shadowing, averaged over the group of subjects. The corresponding t statistic,

$$t = \frac{c^T\hat{\beta}}{\sqrt{\mathrm{var}[c^T\hat{\beta}]}} \tag{42.3}$$

where var[ ] denotes variance, highlights voxels with significantly nonzero differential activity. This shows the *average effect in the group* and is a type of fixed-effects analysis. The resulting Statistical Parametric Map is shown in Fig. 42.2b.

It is also possible to look for differential effects in each subject separately using subject-specific contrasts. For example, to look at the activation from subject 2 one would use the contrast vector

$$c_2 = [0,0,-1,1,0,0,0,0,0,0,0,0,0,0,0,0,0,0,0,0]^T \tag{42.4}$$

The corresponding subject-specific SPMs are shown in Fig. 42.2a.

We note that we have been able to look at subject-specific effects because the design matrix specified a *subject-separable model.* In these models the parameter estimates for each subject are unaffected by data from other subjects. This arises from the block-diagonal structure in the design matrix.

Random-Effects Analysis via Summary Statistics

An RFX analysis can be implemented using the *summary statistic (SS) approach* as follows (Friston *et al.,* 2002; Holmes and Friston, 1998).

1. Fit the model for each subject using different GLMs for each subject or by using a multiple-subject subject-separable GLM (as described in the last section). The latter approach may be procedurally more convenient whilst the former is less computationally demanding. For the purposes of RFX analysis the two approaches are mathematically identical because they will produce the same contrast images.
2. Define the effect of interest for each subject with a contrast vector. Each produces a contrast image containing the contrast of the parameter estimates at each voxel.
3. Feed the contrast images into a GLM that implements a one-sample t test.

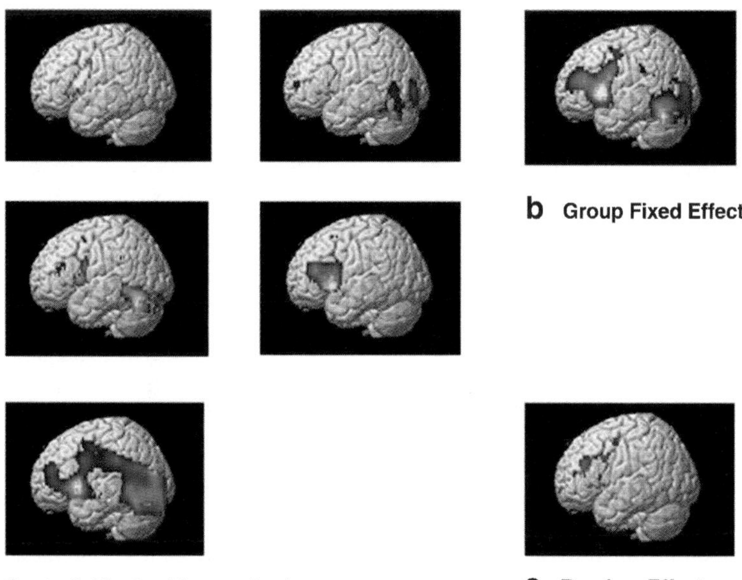

FIGURE 42.2
Analysis of PET data showing active voxels ($p < 0.001$ uncorrected). The maps in (a) show the significance of subject-specific effects, whereas map (b) shows the significance of the average effect over the group. Map (c) shows the significance of the population effect from an RFX analysis.

Modelling in step 1 is referred to as the *first level* of analysis, whereas modelling in step 3 is referred to as the *second level.* A balanced design is one in which all subjects have identical design matrices, and is a requirement for the SS approach to be valid.

If there are, say, two populations of interest and one is interested in making inferences about differences between populations, then a two-sample t test is used at the second level. It is not necessary for the numbers of subjects in each population to be the same, but it is necessary to have the same design matrices for subjects in the same population, i.e., balanced designs at the first level.

In step 3, we have specified that only one contrast per subject be taken to the second level. This constraint may be relaxed if one takes into account the possibility that the contrasts may be correlated or be of unequal variance. This is discussed further in Glaser *et al.* (2001).

An SPM of the RFX analysis is shown in Fig. 42.2(c). We note that, compared to the SPM from the average effect in the group, far fewer voxels are deemed significantly active. This is because RFX analysis takes into account the between-subject variability. If, for example, we were to ask the question "Would a new subject drawn from this population show any significant posterior activity?" the answer would be uncertain. This is because three of the subjects in our sample show such activity but two subjects do not. Thus, based on such a small sample, we would say that our data do not show sufficient evidence against the null hypothesis that there is no population effect in posterior cortex. In contrast, the average effect in the group in Fig. 42.2b is significant over posterior cortex. But this inference is with respect to the group of five subjects, not the population.

We end this section with a disclaimer, which is that the results presented have been presented for tutorial purposes only. This is because between-scan variance is so high in PET that results on single subjects are unreliable. For this reason, we have used uncorrected thresholds for the SPMs and, given that we have no prior anatomical hypothesis, this is not the correct thing to do (Frackowiak *et al.,* 1997) (see Chapter 44). But as our concern is merely to present a tutorial on the difference between RFX and FFX we have neglected these otherwise important points.

VARIANCE COMPONENTS

This section is intended for the reader wishing to understand the statistical basis of the summary statistic approach to RFX and its written for the mathematically inclined. We also show how RFX and FFX differ.

In what follows **E**[ ] denotes the expectation operator, var[ ] denotes the variance and we will make use of the following results. Under a linear transform $y = ax + b,$ the variance of x changes according to

$$\mathrm{var}[ax + b] = a^2\mathrm{var}[x] \tag{42.5}$$

Secondly, if $\mathrm{var}[x_i] = \mathrm{var}[x]$ for all i then

$$\mathrm{var}\left[\frac{1}{N}\sum_{i=1}^{N} x_i\right] = \frac{1}{N}\,\mathrm{var}[x] \tag{42.6}$$

For background reading on expectations, variance transformations and introductory mathematical statistics, see Wackerley *et al.* (1996).

Random Effects Using Maximum Likelihood Estimators

Underlying RFX analysis is a probability model defined as follows. We first envisage that the mean effect in the population (i.e., averaged across subjects) is of size d_{pop} and that the variability of this effect between subjects is σ_b^2. The mean effect for the ith subject (i.e., averaged across scans), d_i, is then assumed to be drawn from a Gaussian with mean d_{pop} and variance σ_b^2. This process reflects the fact that we are drawing subjects at random from a large population. We then take into account the within-subject (i.e., across-scan) variability by modelling the jth observed effect in subject i as being drawn from a Gaussian with mean d_i and variance σ_w^2. Note that σ_w^2 is assumed to be the same for all subjects. This two-stage process is shown graphically in Fig. 42.3.

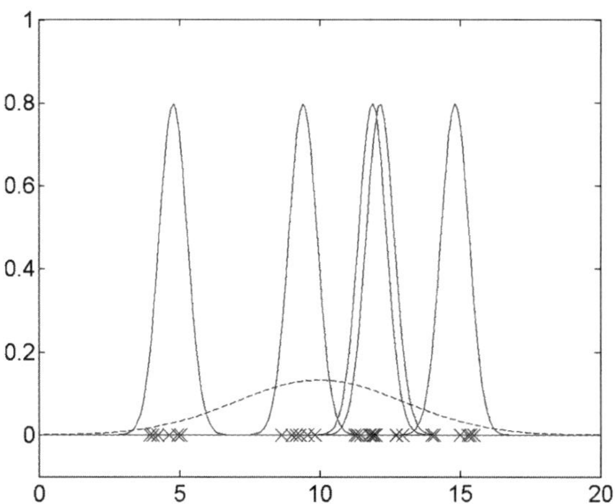

FIGURE 42.3
Synthetic data illustrating the probability model underlying random-effects analysis. The dotted line is the Gaussian distribution underlying the second-level model with mean d_{pop}, the population effect, and variance σ_b^2, the between-subject variance. The mean subject effects, d_i, are drawn from this distribution. The solid lines are the Gaussians underlying the first-level models with means d_i and variances σ_w^2. The crosses are the observed effects d_{ij}, which are drawn from the solid Gaussians.

Given a dataset of effects from N subjects with n replications of that effect per subject, the population contrast is modeled by a two-level process:

$$\begin{aligned} d_{ij} &= d_i + e_{ij} \\ d_i &= d_{pop} + z_i \end{aligned} \tag{42.7}$$

where d_i is the true mean effect for subject i and d_{ij} is the jth observed effect for subject i. For the PET data the effect is a differential effect (the difference in activation between word generation and word shadowing). The first equation captures the within-subject variability and the second equation the between-subject variability.

The within-subject Gaussian error e_{ij} has zero mean and variance $\text{var}[e_{ij}] = \sigma_w^2$. This assumes that the errors are independent over subjects and over replications within subject. The between-subject Gaussian error z_i has zero mean and variance $\text{var}[z_i] = \sigma_b^2$. Collapsing the two levels into one gives

$$d_{ij} = d_{pop} + z_i + e_{ij} \tag{42.8}$$

The maximum-likelihood estimate of the population mean is

$$\hat{d}_{\text{pop}} = \frac{1}{Nn} \sum_{i=1}^{N} \sum_{j=1}^{n} d_{ij} \tag{42.9}$$

This estimate has a mean $\mathbf{E}[\hat{d}_{\text{pop}}] = d_{\text{pop}}$ and a variance given by

$$\begin{aligned} \text{var}[\hat{d}_{\text{pop}}] &= \text{var}\left[\sum_{i=1}^{N} \frac{1}{N} \sum_{j=1}^{n} \frac{1}{n} (d_{\text{pop}} + z_i + e_{ij})\right] \\ &= \text{var}\left[\sum_{i=1}^{N} \frac{1}{N} z_i\right] + \text{var}\left[\sum_{i=1}^{N} \frac{1}{N} \sum_{j=1}^{n} \frac{1}{n} e_{ij}\right] \\ &= \frac{\sigma_b^2}{N} + \frac{\sigma_w^2}{Nn} \end{aligned} \tag{42.10}$$

The variance of the population mean estimate contains contributions from both the within-subject and between-subject variance.

Fixed Effects

Implicit in FFX analysis is a single-level model:

$$d_{ij} = d_i + e_{ij} \tag{42.11}$$

The parameter estimates for each subject are

$$\hat{d}_i = \frac{1}{n}\sum_{j=1}^{n} d_{ij} \tag{42.12}$$

which have a variance given by

$$\begin{aligned} \text{var}[\hat{d}_i] &= \text{var}\left[\sum_{j=1}^{n}\frac{1}{n}d_{ij}\right] \\ &= \frac{\sigma_w^2}{n} \end{aligned} \tag{42.13}$$

The estimate of the group mean is then

$$\hat{d}_{\text{pop}} = \frac{1}{N}\sum_{i=1}^{N}\hat{d}_i \tag{42.14}$$

which has a variance

$$\begin{aligned} \text{var}[\hat{d}_{\text{pop}}] &= \text{var}\left[\sum_{i=1}^{N}\frac{1}{N}\hat{d}_i\right] \\ &= \frac{1}{N}\text{var}[\hat{d}_i] \\ &= \frac{\sigma_w^2}{Nn} \end{aligned} \tag{42.15}$$

The variance of the fixed-effects group mean estimate contains contributions from within-subject terms only. It is not sensitive to between-subject variance. We are not therefore able to make formal inferences about population effects using FFX. We are restricted to informal inferences based on separate case studies or summary images showing the average group effect (e.g., Fig. 42.2a or b).

Random Effects Using Summary Statistics

Implicit in the summary statistic RFX approach is the two-level model:

$$\begin{aligned} \bar{d}_i &= d_i + e_i \\ d_i &= d_{\text{pop}} + z_i \end{aligned} \tag{42.16}$$

where d_i is the true mean effect for subject i, $\bar{d}_i$ is the sample mean effect for subject i and d_{pop} is the true mean effect for the population.

The summary statistic approach is of interest because it is computationally much simpler to implement than the full random-effects model of Eq. (42.7). This is because it is based on the sample mean value, $\bar{d}_i$, rather than on all of the samples d_{ij}. This is important for neuroimaging because the images are so large.

In the first level we consider the variation of the sample mean for each subject around the true mean for each subject. The corresponding variance is $\text{var}[e_i] = \sigma_w^2/n$, where σ_w^2 is the within-subject variance. At the second level we consider the variation of the true subject means about the population mean where $\text{var}[z_i] = \sigma_b^2$, the between-subject variance. We also have $\mathbf{E}[e_i] = \mathbf{E}[z_i] = 0$. Consequently,

$$\bar{d}_i = d_{\text{pop}} + z_i + e_i \tag{42.17}$$

The population mean is then estimated as

$$\hat{d}_{\text{pop}} = \frac{1}{N}\sum_{i-1}^{N}\bar{d}_i \tag{42.18}$$

This estimate has a mean $\mathbf{E}[\hat{d}_{\text{pop}}] = d_{\text{pop}}$ and a variance given by

$$\begin{aligned} \text{var}[\hat{d}_{\text{pop}}] &= \text{var}\left[\sum_{i=1}^{N}\frac{1}{N}\bar{d}_i\right] \\ &= \text{var}\left[\sum_{i=1}^{N}\frac{1}{N}z_i\right] + \text{var}\left[\sum_{i=1}^{N}\frac{1}{N}e_i\right] \\ &= \frac{\sigma_b^2}{N} + \frac{\sigma_w^2}{Nn} \end{aligned} \tag{42.19}$$

Thus, the variance of the estimate of the population mean contains contributions from both the within-subject and between-subject variances. Importantly, both $\mathbf{E}[\hat{d}_{pop}]$ and $\text{var}[\hat{d}_{pop}]$ are identical to the maximum-likelihood estimates derived earlier. This validates the summary statistic approach. Informally, the validity of the summary statistic approach lies in the fact that what is brought forward to the second level is a *sample* mean. It contains an element of within-subject variability which, when operated on at the second level, produces just the right balance of within- and between-subject variance.

DISCUSSION

We have shown how neuroimaging data from multiple subjects can be analysed using FFX or RFX analysis. FFX analysis is used for reporting case studies, and RFX is used to make inferences about the population from which subjects are drawn. For a comparison of these and other methods for combining data from multiple subjects, see Lazar *et al.* (2002).

In neuroimaging, RFX is implemented using the computationally efficient summary statistic approach. We have shown that this is mathematically equivalent to the more computationally demanding maximum-likelihood procedure. For unbalanced designs, however, the maximum-likelihood estimate of the population effect and its variance both change and the summary statistic approach is no longer equivalent. The robustness of the summary statistic approach to violations of these underlying assumptions is a topic covered in more detail in the following chapter.

For more advanced treatments of random-effects analysis,[3] see, e.g., Yandell (1997). These allow, for example, for subject-specific within-subject variances, unbalanced designs, and Bayesian inference (Carlin and Louis, 2000). For a recent application of these ideas to neuroimaging, readers are referred to Chapter 47 in which hierarchical models are applied to single and multiple subject fMRI studies. As groundwork for this more advanced material readers are encouraged to first read the tutorial in Chapter 43.

A general point to note, especially for fMRI, is that because the between-subject variance is larger than the within-subject variance, your scanning time is best used to scan more subjects rather than to scan individual subjects for longer. In practice, this must be traded off against the time required to recruit and train subjects (Worsley *et al.*, 2002).

Further Points

We have so far described how to make inferences about univariate effects in a single population. This is achieved in the summary statistic approach by taking forward a single contrast image per subject to the second level and then using a one sample t test.

This methodology carries over naturally to more complex scenarios where we may have multiple populations or multivariate effects. For two populations, for example, we perform two-sample t tests at the second level. An extreme example of this approach is the comparison of a single case study with a control group. Although this may sound unfeasible, because one population has only a single member, a viable test can in fact be implemented by assuming that the two populations have the same variance.

For multivariate effects we take forward multiple contrast images per subject to the second level and perform an analysis of variance. This can be implemented in the usual way with a GLM but, importantly, we must take into account the fact that we have repeated measures for each subject and that each characteristic of interest may have a different variability. Methods for handling such cases are dealt with in Chapters 39 and 47.

As well as testing for whether univariate population effects are significantly different from hypothesised values (typically zero), it is also possible to test whether they are correlated with other variables of interest. In Ward and Frackowiak (2003), for example, the authors test to see whether task-related activation in the motor system correlates with age.

---

[3] Strictly, what in neuroimaging is known as *random-effects analysis* is known in statistics as *mixed-effects analysis* because the statistical models contain both fixed and random effects.

It is also possible to look for conjunctions at the second level. For example, Gottfried *et al.* (2002) test for areas that are conjointly active for pleasant, unpleasant, and neutral odour valences. For a statistical test involving conjunctions of contrasts it is necessary that the contrast effects be uncorrelated. This can be ensured by taking into account the covariance structure at the second level.

The validity of all of the above approaches relies on the same criteria that underpin the univariate single population summary statistic approach. Namely, that the variance components and estimated parameter values are, on average, identical to those that would be obtained by the equivalent two-level maximum-likelihood model.

References

Carlin, B. P., and Louis, T. A. (2000). *Bayes and Empirical Bayes Methods for Data Analysis.* Chapman and Hall, London.

Frackowiak, R. S. J., Friston, K. J., Frith, C. D., Dolan, R. J., and Mazziotta, J. C. Eds. (1997). *Human Brain Function.* Academic Press, San Diego.

Frison, L., and Pocock, S. J. (1992). Repeated measures in clinical trials: an analysis using mean summary statistics and its implications for design. *Statistics Med.* **11,** 1685–1704.

Friston, K. J., Glaser, D., Henson, R., Kiebel, S., Phillips, C., and Ashburner, J. (2002). Classical and Bayesian inference in neuroimaging: applications. *NeuroImage* **16,** 484–512.

Glaser, D. E., Penny, W. D., Henson, R. N., Rugg, M. D., and Friston, K. J. (2001). Correcting for non-sphericity in imaging data using classical and Bayesian approaches. *NeuroImage* **13**(6), S127.

Gottfried, J. A., Deichmann, R., Winston, J. S., and Dolan, R. J. (2002). Functional heterogeneity in human olfactory cortex: an event-related functional magnetic resonance imaging study. *J. Neurosci.* **22**(24), 10819–10828.

Holmes, A. P., and Friston, K. J. (1998). Generalisability, random effects and population inference. *NeuroImage* **7,** S754.

Lazar, N. A., Luna, B., Sweeney, J. A., and Eddy, W. F. (2002). Combining brains: a survey of methods for statistical pooling of information. *NeuroImage* **16**(2), 538–550.

Wackerley, D. D., Mendenhall, W., and Scheaffer, R. L. (1996). *Mathematical Statistics with Applications.* Duxbury Press.

Ward, N. S., and Frackowiak, R. S. J. (2003). Age related changes in the neural correlates of motor performance. *Brain* **126**, 873–888.

Worsley, K. J., Liao, C. H., Aston, J., Petre, V., Duncan, G. H., Morales, F., and Evans, A. C. (2002). A general statistical analysis for fMRI data. *NeuroImage* **15**(1).

Yandell, B. S. (1997). *Practical Data Analysis for Designed Experiments.* Chapman and Hall, London.

CHAPTER

43

Hierarchical Models

INTRODUCTION

Hierarchical models are central to many current analyses of functional imaging data including random-effects analysis, models using fMRI as priors for EEG source localisation, and spatiotemporal Bayesian modelling of imaging data (Friston *et al.,* 2002a). These hierarchical models posit linear relations between variables with error terms that are Gaussian. The general linear model (GLM), which to date has been so central to the analysis of functional imaging data, is a special case of these hierarchical models consisting of just a single layer.

Model fitting and statistical inference for hierarchical models can be implemented using a Parametric Empirical Bayes (PEB) algorithm described in Chapter 47 and in Friston *et al.* (2002b). The algorithm is sufficiently general to accommodate multiple levels in the hierarchy and allows for the error covariances to take on arbitrary form. This generality is particularly appealing because it renders the method applicable to a wide variety of modelling scenarios. Because of this generality, however, and the complexity of scenarios in which the method is applied, readers wishing to learn about PEB for the first time are advised to read this chapter first.

We provide an introduction to hierarchical models and focus on some relatively simple examples. Each model and PEB algorithm we present is a special case of that described by Friston *et al.* (2002b). Although there are a number of tutorials on hierarchical modelling (Carlin and Louis, 2000; Lee, 1997), what we describe here has been tailored for functional imaging applications. We also note that a tutorial on hierarchical models is, to our minds, also a tutorial on Bayesian inference because higher levels act as priors for parameters in lower levels. Readers are therefore encouraged to also consult background texts on Bayesian inference, such as Gelman *et al.* (1995).

We restrict our attention to two-level models and show how one computes the posterior distributions over the first- and second-level parameters. These are derived, initially, for completely general design and error covariance matrices. We then consider two special cases: (1) models with equal error variances and (2) separable models. We also show how the parameters and covariance components can be estimated using PEB. We then show how a two-level hierarchical model can be used for random-effects analysis. For equal subject error variances at the first level and the same first-level design matrices (i.e., balanced designs), we show that the resulting inferences are identical to those made by the summary statistic (SS) approach (Penny *et al.*, Chapter 42). If either of the criteria are not met then, strictly, the SS approach is not valid. However, we also show that a modified SS approach can be used for unbalanced designs and unequal error variances if the covariance structure of the model at the second level is modified appropriately.

In what follows, the notation $\mathbf{N}(m, \Sigma)$ denotes a uni/multivariate normal distribution with mean m and variance/covariance Σ and lowercase p's denote probability densities. Uppercase letters denote matrices, lowercase denote column vectors, and x^T denotes the transpose of x. We will also make extensive use of the normal density, i.e., if $p(x) = \mathbf{N}(m, \Sigma)$ then

$$p(x) \propto \exp\left[-\frac{1}{2}(x - m)^T \Sigma^{-1}(x - m)\right] \tag{43.1}$$

We also use var[ ] to denote variance, $\otimes$ to denote the Kronecker product, and X^+ to denote the pseudo-inverse.

TWO-LEVEL MODELS

We consider two-level linear Gaussian models of the form

$$\begin{aligned} y &= Xw + e \\ w &= M\mu + z \end{aligned} \tag{43.2}$$

where the errors are zero-mean Gaussian with covariances cov[e] = C and cov[z] = P. The model is shown graphically in Fig. 43.1. The column vectors y and w have K and N entries, respectively. The vectors w and μ are the first- and second-level parameters and X and M are the first- and second-level design matrices. Models of this form have been used in functional imaging. For example, in random-effects analysis the second-level models describe the variation of subject effect sizes about a population effect size, μ. In Bayesian inference with shrinkage priors, the second level models variation of effect size over voxels around a whole brain mean effect size of $\mu = 0$ (i.e., for a given cognitive challenge the response of a voxel chosen at random is, on average, zero). See, for example, Friston *et al.* (2002a).

The aim of Bayesian inference is to make inferences about w and μ (if we don't already know them) based on the posterior distributions $p(w|y)$ and $p(\mu|y)$. These can be derived as follows. We first note that the above equations specify the likelihood and prior probability distributions

$$\begin{aligned} p(y|w) &\propto \exp\left[-\frac{1}{2}(y - Xw)^T C^{-1}(y - Xw)\right] \\ p(w) &\propto \exp\left[-\frac{1}{2}(w - M\mu)^T P^{-1}(w - M\mu)\right] \end{aligned} \tag{43.3}$$

The posterior distribution is then

$$p(w|y) \propto p(y|w)p(w) \tag{43.4}$$

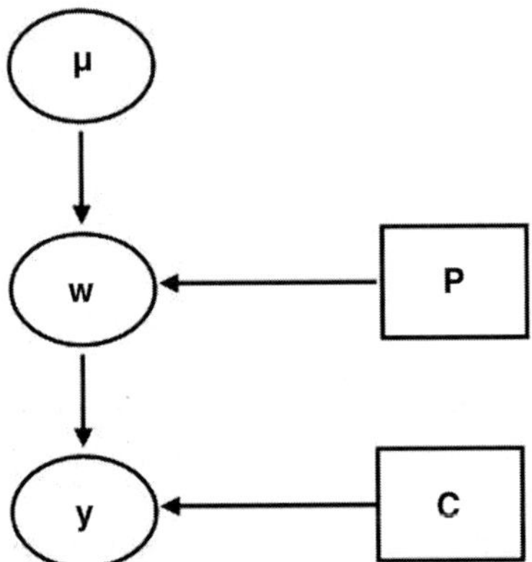

FIGURE 43.1
Two-level hierarchical model. The data y are explained as deriving from an effect w and a zero-mean Gaussian random variation with covariance C. The effects w in turn are random effects deriving from a superordinate effect μ and zero-mean Gaussian random variation with covariance P. The goal of Bayesian inference is to make inferences about μ and w from the posterior distributions $p(\mu|y)$ and $p(w|y)$.

Taking logs and keeping only those terms that depend on w gives

$$\begin{aligned}\log p(w|y) &= -\frac{1}{2}(y - Xw)^T C^{-1}(y - Xw)\\ &\quad -\frac{1}{2}(w - M\mu)^T P^{-1}(w - M\mu) + \ldots \\ &= -\frac{1}{2} w^T(X^T C^{-1}X + P^{-1})w + w^T(X^T C^{-1}y + P^{-1}M\mu) + \ldots\end{aligned} \tag{43.5}$$

Taking logs of the Gaussian density $p(x)$ in Eq. (43.1) and keeping only those terms that depend on x gives

$$\log p(x) = -\frac{1}{2} x^T\Sigma^{-1}x + x^T\Sigma^{-1}m + \ldots \tag{43.6}$$

Comparing Eq. (43.5) with terms in the above equation shows that

$$\begin{aligned}p(w|y) &= \mathbf{N}(m,\Sigma)\\ \Sigma^{-1} &= X^T C^{-1}X + P^{-1}\\ m &= \Sigma(X^T C^{-1}y + P^{-1}M\mu)\end{aligned} \tag{43.7}$$

The posterior distribution over the second-level coefficient is given by Bayes' rule as

$$p(\mu|y) = \frac{p(y|\mu)p(\mu)}{p(y)} \tag{43.8}$$

However, because we do not have a prior $p(\mu)$ this posterior distribution becomes identical to the likelihood term, $p(y|\mu)$, which can be found by eliminating the first-level parameters from our two equations, i.e., by substituting the second-level equation into the first, giving

$$y = XM\mu + Xz + e \tag{43.9}$$

which can be written as

$$y = \tilde{X}\mu + \tilde{e} \tag{43.10}$$

where $\tilde{X} = X\,M$ and $\tilde{e} = X\,z + e$. The solution to Eq. (43.10) then gives

$$\begin{aligned}p(\mu|y) &= \mathbf{N}(\hat{\mu},\Sigma_\mu)\\ \hat{\mu} &= (\tilde{X}^T\tilde{C}^{-1}\tilde{X})^{-1}\tilde{X}^T\tilde{C}^{-1}y\\ \Sigma_\mu &= (\tilde{X}^T\tilde{C}^{-1}\tilde{X})^{-1}\end{aligned} \tag{43.11}$$

where the covariance term

$$\begin{aligned}\tilde{C} &= \text{cov}[\tilde{e}]\\ &= XPX^T + C\end{aligned} \tag{43.12}$$

We have now achieved our first goal, the posterior distributions of first- and second-level parameters being expressed in terms of the data, design, and error covariance matrices. We now consider a number of special cases.

Sensor Fusion

The first special case is the univariate model:

$$\begin{aligned}y &= w + e\\ w &= \mu + z\end{aligned} \tag{43.13}$$

with a single scalar data point, y, and variances $C = 1/\beta$, $P = 1/\alpha$ specified in terms of the data precision β and the prior precision α (the "precision" is the inverse variance). Plugging these values into Eq. (43.7) gives

$$\begin{aligned}p(w|y) &= \mathbf{N}(m,\lambda^{-1})\\ \lambda &= \beta + \alpha\\ m &= \frac{\beta}{\lambda}y + \frac{\alpha}{\lambda}\mu\end{aligned} \tag{43.14}$$

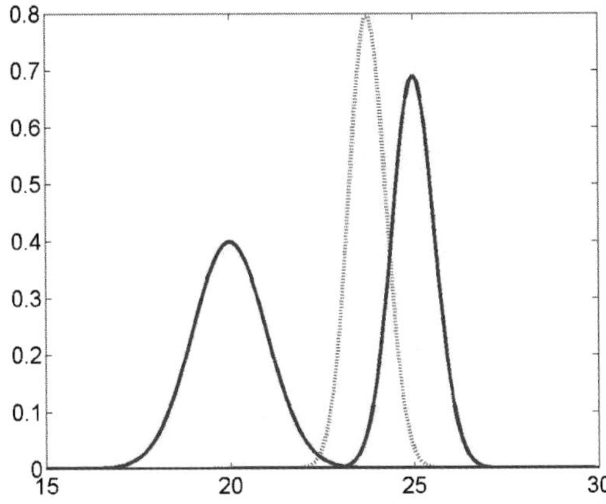

FIGURE 43.2
Bayes' rule for univariate Gaussians. The two solid curves show the probability densities for the prior $p(w) = \mathbf{N}(\mu, \alpha^{-1})$ with $\mu = 20$ and $\alpha = 1$ and the likelihood $p(y|w) = \mathbf{N}(w, \beta^{-1})$ with $w = 25$ and $\beta = 3$. The dotted curve shows the posterior distribution, $p(w|y) = \mathbf{N}(m, \lambda^{-1})$ with $m = 23.75$ and $\lambda = 4$, as computed from Eq. (43.14). The posterior distribution is closer to the likelihood because the likelihood has higher precision.

Despite its simplicity this model possesses two important features of Bayesian learning in linear Gaussian models. The first is that *precisions add*—the posterior precision is the sum of the data precision and the prior precision. The second is that the posterior mean is the sum of the data mean and the prior mean, each weighted by their relative precisions. A numerical example is shown in Fig. 43.2.

Equal Variance

This special case is a two-level multivariate model as in Eq. (43.2) but with isotropic covariances at both the first and second levels. We have $C = \beta^{-1} I_K$ and $P = \alpha^{-1} I_N$. This means that observations are independent and have the same error variance. This is an example of the errors being independent and identically distributed (i.i.d.), where in this case the distribution is a zero-mean Gaussian having a particular variance. In this chapter we also use the term *sphericity* for any model with i.i.d. errors. Models without i.i.d. errors will have nonsphericity. (As an aside, we note that i.i.d. is not actually a requirement of sphericity and readers looking for a precise definition are referred to Winer *et al.* (1991) and to Chapter 39.)

On a further point of terminology, the unknown vectors w and μ will be referred to as *parameters* whereas variables related to error covariances will be called *hyperparameters.* The variables α and β are, therefore, hyperparameters. The posterior distribution is therefore given by

$$\begin{aligned} p(w|y) &= \mathbf{N}(\hat{w}, \hat{\Sigma}) \\ \hat{\Sigma} &= (\beta X^T X + \alpha I_N)^{-1} \\ \hat{w} &= \hat{\Sigma}(\beta X^T y + \alpha M \mu) \end{aligned} \tag{43.15}$$

Note that if $\alpha = 0$ we recover the maximum-likelihood estimate

$$\hat{w}_{ML} = (X^T X)^{-1} X^T y \tag{43.16}$$

This is the familiar Ordinary Least-Squares (OLS) estimate used in the GLM (Holmes *et al.,* 1997). The posterior distribution of the second-level coefficient is given by Eq. (43.11) with

$$\tilde{C} = \beta^{-1} I_K + \alpha^{-1} X X^T \tag{43.17}$$

Separable Model

We now consider "separable models," which can be used, for example, for random-effects analysis. In these models, the first-level splits into N separate submodels. For each submodel i, there are n_i observations y_i giving information about the parameter w_i via the design vector x_i (this would typically be a boxcar or, for event-related designs, a vector of delta functions). The overall first-level design matrix X then has a block-diagonal form $X = \text{blkdiag}(x_1,\ldots,x_i,\ldots,x_N)$ and the covariance is given by $C = \text{diag}[\beta_1 1_{n_1}^T,\ldots,\beta_i 1_{n_i}^T,\ldots,\beta_N 1_{n_N}^T]$ where 1_n is a column vector of 1's with n entries. For example, for $N = 3$ groups with $n_1 = 2$, $n_2 = 3$, and $n_3 = 2$ observations in each group

$$X = \begin{bmatrix} x_1(1) & 0 & 0 \\ x_1(2) & 0 & 0 \\ 0 & x_2(1) & 0 \\ 0 & x_2(2) & 0 \\ 0 & x_2(3) & 0 \\ 0 & 0 & x_3(1) \\ 0 & 0 & x_3(2) \end{bmatrix} \tag{43.18}$$

and $C = \text{diag}[\beta_1, \beta_1, \beta_2, \beta_2, \beta_2, \beta_3, \beta_3]$. The covariance at the second level is $P = \alpha^{-1} I_N$, as before, and we also assume that the second-level design matrix is a column of 1's, $M = 1_N$. The posterior distribution of the first-level coefficient is found by substituting X and C into Eq. (43.7). This gives a distribution that factorises over the different first-level coefficients such that

$$\begin{aligned} p(w|y) &= \prod_{i=1}^{N} p(w_i|y) \\ p(w_i|y) &= N(\hat{w}_i,\hat{\Sigma}_{ii}) \\ \hat{\Sigma}_{ii}^{-1} &= \beta_i x_i^T x_i + \alpha \\ \hat{w}_i &= \hat{\Sigma}_{ii}\beta_i x_i^T y_i + \hat{\Sigma}_{ii}\alpha\mu \end{aligned} \tag{43.19}$$

The posterior distribution of the second-level coefficient is, from Eq. (43.11), given by

$$\begin{aligned} p(\mu|y) &= \mathbf{N}(\hat{u}\,\sigma_\mu^2) \\ \sigma_\mu^2 &= \frac{1}{\sum_{i=1}^{N} x_i^T(\alpha^{-1}x_i x_i^T + \beta_i^{-1})^{-1}x_i} \\ \hat{\mu} &= \sigma_\mu^2 \sum_{i=1}^{N} x_i^T(\alpha^{-1}x_i x_i^T + \beta_i^{-1})^{-1}y_i \end{aligned} \tag{43.20}$$

We note that in the absence of any second-level variability, i.e., $\alpha \to \infty$, the estimate $\hat{\mu}$ reduces to the mean of the first-level coefficients weighted by their precision

$$\hat{\mu} = \frac{\beta_i x_i^T y_i}{\Sigma_i \beta_i x_i^T x_i} \tag{43.21}$$

PARAMETRIC EMPIRICAL BAYES

We showed in the preceding section how to compute the posterior distributions $p(w|y)$ and $p(\mu|y)$. As can be seen from Eqs. (43.7) and (43.11), however, these equations depend on covariances P and C, which in general are unknown. For the equal variance model and the separable model, the hyperparameters α and β_i are generally unknown. Friston *et al.* (2002b) decompose the covariances using

$$\begin{aligned} C &= \sum_j \lambda_j^1 Q_j^1 \\ P &= \sum_j \lambda_j^2 Q_j^2 \end{aligned} \tag{43.22}$$

where Q_j^1 and Q_j^2 are basis functions that are specified by the modeler depending on the application in mind. For example, for analysis of fMRI data from a single subject, two basis functions are used, the first relating to error variance and the second relating to temporal autocorrelation (Friston *et al.*, 2002a). The hyperparameters $\lambda = [\{\lambda_j^1\}, \{\lambda_j^2\}]$ are unknown but can be estimated using the PEB algorithm described in Friston *et al.* (2002b). Variants of this algorithm are known as the *evidence framework* (Mackay, 1992) or *maximum likelihood II*

(ML-II) (Berger, 1985). The PEB algorithm is also referred to as simply *empirical Bayes* but we use the term PEB to differentiate it from the nonparametric empirical Bayes methods described in Carlin and Louis (2000). The hyperparameters are set so as to maximise the evidence (also known as the marginal likelihood)

$$p(y|\lambda) = \int p(y|w,\lambda)\, p(w|\lambda)\, dw \tag{43.23}$$

This is the likelihood of the data after we have integrated out the first-level parameters. For the two multivariate special cases described above, by substituting in our expressions for the prior and likelihood, integrating, taking logs, and then setting the derivatives to zero, we can derive a set of update rules for the hyperparameters. These derivations are provided in the following two sections.

Equal Variance

For the equal variance model the objective function is

$$p(y|\alpha,\beta) = \int p(y|w,\beta)\, p(w|\alpha)\, dw \tag{43.24}$$

Substituting in expressions for the likelihood and prior gives

$$p(y|\alpha,\beta) = \left(\frac{\beta}{2\pi}\right)^{K/2}\left(\frac{\alpha}{2\pi}\right)^{N/2} \int \exp\left[-\frac{\beta}{2}e(w)^T e(w) - \frac{\alpha}{2}z(w)^T z(w)\right] dw$$

where $e(w) = y - Xw$ and $z(w) = w - M\mu$. By rearranging the terms in the exponent (and keeping all of them, unlike earlier where we were only interested in w-dependent terms), the integral can be written as

$$I = \int \exp\left[-\frac{1}{2}(w-\hat{w})^T \hat{\Sigma}^{-1}(w-\hat{w})\right] dw \tag{43.25}$$

$$\exp\left[-\frac{\beta}{2}e(\hat{w})^T e(\hat{w}) - \frac{\alpha}{2}z(\hat{w})^T z(\hat{w})\right]$$

where the second term is not dependent on w. The first factor is then simply given by the normalising constant of the multivariate Gaussian density

$$(2\pi)^{N/2}|\hat{\Sigma}|^{1/2} \tag{43.26}$$

Hence,

$$p(y|\alpha,\beta) = \left(\frac{\beta}{2\pi}\right)^{K/2}\alpha^{N/2}|\hat{\Sigma}|^{1/2}\exp\left[-\frac{\beta}{2}e(\hat{w})^T e(\hat{w}) - \frac{\alpha}{2}z(\hat{w})^T z(\hat{w})\right]$$

where $|\hat{\Sigma}|$ denotes the determinant of $\hat{\Sigma}$. Taking logs gives the *log-evidence:*

$$F = \frac{K}{2}\log\frac{\beta}{2\pi} + \frac{N}{2}\log\alpha + \frac{1}{2}\log|\hat{\Sigma}| - \frac{\beta}{2}e(\hat{w})^T e(\hat{w}) - \frac{\alpha}{2}z(\hat{w})^T z(\hat{w}) \tag{43.27}$$

To find equations for updating the hyperparameters, we must differentiate F with respect to α and β and set the derivative to zero. The only possibly problematic term is the log-determinant, but this can be differentiated by first noting that the inverse covariance is given by

$$\hat{\Sigma}^{-1} = \beta X^T X + \alpha I_N \tag{43.28}$$

If λ_j are the eigenvalues of the first term, then the eigenvalues of $\hat{\Sigma}^{-1}$ are $\lambda_j + \alpha$. Hence,

$$\begin{aligned}
|\hat{\Sigma}^{-1}| &= \prod_j (\lambda_j + \alpha)\\
|\hat{\Sigma}| &= \frac{1}{\prod_j (\lambda_j + \alpha)}\\
\log|\hat{\Sigma}| &= -\sum_j \log(\lambda_j + \alpha)\\
\frac{\partial}{\partial\alpha}\log|\hat{\Sigma}| &= -\sum_j \frac{1}{\lambda_j + \alpha}
\end{aligned} \tag{43.29}$$

Setting the derivative $\partial F/\partial \alpha$ to zero then gives

$$\begin{aligned} \alpha\, z(\hat{w})^T z(\hat{w}) &= N - \sum_j \frac{\alpha}{\lambda_j + \alpha} \\ &= \sum_j \frac{\lambda_j + \alpha}{\lambda_j + \alpha} - \sum_j \frac{\alpha}{\lambda_j + \alpha} \\ &= \sum_j \frac{\lambda_j}{\lambda_j + \alpha} \end{aligned} \tag{43.30}$$

This is an implicit equation in α that leads to the following update rule. We first define the quantity γ, which is computed from the "old" value of α:

$$\gamma = \sum_{j=1}^{N} \frac{\lambda_j}{\lambda_j + \alpha} \tag{43.31}$$

and then let

$$\frac{1}{\alpha} = \frac{z(\hat{w})^T z(\hat{w})}{\gamma} \tag{43.32}$$

The update for β is derived by first noting that the eigenvalues λ_j are linearly dependent on β. Hence,

$$\frac{\partial \lambda_i}{\partial \beta} = \frac{\lambda_i}{\beta} \tag{43.33}$$

The derivative of the log-determinant is then given by

$$\frac{\partial}{\partial \beta} \log|\hat{\Sigma}^{-1}| = \frac{1}{\beta} \sum_j \frac{\lambda_i}{\lambda_i + \alpha} \tag{43.34}$$

which leads to the update

$$\frac{1}{\beta} = \frac{e(\hat{w})^T e(\hat{w})}{K - \gamma} \tag{43.35}$$

The PEB algorithm consists of iterating the update rules in Eqs. (43.31), (43.32), (43.35), and the posterior estimates in Eq. (43.15), until convergence.

The update rules in Eqs. (43.31), (43.32), and (43.35) can be interpreted as follows. For every j for which $\lambda_j >> \alpha$, the quantity γ increases by 1. Because α is the prior precision and λ_j is the data precision (of the jth "eigencoefficient"), γ therefore measures the number of parameters that are determined by the data. Given K data points, the quantity $K - \gamma$ therefore corresponds to the number of degrees of freedom in the dataset. The variances α^{-1} and β^{-1} are then updated based on the sum of squares divided by the appropriate degrees of freedom.

Separable Models

For separable models the objective function is

$$p(y|\alpha,\{\beta_i\}) = \int p(y|w,\{\beta_i\})\, p(w|\alpha)\, dw \tag{43.36}$$

Because the second level here is the same as for the equal variance case, so is the update for alpha. The updates for β_i are derived in a similar manner as before but we also make use of the fact that the first-level posterior distribution factorises [see Eq. (43.19)]. This decouples the updates for each β_i and results in the following PEB algorithm:

$$\begin{aligned} \hat{e}_i &= y_i - \hat{w}_i x_i \\ \hat{z}_i &= \hat{w}_i - \hat{\mu} \\ \lambda_i &= \beta_i x_i^T x_i \\ \gamma_i &= \frac{\lambda_j}{\lambda_j + \alpha} \\ \gamma &= \sum_i \gamma_i \end{aligned}$$

$$\begin{aligned} \beta_i &= (n_i - \gamma_i)/\hat{e}_i^T\hat{e}_i \\ \alpha &= \gamma/\hat{z}^T\hat{z} \\ \hat{w}_i &= (\beta_i x_i^T y_i + \alpha\mu)/(\lambda_i + \alpha) \\ d_i &= (\alpha_i^{-1} x_i x_i^T + \beta_i^{-1} I_{n_i})^{-1} \\ \sigma_\mu^2 &= 1/(\sum_i x_i^T d_i x_i) \\ \hat{\mu} &= \sigma_\mu^2 \sum_i x_i^T d_i y_i \end{aligned} \tag{43.37}$$

Initial values for $\hat{w}_i$ and β_i are set using OLS, $\hat{\mu}$is initially set to the mean of $\hat{w}_i$ and α is initially set to 0. The equations are then iterated until convergence. (In our examples we never required more than 10 iterations.)

The PEB algorithms we have described show how Bayesian inference can take place when the variance components are unknown (earlier we assumed the variance components were known). We now turn to an application.

RANDOM-EFFECTS ANALYSIS

To make contact with the summary statistic and ML approaches (see Penny *et al.,* Chapter 42), we described the statistical model underlying random-effects analysis as follows. The model described in this section is identical to the separable model but with $x_i = 1_n$ and $\beta_i = \beta$. Given a dataset of contrasts from N subjects with n scans per subject, the population contrast can be modelled by the two-level process:

$$\begin{aligned} y_{ij} &= w_i + e_{ij} \\ w_i &= w_{pop} + z_i \end{aligned} \tag{43.38}$$

where y_{ij} (a scalar) is the data from the ith subject and the jth scan at a particular voxel. These data points are accompanied by errors e_{ij} with w_i being the size of the effect for subject i, w_{pop} being the size of the effect in the population, and z_i being the between-subject error. This may be viewed as a Bayesian model where the first equation acts as a likelihood and the second equation acts as a prior. That is

$$\begin{aligned} p(y_{ij}|w_i) &= \mathbf{N}(w_i,\sigma_w^2) \\ p(w_i) &= \mathbf{N}(w_{pop},\sigma_b^2) \end{aligned} \tag{43.39}$$

where σ_b^2 is the between-subject variance and σ_w^2 is the within-subject variance. We can make contact with the hierarchical formalism by making the following identities. We place the y_{ij} in the column vector y in the order—all from subject 1, all from subject 2, etc. (This is described mathematically by the vec operator and is implemented in MATLAB (from Mathworks, Inc., by the colon operator.) We also let $X = I_N \otimes 1_n$ where $\otimes$ is the Kronecker product, and let $w = [w_1, w_2,\ldots, w_N]^T$. With these values the first level in Eq. (43.2) is then the matrix equivalent of Eq. (43.38) (i.e., it holds for all i, j). For $y = Xw + e$ and, e.g., $N = 3$, $n = 2$, we then have

$$\begin{bmatrix} y_{11} \\ y_{12} \\ y_{21} \\ y_{22} \\ y_{31} \\ y_{32} \end{bmatrix} = \begin{bmatrix} 1 & 0 & 0 \\ 1 & 0 & 0 \\ 0 & 1 & 0 \\ 0 & 1 & 0 \\ 0 & 0 & 1 \\ 0 & 0 & 1 \end{bmatrix} \begin{bmatrix} w_1 \\ w_2 \\ w_3 \end{bmatrix} + \begin{bmatrix} e_{11} \\ e_{12} \\ e_{21} \\ e_{22} \\ e_{31} \\ e_{32} \end{bmatrix} \tag{43.40}$$

We then note that $X^TX = nI_N$, $\hat{\Sigma} = \text{diag}(\text{var}[w_1], \text{var}[w_2],\ldots, \text{var}[w_N])$ and the ith element of $X^T{}_Y$ is equal to $\sum_{j=1}^{n} y_{ij}$.

If we let $M = 1_N$, then the second level in Eq. (43.2) is the matrix equivalent of the second level in Eq. (43.38) (i.e., it holds for all i). Plugging in our values for M and X and letting $\beta = 1/\sigma_w^2$ and $\alpha = 1/\sigma_b^2$ gives

$$\text{var}[\hat{w}_{pop}] = \frac{1}{N}\frac{\alpha + \beta n}{\alpha\beta n} \tag{43.41}$$

and

$$\begin{aligned}\hat{w}_{pop} &= \frac{1}{N}\frac{\alpha+\beta n}{\alpha\beta n}\frac{\alpha\beta}{\alpha+\beta n}\sum_{i,j} y_{ij} \\ &= \frac{1}{Nn}\sum_{i,j} y_{ij}\end{aligned} \tag{43.42}$$

So the estimate of the population mean is simply the average value of y_{ij}. The variance can be rewritten as

$$\mathrm{var}[\hat{w}_{pop}] = \frac{\sigma_b^2}{N} + \frac{\sigma_w^2}{Nn} \tag{43.43}$$

This result is identical to the maximum-likelihood and summary statistic results. The equivalence between the Bayesian and ML results derives from the fact that there is no prior at the population level. Hence, $p(Y|\mu) = p(\mu|Y)$ as indicated earlier.

Unequal Variances

The model described in this section is identical to the separable model but with $x_i = 1_{ni}$. If the error covariance matrix is nonisotropic, i.e., $C \neq \sigma_w^2 I$, then the population estimates will change. This can occur, for example, if the design matrices are different for different subjects (so-called "unbalanced-designs") or if the data from some of the subjects is particularly ill fitting. In these cases, we consider the within-subject variances $\sigma_w^2(i)$ and the number of scans n_i to be subject specific.

If we let $M = 1_N$, then the second level in Eq. (43.2) is the matrix equivalent of the second level in Eq. (43.38) (i.e., it holds for all i). Plugging in our values for M and X gives

$$\mathrm{var}[\hat{w}_{pop}] = \left(\sum_{i=1}^{N}\frac{\alpha\beta_i n_i}{\alpha + n_i\beta_i}\right)^{-1} \tag{43.44}$$

and

$$\hat{w}_{pop} = \left(\sum_{i=1}^{N}\frac{\alpha\beta_i n_i}{\alpha + n_i\beta_i}\right)^{-1}\sum_{i=1}^{N}\frac{\alpha\beta_i}{\alpha + n_i\beta_i}\sum_{j=1}^{n_i} y_{ij} \tag{43.45}$$

This reduces to the earlier result if $\beta_i = \beta$ and $n_i = n$. Both of these results are different than the summary statistic approach, which we note is therefore invalid for unequal variances.

Parametric Empirical Bayes

To implement the PEB estimation scheme for the unequal variance case, we first compute the errors $\hat{e}_{ij} = y_{ij} - X\hat{w}_i$, $\hat{z}_i = \hat{w}_i - M\hat{w}_{\text{pop}}$. We then substitute $x_i = 1_{ni}$ into the update rules derived earlier to obtain

$$\sigma_b^2 \equiv \frac{1}{\alpha} = \frac{1}{\gamma}\sum_{i=1}^{N}\hat{z}_i^2 \tag{43.46}$$

$$\sigma_w^2(i) \equiv \frac{1}{\beta_i} = \frac{1}{n_i - \gamma_i}\sum_{j=1}^{n_i}\hat{e}_{ij}^2 \tag{43.47}$$

where

$$\gamma = \sum_{i=1}^{N}\gamma_i \tag{43.48}$$

and

$$\gamma_i = \frac{n_i\beta_i}{\alpha + n_i\beta_i} \tag{43.49}$$

For balanced designs $\beta_i = \beta$ and $n_i = n$ we get

$$\sigma_b^2 \equiv \frac{1}{\alpha} = \frac{1}{\gamma}\sum_{i=1}^{N}\hat{z}_i^2 \tag{43.50}$$

$$\sigma_w^2 \equiv \frac{1}{\beta} = \frac{1}{Nn - \gamma} \sum_{i=1}^{N} \sum_{j=1}^{n} \hat{e}_{ij}^2 \tag{43.51}$$

where

$$\gamma = \frac{n\beta}{\alpha + n\beta} N \tag{43.52}$$

Effectively, the degrees of freedom in the dataset (Nn) are partitioned into those that are used to estimate the between-subject variance, γ, and those that are used to estimate the within-subject variance, $Nn - \gamma$.

The posterior distribution of the first-level coefficients is

$$p(w_i \mid y_{ij}) \equiv p(\hat{w}_i) = \mathbf{N}(\bar{w}_i, \text{var}[\hat{w}_i]) \tag{43.53}$$

where

$$\text{var}[\hat{w}_i] = \frac{1}{\alpha + n_i \beta_i} \tag{43.54}$$

$$\hat{w}_i = \frac{\beta_i}{\alpha + n_i \beta_i} \sum_{j=1}^{n_i} y_{ij} + \frac{\alpha}{\alpha + n_i \beta_i} \hat{w}_{\text{pop}} \tag{43.55}$$

Overall, the EB estimation scheme is implemented by first initialising $\hat{w}_i$, $\hat{w}_{\text{pop}}$ and α, β_i (for example, to values given from the equal error variance scheme). We then compute the errors $\hat{e}_{ij}$, $\hat{z}_i$ and reestimate the α and β_i's using the above equations. The coefficients $\hat{w}_i$ and $\hat{w}_{\text{pop}}$ are then reestimated and the last two steps are iterated until convergence. This algorithm is identical to the PEB algorithm for the separable model but with $x_i = 1_{n_i}$.

SECOND-LEVEL MODELLING

The results at the beginning of the preceding section show that the SS approach is equivalent to PEB for equal first-level error variances and balanced designs, but that SS is otherwise invalid. In this section we show that a modified SS approach that uses a nonisotropic covariance at the second level is equivalent to PEB. Firstly, we rewrite the first-level equation in Eq. (43.2) as

$$w = X^+ (y - e) \tag{43.56}$$

and substitute w into the second level and rearrange to give

$$X^+ y = M\mu + z + X^+ e \tag{43.57}$$

By letting $c = X^+ y$ and $r = z + X^+ e$ we can write the above equation as

$$c = M\mu + r \tag{43.58}$$

where

$$R \equiv \text{cov}[r] = P + X^+ C (X^+)^T \tag{43.59}$$

The estimation of μ can then proceed based solely on c, R, and M:

$$\begin{aligned} p(\mu \mid y) &= \mathbf{N}(\hat{\mu}, \Sigma_\mu) \\ \hat{\mu} &= (M^T R^{-1} M)^{-1} M^T R^{-1} c \\ \Sigma_\mu &= (M^T R^{-1} M)^{-1} \end{aligned} \tag{43.60}$$

This implies that if we bring forward OLS parameter estimates from the first level (i.e., $c = X^+ y$) then we can take into account the, as yet unaccounted for, nonsphericity at the first level by using an appropriately corrected covariance matrix at the second level (the matrix R). Jenkinson *et al.* (2002) have proposed a similar strategy but based on weighted least-squares (WLS) parameter estimates from the first level. The problem with this "plug-in" approach, however, is that P is unknown. Note that SS estimates of hyperparameters in P contain contributions from both within and between subject error, as shown in Penny *et al.* (Chapter 42), so these could not be used directly.

Separable Models

For the case of unequal variances at the first level (described at the beginning of this section), we have $C = \Sigma_{i=1}^{N} \beta_i^{-1} I^i$, $P = \alpha^{-1} I_N$ and $X = I_N \otimes 1_n$. This gives $X^+ = n^{-1} (I_N \otimes 1_n^T)$ and results in a diagonal matrix for R with entries

$$R_{ii} = \sigma_b^2 + \frac{1}{n_i}\sigma_{w(i)}^2 \tag{43.61}$$

The fact that R is diagonal for separable models is no surprise because subjects are drawn independently from the population. Reassuringly, plugging in the above value of R_{ii} into the expression for Σ_μ above gives the same estimate of population variance as before [cf. Eqs. (43.43) and (43.44)].

Thus, in principle, one could bring forward both OLS estimates, c, *and* first-level variances ($\sigma_{w(i)}^2$) to a second-level analysis. However, as we have already mentioned, the hyperparameter of P, i.e., σ_b^2, is unknown.

An alternative strategy is to estimate the hyperparameters R_{ii} using PEB based solely on a second-level model. Ordinarily this would be impossible because there are more hyperparameters and parameters (N + 1) than second-level data points (N). But by pooling data over voxels, as described by Glaser and Friston (2003), this becomes feasible.

EXAMPLE

We now give an example of random effects analysis on simulated data. The purpose is to compare the PEB and SS algorithms. We generated data from a three-subject, two-level model with population mean $\mu = 2$, subject effect sizes $w = [2.2, 1.8, 0.0]^T$, and within-subject variances $\sigma_w^2(1) = 1$, $\sigma_w^2(2) = 1$. For the third subject $\sigma_w^2(3)$ was varied from 1 to 10. The second-level design matrix was $M = [1, 1, 1]^T$ and the first-level design matrix was given by $X = \text{blkdiag}(x_1, x_2, x_3)$ with x_i being a boxcar. This model conforms to the notion of a separable model defined earlier.

Figure 43.3 shows a realisation of the three time series for $\sigma_w^2(3) = 2$. The first two time series contain stimulus-related activity but the third does not. We then applied the PEB algorithm to obtain estimates of the population mean $\hat{\mu}$ and estimated variances, σ_μ^2. For comparison, we also obtained equivalent estimates using the SS approach. We then computed the accuracy with which the population mean was estimated using the criterion $(\hat{\mu} - \mu)^2$. This was repeated for 1000 different datasets generated using the above parameter values, and for 10 different values of $\sigma_w^2(3)$. The results are shown in Fig. 43.4 and 43.5.

First we note that, as predicted by theory, both PEB and SS give identical results when the first-level error variances are equal. When the variance on the "rogue" time series approaches double that of the others, we see different estimates of both $\hat{\mu}$ and σ_μ^2. With increasing rogue error variance, the SS estimates get worse but the PEB estimates get better (with respect to the true values, as shown in Fig. 43.4, and with respect to the variability of the estimate, as shown in Fig. 43.5). This is because the third time series is more readily recognised by PEB as containing less reliable information about the population mean and is increasingly ignored. This gives better estimates $\hat{\mu}$ and a reduced estimation error, σ_μ^2.

We created the above example to reiterate a key point of this chapter, that SS gives identical results to PEB for equal within-subject error variances (homoscedasticity) and unbalanced designs, but not otherwise. In the example, divergent behaviour is observed when the error variances differ by a factor of 2. For studies with more subjects (12 being a typical number), however, this divergence requires a much greater disparity in error variances. In fact we initially found it difficult to generate datasets where PEB showed a consistent improvement over SS! It is therefore our experience that the vanilla SS approach is particularly robust to departures from homoscedasticity. This conclusion is supported by what is known of the robustness of the t test that is central to the SS approach. Lack of homoscedasticity only causes problems when the sample size (i.e., number of subjects) is small. As sample size increases so does the robustness (see, e.g., Yandell, 1997).

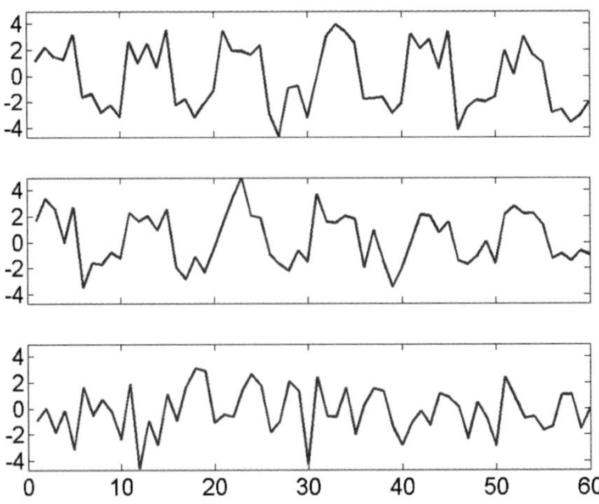

FIGURE 43.3
Simulated data for random-effects analysis. Three representative time series produced from the two-level hierarchical model. The first two time series contain stimulus-related activity but the third does not.

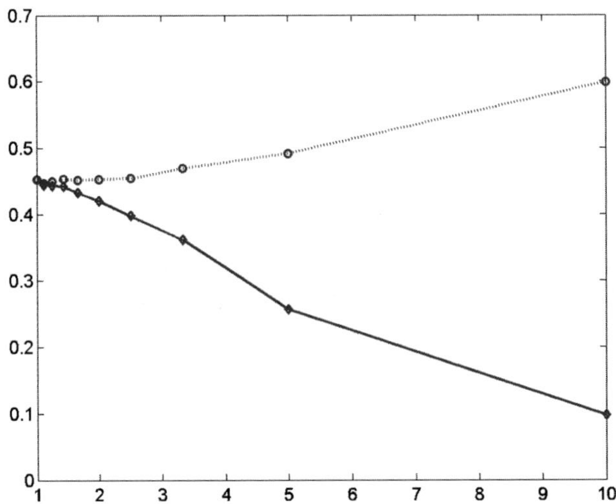

FIGURE 43.4
A plot of the error in estimating the population mean $E = < (\hat{\mu} - \mu)^2 >$ versus the observation noise level for the third subject, $\sigma_w^2(3)$, for the empirical Bayes approach (solid line) and the summary statistic approach (dotted line).

DISCUSSION

We have described Bayesian inference for some particular two-level linear Gaussian hierarchical models. A key feature of Bayesian inference in this context is that the posterior distributions are Gaussian with precisions that are the sum of the data and prior precisions and with means that are the sum of the data and prior means, each weighted according to their relative precision. With zero prior precision, two-level models reduce to a single-level model (i.e., a GLM) and Bayesian inference reduces to the familiar maximum-likelihood estimation scheme. With nonzero and, in general, unknown prior means and precisions these parameters can be estimated using PEB.

We have described two special cases of the PEB algorithm, one for equal variances and one for separable models. Both algorithms are special cases of a general approach described by Friston *et al.* (2002b) and in Chapter 47. In these contexts, we have shown that PEB automatically partitions the total degrees of freedom (i.e., number of data points) into those to be used to estimate the hyperparameters of the prior distribution and those to be used to estimate hyperparameters of the likelihood distribution.

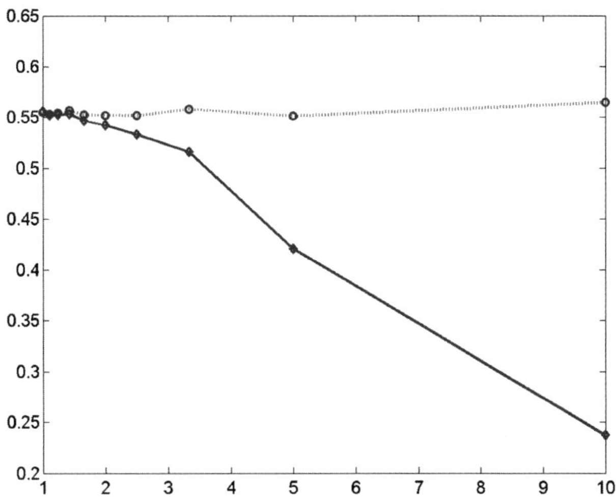

FIGURE 43.5
A plot of the estimated variance of the population mean σ_μ^2 versus the observation noise level for the third subject, $\sigma_w^2(3)$, for the empirical Bayes approach (solid line) and the summary statistic approach (dotted line).

We have shown, both theoretically and via computer simulation, that a random-effect analysis based on PEB and one based on the summary statistic approach are identical given that the first-level error variances are equal. For unequal error variances we have shown, via simulations, how the accuracy of the summary statistic approach falls off.

Finally, we have noted that the standard summary statistic approach assumes an isotropic error covariance matrix at the second level. If, however, this matrix is changed to reflect both first- and second-level covariance terms, then this "modified" summary statistic approach will give identical results to PEB. This requires that we make estimates of the nonsphericity (see Chapter 39) at the second level.

References

Berger, J. O. (1985). *Statistical Decision Theory and Bayesian Analysis.* Springer-Verlag, Berlin.

Carlin, B. P., and Louis, T. A. (2000). *Bayes and Empirical Bayes Methods for Data Analysis.* Chapman and Hall, London.

Friston, K. J., Glaser, D., Henson, R., Kiebel, S., Phillips, C., and Ashburner, J. (2002a). Classical and Bayesian inference in neuroimaging: applications. *NeuroImage* **16,** 484–512.

Friston, K. J., Penny, W., Phillips, C., Kiebel, S., Hinton, G., and Ashburner, J. (2002b). Classical and Bayesian inference in neuroimaging: theory. *NeuroImage* **16,** 465–483.

Gelman, A., Carlin, J. B., Stern, H. S., and Rubin, D. B. (1995). *Bayesian Data Analysis.* Chapman and Hall, London.

Glaser, D. E., and Friston, K. J. (2003). Pooling and covariance component estimation in SPM. Manuscript in preparation.

Holmes, A., Poline, J.-B., and Friston, K. J. (1997). Characterising brain images with the general linear model. In *Human Brain Function,* Frackowiak, R. S. J., Friston, K. J., Frith, C. D., Dolan, R. J., and Mazziotta, J. C. Eds., pp. 59–84. Academic Press, San Diego.

Jenkinson, M., Woolrich, M., Leibovici, D., Smith, S., and Beckmann, C. (2002). Group analysis in fMRI using general multi-level linear modelling. In *HBM: Eighth International Conference on Functional Mapping of the Human Brain,* Sendai, Japan, p. 417.

Lee, P. M. (1997). *Bayesian Statistics: An Introduction,* 2nd ed. John Wiley, New York.

Mackay, D. J. C. (1992). Bayesian interpolation. *Neural Computation* **4**(3), 415–447.

Penny, W. D., Holmes, A., and Friston, K. J. Random effects analysis. Technical report, In Human Brain Function II.

Winer, B. J., Brown, D. R., and Michels, K. M. (1991). *Statistical Principles in Experimental Design.* McGraw-Hill, New York.

Yandell, B. S. (1997). *Practical Data Analysis for Designed Experiments.* Chapman and Hall, London.

SECTION THREE

INFERENCE

CHAPTER

44

Introduction to Random Field Theory

INTRODUCTION

This chapter is an introduction to the multiple comparison problem in functional imaging and the way it can be solved using random field theory (RFT).

In a standard functional imaging analysis, we fit a statistical model to the data, to give us model parameters. We then use the model parameters to look for an effect we are interested in, such as the difference between a task and baseline. To do this, we usually calculate a statistic for each brain voxel that tests for the effect of interest in that voxel. The result is a large volume of statistic values.

We now need to decide if this volume shows any evidence of the effect. To do this, we have to take into account that there are many thousands of voxels and therefore many thousands of statistic values. This is the multiple comparison problem in functional imaging. *Random field theory* is a recent branch of mathematics that can be used to solve this problem.

To explain the use of RFT, we will first go back to the basics of hypothesis testing in statistics. We describe the multiple comparison problem and the usual solution, which is the Bonferroni correction. We explain why spatial correlation in imaging data causes problems for the Bonferroni correction and introduce RFT as a solution. Finally, we discuss the assumptions underlying RFT and the problems that arise when these assumptions do not hold. We hope this chapter will be accessible to those with no specific expertise in mathematics or statistics. Those more interested in mathematical details and recent developments are referred to Chapter 45.

Rejecting the Null Hypothesis

When we calculate a statistic, we often want to decide whether the statistic represents convincing evidence of the effect in which we are interested. Usually we test the statistic against the null hypothesis, which is the hypothesis that there is no effect. If the statistic is not compatible with the null hypothesis, we may conclude that there is an effect. To test against the null hypothesis, we can compare our statistical value to a *null distribution,* which is the distribution of statistic values we would expect if there were no effect. Using the null distribution, we can estimate how likely it is that our statistic could have come about by chance. We may find that the result we found has a 5% chance of resulting from a null distribution. We therefore decide to reject the null hypothesis, and accept the alternative hypothesis that there is an effect. In rejecting the null hypothesis, we must accept a 5% chance that the result has in fact arisen when there is in fact no effect, i.e., the null hypothesis is true. The value of 5% is our expected *type I* error rate, or the chance that we take that we are wrong when we reject the null hypothesis.

For example, when we do a single t test, we compare the t value we have found to the null distribution for the t statistic. Let us say we have found a t value of 2.42, and have 40 degrees of freedom. The null distribution of t statistics with 40 degrees of freedom tells us that the probability of observing a value greater than or equal to 2.42, if there is no effect, is only 0.01. In our case, we can reject the null hypothesis with a 1% risk of type I error.

The situation is more complicated in functional imaging because we have many voxels and therefore many statistic values. If we do not know where in the brain our effect will occur, our hypothesis refers to the whole volume of statistics in the brain. Evidence against the null hypothesis would be that the whole observed *volume* of values is unlikely to have arisen from a null distribution. The question we are asking is now a question about the volume, or *family* of voxel statistics, and the risk of error that we are prepared to accept is the family–wise error (FWE) rate, which is the likelihood that this family of voxel values could have arisen by chance.

We can test a family-wise null hypothesis in a variety of ways, but one useful method is to look for any statistic values that are larger than we would expect if they all had come from a null distribution. The method requires that we find a threshold to apply to every statistic value, so that any values above the threshold are unlikely to have arisen by chance. This is often referred to as *height thresholding,* and it has the advantage that if we find voxels above threshold, we can conclude that there is an effect at these voxel locations; i.e., the test has localising power. Alternative procedures based on cluster-and set-level inferences are discussed in a later section.

A height threshold that can control FWE must take into account the number of tests. We saw above that a single t-statistic value from a null distribution with 40 degrees of freedom has a 1% probability of being greater than 2.42. Now imagine our experiment has generated 1000 t values with 40 degrees of freedom. If we look at any single statistic, then by chance it will have a 1% probability of being greater than 2.42. This means that we would expect 10 t values in our sample of 1000 to be greater than 2.42. So, if we see one or more t values above 2.42 in this family of tests, this is not good evidence against the *family-wise* null hypothesis, which is that all these values have been drawn from a null distribution. We need to find a new threshold, such that, in a family of 1000 t-statistic values, there is a 1% probability of there being *one or more t* values above that threshold. The Bonferroni correction is a simple method of setting this threshold.

BONFERRONI CORRECTION

The Bonferroni correction is based on simple probability rules. Imagine we have taken our t values and used the null t distribution to convert them to probability values. We then apply a probability threshold α to each of our n probability values; in our previous example α was 0.01 and n was 1000. If all the test values are drawn from a null distribution, then each of our n probability values has a probability α of being greater than threshold. The probability of *all* tests being less than α is therefore $(1 - \alpha)^n$. The family-wise error rate (P^{FWE}) is the probability that one or more values will be greater than α, which is simply

$$P^{\text{FWE}} = 1 - (1 - \alpha)^n \tag{44.1}$$

Because α is small this can be approximated by the following simpler expression:

$$P^{\text{FWE}} \leq n\alpha \tag{44.2}$$

Using Eq. (44.2), we can find a single-voxel probability threshold α that will give us our required family-wise error rate, P^{FWE}, such that we have a P^{FWE} probability of seeing any voxel above threshold in all of the n values. We simply solve Eq. (44.2) for α:

$$\alpha = P^{\text{FWE}}/n \tag{44.3}$$

If we have a brain volume of 100,000 t statistics, all with 40 degrees of freedom, and we want a FWE rate of 0.05, then the required probability threshold for a single voxel, using the Bonferroni correction, would be 0.05/100,000 = 0.0000005. The corresponding t statistic is 5.77. If any voxel t statistic is above 5.77, then we can conclude that a voxel statistic of this magnitude has only a 5% chance of arising anywhere in a volume of 100,000 t statistics drawn from the null distribution.

The Bonferroni procedure gives a *corrected p* value; in the case above, the uncorrected p value for a voxel with a t statistic of 5.77 was 0.0000005; the p value corrected for the number of comparisons is 0.05.

The Bonferroni correction is used for calculating FWE rates for some functional imaging analyses. However, in many cases, the Bonferroni correction is too conservative because most functional imaging data have some degree of spatial correlation; i.e., there is correlation between neighbouring statistic values. In this case, there are fewer *independent* values in the statistic volume than there are voxels.

Spatial Correlation

Some degree of spatial correlation is almost universally present in functional imaging data. In general, data from any one voxel in the functional image will tend to be similar to data from nearby voxels, even after the modeled effects have been removed. Thus the errors from the statistical model will tend to be correlated for nearby voxels. The reasons for this include factors inherent in collecting the image, a physiological signal that has not been modeled, and spatial preprocessing applied to the data before statistical analysis.

For PET data, much more than for fMRI, nearby voxels are related because of the way in which the scanner collects and reconstructs the image. Thus, data that do in fact arise from a single voxel location in the brain will also cause some degree of signal change in neighbouring voxels in the resulting image. The extent to which this occurs is a measure of the performance of the PET scanner and is referred to as the *point spread function.*

Spatial preprocessing of functional data introduces spatial correlation. Typically, we will realign images for an individual subject to correct for motion during the scanning session (see Chapter 32), and may also spatially normalise a subject's brain to a template to compare data between subjects (see Chapter 33). These transformations will require the creation of new resampled images that have voxel centres that are very unlikely to be the same as those in the original images. The resampling requires that we estimate the signal for these new voxel locations from the values in the original image, and typical resampling methods require some degree of averaging of neighbouring voxels to derive the new voxel value (see Chapter 32).

It is very common to smooth the functional images before statistical analysis. A proportion of the noise in functional images is independent from voxel to voxel, whereas the signal of interest usually extends over several voxels. This is due both to the possibly distributed nature of neuronal sources and the spatially extended nature of the hemodynamic response (see Chapter 41). According to the matched filter theorem, smoothing will therefore improve the signal-to-noise ratio. For multiple-subject analyses, smoothing may also be useful for blurring the residual differences in location between corresponding areas of functional activation. Smoothing involves averaging over voxels, which will by definition increase spatial correlation.

The Bonferroni Correction and Independent Observations

Spatial correlation refers to the fact that there are fewer independent observations in the data than there are voxels. This means that the Bonferroni correction will be too conservative because the family-wise probability from Eq. (44.1) relies on the individual probability values being independent, so that we can use multiplication to calculate the probability of combined events. For Eq. (44.1), we used multiplication to calculate the probability that all tests will be below threshold with $(1 - \alpha)^n$. Thus the n in the equation must be the number of *independent* observations. If we have n voxels in our data, but there are only n_i independent observations, then Eq. (44.1) becomes $P^{\text{FWE}} = 1 - (1 - \alpha)^{n_i}$, and the corresponding α from Eq. (44.3) is given by $\alpha = P^{\text{FWE}}/n_i$. This is best illustrated by example.

Let us take a single image slice, of 100 by 100 voxels, with a t-statistic value for each voxel. For the sake of simplicity, let the t statistics have very high degrees of freedom, so that we can consider the t-statistic values as being from the normal distribution; i.e., that they are Z scores. We can simulate this slice from a null distribution by filling the voxel values with independent random numbers from the normal distribution, which results in an image such as that shown in Fig. 44.1.

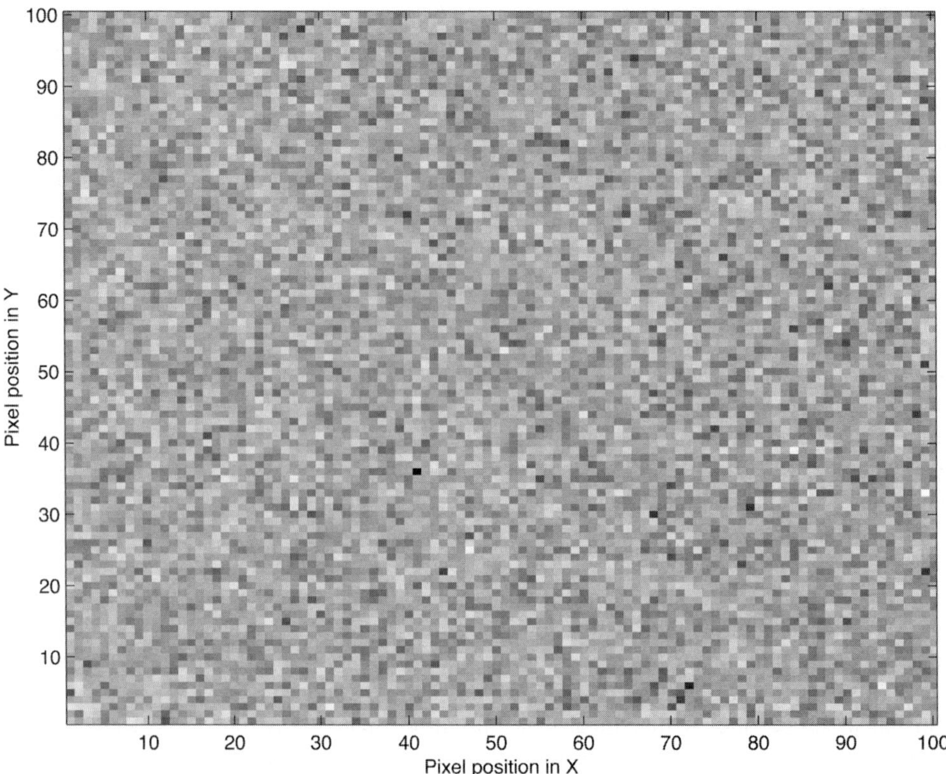

FIGURE 44.1
Simulated image slice using independent random numbers from the normal distribution. Whiter pixels are more positive.

If this image had come from the analysis of real data, we might want to test if any of the numbers in the image are more positive than is likely by chance. The values are independent, so the Bonferroni correction will give an accurate threshold. There are 10,000 Z scores, so the Bonferroni threshold, α, for a FWE rate of 0.05, is 0.05/10000 = 0.000005. This corresponds to a Z score of 4.42. Given the null hypothesis (which is true in this case), we would expect only 5 out of 100 such images to have one or more Z scores more positive than 4.42.

The situation changes if we add spatial correlation. Let us perform the following procedure on the image: Break up the image into squares of 10 by 10 pixels; for each square, calculate the mean of the 100 values contained; replace the 100 random numbers in the square by the mean value.[1] The image that results is shown in Fig. 44.2.

We still have 10,000 numbers in our image, but there are only 10 by 10 = 100 numbers that are independent. The appropriate Bonferroni correction is now 0.05/100 = 0.0005, which corresponds to a Z score of 3.29. We would expect only 5 of 100 of such images to have a square of values greater than 3.29 by chance. If we had assumed all of the values were independent, then we would have used the correction for 10,000 values, i.e., α = 0.000005. Because we actually have only 100 independent observations, Eq. (44.2), with n = 100 and α = 0.000005, tells us that we expect a FWE rate of 0.0005, which is 100 times lower (i.e., more conservative) than the rate we wanted.

Smoothing and Independent Observations

In the preceding section we replaced a square of values in the image with their mean in order to show the effect of reducing the number of independent observations. This procedure is a very simple form of smoothing. When we smooth an image with a smoothing kernel such as a Gaussian, each value in the image is replaced with a weighted average of itself and its

[1] Averaging the random numbers will make them tend to zero; to return the image to a variance of 1, we need to multiply the numbers in the image by 10; this is $\sqrt{n}$, where n is the number of values we have averaged.

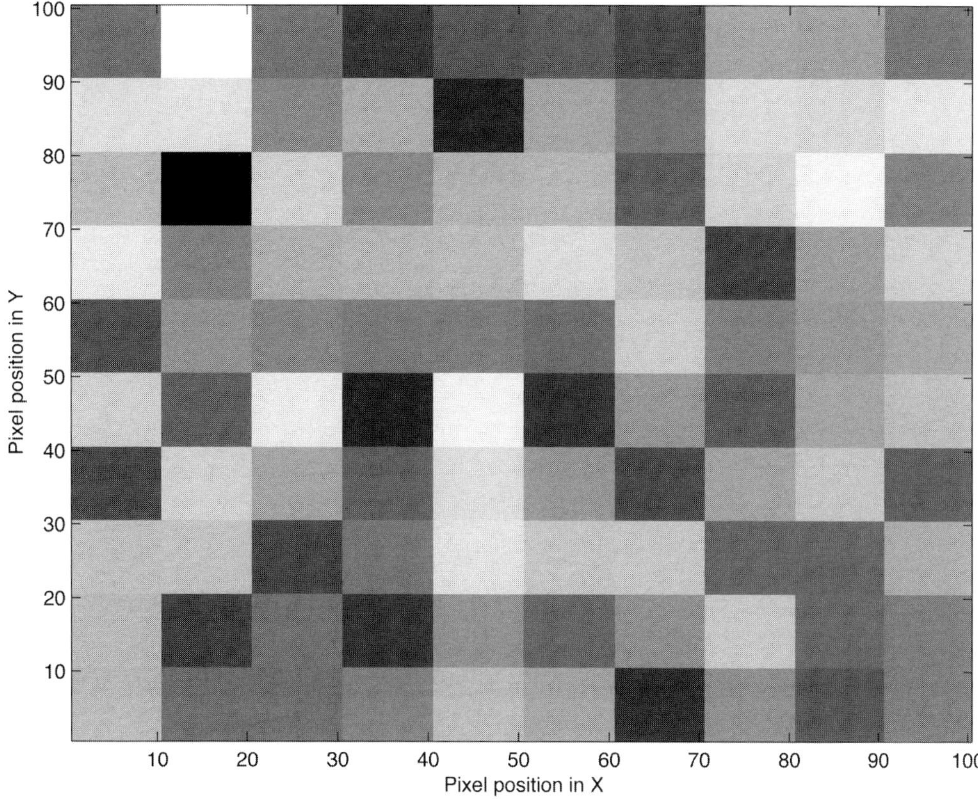

FIGURE 44.2
Random number image from Fig. 44.1 after replacing values in the 10 by 10 squares by the value of the mean within each square.

neighbours. Figure 44.3 shows the image from Fig. 44.1 after smoothing with a Gaussian kernel of full-width at half-maximum (FWHM) of 10 pixels.[2] An FWHM of 10 pixels means that, at five pixels from the center, the value of the kernel is half of its peak value. Smoothing has the effect of blurring the image and reduces the number of independent observations.

The smoothed image contains spatial correlation, which is typical of the output from the analysis of functional imaging data. We now have a problem, because there is no simple way of calculating the number of independent observations in the smoothed data, so we cannot use the Bonferroni correction. This problem can be addressed using random field theory.

RANDOM FIELD THEORY

Random field theory (RFT) is a recent body of mathematics defining theoretical results for smooth statistical maps. The theory has been versatile in dealing with many of the thresholding problems that we encounter in functional imaging. Among many other applications, it can be used to solve our problem of finding the height threshold for a smooth statistical map that gives the required family–wise error rate.

RFT solves this problem by using results that give the expected *Euler characteristic* (EC) for a smooth statistical map that has been thresholded. We discuss the EC in more detail below; for now it is only necessary to note that the expected EC leads directly to the expected number of clusters above a given threshold, and that this in turn gives the height threshold that we need.

[2] As for the procedure where we took the mean of the 100 observations in each square, the smoothed values will no longer have a variance of 1, because the averaging involved in smoothing will make the values tend to zero. As for the square example, we need to multiply the values in the smoothed image by a scale factor to return the variance to 1; the derivation of the scale factor is rather technical and not relevant to our current discussion.

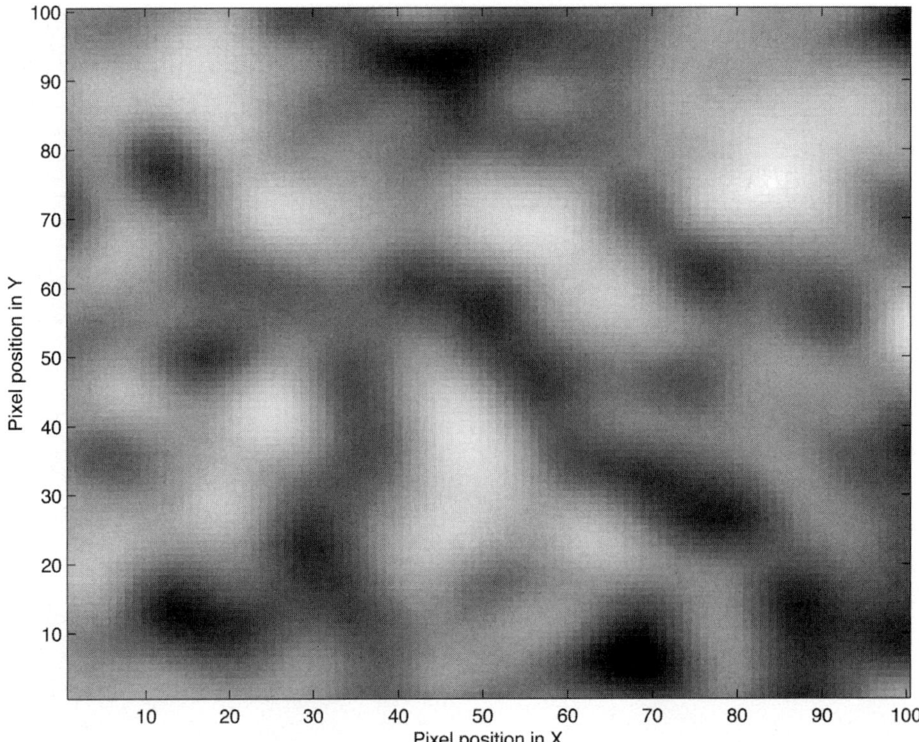

FIGURE 44.3
Random number image from Fig. 44.1 after smoothing with a Gaussian smoothing FWHM kernel of 10 pixels

The application of RFT proceeds in stages. First we estimate the smoothness (spatial correlation) of our statistical map. Then we use the smoothness values in the appropriate RFT equation, to give the expected EC at different thresholds. This allows us to calculate the threshold at which we would expect 5% of equivalent statistical maps arising under the null hypothesis to contain at least one area above threshold.

Smoothness and Resels

Usually we do not know the smoothness of our statistical map. This is so even if the map resulted from smoothed data, because we usually do not know the extent of spatial correlation in the underlying data before smoothing. If we do not know the smoothness, it can be calculated using the observed spatial correlation in the images. For our example (Fig. 44.3), however, we *know* the smoothness, because the data were independent before smoothing. In this case, the smoothness results entirely from the smoothing we have applied. The smoothness can be expressed as the width of the smoothing kernel, which was 10 pixels FWHM in the x and y direction. We can use the FWHM to calculate the number of *resels* in the image. *Resel* was a term introduced by Worsley *et al.* (1992), and is a measure of the number of "resolution elements" in the statistical map. This can be thought of as *similar to* the number of independent observations, but it is not the same, as we will see below. A resel is simply defined as a block of values (in our case, pixels) that is the same size as the FWHM. For the image in Fig. 44.3, the FWHMs were 10 by 10 pixels, so that a resel is a block of 100 pixels. Because there are 10,000 pixels in our image, there are 100 resels. Note that the number of resels depends only on the smoothness (FWHM) and the number of pixels.

The Euler Characteristic

The Euler characteristic is a property of an image after it has been thresholded. For our purposes, the EC can be thought of as the number of blobs in an image after thresholding. For example,

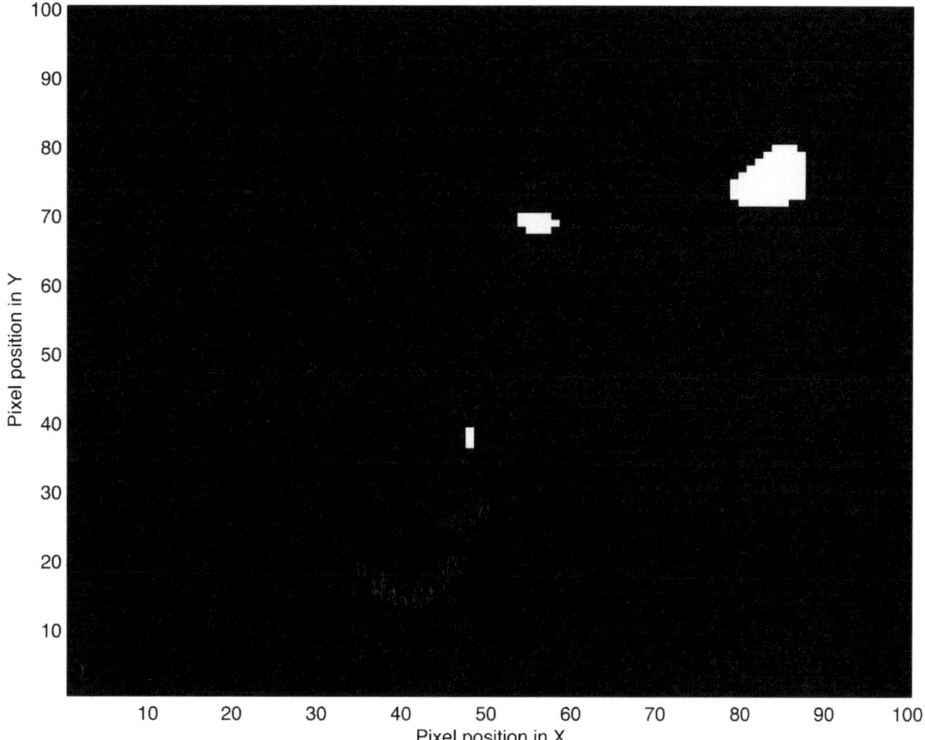

FIGURE 44.4
Smoothed random number image from Fig. 44.3 after thresholding at $Z = 2.5$. Values less than 2.5 have been set to zero (displayed as black). The remaining values have been set to one (displayed as white).

we can threshold our smoothed image (Fig. 44.3) at $Z = 2.5$; all pixels with Z scores of less than 2.5 are set to zero, and the rest are set to one. This results in the image shown in Fig. 44.4.

There are three white blobs in Fig. 44.4, corresponding to three areas with Z scores higher than 2.5. The EC of this image is therefore 3. If we increase the Z-score threshold to 2.75, we find that the two central blobs disappear—because the Z scores were less than 2.75 (Fig. 44.5).

The area in the upper right of the image remains; the EC of the image in Fig. 44.5 is therefore one. At high thresholds the EC is either one or zero. Hence, the average or expected EC, written **E**[EC], corresponds (approximately) to the probability of finding an above threshold blob in our statistic image. That is, the probability of a family wise error is approximately equivalent to the expected Euler characteristic, $P^{FWE} \approx \mathbf{E}[EC]$.

It turns out that if we know the number of resels in our image, it is possible to calculate **E**[EC] at any given threshold. For an image of two dimensions, **E**[EC] is given by Worsley *et al.* (1992). If R is the number of resels and Z_t is the Z-score threshold, then:

$$\mathbf{E}[EC] = R(4 \log_e 2)\,(2\pi)^{-\frac{3}{2}} Z_t e^{-\frac{1}{2} Z_t^2} \quad (44.4)$$

Figure 44.6 shows **E**[EC] for an image of 100 resels, for Z-score thresholds between zero and five. As the threshold drops from one to zero, **E**[EC] drops to zero; this is because the precise definition of the EC is more complex than simply the number of blobs (Worsley *et al.*, 1996). This makes a difference at low thresholds but is not relevant for our purposes because, as explained above, we are only interested in the properties of **E**[EC] at high thresholds, i.e., when it approximates P^{FWE}.

Note also that the graph in Fig. 44.6 does a reasonable job of predicting the EC in our image; at a Z threshold of 2.5 it predicted an EC of 1.9, when we observed a value of 3; at $Z = 2.75$ it predicted an EC of 1.1, for an observed EC of 1.

We can now apply RFT to our smoothed image (Fig. 44.3), which has 100 resels. For 100 resels, Eq. (44.4) gives an **E**[EC] of 0.049 for a Z threshold of 3.8 (cf. the graph in Fig. 44.6). If we have a two-dimensional image with 100 resels, then the probability of getting one or more

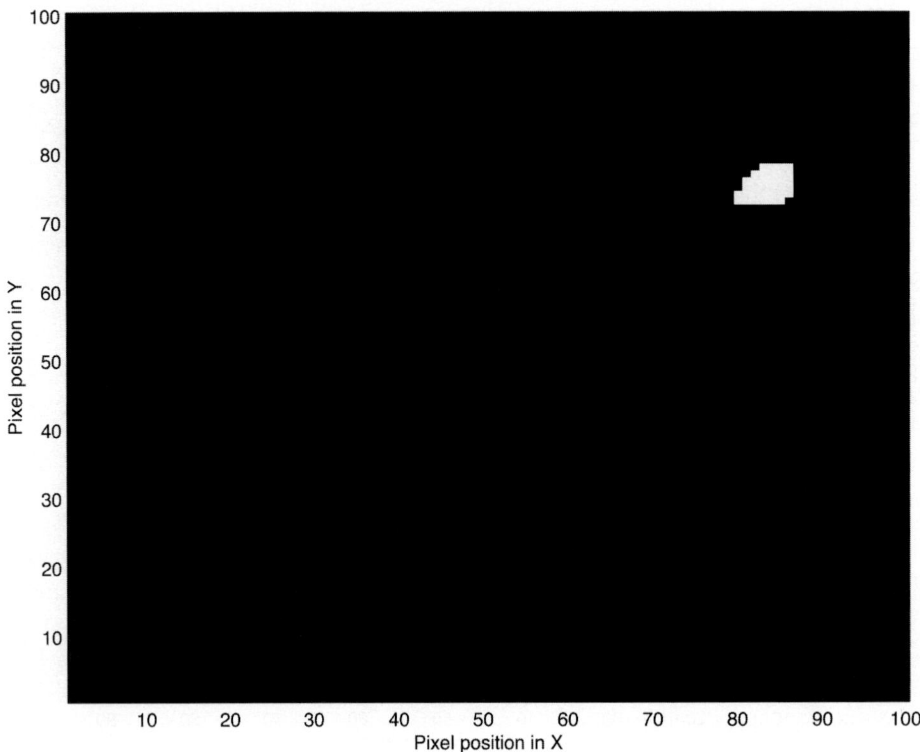

FIGURE 44.5
Smoothed random number image from Fig. 44.3 after thresholding at $Z = 2.75$. Values less than 2.75 have been set to zero (displayed as black). The remaining values have been set to one (displayed as white).

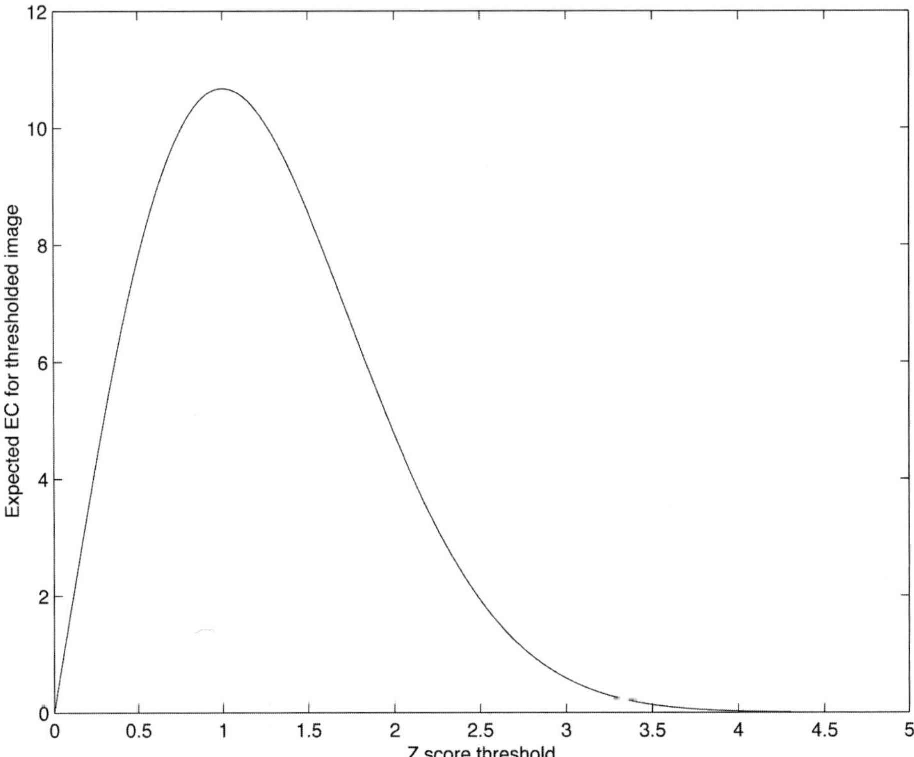

FIGURE 44.6
Expected EC values for an image of 100 resels.

blobs where Z is greater than 3.8 is 0.049. We can use this for thresholding. Let x be the Z-score threshold that gives an **E**[EC] of 0.05. If we threshold our image at x, we can conclude that any blobs that remain have a probability of less than or equal to 0.05 that they have occurred by chance. From Eq. (44.4), the threshold, x, depends only on the number of resels in our image.

Random Field Thresholds and the Bonferroni Correction

The random field correction derived using the EC is not the same as a Bonferroni correction for the number of resels. We stated above that the resel count in an image is not exactly the same as the number of independent observations. If it was the same, then instead of using RFT, we could use a Bonferroni correction based on the number of resels. However, these two corrections give different answers. For $\alpha = 0.05$, the Z threshold according to RFT, for our 100 resel image, is $Z = 3.8$. The Bonferroni threshold for 100 independent tests is 0.05/100, which equates to a Z score of 3.3. Although the RFT math gives us a correction that is similar in principle to a Bonferroni correction, it is not the same. If the assumptions of RFT are met (see "Discussion" section), then the RFT threshold is more accurate than the Bonferroni.

Random Fields and Functional Imaging

Analyses of functional imaging data usually lead to three-dimensional statistical images. So far we have discussed the application of RFT to an image of two dimensions, but the same principles apply in three dimensions. The EC is the number of 3D blobs of Z scores above a certain threshold and a resel is a cube of voxels of size (FWHM in x) by (FWHM in y) by (FWHM in z). The equation for **E**[EC] is different in the 3-D case, but still depends only on the resels in the image.

For the sake of simplicity, we have only considered a random field of Z scores, i.e., numbers drawn from the normal distribution. There are now equivalent results for t, F, and χ^2 random fields (Worsley, 1994). For example, SPM99 software uses formulas for t and F random fields to calculate corrected thresholds for height.

As noted earlier, we usually do not know the smoothness of a statistic volume from a functional imaging analysis, because we do not know the extent of spatial correlation before smoothing. We cannot assume that the smoothness is the same as any explicit smoothing that we have applied and will need to calculate smoothness from the images themselves. In practice, smoothness is calculated using the residual values from the statistical analysis as described in Kiebel *et al.* (1999) and Worsley *et al.* (1999).

Small Volume Correction

We noted above that the results for the expected Euler characteristic depend only on the number of resels contained in the volume of voxels we are analyzing. This is not strictly accurate, although it is a very close approximation when the voxel volume is large compared to the size of a resel (Worsley *et al.*, 1996). In fact, **E**[EC] also depends on the shape and size of the volume. The shape of the volume becomes important when we have a small or oddly shaped region. This is unusual if we are analyzing statistics from the whole brain, but there are often situations where we wish to restrict our search to a smaller subset of the volume, for example, where we have a specific hypothesis as to where our signal is likely to occur.

The reason the shape of the volume may influence the correction is best explained by example. Let us return to the 2-D image of smoothed random numbers (Fig. 44.3). We could imagine that we had reason to believe that signal change will occur only in the center of the image. Our search region will not be the whole image, but might be a box at the image center, with size 30 by 30 pixels (see Fig. 44.7).

The box contains 9 resels. Figure 44.7 shows a grid of X-shaped markers; these are spaced at the width of a resel, i.e., 10 pixels. The box can contain a maximum of 16 of these markers. Now let us imagine we had a more unusually shaped search region. For some reason we might expect that our signal of interest will occur within a frame 2.5 pixels wide around the outside of the image. The frame contains the same number of voxels as the box and, therefore, has the same volume in terms of resels. However, the frame contains many more markers (32), so the frame

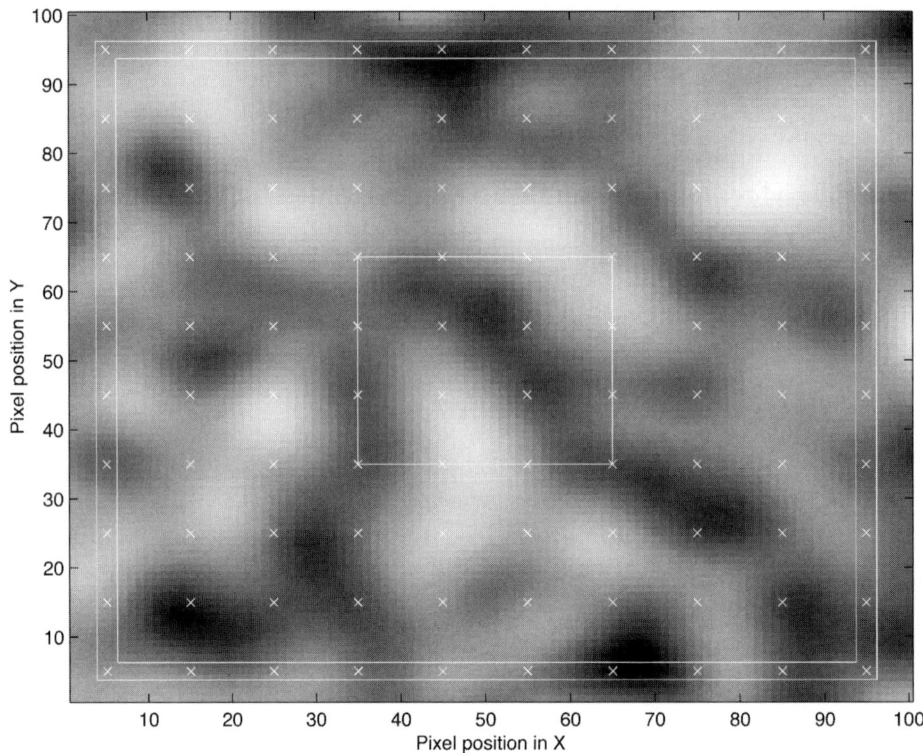

FIGURE 44.7
Smoothed random number image from Fig. 44.3 with two-example search regions: a box (center) and a frame (outer border of image). X-shaped markers are spaced at one-resel widths across the image.

is sampling from the data of more resels than the box. Multiple comparison correction for the frame must therefore be more stringent than for the box.

In fact, **E**[EC] depends on the volume, surface area, and diameter of the search region (Worsley *et al.,* 1996). These parameters can be calculated for continuous shapes for which formulas are available for volume, surface area, and diameter, such as spheres or boxes. Otherwise, the parameters can be estimated from any shape that has been defined in an image. Restricting the search region to a small volume within a statistical map can lead to greatly reduced thresholds for given FWE rates. For Fig. 44.8, we assumed a statistical analysis that resulted in a t-statistic map with 8-mm smoothness in the x, y, and z directions. The t statistic has 200 degrees of freedom, and we have a spherical search region. The graph shows the t-statistic value that gives a corrected p value of 0.05 for spheres of increasing radius.

For a sphere of zero radius, the threshold is simply that for a single t statistic (uncorrected = corrected $p = 0.05$ for $t = 1.65$ with 200 degrees of freedom). The corrected t threshold increases sharply as the radius increases to $\approx$10 mm, and less steeply thereafter.

Uncorrected p Values and Regional Hypotheses

When making inferences about regional effects (e.g., activations) in SPMs, one often has some idea about where the activation should be. In this instance a correction for the entire search volume is inappropriate.

If the hypothesised region contained a single voxel, then inference could be made using an uncorrected p value (because there is no extra search volume to correct for). In practice, however, the hypothesised region will usually contain many voxels and can be characterised, for example, using spheres or boxes centered on the region of interest, and we must therefore use a p value that has been appropriately corrected. As described in the previous section, this corrected p value will depend on the size and shape of the hypothesised region and the smoothness of the statistic image.

Some research groups have used uncorrected p-value thresholds, such as $p < 0.001$, in order to control FWE when there is a regional hypothesis of where the activation will occur. This

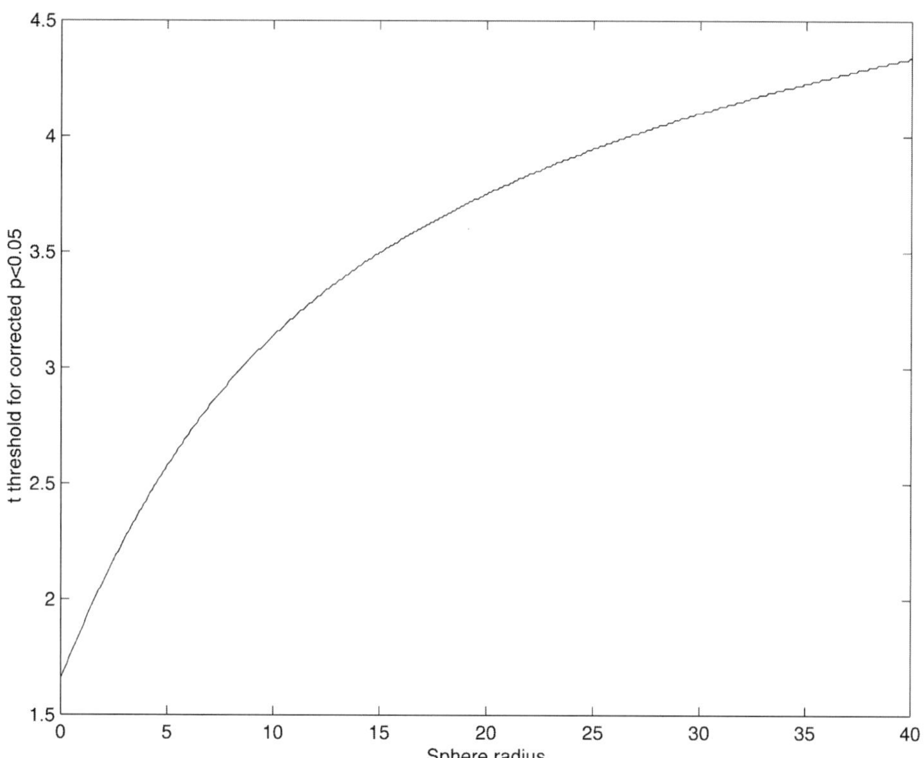

FIGURE 44.8
The t threshold giving a FWE rate of 0.05 for spheres of increasing radius. Smoothness was 8 mm in x, y, and z directions, and the example analysis had 200 degrees of freedom.

approach gives unquantified error control, however, because any hypothesised region is likely to contain more than a single voxel. For example, for 8-mm smoothness, a spherical region with a radius greater than 6.7 mm will require an uncorrected p-value threshold of less than 0.001 for a FWE rate ≤ 0.05. For a sphere of radius 15 mm, an uncorrected p-value threshold of 0.001 gives an **E**[EC] of 0.36, so there is approximately a 36% chance of seeing one or more voxels above threshold even if the null hypothesis is true.

DISCUSSION

In this chapter we have focussed on voxel-level inference based on height thresholds to ask the question "Is activation at a given voxel significantly nonzero?" More generally, however, voxel-level inference can be placed in a larger framework involving cluster-level and set-level inference. These require height and spatial extent thresholds to be specified by the user. Corrected p values can then be derived that pertain to (1) the number of activated regions (i.e., number of clusters above the height and volume threshold)—set-level inferences, (2) the number of activated voxels (i.e., volume) comprising a particular region—cluster-level inferences, and (3) the p value for each voxel within that cluster—voxel-level inferences. These p values are corrected for the multiple dependent comparisons and are based on the probability of obtaining c, or more, clusters with k, or more, voxels, above a threshold u in an SPM of known or estimated smoothness. Chapter 46, for example, describes cluster-level inference in a PET auditory stimulation study. Set-level inferences can be more powerful than cluster-level inferences, and cluster-level inferences can be more powerful than voxel-level inferences. The price paid for this increased sensitivity is reduced localising power. Voxel-level tests permit individual voxels to be identified as significant, whereas cluster- and set-level inferences only allow clusters or sets of clusters to be declared significant. Remember that these conclusions, about the relative power of different inference levels, are based on distributed activations. Focal activation may well be detected with greater sensitivity using voxel-level tests based on peak height. Typically, people use voxel-level inferences and a spatial extent threshold of zero. This reflects the fact that characterisations of functional anatomy are generally more useful when specified with a high degree of anatomical precision.

Two assumptions underlie RFT. The first is that the error fields are a reasonable lattice approximation to an underlying random field with a multivariate Gaussian distribution. The second is that these fields are continuous, with a twice-differentiable autocorrelation function. A common misconception is that the autocorrelation function has to be Gaussian. But this is not the case.

If the data have been sufficiently smoothed and the general linear models correctly specified (so that the errors are indeed Gaussian), then the RFT assumptions will be met. One scenario in which the assumptions may not be met, however, is in a random effects analysis (see Chapter 42) with a small number of subjects. This is because the resulting error fields will not be very smooth and so may violate the "reasonable lattice approximation" assumption. One solution is to reduce the voxel size by subsampling. Alternatively, one can turn to different inference procedures. One such alternative is the nonparametric framework described in Chapter 46 where, for example, inference on statistic images with low degrees of freedom can be improved with the use of pseudo-t statistics, which are much smoother than the corresponding t statistics.

Other inference frameworks are the false discovery rate (FDR) approach and Bayesian inference. While RFT controls the family-wise error, the probability of reporting a false positive anywhere in the volume, FDR controls the proportion of false positives among those that are declared positive. This very different approach is discussed in the next chapter. Finally, Chapter 47 introduces Bayesian inference where, instead of focussing on how unlikely the data are under a null hypothesis, inferences are made on the basis of a posterior distribution that characterises our parameter uncertainty without reference to a null distribution.

Literature

The mathematical basis of RFT is described in a series of peer-reviewed articles in statistical journals (Cao and Worsley, 1999; Sigmund and Worsley, 1995; Worsley, 1994, 1995, 1996). The core paper for RFT as applied to functional imaging is by Worsley *et al.* (1996). This provides estimates of p values for local maxima of Gaussian, t, χ^2, and F fields over search regions of any shape or size in any number of dimensions. This unifies earlier results on 2D (Friston *et al.,* 1991) and 3D (Worsley *et al.,* 1992) images.

The above analysis requires an estimate of the smoothness of the images. Poline *et al.* (1995) estimate the dependence of the resulting SPMs on the estimate of this parameter. Whilst the applied smoothness is usually fixed, Worsley *et al.* (1995) propose a scale-space procedure for assessing the significance of activations over a range of proposed smoothings. Kiebel *et al.* (1999) implement an unbiased smoothness estimator for Gaussian t fields and Gaussianised t fields. Worsley *et al.* (1999) derive a further improved estimator that takes into account some nonstationarity of the statistic field.

Another approach to assessing significance is based, not on the height of activity, but on spatial extent (Friston *et al.,* 1994), as described in the previous section. Friston *et al.* (1995) consider a hierarchy of tests that are regarded as voxel-level, cluster-level, and set-level inferences. If the approximate location of an activation can be specified in advance, then the significance of the activation can be assessed using the spatial extent or volume of the nearest activated region (Friston, 1997). This test is particularly elegant because it does not require a correction for multiple comparisons.

More recent developments in applying RFT to neuroimaging are described in the following chapter. Finally, we refer readers to an online resource, http://www.mrc-cbu.cam.ac.uk/Imaging/randomfields.html, from which much of the material in this chapter was collated.

References

Cao, J., and Worsley, K. J. (1999). The detection of local shape changes via the geometry of Hotelling's T^2 fields. *Ann. Statistics* **27**(3), 925–942.

Friston, K. J. (1997). Testing for anatomically specified regional effects. *Hum. Brain Mapping* **5,** 133–136.

Friston, K. J., Frith, C. D., Liddle, P. F., and Frackowiak, R. S. J. (1991). Comparing functional (PET) images: the assessment of significant change. *J. Cereb. Blood Flow Metab.* **11,** 690–699.

Friston, K. J., Worsley, K. J., Frackowiak, R. S. J., Mazziotta, J. C., and Evans, A. C. (1994). Assessing the significance of focal activations using their spatial extent. *Hum. Brain Mapping* **1,** 214–220.

Friston, K. J., Holmes, A., Poline, J.-B., Price, C. J., and Frith, C. D. (1995). Detecting activations in PET and fMRI: levels of inference and power. *NeuroImage* **40,** 223–235.

Kiebel, S. J., Poline, J.-B., Friston, K. J., Holmes, A. P., and Worsley, K. J. (1999). Robust smoothness estimation in statistical parametric maps using standardised residuals from the general linear model. *NeuroImage* **10,** 756–766.

Poline, J.-B., Friston, K. J., Worsley, K. J., and Frackowiak, R. S. J. (1995). Estimating smoothness in statistical parametric maps: Confidence intervals on *p*-values. *J. Comput. Assist. Tomogr.* **19**(5), 788–796.

Sigmund, D. O., and Worsley, K. J. (1995). Testing for a signal with unknown location and scale in a stationary Gaussian random field. *Ann. Statistics* **23,** 608–639.

Worsley, K. J. (1994). Local maxima and the expected Euler characteristic of excursion sets of χ^2, F and t fields. *Adv. Appl. Prob.* **26,** 13–42.

Worsley, K. J. (1995). Estimating the number of peaks in a random field using the Hadwiger characteristic of excursion sets, with applications to medical images. *Ann. Statistics* **23,** 640–669.

Worsley, K. J. (1996). The geometry of random images. *Chance* **9**(1), 27–40.

Worsley, K. J., Evans, A. C., Marrett, S., and Neelin, P. (1992). A three dimensional statistical analysis for CBF activation studies in the human brain. *J. Cereb. Blood Flow Metab.* **12,** 900–918.

Worsley, K. J., Marrett, S., Neelin, P., Vandal, A. C., Friston, K. J., and Evans, A. C. (1995). Searching scale space for activation in PET images. *Hum. Brain Mapping* **4,** 74–90.

Worsley, K. J., Marrett, S., Neelin, P., Vandal, A. C., Friston, K. J., and Evans, A. C. (1996). A unified statistical approach for determining significant voxels in images of cerebral activation. *Hum. Brain Mapping* **4,** 58–73.

Worsley, K. J., Andermann, M., Koulis, T., MacDonald, D., and Evans, A. C. (1999). Detecting changes in nonisotropic images. *Hum. Brain Mapping* **8,** 98–101.

CHAPTER

45

Developments in Random Field Theory

Random field theory is used in the statistical analysis of SPMs whenever there is a spatial component to the inference. Most important is the question of detecting an effect or activation at an unknown spatial location. Very often we do not know in advance where to look for an effect, and we are interested in searching either the whole brain or part of it. This presents special statistical problems related to the problem of multiple comparisons, or multiple tests. Two methods have been proposed, the first based on the maximum of the T or F statistic, the second based on the spatial extent of the region where these statistics exceed some threshold value. Both involve results from random field theory (Adler, 1981).

MAXIMUM TEST STATISTIC

An obvious method is to select those locations where a test statistic Z (which could be a T, χ^2, F, or Hotelling's T^2 statistic) is large, that is, to threshold the image of Z at a height z. The problem is then to choose the threshold z such that it exclude false positives with a high probability, say, 0.95. Setting z to the usual (uncorrected) $P = 0.05$ critical value of Z (1.64 in the Gaussian case) means that 5% of the unactivated parts of the brain will show false positives. We need to raise z so that the probability of finding any activation in the nonactivated regions is 0.05. This is a type of multiple comparison problem, since we are testing the hypothesis of no activation at a very large number of voxels.

A simple solution is to apply a Bonferroni correction. The probability of detecting any activation in the unactivated locations is bounded by assuming that the unactivated locations cover the entire search region. By the Bonferroni inequality, the probability of detecting any activation is further bounded by

$$P(\max Z > z) \leq N\, P(Z > z) \qquad (45.1)$$

where the maximum is taken over all N voxels in the search region. For a $P = 0.05$ test of Gaussian statistics, critical thresholds of 4–5 are common. This procedure is conservative if the image is smooth, although for fMRI data it often gives very accurate thresholds.

Random field theory gives a less conservative (lower) P value if the image is smooth:

$$P(\max Z > z) \approx \sum_{d=0}^{D} \text{resels}_d \text{EC}_d(z) \qquad (45.2)$$

where D is the number of dimensions of the search region, resels_d is the number of d-dimensional resels (resolution elements) in the search region, and $\text{EC}_d(z)$ is the d-dimensional Euler characteristic density. Approximation (45.2) is based on the fact that the left-hand side is the exact expectation of the Euler characteristic of the region above the threshold z. The Euler characteristic counts the number of clusters if the region has no holes, which is likely to be the case if z is large. Details can be found in Worsley *et al.* (1996a).

Approximation (45.2) is accurate for search regions of any size or shape, even a single point, but it is best for search regions that are not too concave. Sometimes it is better to surround a highly convoluted search region, such as gray matter, by a convex hull with slightly higher volume but less surface area, to get a lower and more accurate P value.

For large search regions, the last term ($d = D$) is the most important. The number of resels is

$$\text{resels}_D = V/\text{FWHM}^D$$

where V is the volume of the search region and FWHM is the effective full-width at half-maximum of a Gaussian kernel used to smooth the data (see Chapter 14). The corresponding EC density for a T statistic image with ν degrees of freedom is

$$\text{EC}_3(z) = \frac{(4\log_e 2)^{\frac{3}{2}}}{(2\pi)^2}\left(\frac{\nu-1}{\nu}z^2 - 1\right)\left(1 + \frac{z^2}{\nu}\right)^{-\frac{1}{2}(\nu-1)}$$

For small search regions, the lower dimensional terms $d < D$ become important. However, the P value of (45.2) is not very sensitive to the shape of the search region, so that assuming a spherical search region gives a very good approximation.

Figure 45.1 shows the threshold z for a $P = 0.05$ test calculated by the two methods. If the FWHM is small relative to the voxel size, then the Bonferroni threshold is actually less than the random field one of (45.2). In practice, it is better to take the minimum of the the two thresholds, (45.1) and (45.2).

EC densities for F fields can be found in Worsley *et al.* (1996a), and for Hotelling's T^2, see Cao and Worsley (1999a). Similar results are also available for correlation random fields, useful for detecting functional connectivity; see Cao and Worsley (1999b).

Extensions of the result of (45.2) to scale-space random fields are given in Worsley *et al.* (1996b). Here the search is over all spatial filter widths as well as over location, so that the width of the signal is estimated as well as its location. The price to pay is an increase in the critical threshold of about 0.5.

MAXIMUM SPATIAL EXTENT OF THE TEST STATISTIC

An alternative test can be based on the spatial extent of clusters of connected components of supra-threshold voxels where $Z > z$ (Friston *et al.*, 1994). Typically z is chosen to be about 3 for

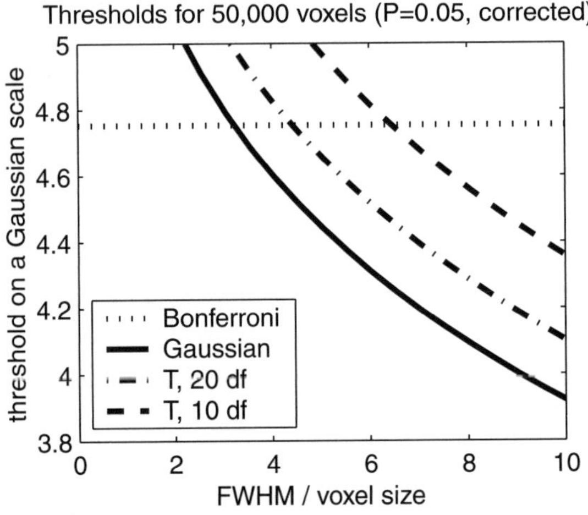

FIGURE 45.1
Thresholds for a volume with $N = 50{,}000$ voxels ($P = 0.05$, corrected). Note that if the FWHM is less than 3.2 voxels, then the Bonferroni method is better than the random field method for a Gaussian statistic. For T statistics with $\nu = 20$ df, this limit is higher (4.4), and much higher (14.4—off the scale) with $\nu = 10$ df.

a Gaussian random field. Once again the image must be a smooth stationary random field. The idea is to approximate the shape of the image by a quadratic with a peak at the local maximum. For a Gaussian random field, the spatial extent S is then approximated by the volume where the quadratic of height H above z cuts the threshold z:

$$S \approx cH^{D/2} \tag{45.3}$$

where

$$c = \text{FWHM}^D(2\pi/z)^{D/2}(4 \log 2)^{-D/2}/\ \Gamma(D/2 + 1)$$

For large z, the upper tail probability of H is well approximated by

$$P(H > h) = P(\max Z > z + h)/P(\max Z > z) \approx \exp(-zh) \tag{45.4}$$

from which we conclude that H has an approximate exponential distribution with mean $1/z$. From this we can find the approximate P value of the spatial extent S of a single cluster:

$$P(S > s) \approx \exp[-z(s/c)^{2/D}] \tag{45.5}$$

The P value for the largest spatial extent is obtained by a simple Bonferroni correction for the expected number of clusters K:

$$P(\max S > s) \approx E(K)\ P(S > s), \quad \text{where } E(K) \approx P(\max Z > z) \tag{45.6}$$

from (45.2).

We can substantially improve the value of the constant c by equating the expected total spatial extent, given by $V\,P(Z > z)$, to that obtained by summing up the spatial extents of all the clusters $S_1,\ldots,S_K$:

$$V\,P(Z > z) = E(S_1 + \ldots + S_K) = E(K)\ E(S)$$

Using the fact that

$$E(S) \approx c\Gamma(D/2 + 1)/z^{D/2}$$

from (45.3), and the expected number of clusters from (45.2), it follows that

$$c \approx \text{FWHM}^D z^{D/2} P(Z > z)/[EC_D(z)\ \Gamma(D/2 + 1)]$$

Cao (1999) has extended these results to T, χ^2, and F fields, but unfortunately there are no theoretical results for nonsmooth fields such as raw fMRI data.

SEARCHING IN SMALL REGIONS

For small prespecified search regions such as the cingulate, the P values for the maximum test statistic are very well estimated by (45.2), but the results in the preceding section only apply to large search regions. Friston (1997) has proposed a fascinating method that avoids the awkward problem of prespecifying a small search region altogether. We threshold the image of test statistics at z, then simply pick the nearest peak to a point or region of interest. The clever part is this. Since we have identified this peak based only on its spatial location and not based on its height or extent, there is now no need to correct for searching over all peaks. Hence, the P value for its spatial extent S is simply $P(S > s)$ from (45.5), and the P value for its peak height H above z is simply $P(H > h)$ from Eq. (45.4).

ESTIMATING THE FWHM

The only data-dependent component required for setting the above thresholds is resels$_D$ and, indirectly, the FWHM. The FWHM often depends on the location: fMRI data are considerably smoother in cortex than white matter (see Fig. 45.2), and for VBM data FWHM varies considerably from one location to another. This means that the random field is not isotropic, so the above random field theory is not valid. Fortunately, there is a simple way of allowing for this by estimating the FWHM separately at each voxel.

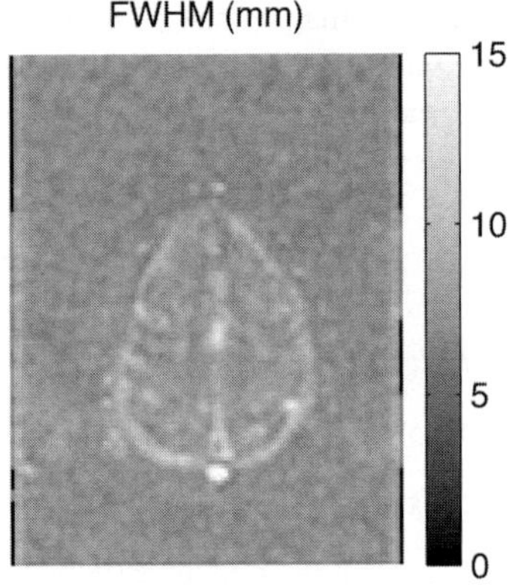

FIGURE 45.2
The estimated FWHM for one slice of fMRI data. Note the ~6-mm FWHM outside the brain due to smoothing imposed by motion correction. The FWHM in cortex is much higher, ~10 mm, while white matter is lower, ~6 mm.

Let $\mathbf{r}$ be the n-vector of least-squares residuals from the (possibly whitened) linear model fitted at each voxel, and let $\mathbf{u}$ be the vector of normalised residuals $\mathbf{u} = \mathbf{r}/(\mathbf{r}'\mathbf{r})^{1/2}$. Let $\dot{\mathbf{u}}$ be the $n \times 3$ spatial derivative of $\mathbf{u}$ in the three-orthogonal directions of the voxel lattice. The estimated FWHM is

$$\widehat{\text{FWHM}} = (4 \log 2)^{1/2} |\dot{\mathbf{u}}'\dot{\mathbf{u}}|^{-1/(2D)} \tag{45.7}$$

and the estimated resels_D is

$$\widehat{\text{resels}_D} = \sum_{\text{volume}} v\widehat{\text{FWHM}}^{-D}$$

where summation is over all voxels in the search region and v is the volume of a single voxel (Worsley *et al.*, 1998). The extra randomness added by estimating resels_D can be ignored if the search region is large.

However, spatially varying FWHM can have a strong effect on the validity of the P value for spatial extent. If the cluster is in a region where FWHM is large, then its extent will be larger by chance alone, and so its P value will be too small. In other words, clusters will look more significant in smooth regions than in rough regions of the image. To correct for this, we simply replace cluster volume by cluster resels, defined as follows:

$$\tilde{S} = \sum_{\text{cluster}} v\widehat{\text{FWHM}}^{-D}$$

where summation is over all voxels in the cluster.

There is one remaining problem: since the above summation is over a small cluster, rather than a large search region, the randomness in estimating FWHM now makes a significant contribution to the randomness of $\tilde{S}$, and hence its P value. Worsley (2002) suggests allowing for this by the approximation

$$\tilde{S} \approx \tilde{c} H^{D/2} \prod_{k=1}^{D+1} X_k^{p_k} \tag{45.8}$$

where $X_1,\ldots, X_{D+1}$ are independent χ^2 random variables. The degrees of freedom of X_k is $\nu - k + 1$ where $\nu = n - p$ and p is the number of regressors in the linear model, raised to the power $p_k = -D/2$ if $k = 1$ and $p_k = 1/2$ if $k > 1$. Again the constant $\tilde{c}$ is chosen so that the expected total resels of all clusters matches the probability of exceeding the threshold times the volume of the search region

$$\tilde{c} \approx z^{D/2} P(Z > z)/[EC_D(z)\, \Gamma\, (D/2 + 1)]$$

Combining this with the approximate distributions of spatial extents for T, χ^2, and F fields from Cao (1999) requires no extra computational effort. H is replaced by a beta random variable in (45.8), multiplied by powers of yet more χ^2 random variables, with appropriate adjustments to $\tilde{c}$.

In practice, the distribution function of $\tilde{S}$ is best calculated by first taking logarithms, so that log S is then a sum of independent random variables. The density of a sum is the convolution of the densities, whose Fourier transform is the sum of the Fourier transforms. It is easier to find the upper tail probability of log $\tilde{S}$ by replacing the density of one of the random variables by its upper tail probability *before* doing the convolution. The obvious choice is the exponential or beta random variable, since its upper tail probability has a simple closed-form expression. This method has been implemented in the stat_threshold.m function of fmristat, available from http://www.math.mcgill.ca/keith/fmristat.

FALSE DISCOVERY RATE

A remarkable breakthrough in multiple testing was made by Benjamini and Hochberg in 1995 who took a completely different approach. Instead of controlling the probability of ever reporting a false positive, they devised a procedure for controlling the *false discovery rate* (FDR), the expected proportion of false positives among those voxels declared positive (the *discoveries*) (see Fig. 45.3). The procedure is extremely simple to implement. Simply calculate the uncorrected P value for each voxel and order them so that the ordered P values are $P_1 \leq P_2 \leq \ldots \leq P_N$. To control the FDR at α, find the largest value k so that $P_k < \alpha k/N$. This procedure is conservative if the voxels are positively dependent, which is a reasonable assumption for most unsmoothed or smoothed imaging data. See Genovese *et al.* (2002) for an application of this method to fMRI data and for further references.

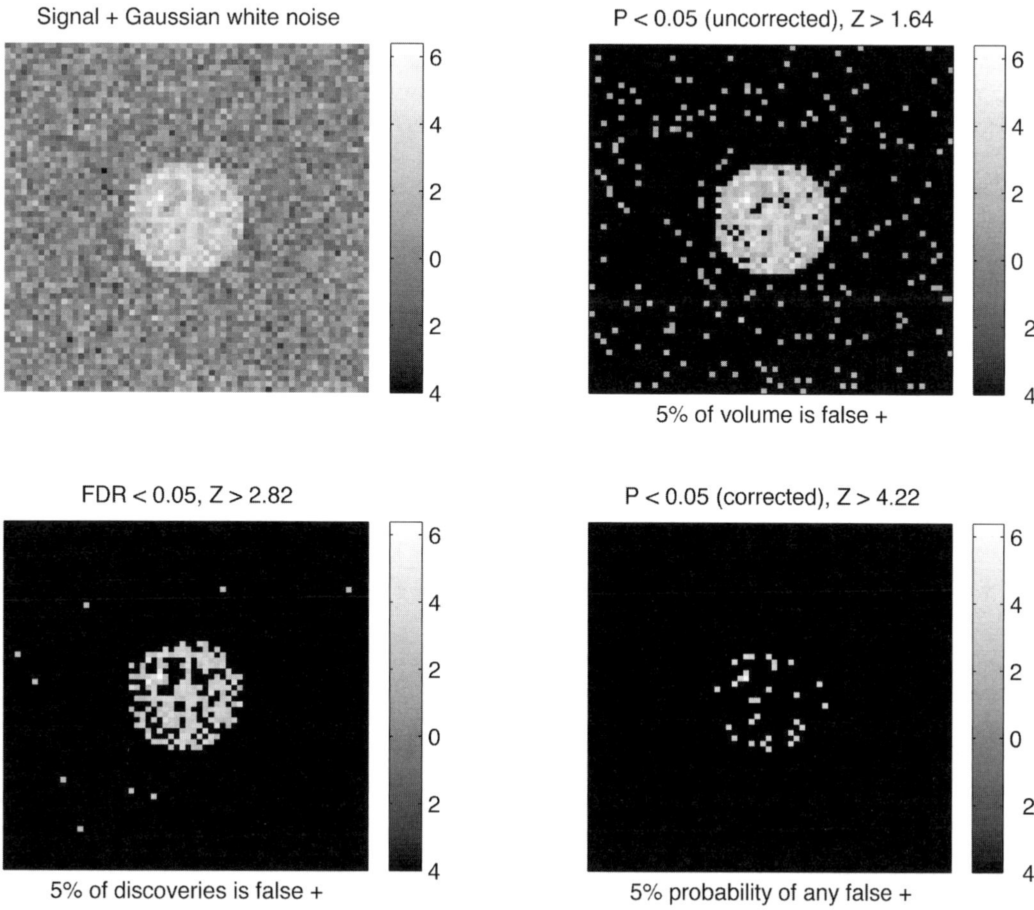

FIGURE 45.3
Illustration of the difference between false discovery rate and Bonferroni/random field methods for thresholding an image.

TABLE 45.1 **Examples of Thresholds of False Discovery Rate, Bonferroni, and Random Field Methods for Thresholding an Image**

Proportion of true + in image	1	0.1	0.01	0.001	0.0001
FDR threshold	1.64	2.56	3.28	3.88	4.41
Number of voxels in image	1	10	100	1000	10000
Bonferroni threshold	1.64	2.58	3.29	3.89	4.42
Number of resels in image	0	1	10	100	1000
Random fields threshold	1.64	2.82	3.46	4.09	4.65

The resulting threshold, corresponding to the value of Z for P_k, depends on the amount of signal in the data, not on the number of voxels or the smoothness. Table 45.1 compares thresholds for the FDR, Bonferroni, and random field methods. Thresholds of 2–3 are typical for brain mapping data with a reasonably strong signal, quite a bit lower than the Bonferroni or random field thresholds.

But we must remember that the interpretation of the FDR is quite different. False positives will be detected; we are simply controlling them so that they make up no more than α of our discoveries. On the other hand, the Bonferroni and random field methods control the probability of *ever* reporting a false discovery (see Fig. 45.3).

CONCLUSION

The idea of using a hypothesis test to detect activated regions does contain a fundamental flaw that all experimenters should be aware of. Think of it this way: if we had enough data, T statistics would increase (as the square root of the number of scans or subjects) until *all* voxels were "activated"! In reality, *every* voxel must be affected by the stimulus, perhaps by a very tiny amount; it is impossible to believe that there is never any signal at all. So thresholding simply excludes those voxels where we do not yet have enough evidence to distinguish their effects from zero. If we had more evidence, perhaps with better scanners, or simply more subjects, we surely would be able to do so. But then we would probably not want to detect activated regions. As for satellite images, the job for statisticians would then be signal *enhancement* rather than signal detection. The distinguishing feature of most brain mapping data is that there is so little signal to enhance. Even with the advent of better scanners this is still likely to be the case, because neuroscientists will surely devise yet more subtle experiments that are always pushing the signal to the limits of detectability.

References

Adler, R. J. (1981). *The Geometry of Random Fields.* New York: Wiley.

Cao, J. (1999). The size of the connected components of excursion sets of χ^2, t and F fields. *Adv. Appl. Prob.* **31,** 577–593.

Cao, J., and Worsley, K. J. (1999a). The detection of local shape changes via the geometry of Hotelling's T^2 fields. *Ann. Statistics* **27,** 925–942.

Cao, J., and Worsley, K. J. (1999b). The geometry of correlation fields, with an application to functional connectivity of the brain. *Ann. Appl. Prob.* **9,** 1021–1057.

Friston, K. J. (1997). Testing for anatomically specified regional effects. *Hum. Brain Mapping* **5,** 133–136.

Friston, K. J., Worsley, K. J., Frackowiak, R. S. J., Mazziotta, J. C., and Evans, A. C. (1994). Assessing the significance of focal activations using their spatial extent. *Hum. Brain Mapping* **1,** 214–220.

Genovese, C. R., Lazar, N. A., and Nichols, T. E. (2002). Thresholding of statistical maps in functional neuroimaging using the false discovery rate. *NeuroImage* **15,** 772–786.

Worsley, K. J. (2002). Non-stationary FWHM and its effect on statistical inference for fMRI data. *NeuroImage* **15** S346.

Worsley, K. J., Marrett, S., Neelin, P., Vandal, A. C., Friston, K. J., and Evans, A. C. (1996a). A unified statistical approach for determining significant signals in images of cerebral activation. *Hum. Brain Mapping* **4,** 58–73.

Worsley, K. J., Marrett, S., Neelin, P., and Evans, A. C. (1996b). Searching scale space for activation in PET images. *Hum. Brain Mapping* **4,** 74–90.

Worsley, K. J., Andermann, M., Koulis, T., MacDonald, D., and Evans, A. C. (1999). Detecting changes in nonisotropic images. *Hum. Brain Mapping* **8,** 98–101.

CHAPTER

46

Nonparametric Permutation Tests for Functional Neuroimaging

INTRODUCTION

The statistical analyses of functional mapping experiments usually proceeds at the voxel level, involving the formation and assessment of a *statistic image:* at each voxel a statistic indicating evidence of the experimental effect of interest, at that voxel, is computed, giving an image of statistics, a *statistic image* or *statistical parametric map* (SPM). In the absence of *a priori* anatomical hypotheses, the entire statistic image must be assessed for significant experimental effects, using a method that accounts for the inherent multiplicity involved in testing at all voxels simultaneously.

Traditionally, this has been accomplished in a classical *parametric* statistical framework. In the methods discussed in Chapters 7 and 8 of this book, the data are assumed to be normally distributed, with mean parameterised by a general linear model. This flexible framework encompasses t tests, F tests, paired t tests, ANOVA (see, e.g., Chapter 7), correlation, linear regression, multiple regression, and ANCOVA, among others. The estimated parameters of this model are contrasted to produce a test statistic at each voxel, which has a Student's t distribution under the null hypothesis. The resulting t-statistic image is then assessed for statistical significance, using distributional results for continuous random fields to identify voxels or regions where there is significant evidence against the null hypothesis (Worsley, 1996; Worsley *et al.,* 1995; Friston *et al.,* 1994, 1996; Poline *et al.,* 1997).

Holmes *et al.* (1996) introduced a nonparametric alternative based on permutation test theory. This method is conceptually simple, relies only on minimal assumptions, deals with the multiple-comparisons issue, and can be applied when the assumptions of a parametric approach are untenable. Further, in some circumstances, the permutation method outperforms parametric approaches. Arndt *et al.* (1996), working independently, also discussed the advantages of similar approaches. Subsequently, Grabrowski *et al.* (1996) demonstrated empirically the potential power of the approach in comparison with other methods. Halber *et al.* (1997), discussed further by Holmes *et al.* (1998), also favor the permutation approach. Nichols and Holmes (2001) review the nonparametric theory and demonstrate how multisubject fMRI can be analyzed. Applications of permutation testing methods to single-subject fMRI require modelling of the temporal autocorrelation in the fMRI time series. Bullmore *et al.* (1996) develop permutation-based procedures for periodic fMRI activation designs using a simple ARMA model for temporal autocorrelations, though they eschew the problem of multiple comparisons. Bullmore *et al.* (2001) use a wavelet transformation to account for more general forms of fMRI correlation. Locascio *et al.* (1997) describe an application to fMRI combining the general linear model

(Friston *et al.,* 1995b), ARMA modelling (Bullmore *et al.,* 1996), and a multiple-comparisons permutation procedure (Holmes *et al.,* 1996). Liu *et al.* (1998) consider an alternative approach, permuting labels. Bullmore *et al.* (1999) apply nonparametric methods to compare groups of structural MR images.

The aim of this chapter is to present the theory of the multiple-comparisons nonparametric permutation for independent data (e.g., PET or intersubject fMRI), including detailed examples. While the traditional approach to multiple comparisons controls the family-wise error rate, the chance of any false positives, another perspective has recently been introduced. The new approach controls the *false discovery rate* (FDR), the fraction of false positives among all detected voxels (Genovese *et al.,* 2001) (see Chapter 15 for a brief description). While this chapter only considers the family-wise error rate, we note that a permutation approach to FDR has been proposed (Yekutieli and Benjamini, 1999).

We begin with an introduction to nonparametric permutation testing, reviewing experimental design and hypothesis testing issues, and illustrating the theory by considering testing a functional neuroimaging dataset at a single voxel. The problem of searching the brain volume for significant activations is then considered, and the extension of the permutation methods to the *multiple-comparisons problem* of simultaneously testing at all voxels is described. With appropriate methodology in place, we conclude with three annotated examples illustrating the approach. Software implementing the approach, called Statistical Nonparametric Mapping (SnPM), is available as an extension of the MATLAB-based SPM package.

PERMUTATION TESTS

Permutation tests are one type of nonparametric test. They were proposed in the early 20th century, but have only recently become popular with the availability of inexpensive, powerful computers to perform the computations involved.

The essential concept of a permutation test is relatively intuitive: for example, consider a simple single-subject PET activation experiment, in which a single subject is scanned repeatedly under "rest" and "activation" conditions. Considering the data at a particular voxel, if there is really no difference between the two conditions, then we would be fairly surprised if most of the "activation" observations were larger than the "rest" observations, and would be inclined to conclude that there was evidence of some activation at that voxel. Permutation tests simply provide a formal mechanism for quantifying this "surprise" in terms of probability, thereby leading to significance tests and p values.

If there is no experimental effect, then the labeling of observations by the corresponding experimental condition is arbitrary, since the same data would have arisen whatever the condition. These *labels* can be any relevant attribute: condition "tags," such as "rest" or "active"; a covariate, such as task difficulty or response time; or a label, indicating group membership. Given the null hypothesis that the labelings are arbitrary, the significance of a statistic expressing the experimental effect can then be assessed by comparison with the distribution of values obtained when the labels are permuted.

The justification for exchanging the labels comes from either weak distributional assumptions or by appeal to the randomisation scheme used in designing the experiment. Tests justified by the initial randomisation of conditions to experimental units (e.g., subjects or scans) are sometimes referred to as *randomisation tests,* or *rerandomisation tests.* Whatever the theoretical justification, the mechanics of the tests are the same. Many authors refer to both generically as *permutation tests,* a policy we shall adopt unless a distinction is necessary.

In this section, we describe the theoretical underpinning for randomisation and permutation tests. Beginning with simple univariate tests at a single voxel, we first present randomisation tests, describing the key concepts at length, before turning to permutation tests. These two approaches lead to exactly the same test, which we illustrate with a simple worked example, before describing how the theory can be applied to assess an entire statistic image. For simplicity of exposition, the methodology is developed using the example of a simple single-subject PET activation experiment. However, the approach is not limited to activation experiments, nor to PET.

Randomisation Test

We first consider randomisation tests, using a single-subject activation experiment to illustrate the thinking: suppose we are to conduct a simple single-subject PET activation experiment, with the regional cerebral blood flow (rCBF) in "active" (A) condition scans to be compared with that in scans acquired under an appropriate "baseline" (B) condition. The fundamental concepts are of experimental *randomisation,* the *null hypothesis, exchangeability,* and the *randomisation distribution.*

Randomisation

To avoid unexpected confounding effects, suppose we randomise the allocation of conditions to scans prior to conducting the experiment. Using an appropriate scheme, we label the scans as A or B according to the conditions under which they will be acquired, and hence specify the *condition presentation order.* This allocation of condition labels to scans is randomly chosen according to the randomisation scheme, and any other possible labeling of this scheme was equally likely to have been chosen.

Null Hypothesis

In the randomisation test, the null hypothesis is explicitly about the acquired data. For example: $\mathcal{H}_0$: "Each scan would have been the same whatever the condition, A or B." The hypothesis is that the experimental conditions did not affect the data differentially, such that had we run the experiment with a different condition presentation order, we would have observed exactly the same data. In this sense we regard the data as fixed, and the experimental design as random (in contrast to regarding the design as fixed, and the data as a realisation of a random process). Under this null hypothesis, the labelings of the scans as A or B is arbitrary, since these labelings arose from the initial random allocation of conditions to scans, and any initial allocation would have given the same data. Thus, we may rerandomise the labels on the data, effectively permuting the labels, subject to the restriction that each permutation could have arisen from the initial randomisation scheme. The observed data are equally likely to have arisen from any of these permuted labelings.

Exchangeability

This leads to the notion of *exchangeability.* Consider the situation before the data are collected, but after the condition labels have been assigned to scans. Formally, the labels on the data (still to be collected) are *exchangeable* if the distribution of the statistic (still to be evaluated) is the same whatever the labeling (Good, 1994). For our activation example, we would use a statistic expressing the difference between the "active" and "baseline" scans. Thus under the null hypothesis of no difference between the A and B conditions, the labels are exchangeable, provided the permuted labeling could have arisen from the initial randomisation scheme. The initial randomisation scheme gives us the probabilistic justification for permuting the labels; the null hypothesis asserts that the data would have been the same.

So with a randomisation test, the randomisation scheme prescribes the possible labelings, and the null hypothesis asserts that the labels are exchangeable within the constraints of this scheme. Thus we define an *exchangeability block* (EB) as a block of scans within which the labels are exchangeable, a definition which mirrors that of randomisation blocks, blocks of observations within which condition order is randomised.

Randomisation Distribution

Consider now some statistic expressing the experimental effect of interest at a particular voxel. For the current example of a PET single-subject activation, this could be the mean difference between the A and the B condition scans, a two-sample t statistic, a t statistic from an ANCOVA, or any appropriate statistic. We are not restricted to the common statistics of classical parametric hypothesis whose null distributions are known under specific assumptions, because the appropriate distribution will be derived from the data.

The computation of the statistic depends on the labeling of the data. For example, with a two-sample t statistic, the labels A and B specify the groupings. Thus, permuting the labels leads to an alternative value of the statistic.

Given exchangeability under the null hypothesis, the observed data are equally likely to have arisen from any of the possible labelings. Hence, the statistics associated with each of the possible labelings are also equally likely. Thus, we have the permutation (or randomisation) distribution of our statistic: the *permutation distribution* is the *sampling distribution* of the statistic under the null hypothesis, given the data observed. Under the null hypothesis, the observed statistic is randomly chosen from the set of statistics corresponding to all possible relabelings. This gives us a way to formalise our "surprise" at an outcome: the probability of an outcome as or more extreme than the one observed, the p value, is the proportion of statistic values in the permutation distribution that is greater or equal to that observed. The actual labeling used in the experiment is one of the possible labelings, so if the observed statistic is the largest of the permutation distribution, the p value is $1/N$, where N is the number of possible labelings of the initial randomisation scheme. Since we are considering a test at a single voxel, these would be *uncorrected p* values in the language of multiple comparisons (see later section).

Randomisation Test: Summary

To summarise, the null hypothesis asserts that the scans would have been the same whatever the experimental condition, A or B. Under this null hypothesis, the initial randomisation scheme can be regarded as arbitrary labeling scans as A or B, under which the experiment would have given the same data, and the labels would be exchangeable. The statistic corresponding to any labeling from the initial randomisation scheme is as likely as any other, since the permuted labeling could equally well have arisen in the initial randomisation. The sampling distribution of the statistic (given the data) is the set of statistic values corresponding to all the possible labelings of the initial randomisation scheme, each value being equally likely.

Randomisation Test: Mechanics

Let N denote the number of possible relabelings and t_i the statistic corresponding to relabeling i. (After having performed the experiment, we refer to *re*labelings for the data, identical to the labelings of the randomisation scheme.) The set of t_i for all possible relabelings constitutes the *permutation distribution.* Let T denote the value of the statistic for the actual labeling of the experiment. As usual in statistics, we use a capital letter for a *random variable.* Variable T is random, since under $\mathcal{H}_0$ it is chosen from the permutation distribution according to the initial randomisation.

Under $\mathcal{H}_0$, all of the t_i are equally likely, so we determine the significance of our observed statistic T by counting the proportion of the permutation distribution as or more extreme than T, giving us our p value. We reject the null hypothesis at significance level α if the p value is less than α. Equivalently, T must be greater than or equal to the $100(1 - \alpha)$th percentile of the permutation distribution. Thus, the *critical value* is the $(c + 1)$th largest member of the permutation distribution, where $c = \lfloor \alpha N \rfloor$, αN rounded down. If T exceeds this critical value, then the test is significant at level α.

Permutation Test

In many situations it is impractical to randomly allocate experimental conditions, or perhaps we are presented with data from an experiment that was not randomised. For instance, we cannot randomly assign subjects to be patients or normal controls. Or, for example, consider a multi-subject fMRI second-level analysis in which a covariate is measured for each subject, and we seek brain regions whose activation appears to be related to the covariate value.

In the absence of an explicit randomisation of conditions to scans, we must make weak distributional assumptions to justify permuting the labels on the data. Typically, all that is required is that distributions have the same shape, that is, are symmetric. The actual permutations that are performed again depend on the degree of exchangeability, which in turn depend on the actual assumptions made. With the randomisation test, the experimenter designs the initial randomisation scheme carefully to avoid confounds. The randomisation scheme reflects an implicitly assumed degree of exchangeability. With the permutation test, the degree of exchangeability must be assumed *post hoc*. Usually, the reasoning that would have led to a particular randomisation scheme can be applied *post hoc* to an experiment, leading to a permutation test with the same degree of exchangeability. Given exchangeability, computation proceeds as for the randomisation test.

Permutation Test: Summary

Weak distributional assumptions are made that embody the degree of exchangeability. The exact form of these assumptions depends on the experiment at hand, as illustrated in the following section and in the examples section.

For a simple single-subject activation experiment, we might typically assume the following: for a particular voxel, "active" and "baseline" scans within a given block have a distribution with the same shape, though possibly different means. The null hypothesis asserts that the distributions for the "baseline" and "active" scans have the same mean and, hence, are the same. Then the labels are arbitrary within the chosen blocks, which are thus the exchangeability blocks. Any permutation of the labels within the exchangeability blocks leads to an equally likely statistic.

The mechanics are then the same as with the randomisation test: for each of the possible relabelings, compute the statistic of interest; for relabeling *i,* call this statistic t_i. Under the null hypothesis, each of the t_i is equally likely, so the p value is the proportion of the t_i's greater than or equal to the statistic T corresponding to the correctly labeled data.

Single-Voxel Example

To make these concepts concrete, consider assessing the evidence of an activation effect at a single voxel of a single-subject PET activation experiment consisting of six scans, three in each of the "active" (A) and "baseline" (B) conditions. Suppose that the conditions were presented alternately, starting with rest, and that the observed data at this voxel are {90.48, 103.00, 87.83, 99.93, 96.06, 99.76} to two decimal places. (These data are from a voxel in the primary visual cortex of the second subject in the PET visual activation experiment presented in the examples section.)

As mentioned before, any statistic can be used, so for simplicity of illustration we use the "mean difference," i.e., $T = \frac{1}{3}\sum_{j=1}^{3}(A_j - B_j)$ where A_j and B_j indicate the value of the jth scan at the particular voxel of interest, under the active and baseline conditions, respectively. Thus, we observe statistic $T = 9.45$.

Randomisation Test

Suppose that the condition presentation order was randomised, the actual ordering of BABABA having being randomly selected from all allocations of three A's and three B's to the six available scans, a simple balanced randomisation within a single randomisation block of size 6. By combinatorics, or some counting, we find that this randomisation scheme has 20 (${}_6C_3 = 20$) possible outcomes.

Then we can justify permuting the labels on the basis of this initial randomisation. Under the null hypothesis $\mathcal{H}_0$: "The scans would have been the same whatever the experimental condition, A or B," the labels are exchangeable, and the statistics corresponding to the 20 possible labelings are equally likely. The 20 possible labelings are as follows:

1:	AAABBB	6:	ABABAB	11:	BAAABB	16:	BABBAA
2:	AABABB	7:	ABABBA	12:	BAABAB	17:	BBAAAB
3:	AABBAB	8:	ABBAAB	13:	BAABBA	18:	BBAABA
4:	AABBBA	9:	ABBABA	14:	BABAAB	19:	BBABAA
5:	ABAABB	10:	ABBBAA	15:	BABABA	20:	BBBAAA

Permutation Test

Suppose there was no initial randomisation of conditions to scans, and that the condition presentation order ABABAB was simply chosen. With no randomisation, we must make weak distribution assumptions to justify permuting the labels, effectively prescribing the degree of exchangeability.

For this example, consider permuting the labels freely among the six scans. This corresponds to *full exchangeability,* a single exchangeability block of size 6. For this to be tenable, we must either assume the absence of any temporal or similar confounds, or model their effect such that they do not affect the statistic under permutations of the labels. Consider the former. This gives 20 possible permutations of the labels, precisely those enumerated for the randomisation justification above. Formally, we're assuming that the voxel values for the "baseline" and "active" scans come from distributions that are the same except for a possible difference in location, or mean. Our null hypothesis is that these distributions have the same mean and, therefore, are the same.

Clearly the mean difference statistic under consideration in the current example is confounded with time for labelings such as AAABBB (#1) and BBBAAA (#20), where a time effect will result in a large mean difference between the A and the B labeled scans. The test is still valid, but possibly conservative. The actual condition presentation order of BABABA is relatively unconfounded with time, but the contribution of confounds to the statistics for alternative labelings such as #1 and #20 will potentially increase the number of statistics greater than the observed statistic.

Computation

Let t_i be the mean difference for labeling i, as enumerated above. Computing for each of the 20 relabelings:

$t_1 = +4.82$	$t_6 = +9.45$	$t_{11} = -1.48$	$t_{16} = -6.86$
$t_2 = -3.25$	$t_7 = +6.97$	$t_{12} = +1.10$	$t_{17} = +3.15$
$t_3 = -0.67$	$t_8 = +1.38$	$t_{13} = -1.38$	$t_{18} = +0.67$
$t_4 = -3.15$	$t_9 = -1.10$	$t_{14} = -6.97$	$t_{19} = +3.25$
$t_5 = +6.86$	$t_{10} = +1.48$	$t_{15} = -9.45$	$t_{20} = -4.82.$

This is our permutation distribution for this analysis, summarised as a histogram in Fig. 46.1. Each of the possible labelings was equally likely. Under the null hypothesis the statistics corresponding to these labelings are equally likely. The p value is the proportion of the permutation distribution greater or equal to T. Here the actual labeling #6 with $t_6 = +9.4$ gives the largest mean difference of all the possible labelings, so the p value is $1/20 = 0.05$. For a test at given α level, we reject the null hypothesis if the p value is less than α, so we conclude that there is significant evidence against the null hypothesis of no activation at this voxel at level $\alpha = 0.05$.

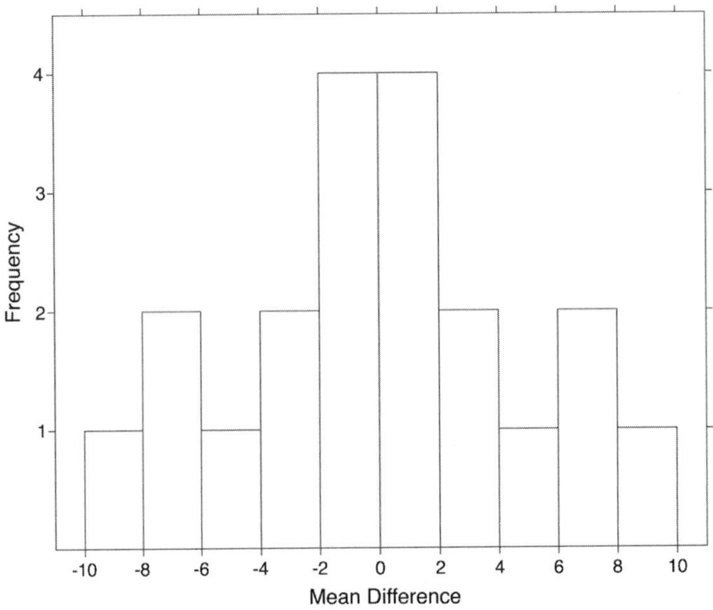

FIGURE 46.1
Histogram of permutation distribution for single-voxel example, using a mean difference statistic. Note the symmetry of the histogram about the y axis. This occurs because for each possible labeling, the opposite labeling is also possible, and yields the same mean difference but in the opposite direction. This trick can be used in many cases to halve the computational burden.

Multiple-Comparisons Permutation Tests

Thus far we have considered using a permutation test at a single voxel: for each voxel we can produce a p value, p^k, for the null hypothesis $\mathcal{H}_0^k$, where the superscript k indexes the voxels. If we have an *a priori* anatomical hypothesis concerning the experimentally induced effect at a single voxel, then we can simply test at that voxel using an appropriate α level test. If we don't have such precise anatomical hypotheses, evidence for an experimental effect must be assessed at each and every voxel. We must take into account the multiplicity of testing. Clearly 5% of voxels are expected to have p values less than $\alpha = 0.05$. This is the essence of the *multiple-comparisons problem.* In the language of multiple comparisons, these p values are *uncorrected* p values. Type I errors must be controlled overall, such that the probability of falsely declaring any region as significant is less than the nominal test level α. This is known as controlling the family-wise error rate, the family being the collection of tests performed over the entire brain. Formally, we require a test procedure maintaining strong control over *family-wise* type I error, giving *adjusted p* values, p values *corrected* for multiple comparisons.

The construction of suitable of suitable multiple comparisons procedures for the problem of assessing statistic images from functional mapping experiments within parametric frameworks has occupied many authors (Friston *et al.,* 1991; Worsley, 1994; Worsley *et al.,* 1992, 1995; Poline and Mazoyer, 1993; Poline *et al.,* 1997; Roland *et al.,* 1993; Forman *et al.,* 1995; Friston *et al.,* 1994, 1996; and Cao, 1999, among others). In contrast to these parametric and simulation-based methods, a nonparametric resampling-based approach provides an intuitive and easily implemented solution (Westfall and Young, 1993). The key realisation is that the reasoning presented above for permutation tests at a single voxel relies on relabeling entire *images,* so the arguments can be extended to image level inference by considering an appropriate *maximal statistic.* If, under the omnibus null hypothesis the labels are exchangeable with respect to the voxel statistic under consideration, then the labels are exchangeable with respect to any statistic summarising the voxel statistics, such as their maxima.

We consider two popular types of test, *single threshold* and *supra-threshold cluster* size tests, but note again the flexibility of these methods to consider any statistic.

Single Threshold Test

With a single threshold test, the statistic image is thresholded at a given *critical threshold,* and voxels with statistic values exceeding this threshold have their null hypotheses rejected. Rejection of the *omnibus hypothesis* (that all the voxel hypotheses are true) occurs if any voxel value exceeds the threshold, a situation clearly determined by the value of the maximum value of the statistic image. Thus, consideration of the maximum voxel statistic deals with the multiple-comparisons problem. For a valid omnibus test, the critical threshold is such that the probability that it is exceeded by the maximal statistic is less than α. Thus, we require the distribution of the maxima of the null statistic image. Approximate parametric derivations based on the theory of strictly stationary continuous random fields are given by Friston *et al.* (1991), Worsley (1994), and Worsley *et al.* (1992, 1995).

The permutation approach can yield the distribution of the maximal statistic in a straightforward manner: rather than compute the permutation distribution of the statistic at a particular voxel, we compute the permutation distribution of the maximal voxel statistic over the volume of interest. We reject the omnibus hypothesis at level α if the maximal statistic for the actual labeling of the experiment is in the top 100α % of the permutation distribution for the maximal statistic. The critical value is the $(c+1)$th largest member of the permutation distribution, where $c = \lfloor \alpha N \rfloor$, αN rounded down. Furthermore, we can reject the null hypothesis at any voxel with a statistic value exceeding this threshold: the critical value for the maximal statistic is the critical threshold for a single threshold test over the same volume of interest. This test can be shown to have *strong* control over *experiment-wise* type I error. A formal proof is given by Holmes *et al.* (1996).

The mechanics of the test are as follows: For each possible relabeling $i = 1,\ldots, N,$ note the maximal statistic $t^{\max}{}_i$, the maximum of the voxel statistics for relabeling i: $t_i^{\max} = \max \{t_i\}_{i=1}^N$. This gives the permutation distribution for $T^{\max}$, the maximal statistic. The critical threshold is the $c + 1$ largest member of the permutation distribution for $T^{\max}$, where $c = \lfloor \alpha N \rfloor$, αN rounded down. Voxels with statistics exceeding this threshold exhibit evidence against the corresponding voxel hypotheses at level α. The corresponding corrected p value for each voxel is the proportion of the permutation distribution for the maximal statistic that is greater than or equal to the voxel statistic.

Supra-Threshold Cluster Tests

Supra-threshold cluster tests start by thresholding the statistic image at a predetermined *primary* threshold, and then assessing the resulting pattern of supra-threshold activity. Supra-threshold cluster size tests assess the size of connected suprathreshold regions for significance, declaring regions greater than a critical size as activated. Thus, the distribution of the maximal supra-threshold cluster size (for the given primary threshold) is required. Simulation approaches have been presented by Poline and Mazoyer (1993) and Roland *et al.* (1993) for PET, and by Forman *et al.* (1995) for fMRI. Friston *et al.* (1994) give a theoretical parametric derivation for Gaussian statistic images based on the theory of continuous Gaussian random fields, Cao (1999) gives results for χ^2, t, and F fields.

Again, as noted by Holmes *et al.* (1996), a nonparametric permutation approach is simple to derive. Simply construct the permutation distribution of the maximal supra-threshold cluster size. For the statistic image corresponding to each possible relabeling, note the size of the largest supra-threshold cluster above the primary threshold. The critical supra-threshold cluster size for this primary threshold is the ($\lfloor \alpha N \rfloor$, + 1)th largest member of this permutation distribution. Corrected p values for each supra-threshold cluster in the observed statistic image are obtained by comparing their size to the permutation distribution.

In general, such supra-threshold cluster tests are more powerful for functional neuroimaging data than the single threshold approach (see Friston *et al.,* 1995b, for a fuller discussion). However, it must be remembered that this additional power comes at the price of reduced localising power: the null hypotheses for voxels within a significant cluster are not tested, so individual voxels cannot be declared significant. Only the omnibus null hypothesis for the cluster can be rejected. Further, the choice of primary threshold dictates the power of the test in detecting different types of deviation from the omnibus null hypothesis. With a low threshold, large supra-threshold clusters are to be expected, so intense focal "signals" will be missed. At higher thresholds these focal activations will be detected, but lower intensity diffuse "signals" may go undetected below the primary threshold.

Poline *et al.* (1997) addressed these issues within a parametric framework by considering the supra-threshold cluster size and height jointly. A nonparametric variation could be to consider the *exceedance mass,* the excess mass of the supra-threshold cluster, defined as the integral of the statistic image above the primary threshold within the supra-threshold cluster (Holmes, 1994; Bullmore *et al.,* 1999). Calculation of the permutation distribution and p values proceeds exactly as before.

Considerations

Before turning to example applications of the nonparametric permutation tests described above, we note some relevant theoretical issues. The statistical literature (referenced below) should be consulted for additional theoretical discussion. For issues related to the current application to functional neuroimaging, see also Holmes (1994), Holmes *et al.* (1996), and Arndt *et al.* (1996).

Nonparametric Statistics

First, note that these methods are neither new nor contentious: Originally expounded by Fisher (1935), Pitman (1937a, b, c), and later Edgington (1964, 1969a, b), these approaches are enjoying a renaissance as computing technology makes the requisite computations feasible for practical applications. Had R. A. Fisher and his peers had access to similar resources, it is possible that large areas of parametric statistics would have gone undeveloped! Modern texts on the subject include Good's *Permutation Tests* (1994), Edgington's *Randomisation Tests* (1995), and Manly's *Randomisation, Bootstrap and Monte-Carlo Methods in Biology* (1997). Recent interest in more general resampling methods, such as the bootstrap, has further contributed to the field. For a treatise on resampling-based multiple-comparisons procedures, see Westfall and Young (1993).

Many standard statistical tests are essentially permutation tests: The "classic" nonparametric tests, such as the Wilcoxon and Mann-Whitney tests, are permutation tests with the data replaced by appropriate ranks, such that the critical values are only a function of sample size and can therefore be tabulated. Fisher's exact test (Fisher and Bennett, 1990) and tests of Spearman and Kendall correlations (Kendall and Gibbons, 1990) are all permutation/randomisation based.

Assumptions

The only assumptions required for a valid permutation test are those to justify permuting the labels. Clearly the experimental design, model, statistic, and permutations must also be appropriate for the question of interest. For a randomisation test, the probabilistic justification follows directly from the initial randomisation of condition labels to scans. In the absence of an initial randomisation, permutation of the labels can be justified via weak distributional assumptions. Thus, only minimal assumptions are required for a valid test. (The notable case when exchangeability under the null hypothesis is not tenable is fMRI time series, due to temporal autocorrelation.)

In contrast to parametric approaches where the statistic must have a known null distributional form, the permutation approach is free to consider any statistic summarising evidence for the effect of interest at each voxel. The consideration of the maximal statistic over the volume of interest then deals with the multiple-comparisons problem.

However, there are additional considerations when using the nonparametric approach with a maximal statistic to account for multiple comparisons. In order for the single threshold test to be equally sensitive at all voxels, the (null) sampling distribution of the chosen statistic should be similar across voxels. For instance, the simple mean difference statistic used earlier in the single-voxel example could be considered as a voxel statistic, but areas where the mean difference is highly variable will dominate the permutation distribution for the maximal statistic. The test will still be valid, but will be less sensitive at those voxels with lower variability. So, although for an individual voxel a permutation test on group mean differences is equivalent to one using a two-sample t statistic (Edgington, 1995), this not true in the multiple-comparisons setting using a maximal statistic.

One approach to this problem is to consider multistep tests, which iteratively identify activated areas, cut them out, and continue assessing the remaining volume. These are described below, but are additionally computationally intensive. Preferable is to use a voxel statistic with approximately homogeneous null permutation distribution across the volume of interest, such as an appropriate t statistic. A t statistic is essentially a mean difference normalised by a variance estimate, effectively measuring the reliability of an effect. Thus, we consider the same voxel statistics for a nonparametric approach as we would for a comparable parametric approach.

Pseudo t Statistics

Nonetheless, we can still do a little better than a straight t statistic, particularly at low degrees of freedom. A t statistic is a change divided by the square root of the estimated variance of that change. When there are few degrees of freedom available for variance estimation, say, less than 20, this variance is estimated poorly. Errors in estimation of the variance from voxel to voxel appear as high-spatial-frequency noise in images of the estimated variance or near-zero variance estimates, which in either case cause noisy t-statistic images. Given that PET and fMRI measure (i.e., are indicators of) blood flow, physiological considerations would suggest that the variance be roughly constant over small localities. This suggests pooling the variance estimate at a voxel with those of its neighbours to give a locally pooled variance estimate as a better estimate of the actual variance. Since the model is of the same form at all voxels, the voxel variance estimates have the same degrees of freedom, and the locally pooled variance estimate is simply the average of the variance estimates in the neighbourhood of the voxel in question. More generally, weighted locally pooled voxel variance estimates can be obtained by smoothing the raw variance image. The filter kernel then specifies the weights and neighbourhood for the local pooling. The *pseudo t*-statistic images formed with smoothed variance estimators are smooth. In essence, the noise (from the variance image) has been smoothed, but not the signal. A derivation of the parametric distribution of the pseudo t requires knowledge of the variance-covariances of the voxel-level variances, and has so far proved elusive. This precludes parametric analyses using a pseudo t statistic, but poses no problems for a nonparametric approach.

Number of Relabelings and Test Size

A constraint on the permutation test is the number of possible relabelings. Since the observed labeling is always one of the N possible labelings, the smallest p value attainable is $1/N$. Thus, for a level $\alpha = 0.05$ test to potentially reject the null hypothesis, there must be at least 20 possible relabelings.

More generally, the permutation distribution is *discrete,* consisting of a finite set of possibilities corresponding to the N possible relabelings. Hence, any p values produced will be multiples of $1/N$. Further, the $100(1-\alpha)$th percentile of the permutation distribution, the critical threshold for a level α test, may lie between two values. Equivalently, α may not be a multiple of $1/N$, such that a p value of exactly α cannot be attained. In these cases, an exact test with size exactly α is not possible. It is for this reason that the critical threshold is computed as the $(c + 1)$th largest member of the permutation distribution, where $c = \lfloor \alpha N \rfloor$, αN rounded down. The test can be described as *almost* exact, since the size is at most $1/N$ less than α.

Approximate Tests

A large number of possible relabelings is also problematic, due to the computations involved. In situations where it is not feasible to compute the statistic images for all relabelings, a subsample of relabelings can be used (Dwass, 1957; see also Edgington, 1969a, for a less mathematical description). The set of N possible relabelings is reduced to a more manageable N' consisting of the true labeling and $N' - 1$ randomly chosen from the set of $N - 1$ possible relabelings. The test then proceeds as before.

Such a test is sometimes known as an *approximate* permutation test, since the permutation distribution is approximated by a subsample, leading to approximate p values and critical thresholds. (These tests are also known as *Monte Carlo permutation tests* or *random permutation tests,* reflecting the random selection of permutations to consider.)

Despite the name, the resulting test is still exact. However, as might be expected from the previous section, using an approximate permutation distribution results in a test that is more conservative and less powerful than one using the full permutation distribution.

Fortunately, as few as 1000 permutations can yield an effective approximate permutation test (Edgington, 1969a). However, for an approximate test with minimal loss of power in comparison to the full test (i.e., with high efficiency), one should consider rather more (Jöckel, 1686), as many as 10,000.

Power

Frequently, nonparametric approaches are less powerful than equivalent parametric approaches when the assumptions of the latter are true. The assumptions provide the parametric approach with additional information that the nonparametric approach must "discover." The more relabelings, the better the power of the nonparametric approach relative to the parametric approach. In a sense the method has more information from more relabelings, and "discovers" the null distribution assumed in the parametric approach. However, if the assumptions required for a parametric analysis are not credible, a nonparametric approach provides the only valid method of analysis.

In the current context of assessing statistic images from functional neuroimaging experiments, the prevalent SPM techniques require a number of assumptions and involve some approximations. Experience suggests that the permutation methods described here do at least as well as the parametric methods, at least on real (PET) data (Arndt *et al.,* 1996). For noisy statistic images, such as t-statistic images with low degrees of freedom, the ability to consider pseudo t statistics constructed with locally pooled (smoothed) variance estimates affords the permutation approach additional power (Holmes, 1994; Holmes *et al.,* 1996; and examples below).

Multistep Tests

The potential for confounds to affect the permutation distribution via the consideration of unsuitable relabelings was considered in an earlier section. Recall also the above comments regarding the potential for the multiple comparison permutation tests to be differentially sensitive across the volume of interest if the null permutation distribution varies dramatically from voxel to voxel. In addition, there is also the prospect that departures from the null hypothesis influence the permutation distribution. Thus far, our nonparametric multiple-comparisons permutation testing technique has consisted of a *single step:* The null sampling distribution (given the data) is the permutation distribution of the maximal statistic computed over all voxels in the volume of interest, potentially including voxels where the null hypothesis is not true. A large departure from the null hypothesis will give a large statistic, not only in the actual labeling of the experiment, but also in other relabelings, similar to the true labeling. This does not affect the overall validity of the test, but may make it more conservative for voxels other than that with the maximum observed statistic.

One possibility is to consider *step-down tests,* in which significant regions are iteratively identified, cut out, and the remaining volume reassessed. The resulting procedure still maintains strong control over family-wise type I error, our criteria for a test with localising power, but will be more powerful (at voxels other than that with the maximal statistic). However, the iterative nature of the procedure multiplies the computational burden of an already intensive procedure. Holmes *et al.* (1996) gave a discussion and efficient algorithms, developed further in Holmes (1994), but found that the additional power gained was negligible for the cases studied.

Recall also the motivations for using a normalised voxel statistic, such as the t statistic: an inappropriately normalised voxel statistic will yield a test differentially sensitive across the image. In these situations the step-down procedures may be more beneficial.

Further investigation of step-down methods and sequential tests more generally are certainly warranted, but are unfortunately beyond the scope of this chapter.

Generalisability

Questions often arise about the scope of inference, or generalisability, of nonparametric procedures. For parametric tests, when a collection of subjects has been randomly selected from a population of interest and intersubject variability is considered, the inference is on the population sampled and not just the sampled subjects. The randomisation test, in contrast, only makes inference on the data at hand: a randomisation test regards the data as fixed and uses the randomness of the experimental design to justify exchangeability. A permutation test, while operationally identical to the randomisation test, *can* make inferences on a sampled population. A permutation test also regards the data as fixed but it additionally assumes the presence of a population distribution to justify exchangeability and, hence, can be used for population inference. The randomisation test is truly assumption free, but has a limited scope of inference.

In practice, since subjects rarely constitute a random sample of the population of interest, we find the issue of little practical concern. Scientists routinely generalise results, integrating prior experience, other findings, existing theories, and common sense in a way that a simple hypothesis test does not admit.

WORKED EXAMPLES

The following sections illustrate the application of the techniques described above to three common experimental designs: single-subject PET "parametric," multisubject PET activation, and multisubject fMRI activation. In each example we illustrate the key steps in performing a permutation analysis:

1. *Null hypothesis.* Specify the null hypothesis.
2. *Exchangeability.* Specify exchangeability of observations under the null hypothesis.
3. *Statistic.* Specify the statistic of interest, usually broken down into specifying a voxel-level statistic and a summary statistic.
4. *Relabelings.* Determine all possible relabelings given the exchangeability scheme under the null hypothesis.
5. *Permutation distribution.* Calculate the value of the statistic for each relabeling, building the permutation distribution.
6. *Significance.* Use the permutation distribution to determine the significance of correct labeling and the threshold for statistical image.

The first three items follow from the experimental design and must be specified by the user; the last three are computed by the software, although we still address them here. When comparable parametric analyses are available (within SPM), we compare the permutation results to the parametric results.

Single-Subject PET: Parametric Design

The first study illustrates how covariate analyses are implemented and how the supra-threshold cluster size statistic is used. This example also shows how randomisation in the experimental design dictates the exchangeability of the observations.

Study Description

The data come from a study of Silbersweig *et al.* (1994). The aim of the study was to validate a novel PET methodology for imaging transient, randomly occurring events, specifically events that were shorter than the duration of a PET scan. This work was the foundation for later work imaging hallucinations in schizophrenics (Silbersweig *et al.,* 1995). We consider one subject from the study, who was scanned 12 times. During each scan the subject was presented with brief auditory stimuli. The proportion of each scan over which stimuli were delivered was chosen randomly, within three randomisation blocks of size 4. A score was computed for each scan, indicating the proportion of activity infused into the brain during stimulation. This scan activity score is our covariate of interest, which we shall refer to as DURATION. This is a type of parametric design, although in this context *parametric* refers not to a set of distributional assumptions, but rather to an experimental design in which the experimental parameter is varied continuously. This is in contradistinction to a factorial design where the experimental probe is varied over a small number of discrete levels.

We also have to consider the global cerebral blood flow (gCBF), which we account for here by including it as a nuisance covariate in our model. This gives a multiple regression, with the slope of the DURATION effect being of interest. Note that regressing out gCBF like this requires an assumption that there is no linear dependence between the score and global activity; examination of a scatterplot and a correlation coefficient of 0.09 confirmed this as a tenable assumption (see Chapter 7 for further discussion of global effects in PET).

Null Hypothesis

Since this is a randomised experiment, the test will be a randomisation test, and the null hypothesis pertains directly to the data, and no assumptions are required:

$$\mathcal{H}_0\text{: The data would be the same whatever the DURATION.}$$

Exchangeability

Because this experiment was randomised, our choice of EB matches the randomisation blocks of the experimental design, which was chosen with temporal effects in mind. The values of DURATION were grouped into three blocks of four, such that each block had the same mean and similar variability, and then randomised within the block. Thus we have three EBs of size 4.

Statistic

We decompose our statistic of interest into two statistics: one voxel-level statistic that generates a statistic image, and a maximal statistic that summarises that statistic image in a single number. An important consideration will be the degrees of freedom. We have one parameter for the grand mean, one parameter for the slope with DURATION, and one parameter for confounding covariate gCBF. Hence 12 observations less three parameters leaves just nine degrees of freedom to estimate the error variance at each voxel.

Voxel-level statistic With only 9 degrees of freedom, this study shows the characteristic noisy variance image (Fig. 46.2). The high-frequency noise from poor variance estimates propagates into the *t*-statistic image, when one would expect an image of evidence against $\mathcal{H}_0$ to be smooth (as is the case for studies with greater degrees of freedom) since the raw images are smooth.

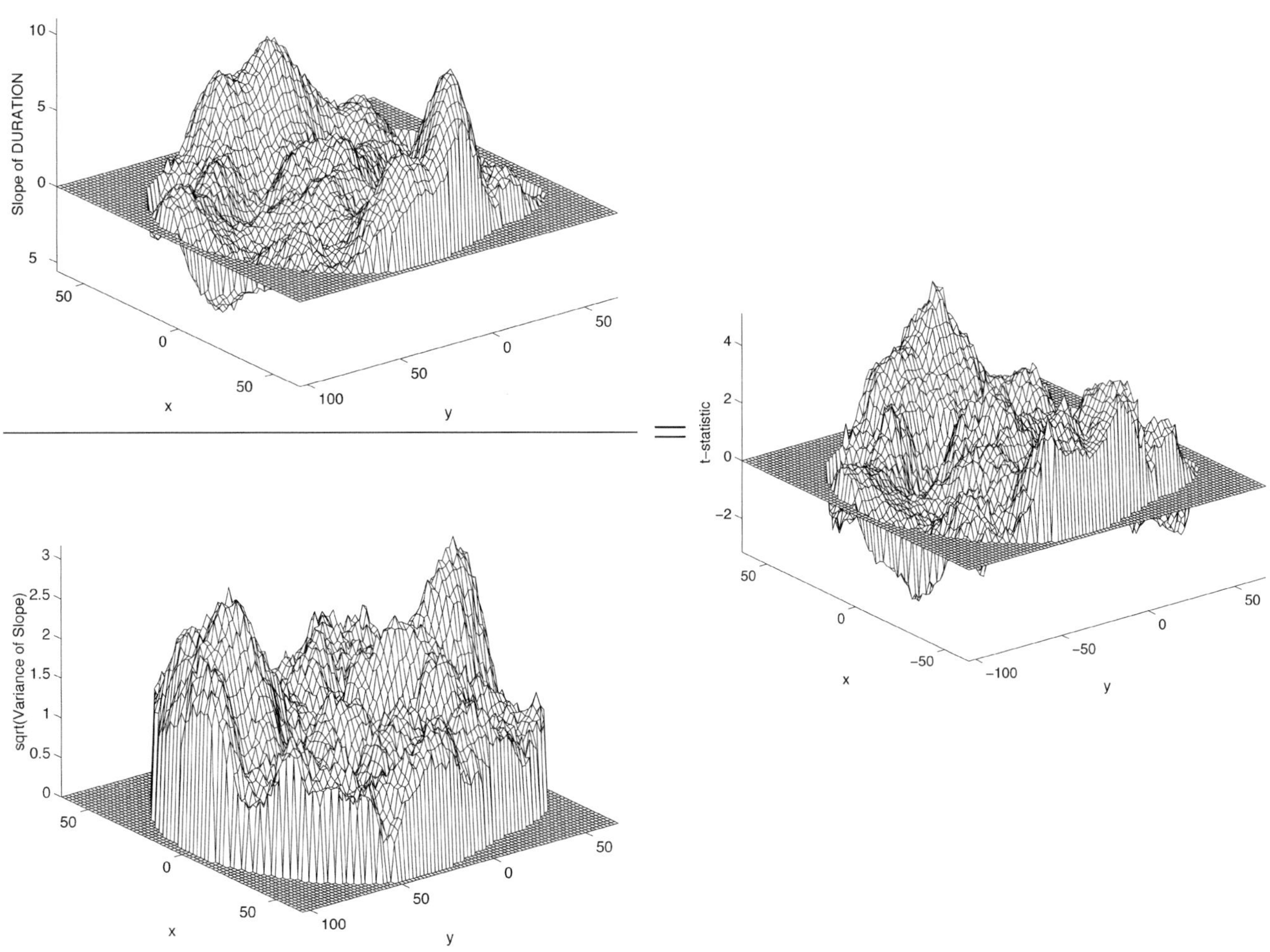

FIGURE 46.2
Mesh plots of parametric analysis, $z = 0$ mm. (Upper left) Slope estimate. (Lower left) Standard deviation of slope estimate. (Right) t image for DURATION. Note how the standard deviation image is much less smooth than the slope image, and how the t image is correspondingly less smooth than the slope image.

We address this situation by smoothing the variance images (see earlier section on pseudo t statistics), replacing the variance estimate at each voxel with a weighted average of its neighbours. We use weights from an 8-mm spherical Gaussian smoothing kernel. The statistic image consisting of the ratio of the slope and the square root of the smoothed variance estimate is smoother than that computed with the raw variance. At the voxel level the resulting statistic does not have a student's t distribution under the null hypothesis, so we refer to it as a *pseudo t* statistic.

Figure 46.3 shows the effect of variance smoothing. The smoothed variance image creates a smoother statistic image, the pseudo t-statistic image. The key here is that the parametric t statistic introduces high-spatial-frequency noise via the poorly estimated standard deviation—by smoothing the variance image we are making the statistic image more like the "signal."

Summary statistic We summarise evidence against $\mathcal{H}_0$ for each relabeling with the maximum statistic, and in this example consider the maximum supra-threshold cluster size (max STCS).

Clusters are defined by connected supra-threshold voxels. Under $\mathcal{H}_0$, the statistic image should be random with no features or structure; hence, large clusters are unusual and indicate the presence of an activation. A primary threshold is used to define the clusters. The selection of the primary threshold is crucial. If set too high, there will be no clusters of any size; if set too low, the clusters will be too large to be useful.

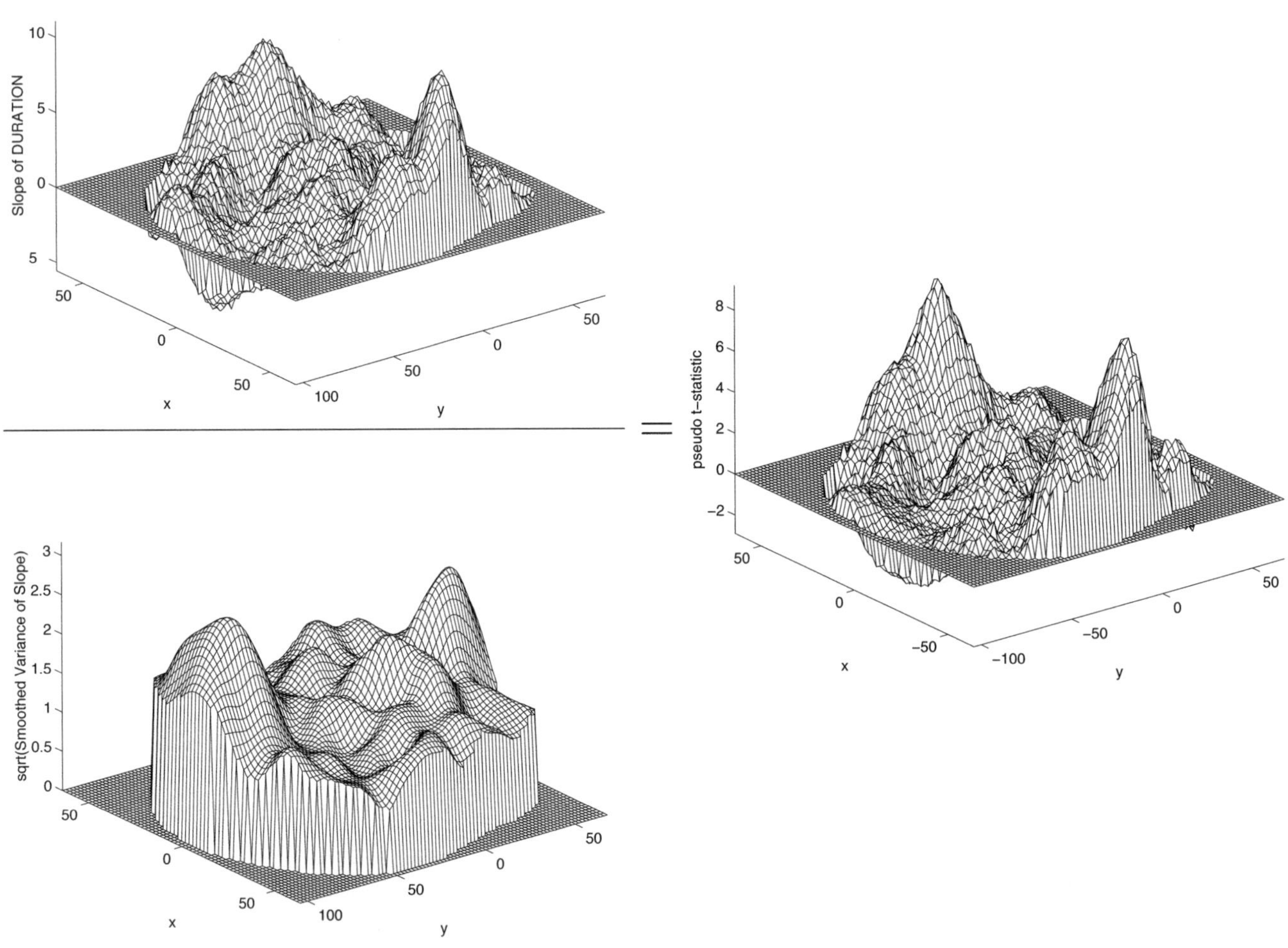

FIGURE 46.3
Mesh plots of permutation analysis, $z = 0$ mm. (Upper left) Slope estimate. (Lower left) Square root of smoothed variance of slope estimate. (Right) Pseudo t image for DURATION. Note that the smoothness of the pseudo t image is similar to that of the slope image (cf. Fig. 46.2).

Relabeling Enumeration

Each of the three previous sections corresponds to a choice that a user of the permutation test has to make. Those choices and the data are sufficient for an algorithm to complete the permutation test. This and the next two sections describe the ensuing computational steps.

To create the labeling used in the experiment, the labels were divided into three blocks of four, and randomly ordered within blocks. There are $4! = 4 \times 3 \times 2 \times 1 = 24$ ways to permute 4 labels, and since each block is independently randomised, there are a total of $4!^3 = 13{,}824$ permutations of the labels.

Computations for 13,824 permutations would be burdensome, so we use an approximate test. We randomly select 999 relabelings to compute the statistic, giving 1000 relabelings including the actual labeling used in the experiment. Recall that while the p values are approximates, the test is still exact.

Permutation Distribution

For each of the 1000 relabelings, the statistic image is computed and thresholded, and the maximal supra-threshold cluster size is recorded. For each relabeling this involves model fitting at each voxel, smoothing the variance image, and creating the pseudo t-statistic image. This is the most computationally intensive part of the analysis, but is not onerous on modern computing hardware. (See the "Discussion of Examples" section for computing times.)

Selection of the primary threshold is a quandary. For the results to be valid, we need to pick the threshold before the analysis is performed. With a parametric voxel-level statistic we could

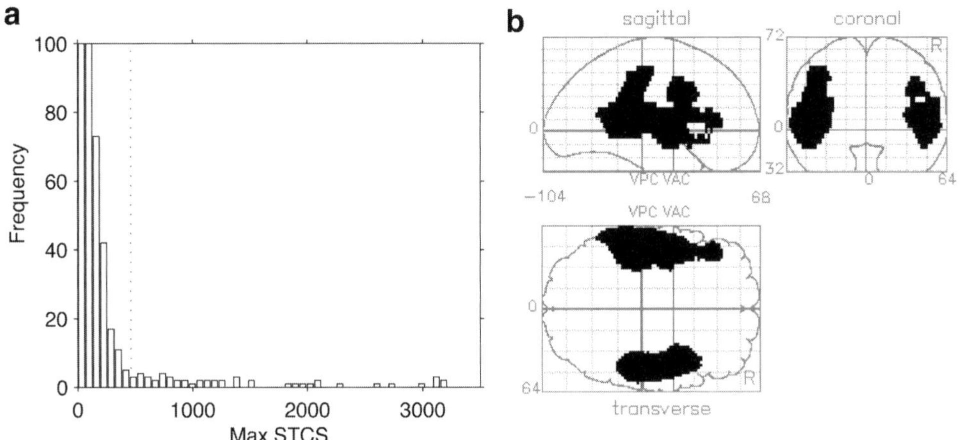

FIGURE 46.4
(a) Distribution of maximum supra-threshold cluster size with a primary threshold of 3. Dotted line shows 95th percentile. The count axis is truncated at 100 to show low-count tail; first two bars have counts 579 and 221. (b) Maximum intensity projection image of significantly large clusters.

use its null distribution to specify a threshold from the uncorrected p value (e.g., by using a t table). Here we cannot take this approach since we are using a nonparametric voxel-level statistic whose null distribution is not known *a priori*. Picking several thresholds is not valid, because this introduces a new multiple-comparisons problem. We suggest gaining experience with similar datasets from *post hoc* analyses: apply different thresholds to get a feel for an appropriate range and then apply such a threshold to the data on hand. Using data from other subjects in this study, we found 3.0 to be a reasonable primary threshold.

Significance Threshold

The distribution of max STCS is used to assess the overall significance of the experiment and the significance of individual clusters: The significance is the proportion of relabelings that had max STCS greater than or equal to the maximum STCS of the correct labeling. Put another way, if max STCS of the correct labeling is at or above the 95th percentile of the max STCS permutation distribution, the experiment is significant at $\alpha = 0.05$. Also, any cluster in the observed image with size greater than the 95th percentile is the significant at $\alpha = 0.05$. Since we have 1000 relabelings, $1000 \times 0.95 = 950$, so the 950th largest max STCS will be our significance threshold.

Results

The permutation distribution of max STCS under $\mathcal{H}_0$ is shown in Fig. 46.4a. Most relabelings have max STCS less than 250 voxels. The vertical dotted line indicates the 95th percentile: the top 5% are spread from about 500 to 3000 voxels.

For the correctly labeled data, the max STCS was 3101 voxels. This is unusually large in comparison to the permutation distribution. Only five relabelings yield max STCS equal to or larger than 3101, so the p value for the experiment is $5/1000 = 0.005$. The 95th percentile is 462, so any supra-threshold clusters with size greater than 462 voxels can be declared significant at level 0.05, accounting for the multiple-comparisons implicit in searching over the brain.

Figure 46.4b is a *maximum intensity projection* (MIP) of the significant supra-threshold clusters. Only these two clusters are significant; that is, there are no other supra-threshold clusters larger than 462 voxels. These two clusters cover the bilateral auditory (primary and associative) and language cortices. They are 3101 and 1716 voxels in size, with p values of 0.005 and 0.015, respectively. Since the test concerns supra-threshold clusters, it has no localising power: significantly large supra-threshold clusters contain voxels with a significant experimental effect, but the test does not identify them.

Discussion

The nonparametric analysis presented here uses maximum STCS on a pseudo t-statistic image. Since the distribution of the pseudo t statistic is not known, the corresponding primary threshold for a parametric analysis using a standard t statistic cannot be computed. This precludes a straightforward comparison of this nonparametric analysis with a corresponding parametric analysis such as that of Friston *et al.* (1994).

Although the need to choose the primary threshold for supra-threshold cluster identification is a problem, the same is true for parametric approaches. The only additional difficulty occurs with pseudo t-statistic images, when specification of primary thresholds in terms of upper-tail probabilities from a Student's t distribution is impossible. Further, parametric supra-threshold cluster size methods (Friston *et al.,* 1994; Poline *et al.,* 1997) utilise asymptotic distributional results and, therefore, require high primary thresholds. The nonparametric technique is free of this constraint, giving exact p values for any primary threshold (although very low thresholds are undesirable due to the large supra-threshold clusters expected and consequent poor localisation of an effect).

Although only supra-threshold cluster size has been considered, any statistic summarising a supra-threshold cluster could be considered. In particular, an exceedance mass statistic could be employed.

Multisubject PET: Activation

For the second example we consider a multisubject, two-condition activation experiment. Here we will use a standard t statistic with a single threshold test, enabling a direct comparison with the standard parametric random field approach.

Study Description

Watson *et al.* (1993) localised the region of visual cortex sensitive to motion, area MT/V5, using high-resolution 3-D PET imaging of 12 subjects. These the data were analyzed by Holmes *et al.* (1996), using proportional scaling global flow normalisation and a repeated measures pseudo t statistic. Here we consider the same data, but use a standard repeated measures t statistic, allowing direct comparison of parametric and nonparametric approaches.

The visual stimulus consisted of randomly placed squares. During the baseline condition the pattern was stationary, whereas during the active condition the squares smoothly moved in independent directions. Prior to the experiment, the 12 subjects were randomly allocated to one of two scan condition presentation orders in a balanced randomisation. Thus six subjects had scan conditions ABABABABABAB; the remaining six had BABABABABABA, which we refer to as AB and BA orders, respectively.

Null Hypothesis

In this example the labels of the scans as A and B are allocated by the initial randomisation, so we have a randomisation test, and the null hypothesis concerns the data directly:

$\mathcal{H}_0$: For each subject, the experiment would have yielded the same data were the conditions reversed.

Exchangeability

Given the null hypothesis, exchangeability follows directly from the initial randomisation scheme: The experiment was randomised at the subject level, with six AB and six BA labels randomly assigned to the 12 subjects. Correspondingly, the labels are exchangeable subject to the constraint that they could have arisen from the initial randomisation scheme. Thus we consider all permutations of the labels that result in 6 subjects having scans labeled AB, and the remaining 6 BA. The initial randomisation could have resulted in any 6 subjects having the AB condition presentation order (the remainder being BA), and under the null hypothesis the data would have been the same, hence, exchangeability.

Statistic

We are interested in the activation magnitude relative to the intersubject variability in activation; hence, we use the statistic associated with a *random-effects* model, which incorporates a random subject by means of a condition interaction term.

Voxel-level statistic A random-effects analysis is easily effected by collapsing the data within subject and computing the statistic across subjects (Worsley *et al.,* 1991; Holmes and Friston, 1999). In this case the result is a repeated-measures t statistic after proportional scaling global flow normalisation. Each scan is proportionally scaled to a common global mean of 50; each subject's data are collapsed into two average images, one for each condition; a paired t statistic is computed across the subjects' "rest"–"active" pairs of average images. By computing this paired t statistic on the collapsed data, both the intersubject and intrasubject (error) components of variance are accounted for appropriately. Because there are 12 subjects there are 12 pairs of average condition images, and the t statistic has 11 degrees of freedom. With just 11 degrees of freedom we anticipate the same problems with noisy variance images as in the previous examples, but in order to make direct comparisons with a parametric approach, we do not consider variance smoothing and pseudo t statistics for this example.

Summary statistic To consider a single threshold test over the entire brain, the appropriate summary statistic is the maximum t statistic.

Relabeling Enumeration

This example is different from the previous one in that we permute across subjects instead of across replications of conditions. Here our EB is not in units of scans, but subjects. The EB size here is 12 subjects, since the six AB and six BA labels can be permuted freely among the 12 subjects. There are $\binom{12}{6} = \frac{12!}{6!(12-6)!} = 924$ ways of choosing 6 of the 12 subjects to have the AB labeling. This is a sufficiently small number of permutations to consider a complete enumeration.

One may consider permuting labels within subjects, particularly in the permutation setting when there is no initial randomisation dictating the exchangeability. However, the bulk of the permutation distribution is specified by these between-subject permutations, and any within-subject permutations just flesh out this framework, yielding little practical improvement in the test at considerable computational cost.

Permutation Distribution

For each of 924 relabelings we calculate the maximum repeated-measures t statistic, resulting in the permutation distribution shown in Fig. 46.5a. Note that for each possible relabeling and t-statistic image, the opposite relabeling is also possible, and gives the negative of the t-statistic image. Thus, it is only necessary to compute t-statistic images for half of the relabelings and to retain their maxima and minima. The permutation distribution is then that of the maxima for half the relabelings concatenated with the negative of the corresponding minima.

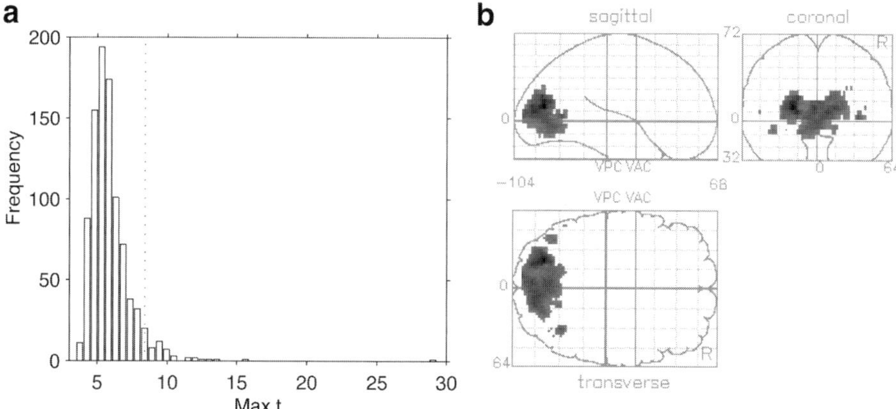

FIGURE 46.5
(a) Permutation distribution of maximum repeated-measures t statistic. Dotted line indicates the 5% level corrected threshold. (b) Maximum intensity projection of t-statistic image, thresholded at critical threshold for a 5% level permutation test analysis of 8.401.

Significance Threshold

As before, the 95th percentile of the maximum t distribution provides both a threshold for omnibus experimental significance and a voxel-level significance threshold appropriate for the multiple-comparisons problem. With 924 permutations, the 95th percentile is at $924 \times 0.05 = 46.2$, so the critical threshold is the 47th largest member of the permutation distribution. Any voxel with intensity greater than this threshold can be declared significant at the 0.05 level.

Results

Figure 46.5a shows the permutation distribution of the maximum repeated-measures t statistic. Most maxima lie between about 4 and 9, though the distribution is skewed in the positive direction.

The outlier at 29.30 corresponds to the observed t statistic, computed with correctly labeled data. Since no other relabelings are higher, the p value is $1/924 = 0.0011$. The 47th largest member of the permutation distribution is 8.40, the critical threshold (marked with a dotted vertical line on the permutation distribution). The t-statistic image thresholded at this critical value is shown in Fig. 46.5b. There is a primary region of 1424 significant voxels covering the V1/V2 region, flanked by two secondary regions of 23 and 25 voxels corresponding to area V5, plus six other regions of 1 or 2 voxels.

For a t-statistic image of 43,724 voxels of size $2 \times 2 \times 4$ mm, with an estimated smoothness of $7.8 \times 8.7 \times 8.7$ mm FWHM, the parametric theory gives a 5% level critical threshold of 11.07, substantially higher than the corresponding 4.61 of the nonparametric result. The thresholded image is shown in Fig. 46.6b; the image is very similar to the nonparametric image (Fig. 46.5b), with the primary region having 617 voxels, and two secondary regions of 7 and 2 voxels. Another parametric result is the well-known, but conservative, Bonferroni correction; here it specifies a 5% threshold of 8.92, which yields a primary region of 1212 voxels and 5 secondary regions with a total of 48 voxels. In Fig. 46.6a, we compare these three approaches by plotting the significance level versus the threshold. The critical threshold based on the expected Euler characteristic (Worsley *et al.,* 1995) for a t-statistic image is shown as a dashed line and the critical values for the permutation test are shown as a solid line. For a given test level (a horizontal line), the test with the smaller threshold has the greater power. At all thresholds in this plot, the nonparametric threshold is below the random field threshold, though it closely tracks the Bonferroni threshold below the 0.05 level. Thus random field theory (see Chapters 14 and 15) appears to be quite conservative here.

Discussion

This example again demonstrates the role of the permutation test as a reference for evaluating other procedures, here the parametric analysis of Friston *et al.* (1995b). The t-field results are

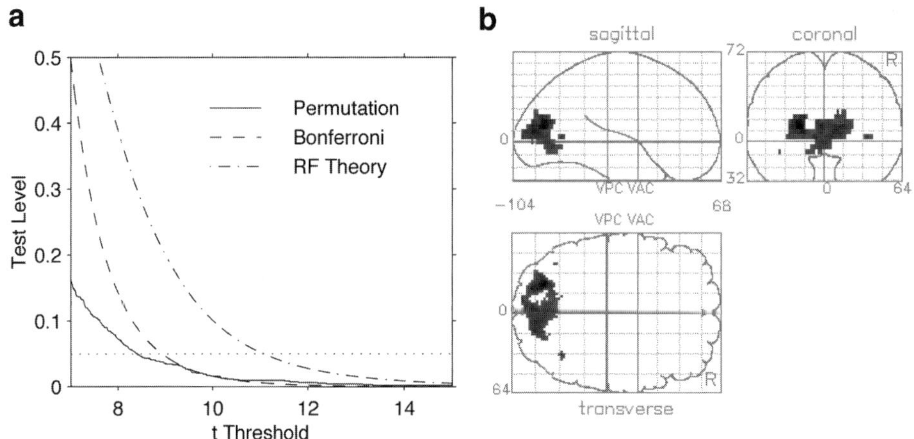

FIGURE 46.6
(a) Test significance (α) levels plotted against critical thresholds, for nonparametric and parametric analyses. (b) Maximum intensity projection of t image, thresholded at parametric 5% level critical threshold of 11.07.

conservative for low degrees of freedom and low smoothness (Keith Worsley, personal communication); the striking difference between the nonparametric and random field thresholds makes this clear.

Figure 46.6a provides a very informative comparison between the two methods. For all typical test sizes ($\alpha \leq 0.05$), the nonparametric method specifies a lower threshold than the parametric method. For these data, this is exposing the conservativeness of the t-field results. For lower thresholds the difference between the methods is even greater, although this is anticipated since the parametric results are based on high threshold approximations.

A randomisation test applied to a random-effects statistic presents an interesting contradiction. While we use a statistic corresponding to a model with a random subject by condition interaction, we are performing a randomisation test that technically excludes inference on a population. However, if we assume that the subjects of this study constitute a random sample of the population of interest, we can ignore the experimental randomisation and perform a permutation test, as we do in the next example.

Multisubject fMRI: Activation

For this third and final example, consider a multisubject fMRI activation experiment. Here we perform a permutation test so that we can make an inference on a population. We will use a smoothed variance t statistic with a single threshold test and will make qualitative and quantitative comparisons with the parametric results.

Before discussing the details of this example, we note that fMRI data present a special challenge for nonparametric methods. Since fMRI data exhibit temporal autocorrelation (Smith *et al.,* 1999), an assumption of exchangeability of scans within subject is not tenable. However, to analyze a group of subjects for population inference we need only assume exchangeability of subjects. Hence, while intrasubject fMRI analyses are not straightforward with the permutation test, multisubject analyses are.

Study Description

Marshuetz *et al.* (2000) studied order effects in working memory using fMRI. The data were analyzed using a random-effects procedure (Holmes and Friston, 1999), as in the last example. For fMRI, this procedure amounts to a generalisation of the repeated-measures t statistic.

There were 12 subjects, each participating in eight fMRI acquisitions. There were two possible presentation orders for each block, and there was randomisation across blocks and subjects. The RT was 2 sec, a total of 528 scans collected per condition. Of the study's three conditions we consider only two, item recognition and control. For item recognition, the subject was presented with five letters and, after a 2-sec interval, presented with a probe letter. They were to respond "yes" if the probe letter was among the five letters and "no" if it was not. In the control condition they were presented with five *X*'s and, 2 sec later, presented with either a *y* or an *n;* they were to press "yes" for *y* and "no" for *n*.

Each subject's data was analyzed, creating a difference image between the item recognition and control effects. These images were analyzed with a one-sample t test, yielding a random-effects analysis that accounts for intersubject differences.

Null Hypothesis

While this study used randomisation within and across subjects and hence permits the use of a randomisation test, we will use a permutation approach to generalise the results to a population.

Again using a random-effects statistic, we only analyze each subject's item vs. control difference image. We make the weak distributional assumption that the values of the subject difference images at any given voxel (across subjects) are drawn from a symmetric distribution. (The distribution may be different at different voxels, as long as it is symmetric). The null hypothesis is that these distributions are centered on zero:

$\mathcal{H}_0$: The symmetric distributions of the (voxel values of the) subjects' difference images have zero mean.

Exchangeability

The conventional assumption of independent subjects implies exchangeability and, hence, a single EB consisting of all subjects.

Exchanging the item and control labels has exactly the effect of flipping the sign of the difference image. So we consider subject labels of "+1" and "–1," indicating an unflipped or flipped sign of the data. Under the null hypothesis, we have data symmetric about zero and, hence, can randomly flip the signs of subject's difference images.

Statistic

In this example we focus on statistic magnitude.

Voxel-level statistic As noted above, this analysis amounts to a one-sample t test on the first-level difference images, testing for a zero-mean effect across subjects. We use a pseudo t test, with a variance smoothing of 4 mm FWHM, comparable to the original within-subject smoothing. In our experience, the use of *any* variance smoothing is more important than the particular magnitude (FWHM) of the smoothing.

Summary statistic Again we are interested in searching the whole brain for significant changes; hence, we use the maximum pseudo t.

Relabeling Enumeration

Based on our exchangeability under the null hypothesis, we can flip the sign on some or all of our subjects' data. There are $2^{12} = 4096$ possible ways of assigning either "+1" or "–1" to each subject. We consider all 4096 relabelings.

Permutation Distribution

For each relabeling we found the maximum pseudo t statistic, yielding the distribution shown in Fig. 46.7a. As in the last example, we have a symmetry in these labels; we need only compute 2048 statistic images and save both the maxima and minima.

Significance Threshold

With 4096 permutations the 95th percentile is $4096 \times 0.05 = 452.3$, and hence the 453rd largest maxima defines the 0.05-level corrected significance threshold.

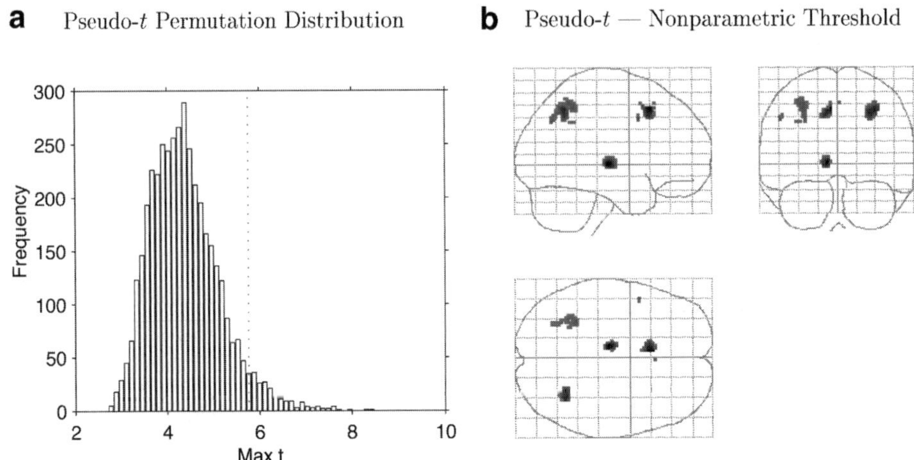

FIGURE 46.7
(a) Permutation distribution of maximum repeated-measures t statistic. Dotted line indicates the 5% level corrected threshold. (b) Maximum intensity projection of pseudo t-statistic image threshold at 5% level, as determined by permutation distribution. (c) Maximum intensity projection of t-statistic image threshold at 5% level as determined by permutation distribution. (d) Maximum intensity projection of t-statistic image threshold at 5% level as determined by random field theory.

Results

The permutation distribution of the maximum pseudo t statistic under $\mathcal{H}_0$ is shown in Fig. 46.7a. It is centered around 4.5 and is slightly positively skewed; all maxima found were between about 3 and 8.

The correctly labeled data yielded the largest maximum, 8.471. Hence the overall significance of the experiment is 1/4096 = 0.0002. The dotted line indicates the 0.05 corrected threshold, 5.763. Figure 46.7b shows the thresholded MIP of significant voxels. There are 312 voxels in eight distinct regions; in particular, there is a pair of bilateral posterior parietal regions, a left thalamus region, and an anterior cingulate region; these are typical of working memory studies (Marshuetz *et al.,* 2000).

It is informative to compare this result to the traditional t statistic, using both a nonparametric and parametric approach to obtain corrected thresholds. We reran this nonparametric analysis using no variance smoothing. The resulting thresholded data are shown in Fig. 46.7c; there are only 58 voxels in three regions that exceeded the corrected threshold of 7.667. Using standard parametric random field methods produced the result in Fig. 46.7d. For 110,776 voxels of size $2 \times 2 \times 2$ mm, with an estimated smoothness of $5.1 \times 5.8 \times 6.9$ mm FWHM, the parametric theory finds a threshold of 9.870; there are only 5 voxels in three regions above this threshold. Note that only the pseudo t statistic detects the bilateral parietal regions. Table 46.1 summarises the three analyses along with the Bonferroni result.

Discussion

In this example we have demonstrated the utility of the nonparametric method for intersubject fMRI analyses. Based solely on independence of the subjects and symmetric distribution of difference images under the null hypothesis, we can create a permutation test that yields inferences on a population.

Multiple subject fMRI studies often have few subjects, many fewer than 20 subjects. By using the smoothed variance t statistic we have gained sensitivity relative to the standard t statistic. Even with the standard t statistic, the nonparametric test proved more powerful, detecting five times as many voxels as active. Although the smoothed variance t is statistically valid, it does not overcome any limitations of *face* validity of an analysis based on only 12 subjects.

We note that this relative ranking of sensitivity (nonparametric pseudo t, nonparametric t, parametric t) is consistent with the other second-level datasets we have analyzed. We believe this is due to a conservativeness of the random t-field results under low degrees of freedom, not just low smoothness.

Discussion of Examples

These examples have demonstrated the nonparametric permutation test for PET and fMRI with a variety of experimental designs and analyses. We have addressed each of the steps in sufficient detail to follow the algorithmic steps that the SnPM software performs. We have shown that the ability to utilise smoothed variances via a pseudo t statistic can offer an approach with increased power over a corresponding standard t-statistic image. Using standard t statistics, we have seen

TABLE 46.1 Comparison of Four Inference Methods for the Item Recognition fMRI Data[a]

Statistic	Inference method	Corrected threshold t	Corrected threshold Pseudo t	Minimum corrected p value	Number of significant voxels
t	Random field	9.870		0.0062	5
t	Bonferroni	9.802		0.0025	5
t	Permutation	7.667		0.0002	58
Pseudo t	Permutation		5.763	0.0002	312

[a] The minimum corrected p-value and number of significant voxels give an overall measure of sensitivity; corrected thresholds can only be compared within statistic type. For this data, the Bonferroni and random field results are very similar, and the nonparametric methods are more powerful; the nonparametric t method detects 10 times as many voxels as the parametric method, and the nonparametric pseudo-t detects 60 times as many.

how the permutation test can be used as a reference against which parametric results can be validated.

However, note that the comparison between parametric and nonparametric results must be made very carefully. Comparable models and statistics must be used, and multiple comparisons procedures with the same degree of control over image-wise type I error used. Further, since the permutation distributions are derived from the data, critical thresholds are specific to the dataset under consideration. Although the examples presented above are compelling, remember that these are only a few specific examples, and further experience with many datasets is required before generalisations can be made. However, the points noted for these specific examples are indicative of our general experience with these methods (Nichols and Hayasaka, in press).

Finally, while we have noted that the nonparametric method has greater computational demands than parametric methods, they are reasonable on modern hardware. The PET examples took 35 and 20 min, respectively, on a 176-MHz Sparc Ultra 1. The fMRI example took 2 hours on a 440-MHz Sparc Ultra 10. The fMRI data took longer due to more permutations (2048 vs. 500) and larger images.

CONCLUSIONS

In this chapter the theory and practicalities of multiple-comparisons nonparametric randomisation and permutation tests for functional neuroimaging experiments have been presented and illustrated with worked examples.

As has been demonstrated, the permutation approach offers various advantages. The methodology is intuitive and accessible. By consideration of suitable maximal summary statistics, the multiple-comparisons problem can easily be accounted for; only minimal assumptions are required for valid inference, and the resulting tests are almost exact, with size at most $1/N$ less than the nominal test level α, where N is the number of relabelings.

The nonparametric permutation approaches described give results similar to those obtained from a comparable SPM approach using a general linear model with multiple comparisons corrections derived from random field theory. In this respect these nonparametric techniques can be used to verify the validity of less computationally expensive parametric approaches. When the assumptions required for a parametric approach are not met, the nonparametric approach described provides a viable alternative analysis method.

In addition, the approach is flexible. Choice of voxel and summary statistic are not limited to those whose null distributions can be derived from parametric assumptions. This is particularly advantageous at low degrees of freedom, when noisy variance images lead to noisy statistic images, and multiple-comparisons procedures based on the theory of continuous random fields are conservative. By assuming a smooth variance structure and by using a pseudo t statistic computed with smoothed variances, the permutation approach gains considerable power.

Therefore we propose that the nonparametric permutation approach is preferable for experimental designs implying low degrees of freedom, including small sample size problems, such as single-subject PET/SPECT, but also PET/SPECT and fMRI multisubject and between-group analyses involving small numbers of subjects, for which analysis must be conducted at the subject level to account for intersubject variability. It is our hope that this chapter, and the accompanying software, will encourage appropriate application of these nonparametric techniques.

Acknowledgments

We thank the authors of the three example datasets analyzed for permission to use their data.

References

Arndt, S., Cizadlo, T., Andreasen, N. C., Heckel, D., Gold, S., and O'Leary, D. S. (1996). Tests for comparing images based on randomisation and permutation methods. *J. Cereb. Blood Flow Metab.* **16**(6), 1271–1279.

Bullmore, E., Brammer, M., Williams, S. C. R., Rabe-Hesketh, S., Janot, N., David, A., Mellers, J., Howard, R., and Sham, P. (1996). Statistical methods of estimation and inference for functional MR image analysis. *Mag. Res. Med.* **35,** 261–277.

Bullmore, E. T., Suckling, J., Overmeyer, S., Rabe-Hesketh, S., Taylor, E., and Brammer, M. J. (1999). Global, voxel, and cluster tests, by theory and permutation, for a difference between two groups of structural MR images of the brain. *IEEE Trans. Med. Imaging* **18**(1), 32–42.

Bullmore, E., Long, C., and Suckling, J. (2001). Colored noise and computational inference in neurophysiological (fMRI) time series analysis: resampling methods in time and wavelet domains. *Hum. Brain Mapping* **12,** 61–78.

Cao, J. (1999). The size of the connected components of excursion sets of χ^2, t and F fields. *Adv. Appl. Prob.* (accepted).

Dwass, M. (1957). Modified randomisation tests for nonparametric hypotheses. *Ann. Math. Statistics* **28,** 181–187.

Edgington, E. S. (1964). Randomisation tests. *J. Psychol.* **57,** 445–449.

Edgington, E. S. (1969a). Approximate randomisation tests. *J. Psychol.* **72,** 143–149.

Edgington, E. S. (1969b). *Statistical Inference: The Distribution Free Approach.* McGraw-Hill, New York.

Edgington, E. S. (1995). *Randomisation Tests,* 3rd ed. Marcel Dekker, New York.

Fisher, R. A. (1935). *The Design of Experiments.* Oliver, Boyd, Edinburgh.

Fisher, R. A., (Auth), and Bennett, J. H. (Ed). (1990). *Statistical Methods, Experimental Design, and Scientific Inference.* Oxford University Press, Oxford, UK.

Forman, S. D., Cohen, J. D., Fitzgerald, M., Eddy, W. F., Mintun, M. A., and Noll, D. C. (1995). Improved assessment of significant activation in functional magnetic resonance imaging (fMRI): use of a cluster-size threshold. *Mag. Res. Med.* **33**(5), 636–647.

Frackowiak, R. S. J., Friston, K. J., Frith, C. D., Dolan, R. J., and Mazziotta, J. C. (1997). *Hum. Brain Function.* Academic Press, San Diego.

Friston, K. J., Frith, C. D., Liddle, P. F., and Frackowiak, R. S. J. (1991). Comparing functional (PET) images: the assessment of significant change. *J. Cereb. Blood Flow Metab.* **11**(4), 690–699.

Friston, K. J., Worsley, K. J., Frackowiak, R. S. J., Mazziotta, J. C., and Evans, A. C. (1994). Assessing the significance of focal activations using their spatial extent. *Hum. Brain Mapping* **1,** 214–220.

Friston, K. J., Holmes, A. P., Poline, J.-B., Grasby, P. J., Williams, S. C. R., Frackowiak, R. S. J., and Turner, R. (1995a). Analysis of fMRI time series revisited. *NeuroImage* **2,** 45–53.

Friston, K. J., Holmes, A. P., Worsley, K. J., Poline, J.-B., and Frackowiak, R. S. J. (1995b). Statistical parametric maps in functional imaging: a general linear approach. *Hum. Brain Mapping* **2,** 189–210.

Friston, K. J., Holmes, A. P., Poline, J.-B., Price, C. J., and Frith, C. D. (1996). Detecting activations in PET and fMRI: levels of inference and power. *NeuroImage* **4**(3 Pt 1), 223–235.

Genovese, C. R., Lazar, N., and Nichols, T. E. (2001). Thresholding of statistical maps in functional neuroimaging using the false discovery rate. *NeuroImage.*

Good, P. (1994). *Permutation Tests. A Practical Guide to Resampling Methods for Testing Hypotheses.* Springer-Verlag, Berlin.

Grabowski, T. J., Frank, R. J., Brown, C. K., Damasio, H., Boles Ponto, L. L., Watkins, G. L., and Hichwa, R. D. (1996). Reliability of PET activation across statistical methods, subject groups, and sample sizes. *Hum. Brain Mapping* **4**(1), 23–46.

Halber, M., Herholz, K., Wienhard, K., Pawlik, G., and Heiss, W. D. (1997). Performance of a randomisation test for single-subject 15-O-Water PET activation studies. *J. Cereb. Blood Flow Metab.* **17,** 1033–1039.

Hochberg, Y., and Tamhane, A. C. (1987). *Multiple Comparison Procedures.* Wiley, New York.

Holmes, A. P. (1994). *Statistical Issues in Functional Brain Mapping.* Ph.D. thesis, University of Glasgow. Available from http://www.fil.ion.ucl.ac.uk/spm/papers/APH_thesis.

Holmes, A. P., and Friston, K. J. (1999). Generalisability, random effects and population inference. *NeuroImage* **7**(4, Pt 2/3), S754. (*Proceedings of Fourth International Conference on Functional Mapping of the Human Brain,* June 7–12, 1998, Montreal, Canada.)

Holmes, A. P., Blair, R. C., Watson, J. D. G., and Ford, I. (1996). Nonparametric analysis of statistic images from functional mapping experiments. *J. Cereb. Blood Flow Metab.* **16**(1), 7–22.

Holmes, A. P., Watson, J. D. G., and Nichols, T. E. (1998). Holmes and Watson, on "Sherlock." *J. Cereb. Blood Flow Metab.* **18**(-), S697. Letter to the editor, with reply.

Jöckel, K.-H. (1686). Finite sample properties and asymptotic efficiency of Monte-Carlo tests. *Ann. Statistics* **14,** 336–347.

Kendall, M., and Gibbons, J. D. (1990). *Rank Correlation Methods* (5th ed.). Edward Arnold.

Liu, C., Raz, J., and Turetsky, B. (1998). (March). An estimator and permutation test for single-trial fMRI data. In *Abstracts of ENAR Meeting of the International Biometric Society.*

Locascio, J. J., Jennings, P. J., Moore, C. I., and Corkin, S. (1997). Time series analysis in the time domain and resampling methods for studies of functional magnetic resonance brain imaging. *Hum. Brain Mapping* **5,** 168–193.

Manly, B. F. J. (1997). *Randomisation, Bootstrap and Monte-Carlo Methods in Biology.* Chapman & Hall, London.

Marshuetz, C., Smith, E. E., Jonides, J., DeGutis, J., and Chenevert, T. L. (2000). Order information in working memory: fMRI evidence for parietal and prefrontal mechanisms. *J. Cog. Neurosci.* **12**(S2), 130–144.

Nichols, T. E., and Hayasaka, S. (in press). Controlling the family wise error rate in functional neuroimaging: A comparative review. *Stat. Meth. Med. Res.*

Nichols, T. E., and Holmes, A. P. (2001). Nonparametric permutation tests for functional neuroimaging: a primer with examples. *Hum. Brain Mapping* **15,** 1–25.

Pitman, E. J. G. (1937a). Significance tests which may be applied to samples from any population. *J. Roy. Stat. Soc. (Suppl.)* **4,** 119–130.

Pitman, E. J. G. (1937b). Signficance tests which may be applied to samples from any population. II. The correlation coefficient test. *J. Roy. Stat. Soc. (Suppl.)* **4,** 224–232.

Pitman, E. J. G. (1937c). Signficance tests which may be applied to samples from any population. III. The analysis of variance test. *Biometrika* **29,** 322–335.

Poline, J. B., and Mazoyer, B. M. (1993). Analysis of individual positron emission tomography activation maps by detection of high signal-to-noise-ratio pixel clusters. *J. Cereb. Blood Flow Metab.* **13**(3), 425–437.

Poline, J. B., Worsley, K. J., Evans, A. C., and Friston, K. J. (1997). Combining spatial extent and peak intensity to test for activations in functional imaging. *NeuroImage* **5**(2), 83–96.

Roland, P. E., Levin, B., Kawashima, R., and Akerman, S. (1993). Three-dimensional analysis of clustered voxels in 15-O-butanol brain activation images. *Hum. Brain Mapping* **1**(1), 3–19.

Silbersweig, D. A., Stern, E., Schnorr, L., Frith, C. D., Ashburner, J., Cahill, C., Frackowiak, R. S. J., and Jones, T. (1994). Imaging transient, randomly occurring neuropsychological events in single subjects with positron emission tomography: an event-related count rate correlational analysis. *J. Cereb. Blood Flow Metab.* **14,** 771–782.

Silbersweig, D. A., Stern, E., Frith, C., Cahill, C., Holmes, A., Grootoonk, S., Seaward, J., McKenna, P., Chua, S. E., Schnorr, L., *et al.* (1995). A functional neuroanatomy of hallucinations in schizophrenia. *Nature* **378**(6553), 176–169.

Smith, A. M., Lewis, B. K., Ruttimann, U. E., Ye, F. Q., Sinnwell, T. M., Yang, Y., Duyn, J. H., and Frank, J. A. (1999). Investigation of low frequency drift in fMRI signal. *NeuroImage* **9,** 526–533.

Watson, J. D. G., Myers, R., Frackowiak, R. S. J., Hajnal, J. V., Woods, R. P., Mazziotta, J. C., Shipp, S., and Zeki, S. (1993). Area V5 of the human brain: evidence from a combined study using positron emission tomography and magnetic resonance imaging. *Cereb. Cortex* **3,** 79–94.

Westfall, P. H., and Young, S. S. (1993). *Resampling-Based Multiple Testing: Examples and Methods for p-Value Adjustment.* Wiley, New York.

Worsley, K. J. (1994). Local maxima and the expected Euler characteristic of excursion sets of χ^2, F and *t* fields. *Adv. Appl. Prob.* **26,** 13–42.

Worsley, K. J. (1996). The geometry of random images. *Chance* **9**(1), 27–40.

Worsley, K. J., and Friston, K. J. (1995). Analysis of fMRI time-series revisited—again. *NeuroImage* **2,** 173–181.

Worsley, K. J., Evans, A. C., Strother, S. C., and Tyler, J. L. (1991). A linear spatial correlation model, with applications to positron emission tomography. *J. Am. Stat. Assoc.* **86,** 55–67.

Worsley, K. J., Evans, A. C., Marrett, S., and Neelin, P. (1992). A three-dimensional statistical analysis for CBF activation studies in human brain. *J. Cereb. Blood Flow Metab.* **12**(6), 1040–1042. See comment in *J. Cereb. Blood Flow Metab.* 1993, **13**(6), 1040–1042.

Worsley, K. J., Marrett, S., Neelin, P., Vandal, A. C., Friston, K. J., and Evans, A. C. (1995). A unified statistical approach for determining significant signals in images of cerebral activation. *Hum. Brain Mapping* **4,** 58–73.

Yekutieli, D., and Benjamini, Y. (1999). Resampling-based false discovery rate controlling multiple test procedures for correlated test statistics. *J. Stat. Planning Inference* **82,** 171–196.

CHAPTER

47

Classical and Bayesian Inference

INTRODUCTION

This chapter revisits hierarchical observation models (see Chapter 43), which are used in functional neuroimaging, in a Bayesian light. It emphasises the common ground shared by classical and Bayesian methods to show that conventional analyses of neuroimaging data can be usefully extended within an *empirical* Bayesian framework. In particular, we formulate the procedures used in conventional data analysis in terms of hierarchical linear models and establish a connection between classical inference and parametric empirical Bayes (PEB) through covariance component estimation. This estimation is based on *expectation maximisation* (EM). The key point is that hierarchical models not only provide for appropriate inference at the highest level but that one can revisit lower levels suitably equipped to make Bayesian inferences. Bayesian inferences eschew many of the difficulties encountered with classical inference and characterise brain responses in a way that is more directly predicated on what one is interested in. The motivation for Bayesian approaches is reviewed and the theoretical background is presented in a way that relates to conventional methods, in particular *restricted maximum likelihood* (ReML).

The first section of this chapter is a theoretical prelude to subsequent sections that deal with applications of the theory to a range of important issues in neuroimaging. These issues include (1) estimating nonsphericity or variance components in fMRI time series that can arise from serial correlations within subject or that are induced by multisubject (i.e., hierarchical) studies; (2) Bayesian models for imaging data, in which effects at one voxel are constrained by responses in others; and (3) Bayesian estimation of nonlinear models of haemodynamic responses. Although diverse, all of these estimation problems are accommodated by the EM framework described in this chapter.

Classical and Bayesian Inference

Since its inception about 10 years ago, *statistical parametric mapping* (SPM) has proved useful for characterising neuroimaging data sequences. However, SPM is limited because it is based on classical inference procedures. In this chapter we introduce a more general framework, which places SPM in a broader context and points to alternative ways of characterising and making inferences about regionally specific effects in neuroimaging. In particular, we formulate the procedures used in conventional data analysis in terms of hierarchical linear models and establish the connection between classical inference and *empirical* Bayesian inference through covariance component estimation. This estimation is based on the EM algorithm.

SPM entails the use of the general linear model and classical statistics, under parametric assumptions, to create a statistic (usually the T statistic) at each voxel. Inferences about regionally specific effects are based on the ensuing image of T statistics, the SPM{T}. The requisite distributional approximations for the peak height, or spatial extent, of voxel clusters, surviving a specified threshold, are derived using Gaussian random field theory (see Chapters 44 and 45). Random field theory enables the use of classical inference procedures—and the latitude afforded by the general linear model—to give a powerful and flexible approach to continuous, spatially extended data. It does so by protecting against family-wise false positives over all the voxels that constitute a search volume; i.e., it provides a way of adjusting the p values, in the same way that a Bonferroni correction does for discrete data (Worsley, 1994; Friston *et al.,* 1995).

Despite its success, statistical parametric mapping has a number of fundamental limitations. In SPM the p value, ascribed to a particular effect, does not reflect the likelihood that the effect is present but simply the probability of getting the observed data in the effect's absence. If sufficiently small, this p value can be used to reject the null hypothesis that the effect is negligible. This classical approach has several shortcomings. First, one can never reject the alternate hypothesis (e.g., that an activation has not occurred) because the probability that an effect is exactly zero is itself zero. This is problematic, for example, in trying to establish double dissociations or indeed functional segregation; one can never say one area responds to colour *but not motion* and another responds to motion *but not colour*. Secondly, because the probability of an effect being zero is vanishingly small, given enough scans or subjects one can always demonstrate a significant effect at every voxel. This fallacy of classical inference is becoming relevant practically, with the thousands of scans entering into some fixed-effect analyses of fMRI data. The issue here is that a trivially small activation can be declared significant if there are sufficient degrees of freedom to render the variability of the activation's estimate small enough. A third problem, which is specific to SPM, is the correction or adjustment applied to the p values to resolve the multiple comparison problem. This has the somewhat nonsensical effect of changing the inference about one part of the brain in a way that is contingent on whether another part is examined. Put simply, the threshold increases with search volume, rendering inference very sensitive to what that inference encompasses. Clearly the probability that any voxel has activated does not change with the search volume and yet the classical p value does.

All of these problems would be eschewed by using the probability that a voxel had activated, or indeed its activation was greater than some threshold. This sort of inference is precluded by classical approaches, which simply give the likelihood of getting *the data, given no activation*. What one would really like is the probability distribution of *the activation given the data*. This is the *posterior* probability used in Bayesian inference. The posterior distribution requires both the *likelihood*, afforded by assumptions about the distribution of errors, and the *prior* probability of activation. These priors can enter as known values or can be estimated from the data, provided we have observed multiple instances of the effect in which we are interested. The latter is referred to as *empirical* Bayes. A key point here is that in many situations we do assess repeatedly the same effect over different subjects, or indeed different voxels, and are in a position to adopt an empirical Bayesian approach. This chapter describes one such approach. In contradistinction to other proposals, this approach is not a novel way of analysing neuroimaging data. The use of a Bayesian formalism in special models for fMRI data has been usefully explored elsewhere, e.g., in spatiotemporal Markov field models (Descombes *et al.,* 1998) and mixture models (Everitt and Bullmore, 1999). See also the compelling work of Hartvig and Jensen (2000), which combines both of these approaches, and of Hfjen-Sfrensen *et al.* (2000) who focus on temporal aspects with hidden Markov models. Generally these approaches assume that voxels are either active or not and use the data to infer their status. Because of this underlying assumption, there is little connection with conventional models that allow for continuous or graded haemodynamic responses. The aim here is to highlight the fact that the conventional models that we use routinely conform to hierarchical observation models that can be treated in a Bayesian fashion. The importance of this rests on (1) the connection between classical and Bayesian inference that ensues and (2) the potential to apply Bayesian procedures that are overlooked from a classical perspective. For example, random-effect analyses of fMRI data (Holmes and Friston, 1998; also Chapter 42 in this text) adopt two-level hierarchical models. In this context, people generally focus on classical inference at the second level, unaware that the same model can support

Bayesian inference at the first. Revisiting the first level, within a Bayesian framework, provides for a much better characterisation of single-subject responses, both in terms of the estimated effects and the nature of the inference.

Overview

The aim of the first section below is to describe hierarchical observation models and establish the relationship between classical *maximum likelihood* (ML) and empirical Bayes estimators. Parametric empirical Bayes can be formulated classically in terms of covariance component estimation (e.g., within-subject vs. between-subject contributions to error). The covariance component formulation is important because it is ubiquitous in fMRI. Different sources of variability in the data induce nonsphericity that has to be estimated before any inferences about an effect can be made. Important sources of nonsphericity in fMRI include serial or temporal correlations among the errors in single-subject studies, or in multisubject studies, the differences among within- and between-subject variability. These issues are used in the second section to emphasise both the covariance component estimation and Bayesian perspectives, in terms of the difference between response estimates based on classical ML estimators and the conditional means from a Bayesian approach.

In the third section, we use the same theory to elaborate on hierarchical models that allow the construction of posterior probability maps (PPMs). Again this employs two-level models but focuses on Bayesian inference at the first level. It complements the preceding fMRI application by showing how priors can be estimated using observations *over voxels* at the second level. The final section addresses the Bayesian identification of dynamic systems in which empirical Bayesian priors are replaced by knowledge about the biophysics that underlies haemodynamic responses (see Chapter 41). This approach can be used to characterise haemodynamic responses at a single voxel or, indeed, the response of a network of coupled brain regions (see Chapter 52).

THEORY

In this section we focus on theory and procedures. The key points are reprised in subsequent sections where they are illustrated using real and simulated data. This section describes how the parameters and hyperparameters of a hierarchical model can be estimated jointly given some data. The distinction between a *parameter* and a *hyperparameter* depends on the context established by the estimation or inference in question. Here parameters are quantities that determine the expected response that is observed. Hyperparameters pertain to the probabilistic behaviour of the parameters. Perhaps the simplest example is provided by a single-sample t test. The parameter of interest is the true effect causing the observations to differ from zero. The hyperparameter corresponds to the variance of the observation error (usually denoted by σ^2). Note that one can *estimate* the parameter, with the sample mean, without knowing the hyperparameter. However, if one wanted to make an *inference* about that estimate, we need to know (or estimate using the residual sum of squares) the hyperparameter. In this chapter all hyperparameters are simply variances of different quantities that cause the measured response (e.g., within-subject variance and between-subject variance). The estimation procedure described below is Bayesian in nature. Because the hyperparameters are estimated from the data, it represents an *empirical* Bayesian approach. However, the aim of this section is to show the close relationship between Bayesian and ML estimation implicit in conventional analyses of imaging data, using the general linear model. Furthermore, we want to place classical and Bayesian inference within the same framework. In this way, we show that conventional analyses are special cases of the more general PEB approach.

First we reprise hierarchical linear observation models that form the cornerstone of the ensuing estimation procedures. These models are then reviewed from the classical perspective of estimating the model parameters using ML and statistical inference using the T statistic. The same model is then considered in a Bayesian light to make an important point: The estimated error variances, at any level, play the role of priors on the variability of the parameters in the level below. At the highest level, the ML and Bayes estimators are the same, as are their standard error and conditional standard deviation. Both classical and Bayesian approaches rest on covariance component estimation, which in turn rests on EM. This is described briefly and presented in detail in the Appendix. The EM algorithm is related to that described in Dempster *et al.* (1981) but extended to cover hierarchical models with any number of levels. The final part of this section addresses Bayesian inference in classical terms of sensitivity and specificity. To do this we "convert" Bayesian inference into classical inference by thresholding the posterior probability to label a region as "activated" or not. This device opens up some interesting questions that are especially relevant to neuroimaging. In classical approaches the same threshold is applied to all voxels in an SPM, to ensure uniform specificity over the brain. Thresholded PPMs, on the other hand, adapt their specificity according to the behaviour of local error terms, engendering a uniform confidence in activations of a given size. This complementary aspect of SPMs and PPMs highlights the relative utility of both approaches in making inferences about regional responses.

For an introduction to EM algorithms in generalised linear models, see Fahrmeir and Tutz (1994). This text provides an exposition of EM algorithm and PEB in linear models, usefully relating EM to classical methods, e.g., ReML (Fahrmeir and Tutz, 1994, p. 225). For an introduction to Bayesian statistics, see Lee (1997). This text adopts a more explicit Bayesian perspective and again usefully connects empirical Bayes with classical approaches, e.g., the Stein "shrinkage" estimator and empirical Bayes estimators used below (Lee, 1997; 1994, p. 232). In most standard texts the hierarchical models considered in the next section are referred to as *random-effects models.*

Hierarchical Linear Observation Models

We will deal with hierarchical linear observation models of the following form:

$$
\begin{aligned}
y &= X^{(1)}\theta^{(1)} + \varepsilon^{(1)} \\
\theta^{(1)} &= X^{(2)}\theta^{(2)} + \varepsilon^{(2)} \\
&\vdots \\
\theta^{(n-1)} &= X^{(n)}\theta^{(n)} + \varepsilon^{(n)}
\end{aligned}
\tag{47.1}
$$

under Gaussian assumptions about the errors $\varepsilon^{(i)} \sim N\{0. C_\varepsilon^{(i)}\}$. The y term is the response variable, usually observed both within units over time and over several units (e.g., subject or voxels), and the $X^{(i)}$ are specified design matrices containing explanatory variables or constraints on the parameters $\theta^{(i-1)}$ of the level below. If the hierarchical model has only one level, it reduces to the familiar general linear model employed in conventional data analysis (see Chapter 37). Two-level models will be familiar to readers who use mixed- or random-effect analyses. In this instance the first-level design matrix models the activation effects, over scans within subjects, in a subject-separable fashion (i.e., in partitions constituting the blocks of a block diagonal matrix). The second-level design matrix models the subject-specific effects over subjects. Usually, but not necessarily, design matrices at all levels are block diagonal matrices with each partition modelling the observations in each unit at that level (e.g., session, subject, or group).

$$
X^{(i)} = \begin{bmatrix} X_1^{(i)} & 0 & \dots & 0 \\ 0 & X_2^{(i)} & & \\ \vdots & & \ddots & \\ 0 & & & X_J^{(i)} \end{bmatrix}
\tag{47.2}
$$

Some examples are shown in Fig. 47.1 (examples of which are used in next section). The design matrix at any level has as many rows as the number of columns in the design matrix of the level below. One can envisage three-level models, which embody activation effects in scans modelled for each session, effects expressed in each session modelled for each subject, and finally effects over subjects.

The Gaussian or parametric assumptions implicit in these models imply that all random sources of variability, in the observed response variable, have a Gaussian distribution. This is appropriate for most models in neuroimaging and makes the relationship between classical approaches and Bayesian treatments (that can be generalised to non-Gaussian densities) much more transparent.

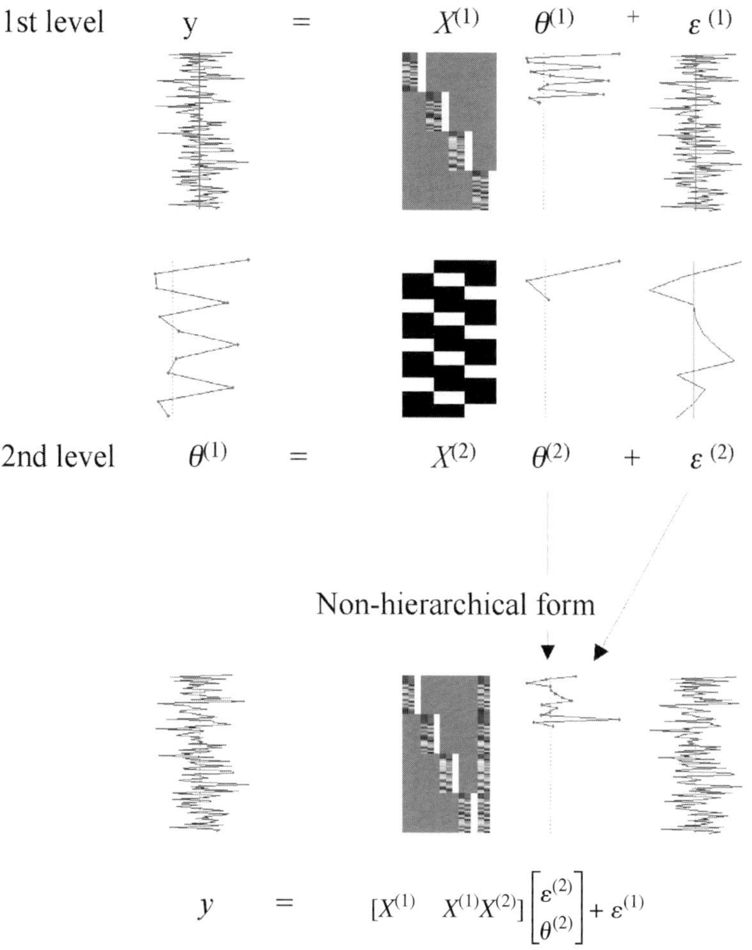

$$y = [X^{(1)} \quad X^{(1)}X^{(2)}]\begin{bmatrix}\varepsilon^{(2)} \\ \theta^{(2)}\end{bmatrix} + \varepsilon^{(1)}$$

FIGURE 47.1
Schematic showing the form of the design matrices in a two-level model and how the hierarchical form (upper panel) can be reduced to a nonhierarchical form (lower panel). The design matrices are shown in image format with an arbitrary colour scale. The response variable, parameters and error terms are depicted as plots. In this example, four subjects or units are observed at the first level. Each subject's response is modeled with the same three effects, one of these being a constant term. These design matrices are part of those used in Friston *et al.* (2002b) to generate simulated fMRI data and are based on the design matrices used in the subsequent empirical event-related fMRI analyses.

Technically, models that conform to Eq. (47.1) fall into the class of conditionally independent hierarchical models when the response variables and parameters are independent across units, conditionally on the hyperparameters controlling the error terms (Kass and Steffey, 1989). These models are also called *parametric empirical Bayes* (PEB) models because the obvious interpretation of the higher level densities as priors led to the development of PEB methodology (Efron and Morris, 1973). Although the procedures considered in this chapter accommodate general models that are not conditionally independent, we refer to the Bayesian procedures below as PEB because the motivation is identical and most of the examples assume conditional independence. Having posited a model with a hierarchical form, the aim is to estimate its parameters and make some inferences about these estimates using their estimated variability or, more generally, their probability distribution. In classical inference one is usually only interested in inferences about the parameters at the highest level to which the model is specified. In a Bayesian context, the highest level is regarded as providing constraints or empirical priors that enable posterior inferences about the parameters in lower levels. Identifying the system of equations in Eq. (47.1) can proceed under two perspectives that are formally identical: a classical statistical perspective and a Bayesian one.

After recursive substitution, to eliminate all but the final level parameters, Eq. (47.1) can be written in an alternative form:

$$y = \varepsilon^{(1)} + X^{(1)}\varepsilon^{(1)} + \ldots + X^{(1)}\ldots X^{(n-1)}\varepsilon^{(n)} + X^{(1)}\ldots X^{(n)}\theta^{(n)} \tag{47.3}$$

In this nonhierarchical form, the components of the response variable comprise linearly separable contributions from all levels. Those components that embody error terms are referred to as *random effects* where the last level parameters enter as *fixed effects*. The covariance partitioning implied by Eq. (47.3) is as follows:

$$E[yy^T] = \underbrace{C_\varepsilon^{(1)}}_{error} + \ldots + \underbrace{X^{(1)}\ldots X^{(i-1)}C_\varepsilon^{(i)}X^{(i-1)T}\ldots X^{(1)T}}_{ith\text{-}level\ random\ effects} + \ldots + \underbrace{X^{(1)}\ldots + X^{(n)}\theta^{(n)}\theta^{(n)T}X^{(n)T}\ldots X^{(1)T}}_{fixed\ effects} \tag{47.4}$$

where $C_\varepsilon^{(i)} = Cov\{\varepsilon^{(i)}\}$. If only one level is specified, the random effects vanish and a fixed-effect analysis ensues. If n is greater than 1, the analysis corresponds to a random-effect analysis (or more exactly a *mixed-effect analysis* that includes random terms). Equation (47.3) can be interpreted in two ways that form, respectively, the basis for a classical

$$\begin{aligned} y &= \tilde{X}\theta^{(n)} + \tilde{\varepsilon} \\ \tilde{X} &= X^{(1)}X^{(2)}\ldots X^{(n)} \\ \tilde{\varepsilon} &= \varepsilon^{(1)} + X^{(1)}\varepsilon^{(2)} + \ldots + X^{(1)}X^{(2)}\ldots X^{(n-1)}\varepsilon^{(n)} \end{aligned} \tag{47.5}$$

and Bayesian estimation

$$\begin{aligned} y &= X\theta + \varepsilon^{(1)} \\ X &= [X^{(1)},\ldots, X^{(1)}X^{(2)}\ldots X^{(n-1)}, X^{(1)}X^{(2)}\ldots X^{(n)}] \\ \theta &= \begin{bmatrix} \varepsilon^{(2)} \\ \vdots \\ \varepsilon^{(n)} \\ \theta^{(n)} \end{bmatrix} \end{aligned} \tag{47.6}$$

In the first, classical formulation of Eq. (47.5) the random effects are lumped together and treated as a composite error, rendering the last level parameters the only ones to appear explicitly. Inferences about nth-level parameters are obtained by simply specifying the model to the order required. In contradistinction, the second formulation, that of Eq. (47.6), treats the error terms as parameters, so that θ comprises the errors at all levels and the final level parameters. Here we have effectively collapsed the hierarchical model into a single level by treating the error terms as parameters (see Fig. 47.1 for a graphical depiction).

Classical Perspective

From the classical perceptive, Eq. (47.5) represents an observation model with response variable y, design matrix $\tilde{X}$, and parameters $\theta^{(n)}$. The objective is to estimate these parameters and make some inference about how large they are based on an estimate of their standard error. Classically, estimation proceeds using the ML estimator of the final level parameters. Under our model assumptions this is the Gauss-Markov estimator:

$$\begin{aligned} \eta_{ML} &= My \\ M &= (\tilde{X}^T C_{\tilde{\varepsilon}}^{-1}\tilde{X})^{-1}\tilde{X}^T C_{\tilde{\varepsilon}}^{-1} \end{aligned} \tag{47.7}$$

where M is an estimator-forming matrix that projects the data onto the estimate. Inferences about this estimate are based on its covariance, against which any contrast (i.e., linear compound specified by the contrast weight vector c) of the estimates can be compared using the T statistic:

$$T = c^T\eta_{ML}/\sqrt{c^T cov\{\eta_{ML}\}c} \tag{47.8}$$

where, from Eqs. (47.5) and (47.7),

$$\begin{aligned} Cov\{\eta_{ML}\} &= MC_{\tilde{\varepsilon}}M^T = (\tilde{X}^T C_{\tilde{\varepsilon}}^{-1}\tilde{X})^{-1} \\ C_{\tilde{\varepsilon}} &= C_\varepsilon^{(1)} + X^{(1)}C_\varepsilon^{(2)}X^{(1)T}\ldots + X^{(1)}\ldots X^{(n-1)}C_\varepsilon^{(n)}X^{(n-1)T}\ldots X^{(1)T} \end{aligned} \tag{47.9}$$

The covariance of the ML estimator represents a mixture of covariances offered up to the highest level by the error at all previous levels. To implement this classical procedure, we need the covariance of the composite errors $C_{\tilde{\varepsilon}} = Cov\{\tilde{\varepsilon}\}$, from all levels, projected down the hierarchy onto the response variable or observation space. In other words, we need the error covariance components of the model. In fact to proceed, in the general case, one has to turn to the second formulation [Eq. (47.6)] and some iterative procedure to estimate these covariance components, in our case an EM algorithm. This dependence, on the same procedures used by PEB methods, reflects the underlying equivalence between classical and empirical Bayes methods.

In some special cases, one does not need to resort to iterative covariance component estimation. This is true, for example, with single-level models. With balanced designs, where $X_1^{(i)} = X_j^{(i)}$ for all i and j, one can replace the response variable with the ML estimates at the penultimate level and proceed as if one had a single-level model. This is the trick harnessed by multistage implementations of random-effect analyses (Holmes and Friston, 1998; see also Chapter 42). Although the ensuing variance estimator is not the same as Eq. (47.9), its expectation is.

In summary, parameter estimation and inference, in hierarchical models, can proceed given estimates of the appropriate covariance components. The reason for introducing inference based on the ML estimate is to motivate the importance of covariance component estimation. In the next section we take a Bayesian approach to the same issue.

Bayesian Perspective

Bayesian inference is based on the conditional probability of the parameters given the data $p(\theta^{(i)} \mid y)$. Under the assumptions above, this *posterior* density is Gaussian and the problem reduces to finding its first two moments, the conditional mean $\eta^{(i)}_{\theta|y}$ and conditional covariance $\eta^{(i)}_{\theta|y}$. These posterior or conditional distributions can be determined for all levels enabling, in contradistinction to classical approaches, inferences at any level using the same hierarchical model. Given the posterior density we can work out the *maximum a posteriori* (MAP) estimate of the parameters (a point estimator equivalent to $\eta^{(i)}_{\theta|y}$ for the linear systems considered here) or the probability that the parameters exceed some specified value. Consider Eq. (47.1) from a Bayesian point of view. Here level i can be thought of as providing *prior* constraints on the expectation and covariances of the parameters below:

$$\begin{aligned} E\{\theta^{(i-1)}\} &= \eta_\theta^{(i-1)} = X^{(i)}\theta^{(i)} \\ Cov\{\theta^{(i-1)}\} &= C_\theta^{(i-1)} = C_\varepsilon^{(i)} \end{aligned} \tag{47.10}$$

In other words, the parameters at level i play the role of supraordinate parameters for level $i - 1$ that control the prior expectation under the constraints specified by $X^{(i)}$. Similarly the prior covariances are simply specified by the error covariances of the level above. For example, given several subjects we can use information about the distribution of activations, over subjects, to inform an estimate pertaining to any single subject. In this case the between-subject variability, from the second level, enters as a *prior* on the parameters of the first level. In many instances we measure the same effect repeatedly in different contexts. The fact that we have some handle on this effect's inherent variability means that the estimate for a single instance can be constrained by knowledge about others. At the final level we can treat the parameters as (1) unknown, in which case their priors are flat[1] (cf. fixed effects) giving an empirical Bayesian approach, or (2) known. In the latter case the connection with the classical formulation is lost because there is nothing to make an inference about at the final level.

The objective is to estimate the conditional means and covariances such that the parameters at lower levels can be estimated in a way that harnesses the information available from higher levels. All of the information we require is contained in the conditional mean and covariance of θ from Eq. (47.6). From the Bayes rule the posterior probability is proportional to the likelihood of obtaining the data, conditional on θ, times the prior probability of θ, that is:

$$p(\theta \mid y) \propto p(y \mid \theta)\, p(\theta) \tag{47.11}$$

[1] Flat or uniform priors denote a probability distribution that is the same everywhere, reflecting a lack of any predilection for specific values. In the limit of very high variance, a Gaussian distribution becomes flat.

where the Gaussian priors $p(\theta)$ are specified in terms of their expectation and covariance:

$$\eta_\theta = E\{\theta\} = \begin{bmatrix} 0 \\ \vdots \\ 0 \\ \eta_\theta^{(n)} \end{bmatrix}, \quad C_\theta = Cov\{\theta\} = \begin{bmatrix} C_\varepsilon^{(2)} & \dots & 0 & 0 \\ \vdots & \ddots & \vdots & \vdots \\ 0 & \dots & C_\varepsilon^{(n)} & 0 \\ 0 & \dots & 0 & C_\theta^{(n)} \end{bmatrix}, \quad \begin{cases} C_\theta^{(n)} = \infty \; unknown \\ C_\theta^{(n)} = 0 \quad known \end{cases} \tag{47.12}$$

Under Gaussian assumptions the likelihood and priors are given by

$$\begin{aligned} p(y\,|\,\theta) &\propto \exp\left\{-\frac{1}{2}(X\theta - y)^T C_\varepsilon^{(1)-1}(X\theta - y)\right\} \\ \mathrm{p}(\theta) &\propto \exp\left\{-\frac{1}{2}(\theta - \eta_\theta)^T C_\varepsilon^{-1}(\theta - \eta_\theta)\right\} \end{aligned} \tag{47.13}$$

Substituting Eq. (47.12) into Eq. (47.10) gives a posterior density with a Gaussian form:

$$p(\theta\,|\,y) \propto \exp\left\{-\frac{1}{2}(\theta - \eta_{\theta|y})^T C_{\theta|y}^{-1}(\theta - \eta_{\theta|y})\right\}$$

where

$$\begin{aligned} C_{\theta|y} &= (X^T C_\varepsilon^{(1)-1} X + C_\theta^{-1})^{-1} \\ \eta_{\theta|y} &= C_{\theta|y}\,(X^T C_\varepsilon^{(1)-1} y + C_\theta^{-1}\eta_\theta) \end{aligned} \tag{47.14}$$

Note that when we adopt an empirical Bayesian scheme, $C_\theta^{(n)} = \infty$ and $C_\theta^{-1}\eta_\theta = 0$ [see Eq. (47.12)]. This means we never have to specify the prior expectation at the last level because it never appears explicitly in Eq. (47.14).

The solution of Eq. (47.14) is ubiquitous in the estimation literature and is presented under various guises in different contexts. If the priors are flat, i.e., $C_\theta^{-1} = 0$, the expression for the conditional mean reduces to the minimum variance linear estimator, referred to as the *Gauss-Markov estimator*. The Gauss-Markov estimator is identical to the ordinary least-squares (OLS) estimator that is obtained after prewhitening. If the errors are assumed to be independently and identically distributed, i.e., $C_\varepsilon^{(1)} = I$, then Eq. (47.14) reduces to the OLS estimator. With nonflat priors, the form of Eq. (47.14) is identical to that employed by *ridge regression* and (weighted) *minimum norm* solutions (e.g., Tikhonov and Arsenin, 1977) commonly found in the inverse problem literature. The Bayesian perspective is useful for minimum norm formulations because it motivates plausible forms for the constraints that can be interpreted in terms of priors.

Equation (47.14) can be expressed in an exactly equivalent but more compact Gauss-Markov form by augmenting the design matrix with an identity matrix and augmenting the data matrix with the prior expectations such that

$$\begin{aligned} C_{\theta|y} &= (\bar{X}^T C_\varepsilon^{-1} \bar{X})^{-1} \\ \eta_{\theta|y} &= C_{\theta|y}(\bar{X}^T C_\varepsilon^{-1} \bar{y}) \end{aligned} \tag{47.15}$$

where

$$\begin{aligned} \bar{y} &= \begin{bmatrix} y \\ \eta_\theta \end{bmatrix} \\ \bar{X} &= \begin{bmatrix} X \\ I \end{bmatrix} \\ C_\varepsilon &= \begin{bmatrix} C_\varepsilon^{(1)} & 0 \\ 0 & C_\theta \end{bmatrix} \end{aligned}$$

Figure 47.2 shows a schematic illustration of the linear model implied by this augmentation. If the priors at the last level are flat, the last level prior expectation can be set to zero. Note from Eq. (47.12) that the remaining prior expectations are zero. This augmented form is computationally more efficient to deal with and simplifies the exposition of the EM algorithm. Furthermore, it highlights the fact that a Bayesian scheme of this sort can be reformulated as the simple weighted least squares or ML problem that Eq. (47.15) represents. The problem now reduces to estimating the error covariances C_ε that determine the weighting. This is exactly where we ended up in the classical approach, namely, reduction to a covariance component estimation problem.

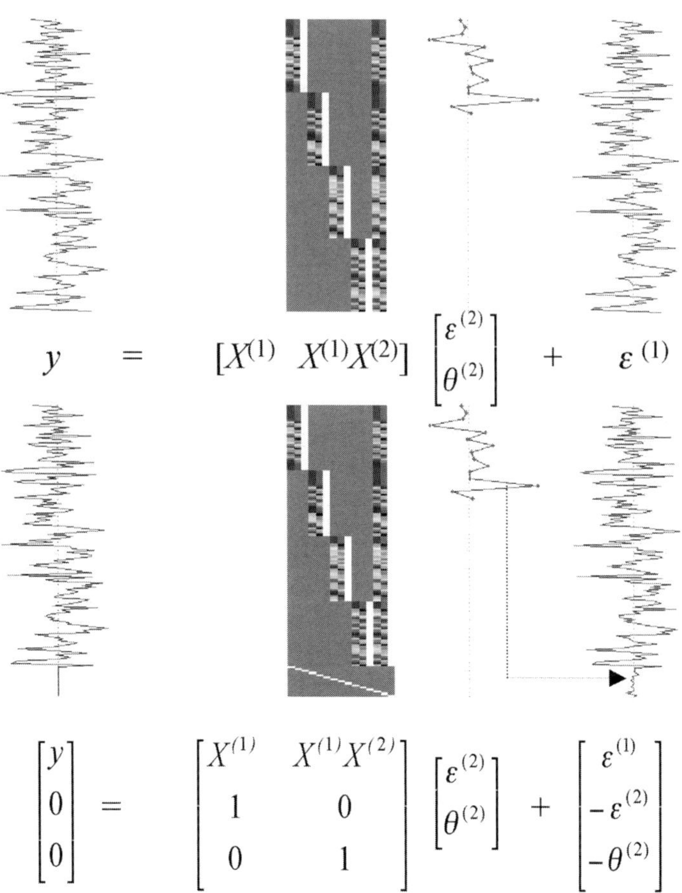

FIGURE 47.2
As for Fig. 47.1 but here showing how the nonhierarchical form is augmented so that the parameter estimates, which include the error terms from all levels and the final level parameters, now appear in the model's residuals. A Gauss-Markov estimator will minimise these residuals in inverse proportion to their prior variance.

Covariance Component Estimation

The classical approach was portrayed earlier as using the error covariances to construct an appropriate statistic. The PEB approach was described as using the error covariances as priors to estimate the conditional means and covariances, recall from Eq. (47.10) that $C_\theta^{(i-1)} = C_\varepsilon^{(i)}$. Both approaches rest on estimating the covariance components. This estimation depends on some parameterisation of these components; in this chapter we use $C_\varepsilon^{(i)} = \Sigma\lambda_j^{(i)}Q_j^{(i)}$ where the $\lambda_j^{(i)}$ are some hyperparameters and the $Q_j^{(i)}$ represent a basis set for the covariance matrices. The bases can be construed as constraints on the prior covariance structures in the same way as the design matrices $X^{(i)}$ specify constraints on the prior expectations. The $Q_j^{(i)}$ term embodies the form of the jth covariance component at the ith level and can model different variances for different levels and different forms of correlations within levels. The bases or constraints Q_j are chosen to model the sort of nonsphericity anticipated. For example, they could specify serial correlations within subject or correlations among the errors induced hierarchically, by repeated measures over subjects (Fig. 47.3 illustrates both of these examples). We illustrate a number of forms for Q_j in the subsequent sections.

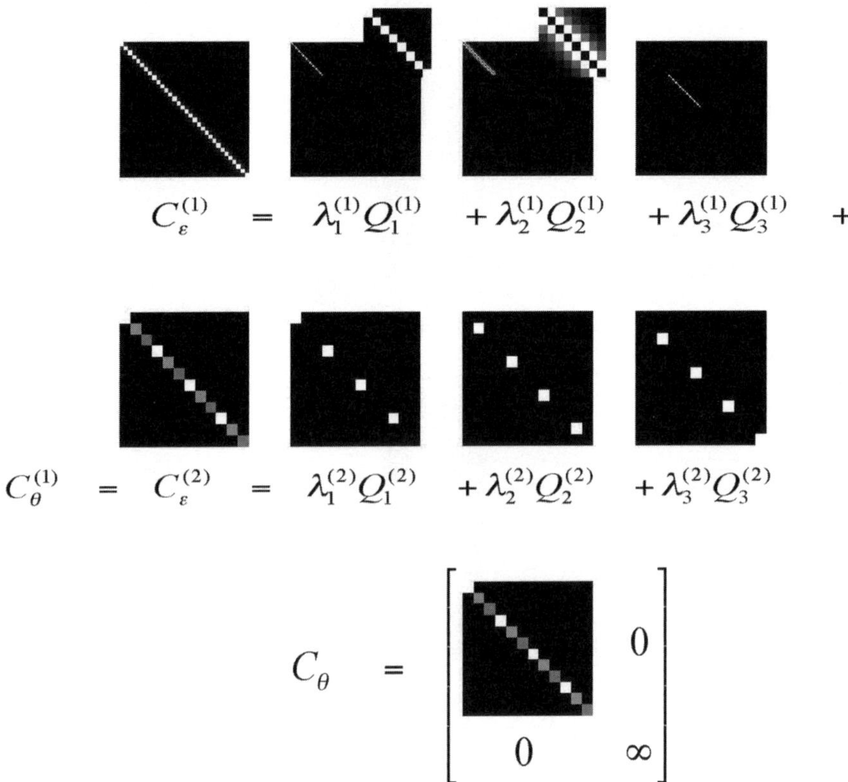

FIGURE 47.3
Schematic illustrating the form of the covariance constraints. These can be thought of as "design matrices" for the second-order behaviour of the response variable. They form a basis set for estimating the error covariance and implicitly the prior covariances. The hyperparameters scale the contribution of each constraint to the error and prior covariances. These covariance constraints correspond to the model in Fig. 47.1. The top row depicts the constraints on the errors. For each subject there are two constraints, one modelling white (i.e., independent) errors and another serial correlation with an AR(1) form. The second-level constraints simply reflect the fact that each of the three parameters estimated on the basis of repeated measures at the first level has its own variance. The estimated priors at each level are assembled with the prior for the last level (here a flat prior) to completely specify the model's priors (lower panel). Constraints of this form are used in Friston *et al.* (2002b) during the simulation of serially correlated fMRI data-sequences and covariance component estimation using real data.

One way of thinking about these covariance constraints is in terms of the Taylor expansion of any function of hyperparameters that produced the actual covariance structure:

$$C(\lambda)_\varepsilon^{(i)} = \sum \lambda_j^{(i)} \frac{\partial C(0)_\varepsilon^{(i)}}{\partial \lambda_j^{(i)}} + \ldots \qquad (47.16)$$

where the basis set corresponds to the partial derivatives of the covariances with respect to the hyperparameters. In variance component estimation, the high-order terms in Eq. (47.16) are generally zero. In this context a linear decomposition of $C_\varepsilon^{(i)}$ is a natural parameterisation because the different sources of conditionally independent variance add linearly and the constraints can be specified directly in terms of these components. In other situations, a different parameterisation may be employed. For example, if the constraints were implementing several independent priors in a nonhierarchical model, a more natural expansion might be in terms of the precision $C_\theta^{-1} = \sum \lambda_j Q_j$. The precision is simply the inverse of the covariance matrix. Here Q_j correspond to precisions specifying the form of independent prior densities. However, in this chapter, we deal only with priors that are engendered by the observation model that induces hierarchically organised, linearly mixed, variance components. Harville (1977, p. 322) comments on the usefulness of making the covariances linear in the hyperparameters.

The augmented form of the covariance constraints is obtained by placing them in the appropriate partition in relation to the augmented error covariance matrix:

$$C_\varepsilon = Q_\theta + \Sigma\lambda_k Q_k$$
$$Q_k = \frac{\partial C_\varepsilon}{\partial \lambda_k} \tag{47.17}$$
$$Q_\theta = \begin{bmatrix} 0 & \dots & 0 & 0 \\ \vdots & \ddots & \vdots & \vdots \\ 0 & \dots & 0 & 0 \\ 0 & \dots & 0 & C_\theta^{(n)} \end{bmatrix}, \quad Q_k = \begin{bmatrix} 0 & & \dots & & 0 & 0 \\ & \ddots & & & & \\ \vdots & & Q_j^{(i)} & & \vdots & \vdots \\ & & & \ddots & & \\ 0 & & \dots & & 0 & 0 \\ 0 & & \dots & & 0 & 0 \end{bmatrix}$$

where the subscript k runs over both levels and the constraints within each level. Having framed the covariance estimation in terms of estimating hyperparameters, we can now use an EM algorithm to estimate them.

Expectation Maximisation

Expectation maximisation is a generic, iterative parameter reestimation procedure that encompasses many iterative schemes devised to estimate the parameters and hyperparameters of a model (Dempster *et al.*, 1977, 1981). It was original introduced as an iterative method to obtain maximum likelihood estimators in incomplete data situations (Hartley, 1958) and was generalised by Dempster *et al.* (1977). More recently, it has been formulated (e.g., Neal and Hinton, 1998) in a way that highlights its elegant nature using a statistical mechanical interpretation. This formulation considers the EM algorithm as a coordinate descent on the *free energy* of a system. The descent comprises an **E**-step, that finds the conditional **E**xpectation of the parameters, holding the hyperparameters fixed and an **M**-step, which updates the **M**aximum-likelihood estimate of the hyperparameters, keeping the parameters fixed.

In brief, EM provides a way to estimate both the parameters and hyperparameters from the data. In other words, it estimates the model parameters when the exact densities of the observation error and priors are unknown. For linear models under Gaussian assumptions the EM algorithm returns (1) the posterior density of the parameters, in terms of their expectation and covariance, and (2) ReML estimates of the hyperparameters. The EM algorithm described in the Appendix [Eq. (47.55)] is depicted schematically in Fig. 47.4. In the context of the linear observation models discussed in this chapter, the EM scheme is the same as using ReML estimates of the hyperparameters, which properly account for the loss of degrees of freedom, incurred by parameter estimation. The operational equivalence between ReML and EM has been established for many years (see Fahrmeir and Tutz, 1994, p. 226). However, it is useful to understand their equivalence because EM algorithms are usually employed to estimate the conditional densities of model parameters when the hyperparameters of the likelihood and prior densities are not known. In contradistinction, ReML is generally used to estimate unknown variance components without explicit reference to the parameters. In the hierarchical linear observation model considered here, the unknown hyperparameters become variance components, which means they can be estimated using ReML. Note that EM algorithms are not restricted to linear observation models or Gaussian priors, and they have found diverse applications in the machine learning community. On the other hand, ReML was developed explicitly for linear observation models under Gaussian assumptions.

In the Appendix we have made an effort to reconcile the free-energy formulation based on statistical mechanics (Neal and Hinton, 1998) with classical ReML (Harville, 1977). This might be relevant for understanding ReML in the context of extensions to the free-energy formulation, afforded by the use of hyperpriors (priors on the hyperparameters). One key insight into the EM approach is that the **M**-step returns not simply the ML estimate of the hyperparameters, but the *restricted* ML, which is properly restricted from a classical perspective.

Having computed the conditional mean and covariances of the parameters we are now in a position to make inferences about the effects at any level using their posterior density.

Augment to embody priors in error covariance

$$\bar{X} = \begin{bmatrix} \prod_{i=1}^{1} X^{(i)} & \cdots & \prod_{i=1}^{n} X^{(i)} \\ I & & 0 \\ \vdots & \ddots & \\ 0 & \cdots & I \end{bmatrix}, \quad \bar{y} = \begin{bmatrix} y \\ 0 \\ \vdots \\ \eta_\theta^{(n)} \end{bmatrix}, \quad C_\theta = \begin{bmatrix} 0 & 0 & 0 \\ & \ddots & \vdots \\ 0 & 0 & 0 \\ 0 & \cdots 0 & C_\theta^{(n)} \end{bmatrix}, \quad Q_1 = \begin{bmatrix} Q_1^{(1)} & 0 & 0 \\ & \ddots & \vdots \\ 0 & 0 & 0 \\ 0 & \cdots 0 & 0 \end{bmatrix}, \quad Q_2 = \ldots$$

Until convergence { **E-Step**

$$C_\varepsilon = C_\theta + \sum \lambda_k Q_k$$
$$C_{\theta|y} = \left(\bar{X}^T C_\varepsilon^{-1} \bar{X}\right)^{-1}$$
$$\eta_{\theta|y} = C_{\theta|y} \bar{X}^T C_\varepsilon^{-1} \bar{y}$$

M-Step

$$P = C_\varepsilon^{-1} - C_\varepsilon^{-1} \bar{X} C_{\theta|y} \bar{X}^T C_\varepsilon^{-1}$$
$$g_i = -\tfrac{1}{2} tr\{PQ_i\} + \tfrac{1}{2} \bar{y}^T P^T Q_i P \bar{y}$$
$$H_{ij} = \tfrac{1}{2} tr\{PQ_i PQ_j\}$$
$$\lambda = \lambda + H^{-1} g$$

}

assemble estimates of error covariance, priors, conditional covariances and means

$$C_\varepsilon = \begin{bmatrix} C_\varepsilon^{(1)} & 0 & 0 \\ & \ddots & \vdots \\ 0 & C_\varepsilon^{(n)} & 0 \\ 0 & \cdots 0 & C_\theta^{(n)} \end{bmatrix}, \quad C_\theta^{(i)} = C_\varepsilon^{(i-1)}$$

$$C_{\theta|y} = \begin{bmatrix} C_{\varepsilon|y}^{(2)} & \cdots & & \\ \vdots & \ddots & & \\ & & C_{\varepsilon|y}^{(n)} & \\ & & & C_{\theta|y}^{(n)} \end{bmatrix}, \quad C_{\theta|y}^{(i)} = C_{\varepsilon|y}^{(n-1)}$$

$$\eta_{\theta|y} = \begin{bmatrix} \eta_{\varepsilon|y}^{(2)} \\ \vdots \\ \eta_{\varepsilon|y}^{(n)} \\ \eta_{\theta|y}^{(n)} \end{bmatrix}, \quad \eta_{\theta|y}^{(i-1)} = X^{(i)} \eta_{\theta|y}^{(i)} + \eta_{\varepsilon|y}^{(i)}$$

FIGURE 47.4
Pseudo-code schematic showing the recursive structure of the EM algorithm (described in the Appendix) as applied in the context of conditionally independent hierarchical models. See main text for a full explanation. This formulation follows Harville (1977).

Conditional and Classical Estimators

Given an estimate of the error covariance of the augmented form of C_e and implicitly the priors that are embedded in it, one can compute the conditional mean and covariance at each level where

$$\eta_{\theta|y} = E\{\theta|y\} = \begin{bmatrix} \eta_{\varepsilon|y}^{(2)} \\ \vdots \\ \eta_{\varepsilon|y}^{(n)} \\ \eta_{\theta|y}^{(n)} \end{bmatrix}, \quad C_{\theta|y} = Cov\{\theta|y\} = \begin{bmatrix} C_{\varepsilon|y}^{(2)} & \cdots & & \\ \vdots & \ddots & & \\ & & C_{\varepsilon|y}^{(n)} & \\ & & & C_{\theta|y}^{(n)} \end{bmatrix} \tag{47.18}$$

The conditional means for each level are obtained recursively with $\eta_{\theta|y}^{(i-1)} = X^{(i)}\eta_{\theta|y}^{(i)} + \eta_{\varepsilon|y}^{(i)}$. The conditional covariances are simply $C_{\theta|y}^{(i-1)} = C_{\varepsilon|y}^{(i)}$ up to the penultimate level and $C_{\theta|y}^{(n)}$ at the final level. The conditional means represent a better "collective" characterisation of the model parameters than the equivalent ML estimates because they are constrained by prior information from higher levels (see discussion below). At the last level the conditional mean and ML estimators are the same. In PEB, inferences about the parameters at subordinate levels are enabled through having an estimate of their posterior density. At the last level the posterior density reduces to the likelihood distribution and inference reverts to a classical one based on the standardised conditional mean.

The standardised conditional mean, or a contrast of means, is the mean normalised by its conditional error. This conditional error is larger than the standard error of the conditional mean with equivalence when the priors are flat (i.e., the conditional variability of a parameter is greater than the estimate of its mean, except at the last level where they are the same):

$$T^{(i)} = c^T\eta_{\theta|y}^{(i)} / \sqrt{c^T C_{\theta|y}^{(i)} c} \tag{47.19}$$

This statistic indicates the number of standard deviations by which the mean of the conditional distribution of the contrast deviates from zero. The critical thing we want to emphasise here is that this statistic is identical to the classical T statistic at the last level. This means that the ML estimate and the conditional mean are the same and the conditional covariance is exactly the same as the covariance of the ML estimate. The convergence of classical and Bayesian inference at the last level rests on this identity and depends on adopting an empirical Bayesian approach. This establishes a close connection between classical random-effect analyses and hierarchical Bayesian models. However, the two approaches diverge if we consider that the real power of Bayesian inference lies in (1) coping with incomplete data or unbalanced designs and (2) looking at the conditional or posterior distributions at lower levels. The relationship between classical and empirical Bayesian inference is developed in the next section.

Classical and Bayesian Inference Compared

In this subsection we establish a relationship between classical and Bayesian inference by applying Bayes in a classical fashion. As noted above, at the last level, PEB inference based on the standardised conditional mean is identical to classical inference based on the T statistic. In this context the ML estimators and the conditional means are the same, as are the conditional covariance and the covariance of the ML estimator. What about inference at intermediate levels? Bayesian inference is based on the conditional or posterior densities (means and covariances) to give the posterior probability that a compound of parameters (i.e., contrast) is greater than some value, say, γ. How does this relate to the equivalent classical inference? Clearly the essence of both inferences are quite distinct. The p value in classical inference pertains to the probability of getting the data under the null hypothesis, whereas in Bayesian inference it is the probability that, given the data, the contrast exceeds γ. However, we can demonstrate the connection between Bayesian and classical inference by taking a classical approach to the former:

Consider the following heuristic argument. Take an observation model with a single parameter and assume that the error and prior covariance of the parameter are known. Classical inference is characterised in terms of specificity and sensitivity given the null $\theta = 0$ and alternate $\theta = A$ hypotheses. Specificity is the probability of correctly accepting the null hypothesis and is $1 - \alpha$, where α is a small false-positive rate. The sensitivity β or power is the probability of correctly rejecting the null hypothesis. Classically, one rejects the null hypothesis whenever the standardised ML estimator exceeds some specified statistical threshold v. The probability of this happening is based on its distribution whose standard deviation is given by Eq. (47.9).

$$\begin{aligned} \alpha &= 1 - \Phi(v) \\ \beta &= 1 - \Phi\left(v - \frac{A}{\sqrt{(X^T C_\varepsilon^{-1} X)^{-1}}}\right) \end{aligned} \tag{47.20}$$

where $\Phi(.)$ is the cumulative density function of the unit normal distribution. Note that one would use Student's T distribution if the error covariance had to be estimated but here we are treating the error variance as known. The terms α and β are the probabilities that the ML estimator divided by its standard deviation would exceed v under the null and alternative hypotheses, respectively. Note that this classical inference disregards any priors on the parameter's variance, assuming them to be infinite. We can now pursue an identical analysis for Bayesian inference. By thresholding the posterior probability (or PPM) a specified confidence (say, 95%) one could declare the surviving voxels as showing a significant effect. This corresponds to thresholding the conditional mean at $\gamma + u\sqrt{C_{\theta|y}}$ where u is a standard Gaussian deviate specifying the level of confidence required. For example, $u = 1.64$ for 95% confidence. One can regard u as a Bayesian threshold. Although thresholding the posterior probability to declare a voxel "activated" is, of course, unnecessary, it is used here as a device to connect Bayesian and classical inference.

Under the null and alternate hypotheses the expectation and variance of the conditional mean are

$$\langle \eta_{\theta|y} \rangle = \begin{cases} 0 & null \\ C_{\theta|y} X^T C_\varepsilon^{-1} XA & alternate \end{cases}$$
$$Cov\{\eta_{\theta|y}\} = C_\eta = C_{\theta|y} X^T C_\varepsilon^{-1} X C_{\theta|y}$$

from which it follows

$$\begin{aligned} \alpha &= 1 - \Phi(w) \\ \beta &= 1 - \Phi\left(w - \frac{C_{\theta|y} X^T C_\varepsilon^{-1} XA}{\sqrt{C_\eta}}\right) \\ &= 1 - \Phi\left(w - \frac{A}{\sqrt{(X^T C_\varepsilon^{-1} X)^{-1}}}\right) \\ w &= \frac{\gamma}{\sqrt{C_\eta}} + \frac{u\sqrt{C_{\theta|y}}}{\sqrt{C_\eta}} \end{aligned} \tag{47.21}$$

where $C_{\theta|y} \geq C_\eta$, with equality when the priors are flat. Comparing Eq. (47.20) and Eq. (47.21) reveals a fundamental difference and equivalence between classical and Bayesian inference. The first thing to note is that the expressions for power and sensitivity have exactly the same form, such that if we chose a threshold u that gave the same specificity as a classical test, then the same sensitivity would ensue. In other words there is no magical increase in power afforded by a Bayesian approach. The classical approach is equally as sensitive given the same specificity.

The essential difference emerges when we consider that the relationship between the posterior probability threshold u and the implied classical threshold w depends on quantities (i.e., error and prior variance) that change over voxels. In a classical approach we would choose some fixed threshold v, say, for all voxels in an SPM. This ensures that the resulting inference has the same specificity everywhere because specificity depends on, and only on, v. To emulate this uniform specificity, when thresholding a PPM, we would have to keep w constant. The critical thing here is that if the prior covariance or observation error changes from voxel to voxel, then either γ or u must change to maintain the same specificity. This means that the nature of the inference changes fundamentally, either in terms of the size of the inferred activation γ or the confidence about that effect u. In short, one can either have a test with uniform specificity (the classical approach) or one can infer an effect of uniform size with uniform confidence (the Bayesian approach) but not both at the same time. For example, given a confidence level determined by u, as the prior variance gets smaller γ must also decrease to maintain the same specificity. Consequently, in some regions a classical inference corresponds to a Bayesian inference about a big effect, and in other regions, where the estimate is intrinsically less variable, the inference is about a small effect. In the limit of estimates that are very reliable, the classical inference pertains to trivially small effects. This is a fallacy of classical inference alluded to in the introduction. There is nothing statistically invalid about this: One might argue that a very reliable activation that is exceedingly small is interesting. However, in many contexts, including neuroimaging, we are generally interested in activations of a nontrivial magnitude and this speaks to the usefulness of Bayesian inference.

In summary, classical inference uses a criterion that renders the specificity fixed. However, this is at the price that the size of the effect, subtending the inferred activation, will change from voxel to voxel or brain region to brain region. By explicitly framing the inference in terms of the posterior probability, Bayesian inference sacrifices a constant specificity to ensure the inference is about the same thing at every voxel. Intuitively one can regard Bayesian inference as adjusting the classical threshold according to the inherent variability of the effect in which one is interested. In regions with high prior variability, the classical threshold is relaxed to ensure that type II errors are avoided. In this context the classical specificity represents the lower bound for Bayesian inference. In other words, Bayesian inference is generally much more specific than classical inference (by several orders of magnitude in the empirical examples presented later) with equivalence when the prior variance becomes very large.

In concluding, note that one does not usually consider issues like specificity from a Bayesian point of view (the null hypothesis plays no role because the real-world behaviour is already specified by the priors). From a purely Bayesian perspective, the specificity and sensitivity of an inference are meaningless because at no point is an activation declared significant (correctly or falsely). It is only when we impose a categorical classification (activated vs. not activated) by thresholding on the posterior probability that specificity and sensitivity become an issue. Ideally, one would report inferences in terms of the conditional density of the activation at every voxel. This is generally impractical in neuroimaging and the posterior probability (that is a function of the conditional density and γ) becomes a useful characterisation. This characterisation is, and should be, the same irrespective of whether we have analysed just one voxel or the entire brain. To threshold the posterior probabilities is certainly tenable for summary or display purposes, but to declare the surviving voxels as "activated" represents a category error. This is because the inherent nature of the inference already specifies that the voxel is probably active with a nontrivial probability of not being activated. However, it is comforting to note that, by enforcing a classical take on Bayesian inference, we do not have to worry too much about the multiple comparison problems because the ensuing inference has an intrinsically high specificity.

Conceptual Issues

This section has introduced three key components that play a role in the estimation of the linear models: Bayesian estimation, hierarchical models, and EM. The summary points below attempt to clarify the relationships among these components. It is worth keeping in mind that there are essentially three sorts of estimation: (1) fully Bayesian, when the priors are known; (2) empirical Bayesian, when the priors are unknown but they can be parameterised in terms of some hyperparameters estimated from the data, and (3) maximum-likelihood estimation, when the priors are assumed to be flat. In the final instance the ML estimators correspond to weighted least squares or minimum norm solutions. All of these procedures can be implemented with an EM algorithm (see Fig. 47.5).

- Model estimation and inference are greatly enhanced by being able to make probabilistic statements about the model parameters given the data, as opposed to probabilistic statements about the data, under some arbitrary assumptions about the parameters (e.g., the null hypothesis), as afforded by classical statistics. The former is predicated on the posterior or conditional distribution of the parameters derived using the Bayes rule.
- Bayesian estimation and inference require priors. If the priors are known then a fully Bayesian estimation can proceed. In the absence of known priors, there may be constraints on the form of the model that can be harnessed using *empirical* Bayes estimates of the associated hyperparameters.
- A model with a hierarchical form embodies implicit constraints on the form of the prior distributions. Hyperparameters that, in conjunction with these constraints, specify the priors can then be estimated with PEB. In short, a hierarchical form for the observation model enables an empirical Bayesian approach.
- If the observation model does not have a hierarchical structure then one knows nothing about the form of the priors, and they are assumed to be flat. Bayesian estimation with flat priors reduces to ML estimation.

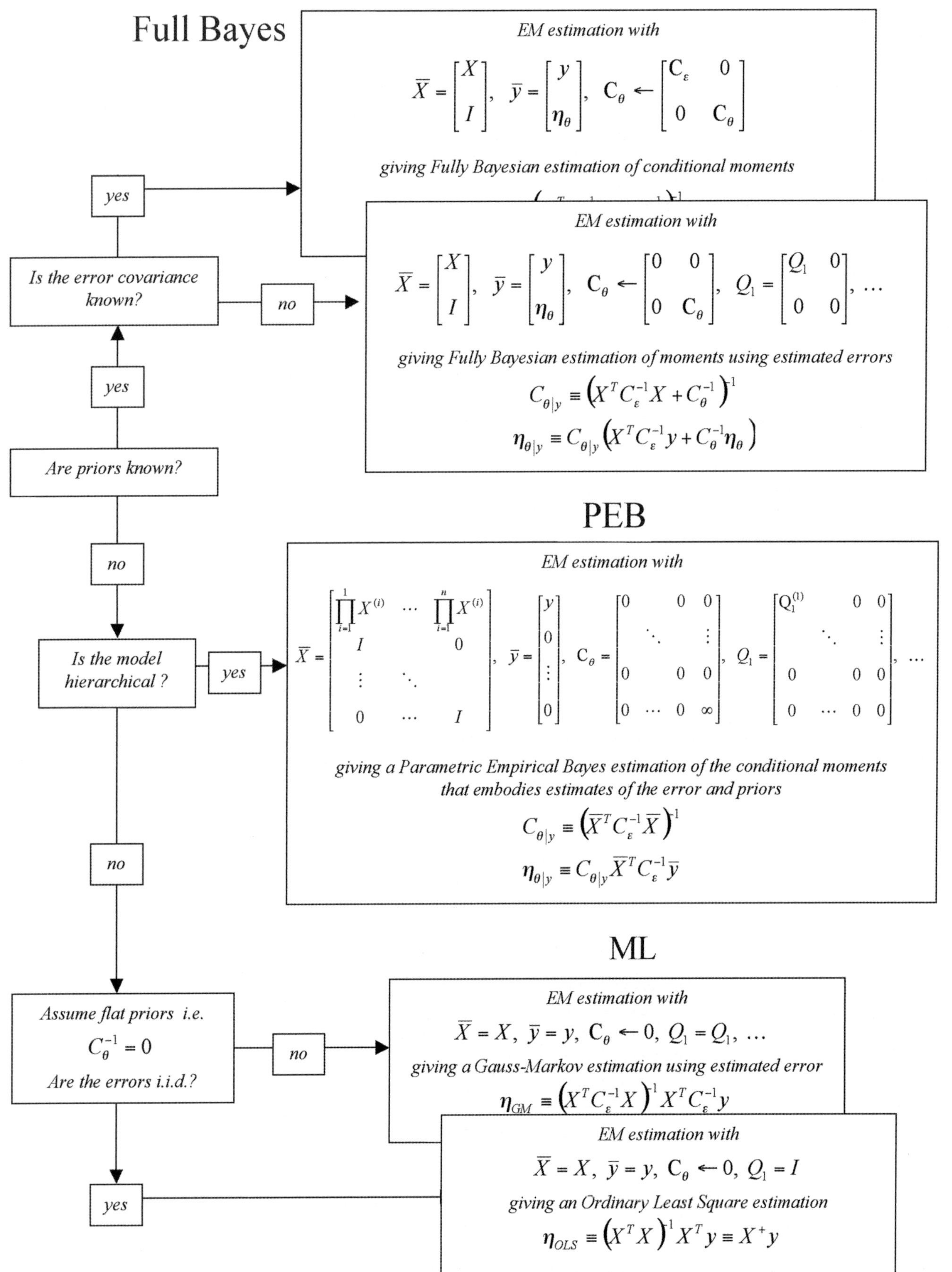

FIGURE 47.5
Schematic showing the relationship among estimation schemes for linear observation models under parametric assumptions. This figure highlights the universal role of the EM algorithm, showing that all conventional estimators can be cast in terms of, or implemented with, the EM algorithm in Fig. 47.4.

- In the context of an empirical Bayesian approach, the priors at the last level are generally unknown and enter as flat priors. This is equivalent to treating the parameters at the last level as fixed effects (i.e., effects with no intrinsic or random variability). One consequence of this is that the conditional mean and the ML estimate, at the last level, are identical.
- In terms of inference, at the last level, PEB and classical approaches are formally identical. At subordinate levels, PEB can use the posterior densities to provide for Bayesian inference about the effects of interest. This is precluded from a classical perspective because there are no priors.
- EM provides a generic framework in which fully Bayes, PEB, or ML estimation can proceed. Its critical utility is the estimation of covariance components, given some data, through the ReML estimation of hyperparameters mixing these covariance components. An EM algorithm can be used to estimate the error covariance in the context of known priors or to estimate both the error and priors by embedding the latter in the former. This embedding is achieved by augmenting the design matrix and data (see Figs. 47.2 and 47.4).
- In the absence of priors, or hierarchical constraints on their form, EM can be used in a ML setting to estimate the error covariance to enable Gauss-Markov estimates (see Fig. 47.5). These estimators are the optimum weighted least-squares estimates in the sense that they have the minimum variance of all unbiased linear estimators. In the limiting case for which the covariance constraints reduce to a single basis (synonymous with known correlations or a single hyperparameter), the EM algorithm converges in a single iteration and emulates a classical sum-of-square estimation of error variance. When this single basis is the identity matrix (i.e., i.i.d. errors), an EM algorithm simply implements an OLS estimation.

In this section we have reviewed hierarchical observation models of the sort commonly encountered in neuroimaging. Their hierarchical nature induces different sources of variability in the observations at different levels (i.e., variance components) that can be estimated using EM. The use of EM, for variance component estimation, is not limited to hierarchical models, but finds a useful application whenever nonsphericity of the errors is specified with more than one hyperparameter (e.g., serial correlations in fMRI). This application will be illustrated next. The critical thing about hierarchical models is that they conform to a Bayesian scheme in which variance estimates at higher levels can be used as constraints on the estimation of effects at lower levels. This perspective rests on exactly the same mathematics that pertains to variance component estimation in nonhierarchical models but allows one to frame the estimators in conditional or Bayesian terms. An intuitive understanding of the conditional estimators, at a given level, is that they "shrink" toward their average, in proportion to the error variance at that level, relative to their intrinsic variability (error variance at the supraordinate level). Lee (1997, p. 232) provides a discussion of PEB and Stein "shrinkage" estimators.

In what sense are these Bayes predictors a better characterisation of the model parameters than the equivalent ML estimates? In other words, what are the gains in using a shrinkage estimator? This is a topic that has been debated at great length in the statistics literature and even in the popular press. See the *Scientific American* article "Stein's Paradox in Statistics" by Efron and Morris (1977). The answer depends on ones definition of *better,* or in technical terms, the *loss function.* If the aim is to find the best predictor for a specific subject, then one can do no better than the ML estimator for that subject. Here the loss function is simply the squared difference between the estimated and real effects for the subject in question. Conversely, if the loss function is averaged over subjects, then the shrinkage estimator is best. This has been neatly summarised in a discussion chapter read before the Royal Statistical Society entitled "Regression, Prediction and Shrinkage" by Copas (1983). The vote of thanks was given by Dunsmore, who said:

> *Suppose I go to the doctor with some complaint and ask him to predict the time* **y** *to remission. He will take some explanatory measurements* **x** *and provide some prediction for* **y**. *What I am interested in is a prediction for my* **x**, *not for any other* **x** *that I might have had—but did not. Nor am I really interested in his necessarily using a predictor which is "best" over all possible* **x***'s. Perhaps rather selfishly, but I believe justifiably, I want the best predictor for my* **x**. *Does it necessarily follow that the best predictor for my* **x** *should take the same form as for some other* **x**? *Of course this can cause problems for the esteem of the*

*doctor or his friendly statistician. Because we are concerned with actual observations the goodness or otherwise of the prediction will eventually become apparent. In this case the statistician will not be able to hide behind the screen provided by averaging over all possible future **x**'s.*

Copas then replied:

*Dr. Dunsmore raises two general points that repay careful thought. Firstly, he questions the assumption made at the very start of the chapter that predictions are to be judged in the context of a population of future **x**'s and not just at some specific **x**. To pursue the analogy of the doctor and the patient, all I can say is that the chapter is written from the doctor's point of view and not from the patient's! No doubt the doctor will feel he is doing a better job if he cures 95% of patients rather than only 90%, even though a particular patient (Dr. Dunsmore) might do better in the latter situation than the former. As explained in the chapter, pre-shrunk predictors do better than least squares for most **x**'s at the expense of doing worse at a minority of **x**'s. Perhaps if we think our symptoms are unusual we should seek a consultant who is prepared to view our complaint as an individual research problem rather than rely on the blunt instrument of conventional wisdom.*

The implication for Bayesian estimators, in the context of neuroimaging, is that they are the best for each subject (or voxel) *on average over subjects (or voxels)*. In this sense Bayesian or conditional estimates of individual effects are only better on average, over the individual effects estimated. The issues, framed by Keith Worsley above, speak to the important consideration that Bayesian estimates, of the sort discussed in this chapter, are only "better" in a collective sense. One example of this collective context is presented below, where between-voxel effects are used to "shrink" within-voxel estimates that are then reported together in a PPM.

The estimators and inference from a PEB approach do not inherently increase the sensitivity or specificity of the analysis. The most appropriate way to do this would be to simply increase sample size. PEB methodology can be better regarded as providing a set of estimates or predictors that are internally consistent within and over hierarchies of the observation model. Furthermore, they enable Bayesian inference (comments about the likelihood of an effect given the data) that complement classical inference (comments about the likelihood of the data). Bayesian inference does not necessarily decide whether an activation is present or not, it simply estimates the probability of an activation, specified in terms of the size of the effect. Conversely, classical inference is predicated on a decision. (Is the null hypothesis true or is the size of the effect different from zero?) The product of classical inference is a decision or declaration, which induces a sensitivity and specificity of the inference. In this section we have used classical notions of sensitivity and specificity to link the two sorts of inference by thresholding the posterior probability. However, one is not compelled to threshold maps of posterior probability. Indeed, one of the motivations, behind Bayesian treatments, is to eschew the difficult compromise between sensitivity and specificity engendered by classical inference in neuroimaging.

ESTIMATION MAXIMISATION AND VARIANCE COMPONENT ESTIMATION

In this section we present a series of models that exemplify the diversity of problems that can be addressed with EM. In hierarchical linear observation models, both classical and empirical Bayesian approaches can be framed in terms of *covariance component estimation* (e.g., variance partitioning). To illustrate the use of EM in covariance component estimation, we focus on two important problems in fMRI: nonsphericity induced by (1) serial or temporal correlations among errors and (2) variance components caused by the hierarchical nature of multisubject studies. In hierarchical observation models, variance components at higher levels can be used as constraints on the parameter estimates of lower levels. This enables the use of PEB estimators, as distinct from classical ML estimates. We develop this distinction to address the difference between response estimates based on ML and the conditional means.

Empirical Bayes enables the joint estimation of an observation model's parameters (e.g., activations) and its hyperparameters that specify the observation's variance components (e.g., within- and between-subject variability). The estimation procedures conform to EM, which, considering just the hyperparameters in linear observation models, is formally identical to ReML. If there is only one variance component, these iterative schemes simplify to conventional, noniterative sum-of-squares variance estimates. However, there are many situations in which a number of hyperparameters have to be estimated. For example, when the correlations among errors are unknown but can be parameterised with a small number of hyperparameters (cf. serial correlations in fMRI time series). Another important example in fMRI is the multisubject design in which the hierarchical nature of the observation induces different variance components at each level. The aim of this section is to illustrate how variance component estimation, with EM, can proceed in both single-level and hierarchical contexts. In particular, the examples emphasise that although the mechanisms inducing nonsphericity can be very different, the variance component estimation problems they represent, and the analytic approaches called for, are identical.

We use two fMRI examples. In the first we deal with the issue of variance component estimation using serial correlations in single-subject fMRI studies. Because there is no hierarchical structure to this problem, there is no Bayesian aspect. However, in the second example, we add a second level to the observation model for the first to address intersubject variability. Endowing the model with a second level affords the opportunity to use empirical Bayes. This enables a quantitative comparison of classical and conditional single-subject response estimates.

Variance Component Estimation in fMRI: A Single-Level Model

In this section we review serial correlations in fMRI and use simulated data to compare ReML estimates, obtained with EM, to estimates of correlations based simply on the model residuals. The importance of modelling temporal correlations, for classical inference based on the T statistic, is discussed in terms of correcting for nonsphericity in fMRI time series. This section concludes with a quantitative assessment of serial correlations within and between subjects.

Serial Correlations in fMRI

In this section we restrict ourselves to a single-level model and focus on the covariance component estimation afforded by EM. We have elected to use a simple but important covariance estimation problem to illustrate one of the potential uses of the scheme described in the appendix. Namely, serial correlations in fMRI embodied in the error covariance matrix for the first (and only) level of this observation model $C_e^{(1)}$. Serial correlations have a long history in the analysis of fMRI time series. fMRI time series can be viewed as a linear admixture of signal and noise. Noise has many contributions that render it rather complicated in relation to other neurophysiological measurements. These include neuronal and non-neuronal sources. Neuronal noise refers to neurogenic signals not modelled by the explanatory variables and has the same frequency structure as the signal itself. Non-neuronal components have both white (e.g., RF noise) and colored components (e.g., pulsatile motion of the brain caused by cardiac cycles and local modulation of the static magnetic field B_0 by respiratory movement). These effects are typically low frequency or wideband and induce long-range correlations in the errors over time. These serial correlations can either be used to whiten the data (Bullmore *et al.*,1996; Purdon and Weisskoff, 1998) or are entered into the nonsphericity corrections described in previous chapters (Worsley and Friston, 1995). Both approaches depend on an accurate estimation of the serial correlations. To estimate correlations among the errors $C(\lambda)_\varepsilon$, in terms of some hyperparameters λ, one needs both the residuals of the model r and the conditional covariance of the parameter estimates that produced those residuals. These combine to give the required error covariance [cf. Eq. (47.58) in the Appendix].

$$C(\lambda)_\varepsilon = rr^T + XC_{\theta|y}X^T \tag{47.22}$$

where $XC_{\theta|y}X^T$ represents the conditional covariance of the parameter estimates $C_{\theta|y}$ "projected" onto the measurement space, by the design matrix X. The problem is that the covariance of the parameter estimates *is itself a function of the error covariance*. This circular problem is solved by the recursive parameter reestimation implicit in EM. It is worth noting that estimators of serial correlations based solely on the residuals (produced by any estimator) will be biased. This bias results from ignoring the second term in Eq. (47.22), which accounts for the component of error covariance due to uncertainty about the parameter estimates themselves. It is likely that any valid recursive scheme for estimating serial correlations in fMRI time series conforms to EM (or ReML) even if the connection is not made explicit. Worsley *et al.* (2002) provide a noniterative approach to AR(p) models.

In summary, the covariance estimation afforded by EM can be harnessed to estimate serial correlations in fMRI time series that coincidentally provides the most efficient (i.e., Gauss-Markov) estimators of the effect in which one is interested. In this section we apply the EM algorithm described in Friston *et al.* (2002a) to simulated fMRI data sequences and take the opportunity to establish the connections among some commonly employed inference procedures based on the T statistic. This example concludes with an application of EM to empirical data to demonstrate quantitatively the relative variability in serial correlations over voxels and subjects.

Estimating Serial Correlations

For each fMRI session we have a single-level observation model that is specified by the design matrix $X^{(1)}$ and constraints on the observation's covariance structure $Q_i^{(1)}$, in this case serial correlations among the errors:

$$\begin{aligned} y &= X^{(1)}\theta^{(1)} + \varepsilon^{(1)} \\ Q_1^{(1)} &= I \\ Q_2^{(1)} &= KK^T, \qquad k_{ij} = \begin{cases} e^{j-i} & i > j \\ 0 & i \leq j \end{cases} \end{aligned} \tag{47.23}$$

where y is the measured response with errors $\varepsilon^{(1)} \sim N\{0, C_e^{(1)}\}$ and I is the identity matrix. Here $Q_1^{(1)}$ and $Q_2^{(1)}$ represent covariance components of $C_e^{(1)}$ that model a white noise and an autoregressive AR(1) process with an AR coefficient of $1/e = 0.3679$. Notice that this is a very simple model of autocorrelations; by fixing the AR coefficient there are just two hyperparameters that allow for different mixtures of an AR(1) process and white noise [cf. the three hyper-parameters needed for a full AR(1) plus white noise model]. The AR(1) component is modelled as an exponential decay of correlations over nonzero lag.

These bases were chosen given the popularity of AR plus white noise models in fMRI (Purdon and Weisskoff, 1998). Clearly this basis set can be extended in any fashion using Taylor expansions to model deviations of the AR coefficient from $1/e$ or indeed model any other form of serial correlations. Nonstationary autocorrelations can be modelled by using non-Toeplitz forms for the bases that allow the elements in the diagonals of $Q_i^{(1)}$ to vary over observations. This might be useful, for example, in the analysis of event-related potentials, where the structure of errors may change with peristimulus time.

In the examples below, the covariance constraints were scaled to a maximum of one. This means that the second hyperparameter can be interpreted as the covariance between one scan and the next. The basis set enters, along with the data, into the EM algorithm (see Appendix) to provide ML estimates of the parameters $\theta^{(1)}$ and ReML estimates of the hyperparameters $\lambda^{(1)}$.

An example, based on simulated data, is shown in Fig. 47.6. In this example the design matrix comprised a boxcar regressor and the first 16 components of a discrete cosine set. The simulated data corresponded to a compound of this design matrix (see figure legend) plus noise, coloured using hyperparameters of 1 and 0.5 for the white and AR(1) components, respectively. The top panel shows the data (dots), the true and fitted effects (broken and solid lines). For comparison, fitted responses based on both ML and OLS are provided. The insert in the upper panel shows that these estimators are very similar but not identical. The lower panel shows the true (dashed) and estimated (solid) autocorrelation function based on $C_e^{(1)} = \lambda_1^{(1)}Q_1^{(1)} + \lambda_2^{(1)}Q_2^{(1)}$. They are nearly identical. For comparison, the sample autocorrelation function (dotted line) and an estimate based directly on the residuals [i.e., ignoring the second term of Eq. (47.1)] (dot-dash line) are provided. The underestimation, which ensues when using the residuals, is evident in the insert that shows the true hyperparameters (black), those estimated properly using ReML (white) and those based on the residuals alone (grey). By failing to account for the uncertainty about the parameter estimates, the hyperparameters based only on the residuals are severe underestimates. The sample autocorrelation function even shows negative correlations. This is a result of fitting

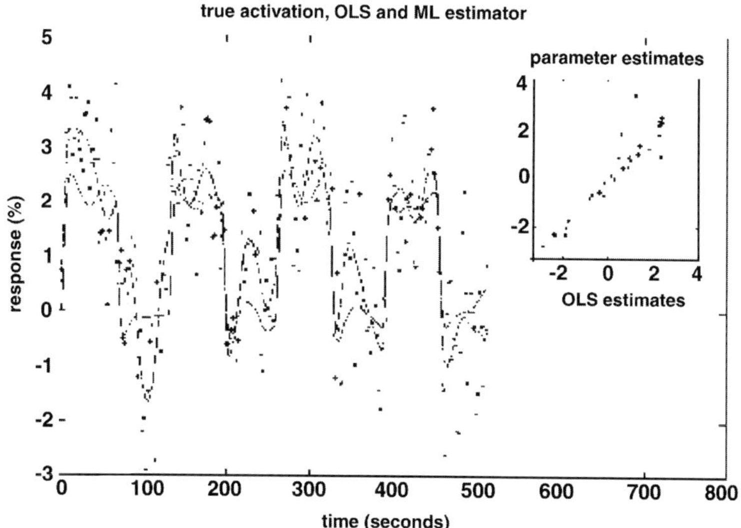

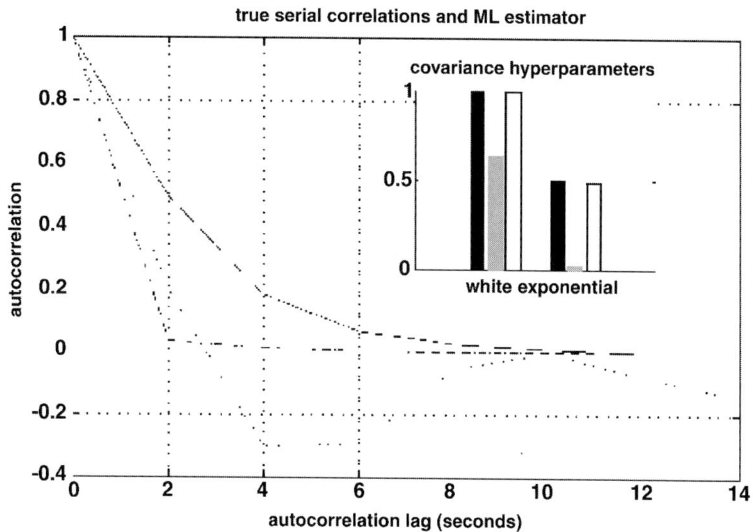

FIGURE 47.6
(Top panel) True response (activation plus random low-frequency components) and that based on the OLS and ML estimators for a simulated fMRI experiment. The insert shows the similarity between the OLS and ML predictions. (Lower panel) True (dashed) and estimated (solid) autocorrelation functions. The sample autocorrelation function of the residuals (dotted line) and the best fit in terms of the covariance constraints (dot-dashed) are also shown. The insert shows the true covariance hyperparameters (black), those obtained just using the residuals (gray), and those estimated by the EM algorithm (white). Note that, in relation to the EM estimates, those based directly on the residuals severely underestimate the actual correlations. The simulated data comprised 128 observations with an interscan interval of 2 sec. The activations were modeled with a boxcar (duty cycle of 64 sec) convolved with a canonical haemodynamic response function and scaled to a peak height of 2. The constant terms and low-frequency components were simulated with a linear combination of the first 16 components of a discrete cosine set, each scaled by a random unit Gaussian variate. Serially correlated noise was formed by filtering unit Gaussian noise with a convolution kernel based on covariance hyperparameters of 1.0 (uncorrelated or white component) and 0.5 [AR(1) component].

the low-frequency components of the design matrix. One way of understanding this is to note that the autocorrelations among the residuals are not unbiased estimators of $C_e^{(1)}$ but $RC_e^{(1)}R^T$, where R is the residual-forming matrix. In other words, the residuals are not the true errors but what is left after projecting them onto the null space of the design matrix.

The full details of this simulated single-session, boxcar design fMRI study are provided in the figure legend.

Inference in the Context of Nonsphericity[2]

This subsection explains why covariance component estimation is so important for inference. In short, although the parameter estimates may not depend on sphericity, the standard error—and ensuing statistics—do. The impact of serial correlations on inference was noted early in the fMRI analysis literature (Friston *et al.,* 1994) and led to the generalised least-squares (GLS) scheme described in Worsley and Friston (1995). In this scheme one starts with any observation model that is premultiplied by some weighting or convolution matrix S to give

$$Sy = SX^{(1)}\theta^{(1)} + S\varepsilon^{(1)} \tag{47.24}$$

The GLS parameter estimates and their covariance are as follows:

$$\begin{aligned} \eta_{LS} &= Ly \\ \mathrm{Cov}\{\eta_{LS}\} &= LC\varepsilon^{(1)}L^T \\ L &= (SX^{(1)})^{+}Sy \end{aligned} \tag{47.25}$$

These estimators minimise the GLS index $(y - X^{(1)}\eta_{LS})^T SS^T (y - X^{(1)}\eta_{LS})$. This family of estimators is unbiased but not necessarily a ML estimate. The Gauss-Markov estimator is the minimum variance and ML estimator that is obtained as a special case when $S = C_\varepsilon^{(1)-1/2}$. The T statistic corresponding to the GLS estimator is distributed with v degrees of freedom where (Worsley and Friston, 1995)

$$\begin{aligned} T &= \frac{c^T\eta_{LS}}{\sqrt{c^T Cov\{\eta_{LS}\}c}} \\ v &= \frac{tr\{RSC_\varepsilon^{(1)}S\}^2}{tr\{RSC_\varepsilon^{(1)}SRSC_\varepsilon^{(1)}S\}} \\ R &= 1 - X^{(1)}L \end{aligned} \tag{47.26}$$

The effective degrees of freedom are based on an approximation due to Satterthwaite (1941). This formulation is formally identical to the nonsphericity correction elaborated by Box (1954), which is commonly known as the Geisser-Greenhouse correction in classical analysis of variance (ANOVA) (Geisser and Greenhouse, 1958).

The key point here is that EM can be employed to give ReML estimates of correlations among the errors that enter into Eq. (47.26) to enable classical inference, properly adjusted for nonsphericity, *about any GLS estimator*. EM finds a special role in enabling inferences about GLS estimators in statistical parametric mapping. When the relative values of hyperparameters can be assumed to be stationary over voxels, ReML estimates can be obtained using the sample covariance of the data over voxels, in a single EM [see Eq. (47.61) in the Appendix]. After renormalisation, the ensuing estimate of the nonsphericity $\Sigma = Q^{(1)} = \sum\lambda_k Q_k^{(1)}$ specifies the serial correlations in terms of a single basis. Voxel-specific hyperparameters can now be estimated in a noniterative fashion in the usual way, because there is only one hyperparameter to estimate.

Application to Empirical Data

In this subsection we address the variability of serial correlations over voxels within subject and over subjects within the same voxel. Here we are concerned only with the form of the correlations The next subsection addresses between-subject error variance per se.

Using the model specification in Eq. (47.23), serial correlations were estimated using EM in 12 randomly selected voxels from the same slice from a single subject. The results are shown in Fig. 47.7, left panel, demonstrating that the correlations from one scan to the next can vary between about 0.1 and 0.4. The data sequences and experimental paradigm are described in the legend for Fig. 47.7. Briefly, these data came from an event-related study of visual word processing in which *new* and *old* words (i.e., encoded during a prescanning session) were presented in a random order with a stimulus onset asynchrony (SOA) of about 4 sec. Although the serial correlations within subject vary somewhat, there is an even greater variability from subject to subject at the same voxel. The right panel of Fig. 47.7 shows the autocorrelation functions

[2] An i.i.d. process is identically and independently distributed and has a probability distribution whose isocontours conform to a *sphere*. Any departure from this is referred to as *nonsphericity*.

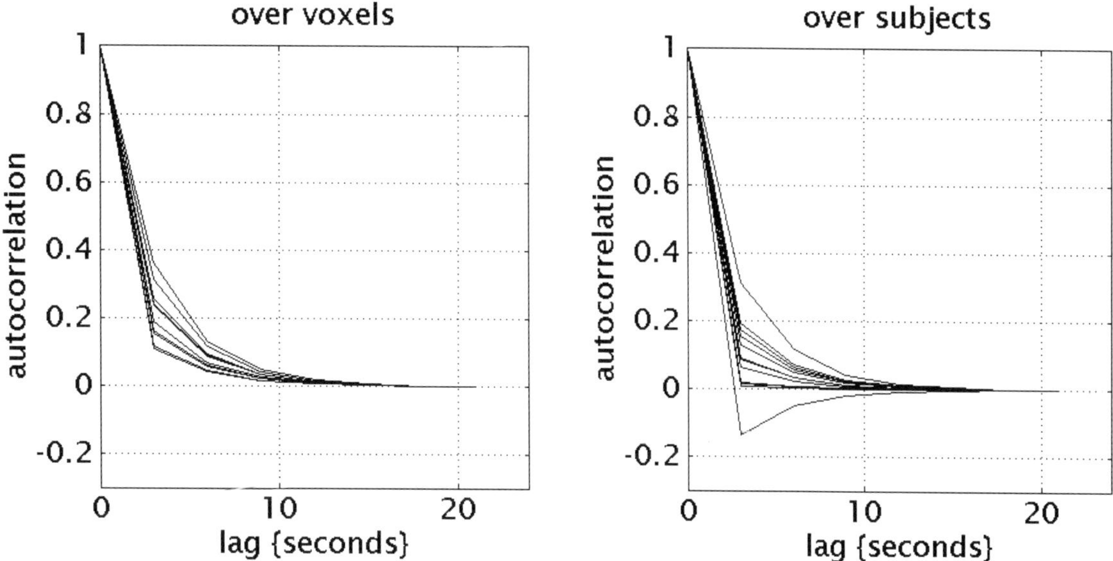

FIGURE 47.7
Estimates of serial correlations expressed as autocorrelation functions based on empirical data. (Left panel) Estimates from 12 randomly selected voxels from a single subject. (Right panel) Estimates from the same voxel over 12 different subjects. The voxel was in the cingulate gyrus. The empirical data are described in Henson *et al.* (2000). They comprised 300 volumes, acquired with EPI at 2 T and a TR of 3 sec. The experimental design was stochastic and event related, looking for a differential response evoked by *new* relative to *old* (studied prior to the scanning session) words. Either a new or old word was presented visually with a mean stimulus onset asynchrony (SOA) of 4 sec (SOA varied randomly between 2.5 and 5.5 sec). Subjects were required to make an old vs. new judgment for each word. The design matrix for these data comprised two regressors (early and late) for each of the four trial types (old vs. new and correct vs. incorrect) and the first 16 components of a discrete cosine set (as in the simulations)

estimated separately for 12 subjects at a single voxel. In this instance, the correlations between one scan and the next range from about –0.1 to 0.3 with a greater dispersion relative to the within-subject autocorrelations.

Summary

These results are provided to illustrate one potential application of covariance component estimation, not to provide an exhaustive characterisation of serial correlations. This sort of application may be important when it comes to making assumptions about models for serial correlations at different voxels or among subjects. We have chosen to focus on a covariance estimation problem that requires an iterative parameter reestimation procedure in which the hyperparameters controlling the covariances depend on the variance of the parameter estimates and vice versa. We could have considered other important applications of covariance component estimation although not all require an iterative scheme. One example is the estimation of condition-specific error variances in PET and fMRI. In conventional SPM analyses, one generally assumes that the error variance expressed in one condition is the same as that in another. This represents a sphericity assumption over conditions and allows one to pool several conditions when estimating the error variance. Assumptions of this sort, and related sphericity assumptions in multisubject studies, can be easily addressed in unbalanced designs or even in the context of missing data, using EM.

Variance Component Estimation in fMRI: Two-Level Models

In this subsection we augment the model above with a second level. This engenders a number of important issues, including the distinction between fixed- and random-effect inferences about the subjects' responses and the opportunity to make Bayesian inferences about single-subject responses. As above, we start with model specification, proceed to simulated data, and conclude with an empirical example. In this example, the second level represents observations over subjects. Analyses of simulated data are used to illustrate the distinction between fixed- and random-effect inferences by looking at how their respective T values depend on the variance components and design factors. The fMRI data are the same as used above and comprise event-related time series from 12 subjects. We chose a dataset that would be difficult to analyse rigorously using software available routinely. These data not only evidence serial correlations but also the number of trial-specific events varied from subject to subject, giving an unbalanced design.

Model Specification

The observation model here comprises two levels with the opportunity for subject-specific differences in error variance and serial correlations at the first level and parameter-specific variance at the second. The estimation model here is simply an extension of that used in the previous subsection to estimate serial correlations. Here it embodies a second level that accommodates observations over subjects.

level one

$$y = X^{(1)}\theta^{(1)} + \varepsilon^{(1)}$$

$$\begin{bmatrix} y_1 \\ \vdots \\ y_s \end{bmatrix} = \begin{bmatrix} X_1^{(1)} & \cdots & 0 \\ \vdots & \ddots & \vdots \\ 0 & \cdots & X_s^{(1)} \end{bmatrix} \begin{bmatrix} \theta_1^{(1)} \\ \vdots \\ \theta_s^{(1)} \end{bmatrix} + \varepsilon^{(1)}$$

$$Q_1^{(1)} = \begin{bmatrix} I_t & \cdots & 0 \\ \vdots & \ddots & \vdots \\ 0 & \cdots & 0 \end{bmatrix}, \ldots, \quad Q_s^{(1)} = \begin{bmatrix} 0 & \cdots & 0 \\ \vdots & \ddots & \vdots \\ 0 & \cdots & I_t \end{bmatrix}$$

$$Q_{s+1}^{(1)} = \begin{bmatrix} KK^T & \cdots & 0 \\ \vdots & \ddots & \vdots \\ 0 & \cdots & 0 \end{bmatrix}, \ldots, \quad Q_{2s}^{(1)} = \begin{bmatrix} 0 & \cdots & 0 \\ \vdots & \ddots & \vdots \\ 0 & \cdots & KK^T \end{bmatrix} \qquad (47.27)$$

level two

$$\theta^{(1)} = X^{(2)}\theta^{(2)} + \varepsilon^{(2)}$$

$$X^{(2)} = I_s \otimes I_p$$

$$Q_1^{(2)} = I_s \otimes \begin{bmatrix} 1 & \cdots & 0 \\ \vdots & \ddots & \vdots \\ 0 & \cdots & 0 \end{bmatrix}, \ldots, \quad Q_p^{(2)} = I_s \otimes \begin{bmatrix} 0 & \cdots & 0 \\ \vdots & \ddots & \vdots \\ 0 & \cdots & 1 \end{bmatrix}$$

for s subjects each scanned on t occasions and p parameters. The Kronecker tensor product $A \otimes B$ simply replaces the element of A with $A_{ij}B$. An example of these design matrices and covariance constraints were shown earlier in Figs. 47.1 and 47.3, respectively. Note that there are $2s$ error covariance constraints, one set for the white noise components and one for AR(1) components. Similarly, there are as many prior covariance constraints as there are parameters at the second level.

Simulations

In the simulations we used 128 scans for each of 12 subjects. The design matrix comprised three effects, modelling an event-related haemodynamic response to frequent but sporadic trials (in fact, the instances of correctly identified "old" words from the empirical example below) and a constant term. Activations were modelled with two regressors, constructed by convolving a series of delta functions with a canonical haemodynamic response function (HRF)[3] and the same function delayed by 3 sec. The delta functions indexed the occurrence of each event. These regressors model event-related responses with two temporal components, which we will refer to as "early" and "late" (cf. Henson *et al.*, 2000). Each subject-specific design matrix therefore comprised three columns, giving a total of 36 parameters at the first level and 3 at the second (the third being a constant term). The HRF basis functions were scaled so that a parameter estimate of one corresponds to a peak response of unity. After division by the grand mean, and multiplication by 100, the units of the response variable and parameter estimates were rendered adimensional and correspond to percent whole brain mean over all scans. The simulated data were generated using Eq. (47.27) with unit Gaussian noise coloured using a temporal, convolution matrix $(\Sigma\lambda_k^{(1)}Q_k^{(1)})^{1/2}$ with first-level hyperparameters $\lambda_k^{(1)}$ 0.5 and –0.1 for each subject's

[3] The canonical HRF was the same as that employed by SPM. It comprises a mixture of two gamma variates modelling peak and undershoot components and is based on a principal component analysis of empirically determined haemodynamic responses, over voxels, as described in Friston *et al.* (1998).

white and AR(1) error covariance components respectively. The second-level parameters and hyperparameters were $\theta^{(2)} = [0.5, 0,0]^T$, $\lambda^{(2)} = [0.02, 0.006,0]^T$. These model substantial early responses with an expected value of 0.5% and a standard deviation over subjects of 0.14% (i.e., square root of 0.02). The late component was trivial with zero expectation and a standard deviation of 0.077%. The third or constant terms were discounted with zero mean and variance. These values were chosen because they are typical of real data (see below).

Figures 47.8 and 47.9 show the results after subjecting the simulated data to EM to estimate the conditional mean and covariances of the subject-specific evoked responses. Figure 47.8 shows the estimated hyperparameters and parameters (black) alongside the true values (white). The first-level hyperparameters controlling within-subject error (i.e., scan-to-scan variability) are estimated in a reasonably reliable fashion but note that these estimates show a degree of variation about the veridical values (see "Conclusion" section). In this example the second-level hyperparameters are overestimated but remarkably good, given only 12 subjects. The parameter estimates at the first and second levels are again very reasonable, correctly attributing the majority of the experimental variance to an early effect. Figure 47.8 should be compared with Fig. 47.10, which shows the equivalent estimates for real data.

The top panel in Fig. 47.9 shows the ML estimates that would have been obtained if we had used a single-level model. These correspond to response estimates from a conventional fixed-effects analysis. The insert shows the classical fixed-effect T values, for each subject, for contrasts testing early and late response components. Although these T values properly reflect the prominence of early effects, their variability precludes any threshold that could render the early components significant and yet exclude false positives pertaining to the late component. The lower panel highlights the potential of revisiting the first level, in the context of a hierarchical model. It shows the equivalent responses based on the conditional mean and the posterior inference (insert) based on the conditional covariance. This allows us to reiterate some points made in the previous section. First, the parameter estimates and ensuing response estimates are informed by information abstracted from higher levels. Second, this prior information enables Bayesian inference about the probability of an activation that is specified in neurobiologically meaningful terms.

In Fig. 47.9 the estimated responses are shown (solid lines) with the actual responses (broken lines). Note how the conditional estimates show a regression or "shrinkage" to the conditional mean. In other words, their variance shrinks to reflect, more accurately, the variability in real responses. In particular, the spurious variability in the apparent latency of the peak response in the ML estimates disappears when using the conditional estimates. This is because the contribution of the late component, which induces latency differences, is suppressed in the conditional estimates. This, in turn, reflects the fact that the variability in its expression over subjects is small relative to that induced by the observation error. Simulations like these suggest that characterisations of intersubject variability using ML approaches can severely overestimate the true variability. This is because the ML estimates are unconstrained and simply minimise observation error without considering how likely the ensuing intersubject variability is.

The posterior probabilities (insert) are a function of the conditional mean $\eta^{(1)}_{\theta|y}$ and covariance $C^{(1)}_{\theta|y}$ and a size threshold $\gamma = 0.1$ that specifies an "activation":

$$1 - \Phi\left(\frac{\gamma - c_j^T \eta^{(1)}_{\theta|y}}{\sqrt{c_j^T C^{(1)}_{\theta|y} c_j}}\right) \tag{47.28}$$

The contrast weight vectors were $c_{early} = [1,0,0]^T$ and $c_{late} = [0,1,0]^T$. As expected, the probability of the early response being greater than γ was uniformly high for all 12 subjects, whereas the equivalent probability for the late component was negligible. Note that, in contradistinction to the classical inference, there is now a clear indication that each subject expressed an early response but no late response.

Empirical Analyses

Here the analysis is repeated using real data and the results are compared to those obtained using simulated data. The empirical data are described in Henson *et al.* (2000). Briefly, they comprised 128+ scans in 12 subjects. Only the first 128 scans were used below. The experimental design

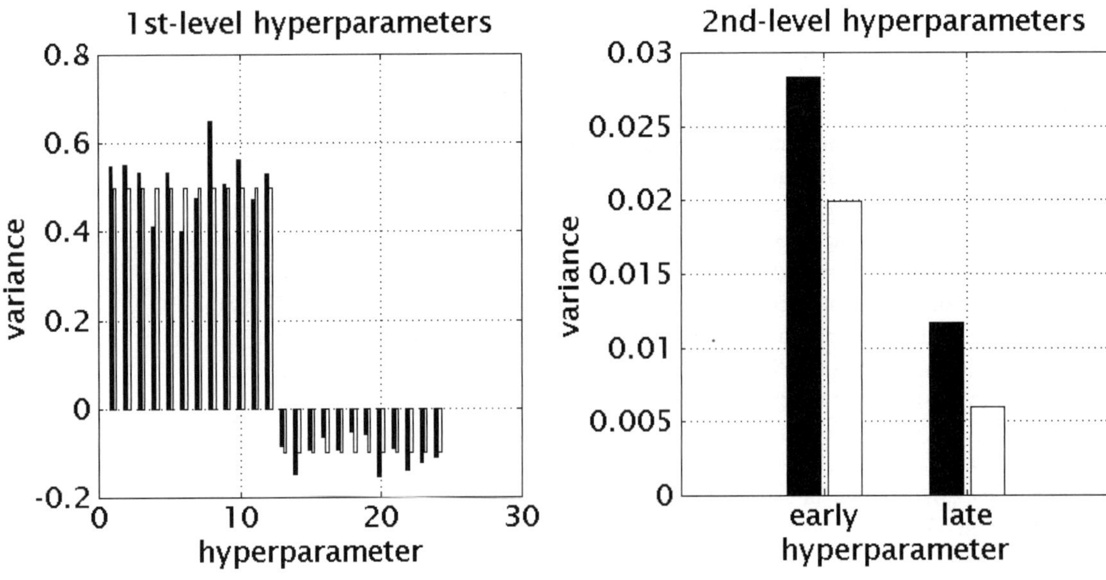

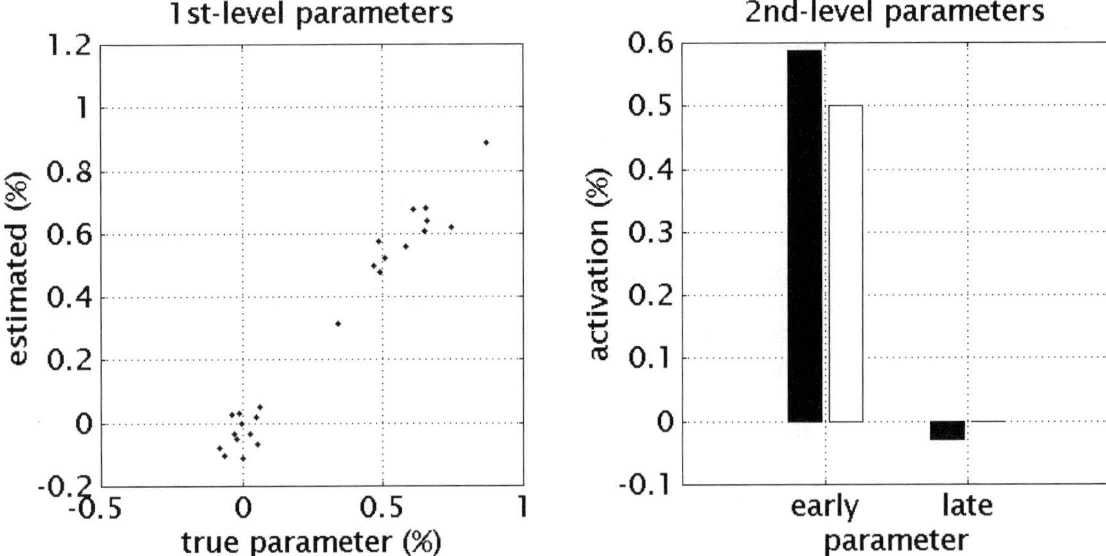

FIGURE 47.8
The results of an analysis of simulated event-related responses in a single voxel. Parameter and hyperparameter estimates based on a simulated fMRI study are shown in relation to the true values. The simulated data comprised 128 scans for each of 12 subjects with a mean peak response over subjects of 0.5%. The construction of these data is described in the main text. Stimulus presentation conformed to the presentation of "old" words in the empirical analysis described in the main text. Serial correlations were modeled as in the main text. (Upper left) First-level hyperparameters. The estimated subject-specific values (black) are shown alongside the true values (white). The first 12 correspond to the "white" term or variance. The second 12 control the degree of autocorrelation and can be interpreted as the covariance between one scan and the next. (Upper right) Hyperparameters for the early and late components of the evoked response. (Lower left) The estimated subject-specific parameters pertaining to the early and late response components are plotted against their true values. (Lower right) The estimated and true parameters at the second level representing the conditional mean of the distribution from which the subject-specific effects are drawn.

was stochastic and event related, looking for differential responses evoked by *new* relative to *old* (studied prior to the scanning session) words. Either a new or old word was presented every 4 sec or so (SOA varied between 2.5 and 5.5 sec). In this design one is interested only in the differences between evoked responses to the two stimulus types. This is because the efficiency of the design to detect the effect of stimuli per se is negligible with such a short SOA. Subjects were

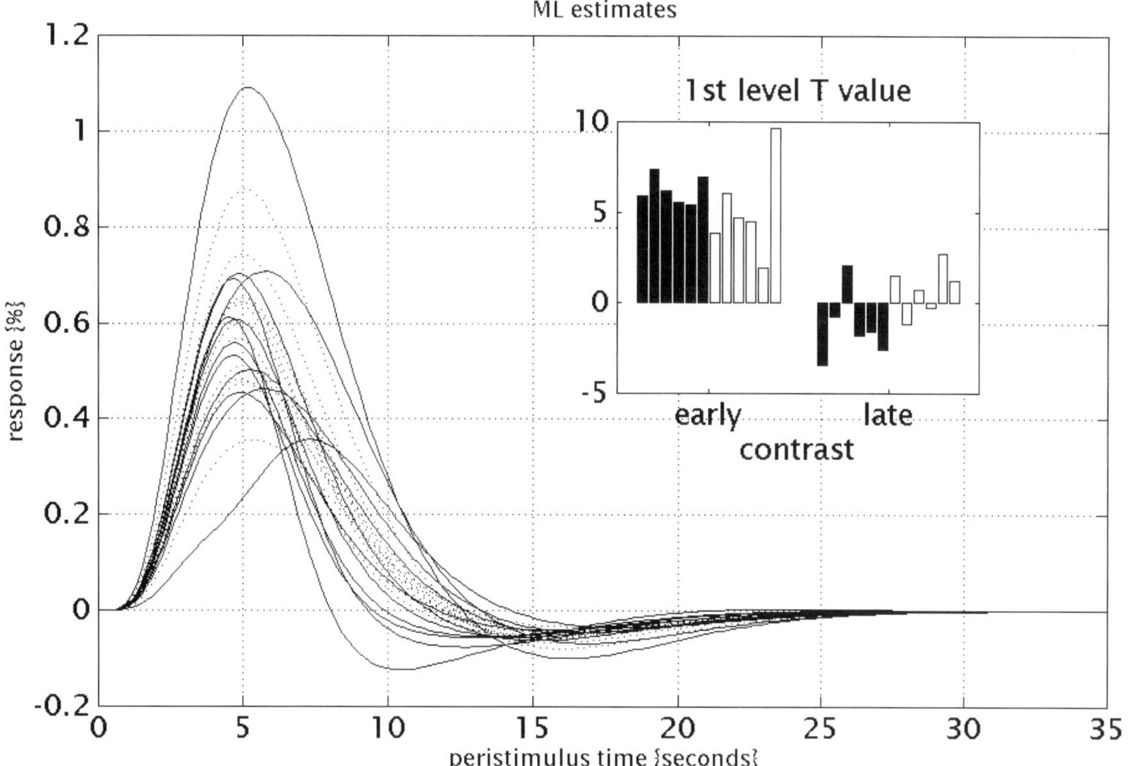

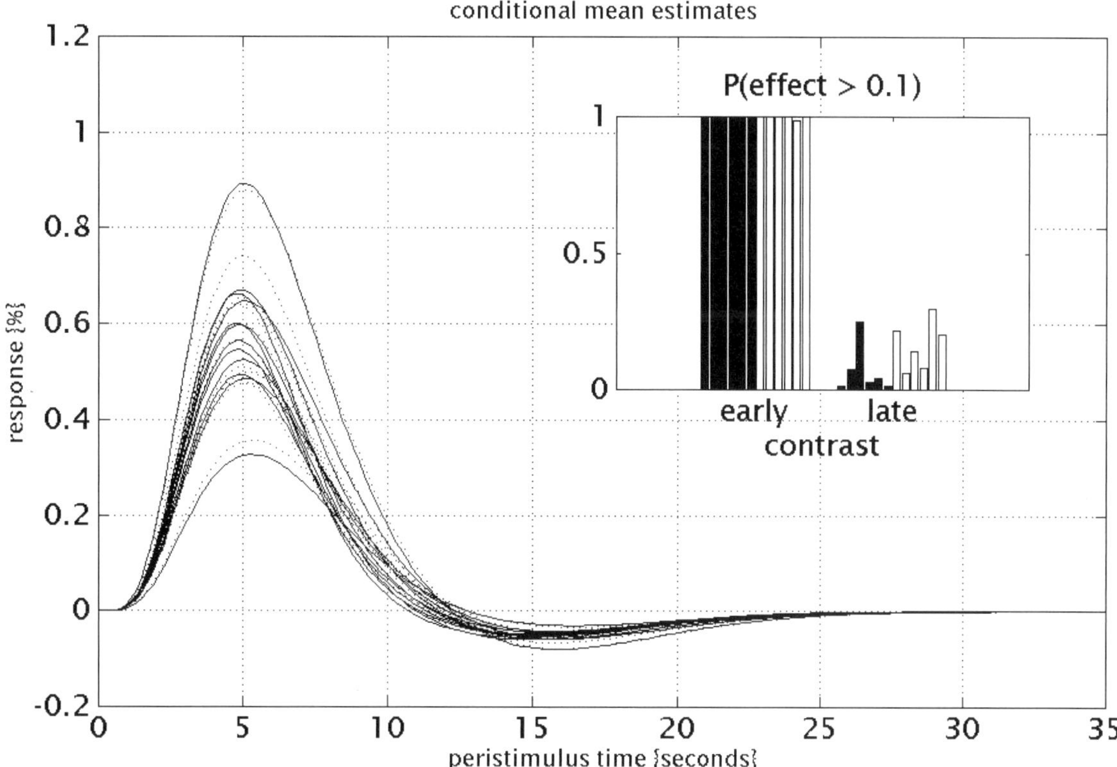

FIGURE 47.9

Response estimates and inferences about the estimates presented in Fig. 47.8. (Upper panel) True (dotted) and ML (solid) estimates of event-related responses to a stimulus over 12 subjects. The units of activation are adimensional and correspond to percent of whole brain mean. The insert shows the corresponding subject-specific T values for contrasts testing for early and late responses. (Lower panel) The equivalent estimates based on the conditional means. It can be seen that the conditional estimates are much "tighter" and reflect better the intersubject variability in responses. The insert shows the posterior probability that the activation was greater than 0.1%. Because the responses were modeled with early and late components (basis functions corresponding to canonical haemodynamic response functions, separated by 3 sec) separate posterior probabilities could be computed for each. The simulated data comprised only early responses as reflected in the posterior probabilities.

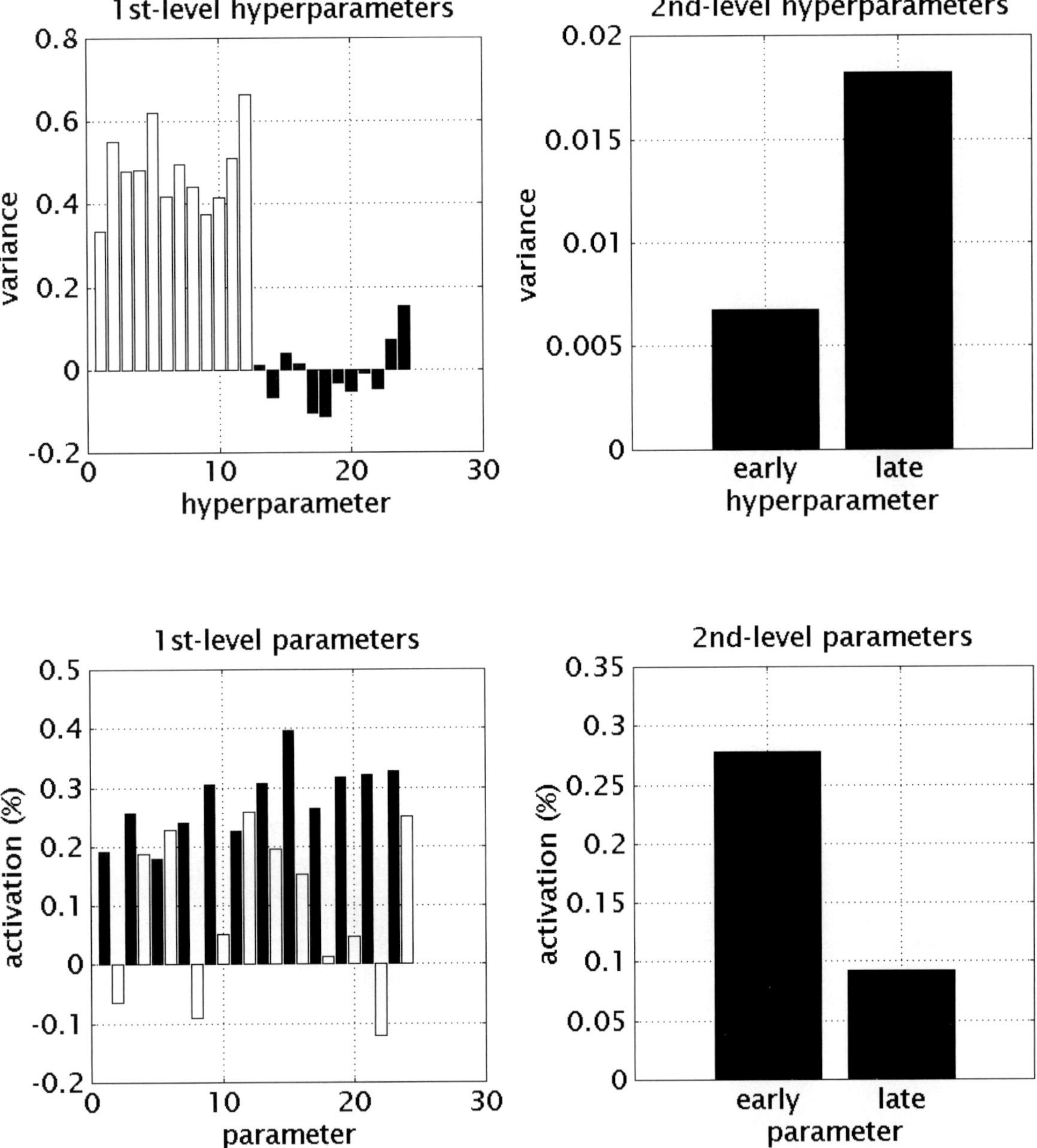

FIGURE 47.10
Estimation of differential event-related responses in real data. The format of this figure is identical to that of Fig. 47.8. The only differences are that these results are based on real data where the response is due to the difference between studied or familiar (old) words and novel (new) words. In this example we used the first 128 scans from 12 subjects. Clearly in this figure we cannot include true effects.

required to make an old vs. new judgment for each word. Drift (the first eight components of a discrete cosine set) and the effects of incorrect trials were treated as confounds and removed using linear regression.[4] The first-level subject-specific design matrix partitions comprised four regressors with early and late effects for both old and new words.

The analyses proceeded in exactly the same way as for the simulated data. The only difference was that the contrast tested for *differences* between the two word types (i.e., $c = [1,0,-1,0]^T$ for an old minus new early effect). The hyperparameter and parameter estimates, for a voxel in the cingulate gyrus (BA 31; –3, –33, 39 mm), are shown in Fig. 47.10, adopting the same format as

[4] Strictly speaking the projection matrix implementing this adjustment should also be applied to the covariance constraints but this would (1) render the constraints singular and (2) ruin their sparsity structure. We therefore omitted this and ensured in simulations that the adjustment had a negligible effect on the hyperparameter estimates.

in Fig. 47.8. Here we see that the within-subject error varies much more in the empirical data with the last subject showing almost twice the error variance of the first subject. As above, the serial correlations vary considerably from subject to subject and are not consistently positive or negative. The second-level hyperparameters showed the early component of the differential response to be more reliable over subjects than the late component (0.007 and 0.19, respectively). All but two subjects had a greater early response, relative to late, which on average was about 0.28%. In other words, activation differentials, on the order of 0.3%, occurred in the context of an observation error with a standard deviation of 0.5% (see Fig. 47.10). The inter-subject variability was about 30% of the mean response amplitude. A component of the variability in within-subject error is due to uncertainty in the ReML estimates of the hyperparameters (see Friston *et al.*, 2002a), but this degree of inhomogeneity is substantially more than in the simulated data (where subjects had equal error variances). It is interesting to note that, despite the fact that the regressors for the early and late components had exactly the same form, the between-subject error for one was less than half that of the other. Results of this sort speak to the prevalence of nonsphericity (in this instance, heteroscedasticity or unequal variances) and a role for the analyses illustrated here.

The response estimation and inference are shown in Fig. 47.11. Again we see the characteristic "shrinkage" when comparing the ML to the conditional estimates. It can be seen that all subjects, apart from the first and third, had more than a 95% chance of expressing an early differential of 0.1% or more. The late differential response was much less consistent, although one subject expressed a difference with about 84% confidence.

Summary

The examples presented above allow us to reprise a number of important points made in the previous section (see also Friston *et al.,* 2002a). In conclusion the main points are as follows:

- There are many instances when an iterative parameter reestimation scheme is required (e.g., when dealing with serial correlations or missing data). These schemes are generally variants of EM.
- Even before considering the central role of covariance component estimation in hierarchical or empirical Bayes models, it is an important aspect of model estimation in its own right, particularly in estimating nonsphericity among observation errors. Parameter estimates can either be obtained directly from an EM algorithm, in which case they correspond to the ML or Gauss-Markov estimates, or the hyperparameters can be used to determine the error correlations, which reenter a GLS scheme, as a nonsphericity correction.
- Hierarchical models enable a collective improvement in response estimates by using conditional, as opposed to ML, estimators. This improvement ensues from the constraints derived from higher levels that enter as priors at lower levels.

In the next section we revisit two-level models but consider hierarchical observations over voxels as opposed to subjects.

POSTERIOR PROBABILITY MAPPING

Introduction

This section describes the construction of *posterior probability maps* that enable conditional or Bayesian inferences about regionally specific effects in neuroimaging. Posterior probability maps are images of the probability or confidence that an activation exceeds some specified threshold, given the data. PPMs represent a complementary alternative to SPMs, which are used to make classical inferences. However, a key problem in Bayesian inference is the specification of appropriate priors. This problem can be finessed using *empirical Bayes* in which prior variances are estimated from the data, under some simple assumptions about their form. Empirical Bayes requires a hierarchical observation model, in which higher levels can be regarded as providing prior constraints on lower levels. In neuroimaging, observations of the

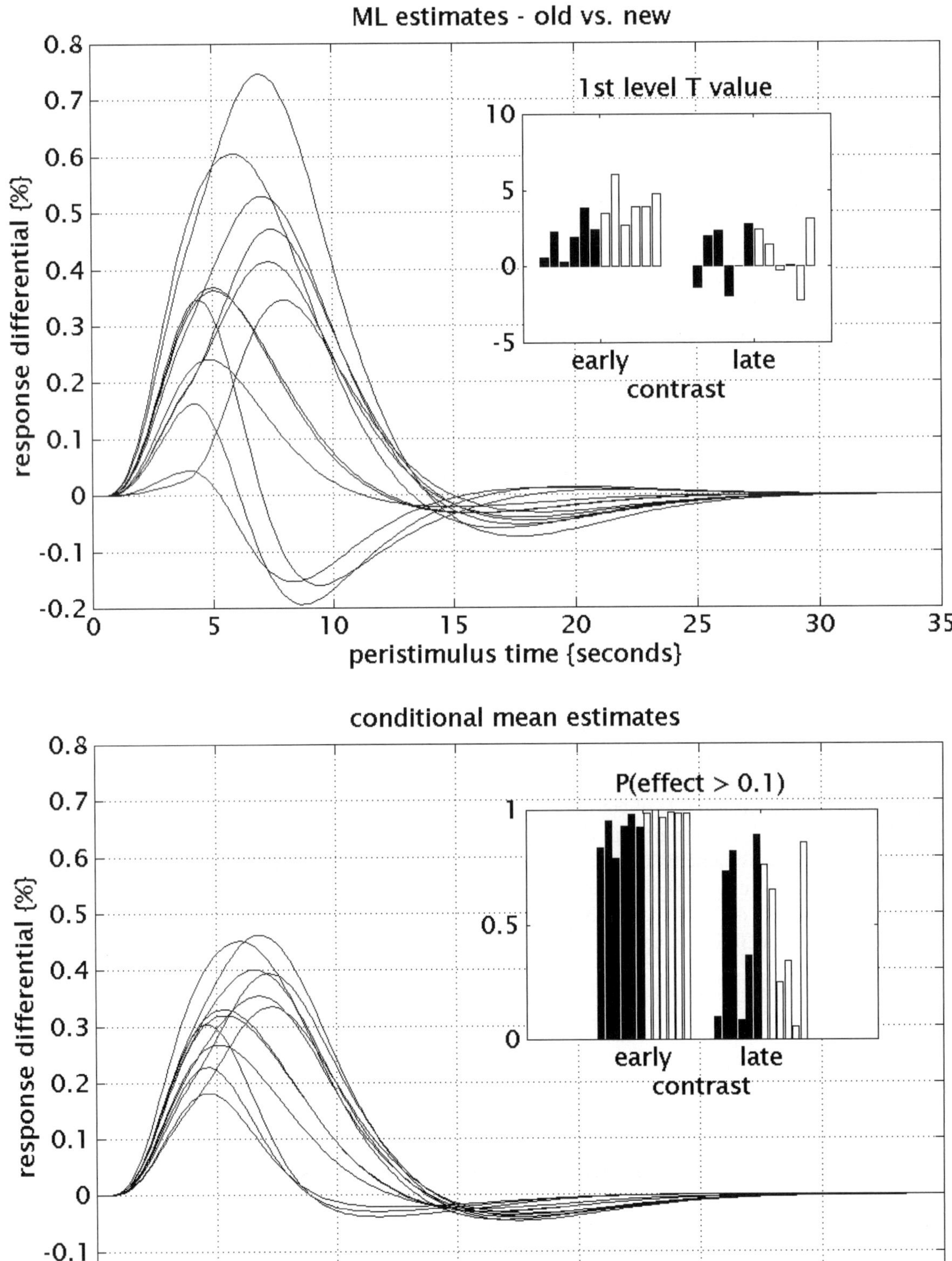

FIGURE 47.11
The format of this figure is identical to that of Fig. 47.9. The only differences are that these results are based on real data where the response is due to the difference between studied or familiar (old) words and novel (new) words. The same regression of conditional responses to the conditional mean is seen when the ML and conditional estimates are compared. In relation to the simulated data, there is more evidence for a late component but no late activation could be inferred for any subject with any degree of confidence. The voxel from which these data were taken was in the cingulate gyrus (BA 31) at −3, −33, and 39 mm.

same effect over voxels provide a natural, two-level hierarchy that enables an empirical Bayesian approach. In this section we present the motivation and the operational details of a simple empirical Bayesian method for computing PPMs. We then compare Bayesian and classical inference through the equivalent PPMs and SPMs testing for the same effect in the same data.

To date, inference in neuroimaging has been restricted largely to classical inferences based on SPMs. The alternative approach is to use Bayesian or conditional inference based on the posterior distribution of the activation given the data (Holmes and Ford, 1993). This necessitates the specification of priors (i.e., the probability distribution of the activation). Bayesian inference requires the posterior distribution and therefore rests on a posterior density analysis. A useful way to summarise this posterior density is to compute the probability that the activation exceeds some threshold. This computation represents a Bayesian inference about the effect, in relation to the specified threshold. We now describe an approach to computing posterior probability maps for activation effects or, more generally, treatment effects in imaging data sequences. This approach represents, probably, the most simple and computationally expedient way of constructing PPMs.

As established in the previous sections, the motivation for using conditional or Bayesian inference is that it has high face validity. This is because the inference is about an effect, or activation, being greater than some specified size that has some meaning in relation to underlying neurophysiology. This contrasts with classical inference, in which the inference is about the effect being significantly different than zero. The problem for classical inference is that trivial departures from the null hypothesis can be declared significant, with sufficient data or sensitivity. Furthermore, from the point of view of neuroimaging, posterior inference is especially useful because it eschews the multiple-comparison problem. Posterior inference does not have to contend with the multiple-comparison problem because there are no false positives. The probability that activation has occurred, given the data, at any particular voxel is the same, irrespective of whether one has analysed that voxel or the entire brain. For this reason, posterior inference using PPMs may represent a relatively more powerful approach than classical inference in neuroimaging. The reason why the p values do not need to be adjusted is because we assume independent prior distributions for the activations over voxels. In this simple Bayesian model, the Bayesian perspective is similar to that of the frequentist who makes inferences on a per-comparison basis (see Berry and Hochberg, 1999, for a detailed discussion).

Priors and Bayesian Inference

PPMs require the posterior distribution or conditional distribution of the activation (a contrast of conditional parameter estimates) given the data. This posterior density can be computed, under Gaussian assumptions, using the Bayes rule. Bayes rule requires the specification of a likelihood function and the prior density of the model's parameters. The models used to form PPMs, and the likelihood functions, are exactly the same as in classical SPM analyses. The only extra bit of information that is required is the prior probability distribution of the parameters of the general linear model employed. Although it would be possible to specify these in terms of their means and variances using independent data, or some plausible physiological constraints, there is an alternative to this fully Bayesian approach. The alternative is empirical Bayes in which the variances of the prior distributions are estimated directly from the data. Empirical Bayes requires a *hierarchical observation model* where the parameters and hyperparameters at any particular level can be treated as priors on the level below. There are numerous examples of hierarchical observation models. For example, the distinction between fixed- and mixed-effects analyses of multisubject studies relies on a two-level hierarchical model. However, in neuroimaging there is a natural hierarchical observation model that is common to all brain mapping experiments. This is the hierarchy induced by looking for the same effects at every voxel within the brain (or gray matter). The first level of the hierarchy corresponds to the experimental effects at any particular voxel and the second level of the hierarchy comprises the effects over voxels. Put simply, the variation in a particular contrast, over voxels, can be used as the prior variance of that contrast at any particular voxel.

The model used here is one in which the spatial relationship among voxels is discounted. The advantage of treating an image like a "gas" of unconnected voxels is that the estimation of between-voxel variance in activation can be finessed to a considerable degree [see Eq. (47.61) in the Appendix and following discussion). This renders the estimation of posterior densities tractable because the between-voxel variance can then be used as a prior variance at each voxel. We therefore focus on this simple and special case and on the "pooling" of voxels to give precise ReML estimates of the variance components required for Bayesian inference. The main focus of this section is the pooling procedure, which affords a computational saving necessary to produce PPMs of the whole brain. In what follows we describe how this approach is implemented and provide some examples of its application.

Theory Conditional Estimators and the Posterior Density

In this subsection we describe how the posterior distribution of the parameters of any general linear model can be estimated at each voxel from imaging data sequences. Under Gaussian assumptions about the errors $\varepsilon \sim N\{0, C_\varepsilon\}$ of a general linear model with design matrix X the responses are modelled as follows:

$$y = X\theta + \varepsilon \tag{47.29}$$

The conditional or posterior covariances and mean of the parameters θ are given by (Friston *et al.,* 2002a)

$$\begin{aligned} C_{\theta|y} &= (X^T C_\varepsilon^{-1} X + C_\theta^{-1})^{-1} \\ \eta_{\theta|y} &= C_{\theta|y} X^T C_\varepsilon^{-1} y \end{aligned} \tag{47.30}$$

where C_θ is the prior covariance and assuming a prior expectation of zero. Once these moments are known, the posterior probability that a particular effect or contrast specified by a contrast weight vector c exceeds some threshold γ is easily computed:

$$p = 1 - \Phi\left(\frac{\gamma - c^T \eta_{\theta|y}}{\sqrt{c^T C_{\theta|y} c}}\right) \tag{47.31}$$

where $\Phi(\cdot)$ is the cumulative density function of the unit normal distribution. An image of these posterior probabilities constitutes a PPM.

Estimating the Error Covariance with ReML

Clearly, to compute the conditional moments in Eq. (47.30) one needs to know the error and prior covariances C_ε and C_θ. In the next section we describe how the prior covariance C_θ can be estimated. For the moment, assume the prior covariance is known. In this case the error covariance can be estimated in terms of a hyperparameter λ_ε where $C_\varepsilon = \lambda_\varepsilon V$, and V is the correlation or nonsphericity matrix of the errors (see below). This hyperparameter is estimated simply by using ReML as described in the Appendix.[5]

Until *convergence* {

E-Step

$$C_\varepsilon = \lambda_\varepsilon V$$
$$C_{\theta|y} = (X^T C_\varepsilon^{-1} X + C_\theta^{-1})^{-1}$$

M-Step

$$P = C_\varepsilon^{-1} - C_\varepsilon^{-1} X C_{\theta|y} X^T C_\varepsilon^{-1}$$
$$g = -\frac{1}{2}\, tr\{PV\} + \frac{1}{2}\, tr\{P^T V P y y^T\}$$
$$H = -\frac{1}{2}\, tr\{PVPV\}$$
$$\lambda_\varepsilon \leftarrow \lambda_\varepsilon + H^{-1} g$$

} (47.32)

In brief, P represents the residual forming matrix, premultiplied by the inverse of the error covariance. It is this projector matrix that "restricts" the estimation of variance components to

[5] Note that the augmentation step shown in Fig. 47.4 is unnecessary because the prior covariance enters explicitly into the conditional covariance.

the null space of the design matrix. The g and H terms are the first- and expected second-order derivatives (i.e., gradients and expected negative curvature) of the ReML objective function. The **M**-step can be regarded as a Fisher scoring scheme that maximises the ReML objective function. Given that there is only one hyperparameter to estimate, this scheme converges very quickly (two to three iterations for a tolerance of 10^{-6}).

Estimating the Prior Density with Empirical Bayes

Simply computing the conditional moments using Eq. (47.30) corresponds to a fully Bayesian analysis at each and every voxel. However, there is an outstanding problem in the sense that we do not know the prior covariances of the parameters. It is at this point that we introduce the hierarchical perspective that enables an empirical Bayesian approach. If we now consider Eq. (47.29) as the first level of the two-level hierarchy, in which the second level corresponds to observations over voxels, we have a hierarchical observation model for all voxels that treats some parameters as random effects and others as fixed. The random effects θ_1 are those that we are interested in, and the fixed effects θ_0 are nuisance variables or confounds (e.g., drifts or the constant term) modelled by the regressors in X_0 where $X = [X_1,X_0]$ and

$$\begin{aligned} y &= [X_1, X_0]\begin{bmatrix}\theta_1\\ \theta_0\end{bmatrix} + \varepsilon^{(1)} \\ \theta_1 &= 0 + \varepsilon^{(2)} \end{aligned} \tag{47.33}$$

This model posits that there is a voxel-wide prior distribution for the parameters θ_1 with zero mean and unknown covariance $E\{\varepsilon^{(2)}\varepsilon^{(2)T}\} = \sum_i \lambda_i Q_i$. The bases Q_i specify the prior covariance structure of the interesting effects and would usually comprise a basis for each parameter whose ith leading diagonal element was one and zero elsewhere. This implies that if we selected a voxel at random from the search volume, the ith parameter at that voxel would conform to a sample from a Gaussian distribution of zero expectation and variance λ_i. The reason this distribution can be assumed to have zero mean is that parameters of interest reflect region-specific effects that, by definition sum to zero over the search volume.[6] By concatenating the data from all voxels and using Kronecker tensor products of the design matrices and covariance bases, it is possible to create a very large hierarchical observation model that could be subject to EM (see, for example, Friston *et al.* 2002b, Section 3.2). However, given the enormous number of voxels in neuroimaging this is computationally prohibitive. A mathematically equivalent but more tractable approach is to consider the estimation of the prior hyperparameters as a variance component estimation problem after collapsing Eq. (47.33) to a single-level model:

$$\begin{aligned} y &= X_0\theta_0 + \xi \\ \xi &= X_1\varepsilon^{(2)} + \varepsilon^{(1)} \end{aligned} \tag{47.34}$$

This is simply a rearrangement of Eq. (47.33) to give a linear model with a compound error covariance that includes the observation error covariance and m components for each parameter in θ_1. These components are induced by variation of the parameters over voxels:

$$\begin{aligned} C_\xi &= E\{\xi\xi^T\} = \Sigma\lambda_k Q_k \\ Q &= \{X_1Q_1X_1^T,\ldots,X_1Q_mX_1^T,V\} \\ \lambda &= [\lambda_1,\ldots,\lambda_m,\lambda_\varepsilon]^T \end{aligned} \tag{47.35}$$

This equation says that the covariance of the compound error can be linearly decomposed into m components (usually one for each parameter) and the error variance. The form of the observed covariances, due to variation in the parameters, is determined by the design matrix X and Q_i that model variance components in parameter space.

Equation (47.35) affords a computationally expedient way to estimate the prior covariances for the parameters that are then entered into Eq. (47.30) to provide for voxel-specific error hyperparameter estimates and conditional moments. In brief, the hyperparameters are estimated by pooling the data from all voxels to provide ReML estimates of the variance components of

[6] In the SPM2 implementation, we allow for any mean of the parameters at the second level by subtracting the mean over voxels from the data. This mean represents an estimate of the prior expectation projected onto the observation space by the design matrix.

C_ξ according to Eq. (47.35). The nice thing about this pooling is that the hyperparameters of the parameter covariances are, of course, the same for all voxels. This is not the case for the error covariance hyperparameters that may change from voxel to voxel. The pooled estimate of λ_ε can be treated as an estimate of the average λ_ε over voxels. The hyperparameters are estimated by iterating as follows:

Until convergence { **E**-Step

$$C_\xi = \Sigma\lambda_k Q_k$$
$$C_{\theta|y} = (X_0^T C_\varepsilon^{-1} X_0)^{-1}$$

M-Step

$$P = C_\xi^{-1} - C_\xi^{-1} X_0 C_{\theta|y} X_0{}^T C_\xi^{-1}$$
$$g_i = -\frac{1}{2}\, tr\{PQ_i\} + \frac{1}{2}\, tr\{P^T Q_i P Y Y^T / n\}$$
$$H_{ij} = -\frac{1}{2}\, tr\{PQ_i PQ_j\}$$
$$\lambda \leftarrow \lambda + H^{-1} g$$

}

(47.36)

We can see that this equation has exactly the form as Eq. (47.32) used for the analysis at each voxel. The differences are as follows: (1) yy^T has been replaced by its sample mean over voxels YY^T/n. (2) There are no priors because the parameters controlling the expression of confounding effects or nuisance variables are treated as fixed effects. This is equivalent to setting their prior variance to infinity (i.e., flat priors) so that $C_{\theta_0}^{-1} \to 0$. (3) Finally, the regressors in X_1 have disappeared from the design matrix because these effects are embodied in the covariance components of the compound error. As above, the inclusion of confounds restricts the hyperparameter estimation to the null space of X_0, hence, *restricted* maximum likelihood. In the absence of confounds, the hyperparameters would simply be ML estimates that minimise the difference between the estimated and observed covariance of the data, averaged over voxels. The ensuing ReML estimates are very high precision estimators. Their precision increases linearly with the number of voxels n and is in fact equal to nH. These hyperparameters now enter as priors into the voxel-specific estimation along with the flat priors for the nuisance variables:

$$C_\theta = \begin{bmatrix} \Sigma\lambda_i Q_i & \cdots & 0 & \\ \vdots & \infty & & \\ & & \ddots & \\ 0 & & & \infty \end{bmatrix} \tag{47.37}$$

We now have a very precise estimate of the prior covariance that can be used to revisit each voxel to compute the conditional or posterior density using Eqs. (47.30) and (47.32). Finally, the conditional moments enter Eq. (47.31) to give the posterior probability for each voxel. Figure 47.12 shows a schematic illustration of this scheme.

Summary

All neuroimaging experiments are characterised by a natural hierarchy, in which the second level is provided by variation over voxels. Although it would be possible to form a very large two-level observation model and estimate the conditional means and covariances of the parameters at the first level, this would involve dealing with matrices of size $(ns) \times (ns)$ (number of voxels n times the number of scans s). The same conditional estimators can be computed using the two-step approach described above. First, the data covariance components induced by parameter variation over voxels and observation error are computed using ReML estimates of the associated covariance hyperparameters. Second, each voxel is revisited to compute voxel-specific error variance hyperparameters and the conditional moments of the parameters, using the empirical priors from the first step (see Fig. 47.12). Both of these steps deal only with matrices of size $n \times n$. The voxel-specific estimation sacrifices the simplicity of a single large iterative scheme

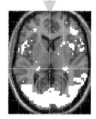

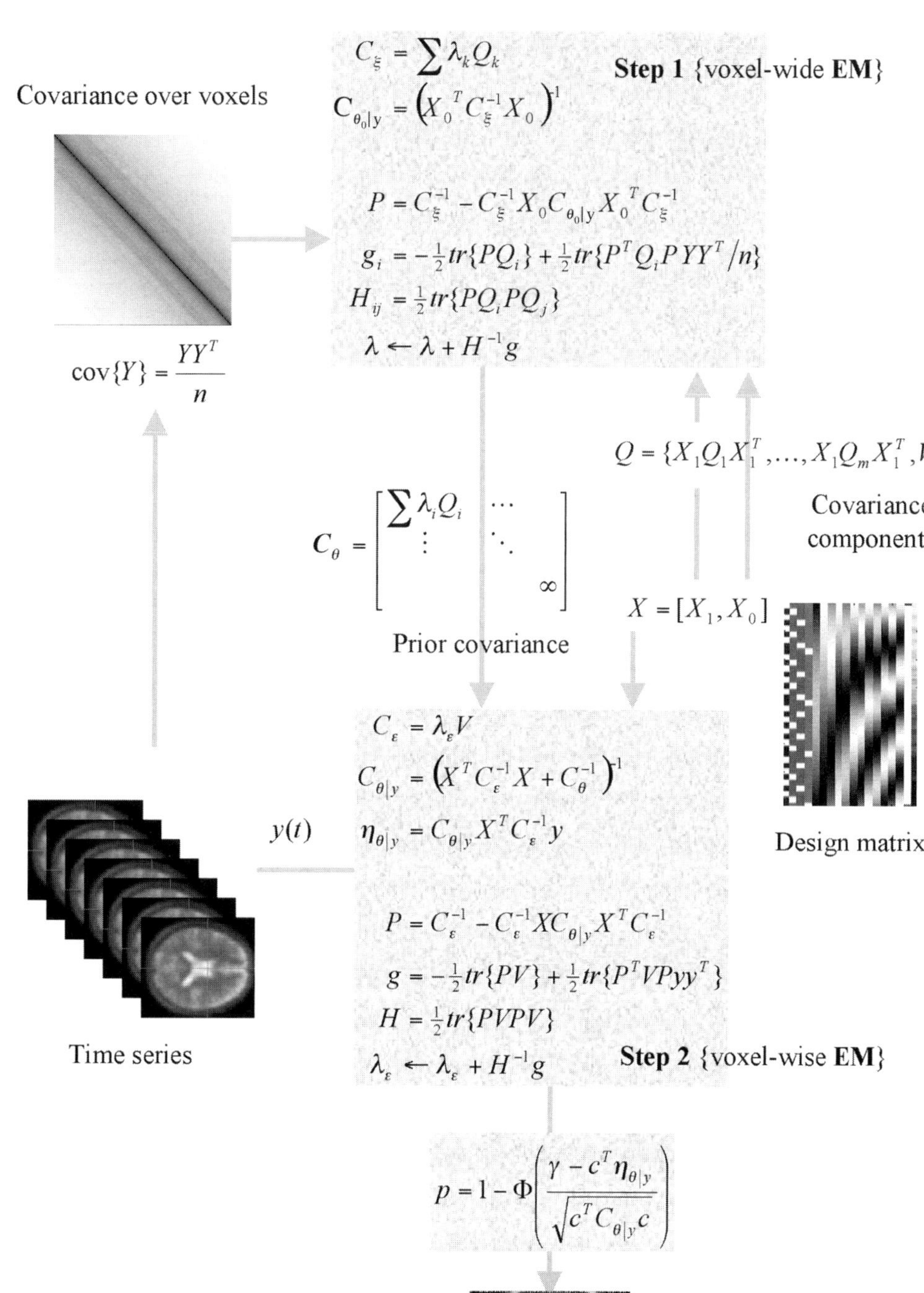

Covariance over voxels
Step 1 {voxel-wide EM}
$C_\xi = \sum \lambda_k Q_k$
$C_{\theta_0|y} = (X_0^T C_\xi^{-1} X_0)^{-1}$
$P = C_\xi^{-1} - C_\xi^{-1} X_0 C_{\theta_0|y} X_0^T C_\xi^{-1}$
$g_i = -\frac{1}{2} tr\{PQ_i\} + \frac{1}{2} tr\{P^T Q_i P YY^T / n\}$
$H_{ij} = \frac{1}{2} tr\{PQ_i PQ_j\}$
$\lambda \leftarrow \lambda + H^{-1} g$
$\mathrm{cov}\{Y\} = \frac{YY^T}{n}$
$Q = \{X_1 Q_1 X_1^T, \ldots, X_1 Q_m X_1^T, V\}$
Covariance components
$C_\theta = \begin{bmatrix} \sum \lambda_i Q_i & \cdots & \\ \vdots & \ddots & \\ & & \infty \end{bmatrix}$
Prior covariance
$X = [X_1, X_0]$
Design matrix
$C_\varepsilon = \lambda_\varepsilon V$
$C_{\theta|y} = (X^T C_\varepsilon^{-1} X + C_\theta^{-1})^{-1}$
$y(t)$
$\eta_{\theta|y} = C_{\theta|y} X^T C_\varepsilon^{-1} y$
$P = C_\varepsilon^{-1} - C_\varepsilon^{-1} X C_{\theta|y} X^T C_\varepsilon^{-1}$
$g = -\frac{1}{2} tr\{PV\} + \frac{1}{2} tr\{P^T VPyy^T\}$
$H = \frac{1}{2} tr\{PVPV\}$
$\lambda_\varepsilon \leftarrow \lambda_\varepsilon + H^{-1} g$
Time series
Step 2 {voxel-wise EM}
$p = 1 - \Phi\left(\frac{\gamma - c^T \eta_{\theta|y}}{\sqrt{c^T C_{\theta|y} c}}\right)$
PPM

FIGURE 47.12
Schematic summarising the two-step procedure for (step 1) ReML estimation of the prior covariance based on the data covariance, pooled over voxels, and (step 2) a voxel-by-voxel estimation of the posterior expectation and covariance of the parameters, required for inference. See the main text for a detailed explanation of the equations.

for lots of quicker iterative schemes at each voxel. This exploits the fact that the same first-level design matrix is employed for all voxels.

Empirical Demonstration

In this section we compare and contrast Bayesian and classical inference using PPMs and SPMs based on real data. The first data we use are the PET verbal fluency data that have been used to illustrate methodological advances in SPM over the years. In brief, these data were required from five subjects each scanned 12 times during the performance of one of two word generation tasks. The subjects were asked to either repeat a heard letter or to respond with a word that began with the heard letter. These tasks were performed in alternation over the 12 scans and the order randomised over subjects. The second dataset comprised data from a study of attention to visual motion (Büchel and Friston, 1997). The data used in this chapter came from the first subject studied. This subject was scanned at 2 T to give a time series of 360 images comprising 10 block epochs of different visual motion conditions. These conditions included a fixation condition, visual presentation of static dots, visual presentation of radially moving dots under attention and no-attention conditions. In the attention condition subjects were asked to attend to changes in speed (which did not actually occur). These data were reanalysed using a conventional SPM procedure and using the empirical Bayesian approach described in the previous section. The ensuing SPMs and PPMs are presented below for the PET and fMRI data, respectively. The contrast for the PET data compared the word generation with the word shadowing condition and the contrast for the fMRI data tested for the effect of visual motion above and beyond that due to photic stimulation with stationary dots.

Inference for the PET Data

The upper panel of Fig. 47.13 shows the PPM for a deactivating effect of verbal fluency. There are two thresholds for the PPM. The first and more important is γ in Eq. (47.31). This defines what we mean by *activation* and, by default, is set at one deviation of the prior variance of the contrast, in this instance, 2.2. This corresponds to a change in rCBF of 2.2 adimensional units (equivalent to ml/dl/min). The second threshold is more trivial and simply enables the use of maximum intensity projections. This is the probability the voxel has to exceed in order to be displayed. In the PPM shown, this was set at 95%. This means that all voxels shown have greater than 95% probability of being deactivated by 2.2 or more. The PPM can be regarded as a way of summarising one's confidence that an effect is present (cf. the use of confidence intervals where the lower bound on the interval is set at γ). Note that posterior inference would normally require the reporting of the conditional probability whether it exceeded some arbitrary threshold or not. However, for the visual display of posterior probability maps, it is useful to remove voxels that fall below some threshold.

Figure 47.14 provides a quantitative representation of Bayesian inference afforded by PPMs. In the upper panel the posterior expectation for the 12 condition-specific effects are shown, encompassed by the 95% confidence intervals (bars) based on the posterior covariance. It can be seen that in the fifth condition (the third word shadowing condition) one could be almost certain the activation is greater than zero. The prior and posterior densities for this activation are shown in the lower panel. These are the probability distributions before and after observing the data. Note that the posterior variance is always smaller than the prior variance, depending on how noisy the data are.

The corresponding SPM is shown in Fig. 47.13b. The SPM has been thresholded at 0.05 adjusted for the search volume using a Gaussian field correction. A remarkable correspondence is seen between the activation profiles inferred by the PPM and the SPM. The similarity between the PPM and the SPM for these data should not be taken as characteristic. The key difference between Bayesian inference, based on the confidence we have about activation, and classical inference, based on rejecting the null hypothesis, is that the latter depends on the search volume. The classical approach, when applied in a mass univariate setting (i.e., over a family of voxels), induces a multiple-comparison problem that calls for a procedure to control for family-wise false positives. In the context of imaging data, this procedure is a Gaussian field adjustment to the threshold. This adjustment depends on the search volume. The consequence is that if we

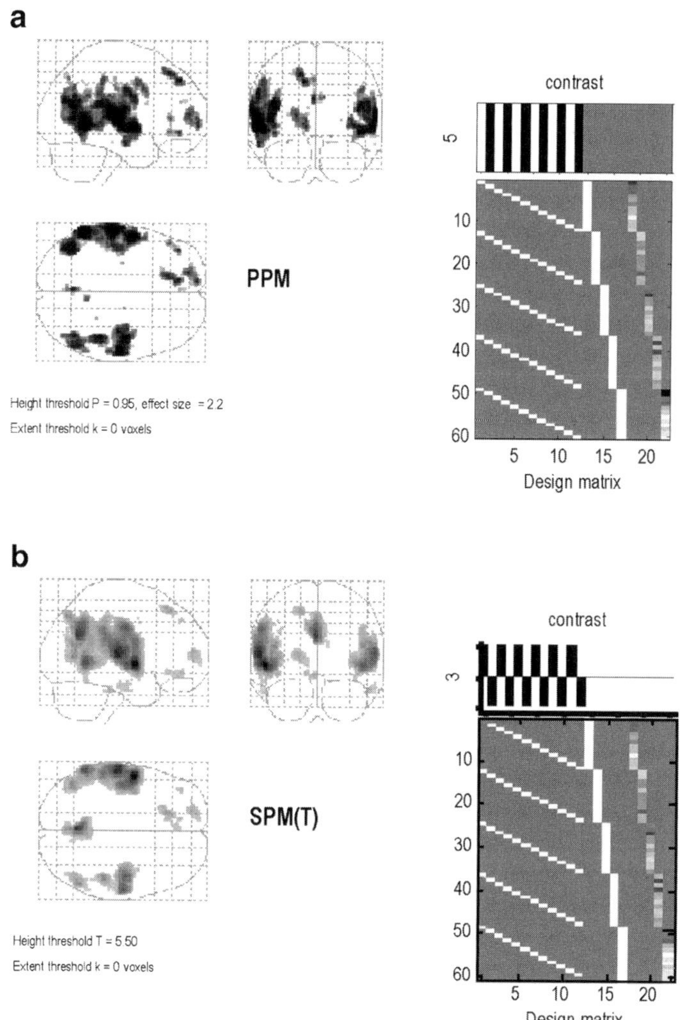

FIGURE 47.13
Bayesian and classical and inference for the PET study of word generation. (a) PPM for a contrast reflecting the difference between word shadowing and word generation, using an activation threshold of 2.2 and a confidence of 95%. The design matrix and contrast for this model are shown (right) in image format. We have modeled each scan as a specific effect that has been replicated over subjects. (b) Classical SPM of the t statistic for the same contrast. This SPM has been thresholded at $p = 0.05$, corrected using a Gaussian field adjustment.

increased the search volume the threshold would rise and some of the voxels seen in the SPM would disappear. Because the PPM does not label any voxel as "activated," there is no multiple comparison problem and the 95% confidence threshold is the same irrespective of search volume. This difference between PPMs and SPMs is highlighted in the analysis of the fMRI data. Here, the search volume is increased by reducing the smoothness of the data. We do this by switching from PET to fMRI. Smoothness controls the "statistical" search volume, which is generally much greater for fMRI than for PET.

Inference for the fMRI Data

The difference between the PPM and SPM for the fMRI analysis is immediately apparent on inspection of Figs. 47.15 and 47.16. Here the default threshold for the PPM was 0.7% (equivalent to percentage whole brain mean signal). Again only voxels that exceed 95% confidence are shown. These are restricted to visual and extrastriate cortex involved in motion processing. The critical thing to note here is that the corresponding SPM identifies a smaller number of voxels than the PPM. Indeed the SPM appears to have missed a critical and bilaterally represented part of the V5 complex (circled cluster on the PPM in the lower panel of Fig. 47.15). The SPM is more conservative because the correction for multiple comparisons in these data

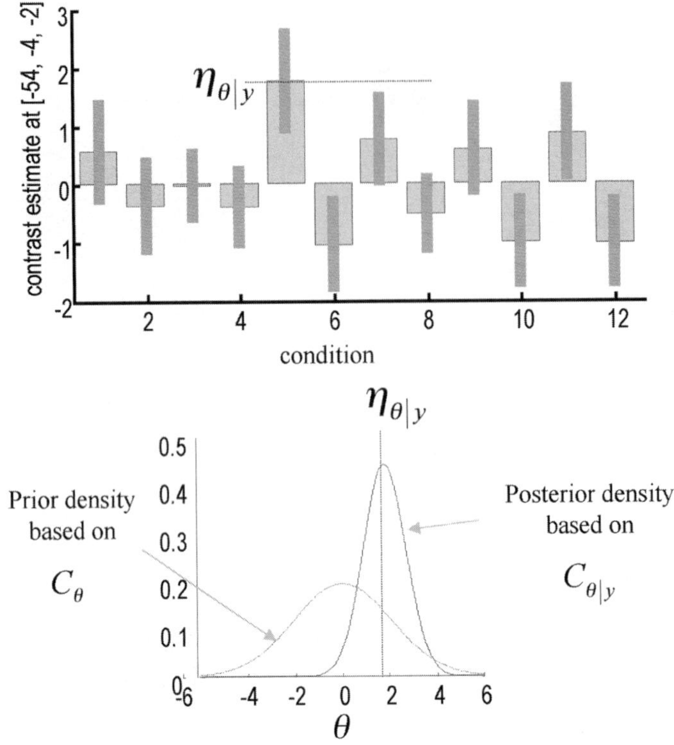

FIGURE 47.14
Illustrative results for a single voxel: the maximum in the left temporal region of the PPM in the previous figure (–54, –4, and –2 mm). (Upper panel) These are the conditional or posterior expectations and 95% confidence intervals for the activation effect associated with each of the 12 conditions. Note that the odd conditions (word shadowing) are generally higher. In condition 5 one would be more than 95% certain the activation exceeded 2.2. (Lower panel) The prior and posterior densities for the parameter estimate for condition 5.

is very severe, rendering classical inference relatively insensitive. It is interesting to note that dynamic motion in the visual field has such widespread (if small) effects at a haemodynamic level.

PPMs and FDR

There is an interesting connection between false discovery rate (FDR) control and thresholded PPMs. Subjecting PPMs to a 95% threshold means that surviving voxels have, at most, a 5% probability of not exceeding the default threshold γ. In other words, if we declared these voxels as "activated," 5% of the voxels could be false activations. This is exactly the same as FDR in the sense that the FDR is the proportion of voxels that are declared significant but are not. Note that many voxels will have a posterior probability that is more than 95%. Therefore, the 5% is an upper bound on the FDR. This interpretation rests explicitly on thresholding the PPM and labelling the excursion set as "activated." It is reiterated that this declaration is unnecessary and only has any meaning in relation to classical inference. However, thresholded PPMs do have this interesting connection to SPMs in which the FDR has been controlled.

Conclusion

In this section we looked at a simple way to construct posterior probability maps using empirical Bayes. Empirical Bayes can be used because of the natural hierarchy in neuroimaging engendered by looking for the same thing over multiple voxels. The approach provides simple shrinkage priors based on between-voxel variation in parameters controlling effects of interest. A computationally expedient way of computing these priors using ReML has been presented that pools over voxels. This pooling device offers enormous computational savings through simplifying the matrix algebra and enabling the construction of whole brain PPMs. The same

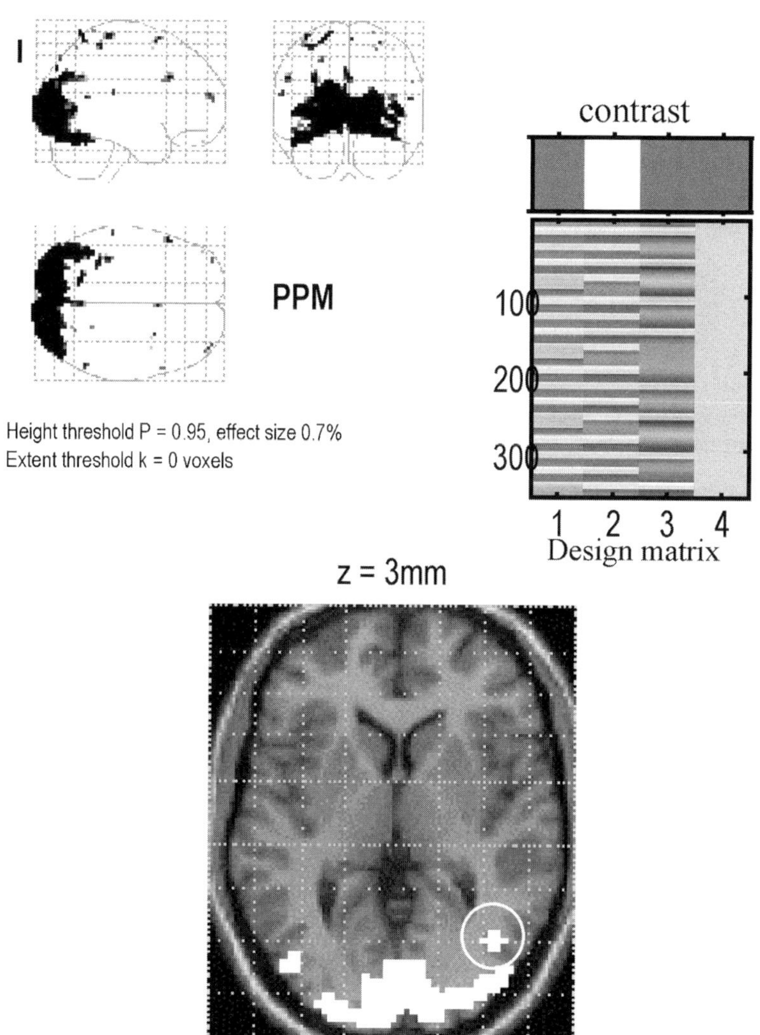

FIGURE 47.15
PPM for the fMRI study of attention to visual motion. The display format in the lower panel uses an axial slice through extrastriate regions but the thresholds are the same as those employed in maximum intensity projections (upper panels). The activation threshold for the PPM was 0.7. As can be imputed from the design matrix, the statistical model of evoked responses comprised boxcar regressors convolved with a canonical haemodynamic response function.

device has found an interesting application in the ReML estimation of prior variance components in space, by pooling over time bins, in the EEG source reconstruction problem (Phillips *et al.*, 2003).

A key consideration when using empirical Bayes in this setting is determining which voxels to include in the hierarchy. There is no right or wrong answer here (cf. the search volume in classical inference with SPMs). The most important thing to bear in mind is that the conditional estimators of an activation or effect are those that minimise some cost function. This cost function can be regarded as the ability to predict the observed response with minimum error, on average, over the voxels included in the hierarchical model. In other words, the voxels over which the priors are computed define the space one wants, on average, the best estimates for. In this work we have simply used potentially responsive voxels within the brain as defined by thresholding the original images (to exclude extracranial regions).

In the next section we turn to Bayesian inferences based on full Bayes where the priors come not from empirical estimates based on hierarchical observations over voxels, but from biophysical parameters mediating the response at a single voxel.

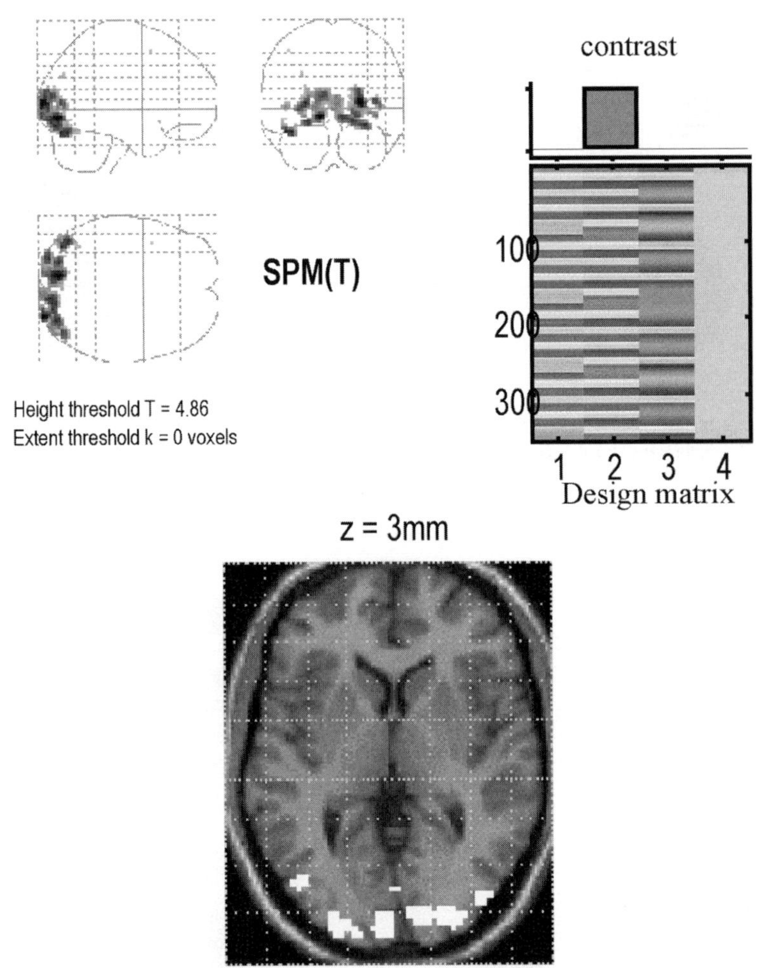

FIGURE 47.16
As for Fig. 47.15, but this time showing the corresponding SPM using a corrected threshold at $p = 0.05$.

BAYESIAN IDENTIFICATION OF DYNAMIC SYSTEMS

This section presents a method for estimating the conditional or posterior distribution of the parameters of deterministic dynamic systems. The procedure conforms to an EM search for the maximum of the conditional or posterior density. The inclusion of priors in the estimation procedure ensures robust and rapid convergence and the resulting conditional densities enable Bayesian inference about the model parameters. The method is demonstrated using an input–state–output model of the haemodynamic coupling between experimentally designed causes or factors in fMRI studies and the ensuing BOLD response (see Chapter 41). This example represents a generalisation of current fMRI analysis models that accommodates nonlinearities and in which the parameters have an explicit physical interpretation.

This section is about the identification of deterministic nonlinear dynamic models. *Deterministic* here refers to models in which the dynamics are completely determined by the state of the system. Random or stochastic effects enter only at the point at which the system's outputs or responses are observed.[7] We focus here on a particular model of how changes in neuronal activity translate into haemodynamic responses. By considering a voxel as an input–state–output system one can model the effects of an input (i.e., stimulus function) on some state variables (e.g., flow, volume, deoxyhemoglobin content) and the ensuing output (i.e., BOLD response).

[7] There is another important class of models in which stochastic processes enter at the level of the state variables themselves (i.e., deterministic noise). These are referred to as *stochastic dynamic models*.

The scheme adopted here uses Bayesian estimation, which is used to identify the posterior or conditional distribution of the parameters, given the data. Knowing the posterior distribution allows one to characterise an observed system in terms of the parameters that maximise their posterior probability (i.e., those parameters that are most likely given the data) or, indeed, make inferences about whether the parameters are bigger or smaller than some specified value.

By demonstrating the approach using haemodynamic models, we can establish the notion that biophysical and physiological models of evoked brain responses can be used to make Bayesian inferences about experimentally induced regionally specific activations. Including parameters that couple experimentally changing stimulus or task conditions to the system's states enables this inference. The posterior or conditional distribution of these parameters can then be used to make inferences about the efficacy of experimental inputs in eliciting measured responses. Because the parameters we want to make an inference about have an explicit physical interpretation, in the context of the haemodynamic model used, the face validity of the ensuing inference is more grounded in physiology. Furthermore, because the "activation" is parameterised in terms of processes that have natural biological constraints, these constraints can be used as priors in a Bayesian scheme.

Previous sections have focussed on *empirical* Bayesian approaches in which the priors were derived from the data being analysed. In this section we use a *fully* Bayesian approach, where the priors are assumed to be known and apply it to the haemodynamic model described in Friston *et al.* (2000) and Chapter 41. Friston *et al.* (2000) presented a haemodynamic model that embedded the balloon/windkessel (Buxton *et al.*, 1998, Mandeville *et al.*, 1999) model of flow to BOLD coupling to give a complete dynamic model of how neuronally mediated signals cause a BOLD response. In this work we restricted ourselves to single input–single output (SISO) systems by considering only one input. Here we demonstrate a general approach to nonlinear system identification using an extension of these SISO models to multiple input–single output (MISO) systems. This allows for a response to be caused by multiple experimental effects and we can assign a causal efficacy to any number of explanatory variables (i.e., stimulus functions). In Chapter 52, we will generalise to multiple input–multiple output systems (MIMO) such that interactions among brain regions at a neuronal level can be addressed.

An important aspect of the proposed model is that it can be reduced, exactly, to the model used in classical SPM-like analyses, in which one uses the stimulus functions, convolved with a canonical haemodynamic response function, as explanatory variables in a general linear model. This classical analysis is a special case that is obtained when the model parameters of interest (the efficacy of a stimulus) are treated as fixed effects with flat priors, and the remaining biophysical parameters are entered as known canonical values with infinitely small prior variance (i.e., high precision). In this sense the current approach can be viewed as a Bayesian generalisation of that normally employed. The advantages of this generalisation rest on (1) the use of a nonlinear observation model and (2) Bayesian estimation of that model's parameters. The fundamental advantage of a nonlinear MISO model over linear models is that only the parameters linking the various inputs to haemodynamics are input or trial specific. The remaining parameters, pertaining to the haemodynamics per se, are the same for each voxel. In conventional analyses the haemodynamic response function for each input is estimated in a linearly separable fashion (usually in terms of a small set of temporal basis functions) despite the fact that the form of the impulse response function to each input is likely to be the same. In other words, a nonlinear model properly accommodates the fact that many of the parameters shaping input-specific haemodynamic responses are shared by all inputs. For example, the components of a compound trial (e.g., cue and target stimuli) might not interact at a neuronal level but may show subadditive effects in the measured response, due to nonlinear haemodynamic saturation. In contradistinction to conventional linear analyses, the analysis proposed in this section could, in principle, disambiguate between interactions at the neuronal and haemodynamic levels. The second advantage is that Bayesian inferences about input-specific parameters can be framed in terms of whether the efficacy for a particular cause exceeded some specified threshold or, indeed the probability that it was less than some threshold (i.e., infer that a voxel did *not* respond). The latter is precluded in classical inference. These advantages should be weighed against the difficulties of establishing a valid model and the computational expense of identification.

This section is divided into four parts. In the first we reprise briefly the haemodynamic model and motivate the four differential equations that it comprises. We touch on the Volterra formulation of nonlinear systems to show that the output can always be represented as a nonlinear function of the input and the model parameters. This nonlinear function is used as the basis of the observation model that is subject to Bayesian identification. This identification require priors that, here, come from the distribution, over voxels, of parameters estimated in Friston *et al.* (2000). The second part describes these priors and how they were determined. Having specified the form of the nonlinear observation model and the prior densities on the model's parameters, the third section describes the estimation of their posterior densities. The ensuing scheme can be regarded as a Gauss-Newton search for the maximum posterior probability (as opposed to the maximum likelihood as in conventional applications) that embeds the EM scheme in the Appendix. This description concludes with a note on integration, required to evaluate the local gradients of the objective function. This, effectively generalises the EM algorithm for linear systems so that is can be applied to nonlinear models.

Finally we demonstrate the approach using empirical data. First, we revisit the same data used to construct the priors using a single input. We then apply the technique to the same study of visual attention used in the previous section, to make inferences about the relative efficacy of multiple experimental effects in eliciting a BOLD response.

The Haemodynamic Model

The haemodynamic model considered here was presented in detail in Friston *et al.* (2000) and Chapter 41. Although relatively simple it is predicated on a substantial amount of previous careful theoretical work and empirical validation [e.g., Buxton *et al.,* 1998; Mandeville *et al.,* 1999; Hoge *et al.,* 1999; Mayhew *et al.,* 1998]. The model is a SISO system with a stimulus function as input, which is supposed to elicit a neuronally mediated flow-inducing signal, and a BOLD response as output. The model has six parameters and four state variables each with its corresponding differential equation. The differential or state equations express how each state variable changes over time as a function of the others. These state equations and the output nonlinearly (a static nonlinear function of the state variables that gives the output) specify the form of the model. The parameters determine any specific realisation of the model. In what follows we review the state equations, the output nonlinearity, extension to a MISO system, and the Volterra representation.

State Equations

Assuming that the dynamic system linking synaptic activity and rCBF is linear (Miller *et al.,* 2000) we start with

$$\dot{f}_{in} = s \tag{47.38}$$

where f_{in} is inflow and s is some flow-inducing signal. The signal is assumed to subsume many neurogenic and diffusive signal subcomponents and is generated by neuronal responses to the input (the stimulus function) $u(t)$:

$$\dot{s} = \varepsilon u(t) - \kappa_s s - \kappa_f (f_{in} - 1) \tag{47.39}$$

where ε, κ_s and κ_f are parameters that represent the efficacy with which input causes an increase in signal, the rate constant for signal decay or elimination, and the rate constant for auto-regulatory feedback from blood flow. The existence of this feedback term can be inferred from (1) poststimulus undershoots in rCBF and (2) the well-characterised vasomotor signal in optical imaging (Mayhew *et al.,* 1998). Inflow determines the rate of change of volume through

$$\begin{aligned} \tau\dot{v} &= f_{in} - f_{out}(v) \qquad (37.40)\\ f_{out}(v) &= v^{1/\alpha} \end{aligned}$$

This says that normalised venous volume changes reflect the difference between inflow f_{in} and outflow f_{out} from the venous compartment with a time constant (transit time) τ. Outflow is a function of volume that models the balloon-like capacity of the venous compartment to expel blood at a greater rate when distended (Buxton *et al.,* 1998). It can be modelled with a single parameter (Grubb *et al.,* 1974) α based on the windkessel model (Mandeville *et al.,* 1999).

The change in normalised total deoxyhemoglobin voxel content q reflects the delivery of deoxyhemoglobin into the venous compartment minus that expelled (outflow times concentration):

$$\tau\dot{q} = f_{in}\frac{E(f_{in},E_0)}{E_0} - f_{out}(v)q/v$$
$$E(f_{in},E_0) = 1-(1-E_0)^{1/f_{in}} \tag{47.41}$$

where $E(f_{in}, E_0)$ is the fraction of oxygen extracted from inflowing blood. This is assumed to depend on oxygen delivery and is consequently flow-dependent. This concludes the state equations, where there are six unknown parameters: efficacy ε, signal decay κ_s, autoregulation κ_f, transit time τ, Grubb's exponent α, and resting net oxygen extraction by the capillary bed E_0.

Output Nonlinearity

The BOLD signal $y(t) = \lambda(v, q, E_0)$ is taken to be a static nonlinear function of volume (v), and deoxyhemoglobin content (q):

$$y(t) = \lambda(v,q) = V_0(k_1(1-q) + k_2(1-q/v) + k_3(1-v)) \tag{47.42}$$
$$k_1 = 7E_0$$
$$k_2 = 2$$
$$k_3 = 2E_0 - 0.2$$

where V_0 is resting blood volume fraction. This signal comprises a volume-weighted sum of extravascular and intravascular signals that are functions of volume and deoxyhemoglobin content. A critical term in Eq. (47.42) is the concentration term $k_2(1 - q/v)$, which accounts for most of the nonlinear behaviour of the haemodynamic model. The architecture of this model is summarised in Fig. 47.17.

Extension to a MISO

The extension to a multiple input system is trivial and involves extending Eq. (47.39) to cover n inputs:

$$\dot{s} = \varepsilon_1 u(t)_1 + \ldots + \varepsilon_n u(t)_n - \kappa_s s - \kappa_f(f_{in} - 1) \tag{47.43}$$

The model now has $5 + n$ parameters: five biophysical parameters κ_s, κ_f, τ, α and E_0 and n efficacies $\varepsilon_1,\ldots\varepsilon_n$. Although all of these parameters have to be estimated we are only interested in making inferences about the efficacies. Note that the biophysical parameters are the same for all inputs.

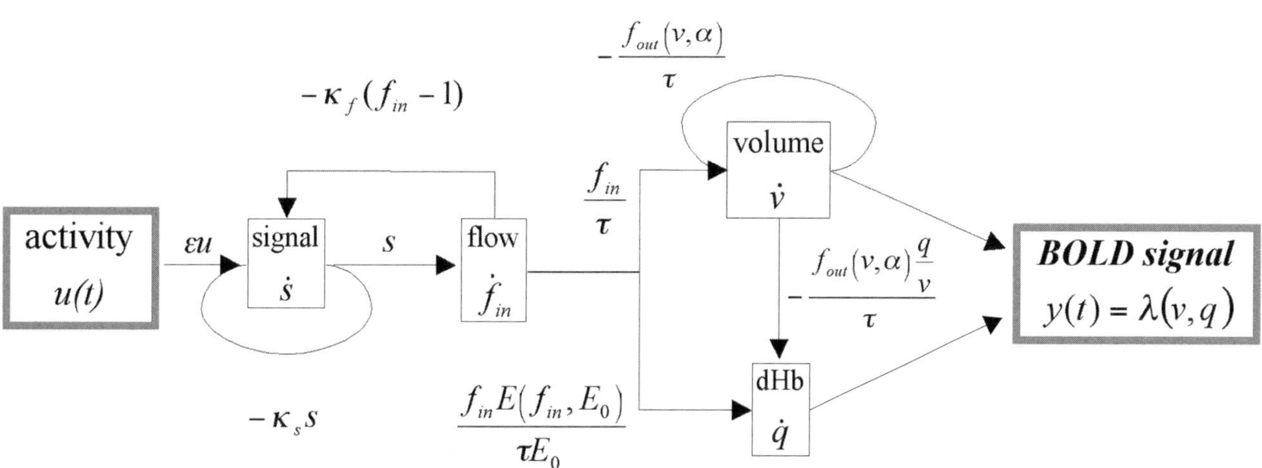

FIGURE 47.17
Schematic illustrating the architecture of the haemodynamic model. This is a fully nonlinear single-input $u(t)$, single-output $y(t)$ state model with four state variables s, f_{in}, v and q. The form and motivation for the changes in each state variable, as functions of the others, is described in the main text.

The Volterra Formulation

In our haemodynamic model, the state variables are $X = \{x_1,\ldots,x_4\}^T = \{s,f_{in},v,q\}^T$ and the parameters are $\theta = (\theta_1,\ldots,\theta_{5+n}\}^T = \{\kappa_s,\kappa_f,\tau,\alpha,E_0,\varepsilon_1,\ldots,\varepsilon_n\}^T$. The state equations and output nonlinearity specify a MISO model:

$$
\begin{aligned}
\dot{X}(t) &= f(X,u(t)) \\
y(t) &= \lambda(X(t)) \\
\dot{x}_1 &= f_1(X,u(t) = \varepsilon_1 u(t)_1 + \ldots + \varepsilon_n u(t)_n - \kappa_s x_1 - \kappa_f(x_2 - 1) \\
\dot{x}_2 &= f_2(X,u(t)) = x_1 \\
\dot{x}_3 &= f_3(X,u(t) = \frac{1}{\tau}(x_2 - f_{out}(x_3,\alpha)) \\
\dot{x}_4 &= f_4(X,u(t) = \frac{1}{\tau}\left(x_2\frac{E(x_2,E_0)}{E_0} - f_{out}(x_3,\alpha)\frac{x_4}{x_3}\right) \\
y(t) &= \lambda(x_1,\ldots,x_4) = V_0\big(k_1(1 - x_4) + k_2(1 - x_4/x_3) + k_3(1 - x_3)\big)
\end{aligned}
\tag{47.44}
$$

This is the state-space representation. The alternative Volterra formulation represents the output $y(t)$ as a nonlinear convolution of the input $u(t)$, critically without reference to the state variables $X(t)$ (see Bendat , 1990). This series can be considered a nonlinear convolution that is obtained from a functional Taylor expansion of $y(t)$ about $X(0)$ and $u(t) = 0$. For a single input this can be expressed as follows:

$$
\begin{aligned}
y(t) &= h(\theta,u) \\
&= \kappa_0 + \sum_{i=1}^{\infty} \int_0^{\infty} \ldots \int_0^{\infty} \kappa_i(\sigma_1,\ldots\sigma_i)u(t - \sigma_1)\ldots u(t - \sigma_i)d\sigma_1,\ldots d\sigma_i \\
\kappa_i(\sigma_1,\ldots\sigma_i) &= \frac{\partial^i y(t)}{\partial u(t - \sigma_1)\ldots u(t - \sigma_i)}
\end{aligned}
\tag{47.45}
$$

where κ_i is the ith generalised convolution kernel (Fliess *et al.,* 1983). Equation (47.45) now expresses the output as a function of the input and the parameters whose posterior distribution we require. The Volterra kernels are a time-invariant characterisation of the input–output behaviour of the system and can be thought of as generalised high-order convolution kernels that are applied to a stimulus function to emulate the observed BOLD response. Integrating Eq. (47.45) and applying the output nonlinearity to the state variables is the same as convolving the inputs with the kernels. Both give the system's response in terms of the output. In what follows, the response is evaluated by integrating Eq. (47.45). This means the kernels are not required. However, the Volterra formulation is introduced for several reasons. First, it demonstrates that the output is a nonlinear function of the inputs $y(t) = h(\theta, u)$. This is critical for the generality of the estimation scheme below. Second, it provides an important connection with conventional analyses using the general linear model (see below). Finally, we use the kernels to characterise evoked responses.

The Priors

Bayesian estimation requires informative priors on the parameters. Under Gaussian assumptions, these prior densities can be specified in terms of their expectation and covariance. These moments are taken here to be the sample mean and covariance, over voxels, of the parameter estimates reported in Friston *et al.* (2000). Normally priors play a critical role in inference; indeed the traditional criticism levelled at Bayesian inference reduces to reservations about the validity of the priors employed. However, in the application considered here, this criticism can be discounted. This is because the priors, on those parameters about which inferences are made, are relatively flat. Only the five biophysical parameters have informative priors.

In Friston *et al.* (2000) the parameters were identified as those that minimised the sum of squared differences between the Volterra kernels implied by the parameters and those derived directly from the data. This derivation used OLS estimators, exploiting the fact that Volterra formulation is linear in the unknowns, namely, the kernel coefficients. The kernels can be thought of as a reparameterisation of the model that does not refer to the underlying state representation. In other words, for every set of parameters there is a corresponding set of kernels (see Friston *et al.*, 2000 and Chapters 41 and 53, for the derivation of the kernels as a function of the parameters). The data and Volterra kernel estimation are described in detail in Friston *et al.* (1998). In brief, we obtained fMRI time series from a single subject at 2 T using a Magnetom VISION (by Siemens, Erlangen) whole body MRI system, equipped with a head volume coil. Multislice T_2*-weighted fMRI images were obtained with a gradient echoplanar sequence using an axial slice orientation (TE = 40 ms, TR = 1.7 sec, 64 × 64 × 16 voxels). After discarding initial scans (to allow for magnetic saturation effects) each time series comprised 1200 volume images with 3-mm isotropic voxels. The subject listened to monosyllabic or bisyllabic concrete nouns (i.e., *dog, radio, mountain, gate*) presented at 5 different rates (10, 15, 30, 60, and 90 words per minute) for epochs of 34 sec, intercalated with periods of rest. The presentation rates were repeated according to a Latin square design.

The distribution of the five biophysical parameters, over 128 voxels, was computed to give our prior expectation η_θ and covariance C_θ. Signal decay κ_s had a mean of about 0.65 per sec, giving a half-life of $t_{1/2} = \ln 2/\kappa_s \approx 1$ sec. Mean feedback rate κ_f was about 0.4 per sec. Mean transit time τ was 0.98 sec. Under steady-state conditions, Grubb's parameter α is about 0.38. The mean over voxels was 0.326. Mean resting oxygen extraction E_0 was about 34%, and the range observed conformed exactly with known values for resting oxygen extraction fraction (between 20% and 55%). Figure 47.18 shows the covariances among the biophysical parameters along with the correlation matrix (left-hand panel). The correlations suggest a high correlation between transit time and the rate constants for signal elimination and autoregulation.

The priors for the efficacies were taken to be relatively flat with an expectation of zero and a variance of 16 per second. The efficacies were assumed to be independent of the biophysical parameters with zero covariance. A variance of 16, or standard deviation of 4, corresponds to time constants in the range of 250 ms. In other words, inputs can elicit flow-inducing signal over a wide range of time constants from infinitely slowly to very fast (250 ms) with about the same probability. A "strong" activation usually has an efficacy in the range of 0.5–0.6 per second. Notice that from a dynamic perspective "activation" depends on the speed of the response, not the percentage change. Equipped with these priors we can now pursue a fully Bayesian approach to estimating the parameters using new datasets and multiple input models:

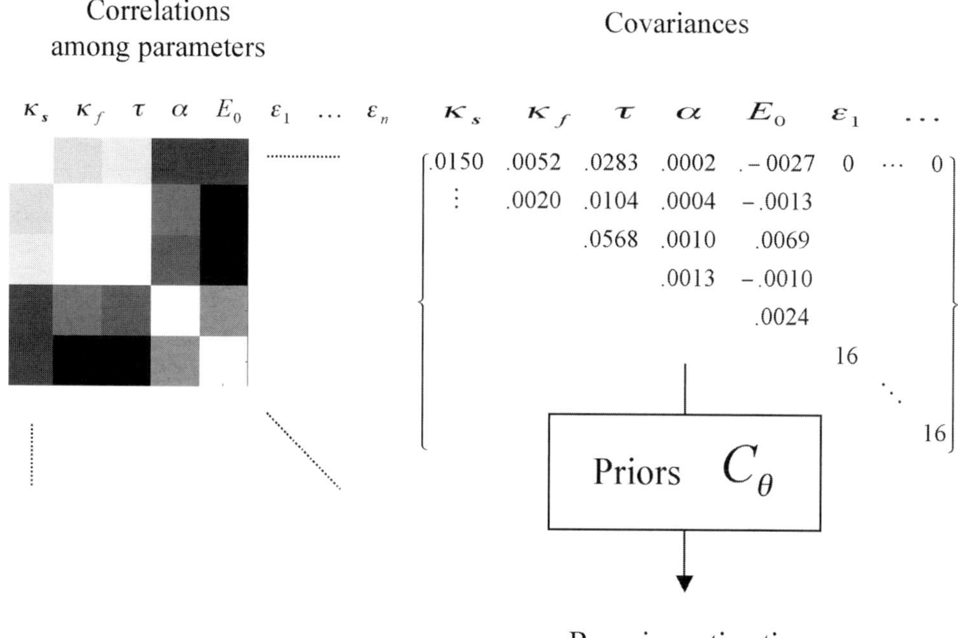

FIGURE 47.18
Prior covariances for the five biophysical parameters of the haemodynamic model in Fig. 47.17. (Left panel) Correlation matrix showing the correlations among the parameters in image format (white = 1). (Right panel) Corresponding covariance matrix in tabular format. These priors represent the sample covariances of the parameters estimated by minimising the difference between the Volterra kernels implied by the parameters and those estimated, empirically using OLS as described in Friston *et al.* (2000).

System Identification

This subsection describes Bayesian inference procedures for nonlinear observation models, with additive noise, of the following form:

$$y = h(\theta,u) + e \tag{47.46}$$

under Gaussian assumptions about the parameters θ and errors $e \sim N\{0, C_\varepsilon\}$. These models can be adopted for any analytic dynamic system due to the existence of the equivalent Volterra series expansion above. Assuming that the posterior density of the parameters is approximately Gaussian, the problem reduces to finding its first two moments, the conditional mean $\eta_{\theta|y}$ and covariance $C_{\theta|y}$.

The observation model can be made linear by expanding Eq. (47.46) about a working estimate $\eta_{\theta|y}$ of the conditional mean:

$$\begin{aligned} h(\theta,u) &\approx h(\eta_{\theta|y}) + J(\theta - \eta_{\theta|y}) \\ J &= \frac{\partial h(\eta_{\theta|y})}{\partial\theta} \end{aligned} \tag{47.47}$$

such that $y - h(\eta_{\theta|y}) \approx J(\theta - \eta_{\theta|y}) + \varepsilon$. This linear model can now be placed in the EM scheme described in the Appendix to give the following:

Until convergence {

E-step

$$\begin{aligned}
J &= \frac{\partial h(\eta_{\theta|y})}{\partial\theta} \\
\bar{y} &= \begin{bmatrix} y - h(\eta_{\theta|y}) \\ \eta_\theta - \eta_{\theta|y} \end{bmatrix}, \quad \bar{J} = \begin{bmatrix} J \\ I \end{bmatrix}, \quad \bar{C}_\varepsilon = \begin{bmatrix} \Sigma\lambda_i Q_i & 0 \\ 0 & C_\theta \end{bmatrix} \\
C_{\theta|y} &= (\bar{J}^T\bar{C}_\varepsilon^{-1}\bar{J})^{-1} \\
\eta_{\theta|y} &\leftarrow \eta_{\theta|y} + C_{\theta|y}\bar{J}^T\bar{C}_\varepsilon^{-1}\bar{y}
\end{aligned}$$

M-Step

$$\begin{aligned}
P &= \bar{C}_\varepsilon^{-1} - \bar{C}_\varepsilon^{-1}\bar{J}C_{\theta|y}\bar{J}^T\bar{C}_\varepsilon^{-1} \\
\frac{\partial F}{\partial\lambda_i} &= -\frac{1}{2}\, tr\{PQ_i\} + \frac{1}{2}\bar{y}^T P^T Q_i P\bar{y} \\
\left\langle\frac{\partial^2 F}{\partial\lambda_{ij}^2}\right\rangle &= -\frac{1}{2} tr\{PQ_i PQ_j\} \\
\lambda &\leftarrow \lambda - \left\langle\frac{\partial^2 F}{\partial\lambda^2}\right\rangle^{-1}\frac{\partial F}{\partial\lambda}
\end{aligned} \tag{47.48}$$

}

This EM scheme is effectively a *Gauss-Newton* search for the posterior mode or MAP estimate of the parameters. The relationship between the **E**-step and a conventional Gauss-Newton ascent can be seen easily in terms of the derivatives of their respective objective functions. For conventional Gauss-Newton schemes, this function is the *log likelihood:*

$$\begin{aligned}
l &= \ln p(y|\theta) = -\frac{1}{2}(y - h(\theta))^T C_\varepsilon^{-1}(y - h(\theta)) + const. \\
\frac{\partial l}{\partial\theta}(\eta_{ML}) &= J^T C_\varepsilon^{-1}(y - h(\eta_{ML})) \\
-\frac{\partial^2 l}{\partial\theta^2}(\eta_{ML}) &\approx J^T C_\varepsilon^{-1} J \\
\eta_{ML} &\leftarrow \eta_{ML} + (J^T C_\varepsilon^{-1} J)^{-1} J^T C_\varepsilon^{-1}(y - h(\eta_{ML}))
\end{aligned} \tag{47.49}$$

This is a conventional Gauss-Newton scheme. By simply augmenting the log likelihood with the log prior we get the *log posterior:*

$$
\begin{aligned}
l &= \ln p(\theta|y) = \ln p(y|\theta) + \ln p(\theta) \\
&= -\frac{1}{2}(y - h(\theta))^T C_\varepsilon^{-1} y - h(\theta) - \frac{1}{2}(\eta_\theta - \theta)^T C_\theta^{-1}(\eta_\theta - \theta) + const. \\
\frac{\partial l}{\partial \theta}(\eta_{\theta|y}) &= J^T C_\varepsilon^{-1}(y - h(\eta_{\theta|y})) + C_\theta^{-1}(\eta_\theta - \eta_{\theta|y}) \\
-\frac{\partial^2 l}{\partial \theta^2}(\eta_{\theta|y}) &\approx J^T C_\varepsilon^{-1} J + C_\theta^{-1} \\
\eta_{\theta|y} &\leftarrow \eta_{\theta|y} + (J^T C_\varepsilon^{-1} J + C_\theta^{-1})^{-1}(J^T C_\varepsilon^{-1}(y - h(\eta_{\theta|y})) + C_\theta^{-1}(\eta_\theta - \eta_{\theta|y})
\end{aligned}
\tag{47.50}
$$

which is identical to the expression for the conditional expectation in the **E**-Step.

In summary, the only difference between the **E**-step and a conventional Gauss-Newton search is that priors are included in the objective log probability function, thus converting it from a log likelihood into a log posterior. The use of an EM algorithm rests on the need to find not only the conditional mean but also the hyperparameters of unknown variance components. The **E**-step finds (1) the current MAP estimate that provides the next expansion point for the Gauss-Newton search and (2) the conditional covariance required by the **M**-Step. The **M**-step then updates the ReML estimates of the covariance hyperparameters that are required to compute the conditional moments in the **E**-step. Technically Eq. (47.48) is a *generalised* EM (GEM) because the **M**-step increases the log likelihood of the hyperparameter estimates, as opposed to maximising it.

Relationship to Established Procedures

The procedure presented above represents a fairly obvious extension to conventional Gauss-Newton searches for the parameters of nonlinear observation models. The extension has two components. First, there is the maximisation of the *posterior* density that embodies priors, as opposed to the likelihood. This allows for the incorporation of prior information into the solution and ensures uniqueness and convergence. The second component is the estimation of unknown covariance components. This is important because it accommodates nonsphericity in the error terms. The overall approach engenders a relatively simple way of obtaining Bayes estimators for nonlinear systems with unknown additive observation error. Technically, the algorithm represents a *posterior mode estimation* for nonlinear observation models using EM. It can be regarded as approximating the posterior density of the parameters by replacing the conditional mean with the mode and the conditional precision with the curvature (at the current expansion point). Covariance hyperparameters are then estimated that maximise the expectation of the log likelihood of the data over this approximate posterior density.

Posterior mode estimation is an alternative to full posterior density analysis, which avoids numerical integration (Fahrmeir and Tutz , 1994, p. 58) and has been discussed extensively in the context of *generalised linear models* (e.g., Santner and Duffy, 1989). The departure from Gaussian assumptions in generalised linear models comes from non-Gaussian likelihoods, as opposed to nonlinearities in the observation model considered here, but the issues are similar. Posterior mode estimation usually assumes that the error covariances and priors are known. If the priors are unknown constants, then empirical Bayes can be employed to estimate the required hyperparameters.

It is important not to confuse this application of EM with Kalman filtering. Although Kalman filtering can be formulated in terms of EM and, indeed, posterior mode estimation, Kalman filtering is used with completely different observation models, that is, *state-space models*. State-space or dynamic models comprise a *transition* equation and an *observation* equation (cf. the state equation and output nonlinearity above) and cover systems in which the underlying state is hidden and is treated as a stochastic variable. This is not the sort of model considered here, in which the inputs (experimental design) and the ensuing states are known. This means that the conditional densities can be computed for the entire time series simultaneously. (Kalman filtering updates the conditional density recursively by stepping through the time series.) If we treated the inputs as unknown and random, then the state equation could be rewritten as a stochastic differential equation (SDE) and a transition equation derived from it, using local linearity assumptions. This would form the basis of a state-space model (see Chapter 53). This approach may be useful for accommodating deterministic noise in the haemodynamic model, but, in this treatment, we consider the inputs to be fixed. This means that the only random effects enter at the level of the observation or output nonlinearity. In other words, we are assuming that the measurement error in fMRI is the principal source of randomness in our measurements and that haemodynamic responses per se are determined by known inputs. This is the same assumption used in conventional analyses of fMRI data.

A Note on Integration

To iterate Eq. (47.48), the local gradients $J = \partial h/\partial\theta$ have to be evaluated. This involves evaluating $h(\theta,u)$ around the current expansion point with the generalised convolution of the inputs for the current conditional parameter estimates according to Eq. (47.45) or, equivalently, the integration of Eq. (47.44). The latter can be accomplished efficiently by capitalising on the fact that stimulus functions are usually sparse. In other words, inputs arrive as infrequent events (e.g., event-related paradigms) or changes in input occur sporadically (e.g., boxcar designs). We can use this to evaluate $y(t) = h(\eta_{\theta|y}, u)$at the times the data were sampled using a bilinear approximation to Eq. (47.44). The Taylor expansion of $\dot{X}(t)$ about $X(0) = X_0 = [0,1,1,1]^T$

$$\dot{X}(t) \approx f(X_0, 0) + \frac{\partial f(X_0, 0)}{\partial X}(X - X_0) + \sum_i u(t)_i \left(\frac{\partial^2 f(X_0, 0)}{\partial X \partial u_i} (X - X_0) + \frac{\partial f(X_0, 0)}{\partial u_i} \right)$$

has a bilinear form, following a change of variables, which is equivalent to adding an extra state variable $x_0(t) = 1$:

$$\begin{aligned} \dot{\tilde{X}}(t) &\approx A\tilde{X} + \sum_i u(t)_i B_i \tilde{X} \\ \tilde{X} &= \begin{bmatrix} 1 \\ X \end{bmatrix} \\ A &= \begin{bmatrix} 0 & 0 \\ \left(f(X_0, 0) - \frac{\partial f(X_0, 0)}{\partial X} X_0 \right) & \frac{\partial f(X_0, 0)}{\partial X} \end{bmatrix} \\ B_i &= \begin{bmatrix} 0 & 0 \\ \left(\frac{\partial f(X_0, 0)}{\partial u_i} - \frac{\partial^2 f(X_0, 0)}{\partial X \partial u_i} X_0 \right) & \frac{\partial^2 f(X_0, 0)}{\partial X \partial u_i} \end{bmatrix} \end{aligned} \tag{47.51}$$

This bilinear approximation is important because the Volterra kernels of bilinear systems have closed-form expressions. This means that the kernels can be derived analytically—and quickly—to provide a characterisation of the impulse response properties of the system. The integration of Eq. (47.51) is predicated on its solution over periods $\Delta t_k = t_{k+1} - t_k$ within which the inputs are constant:

$$\begin{aligned} \tilde{X}(t_{k+1}) &\approx e^{J\Delta t_k} \tilde{X}(t_k) \\ y(t_{k+1}) &\approx \lambda(X(t_{k+1})) \\ J &= A + \sum_i u(t_k)_i B_i \end{aligned} \tag{47.52}$$

This quasi-analytical integration scheme can be an order of magnitude quicker than straightforward numerical integration, depending on the sparsity of inputs.

Relation to Conventional fMRI Analyses

Note that if we treated the five biophysical parameters as known canonical values and discounted all but the first-order terms in the Volterra expansion of Eq. (47.45), the following linear model would result:

$$\begin{aligned} h(u,\theta) &= \kappa_0 + \sum_{i=1}^{n} \int_0^t \kappa_1(\sigma) u(t-\sigma)_i d\sigma = \sum_{i=1}^{n} \kappa_1 * u(t)_i \\ &\approx \kappa_0 + \sum_{i=1}^{n} \left(\frac{\partial \kappa_1}{\partial \varepsilon_i} * u(\mathrm{t})_i \right) \varepsilon_i \end{aligned} \tag{47.53}$$

where * denotes convolution, and the second expression is a first-order Taylor expansion around the expected values of the parameters.[8] This is exactly the same as the general linear model

[8] Note that in this first-order Taylor approximation $\kappa_1 = 0$ when expanding around the prior expectations of the efficacies = 0. Furthermore, all first-order partial derivatives $\partial\kappa_1/\partial\theta_i = 0$ unless they are with respect to an efficacy.

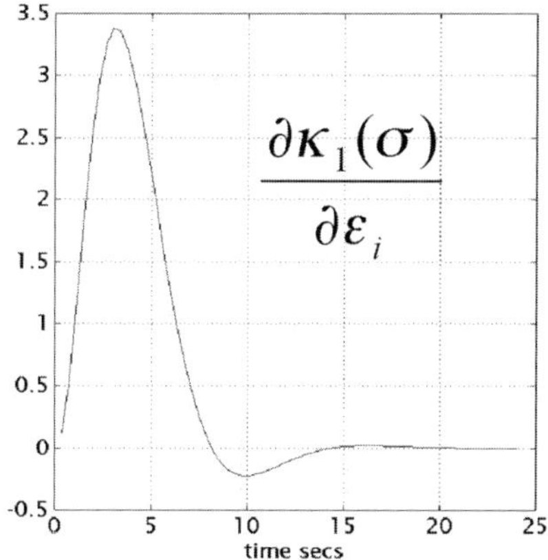

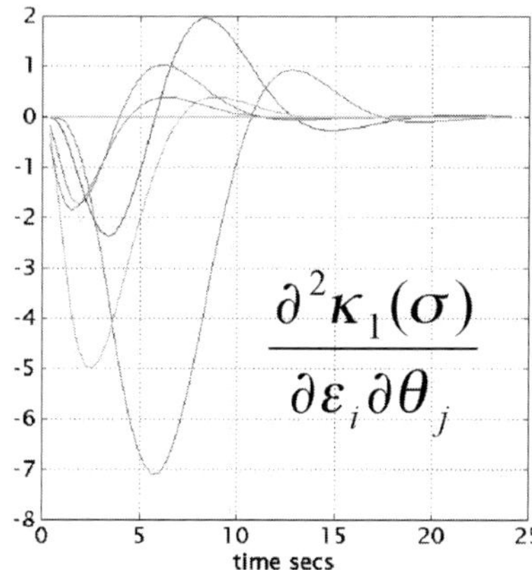

FIGURE 47.19
Partial derivatives of the kernels with respect to parameters of the model evaluated at their prior expectation. (Upper panel) First-order partial derivative with respect to efficacy. (Lower panels) Second-order partial derivatives with respect to efficacy and the biophysical parameters. When expanding around the prior expectations of the efficacies = 0 the remaining first- and second-order partial derivatives with respect to the parameters are zero.

adopted in conventional analysis of fMRI time series, if we elect to use just one canonical HRF to convolve our stimulus functions with. In this context the HRF plays the role of $\partial\kappa_1/\partial\varepsilon_i$ in Eq. (47.53). This partial derivative is shown in Fig. 47.19 (upper panel) using the prior expectations of the parameters, and it conforms closely to the sort of HRF used in practice. Now, by treating the efficacies as fixed effects (i.e., with flat priors) the MAP and ML estimators reduce to the same thing and the conditional expectation reduces to the Gauss-Markov estimator

$$\eta_{ML} = (J^T C_\varepsilon^{-1} J)^{-1} J^T C_\varepsilon^{-1} y$$

where J is the design matrix. This is precisely the estimator used in conventional analyses when whitening strategies are employed.

Consider now the second-order Taylor approximation to Eq. (47.53) that is obtained when we do not know the exact values of the biophysical parameters and they are treated as unknown:

$$h(\theta,u) \approx \kappa_0 + \sum_{i=1}^{n}\left[\left(\frac{\partial\kappa_1}{\partial\varepsilon_i}*u(t)_i\varepsilon_i + \frac{1}{2}\sum_{j=1}^{5}\left(\frac{\partial^2\kappa_1}{\partial\varepsilon_i\partial\theta_i}*u(t)_i\right)\varepsilon_i\theta_i\right)\right] \tag{47.54}$$

This expression[9] is the general linear model proposed in Friston *et al.* (1998) and implemented in our software. In this instance the explanatory variables comprise the stimulus functions, each convolved with a small temporal basis set corresponding to the canonical $\partial\kappa_1/\partial\varepsilon_i$

[9] Note that in this second-order Taylor approximation all second-order partial derivatives $\partial^2\kappa_1/\partial\theta_i\partial\theta_j = 0$ unless they are with respect to an efficacy and one of the biophysical parameters.

and its partial derivatives with respect to the biophysical parameters. Examples of these second-order partial derivatives are provided in the lower panel of Fig. 47.19. The unknowns in this general linear model are the efficacies ε_i and the interaction between the efficacies and the biophysical parameters $\varepsilon_i\theta_i$. Of course, the problem with this linear approximation is that generalised least-squares estimates of the unknown coefficients $\beta = \{\varepsilon_i,\ldots,\varepsilon_n,\varepsilon_1\theta_1,\ldots,\varepsilon_n\theta_1, \varepsilon_n\theta_2,\ldots]^T$ are not constrained to factorise into stimulus-specific efficacies ε_i and biophysical parameters θ_j that are the same for all inputs. Only a nonlinear estimation procedure can do this.

In the usual case of using a temporal basis set (e.g., a canonical form and various derivatives) one obtains a ML or generalised least-squares estimate of functions of the parameters in some subspace defined by the basis set. Operationally this is like specifying priors but of a very particular form. This form can be thought of as uniform priors over the support of the basis set and zero elsewhere. In this sense basis functions implement hard constraints that may not be very realistic but provide for efficient estimation. The soft constraints implied by the Gaussian priors in the EM approach are more plausible but are computationally more expensive to implement.

Summary

This subsection has described a nonlinear EM algorithm that can be viewed as a Gauss-Newton search for the conditional distribution of the parameters of a deterministic dynamic system, with additive Gaussian error. It was shown that classical approaches to fMRI data analysis are special cases that ensue when considering only first-order kernels and adopting flat or uninformative priors. Put another way, the scheme can be regarded as a generalisation of existing procedures that is extended in two important ways. First, the model encompasses nonlinearities and, second, it moves the estimation from a classical into a Bayesian frame.

An Empirical Illustration

Single Input Example

In this, the first of the two examples, we revisit the original dataset on which the priors were based. This constitutes a single-input study where the input corresponds to the aural presentation of single words, at different rates, over epochs. The data were subject to a conventional event-related analysis where the stimulus function comprised trains of spikes indexing the presentation of each word. The stimulus function was convolved with a canonical HRF and its temporal derivative. The data were high-pass filtered by removing low-frequency components modelled by a discrete cosine set. The resulting SPM{T}, testing for activations due to words, is shown in Fig. 47.20 (left panel) thresholded at $p = 0.05$ (corrected).

A single region in the left superior temporal gyrus was selected for analysis. The input comprised the same stimulus function used in the conventional analysis and the output was the first eigenvariate of high-pass filtered time series, of all voxels, within a 4-mm sphere, centred on the most significant voxel in the SPM{T} (marked by an arrow in Fig. 47.20). The error covariance basis set Q comprised two bases; an identity matrix modelling white or an i.i.d. component and a second with exponentially decaying off-diagonal elements modelling an AR(1) component [see Friston *et al.,* 2002b, and Eq. (47.23)]. This models serial correlations among the errors. The results of the estimation procedure are shown in the right-hand panel of Fig. 47.20 in terms of (1) the conditional distribution of the parameters and (2) the conditional expectation of the first- and second-order kernels. The kernels are a function of the parameters and their derivation using a bilinear approximation is described in Friston *et al.* (2000). The upper right panel shows the first-order kernels for the state variables (signal, inflow, deoxyhemoglobin content, and volume). These can be regarded as impulse response functions detailing the response to a transient input. The first- and second-order output kernels for the BOLD response are shown in the lower right panels. They concur with those derived empirically in Friston *et al.* (2000). Note the characteristic undershoot in the first-order kernel and the pronounced negativity in the upper left of the second-order kernel, flanked by two off-diagonal positivities at around 8 sec. These lend the hemodynamics a degree of refractoriness when presenting paired stimuli less than a few seconds apart and a superadditive response with about an 8-sec separation. The left-hand panels show the conditional or posterior distributions. The density for the efficacy is presented in the upper panel and those for the five biophysical parameters are shown in the lower

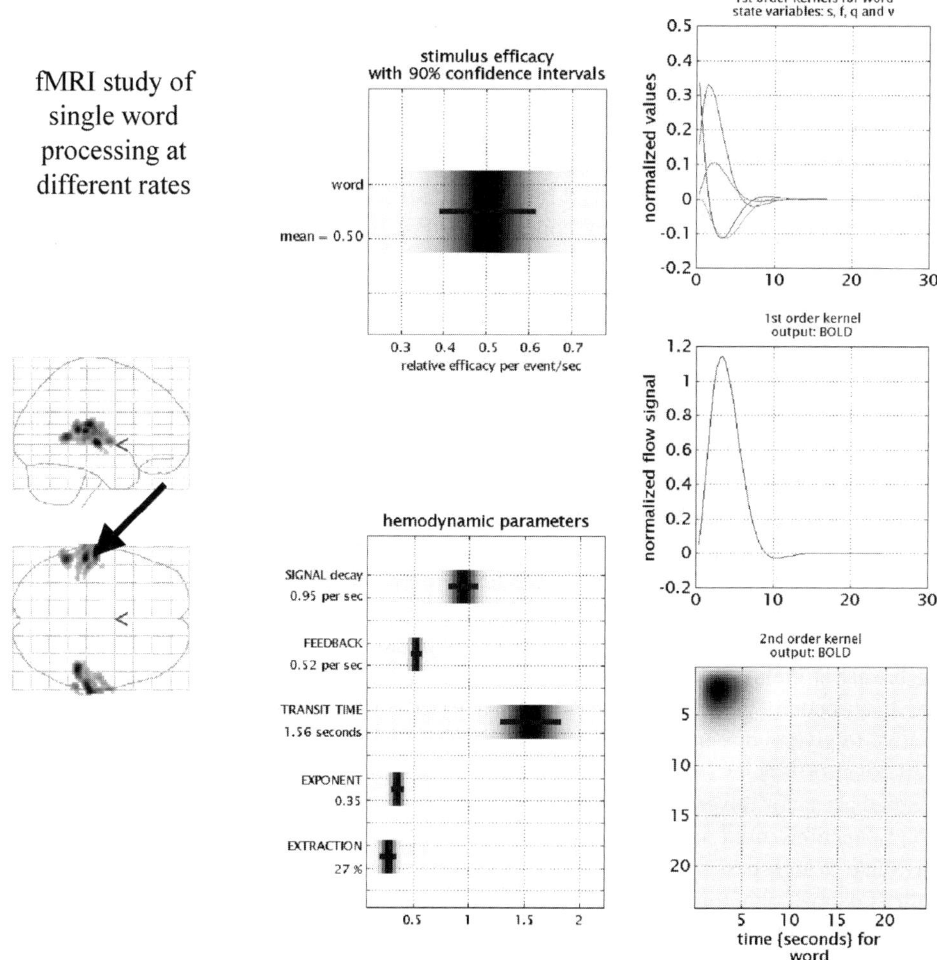

FIGURE 47.20
A SISO example. (Left panel) Conventional SPM{T} testing for an activating effect of word presentation. The arrow shows the center of the region (a sphere of 4-mm radius) whose response was entered into the Bayesian estimation procedure. The results for this region are shown in the right-hand panel in terms of (1) the conditional distribution of the parameters and (2) the conditional expectation of the first- and second-order kernels. The upper right panel shows the first-order kernels for the state variables (signal, inflow, deoxyhemoglobin content, and volume). The first- and second-order output kernels for the BOLD response are shown in the lower right panels. The left-hand panels show the conditional or posterior distributions. That for efficacy is presented in the upper panel and those for the five biophysical parameters in the lower panel. The shading corresponds to the probability density and the bars to 90% confidence intervals.

panel using the same format. The shading corresponds to the probability density and the bars to 90% confidence intervals. The values of the biophysical parameters are all within a very acceptable range. In this example, the signal elimination and decay appear to be slower than normally encountered, with the rate constants being significantly larger than their prior expectations. Grubb's exponent here is closer to the steady-state value of 0.38 than the prior expectation of 0.32. Of greater interest is the efficacy. It can be seen that the efficacy lies between 0.4 and 0.6 and is clearly greater than 0. This would be expected given we chose the most significant voxel from the conventional analysis. Notice that there is no null hypothesis here and we do not even need a p value to make the inference that words evoke a response in this region. An important facility, with inferences based on the conditional distribution and precluded in classical analyses, is that one can infer a cause did not elicit a response. This is demonstrated in the second example.

Multiple Input Example

In this example we turn to a dataset used in previous sections, in which there are three experimental causes or inputs. This was a study of attention to visual motion. Subjects were studied with fMRI under identical stimulus conditions (visual motion subtended by radially moving dots) while manipulating the attentional component of the task (detection of velocity changes). The data were acquired from normal subjects at 2 T using a Magnetom VISION (by Siemens, Erlangen) whole body MRI system, equipped with a head volume coil. Here we analyse data from the first subject. Contiguous multislice T_2*-weighted fMRI images were obtained with a gradient echoplanar sequence (TE = 40 ms, TR = 3.22 sec, matrix size = $64 \times 64 \times 32$, voxel size = $3 \times 3 \times 3$ mm). Each subject had four consecutive 100-scan sessions comprising a series of 10-scan blocks under five different conditions D F A F N F A F N S. The first condition (D) was a dummy condition to allow for magnetic saturation effects. F (Fixation) corresponds to a low-level baseline where the subjects viewed a fixation point at the centre of a screen. In condition A (Attention) subjects viewed 250 dots moving radially from the centre at 4.7 degrees per second and were asked to detect changes in radial velocity. In condition N (No attention) the subjects were asked simply to view the moving dots. In condition S (Stationary) subjects viewed stationary dots. The order of A and N was swapped for the last two sessions. In all conditions subjects fixated the centre of the screen. In a prescanning session the subjects were given five trials with five speed changes (reducing to 1%). During scanning there were no speed changes. No overt response was required in any condition.

This design can be reformulated in terms of three potential causes, photic stimulation, visual motion, and directed attention. The F epochs have no associated cause and represent a baseline. The S epochs have just photic stimulation. The N epochs have both photic stimulation and motion, whereas the A epochs encompass all three causes. We performed a conventional analysis using boxcar stimulus functions encoding the presence or absence of each of the three causes during each epoch. These functions were convolved with a canonical HRF and its temporal derivative to give two repressors for each cause. The corresponding design matrix is shown in the left panel of Fig. 47.21. We selected a region that showed a significant attentional effect in the lingual gyrus for Bayesian inference. The stimulus functions modelling the three inputs were the box functions used in the conventional analysis. The output corresponded to the first eigenvariate of high-pass filtered time series from all voxels in a 4-mm sphere centred on 0, –66, –3 mm (Talairach and Tournoux, 1998). The error covariance basis set was simply the identity matrix.[10] The results are shown in the right-hand panel of Fig. 47.21 using the same format as Fig. 47.20. The critical thing here is that there are three conditional densities, one for each of the input efficacies. Attention has a clear activating effect with more than a 90% probability of being greater than 0.25 per second. However, in this region neither photic stimulation per se or motion in the visual field evokes any real response. The efficacies of both are less than 0.1 and are centred on 0. This means that the time constants of the response to visual stimulation would range from about 10 sec to never. Consequently, these causes can be discounted from a dynamic perspective. In short, this visually unresponsive area responds substantially to attentional manipulation *showing a true functional selectivity*. This is a crucial statement because classical inference does not allow one to infer that any region does not respond and therefore precludes a formal inference about the selectivity of regional responses. The only reason one can say "this region responds *selectively* to attention" is because Bayesian inference allows one to say "it does *not* response to photic stimulation with random dots or motion."

Conclusion

In this section we have looked at a method that conforms to an EM implementation of the Gauss-Newton method, for estimating the conditional or posterior distribution of the parameters of a deterministic dynamic system. The inclusion of priors in the estimation procedure ensures robust and rapid convergence and the resulting conditional densities enable Bayesian inference about the model's parameters. We have examined the coupling between experimentally designed causes or factors in fMRI studies and the ensuing BOLD response. This application represents a generalisation of existing linear models to accommodate nonlinearities in the transduction of

[10] We could motivate this by noting that the TR is considerably longer in these data than in the previous example. However, in reality, serial correlations were ignored because the loss of sparsity in the associated inverse covariance matrices considerably increases computation time and we wanted to repeat the analysis many times (see Friston, 2002).

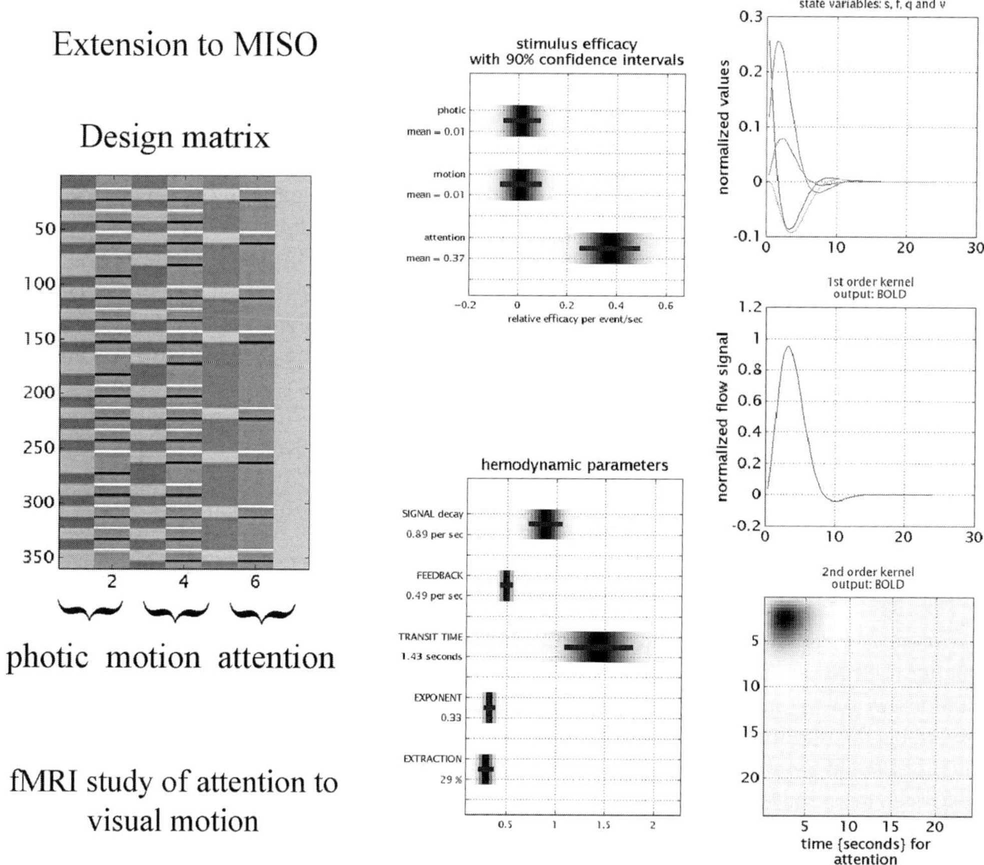

FIGURE 47.21
A MISO example using visual attention to motion. The left panel shows the design matrix used in the conventional analysis and the right panel shows the results of the Bayesian analysis of a lingual extrastriate region. This panel has the same format as Fig. 47.20.

experimental causes to measured output in fMRI. Because the model is predicated on biophysical processes the parameters have a physical interpretation. Furthermore, the approach extends classical inference about the likelihood of the data to more plausible inferences about the parameters of the model given the data. This inference provides confidence intervals based on the conditional density.

Perhaps the most important extension of the scheme described in this section is to MIMO systems where we deal with multiple regions or voxels at the same time. The fundamental importance of this extension is that one can incorporate interactions among brain regions at the neuronal level. This provides a promising framework for the dynamic causal modelling of functional integration in the brain (see Chapter 52).

APPENDIX

EM Algorithm

This appendix describes EM using a statistical mechanics perspective adopted by the machine learning community (Neal and Hinton, 1998). The second section of the appendix connects this formulation with classical ReML methods. We show that, in the context of linear observation models, the negative free energy is the same as the objective function maximised in classical schemes such as ReML.

The EM algorithm is ubiquitous in the sense that many estimation procedures can be formulated as such, from mixture models through to factor analysis. Its objective is to maximise the likelihood of the observed data $p(y|\lambda)$, conditional on some hyperparameters, in the presence of unobserved variables or parameters θ. This is equivalent to maximising the log likelihood as follows:

$$\begin{aligned} \ln p(y|\lambda) &= \ln \int p(\theta, y|\lambda)d\theta \geq \\ F(q, \lambda) &= \int q(\theta)\ln p(\theta,y|\lambda)d\theta - \int q(\theta)\ln q(\theta)d\theta \end{aligned} \tag{47.55}$$

where $q(\theta)$ is *any* distribution over the model parameters (Neal and Hinton, 1998). Equation (47.55) rests on the Jensen inequality that follows from the concavity of the log function, which renders the log of an integral greater than the integral of the log. The term F corresponds to the negative free energy in statistical thermodynamics and comprises two terms, related to the energy (first term) and entropy (second term). The EM algorithm alternates between maximising F, and implicitly the likelihood of the data, with respect to the distribution $q(\theta)$ and the hyperparameters λ, holding the other fixed:

$$\textbf{E}\text{-step:} \qquad q(\theta) \leftarrow \arg\max_{q} F(q(\theta),\lambda)$$

$$\textbf{M}\text{-step:} \qquad \lambda \leftarrow \arg\max_{\lambda} F(q(\theta),\lambda)$$

This iterative alternation performs a coordinate ascent on F. It is easy to show that the maximum in the **E**-step is obtained when $q(\theta) = p(\theta|y,\lambda)$, at which point (47.55) becomes an equality. The **M**-step finds the ML estimate of the hyperparameters, i.e., the values of λ that maximise $p(y|\lambda)$ by integrating $p(\theta,y|\lambda)$ over the parameters, using the current estimate of their conditional distribution. In short, the **E**-step computes sufficient statistics (in our case the conditional mean and covariance) relating to the distribution of the unobserved parameters to enable the **M**-step to optimise the hyperparameters, in a maximum-likelihood sense, using this distribution. These new hyperparameters reenter into the estimation of the conditional distribution and so on until convergence.

The E-Step

In our hierarchical model, with Gaussian (i.e., parametric) assumptions, the **E**-step is trivial and corresponds to taking the conditional mean and covariance according to Eq. (47.15). These are then used, with the data, to estimate the hyperparameters of the covariance components in the **M**-step.

The M-Step

Given that we can reduce the problem to estimating the error covariances with the augmented expressions for the conditional mean and covariance [Eq. (47.15)], we only need to estimate the hyperparameters of the error covariances (which contain the prior covariances). Specifically, we require the hyperparameters that maximise the first term in the expression for F above. From Eq. (47.15),

$$\log p(\theta,y|\lambda) = -\frac{1}{2}\ln|C_\varepsilon| - \frac{1}{2}(\bar{y} - \bar{X}\theta)^T C_\varepsilon^{-1}(\bar{y} - \bar{X}\theta) + const.$$

$$\begin{aligned} \int q(\theta)\ln p(\theta,y|\lambda)d\theta &= -\frac{1}{2}\ln|C_\varepsilon| - \frac{1}{2}r^T C_\varepsilon^{-1} r - \frac{1}{2}\left\langle(\theta - \eta_{\theta|y})^T \bar{X}^T C_\varepsilon^{-1}\bar{X}(\theta - \eta_{\theta|y})\right\rangle_q + const. \\ &= -\frac{1}{2}\ln|C_\varepsilon| - \frac{1}{2}r^T C_\varepsilon^{-1} r - \frac{1}{2}tr\{C_{\theta|y}\bar{X}^T C_\varepsilon^{-1}\bar{X}\} + const. \end{aligned} \tag{47.56}$$

$$\int q(\theta)\log q(\theta) = -\frac{1}{2}\ln|C_{\theta|y}| + const.$$

$$F = -\frac{1}{2}\ln|C_\varepsilon^{-1}| - \frac{1}{2}r^T C_\varepsilon^{-1} r - \frac{1}{2}tr\{C_{\theta|y}\bar{X}^T C_\varepsilon^{-1}\bar{X}\}\ \frac{1}{2}\ln|C_{\theta|y}| + const.$$

where the residuals $r = \bar{y} - \bar{X}\eta_{\theta|y}$. We now simply take the derivatives of F with respect to the hyperparameters and use some nonlinear search to find the maximum. Note that the second entropy term does not depend on the hyperparameters. There is an interesting intermediate derivative. From Eq. (47.56),

$$\frac{\partial F}{\partial C_\varepsilon^{-1}} = \frac{1}{2}C_\varepsilon - \frac{1}{2}rr^T - \frac{1}{2}\bar{X}C_{\theta|y}\bar{X}^T \tag{47.57}$$

Setting this derivative to zero (at the maximum of F) requires

$$C(\lambda)_\varepsilon = rr^T + \bar{X}C_{\theta|y}\bar{X}^T \tag{47.58}$$

(cf. Dempster *et al.,* 1981, p. 350). Equation Eq. (47.58) says that the error covariance estimate has two components: that due to differences between the data observed and predicted by the conditional expectation of the parameters and another component due to the variation of the parameters about their conditional mean. More generally one can adopt a Fischer scoring algorithm and update the hyperparameters $\lambda \leftarrow \lambda + \Delta\lambda$ using the first and expected second partial derivatives of the negative free energy:

$$\begin{aligned}
\Delta\lambda &= H^{-1}g \\
g_i &= \frac{\partial F}{\partial \lambda_i} = tr\left\{-\frac{\partial F}{\partial C_\varepsilon^{-1}}C_\varepsilon^{-1}Q_iC_\varepsilon^{-1}\right\} \\
&= -\frac{1}{2}tr\{PQ_i\} + \frac{1}{2}\bar{y}^TP^TQ_iP\bar{y} \\
\frac{\partial^2 F}{\partial \lambda_{ij}^2} &= \frac{\partial g_i}{\partial \lambda_j} = \frac{1}{2}\,tr\{PQ_iPQ_j\} - \bar{y}^TPQ_iPQ_jP\bar{y} \\
H_{ij} &= E\left\{-\frac{\partial^2 F}{\partial \lambda_{ij}^2}\right\} = \frac{1}{2}tr\{PQ_iPQ_j\} \\
P &= C_\varepsilon^{-1} - C_\varepsilon^{-1}\bar{X}C_{\theta|y}\bar{X}^TC_\varepsilon^{-1}X
\end{aligned} \tag{47.59}$$

Fisher scoring corresponds to augmenting a simple Newton-Raphson scheme by replacing the second derivatives or "curvature" observed at the particular response y with its expectation over realisations of the data. The ensuing matrix H is referred to as *Fisher's information matrix.*[11] The computation of the gradient vector g can be made computationally efficient by capitalising on any sparsity structure in the constraints and by bracketing the multiplications appropriately. Equation (47.59) is general in that it accommodates almost any form for the covariance constraints through a Taylor expansion of $C\{\lambda\}_\varepsilon$. In many instances the bases can be constructed so that they do not "overlap" or interact through the design matrix, i.e., $PQ_iPQ_j = 0$, and estimates of the hyperparameters can be based directly on the first partial derivatives in Eq. (47.59) by solving for $g = 0$. For certain forms of $C\{\lambda\}_\varepsilon$, the hyperparameters can be calculated very simply.[12] However, we work with the general solution above that encompasses all of these special cases.

Once the hyperparameters have been updated they are entered into Eq. (47.19) to give the new covariance estimate, which in turn is entered into Eq. (47.15) to give the new conditional estimates, which themselves reenter Eq. (47.59) to give new updates until convergence. A pseudo-code illustration of the complete algorithm is presented in Fig. 47.4. Note that in this

[11] The derivation of the expression for the Information matrix uses standard linear algebra results and is most easily seen by (1) differentiating the form for g in Eq. (47.61) by noting

$$\frac{\partial P}{\partial \lambda_j} = -PQ_jP$$

and (2) taking the expectation, using $\langle tr\{PQ_iP\bar{y}\bar{y}^TPQ_j\}\rangle_q = tr\{PQ_iPC_\varepsilon PQ_j\} = tr\{PQ_iPQ_j\}$

[12] Note that if there is only one hyperparameter then $g = 0$ can be solved directly:

$$\begin{aligned}
tr\{PQ\} &= \bar{y}PQP\bar{y} \Rightarrow \\
\lambda &= \frac{r^TQ^{-1}r}{tr\{R\}}
\end{aligned}$$

where $C_\varepsilon = \lambda Q$ and $R = I - \bar{X}(\bar{X}^TQ^{-1}\bar{X})^{-1}\bar{X}^TQ^{-1}$ is a residual forming matrix. This is the expression used in classical schemes, given the correlation matrix Q, to estimate the error covariance using the sum of squared decorrelated residuals.

implementation one is effectively performing a single Fisher scoring iteration for each **M**-step. One could postpone each **E**-step until this search converged, but a single step is sufficient to perform a coordinate ascent on F. Technically, this renders Eq. (47.59) a generalised EM or GEM algorithm.

Note that the search for the maximum of F does not have to employ a Fisher scoring scheme or indeed the parameterisation of C_ε used in Eq. (47.18). Other search procedures such as quasi-Newton searches are commonly employed (Fahrmeir and Tutz, 1994). Harville (1977) originally considered Newton-Raphson and scoring algorithms, and Laird and Ware (1982) recommend several versions of the EM algorithm. One limitation of the hyperparameterisation described above is that does not guarantee that C_ε is positive definite. This is because the hyperparameters can take negative values with extreme degrees of nonsphericity. The EM algorithm employed by MULTISTAT (Worsley *et al.,* 2002), for variance component estimation in multisubject fMRI studies uses a slower but more stable EM algorithm that ensures positive definite covariance estimates. The common aspect of all of these algorithms is that they (explicitly or implicitly) maximise F (or minimise free energy). As shown next, this is equivalent to the method of restricted maximum likelihood.

Relationship to ReML

ReML was introduced by Patterson and Thompson in 1971 as a technique for estimating variance components that accounts for the loss in degrees of freedom that result from estimating fixed effects (Harville , 1977). It is commonly employed in standard statistical packages (e.g., SPSS). Under the present model assumptions, ReML is formally identical to EM. One can regard ReML as embedding the **E**-step into the **M**-step to provide a single log-likelihood objective function: Substituting the $C_{\theta|y} = (\bar{X}^T C_\varepsilon^{-1} \bar{X})^{-1}$ from Eq. (47.15) into the expression for the negative free energy Eq. (47.56) gives

$$F = -\frac{1}{2}\ln|C_\varepsilon| - \frac{1}{2}r^T C_\varepsilon^{-1} r - \frac{1}{2}\ln|\bar{X}^T C_\varepsilon^{-1}\bar{X}| + const. \tag{47.60}$$

which is the ReML objective function (see Harville, 1977, p. 325). Critically the derivatives of Eq. (47.60), with respect to the hyperparameters, are exactly the same as those given in Eq. (47.59).[13] Operationally, Eq. (47.59) can be rearranged to give a ReML scheme by removing any explicit reference to the conditional covariance:

$$\begin{aligned} gi &= -\frac{1}{2}tr\{PQ_i\} + \frac{1}{2}tr\{P\bar{y}\bar{y}^T P^T Q_i\} \\ H_{ij} &= \frac{1}{2}tr\{PQ_i PQ_j\} \\ P &= C_\varepsilon^{-1} - C_\varepsilon^{-1}\bar{X}(\bar{X}^T C_\varepsilon^{-1}\bar{X})^{-1}\bar{X}^T C_\varepsilon^{-1} \end{aligned} \tag{47.61}$$

These expressions are formally identical to those described in Section 5 of Harville (1977, p. 326). Because Eq. (47.61) does not depend explicitly on the conditional density, one could think of ReML as estimating the hyperparameters in a subspace that is *restricted* in the sense that the estimates are conditionally independent of the parameters. Harville (1977) provides a discussion of expressions, comparable to the terms in Eq. (47.61), that are easier to compute for particular hyperparameterisations of the variance components.

The particular form of Eq. (47.61) has a very useful application when y is a multivariate data matrix and the hyperparameters are the same for all columns (i.e., voxels). Here, irrespective of the voxel-specific parameters, the voxel-wide hyperparameters can be obtained efficiently by iterating Eq. (47.61) using the sample covariance matrix yy^T. This is possible because the conditional parameter estimates are not required in the ReML formulation. This is used in the current version of the SPM software to estimate voxel-wide nonsphericity.

[13] Note that

$$\frac{\partial \ln|\bar{X}^T C_\varepsilon^{-1}\bar{X}|}{\partial\lambda_i} = tr\left\{(\bar{X}^T C_\varepsilon^{-1}\bar{X})^{-1}\frac{\partial \bar{X}^T C_\varepsilon^{-1}\bar{X}}{\partial\lambda_i}\right\} = -tr\{C_{\theta|y}\bar{X}^T C_\varepsilon^{-1} Q_i C_\varepsilon^{-1}\bar{X}\}$$

References

Bendat, J. S. (1990). *Nonlinear System Analysis and Identification from Random Data.* John Wiley and Sons, New York.

Berry, D. A., and Hochberg, Y. (1999). Bayesian perspectives on multiple comparisons. *J. Statistical Planning Inference* **82**, 215–227.

Büchel, C., and Friston, K. J. (1997). Modulation of connectivity in visual pathways by attention: cortical interactions evaluated with structural equation modelling and fMRI. *Cerebral Cortex* **7,** 768–778.

Box, G. E. P. (1954). Some theorems on quadratic forms applied in the study of analysis of variance problems, I. Effect of inequality of variance in the one-way classification. *Ann. Math. Stats.* **25**, 290–302.

Bullmore, E. T., Brammer, M. J., Williams, S. C. R., Rabe-Hesketh, S., Janot, N., David, A., Mellers, J., Howard, R., and Sham, P. (1996). Statistical methods of estimation and inference for functional MR images. *Mag. Res. Med.* **35**, 261–277.

Buxton, R. B., Wong, E. C., and Frank, L. R. (1998). Dynamics of blood flow and oxygenation changes during brain activation: the balloon model. *MRM* **39,** 855–864.

Copas, J. B. (1983). Regression prediction and shrinkage. *J. Roy. Statistical. Soc. Ser. B* **45**;311–354.

Dempster, A. P., Laird, N. N., and Rubin, D. B. (1977). Maximum likelihood from incomplete data via the EM algorithm. *J. Roy. Stat. Soc. Ser.* B **39**;1–38.

Dempster, A. P., Rubin, D. B., and Tsutakawa, R. K. (1981). Estimation in covariance component models. *J. Am. Statistical Assoc.* **76,** 341–353.

Descombes, X., Kruggel, F., and von Cramon, D. Y. (1998). fMRI signal restoration using a spatio-temporal Markov random field preserving transitions. *NeuroImage* **8,** 340–349.

Efron, B., and Morris, C. (1973). Stein's estimation rule and its competitors—an empirical Bayes approach. *J. Am. Stats. Assoc.* **68**, 117–130.

Efron, B., and Morris, C. (1977). Stein's paradox in statistics. *Sci. Am.* May, pp. 119–127.

Everitt, B. S., and Bullmore, E. T. (1999). Mixture model mapping of brain activation in functional magnetic resonance images. *Hum. Brain Mapping* **7**, 1–14.

Fahrmeir, L., and Tutz, G. (1994). *Multivariate Statistical Modelling Based on Generalised Linear Models,* pp. 355–356.Springer-Verlag, New York.

Fliess, M., Lamnabhi, M., and Lamnabhi-Lagarrigue, F. (1983). An algebraic approach to nonlinear functional expansions. *IEEE Trans. Circuits Syst.* **30,** 554–570.

Friston, K. J. (2002). Bayesian estimation of dynamical systems: an application to fMRI. *NeuroImage* **16,** 465–483.

Friston, K. J., Jezzard, P. J., and Turner, R. (1994). Analysis of functional MRI time-series *Hum. Brain Mapping* **1**, 153–171.

Friston, K. J., Holmes, A. P., Worsley, K. J., Poline, J.-B., Frith, C. D., and Frackowiak, R. S. J. (1995). Statistical parametric maps in functional imaging: a general linear approach. *Hum. Brain Mapping* **2,**189–210.

Friston, K. J., Josephs, O., Rees, G., and Turner, R. (1998). Nonlinear event-related responses in fMRI. *Mag. Res. Med.* **39**, 41–52.

Friston, K. J., Mechelli, A., Turner, R., and Price, C. J. (2000). Nonlinear responses in fMRI: the balloon model, Volterra kernels and other hemodynamics. *NeuroImage* **12,** 466–477.

Friston, K. J., Penny, W., Phillips, C., Kiebel, S., Hinton, G., and Ashburner, J. (2002a). Classical and Bayesian inference in neuroimaging: theory. *NeuroImage* **16,** 465–483.

Friston, K. J., Glaser, D. E., Henson, R. N. A., Kiebel, S., and Phillips, C., and Ashburner, J. (2002b). Classical and Bayesian inference in neuroimaging: applications. *NeuroImage* **16,** 484–512.

Geisser, S., and Greenhouse, S. W. (1958). An extension of Box's results on the use of the F distribution in multivariate analysis. *Ann. Math. Stats.* **29,** 885–891.

Grubb, R. L., Rachael, M. E., Euchring, J. O., and Ter-Pogossian, M. M. (1974). The effects of changes in PCO_2 on cerebral blood volume, blood flow and vascular mean transit time. *Stroke* **5,** 630–639.

Hartley, H. (1958). Maximum likelihood estimation from incomplete data. *Biometrics* **14**, 174–194.

Hartvig, N. V., and Jensen, J. L. (2000). Spatial mixture modelling of fMRI data. *Hum. Brain Mapping*, **11**, 233–248.

Harville, D. A. (1977). Maximum likelihood approaches to variance component estimation and to related problems. *J. Am. Stat. Assoc.* **72**, 320–338.

Henson, R. N. A., Rugg, M. D., Shallice, T., and Dolan, R. J. (2000). Confidence in recognition memory for words: Dissociating right prefrontal roles in episodic retrieval. *J. Cog. Neurosci.*, **12**, 913–923.

Hoge, R. D., Atkinson, J., Gill, B., Crelier, G. R., Marrett, S., and Pike, G. B. (1999). Linear coupling between cerebral blood flow and oxygen consumption in activated human cortex. *Proc. Natl. Acad. Sci. USA* **96,** 9403–9408.

Hfjen-Sfrensen, P., Hansen, L. K., and Rasmussen, C. E. (2000). Bayesian modelling of fMRI time-series. In *Advances in Neural Information Processing Systems,* Vol. 12, Solla, S. A., Leen, T. K., and Muller K. R., Eds., pp. 754–760. MIT Press, Cambridge, MA.

Holmes, A., and Ford, I. (1993). A Bayesian approach to significance testing for statistic images from PET. In *Quantification of Brain Function, Tracer Kinetics and Image Analysis in Brain PET.* Uemura, K., Lassen, N. A., Jones, T., and Kanno, I., Eds., pp. 521–534. Excerpta Medica, Int. Cong. Ser. No. 1030.

Holmes, A. P., and Friston, K. J. (1998). Generalisability, random effects and population inference. *NeuroImage* S754.

Kass, R. E., and Steffey, D. (1989). Approximate Bayesian inference in conditionally independent hierarchical models (parametric empirical Bayes models*). J. Am. Stat. Assoc.* **407**, 717–726.

Laird, N. M., and Ware, J. H. (1982). Random effects models for longitudinal data. *Biometrics* **38**, 963–974.

Lee, P. M. (1997). *Bayesian Statistics an Introduction.* John Wiley and Sons, New York.

Neal, R. M., and Hinton, G. E. (1998). A view of the EM algorithm that justifies incremental, sparse and other variants. In *Learning in Graphical Models,* Jordan, M. I., Ed., pp. 355–368. Kluwer Academic Press, The Netherlands.

Mandeville, J. B., Marota, J. J., Ayata, C., Zararchuk, G., Moskowitz, M. A., Rosen, B., and Weisskoff, R. M. (1999). Evidence of a cerebrovascular postarteriole windkessel with delayed compliance. *J. Cereb. Blood Flow Metab.* **19,** 679–689.

Mayhew, J., Hu, D., Zheng, Y., Askew, S., Hou, Y., Berwick, J., Coffey, P. J., and Brown, N. (1998). An evaluation of linear models analysis techniques for processing images of microcirculation activity *NeuroImage* **7,** 49–71.

Miller, K. L., Luh, W. M., Liu, T. T., Martinez, A., Obata, T., Wong, E. C., Frank, L. R., and Buxton, R. B. (2000). Characterising the dynamic perfusion response to stimuli of short duration. *Proc. ISRM* **8,** 580.

Phillips, C., Mattout, J., Rugg, M. D., Maquet, P., and Friston, K. J. (2003). Restricted maximum likelihood solution of the source localisation problem in EEG. Submitted for publication.

Purdon, P. L., and Weisskoff, R. (1998). Effect of temporal autocorrelations due to physiological noise stimulus paradigm on voxel-level false positive rates in fMRI. *Hum. Brain Mapping* **6**, 239–249.

Santner, T. J., and Duffy, D. E. (1989). *The Statistical Analysis of Discrete Data.* Springer, New York.

Satterthwaite, E. F. (1941). Synthesis of variance. *Psychometrika* **6**, 309–316.

Talairach, J., and Tournoux, P. (1988). *A Co-Planar Stereotaxic Atlas of a Human Brain.* Thieme, Stuttgart.

Tikhonov, A. N., and Arsenin, V. Y. (1977). *Solution of Ill Posed roblems.* Winston and Sons, Columbia, MD.

Worsley, K. J., and Friston, K. J. (1995). Analysis of fMRI time-series revisited—again *NeuroImage* **2,** 173–181.

Worsley, K. J. (1994). Local maxima and the expected Euler characteristic of excursion sets of chi squared, F and *t* fields. *Advances Appl. Prob.* **26,** 13–42.

Worsley, K. J., Liao, C., Aston, J., Petre, V., Duncan, G. H., and Evans, A. C. (2002). A general statistical analysis for fMRI data. *NeuroImage.*, **15**, 1–15.

SECTION FOUR

FUNCTIONAL INTEGRATION

C H A P T E R

48

Functional Integration in the Brain

INTRODUCTION

This section is about functional integration in the brain. This first chapter in this section introduces the neurobiological background of functional integration in terms of neuronal information processing in cortical hierarchies. This serves to frame the sorts of question than can be addressed with analyses of functional and effective connectivity. In fact, we take the empirical Bayesian theory described in the previous chapter as a possible basis for understanding integration among the levels of hierarchically organised cortical systems. The next two chapters (Chapters 49 and 50) deal with the fundaments of functional and effective connectivity, that are revisited in the next two chapters. Chapters 51 and 52 deal with two complementary perspectives on models of functional integration, namely, the Volterra or generalised convolution formulation and the state-space representation used by dynamic causal modelling. In the final chapter in this section, Chapter 53, we reconcile various approaches, looking more closely at the underlying mathematics.

Self-supervised models of how the brain represents and categorises the causes of its sensory input can be divided into those that minimise the mutual information (i.e., redundancy) among evoked responses and those that minimise the prediction error. This chapter describes one such model and its implications for the functional anatomy of sensory cortical hierarchies in the brain. We then consider how analyses of effective connectivity can be used to look for architectures that are sufficient for perceptual learning and synthesis.

Many models of representational learning require prior assumptions about the distribution of sensory causes. However, as seen in the previous chapter, the notion of empirical Bayes suggests that these assumptions are not necessary and that priors can be learned in a hierarchical context. The main point made in this chapter is that backward connections, mediating internal or generative models of how sensory inputs are caused, are essential and that feedforward architectures, on their own, are not sufficient. Moreover, nonlinearities in generative models require these connections to be modulatory so that estimated causes in higher cortical levels can interact to predict responses in lower levels. This is important in relation to functional asymmetries in forward and backward connections that have been demonstrated empirically.

Ascertaining whether backward influences are expressed functionally requires measurements of functional integration among brain systems. This chapter summarises approaches to integration in terms of functional and effective connectivity and uses the theoretical considerations above to illustrate the sorts of questions that can be addressed. Specifically, we will show that functional neuroimaging can be used to test for interactions between bottom-up and top-down inputs to an area.

In concert with the growing interest in contextual and extra-classical receptive field effects in electrophysiology (i.e., how the receptive fields of sensory neurons change according to the context in which a stimulus is presented), a similar paradigm shift is emerging in imaging neuroscience. Namely, the appreciation that functional specialisation exhibits similar extra-classical phenomena, in which a cortical area may be specialised for one thing in one context but something else in another. These extra-classical phenomena have implications for theoretical ideas about how the brain might work. This chapter uses theoretical models of representational learning as a vehicle to illustrate how imaging can be used to address important questions about functional brain architectures.

We start by reviewing two fundamental principles of brain organisation, namely, *functional specialisation* and *functional integration,* and how they rest on the anatomy and physiology of cortico-cortical connections in the brain. The second section deals with the nature and learning of representations from a theoretical or computational perspective. The key focus of this section is on the functional architectures implied by the model. Generative models based on predictive coding rest on hierarchies of backward and lateral projections and, critically, confer a necessary role on backward connections.

Empirical evidence from electrophysiological studies of animals and functional neuro-imaging studies of human subjects is presented in the third and fourth sections to illustrate the context-sensitive nature of functional specialisation and how its expression depends on integration among remote cortical areas. The third section looks at extra-classical effects in electro-physiology, in terms of the predictions afforded by generative models of brain function. The theme of context-sensitive evoked responses is generalised to a cortical level and human functional neuroimaging studies in the subsequent section. The critical focus of this section is evidence for the interaction of bottom-up and top-down influences in determining regional brain responses. These interactions can be considered signatures of backward connections. The final section reviews some of the implications of the preceding sections for lesion studies and neuropsychology. *Dynamic diaschisis* is described, in which aberrant neuronal responses can be observed as a consequence of damage to distal brain areas providing enabling or modulatory afferents. This section uses neuroimaging in neuropsychological patients and discusses the implications for constructs based on the lesion-deficit model.

FUNCTIONAL SPECIALISATION AND INTEGRATION

Background

The brain appears to adhere to two fundamental principles of functional organisation, functional integration and functional specialisation, in which the integration within and among specialised areas is mediated by effective connectivity. The distinction relates to that between "local-isationism" and "(dis)connectionism" that dominated thinking about cortical function in the 19th century. Since the early anatomical theories of Gall, the identification of a particular brain region with a specific function has become a central theme in neuroscience. However, functional localisation per se was not easy to demonstrate. For example, a meeting that took place on August 4, 1881, addressed the difficulties of attributing function to a cortical area, given the dependence of cerebral activity on underlying connections (Phillips *et al.,, 19*84). This meeting was entitled "Localisation of Function in the Cortex Cerebri." Goltz, although accepting the results of electrical stimulation in dog and monkey cortex, considered that the excitation method was inconclusive, in that the behaviours elicited might have originated in related pathways, or current could have spread to distant centres. In short, the excitation method could not be used to infer functional localisation because localisationism discounted interactions, or functional integration, among different brain areas. It was proposed that lesion studies could supplement excitation experiments. Ironically, it was observations on patients with brain lesions some years later (see Absher and Benson, 1993) that led to the concept of "disconnection syndromes" and the refutation of localisationism as a complete or sufficient explanation of cortical organisation. Functional localisation implies that a function can be localised in a cortical area, whereas specialisation suggests that a cortical area is specialised for some aspects of perceptual or motor processing, where this *specialisation* can be anatomically *segregated* within the cortex. The cortical infrastructure supporting a single function may then involve many specialised areas whose union is mediated by the functional integration among them. Functional specialisation and integration are not exclusive, they are complementary. Functional specialisation is only meaningful in the context of functional integration and vice versa.

Functional Specialisation and Segregation

The functional role, played by any component (e.g., cortical area, subarea, neuronal population or neuron) of the brain, is defined largely by its connections. Certain patterns of cortical projections are so common that they could amount to rules of cortical connectivity. "These rules revolve around one, apparently, overriding strategy that the cerebral cortex uses—that of functional segregation" (Zeki, 1990). Functional segregation demands that cells with common functional properties be grouped together. This architectural constraint in turn necessitates both convergence and divergence of cortical connections. Extrinsic connections, between cortical regions, are not continuous but occur in patches or clusters. This patchiness has, in some instances, a clear relationship to functional segregation. For example, the secondary visual area V2 has a distinctive cytochrome oxidase architecture, consisting of thick stripes, thin stripes, and interstripes. When recordings are made in V2, directionally selective (but not wavelength or colour selective) cells are found exclusively in the thick stripes. Retrograde (i.e., backward) labelling of cells in V5 is limited to these thick stripes. All available physiological evidence suggests that V5 is a functionally homogeneous area that is specialised for visual motion. Evidence of this nature supports the notion that patchy connectivity is the anatomical infrastructure that underpins functional segregation and specialisation. If it is the case that neurons in a given cortical area share a common responsiveness (by virtue of their extrinsic connectivity) to some sensorimotor or cognitive attribute, then this functional segregation is also an anatomical one. Challenging a subject with the appropriate sensorimotor attribute or cognitive process should lead to activity changes in, and only in, the areas of interest. This is the model on which the search for regionally specific effects with functional neuroimaging is based.

The Anatomy and Physiology of Cortico-Cortical Connections

If specialisation rests on connectivity, then important organisational principles should be embodied in the neuroanatomy and physiology of extrinsic connections. Extrinsic connections couple different cortical areas, whereas intrinsic connections are confined to the cortical sheet. Certain features of cortico-cortical connections provide strong clues about their functional role. In brief, there appears to be a hierarchical organisation that rests on the distinction between *forward* and *backward* connections. The designation of a connection as forward or backward depends primarily on its cortical layers of origin and termination. Some characteristics of cortico-cortical connections are presented below and are summarised in Table 48.1. The list is not exhaustive, nor properly qualified, but serves to introduce some important principles that have emerged from empirical studies of visual cortex.

- Hierarchical *organisation*. The organisation of the visual cortices can be considered as a hierarchy of cortical levels with reciprocal extrinsic cortico-cortical connections among the constituent cortical areas (Felleman and Van Essen, 1991). The notion of a hierarchy depends on a distinction between reciprocal forward and backward extrinsic connections.
- *Reciprocal connections.* Although reciprocal, forward and backward connections show both a microstructural and functional asymmetry. The terminations of both show laminar specificity. Forward connections (from a low to a high level) have sparse axonal bifurcations and are topographically organised, originating in supragranular layers and terminating largely in layer IV. Backward connections, on the other hand, show abundant axonal bifurcation and a more diffuse topography. Their origins are bilaminar/infragranular and they terminate predominantly in supragranular layers (Rockland and Pandya, 1979; Salin and Bullier, 1995). Extrinsic connections show an orderly convergence and divergence of connections from one cortical level to the next. At a macroscopic level, one point in a given cortical area will connect to a region 5–8 mm in diameter in another. An important distinction between forward

TABLE 48.1 Some Key Characteristics of Extrinsic Cortico-Cortical Connections in the Brain

Hierarchical Organisation
- The organisation of the visual cortices can be considered as a hierarchy (Felleman and Van Essen, 1991).
- The notion of a hierarchy depends on a distinction between forward and backward extrinsic connections.
- This distinction rests on different laminar specificity (Rockland and Pandya, 1979; Salin and Bullier, 1995).
- Backward connections are more numerous and transcend more levels.
- Backward connections are more divergent than forward connections (Zeki and Shipp, 1988).

Forwards Connections	Backwards Connections
Sparse axonal bifurcations	Abundant axonal bifurcation
Topographically organised	Diffuse topography
Originate in supragranular layers	Originate in bilaminar/infragranular layers
Terminate largely in layer IV	Terminate predominantly in supragranular layers
Postsynaptic effects through fast AMPA (1.3- to 2.4-ms decay) and $GABA_A$ (6-ms decay) receptors.	Modulatory afferents activate slow (50-ms decay) Voltage-sensitive NMDA receptors

and backward connections is that backward connections are more divergent. For example, the divergence region of a point in V5 (i.e., the region receiving backward afferents from V5) may include thick and interstripes in V2, whereas its convergence region (i.e., the region providing forward afferents to V5) is limited to the thick stripes (Zeki and Shipp, 1988). Backward connections are more abundant than forward connections and transcend more levels. For example the ratio of forward efferent connections to backward afferents in the lateral geniculate is about 1:10/20. Another important distinction is that backward connections will traverse a number of hierarchical levels, whereas forward connections are more restricted. For example, there are backward connections from TE and TEO to V1, but no monosynaptic connections from V1 to TE or TEO (Salin and Bullier, 1995).

- *Functionally asymmetric forward and backward connections.* Functionally, reversible inactivation (e.g., Sandell and Schiller, 1982; Girard and Bullier, 1989) and neuroimaging (e.g., Büchel and Friston, 1997) studies suggest that forward connections are driving, always eliciting a response, whereas backward connections can also be modulatory. In this context, modulatory means backward connections modulate responsiveness to other inputs. The notion that forward connections are concerned with the promulgation and segregation of sensory information is consistent with (1) their sparse axonal bifurcation, (2) patchy axonal terminations, (3) and topographic projections. In contradistinction, backward connections are generally considered to have a role in mediating contextual effects and in the coordination of processing channels. This is consistent with (1) their frequent bifurcation, (2) diffuse axonal terminations, (3) and more divergent topography (Salin and Bullier, 1995; Crick and Koch, 1998). Forward connections meditate their postsynaptic effects through fast AMPA (1.3- to 2.4-ms decay) and $GABA_A$ (6-ms decay) receptors. Modulatory effects can be mediated by NMDA receptors. NMDA receptors are voltage sensitive, showing nonlinear and slow dynamics (~50-ms decay). They are found predominantly in supragranular layers where backward connections terminate (Salin and Bullier, 1995). These slow time constants again point to a role in mediating contextual effects that are more enduring than phasic sensory-evoked responses.

Many mechanisms are responsible for establishing connections in the brain. Connectivity results from interplay between genetic, epigenetic, and activity- or experience-dependent mechanisms. *In utero*, epigenetic mechanisms predominate, such as the interaction between the topography of the developing cortical sheet, cell migration, and gene expression and the mediating role of gene–gene interactions and gene products such as cell adhesion molecules (CAMs). Following birth, connections are progressively refined and remodelled with a greater emphasis on activity- and use-dependent plasticity. These changes endure into adulthood with ongoing reorganisation and experience-dependent plasticity that subserves behavioural adaptation and learning throughout life. In brief, there are two basic determinants of connectivity: (1) *structural plasticity*, reflecting the interactions between the molecular biology of gene expression, cell migration, and neurogenesis in the developing brain; and (2) *synaptic plasticity*, the activity-dependent modelling of the pattern and strength of synaptic connections. This plasticity involves changes in the form, expression, and function of synapses that endure throughout life. Plasticity is an important functional attribute of connections in the brain and is thought to subserve perceptual and procedural learning and memory. A key aspect of this plasticity is that it is generally associative.

- *Associative plasticity.* Synaptic plasticity may be transient [e.g., short-term potentiation (STP) or depression (STD) or enduring, long-term potentiation (LTP) or (LTD)] with many different time constants. In contrast to short-term plasticity, long-term changes rely on protein synthesis, synaptic remodelling, and infrastructural changes in cell processes (e.g., terminal arbors or dendritic spines) that are mediated by calcium-dependent mechanisms. An important aspect of NMDA receptors, in the induction of LTP, is that they confer associatively on changes in connection strength. This is because their voltage sensitivity only allows calcium ions to enter the cell when there is conjoint presynaptic release of glutamate and sufficient postsynaptic depolarisation (i.e., the temporal association of pre- and postsynaptic events). Calcium entry renders the postsynaptic specialisation eligible for future potentiation by promoting the formation of synaptic "tags" (e.g., Frey and Morris, 1998) and other calcium-dependent intracellular mechanisms.

In summary, the anatomy and physiology of cortico-cortical connections suggest that forward connections are driving and commit cells to a prespecified response given the appropriate pattern of inputs. Backward connections, on the other hand, are less topographic and are in a position to modulate the responses of lower areas to driving inputs from either higher or lower areas (see Table 48.1). For example, in the visual cortex Angelucci *et al.* (2002a) used a combination of anatomical and physiological recording methods to determine the spatial scale and retinotopic logic of intra-areal V1 horizontal connections and interareal feedback connections to V1. "Contrary to common beliefs, these [monosynaptic horizontal] connections cannot fully account for the dimensions of the surround field [of macaque V1 neurons]. The spatial scale of feedback circuits from extrastriate cortex to V1 is, instead, commensurate with the full spatial range of centre-surround interactions. Thus these connections could represent an anatomical substrate for contextual modulation and global-to-local integration of visual signals."

Brain connections are not static but are changing at the synaptic level all the time. In many instances, this plasticity is associative. Backward connections are abundant in the brain and are in a position to exert powerful effects on evoked responses, in lower levels, that define the specialisation of any area or neuronal population. Modulatory effects imply that the postsynaptic response evoked by presynaptic input is modulated, or interacts with, another. By definition this interaction must depend on nonlinear synaptic or dendritic mechanisms.

Functional Integration and Effective Connectivity

Electrophysiology and imaging neuroscience have firmly established functional specialisation as a principle of brain organisation in man. The functional integration of specialised areas has proven more difficult to assess. Functional integration refers to the interactions among specialised neuronal populations and how these interactions depend on the sensorimotor or cognitive context. Functional integration is usually assessed by examining the correlations among activity in different brain areas, or trying to explain the activity in one area in relation to activities elsewhere. *Functional connectivity* is defined as correlations between remote neurophysiological events.[1] However, correlations can arise in a variety of ways. For example, in multiunit electrode recordings, they can result from stimulus-*locked* transients evoked by a common input or reflect stimulus-*induced* oscillations mediated by synaptic connections (Gerstein and Perkel, 1969). Integration within a distributed system is better understood in terms of *effective connectivity*. Effective connectivity refers explicitly to the influence that one neuronal system exerts over another, either at a synaptic (i.e., synaptic efficacy) or population level. It has been proposed that "the [electrophysiological] notion of effective connectivity should be understood as the

[1] More generally, any statistical dependency as measured by the mutual information.

experiment- and time-dependent, simplest possible circuit diagram that would replicate the observed timing relationships between the recorded neurons" (Aertsen and Preißl, 1991). This speaks to two important points: (1) Effective connectivity is dynamic, i.e., activity and time dependent, and (2) it depends on a model of the interactions. An important distinction, among models employed in functional neuroimaging, is whether these models are linear or nonlinear. Recent characterisations of effective connectivity have focused on nonlinear models that accommodate the modulatory or nonlinear effects mentioned above. A more detailed discussion of these models is provided in subsequent chapters, after the motivation for their application is established below. In this chapter, the terms *modulatory* and *nonlinear* are used almost synonymously. Modulatory effects imply the postsynaptic response evoked by one input is modulated, or interacts with, another. By definition this interaction must depend on nonlinear synaptic mechanisms.

In summary, the brain can be considered as an ensemble of functionally specialised areas that are coupled in a nonlinear fashion by effective connections. Empirically, it appears that connections from lower to higher areas are predominantly driving, whereas backward connections, which mediate top-down influences, are more diffuse and are capable of exerting modulatory influences. In the next section we describe a theoretical perspective, provided by "generative models," that highlights the functional importance of backward connections and nonlinear interactions.

REPRESENTATIONAL LEARNING

This section describes the heuristics behind self-supervised learning based on *empirical Bayes.* This approach is considered within the framework of *generative models* and follows Dayan and Abbott (2001, pp. 359–397) to which the reader is referred for more detailed background. A more heuristic discussion of these issues can be found in Friston (2002).

An important focus of this section is the interaction among causes of sensory input. These interactions create a problem of contextual invariance. In brief, it will be shown that this problem points to the adoption of generative models in which interactions among causes of a percept are modelled explicitly in backward connections. First, we will reprise empirical Bayes in the context of brain function per se. Having established the requisite architectures for representational learning, neuronal implementation is considered in sufficient depth to make predictions about the structural and functional anatomy that would be needed to implement empirical Bayes in the brain. We conclude by relating theoretical predictions with the four neurobiological principles listed in the previous section.

The Nature of Inputs, Causes, and Representations

Here a representation is taken to be a neuronal event that represents some "cause" in the sensorium. Causes are simply the states of processes generating sensory data or input. It is not easy to ascribe meaning to these states without appealing to the way we categorise things, perceptually or conceptually. High-level conceptual causes may be categorical in nature, such as the identity of a face in the visual field or the semantic category to which a perceived object belongs. In a hierarchical setting, high-level causes may induce priors on lower level causes that are more parametric in nature. For example, the perceptual cause "moving quickly" may show a one-to-many relationship with representations of different velocities in V5 (MT) units. Causes have relationships to each other (e.g., "is part of") that often have a hierarchical structure. This hierarchical ontology is attended by ambiguous many-to-one and one-to-many mappings (e.g., a table has legs but so do horses; a wristwatch is a watch irrespective of the orientation of its hands). This ambiguity can render the problem of inferring causes from sensory information underdetermined or ill posed.

Even though causes may be difficult to describe they are easy to define operationally. Causes are the variables or states that are necessary to specify the products of a process generating sensory information. To keep things simple, let us frame the problem of representing causes in terms of a deterministic nonlinear generative function:

$$u = G(v, \theta) \tag{48.1}$$

where v is a vector of underlying causes in the environment (e.g., the velocity of a particular object or the direction of radiant light), and u represents some sensory inputs. The term $G(v, \theta)$ is a function that generates inputs from the causes. Nonlinearities in Eq. (48.1) represent interactions among the causes. Second-order interactions are formally identical to interaction terms in conventional statistical models of observed data. These can often be viewed as contextual effects, where the expression of a particular cause depends on the context established by another. For example, the extraction of motion from the visual field depends on there being sufficient luminance or wavelength contrast to define the surface moving. Another ubiquitous example, from early visual processing, is the occlusion of one object by another. In the absence of interactions we would see a linear superposition of both objects but the visual input, caused by the nonlinear mixing of these two causes, renders one occluded by the other. At a more cognitive level, the cause associated with the word *HAMMER* will depend on the semantic context (which determines whether the word is a verb or a noun). These contextual effects are profound and must be discounted before the representations of the underlying causes can be considered veridical.

The problem the brain has to contend with is to find a function of the input that recognises or represents the underlying causes. To do this, the brain must effectively undo the interactions to disclose contextually invariant causes. In other words, the brain must perform some form of nonlinear unmixing of causes and context without knowing either. The key point here is that this nonlinear mixing may not be invertible and that the estimation of causes from input may be fundamentally ill posed. For example, no amount of unmixing can discern the parts of an object that are occluded by another. The mapping $u = v^2$ provides a trivial example of this non-invertibility. Knowing u does not uniquely determine v. The corresponding indeterminacy, in probabilistic learning, rests on the combinatorial explosion of ways in which stochastic generative models can generate input patterns (Dayan *et al.,* 1995). The combinatorial explosion represents another example of the uninvertible many-to-one relationship between causes and inputs.

In probabilistic learning one allows for stochastic components in the generation of inputs, and recognising a particular cause becomes probabilistic. Here the issue of deterministic invertibility is replaced by the existence of an inverse conditional probability (i.e., recognition) density that can be parameterised. Although not a mathematical fundament, parameterisation is critical for the brain because it has to encode the parameters of these densities with biophysical attributes of its nervous tissue. In what follows we consider the implications of this problem. In brief, we will show that one needs separate (approximate) recognition and generative models that induce the need for both forward and backward influences. Separate recognition and generative models resolve the problem caused by generating processes that are difficult to invert and speak to a possible role for backward connections in the brain.

Generative Models and Representational Learning

Generative models afford a generic formulation of representational leaning in a supervised or self-supervised context. There are many forms of generative models that range from conventional statistical models (e.g., factor and cluster analysis) to those motivated by Bayesian inference and learning (e.g., Dayan *et al.,* 1995, Hinton *et al.,* 1995). The goal of generative models is "to learn representations that are economical to describe but allow the input to be reconstructed accurately" (Hinton *et al.,* 1995). Representational learning is framed in terms of estimating probability densities of the causes. This is referred to as *posterior density analysis* in the estimation literature and *posterior mode analysis* if the inference is restricted to estimating the most likely cause (See Chapter 47). Although density learning is formulated at a level of abstraction that eschews many issues of neuronal implementation (e.g., the dynamics of real-time learning), it provides a unifying framework that connects the various schemes considered below.

Inference vs. Learning

Equation (48.1) relates the unknown state of the causes v and some unknown parameters θ, to observed inputs u. The objective is to make *inferences* about the causes and *learn* the parameters.

Inference may be simply estimating the most likely state of the causes and is based on the products of learning. A useful way of thinking about the distinction between inference and learning is in terms of how one accounts for the patterns or distribution of inputs encountered. Figure 48.1 shows a very simply example with a univariate cause and a bivariate observation. Observations are denoted by dots in the right-hand panel and cluster around a curvilinear line. A parsimonious way of generating dots like these would be move up and down the line and add a small amount of observation error. The position on the line corresponds to the state of the single cause and the probability of selecting a particular position to the probability density of the causes on the right. *Inference* means ascertaining the probability of each potential cause given an observation. *Estimation* refers to estimating the most likely cause, denoted in Fig. 48.1 by $\dot{v}$. This estimate is the closest point on the line to the observation that *a priori* has a reasonable probability of being selected. This simple example introduces the notion of representing observations in terms of points that lie on a low-dimensional manifold in observation space, in this case a line. The dimensions of this manifold are the causes. The shape and position of the manifold depends on the parameters θ. These have to be known or learned before inference about any particular observation can proceed. This learning requires multiple observations so that the manifold can be placed to transect the highest density of observations. In short, representational learning can be construed as learning a low-dimensional manifold onto which data can be projected with minimum loss of information. This manifold is an essential component of generative models.

The goal of learning is to acquire a recognition model for inference that is effectively the inverse of a generative model. Learning a generative model corresponds to making the density of the inputs, implied by a generative model $p(u;\theta)$, as close as possible to those observed $p(u)$. The generative model is specified in terms of a *prior* distribution over the causes $p(v;\theta)$ and the *generative* distribution or likelihood of the inputs given the causes $p(u \mid v;\theta)$. Together, these define the marginal distribution that has to be matched to the input distribution:

$$p(u;\theta) = \int p(u \mid v;\theta)\, p(u;\theta) dv \tag{48.2}$$

See Fig. 48.1. Once the parameters of the generative model have been learned, through this matching, the posterior density of the causes, given the inputs, are provided by the recognition model, which is defined in terms of the *recognition* distribution:

$$p(u \mid v;\theta) = \frac{p(u \mid v;\theta)p(v;\theta)}{p(u;\theta)} \tag{48.3}$$

However, as considered above, the generative model may not be easily inverted and it may not be possible to parameterise the recognition distribution. This is crucial because the endpoint

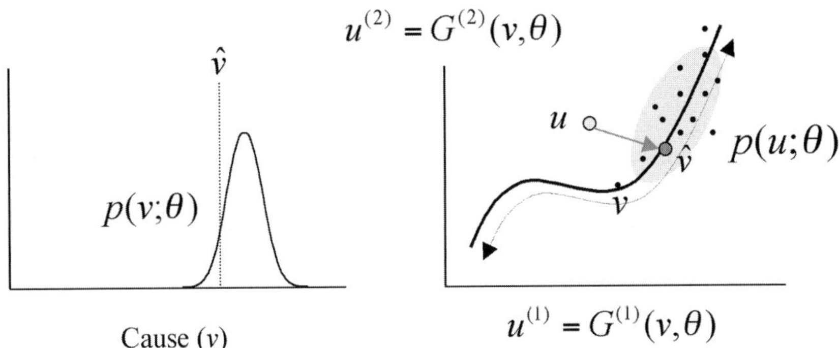

FIGURE 48.1
Schematic of a simple model with a univariate cause and a bivariate observation. Observations are denoted by dots in the right-hand panel and cluster around a curvilinear line. A parsimonious way of generating dots like these would be move up and down the line and add a small amount of random error. The position on the line corresponds to the state of the single cause and the probability of selecting a particular position the probability density of the causes on the right.

of learning is the acquisition of a useful recognition model that can be applied to sensory inputs. One solution is to posit an approximate recognition distribution $q(v;u, \phi)$ that is consistent with the generative model and that can be learned at the same time. The approximate recognition distribution has some parameters ϕ, for example, the strength of forward connections or its mode (i.e., most likely value). The first question addressed in this section is whether forward connections are sufficient for representational leaning.

Density Estimation and EM

In density learning, representational learning has two components that are framed in terms of expectation maximisation (EM) (Dempster *et al.,* 1977). Iterations of an **E**-step ensure that the recognition approximates the inverse of the generative model, and the **M**-step ensures that the generative model can predict the observed inputs. Probabilistic recognition proceeds by using $q(v;u, \phi)$ to determine the probability that v caused the observed sensory inputs. EM provides a useful procedure for density estimation that helps relate many different models within a framework that has direct connections with statistical mechanics. Both steps of the EM algorithm involve maximising a function of the densities that corresponds to the negative free energy in physics:

$$
\begin{aligned}
F &= \langle l(u) \rangle_u \\
l &= \int q(v;u,\phi) \ln \frac{p(v,u;\theta)}{p(v;u,\phi)} dv \\
&= \langle \ln p(v,u;\theta) \rangle_q - \langle \ln q(v;u,\phi) \rangle_q \\
&= \ln p(u;\theta) - KL\{q(v;u,\phi), p(v \mid u;\theta)\}
\end{aligned}
\tag{48.4}
$$

This objective function comprises two terms. The first is the expected log likelihood of the inputs under the generative model. The second term is the Kullback-Leibler (KL) divergence[2] between the approximating and true recognition densities. Critically, the KL term is always positive, rendering F a lower bound on the expected log likelihood of the inputs. Maximising F encompasses two components of representational learning: (1) It increases the likelihood of the inputs produced by the generative model and (2) it minimises the discrepancy between the approximate recognition model and that implied by the generative model. The **E**-step increases F with respect to the recognition parameters ϕ, ensuring a veridical approximation to the recognition distribution implied by the generative parameters ϕ. The **M**-step changes ϕ, enabling the generative model to reproduce the inputs:

$$
\begin{aligned}
&\mathbf{E} \quad \phi = \max_{\phi} F \\
&\mathbf{M} \quad \theta = \max_{\theta} F
\end{aligned}
\tag{48.5}
$$

There are a number of ways of motivating the free-energy formulation in Eq. (48.4). A useful one, in this context, rests on the problem posed by noninvertible models. This problem is finessed by assuming it is sufficient to match the joint probability of inputs and causes under the generative model $p(v,u;\theta) = p(u \mid v;\theta)\, p(v;\theta)$ with that implied by recognising the causes of inputs encountered $p(v,u;\phi) = q(v;u,\phi)\, p(u)$. Both of these distributions are well defined even when $p(v \mid u;\theta)$ is not easily parameterised. This matching minimises the divergence:

$$
\begin{aligned}
KL\{p(v,u;\phi), p(v,u;\theta) &= \int q(v;u,\phi) p(u) \ln \frac{q(v,u;\phi)\, p(u)}{p(v,u;\theta)} dvdu \\
&= -F - H(u)
\end{aligned}
\tag{48.6}
$$

This is equivalent to maximising F because the entropy of the inputs $H(u)$ is fixed. This perspective is used in Fig. 48.2 to illustrate the **E-** and **M**-steps schematically. The **E**-step adjusts the recognition parameters to match the two joint distributions, whereas the **M**-step does exactly the same thing but by changing the generative parameters. The dependency of the generative parameters, on the input distribution, is mediated vicariously in the **M**-step through the recog-

[2] A measure of the distance or difference between two probability densities.

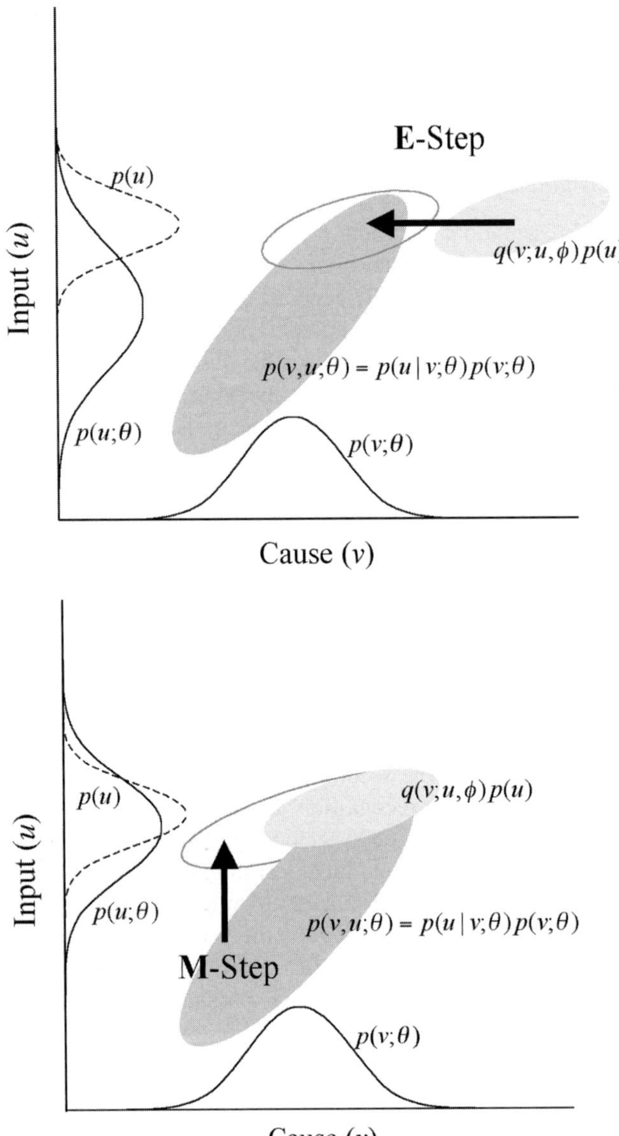

FIGURE 48.2
Schematic illustrating the two components of EM. In the **E**-step the joint distribution of causes and inputs under the recognition model changes to approximate that under the generative model. This refines the recognition model. In the **M**-step the joint distribution under the generative model changes to approximate that under the recognition model. This reduces the difference between the distribution of inputs implied by the generative model and that observed.

nition. In the setting of invertibility, where $q(v;u,\phi) = p(v \mid u;\theta)$, the divergence in Eq. (48.6) reduces to $\mathrm{K}\{p(u), p(u;\theta)\}$. As above, the **M**-step then finds parameters that allow the model to simply match the observed input distribution (i.e., maximise the expected likelihood).

Invertibility

This formulation of representational leaning is critical for the thesis of this section because it suggests that backward and lateral connections, parameterising a generative model, are essential when the model is not invertible. If the generative model is invertible, then the KL term in Eq. (48.4) can be discounted by setting $q(v;u,\phi) = p(v \mid u;\theta)$ with Eq. (48.3), and learning reduces to the **M**-step (i.e., maximising the expected likelihood):

$$\mathrm{F} = \langle \ln p(u;\theta) \rangle_u \tag{48.7}$$

In principle, this could be done using a feedforward architecture corresponding to the inverse of the generative model. However, when processes generating inputs are noninvertible (in terms of the parameterisation of the recognition density), a generative model and approximate recognition model are required that are updated in the **M**- and **E**-steps, respectively. In short, noninvertibility enforces an explicit parameterisation of the generative model in representational learning. In the brain this parameterisation may be embodied in backward connections.

Deterministic Recognition

Another special case arises when the recognition is deterministic. The recognition becomes deterministic when $q(v;u,\phi)$ is a Dirac δ function over its mode. In this instance, posterior density analysis reduces to a posterior mode analysis at which point inference and estimation coincide. They are equivalent in the sense that inferring the posterior distribution of causes is the same as estimating the most likely cause given the inputs (the maximum *a posteriori* or MAP estimator). Here the integral in Eq. (48.4) disappears, leaving the joint probability of the inputs and their cause to be maximised:

$$\begin{aligned} F &= \langle \ln p(v(u),u;\theta) \rangle_u \\ &= \langle \ln p(u \mid v(u);\theta) + \ln p(v(u);\theta) \rangle_u \end{aligned} \tag{48.8}$$

Notice, again, that this objective function does not require $p(v \mid u;\theta)$ and eschews the inversion in Eq. (48.3). (An illustration of the **E**-step for deterministic recognition is shown later in Fig. 48.4, lower panel.) Here, the distinction between deterministic and stochastic relates to inference and refers to the form of the recognition density. Note that learning could also employ a deterministic or stochastic ascent on F. We will deal largely with deterministic learning schemes.

Summary

EM enables exact and approximate maximum-likelihood density estimation for a whole variety of generative models that can be specified in terms of prior and generative distributions. Dayan and Abbott (2001) work through a series of didactic examples, from cluster analysis to independent component analyses, within this unifying framework. For example, factor analysis corresponds to the following generative model:

$$\begin{aligned} p(v;\theta) &= N(v:0,1) \\ p(u \mid v;\theta) &= N(u:\theta v,\Sigma) \end{aligned} \tag{48.9}$$

Namely, the underlying causes of inputs are independent normal variates that are mixed linearly and added to Gaussian noise to form inputs. In the limiting case of $\Sigma \to 0$, the ensuing model becomes deterministic and conforms to PCA. By simply assuming non-Gaussian priors, one can specify generative models for sparse coding of the sort proposed by Olshausen and Field (1996):

$$\begin{aligned} p(v;\theta) &= \prod p(v_i;\theta) \\ p(u \mid v;\theta) &= N(u:\theta v,\Sigma) \end{aligned} \tag{48.10}$$

where $p(v_i;\theta)$ are chosen to be suitably sparse (i.e., heavy tailed) with a cumulative density function that corresponds to the squashing function described in Chapter 49. The deterministic equivalent of sparse coding is ICA, which is obtained when $\Sigma \to 0$. The relationships among different models are rendered apparent under the perspective of generative models. In what follows we consider a hierarchical models and the requisite EM steps. We then consider whether they could be implemented plausibly in the brain.

Cortical Hierarchies and Empirical Bayes

Empirical Bayes harnesses the hierarchical structure of a generative model, treating the estimates at one level as prior expectations for the subordinate level (Efron and Morris, 1973). This provides a natural framework within which to treat cortical hierarchies in the brain, each providing constraints on the level below. This approach models the world as a hierarchy of systems where supraordinate causes induce—and moderate—changes in subordinate causes. For

Jack and Jill went up the hill
The last event was cancelled

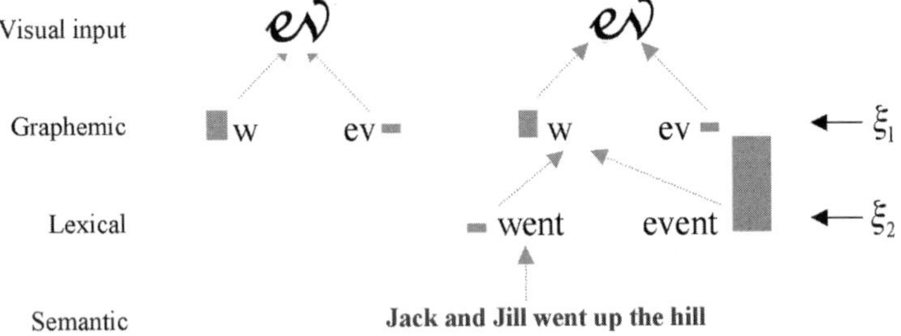

FIGURE 48.3
Schematic illustrating the role of priors in biasing toward one representation of an input or another. (Upper panel) On reading the first sentence "Jack and Jill went up the hill" we perceive the word *event* as *went* despite the fact it is *event* (as in the second sentence). However, in the absence of any hierarchical inference, the best explanation for the pattern of visual stimulation incurred by the text is the grapheme *ev*. This would correspond to the ML estimate and would be the most appropriate in the absence of prior information, from the lexical and semantic context, about which is the most likely grapheme. However, within hierarchical inference the semantics (provided by the sentence) provides top-down predictions about the word, which in turn predicts the graphemes and finally the visual input. The posterior estimate is accountable to all of these levels. When the semantic prior biases in favour of *went* and *w*, we tolerate a small error as a lower level of visual analysis to minimise the overall prediction error. (Lower panel, left) The grapheme *ev* is selected as the most likely cause of visual input. (Lower panel, right) The letter *w* is selected, because it is (1) a reasonable explanation for the sensory input and (2) it conforms to prior expectations induced by lexico-semantic context. The bars represent prediction error, which is minimised over all levels to attain the most likely cause.

example, the presence of a particular object in the visual field changes the incident light falling on a particular part of the retina. A more intuitive example is provided in Fig. 48.3. These priors offer contextual guidance toward the most likely cause of the input. Note that predictions at higher levels are subject to the same constraints; only the highest level, if there is one in the brain, is free to be directed solely by bottom-up influences (although there are always implicit priors). If the brain has evolved to recapitulate the casual structure of its environment, in terms of its sensory infrastructures, it is interesting to reflect on the possibility that our visual cortices reflect the hierarchical casual structure of our environment.

The Nature of Hierarchical Models

Consider any level i in a hierarchy whose causes v_i are induced by corresponding causes in the level above v_{i+1}. The hierarchical form of the implicit generative model is

$$\begin{aligned} u &= G_1(v_2,\theta_1) + \varepsilon_1 \\ v_2 &= G_2(v_3,\theta_2) + \varepsilon_2 \\ v_3 &= \ldots \end{aligned} \tag{48.11}$$

with $u = v_1$ [cf. Eq. (48.1)]. Technically, these models fall into the class of conditionally independent hierarchical models when the stochastic terms are independent at each level (Kass and Steffey, 1989). These models are also called *parametric empirical Bayes* (PEB) models because the obvious interpretation of the higher level densities as priors led to the development of PEB methodology (Efron and Morris, 1973). Often, in statistics, these hierarchical models comprise just two levels, which is a useful way to specify simple shrinkage priors on the parameters of single-level models. We will assume the stochastic terms are Gaussian with covariance $\Sigma_i = \Sigma(\lambda_i)$. Therefore, θ_i and λ_i parameterise the means and covariances of the likelihood at each level:

$$p(v_1 \mid v_{i+1};\theta) = N(v_i : G_i(v_{i+1},\theta_i),\Sigma_i) \tag{48.12}$$

This likelihood of v_i also plays the role of a prior on v_{i-1} that is jointly maximised with the likelihood of the level below $p(v_{i-1} \mid v_i;\theta)$. This is the key to understanding the utility of

Hierarchical models

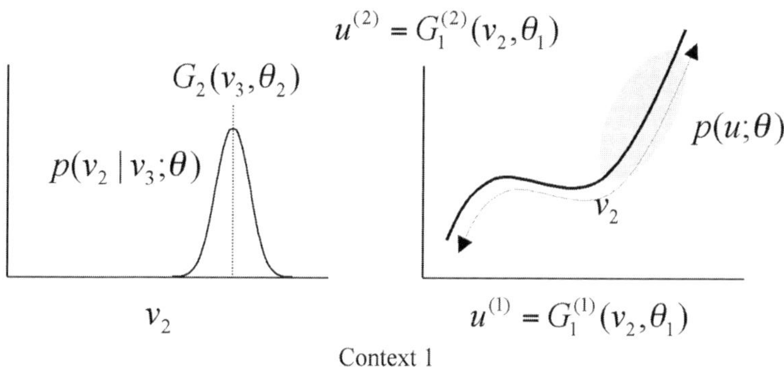

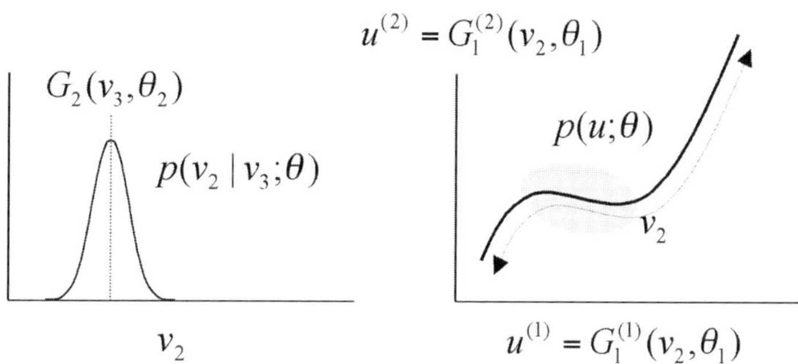

FIGURE 48.4
Hierarchical models embody context sensitivity not found in single-level models (cf. Fig. 48.1). High-level causes v_{i+1} determine the prior expectation of causes v_i in the subordinate level. Changes in v_{i+1} can completely change the marginal $p(v_{i-1};\theta)$ and recognition $p(v_i|v_{i-1};\theta)$ distributions on which inference in based.

hierarchical models: by learning the parameters of the generative distribution of level i one is implicitly learning the parameters of the prior distribution for level i–1. This enables this learning of prior densities.

The hierarchical nature of these models lends an important context sensitivity to recognition densities not found in single-level models. This is illustrated in Fig. 48.4, which should be compared with Fig. 48.1. The key point here is that high-level causes v_{i+1} determine the prior expectation of causes v_i in the subordinate level. This can completely change the marginal and recognition $p(v_i \mid v_{i-1};\theta)$ distributions on which inference in based. From the manifold perspective on inference, the part of the manifold $G_{i-1}(v_i;\theta_{i-1})$ highlighted by prior expectations changes from input to input in a context-dependent way (see Fig. 48.4). The context established by priors is not determined by preceding events but is immediate and conferred by higher hierarchical levels. For example, in Fig. 48.3, the semantic context induced by reading one of the sentences has a profound effect on the most likely graphemic cause of the visual input subtended by *ev*. The dual role of $p(v_i \mid v_{i+1};\theta)$ as a likelihood or generative density for level i and a prior density for level $i - 1$ is recapitulated by a dual role for MAP estimates of v_i. From a bottom-up perspective, these correspond to parameters (modes) of the recognition densities. However, from a top-down perspective they also act as parameters of the generative model by interacting with θ_{i-1} in $G_{i-1}(v_i,\theta_{i-1})$ to give the prior expectation of v_{i-1}.

Although λ_i are parameters of the forward model we have referred to as hyperparameters in previous chapters, in classical statistics they correspond to variance components. We preserve the distinction between θ_i and λ_i because they may correspond to backward and lateral connections strengths, respectively.

Implementation

The biological plausibility of the empirical Bayes in the brain can be established fairly simply. To do this, a hierarchical scheme is described in some detail. For the moment, we will address neuronal implementation at a purely theoretical and somewhat heuristic level, using the framework developed above.

For simplicity, we will assume deterministic recognition such that $q(\phi(u); u) = 1$. In this setting, with conditional independence, F comprises a series of log likelihoods:

$$\begin{aligned} l(u) &= \langle \ln p(u,v;\theta)\rangle_q = \ln p(u,\phi_2,\ldots;\theta) \\ &= \ln p(u \mid \phi_2;\theta) + \ln(\phi_2 \mid \phi_3;\theta) + \ldots \\ &= -\frac{1}{2}\xi_1^T\xi_1 - \frac{1}{2}\xi_2^T\xi_2 - \ldots - \frac{1}{2}\ln|\Sigma_1| - \frac{1}{2}\ln|\Sigma_2| - \ldots \\ \xi_i &= \phi_i - G_i(\phi_{i+1},\theta_i) - \lambda_i\xi_i \\ &= (1+\lambda_i)^{-1}(\phi_i - G_i(\phi_{i+1},\theta_i)) \end{aligned} \tag{48.13}$$

Here $\Sigma_i^{1/2} = 1 + \lambda_i$. In the setting of neuronal models, the (whitened) prediction error is encoded by the activities of units denoted by ξ_i. These error units receive a prediction from units in the level above[3] and connections from the principal units ϕ_i being predicted. Horizontal interactions among the error units serve to decorrelate them, where the symmetric lateral connection strengths λ_i hyperparameterise the covariances of the errors Σ_i, which are the prior covariances for level $i - 1$.

The estimators ϕ_i and the connection strength parameters perform a gradient ascent on the compound log probability:

$$\begin{aligned} &\mathbf{E} \qquad \dot{\phi}_{i+1} = \frac{\partial l(u)}{\partial \phi_{i+1}} = -\frac{\partial \xi_i^T}{\partial \phi_{i+1}}\xi_i - \frac{\partial \xi_{i+1}^T}{\partial \phi_{i+1}}\xi_{i+1} \\ &\mathbf{M} \qquad \dot{\theta}_i = \frac{\partial F}{\partial \theta_i} = -\left\langle \frac{\partial \xi_i^T}{\partial \theta_i}\xi \right\rangle_u \\ &\qquad\quad\;\; \dot{\lambda}_i = \frac{\partial F}{\partial \lambda_i} = -\left\langle \frac{\partial \xi_i^T}{\partial \lambda_i}\xi \right\rangle_u - (1+\lambda_i)^{-1} \end{aligned} \tag{48.14}$$

Each of the learning components has a relatively simple neuronal interpretation (see below).

Implications for Neuronal Implementation

The scheme implied by Eq. (48.14) has four clear implications or predictions about the functional architectures required for its implementation. We now review these in relation to cortical organisation in the brain. A schematic summarising these points in provided in Fig. 48.5. In short, we arrive at exactly the same four points presented in the previous section:

- *Hierarchical organisation.* Hierarchical models enable empirical Bayesian learning of prior densities and provide a plausible model for sensory inputs. Single-level models that do not show any conditional independence (e.g., those used by connectionist and infomax schemes) depend on prior constraints for unique inference and do not call on a hierarchical cortical organisation. On the other hand, if the causal structure of generative processes is hierarchical, this will be reflected, literally, by the hierarchical architectures trying to minimise prediction error, not just at the level of sensory input but at all levels (notice the deliberate mirror symmetry in Fig. 48.5). The nice thing about this architecture is that the responses of units at the ith level ϕ_i depend only on the error for the current level and the immediately preceding level. This follows from conditional independence and is important because it permits a biologically plausible implementation, where the connections driving the error minimisation only run forward from one level to the next.
- *Reciprocal connections.* As established at the beginning of this section, the noninvertibility of processes generating sensory data induces a need for both forward and backward connections.

[3] Clearly, in the brain, backward connections are not inhibitory but, after mediation by inhibitory interneurons, their effective influence could be rendered so.

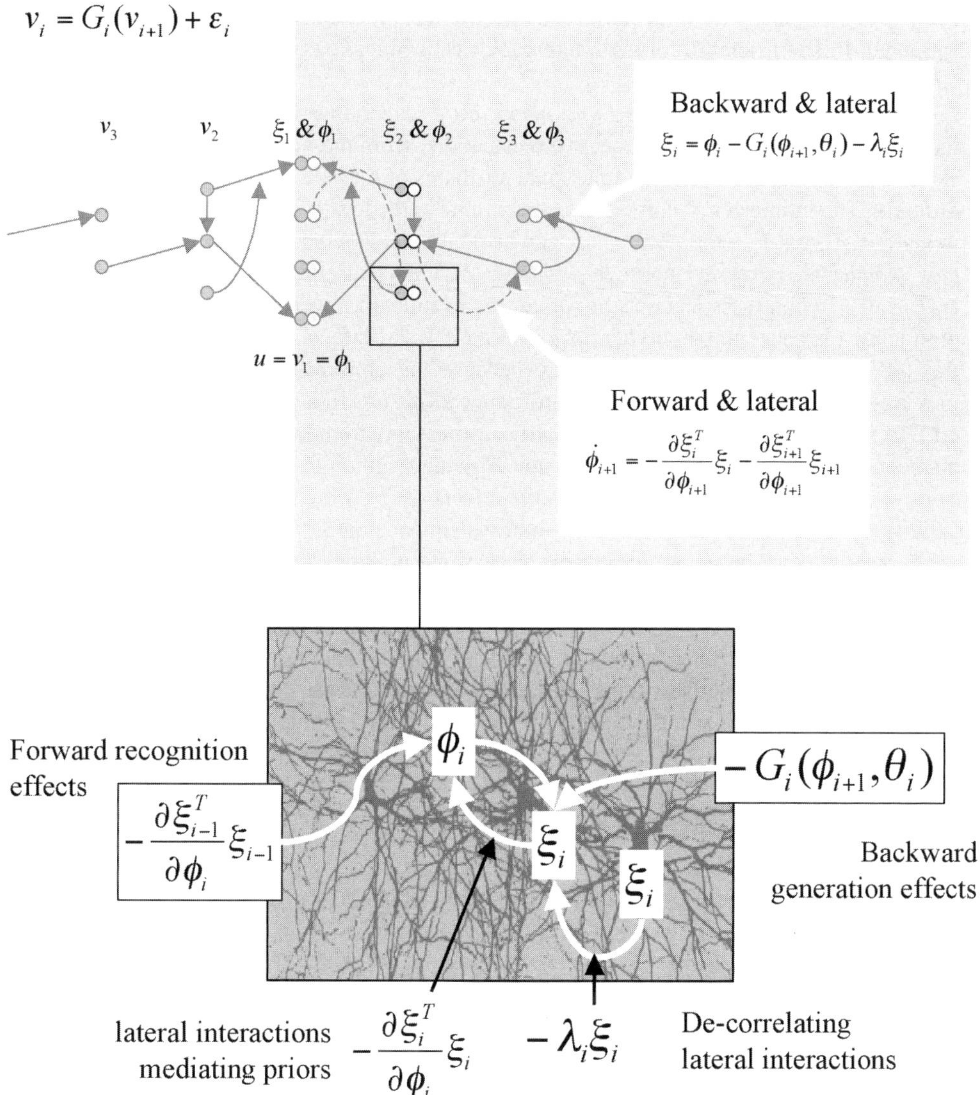

FIGURE 48.5
(Upper panel) Schematic depicting a hierarchical extension to the predictive coding architecture. Hierarchical arrangements within the model serve to provide predictions or priors to representations in the level below. The open circles are the error units and the filled circles are the states encoding the conditional expectation of causes in the environment. These change to minimise both the discrepancies between their predicted value and the mismatch incurred by their own prediction of the level below. These two constraints correspond to prior and likelihood terms, respectively (see main text). (Lower panel) A more detailed picture of the influences on principal and error units.

In the hierarchical model, the dynamics of principal units ϕ_{i+1} are subject to two, locally available influences: a likelihood or recognition term mediated by forward afferents from the error units in the level below and an empirical prior conveyed by error units in the same level. Critically, the influences of the error units in both levels are meditated by linear connections with a strength that is exactly the same as the (negative) effective connectivity of the *reciprocal* connections from ϕ_{i+1} to ξ_i and ξ_{i+1}. Functionally, forward and lateral connections are reciprocated, whereas backward connections generate predictions of lower level responses. Effective connectivity is simply the change in a neuronal unit (neuron, assembly or cortical area) induced by inputs from another (Friston, 1995). In this case $\partial\xi_i/\partial\phi_{i+1}$ and $\partial\xi_{i+1}/\partial\phi_{i+1}$.

Effective connectivity in the forward direction is the reciprocal (negative transpose) of that in the backward direction $\partial\xi_i/\partial\phi_{i+1} = -\partial G_i(\phi_{i+1}, \beta_i)_i/\partial v_{i+1}$ that is a function of the generative parameters. Lateral connections, within each level, mediate the influence of error units on the principal units, and intrinsic connections λ_i among the error units decorrelate them, allowing competition among prior expectations with different precisions (precision is the inverse of variance). In short, lateral, forward, and backward connections are all reciprocal, consistent with anatomical observations.

- *Functionally asymmetric forward and backward connections.* The forward connections are the reciprocal of the backward effective connectivity from the higher level to the lower level, extant at that time. However, the functional attributes of forward and backward influences are different. The influences of units ϕ_{i+1} on error units in the lower level ξ_i instantiate the forward model $\xi_i = \phi_i - G_i(\phi_{i+1}, \theta_i) - \lambda_i\xi_i$. These can be nonlinear, in which each unit in the higher level *may modulate or interact with the influence of others*, according to the nonlinearities in $G_i(\phi_{i+1}, \theta_i)$. In contradistinction, the influences of units in lower levels do not interact when producing changes in the higher level because their effects are linearly separable [see Eq. (48.14)]. This is a key observation because the empirical evidence, reviewed in the previous section, suggests that backward connections are in a position to interact (through NMDA receptors expressed predominantly in the supragranular layers receiving backward connections). Forward connections are not. Note that, although the implied forward connections $-\partial\xi_i/\partial\phi_{i+1}{}^T$ mediate linearly separable effects of ξ_i on ϕ_{i+1}, these connections might be activity and time dependent because of their dependence on ϕ_{i+1}. In summary, nonlinearities, in the way sensory inputs are produced, necessitate nonlinear interactions in the generative model that are mediated by backward influences but do not require forward connections to be modulatory.
- *Associative plasticity.* Changes in the parameters correspond to plasticity in the sense that the parameters control the strength of backward and lateral connections. The backward connections parameterise the prior expectations of the forward model, and the lateral connections hyperparameterise the prior covariances. Together they parameterise the Gaussian densities that constitute the priors (and likelihoods) of the model. The plasticity implied can be seen more clearly with an explicit parameterisation of the connections. For example, let $G_i(v_{i+1}, \theta_i) = \theta_i v_{i+1}$. In this instance,

$$\begin{aligned} \dot{\theta}_i &= (1 + \lambda_i)^{-1}\left\langle \xi_i \phi_{i+1}^T \right\rangle_u \\ \dot{\lambda}_i &= (1 + \lambda_i)^{-1}\left(\left\langle \xi_i \xi_i^T \right\rangle_u - 1\right) \end{aligned} \tag{48.15}$$

This is just Hebbian or associative plasticity where the connection strengths change in proportion to the product of pre- and postsynaptic activity. An intuition about Eq. (48.15) is obtained by considering the conditions under which the expected change in parameters is zero (i.e., after learning). For the backward connections this implies that there is no component of prediction error that can be explained by estimates at the higher level $\langle \xi_i \phi_{i+1}^T \rangle = 0$. The lateral connections stop changing when the prediction error has been whitened $\langle \xi_i \xi_i^T \rangle = 1$.

It is evident that the predictions of the theoretical analysis coincide almost exactly with the empirical aspects of functional architectures in visual cortices highlighted by the previous section (hierarchical organisation, reciprocity, functional asymmetry, and associative plasticity). Although somewhat contrived, it is pleasing that purely theoretical considerations and neurobiological empiricism converge so precisely.

GENERATIVE MODELS AND THE BRAIN

In summary, generative models lend themselves naturally to a hierarchical treatment, which considers the brain as an empirical Bayesian device. The dynamics of the units or populations are driven to minimise prediction error at all levels of the cortical hierarchy and implicitly render themselves posterior modes of the causes given the data. The overall scheme implied by Eq. (48.14) sits comfortably with the hypothesis (Mumford, 1992): "On the role of the reciprocal, topographic pathways between two cortical areas, one often a 'higher' area dealing with more abstract information about the world, the other 'lower,' dealing with more concrete data. The higher area attempts to fit its abstractions to the data it receives from lower areas by sending back to them from its deep pyramidal cells a template reconstruction best fitting the lower level view. The lower area attempts to reconcile the reconstruction of its view that it receives from higher areas with what it knows, sending back from its superficial pyramidal cells the features in its data which are not predicted by the higher area. The whole calculation is done with all areas working simultaneously, but with order imposed by synchronous activity in the various top-down, bottom-up loops."

Context, Causes, and Representations

The Bayesian perspective suggests something quite profound for the classical view of receptive fields. If neuronal responses encompass a bottom-up likelihood term and top-down priors, then responses evoked by bottom-up input should change with the context established by prior expectations from higher levels of processing. Consider the example in Fig. 48.3. Here a unit encoding the visual form of *went* responds when we read the first sentence at the top of this figure. When we read the second sentence "The last event was cancelled," it would not. If we recorded from this unit we might infer that our *went* unit was, in some circumstances, selective for the word *event.* This might be difficult to explain without an understanding of hierarchical inference and the semantic context in which the stimulus was presented. In short, under a predictive coding scheme, the receptive fields of neurons should be context sensitive. The remainder of this subsection deals with empirical evidence for these extra-classical receptive field effects.

Generative models suggest that the role of backward connections is to provide contextual guidance to lower levels through a prediction of the lower level's inputs. When this prediction is incomplete or incompatible with the lower area's input, an error is generated that engenders changes in the area above until reconciliation. When, and only when, the bottom-up driving inputs are in harmony with top-down prediction, error is suppressed and a consensus between the prediction and the actual input is established. Given this conceptual model, a stimulus-related response or "activation" corresponds to some transient error signal that drives the appropriate change in higher areas until a veridical higher level representation emerges and the error is "cancelled" by backward connections. Clearly the prediction error will depend on the context, and consequently the backward connections confer context sensitivity on the functional specificity of the lower area. In short, the activation does not just depend on bottom-up input, but on the difference between bottom-up input and top-down predictions.

The prevalence of nonlinear or modulatory top-down effects can be inferred from the fact that context interacts with the content of representations. Here context is established simply through the expression of causes other than the one in question. Backward connections from one higher area can be considered as providing contextual modulation of the prediction from another area. Because the effect of context will only be expressed when the thing being predicted is present, these contextual afferents should not elicit a response by themselves. Effects of this sort, which change the responsiveness of units but do not elicit a response, are a hallmark of modulatory projections. In summary, hierarchical models offer a scheme that allows for contextual effects; first through biasing responses toward their prior expectation and, second, by conferring a context sensitivity on these priors through the modulatory component of backward projections. Next we consider the nature of real neuronal responses and whether they are consistent with this perspective.

Extra-Classical and Context-Sensitive Effects

Classical models (e.g., classical receptive fields) assume that evoked responses will be expressed invariably in the same units or neuronal populations irrespective of the context. However, real neuronal responses are not invariant but depend on the context in which they are evoked. For example, visual cortical units have dynamic receptive fields that can change from moment to moment [cf. the nonclassical receptive field effects modelled by Rao and Ballard (1999)]. A useful synthesis of data for the macaque visual system that highlights the anatomical and physiological substrates of context-dependent responses can be found in Angelucci *et al.*

(2002b). A key conclusion of the authors is that "feedback from extrastriate cortex (possibly together with overlap or interdigitation of coactive lateral connectional fields within V1) can provide a large and stimulus-specific surround modulatory field. The stimulus specificity of the interactions between the centre and surround fields, may be due to the orderly, matching structure and different scales of intra-areal and feedback projection excitatory pathways."

Numerous examples of context-sensitive neuronal responses exist. Perhaps the simplest is short-term plasticity. *Short-term plasticity* refers to changes in connection strength, either potentiation or depression, following presynaptic inputs (e.g., Abbott *et al.,* 1997). In brief, the underlying connection strengths, which define what a unit represents, are a strong function of the immediately preceding neuronal transient (i.e., preceding representation). A second, and possibly richer, example is that of attentional modulation, which can change the sensitivity of neurons to different perceptual attributes (e.g., Treue and Maunsell, 1996). It has been shown, both in single unit recordings in primates (Treue and Maunsell, 1996) and in human functional fMRI studies (Büchel and Friston, 1997), that attention to specific visual attributes can profoundly alter the receptive fields or event-related responses to the same stimuli.

These sorts of effects are commonplace in the brain and are generally understood in terms of the dynamic modulation of receptive field properties by backward and lateral afferents. There is clear evidence that lateral connections in visual cortex are modulatory in nature (Hirsch and Gilbert, 1991), speaking to an interaction between the functional segregation implicit in the columnar architecture of V1 and the neuronal dynamics in distal populations. These observations suggest that lateral and backward interactions may convey contextual information that shapes the responses of any neuron to its inputs (e.g., Kay and Phillips, 1996; Phillips and Singer, 1997) to confer on the brain the ability to make conditional inferences about sensory input. McIntosh (2000) develops the idea from a cognitive neuroscience perspective "that a particular region in isolation may not act as a reliable index for a particular cognitive function. Instead, the *neural context* in which an area is active may define the cognitive function." His argument is predicated on careful characterisations of effective connectivity using neuroimaging.

Conclusion

In conclusion, the representational capacity and inherent function of any neuron, neuronal population, or cortical area in the brain is dynamic and context sensitive. Functional integration, or interactions among brain systems, which employ driving (bottom-up) and backward (top-down) connections, mediate this adaptive and contextual specialisation. Most models of representational learning require prior assumptions about the distribution of causes. However, empirical Bayes suggests that these assumptions can be relaxed and that priors can be learned in a hierarchical context. We have tried to show that this hierarchical prediction can be implemented in brainlike architectures and in a biologically plausible fashion.

A key point, made above, is that backward connections, mediating internal or generative models of how sensory inputs are caused, are essential if the processes generating inputs are difficult to invert. This noninvertibility demands an explicit parameterisation of both the generative model (backward connections) and approximate recognition (forward connections). This suggests that feedforward architectures are not sufficient for representational learning or perception. Moreover, nonlinearities in generative models, which make backward connections necessary, require these connections to be modulatory, so that estimated causes in higher cortical levels can interact to predict responses in lower levels. This is important in relation to asymmetries in forward and backward connections that have been characterised empirically.

The arguments in this section were developed under hierarchical models of brain function, where high-level systems provide a prediction of the inputs to lower levels. Conflict between the two is resolved by changes in the high-level representations, which are driven by the ensuing error in lower regions, until the mismatch is "cancelled." From this perspective the specialisation of any region is determined both by bottom-up driving inputs and by top-down predictions. Specialisation is therefore not an intrinsic property of any region but depends on both forward and backward connections with other areas. Because the latter have access to the context in which the inputs are generated, they are in a position to modulate the selectivity or specialisation of lower areas. The implications for classical models (e.g., classical receptive fields in electrophysiology, classical specialisation in neuroimaging, and connectionism in cognitive models) are severe and suggest that these models may provide incomplete accounts of real brain architectures. On the other hand, representational learning, in the context of hierarchical generative models, not only accounts for extra-classical phenomena seen empirically but enforces a view of the brain as an inferential machine through its empirical Bayesian motivation.

ASSESSING FUNCTIONAL ARCHITECTURES WITH BRAIN IMAGING

Clearly, it would be nice to demonstrate the existence of backward influences with neuroimaging. This is a slightly deeper problem than might be envisaged. This is because making causal inferences about effective connectivity is not straightforward (see Pearl, 2000). It might be thought that showing that regional activity was partially predicted by activity in a higher level would be sufficient to confirm the existence of backward influences, at least at a population level. The problem is that this statistical dependency does not permit any causal inference. Statistical dependencies could easily arise in a purely forward architecture because the higher level activity is predicated on activity in the lower level. One resolution of this problem is to perturb the higher level directly, using transmagnetic stimulation or pathological disruptions (see below). However, discounting these interventions, one is left with the difficult problem of inferring backward influences, based on measures that could be correlated because of forward connections. Although causal modelling techniques are available that can address this problem, we take a simpler approach and note that interactions between bottom-up and top-down influences cannot be explained by a purely feedforward architecture. This is because the top-down influences have no access to the bottom-up inputs. An interaction, in this context, can be construed as an effect of backward connections on the driving efficacy of forward connections. In other words, the response evoked by the same driving bottom-up inputs depends on the context established by top-down inputs. This interaction is used below simply as evidence for the existence of backward influences. Some instances of predictive coding emphasise this phenomenon. For example, the "Kalman filter model demonstrates how certain forms of attention can be viewed as an emergent property of the interaction between top-down expectations and bottom-up signals" (Rao, 1999).

The remainder of this chapter focuses on the evidence for these interactions. From the point of view of functionally specialised responses, these interactions manifest as context sensitive or contextual specialisation, where modality-, category- or exemplar-specific responses, driven by bottom-up inputs, are modulated by top-down influences induced by perceptual set. The first half of this section adopts this perceptive. The second part of this section uses measurements of effective connectivity to establish interactions between bottom-up and top-down influences. All examples presented below rely on attempts to establish interactions by trying to change sensory-evoked neuronal responses through putative manipulations of top-down influences. These include inducing independent changes in perceptual set, cognitive (attentional) set, and, in the last section, through the study of patients with brain lesions.

Context-Sensitive Specialisation

If functional specialisation is context dependent, then one should be able to find evidence for functionally specific responses, using neuroimaging, that are expressed in one context and not in another. The first part of this section provides an empirical example. If the contextual nature of specialisation is mediated by backward modulatory afferents, then it should be possible to find cortical regions in which functionally specific responses, elicited by the same stimuli, are modulated by activity in higher areas. The second example shows that this is indeed possible. Both of these examples depend on multifactorial experimental designs.

Multifactorial Designs

Factorial designs combine two or more factors within a task or tasks. Factorial designs can be construed as performing subtraction experiments in two or more different contexts. The

Regionally-specific interactions

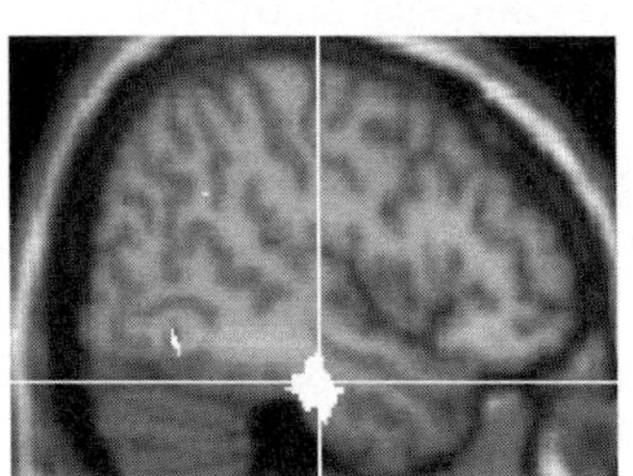

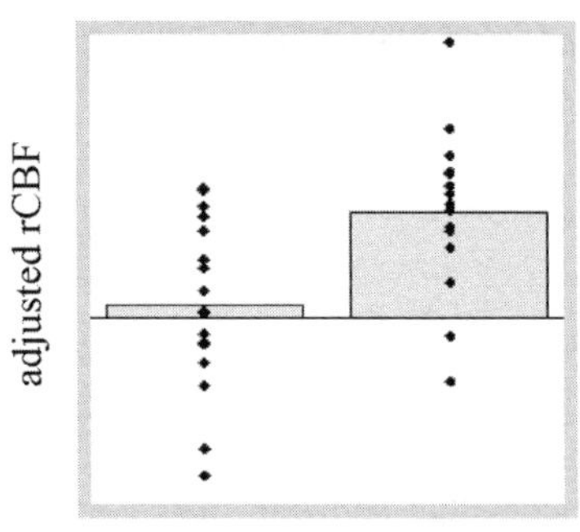

FIGURE 48.6
This example of regionally specific interactions comes from an experiment in which subjects were asked to view coloured nonobject shapes or coloured objects and say "yes," or to name either the coloured object or the colour of the shape. (Left) A regionally specific interaction in the left inferotemporal cortex. The SPM threshold is $p > 0.05$ (uncorrected). (Right) The corresponding activities in the maxima of this region are portrayed in terms of object recognition-dependent responses with and without naming. It is seen that this region shows object recognition responses when, and only when, there is phonological retrieval. The "extra" activation with naming corresponds to the interaction. These data were acquired from six subjects scanned 12 times using PET.

differences in activations, attributable to the effects of context, are simply the interaction. Consider an implicit object recognition experiment, for example, naming (of the object's name or the nonobject's colour) and simply saying "yes" during passive viewing of objects and nonobjects. The factors in this example are implicit object recognition with two levels (objects vs. nonobjects) and phonological retrieval (naming vs. saying "yes"). The idea here is to look at the interaction between these factors, or the effect that one factor has on the responses elicited by changes in the other. Noting that object-specific responses are elicited (by asking subjects to view objects relative to meaningless shapes), with and without phonological retrieval, reveals the factorial nature of this experiment. This "2 × 2" design allows one to look specifically at the interaction between phonological retrieval and object recognition. This analysis identifies not regionally specific activations but regionally specific *interactions*. When we actually performed this experiment, these interactions were evident in the left posterior, inferior temporal region and can be associated with the integration of phonology and object recognition (see Fig. 48.6 and Friston *et al.,* 1996, for details). Alternatively, this region can be thought of as expressing recognition-dependent responses that are realised in, and only in, the context of having to name the object seen. These results can be construed as evidence of contextual specialisation for object-recognition that depends on modulatory afferents (possibly from temporal and parietal regions) that are implicated in naming a visually perceived object. There is no empirical evidence in these results to suggest that the temporal or parietal regions are the source of this top-down influence, but in the next example the source of modulation is addressed explicitly using psychophysiological interactions.

Psychophysiological Interactions

Psychophysiological interactions speak directly to the interactions between bottom-up and top-down influences, where one is modelled as an experimental factor and the other constitutes a measured brain response. In an analysis of psychophysiological interactions, one is trying to explain a regionally specific response in terms of an interaction between the presence of a sensorimotor or cognitive process and activity in another part of the brain (Friston *et al.,* 1997). The supposition here is that the remote region is the source of backward modulatory afferents that confer functional specificity on the target region. For example, by combining information

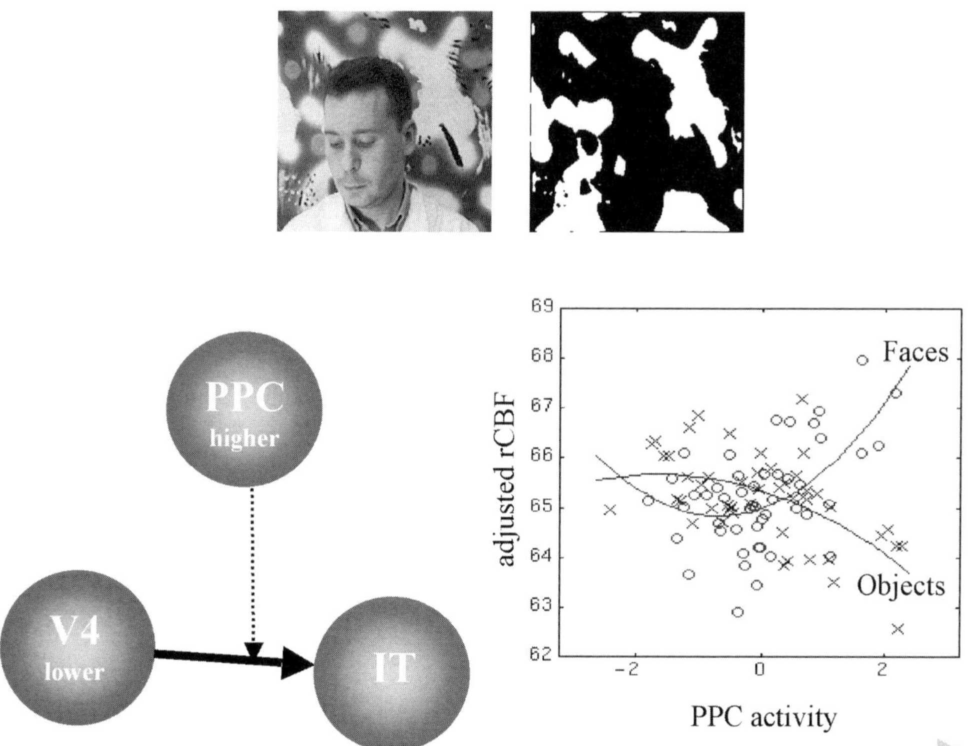

FIGURE 48.7
(Top) Examples of the stimuli presented to subjects. During the measurement of brain responses only degraded stimuli where shown (e.g., the right-hand picture). In half the scans the subject was given the underlying cause of these stimuli, through presentation of the original picture (e.g., left) before scanning. This priming induced a profound difference in perceptual set for the primed, relative to nonprimed, stimuli. (Bottom left) Schematic depicting the underlying conceptual model in which driving afferents from ventral form areas (here designated as V4) that excite inferotemporal (IT) responses, subject to permissive modulation by PPC projections. (Bottom right) Activity observed in a right inferotemporal region, as a function of mean corrected PPC activity. This region showed the most significant interaction between the presence of faces in visually presented stimuli and activity in a reference location in the posterior medial parietal cortex (PPC). This analysis can be thought of as finding those areas that are subject to top-down modulation of face-specific responses by medial parietal activity. The crosses correspond to activity while viewing nonface stimuli and the circles to faces. The essence of this effect can be seen by noting that this region differentiates between faces and nonfaces when, and only when, medial parietal activity is high. The lines correspond to the best second-order polynomial fit. These data were acquired from six subjects using PET.

about activity in the posterior parietal cortex, mediating attentional or perceptual set pertaining to a particular stimulus attribute, can we identify regions that respond to that stimulus when, and only when, activity in the parietal source is high? If such an interaction exists, then one might infer that the parietal area is modulating responses to the stimulus attribute for which the area is selective. This has clear ramifications in terms of the top-down modulation of specialised cortical areas by higher brain regions.

The statistical model employed in testing for psychophysiological interactions is a simple regression model of effective connectivity that embodies nonlinear (second-order or modulatory) effects. As such, this class of model speaks directly to functional specialisation of a nonlinear and contextual sort. Figure 48.7 illustrates a specific example (see Dolan *et al.,* 1997 for details). Subjects were asked to view degraded faces and nonface (object) controls. The interaction between activity in the parietal region and the presence of faces was expressed most significantly in the right inferotemporal region not far from the homologous left inferotemporal region implicated in the object naming experiment above. Changes in parietal activity were induced experimentally by preexposure of the undegraded stimuli before some scans but not others to prime them. The data in the right panel of Fig. 48.7 suggest that the inferotemporal region shows face-specific responses, relative to nonface objects, when, and only when, parietal activity is high. These results can be interpreted as a priming-dependent face-specific response in inferotemporal regions that are mediated by interactions with medial parietal cortex. This is a clear example of contextual specialisation that depends on top-down effects.

Effective Connectivity

The previous examples, demonstrating contextual specialisation, are consistent with functional architectures implied by generative models. However, they do not provide definitive evidence for an interaction between top-down and bottom-up influences. In this subsection we look for direct evidence of these interactions using functional imaging. This rests on being able to measure effective connectivity in a way that is sensitive to interactions among inputs. This requires a plausible model of coupling among brain regions that can accommodate nonlinear effects. We will illustrate the use of a model that is based on the Volterra expansion described in Chapter 50 and expanded on in the subsequent chapter.

Nonlinear Coupling among Brain Areas

Linear models of effective connectivity assume that the multiple inputs to a brain region are linearly separable. This assumption precludes activity-dependent connections that are expressed in one context and not in another. The resolution of this problem lies in adopting nonlinear models like the Volterra formulation that include interactions among inputs. These interactions can be construed as a context- or activity-dependent modulation of the influence that one region exerts over another (Büchel and Friston, 1997). In the Volterra model, second-order kernels model modulatory effects. Within these models the influence of one region on another has two components: (1) the direct or *driving* influence of input from the first (e.g., hierarchically lower) region, irrespective of the activities elsewhere, and (2) an activity-dependent, *modulatory* component that represents an interaction with inputs from the remaining (e.g., hierarchically higher) regions. These are mediated by the first- and second-order kernels, respectively. The example provided in Fig. 48.8 addresses the modulation of visual cortical responses by attentional mechanisms (e.g., Treue and Maunsell, 1996) and the mediating role of activity-dependent changes in effective connectivity. This is the same example used in the introduction and in subsequent chapters.

The lower panel in Fig. 48.8 shows a characterisation of this modulatory effect in terms of the increase in V5 responses, to a simulated V2 input, when posterior parietal activity is zero (broken line) and when it is high (solid lines). In this study subjects were studied with fMRI under identical stimulus conditions (visual motion subtended by radially moving dots) while manipulating the attentional component of the task (detection of velocity changes). The brain regions and connections comprising the model are shown in the upper panel. The lower panel shows a characterisation of the effects of V2 inputs on V5 and their modulation by posterior parietal cortex (PPC) using simulated inputs at different levels of PPC activity. It is evident that V2 has an activating effect on V5 and that PPC increases the responsiveness of V5 to these inputs. The insert shows all the voxels in V5 that evidenced a modulatory effect ($p > 0.05$ uncorrected). These voxels were identified by thresholding statistical parametric maps of the F statistic testing for the contribution of second-order kernels involving V2 and PPC, while treating all other components as nuisance variables. The estimation of the Volterra kernels and statistical inference procedure is described in Friston and Büchel (2000).

This sort of result suggests that backward parietal inputs may be a sufficient explanation for the attentional modulation of visually evoked extrastriate responses. More importantly, they are consistent with the functional architecture implied by predictive coding because they establish the existence of functionally expressed backward connections. V5 cortical responses evidence an interaction between bottom-up input from early visual cortex and top-down influences from parietal cortex. In the final section the implications of this sort of functional integration are addressed from the point of view of the lesion-deficit model and neuropsychology.

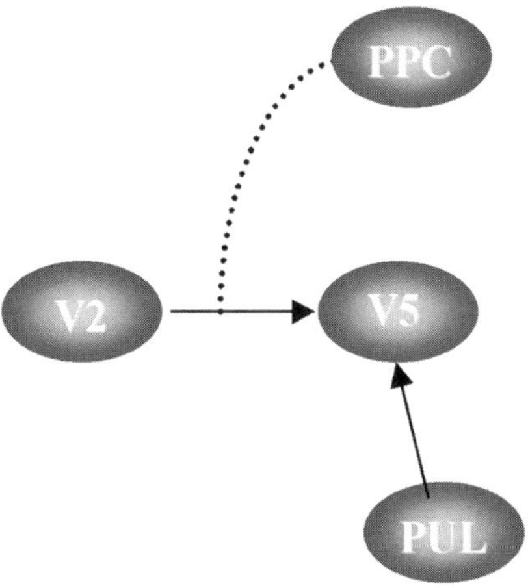

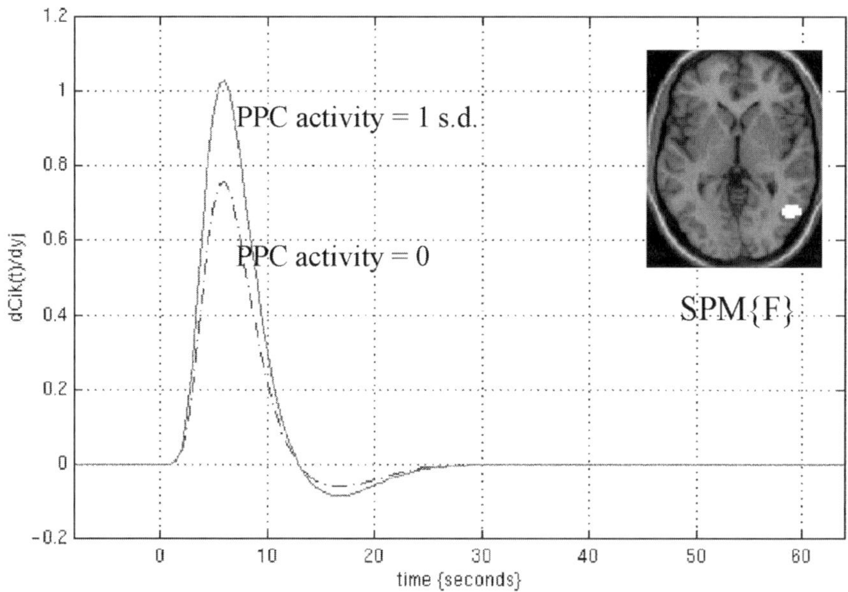

FIGURE 48.8
(Top) Brain regions and connections comprising the model. (Bottom) Characterisation of the effects of V2 inputs on V5 and their modulation by posterior parietal cortex (PPC). The broken lines represent estimates of V5 responses when PPC activity is zero, according to a second-order Volterra model of effective connectivity with inputs to V5 from V2, PPC and the pulvinar (PUL). The solid curves represent the same response when PPC activity is one standard deviation of its variation over conditions. It is evident that V2 has an activating effect on V5 and that PPC increases the responsiveness of V5 to these inputs. The insert shows all the voxels in V5 that evidenced a modulatory effect ($p > 0.05$ uncorrected). These voxels were identified by thresholding a SPM of the F statistic testing for the contribution of second-order kernels involving V2 and PPC (treating all other terms as nuisance variables). The data were obtained with fMRI under identical stimulus conditions (visual motion subtended by radially moving dots) while manipulating the attentional component of the task (detection of velocity changes).

FUNCTIONAL INTEGRATION AND NEUROPSYCHOLOGY

If functional specialisation depends on interactions among cortical areas, then one might predict changes in functional specificity in cortical regions that receive enabling or modulatory afferents from a damaged area. A simple consequence is that aberrant responses will be elicited in regions hierarchically below the lesion if, and only if, these responses depend on inputs from the lesion site. However, there may be other contexts in which the region's responses are perfectly normal (relying on other, intact, afferents). This leads to the notion of a context-dependent region-specific abnormality, caused by, but remote from, a lesion (i.e., an abnormal response that is elicited by some tasks but not others). We have referred to this phenomenon as *dynamic diaschisis* (Price *et al.*, 2001). See Part I, Section 5, for a more psychologically finessed discussion.

Dynamic Diaschisis

Classical diaschisis, demonstrated by early anatomical studies and more recently by neuroimaging studies of resting brain activity, refers to regionally specific reductions in metabolic activity at sites that are remote from, but connected to, damaged regions. The clearest example is *crossed cerebellar diaschisis* (Lenzi *et al.*, 1982) in which abnormalities of cerebellar metabolism are seen characteristically following cerebral lesions involving the motor cortex. Dynamic diaschisis describes the context-sensitive and task-specific effects that a lesion can have on the *evoked responses* of a distant cortical region. The basic idea behind dynamic diaschisis is that an otherwise viable cortical region expresses aberrant neuronal responses when, and only when, those responses depend on interactions with a damaged region. This can arise because normal responses in any given region depend on inputs from, and reciprocal interactions with, other regions. The regions involved will depend on the cognitive and sensorimotor operations engaged at any particular time. If these regions include one that is damaged, then abnormal responses may ensue. However, in some situations the same region may respond normally, for instance, when its dynamics depend only on integration with undamaged regions. If the region can respond normally in some situations, then forward driving components must be intact. This suggests that dynamic diaschisis will only present itself when the lesion involves a hierarchically equivalent or higher area.

An Empirical Demonstration

We investigated this possibility in a functional imaging study of four aphasic patients, all with damage to the left posterior inferior frontal cortex, classically known as *Broca's area* (see Fig. 48.9, upper panels). These patients had speech output deficits but relatively preserved comprehension. Generally, functional imaging studies can only make inferences about abnormal neuronal responses when changes in cognitive strategy can be excluded. We ensured this by engaging the patients in an explicit task that they were able to perform normally. This involved a keypress response when a visually presented letter string contained a letter with an ascending visual feature (e.g.: *h, k, l,* or *t*). While the task remained constant, the stimuli presented were either words or consonant letter strings. Activations detected for words, relative to letters, were attributed to implicit word processing. Each patient showed normal activation of the left posterior middle temporal cortex that has been associated with semantic processing (Price, 1998). However, none of the patients activated the left posterior inferior frontal cortex (damaged by the stroke) or the left posterior inferior temporal region (undamaged by the stroke) (see Fig. 48.4b). These two regions are crucial for word production (Price, 1998). Examination of individual responses in this area revealed that all normal subjects showed increased activity for words relative to consonant letter strings while all four patients showed the reverse effect. The abnormal responses in the left posterior inferior temporal lobe occurred even though this undamaged region lies adjacent and posterior to a region of the left middle temporal cortex that activated normally (see middle column of Fig. 48.9b). Critically, this area is thought to be involved in an earlier stage of word processing than the damaged left inferior frontal cortex (i.e., it is hierarchically lower than the lesion). From these results we can conclude that, during the reading task, responses in the left basal temporal language area rely on afferent inputs from the left posterior inferior frontal cortex. When the first patient was scanned again, during an explicit semantic task, the left posterior inferior temporal lobe responded normally. The abnormal implicit reading related responses were therefore task specific.

These results serve to illustrate the concept of dynamic diaschisis; namely, the anatomically remote and context-specific effects of focal brain lesions. Dynamic diaschisis represents a form of functional disconnection in which regional dysfunction can be attributed to the loss of enabling inputs from hierarchically equivalent or higher brain regions. Unlike classical or

Dynamic diaschisis

a) Lesion sites in four patients

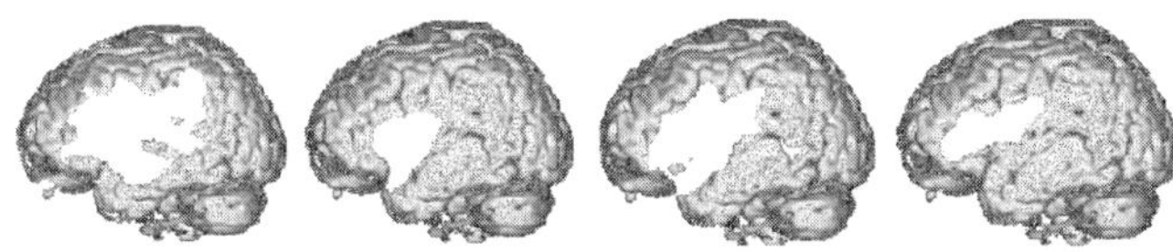

b) Patterns of activation

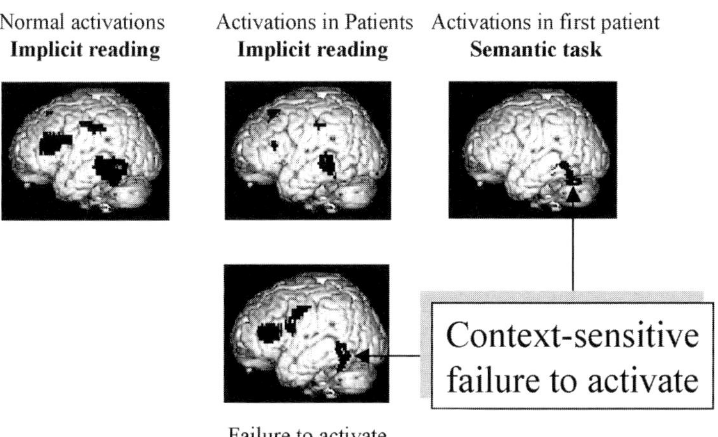

FIGURE 48.9
(a) Renderings illustrating the extent of cerebral infarcts in four patients, as identified by voxel-based morphometry. Regions of reduced gray matter (relative to neurologically normal controls) are shown in white on the left hemisphere. The SPMs were thresholded at $P > 0.001$ uncorrected. All patients had damage to Broca's area. The first (upper left) patient's left middle cerebral artery infarct was most extensive, encompassing temporal and parietal regions as well as frontal and motor cortex. (b) SPMs illustrating the functional imaging results with regions of significant activation shown in black on the left hemisphere. Results are shown for (1) normal subjects reading words (left), (2) activations common to normal subjects and patients reading words using a conjunction analysis (middle-top), (3) areas where normal subjects activate significantly more than patients reading words, using the group times condition interaction (middle-lower), and (4) the first patient activating normally for a semantic task. Context-sensitive failures to activate are implied by the abnormal activations in the first patient, for the implicit reading task, despite a normal activation during a semantic task.

anatomical disconnection syndromes, its pathophysiological expression depends on the functional brain state at the time responses are evoked. Dynamic diaschisis may be characteristic of many regionally specific brain insults and may have implications for neuropsychological inference.

CONCLUSION

In conclusion, the representational capacity and inherent function of any neuron, neuronal population, or cortical area in the brain is dynamic and context sensitive. Functional integration, or interactions among brain systems, that employ driving (bottom up) and backward (top-down) connections, mediate this adaptive and contextual specialisation. A critical consequence is that hierarchically organised neuronal responses, in any given cortical area, can represent different things at different times. Although most models of representational learning require prior assumptions about the distribution of causes, the empirical Bayes approach suggests that these assumptions can be relaxed and that priors can be learned in a hierarchical context. We have tried to show that this hierarchical prediction can be implemented in brainlike architectures and in a biologically plausible fashion. The arguments in this chapter were developed under generative models of brain function, where higher level systems provide a prediction of the inputs to lower level regions. Conflict between the two is resolved by changes in the higher level representations, which are driven by the ensuing error in lower regions, until the mismatch is "cancelled." From this perspective the specialisation of any region is determined both by bottom-up driving inputs and by top-down predictions. Specialisation is therefore not an intrinsic property of any region but depends on both forward and backward connections with other areas. Because the latter have access to the context in which the inputs are generated, they are in a position to modulate the selectivity or specialisation of lower areas.

The emphasis on theoretical neurobiology has been used to expose the usefulness of being able to measure effective connectivity and the importance of modulatory or nonlinear coupling in the brain. These nonlinear aspects of effective connectivity will be a recurrent theme in subsequent chapters that discuss functional and effective connectivity from an operational point of view.

References

Abbot, L. F., Varela, J. A., Karmel, S., and Nelson, S. B. (1997). Synaptic depression and cortical gain control. *Science* **275,** 220–223.

Absher, J. R., and Benson, D. F. (1993). Disconnection syndromes: an overview of Geschwind's contributions. *Neurology* **43**, 862–867.

Aertsen, A., and Preißl, H. (1991). Dynamics of activity and connectivity in physiological neuronal Networks. In *Non Linear Dynamics and Neuronal Networks,* Schuster, H. G., Ed., pp. 281–302. VCH Publishers, New York.

Angelucci, A., Levitt, J. B., Walton, E. J., Hupe, J. M., Bollier, J., and Lund, J. S. (2002a). Circuits for local and global signal integration in primary visual cortex. *J. Neurosci.*, **22**, 8633–8646.

Angelucci, A., Levitt, J. B., and Lunde, J. S. (2002b). Anatomical origins of the classical receptive field and modulatory surround field of single neurons in macaque visual cortical area VI. *Prog. Brain Res.*, **136**, 373–388.

Büchel, C., and Friston, K. J. (1997). Modulation of connectivity in visual pathways by attention: cortical interactions evaluated with structural equation modelling and fMRI. *Cerebral Cortex* **7**, 768–778.

Crick, F., and Koch, C. (1998). Constraints on cortical and thalamic projections: the no-strong-loops hypothesis. *Nature* **391**, 245–250.

Dayan, P., Hinton, G. E., and Neal, R. M. (1995). The Helmholtz machine. *Neural Computation* **7**, 889–904.

Dayan, P., and Abbott, L. F. (2001). The cortical neuroscience. *Computational and Mathematical Modelling of Neural Systems*, MIT Press, Boston.

Dempster, A. P., Laird, N. M., and Rubin. L. B. (1977). Maximum likelihood from incomplete data via the EM algorithm. *J. Roy. Stat. Soc. Ser. B* **39,** 1–38.

Dolan, R. J., Fink, G. R., Rolls, E., Booth, M., Holmes, A., Frackowiak, R. S. J., Friston, K. J. (1997). How the brain learns to see objects and faces in an impoverished context. *Nature* **389**, 596–598.

Efron, B., and Morris, C. (1973). Stein's estimation rule and its competitors—an empirical Bayes approach. *J. Am. Stats. Assoc.* **68,** 117–130.

Felleman, D. J., and Van Essen, D. C. (1991). Distributed hierarchical processing in the primate cerebral cortex. *Cerebral Cortex* **1**, 1–47.

Frey, U., and Morris, R. G. (1988). Synaptic tagging: implications for late maintenance of hippocampal long-term potentiation. *Trends Neurosci.*, **21**, 181–188.

Friston, K. J. (1995). Functional and effective connectivity in neuroimaging: A synthesis. *Hum. Brain Mapping* **2,** 56–78.

Friston, K. J., and Büchel, C. (2000). Attentional modulation of V5 in human. *Proc. Natl. Acad. Sci. USA* **97**, 7591–7596.

Friston, K. J., Price, C. J., Fletcher, P., Moore, C., Frackowiak, R. S. J., and Dolan, R. J. (1996). The trouble with cognitive subtraction. *NeuroImage* **4**, 97–104.

Friston, K. J., Büchel, C., Fink, G. R., Morris, J., Rolls, E., and Dolan, R. J. (1997). Psychophysiological and modulatory interactions in neuroimaging. *NeuroImage* **6**, 218–229.

Friston, K. J. (2002). Functional integration and inference in the brain. *Prog. Neurobiol.*, **68**, 113–143.

Gerstein, G. L., and Perkel, D. H. (1969). Simultaneously recorded trains of action potentials: analysis and functional interpretation. *Science* **164**, 828–830.

Girard, P., and Bullier, J. (1989). Visual activity in area V2 during reversible inactivation of area 17 in the macaque monkey. *J. Neurophysiol.* **62**, 1287–1301.

Hinton, G. E., Dayan, P., Frey, B. J., and Neal, R. M. (1995). The "Wake-Sleep" algorithm for unsupervised neural networks. *Science* **268**, 1158–1161.

Hirsch, J. A., and Gilbert, C. D. (1991). Synaptic physiology of horizontal connections in the cat's visual cortex. *J. Neurosci.* **11**, 1800–1809.

Kass, R. E., and Steffey, D. (1989). Approximate Bayesian inference in conditionally independent hierarchical models (parametric empirical Bayes models). *J. Am. Stat. Assoc.* **407**, 717–726.

Kay, J., and Phillips, W. A. (1996). Activation functions, computational goals and learning rules for local processors with contextual guidance. *Neural Computation* **9**, 895–910.

Lenzi, G. L., Frackowiak, R. S. J., Jones, T. (1982). Cerebral oxygen metabolism and blood flow in human cerebral ischaemic infarction. *J. Cereb. Blood Flow Metab.* **2**, 321–335.

Mumford, D. (1992). On the computational architecture of the neocortex. II. The role of cortico-cortical loops. *Biol. Cybern.* **66**, 241–251.

McIntosh, A. R. (2000). Towards a network theory of cognition. *Neural Networks* **13**, 861–870.

Olshausen, B. A., and Field, D. J. (1996). Emergence of simple-cell receptive field properties by learning a sparse code for natural images. *Nature* **381**, 607–609.

Pearl, J. (2000). *Causality, Models, Reasoning and Inference.* Cambridge University Press, UK.

Phillips, C. G., Zeki, S., and Barlow, H. B. (1984). Localisation of function in the cerebral cortex Past present and future. *Brain* **107**, 327–361.

Phillips, W. A., and Singer, W. (1997). In search of common foundations for cortical computation. *Behav. Brain Sci.* **20**, 57–83.

Price, C. J. (1998). The functional anatomy of word comprehension and production. *Trends. Cog. Sci.* **2**, 281–288.

Price, C. J, Warburton, E. A., Moore, C. J., Frackowiak, R. S. J., and Friston, K. J. (2001). Dynamic diaschisis: anatomically remote and context-specific human brain lesions. *J. Cog. Neurosci.* **13**, 419–429.

Rao, R. P. (1999). An optimal estimation approach to visual perception and learning. *Vision Res.* **39,** 1963–89.

Rao, R. P., and Ballard, D. H. (1999). Predictive coding in the visual cortex: A functional interpretation of some extra-classical receptive field effects. *Nature Neurosci.* **2,** 79–87.

Rockland, K. S., and Pandya, D. N. (1979). Laminar origins and terminations of cortical connections of the occipital lobe in the rhesus monkey. *Brain Res.* **179**, 3–20.

Salin, P.-A., and Bullier, J. (1995). Corticocortical connections in the visual system: Structure and function. *Psychol. Bull.* **75**, 107–154.

Sandell, J. H., and Schiller, P. H. (1982). Effect of cooling area 18 on striate cortex cells in the squirrel monkey. *J. Neurophysiol.* **48**, 38–48.

Treue, S., and Maunsell, H. R. (1996). Attentional modulation of visual motion processing in cortical areas MT and MST. *Nature* **382**, 539–41.

Zeki, S. (1990). The motion pathways of the visual cortex. In *Vision: Coding and Efficiency,* Blakemore, C., Ed., pp. 321–345. Cambridge University Press, UK.

Zeki, S., and Shipp, S. (1988). The functional logic of cortical connections. *Nature* **335**, 311–317.

CHAPTER

49

Functional Connectivity

Eigenimages and Multivariate Analyses

INTRODUCTION

This chapter is concerned with the characterisation of imaging data from a multivariate perspective. This means that the observations at each voxel are considered jointly with explicit reference to the interactions among brain regions. The concept of functional connectivity is reviewed and provides the basis for understanding what eigenimages represent and how they can be interpreted. Having considered the nature of eigenimages and variations on their applications, we then turn to a related approach that, unlike eigenimage analysis, is predicated on a statistical model. This approach is called *multivariate analysis of variance* (MANCOVA) and uses canonical variate analysis to create canonical images. The integrated and distributed nature of neurophysiological responses to sensorimotor or cognitive challenge makes a multivariate perspective particularly appropriate, if not necessary, for functional integration.

A Functional Integration and Connectivity

A landmark meeting that took place on the morning of August 4, 1881, highlighted the difficulties of attributing function to a cortical area, given the dependence of cerebral activity on underlying connections (Phillips *et al., 1*984). Goltz, although accepting the results of electrical stimulation in dog and monkey cortex, considered the excitation method inconclusive, in that the movements elicited might have originated in related pathways or current could have spread to distant centres. Despite advances during the past century, the question remains: Are the physiological changes elicited by sensorimotor or cognitive challenges explained by functional segregation or by integrated and distributed changes mediated by neuronal connections? The question itself calls for a framework within which to address these issues. *Functional and effective connectivity* are concepts critical to this framework.

Origins and Definitions

In the analysis of neuroimaging time series, functional connectivity is defined as the *correlations between spatially remote neurophysiological events*. This definition provides a simple characterisation of functional interactions. The alternative is effective connectivity (i.e., *the influence one neuronal system exerts over another*). These concepts originated in the analysis of separable spike trains obtained from multiunit electrode recordings (Gerstein and Perkel, 1969). Functional connectivity is simply a statement about the observed correlations; it does not comment on how these correlations are mediated. For example, at the level of multiunit microelectrode recordings, correlations can result from *stimulus-locked transients,* evoked by a common afferent input, or reflect *stimulus-induced oscillations,* phasic coupling of neural assemblies mediated by synaptic connections. Effective connectivity is closer to the notion of a connection and can be defined as *the influence one neural system exerts over another*, either at a synaptic (cf. synaptic efficacy) or cortical level. Although functional and effective connectivity can be invoked at a conceptual level in both neuroimaging and electrophysiology, they differ fundamentally at a practical level. This is because the timescales and nature of neurophysiological measurements are very different (seconds vs. milliseconds and haemodynamic vs. spike trains). In electrophysiology it is often necessary to remove the confounding effects of stimulus-locked transients (that introduce correlations *not* causally mediated by direct neural interactions) in order to reveal an underlying connectivity. The confounding effect of stimulus-evoked transients is less problematic in neuroimaging because promulgation of dynamics from primary sensory areas onwards *is* mediated by neuronal connections (usually reciprocal and interconnecting). However, remember that functional connectivity is not necessarily due to effective connectivity (e.g., common neuromodulatory input from ascending aminergic neurotransmitter systems or thalamocortical afferents) and, where it is, effective influences may be indirect (e.g., polysynaptic relays through multiple areas).

EIGENIMAGES, MULTIDIMENSIONAL SCALING, AND OTHER DEVICES

In what follows we introduce a number of techniques (eigenimage analysis, multidimensional scaling, partial least squares, and generalised eigenimage analysis) using functional connectivity as a reference. Emphasis is placed on the relationships between these techniques. For example, eigenimage analysis is equivalent to principal component analysis, and the variant of multi-dimensional scaling considered here is equivalent to principal coordinates analysis. Principal components and coordinates analyses are predicated on exactly the same eigenvector solution and from a mathematical perspective are essentially the same thing.

Measuring Patterns of Correlated Activity

Here we introduce a simple way of measuring the amount a pattern of activity (representing a connected brain system) contributes to the functional connectivity or variance-covariances observed in the imaging data. Functional connectivity is defined in terms of statistical dependencies among neurophysiological measurement. If we assume that these measurements conform to Gaussian assumptions, then we need only characterise their correlations or covariance (correlations are normalised covariances).[1] The point-to-point functional connectivity between one voxel and another is not usually of great interest. The important aspect of a covariance structure is the pattern of correlated activity subtended by an enormous number of pairwise covariances. In measuring such patterns it is useful to introduce the concept of a *norm*. Vector and matrix norms serve the same purpose as absolute values for scalar quantities. In other words, they furnish a measure of distance. One frequently used norm is the 2-norm, which is the length of a vector. The vector 2-norm can be used to measure the degree to which a particular pattern of brain activity contributes to a covariance structure. If a pattern is described by a column vector (p), with an element for each voxel, then the contribution of that pattern to the covariance structure can be measured by the 2-norm of $Mp = ||Mp||$ where M is a mean corrected matrix of data with one row for each successive scan and one column for each voxel:

$$||Mp||^2 = p^T M^T MP \qquad (49.1)$$

(where the superscript T denotes transposition). Put simply the 2-norm is a number that reflects the amount of variance-covariance or functional connectivity that can be accounted for by a particular distributed pattern. Note that the 2-norm only measures the pattern of interest. There

[1]Clearly, neuronal processes are not necessarily Gaussian. However, we can still characterise the second-order dependencies with the correlations. Higher order dependencies would involve computing cumulants as described in the final chapter of this section.

may be many other important patterns of functional connectivity. This fact begs the question "What are the most prevalent patterns of coherent activity?" To answer this question, one turns to eigenimages or spatial modes.

Eigenimages and Spatial Modes

In this section the concept of eigenimages or spatial modes is introduced in terms of patterns of activity defined above. We show that spatial modes are simply those patterns that account for the most variance-covariance (i.e., have the largest 2-norm).

Eigenimages or spatial modes are most commonly obtained using singular value decomposition (SVD). SVD is an operation that decomposes an original time series (M) into two sets of orthogonal vectors (patterns in space and patterns in time) V and U where:

$$\begin{aligned}[U,S,V] &= SVD(M) \\ M &= USV^T\end{aligned} \tag{49.2}$$

Here, U and V are unitary orthogonal matrices $U^TU = 1$, $V^TV = 1$, and $V^TU = 0$ (the sum of squares of each column is unity and all the columns are uncorrelated) and S is a diagonal matrix (only the leading diagonal has nonzero values) of decreasing singular values. The singular value of each eigenimage is simply its 2-norm. Because SVD maximises the first singular value, the first eigenimage is the pattern that accounts for the greatest amount of the variance-covariance structure. In summary, SVD and equivalent devices are powerful ways of decomposing an imaging time series into a series of orthogonal patterns that embody, in a step-down fashion, the greatest amounts of functional connectivity. Each eigenvector (column of V) defines a distributed brain system that can be displayed as an image. The distributed systems that ensue are called *eigenimages* or *spatial modes* and have been used to characterise the spatiotemporal dynamics of neurophysiological time series from several modalities, including multiunit electrode recordings (Mayer-Kress *et al.,* 1991), EEG (Friedrich *et al.,* 1991), MEG (Fuchs *et al., 1*992), PET (Friston *et al.,* 1993a), and functional MRI (Friston *et al.,* 1993b). Interestingly in fMRI the application of eigenimage analysis that has attracted the most interest is in characterising functional connections while the brain is at "rest" (see Biswal *et al.,* 1995).

Many readers will notice that the eigenimages associated with the functional connectivity or covariance matrix are simply principal components of the time series. In the EEG literature one sometimes comes across the Karhunen-Loeve expansion, which is employed to identify spatial modes. If this expansion is in terms of eigenvectors of covariances (and it usually is), then the analysis is formally identical to the one presented above.

One might ask what the column vectors of U in Eq. (49.2) correspond to. These vectors are the time-dependent profiles associated with each eigenimage known as *eigenvariates*. They reflect the extent to which an eigenimage is expressed in each experimental condition or over time. Figure 49.1 shows a simple schematic illustrating the decomposition of a time series into orthogonal modes. This is sometimes called *spectral decomposition.* Eigenvariates play an important role in the functional attribution of distributed systems defined by eigenimages. This point and others will be illustrated next.

Mapping Function into Anatomical Space: Eigenimage Analysis

To illustrate the approach, we will use the PET word generation study used in Friston *et al.* (1993a). The data were obtained from five subjects scanned 12 times while performing one of two verbal tasks in alternation. One task involved repeating a letter presented aurally at one per 2 sec (*word shadowing*). The other was a paced verbal fluency task, in which subjects responded with a word that began with the heard letter (*word generation*). To facilitate intersubject pooling, the data were realigned and spatially normalised and smoothed with an isotropic Gaussian kernel (FWHM of 16 mm). The data were then subject to an ANCOVA (with 12 conditions, subject effects, and global activity as a confound). Voxels were selected using a conventional SPM{F} to identify those significant at $p > 0.05$ (uncorrected). The time series of condition-specific effects, from each of these voxels, were entered into a mean corrected data matrix M with 12 rows (one for each condition) and one column for each voxel.

Eigenimages

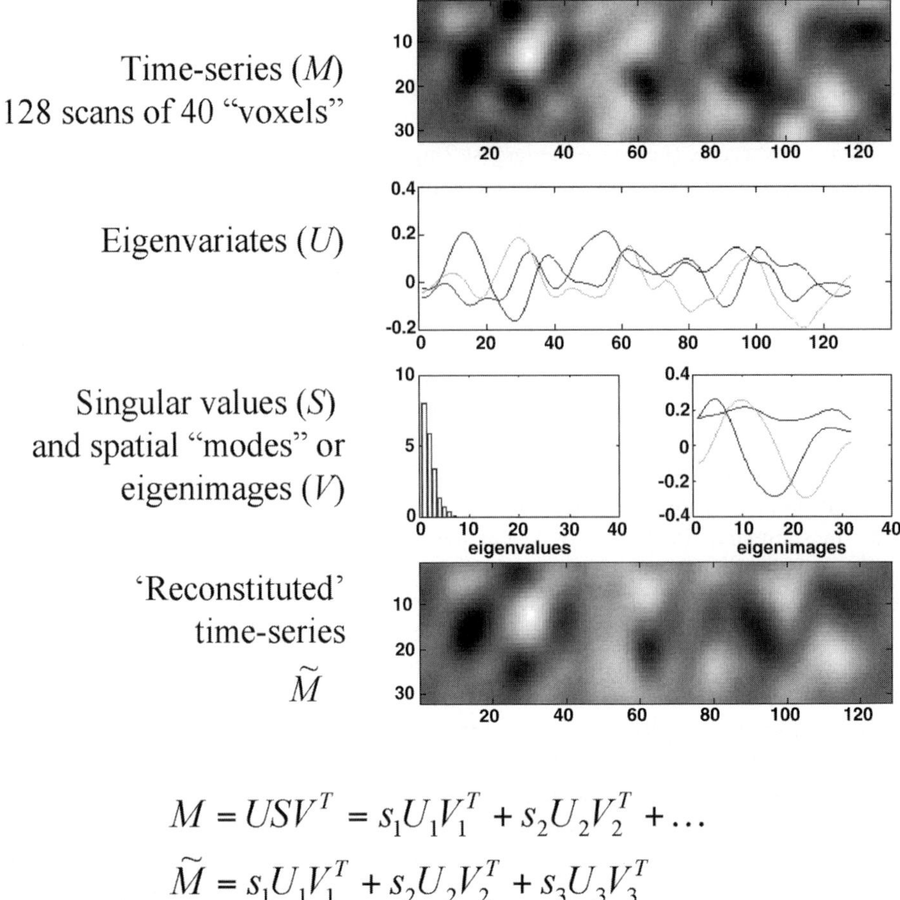

$$M = USV^T = s_1U_1V_1^T + s_2U_2V_2^T + \ldots$$

$$\tilde{M} = s_1U_1V_1^T + s_2U_2V_2^T + s_3U_3V_3^T$$

FIGURE 49.1
Schematic illustrating a simple spectral decomposition or singular decomposition of a multivariate time series. The original time series is shown in the upper panel with time running along the x axis. The first three eigenvariates and eigenvectors are shown in the middle panels together with the spectrum (hence, spectral decomposition) of singular values. The eigenvalues are the square of the singular values $\lambda = SS^T$. The lower panel shows the data reconstructed using only three principal components. Because they capture most of the variance, the reconstructed sequence is very similar to the original time series.

Matrix M was subject to SVD as described above. The distribution of eigenvalues (Fig. 49.2, lower left) suggests that only two eigenimages are required to account for most of the observed variance-covariance structure. The first mode accounted for 64% and the second for 16% of the variance. The first eigenimage V_1 is shown in Fig. 49.2 (top) along with the corresponding eigenvariate U_1 (lower right). The first eigenimage has positive loadings in the anterior cingulate, the left DLPFC, Broca's area, the thalamic nuclei, and the cerebellum. Negative loadings were seen bitemporally and in the posterior cingulate. According to this analysis, the first eigenimage is prevalent in the verbal fluency tasks with negative scores in word shadowing. The second spatial mode (not shown) had its highest positive loadings in the anterior cingulate and bitemporal regions (notably Wernicke's area on the left). This mode appeared to correspond to a highly nonlinear, monotonic time effect with greatest prominence in earlier conditions.

The *post hoc* functional attribution of these eigenimages is usually based on their eigenvariates (U). The first mode may represent an *intentional* system critical for the intrinsic generation of words in the sense that the key cognitive difference between verbal fluency and

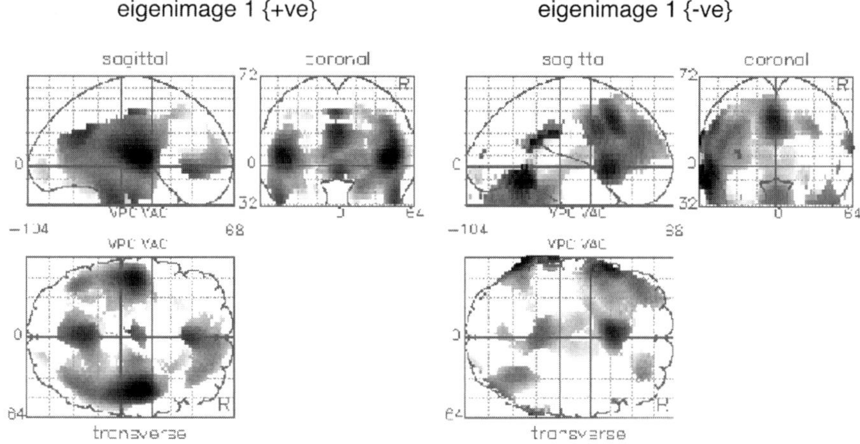

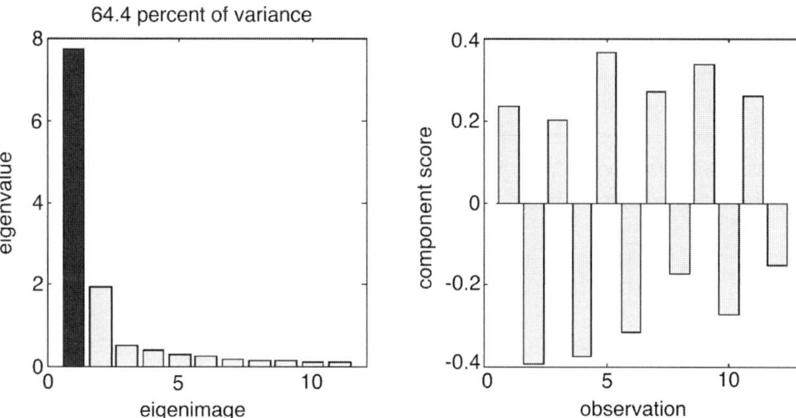

FIGURE 49.2
Eigenimage analysis of the PET activation study of word generation. (Top) Positive and negative components of the first eigenimage (i.e., first column of V). The maximum intensity projection display format is standard and provides three views of the brain (from the back, from the right, and from the top). (Bottom left) Eigenvalues (singular values squared) of the functional connectivity matrix reflecting the relative amounts of variance accounted for by the 11 eigenimages associated with these data. Only two eigenvalues are greater than unity and to all intents and purposes the changes characterising this time series can be considered two dimensional. (Bottom right) The temporal eigenvariate reflecting the expression of this eigenimage over the 12 conditions (i.e., the first column of U).

word shadowing is the intrinsic generation as opposed to extrinsic specification of word representations and implicit mnemonic processing. The second system, which includes the anterior cingulate, may be involved in habituation, possibly of attentional or perceptual set.

There is nothing "biologically" important about the particular spatial modes obtained in this fashion, in the sense that one could "rotate" the eigenvectors such that they would still be orthogonal and yet give different eigenimages. The uniqueness of the particular solution given by SVD is that the first eigenimage accounts for the largest amount of variance-covariance and the second for the greatest amount that remains and so on. The reason that the eigenimages in the example above lend themselves to such a simple interpretation is that the variance introduced by experimental design (intentional) was substantially greater than that due to time (attentional), and both these sources were greater than any other effect. Other factors that ensure a parsimonious characterisation of a time series, with small numbers of well-defined modes include (1) smoothness in the data and (2) using only voxels that showed a nontrivial amount of change during the scanning session.

Mapping Anatomy into Functional Space: Multidimensional Scaling

In the previous section the functional connectivity matrix was used to define associated eigenimages or spatial modes. In this section functional connectivity is used in a different way, namely, to constrain the proximity of two cortical areas in some functional space (Friston *et al.*, 1996a). The objective here is to transform anatomical space so that the distance between cortical areas is directly related to their functional connectivity. This transformation defines a new space whose topography is purely functional in nature. This space is constructed using multidimensional scaling or principal coordinates analysis (Gower, 1966).

Multidimensional scaling (MDS) is a descriptive method for representing the structure of a system. It is based on pairwise measures of similarity or confusability (Torgerson, 1958; Shepard, 1980). The resulting multidimensional spatial configuration of a system's elements embody, in their proximity relationships, comparative similarities. The technique was developed primarily for the analysis of perceptual spaces. The proposal that stimuli be modelled by points in space, so that perceived similarity is represented by spatial distances, goes back to the days of Isaac Newton (1794).

Imagine k measures from n voxels plotted as n points in a k-dimensional space (k-space). If they have been normalised to zero mean and unit sum of squares, these points will fall on a $k-1$ dimensional sphere. The closer any two points are to each other, the greater their correlation or functional connectivity (in fact, the correlation is a cosine of the angle subtended at the origin). The distribution of these points embodies the functional topography. A view of this distribution, which reveals the greatest structure, is simply obtained by rotating the points to maximise their apparent dispersion (variance). In other words, one looks at the subspace with the largest "volume" spanned by the principal axes of the n points in k-space. These principal axes are given by the eigenvectors of MM^T, i.e., the column vectors of U_1. From Eq. (49.2),

$$\begin{aligned} MM^T &= U\lambda U^T \\ \lambda &= SS^T \end{aligned} \tag{49.3}$$

Let Q be the matrix of desired coordinates derived by simply projecting the original data onto axes defined by U, where $Q = M^T U$. Voxels that have a correlation of unity will occupy the same point in MDS space. Voxels that have uncorrelated dynamics will be $\pi/2$ apart. Voxels that are negatively but totally correlated (correlation $= -1$) will be maximally separated on the opposite sides of the MDS hyperspace. Profound negative correlations denote a functional association that is modelled in MDS functional space as diametrically opposed locations on the hypersphere. In other words, two regions with profound negative correlations will form two "poles" in functional space.

Following normalisation to unit sum of squares over each column M (the adjusted data matrix from the word generation study above), the data were subjected to singular value decomposition according to Eq. (49.2) and the coordinates Q of the voxels in MDS functional space were computed. Recall that only two eigenvalues exceed unity (Fig. 49.2, right), suggesting a functional space that is essentially two dimensional. The locations of voxels in this two-dimensional subspace are shown in Fig. 49.3 (lower row) by rendering voxels from different regions in different colors. The anatomical regions corresponding to the different colors are shown in the upper row. Anatomical regions were selected to include those parts of the brain that showed the greatest variance during the 12 conditions. Anterior regions (Fig. 49.3, right) included the mediodorsal thalamus (blue), the dorsolateral prefrontal cortex (DLPFC), Broca's area (red), and the anterior cingulate (green). Posterior regions (Fig. 49.3, left) included the superior temporal regions (red), the posterior superior temporal regions (blue), and the posterior cingulate (green). The corresponding functional spaces (Fig. 49.3, lower rows) reveal a number of things about the functional topography elicited by this set of activation tasks. First, each anatomical region maps into a relatively localised portion of functional space. This preservation of local contiguity reflects the high correlations within anatomical regions, due in part to smoothness of the original data and to high degrees of intraregional functional connectivity. Secondly, the anterior regions are almost in juxtaposition as are posterior regions. However, the confluence of anterior and posterior regions forms two diametrically opposing poles (or one axis). This configuration

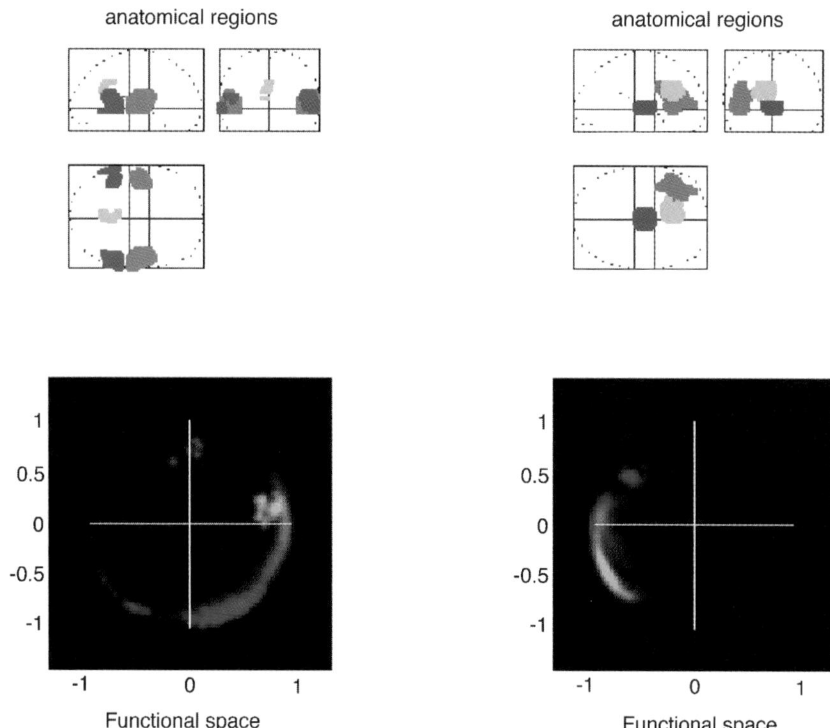

FIGURE 49.3
Classical or metric scaling analysis of the functional topography of intrinsic word generation in normal subjects. (Top) Anatomical regions categorised according to their colour. The designation was by reference to the atlas of Talairach and Tournoux (1988). (Bottom) Regions plotted in a functional space following the scaling transformation. In this space the proximity relationships reflect the functional connectivity among regions. The colour of each voxel corresponds to the anatomical region to which it belongs. The brightness reflects the local density of points corresponding to voxels in anatomical space. This density was estimated by binning the number of voxels in 0.02 "boxes" and smoothing with a Gaussian kernel of FWHM of 3 boxes. Each colour was scaled to its maximum brightness.

suggests an anterior-posterior axis with prefrontotemporal and cingulocingulate components. One might have predicted this configuration by noting that the anterior regions had high positive loadings on the first eigenimage (see Fig. 49.2), while the posterior regions had high negative loadings. Thirdly, within the anterior and posterior sets of regions certain generic features are evident. The most striking is the particular ordering of functional interactions. For example, the functional connectivity between posterior cingulate (green) and superior temporal regions (red) is high, as is true for the superior temporal (red) and posterior temporal regions (blue). Yet the posterior cingulate and posterior temporal regions show very little functional connectivity (they are $\pi/2$ apart or, equivalently, subtend 90 degrees at the origin).

These results are consistent with known anatomical connections. For example, DLPFC anterior cingulate connections, DLPFC temporal connections, bitemporal commissural connections, and mediodorsal thalamic DLPFC projections have all been demonstrated in nonhuman primates (Goldman-Rakic, 1988). The mediodorsal thalamic region and DLPFC are so correlated that one is embedded within the other (purple area). This is pleasing given the known thalamocortical projections to DLPFC.

Functional Connectivity between Systems: Partial Least Squares

Hitherto, we have been dealing with functional connectivity between two voxels. The same notion can be extended to functional connectivity between two systems by noting that there is no fundamental difference between the dynamics of one voxel and the dynamics of a distributed system or pattern. The functional connectivity between two systems is simply the correlation or covariance between their time-dependent activity. The time-dependent activity of a system or pattern p_i is given by

$$\begin{aligned} v_i &= MP_i \\ C_{ij} &= v_i^T v_j = p_i^T M^T M p_j \end{aligned} \tag{49.4}$$

where C_{ij} is the functional connectivity between the systems described by vectors p_i and p_j. Consider functional connectivity between two systems in separate parts of the brain, for example, the right and left hemispheres. Here the data matrices (M_i and M_j) derive from different sets of voxels and Eq. (49.4) becomes

$$C_{ij} = v_i^T v_j = p_i^T M_i^T M_j p_j \tag{49.5}$$

If one wanted to identify the intrahemispheric systems that showed the greatest interhemispheric functional connectivity (i.e., covariance), one would need to identify the pair of vectors p_i and p_j that maximise C_{ij} in Eq. (49.5). SVD finds another powerful application in doing just this where

$$\begin{aligned} [U,S,V] &= SVD(M_i^T M_j) \\ M_i^T M_j &= USV^T \\ U^T M_i^T M_j V &= S \end{aligned} \tag{49.6}$$

The first columns of U and V represent the singular images that correspond to the two systems with the greatest amount of functional connectivity (the singular values in the diagonal matrix S). In other words SVD of the (generally asymmetric) cross-covariance matrix, based on time series from two anatomically separate parts of the brain, yields a series of paired vectors (paired columns of U and V) that, in a step-down fashion, define pairs of brain systems that show the greatest functional connectivity. This particular application of SVD is also known as *partial least squares* and has been proposed for analysis of designed activation experiments in which the two data matrices comprise (1) an imaging time series and (2) a set of behavioural or task parameters (Macintosh *et al.,* 1996). In this application the paired singular vectors correspond to (1) a singular image and (2) a set of weights that give the linear combination of task parameters that show the maximal covariance with the corresponding singular image.

Differences in Functional Connectivity: Generalised Eigenimages

In this section we introduce an extension of eigenimage analysis using the solution to the generalised eigenvalue problem. This problem involves finding the eigenvector solution that involves two functional connectivity or covariance matrices and can be used to find the eigenimage that is maximally expressed in one time series relative to another. In other words, it can find a pattern of distributed activity that is most prevalent in one dataset and least expressed in another. The example used to illustrate this idea is frontotemporal functional disconnection in schizophrenia (see Friston *et al.,* 1996b).

The notion that schizophrenia represents a disintegration or fractionation of the psyche is as old as its name, introduced by Bleuler (1911) to convey a "splitting" of mental faculties. Many of Bleuler's primary processes, such as "loosening of associations," emphasise a fragmentation and loss of coherent integration. In what follows we assume that this mentalistic "splitting" has a physiological basis and, furthermore, that both the mentalistic and physiological disintegration have precise and specific characteristics that can be understood in terms of functional connectivity.

The idea is that although localised pathophysiology in cortical areas may be a sufficient explanation for some signs of schizophrenia it does not suffice as a rich or compelling explanation for the symptoms of schizophrenia. The conjecture is that symptoms such as hallucinations and delusions are better understood in terms of abnormal interactions or impaired integration between different cortical areas. This dysfunctional integration, expressed at a physiological level as abnormal functional connectivity, is measurable with neuroimaging and observable at a cognitive level as a failure to integrate perception and action that manifests as clinical symptoms. The distinction between a regionally specific pathology and a pathology of interaction can be seen in terms of a first-order effect (e.g., hypofrontality) and a second-order effect that only exists in the relationship between activity in the prefrontal cortex and some other (e.g., temporal) region. In a similar way psychological abnormalities can be regarded as first order (e.g., a poverty of intrinsically cued behaviour in psychomotor poverty) or second order (e.g., a failure to integrate intrinsically cued behaviour and perception in reality distortion).

Generalised Eigenvalue Solution

Suppose that we want to find a pattern embodying the greatest amount of functional connectivity in control subjects, relative to schizophrenic subjects (e.g., frontotemporal covariance). To achieve this, we identify an eigenimage that reflects the most functional connectivity in control subjects relative to a schizophrenic group (*d*). This eigenimage is obtained by using a generalised eigenvector solution:

$$\begin{aligned} C_i^{-1}C_jd &= d\lambda \\ C_jd &= C_id\lambda \end{aligned} \qquad (49.7)$$

where C_i and C_j are the two functional connectivity matrices. The generalised eigenimage d is essentially a single pattern that maximises the ratio of the 2-norm measures [Eq. (49.1)] when applied to C_i and C_j. Generally speaking, these matrices could represent data from two groups of subjects or from the same subjects scanned under different conditions. In the present example we use connectivity matrices from control subjects and people with schizophrenia showing pronounced psychomotor poverty.

The data were acquired from two groups of six subjects. Each subject was scanned six times during the performance of three word generation tasks (A B C C B A). Task A was a verbal fluency task, requiring subjects to respond with a word that began with a heard letter. Task B was a semantic categorisation task in which subjects responded "man-made" or "natural," depending on a heard noun. Task C was a word-shadowing task in which subjects simply repeated what was heard. In the current context, the detailed nature of the tasks is not very important. They were used to introduce variance and covariance in activity that could support an analysis of functional connectivity.

The groups comprised six control subjects and six schizophrenic patients. The schizophrenic subjects produced fewer than 24 words on a standard (1-min) FAS verbal fluency task (generating words beginning with the letters *F, A,* and *S*). The results of a generalised eigenimage analysis are presented in Fig. 49.4. As expected the pattern that best captures differences between the two groups involves prefrontal and temporal cortices. Negative correlations between left DLPFC and bilateral superior temporal regions are found (Fig. 49.4; upper panels). The amount to which this pattern was expressed in each individual group is shown in the lower panel using the appropriate 2-norm $||d^TC_id||$. We can see that this eigenimage, while prevalent in control subjects, is uniformly reduced in schizophrenic subjects.

Summary

In the preceding sections we have seen how eigenimages can be framed in terms of functional connectivity and the relationships among eigenimage analysis, multidimensional scaling, partial least squares, and generalised eigenimage analysis. In the next section we use the generative model's perspective, described in the previous chapter, to take component analysis into the nonlinear domain.

NONLINEAR PCA AND ICA

Generative Models

Recall from the previous chapter how generative models of data could be framed in terms of a *prior* distribution over causes $p(v;\theta)$ and a *generative* distribution or likelihood of the inputs given the causes $p(u|v;\theta)$. For example, factor analysis corresponded to a generative model as follows:

$$\begin{aligned} p(v;\theta) &= N(v:0,1) \\ p(u|v;\theta) &= N(u:\theta v,\Sigma) \end{aligned} \qquad (49.8)$$

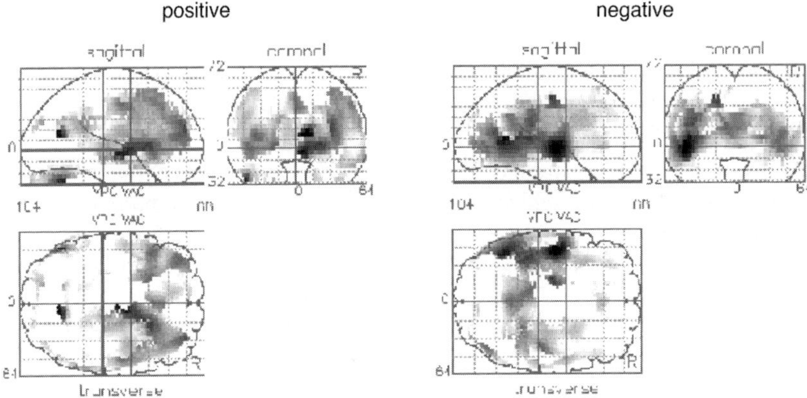

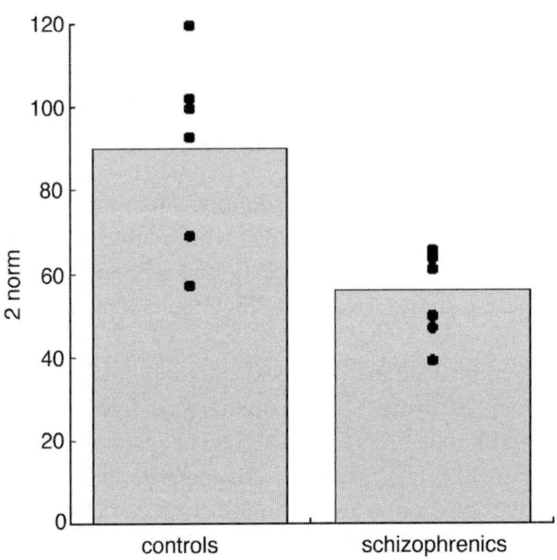

FIGURE 49.4
Generalised eigenimage analysis of schizophrenic and control subjects. (Top left and right) Positive and negative loadings of the first eigenimage that is maximally expressed in the control group and minimally expressed in the schizophrenic group. This analysis used PET activation studies of word generation with six scans per subject and six subjects per group. The activation study involved three word generation conditions (word shadowing, semantic categorisation, and verbal fluency) each of which was presented twice. The gray scale is arbitrary and each image has been normalised to the image maximum. The display format is standard and represents a maximum intensity projection. This eigenimage is relatively less expressed in the schizophrenic data. This point is made by expressing the amount of functional connectivity attributable to the eigenimage in (each subject in) both groups, using the appropriate 2-norm (bottom panel).

Namely, the underlying causes of inputs are independent normal variates that are mixed linearly and added to Gaussian noise to form inputs. In the limiting case of $\Sigma \to 0$, the model becomes deterministic and conforms to PCA. By simply assuming non-Gaussian priors one can specify generative models for sparse coding:

$$\begin{aligned} p(v;\theta) &= \prod p(v_i;\theta) \\ p(u \mid v;\theta) &= N(u : \theta v, \Sigma) \end{aligned} \tag{49.9}$$

where $p(v_i;\theta)$ are chosen to be suitably sparse (i.e., heavy tailed) with a cumulative density function that corresponds to the squashing function below. The deterministic equivalent of sparse coding is ICA that is obtained when $\Sigma \to 0$. These formulations allow us to consider simple extensions of PCA by looking at nonlinear versions of the underlying generative model.

Nonlinear PCA

Despite its exploratory power, eigenimage analysis is fundamentally limited because the particular modes obtained are uniquely determined by constraints that are biologically implausible. This represents an inherent limitation on the interpretability and usefulness of eigenimage analysis. The two main limitations of conventional eigenimage analysis are that the decomposition of any observed time series is in terms of linearly separable components. Secondly, the spatial modes are somewhat arbitrarily constrained to be orthogonal and account, successively, for the largest amount of variance. From a biological perspective, the linearity constraint is a severe one because it precludes interactions among brain systems. This is an unnatural restriction on brain activity, where one expects to see substantial interactions that render the expression of one mode sensitive to the expression of others. Nonlinear PCA attempts to circumvent these sorts of limitations.

The generative model implied by Eq. (49.8), when $\Sigma \rightarrow 0$, is linear and deterministic:

$$\begin{aligned} p(v;\theta) &= N(v:0,1) \\ u &= \theta v \end{aligned} \tag{49.10}$$

Here the causes v correspond to the eigenvariates and the model parameters to scaled eigenvectors $\theta = VS$. The u term is the observed data or image that comprised each row of M above. This linear generative model $G(v,\theta) = \theta v$ can now be generalised to any static nonlinear model by taking a second-order approximation:

$$\begin{aligned} p(v;\theta) &= N(v:0,1) \\ u &= G(v,\theta) \\ &= \sum_i V_i v_i + \frac{1}{2}\sum_{ij} V_{ij} v_i v_j + \ldots \\ V_i &= \frac{\partial G}{\partial v} \\ V_{ij} &= \frac{\partial^2 G}{\partial v_i \partial v_j} \end{aligned} \tag{49.11}$$

This nonlinear model has two sorts of modes. First-order modes V_i that mediate the effect of any orthogonal cause on the response (i.e., maps the causes onto voxels directly) and second-order modes V_{ij} that map interactions among causes onto the measured response. These second-order modes could represent the distributed systems implicated in the interaction between various experimentally manipulated causes. See the example below.

The identification of the first- and second-order modes proceeds using expectation maximisation (EM) as described in the previous chapter. In this instance the algorithm can be implemented as a simple neural net with forward connections from the data to the causes and backward connections from the causes to the predicted data. The **E**-step corresponds to *recognition* of the causes by the forward connections using the current estimate of the first-order modes and the **M**-step adjusts these connections to minimise the prediction error of the generative model in Eq. (49.11), using the recognised causes. These schemes (e.g., Kramer, 1991; Karhunen and Joutsensalo, 1994; Friston *et al.,* 2000) typically employ a "bottleneck" architecture that forces the inputs through a small number of nodes (see the insert in Fig. 49.5). The output from these nodes then diverges to produce the predicted inputs. After learning, the activity of the bottleneck nodes can be treated as estimates of the causes. These representations are obtained by projection of the input onto a low-dimensional curvilinear manifold that is defined by the activity of the bottleneck. Before looking at an empirical example we will briefly discuss ICA.

Independent Component Analysis

ICA represents another way of generalising the linear model used by PCA. This is achieved, not through nonlinearities, but by assuming non-Gaussian priors. The non-Gaussian form can be specified by a nonlinear transformation of the causes $\tilde{v} = \sigma(v)$ that renders then normally distributed, such that when $\Sigma \rightarrow 0$, in Eq. (49.9) we get

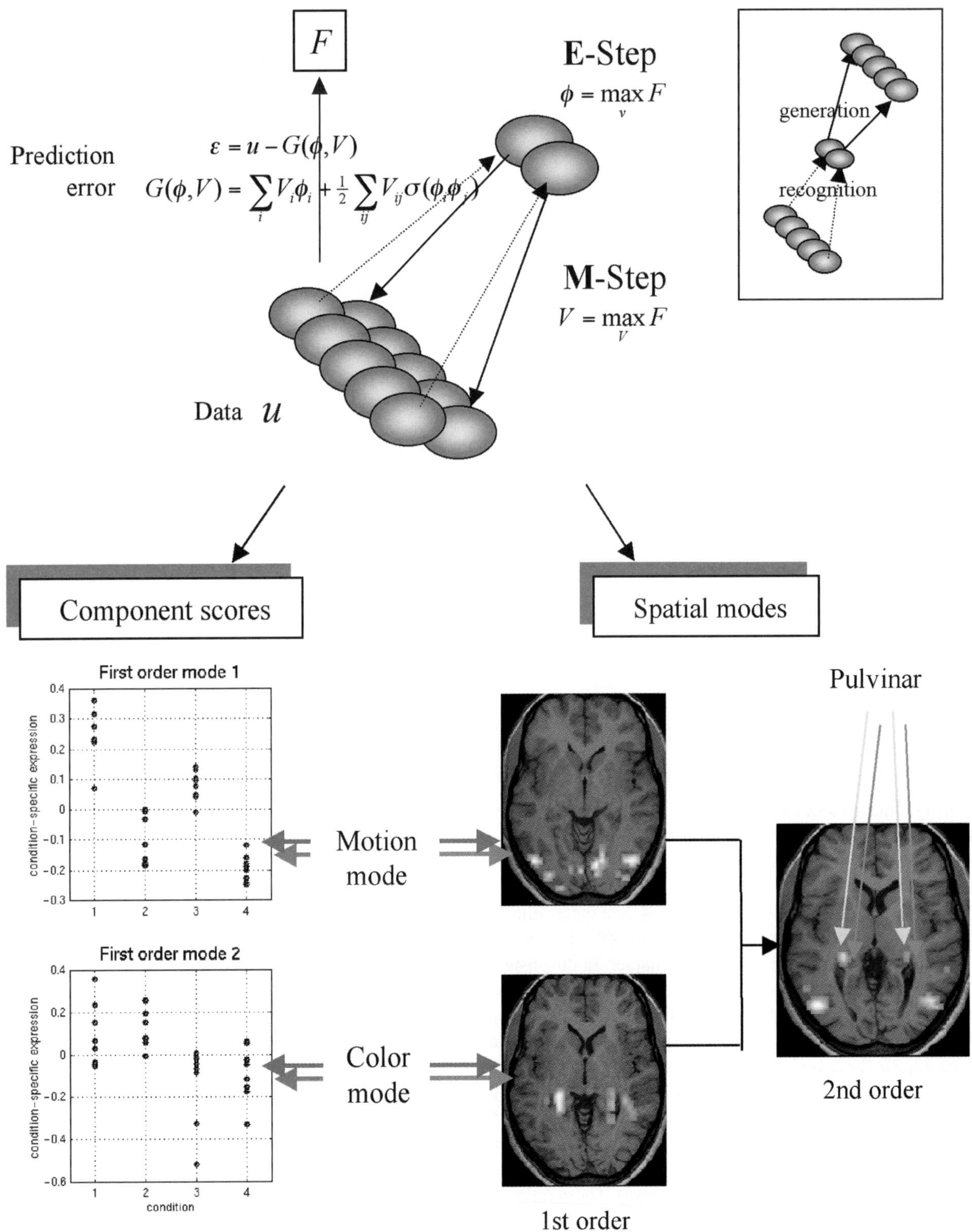

FIGURE 49.5
(Top) Schematic of the neural net architecture used to estimate causes and modes. Feedforward connections from the input layer to the hidden layer provide an estimate of the causes using some recognition model (the **E**-Step). This estimate minimises prediction error under the constraints imposed by prior assumption about the causes. The modes or parameters are updated in an **M**-step. The architecture is quite ubiquitous and when "unwrapped" discloses the hidden layer as a "bottleneck" (see insert). These "bottleneck" architectures are characteristic of manifold learning algorithms like nonlinear PCA. (Bottom left) Condition-specific expression of the two first-order modes ensuing from the visual processing fMRI study. These data represent the degree to which the first principal component of epoch-related responses over the 32 photic stimulation/baseline pairs was expressed. These condition-specific responses are plotted in terms of the four conditions for the two modes. 1 and 3, motion present; 2 and 4, stationary dots; 1 and 2, isoluminant, chromatic contrast stimuli; 3 and 4, isochromatic, luminance contrast stimuli. (Bottom right) The axial slices have been selected to include the maxima of the corresponding spatial modes. In this display format, the modes have been thresholded at 1.64 of each mode's standard deviation over all voxels. The resulting excursion set has been superimposed onto a structural T_1-weighted MRI image.

$$
\begin{aligned}
p(\tilde{v};\theta) &= N(\tilde{v};0,1)\\
u &= \theta\sigma^{-1}(\tilde{v})\\
\tilde{v} &= \sigma(\theta^{-1}u)
\end{aligned}
\tag{49.12}
$$

This is not the conventional way to present ICA but is used here to connect the models for PCA and ICA. The form of the nonlinear squashing function $\tilde{v} = \sigma(v)$ embodies our prior assumptions about the marginal distribution of the causes. These are usually supra-Gaussian. Simple algorithms exist that implicitly minimise the objective function F (see previous chapter) using the covariances of the data. In neuroimaging, this enforces an ICA of independent spatial modes, because there are more voxels than scans (McKeown *et al.*, 1998). In EEG there are more time bins than channels and the independent components are temporal in nature. The distinction between *spatial* and *temporal* ICA depends on whether one regards Eq. (49.12) as generating data over space or time. Friston (1998) discusses their relative merits. The important thing about ICA, relative to PCA, is that the prior densities model independent causes not just uncorrelated causes. This difference is expressed in terms of statistical dependencies beyond second order. Stone (2002) provides an introduction to these issues.

An Example

This example comes from Friston *et al.* (2000)[2] and is based on an fMRI study of visual processing that was designed to address the interaction between colour and motion systems. We had expected to demonstrate that a "colour" mode and "motion" mode would interact to produce a second-order mode reflecting (1) reciprocal interactions between extrastriate areas functionally specialised for colour and motion, (2) interactions in lower visual areas mediated by convergent backward efferents, or (3) interactions in the pulvinar mediated by corticothalamic loops).

Data Acquisition and Experimental Design

A young subject was scanned under four different conditions, in six scan epochs, intercalated with a low-level (visual fixation) baseline condition. The four conditions were repeated eight times in a pseudo-random order, giving 384 scans in total or 32 stimulation/baseline epoch pairs. The four experimental conditions comprised the presentation of (1) radially moving dots and (2) stationary dots, using (1) luminance contrast and (2) chromatic contrast in a 2×2 factorial design. Luminance contrast was established using isochromatic stimuli (red dots on a red background or green dots on a green background). Hue contrast was obtained by using red (or green) dots on a green (or red) background and establishing isoluminance with flicker photometry. In the two movement conditions the dots moved radially from the centre of the screen at 8 degrees per second to the periphery, where they vanished. This creates the impression of optical flow. By using these stimuli we hoped to excite activity in a visual motion system and one specialised for colour processing. Any interaction between these systems would be expressed in terms of motion-sensitive responses that depended on the hue or luminance contrast subtending that motion.

Nonlinear PCA

The data were reduced to an eight-dimensional subspace using SVD and entered into a nonlinear PCA using two causes. The functional attribution of the resulting sources was established by looking at the expression of the corresponding first-order modes over the four conditions (right lower panels in Fig. 49.5). This expression is simply the score on the first principal component over all 32 epoch-related responses for each cause. The first mode is clearly a motion-sensitive mode but one that embodies some colour preference in the sense that the motion-dependent responses of this system are accentuated in the presence of colour cues. This was not quite what we had anticipated; the first-order effect contains what would functionally be called an interaction

[2]Although an example of nonlinear PCA, the generative model actually used finessed Eq. (49.10) with a nonlinear function of the second-order terms:

$$u = G(v) = \sum_i V_i v_i + \frac{1}{2}\sum_{ij} V_{ij}\sigma(v_i v_j)$$

This endows the causes with a unique scaling.

between motion and colour processing. The second source appears to be concerned exclusively with colour processing. The corresponding anatomical profiles are shown in Fig. 49.5 (left panels). The first-order mode, which shows both motion and related-related responses, shows high loadings in bilateral motion-sensitive complex V5 (Brodmann areas 19 and 37 at the occiptotemporal junction) and areas traditionally associated with colour processing (V4, the lingual gyrus). The second first-order mode is most prominent in the hippocampus, parahippocampal, and related lingual cortices on both sides. In summary, the two first-order modes comprise (1) an extrastriate cortical system including V5 and V4 that responds to motion, preferentially when motion is supported by colour cues, and (2) a (para)hippocampal/lingual system that is concerned exclusively with colour processing, above and beyond that accounted for by the first system. The critical question is where do these modes interact?

The interaction between the extrastriate and (para)hippocampal/lingual systems conforms to the second-order mode in the lower panels. This mode highlights the pulvinar of the thalamus and V5 bilaterally. This is a pleasing result in that it clearly implicates the thalamus in the integration of extrastriate and (para)hippocampal systems. This integration is mediated by recurrent (sub)corticothalamic connections. It is also a result that would not have been obtained from a conventional SPM analysis. Indeed we looked for an interaction between motion and colour processing and did not see any such effect in the pulvinar.

Summary

We have reviewed eigenimage analysis and generalisations based on nonlinear and non-Gaussian generative models. All of the techniques discussed above are essentially descriptive, in that they do not allow one to make any statistical inferences about the characterisations obtained. In the second half of this chapter, we turn to multivariate techniques that do embody statistical inference and explicit hypothesis testing. We introduce *canonical images* that can be thought of as statistically informed eigenimages pertaining to a particular effect introduced by experimental design. We have seen that, using the generalised eigenvalue solution, patterns can be identified that are maximally expressed in one covariance structure relative to another. Consider now the use of this approach where the first covariance matrix reflected the effects we were interested in, and the second embodied covariances due to error. This corresponds to canonical image analysis and is considered in the following sections.

MANCOVA AND CANONICAL IMAGE ANALYSIS

Introduction

In the following sections we review multivariate approaches to the analysis of functional imaging studies. The exemplar analysis described uses standard multivariate techniques to make statistical inferences about activation effects and to describe their important features. Specifically, we introduce multivariate analysis of covariance (MANCOVA) and canonical variates analysis (CVA) to characterise activation effects. This approach characterises the brain's response in terms of functionally connected and distributed systems in a fashion similar to that of eigenimage analysis. Eigenimages figure in the current analysis in the following way. A problematic issue in multivariate analysis of functional imaging data is that the number of samples (i.e., scans) is usually very small in relation to the number of components (i.e., voxels) of the observations. This issue is resolved by analysing the data, not in terms of voxels, but in terms of eigenimages, because the number of eigenimages is much smaller than the number of voxels. The importance of the multivariate analysis that ensues can be summarised as follows: (1) Unlike eigenimage analysis, it provides for statistical inferences (based on classical p values) about the significance of the brain's response in terms of some hypothesis. (2) The approach implicitly takes into account spatial correlations in the data without making any assumptions. (3) The canonical variate analysis produces generalised eigenimages (canonical images) that capture the activation effects, while suppressing the effects of noise or error. (4) The theoretical basis is well established and can be found in most introductory texts on multivariate analysis (see also Friston *et al.*, 1996c).

Although useful, in a descriptive sense, eigenimage analysis and related approaches are not generally considered to be "statistical" methods that can be used to make statistical inferences; they are mathematical devices that simply identify prominent patterns of correlations or functional connectivity. It must be said, however, that large-sample, asymptotic, multivariate normal theory could be used to make some inferences about the relative contributions of each eigenimage (e.g., tests for nonsphericity) if a sufficient number of scans were available. In what follows we observe that MANCOVA with CVA combines some features of statistical parametric mapping and eigenimage analysis. Unlike statistical parametric mapping, MANCOVA is multivariate. In other words, it considers as one observation all voxels in a single scan. The importance of this multivariate approach is that effects, due to activations, confounding effects and error effects, are assessed both in terms of effects at each voxel *and interactions among voxels*. This means one does not have to assume anything about spatial correlations (cf. stationariness with Gaussian field models) to assess the significance of an activation effect. Unlike statistical parametric mapping, these correlations are explicitly included in the analysis. The price one pays for adopting a multivariate approach is that inferences cannot be made about regionally specific changes (cf. statistical parametric mapping). This is because the inference pertains to all components (voxels) of a multivariate variable (not a particular voxel or set of voxels). Furthermore, because the spatial nonsphericity has to be estimated without knowing the observations came from continuous spatially extended processes, the estimates are less efficient and inferences are less powerful.

In general, multivariate analyses are implemented in two steps. First, the significance of a hypothesised effect is assessed in terms of a p value and, second, if justified, the exact nature of the effect is determined. The analysis here conforms to this two-stage procedure. When the brain's response is assessed to be significant using MANCOVA, the nature of this response remains to be characterised. CVA is an appropriate way to do this. The canonical images obtained with CVA are similar to eigenimages but are based on both the activation and error. CVA is closely related to denoising techniques in EEG and MEG time series analyses that use a generalised eigenvalue solution. Another way of looking at canonical images is to think of them as eigenimages that reflect functional connectivity due to activations, when spurious correlations due to error are explicitly discounted.

Dimension Reduction and Eigenimages

The first step in multivariate analysis is to ensure that the dimensionality (number of components or voxels) of the data is smaller than the number of observations. Clearly for images this is not the case, because there are more voxels than scans; therefore, the data have to be transformed. The dimension reduction proposed here is straightforward and uses the scan-dependent expression Y of eigenimages as a reduced set of components for each multivariate observation (scan), where

$$\begin{aligned}[U,S,V] &= SVD(M) \\ Y &= US\end{aligned} \tag{49.13}$$

As above M is a large matrix of adjusted voxel values with one column for each voxel and one row for each scan. Here "adjusted" implies mean correction and removal of any confounds using linear regression. The eigenimages constitute the columns of U, another unitary orthonormal matrix, and their expression over scans corresponds to the columns of the matrix Y, which has one column for each eigenimage and one row for each scan. In our work we use only the j columns of Y and U associated with eigenvalues greater than unity (after normalising each eigenvalue by the average eigenvalue).

General Linear Model Revisited

Recall the general linear model from previous chapters:

$$Y = X\beta + \varepsilon \tag{49.14}$$

where the errors are assumed to be independent and identically normally distributed. The design matrix X has one column for every effect (factor or covariate) in the model. The design matrix can contain both covariates and indicator variables reflecting an experimental design. The β represents the parameter matrix with one column vector of parameters for each mode. Each column of X has an associated unknown parameter. Some of these parameters will be of interest, the remaining parameters will not. We will partition the model accordingly:

$$Y = X_1\beta_1 + X_0\beta_0 + \varepsilon \tag{49.15}$$

where X_1 represents a matrix of 0's or 1's depending on the level or presence of some interesting condition or treatment effect (e.g., the presence of a particular cognitive component) or the columns of X_1 might contain covariates of interest that could explain the observed variance in Y (e.g., dose of apomorphine or "time on target"). The term X_0 corresponds to a matrix of indicator variables denoting effects that are not of any interest (e.g., of being a particular subject or block effect) or covariates of no interest (i.e., "nuisance variables" such as global activity or confounding time effects).

Statistical Inference

Significance is assessed by testing the null hypothesis that the effects of interest do not significantly reduce the error variance when compared to the remaining effects alone (or alternatively the null hypothesis that β_1 is zero). The null hypothesis is tested in the following way. The sum of squares and products matrix (SSPM) due to error is obtained from the difference between actual and estimated values of the response:

$$S_R = (Y - X\hat{\beta})^T (Y - X\hat{\beta}) \tag{49.16}$$

where the sums of squares and products due to effects of interest is given by

$$S_T = (X_1\hat{\beta}_1)^T (X_1\hat{\beta}_1) \tag{49.17}$$

The error sum of squares and products under the null hypothesis, i.e., after discounting the effects of interest, are given by

$$S_0 = (Y - X_0\hat{\beta}_0)^T (Y - X_0\hat{\beta}_0) \tag{49.18}$$

The significance can now be tested with

$$\lambda = \frac{S_R}{S_0} \tag{49.19}$$

This is Wilk's statistic (known as Wilk's lambda). A special case of this test is Hotelling's T^2 test and applies when one simply compares one condition with another, i.e., X_1 has only one column (Chatfield and Collins, 1980). Under the null hypothesis, after transformation, λ has a chi-squared distribution with degrees of freedom jh. The transformation is given by

$$-(v - ((j - h + 1)/2)\ln \lambda \sim \chi^2_{jh} \tag{49.20}$$

where v are the degrees of freedom associated with error terms, equal to the number of scans (n) minus the number of effects modelled = n − rank(X), j is the number of eigenimages in the j-variate response variable, and the h are the degrees of freedom associated with effects of interest = rank(X_1).

Characterising the Effect

Having established that the effects of interest are significant (e.g., differences among two or more activation conditions) the final step is to characterise these effects in terms of their spatial topography. This characterisation uses CVA. The objective is to find a linear combination (compound or contrast) of the components of Y, in this case the eigenimages, that best expresses the activation effects when compared to error effects. More exactly we want to find c_1 such that the variance ratio

$$\frac{c_1^T S_T c_1}{c_1^T S_R c_1} \tag{49.21}$$

is maximised. Let $z_1 = Yc_1$ where z_1 is the first canonical variate and c_1 is a canonical image (defined in the space of the spatial modes) that maximises this ratio. c_2 is the second canonical image that maximises the ratio subject to the constraints $c_i^T c_j = 0$ (and so on). The matrix of canonical images c = $[c_1,\ldots,c_h]$ is given by solution of the generalised eigenvalue problem:

$$S_T c = S_R c \lambda \tag{49.22}$$

where λ is a diagonal matrix of eigenvalues. Voxel-space canonical images are obtained by rotating the canonical image in the columns of c back into voxel space with the original eigenimages $C = Vc$. The columns of C now contain the voxel values of the canonical images. The kth column of C (the kth canonical image) has an associated canonical value equal to the kth leading diagonal element of λ times r/h. Note that the "activation" effect is a multivariate one, with j components or canonical images. Normally only a few of these components have large canonical values and only these need to be reported. There are procedures based on distributional approximations of λ that allow inferences about the dimensionality of a response (number of canonical images). We refer the interested reader to Chatfield and Collins (1980) for further details.

Relationship to Eigenimage Analysis

When applied to adjusted data, eigenimages correspond to the eigenvectors of S_T. These have an interesting relationship to the canonical images: On rearranging Eq. (49.22), we note that the canonical images are eigenvectors of $S_R^{-1} S_T$. In other words, an eigenimage analysis of an activation study returns the eigenvectors that express the most variance due to the effects of interest. A canonical image, on the other hand, expresses the greatest amount of variance due to the effects of interest *relative to error*. In this sense, a CVA can be considered to be an eigenimage analysis that is "informed" by the estimates of error and their correlations over voxels.

An Illustrative Approach

In this section we consider an application of the above theory to the word generation study in normal subjects, used in previous sections. We assessed the significance of condition-dependent effects by treating each of the 12 scans as a different condition. Note that we do not consider the word generation (or word shadowing) conditions as replications of the same condition. In other words, the first time one performs a word generation task is a different condition from the second time ,and so on. The alternative hypothesis adopted here states that there is a significant difference among the 12 conditions, but does not constrain the nature of this difference to a particular form. The most important differences will emerge from the CVA. Clearly one might hope that these differences will be due to word generation, but they might not be. This hypothesis should be compared with a more constrained hypothesis that considers the conditions as six replications of word shadowing and word generation. This latter hypothesis is more directed and explicitly compares word shadowing with word generation. This comparison could be tested in a single subject. The point is that the generality afforded by the current framework allows one to test very constrained (i.e., specific) hypotheses or rather general hypotheses about some unspecified activation effect.[3] We choose the latter case here because it places more emphasis on canonical images as descriptions of what has actually occurred during the experiment.

The design matrix partition for effects of interest X_1 had 12 columns representing the 12 different conditions. We designated subject effects, time, and global activity as uninteresting confounds X_0. The adjusted data were reduced to 60 eigenvectors as described above. The first 14 eigenvectors had normalised eigenvalues greater than unity and were used in the subsequent analysis. The resulting matrix data Y, with 60 rows (one for each scan) and 14 columns (one for each eigenimage), was subject to MANCOVA. The significance of the condition effects was assessed with Wilk's lambda. The threshold for condition or activation effects was set at $p = 0.02$. In other words the probability of there being no differences among the 12 conditions was 2%.

[3] This is analogous to the use of the SPM{F}, relative to more constrained hypotheses tested with SPM{T}, in conventional mass-univariate approaches.

canonical image 1 {+ve}

canonical image 1 {-ve}

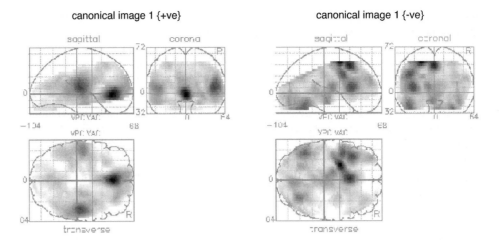

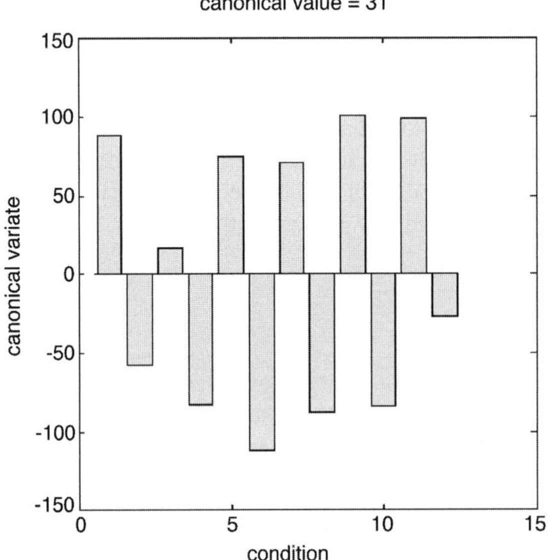

FIGURE 49.6
(Top) The first canonical image displayed as maximum intensity projections of the positive and negative components. The display format is standard and provides three views of the brain from the front, the back, and the right-hand side. The gray scale is arbitrary and the space conforms to that described in the atlas of Talairach and Tournoux (1988). (Bottom) The expression of the first canonical image (i.e., the canonical variate) averaged over conditions. The odd conditions correspond to word shadowing and the even conditions correspond to word generation. This canonical variate is clearly sensitive to the differences evoked by these two tasks.

Canonical Variates Analysis

The first canonical image and its canonical variate are shown in Fig. 49.6. The upper panels show this system to include anterior cingulate and Broca's area, with more moderate expression in the left posterior inferotemporal regions (right). The positive components of this canonical image (left) implicate ventromedial prefrontal cortex and bitemporal regions (right greater than left). One important aspect of these canonical images is their highly distributed yet structured nature, reflecting the distributed integration of many brain areas. The canonical variate expressed in terms of mean condition effects is seen in the lower panel of Fig. 49.6. It is pleasing to note that the first canonical variate corresponds to the difference between word shadowing and verbal fluency.

Recall that the eigenimage in Fig. 49.2 reflects the main pattern of correlations evoked by the mean condition effects and should be compared with the first canonical image in Fig. 49.6. The differences between these characterisations of activation effects are informative: The eigenimage is totally insensitive to the reliability or error attributable to differential activation from subject to subject, whereas the canonical image does reflect these variations. For example, the absence of the posterior cingulate in the canonical image and its relative prominence in the eigenimage suggests that this region is implicated in some subjects but not in others. The subjects that engage the posterior cingulate must do so to some considerable degree because the average effects (represented by the eigenimage) are quite substantial. Conversely, the medial prefrontal cortical deactivations are a more pronounced feature of activation effects than would have been inferred on the basis of the eigenimage analysis. These observations beg the question "Which is the best characterisation of functional anatomy?" Obviously there is no simple answer, but the question speaks to an important point. A canonical image characterises a response *relative to error,* by partitioning the observed variance into effects of interest and a residual variation about these effects. Experimental design, a hypothesis, and the inferences that are sought determine this partitioning. An eigenimage does not embody any concept of error and is not constrained by any hypothesis.

Multivariate Models

CVA rests on i.i.d. assumptions about the errors over time. Violation of these assumptions has motivated the study of multivariate linear models (MLMs) for neuroimaging that allow for temporal nonsphericity (see Worsley *et al.,* 1997). Although MLMs are important, this book has chosen to focus more on univariate models. There is a reason for this: Any MLM can be reformulated as a univariate model by simply vectorising the multivariate response. For example, the MLM

$$\begin{aligned} Y &= X\beta + \varepsilon \\ [y_1,\ldots y_j\} &= X[\beta_1,\ldots\beta_j] + [\varepsilon_1,\ldots\varepsilon_j] \end{aligned} \tag{49.23}$$

can be rearranged to give a univariate model:

$$\begin{aligned} vec(Y) &= (1 \otimes X)\, vec(\beta) + vec(\varepsilon) \\ \begin{bmatrix} y_1 \\ \vdots \\ y_j \end{bmatrix} &= \begin{bmatrix} X & & \\ & \ddots & \\ & & X \end{bmatrix} \begin{bmatrix} y_1 \\ \vdots \\ y_j \end{bmatrix} + \begin{bmatrix} \varepsilon_1 \\ \vdots \\ \varepsilon_j \end{bmatrix} \end{aligned} \tag{49.24}$$

where $\otimes$ denotes the Kronecker tensor product. Here $cov(vec(\varepsilon)) = \Sigma \otimes V$, where Σ are the covariances among components and V encodes the temporal correlations. In MLMs Σ is unconstrained and requires full estimation (in terms of S_R). Therefore, any MLM and its univariate version are exactly equivalent if we place constraints on the nonsphericity of the errors that ensure it has the form $\Sigma \otimes V$. This speaks to an important point: Any multivariate analysis can proceed in a univariate setting with appropriate constraints on the nonsphericity. In fact, MLMs are special cases that assume the covariances factorise into $\Sigma \otimes V$ and Σ is unconstrained. In neuroimaging there are obvious constraints on the form of Σ because this embodies the spatial covariances. Random field theory harnesses these constraints. MLMs do not and are therefore less sensitive.

SUMMARY

This chapter has described multivariate approaches to the analysis of functional imaging studies. These use standard multivariate techniques to describe or make statistical inferences about distributed activation effects and characterise important features of functional connectivity. The multivariate approach differs fundamentally from statistical parametric mapping, because the concept of a separate voxel or region of interest ceases to have meaning. In this sense inference is about the whole image volume not any component of it. This feature precludes statistical inferences about regional effects made without reference to changes elsewhere in the brain. This fundamental difference ensures that mass-univariate and multivariate approaches are likely to be regarded as distinct and complementary approaches to functional imaging data (see Kherif *et al.,* 2002).

In this chapter we have used correlations among brain measurements to identify systems that respond in a coherent fashion. This identification proceeds without reference to the mechanisms that may mediate distributed and integrated responses. In the next chapter we turn to models of effective connectivity that ground the nature of these interactions.

References

Biswal, B., Yetkin, F. Z., Haughton, V. M., and Hyde, J. S. (1995). Functional connectivity in the motor cortex of resting human brain using echo-planar MRI. *Mag. Res. Med.* **34,** 537–541.

Bleuler, E. (1911). Dementia Praecox or the group of schizophrenias. Translated into English 1987 in *The Clinical Roots of the Schizophrenia Concept,* Cutting, J., and Shepherd, M., Eds. Cambridge University Press, UK.

Chatfield, C., and Collins, A. J. (1980). *Introduction to Multivariate Analysis,* pp. 189–210. Chapman and Hall, London.

Friedrich, R., Fuchs, A., and Haken, H. (1991). Modelling of spatio-temporal EEG patterns. In *Mathematical Approaches to Brain Functioning Diagnostics*, Dvorak, I., and Holden, A. V., Eds. Manchester University Press, New York.

Fuchs, A., Kelso, J. A. S., and Haken, H. (1992). Phase transitions in the human brain: spatial mode dynamics. *Int. J. Bifurcation Chaos* **2,** 917–939.

Friston, K. J. (1998). Modes or models: a critique on independent component analysis for fMRI. *Trends Cog. Sci.* **2,** 373–374.

Friston, K. J., Frith, C. D., Liddle, P. F., and Frackowiak, R. S. J. (1993a). Functional connectivity: the principal component analysis of large (PET). data sets. *J. Cereb. Blood Flow Metab.* **13,** 5-14.

Friston, K. J., Jezzard, P., Frackowiak, R. S. J., and Turner, R. (1993b). Characterising focal and distributed physiological changes with MRI and PET. In *Functional MRI of the Brain,* pp. 207&n dash;216. Society of Magnetic Resonance in Medicine, Berkeley CA.

Friston, K. J., Frith, C. D., Fletcher, P., Liddle, P. F., and Frackowiak, R. S. J. (1996a). Functional topography: multidimensional scaling and functional connectivity in the brain *Cerebral Cortex* **6,** 156–164.

Friston, K. J., Herold, S., Fletcher, P., Silbersweig, D., Cahill, C., Dolan, R. J., Liddle, P. F., Frackowiak, R. S. J., and Frith, C. D.(1996b). Abnormal fronto-temporal interactions in schizophrenia In *Biology of Schizophrenia and Affective Disease,* Watson, S. J., Ed., *ARNMD Ser.* **73,** 421–429.

Friston, K. J., Poline, J.-B., Holmes, A. P., Frith, C. D., and Frackowiak, R. S. J. (1996c). A multivariate analysis of PET activation studies. *Hum. Brain Mapping* **4,** 140–151.

Friston, K. J, Phillips, J., Chawla, D., and Büchel, C. (2000). Nonlinear PCA: characterising interactions between modes of brain activity. *Phil. Trans. Roy. Soc. Lond. B* **355,** 135–146.

Gerstein, G. L., and Perkel, D. H. (1969). Simultaneously recorded trains of action potentials: analysis and functional interpretation. *Science* **164,** 828–830.

Goldman-Rakic, P. S. (1988). Topography of cognition: parallel distributed networks in primate association cortex. *Ann. Rev. Neurosci.* **11,** 137–156.

Gower, J. C. (1966). Some distance properties of latent root and vector methods used in multivariate analysis. *Biometrika* **53,** 325–328.

Karhunen, J., and Joutsensalo, J. (1994). Representation and separation of signals using nonlinear PCA type learning. *Neural Networks* **7,** 113–127.

Kherif, F., Poline, J. B., Flandin, G., Benali, H., Simon, O., Dehaene, S., and Worsley, K. J. (2002). Multivariate model specification for fMRI data. *NeuroImage* **16,** 1068–83.

Kramer, M. A. (1991). Nonlinear principal component analysis using auto-associative neural networks. *AIChE J.* **37,** 233–243.

Mayer-Kress, G., Barczys, C., and Freeman, W. (1991). Attractor reconstruction from event-related multi-electrode EEG data. In *Mathematical Approaches to Brain Functioning Diagnostics,* Dvorak, I., and Holden, A. V., Eds. Manchester University Press, New York.

McIntosh, A. R., Bookstein, F. L., Haxby, J. V., and Grady, C. L. (1996). Spatial pattern analysis of functional brain images using partial least squares. *NeuroImage* **3,** 143–157.

McKeown, M. J., Makeig, S., Brown, G. G., Jung, T. P., Kindermann, S. S., Bell, A. J., and Sejnowski, T. J. (1998). Analysis of fMRI data by blind separation into independent spatial components. *Hum. Brain Mapping* **6,** 160–188..

Newton, I. (1794). *Opticks.* Book 1, Part 2, Prop. 6. Smith and Walford, London.

Phillips, C. G., Zeki, S., and Barlow, H. B. (1984). Localisation of function in the cerebral cortex. Past, present and future. *Brain* **107,** 327–361.

Shepard, R. N. (1980). Multidimensional scaling, tree-fitting and clustering. *Science* **210,** 390–398.

Stone, J. V. (2002). Independent component analysis: an introduction, *Trends Cog. Sci.* **6**; 59–64.

Talairach, J., and Tournoux, P. (1988). *A Co-Planar Stereotaxic Atlas of a Human Brain.* Thieme, Stuttgart.

Torgerson, W. S. (1958). *Theory and Methods of Scaling.* Wiley, New York.

Worsley, K. J., Poline, J. B., Friston, K. J., and Evans, A. C. (1997).Characterising the response of PET and fMRI data using multivariate linear models. *NeuroImage* **6**;305–319.

CHAPTER

50

Effective Connectivity

INTRODUCTION

In the previous chapter we dealt with functional connectivity and different ways of summarising patterns of correlations among brain systems. In this chapter we turn to effective connectivity and the models of mechanisms that might mediate these correlations.

Brain function depends on interactions among brain components that range from individual cell compartments to neuronal populations. As described in Chapter 48, anatomical and physiological studies of connectivity *in vivo* speak to a hierarchy of specialised regions that process increasingly abstract features, from simple edges in V1, through colour and motion in V4 and V5, respectively, to face recognition in the fusiform gyrus. The implicitly specialised regions are connected, allowing distributed and reentrant neuronal information processing. The selective responses, or specialisation, of a region is a function of its connectivity. An important theme is this chapter is that these connections can change and show context sensitivity. We refer to these changes as *plasticity,* to describe physiological changes in the influence different brain systems have on each other. The formation of distributed networks, through dynamic interactions, is the basis of functional integration, which is itself, time and context dependent. Changes in connectivity are important for development, learning, perception, and adaptive response to injury.

Given the importance of changes in connectivity, we consider two classes of experimental factors or input to the brain. The first class evokes responses directly, but the second has a more subtle effect and can induce input-dependent changes in connectivity that modulates responses to the first. We will refer to the second class of inputs as *contextual.* For example, augmented neuronal responses associated with attending to a stimulus can be attributed to the changes induced in connectivity by attention. The distinction between inputs that evoke responses and those that modulate effective connectivity is the motivation for developing models that accommodate contextual changes in connection strength.

This chapter is divided into four sections. First, we motivate a systems identification approach, in which brain responses are parameterised within the framework of a mathematical model. The state-space representation is used to illustrate coupling within a system and interactions with experimental factors. To demonstrate how connectivity can be modulated experimentally, and how the notion of effective connectivity emerges as a natural metric, a bilinear state-space model (BSSM) is derived to approximate generic nonlinear networks. We then describe the theory behind different approaches to estimating functional integration, looking at static and dynamic models. We conclude with some remarks on strategies and the features of models that have proved useful in modelling connectivity to date.

Notation

Lowercase letters are used for scalars and vectors and uppercase for matrices. If x is a normally distributed random variable with mean μ and variance σ^2, we write $x \sim N(\mu,\sigma^2)$. A time series of observations at voxel i is written y^i. An image at time t is written y_t , and the value of the ith voxel at time t is y^i_t. The total number of voxels and scans are N and T, respectively. We use $\exp(X)$, X^T, X^{-1}, and X^+ to denote the matrix exponential, transpose, inverse, and pseudo-inverse, respectively. We also write $x \times y$ to denote the Hadamard product between two vectors (in Matlab this is an array or element-by-element multiplication with $x.*y$). The first-order derivative of the time-dependent variable $x(t)$ with respect to time $[\partial x(t)/\partial t]$ is denoted by $\dot{x}$.

IDENTIFICATION OF DYNAMIC SYSTEMS

System identification (SI) is the use of observed data to estimate the parameters of mathematical models representing a physical system. The mathematical models may be linear or nonlinear, in discrete or continuous time, and parameterised in the time or frequency domain. The aim is to construct a mathematical description of a system's response to input. Models may be divided into two main categories: those that invoke hidden states and those that quantify relationships between inputs and outputs without hidden states, effectively treating the system as a black box (see Juang, 2001, for a comprehensive account). Examples of the former include state-space models (SSM) and hidden Markov models (HMM), whereas the latter include generalised convolution models (Bendat, 1998) and autoregressive models (Chatfield, 1996).

The two main requirements of a biologically plausible model of functional integration are that it be dynamic and nonlinear. Dynamic, because the brain is a physical system extended in time, meaning that the state of the brain now effects its state in the future. We look later at the benefits and problems that stem from relaxing this requirement. In addition, biological systems depend on nonlinear phenomena for much of their characteristic behaviour (Scott, 1999). Examples include the neuronal dynamics of action potentials (Dayan and Abbott, 2001), population dynamics in coevolutionary systems (Glass and Kaplan, 2000), and limit cycles in physiological systems (Glass, 2001). The motivation for appealing to nonlinear dynamic models is that their nonadditive characteristics enable them to reproduce highly complex behaviour, of the sort we observe in biological systems. However, nonlinear models are often mathematically intractable, calling for approximation techniques.

Linear dynamic models, on the other hand, can be analysed in closed form. Consequently, a large body of theory exists for handling them. This is due to their adherence to the principle of superposition, which means that the system's response to input is additive. There are no interactions between different inputs or between inputs and the intrinsic states of the system such that the response is a weighted linear mixture of inputs. A system that violates this principle would respond in a nonadditive manner, i.e., with more or less than a linear combination of inputs. Such a system is, by definition, nonlinear. However, we pay a price for the ease with which linear models can be analysed, because their behavioural repertoire is limited to exponential decay and growth, oscillation, or a combination of these. Examples of subadditive responses are ubiquitous in physiology (e.g., saturation). With increasing input many biological systems (e.g., biochemical reactions or synaptic input) reach a saturation point where further input does not generate a further response.

A useful compromise is to make linear approximations to a generic nonlinear model. These models have the advantage that they capture essential nonlinear features while remaining mathematically tractable. This strategy has engendered bilinear models (Rao, 1992), in which nonlinear interaction terms are limited to interactions that can be modelled as the product of two variables (input or intrinsic states). Despite constraints on higher order nonlinearities, bilinear models can easily model plasticity in effective connections.

We use a bilinear state-space representation to illustrate the concepts of linear and bilinear coupling and how they may be used to model effective connectivity. The introduction of unknown variables (hidden states) may appear to complicate the problem, but this is not the case because long-range order, within observed time series, can be modelled through interactions among the states.

Approximating Nonlinear Functions

Any sufficiently smooth function, $f(x)$, of a scalar quantity x may be approximated in the neighbourhood of an expansion point, x_0, using the Taylor series expansion as follows:

$$f(x) \approx f(x_0) + \frac{df(x_0)}{dx}(x - x_0) + \frac{d^2f(x_0)}{dx^2}\frac{(x - x_0)^2}{2!} + \ldots + \frac{d^nf(x_0)}{dx^n}\frac{(x - x_0)^n}{n!} \tag{50.1}$$

where the nth-order derivatives are evaluated at x_0. These values are coefficients that scale the contribution of their respective terms. The derivatives are used as they map a local change in $(x - x_0)^n$ onto a change in $f(x)$. The degree of nonlinearity of f determines the rate of convergence, with weakly nonlinear functions converging rapidly. The series converges to the *exact* function with inclusion of higher order terms. A simple example is shown in Fig. 50.1.

When these ideas are extended to bivariate nonlinear functions, where $f(x,u)$ depends on two quantities x and u, the corresponding Taylor series includes increasingly complex (high-order) terms (products of x and u). The linear and bilinear approximations are given by f_L and f_{BL}:

$$\begin{aligned} f_L(x,u) &= ax + cu \\ a &= \frac{\partial f}{\partial x} \\ c &= \frac{\partial f}{\partial u} \\ f_{BL}(x,u) &= ax + bxu + cu \\ b &= \frac{\partial^2 f}{\partial x \partial u} \end{aligned} \tag{50.2}$$

For clarity, the expansion point $x_0 = 0$ and the series have been centred so that $f(x_0) = f(u_0) = 0$. The approximation, f_L, depends on linear terms in x and u scaled by coefficients a and c, calculated from first-order derivatives. The first-order terms of f_{BL} are the same as f_L, however, the third term is composed of the product of x and u, which is scaled by b, the second-order

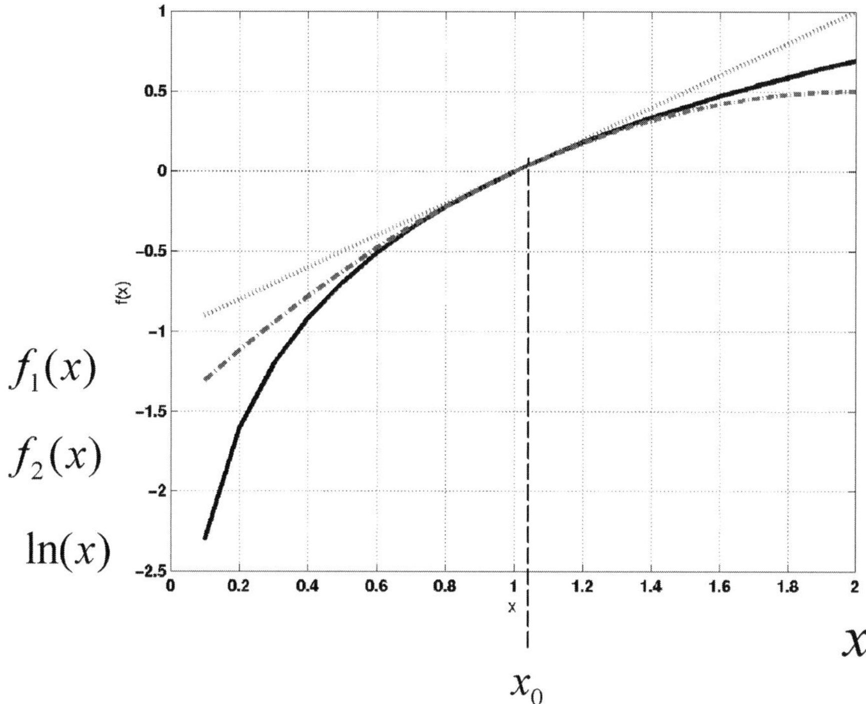

FIGURE 50.1
Approximations to $f(x) = \ln(x)$ about $x_0 = 1$ using Taylor series expansions, where $f_1(x) = x - 1$ and $f_2(x) = (x - 1) - 1/2\,(x - 1)^2$ are the first- and second-order approximations. The improvement about x_0 for higher order approximations is apparent.

derivative with respect to both variables. This term introduces nonlinearity into f_{BL}. Note that the bilinear form does not include quadratic functions of x or u. The resulting approximation has the appealing property of being both linear in x and u, but allowing for a modulation of x by u. Changes in $f(x,u)$ are no longer only a linear sum of changes in x and u, but now include a contribution from a new variable xu.

We can now replace the scalar quantities with vectors where $x = [x_1,\ldots,x_n]^T$ and $x = [u_1,\ldots,u_m]^T$. The x represents an $n \times 1$ vector containing n different state variables and u is an $m \times 1$ vector containing m input variables. The linear and bilinear approximations can be written in matrix form, as follows:

$$f_L(x,u) = Ax + Cu \tag{50.3}$$
$$f_{BL}(x,u) = Ax + \sum_i u_j B^j x + Cu$$

The coefficients are matrices as opposed to scalar terms. They look more complicated, but the same operation is being applied to all the elements of the matrix coefficients. Matrixes A and B^j are $n \times n$ and C is $n \times m$. For example,

$$A = \frac{\partial f}{\partial x} = \begin{bmatrix} \frac{\partial f_1}{\partial x_1} & \cdots & \frac{\partial f_1}{\partial x_n} \\ \vdots & \ddots & \vdots \\ \frac{\partial f_n}{\partial x_1} & \vdots & \frac{\partial f_n}{\partial x_n} \end{bmatrix} \tag{50.4}$$

Linear Dynamic Models

The equations above can be used to model the dynamics of a physical system. Figure 50.2 shows a simple illustration. A physical system can be modelled by a number of states and inputs. The states are contained in x, called the *state vector,* and inputs in u, the *input vector.* Generally, x and u can vary with time, denoted by $x(t)$ and $u(t)$. The number of states and inputs in the model are given by n and m, respectively. Each state defines a coordinate in state-space within which the behaviour of the system is represented as a trajectory. The temporal evolution of the states is modelled by a state equation, which is the first-order temporal derivative of the state vector, written as $\dot{x}(t)$ and can therefore be approximated by a Taylor series as above:

$$\dot{x} = f_L(x,u) = Ax + Cu \tag{50.5}$$

A linear dynamic system (LDS) is shown in Fig. 50.3. The figure consists of two states, $x_1(t)$ and $x_2(t)$, and external inputs, $u_1(t)$ and $u_2(t)$, coupled through a state equation parameterised by matrices A and C. Because the model contains two states and two inputs, these matrices are both 2×2.

Matrix A contains parameters that determine interactions among states (labelled interstate in Fig. 50.3) and the influence a state's own activity has on itself (for example, the damping term in a linearly damped harmonic oscillator), whereas the elements of C couple inputs with states. The state equation describes the influences among states and their response to input, thereby providing a complete description of the dynamics of the system, otherwise known as the system's equation of motion. These models are sometimes called linear time-invariant (LTI) systems as A and C do not change with time. Eq. (50.5) can be rewritten as

$$z(t) = Jz(t) \tag{50.6}$$

where $z(t)$ is an $(n + 1) \times 1$ vector and J is an $(n + 1) \times (n + 1)$ matrix. This is a linear equation, which can be solved using standard linear techniques (Boas, 1983), such as the matrix exponential method (see the Appendix at the end of this chapter).

Bilinear Dynamic Models

Linear models have dominated scientific models, despite much nonlinearity around us, because they are good first approximations to many phenomena. However, they remain restricted and

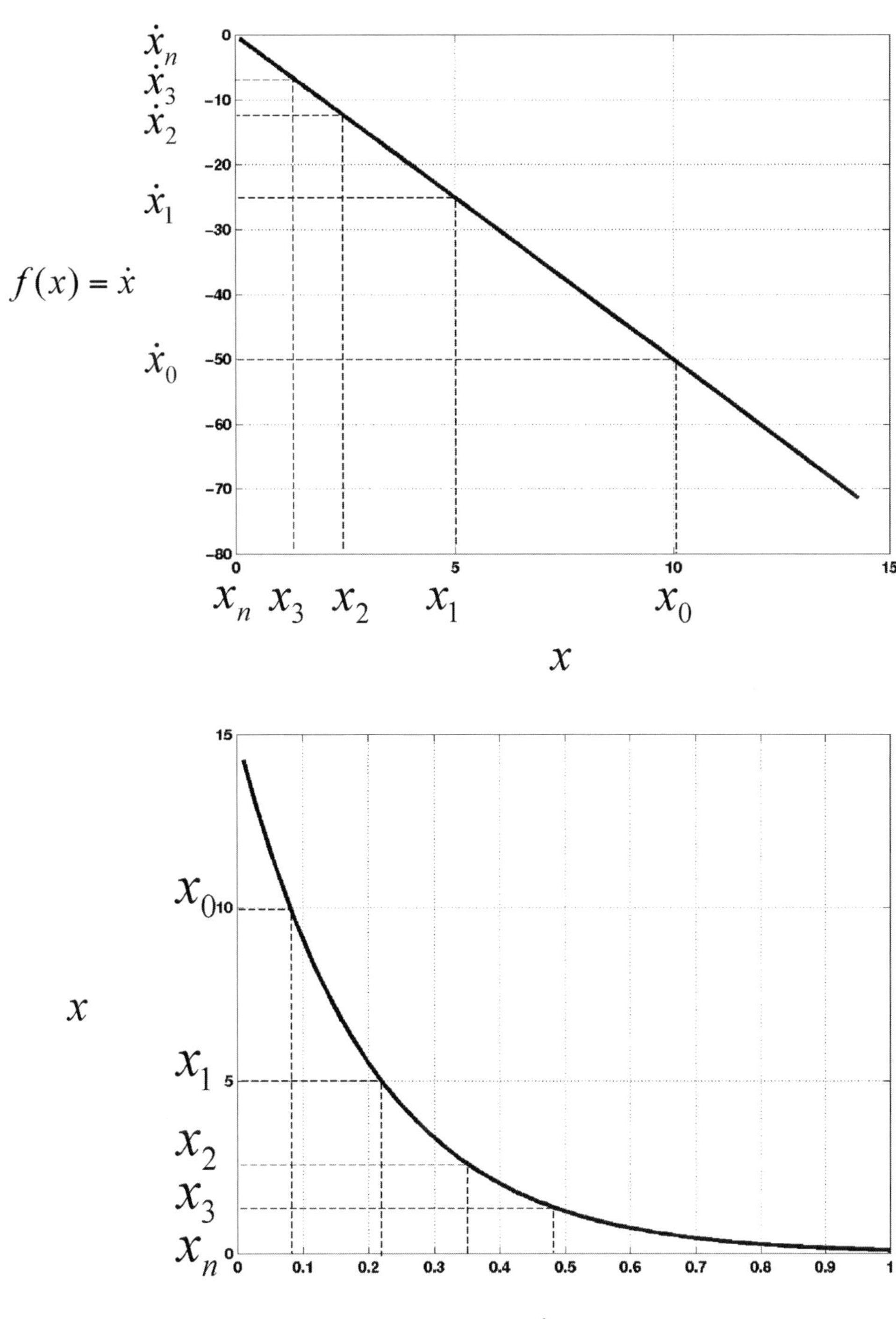

FIGURE 50.2
The function $f(x)$ models a simple one-state (x) linear dynamic system, i.e., $\dot{x} = f(x)$. The state starts at the value x_0 where it *decreases* [i.e., the value of $f(x) > 0$] at the rate $\dot{x}_0$. After a period of time, the state has decreased to x_1 with a rate of $\dot{x}_1$. The state continues to change until $f(x) = 0$, when $\dot{x}_1 = 0$. The overall behaviour of the model is that the state decreases exponentially with time. A familiar example is radioactive decay, where the state is the number of radioactive atoms. Their rate of decay is not uniform, but varies linearly with the number of atoms.

sometimes unrealistic descriptions. The use of bilinear models represents a substantial break with linearity. The model in Fig. 50.4 has been augmented to illustrate the simple steps needed to formulate a bilinear model. The state equation can be modelled by an equation of the same form as f_{BL}, whose essential feature is the bilinear interaction involving the product of an input with a state. This can be written

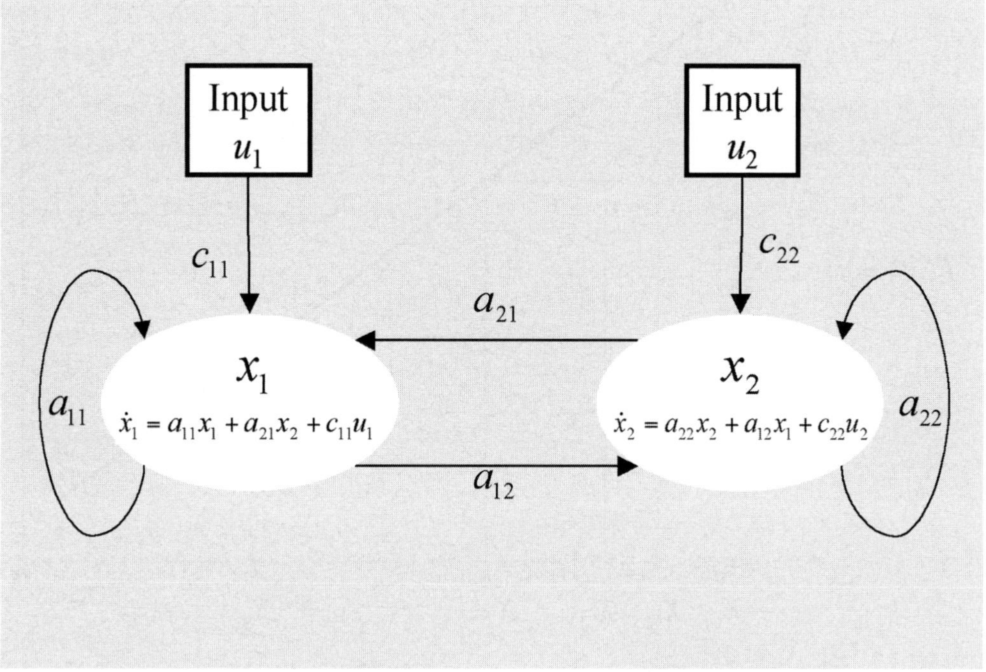

Intrinsic connectivity | Connectivity to extrinsic input

$$\begin{bmatrix} \dot{x}_1 \\ \dot{x}_2 \end{bmatrix} = \begin{bmatrix} a_{11} & a_{12} \\ a_{21} & a_{22} \end{bmatrix} \begin{bmatrix} x_1 \\ x_2 \end{bmatrix} + \begin{bmatrix} c_{11} & 0 \\ 0 & c_{22} \end{bmatrix} \begin{bmatrix} u_1 \\ u_2 \end{bmatrix}$$

Inter-state & self

$$\dot{x} = Ax + Cu$$

FIGURE 50.3
A linear dynamic system with two states, x_1 and x_2, and inputs, u_l and u_2, determined by the time-invariant matrices A and C in the state equation. The state equation contains terms for intrinsic connectivity and how states are connected to external inputs. These are parameterised by the elements in matrices A and C, respectively. Matrix A contains elements that model influences among states (interstate) and on themselves (for example, the damping term in the model of a linearly damped harmonic oscillator).

$$\begin{aligned} \dot{x} &= f_{BL}(x,u) \\ &= (A + \sum_{j=1}^{m} u_j B^j)x + Cu \\ &= \tilde{A}x + Cu \end{aligned} \tag{50.7}$$

The critical difference is the addition of B that is now modulated by $u(t)$, which, when added to A, models input-dependent changes to the intrinsic connectivity of the network. This is illustrated in Fig. 50.4 where the coupling coefficient a_{21} is modulated by the product $b_{21}^2 u_2$. The modified matrix $\tilde{A}$ operates on the state vector and determines the response of the model. The difference is that $\tilde{A}$ changes with time because it is a function of time-varying input, which distinguishes it from the LTI model above.

It helps to consider a specific example. If u_2 is binary, the model in Fig. 50.4 effectively consists of two LTI models. The model's behaviour, i.e., $x(t)$, will be characterised by two linear

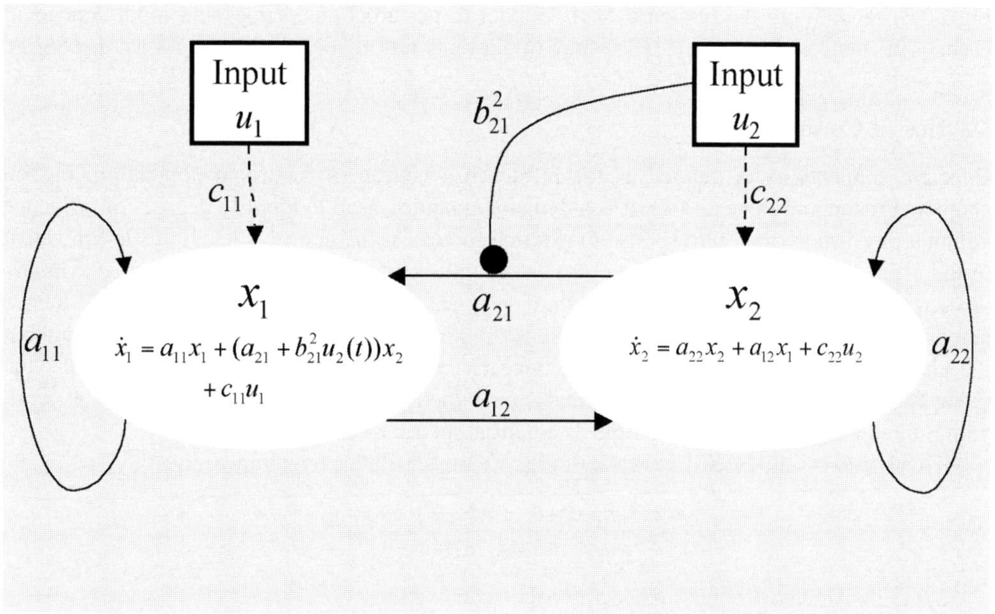

$$\begin{bmatrix} \dot{x}_1 \\ \dot{x}_2 \end{bmatrix} = \left(\begin{bmatrix} a_{11} & a_{12} \\ a_{21} & a_{22} \end{bmatrix} + \begin{bmatrix} 0 & 0 \\ b_{21}^2 & 0 \end{bmatrix} u_2 \right) \begin{bmatrix} x_1 \\ x_2 \end{bmatrix} + \begin{bmatrix} c_{11} & 0 \\ 0 & c_{22} \end{bmatrix} \begin{bmatrix} u_1 \\ u_2 \end{bmatrix}$$

$$\dot{x} = \widetilde{A}x + Cu$$

$$\widetilde{A} = A + \sum_{j=1}^{m} u_j B^j$$

Induced connectivity

FIGURE 50.4
A bilinear dynamic model similar to Fig. 50.3. However, input u_2 can interact with coupling coefficients a_{21} rendering matrix $\widetilde{A}(t)$ time dependent. This induces input-dependent modulation of the coupling parameters, with the consequence of different responses to other inputs, i.e., u_1. All connections that are not shown correspond to zero elements in the matrices.

systems switching from one to the other. The moment the system switches from one linear mode will be determined by changes in u_2. For instance, if the two linear models were linearly damped harmonic oscillators, each with markedly different characteristic behaviours, i.e., period of oscillation, a switch from one state to another would be accompanied by changes in the oscillation of the states. In short, the dynamics of x represents a simple two-state system.

The benefit of constraining the model to include only bilinear terms is that we have circumvented the issue of intractability of nonlinear models, yet have retained a uniquely nonlinear feature: input-dependent modulation of intrinsic dynamics. Inputs can now be divided into two classes: perturbing and contextual. Perturbing inputs (e.g., u_1 in Fig. 50.3) influence states directly, without modulating model parameters. The effects of these inputs are distributed according to the intrinsic connections of the model, whereas contextual inputs (e.g., u_2 in

Fig. 50.3) reconfigure the response of the model to perturbations. Time- and input-dependent changes in connectivity are a central feature of plasticity and are the motivation for using BSSMs.

Metrics of Connectivity

Effective connectivity is defined as the influence a neuron (or neuronal population) has on another (Friston and Price, 2001). It is a dynamic quantity, used to identify degrees of influence within a physical system, in response to external forces. At the neuronal level, this is equivalent to the effect presynaptic activity has on postsynaptic responses, otherwise known as *synaptic efficacy.* Models of effective connectivity are designed to identify a suitable metric of influence among interconnected components (or regions of interest) in the brain. We shall see, throughout the chapter, how measures of effective connectivity identify dynamic structure within data, induced through experimental design and constrained by the operational principles at work within the brain, and how they emerge as a natural metric of plasticity.

Given the two-state BSSM network in Fig. 50.4, each state's equation is given by

$$\dot{x}_1 = a_{11}x_1 + (a_{21} + b^2_{21}u_2)x_2 + c_{11}u_1$$
$$\dot{x}_2 = a_{22}x_2 + a_{12}x_1 + c_{22}u_2$$

Taking derivatives of $\dot{x}$ with respect to each state, we get

$$\frac{\partial \dot{x}_1}{\partial x_2} = k_{21}(x,u) = a_{21} + b^2_{21}u_2$$

$$\frac{\partial \dot{x}_2}{\partial x_1} = k_{12}(x,u) = a_{12}$$

This operation discloses the coupling between the two regions (states), i.e., the direct influence one region has on another. Generally, this may be linear or nonlinear, however, it is reduced to a simple function in a bilinear model, described by k_{12} and k_{21}. The coupling from x_1 to x_2 is linear, represented by a constant term, a_{12}. However, the interaction between u_2 and x_2 induces nonlinearities in the network, rendering k_{21} a function of u_2. The degree of influence x_2 has on x_1 therefore depends on u_2. This effect may be quantified by taking derivatives with respect to u_2, the contextual input:

$$\frac{\partial^2 \dot{x}_1}{\partial x_2 \partial u_2} = h(x,u) = b^2_{21}$$

As for the first-order derivative, $h(x,u)$, a second-order derivative may be a nonlinear function of the states and input for an arbitrarily nonlinear equation of motion. However, it reduces to a constant term in the bilinear model.

The first- and second-order derivatives quantify dynamic characteristics within a network. Therefore, they are equivalent to first- and second-order effective connectivity or obligatory and modulatory influences (Büchel and Friston, 2000). This distinction highlights two important issues: the difference between perturbing and contextual input and how to derive a practical measure of connectivity. As illustrated in Fig. 50.4, external input can be categorised by way of its effect on the intrinsic states of a system. Either input modulates a systems intrinsic connectivity or it perturbs the states directly. The former we have coined *contextual* and the latter *perturbing.* Both evoke a response. However, contextual inputs enable the model to represent contextual changes by modulation of the intrinsic connectivity. This is a subtle but crucial difference. Practically, models of this nature can be used to infer levels of effective connectivity through estimating parameters such as a_{12} and b^2_{21} from real data.

A caveat is necessary at this point. All models require some form of *a priori* knowledge. Factoring this into a model fairly will always be cause for some debate. This is because what is "fair" for one model may not be for another. However, for progress to be made, a strategy has to be formulated and appraised to assess its value in the context of the data. Models of effective connectivity generally require an anatomical model to specify *which* regions are connected. A simplified but sufficient anatomical model can be based on lesion studies or anatomical data from animal models. A mathematical model, such as that described above, i.e., an equation of motion representing the brain as a connected physical system, is necessary to model *how* the different regions in the anatomical model interact. These mathematical models can become very complicated and mathematically intractable. Models can be simplified by approximating methods, as we saw with the bilinear model, and making assumptions, such as ignoring temporally distant effects of neuronal events, i.e., assuming only instantaneous effects of disparate brain regions on each other. This may sound a little abstract at the moment, but we will see later how this assumption allows us to make progress by rendering the models tractable. Even though simple models may be criticised for being biologically implausible, progress can be incremental. In the next section, we discuss various models for measuring connectivity from PET and fMRI data, highlighting their heuristics, and assumptions.

Relevance to Neurophysiology

Figure 50.5 portrays a model of the visual and attention systems. The model posits photic stimulation as an input, or cause in the environment, which perturbs the brain evoking a response that depends on its current state of connectivity. This connectivity embodies a context, such as attentional set or memory (i.e., whether the stimulus is salient). Perceptual learning, or changes in attention, induce a reconfiguration of synaptic efficacies and connectivity in terms of ensemble responses (see Chapter 52). In the model, these are examples of contextual input that enable the brain to respond differently to the same perturbing stimulus, i.e., the difference between a novel visual image or the recognition of a stimulus that has recently become salient.

Having described the basis for modelling the brain as a physical interconnected system and establishing a fundamental distinction between inputs that change states and those that change (parameter) connections, we now turn to some specific examples. We start with simple models and work back toward the dynamic models described in this section.

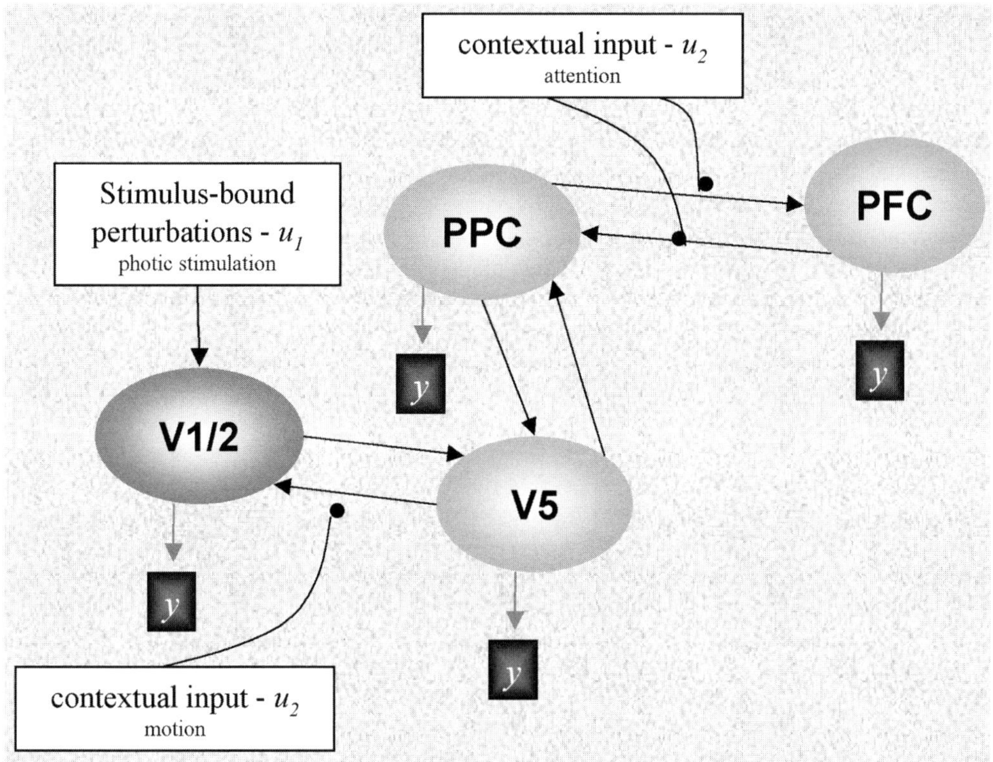

FIGURE 50.5
A model of functional integration between the visual and attention systems. Sensory input has a direct effect on the primary visual cortex, whereas contextual inputs, such as motion or attention to the stimulus, modulate pathways between nodes in the extended network. In this way, contextual input (e.g., induced by instructional set) may activate (or deactivate) pathways, which in turn determine the response of the system to stimulus-bound inputs.

LINEAR MODELS OF EFFECTIVE CONNECTIVITY

The objective of an effective connectivity analysis is to estimate parameters that represent influences among regions that may change over time and with respect to experimental tasks. Neuroimaging data are usually processed into a voxel-based time-series of an index of neuronal activity (rCBF or BOLD for PET and fMRI, respectively). Structure exists in the experimental design, neurophysiological data, and, critically, the theoretical assumptions used to model the observed responses. For example, the spatial and temporal order within the data provide essential insights into the underlying generative processes and is clearly the rationale of an empirical approach. Models also contain structure, because they represent the theoretical constructs and assumptions needed to identify operational principles responsible for generating the data.

Identifying a complete and biologically plausible mathematical model requires a high level of sophistication. However, some progress can be made by modelling relationships in the data alone (among voxels or regions), without invoking hidden states and ignoring the consequent temporal correlations. This last simplification makes the mathematics much easier but discards temporal information and is biologically unrealistic. We will call these models *static* because they model interactions among regions as occurring instantaneously and do not encompass the influence previous states have on current responses. Static models are reviewed before turning to more realistic, *dynamic* models. Both are important in the development of a plausible metric of effective connectivity, the former establishing an historical benchmark to validate the latter. In what follows we describe the development of approaches, demonstrated through different models, designed to represent dynamic interactions as measured through neuroimaging data.

Linear Models

After measuring an index of neuronal activity at each voxel in the brain, over the duration of an experiment, the next step is to determine, on the basis of these data, if there is any reason to believe that different regions of the brain influence each other.

Our first model is linear and assumes that y_t^i is statistically independent of $y_{t-\tau}^i$ for arbitrary τ. This is a valid assumption for PET data because the sampling rate is slow relative to neuronal dynamics. In fact, data are acquired while holding brain states constant using an appropriate task or stimulus. Each measurement is therefore assumed to represent some average brain state. Mathematically, this means the rate of change of the states is assumed to be zero. For fMRI time series, however, this assumption is generally violated (and certainly for electrophysiological measurements). As the sampling rate of measurement increases, so does the dynamic character of the data. This is the motivation for dynamic models of fMRI responses.

In static linear models, the activity of each voxel is modelled as a linear mixture activity in all voxels plus some error. This can be written as follows:

$$
\begin{aligned}
y_t^i &= \beta_{1i}y_t^1 + \beta_{2i}y_t^2 + \ldots + \varepsilon_t^i \\
&= y_t\beta_i + \varepsilon_t^i \\
\beta_i &= \begin{bmatrix} \beta_{1i} \\ \vdots \\ \beta_{Ni} \end{bmatrix} \\
\hline
y_t &= y_t\beta + \varepsilon_t \\
y_t &= [y_t^1, \ldots, y_t^N] \\
\beta &= [\beta_1, \ldots, \beta_N] \\
\hline
Y &= Y\beta + \varepsilon \\
Y &= \begin{bmatrix} y_1 \\ \vdots \\ y_T \end{bmatrix}
\end{aligned}
\tag{50.8}
$$

for one region at one time, all regions at one time, and all the data, respectively. The problem with this formulation is that the trivial solution $\beta_{ii} = 1$ completely accounts for the data. We will see later how structural equation modelling deals with this by setting self-connections to zero.

$$M = s_1 U_1 V_1^T + U_2 V_2^T + \ldots U_m V_m^T$$

$$\widetilde{M} = \sum_{i=1}^{r} s_i U_i V_i^T = \sum_{i=1}^{r} s_i M_i$$

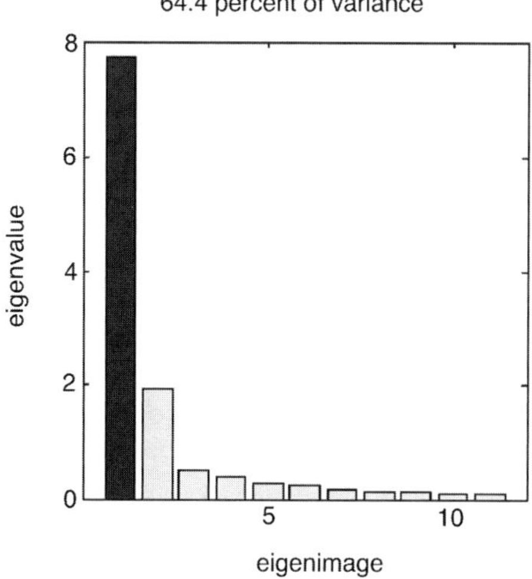

FIGURE 50.6
(Top) Singular value decomposition. The SVD technique converts an arbitrary matrix, such as M, into an equivalent form, consisting of a mixture of eigenimages (eigenvectors) and scaled by a variance component. (Bottom) Eigenspectrum of a typical PET dataset is shown to demonstrate that the majority of variance is captured by the first few eigenvectors.

However, one also can finesse this problem using singular value decomposition (SVD). Multivariate techniques like SVD are usually thought of as summarising the covariance structure of data or functional connectivity (see the previous chapter). The ensuing eigenimages can be regarded as spatial modes that are functionally disconnected from each other.

Figure 50.6 illustrates an SVD of an arbitrary matrix M (of size $n \times$ m, where $n >$ m) into an equivalent form using the relation $MV = US$, where V is a set of eigenvectors that form a natural coordinate system.

A plot of the variance components of an SVD for a typical PET dataset (that used in the previous chapter), is shown in Fig. 50.6. The spectrum shows a rapid decrease in the eigenvalues after the first few components (Friston *et al.,* 1993). This indicates spatiotemporal order within the data.[1] Such order is a consequence of coherent modes of distributed activity induced by task-related changes that are responsible for generating the data. One could regard the eigenvalues $\lambda = SS^T$ as indices of self-functional connectivity. However, static linear models also afford a perspective on effective connectivity. One can take these eigenimages to represent their influence on a voxel-specific measurement at the ith voxel. If the expression of the modes is given by $Y = US$, then

$$y^i = Y\beta_i = USV_i^T$$
$$\beta_i = V_i^T$$

[1] A white noise process would have a homogeneous eigenvalue spectrum.

where V_i^T is the ith row of V. Compare this with Eq. (50.8). In other words, the eigenimages can be interpreted as the effective connectivity between the voxel in question and the mode corresponding to the eigenimage.

In summary, this perspective on eigenimage analysis furnishes a measure of connectivity between the voxel i and the rest of the brain in terms of spatiotemporal eigenmodes, as opposed to separate voxels. However, this interpretation is limited to LTI connection strengths. Next we describe how linear models can be used to approximate nonlinear systems by including interaction, or bilinear, terms.

Modelling Nonlinearities

Linear models cannot be used to estimate *changes* in connectivity (induced by modulatory interactions among populations of neurons or contextual inputs). However, by introducing interaction terms one can attain a dynamic representation. This requires a simple extension to Eq. (50.8): the addition of a new variable, calculated from the product of two voxels or regions (indexed by j and k). We will refer to this new variable as the *bilinear term,* written as $y_t^j y_t^k$ for scalar and $y^j \times y^k$ (the Hadamard product) for vectors. The idea is that now the model can be used to estimate the effect this new term has on activity in the ith voxel:

$$y_t^i = y_t^j b_1 + y_t^j y_t^k b_2 + e_t^i \tag{50.9}$$

where b_1 and b_2 are model parameters, which scale the effect of their respective terms. The quantity b_1 is equivalent to an element in β_{ji} [Eq. (50.8)], however, b_2 is different because it parameterises the effect of a bilinear term $y_t^j y_t^k$. These two coefficients are the obligatory and modulatory effects discussed earlier. Obligatory connections have a direct driving effect, but modulatory connections are subtler and introduce context into the model. This is best illustrated with an example.

The model in Fig. 50.7a is a simple nonlinear model. It consists only of two variables but this is sufficient to illustrate nonlinearity and how we can measure it. It consists of an input x, which generates an output y. The nonlinearity is due to an interaction between the input and output; i.e., the model's response y depends on its current (intrinsic) activity y. This simple model consists of a linear and bilinear term parameterised by b_1 and b_2 respectively:

$$y = xb_1 + xyb_2 \tag{50.10}$$

If the model contained the first term only, it would be linear and the relationship between input and output would be represented by a straight line in a plot of x and y. The addition of the second term introduces markedly nonlinear behaviour. Plotting x and y for different values of b_2 demonstrates this. The input–output behaviour depends on b_2 and is reflected in the two different curves in Fig. 50.7b. It helps to focus on the model's response to a fixed input. It is easily appreciated that the sensitivity of y to x (the slope) depends on b_2. The key point is that data generated from such a process is not distributed in a linear fashion, i.e., the dependence of y on x is not modelled with a straight line. We will describe next a piece-wise local linear approximation to modelling this very simple sort of nonlinearity.

First we need to consider how to estimate the parameters in Eq. (50.10) from measurements of x and y. If we assume that the nonlinearities are weak about a local region of the data then the model can be approximated by

$$y_l \approx x(b_1 + \langle y_l \rangle b_2) = xb_l \tag{50.11}$$

where y_l is a vector containing values of y within a local range of the $\langle y_l \rangle$ data and is its average. If we assume that b_1 and b_2 are constant within this region, then $b_1 + \langle y \rangle b_2$ is also constant (abbreviated to b_l) and can be estimated from values of x and y_l. If y is partitioned into n divisions, then this procedure can be repeated for all n domains. Differences in values of b_l for different regions indicate nonlinearity in the data.

Let us turn now to the illustration in Fig. 50.8. These data have been generated from the model in Fig. 50.7, with $b_2 = 0.8$, with added noise. The data are distributed, roughly, into two subgroups. Modelling the data as a linear process does not capture this feature. The characterisation

a

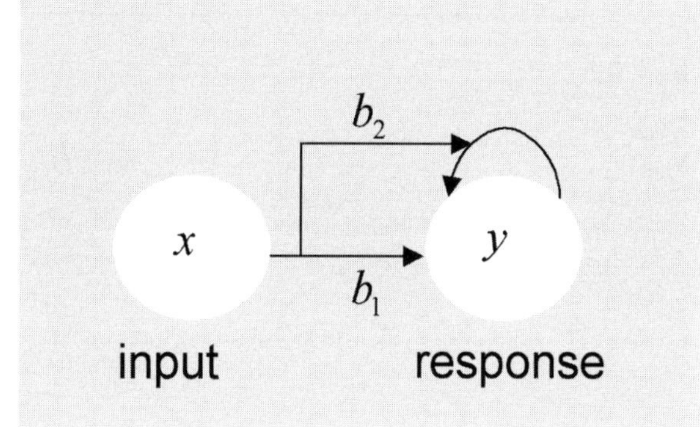

b

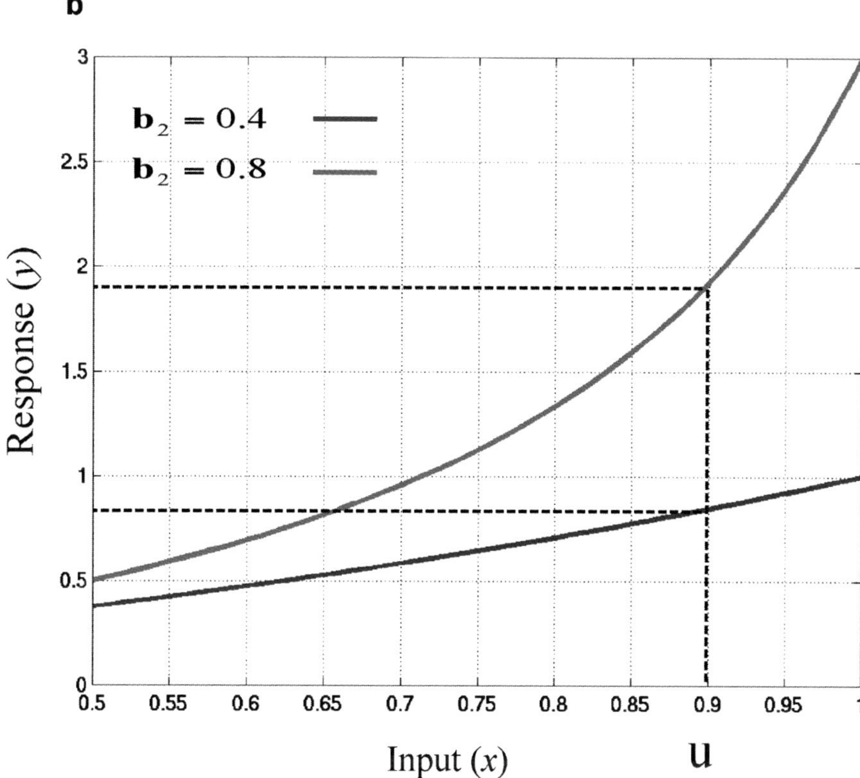

FIGURE 50.7
Piece-wise local linear approximation of a simple nonlinear relation between x (input) and y (response). (a) A simple nonlinear model is shown. Nonlinearity in the response is generated from a bilinear term xy, which models a nonadditive interaction between input and intrinsic activity. The model is noise free for simplicity. The interaction term is scaled by b_2, effectively quantifying the model's sensitivity to input at different levels of intrinsic activity. (b) Plots of input and output data at different values of b_2 disclose the model's sensitivity to b_2. At a fixed input, $x = u$, the response varies dependent on its value. The key point is that data generated from such processes are not distributed in a linear fashion.

can be finessed by partitioning the data on the basis of "high" and "low" levels of response (denoted by y_{high} and y_{low}). A linear model, given by Eq. (50.11), can then be used for each partition:

$$\begin{aligned} y_{high} &\approx x(b_1 + \langle y_{high} \rangle b_2) = xb_{high} \\ y_{low} &\approx x(b_1 + \langle y_{low} \rangle b_2) = xb_{low} \end{aligned} \tag{50.11}$$

where we have assumed b_1 and b_2 are constant within the domains of high or low activity. We then use the two partitions of y and x to estimate values of b_{high} and b_{low}, where

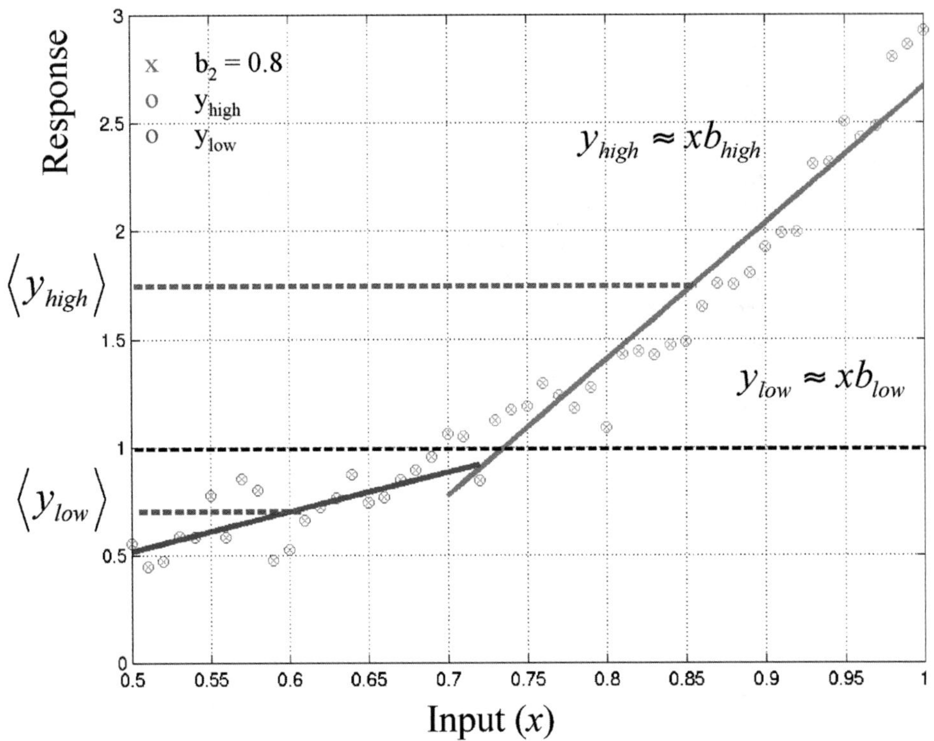

$$y_l \approx x(b_1 + b_2\langle y\rangle)$$
$$= xb_l$$

FIGURE 50.8
Data have been generated from the model in Fig. 50.7 ($b_2 = 0.8$) and noise added. This illustrates how an index of nonlinearity can be constructed by partitioning the data. Data in y are divided into two ranges, where all values of y greater than 1 were grouped into y_{high} and all values lower than 1 into y_{low}. The linear relationship between x and y within each of these ranges can be estimated using the approximation at the bottom of the figure. The value of b_l reflects local sensitivity to global nonlinearities. An index of linear and nonlinear features of the data can be approximated through estimates of b_1 and b_2.

$$b_1 = \frac{\langle y_{high}\rangle b_{low} - \langle y_{low}\rangle b_{high}}{\langle y_{high}\rangle - \langle y_{low}\rangle}$$
$$b_2 = \frac{b_{low} - b_{high}}{\langle y_{low}\rangle - \langle y_{high}\rangle} \tag{50.13}$$

These coefficients serve as an index of linearity (b_1) and nonlinearity (b_2), and can be estimated from measured data. Applying these ideas to neuroimaging data, b_1 and b_2 represent measures of obligatory and modulatory connectivity. This approach of approximating nonlinear interactions was used by Friston *et al.* (1995) to demonstrate asymmetrical nonlinear interactions between V1 and V2 from fMRI data during visual stimulation.

The inclusion of a bilinear term enabled us to introduce nonlinear behaviour into our model. The method of piece-wise linear approximation provided a way to measure this nonlinearity. However, the bilinear term was only implicit. Next, we model the bilinear term explicitly in a general linear model. These models have been called *psychophysiological* (and *physio-physiological*) interaction (PPI) models.

Psychophysiological Interactions

The partitioning of data required above may seem arbitrary. A way around this is to embed the interaction term into one linear model. Büchel *et al.* (1996) discussed a series of increasingly high-order interaction terms in a general linear model, each of which is constructed from the products of individual variables. These are introduced as new explanatory variables and provide a means of modelling the difference in regression slopes without partitioning or splicing the data by hand. In this way, standard linear regression techniques, implemented in SPM, can be used to estimate the magnitude and significance of these bilinear effects directly.

Changing the symbols representing the *j*th and *k*th voxels in the previous equation to u_1 and u_2, denoting input to a system whose response is y^i, the prototype linear model is

$$\begin{aligned} y^i &= X_L\beta_L + e^i \\ &= [u_1,u_2,X_0]\beta_L + e^i \end{aligned} \tag{50.14}$$

The equation has been simplified by dividing the explanatory variables into those of interest and X_0, which contains all the other covariates. The model's parameters quantify the influence each explanatory variable has on y^i and can be estimated using standard linear techniques. Extending the model to include a bilinear variable, denoted by $u_1 \times u_2$ (the Hadamard product), gives

$$\begin{aligned} y^i &= X_{BL}\beta_{BL} + e^i \\ &= [u_1 \times u_2,u_1,u_2,X_0]\begin{bmatrix} \beta_I \\ \beta_L \end{bmatrix} + e^i \end{aligned} \tag{50.15}$$

The model is divided into bilinear and linear terms. The corresponding parameters, β_I and β_L, can be estimated as before. Both the main effect and interaction terms are included because the main effect of each covariate has to be modelled to properly assess the additional explanatory power afforded by the bilinear or PPI term. Standard hypothesis testing of the bilinear term (testing $H_0 : \beta_I = 0$) can be used to estimate the significance of its effect. In this analysis, the data do not have to be divided, because input-dependent changes in regression slope are modelled by the bilinear term.

Figure 50.9 illustrates two examples of bilinear effects in real data. The study was a fMRI experiment investigating the modulatory effects of attention on visual responses to radial motion (see the figure legend and Büchel and Friston, 1997, for experimental details). The aim of both models was to quantify a top-down modulatory effect of attention on V1 to V5 connectivity. The left-hand model combines psychological data (attentional set) with physiological data (V1 and V5 activity) to model the interaction, whereas the right-hand model uses a physiological measure (PPC activity) as a surrogate for the psychological effect. These analyses correspond to psychophysiological and physio-physiological interactions, respectively. Both demonstrate a significant modulatory effect of attention (Büchel and Friston, 1997; Friston *et al.,* 1997). The lower diagram in Fig. 50.9 is a regression analysis of the same data, divided according to attentional set, to demonstrate the difference in regression slopes.

In this example, attention was modelled as a "contextual" variable, while visual stimulation perturbed the system. The latter evoked a response within the context of the former. Using the example in Fig. 50.9, visual stimuli evoke different responses depending on attentional set, modelled as a change in connectivity. Attention appears to reconfigure connection strengths among prefrontal and sensory cortical areas (Mesulam, 1998). The bilinear effect may take any appropriate form in PPI models, including, for example, psychological, physiological, or pharmacological indices. These models emphasise the use of factorial experimental designs (Friston *et al.*, 1997) and allow us to consider experimental inputs in a different light, distinguishing contextual input (one factor) from direct perturbation (another factor). PPI models have provided important evidence for the interactions among distributed brain systems and enabled inferences about task-dependent plasticity using a relatively simple procedure.

The next model we consider was developed explicitly with path analysis in mind and adopts a different approach to the estimation of model parameters. This approach rests on the specification of priors or constraints on the connectivity.

a

Psychophysiological

$$V5 = (V1 \times U)\beta_{PPI} + [V1 \quad U]\beta + e$$

U = attentional set

Physio-physiological

$$V5 = (V1 \times PPC)\beta_{PPI} + [V1 \quad PPC]\beta + e$$

β_{PPI} β_M β_{PPI} β_M

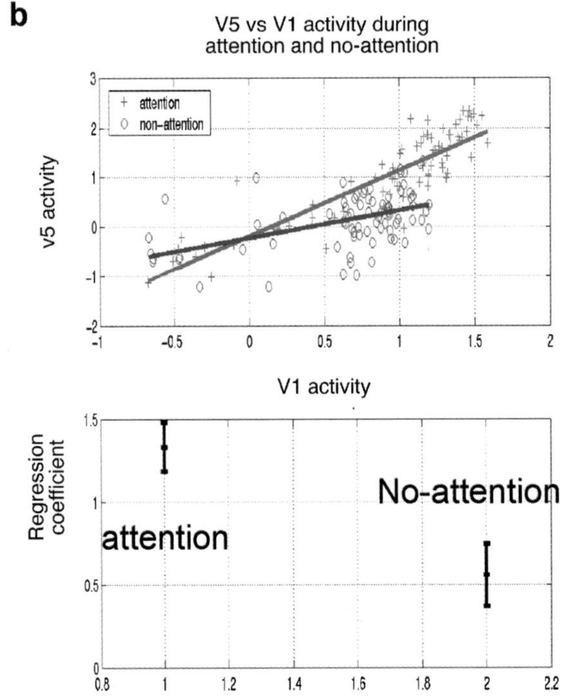

FIGURE 50.9
(a) Extended statistical model including interaction terms used to model psychophysiological and physio-physiological interactions (PPI). Subjects were asked to make a judgment regarding changes in velocity of a radially moving stimulus or to just observe the stimulus. The velocity of the actual stimulus remained constant, so that only the attentional set was manipulated. Comparisons of connectivity among the primary visual cortex (V1/2 complex and V5) and posterior parietal cortex (PPC) during the different cognitive states were assessed. Bilinear terms are denoted by PPI. The model on the left examines the modulatory influence of attentional set (U) on V1 and V5 coupling, whereas the one on the right assesses PPC activity-dependent modulation of the same connection. (b) This panel demonstrates the change in sensitivity of V5 to V1 input, depending on attentional set, using the method illustrated in Fig. 50.8, i.e., partitioning the data and regressing V5 on V1. The lower graph shows the difference in regression slopes and their variance (2 standard deviations).

Structural Equation Modelling

Structural equation modelling (SEM), or path analysis, is a multivariate tool that is used to test hypotheses regarding the influences among interacting variables. Its roots go back to the 1920s when path analysis was developed to quantify unidirectional causal flow in genetic data and developed further by social scientists in the 1960s (Maruyama, 1998). It received criticism for the limitations inherent in the least-squares method of estimating model parameters, which motivated a general linear modelling approach from the 1970s onward. It is now available in commercial software packages including LISREL, EQS, and AMOS. Maruyama (1998) provides an introduction to the basic ideas. Researchers in functional imaging started to use it in the early 1990s (McIntosh and Gonzalez-Lima, 1991, 1992a,b, 1994). It was applied first to animal autoradiographic data and later to human PET data, where, among other experiments, it was used to identify task-dependent differential activation of the dorsal and ventral visual pathways (McIntosh *et al.,* 1994). Many investigators have used SEM since then. An example of its use to identify attentional modulation of effective connectivity between prefrontal and premotor cortices can found in Rowe *et al.* (2002).

A SEM relates to the general linear model above in that it has the same form. There are, however, a number of modifications, some of which are illustrated in Fig. 50.10. The coupling matrix β, has been "pruned" to include only paths of interest. Critically, self-connections are precluded. The data matrix, Y, contains responses from regions of interest and possibly experimental or bilinear terms. The model is

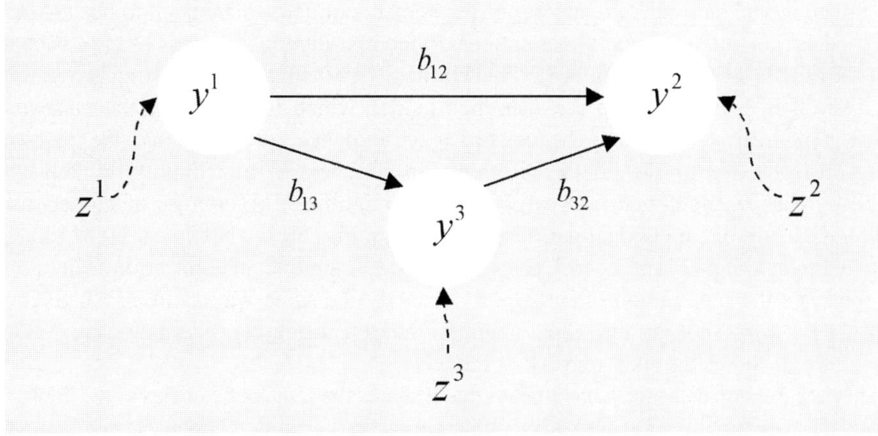

$$\begin{bmatrix} y_t^1 & y_t^2 & y_t^3 \end{bmatrix} = \begin{bmatrix} y_t^1 & y_t^2 & y_t^3 \end{bmatrix} \begin{bmatrix} 0 & b_{12} & b_{13} \\ 0 & 0 & 0 \\ 0 & b_{32} & 0 \end{bmatrix} + \begin{bmatrix} z_t^1 & z_t^2 & z_t^3 \end{bmatrix}$$

$$y_t = y_t\beta + z_t$$
$$z_t \sim N(0, \Sigma)$$

FIGURE 50.10
A SEM is used to estimate path coefficients for a specific network of connections, by "pruning" the coupling matrix. The figure illustrates that a particular connectivity is specified, which is usually based on a prior anatomical model. y may contain physiological data, psychological data, or interaction terms (to estimate to the influence of "contextual" input on first-order coupling). The innovations z are assumed to be independent, and can be interpreted as driving inputs to each node.

$$y_t = y_t\beta + z_t \tag{50.16}$$

The regional time-series y_t are known but β contains free parameters to be estimated. To simplify the model, the residuals z are assumed to be independent. They are interpreted as driving each region stochastically from one measurement to another and, to reflect this, are sometimes called *innovations.*

The free parameters are estimated using the covariance structure of the data, instead of minimising the sum of squared errors as described above. The rationale is that the former reflects the global behaviour of the data, i.e., capturing relationships among variables, in contrast to the latter, which reflects the goodness of fit from the point of view of each region. Practically, a cost function is constructed from the actual and implied covariance, which is used as an objective function to estimate parameters. The implied covariance, $\langle y_t^T y_t \rangle$, is easily computed by re-arranging Eq. (50.16) and assuming some value for the covariance of the innovations, $\langle z_t^T z_t \rangle$:

$$\begin{aligned} y_t(1-\beta) &= z_t \\ y_t &= z_t(1-\beta)^{-1} \\ \langle y_t^T y_t \rangle &= (1-\beta)^{-1T} \langle z_t^T z_t \rangle (1-\beta)^{-1} \end{aligned} \tag{50.17}$$

Details are provided in the Appendix. A gradient descent such as a Newton-Raphson scheme can be used to estimate parameters, where starting values can be estimated using an ordinary least-squares (OLS) approach (McIntosh and Gonzalez-Lima, 1994).

Inferences about path coefficients rest on the notion of nested, or stacked, models. A nested model consists of a free model within which any number of constrained models are "nested." In a free model, all parameters are free to take values that optimise the objective function, whereas a constrained model has one, or a number of parameters omitted, constrained to be zero or equal across models (i.e., attention and nonattention). By comparing the goodness of fit of each model against the others, χ^2 statistics can be derived (Bollen, 1989). Hypotheses testing proceeds using this statistic. For example, given a constrained model, which is defined by the *omission* of a pathway, hypothesis testing may be construed as evidence for or against the pathway by "nesting" it in the free model. If the difference in goodness of fit is highly unlikely to have occurred by chance, the connection can be declared significant. Examples of models used by Büchel *et al.* using the attentional dataset are shown in Fig. 50.11. Nonlinear SEM models are constructed by adding a bilinear term as an extra node. A significant connection from a bilinear term represents the modulation of influence in exactly the same way as in a PPI. Büchel and Friston (1997) used SEM on the visual attention dataset, validating the method by confirming conclusions reached using other regression models.

SEM is a regression analysis, which means that it shares the same deficiencies as the linear model approach described above, i.e., temporal information is discounted.[2] However, it has enjoyed relative success and become established during the past decade due, in part, to its commercial availability as well as its intuitive appeal. However, it usually requires a number of rather ad hoc procedures, such as partitioning the data to create nested models, or pruning the coupling matrix to render the solution tractable. These problems are confounded with an inability to capture nonlinear features and temporal dependencies. By moving to more sophisticated models, we acknowledge the effect of the history of input and embed *a priori* knowledge into models at a more plausible and mechanistic level. These issues are addressed in the following section.

DYNAMIC MODELS

The static models described above discount temporal information. Consequently, permuted datasets produce the same path coefficients as the original permutation. Models that use the order in which data are produced are more natural candidates for the brain and include those that attempt to model its equations of motion, e.g., state-space models and generalised convolution models. In this section we will review Kalman filtering, autoregression, and generalised convolution models.

[2] Some versions of SEM do model dynamic information; see (Cudeck, 2002) for details of dynamic factor analysis.

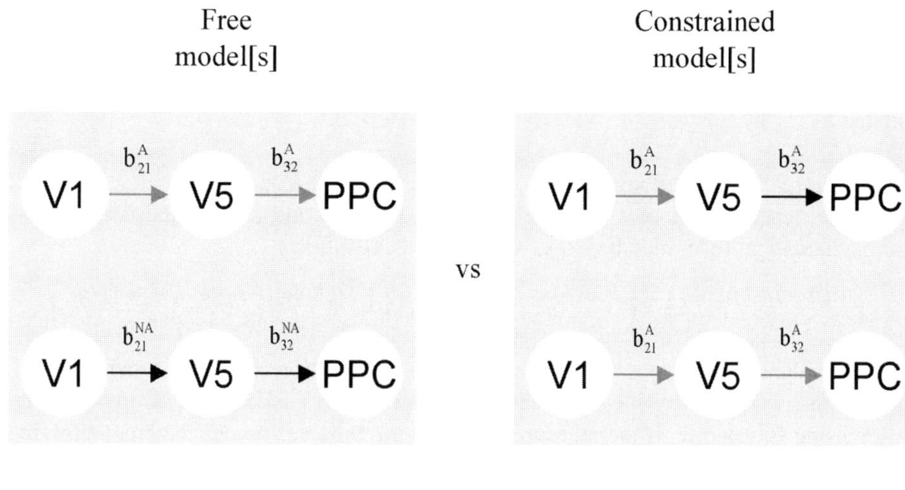

$$H_0 : b_{21}^{A} = b_{21}^{NA}, \quad b_{32}^{A} = b_{32}^{NA}$$

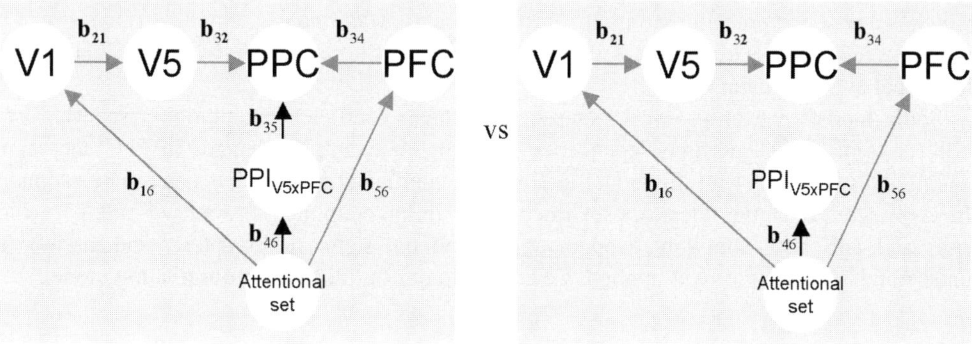

$$H_0 : b_{35} = 0$$

FIGURE 50.11
Inference about connection strengths proceeds using nested models. Parameters from free and constrained models are compared with a χ^2 statistic. Two examples are given, first comparing coupling coefficients during attention and nonattention and testing if they are the same. The second tests for the significance of a connection strength between an interaction term and PPC activity (see Büchel and Friston, 1997).

Kalman Filter

The Kalman filter is used extensively in engineering to model dynamic data (Juang, 2001). It is based on a state-space model that invokes an extra set of hidden variables to generate data. These models are powerful because long-range order, within observed data, is modelled through interactions among hidden states, instead of mapping input directly onto output (see below). It is an "online" procedure consisting of two steps: prediction and correction. The hidden states are estimated (prediction step) using the current information, which is updated (correction step) on receipt of each new measurement. These two steps are repeated recursively as new information arrives. A simple example demonstrates intuitively how the filter works. This example is taken from the source in Ghahramani (2002).

Consider a series of data points, which we receive one at a time. Say we wanted to calculate a running average with each new data point. Given that the tth variable is x_t and the estimate of the mean (which we will call the *state*) after t values of $\hat{x}_t$ is

$$\hat{x}_t = \frac{1}{t} \sum_t x_t$$

for t-1 samples $$\hat{x}_{t-1} = \frac{1}{t-1} \sum_{t-1} x_{t-1}$$

$\hat{x}_t$ is related to $\hat{x}_{t-1}$ by $$\hat{x}_t = \frac{t-1}{t} \hat{x}_{t-1} + \frac{1}{t} x_t$$

This can be rearranged, giving $\hat{x}_t = \hat{x}_{t-1} + K(x_t - \hat{x}_{t-1})$, where K is the Kalman gain = 1/t. This illustrates the general form of a Kalman filter: a prediction and a weighted correction. This general mathematical form may be expressed in words as follows:

$$\begin{pmatrix} \textit{Current estimate} \\ \hat{x}_t \end{pmatrix} = \begin{pmatrix} \textit{Previous estimate} \\ \hat{x}_{t-1} \end{pmatrix} + \begin{pmatrix} \textit{Weighted (K) prediction error} \\ (\hat{x}_t - \hat{x}_{t-1}) \end{pmatrix}$$

The filter balances two types of information from a prediction (based on previous data) and an observation, weighted by their respective precisions. This is performed optimally as the weighting using Bayes rule. If the measured data are not reliable, K goes to zero, weighting the prediction error less and relying more on the preceding prediction to afford a current one. Conversely, if the dependence on sequential state values is unreliable, then K is large. This emphasises information provided by the data when constructing an estimate of the current state.

Quantities that require calculation in the forward recursion are Kalman gain, mean and covariance of prediction, and correction matrices. A backward recursive algorithm called the *Kalman smoother* calculates the mean and covariance of the states at time t, given all the data, which is a post hoc procedure to improve the estimates. Maximum-likelihood estimators can be used to calculate these quantities. A demonstration of the filter is shown in Fig. 50.12, applied to the visual attention data.

Static models can only model “snapshots” of path coefficients (although a snapshot of a bilinear term introduces time dependence through, for example, changes in PFC activity or attentional set). In contrast, by modelling the path coefficient as a hidden state, to be estimated from observed data, the filter exposes fluctuations in the coupling, between V1 and V5, which rises and falls with attention (even though attentional status never entered the model). To understand how the filter was applied, we start with our familiar linear observation model:

$$\begin{aligned} y_t &= x_t \beta_t + \varepsilon_t \\ \varepsilon_t &\sim N(0,R) \end{aligned} \tag{50.18}$$

To simplify notation, y and x are univariate and are both known, e.g., BOLD activity from V1 and V5. The term β is modelled as a state variable, observed vicariously through the BOLD responses; it is allowed to change with time (influenced by its own internal states and input) according to the update equation:

$$\begin{aligned} \beta_t &= \beta_{t-1} + \eta_t \\ \eta_t &\sim N(0,Q) \end{aligned} \tag{50.19}$$

where the subscript indexes the scan number, because β_t can vary from scan to scan. Given this extra state variable, the Kalman filter can be used to estimate its dynamics. Figure 50.12 illustrates the model and plots the time-dependent path coefficient, β_t, for V1 to V5 connectivity. Note that if $\eta_t = 0$ then $\beta_t = \beta_{t-1}$. This is the static estimate from an ordinary regression analysis.

The results of this analysis, also known as variable parameter regression, agree with previous analyses, in that task-dependent variation is seen in interregional connectivity. This variation has the same form as that described by a BSSM of contextual input, but the variation is treated as random and unknown [see Eq. (50.19)]. However, in general, these changes in connectivity are induced experimentally by known and deterministic causes.

In Chapter 52 we return to state-space models and reanalyse the attentional dataset in a way that allows designed manipulations of attention to affect the model's hidden states. In dynamic casual modelling the states are dynamic variables (e.g., neuronal activity) and the effective connectivity corresponds to fixed parameters than can interact with time-varying states and inputs.[3] The remainder of this chapter focuses on approaches that do not refer to hidden states, such as autoregression and generalised convolution models.

[3] This should be contrasted with the above application in which the connectivity itself was presumed to be a time-varying state.

in a least-squares sense, without necessarily capturing the dynamics of the system any better than a more parsimonious, optimal model. A procedure for choosing an optimal value of p is therefore necessary. This can be achieved using a Bayesian approach (Penny and Roberts, 2002). A Bayesian framework also allows for inferences about connection strengths to be made based on posterior probabilities (see Chapter 47).

MAR was used to model the visual attention data. The results are shown in Fig. 50.14. Two models were estimated using three regions in each. The motive was to validate the method against established procedures that demonstrated a modulatory influence of PFC on V5 to PPC connectivity and PPC on V1 to V5 connectivity. The posterior densities of the weight matrix W are shown using their conditional means and variances. The probability that an individual parameter is different from zero can be inferred from these posterior distributions. Parameters whose conditional density encompasses zero are less likely to have any influence. Conversely, the more distal a density mass is from zero, the greater our certainty that the model supports an effect. Nonzero parameters that characterise second-order connectivity are circled in the figure.

MAR models have not been used as extensively as other models of effective connectivity. However they are an established technique for quantifying temporal dependencies within time series (Chatfield, 1996). They are simple and intuitive models requiring no *a priori* knowledge of connectivity, as in SEM. However, this could also be construed as a shortcoming, in that simple MAR models cannot harness *a priori* knowledge.

Generalised Convolution Models

Up until now we have considered models based on the general linear model and simple state-space models. The former may be criticised for not embracing temporal information within data, which the Kalman filter (an example of the latter) resolved by invoking hidden states. An alternative approach is to exclude hidden states and formulate a function that maps the history of input directly onto output. This can be achieved by characterising the response (output) of a physical system over time to an idealised input (an impulse), called an *impulse response function* (IRF) or *transfer function* (TF). In the time domain this function comprises a kernel that quantifies the idealised response. This is convenient because it bypasses any characterisation of possible internal states generating the data. However, it renders the system a "black box," within which we have no model. This is both the method's strength and weakness.

Once the IRF has been characterised from experimental data, it can be used to model responses to arbitrary inputs. For linear systems, which adhere to the principle of superposition, this reduces to convolving the input with the IRF. The modelled response depends on the input, without any reference to the interactions that may have produced it. An example, familiar to neuroimaging, is the haemodynamic response function (HRF) used to model the haemodynamic response of the brain to experimental tasks. However, we are interested in nonlinear models, which are obtained by generalising the notion of convolution models to include high-order interactions among inputs, an approach originally developed by Volterra in 1930 (Rieke *et al.*, 1997).

The generalised nonlinear state and observation equations are, respectively,

$$\begin{aligned} \dot{x}(t) &= f(x(t),u(t)) \\ y(t) &= g(x(t),u(t)) \end{aligned} \tag{50.22}$$

These can be reformulated to relate output, to input $u(t)$, without reference to the states $x(t)$. Where h is a nonlinear function, which can be expanded into a series of functionals (functions of functions, see below), we get

$$\begin{aligned} y(t) = h_0 &+ \int_{-\infty}^{\infty} h_1(\tau_1)u(t-\tau_1)\partial\tau_1 + \int_{-\infty}^{\infty}\int_{-\infty}^{\infty} h_2(\tau_1,\tau_2)u(t-\tau_2)\partial\tau_1\partial\tau_2 + \ldots \\ &+ \int_{-\infty}^{\infty} h_n(\tau_1,\ldots,\tau_n)u(t-\tau_1)\ldots u(t-\tau_n)\partial\tau_1\ldots\partial\tau_n \end{aligned} \tag{50.23}$$

where n is the order of the series and may take any positive integer to infinity. This is known as a *Volterra series.* Under certain conditions, h converges as n increases (Fliess *et al.*, 1983) and can provide a complete description of a system given enough terms. To understand this, we

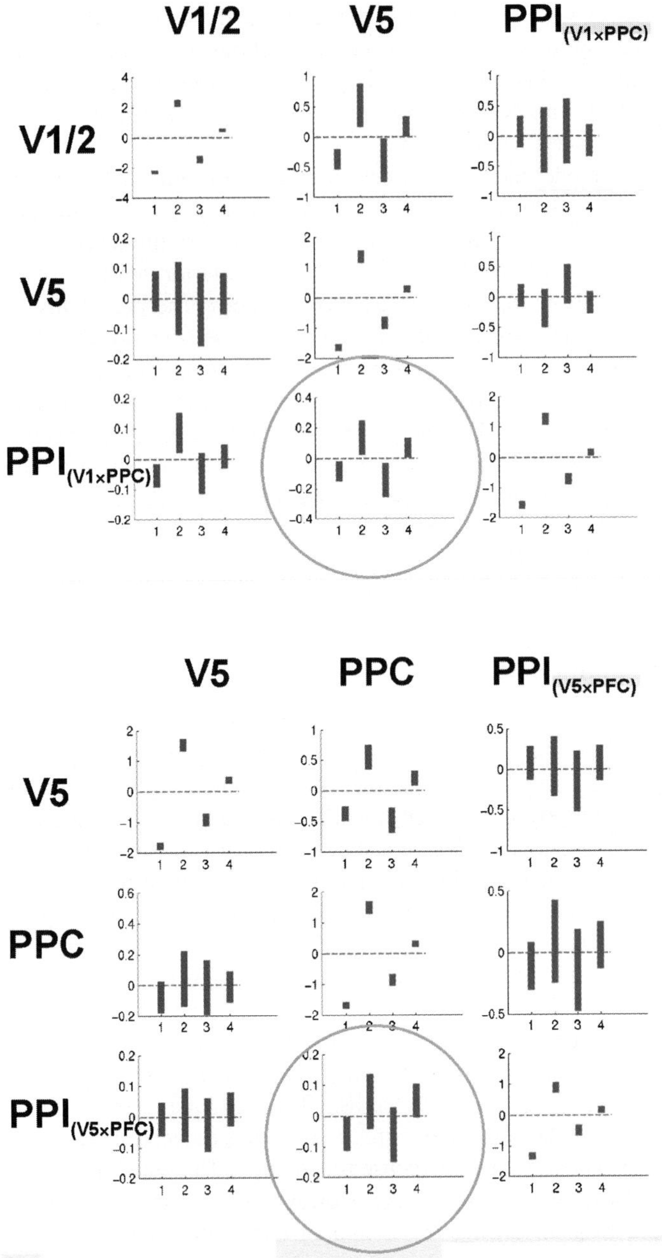

FIGURE 50.14
Results of two MAR models applied to the visual attention dataset. Each panel contains posterior density estimates of W over time lags (x axis) for each connection. The mean and 2 standard deviations for each posterior density are shown. Diagonal elements quantify autocorrelations and the off-diagonals quantify the cross-correlations. The regions used in each model are V1/2, V5, and $PPI_{V1\times PPC}$ and V5, PPC, and $PPI_{V5\times PFC}$. The models support coupling between the interaction terms and V5 and PPC, respectively.

need to consider the Taylor series expansion as a means of constructing an approximation to a general nonlinear function (see Fig. 50.1). Any sufficiently smooth nonlinear function can be approximated, within the neighbourhood of an expansion point x_0, by scaling increasingly higher order terms of coefficients computed from derivatives of the function about x_0 [see Eq. (50.1)]. The Volterra series is a Taylor series expansion, in which high-order terms are constructed from variables modelling interactions and scaled by time-varying coefficients. The Volterra series is a power-series expansion where the coefficients of Eq. (50.1) are now functions, known as *kernels*. The kernels are functions of time, and because the series involves functions of functions they are known as *functionals*.

An increase in accuracy of the approximation is achieved by considering higher order terms, as demonstrated by deriving linear and bilinear SSMs. The same is true of the linear and bilinear convolution models:

$$y(t) \approx h_0 + \int h_1(\tau_1)u(t - \tau_1)\partial\tau_1$$

$$y(t) \approx h_0 + \int h_1(\tau_1)u(t - \tau_1)\partial\tau_1 + \int\int h_2(\tau_1,\tau_2)u(t - \tau_1)u(t - \tau_2)\partial\tau_1\partial\tau_2$$

The HRF is derived from a linear convolution model. The systems IRF and the occurrences of experimental trials are therefore represented by h_1 and $u(t)$, respectively. The linear model is distinguished by its compliance with the principle of superposition: Given two input impulses, the response is simply the sum of the two responses. By including the second-order kernel, nonadditive responses can be modelled. Practically, this means that the timing of inputs is important in that different pairs of inputs may produce different responses. The Volterra approach is a generalisation of the convolution method, which convolves increasingly higher order interactions with multidimensional kernels to approximate the nonadditive component of a systems response.

Kernels scale the effect each input, in the past, has on the current value of $y(t)$. As such, Volterra series have been described as *power series with memory.* Sequential terms embody increasingly complex interactions among inputs up to arbitrary order. The series converges with increasing terms, which, for weakly nonlinear systems, is assumed to occur after the second-order term. Nonlinear behaviour is modelled using these interactions, scaled throughout their history. A diagram of a bilinear convolution model is shown in Fig. 50.15.

The first- and second-order kernels quantify the linear and bilinear responses; consequentially, they are equivalent to first- and second-order effective connectivity respectively (Friston, 2000). The kernels are also related mathematically to the bilinear state-space representation (see Chapter 53). For every state-space representation there is an equivalent set of kernels and an equivalent generalised convolution representation.

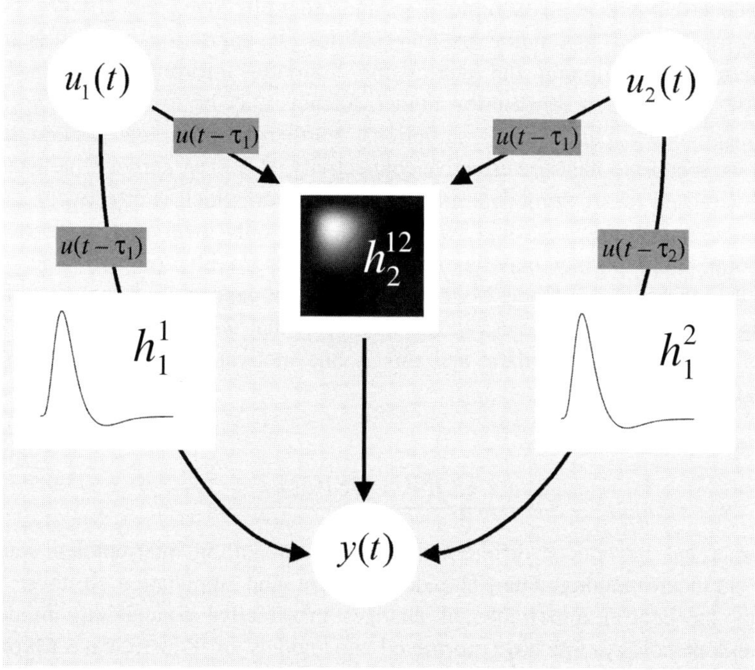

FIGURE 50.15
A bilinear convolution model of a simple network consisting of two inputs and an output. Linear contributions from each input are estimated by the first-order kernels h_1. However, nonadditive responses, due to nonlinear interactions within the system, are modelled by the second-order kernel, h_2.

Having established that Volterra kernels are a metric of effective connectivity, we need to estimate them from experimental data. By reformulating the model using an appropriate basis set, kernels can be reconstructed from estimated coefficients. The HRF is modelled well by gamma functions and this is the reason for choosing them to approximate Volterra kernels. The Volterra kernels, for a general dynamic system (of any arbitrary form or complexity), are difficult to compute unless the underlying generative process leading to the data is well characterised, as is the HRF.

A bilinear convolution model can be reformulated by convolving the basis set with the inputs:

$$x_i(t) = \int b_i(\tau_1)u(t-\tau_1)\partial\tau_1$$

These are then used as explanatory variables in a GLM as follows:

$$y(t) = g_0 + \sum_{i=1}^{n} g_i x_i(t) + \sum_{i=1}^{n}\sum_{j=1}^{n} g_{ij} x_i(t) x_j(t) \tag{50.24}$$

where $y(t)$ and $x_i(t)$ are known and g_0, g_i and g_{ij} are to be estimated. The kernels are given by

$$\begin{aligned} h_0 &= g_0 \\ h_2(\tau_1) &= \sum_{i=1}^{n} g_i b_i(\tau_1) \\ h_2(\tau_1,\tau_2) &= \sum_{i=1}^{n}\sum_{j=1}^{n} g_{ij} b_i(\tau_1) b_j(\tau_2) \end{aligned} \tag{50.25}$$

The unknowns in Eq. (50.24) can be estimated using a GLM and used to reconstruct the original kernels from Eq. (50.25). This method was applied to the attentional dataset used previously. The model consisted of inputs from three regions—putamen, V1/2 complex, and PPC—to V5, as shown in Fig. 50.16. BOLD recordings from these regions were used as an index of neuronal activity, representing input to V5. The lower panel illustrates responses to simulated inputs, using the empirically determined kernels. It shows the response of V5 to an impulse from V2 and provides a direct comparison of V5 responses to the same input from V2, but with and without PFC activity. The influence of PFC is clear. This is due to its modulatory influence on V2 to V5 connectivity and is an example of second-order effective connectivity.

The Volterra method has many useful qualities. It approximates nonlinear behaviour without arbitrarily partitioning the data using temporal information within the familiar framework of a generalised convolution model. Kernels may be estimated using a GLM and inferences made under parametric assumptions. Furthermore, kernels contain the dynamic information we require to measure effective connectivity. However, kernels characterise an ideal response, generalised to accommodate nonlinear behaviour, which is effectively a summary of the system as a whole. Note also that Volterra series are only local approximations around an expansion point. Although they may be extremely good approximations for some systems, they may not be for others. For instance, Volterra series cannot capture the behaviour of periodic or chaotic dynamics. A major weakness of the method is that we have no notion of the internal mechanisms that generated the data, and this is one motivation for returning to state-space models (see Chapter 52).

CONCLUSION

This chapter has introduced different methods of modelling interregional coupling using information in neuroimaging data. The development and application of these methods is motivated by the central importance of changes in effective connectivity in development, cognition, and pathology. We have portrayed the models in a historical fashion; from the first linear observation models to bilinear terms of regression and convolution models. In the next two chapters, we will revisit Volterra-based and bilinear state-space models. The emphasis has been on the bilinearity within imaging data and how different models attempt to extract this information. Bilinear models are a practical extension to linear models, capturing plasticity

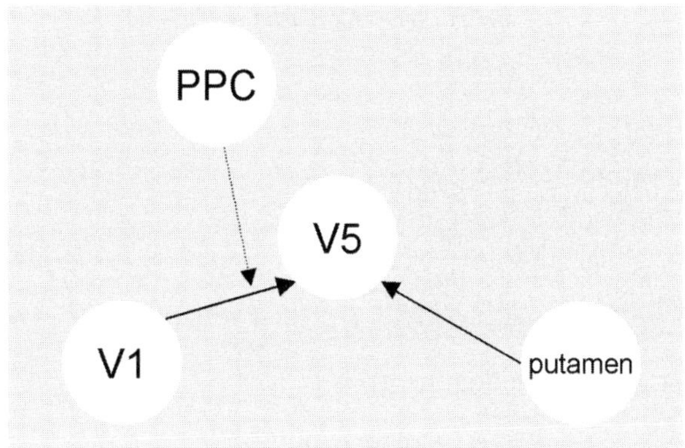

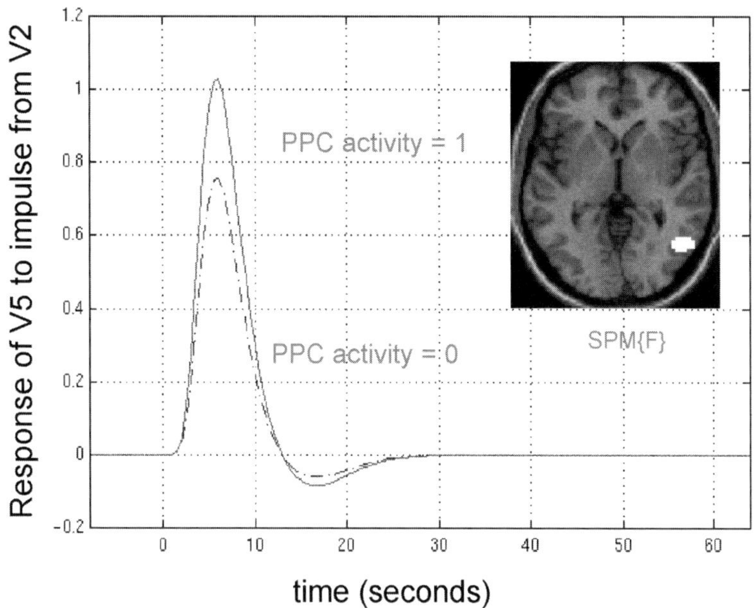

FIGURE 50.16
(Top) Brain regions and connections comprising the model. (Bottom) Characterisation of the effects of V2 inputs on V5 and their modulation by PPC. The broken lines represent estimates of V5 responses when PPC activity is zero, according to a second-order Volterra model of effective connectivity with inputs to V5 from V2, PPC, and the pulvinar (PUL). The solid curve represents the same response when PPC activity is 1 standard deviation of its between-condition variation. It is evident that V2 has an activating effect on V5 and that PPC increases the responsiveness of V5 to these inputs. The insert shows all voxels in V5 that evidenced a modulatory effect ($p > 0.05$ uncorrected). These voxels were identified by thresholding a statistical parametric map of the F statistic testing for the contribution of second-order kernels involving V2 and PPC (treating all other terms as nuisance variables). The data were obtained from with fMRI under identical stimulus conditions (visual motion subtended by radially moving dots) while manipulating the attentional component of the task (detection of velocity changes).

induced by environmental and neurophysiological changes, while retaining mathematical tractability.

APPENDIX

Matrix Exponential Method for Integrating State Equations

Variables x, u, and z are time dependent (i.e., they are functions of time), however, for simplicity, the time dependence has been omitted. Consider any differential equation:

$$\dot{x} = f(x,u) \approx Ax + uBx + Cu + D$$
$$A = \frac{\partial f}{\partial x}$$
$$B = \frac{\partial^2 f}{\partial x \partial u} \tag{50.26}$$
$$C = \frac{\partial f}{\partial u}$$
$$D = f(0,0)$$

A time-dependent general solution for $z(t)$ is

$$z(t + \Delta t) = \exp(J\Delta t)z(t)$$
$$z = \begin{bmatrix} 1 \\ x \end{bmatrix}$$
$$J = M + Nu \tag{50.27}$$
$$M = \begin{bmatrix} 0 & 0 \\ D & A \end{bmatrix}$$
$$N = \begin{bmatrix} 0 & 0 \\ C & B \end{bmatrix}$$

for *constant input.* The value of $z(t)$ can be calculated iteratively over epochs of time during which u is stationary. The stability of the solution depends on the eigenvalues of J, with negative values resulting in stable solutions (Boas, 1983).

SEM Objective Function

The observed covariance calculated from the data is

$$S = \frac{1}{N-1} Y^T Y \tag{50.28}$$

where N is the number of observations. The covariance implied by the SEM is

$$\Sigma = (1 - \beta)^{-1T} \langle z_t^T z \rangle (1 - \beta)^{-1} \tag{50.29}$$

where $\langle z_t^T z \rangle$ is diagonal, because the innovations are assumed to be independent. An objective function comparing S and Σ is the maximum-likelihood function below. Note that a weighted least-squares function can be used for non-Gaussian data (Büchel and Friston, 1997) to reduce the discrepancy between the implied and estimated covariance matrices:

$$F_{ML} = \log|\Sigma| - trace(S\Sigma^{-1}) - \log|S| - p \tag{50.30}$$

References

Bendat, J. S. (1998). *Nonlinear Systems Techniques and Applications.* John Wiley & Sons, New York.

Boas, M. L. (1983). *Mathematical Models in the Physical Sciences.* John Wiley & Sons, New York.

Bollen, K. A. (1989). *Structural Equations with Latent Variables.* John Wiley & Sons, New York.

Büchel, C., and Friston, K. J. (1997). Modulation of connectivity in visual pathways by attention: cortical interactions evaluated with structural equation modelling and fMRI. *Cereb. Cortex* **7,** 768–778.

Büchel, C., and Friston, K. (2000). Assessing interactions among neuronal systems using functional neuroimaging. *Neural Netw.* **13,** 871–882.

Büchel, C., Wise, R. J., Mummery, C. J., Poline, J. B., and Friston, K .J. (1996). Nonlinear regression in parametric activation studies. *NeuroImage* **4,** 60–66.

Büchel, C., and Friston, K. J. (1997). Characterising functional integration. In *Human Brain Function,* Frackowiak, R. S. J., ed., pp. 108–127. Academic Press, San Diego.

Chatfield, C. (1996). *The Analysis of Time Series: An Introduction.* CRC Press, Boca Raton, FL.

Dayan, P., and Abbott, L. (2001). *Theoretical Neuroscience.* The MIT Press, Cambridge, MA.

Fliess, M., Lamnabhi, M., and Lamnabhi-Lagarrigue, F. (1983). An algebraic approach to nonlinear functional expansions. *IEEE Trans. Circ. Syst.* **30,** 554–570.

Friston, K. J. (2000). The labile brain. I. Neuronal transients and nonlinear coupling. *Philos. Trans. Roy. Soc. London B Biol. Sci.* **355,** 215–236.

Friston, K. J., and Price, C. J. (2001). Dynamic representations and generative models of brain function. *Brain Res. Bull.* **54,** 275–285.

Friston, K. J., Frith, C. D., and Frackowiak, R. S. J. (1993). Time-dependent changes in effective connectivity measured with PET. *Hum. Brain Mapping* **1,** 69–79.

Friston, K. J., Ungerleider, L. G., Jezzard, P., and Turner, R. (1995). Characterizing modulatory interactions between areas V1 and V2 in human cortex: a new treatment of functional MRI data. *Hum. Brain Mapping* **2,** 211–224.

Friston, K. J., Buechel, C., Fink, G. R., Morris, J., Rolls, E., and Dolan, R. J. (1997). Psychophysiological and modulatory interactions in neuroimaging. *NeuroImage* **6,** 218–229.

Ghahramani, Z. (2002). Unsupervised Learning course (lecture 4). Available at http://www.gatsby.ucl.ac.uk/~zoubin/index.html.

Glass, L. (2001). Synchronisation and rhythmic processes in physiology 3. *Nature* **410,** 277–284.

Glass, L., and Kaplan, D. (2000). *Understanding Nonlinear Dynamics*, Springer Verlag, New York.

Harrison, L. M., Penny, W., and Friston, K. J. (2003). Multivariate autoregressive modelling of fMRI time series. *NeuroImage*, **19**, 1477–1491.

Juang, J.-N. (2001). *Identification and Control of Mechanical Systems.* Cambridge University Press, Cambridge, UKIL.

Maruyama, G. M. (1998). *Basics of Structural Equation Modelling.* Sage Publications, Los Angeles.

McIntosh, A. R., and Gonzalez-Lima, F. (1991). Structural modelling of functional neural pathways mapped with 2-deoxyglucose: effects of acoustic startle habituation on the auditory system 7. *Brain Res.* **547,** 295–302.

McIntosh, A. R., and Gonzalez-Lima, F. (1992a). The application of structural equation modelling to metabolic mapping of functional neural systems. In *Advances in Metabolic Mapping Techniques for Brain Imaging of Behavioural and Learning Functions,* pp. 219–255. Kluwer Academic Publishers, The Netherlands.

McIntosh, A. R., and Gonzalez-Lima, F. (1992b). Structural modelling of functional visual pathways mapped with 2-deoxyglucose: effects of patterned light and footshock 5. *Brain Res.* **578,** 75–86.

McIntosh, A. R., and Gonzalez-Lima, F. (1994). Structural equation modelling and its application to network analysis in functional brain imaging. *Hum. Brain Mapping* **2,** 2–22.

McIntosh, A. R., Grady, C. L., Ungerleider, L. G., Haxby, J. V., Rapoport, S. I., and Horwitz, B. (1994). Network analysis of cortical visual pathways mapped with PET. *J. Neurosci.* **14,** 655–666.

Mesulam, M. M. (1998). From sensation to cognition. *Brain* **121,** 1013–1052.

Penny, W., and Roberts, S. J. (2002). Bayesian multivariate autoregressive models with structured priors. *IEE Proc. Vis. Image Signal Process.* **149,** 33–41.

Rao, T. S. (1992). Identification of bilinear time series models 5. *Statistica Sinica* **2,** 465–478.

Rieke, F., Warland, D., de Ruyter van Steveninck, R., and Bialek, W. (1997). Foundations. In *Spikes: Exploring the Neural Code,* pp. 38–48. The MIT Press, Cambridge, MA.

Rowe, J., Friston, K., Frackowiak, R., and Passingham, R. (2002). Attention to action: specific modulation of corticocortical interactions in humans. *NeuroImage* **17,** 988–998.

Scott, A. (1999). *Nonlinear Science: Emergence & Dynamics of Coherent Structures.* Oxford University Press, Oxford, UK.

CHAPTER

51

Volterra Kernels and Effective Connectivity

INTRODUCTION

The purpose of this brief chapter is to establish the Volterra formulation of effective connectivity from a conceptual and neurobiological point of view. Recall from the previous chapter that the generalised convolution representation of dynamic systems, afforded by Volterra expansions, is just another way of describing the input–output behaviour of systems that havc an equivalent state-space representation. In the next chapter we will deal with state-space representations in more detail. Before proceeding to explicit input–state–output models we will look at why the Volterra formulation can be so useful.

The Brain and Dynamic Systems

The brain can be regarded as an ensemble of connected dynamic systems and, as such, it conforms to some simple principles relating to the inputs and outputs of its constituent parts. The ensuing implications, for the way we think about, and measure, neuronal interactions can be quite profound. These range from implications for which aspects of neuronal activity are important to measure and how to characterise coupling among neuronal populations, to implications pertaining to the dynamic instability and complexity that are necessary for adaptive self-organisation.

This chapter focuses on the first issue by looking at neuronal interactions, coupling, and implicit neuronal codes from a dynamic perspective. By considering the brain in this light, one can show that a sufficient description of neuronal activity must comprise activity at the current time *and its recent history*. This history constitutes a neuronal transient. Such transients represent an essential metric of neuronal interactions and, implicitly, a code employed in the functional integration of brain systems. The nature of transients, expressed conjointly in different neuronal populations, reflects the underlying coupling among brain systems. A complete description of this coupling, or *effective connectivity*, can be expressed in terms of generalised convolution kernels (Volterra kernels) that embody high-order or nonlinear interactions. This coupling may be *synchronous*, and possibly oscillatory, or *asynchronous*. A critical distinction between synchronous and asynchronous coupling is that the former is essentially linear and the latter is nonlinear. The nonlinear nature of asynchronous coupling enables context-sensitive interactions that characterise real brain dynamics, suggesting that it plays an important role in functional integration.

Brain states are inherently labile, with a complexity and transience that renders their invariant characteristics elusive. The position adopted in this chapter is that the best approach is to embrace these dynamic aspects. Its aim is to introduce the notion of neuronal transients and the underlying framework (Friston, 2000). The central tenet is that the dynamics of neuronal systems can be viewed as a succession of transient spatiotemporal patterns of activity. These transients are shaped by the brain's anatomical infrastructure, principally connections, which have been selected to ensure the adaptive nature of the resulting dynamics. Although rather obvious, this formulation embodies one fundamental point; namely, that any description of brain state should have an explicit temporal dimension. In other words, measures of brain activity are only meaningful when specified over periods of time. This is particularly important in relation to fast dynamic interactions among neuronal populations that are characterised by synchrony. Synchronisation has become popular in the past years (e.g., Gray and Singer, 1989; Eckhorn *et al.,* 1988; Engel *et al.*, 1991) and yet represents only one possible sort of interaction.

This chapter is divided into four sections. In the first we review the conceptual basis of neuronal transients. This section uses an equivalence between two mathematical formulations of nonlinear systems to show that descriptions of brain dynamics, in terms of (1) neuronal transients and (2) the coupling among interacting brain systems, is complete and sufficient. The second section uses this equivalence to motivate a taxonomy of neuronal codes and establish the relationship among neuronal transients, asynchronous coupling, *dynamic correlations,* and nonlinear interactions. In the third section, we illustrate nonlinear coupling using magnetoencephalography (MEG) data. The final section discusses some neurobiological mechanisms that might mediate nonlinear coupling.

NEURONAL TRANSIENTS

The assertion that meaningful measures of brain dynamics have a temporal domain is neither new nor contentious (e.g., von der Malsburg, 1985; Engel *et al.*, 1991; Aertsen *et al.*, 1994; Freeman and Barrie, 1994; Abeles *et al.*, 1995; deCharms and Merzenich, 1996). A straightforward analysis demonstrates its veracity: Suppose that one wanted to posit some variables x that represented a complete and self-consistent description of brain activity. In short, everything needed to determine the evolution of the brain's state, at a particular place and time, was embodied in these measurements. Consider a component of the brain (e.g., a neuron or neuronal population). If such a set of variables existed for this component system they would satisfy some immensely complicated nonlinear state equation:

$$\frac{\partial x(t)}{\partial t} = f(x(t), u(t)) \tag{51.1}$$

where x is a huge vector of state variables that range from depolarisation at every point in the dendritic tree to the phosphorylation status of every relevant enzyme, from the biochemical status of every glial cell compartment to every aspect of gene expression. The $u(t)$ term represents a set of inputs conveyed by afferent from other regions. Equation (51.1) simply says that the changes in the state variables are nonlinear functions of the variables themselves and some inputs. The vast majority of these variables are hidden and not measurable directly. However, a small number of derived measurements y can be made:

$$y(t) = \lambda(x(t)) \tag{51.2}$$

such as activities of whole cells or populations. These activities could be measured in many ways, for example firing at the initial segment of an axon or local field potentials. The problem is that a complete and sufficient description appears unattainable, given that the underlying state variables cannot be observed directly. This is not the case. The resolution of this apparent impasse rests on two things: (1) a fundamental mathematical equivalence relating the inputs and outputs of a dynamic system and (2) the fact that these measurable outputs constitute the inputs to other cells or populations.

Convolution and State-Space Representations

Assume that every neuron in the brain is modelled by a nonlinear dynamic system of the sort described by Eq. (51.1). Under this assumption it can be shown that *the output is a function of the recent history of its inputs*:

$$y(t) = h(u(t - \sigma)) \tag{51.3}$$

where $u(t - \sigma)$ represents the inputs in the recent past. Furthermore, this relationship can be expressed as a Volterra series of the inputs (see the Appendix at the end of the chapter). The critical thing here is that we never need to know the underlying and "hidden" variables that describe the details of each cell's electrochemical and biochemical status. We only need to know the history of its inputs, which, of course, are the outputs of other cells. Equation (51.3) is, in principle, a sufficient description of brain dynamics and involves the variables $u(t - \sigma) = y(t - \sigma)$, which represent activity at all times σ preceding the moment in question. These are simply neuronal transients. The degree of transience depends on how far back in time it is necessary to go to fully capture the brain's dynamics. The sensible nature of Eq. (51.3) can be readily seen. For example, if we wanted to determine the behaviour of a cell in V1 (primary visual cortex), then we would need to know the activity of all connected cells in the immediate vicinity over the last millisecond or so to account for propagation delays down afferent axons. We would also need to know the activity in distant sources, like the lateral geniculate nucleus and higher cortical areas, some 10 or more milliseconds ago. In short, we need the recent history of all inputs.

Transients can be expressed in terms of firing rates (e.g., chaotic oscillations; see Freeman and Barrie, 1994) or individual spikes (e.g., syn-fire chains; see Abeles *et al.,* 1995). Transients are not just a mathematical abstraction; they have real implications at a number of levels. For example, the emergence of fast oscillatory interactions among simulated neuronal populations depends on the time delays implicit in axonal transmission and the time constants of post-synaptic responses. Another slightly more subtle aspect of this formulation is that changes in synaptic efficacy, such as short-term potentiation or depression, take some time to be mediated by intracellular mechanisms. This means that the interaction between inputs at different times, which models these activity-dependent effects, again depends on the relevant history of activity.

Levels of Description

The above arguments lead to a conceptual model of the brain that comprises a collection of dynamic systems (e.g., cells or populations of cells), each represented as an input–state–output model, where the state remains forever hidden. However, the inputs and outputs are accessible and are causally related where the output of one system constitutes the input to another. A complete description, therefore, comprises the nature of these relationships (the Volterra series corresponding to the function h) and the neuronal transients. This constitutes a *mesoscopic* level of description that permits a degree of "black-boxness" but with no loss of information.

The equivalence, in terms of specifying the behaviour of a neuronal system, between microscopic and mesoscopic levels of description is critical. In short, the equivalence means that all information inherent in unobservable microscopic variables that determine the response of a neuronal system is embodied in the history of its observable inputs and outputs. Although the microscopic level of description may be more mechanistically informative, from the point of view of response prediction, neuronal transients are an entirely equivalent representation.[1]

Effective Connectivity and Volterra Kernels

The first conclusion so far is that neuronal transients are necessary to specify brain dynamics. The second conclusion is that a complete model of the influence one neuronal population exerts over another should take the form of a Volterra series.[2] This implies that a complete characterisation of these influences (i.e., effective connectivity) comprises the Volterra kernels that are

[1] We have focused on the distinction between microscopic and mesoscopic levels of description. The *macroscopic* level is reserved for approaches, exemplified by synergistics (Haken, 1983), that characterise the spatiotemporal evolution of brain dynamics in terms of a small number of macroscopic order parameters [see Kelso (1995) for an engaging exposition]. Order parameters are created and determined by the cooperation of microscopic quantities and yet, at the same time, govern the behaviour of the whole system. See Jirsa *et al.* (1995) for a nice example.

[2] An important qualification here is that each system is "controllable." Systems that are not "controlled" have quasi-periodic or chaotic behaviours that are maintained by interactions among the states of the system. Although an important issue at the microscopic level, it is fairly easy to show that the mean field approximation to any ensemble of subsystems is controllable.

applied to the inputs to yield the outputs. Effective connectivity refers explicitly to "the influence that one neural system exerts over another, either at a synaptic (i.e., synaptic efficacy) or population level" (Friston, 1995a). It has been proposed (Aertsen and Preißl, 1991) that "the notion of effective connectivity should be understood as the experiment- and time-dependent, simplest possible circuit diagram that would replicate the observed timing relationships between the recorded neurons" (see the previous chapter).

If effective connectivity is the influence that one neural system exerts over another it should be possible, given the effective connectivity and the afferent activity, to predict the response of a recipient population. This is precisely what Volterra kernels do. Any model of effective connectivity can be expressed as a Volterra series and any measure of effective connectivity can be reduced to a set of Volterra kernels (see the Appendix). An important aspect of effective connectivity is its context sensitivity. Effective connectivity is simply the "effect" that input has on the output of a target system. This effect will be sensitive to other inputs, its own history, and, of course, the microscopic state and causal architecture intrinsic to the target population. This intrinsic dynamic structure is embodied in the Volterra kernels. In short, Volterra kernels are synonymous with effective connectivity because they characterise the measurable effect that an input has on its target. An example of using Volterra kernels—for characterising context-sensitive changes in effective connectivity—was provided in the previous chapter (see Fig. 50.16). This example used hemodynamic responses to changes in neuronal activity as measured with functional magnetic resonance imaging (fMRI).

NEURONAL CODES

Functional integration refers to the concerted interactions among neuronal populations that mediate perceptual binding, sensorimotor integration, and cognition. It pertains to the mechanisms of, and constraints under which, the state of one population influences that of another. It has been suggested by many that functional integration, among neuronal populations, uses transient dynamics that represent a temporal "code." A compelling proposal is that population responses, encoding a percept, become organised in time, through reciprocal interactions, to discharge in synchrony (von der Malsburg, 1985; Singer, 1994). The use of the term *encoding* here speaks directly to the notion of codes. Here a neuronal code is taken to be a metric that reveals interactions among neuronal systems by enabling some prediction of the response in one population given the same sort of measure in another.[3] Clearly, from the previous section, neuronal transients represent the most generic form of code because, given the Volterra kernels, the output can, in principle, be predicted exactly. Neuronal transients have a number of attributes (interspike interval, duration, mean level of firing, predominant frequency, etc.), and any of these could be contenders for a more parsimonious code. The problem of identifying possible codes can be reduced to identifying the form that the Volterra kernels in the Appendix can take. If we know their form, then we can say which aspects of the input will cause a response. Conversely, it follows that the different forms of kernels should specify the various codes that might be encountered. This is quite an important point and leads to a clear formulation of what can and cannot constitute a code. We now review different codes in terms of the different sorts of kernels that could mediate them.

Instantaneous vs. Temporal Codes

The first kernel characteristic that engenders a coding taxonomy is kernel depth. The limiting case here is when the kernels support shrinks to a point in time. This means that the only relevant history is the immediate activity of inputs (all earlier activities are "ignored" by the kernel). In this case the activity in any unit is simply a nonlinear function of current activities elsewhere. An example of this is instantaneous rate coding.

[3] Although the term *code* is not being used to denote anything that "codes" for something in the environment, it could be used to define some aspect of an evoked transient that expresses a high mutual information with a stimulus parameter (e.g., Tovee *et al.*, 1993).

Rate coding considers spike-trains as *stochastic processes* whose first-order moments (i.e., mean activity) describe neuronal interactions. These moments may be in terms of spikes themselves or other compound events (e.g., the average rate of bursting; see Bair *et al.*, 1994). Interactions based on rate coding are usually assessed in terms of cross-correlations. From the dynamic perspective, instantaneous rate codes are considered insufficient. This is because they predict nothing about a cell, or population, response unless one knows the microscopic state of that cell or population.

The distinction between rate and temporal coding (see Shadlen and Newsome, 1995; de Ruyter van Steveninck *et al.*, 1997) centres on whether the precise timing of individual spikes is sufficient to facilitate meaningful neuronal interactions. In temporal coding the exact time at which an individual spike occurs is the important measure and the spike-train is considered as a *point process*. There are clear examples of temporal codes that have predictive validity; for example, the primary cortical representation of sounds by the coordination of action potential timing (deCharms and Merzenich, 1996). These codes depend on the relative timing of action potentials and, implicitly, an extended temporal frame of reference. They therefore fall into the class of transient codes, where selective responses to particular interspike intervals are modelled by temporally extended second-order kernels. A nice example is provided by de Ruyter van Steveninck *et al.* (1997) who show that the temporal patterning of spike-trains, elicited in fly motion-sensitive neurons by natural stimuli, can carry twice the amount of information than an equivalent Poisson rate code.

Transient Codes: Synchronous vs. Asynchronous

The second distinction, assuming the kernels have a nontrivial depth, is whether they comprise high-order terms or not. Expansions that encompass just first-order terms are only capable of meditating linear or synchronous interactions. Higher order kernels confer nonlinearity on the influence of an input that leads to asynchronous interactions. Mathematically, if there are only first-order terms then the Fourier transform of the Volterra kernel completely specifies the relationship (the transfer function) between the spectral density of input and output in a way that precludes interactions among frequencies, or indeed inputs. In other words, the expression of any frequency in a recipient cell is predicted exactly by the expression of the same frequency in the source (after some scaling by the transfer function).

Synchronous Codes

The proposal most pertinent to these forms of code is that population responses, participating in the encoding of a percept, become organised in time through reciprocal interactions so that they come to discharge in synchrony (von der Malsburg, 1985; Singer, 1994) with regular periodic bursting. Note that synchronisation does not necessarily imply oscillations. However, synchronised activity is usually inferred operationally by oscillations implied by the periodic modulation of cross-correlograms of separable spike-trains (e.g., Gray and Singer, 1989; Eckhorn *et al.,* 1988) or measures of coherence in multichannel electrical and neuromagnetic time series (e.g., Llinas *et al.*, 1994). The underlying mechanism of these frequency-specific interactions is usually attributed to phase-locking among neuronal populations (e.g., Sporns *et al.*, 1989; Aertsen and Preißl, 1991). The key aspect of these measures is that they refer to the extended temporal structure of synchronised firing patterns, either in terms of spiking (e.g., synfire chains; Abeles *et al.*, 1995; Lumer *et al.*, 1997) or oscillations in the ensuing population dynamics (e.g., Singer, 1994).

Many aspects of functional integration and feature linking in the brain are thought to be mediated by synchronised dynamics among neuronal populations (Singer, 1994). Synchronisation reflects the direct, reciprocal exchange of signals between two populations, whereby the activity in one population influences the second, such that the dynamics become entrained and mutually reinforcing. In this way the binding of different features of an object may be accomplished in the temporal domain through the transient synchronisation of oscillatory responses. This "dynamic linking" defines their short-lived functional association. Physiological evidence is compatible with this theory (e.g., Engel *et al.*, 1991; Fries *et al.*, 1997). Synchronisation of oscillatory responses occurs within as well as among visual areas, for example, between homologous areas of the left and right hemispheres and between areas at different levels of the visuomotor pathway (Engel *et al.*, 1991). Synchronisation in the visual cortex appears to depend on stimulus properties, such as continuity, orientation, and motion coherence.

The problem with synchronisation is that there is nothing essentially dynamic about synchronous interactions per se. As argued by Erb and Aertsen (1992) "the question might not be so much how the brain functions by virtue of oscillations, as most researchers working on cortical oscillations seem to assume, but rather how it manages to do so in spite of them." To establish dynamic cell assemblies, it is necessary to create and destroy synchronised couplings. It is precisely these dynamic aspects that speak to changes in synchrony (e.g., Desmedt and Tomberg, 1994) and the asynchronous transitions between synchronous states as the more pertinent phenomenon. In other words, it is the successive reformulation of dynamic cell assemblies, through nonlinear or asynchronous interactions, that is at the heart of "dynamic linking" (Singer, 1994).

Asynchronous Codes

An alternative perspective on neuronal codes is provided by *dynamic correlations* (Aertsen *et al.*, 1994) as exemplified in Vaadia *et al.* (1995). A fundamental phenomenon, observed by Vaadia *et al.* (1995), is that, following behaviourally salient events, the degree of coherent firing between two neurons can change profoundly and systematically over the ensuing second or so. One implication is that a complete model of neuronal interactions has to accommodate dynamic changes in correlations, modulated on timescales of 100–1,000 ms. Neuronal transients provide a simple explanation for this temporally modulated coherence or dynamic correlation. Imagine that two neurons respond to an event with a similar transient. For example, if two neurons respond to an event with decreased firing for 400 ms, and this decrease was correlated over epochs, then positive correlations between the two firing rates would be seen for the first 400 ms of the epoch, and then fade away, exhibiting a dynamic modulation of coherence. In other words, a transient modulation of covariance can be equivalently formulated as covariance in the expression of transients. The generality of this equivalence can be established using singular value decomposition (SVD) of the joint-peristimulus time histogram (J-PSTH) as described in Friston (1995b). This is simply a mathematical device to show that dynamic changes in coherence are equivalent to the coherent expression of neural transients. In itself it is not important, in the sense that dynamic correlations are just as valid a characterisation as neuronal transients and indeed may provide more intuitive insights into how this phenomenon is mediated (e.g., Riehle *et al.*, 1997). A more important observation is that J-PSTHs can be asymmetric about the leading diagonal. This suggests that coupled transients in two units can have a different patterning of activity. This can only be explained by asynchronous or nonlinear coupling.

Summary

In summary, the critical distinction between synchronous and asynchronous coupling is the difference between linear and nonlinear interactions among units or populations.[4] This difference reduces to the existence of high-order Volterra kernels in the mediating the input–output behaviour of coupled cortical regions. There is a close connection between asynchronous/nonlinear coupling and the expression of distinct transients in two brain regions: Both would be expressed as dynamic correlations or, in the EEG, as event-related changes in synchronisation (e.g., induced oscillations). If the full transient model is correct, then important transactions among cortical areas will be overlooked by techniques that are predicated on rate coding (correlations, covariance patterns, spatial modes, etc.) or synchronisation models (e.g., coherence analysis and cross-correlograms). Clearly the critical issue here is whether there is direct

[4] The term *generalised synchrony* has been introduced to include nonlinear interdependencies (see Schiff *et al.*, 1996). Generalised synchrony subsumes synchronous and asynchronous coupling. An elegant method for making inferences about generalised synchrony is described in Schiff *et al.* (1996). This approach is particularly interesting from our point of view because it calls on the recent history of the dynamics through the use of temporal embedding to reconstruct the attractors analysed.

evidence for nonlinear or asynchronous coupling that would render high-order Volterra kernels necessary.

EVIDENCE FOR NONLINEAR COUPLING

Why is asynchronous coupling so important? The reason is that asynchronous interactions embody all of the nonlinear interactions implicit in functional integration and it is these that mediate the context-sensitive nature of neuronal interactions. Nonlinear interactions among cortical areas render the effective connectivity among them inherently dynamic and contextual. Compelling examples of context-sensitive interactions include the attentional modulation of evoked responses in functionally specialised sensory areas (e.g., Treue and Maunsell, 1996) and other contextually dependent dynamics (see Phillips and Singer, 1997). Whole classes of empirical phenomena such as extraclassical receptive field effects rely on nonlinear or asynchronous interactions.

Nonlinear Coupling and Asynchronous Interactions

If the temporal structures of recurring transients in two parts of the brain are distinct, then the prevalence of certain frequencies in one cortical area should predict the expression of *different* frequencies in another. In contrast, synchronisation posits the expression of the *same* frequencies. Correlations among different frequencies therefore provide a basis for discriminating between synchronous and asynchronous coupling.

Consider time series from two neuronal populations or cortical areas. Synchrony requires the expression of a particular frequency (e.g., 40 Hz) in one time series to be coupled with the expression of the same frequency in the other. In other words, the modulation of this frequency in one area can be explained or predicted by its modulation in the second. Conversely, asynchronous coupling suggests that the power at a reference frequency, say, 40 Hz, can be predicted by the spectral density in the second time series at frequencies other than 40 Hz. These predictions can be tested empirically using standard time-frequency and regression analyses as described in Friston (2000). Figure 51.1 shows an example of this sort of analysis, revealing the dynamic changes in spectral density between 8 and 64 Hz over 16 sec. The cross-correlation matrix of the time-dependent expression of different frequencies in the parietal and prefrontal regions is shown in the lower left panel. There is anecdotal evidence here for both synchronous and asynchronous coupling. Synchronous coupling, based on the comodulation of the same frequencies, is manifest as hot spots along, or near, the leading diagonal of the cross-correlation matrix (e.g., around 20 Hz). More interesting are correlations between high frequencies in one time series and low frequencies in another. In particular, note that the frequency modulation at about 34 Hz in the parietal region (second time series) could be explained by several frequencies in the prefrontal region. The most profound correlations are with lower frequencies in the first time series (26 Hz). Using a simple regression framework, statistical inferences can be made about the coupling within and between different frequencies (see Friston, 2000, for details). A regression analysis shows that coupling at 34 Hz has significant synchronous and asynchronous components, whereas the coupling at 48 Hz is purely asynchronous (middle and right peaks in the graphs), i.e., a coupling between beta dynamics in the premotor region and gamma dynamics in the parietal region.

THE NEURAL BASIS OF NONLINEAR COUPLING

In Friston (1997) it was suggested that, from a neurobiological perspective, the distinction between nonlinear (asynchronous) and linear (synchronous) interactions could be viewed in the following way. Synchronisation emerges from the reciprocal exchange of signals between two populations, where each *drives* the other, such that the dynamics become entrained and mutually reinforcing. In asynchronous coding the afferents from one population exert a *modulatory* influence, not on the activity of the second, but on the interactions within it (e.g., a modulation

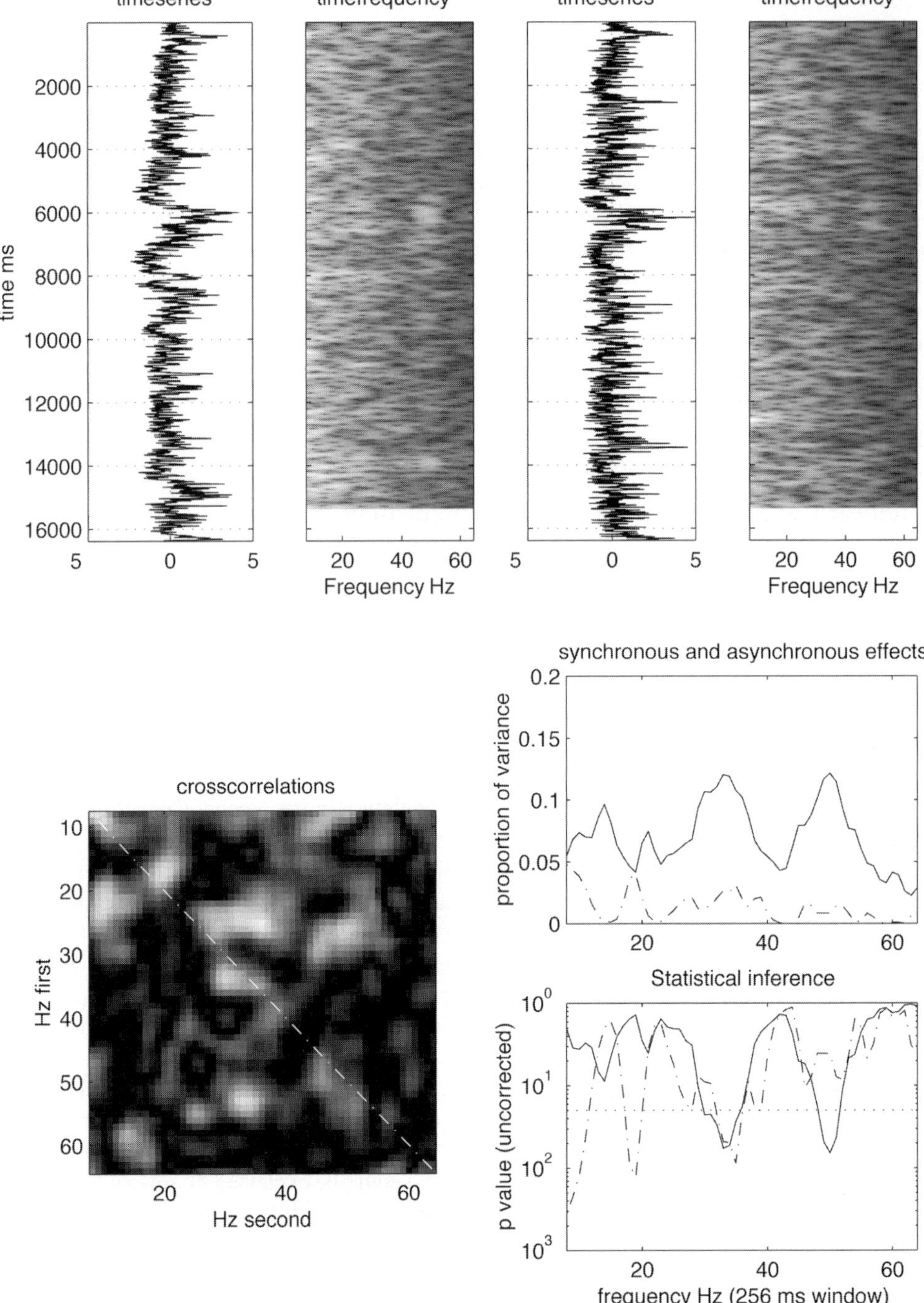

FIGURE 51.1
Time-frequency and regression analysis of MEG time series designed to characterise the relative contribution of synchronous and asynchronous coupling. Neuromagnetic data were acquired from a normal subject using a KENIKRON 37-channel MEG system at 1-ms intervals for periods of up to 2 min. During this time the subject made volitional joystick movements to the left, every 2 sec or so. Paired epochs were taken from a left prefrontal and left parietal region. (Top) The two times series (plots) and their corresponding time-frequency profiles (images). The first time series comes from the left prefrontal region. The second comes from the left superior parietal region. (Lower left) This is a simple characterisation of the coupling among frequencies in the two regions and represents the squared cross-correlations of the time-varying expression of different frequencies from the upper panels. (Lower right) These are the results of a linear regression analysis that partitions the variance in the second (parietal) time series into components that can be attributed to synchronous (broken lines) and asynchronous (solid lines) contributions from the first (prefrontal) time series. The upper graph shows the relative contribution in terms of the proportion of variance explained and in terms of the significance using a semi-log plot of the corresponding p values (lower graph). The dotted line in the latter corresponds to $p = 0.05$.

This example was chosen because it illustrates three sorts of coupling (synchronous, asynchronous, and mixed). From inspection of the cross-correlation matrix, it is evident that power in the beta range (20 Hz) in the second time series is correlated with similar frequency modulation in the first, albeit at a slightly lower frequency. The resulting correlations appear just off the leading diagonal (broken line) on the upper left. The proportion of variance explained by synchronous and asynchronous coupling is roughly the same and, in terms of significance, synchrony supervenes (see upper graph). In contrast, the high correlations, between 48 Hz in the second time series and 26 Hz in the first, are well away from the leading diagonal, with little evidence of correlations within either of these frequencies. The regression analysis confirms that, at this frequency, asynchronous coupling prevails. The variation at about 34 Hz in the parietal region could be explained by several frequencies in the prefrontal region. A formal analysis shows that both synchronous and asynchronous coupling coexist at this frequency (i.e., the middle peak in the graphs).

of effective connectivity or synaptic efficacies within the target population), leading to changes in the dynamics intrinsic to the second population. In this model there is no necessary synchrony between the intrinsic dynamics that ensue and the temporal pattern of modulatory input. To test this hypothesis, one would need to demonstrate that asynchronous coupling emerges when extrinsic connections are changed from driving connections to modulatory connections. Clearly this cannot be done in the real brain. However, we can use computational techniques to create a biologically realistic model of interacting populations and test this hypothesis directly.

Interactions between Simulated Populations

Two populations were simulated using the model described in Friston (2000). This model simulates entire neuronal populations in a deterministic fashion based on known neurophysiological mechanisms. In particular, we modelled three sorts of synapse, fast inhibitory (GABA), fast excitatory (AMPA), and slower voltage-dependent synapses (NMDA). Connections intrinsic to each population used only GABA and AMPA-like synapses. Simulated glutaminergic extrinsic connections between the two populations used either driving AMPA-like synapses or modulatory NMDA-like synapses. Transmission delays for extrinsic connections were fixed at 8 ms. By using realistic time constants, the characteristic oscillatory dynamics of each population were expressed in the gamma range.

The results of coupling two populations with unidirectional AMPA-like connections are shown in the top of Fig. 51.2 in terms of the simulated local field potentials (LFPs). Occasional transients in the driving population were evoked by injecting a depolarising current, of the same magnitude, at random intervals (dotted lines). The tight synchronised coupling that ensues is evident. This example highlights the point that near-linear coupling can arise even in the context of loosely coupled, highly nonlinear neuronal oscillators of the sort modelled here. Contrast these entrained dynamics under driving connections with those that emerge when the connection is modulatory or NMDA-like (lower panel in Fig. 51.2). Here there is no synchrony and, as predicted, fast transients of an oscillatory nature are facilitated by the input from the first population that has a lower frequency (cf. the MEG analyses above). This is a nice example of asynchronous coupling that is underpinned by nonlinear modulatory interactions between neuronal populations. The nature of the coupling can be characterised using the time-frequency analysis (identical in every detail) applied to the neuromagnetic data of the previous section. The results for the NMDA simulation are presented in Fig. 51.3. The cross-correlation matrix resembles that obtained with the MEG data in Fig. 51.1. Both in terms of the variance, and inference, asynchronous coupling supervenes at most frequencies but, as in the real data, mixed coupling is also evident. These results can be taken as a heuristic conformation of the notion that modulatory, in this case voltage-dependent, interactions are sufficiently nonlinear to account for the emergence of asynchronous coupling.

Modulatory Interactions and Nonlinear Coupling

In summary, asynchronous coupling is synonymous with nonlinear coupling. Nonlinear coupling can be framed in terms of the modulation of intrinsic interactions, within a cortical area or neuronal population, by extrinsic input offered by afferents from other parts of the brain. This mechanism predicts that the modulation of fast (e.g., gamma) activity in one cortical area can be predicted by much slower changes in other areas. This form of coupling is very different from coherence or other measures of synchronous coupling and concerns the relationship between the first-order dynamics in one area and the second-order dynamics (spectral density) expressed in another. In terms of the above NMDA simulation, transient depolarisation in the modulating population causes a short-lived increased input to the second. These afferents impinge on voltage-sensitive NMDA-like synapses with time constants (in the model) of about 100 ms. These synapses open and slowly close again, remaining open long after an afferent volley. Because of their voltage-sensitive nature this input will have no effect on the dynamics intrinsic to the second population unless there is already a substantial degree of depolarisation. If there is then, through self-excitation and inhibition, the concomitant opening of fast excitatory and inhibitory channels will generally increase membrane conductance, decrease the effective

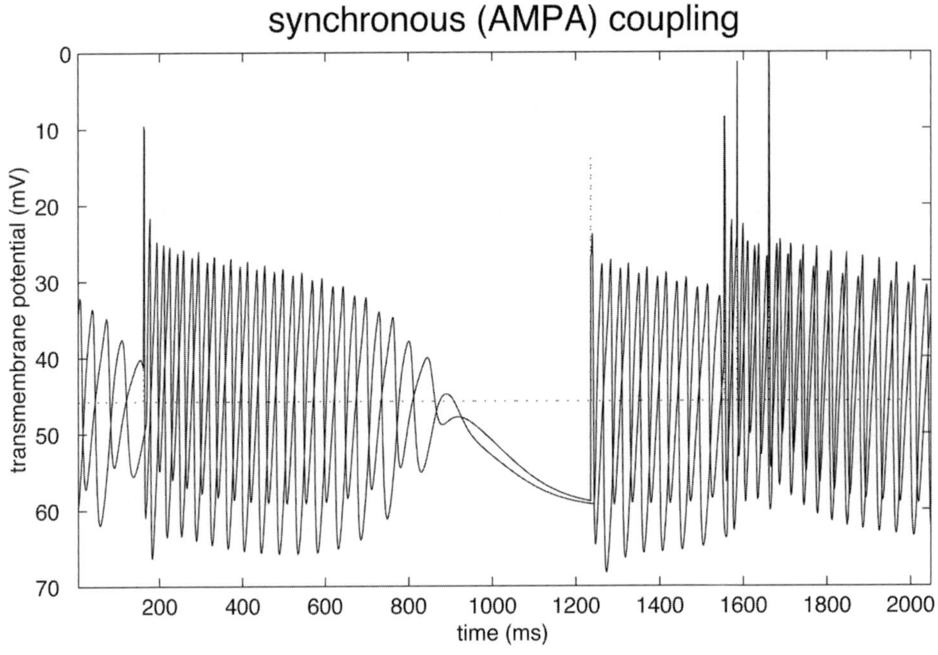

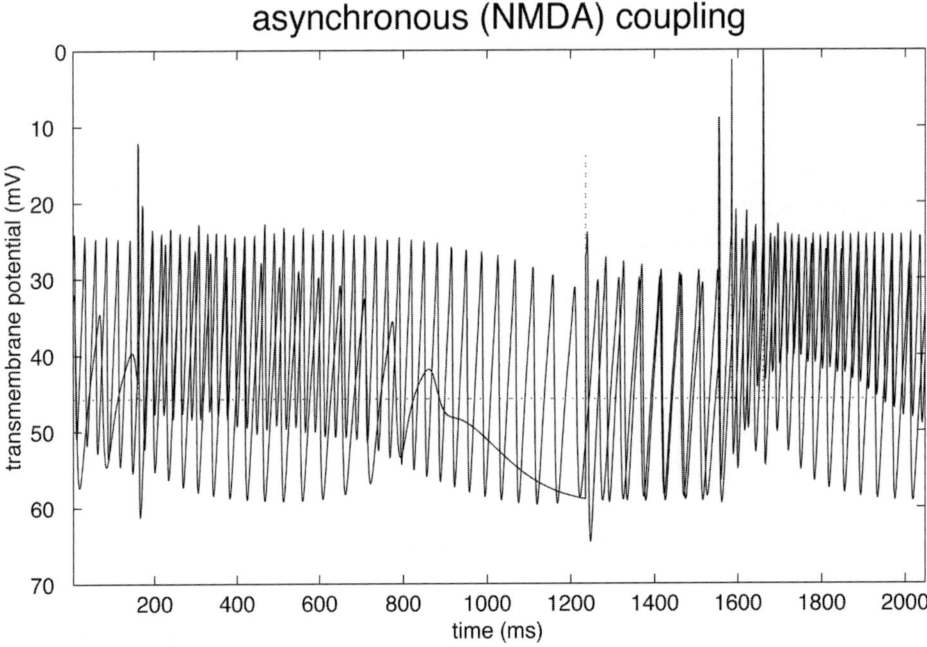

FIGURE 51.2
Simulated LFPs of two coupled populations using two different sorts of postsynaptic responses (AMPA and NMDA-like) to connections from the first to the target population. The dotted line shows the depolarisation effected by sporadic injections of current into the first population. The key thing to note is that under AMPA-like or driving connections the second population is synchronously entrained by the first. When the connections are modulatory or voltage-dependent (NMDA), the effects are much more subtle and resemble a frequency modulation. These data were simulated using a biologically plausible model of excitatory and inhibitory subpopulations. The model was deterministic with variables pertaining to the collective, probabilistic behaviour of the subpopulations (cf. a mean field treatment). See Friston (2000) for details.

membrane time constants, and lead to fast oscillatory transients. This is what we observe in the lower panel of Fig. 51.2. In relation to the MEG analyses, the implied modulatory mechanisms, which may underpin this effect, are entirely consistent with the anatomy, laminar specificity, and functional role attributed to prefrontal efferents (Rockland and Pandya, 1979; Selemon and Goldman-Rakic, 1988).

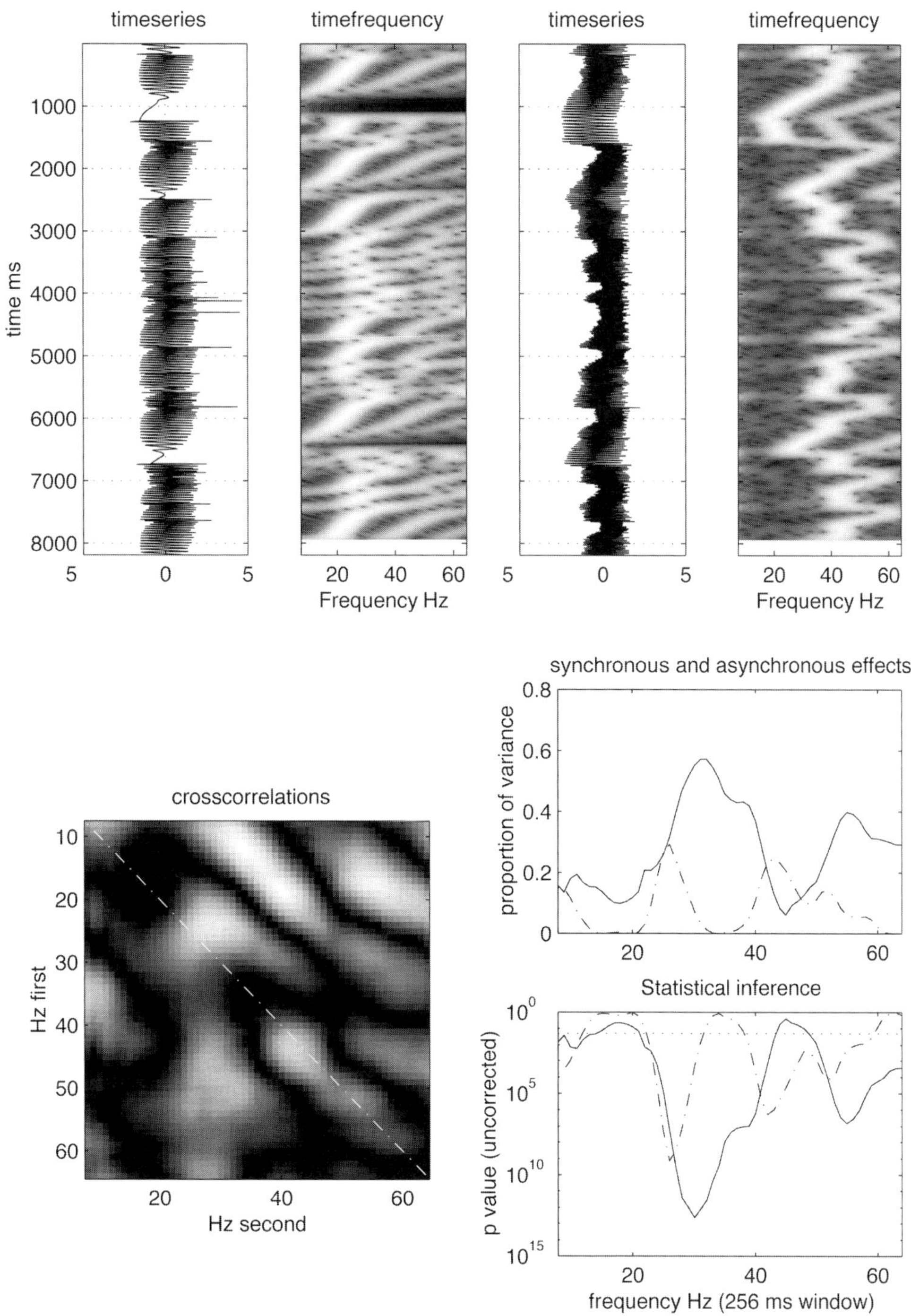

FIGURE 51.3
As for Fig. 51.1, but here using the simulated data employing voltage-dependent NMDA-like connections. The coupling here includes some profoundly asynchronous (nonlinear) components involving frequencies in the gamma range implicated in the analyses of the real (MEG) data shown in Fig. 51.1. In particular, note the asymmetrical cross-correlation matrix and the presence of asynchronous and mixed coupling implicit in the *p*-value plots on the lower right.

CONCLUSION

In this chapter we have dealt with some interesting and interrelated aspects of effective connectivity, neuronal codes, nonlinear coupling, neuronal transients, and dynamic correlations (e.g., induced oscillations). The key points can be summarised as follows:

- Starting with the premise that the brain can be represented as an ensemble of connected input–state–output systems (e.g., cellular compartments, cells or populations of cells), there exists an equivalent input–output formulation in terms of a Volterra series. This is simply a functional expansion of each system's inputs that produces its outputs (where the outputs to one system constitute the inputs to another).
- The existence of this expansion suggests that the history of inputs, or neuronal transients, and the Volterra kernels are a complete and sufficient specification of brain dynamics (to the extent they are controllable). This is the primary motivation for framing dynamics in terms of neuronal transients and using Volterra kernels to model effective connectivity.
- The Volterra formulation provides constraints on the form to which neuronal interactions and implicit codes must conform. There are two limiting cases: (1) when the kernel decays very quickly and (2) when high-order kernels disappear. The first case corresponds to instantaneous codes (e.g., rate codes) and the second to synchronous interactions (e.g., synchrony codes).
- High-order kernels in the Volterra formulation of effective connectivity speak to nonlinear interactions and implicitly to asynchronous coupling. Asynchronous coupling implies coupling among the expression of different frequencies.
- Coupling among different frequencies is easy to demonstrate using neuromagnetic measurements of real brain dynamics. This implies that nonlinear, asynchronous coupling is a prevalent component of functional integration.
- High-order kernels correspond to modulatory interactions that can be construed as a nonlinear effect of inputs that interact bilinearly with the intrinsic states of the recipient system. This implies that driving connections may be linear and engender synchronous interactions. Conversely, modulatory connections, being nonlinear, may be revealed by asynchronous coupling and be expressed in high-order kernels.

APPENDIX: DYNAMIC SYSTEMS AND VOLTERRA KERNELS

Input–State–Output Systems and Volterra Series

Neuronal systems are inherently nonlinear and lend themselves to modelling with nonlinear dynamic systems. However, due to the complexity of biological systems, it is difficult to find analytic equations that describe them adequately. Even if these equations were known the state variables are often not observable. An alternative approach to identification is to adopt a very general model (Wray and Green, 1994) and focus on the inputs and outputs. Consider the single input–single output (SISO) system:

$$\begin{aligned}\dot{x}(t) &= f(x(t), u(t)) \\ y(t) &= \lambda(x(t))\end{aligned} \tag{51.4}$$

The Fliess fundamental formula (Fliess *et al.*, 1983) describes the causal relationship between the outputs and the recent history of the inputs. This relationship can be expressed as a Volterra series that expresses the output $y(t)$ as a nonlinear convolution of the inputs $u(t)$, critically without reference to the state variables $x(t)$. This series is simply a functional Taylor expansion of $y(t)$ in Eq. (51.3), per the main text.

$$\begin{aligned}y(t) = h(u(t-\sigma)) &= \sum_{i=1}^{\infty} \int_0^t \ldots \int_0^t \kappa_i(\sigma_1 \ldots \sigma_i) \ldots u(t-\sigma_i) d\sigma_1 \ldots d\sigma_i \\ \kappa_i(\sigma_1 \ldots \sigma_i) &= \frac{\partial^i y(t)}{\partial u(t-\sigma_1) \ldots \partial u(t-\sigma_i)}\end{aligned} \tag{51.3}$$

where $\kappa_i(\sigma_1 \ldots \sigma_i)$ is the ith-order kernel. Volterra series have been described as a "power series with memory" and are generally thought of as a high-order or "nonlinear convolution" of the inputs to provide an output. See Bendat (1990) for a fuller discussion.

Volterra Kernels and Effective Connectivity

Volterra kernels are essential in characterising the effective connectivity or influences that one neuronal system exerts over another because they represent the causal input–output characteristics of the system in question. Neurobiologically they have a simple and compelling interpretation: *They are synonymous with effective connectivity*. From (51.5),

$$\kappa_1(\sigma_1) = \frac{\partial y(t)}{\partial u(t - \sigma_1)}, \quad \kappa_2(\sigma_1,\sigma_2) = \frac{\partial^2 y(t)}{\partial u(t - \sigma_1)\partial u(t - \sigma_2)}, \ \ldots$$

It is evident that the first-order kernel embodies the response evoked by a change in input at $t - \sigma_1$. In other words, it is a time-dependant measure of *driving* efficacy. Similarly, the second-order kernel reflects the *modulatory* influence of the input at $t - \sigma_1$ on the response evoked by input at $t - \sigma_2$—and so on for higher orders.

References

Abeles, M., Bergman, H., Gat, I., Meilijson, I., Seidmann, E., Tishby, N., and, Vaadia, E. (1995). Cortical activity flips among quasi-stationary states. *Proc. Natl. Acad. Sci. USA* **92,** 8616–8620.

Aertsen, A., Erb, M., and Palm, G. (1994). Dynamics of functional coupling in the cerebral cortex: an attempt at a model-based interpretation, *Physica D* **75,** 103–128.

Aertsen, A., and Preißl, H. (1991). Dynamics of activity and connectivity in physiological neuronal networks. In *Non Linear Dynamics and Neuronal Networks,* Schuster, H. G., Ed., pp. 281–302. VCH Publishers, New York.

Bair, W., Koch, C., Newsome, W., and Britten, K. (1994). Relating temporal properties of spike trains from area MT neurons to the behaviour of the monkey. In *Temporal Coding in the Brain,* Buzsaki, L. R., Singer, W., Berthoz, A., and Christen, T., Eds., pp. 221–250. Springer Verlag, Berlin.

Bendat, J. S. (1990). *Nonlinear System Analysis and Identification from Random Data.* John Wiley and Sons, New York.

Büchel, C., and Friston, K. J. (1997). Modulation of connectivity in visual pathways by attention: cortical interactions evaluated with structural equation modelling and fMRI. *Cerebral Cortex* **7,** 768–778.

deCharms, R. C., and Merzenich, M. M. (1996). Primary cortical representation of sounds by the coordination of action potential timing. *Nature* **381,** 610–613.

de Ruyter van Steveninck, R. R., Lewen, G. D., Strong, S. P., Koberie, R., and Bialek, W. (1997). Reproducibility and variability in neural spike trains. *Science* **275,** 1085–1088.

Desmedt, J. E., and Tomberg, C. (1994). Transient phase-locking of 40-Hz electrical oscillations in prefrontal and parietal human cortex reflects the process of conscious somatic perception. *Neurosci. Lett.* **168,** 126–129.

Eckhorn, R., Bauer, R., Jordan, W., Brosch, M., Kruse, W., Munk, M., and Reitboeck, H. J. (1988). Coherent oscillations: a mechanism of feature linking in the visual cortex?. Multiple electrode and correlation analysis in the cat. *Biol. Cybern.* **60,** 121–130.

Erb, M., and Aertsen, A. (1992). Dynamics of activity in biology-oriented neural network models: stability analysis at low firing rates. In *Information Processing in the Cortex. Experiments and Theory,* Aertsen, A., and Braitenberg, V., Eds., pp. 201–223. Springer-Verlag, Berlin.

Engel, A. K., Konig, P., and Singer, W. (1991). Direct physiological evidence for scene segmentation by temporal coding. *Proc. Natl. Acad. Sci USA* **88,** 9136–9140.

Fliess, M., Lamnabhi, M., and Lamnabhi-Lagarrigue, F. (1983). An algebraic approach to nonlinear functional expansions. *IEEE Trans. Circuits Syst.* **30,** 554–570.

Freeman, W, and Barrie, J. (1994). Chaotic oscillations and the genesis of meaning in cerebral cortex. In *Temporal Coding in the Brain,* Buzsaki, L. R., Singer, W., Berthoz, A., and Christen, T., Eds., pp. 13–38. Springer Verlag, Berlin.

Fries, P., Roelfsema, P. R., Engel, A., Konig, P., and Singer, W. (1997). Synchronisation of oscillatory responses in visual cortex correlates with perception in inter-ocular rivalry. *Proc. Natl. Acad. Sci. USA* **94,** 12699–12704.

Friston, K. J. (1995a). Functional and effective connectivity in neuroimaging: a synthesis. *Hum. Brain Mapping* **2,** 56–78.

Friston, K. J. (1995b). Neuronal transients. *Proc. Roy. Soc. Series B* **261,** 401–405.

Friston, K. J. (1997). Transients metastability and neuronal dynamics. *NeuroImage* **5,** 164–171.

Friston, K. J. (2000). The labile brain I: neuronal transients and nonlinear coupling. *Phil. Trans. R. Soc. London* **355,** 215–236.

Gray, C. M., and Singer, W. (1989). Stimulus specific neuronal oscillations in orientation columns of cat visual cortex *Proc. Natl. Acad. Sci USA* **86,** 1698–1702.

Haken, H. (1983). *Synergistics: An Introduction,* 3rd ed. Springer Verlag, Berlin.

Jirsa, V. K., Friedrich, R., and Haken, H. (1995). Reconstruction of the spatio-temporal dynamics of a human magnetoencephalogram. *Physica D* **89,** 100–122.

Kelso, J. A. S. (1995). *Dynamic Patterns: The Self-Organisation of Brain and Behaviour.* The MIT Press, Cambridge, MA.

Llinas, R., Ribary, U., Joliot, M., and Wang, X.-J. (1994). Content and context in temporal thalamocortical binding. In *Temporal Coding in the Brain,* Buzsaki, L. R., Singer, W., Berthoz, A., and Christen, T., Eds., pp. 251–272. Springer Verlag, Berlin.

Lumer, E. D., Edelman, G. M., and Tononi, G. (1997). Neural Dynamics in a model of the thalamocortical System II. The role of neural synchrony tested through perturbations of spike timing. *Cerebral Cortex* **7,** 228 –236.

Phillips, W. A., and Singer, W. (1997). In search of common foundations for cortical computation. *Behav. Brain Sci.* **20,** 57–83.

Riehle, A., Grun, S., Diesmann, M., and Aertsen, A. (1997). Spike synchronisation and rate modulation differentially involved in motor cortical function. *Science* **278,** 1950–1953.

Rockland, K. S., and Pandya, D. N. (1979). Laminar origins and terminations of cortical connections of the occipital lobe in the rhesus monkey. *Brain Res.* **179,** 3–20.

Schiff, S. J., So, P., Chang, T., Burke, R. E., and Sauer, T. (1996). Detecting dynamical interdependence and generalised synchrony through mutual prediction in a neuronal ensemble. *Phys. Rev. E* **54,** 6708–6724.

Selemon, L. D., and Goldman-Rakic, P. S. (1988). Common cortical and subcortical targets of the dorsolateral prefrontal and posterior parietal cortices in the rhesus monkey: evidence for a distributed neural network subserving spatially guided behaviour. *J. Neurosci.* **8,** 4049–4068.

Shadlen, M. N., and Newsome, W. T. (1995). Noise, neural codes and cortical organisation. *Curr. Opin. Neurobiol.* **4,** 569–579.

Singer, W. (1994). Time as coding space in neocortical processing: a hypothesis. In *Temporal Coding in the Brain,* Buzsaki, L. R., Singer, W., Berthoz, A., and Christen, T., Eds., pp. 51–80. Springer Verlag, Berlin.

Sporns, O., Gally, J. A., Reeke, G. N., and Edelman, G. M. (1989). Reentrant signaling among simulated neuronal groups leads to coherence in their oscillatory activity *Proc. Natl. Acad. Sci USA* **86,** 7265–7269.

Tovee, M. J., Rolls, E. T., Treves, A., and Bellis, R. P. (1993). Information encoding and the response of single neurons in the primate temporal visual cortex. *J. Neurophysiol.* **70,** 640–654.

Treue, S., and Maunsell, H. R. (1996). Attentional modulation of visual motion processing in cortical areas MT and MST. *Nature* **382,** 539–541.

Vaadia, E., Haalman, I., Abeles, M., Bergman, H., Prut, Y., Slovin, H., and Aertsen, A. (1995). Dynamics of neuronal interactions in monkey cortex in relation to behavioural events. *Nature* **373,** 515–518.

von der Malsburg, C. (1985). Nervous structures with dynamical links. *Ber Bunsenges. Phys. Chem.* **89,** 703–710.

Wray, J., and Green, G. G. R. (1994). Calculation of the Volterra kernels of non-linear dynamic systems using an artificial neuronal network. *Biol. Cybern.* **71,** 187–195.

CHAPTER

52

Dynamic Causal Modelling

INTRODUCTION

In this chapter we apply the system identification techniques described in Chapter 47 to the bilinear state-space models of effective connectivity introduced in Chapter 50. By using a bilinear approximation to the dynamics of any system, the parameters of the implicit causal model reduce to three sets. These comprise parameters that (1) mediate the influence of extrinsic inputs on the states, (2) mediate intrinsic coupling among the states, and (3) allow the inputs to modulate that coupling (bilinear parameters).

We describe this approach for the analysis of effective connectivity using experimentally designed inputs and fMRI responses. In this context, the coupling parameters correspond to effective connectivity and the bilinear parameters reflect the changes in connectivity induced by inputs. The ensuing framework allows one to characterise fMRI experiments, conceptually, as an experimental manipulation of integration among brain regions (by contextual or trial-free inputs, such as time or attentional set) that is revealed using evoked responses (to perturbations or trial-bound inputs like stimuli).

As with previous analyses of effective connectivity, the focus is on experimentally induced changes in coupling (cf. psychophysiologic interactions). However, unlike previous approaches in neuroimaging, the causal model ascribes responses to designed deterministic inputs, as opposed to treating inputs as unknown and stochastic.

Background

This chapter is about modelling interactions among neuronal populations, at a cortical level, using neuroimaging (hemodynamic or electromagnetic) time series. It presents the motivation and procedures for dynamic causal modelling of evoked brain responses. The aim of this modelling is to estimate, and make inferences about, the coupling among brain areas and how that coupling is influenced by changes in experimental context (e.g., time or cognitive set). Dynamic causal modelling represents a fundamental departure from existing approaches to effective connectivity because it employs a more plausible generative model of measured brain responses that embraces their nonlinear and dynamic nature.

The basic idea is to construct a reasonably realistic neuronal model of interacting cortical regions or nodes. This model is then supplemented with a forward model of how neuronal or synaptic activity is transformed into a measured response. This enables the parameters of the neuronal model (i.e., effective connectivity) to be estimated from observed data. These supplementary models may be forward models of electromagnetic measurements or hemodynamic models of fMRI measurements. In this chapter we focus on fMRI. Responses are evoked by known deterministic inputs that embody designed changes in stimulation or context. This is accomplished by using a dynamic input–state–output model with multiple inputs and outputs. The inputs correspond to conventional stimulus functions that encode experimental manipulations. The state variables cover both the neuronal activities and other neurophysiological or biophysical variables needed to form the outputs. The outputs are measured electromagnetic or hemodynamic responses over the brain regions considered.

Intuitively, this scheme regards an experiment as a designed perturbation of neuronal dynamics that are promulgated and distributed throughout a system of coupled anatomical nodes to change region-specific neuronal activity. These changes engender, through a measurement-specific forward model, responses that are used to identify the architecture and time constants of the system at the neuronal level. This represents a departure from conventional approaches (e.g., structural equation modelling and autoregression models; McIntosh and Gonzalez-Lima, 1994; Büchel and Friston, 1997; Harrison *et al.,* 2003), in which one assumes the observed responses are driven by endogenous or intrinsic noise (i.e., innovations). In contradistinction, dynamic causal models assume that the responses are driven by designed changes in inputs. An important conceptual aspect of dynamic causal models, for neuroimaging, pertains to how the experimental inputs enter the model and cause neuronal responses. We have established in previous chapters that experimental variables can illicit responses in one of two ways. First, they can elicit responses through direct influences on specific anatomical nodes. This would be appropriate, for example, in modelling sensory-evoked responses in early visual cortices. The second class of input exerts its effect vicariously, through a modulation of the coupling among nodes. These sorts of experimental variables would normally be more enduring, for example, attention to a particular attribute or the maintenance of some perceptual set. These distinctions are seen most clearly in relation to existing analyses and experimental designs.

DCM and Existing Approaches

The central idea behind dynamic causal modelling (DCM) is to treat the brain as a deterministic nonlinear dynamic system that is subject to inputs and produces outputs. Effective connectivity is parameterised in terms of coupling among unobserved brain states (e.g., neuronal activity in different regions). The objective is to estimate these parameters by perturbing the system and measuring the response. This is in contradistinction to established methods for estimating effective connectivity from neurophysiological time series, which include structural equation modelling and models based on multivariate autoregressive processes. In these models, there is no designed perturbation and the inputs are treated as unknown and stochastic. Multivariate autoregression models and their spectral equivalents, like coherence analysis, not only assume the system is driven by stochastic innovations, but are restricted to linear interactions. Structural equation modelling assumes the interactions are linear and, furthermore, instantaneous in the sense that structural equation models are not time-series models. In short, dynamic causal modelling is distinguished from alternative approaches not just by accommodating the nonlinear and dynamic aspects of neuronal interactions, but by framing the estimation problem in terms of perturbations that accommodate experimentally designed inputs. This is a critical departure from conventional approaches to causal modelling in neuroimaging and, importantly, brings the analysis of effective connectivity much closer to the analysis of region-specific effects. Dynamic causal modelling calls on the same experimental design principles to elicit region-specific interactions that we use in conventional experiments to elicit region-specific activations. In fact, as shown later, the convolution model, used in the standard analysis of fMRI time series, is a special and simple case of DCM that ensues when the coupling among regions is discounted. In DCM the causal or explanatory variables that comprise the conventional design matrix become the inputs and the parameters become measures of effective connectivity. Although DCM can be framed as a generalisation of the linear models used in conventional analyses to cover bilinear models (see below), it also represents an attempt to embed more plausible forward models of how neuronal dynamics respond to inputs and produce measured responses. This reflects the growing appreciation of the role that neuronal models may have to play in understanding measured brain responses (see Horwitz *et al.,* 2001, for a discussion).

This chapter can be regarded as an extension of previous work on the Bayesian identification of hemodynamic models (Friston, 2002) to cover multiple regions. In Chapter 47 we focussed on the biophysical parameters of a hemodynamic response in a single region. The most important parameter was the efficacy with which experimental inputs could elicit an activity-dependent vasodilatory signal. In this chapter neuronal activity is modelled explicitly, allowing for interactions among the activities of multiple regions in generating the observed hemodynamic response. The estimation procedure employed for DCM is formally identical to that described in Chapter 47.

DCM and Experimental Design

DCM is used to test the specific hypothesis that motivated the experimental design. It is not an exploratory technique; as with all analyses of effective connectivity, the results are specific to the tasks and stimuli employed during the experiment. In DCM, designed inputs can produce responses in one of two ways. Inputs can elicit changes in the state variables (i.e., neuronal activity) directly. For example, sensory input could be modelled as causing direct responses in primary visual or auditory areas. The second way in which inputs affect the system is through changing the effective connectivity or interactions. Useful examples of this sort of effect would be the attentional modulation of connections between parietal and extrastriate areas. Another ubiquitous example of this second sort of contextual input would be time. Time-dependent changes in connectivity correspond to plasticity. It is useful to regard experimental factors as inputs that belong to the class that produces evoked responses or to the class of contextual factors that induces changes in coupling (although, in principle, all inputs could do both). The first class comprises trial- or stimulus-bound perturbations, whereas the second establishes a context in which effects of the first sort evoke responses. This second class is typically trial free and induced by task instructions or other contextual changes. Measured responses in high-order cortical areas are mediated by interactions among brain areas elicited by trial-bound perturbations. These interactions can be modulated by other set-related or contextual factors that modulate the latent or intrinsic coupling among areas. Figure 52.1 illustrates this schematically. The important implication here, for experimental design in DCM, is that it should be multifactorial, with at least one factor controlling sensory perturbation and another factor manipulating the context in which the sensory-evoked responses are promulgated throughout the system (cf. psychophysiological interaction studies of Friston *et al.,* 1997).

In this chapter we use bilinear approximations to any DCM. The bilinear approximation reduces the parameters to three sets that control three distinct things. First, the direct or extrinsic influence of inputs on brain states in any particular area. Second; the intrinsic or latent connections that couple responses in one area to the state of others and, finally, change in this intrinsic coupling induced by inputs. Although, in some instances, the relative strengths of intrinsic connections may be of interest, most analyses of DCMs focus on the changes in connectivity embodied in the bilinear parameters. The first set of parameters is generally of little interest in the context of DCM but is the primary focus in classical analyses of regionally specific effects. In classical analyses, the only way experimental effects can be expressed is though a direct or extrinsic influence on each voxel because mass-univariate models (e.g., SPM) preclude connections and their modulation.

DCM is used primarily to answer questions about the modulation of effective connectivity through inferences about the bilinear parameters described above. They are bilinear in the sense that an input-dependent change in connectivity can be construed as a second-order interaction between the input and activity in a source region, when causing a response in a target region. The key role of bilinear terms reflects the fact that the more interesting applications of effective connectivity address changes in connectivity induced by cognitive set or time. In short, DCM with a bilinear approximation allows one to claim that an experimental manipulation has "activated a pathway" as opposed to a cortical region. Bilinear terms correspond to psychophysiological interaction terms in classical regression analyses of effective connectivity (Friston *et al.,* 1997) and those formed by moderator variables (Kenny and Judd, 1984) in structural equation modelling (Büchel and Friston, 1997). This bilinear aspect speaks again to the

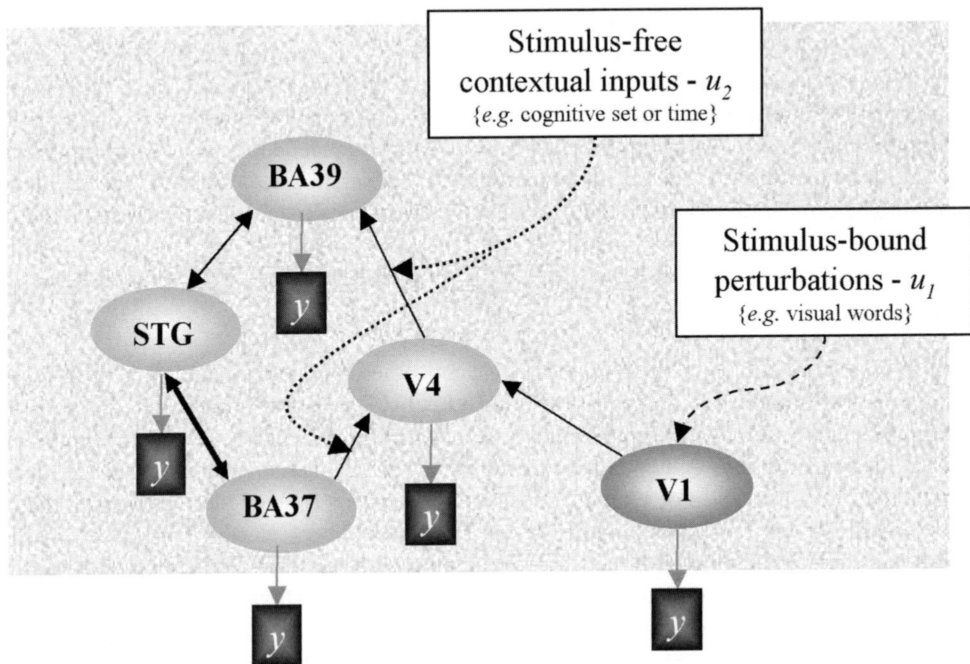

FIGURE 52.1
Schematic illustrating the concepts underlying dynamic causal modelling. In particular, this figure highlights the two distinct ways in which inputs or perturbations can illicit responses in the regions or nodes that comprise the model. In this example there are five nodes, including visual areas V1 and V4 in the fusiform gyrus and areas 39 and 37 and the superior temporal gyrus STG. Stimulus-bound perturbations designated u_1 act as extrinsic inputs to the primary visual area V1. Stimulus-free or contextual inputs u_2 mediate their effects by modulating the coupling between V4 and BA39 and between BA37 and V4. For example, the responses in the angular gyrus (BA39) are caused by inputs to V1 that are transformed by V4, where the influences exerted by V4 are sensitive to the second input. The dark square boxes represent the components of the DCM that transform the state variables z_i in each region (neuronal activity) into a measured (hemodynamic) response y_i.

importance of multifactorial designs that allow these interactions to be measured and the central role of the context in which region-specific responses are formed (see McIntosh, 2000).

DCM and Inference

Because DCMs are not restricted to linear or instantaneous systems, they are necessarily complicated and, potentially, need a large number of free parameters. This is why they have greater biological plausibility in relation to alternative approaches. However, this makes the estimation of the parameters more dependent on constraints. A natural way to embody the requisite constraints is within a Bayesian framework. Consequently, dynamic causal models are estimated using Bayesian or conditional estimators and inferences about particular connections are made using the posterior or conditional density. In other words, the estimation procedure provides the probability distribution of a coupling parameter in terms of its mean and standard deviation. Having established this posterior density, the probability that the connection exceeds some specified threshold is easily computed. Bayesian inferences like this are more straightforward and interpretable than corresponding classical inferences and, furthermore, they eschew the multiple comparison problem. The posterior density is computed using the likelihood and prior densities. The likelihood of the data, given some parameters, is specified by the DCM. (In one sense all models are simply ways of specifying the likelihood of an observation.) The prior densities on the connectivity parameters offer suitable constraints to ensure robust and efficient estimation. These priors harness some natural constraints about the dynamics of coupled systems (see below), but also allow the user to specify which connections are likely to be present and which are not. An important use of prior constraints of this sort is seen in the restriction of where inputs can elicit extrinsic responses. It is interesting to reflect that conventional analyses suppose that all inputs have unconstrained access to all brain regions. This is because classical models assume activations are caused directly by experimental factors, as opposed to being mediated by afferents from other brain areas.

Additional constraints, on the intrinsic connections and their modulation by contextual inputs, can also be specified but they are not necessary. These additional constraints can be used to finesse a model by making it more parsimonious, allowing one to focus on a particular connection. We provide examples of this below. Unlike structural equation modelling, there are no limits on the number of connections that can be modelled because the assumptions and estimations scheme used by dynamic causal modelling are completely different, relying on known inputs.

Overview

This chapter comprises a theoretical section and three sections demonstrating the use and validity of DCM. In the theoretical section, we present the conceptual and mathematical fundaments that are used in the remaining sections. The later sections address the face, predictive, and construct validity of DCM, respectively. Face validity entails determining that the estimation and inference procedure identifies what it is supposed to. The subsequent section on predictive validity uses empirical data from an fMRI study of single word processing at different rates. These data were obtained consecutively in a series of contiguous sessions. This allowed us to repeat the DCM using independent realisations of the same paradigm. Predictive validity, over the multiple sessions, was assessed in terms of the consistency of the effective connectivity estimates and their posterior densities. The final section on construct validity revisits changes in connection strengths among parietal and extrastriate areas induced by attention to optic flow stimuli. We have established previously attentionally mediated increases in effective connectivity using both structural equation modelling and a Volterra formulation of effective connectivity (Büchel and Friston, 1997; Friston and Büchel, 2000). Our aim here is to show that dynamic causal modelling led us to the same conclusions. This chapter ends with a brief discussion of dynamic causal modelling and its limitations and potential applications.

THEORY

In this section we present the theoretical motivation and operational details on which DCM rests. In brief, DCM is a fairly standard nonlinear system identification procedure using Bayesian estimation of the parameters of deterministic input–state–output dynamic systems. In this chapter the system can be construed as a number of interacting brain regions. We focus here on a particular form for the dynamics that corresponds to a bilinear approximation to any analytic system. However, the idea behind DCM is not restricted to bilinear forms.

This section is divided into three parts. First, we describe the DCM itself, then consider the nature of priors on the parameters of the DCM, and finally summarise the inference procedure using the posterior distribution of these parameters. The estimation conforms to the posterior density analysis under Gaussian assumptions described in Chapter 47. In this previous chapter we were concerned primarily with estimating the efficacy with which input elicits a vasodilatory signal, presumably mediated by neuronal responses to the input. The causal models in this chapter can be regarded as a collection of hemodynamic models, one for each area, in which the experimental inputs are supplemented with neural activity from other areas. The parameters of interest now embrace not only the direct efficacy of experimental inputs but also the efficacy of neuronal input from distal regions, i.e., effective connectivity (see Fig. 52.1).

The posterior density analysis finds the maximum or mode of the posterior density of the parameters (i.e., the most likely coupling parameters given the data) by performing a gradient assent on the log posterior. The log posterior requires both likelihood and prior terms. The likelihood obtains from Gaussian assumptions about the errors in the observation model implied by the DCM. This likelihood or forward model is described in the next subsection. By combining the ensuing likelihood with priors on the coupling and hemodynamic parameters, described in the second subsection, one can form an expression for the posterior density that is used in the estimation.

Dynamic Causal Models

The dynamic causal model is a multiple-input/multiple-output (MIMO) system that comprises m inputs and l outputs with one output per region. The m inputs correspond to designed causes (e.g., boxcar or stick stimulus functions). The inputs are exactly the same as those used to form design matrices in conventional analyses of fMRI and can be expanded in the usual way when necessary (e.g., using polynomials or temporal basis functions). In principle, each input could have direct access to every region. However, in practice, the extrinsic effects of inputs are usually restricted to a single input region. Each of the l regions produces a measured output that corresponds to the observed BOLD signal. These l time series would normally be taken as the average or first eigenvariate of key regions, selected on the basis of a conventional analysis. Each region has five state variables. Four of these are of secondary importance and correspond to the state variables of the hemodynamic model first presented in Friston *et al.* (2000) and described in previous chapters. These hemodynamic states comprise a vasodilatory signal, normalised flow, normalised venous volume, and normalised deoxyhemoglobin content. These variables are required to compute the observed BOLD response and are not influenced by the states of other regions.

Central to the estimation of effective connectivity or coupling parameters are the first state variables of each region. These correspond to average neuronal or synaptic activity and are a function of the neuronal states of other brain regions. We deal first with the equations for the neuronal states and then briefly reprise the differential equations that constitute the hemodynamic model for each region.

Neuronal State Equations

Restricting ourselves to the neuronal states $z = [z_1,\ldots,z_l]^T$, one can posit any arbitrary form or model for effective connectivity:

$$\dot{z} = F(z,u,\theta) \tag{52.1}$$

where F is some nonlinear function describing the neurophysiological influences that activity in all l brain regions z and inputs u exert on changes in the others. The θ are the parameters of the model whose posterior density we require for inference. It is not necessary to specify the form of Eq. (52.1) because its bilinear approximation provides a natural and useful reparameterisation in terms of effective connectivity. The bilinear form of Eq. (52.1) is

$$\begin{aligned}
\dot{z} &\approx Az + \textstyle\sum u_j B^j z + Cu \\
&= (A + \textstyle\sum u_j B^j)z + Cu \\
A &= \frac{\partial F}{\partial z} = \frac{\partial \dot{z}}{\partial z} \\
B_j &= \frac{\partial^2 F}{\partial z \partial u_j} = \frac{\partial}{\partial u_j}\frac{\partial \dot{z}}{\partial z} \\
C &= \frac{\partial F}{\partial u}
\end{aligned} \tag{52.2}$$

The Jacobian or connectivity matrix A represents the first-order connectivity among the regions in the absence of input. Effective connectivity is the influence that one neuronal system exerts over another in terms of inducing a response $\partial\dot{z}/\partial z$. In DCM a response is defined in terms of a change in activity with time $\dot{z}$. This latent connectivity can be thought of as the intrinsic coupling in the absence of experimental perturbations. Notice that the state, which is perturbed, depends on the experimental design (e.g., baseline or control state) and therefore the intrinsic coupling is specific to each experiment. The matrices B^j are effectively the change in intrinsic coupling induced by the jth input. They encode the input-sensitive changes in $\partial\dot{z}/\partial z$ or, equivalently, the modulation of effective connectivity by experimental manipulations. Because B^j are second-order derivatives, these terms are referred to as *bilinear*. Finally, the matrix C embodies the extrinsic influences of inputs on neuronal activity. The parameters $\theta^c = \{A,B^j,C\}$ are the connectivity or coupling matrices that we wish to identify and define the functional architecture and interactions among brain regions at a neuronal level. Figure 52.2 shows an

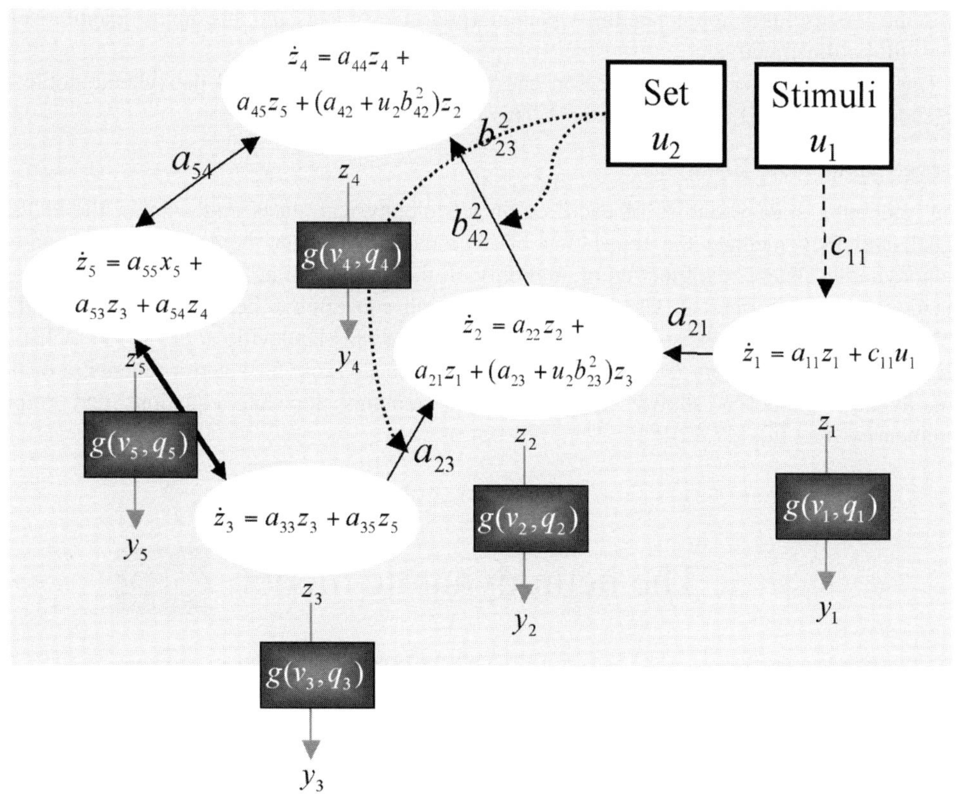

latent connectivity induced connectivity

$$\begin{bmatrix}\dot z_1\\ \vdots \\ \dot z_5\end{bmatrix} = \left\{ \begin{bmatrix} a_{11} & & \cdots & & 0 \\ a_{21} & a_{22} & a_{23} & & \\ \vdots & & a_{33} & & a_{35} \\ & a_{42} & & a_{44} & a_{45} \\ 0 & \cdots & a_{53} & a_{54} & a_{55}\end{bmatrix} + u_2 \begin{bmatrix} 0 & & \cdots & & 0\\ & & b^2_{23} & & \\ \vdots & & \ddots & & \vdots \\ & b^2_{42} & & & \\ 0 & & \cdots & & 0\end{bmatrix}\right\} \begin{bmatrix} z_1 \\ \vdots \\ z_5\end{bmatrix} + \begin{bmatrix} c_{11} & 0 \\ \vdots & \vdots \\ 0 & 0\end{bmatrix}\begin{bmatrix}u_1\\u_2\end{bmatrix}$$

Forward, backward & self

$$\dot{z} = (A + \sum_j u_j B^j)z + Cu$$

The bilinear model

FIGURE 52.2
This schematic (upper panel) recapitulates the architecture in Fig. 52.1 in terms of the differential equations implied by a bilinear approximation. The equations in each of the white areas describe the change in neuronal activity z_i in terms of linearly separable components that reflect the influence of other regional state variables. Note particularly, how the second contextual inputs enter these equations. They effectively increase the intrinsic coupling parameters (a_{ij}) in proportion to the bilinear coupling parameters (b^k_{ij}). In this diagram the hemodynamic component of the DCM illustrates how the neuronal states enter a region-specific hemodynamic model to produce the outputs y_i, which are a function of the region's biophysical states reflecting deoxyhemoglobin content and venous volume (q_i and v_i). The lower panel reformulates the differential equations in the upper panel into a matrix format. These equations can be summarised more compactly in terms of coupling parameter matrices A, B^j, and C. This form of expression is used in the main text and shows how it relates to the underlying differential equations that describe the state dynamics.

example of a specific architecture to demonstrate the relationship between the matrix form of the bilinear model and the underlying state equations for each region. Notice that the units of connections are per unit time and therefore correspond to rates. Because we are in a dynamic setting, a strong connection means an influence that is expressed quickly or with a small time constant. It is useful to appreciate this when interpreting estimates and thresholds quantitatively. This will be illustrated later.

The neuronal activity in each region causes changes in volume and deoxyhemoglobin to engender the observed BOLD response y. This is described next.

Hemodynamic State Equations

The remaining state variables of each region are biophysical states engendering the BOLD signal, and they mediate the translation of neuronal activity into hemodynamic responses. Hemodynamic states are a function of, and only of, the neuronal state of each region. The state equations were described in Chapters 41 and 47 and constitute a hemodynamic model that embeds the balloon-Windkessel model (Buxton *et al.*, 1998; Mandeville *et al.*, 1999). A list of the biophysical parameters $\theta^h = \{\kappa,\gamma,\tau,\alpha,\rho\}$ is provided in Table 52.1 and a schematic of the hemodynamic model is shown in Fig. 52.3 that contains the state equations and output nonlinearity [i.e., Eq. (47.42)].

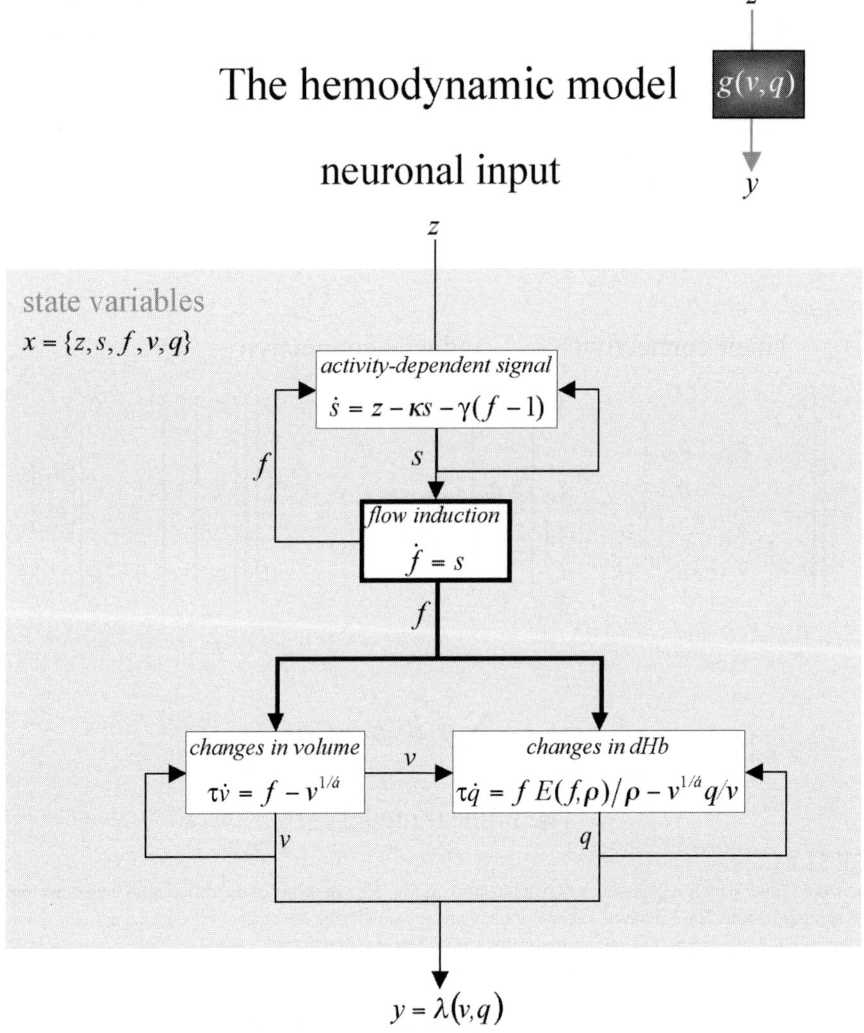

FIGURE 52.3
This schematic shows the architecture of the hemodynamic model for a single region (regional subscripts have been dropped for clarity). Neuronal activity induces a vasodilatory and activity-dependent signal s that increases the flow f. Flow causes changes in volume and deoxyhemoglobin (v and q). These two hemodynamic states enter the output nonlinearity [Eq. (52.3)] to give the observed BOLD response y. This transformation from neuronal states z_i to hemodynamic response y_i is encoded graphically by the dark grey boxes in the previous figure and in the insert at the top of this figure.

The Model

Combining the neuronal states $x = \{z,s,f,v,q\}$ with the hemodynamic states gives us a full forward model specified by the neuronal state Eq. (52.2) and the hemodynamic equations in Fig. 52.3:

$$\begin{aligned} \dot{x} &= f(x,u,\theta) \\ y(t) &= \lambda(x) \end{aligned} \tag{52.3}$$

with parameters $\theta = \{\theta^c, \theta^h\}$. For any set of parameters and inputs, the state equation can be integrated and passed through the output nonlinearity to give the predicted response $h(u,\theta)$. This integration can be made quite expedient by capitalising on the sparsity of stimulus functions commonly employed in fMRI designs (see Chapter 47). Integrating Eq. (52.3) is equivalent to a generalised convolution of the inputs with the system's Volterra kernels. These kernels are easily derived from the Volterra expansion of Eq. (52.3) (Bendat,, 1990):

$$\begin{aligned} h(u,\theta) &= \sum_k \int_0^t \ldots \int_0^t \kappa_i^k(\sigma_1 \ldots \sigma_k) u(t-\sigma_1) \ldots u(t-\sigma_k) d\sigma_1 \ldots d\sigma_k \\ \kappa_i^k(\sigma_1 \ldots \sigma_k) &= \frac{\partial^k y_i(t)}{\partial u(t-\sigma_1) \ldots \partial u(t-\sigma_k)} \end{aligned} \tag{52.4}$$

either by numerical differentiation or analytically through bilinear approximations (see Friston, 2002). The term κ_i^k represents the kth-order kernel for region i. For simplicity, Eq. (52.4) has been written for a single input. The kernels are simply a reparameterisation of the model. We use these kernels to characterise regional impulse responses at neuronal and hemodynamic levels later.

The forward model can be made into an observation model by adding error and confounding or nuisance effects $X(t)$ to give $y = h(u,\theta) + X\beta + \varepsilon$. Here β are the unknown coefficients of the confounds. In the examples used below, $X(t)$ comprised a low-order discrete cosine set, modelling low-frequency drifts and a constant term. Following the approach described in Chapter 47, we note

$$\begin{aligned} y - h(u,\eta_{\theta|y}) &\approx J\Delta\theta + X\beta + \varepsilon \\ &= [J, X] \begin{bmatrix} \Delta\theta \\ \beta \end{bmatrix} + \varepsilon \\ \Delta\theta &= \theta - \eta_{\theta|y} \end{aligned} \tag{52.5}$$

This local linear approximation then enters an EM scheme as described in previous chapters:

Until convergence {

E-step

$$\begin{aligned} J &= \frac{\partial h(\eta_{\theta|y})}{\partial \theta} \\ \bar{y} &= \begin{bmatrix} y - h(\eta_{\theta|y}) \\ \eta_\theta - \eta_{\theta|y} \end{bmatrix}, \quad \bar{J} = \begin{bmatrix} J & X \\ 1 & 0 \end{bmatrix}, \quad \bar{C}_\varepsilon = \begin{bmatrix} \Sigma\lambda_i Q_i & 0 \\ 0 & C_\theta \end{bmatrix} \\ C_{\theta|y} &= (\bar{J}^T \bar{C}_\varepsilon^{-1} \bar{J})^{-1} \\ \begin{bmatrix} \Delta\eta_{\theta|y} \\ \eta_{\beta|y} \end{bmatrix} &= C_{\theta|y}(\bar{J}^T \bar{C}_\varepsilon^{-1} \bar{y}) \\ \eta_{\theta|y} &\leftarrow \eta_{\theta|y} + \Delta\eta_{\theta|y} \end{aligned} \tag{52.6}$$

M-Step

$$\begin{aligned} P &= \bar{C}_\varepsilon^{-1} - \bar{C}_\varepsilon^{-1} \bar{J} C_{\theta|y} \bar{J}^T \bar{C}_\varepsilon^{-1} \\ \frac{\partial F}{\partial \lambda_i} &= -\tfrac{1}{2}\mathrm{tr}\{PQ_i\} + \tfrac{1}{2}\bar{y}^T P^T Q_i P \bar{y} \\ \left\langle \frac{\partial^2 F}{\partial \lambda_{ij}^2} \right\rangle &= -\tfrac{1}{2}\mathrm{tr}\{PQ_i PQ_j\} \\ \lambda &\leftarrow \lambda - \left\langle \frac{\partial^2 F}{\partial \lambda^2} \right\rangle^{-1} \frac{\partial F}{\partial \lambda} \quad \} \end{aligned}$$

These expressions are formally the same as Eqs. (47.47) and (47.48) in Chapter 47, but for the addition of confounding effects in X. These confounds are treated as fixed effects with infinite prior variance, which does not need to appear explicitly in Eq. (52.6).

Note that the prediction and observations encompass the entire experiment. They are therefore large $ln \times 1$ vectors whose elements run over regions and n time points. Although the response variable could be viewed as a multivariate times series, it is treated as a single observation vector, whose error covariance embodies both temporal and interregional correlations: $C_\varepsilon = V \otimes \Sigma(\lambda) = \Sigma\lambda_i Q_i$. This covariance is parameterised by some covariance hyperparameters λ. In the examples below these correspond to region-specific error variances assuming the same temporal correlations $Q_i = V \otimes \Sigma_i$ in which Σ_i is a $l \times l$ sparse matrix with the ith leading diagonal element equal to 1.

Equation (52.6) enables us the estimate the conditional moments of the coupling parameters (and the hemodynamics parameters) plus the hyperparameters controlling observation error. However, to proceed we need to specify the priors.

Priors

In this context we use a fully Bayesian approach because (1) there are clear and necessary constraints on neuronal dynamics that can be used to motivate priors on the coupling parameters and (2) empirically determined priors on the biophysical hemodynamic parameters are relatively easy to specify. We deal first with priors on the coupling parameters.

Priors on the Coupling Parameters

It is self-evident that neuronal activity cannot diverge exponentially to infinite values. Therefore, we know that, in the absence of input, the dynamics must return to a stable mode. This means that the largest real component of the eigenvalues of the intrinsic coupling matrix cannot exceed zero. We use this constraint to establish a prior density on the coupling parameters A, which ensures that the system is dissipative.

If the largest real eigenvalue (Lyapunov exponent) is less than zero, the stable mode is a point attractor. If the largest Lyapunov exponent is zero, the system will converge to a periodic attractor with oscillatory dynamics. Therefore, it is sufficient to establish a probabilistic upper bound on the interregional coupling strengths, imposed by Gaussian priors that ensure the largest Lyapunov exponent is unlikely to exceed zero. If the prior densities of each connection are independent, then the prior density can be specified in terms of a variance for the off-diagonal elements of A. This variance can then be chosen to render the probability of the principal exponent exceeding zero, less than some suitably small value.

The specification of priors on the connections can be finessed by a reparameterisation of the coupling matrices A and B^j:

$$A \to \sigma A = \sigma \begin{bmatrix} -1 & a_{12} & \cdots \\ a_{21} & -1 & \\ \vdots & & \ddots \end{bmatrix} \qquad (52.7)$$

$$B^j \to \sigma B^j = \sigma \begin{bmatrix} b^j_{11} & b^j_{12} & \cdots \\ b^j_{21} & \ddots & \\ \vdots & & \end{bmatrix}$$

This factorisation into a scalar and normalised coupling matrix renders the normalised couplings adimensional, such that strengths of connections among regions are relative to their self-connections. From this point on, we deal with normalised parameters. This particular factorisation enforces the same self-connection or temporal scaling σ in all regions. This is sensible given that neuronal transients are likely to decay at a similar rate in different regions (different factorisations could be employed in a different context).

Consider any set of $l(l-1)$ interregional connections with sum of squared values $\xi = \Sigma a_{ij}^2$. For any given value of ξ the largest Lyapunov exponent λ_a is obtained when the connection strengths are equal $a_{ij} = a$, for all $i \neq j$ in which case

$$\begin{aligned} \lambda_a &= (l-1)a - 1 \\ \xi &= l(l-1)a^2 \end{aligned} \qquad (52.8)$$

This means that as the sum of squared connection strengths reaches $\xi = l/(l-1)$, the maximum exponent attainable approaches zero. Consequently, if ξ is constrained to be less than this threshold, we can set an upper bound on the probability that the principal exponent exceeds zero. The term ξ is constrained through the priors on a_{ij}. If each connection has a prior Gaussian density with zero expectation and variance C_a, then the sum of squares has a scaled chi-squared distribution $\xi/C_a \sim \chi^2_{l(l-1)}$ with degrees of freedom $l(l-1)$, and C_a is chosen to make $p(\xi > l/(l-1))$suitably small, i.e.:

$$C_a = \frac{l/(l-1)}{\phi_\chi^{-1}(1-p)} \tag{52.9}$$

where ϕ_χ is the cumulative $\chi^2_{l(l-1)}$ distribution and p is the required probability. As the number of regions increases, the prior variance on connections decreases.

In addition to constraints on the normalised connections, the factorisation in Eq. (52.7) requires the temporal scaling parameter σ to be greater than zero. This is simply achieved through a noncentral prior density specified in terms of its moments such that $\sigma \sim N(\eta_\sigma, C_\sigma)$ where the expectation η_σ controls the characteristic time constant of the system and the variance C_σ is chosen to ensure $p(\sigma > 0)$ is small, i.e.:

$$C_a = \left(\frac{\eta_\sigma}{\phi_N^{-1}(1-p)}\right)^2 \tag{52.10}$$

where ϕ_N is the cumulative normal distribution and p the required probability.

In summary, priors on the connectivity parameters ensure that the system remains stable. The spectrum of eigenvalues of the intrinsic coupling matrix determines the time constants of orthogonal modes or patterns of regional activity. These are scaled by σ, whose prior expectation controls the characteristic time constants (i.e., those observed in the absence of coupling). We assume a value of 1 sec. The prior variance on this scaling parameter is chosen such that the probability that it is less than zero is suitably small (in our case 10^{-2}). The ensuing prior density can be expressed as a function of the implicit half-life $\tau_z(\sigma) = \ln 2/\sigma$ by noting $p(\tau_z) = p(\sigma)\partial\sigma/\partial\tau_z$ (see Fig. 52.4). This portrayal of the prior density shows that we expect regional transients with time constants in the range of a few hundred milliseconds to several seconds.

The prior distribution of individual connection strengths is assumed to be identically and independently distributed with a prior expectation of zero and a variance C_a that ensures the

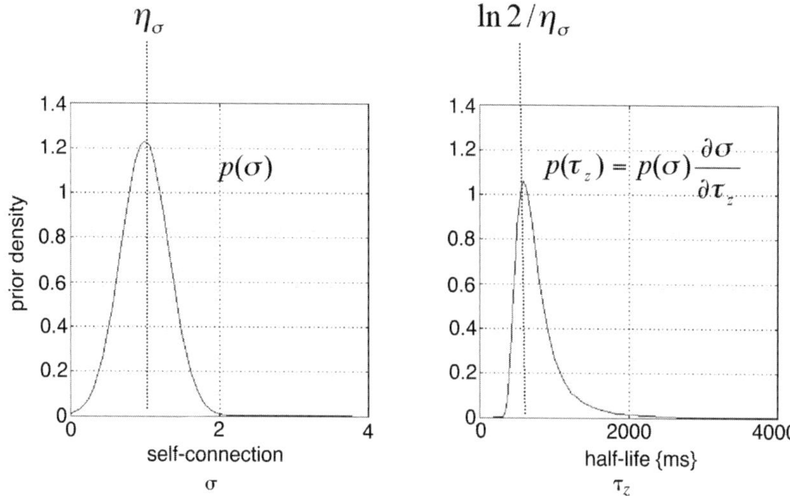

FIGURE 52.4
Prior probability density functions for the temporal scaling parameter or self-connection σ. This has a Gaussian form (left panel) that translates into a skewed distribution, when expressed in terms of the characteristic half-life of neural transients τ_z in any particular region (right panel). This prior distribution implies that neuronal activity will decay with a half-life of roughly 500 ms, falling in the range of 300 ms to 2 sec.

$$A = \begin{bmatrix} -1 & a_{12} & \frac{1}{2} \\ a_{21} & -1 & \frac{1}{2} \\ \frac{1}{2} & \frac{1}{2} & -1 \end{bmatrix}$$

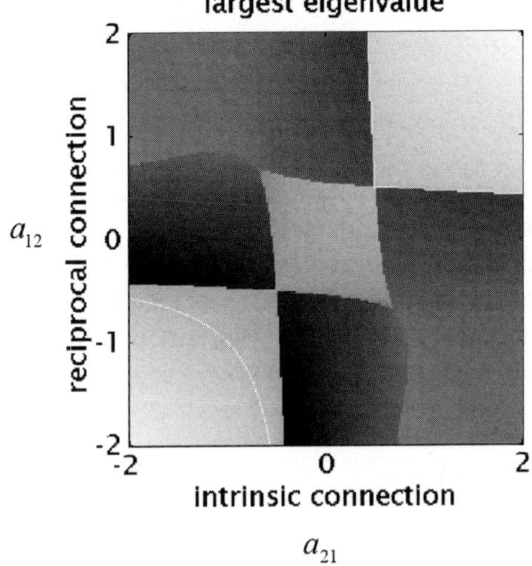

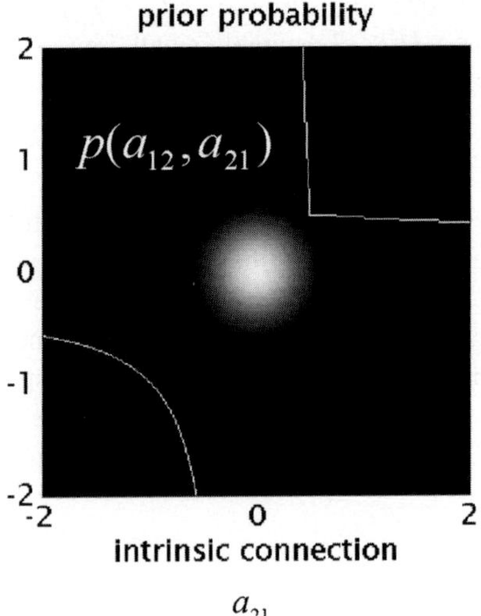

FIGURE 52.5
Prior probability density on the intrinsic coupling parameters for a specific intrinsic coupling matrix A. The left-hand panel shows the real value of the largest eigenvalue of A (the principal Lyapunov exponent) as a function of the connection from the first to the second region and the reciprocal connection from the second to the first. The remaining connections were held constant at 0.5. This density can be thought of as a slice through a multidimensional spherical distribution over all connections. The right panel shows the prior probability density function and the boundaries at which the largest real eigenvalue exceeds zero (dotted white lines). The variance or dispersion of this probability distribution is chosen to ensure that the probability of excursion into unstable domains of parameter space is suitably small. These domains are the upper right and lower left bounded regions.

principal exponent has a very small probability of being greater than zero (here 10^{-2}). This variance decreases with the number of connections or regions. To provide an intuition about how these priors keep the system from diverging exponentially, a quantitative example is shown in Fig. 52.5. Figure 52.5 shows the prior density of two connections that renders the probability of a positive exponent less than 10^{-2}. We can see that this density lies in a domain of parameter space encircled by regions in which the maximum Lyapunov exponent exceeds zero (bounded by dotted white lines). See the figure legend for more details.

Priors on the bilinear coupling parameters have the same form (zero mean and variance) as those for the intrinsic coupling parameters. For consistency, these parameters are also normalised by σ and are consequently adimensional. Conversely, priors on the influences of extrinsic input are not scaled and are relatively uninformative with zero expectation and unit variance. As noted in the introduction, additional constraints can be implemented by precluding certain connections. This is achieved by setting their variance to zero.

Hemodynamic Priors

The hemodynamic priors are based on those used in Friston (2002) and in Chapter 47. In brief, the mean and variance of posterior estimates of the five biophysical parameters were computed over 128 voxels using the single word presentation data presented in the next section. These means and variances (see Table 52.1) were used to specify Gaussian priors on the hemodynamic parameters.

Combining the prior densities on the coupling and hemodynamic parameters allows us to express the prior probability of the parameters in terms of their prior expectation η_θ and covariance C_θ:

TABLE 52.1 Priors on biophysical parameters

Parameter	Description	Prior mean η_θ	Prior variance C_θ
κ	Rate of signal decay	0.65 per sec	0.015
γ	Rate of flow-dependent elimination	0.41 per sec	0.002
τ	Hemodynamic transit time	0.98 sec	0.0568
α	Grubb's exponent	0.32	0.0015
ρ	Resting oxygen extraction fraction	0.34	0.0024

$$\theta = \begin{bmatrix} \sigma \\ a_{ij} \\ b_{ij} \\ c_{ik} \\ \theta^h \end{bmatrix}, \quad \eta_\theta = \begin{bmatrix} 1 \\ 0 \\ 0 \\ 0 \\ \eta_\theta^h \end{bmatrix}, \quad C_\theta = \begin{bmatrix} C_\sigma & & & & \\ & C_A & & & \\ & & C_B & & \\ & & & 1 & \\ & & & & C_h \end{bmatrix} \tag{52.11}$$

where the prior covariances C_A and C_B contain leading diagonal elements C_a for all connections that are allowed to vary. Having specified the priors, we are now in a position to form the posterior and proceed with estimation using Eq. (52.6).

Inference

As noted above, the estimation scheme is a posterior density analysis under Gaussian assumptions. In short, the estimation scheme provides the approximating Gaussian posterior density of the parameters $q(\theta)$ in terms of its expectation $\eta_{\theta|y}$ and covariance $C_{\theta|y}$. The expectation is also known as the posterior mode or *maximum a posteriori* (MAP) estimator. The marginal posterior probabilities are then used for inference that any particular parameter or contrast of parameters $c^T\eta_{\theta|y}$ (e.g., average) exceeded a specified threshold γ:

$$p = \phi_N\left(\frac{c^T\eta_{\theta|y} - \gamma}{\sqrt{c^T C \eta_{\theta|y} c}}\right) \tag{52.12}$$

As above ϕ_N is the cumulative normal distribution. In this chapter, we are primarily concerned with the coupling parameters θ^c and, among these, the bilinear terms. The units of these parameters are hertz or per second (or adimensional if normalised) and the thresholds are specified as such. In dynamic modelling, strength corresponds to a fast response with a small time constant.

Relationship to Conventional Analyses

It is interesting to note that conventional analyses of fMRI data using linear convolution models are a special case of dynamic causal models using a bilinear approximation. This is important because it provides a direct connection between DCM and classical models. If we allow inputs to be connected to all regions and discount interactions among regions by setting the prior variances on A and B to zero, we produce a set of disconnected brain regions or voxels that respond to, and only to, extrinsic input. The free parameters of interest reduce to the values of C, which reflects the ability of input to excite neural activity in each voxel. By further setting the prior variances on the self-connections (i.e., scaling parameter) and those on the hemodynamic parameters to zero, we end up with a single-input/single-output model at each and every brain region that can be reformulated as a convolution model as described in Friston (2002). For voxel i and input j the parameter can be estimated by simply convolving the input with $\partial\kappa_i^1/\partial c_{ij}$ where κ_i^1 is the first-order kernel meditating the influence of input j on output i. The convolved inputs are then used to form a general linear model that can be estimated using least squares in the usual way. This is precisely the approach adopted in classical analyses, in which $\partial\kappa_i^1/\partial c_{ij}$ is the hemodynamic response function. The key point here is that the general linear models used in typical data analyses are special cases of bilinear models that embody more assumptions. These assumptions enter through the use of highly precise priors that discount interactions among regions and prevent any variation in biophysical responses. Having described the theoretical aspects of DCM we now turn to applications and assessing DCM validity.

FACE VALIDITY: SIMULATIONS

In this section we use simulated data to establish the utility of the bilinear approximation and the robustness of the estimation scheme described in the previous section. We deliberately chose an architecture that would be impossible to characterise using existing methods based on regression models (e.g., structural equation modelling). This architecture embodies loops and reciprocal connections and poses the problem of vicarious input—the ambiguity between the direct influences of one area and influences that are mediated through others.

The Simulated System

The architecture is depicted in Fig. 52.6 and has been labelled so that it is consistent with the DCM characterised empirically in the next section. The model comprises three regions: a primary (A1) and secondary (A2) auditory area and a higher level region (A3). There are two inputs. The first is a sensory input encoding the presentation of epochs of words at different frequencies. The second input is contextual in nature and is simply an exponential function of the time elapsed since the start of each epoch (with a time constant of 8 sec). These inputs were based on a real experiment and are the same as those used in the empirical analyses of the next section. The scaling of the inputs is important for the quantitative evaluation of the bilinear and extrinsic coupling parameters. The convention adopted here is that inputs encoding events approximate delta functions such that their integral over time corresponds to the number of events that have occurred. For event-free inputs, like the maintenance of a particular instructional set, the input is scaled to a maximum of unity, so that the integral reflects the number of seconds over which the input was prevalent. The inputs were specified in time bins that were a sixteenth of the interval between scans (repetition time; TR = 1.7 sec).

The auditory input is connected to the primary area; the second input has no direct effect on activity but modulates the forward connections from A1 to A2 so that its influence shows adaptation during the epoch. The second auditory area receives input from the first and sends signals to the higher area (A3). In addition to reciprocal backward connection, in this simple auditory hierarchy, a connection from the lowest to the highest area has been included. Finally, the first input (word presentation) modulates the self-connections of the third region. This influence has been included to show how bilinear effects can emulate nonlinear responses. A bilinear modulation of the self-connection can augment or attenuate decay of synaptic activity rendering the average response to streams of stimuli rate dependent. This is because the bilinear effect will only be expressed if sufficient synaptic activity persists after the previous stimulus. This, in turn, depends on a sufficiently fast presentation rate. The resulting response emulates a saturation at high presentation rates or small stimulus onset asynchronies that have been observed empirically. Critically, we are in a position to disambiguate between neuronal saturation, modelled by this bilinear term, and hemodynamic saturation, modelled by nonlinearities in the hemodynamic component of this DCM. A significant bilinear self-connection implies neuronal saturation above and beyond that attributable to hemodynamics. Figure 52.7 illustrates this neuronal saturation by plotting the simulated response of A3 in the absence of saturation $B^1 = 0$ against the simulated response with $b^1_{3,3} = -0.4$. It is evident that a nonlinear subadditive effect exists at high response levels. Note that true neuronal saturation of this sort is mediated by second-order interactions among the states (i.e., neuronal activity). However, as shown in Fig. 52.7, we can emulate these effects by using the first extrinsic input as a surrogate for neuronal inputs from other areas in the bilinear component of the model.

Using this model we simulated responses using the values for A, B^1, B^2, and C given in Fig. 52.6 and the prior expectations for the biophysical parameters given in Table 52.1. The values of the coupling parameters were chosen to emulate those typically seen in practice. This ensured that the simulated responses were realistic in relation to simulated noise. After

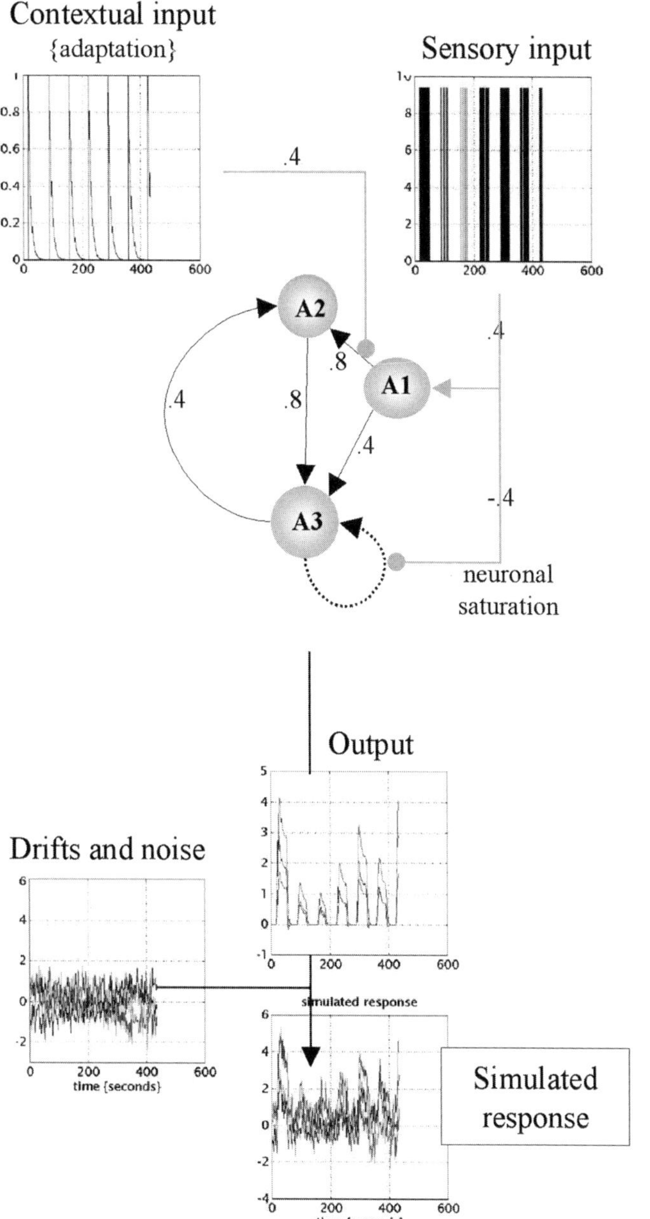

FIGURE 52.6
This is a schematic of the architecture used to generate simulated data. Nonzero intrinsic connections are shown as directed black arrows with the strength or true parameter alongside. Here, the perturbing input is the presentation of words (sensory inputs) and acts as an intrinsic influence on A1. In addition, this input modulates the self-connection of A3 to emulate saturation like-effects (see main text and Fig. 52.7). The contextual input is a decaying exponential of within-epoch time and positively modulates the forward connection from A1 to A2. The lower panel shows how responses were simulated by mixing the output of the system described above with drifts and noise as described in the main text.

downsampling these deterministic responses every 1.7 sec (the TR of the empirical data used in the next section), we added known noise to produce simulated data. These data comprised a time series of 256 observations with independent or serially correlated Gaussian noise based on an AR(1) process. Unless otherwise stated, the noise had 0.5 standard deviation and was i.i.d. (independently and identically distributed). The drift terms were formed from the first six components of a discrete cosine set mixed linearly with normal random coefficients, scaled by one over the order. This emulates a $1/f^2$ plus white noise spectrum for the noise and drifts. (See the lower panel of Fig. 52.6 for an exemplar data simulation with an i.i.d. noise of unit variance.)

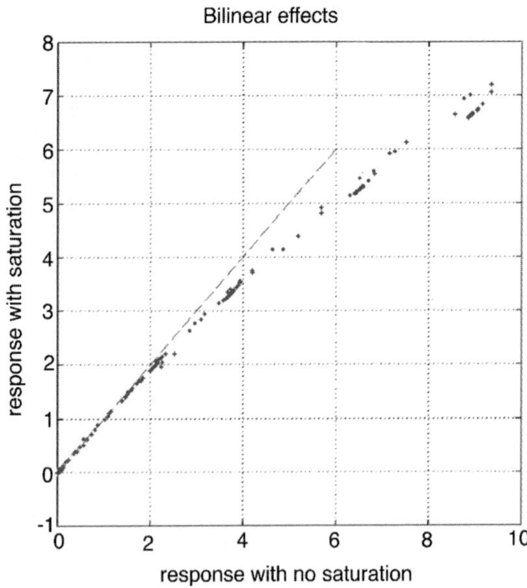

FIGURE 52.7
This is a plot of the simulated response with saturation against the equivalent response with no saturation. These simulated responses were obtained by setting the bilinear coupling parameter b^1_{33} labelled "neuronal saturation" in the previous figure to −0.4 and 0, respectively. The key thing to observe is a saturation of responses at high levels. The dashed line depicts the response expected in the absence of saturation. This illustrates how bilinear effects can introduce nonlinearities into the response.

Exemplar Analysis

The analysis described in the previous section was applied to the data shown in Fig. 52.6. The priors on coupling parameters were augmented by setting the variance of the off-diagonal elements of B^1 (saturation) and all but two connections in B^2 (adaptation) to zero. These two connections were the first and second forward connections of this cortical hierarchy. The first had simulated adaptation, whereas the second did not. Extrinsic input was restricted to the primary area A1 by setting the variances of all but c_{11} to zero. We placed no further constraints on the intrinsic coupling parameters. This is equivalent to allowing full connectivity. This would be impossible with structural equation modelling. The results are presented in Fig. 52.8 in terms of the MAP or conditional expectations of the coupling parameters (upper panels) and the associated posterior probabilities (lower panels) using Eq. (52.12). We can see that the intrinsic coupling parameters are estimated reasonably accurately with a slight overestimation of the backward connection from A3 to A2. The bilinear coupling parameters modelling adaptation are shown in the lower panels, and the estimators have correctly identified the first forward connection as the locus of greatest adaptation. The posterior probabilities suggest inferences about the coupling parameters that would lead us to the veridical architecture if we considered only connections whose half-life exceeded 4 sec with 90% confidence or more.

The MAP estimates allow us to compute the MAP kernels associated with each region both in terms of neuronal output and hemodynamics response using Eq. (52.6). The neuronal and hemodynamic kernels for the three regions are shown in Fig. 52.9 (upper panels). It is interesting to note that the regional variation in the form of the neuronal kernels is sufficient to induce differential onset and peak latencies, on the order of a second or so, in the hemodynamic kernels despite the fact that neuronal onset latencies are the same. This difference in form is due to the network dynamics as activity is promulgated up the system and is recursively reentered into lower levels. Notice also that the neuronal kernels have quite protracted dynamics compared to the characteristic neuronal time constants of each area (about a second). This enduring activity, particularly in the higher two areas, is a product of the network dynamics. The MAP estimates also enable us to compute the predicted response (lower left panel) in each region and compare it to the true response without observation noise (lower right panel). This comparison shows that the actual and predicted responses are very similar.

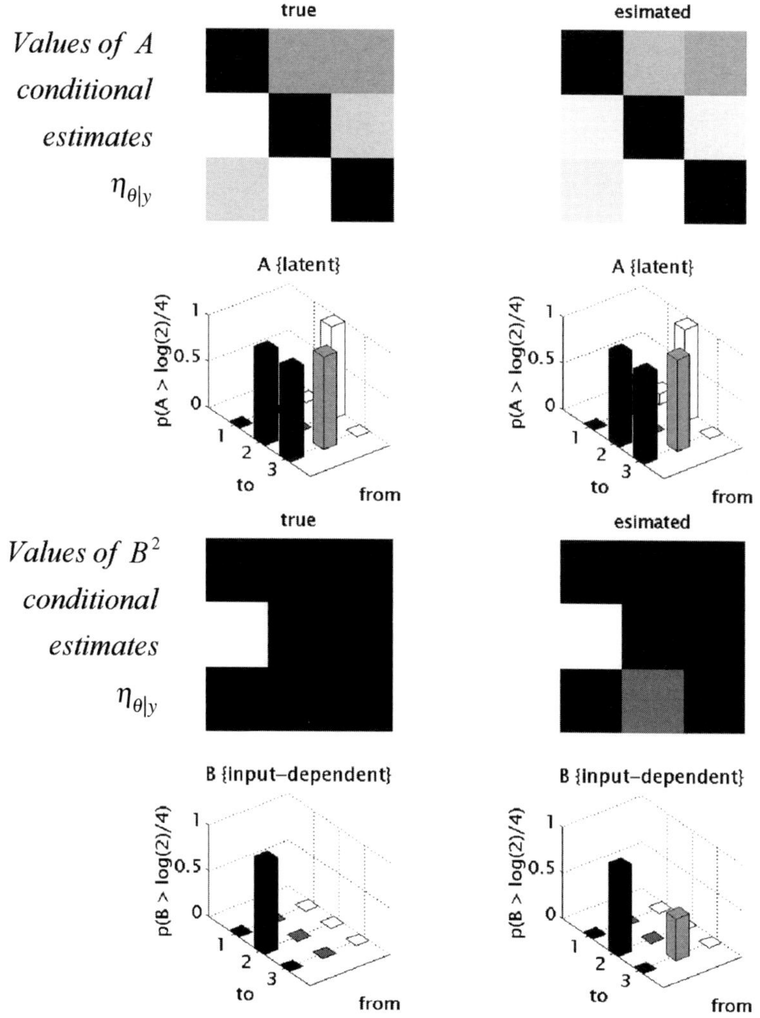

FIGURE 52.8
Results summarising the conditional estimation based on the simulated data of Fig. 52.6. The upper panels show the conditional estimates and posterior probabilities pertaining to the intrinsic coupling parameters. The lower panels show the equivalent results for bilinear coupling parameters mediating the effect of within-epoch time. Conditional or MAP estimates of the parameters are shown in image format with arbitrary scaling. The posterior probabilities that these parameters exceeded a threshold of ln(2)/4 per second are shown as three-dimensional bar charts. True values and probabilities are shown on the left, whereas the estimated values and posterior probabilities are shown on the right. This illustrates that the conditional estimates are a reasonable approximation to the true values and, in particular, the posterior probabilities conform to the true probabilities if we consider values of 90% or more.

In Friston *et al.* (2002a) we repeated this estimation procedure to explore the face validity of the estimation scheme over a range of hyperparameters such as noise levels, slice timing artifacts, extreme values of the biophysical parameters, and so on. In general, the scheme proved to be robust to most violations assessed. Here we will just look at the effects of error variance on estimation because this speaks to some important features of Bayesian estimation in this context and the noise levels that can be tolerated.

Effects of Noise

In this subsection we investigate the sensitivity and specificity of posterior density estimates to the level of observation noise. Data were simulated as described above and mixed with various levels of white noise. For each noise level, the posterior densities of the coupling parameters were estimated and plotted against the noise hyperparameter (expressed as its standard deviation) in terms of the posterior mean and 90% confidence intervals. Figure 52.10 shows

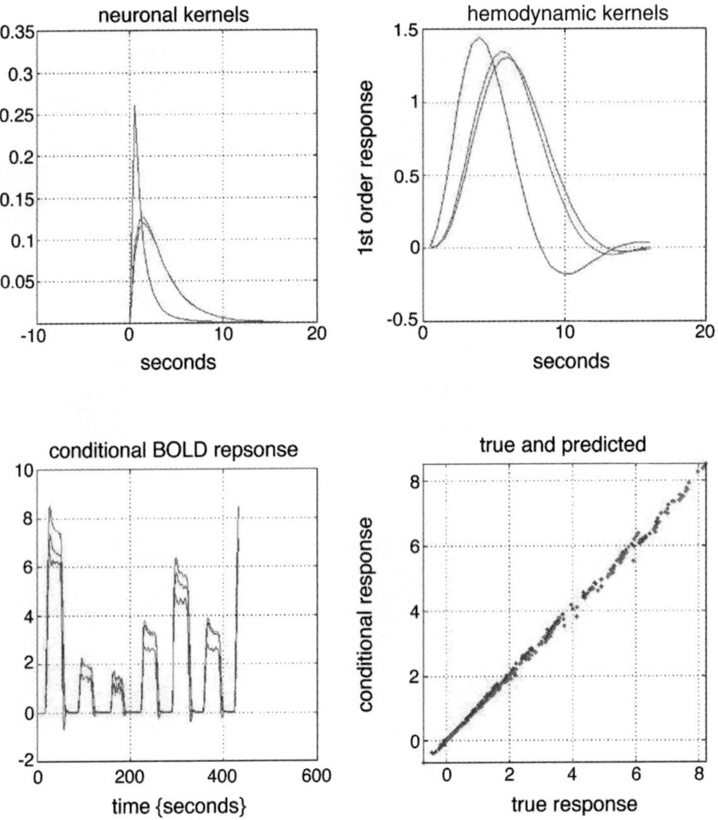

FIGURE 52.9
These results are based on the conditional or MAP estimates of the previous figure. The upper panels show the implied first-order kernels for neuronal responses (upper left) and equivalent hemodynamic responses (upper right) as a function of peristimulus time for each of the three regions. The lower panels show the predicted response based on the MAP estimators and a comparison of this response to the true response. The agreement is self-evident.

some key coupling parameters that include both zero and nonzero connection strengths. The solid lines represent the posterior expectation or MAP estimator and the dashed lines indicate the true value. The grey areas encompass the 90% confidence regions. Characteristic behaviours of the estimation are apparent from these results. As one might intuit, increasing the level of noise increases the uncertainty in the posterior estimates as reflected by an increase in the conditional variance and a widening of the confidence intervals. This widening is, however, bounded by the prior variances to which the conditional variances asymptote, at very high levels of noise. Concomitant with this effect is "shrinkage" of some posterior means to their prior expectation of zero. Put simply, when the data become very noisy, the estimation relies more heavily on priors and the prior expectation is given more weight. This is why priors of the sort used here are referred to as *shrinkage priors.* These simulations suggest that for this level of evoked response, noise levels between 0 and 2 permit the connection strengths to be identified with a fair degree of precision and accuracy. Noise levels in typical fMRI experiments are about 0.5–1.5. The units of signal and noise are adimensional and correspond to percentage whole brain mean. Fortunately, noise did not lead to false inferences in the sense that the posterior densities always encompassed the true values even at high levels of noise (Fig. 52.10).

PREDICTIVE VALIDITY: ANALYSIS OF SINGLE WORD PROCESSING

In this section we illustrate the predictive validity of DCM by showing that reproducible results can be obtained from independent data. The data set we used was especially designed for these sorts of analyses, comprising more than 1200 scans with a relatively short TR of 1.7 sec. This necessitated a limited field of coverage but provided relatively high temporal acuity. The

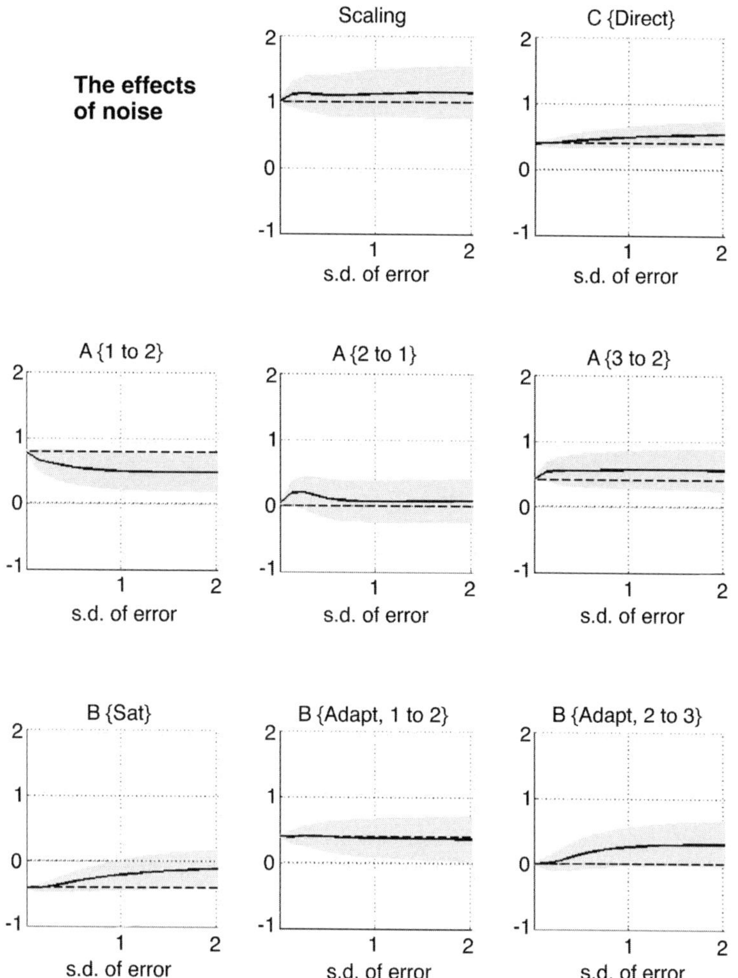

FIGURE 52.10
Posterior densities as a function of noise levels: The analysis, summarised in the previous two figures, was repeated for simulated data sequences at different levels of noise ranging from 0 to 2 units of standard deviation. Each graph shows the conditional expectation or MAP estimate of a coupling parameter (solid line) and the 90% confidence region (grey region). The true value for each parameter is also shown (dashed line). The top row shows the temporal scaling parameter and the extrinsic connection between the first input and the first area. The middle row shows some intrinsic coupling parameters and the bottom row bilinear parameters. As anticipated, the conditional variance of these estimators increases with noise, as reflected by a divergence of the confidence region with increasing standard deviation of the error.

paradigm was a passive listening task, using epochs of single words presented at different rates. These data have been used previously to characterise nonlinear aspects of hemodynamics (e.g., Friston *et al.,* 1998, 2000, 2002a). Details of the experimental paradigm and acquisition parameters are provided in the legend to Fig. 52.11. These data were acquired in consecutive sessions of 120-scan sets, enabling us to analyse the entire time series or each session independently. We first present the results obtained by concatenating all of the sessions into a single data sequence. We then revisit the data, analysing each session independently to provide 10 independent conditional estimates of the coupling parameters to assess reproducibility and mutual predictability.

Analysis of the Complete Time Series

Three regions were selected using maxima of the SPM{F} following a conventional SPM analysis (see Fig. 52.11). The three maxima were those that were closest to the primary and secondary auditory areas and Wernicke's area in accord with the anatomical designations provided in the atlas of Talairach and Tournoux (1988). Region-specific time series comprised the first eigenvariate of all voxels within a 4-mm radius sphere centred on each location. The

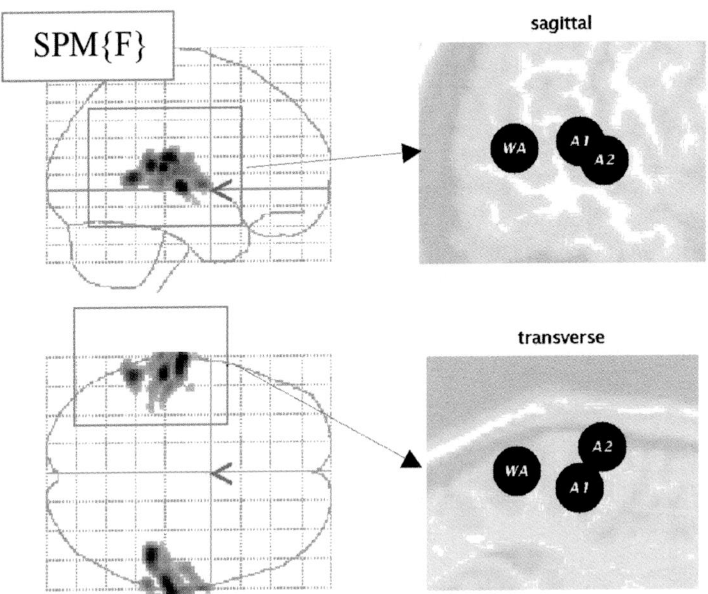

FIGURE 52.11
Region selection for the empirical word processing example: statistical parametric maps of the F ratio, based on a conventional SPM analysis, are shown in the left panels and the spatial locations of the selected regions are shown on the right. These are superimposed on a T_1-weighted reference image. The regional activities shown in the next figure correspond to the first eigenvariates of a 4-mm-radius sphere centred on the following coordinates in the standard anatomical space of Talairach and Tournoux: primary auditory area A1: −50, −26, and 8 mm; secondary auditory area A2: −64, −18, and 2 mm; and Wernicke's area WA: −56, −48, and 6 mm. In brief, we obtained fMRI time series from a single subject at 2 T using a Magnetom VISION (Siemens, Erlangen) whole body MRI system, equipped with a head volume coil. Contiguous multislice T_2*-weighted fMRI images were obtained with a gradient echo-planar sequence using an axial slice orientation (TE = 40 ms, TR = 1.7 sec, 64 × 64 × 16 voxels). After discarding initial scans (to allow for magnetic saturation effects) each time series comprised 1200 volume images with 3-mm isotropic voxels. The subject listened to monosyllabic or bisyllabic concrete nouns (i.e., *dog, mountain, gate*) presented at five different rates (10, 15, 30, 60, and 90 words per minute) for epochs of 34 sec, intercalated with periods of rest. The five presentation rates were successively repeated according to a Latin square design. The data were processed within SPM99 (Wellcome Department of Cognitive Neurology, http://www.fil.ion.ucl.ac.uk/spm). The time series were realigned, corrected for movement-related effects, and spatially normalised. The data were smoothed with a 5-mm isotropic Gaussian kernel. The SPM{F} above was based on a standard regression model using word presentation rate as the stimulus function and convolving it with a canonical hemodynamic response and its temporal derivative to form regressors.

anatomical locations are shown in Fig. 52.11. As in the simulations, there were two inputs corresponding to a delta function for the occurrence of an aurally presented word and a parametric input modelling within-epoch adaptation. The outputs of the system were the three eigenvariate time series from each region. As in the previous section, we allowed for a fully connected system. In other words, each region was potentially connected to every other region. Generally, one would impose constraints on highly unlikely or implausible connections by setting their prior variance to zero. However, we wanted to demonstrate that dynamic causal modelling can be applied to connectivity graphs that would be impossible to analyse with structural equation modelling. The auditory input was connected to A1. In addition, auditory input was entered bilinearly to emulate saturation, as in the simulations. The contextual input, modelling putative adaptation, was allowed to exert influences over all intrinsic connections. From a neurobiological perspective, an interesting question is whether plasticity can be demonstrated in forward connections or backward connections. Plasticity, in this instance, entails a time-dependent increase or decrease in effective connectivity and would be inferred by significant bilinear coupling parameters associated with the second input.

The inputs, outputs, and priors on the DCM parameters were entered into the Bayesian estimation procedure as described above. Drifts were modelled with the first 40 components of

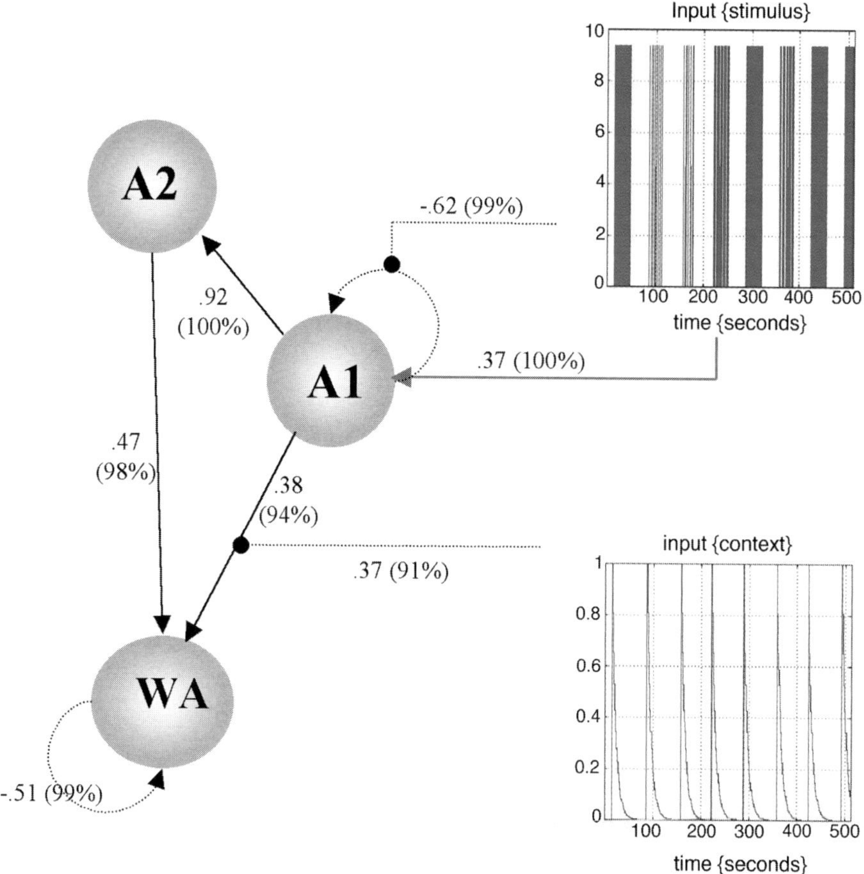

FIGURE 52.12
Results of a DCM analysis applied to the data described in the previous figure. The display format follows that of Fig. 52.6. The coupling parameters are shown alongside the corresponding connections. The values in brackets are the percentage confidence that these values exceed a threshold of ln(2)/8 per sec.

a discrete cosine set, corresponding to X in Eq. (52.6). The results of this analysis, in terms of the posterior densities and ensuing Bayesian inference, are presented in Figs. 52.12 and 52.13. Bayesian inferences were based on the probability that the coupling parameters exceeded 0.0866. This corresponds to a half-life of 8 sec. Intuitively, this means that we only consider the influences of one region on another to be meaningfully large if this influence is expressed within a time frame of 8 sec or less. The results show that the most probable architecture, given the inputs and data, conforms to a simple hierarchy of forward connections where A1 influences A2 and WA, whereas A2 sends connections just to WA (Fig. 52.12). Although backward connections between WA and A2 were estimated to be greater than our threshold with 82% confidence, they are not shown in Fig. 52.12 (which is restricted to posterior probabilities of 90% or more). Saturation could be inferred in A1 and WA with a high degree of confidence with b^1_{11} and b^1_{33} being greater than 0.5. Significant plasticity or time-dependent changes were expressed predominantly in the forward connections, particularly that between A1 and A3, i.e., $b^2_{13} = 0.37$. The conditional estimates are shown in more detail in Fig. 52.13 along with the conditional fitted responses and associated kernels. A full posterior density analysis for a particular contrast of effects is shown in Fig. 52.13a (lower panel). This contrast tested for the average plasticity over all forward and backward connections and demonstrates that we can be virtually certain plasticity was greater than zero.

This analysis illustrates three things. First, the DCM has defined a hierarchical architecture that is a sufficient explanation for the data and is, indeed, the most likely given the data. This

a

MAP estimates $\eta_{\theta|y}$

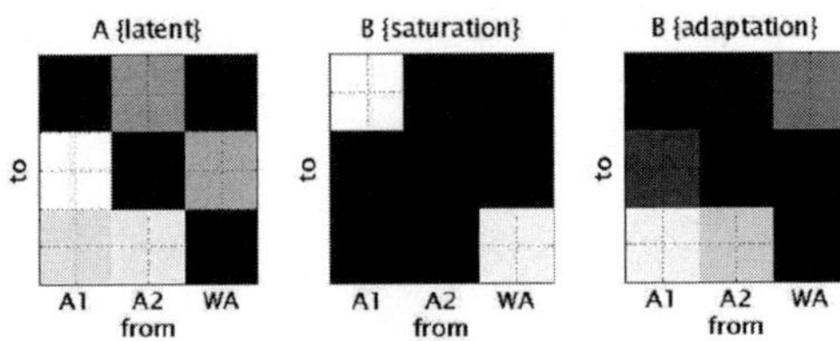

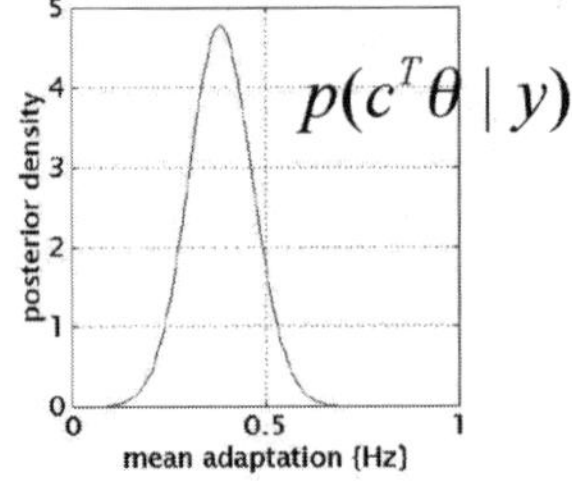

b

Responses

Kernels

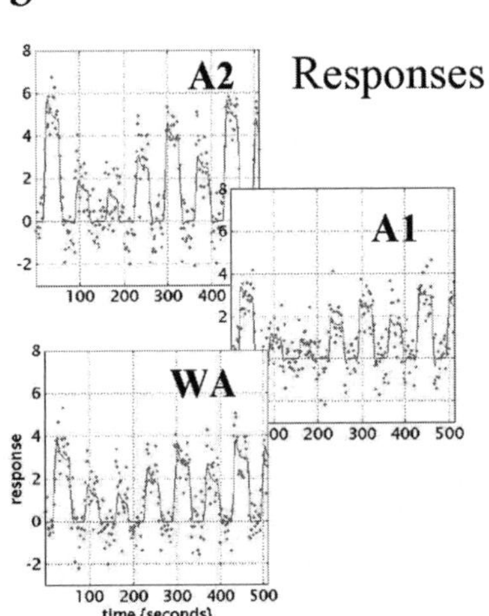

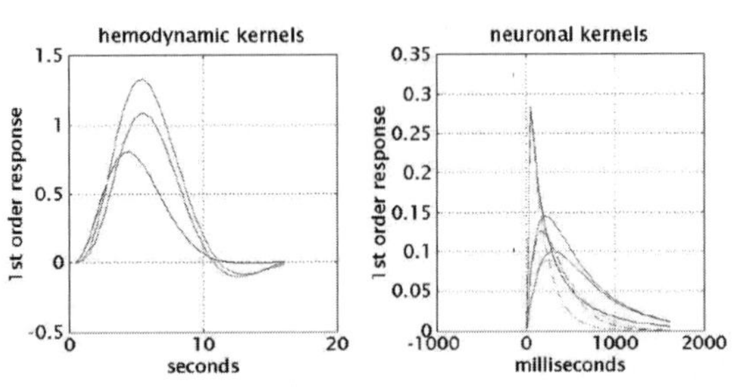

FIGURE 52.13
This figure provides a more detailed characterisation of the conditional estimates. The images in the top row are the MAP estimates for the intrinsic and bilinear coupling parameters, pertaining to saturation and adaptation. The middle panel shows the posterior density of a contrast of all bilinear terms mediating adaptation, namely, the modulation of intrinsic connections by the second time-dependent experimental effect. The predicted responses based on the conditional estimators are shown for each of the three regions on the lower left (solid lines) with the original data (dots) after removal of confounds. A reparameterisation of the conditional estimates, in terms of the first-order kernels, is shown on the lower right. The hemodynamic (left) and neuronal (right) kernels should be compared with the equivalent kernels for the simulated data in Fig. 52.9.

hierarchical structure was not part of the prior constraints because we allowed for a fully connected system. Second, the significant bilinear effects of auditory stimulation suggest that there is measurable neuronal saturation above and beyond that attributable to hemodynamic nonlinearities. This is quite significant because such disambiguation is usually impossible given just hemodynamic responses. Finally, we were able to show time-dependent decreases in effective connectivity in forward connections from A1. Although this experiment was not designed to test for plasticity, the usefulness of DCM, in studies of learning and priming, should be self-evident.

Reproducibility

The analysis above was repeated identically for each and every 120-scan session to provide 10 sets of Bayesian estimators. Drifts were modelled with the first four components of a discrete cosine set. The estimators are presented graphically in Fig. 52.14 and demonstrate extremely consistent results. In the upper panels, the intrinsic connections are shown to be very similar in their profile, again reflecting a hierarchical connectivity architecture. The conditional means and 90% confidence regions for two connections are shown in Fig. 52.14a. These connections included the forward connection from A1 to A2 that is consistently estimated to be very strong. The backward connection from WA to A2 was weaker but was certainly greater than zero in every analysis. Equivalent results were obtained for the modulatory effects or bilinear terms, although the profile was less consistent (Fig. 52.14b). However, the posterior density of the contrast testing for average time-dependent adaptation or plasticity is relatively consistent and again almost certainly greater than zero in each analysis.

To illustrate the stability of hyperparameter estimates, over the 10 sessions, the standard deviations of observation error are presented for each session over the three areas in Fig. 52.15. As is typical of studies at this field strength, the standard deviation of noise is about 0.8% to 1% whole brain mean. It is pleasing to note that the session-to-session variability in hyperparameter estimates was relatively small in relation to region-to-region differences.

In summary, independent analyses of data acquired under identical stimulus conditions, on the same subject, in the same scanning session, yield remarkably similar results. These results are biologically plausible and speak to the interesting notion that time-dependent changes, following the onset of a stream of words, are prominent in forward connections among auditory areas.

CONSTRUCT VALIDITY: ANALYSIS OF ATTENTIONAL EFFECTS ON CONNECTIONS

In this final section we address the construct validity of DCM. In previous chapters we have seen that attention positively modulates the backward connections in a distributed system of cortical regions mediating attention to radial motion. We use the same data in this section. In brief, subjects viewed optic flow stimuli comprising radially moving dots at a fixed velocity. In some epochs, subjects were asked to detect changes in velocity that did not actually occur. This attentional manipulation was validated post hoc using psychophysics and the motion after-effect. Analyses using structural equation modelling (Büchel and Friston, 1997) and a Volterra formulation of effective connectivity (Friston and Büchel, 2000) have established a hierarchical backward modulation of effective connectivity where a higher area increases the effective connectivity among two subordinate areas. These analyses have been extended using variable parameter regression and Kalman filtering (Büchel and Friston, 1998) to look at the effect of attention directly on interactions between V5 and the posterior parietal complex. In this context, the Volterra formulation can be regarded as a highly finessed regression model that embodies nonlinear terms and some dynamic aspects of fMRI time series. However, even simple analyses, such as those employing psychophysiological interactions, point to the same conclusion that attention generally increases the effective connectivity among extrastriate and parietal areas. In short, we have established that the superior posterior parietal cortex (SPC) exerts a modulatory role on V5 responses using Volterra-based regression models (Friston and Büchel, 2000) and that the inferior frontal gyrus (IFG) exerts a similar influence on SPC using structural equation modelling (Büchel and Friston, 1997). The aim of this section is to show that DCM leads one to the same conclusions but using a completely different approach.

Analysis

The experimental paradigm and data acquisition parameters are described in the legend to Fig. 52.16. This figure also shows the location of the regions that entered into the DCM (insert, Fig. 52.16b). These regions were based on maxima from conventional SPMs that were testing for the effects of photic stimulation, motion, and attention. As in the previous section, regional time courses were taken as the first eigenvariate of spherical volumes of interest centred on the maxima shown in the figure. The inputs, in this example, comprise one sensory perturbation and two contextual inputs. The sensory input was simply the presence of photic stimulation, and the

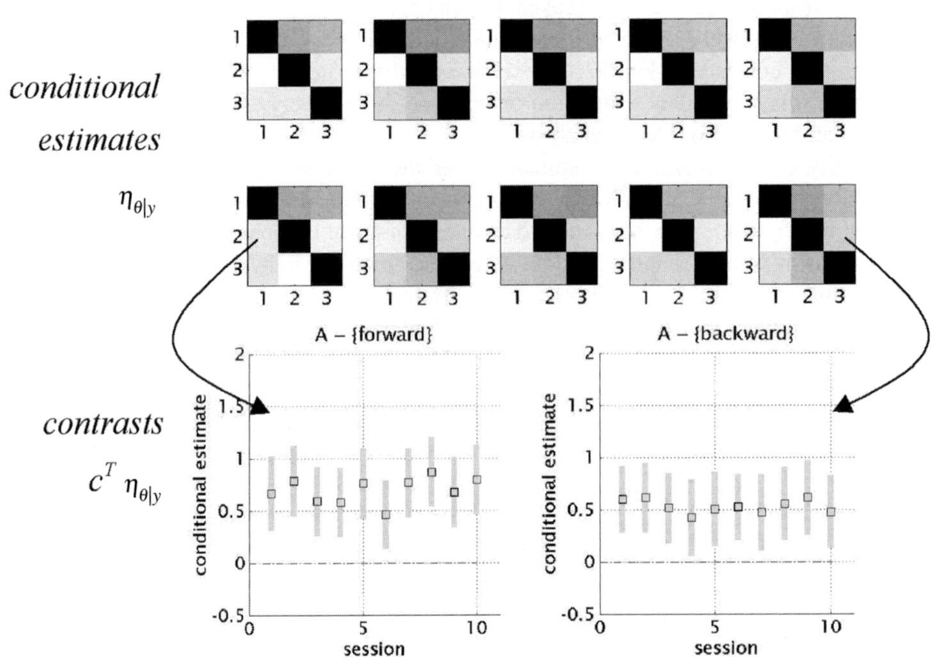

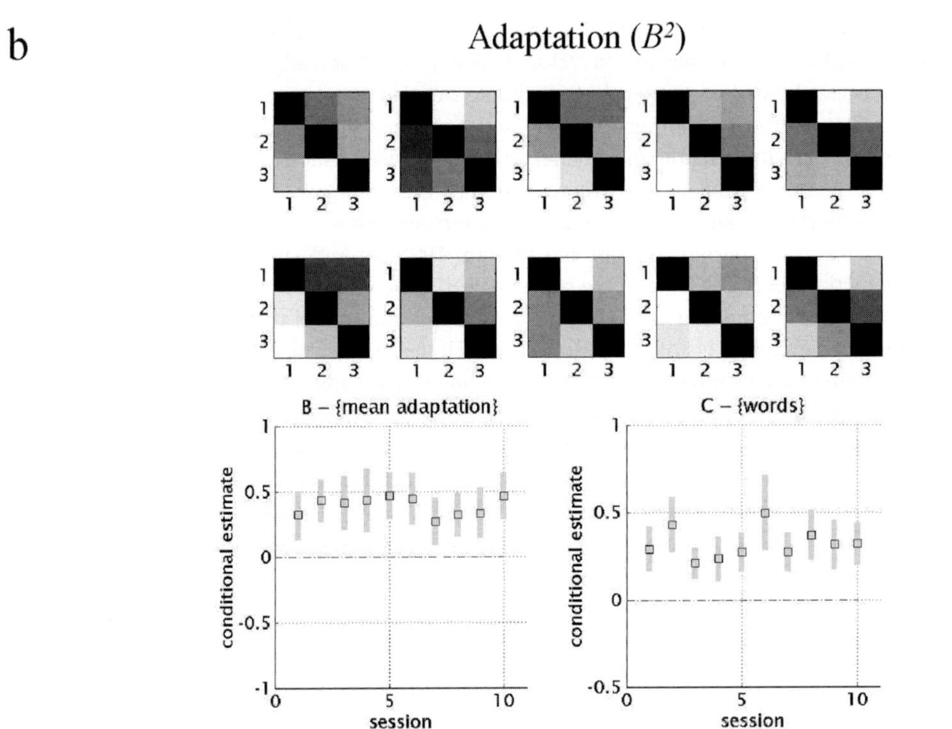

FIGURE 52.14

Results of the reproducibility analyses. (a) Results for the intrinsic parameters. The profile of conditional estimates for the 10 independent analyses described in the main text are shown in image format, all scaled to the maximum. The posterior densities, on which these estimates are based, are shown for two selected connections in the lower two graphs. These densities are displayed in terms of their expectation and 90% confidence intervals (grey bars) for the forward connection from A1 to A2. The equivalent densities are shown for the backward connection from WA to A2. Although the posterior probability that the latter connections exceeded the specified threshold was less than 90%, it can be seen that this connection is almost certainly greater than zero. (b) Equivalent results for the bilinear coupling matrices mediating adaptation. The lower panels here refer to the posterior densities of a contrast testing for the mean of all bilinear parameters (left) and the extrinsic connection to A1 (right).

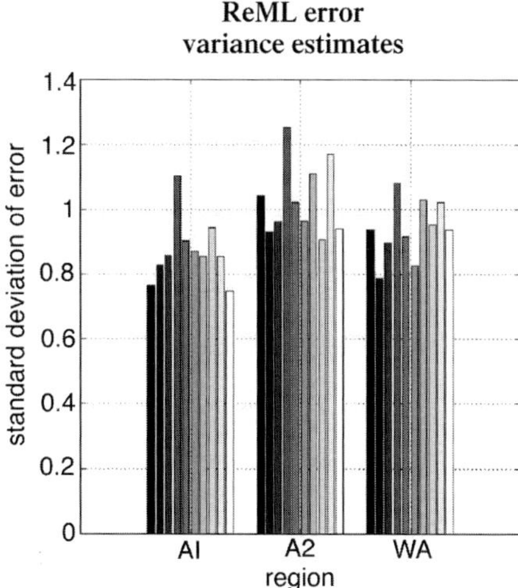

FIGURE 52.15
ReML hyperparameter variance estimates for each region and analysis. These estimates provide an anecdotal characterisation of the within- and between-area variability, in hyperparameter estimates, and show that they generally lie between 0.8 and 1 (adimensional units corresponding to percent whole brain mean).

first contextual one was the presence of motion in the visual field. The second contextual input, encoding attentional set, was unity during attention to speed changes and zero otherwise. The outputs corresponded to the four regional eigenvariates in Fig. 52.16b. The intrinsic connections were constrained to conform to a hierarchical pattern in which each area was reciprocally connected to its supraordinate area. Photic stimulation entered at, and only at, V1. The effect of motion in the visual field was modelled as a bilinear modulation of the V1 to V5 connectivity and attention was allowed to modulate the backward connections from IFG and SPC.

The results of the DCM are shown in Fig. 52.16a. Of primary interest here is the modulatory effect of attention that is expressed in terms of the bilinear coupling parameters for this third input. As hoped, we can be highly confident that attention modulates the backward connections from IFG to SPC and from SPC to V5. Indeed, the influences of IFG on SPC are negligible in the absence of attention (dotted connections in Fig. 52.16a). It is important to note that the only way in which attentional manipulation can effect brain responses is through this bilinear effect. Attention-related responses are seen throughout the system (attention epochs are marked with arrows in the plot of IFG responses in Fig. 52.16b). This attentional modulation is accounted for, sufficiently, by changing just two connections. This change is, presumably, instantiated by an instructional set at the beginning of each epoch. The second thing this analysis illustrates is how functional segregation is modelled in DCM. Here one can regard V1 as a "segregating" motion from other visual information that distributes it to the motion-sensitive area V5. This segregation is modelled as a bilinear "enabling" of V1 to V5 connections when, and only when, motion is present. Note that in the absence of motion the intrinsic V1 to V5 connection was trivially small (in fact the MAP estimate was –0.04). The key advantage of entering motion through a bilinear effect, as opposed to a direct effect on V5, is that we can finesse the inference that V5 shows motion-selective responses with the assertion that these responses are mediated by afferents from V1.

The two bilinear effects above represent two important aspects of functional integration that DCM was designed to characterise.

CONCLUSION

In this chapter we have presented dynamic causal modelling. DCM is a causal modelling procedure for dynamical systems in which causality is inherent in the differential equations that specify the model. The basic idea is to treat the system of interest, in this case the brain, as an input–state–output system. By perturbing the system with known inputs, measured responses are

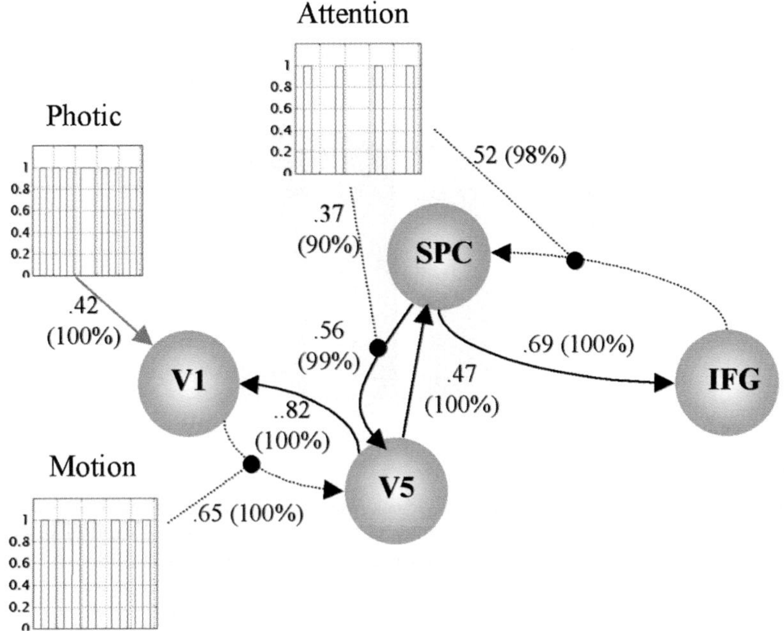
a
Attention
Photic
Motion
SPC
V1
V5
IFG
.52 (98%)
.37 (90%)
.42 (100%)
.56 (99%)
.69 (100%)
.47 (100%)
.82 (100%)
.65 (100%)

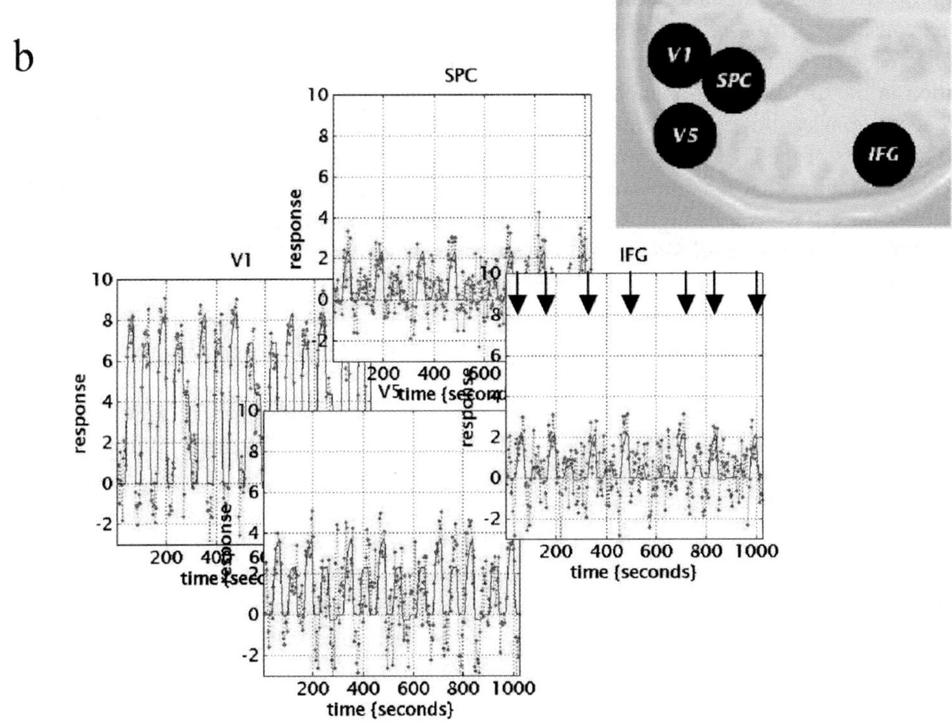
b
SPC
V1
V5
IFG
response
time {seconds}

FIGURE 52.16
Results of the empirical analysis of the attention study. (a) Functional architecture based on the conditional estimates displayed using the same format as Fig. 52.12. The most interesting aspects of this architecture involved the role of motion and attention in exerting bilinear effects. Critically, the influence of motion is to enable connections from V1 to the motion-sensitive area V5. The influence of attention is to enable backward connections from the IFG to the SPC. Furthermore, attention increases the latent influence of SPC on the V5 area. Dotted arrows connecting regions represent significant bilinear affects in the absence of significant intrinsic coupling. (b) Fitted responses based on the conditional estimates and the adjusted data are shown using the same format as in Fig. 52.13. The insert shows the location of the regions, again adopting the same format as is used in previous figures. The location of these regions centred on the primary visual cortex V1: 6, −84, −6 mm; motion-sensitive area V5: 45, −81, and 5 mm; SPC: 18, −57, and 66 mm; and IFG: 54, 18, and 30 mm. The volumes from which the first eigenvariates were calculated corresponded to 8-mm-radius spheres centred on these locations.

Subjects were studied with fMRI under identical stimulus conditions (visual motion subtended by radially moving dots) while manipulating the attentional component of the task (detection of velocity changes). The data were acquired from normal subjects at 2 T using a Magnetom VISION (Siemens, Erlangen) whole body MRI system, equipped with a head volume coil. Here we analyse data from the first subject. Contiguous multislice T_2*-weighted fMRI images were obtained with a gradient echo-planar sequence (TE = 40 ms, TR = 3.22 sec, matrix size = 64 × 64 × 32; voxel size 3 × 3 × 3 mm). Each subject had four consecutive 100-scan sessions comprising a series of 10-scan blocks under five different conditions: D F A F N F A F N S. The first condition (D) was a dummy condition to allow for magnetic saturation effects. Condition F (Fixation) corresponds to a low-level baseline where the subjects viewed a fixation point at the centre of a screen. In condition A (Attention) subjects viewed 250 dots moving radially from the centre at 4.7 degrees per second and were asked to detect changes in radial velocity. In condition N (No attention) the subjects were asked simply to view the moving dots. In condition S (Stationary) subjects viewed stationary dots. The order of A and N was swapped for the last two sessions. In all conditions subjects fixated the centre of the screen. In a prescanning session the subjects were given five trials with five speed changes (reducing to 1%). During scanning there were no speed changes. No overt response was required in any condition.

used to estimate various parameters that govern the evolution of brain states. Although there are no restrictions on the parameterisation of the model, a bilinear approximation affords a simple reparameterisation in terms of effective connectivity. This effective connectivity can be latent or intrinsic or, through bilinear terms, can model input-dependent changes in effective connectivity. Parameter estimation proceeds using fairly standard approaches to system identification that rest on Bayesian inference.

Dynamic causal modelling represents a fundamental departure from conventional approaches to modelling of effective connectivity in neuroscience. The critical distinction between DCM and other approaches, such as structural equation modelling or multivariate autoregressive techniques, is that the input is treated as known, as opposed to stochastic. In this sense, DCM is much closer to conventional analyses of neuroimaging time series because the causal or explanatory variables are known fixed quantities. The use of designed and known inputs in characterising neuroimaging data with the general linear model or DCM is a more natural way to analyse data from designed experiments. Given that the vast majority of imaging neuroscience relies on designed experiments, we consider DCM a potentially useful complement to existing techniques. We develop this point and the relationship of DCM to other approaches in the following chapter.

References

Bendat, J. S. (1990). *Nonlinear System Analysis and Identification from Random Data.* John Wiley and Sons, New York.

Büchel, C., and Friston, K. J. (1997). Modulation of connectivity in visual pathways by attention: cortical interactions evaluated with structural equation modelling and fMRI. *Cerebral Cortex* **7,** 768–778.

Büchel, C., and Friston, K. J. (1998). Dynamic changes in effective connectivity characterised by variable parameter regression and Kalman filtering. *Hum. Brain Mapping,* **6,** 403–408.

Buxton, R. B., Wong, E. C., and Frank, L. R. (1998). Dynamics of blood flow and oxygenation changes during brain activation: the balloon model. *MRM* **39,** 855–864.

Friston, K. J., Buechel, C., Fink, G. R., Morris, J., Rolls, E., and Dolan, R. J. (1997). Psychophysiological and modulatory interactions in neuroimaging. *NeuroImage* **6,** 218–229.

Friston, K. J., Josephs, O., Rees, G., and Turner, R. (1998). Nonlinear event-related responses in fMRI. *Mag. Res. Med.* **39**, 41–52.

Friston, K. J., and Büchel, C. (2000). Attentional modulation of effective connectivity from V2 to V5/MT in humans. *Proc. Natl. Acad. Sci. USA* **97,** 7591–7596.

Friston, K. J., Mechelli, A., Turner, R., and Price, C. J. (2000). Nonlinear responses in fMRI: the balloon model, Volterra kernels and other hemodynamics. *NeuroImage* **12,** 466–477.

Friston, K. J. (2002). Bayesian estimation of dynamical systems: An application to fMRI. *NeuroImage* **16,** 513–530.

Friston, K.J., Harrison, L., and Penny, W. (2002a). Dynamic causal modelling. *NeuroImage*, **19**, 1273–1302.

Friston, K. J., Penny, W., Phillips, C., Kiebel, S., Hinton, G., and Ashburner, J. (2002b). Classical and Bayesian inference in neuroimaging: theory. *NeuroImage* **16,** 465–483.

Harrison, L. M., Penny, W., and Friston, K. J. (2003). Multivariate autoregressive modelling of fMRI time series. *NeuroImage*, **19**, 1477–1491.

Horwitz, B., Friston, K. J., and Taylor, J. G. (2001). Neural modeling and functional brain imaging: an overview. *Neural Networks* **13,** 829–846.

Kenny, D. A., and Judd, C. M. (1984). Estimating nonlinear and interactive effects of latent variables. *Psychol. Bull.* **96,** 201–210.

Mandeville, J. B., Marota, J. J., Ayata, C., Zararchuk, G., Moskowitz, M. A., Rosen, B., and Weisskoff, R. M. (1999). Evidence of a cerebrovascular postarteriole windkessel with delayed compliance. *J. Cereb. Blood Flow Metab.* **19,** 679–689.

McIntosh, A. R. (2000). Towards a network theory of cognition. *Neural Networks* **13,** 861–870.

McIntosh, A. R., and Gonzalez-Lima, F. (1994). Structural equation modelling and its application to network analysis in functional brain imaging. *Hum. Brain Mapping* **2,** 2–22.

Talairach, J., and Tournoux, P. (1988). *A Co-Planar Stereotaxic Atlas of a Human Brain.* Thieme, Stuttgart.

CHAPTER

53

Mathematical Appendix

INTRODUCTION

Overview

This chapter presents a theoretical review of models that are used for effective connectivity. In this discussion we focus on the nature and form of the models themselves and less on estimation or inference issues. The aim is to relate the various models commonly employed and to make their underlying assumptions and requirements more transparent.

As we have seen in the preceding chapters, a number of different models are available for estimating effective connectivity using neuroimaging time series (PET, fMRI, EEG, and MEG). By definition, effective connectivity depends on a model, through which it is defined operationally (Friston, 1995). This chapter reviews the principal models that could be adopted and how they relate to each other. We consider dynamic causal models (DCMs), generalised convolution models (GCMs), bicoherence, structural equation models (SEMs), and multivariate autoregression models (MARs). In brief, we will show that they are all special cases of each other and try to emphasise their points of contact. However, some fundamental distinctions arise that guide the selection of the appropriate models in different situations.

Single or Multiple Regions?

The first distinction rests on whether the model is used to explain the coupling between the inputs and the responses of one cell, assembly, or region, or whether the model encompasses interactions among the states of multiple regions. In terms of models, this distinction is between input–output models [e.g., multiple-input/single-output models (MISO) and multiple-input/multiple-output models (MIMO)] and explicit input–state–output models. Usually the input–output approach is concerned with the nonlinear transformation of inputs, by a region, to produce its outputs. The implicit states correspond to hidden states of a single region, and the effective connectivity concerns the *vertical* link between inputs and outputs (see Fig. 53.1a). In contradistinction, the input–state–output approach is generally concerned with characterising the *horizontal* coupling among variables that represent the states of different regions. These states are observed vicariously though the outputs (see Fig. 53.1b). Examples of input–output models include the Volterra formulation of effective connectivity and related coherence analyses in the spectral domain. An example of a model that tries to estimate horizontal coupling among hidden states is DCM. A critical aspect of vertical, input–output models of effective connectivity is that they can proceed without reference to the hidden states. Conversely, the horizontal interactions require indirect access to the states or some strong assumptions about how they produce outputs.

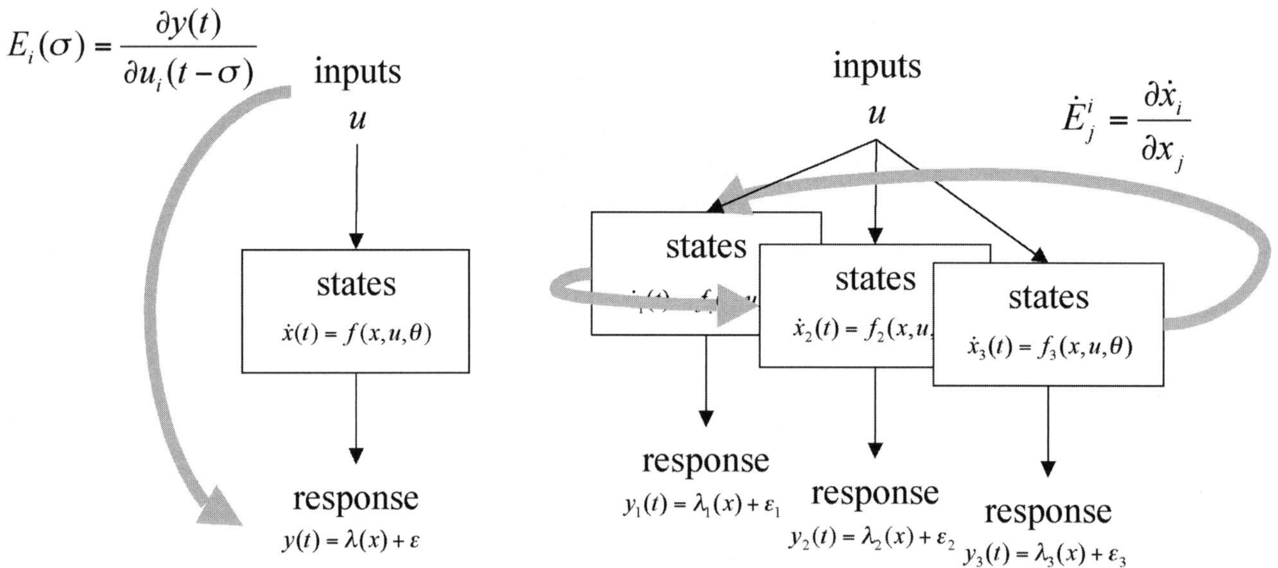

FIGURE 53.1
Schematic depicting the difference between analyses of effective connectivity that address the input–output behaviour of a single region and those that refer explicitly to interaction among the states of multiple regions.

In short, analyses of effective connectivity can be construed as trying to characterise the input–output behaviour of a single region or the coupling among the states of several regions using an explicit input–state–output model. Below we start by reviewing input–output models and then turn to input–state–output models.

Deterministic or Stochastic Inputs?

The second key distinction is between models, where the input is known and fixed (e.g., DCM) and those in which it is not (MAR and SEM). Only the former class of models affords direct measures of effective connectivity. The remaining models are useful for establishing the presence of coupling under certain assumptions about the input (usually that it is white noise that drives the system). This distinction depends on whether the inputs enter as known and deterministic quantities (e.g., experimentally designed causes of evoked responses) or whether we know (or can assume) something about the density function of the inputs (i.e., its statistics up to second or higher orders). Most models of the stochastic variety assume the inputs are Gaussian, i.i.d., and stationary. Some stochastic models (e.g., coherence) use local stationarity assumptions to estimate high-order moments from observable but noisy inputs. For example, polyspectral analysis represents an intermediate case in which the inputs are observed but only their statistics are used. However, the key distinction is not whether one has access to the inputs but whether those inputs have to be treated as stochastic or not. Stationarity assumptions in stochastic models are critical because they preclude full analyses of evoked neuronal responses or transients that, by their nature, are nonstationary. Despite this, in some situations the input is not observable or under experimental control. These situations preclude the estimation of the parameters of DCMs. Approaches such as MAR and SEM can be used to proceed if the inputs can be regarded as stationary. The distinction between deterministic and stochastic inputs is critical in the sense that it would be inappropriate to adopt one class of model in a context that calls for the other.

Connections or Statistical Dependencies?

The final distinction is in terms of what is being estimated or inferred. Recall that functional connectivity is defined by the presence of statistical dependencies among remote neurophysiological measurements. Conversely, effective connectivity is a parameter of a model that specifies the causal influences among brain systems. It is useful to distinguish *inferences* about statistical dependencies and *estimation* of effective connectivity in terms of the distinction between functional and effective connectivity. Examples of approaches that try to establish static dependencies include coherence analyses and MAR. This is because these techniques do not presume any model of how hidden states interact to produce responses. They are interested only in establishing dependencies (usually linear) among outputs over different frequencies or time lags. Although MAR may employ some model to assess dependencies, this is a model of dependencies among outputs. There is no assertion that outputs *cause* outputs. Conversely, SEM and DCM try to estimate the model parameters and constitute analyses of effective connectivity proper. Generalised convolution approaches fall into this class because they rest on the *estimation* of kernels that are an equivalent representation of some input–state–output model parameters.

Effective Connectivity

Effective connectivity is the influence that one neuronal system exerts over another at a synaptic or ensemble level. This should be contrasted with functional connectivity, which implies a statistical dependence between two neuronal systems that could be mediated in any number of ways. Operationally, effective connectivity can be expressed as the response induced in an ensemble, unit, or region by input from others, in terms of partial derivatives of the target activity x_i, with respect to the source activities. First E^i_j and second order E^i_{jk} connectivities are then as follows:

$$E^i_j(\sigma_1) = \frac{\partial x_i(t)}{\partial x_j(t-\sigma_1)}, \quad E^i_{jk}(\sigma_1,\sigma_2) = \frac{\partial^2 x_i(t)}{\partial x_j(t-\sigma_1)\partial x_k(t-\sigma_2)}, \quad \ldots \tag{53.1}$$

First-order connectivity embodies the response evoked by a change in input at $t - \sigma_1$. In other words, it is a time-dependant measure of *driving* efficacy. Second-order connectivity reflects the *modulatory* influence of the input at $t - \sigma_1$ on the response evoked at $t - \sigma_2$—and so on for higher orders. Note that in this general formulation, effective connectivity is a function of current input and inputs over the recent past.[1] Furthermore, implicit in Eq. (53.1) is the fact that effective connectivity is causal, unless σ_1 is allowed to be negative. It is useful to introduce the dynamic equivalent, in which the response of the target is measured in terms of *changes in* activity:

$$\dot{E}^i_j = \frac{\partial \dot{x}_i}{\partial x_j}, \quad \dot{E}^i_{jk} = \frac{\partial^2 \dot{x}_i}{\partial x_j \partial x_k} \ldots \tag{53.2}$$

where $\dot{x}_i = \partial x_i/\partial t$. In this dynamic form all influences are causal and instantaneous. Before considering specific models of effective connectivity we briefly review their basis (see Chapter 50).

Dynamical Systems

The most general and plausible model of neuronal systems is a nonlinear dynamical model that corresponds to an analytic MIMO system. The state and output equations of an analytic dynamical system are

$$\begin{aligned} \dot{x}(t) &= f(x(t),u(t),\theta) \\ y(t) &= \lambda(x(t)) + \varepsilon \end{aligned} \tag{53.3}$$

Typically the inputs correspond to designed experimental effects (e.g., stimulus functions in fMRI), or represent stochastic drives or system perturbations. Stochastic observation error $\varepsilon \sim N(0,\Sigma)$ enters linearly in this model. For simplicity, the expressions below deal with single-input/single-output (SISO) systems and will be generalised later. The measured response y is some nonlinear function of the states of the system x. These state variables are usually un-

[1] In contrast, functional connectivity is model free and simply reflects the mutual information . In this chapter, we are concerned only with models of effective connectivity.

observed or hidden (the configurational status of all ion channels, the depolarisation of every dendritic compartment, etc.). The parameters of the state equation embody effective connectivity, either in terms of mediating the coupling between inputs and outputs (MISO models of a single region) or through the coupling among state variables (MIMO models of multiple regions). The objective is to estimate and make inferences (usually Bayesian) about these parameters, given the outputs and possibly the inputs. Sometimes this requires one to specify the form of the state equation. A ubiquitous and useful form is the bilinear approximation to Eq. (53.3); expanding around x_0

$$\begin{aligned} \dot{x}(t) &\approx Ax + uBx + Cu \\ y &= Lx \end{aligned} \tag{53.4}$$

$$A = \frac{\partial f}{\partial x}, \quad B = \frac{\partial^2 f}{\partial x \partial u}, \quad C = \frac{\partial f}{\partial u}, \quad L = \frac{\partial \lambda}{\partial x}$$

For simplicity, we have assumed $x_0 = 0$ and $f(0) = \lambda(0) = 0$. This bilinear model is sometimes expressed in a more compact form by augmenting the states with a constant as follows:

$$\begin{aligned} \dot{X} &= (M + uN)X \\ y &= HX \end{aligned} \tag{53.5}$$

$$X = \begin{bmatrix} 1 \\ x \end{bmatrix}, \quad M = \begin{bmatrix} 0 & 0 \\ f(0) & A \end{bmatrix}, \quad N = \begin{bmatrix} 0 & 0 \\ C & B \end{bmatrix}, \quad H = [\lambda(0) \quad L]$$

(see Friston, 2002). Here the model's parameters comprise the matrices $\theta \in \{A,B,C,L\}$. We will use the bilinear parameterisation when dealing with MIMO models and their derivatives below. We will first deal with MISO models, with and without deterministic inputs.

INPUT–OUTPUT MODELS FOR SINGLE REGIONS

Models for Deterministic Inputs: The Volterra Formulation

In this section we review the Volterra formulation of dynamic systems. This formulation is important because it allows the input–output behaviour of a system to be characterised in terms of kernels that can be estimated without knowing the states of the system.

The Fliess fundamental formula (Fliess *et al.*, 1983) describes the causal relationship between the outputs and the history of the inputs in Eq. (53.3). This relationship conforms to a Volterra series, which expresses the output $y(t)$ as a generalised convolution of the input $u(t)$, critically without reference to the state variables $x(t)$. This series is simply a functional Taylor expansion of the outputs with respect to the inputs (Bendat, 1990). The reason it is a *functional* expansion is that the inputs are a function of time:

$$\begin{aligned} y(t) &= h(u,\theta) + \varepsilon \\ h(u,\theta) &= \sum_i \int_0^t \ldots \int_0^t \kappa_i(\sigma_1,\ldots,\sigma_i)u(t-\sigma_1),\ldots,u(t-\sigma_i)d\sigma_1,\ldots,d\sigma_i \\ \kappa_i(\sigma_1,\ldots,\sigma_i) &= \frac{\partial^i y(t)}{\partial u(t-\sigma_1),\ldots,\partial u(t-\sigma_i)} \end{aligned} \tag{53.6}$$

where $\kappa_i(\sigma_1,\ldots,\sigma_i)$ is the ith-order kernel. In Eq. (53.6) the integrals are restricted to the past or history of the inputs. This renders Eq. (53.6) causal. In some situations an acausal formulation may be appropriate (e.g., one in which the kernels have nonzero values for future inputs; see Friston and Büchel, 2000). One important thing about Eq. (53.6) is that it is linear in the unknowns, enabling unbiased estimates of the kernels using least squares. In other words, Eq. (53.6) can be treated as a general linear observation model enabling all of the usual estimation and inference procedures (see Chapter 50 for an example). Volterra series are generally thought of as a high-order or generalised nonlinear convolution of the inputs to provide an output. To ensure estimability of the kernels, they can be expanded in terms of some appropriate basis functions $q_j^i(\sigma_1,\ldots,\sigma_i)$to give the general linear model:

$$
\begin{aligned}
y(t) &= \sum_{ij} \beta_j^i h_j^i(u) + \varepsilon \\
h_j^i(u) &= \int_0^t \ldots \int_0^t q_j^i(\sigma_1,\ldots,\sigma_i)u(t-\sigma_1),\ldots,u(t-\sigma_i)d\sigma_1,\ldots,d\sigma_i \\
\kappa_i(\sigma_1,\ldots,\sigma_i) &= \sum_j \beta_j^i q_j^i(\sigma_1,\ldots,\sigma_i)
\end{aligned} \tag{53.7}
$$

The Volterra formulation is useful as a way of characterising the influence of inputs on the responses of a region. The kernels can be regarded as a reparameterisation of the bilinear form in Eq. (53.4) that encodes the impulse response to input. The kernels for the states are

$$
\begin{aligned}
\kappa_0 &= X(0) \\
\kappa_1(\sigma_1) &= e^{\sigma_1 M} N e^{-\sigma_1 M} X(0) \\
\kappa_2(\sigma_1,\sigma_2) &= e^{\sigma_2 M} N e^{(\sigma_1-\sigma_2)M} N e^{-\sigma_1 M} X(0) \\
\kappa_2(\sigma_1,\sigma_2,\sigma_3) &= \ldots
\end{aligned} \tag{53.8}
$$

The kernels associated with the output follow from the chain rule:

$$
\begin{aligned}
h_0 &= H\kappa_0 \\
h_1(\sigma_1) &= H\kappa_1(\sigma_1) \\
h_2(\sigma_1,\sigma_2) &= \ldots
\end{aligned} \tag{53.9}
$$

(see Friston, 2002, for details). If the system is fully nonlinear, then the kernels can be considered local approximations. If the system is bilinear, they are globally exact. It is important to remember that the estimation of the kernels does not assume any form for the state equation and completely eschews the states. This is the power of as well as weakness of Volterra-based analyses.

The Volterra formulation can be used directly in the assessment of effective connectivity if we assume the measured response of one region (j) constitutes the input to another (i); that is, $u_i(x) = y_j(t)$. In this case the Volterra kernels have a special interpretation; they are synonymous with effective connectivity. From Eq. (53.6) the first-order kernels are

$$
\kappa_1(\sigma_1) = \frac{\partial y_i(t)}{\partial y_j(t-\sigma_1)} = E_j^i(\sigma_1) \tag{53.10}
$$

Extensions of Eq. (53.6) to MISO models are trivial and allow high-order interactions among inputs to a single region to be characterised. This approach was used in Friston and Büchel (2000) to examine parietal modulation of V2 inputs to V5, by estimating and making inferences about the appropriate second-order kernel. The advantage of the Volterra approach is that nonlinearities can be modelled and estimated in the context of highly nonlinear transformations within a region and yet the estimation and inference proceed in a standard linear least-squares setting. However, one has to assume that the inputs conform to measured responses elsewhere in the brain. This may be tenable for EEG but the hemodynamic responses measured by fMRI make this a more questionable approach. Furthermore, there is no causal model of the interactions among areas that would otherwise offer useful constraints on the estimation. The direct application of Volterra estimation, in this fashion, simply examines each node, one at a time, assuming the activities of other nodes are veridical measurements of the inputs to the node in question. In summary, although the Volterra kernels are useful characterisations of the input–output behaviour of single regions, they are not constrained by any model of interactions among regions. Before turning to DCMs, which embody these interactions, we deal with the SISO situation in which the input is treated as stochastic.

Models for Stochastic Inputs: Coherence and Polyspectral Analysis

In this section we deal with systems in which the input is stochastic. The aim is to estimate the kernels (or their spectral equivalents) given only statistics about the joint distribution of the inputs and outputs. When the inputs are unknown one generally makes assumption about their distributional properties and assumes (local) stationariness. Alternatively, the inputs may be measurable but too noisy to serve as inputs in Eq. (53.7). In this case they can be used to estimate the input and output densities in terms of higher order cumulants or polyspectral density. The nth-order cumulate of the input is

$$c_u\{\sigma_1,\ldots,\sigma_{i-1}\} = \langle u(t)u(t-\sigma_1),\ldots,u(t-\sigma_{n-1})\rangle \tag{53.11}$$

where we have assumed here and throughout that $E\{u(t)\} = 0$. It can be seen that cumulants are a generalisation of autocovariance functions. The second-order cumulant is simply the autocovariance function of lag and summarises the stationary second-order behaviour of the input. Cumulants allow one to formulate Eq. (53.6) in terms of the second-order statistics of input and outputs. For example,

$$\begin{aligned} c_{yu}(\sigma_a) &= \langle y(t)u(t-\sigma_a)\rangle \\ &= \sum_i \int_0^t \ldots \int_0^t \kappa_i(\sigma_1,\ldots,\sigma_i)\langle u(t-\sigma_a)u(t-\sigma_1)\ldots u(t-\sigma_i)\rangle d\sigma_1\ldots d\sigma_i \\ &= \sum_i \int_0^t \ldots \int_0^t \kappa_i(\sigma_1,\ldots,\sigma_i)c_u(\sigma_a-\sigma_1,\ldots,\sigma-\sigma_i)d\sigma_1\ldots d\sigma_i \end{aligned} \tag{53.12}$$

which says that the cross-covariance between the output and the input can be decomposed into components that are formed by convolving the ith-order kernel with the input's $(i+1)$th cumulant. The important thing about this is that all cumulants, greater than second order, of Gaussian processes are zero. This means that if we can assume the input is Gaussian then

$$c_{yu}(\sigma_a) = \int_0^t \kappa_i(\sigma_1)c_u(\sigma_a-\sigma_1)d\sigma_1 \tag{53.13}$$

In other words, the cross-covariance between the input and output is simply the autocovariance function of the inputs convolved with the first-order kernel. Although it is possible to formulate the covariance between inputs and outputs in terms of cumulants, the more conventional formulation is in frequency space using polyspectra. The nth polyspectrum is the Fourier transform of the corresponding cumulant:

$$g_u(\omega_1,\ldots,\omega_{n-1}) = \left(\tfrac{1}{2\pi}\right)^{n-1}\int\ldots\int c_u\{\sigma_1,\ldots,\sigma_{n-1}\}e^{-j(\omega\sigma_1,\ldots,\omega\sigma_{n-1})}d\sigma_1\ldots d\sigma_{n-1} \tag{53.14}$$

Again, polyspectra are simply a generalisation of spectral densities. For example, the second polyspectrum is spectral density and the third polyspectrum is bispectral density. It can be seen that these relationships are generalisations of the Wiener–Khinchine theorem, relating the autocovariance function and spectral density through the Fourier transform. Introducing the spectral density representation,

$$u(t) = \int s_u(\omega)e^{-j\omega}d\omega \tag{53.15}$$

we can now rewrite the Volterra expansion, Eq. (53.6), as

$$h(u,\theta) = \sum_i \int_{-\pi}^{\pi}\ldots\int_{-\pi}^{\pi} e^{j(\omega_1+,\ldots,+\omega_i)t}\Gamma_1(\omega_1,\ldots,\omega_i)s_u(\omega_1),\ldots,s_u(\omega_i)d\omega_1,\ldots,d\omega_i \tag{53.16}$$

where the functions

$$\begin{aligned} \Gamma_1(\omega_1) &= \int_0^\infty e^{-j\omega_1\sigma_1}\kappa_1(\sigma_1)d\sigma_1 \\ \Gamma_2(\omega_1,\omega_2) &= \int_0^\infty\int_0^\infty e^{-j(\omega_1\sigma_1+\omega_2\sigma_2)}\kappa_2(\sigma_1,\sigma_2)d\sigma_1 d\sigma_2 \\ &\ldots \end{aligned}$$

are the Fourier transforms of the kernels. These functions are called *generalised transfer functions* and mediate the expression of frequencies in the output given those in the input. Critically, the influence of higher order kernels, or equivalently generalised transfer functions, means that a given frequency in the input can induce a *different* frequency in the output. A simple example of this would be squaring a sine-wave input to produce an output of twice the frequency. In the Volterra approach, the kernels were identified in the time domain using the inputs and outputs directly. In this section system identification means estimating their Fourier transforms (i.e., the transfer functions) using second-order and higher order statistics of the inputs and outputs. Generalised transfer functions are usually estimated through estimates of polyspectra. For example, the spectral form for Eq. (53.13) and its high-order counterparts are

$$\begin{aligned} g_{uy}(-\omega_1) &= \Gamma_1(\omega_1)g_u(\omega_1) \\ g_{uuy}(-\omega_1,-\omega_2) &= 2\Gamma_2(\omega_1,\omega_2)g_u(\omega_1)g_u(\omega_2) \\ &\vdots \\ g_{u\ldots y}(-\omega_1),\ldots,-\omega_n) &= n!\Gamma_n(\omega_1,\ldots,\omega_n)g_u(\omega_1)\ldots g_u(\omega_n) \end{aligned} \tag{53.17}$$

Given estimates of the requisite cross-polyspectra, these equalities can be used to provide estimates of the transfer functions (see Fig. 53.2). These equalities hold when the Volterra expansion contains just the nth-order term and the equalities are a generalisation of the classical results for the transfer function of a linear system [first equality in Eq. (53.17)]. The importance of these results, in terms of effective connectivity, is the implicit meaning conferred on *coherence* and *bicoherence* analyses. Coherence is simply the second-order cross-spectrum $g_{uy}(\omega)$ between the input and output and is related to first-order effects (i.e., the first-order kernel or transfer function) through Eq. (53.17). Coherence is therefore a surrogate marker for first-order or linear connectivity. Bicoherence or the cross-bispectrum $g_{uy}(\omega_1,\omega_2)$ is the third-order cross-polyspectrum and implies a nonzero second-order kernel or transfer function. Bispectral analysis was used (in a simplified form) to demonstrate nonlinear coupling between parietal and frontal regions using MEG in Chapter 51. In this example cross-bispectra were estimated, in a simple fashion, using time-frequency analyses.

Summary

In summary, Volterra kernels (generalised transfer functions) characterise the input–output behaviour of a system. The nth-order kernel is equivalent to nth-order effective connectivity when the inputs and outputs conform to processes that mediate interactions among neuronal systems. If the inputs and outputs are known, or can be measured precisely, the estimation of the kernels is straightforward. In situations where inputs and outputs are less precisely observed, kernels can be estimated indirectly through their generalised transfer functions using cross-polyspectra. The robustness of kernel estimation, conferred by expansion in terms of temporal basis functions, is recapitulated in the frequency domain by smoothness constraints during estimation of the polyspectra. The spectral approach is limited because it assumes (1) the system contains only the kernel of the order estimated and (2) stationariness. The intuition behind the first limitation relates to the distinction between parameter estimation and variance partitioning in standard regression analyses. Although it is perfectly possible to estimate the parameters of a regression model given a set of nonorthogonal explanatory variables, it is not possible to uniquely partition variance in the output caused by these explanatory variables.

INPUT–STATE–OUTPUT MODELS FOR MULTIPLE REGIONS

In this section we address models for multiple interconnected regions where one can measure the responses of these regions to input that may or may not be known. Although it is possible to extend the techniques of the previous sections to cover MIMO systems, the ensuing inferences about the influence of input to one region on the response of another are not sufficiently specified to constitute an analysis of effective connectivity. This is because these influences may be mediated in many ways and are not parameterised in terms of the effective connectivity among the regions themselves. In short, one is not interested in the vertical relationship between multiple inputs and multiple outputs, but in the horizontal interactions among the state variables of each region (Fig. 53.1). A parameterisation that encodes this interregional coupling is therefore required. All of the models discussed below assume some form or model for the interactions among the state variables and attempt to estimate the parameters of this model, sometimes without actually observing the states themselves.

Models for Known Inputs: Dynamic Causal Modelling

The most direct and generic approach is to estimate directly the parameters of Eq. (53.3) and use them to compute effective connectivity as described in Eqs. (53.1) and (53.2). Although there are many forms one could adopt for Eq. (53.3), we focus on the bilinear approximation, which is possibly the most parsimonious but useful nonlinear approximation available. Furthermore, as shown below, the bilinear approximation reparameterises the state equations of the model directly in terms of effective connectivity. Dynamic causal modelling does not necessarily entail the use of a bilinear model. Indeed DCMs can be specified to any degree of biological complexity and realism supported by the data. However, bilinear approximations represent the simplest form to which all DCMs can be reduced. This reduction allows analytic derivation of kernels and other computations, like integrating the state equation, to proceed in an efficient fashion.

Each region may comprise several state variables whose casual interdependencies are summarised by the bilinear form in Eq. (53.4). Here the key connectivity parameters of the state equation are the matrices M and N. For a given set of inputs or experimental context, the bilinear approximation to any set of state equations is

$$\begin{aligned} \dot{X}(t) &= JX(t) \\ X(t+\sigma) &= e^{J\sigma}X(t) \\ J &= M + \sum_i N_i u_i \end{aligned} \qquad (53.18)$$

Notice that there are now as many N matrices as there are multiple inputs. The bilinear form reduces the model to first-order connections that can be modulated by the inputs. In MIMO models the effective connectivity is among the states such that first-order effective connectivities are simply

$$\begin{aligned} \dot{E} &= \frac{\partial \dot{X}}{\partial X} = J \\ E &= \frac{\partial X(t)}{\partial X(t+\sigma)} = e^{J\sigma} \end{aligned} \qquad (53.19)$$

[This includes connections with the constant term in Eq. (53.5).] Note that these are context sensitive in the sense that the Jacobian J is a function of experimental context or inputs $u(t) = [u_1(t),\ldots u_m(t)]$. A useful way to think about the bilinear parameter matrices is to regard them as the intrinsic or latent dynamic connectivity, in the absence of input, and changes induced by each input (see the previous chapter for a fuller description):

$$\begin{aligned} \dot{E}(0) &= M = \begin{bmatrix} 0 & 0 \\ f(0) & A \end{bmatrix} \\ \frac{\partial \dot{E}}{\partial u_i} &= N_i = \begin{bmatrix} 0 & 0 \\ C_i & B_i \end{bmatrix} \end{aligned} \qquad (53.20)$$

The latent dynamic connectivity among the states is A. Often one is more interested in the B_i as embodying changes in this connectivity induced by a different cognitive set, time, or drugs. Note that C_i is treated as the input-dependent component of the connection from the constant term or drive. Clearly, it would be possible to introduce other high-order terms to model interactions among the states, but we restrict ourselves to bilinear models for simplicity.

The fundamental advantage of DCM over alternative strategies is that the casual structure is made explicit by parameterising the state equation. The estimation of effective connectivity and ensuing inferences are usually made through posterior mode analysis based on normality assumptions about the errors and some suitable priors on the parameters. The parameters of the bilinear form are $\theta = \{A,B,C,L\}$. If the priors are also specified under Gaussian assumptions, in terms of their expectation η_θ and covariance C_θ, a Gauss–Newton EM scheme can be adopted to find the posterior mode $\eta_{\theta|y}$ (see the previous chapter for details).

In essence, dynamic causal modelling comprises the following:

1. Specification of the state and output equations of an ensemble of region-specific state variables. A bilinear approximation to the state equation reduces the model to first-order coupling and bilinear terms that represent the modulation of that coupling by inputs.

2. Posterior density analysis of the model parameters then allows one to estimate and make inferences about interregional connections and the effect of experimental manipulations on those connections.

As mentioned above, the state equations do not have to conform to the bilinear form. The bilinear form can be computed automatically given any state equation. This is important because the priors may be specified more naturally in terms of the original biophysical parameters of the DCM, as opposed to the bilinear form. The choice of the state variables clearly has to accommodate their role in mediating the effect of inputs on responses and the interactions among areas. In the simplest case the states variables could be reduced to mean neuronal activity per region, plus any biophysical state variables needed to determine the output (e.g., the states of hemodynamic models for fMRI). Implicit in choosing such state variables is the assumption that they model all of the dynamics to the level of detail required. Mean field models and neural mass models are useful here in motivating the number of state variables and the associated state equations. Constraints on the parameters of the model are implemented through their priors. These restrict the parameter estimates to plausible ranges. An important constraint is that the system is dissipative and does not diverge exponentially in the absence of input. In other words, the priors ensure that the largest eigenvalue of J is less than zero.

Summary

In summary, DCM is the most general and direct approach to identifying the effective connectivity among the states of MIMO systems. The identification of DCMs usually proceeds using Bayesian schemes to estimate the posterior mode or most likely parameters of the model given the data. Posterior mode analysis requires only the state equations and priors to be specified. The state equations can be arbitrarily complicated and nonlinear. However, a bilinear approximation to the causal influences among state variables serves to reduce the complexity of the model and parameterises the model directly in terms of first-order connectivity and its changes with input (the bilinear terms). In the next section we deal the situations in which the input is unknown. This precludes DCM because the likelihood of the responses cannot be computed unless we know what caused them.

Models for Stochastic Inputs: SEM and Regression Models

When the inputs are treated as unknown, and the statistics of the outputs are only considered to second order, one is effectively restricted to linear or first-order models of effective connectivity. Although it is possible to deal with discrete-time bilinear models, with white noise inputs, they have the same covariance structure as ARMA (autoregressive moving average) models of the same order (Priestly, 1988, p. 66). This means that, in order to distinguish between linear and nonlinear models, one would need to study moments higher than second order (cf. the third-order cumulants in bicoherence analyses). Consequently, we focus on linear models of effective connectivity under white stationary inputs. These inputs are the innovations introduced in Chapter 53. There are two important classes of model here: structural equation models and ARMA models. Both are finite parameter linear models that are distinguished by their dependency on dynamics. In SEM the interactions are assumed to be instantaneous, whereas in ARMA the dynamic aspect is retained explicitly in the model.

SEM can be derived from DCMs by assuming the inputs vary slowly in relation to neuronal and hemodynamics. This is appropriate for PET experiments and possibly some epoch-related fMRI designs but not for event-related designs in ERP or fMRI. Note that this assumption pertains to the inputs or experimental design, not to the time constants of the outputs. In principle, it would be possible to apply DCM to a PET study.

Consider a linear DCM where we can observe the states precisely and where there is only one state variable per region:

$$\begin{aligned} \dot{x} &= f(x,u) \\ &= Ax + u = (A^0 - 1)x + u \\ y &= \lambda(x) = x \end{aligned} \tag{53.21}$$

Here we have discounted observation error but allow stochastic inputs $u \sim N(0,Q)$. To make the connection to SEMs more explicit, we have expanded the connectivity matrix into off-diagonal connections and a leading diagonal matrix, modelling unit decay $A = A^0 - 1$. For simplicity, we have absorbed C into the covariance structure of the inputs Q. Because the inputs are changing slowly relative to the dynamics, the change in states will be zero at the point of observation and we obtain the regression model used by SEM:

$$\begin{aligned} \dot{x} &= 0 \Rightarrow \\ (1 - A^0)x &= u \\ x &= (1 - A^0)^{-1}u \end{aligned} \tag{53.22}$$

This should be compared with Eq. (50.17) in Chapter 50. The more conventional motivation for Eq. (53.22) is to start with an instantaneous regression equation $x = A^0x + u$ that is formally identical to the second line above. Although this regression model obscures the connection with dynamic formulations, it is important to consider because it is the basis of commonly employed methods for estimating effective connectivity in neuroimaging to data. These are simple regression models and SEM.

Simple Regression Models

The equation $x = A^0x + u$ can be treated as a general linear model by focussing on one region at a time, for example, the first, to give

$$x_1 = [x_2, \ldots, x_n] \begin{bmatrix} A_{12} \\ \vdots \\ A_{1n} \end{bmatrix} + u_1 \tag{53.23}$$

[cf. Eq. (50.8) in Chapter 50]. The elements of A can then be solved in a least-squares sense by minimising the norm of the unknown stochastic inputs u for that region (i.e., by minimising the unexplained variance of the target region given the states of the remainder). This approach was proposed in Friston (1995) and has the advantage of providing precise estimates of connectivity with high degrees of freedom. However, these least-square estimators assume, rather implausibly, that the inputs are orthogonal to the states and, more importantly, do not ensure the inputs to different regions conform to the known covariance Q. Furthermore, there is no particular reason that the input variance should be minimised just because it is unknown. Structural equation modelling overcomes these limitations at the cost of degrees of freedom for efficient estimation

Structural Equation Modelling

In SEM estimates of A^0 minimise the difference (KL divergence) between the observed covariance among the observable states and that implied by the model and assumptions about the inputs:

$$\begin{aligned} \langle xx^T \rangle &= \langle (1 - A^0)^{-1}uu^T(1 - A^0)^{-1T} \rangle \\ &= (1 - A^0)^{-1}Q(1 - A^0)^{-1T} \end{aligned} \tag{53.24}$$

This is critical because the connectivity estimates implicitly minimise the discrepancy between the observed and implied covariances among the states induced by stochastic inputs. This is in contradistinction to the instantaneous regression approach (above) or ARMA analyses (below) in which the estimates simply minimise unexplained variance on a region-by-region basis.

Quasi-Bilinear Models: PPIs and Moderator Variables

There is a useful extension to the regression model implicit in Eq. (53.22) that includes bilinear terms formed from known inputs that are distinct from stochastic inputs inducing covariance in the states. Let these known inputs be denoted by v. These usually represent some manipulated experimental context such as cognitive set (e.g., attention) or time. These deterministic inputs are also known as *moderator variables* in SEM. The underlying quasi-bilinear DCM, for one such input, is

$$\dot{x} = (A^0 - 1)x + Bvx + u \tag{53.25}$$

Again, assuming the system has settled at the point of observation

$$\begin{aligned} \dot{x} &= 0 \\ (1 - A^0 - Bv)x &= u \\ x &= A^0x + Bvx + u \end{aligned} \tag{53.26}$$

This regression equation can be used to form least-squares estimates as in Eq. (53.23) in which case the additional bilinear regressors vx are known as *psychophysiological interaction* (PPI) terms (for obvious reasons). The corresponding SEM or path analysis usually proceeds by creating extra "virtual" regions whose dynamics correspond to the bilinear terms. This is motivated by rewriting the last expression in Eq. (53.26) as

$$\begin{bmatrix} x \\ vx \end{bmatrix} = \begin{bmatrix} A^0 & B \\ 0 & 1 \end{bmatrix} \begin{bmatrix} x \\ vx \end{bmatrix} + \begin{bmatrix} u \\ 0 \end{bmatrix} \tag{53.27}$$

It is important to note that psychophysiological interactions and moderator variables in SEM are exactly the same thing and both speak to the importance of bilinear terms in casual models. Their relative success in the neuroimaging literature is probably due to the fact that they model changes in effective connectivity that are generally much more interesting than the connection strengths *per se*. Examples are changes induced by attentional modulation, changes during procedural learning, and changes mediated pharmacologically. In other words, bilinear components afford ways of characterising *plasticity* and as such play a key role in methods for functional integration. It is for this reason we focussed on bilinear approximations as a minimal DCM in the previous section.

Summary

In summary, SEM is a simple and pragmatic approach to effective connectivity when (1) dynamical aspects can be discounted, (2) a linear model is sufficient, (3) the state variables can be measured precisely, and (4) the input is unknown but stochastic and stationary. These assumptions are imposed by ignorance about the inputs. Some of these represent rather severe restrictions that limit the utility of SEM in relation to DCM or state-space models considered next. The most profound criticism of simple regression and SEM in imaging neuroscience is that they are models for interacting brain systems in the context of unknown input. The whole point of designed experiments is that the inputs are known and under experimental control. This renders the utility of SEM for designed experiments somewhat questionable.

MULTIVARIATE ARMA MODELS

ARMA models can be generally represented as *state-space* (or *Markovian*) models that provide a compact description of any finite parameter linear model. From this state-space representation, MAR models can be derived and estimated using a variety of well-established techniques. We focus on how the state-space representation of linear models of effective connectivity can be derived from the dynamic formulation and the assumptions required in this derivation.

As in the previous section, let us assume a linear DCM in which inputs comprise stationary white noise $u \sim N(0,Q)$ that are offered to each region in equal strength (i.e., $C = 1$). This renders Eq. (53.3) a linear stochastic differential equation (SDE):

$$\begin{aligned} \dot{x} &= Ax + u \\ y &= Lx \end{aligned} \tag{53.28}$$

The value of x at some future lag comprises a deterministic and a stochastic component η that is obtained by regarding the effects of the input as a cumulation of local linear perturbations:

$$\begin{aligned} x(t + \tau) &= e^{\tau A}x(t) + \eta \\ \eta &= \int_0^\tau e^{\sigma A}u(t + \sigma)d\sigma \end{aligned} \tag{53.29}$$

Using the assumption that the input is serially uncorrelated,

$$\langle u(t+\sigma_1)u(t+\sigma_2)^T\rangle = \begin{cases} Q, & \sigma_1 = \sigma_2 \\ 0, & \sigma_1 \neq \sigma_2 \end{cases}$$

the covariance of the stochastic part is

$$\begin{aligned} W &= \langle \eta\eta^T \rangle \\ &= \left\langle \int_0^\tau e^{\tau_1 A} u(t+\sigma_1)d\sigma_1 \int_0^\tau u(t+\sigma_2)^T e^{\tau_2 A^T} d\sigma_2 \right\rangle \\ &= \int_0^\tau e^{\sigma A} \langle u(t+\sigma)u(t+\sigma)^T \rangle e^{\sigma A^T} d\sigma \\ &= \int_0^\tau e^{\sigma A} Q e^{\sigma A^T} d\sigma \end{aligned} \tag{53.30}$$

We can see that when the lag is small $e^{\sigma A} \rightarrow 1$ and $W \approx Q$.

Equation (53.29) is simply a MAR(1) model that could be subject to the usual analysis procedures:

$$x_{t+1} = e^{\tau A} x_t + \eta_t \tag{53.31}$$

By incorporating the output transformation and observation error we can augment this AR(1) model to a full state-space model with system matrix $F = e^{\tau A}$, input matrix $G = \sqrt{W}$, and observation matrix L:

$$\begin{aligned} x_t &= Fx_{t-1} + Gz_t \\ y_t &= Lx_t + \varepsilon_t \end{aligned} \tag{53.32}$$

where z is some white innovation that models dynamically transformed stochastic input u. This formulation would be appropriate if the state variables were not directly accessible and observation noise ε_t was large in relation to system noise z_t.

A first-order AR(1) model is sufficient to completely model effective connectivity if we could observe all of the states with reasonable precision. In situations where only some of the states are observed, it is possible to compensate for lack of knowledge about the missing states by increasing the order of the model:

$$\begin{aligned} x_t &= F_1 x_{t-1} + \ldots + F_p x_{t-p} + Gz_t \\ y_t &= Lx_t + \varepsilon_t \end{aligned} \tag{53.33}$$

Similar devices are using in the reconstruction of attractor using temporal embedding at various lags. Note that increasing the order does not render the model nonlinear, it simply accommodates the possibility that each region's dynamics may be governed by more than one state variable. However, increasing model order loses any direct connection with formal models of effective connectivity because it is not possible to transform an AR(p) model into a unique DCM. Having said that, AR(p) models may be very useful in establishing the presence of coupling even if the exact form of the coupling is not specified (cf. Volterra characterisations).

In summary, discrete-time linear models of effective connectivity can be reduced to multivariate AR(1) or, more generally, ARMA(1,1) models, whose coefficients can be estimated given only the states (or outputs) by assuming the inputs are white Gaussian and enter with the same strength at each node. They therefore operate under the same assumptions as SEM but are true time-series models. The problem is that MAR coefficients in F can only be interpreted as effective connections when (1) the dynamics are linear and (2) all the states can be observed through the observation matrix. In this case,

$$E = \frac{\partial x_t}{\partial x_{t-1}} = F = e^{\tau A} \tag{53.34}$$

Compare with Eq. (53.19). However, high-order MAR(p) do represent a useful way of establishing statistical dependencies among the responses, irrespective of how they are caused.

CONCLUSION

We have reviewed a series of models, all of which can be formulated as special cases of DCMs. Two fundamental distinctions organise these models. The first is whether they pertain to the coupling of inputs and outputs by the nonlinear transformations enacted among hidden states of a single region or whether one is modelling the lateral interactions among the state variables of several systems, each with its own inputs and outputs. The second distinction (see Fig. 53.2) is that between models that require the inputs to be fixed and deterministic as in designed experiments and those for which the input is not under experimental control but can be assumed to be well behaved (usually i.i.d. Gaussian). Given only information about density of the inputs, or the joint density of the inputs and outputs, imposes limitations on the model of effective connectivity adopted. Unless one embraces moments greater than second order only linear models can be estimated.

Many methods for nonlinear system identification and casual modelling have been developed in situations where the system's input was not under experimental control and, in the case of SEM, not necessarily for time-series data. Volterra kernels and DCMs may be especially useful in neuroimaging because we deal explicitly with time-series data generated by designed experiments.

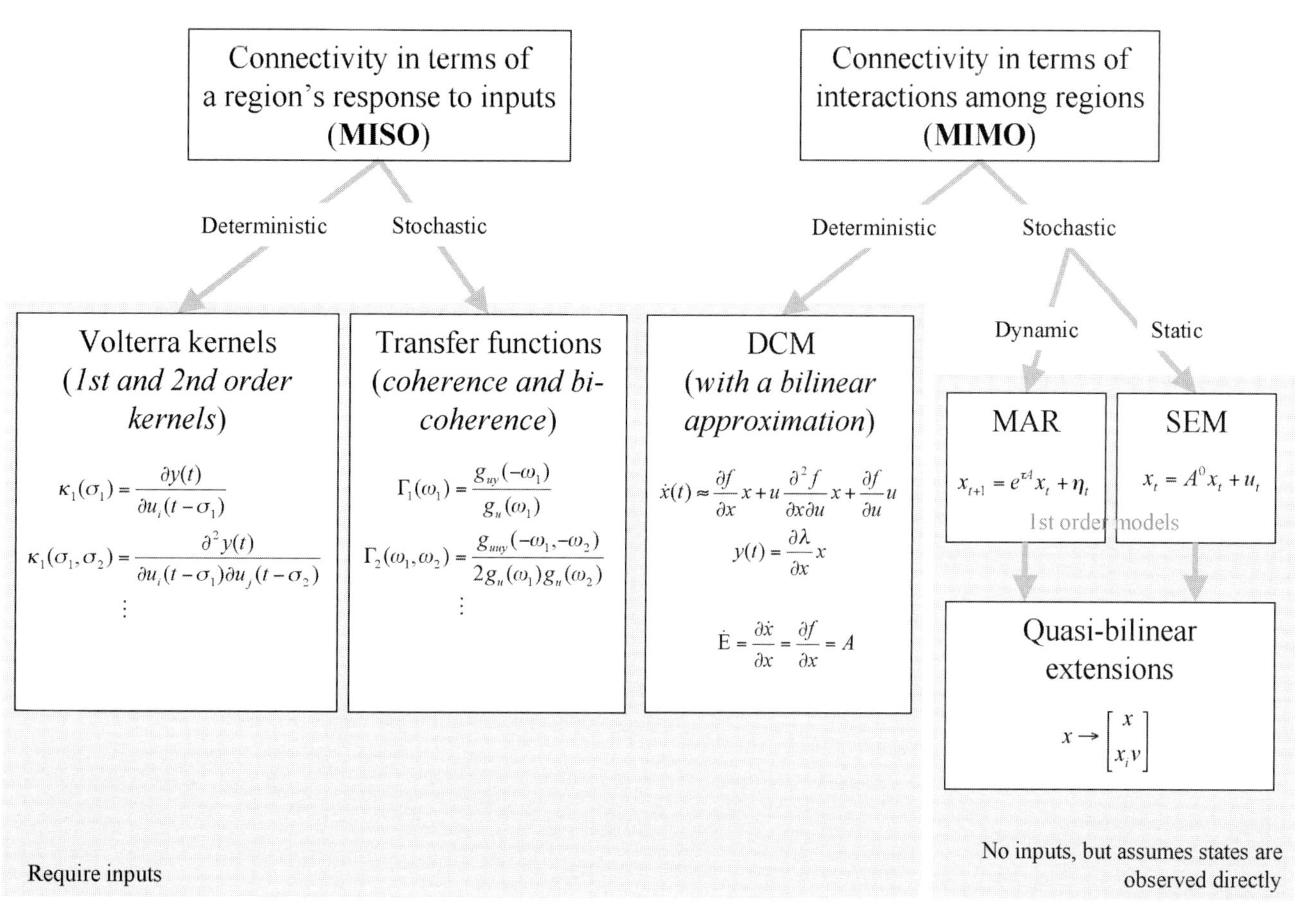

FIGURE 53.2
Overview of the models considered in this chapter. They have been organised to reflect their dependence on whether the inputs are known or not and whether the model is a time-series model or not.

References

Bendat, J. S. (1990). *Nonlinear System Analysis and Identification from Random Data.* John Wiley and Sons, New York.

Fliess, M., Lamnabhi, M., and Lamnabhi-Lagarrigue, F. (1983). An algebraic approach to nonlinear functional expansions. *IEEE Trans. Circuits Syst.* **30,** 554–570.

Friston, K. J. (1995). Functional and effective connectivity in neuroimaging: a synthesis. *Hum. Brain Mapping* **2,** 56–78.

Friston, K. J., and Büchel, C. (2000). Attentional modulation of V5 in human. *Proc. Natl. Acad. Sci. USA* **97,** 7591–7596.

Friston, K. J. (2002). Bayesian estimation of dynamical systems: an application to fMRI. *NeuroImage* **16,** 465–483.

Priestly, M. B. (1988). *Non-Linear and Non-Stationary Time-Series Analysis*. Academic Press, London.

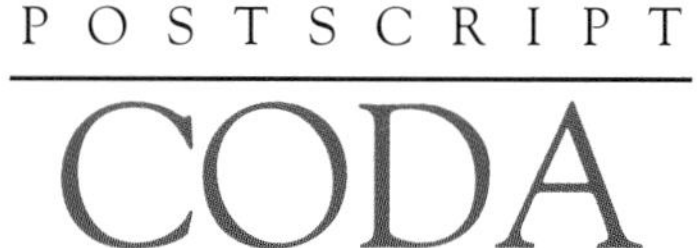

Mapping Brain Mappers: An Ethnographic Coda

SCIENTIFIC TRIBES

For more than two decades, anthropologists, sociologists, and ethnographers have increasingly turned their attention to a novel class of hitherto undescribed tribes (Bourdieu, 1975; Knorr-Cetina, 1981, 1999; Latour and Woolgar, 1979; Nader, 1996; Pickering, 1992). In stark contrast with the traditional objects of ethnographic inquiry, these people are not usually found in remote and isolated locations such as barren mountain valleys, deep jungles, or distant islands. On the contrary, they normally reside if not in, then near the political, economical, and cultural centres of the world, and they are strongly interconnected through multidimensional webs of material, symbolic. and personal links.

Apart from these differences in the spatial and connective topography, these new subjects, who may loosely be grouped under the heading of *scientists,* share many traits with the traditional ethnographic objects. They appear to create and constitute semiautonomous, self-organised fields within the modern world—vehemently guarding their particular criteria of inclusion and exclusion and their principles of truth. They usually see themselves as an integral part of a distinct tradition, defined in part by the forefathers who they acknowledge.

As with all other lineages, the forefathers they actively identify with constitute but one selection of the potential sum of previous connections (Bourdieu, 1977). This suggests that the adherence to a tradition and the acknowledgement of a certain lineage is an active process of self-identification as much as a passive reproduction of that "which is and always has been." In this respect also, these novel objects and subjects of ethnographic inquiry are very much like the traditional objects of study (Otto and Pedersen, 2000). Through this highly particular selection of legacy and inheritance,[1] they construct a distinct identity both in relation to other, parallel scientific fields and to society at large.

BRAIN MAPPING CULTURE

Brain imaging is one of the youngest and most rapidly developing scientific fields. It emerges at the intersection of a variety of well-established disciplines, from anatomy, neurobiology, and psychology to physics, computer science, and theoretical biology, while touching on philosophy

[1] Who would you choose of the following: Darwin, Descartes, Freud, Goethe, Helmholtz, Lamarck, Pavlov, Vygotsky, Wernicke, or Wundt? What would be the genealogy of the gurus and the heretics in the field, and what about the outsiders?

and perhaps even religion. Its working methods and ideas are as bizarre and counterintuitive as some of the most extreme human practices and cosmologies described by anthropologists. Brain mappers turn individual persons into experimental subjects and put them into narrow tunnels. They expose them to strange stimuli and bombard them with invisible rays and forces. Finally, they claim that this can reveal the true, objective nature of the workings, not only of their subjects' minds, but of everybody's mind. This redraws the boundary between nature and culture by showing humans to be very much like animals—anatomically, physiologically, and functionally—and yet also to be very unique with highly particular and specific abilities like mind-reading, cheating, and feeling empathy.

The field is conceptually both empirical and imperialist as it expands its examinations into areas hitherto claimed by other scientific traditions. It scrutinises every conceivable variety of human interest from beauty, love, and aesthetics via culture, language, and religion to fear, sex, and hunger. While it attempts to tear apart well-established ideas and thought constructions, it is itself struggling with cosmology making as it replaces old narratives with new ones.

Does a novel, heterogeneous field like human brain mapping qualify as a distinct culture? People in brain imaging seem at times to think so. Visiting anthropologists and ethnographers routinely hear them refer to their own interactions in laboratories, at conferences, and on the Internet as taking place "within their own culture." For a numbers of reasons internal to their tradition (Kuper, 1999) anthropologists have, however, during the last decades been increasingly hesitant to use the notion of culture as an analytical concept. One of the problems is that culture is no longer something anthropologists may simply study as a passive phenomenon that people just have. "Culture" is increasingly something that groups of people everywhere—from the boardrooms of multinational corporations to the plenitude of postcolonial "ethnic" groupings to the various subniches of modern cosmopolitan life—claim to possess. Should anthropologists believe that there really is a distinct brain mapper culture, just because brain mappers themselves claim to have one? At present there is no agreed answer within the anthropological tradition. The problem is, as suggested by the historian of science Ian Hacking (1999), that most human categories are interactive kinds that, in contrast with the indifferent kinds of most natural sciences, are changed by being described. The short argument is that representing is a way of intervening and people generally react to being intervened with. This complicates the object–observer relationship. Consequently, anthropologists have been on the lookout for other conceptual interfaces that may encompass those elements of interaction and intervening. This is fundamental to the discipline's call for participant-observation.

One suggestion is for anthropologists to leave "culture" to the natives, forget it as an analytical concept, and turn their attention to something else, for instance, knowledge (Barth, 2002; Roepstorff, 2001b). This analytical stance presents knowledge as an empirical problem to be examined: What is it that a certain group considers to be knowledge? Who would actually take this to be true and/or useful? How do they go about establishing this as knowledge?

BRAIN MAPPER FACTS, THOUGHT COLLECTIVES, AND STYLES

One of the forefathers of this empirical approach to the study of scientific knowledge was the Polish-Jewish serologist Ludwik Fleck (1896–1961). His interwar monograph *Genesis and Development of a Scientific Fact* (Fleck, 1979; originally published in German in, 1935) did not receive much attention at the time of publication, and it disappeared into oblivion after World War II. At a time when most sociologists, philosophers, and ethnographers "exhibit an excessive respect, bordering on pious reverence for scientific facts" (Fleck, 1979, p. 47), Fleck stated that scientific facts were not radically different from all other facts. Rather, he argued, facts were always made within thought collectives endowed with particular thought styles. Fleck claimed that most thought collectives, regardless of whether they were scientific, artistic, "primitive," etc., came to share a general topography as they stabilised. Around "thought formations," i.e., central ideas, theories, and other works of the mind, two circles of thought collective members spontaneously form: a small esoteric one and a larger exoteric one. There is usually a hierarchical initiation into the esoteric circle, and the exoteric circle has no direct link with the thought formation. Instead, the relation is mediated through the esoteric circle. This means that for most members of the thought collective, the relation to central ideas and tenets relies on trust in the initiated. A thought collective usually consists of several intersecting circles of this kind, and most individuals belong to several exoteric and fewer, if any, esoteric circles. According to Fleck, each of these esoteric circles is characterised by a certain style displayed in how observations are made and used, in what is considered obvious, and in how findings are presented.

As the brain imaging field has evolved and stabilised during the last decade or so, its topology seems increasingly comparable to Fleck's analysis of scientific thought collectives. The book, which you are currently reading, is a representation of some of the central thought formations in the brain imaging field. A small esoteric circle of initiated contributors reverberates around it, surrounded by a larger circle of exoteric participants. The latter may very well use the methods and ideas represented, but they usually have to trust the esoteric circle and the effectiveness of its methods. The contours of this exoteric circle can be roughly sketched by analysing principal components in patterns of references (Nielsen, 2001) or by mapping the subscribers and participants in the Internet-based debate forums and helplines.

In Canada, the United States, continental Europe, Scandinavia, and Asia, similar esoteric centres partly share and partly create their own esoteric and exoteric members and conglomerates of ideas, techniques, and methods. Researchers, students, technologies, and ideas are shuttling back and forth between these centres. At the grand international meetings, such as the Human Brain Mapping conference, these minicollectives, which over the year may exist mainly in the virtual space of the Internet, get very concrete as people, apparently spontaneously, form small groups at receptions and dinners. They exchange news, gossip, and stories of who-is-where and how-things-are-going.[2] As with clan-like organisations everywhere, most recently seen in Afghanistan, the boundaries between the various centres are not fixed. Rather, the groupings and alliances depend very much on the scale and the context. In one situation, it is "me against my brother"; on other occasions, "we" unite to fight "our cousins," only to group with them against those from "the next village," "the next clan," or "the next country." The most important outer boundary is probably the category of "scientists" in general. Although it may appear rather diffuse, it is more or less united by an ambition to inscribe oneself in *Science* or *Nature* understood both as concrete journals and as those abstract entities indicated by the names.

One of Fleck's central claims was that facts, once established, become " 'signs of resistance' shutting off some pathways of thought while allowing others to develop. As such, facts come to constitute an interlaced network in accordance with a certain thought style. This style helps to orient the fact -making process by providing a "directed perception with corresponding mental and objective assimilation of what has been so perceived. ... [It is] characterised by common features in the problems of interest ..., by the judgement which the thought collective considers obvious, and by the methods which it applies as a means of acquiring knowledge ... accompanied by a technical and literary style characteristic of the given system of knowledge" (Fleck, 1979, p. 99) .[3]

This element of style-boundness is not necessarily a hindrance to the actual research process. Working within and according to a particular style is essential not only for focussing attention, but also for establishing a thought collective—a peer group—that one may refer one's findings to for evaluation and recognition. In that respect also, brain imaging appears to be coming of age.

During the last decade, the methods applied as a means of acquiring knowledge in brain imaging have become increasingly standardised (Beaulieu, 2002). Articles published in the very best general journals, such as *Nature, Science, PNAS, New England Journal of Medicine,* the *Lancet,* and *Neuron,* demonstrate that PET and MR scanners are widely accepted in the general scientific field as valuable and valid tools for examining structural and functional parameters and for probing cognitive and psychological questions. Along with this general acceptance, the

[2] That the social organisation of researchers follows a pattern known from other thought collectives such as clerical organisations is evident from the metaphors used to describe central groups, persons and elements (e.g. "popes," "heretics," "the bible," "the monastery," "disciples," etc.). One of the esoteric centres in brain mapping is even physically located in "St. John's House," and pitched over the entrance, the Baptist's open hand blesses each person entering the building.

[3] After consulting the German original (Fleck, 1980, p. 130), a few changes have been made to the English translation in that *Erkenntnissmittel* is rendered as "a means of acquiring knowledge," rather than "a means of cognition," and *evident* as "obvious" rather than "evident."

methods are constantly being refined and reworked in the specialist journals of the field, such as *NeuroImage, Human Brain Mapping,* and the *Journal of Cerebral Blood Flow and Metabolism.* The implementation of basic principles of analysis in publicly available software packages allows for a rapid semiautomatic transformation of the massive sets of raw data into a few significant "blobs." This standardised path of analysis, with its sequence of alignment, normalisation, smoothing, filtering, modelling, and statistical analysis, ensures that a judgement that the thought collective considers obvious is rigorously applied to the data. This procedure allows for a directed perception of the data that separates the "blobs," which should be reported, from those "below-threshold-activations," which should not be publicly discussed and commented on. The former may then be mentally and objectively assimilated into the network of already established facts where they form new signs of resistance to be taken into account by the researchers.

LABORATORIES AND EXPERIMENTS

The basic idea in brain imaging is wonderfully simple. First you take a living brain, preferably human, and put it inside a scanner. Then you expose it to various kinds of stimuli and tasks, while you use the scanner and sophisticated mathematical models to pinpoint approximately where and when something measurable happened in the brain. There are, of course, all sorts of methodological difficulties and practical shortcomings, but the net result is that a whole range of internal, functional, and cognitive processes may suddenly be effectively studied experimentally in an almost traditional laboratory setting. But what is it that makes laboratories such powerful places?

The sociologist of science Karin Knorr-Cetina has claimed that a particular order is set up in laboratories "built upon upgrading the ordinary and mundane components of social life." They are places that "recast objects of investigation by inserting them into new temporal and territorial regimes" (Knorr-Cetina, 1999, p. 43). Laboratories are not a world apart; they are hyperversions of their contemporary society—places where apparently well-known phenomena, objects, and processes are reconfigured to allow for experiments to be made. Experiments generally treat the studied objects as "decomposable entities from which effects can be extracted through appropriate treatments" (Knorr-Cetina, 1999, p. 37). In this respect also the brain imaging field is an almost ideal exemplar of a general case, with one very important modification: A rather peculiar class of objects is studied.

The objects of a typical brain imaging experiment are concrete persons, who all agree to play a very particular role as an experimental subject who adheres to a highly structured script (Jack and Roepstorff, 2002; Roepstorff, 2001a). This role requires the person to enter into a highly confined space to be exposed to all sorts of invisible forces such as radioactivity, magnetic fields, and radio pulses. While staying virtually immobile, the person has to focus attention on various strange stimuli while responding in highly restricted ways that were specified before entering the scanner. Such is the amazing power of human curiosity, compliance, and helpfulness that many people happily agree to play this unusual role in the most conscientious manner while receiving in return just a picture of their brain and some symbolic monetary compensation.

It is the brains of these individuals, who agree to act as homogenous subjects stereotypically responding to stimuli, that form the objects in which effects are being studied. The effects are a result of the subjects' adherence to a strict regime, an experimental paradigm. The idea is that the precise temporal organisation of the paradigm and the fixed location of the brain make it possible to measure parameters that reflect the activity in the brain at a particular moment. These differential brain activities are related to the effects generated in the brain as a result of the paradigm—at least if the individual in the scanner has been a good and compliant subject and if the technique works well. The data then pass through long chains of mathematical transformations as discussed elsewhere in this book. At each step they lose locality, particularity, and materiality while simultaneously gaining compatibility, standardisation, and relative universality.

This simultaneous process of gain and loss, of reduction and amplification is a standard procedure in a knowledge-making process (Latour, 1999, pp. 68–73), and it is imperative that it be potentially reversible. The results are to be trusted because of the possibility of moving back and forth along this chain, because it is possible to reconstruct all steps between what enters a scanner—individual persons taking on a role as experimental subjects—and what comes out of the laboratory—objectivity to be inscribed in *Science* and *Nature* (Roepstorff, 2002).

The importance of this potential reversibility is clear from the literary style employed in brain imaging articles. Numerous references to previous works serve to show that even if the authors may not have studied or understood every step themselves, other persons that can be trusted have. This mechanism is part of the explanation behind the enormous importance given to science-citation-index-measurements not only by funding bodies, but also by the scientists themselves. A highly cited scientist is very likely to be an esoteric member of a thought collective. He is one to be trusted or, alternatively, to be disagreed with if one belongs to a different circle; and being esoteric in Fleck's sense is perhaps the strongest recognition a scientist can obtain.

ARE BRAIN MAPPER FACTS TRUE?

If we accept the reversibility of transformations as one important criterion for truth, are brain imaging results, then, to be trusted? Yes, the brain mapper will claim. Each step from the data being registered by the scanner to the representation of the significant findings in a colourful picture is carefully documented and scrutinised. It employs well-established methods from various fields, elegantly put together in one common process. The facts are therefore in principle to be trusted, although there may be some people out there who do not really understand what they are doing, thereby producing findings that are not altogether reliable.

Some neuroscientists disagree with this claim. They point out, e.g., that the metabolic and vascular measurements made with PET and fMRI are far downstream from the actual neural processes, and that the techniques are unable to discriminate between central neuronal mechanisms such as inhibition and excitation. They argue that the spatial and temporal resolutions are magnitudes above the relevant dimensions of neuronal processes. These claims question whether the "chain of transformations" followed by brain mappers begins in the right place. They suggest that one should begin much earlier: One should deal with the direct process whereby well-defined neurons or groups of neurons exchange signals mediated by subtle chemical and electrical changes.

The brain mapper's classic counter-answer is, of course, pragmatic:

We know that, but we have to start somewhere, and we will soon be able to approach to this level using the right tracers and scanner setups.

The outside observer, who cannot appreciate the technical details in these discussions, may want to extend the chain in a very different direction:

You guys may be very good at analysing what comes out of the scanner, but this is not where the experiment begins, is it? You start out with persons who are given a set of implicit and explicit instructions. If the person agrees to do it, this may, then, allow you to set up the task and the stimulus-response paradigm that the scanner is probing. You may of course analyse the data as if the task was all that went on. However, this task rides piggyback on a set of other processes that philosophers, semioticians, and phenomenologists have discussed for ages: questions of "subjective experience," sharing of meaning, exchange of interpretive frames, etc. You, on the other hand, act as if all there is in the scanner is a general brain-in-a-vat, and this is a highly unrealistic account of your own experiments. More importantly, the resulting general model of human brain function and of "human nature," which you are producing, isn't really that trustworthy. You ignore that it takes an awful lot of interpersonal exchange, sharing of meaning, institutions, technologies, and resources—in other words "culture"—to produce a picture of man as pure nature for the 21st century: a general and universal brain.

The brain mapper's standard answer to this claim seems to be:

We know that, but we have to start with the small questions. There are already people doing something they call neurophenomenology (Varela, 1996), neurosemiotics (Deacon, 1997), and neurodeconstruction (Globus, 1995), and it is not clear that it really leads them anywhere. What you are describing is, of course, the problem of consciousness, and as you probably know already, we have been studying that for quite a while. So if you have anything to say about these issues, why don't you just join the Association for the Scientific Study of Consciousness and try to come through with your slightly wacky ideas?

The brain mappers seem, in other words, to have very strong, straightforward arguments against criticisms. One of the merits of this position is that it ties together in a novel fashion well-established mainstream techniques. This allows a strong conceptual correspondence between the findings and already established bodies of knowledge. The net result becomes an extension of a standard scientific method. It allows for a biological gaze (Keller, 1996) that moves into entirely new fields that were not previously available for scientific representations. In this, the development of the techniques is reminiscent of the development of the microscope, which, by granting visibility to the smallest details, redefined the perception of life and death (Keller, 1996). Although the end result of brain imaging may look like a snapshot, the representation is digital all through. The relationship between the representation and the represented is therefore much more complicated than an old-fashioned photograph because it is generated by these long chains of transformations that are limited and guided by conventions as much as by physical constraints.

In this interesting combination of methods and concepts, of rigidity and flexibility, lies a strength of brain imaging. Almost any conceivable critique can be responded to in the same effective manner:

What you take to be a point of criticism will for us be a starting point for an examination, if we see a reliable difference somewhere in the brain, you are probably on to something, if not....

STYLISED CHOICES

The standard analytical trajectory is, of course, not the only one available, possible, or publishable. Each of the normal analytical steps (normalising, grouping subjects, smoothing, applying a linear model, establishing essentially random levels of significance, correcting for multiple comparison, etc.) has at times been claimed to be nonobvious, perhaps even faulty. Several researchers, who have used different ways, programs, or methods of analysis, recount how getting their results through the review process has been complicated by a demand to compare their findings to the ones generated by the now widely established modes, models, and programs of analysis.

Such discussions are an important part of any science. In contrast to another highly competitive arena, sports, a major part of the work in scientific fields is not about playing by the rules, but about defining, developing, and maintaining those rules governing the scientific process. This question is particularly pertinent in a novel, highly complicated field like brain imaging where "facts" are established as a result of a very complicated analytical process. A "proper" analysis therefore involves a set of choices. They are sometimes made deliberately; sometimes they are automatically and almost "unconsciously" taken by the established methods and standard software programmes. Issues like the following have important implications for which facts one allows the scanners to produce:

- Although mathematically elegant, is it reasonable to stretch and turn brain representations as if they were homogeneously made of a flexible material?
- Should multisubject experiments be described according to a fixed-effects model, where the statistical analysis acts as if all scans came from one standardised brain without taking the different individuals into account? Should a random-effects model, where effects within each subject are taken into account, be preferred? Is the choice between the two really a matter of "generalising to the population at large" and is it a sound practice to generalise the findings when the experimental subjects are usually recruited from a narrow subset?
- The standard analytical and experimental framework, built on contrasting conditions and comparisons across subjects, is particularly well tailored to identifying "blobs," that is, areas of discrete, significant activity. However, how does this square with the often-held claim that connectivity is the key to the complexities of the brain? Is it like seeing the tip of the iceberg where lowering the statistical threshold is like increasing the salinity of the water? New configurations and connections may suddenly show up until there is nothing but ice in sight.
- Although the statistical arguments for multiple comparison correction are convincing, is it

acceptable to allow for other significance criteria in areas where activation has been suggested by an *a priori* hypothesis? Would that require establishing a central committee where one should send one's predictions in a sealed envelope before the experiment is carried out?
- Given that findings are intrinsically woven into the very experimental and analytical process, should one establish large databases of raw data that should ideally, like everything else raw, be free of style and therefore open for any treatment, cooking, and analysis? Is it possible to talk of "raw data" when the problems and merits of style enter even before the scanner is used in, for instance, the selection of a research question and in the design of the experiment?
- Can one treat mental properties as if they were clearly defined objects that can be compared by subtraction?
- Does it make any sense to talk of baseline scans, when everybody who has been inside a scanner knows that the actual experience of being there is particular and highly individual?

These and similar issues are currently being discussed in the brain imaging field. As each of them finds an answer, be that pragmatic, technological, or theoretical, the styles of brain imaging continuously change, if only so slightly, and new lines will be added to the long informal script of do's and don'ts that any aspiring brain imager is initiated into during training and acculturation in the field. In that process, an increasingly dense pattern of brain imaging facts will be spun, metaphorically speaking, in ways that remind us of the way neurons build brains: They use as scaffolding those facts and connections already established, and they become attracted to a particular trajectory by the current thought style which, like a neuronal growth factor, seductively calls out: "Look for new connections in this direction!"

NEUROSCIENCE AS A MODEL SCIENCE FOR THE 21ST CENTURY?

As with neurons growing in brains, the resulting network of facts is a highly particular one. It is neither arbitrary nor general, but at any particular moment an actualisation of a historical process that represents a dynamic equilibrium between the unfolding of internal logic and outside influence: an inside and an outside that are both being continuously modified as the network develops. The links between brains and knowledge, facts and neurons, styles and growth factors are, of course, metaphorical, but the structural and semantic similarities, which render the metaphor possible, suggest that the conceptual problems with which one is currently struggling in neuroscience share affinities with problems found in other areas.

Transfer of models between scientific traditions does not happen simply because explanations and rules from one field are directly applicable to other fields.[4] It seems, rather, that one field may become paradigmatic because central conceptual problems, shared by many different contemporary thought collectives working in very different styles, are highlighted, purified, and scrutinised more than in most other fields. This was the case with questions of observability, causality, complementarity, and relativity in physics in the beginning of the 20th century. These concepts were debated in most other scientific traditions during the century we have just left, a century where physics was the unachievable gold standard for most other scientific enterprises.

At present, questions of networks, connectivity, agency, and emergence appear to be on the agenda over a wide range of disciplines spanning the traditional borderlines between science and humanities. Arguably, these concepts are absolutely central in the neurosciences in general and in brain imaging in particular to the extent that they constantly feature as variables in models and experiments. This development could make neuroscience one of the paradigmatic sciences for the 21st century, and it is likely that models and concepts developed in this field will be applied and used, somewhat metaphorically, across a wide range of fields of inquiry.

If Fleck, Latour, Knorr-Cetina, and other sociologists and anthropologists of science are right in their analyses, then the shape and direction in the development of an actual body of knowledge is not only determined by the technological possibilities; the tangible style also plays a major part. With it come questions about the appropriate, the elegant, the laudable, the tardy, the primitive, and the vulgar.

---

[4] The famous hoax in the so-called Sokal scandal played on this by demonstrating the ridicule of naively importing concepts from one field to another (Sokal, 1996).

Because the explicit criteria of truth are mainly probed, tested, and developed within a particular group, within a particular style, they are in practice relatively inaccessible to outsiders. Outsiders have no way of validating whether, for instance, in a given article, the right hemodynamic response function has been used to fit the data or whether the right pulse sequence and gradient manipulations were used in the MRI scanner. To a large extent, an outsider to a scientific field has to trust, first, that things are done properly and, second, that there are internal mechanisms for checking and validating whether this was indeed the case. Settling the truth and finding the facts is, in other words, an internal process. However, the question of style seems much more easily picked up by outsiders, just as a visitor to a foreign country may immediately perceive peculiarities in ways of dressing and behaving that to the local have become second nature and invisible. Two issues are a stake when different styles meet. The first concerns the effects when "facts" move outside their original context and into wider circulation as currently happens to brain maps. The second question is what happens when separate scientific traditions—different thought collectives and styles—begin to share a common research field as has happened with "the scientific study of consciousness."

FACTS IN CIRCULATION

Every first-year student in a brain mapping lab has learned to be very sceptical about these beautiful brain images. He is taught to see them as carefully selected representations of the outcome of complicated experiments. They are not photograph-like snapshots but ideograms or cartoons illustrating an idea or a principle. This is, however, rarely the way the pictures are received and used outside the brain imaging world where colourful pictures of activated brains are widely disseminated in magazines, newspapers, and TV programmes.

This process of communicating knowledge "which can by no means be compared with a simple translocation of a rigid body in Euclidean Space" (Fleck, 1979, p. 110) follows principles very different from the ones that established the facts in the first place. It is as if the pictures are stripped of their usual interpretations once they enter the world of catchy stories and popular science. They are no longer read as conventional representations that result from a long series of choices and transformations. Instead, they seem to take on an iconic quality of apparently stable categories like "a male brain," "a female brain," "a schizophrenic brain," "a depressed brain," or "a malingering brain." It is as if the complex colour coding of selected statistical parameters is suddenly taken to be an inherent property of indifferent and stable categories.

This issue becomes increasingly important once brain imaging leaves the confines of intellectual discourse to be implemented in various practices. What happens when the statistical maps are suddenly used to categorise individuals? Are the facts and categories underlying the colourful pictures so stable that they may and should enter the courtroom as evidence for or against a particular case (Dumit, 1999)? Can facts from neuroscience be generalised to such an extent that they may enter into teaching to form a neuropedagogical basis for the upbringing of future generations? Is it meaningful to use individual functional maps for diagnosis and prognosis (Beaulieu, 2000)? Should one rather complicate the story by asking for more research into basic questions and mechanisms before the facts are allowed to be circulated and implemented in three of the most important human institutions: the court, the school, and the hospital?

Many brain mappers appear to take a slightly ambivalent position on these matters. It is as if they evaluate the benefits of publicity on the one hand and the drawbacks of simplification on the other. The potential gain of fame is large in a market where many different agents fight over research money. So are the perils of losing that trust in the esoteric knowledge, which is the final rationale not only for funding, but for the very legitimacy of the scientific endeavour.

SCIENTIFIC TABOOS AND A FEW WORDS ABOUT CONSCIOUSNESS

For those readers who are dismayed not to have found one sentence in this final chapter containing the word consciousness, here it is!
(Final sentence in Human Brain Function, 1st ed.)

It is well known that mentioning particular words, whether names, nouns, verbs, or concepts, may become inappropriate within certain societies or subgroups. The phenomenon has been described from the tropics to the Arctic, and in the linguistic literature such concepts or names have become known as tabu words (Hjelmslev, 1970). This terminology can be traced to the explorer James Cook, who during his travels noted that derivatives of the word *tapu* were used throughout Polynesia to designate something or someone set apart or consecrated for a special purpose (Holden, 2000). Over the years, anthropologists struggled with the meaning of the term, and it was increasingly used as a noun to mean something forbidden, prohibited, sacred, or devoted (Steiner, 1956).

The cognitive psychologist and historian of psychology Bernard Baars has recently suggested that the role of consciousness in 20th-century scientific thought can be likened to a taboo. He has documented that many researchers in mainstream psychology, psychiatry, and philosophy felt it impossible to use the C-word in a scientific article. To secure positions and get results published, self-censorship was quite common. Certainly, the quote opening this section suggests that a number of linguistic strategies, such as euphemisms and mentioning the word without really mentioning it at all, have been used in scientific works when trying to circumscribe the C-word.

The main thrust in Baars' argument is that the scientific taboo on consciousness has to be seen in relation to a parallel focus on consciousness within other intellectual traditions in the 20th century such as literature and arts. This is demonstrated in an autobiographical sketch of B. F. Skinner, who apparently—before he became a behaviourist—aspired to be a stream-of-consciousness writer. He continued to live out a dissociation between the taboo and the thing in his personal writings (Baars, 2002). This narrative falls nicely in line with recent anthropological thinking about taboos. It has been argued that the proper translation of the Polynesian word *tapu* is neither "sacred" nor "forbidden" but rather "off limits" (Keesing, 1985). Something is *tapu,* off limits, only if some agent defines it as such, only given a certain perspective and always to someone. It cannot be *tapu* in and of itself. Being *tapu* implies a context. "A place, act or thing that is *tapu* this afternoon from the perspective of some people and in the context of a particular ritual or circumstance may be *noa* [within limits; A. R.] or *tapu* for different people tomorrow" (Keesing, 1985, p. 205).

The recent upsurge of interest in tying questions of consciousness to a neuronal correlate indicates that the context for the "taboo on consciousness" may already have changed. Brain imaging seems to have played a major role. The classic objection against introspective evidence and conscious processes was that such phenomena could not be measured. They were therefore inherently "subjective" and bound to the individual. That rendered them "off limits" for an objective scientific description that, according to some of the defining agents, should aim at an epistemology "without a knowing subject" (Popper, 1972) representing reality in "a view from nowhere" (Nagel, 1986).

Brain imaging may indeed have assisted in changing this context. First, a whole range of experiments now demonstrate that mentally performing a task, such as imagery, preparing for motion, or problem solving, appears to activate very much the same areas as doing the activity "in the outside world." This lends respectability to notions like introspection and imagery, which much of psychology has deemed subjective (Baars, 2003). At the same time, brain imaging allows for a set of experiments where stimulus and response are identical, while what changes is the attitude, stance, or interpretive frame that the person takes toward the stimuli (Gallagher *et al.,* 2002). These experimental paradigms, which give perfectly objective findings, can only be understood with reference to conscious states that may often best be probed via apparently "subjective" reports (Jack and Roepstorff, 2002).

What will happen when experimental psychology that has been "characterised by lingering nervousness when it came to anything touching on consciousness" (McCrone, 1999, p. 20) is suddenly challenged by apparently paradigmatic scientific methods, which address issues such as consciousness and subjectivity, which were hitherto "off limits"?

To an anthropologist of knowledge, this represents a highly interesting meeting of thought styles, and one may envision a number of different scenarios. The first is an imperialist takeover, in which one style simply eradicates the other. The second possibility is a constant conflict, which creates a conceptual "Berlin Wall," in which one set of rules apply on one side and another set of rules on the other side of an arbitrary borderline, the position of which is determined by the history and the present force of the combatants. A third alternative is a melange, like a Creole language or the English kitchen, where elements from various styles fuse in a characteristic manner. If everything else fails in the present attempt to "solve the question of consciousness scientifically," it will at least produce interesting case material for historians and philosophers of thought to come.

INTERACTING MINDS AS THE "DEFAULT ASSUMPTION"

One of the sharp borderlines in the study of consciousness has been drawn between two different perspectives on knowledge: the objective, third -erson perspective of the scientific enterprise, and the first-person, subjective perspective of an experiencing subject. Overcoming this schism became known as "the hard problem" in consciousness studies in the 1990s (Chalmers, 1996). Philosophers routinely call on versions of this hard problem when they deny that brain mapping can add any novel knowledge on consciousness, "since it will never be able to get at the experience of the redness of a rose." Conversely, there is within brain mapping strong resistance to anything that smacks of subjectivity. Indeed, the processes of brain imaging may be described as a transformation of subjects into objectivity while completely bypassing questions of subjectivity (Roepstorff, 2002).

There is, however, a phenomenon that appears to resist being placed on either side of the hard question's Berlin wall, and yet it is almost mandatory for how experimental paradigms are established in the first place (Roepstorff, 2001a). Most cognitive brain mapping experiments are designed such that a person only needs a few instructions[5] in order to respond in a highly specific way to a stimulus. Ideally, these instructions limit and direct the exact "role" that the subject is going to perform while in the scanner. By an extension of this theatre metaphor, they provide the script that the subject enacts. However, as everybody who has been an experimental subject knows, the instructions do not always achieve what is wanted. A subject may fail to understand or deliberately choose to enact a different script from that intended (Jack and Roepstorff, 2002; Roepstorff, 2001a).

How is one to understand this process? Is the script a subject or an object? Is the effect subjective or objective? Should it be understood from a first-person or a third-person perspective? Linguistically, we are used to thinking of three categories of persons. The first-person experiencing *I,* the third-person objectified *he, she,* or *it,* and the second-person interacting *you.* The actual process of getting people into the scanner and convincing them to respond to strange stimuli seems impossible to understand without a deliberate interaction of persons requiring a second-person perspective. This exchange between two concrete persons, the subject and the experimenter, is a necessary prerequisite for setting up the paradigm that allows both for the generation of the objective facts and the generation of the subjective experience. This element of interacting minds, which are "second persons" relative to each other, is hardly discussed within cognitive brain mapping (but see Frith and Frith, 1999). It also seems to fall outside the philosopher's hard question. However, it appears to be a necessary prerequisite for setting up most brain mapping experiments.

For the anthropologist visiting a brain imaging laboratory, the interacting minds around him present the very first problem. He is surrounded in the field by subjects and informants, who constantly exchange points of views, frames of minds, interpretive stances, and real and virtual objects. Most of the fieldwork is about learning how to enter slowly and usually somewhat incompetently into a few of these interactions. Interacting people is therefore the default assumption and even questions of "why people have culture and history" seem to hinge on this ability (Premack and Premack, 1994). It appears, therefore, very exotic that his subjects, the brain mappers, are not concerned about this fact, which is so obvious in his thought style. And again the brain mappers may answer as follows:

[5] This is a very important difference between cognitive experiments with humans and animals seen, for instance, in a recent attempt at scanning monkeys and people performing "the same experiment." The monkeys had to be trained for months to perform a simplified Wisconsin Card Sorting task, while the human subjects were simply told what to do (Nakahara *et al.*, 2002; Roepstorff and Frith, 2003).

What you take to be a point of criticism will for us be a starting point for an examination, if we see a reliable difference somewhere in the brain, you are probably on to something, if not....

As pointed out by Chris Frith, it is indeed easily conceivable to turn this objection of the outsider into a research question. The proposal is apparently simple: On the inside of brains, "consciousness" presents itself as a problem of squeezing the massively parallel and largely unconscious processes of the brain into a relatively small global workspace (Baars, 1988). On the outside of brains, communication presents itself as a problem to the hard question because interacting people almost automatically exchange and share mental representations and perhaps even synchronised brain states (Roepstorff, 2001a). But perhaps one of the characteristics of human consciousness is that it may be shared, both within the brain—between different brain modules—and between brains—between different people. This suggestion seems to propose a redefinition of the question of consciousness. Perhaps we should now conceive of—and study—it as an inherent property of interacting persons rather than as an intangible characteristic of an abstract, isolated brain (Roepstorff, 2003; Roepstorff and Frith, 2003).

CONNECTING INSIDES AND OUTSIDES?

Accepting interacting minds as a default assumption in cognitive brain mapping appears to make problematic an absolute opposition between the "inside" and "outside" of a brain. Instead, it seems to propose a shift in attention from absolute entities to the links and relations that connect the elements of an almost metaphysical dichotomy.

This postscript has attempted to draft contours of the field of brain mapping from the perspective of an anthropological outsider. The description appears to suggest that even in a scientific field it is very difficult to uphold an absolute opposition between "the inside" and "the outside" (Roepstorff, 2001c). In the context of the book you are currently reading, this postscript itself defies a rigid identification as either "in" or "out," caught as it is somewhere between an attempt to introduce a reflexive voice into the discourse and "going native."

The parallel between very different "insides" and "outsides" is, of course, a literary construct. However, this does not necessarily render it arbitrary. It seems to characterise many anthropological and sociological studies of the sciences that they may start out with clear-cut entities like "nature and culture" or "brain and mind" but end up by identifying links that are simultaneously "real, like nature, narrated, like discourse, and collective like society" (Latour, 1993, p. 6).

The field of brain imaging appears at present to be in a very interesting state. On one hand, its draws on a well-established canon of scientific methodologies to lend credibility to its results, and it applies these to novel fields in ways that may at times appear imperialistic. This may lead to easy accusations of "biological reductionism," but this seems to miss the point. Arguably, the main impact of the colourful maps and of the underlying "facts" may be productive rather than reductive (Beaulieu, 2003). Not only are novel links established between the mind and the brain, they may also serve to connect scientific practice with everyday life in ways that are still very unclear. Brain imaging seems thereby to place itself right in the middle of a metaphysical mess where facts are simultaneously "real, like nature, narrated, like discourse, and collective like society."

In that sense, brain imaging is an ideal contemporary exemplar of processes that have been around for as long as that peculiar modern institution called *science.* At least since Boyle and Hobbes almost 350 years ago fought over the interpretation of the most high-tech scientific results of their time—the experiments with the air pump—events taking place in laboratories using the most sophisticated technologies available have had major conceptual and practical consequences outside the laboratory (Shapin and Shaffer, 1985). However, the willingness of many brain mappers to invite anthropologists, sociologists, philosophers, and other "outsiders" into their laboratories, their research process, and their textbooks seems to be a novelty, which may indeed be exemplary for what science could look like in the 21st century. It will be interesting to see who the members of the thought collectives will be, which judgements they will consider obvious, what methods they will apply as a means of acquiring knowledge, and which technical and literary style they will be arguing in over the years to come.

References

Baars, B. J. (1988). *A Cognitive Theory of Consciousness.* Cambridge University Press, Cambridge, UK.

Baars, B. J. (2002). The double life of B. F. Skinner. Inner conflict, dissociation and the scientific taboo against consciousness. *J. Consciousness Studies*, **10**(1), 5–25.

Baars, B. J. (2003). When brain proves mind. In Trusting the Subject, special issue of *J. Consciousness Studies* (in press).

Barth, F. (2002). An anthropology of knowledge. *Curr. Anthropol.* **43,** 1–18.

Beaulieu, A. (2000). The brain at the end of the rainbow: brain scans and diagnostic promises. In *Wild Science,* Sawchuk, K., and Marchessault, J. (Eds.), pp. 39–52. Routledge, London.

Beaulieu, A. (2002). A space for measuring mind and brain: interdisciplinarity and digital tools in the development of brain mapping and functional mapping, 1980–1990. *Brain Cog.* **49**(1), 13–33.

Beaulieu, A. (2003). Brains, maps and the new territory of psychology. *Theory Psychol.*, **13**(4), 561–568.

Bourdieu, P. (1975). The specificity of the scientific and the social conditions of the progress of reason. *Social Sci. Info.* **14,** 19–47.

Bourdieu, P. (1977). *Outline of a Theory of Practice* (R. Nice, Trans.). Cambridge University Press, Cambridge, UK.

Chalmers, D. J. (1996). *The Conscious Mind. In Search of a Fundamental Theory.* Oxford University Press, Oxford, UK.

Deacon, T. W. (1997). *The Symbolic Species. The Co-Evolution of Language and Brain.* W. W. Norton, New York.

Dumit, J. (1999). Objective brains, prejudicial images. *Sci. Context* **12,** 173–201.

Fleck, L. (1979). *Genesis and Development of a Scientific Fact.* University of Chicago Press, Chicago.

Fleck, L. (1980/1935). *Die Entstehung und Entwicklung einer Wissenschaftlichen Tatsache.* Suhrkamp, Frankfurt am Main.

Frith, C. D., and Frith, U. (1999). Interacting minds—a biological basis. *Science* **286,** 1692–1695.

Gallagher, H., Jack, A. I., Roepstorff, A., and Frith, C. D. (2002). Imagining the intentional stance. *NeuroImage*, **16,** 814–821.

Globus, G. G. (1995). *The Postmodern Brain.* John Benjamins Publishing Company, Amsterdam/Philadelphia.

Hacking, I. (1999). *The Social Construction of What?* Harvard University Press, Cambridge, MA.

Hjelmslev, L. (1970). *Language, An Introduction.* University of Michigan Press, Ann Arbor.

Holden, L. (2000). *Encyclopaedia of Taboos.* ABC-CLIO, Oxford.

Jack, A. I., and Roepstorff, A. (2002). Introspection and cognitive brain mapping: from stimulus-response to script-report. *Trends Cog. Sci.* **6,** 333–339.

Keesing, R. M. (1985). Conventional metaphors and anthropological metaphysics. The problematic of cultural translation. *J. Anthropol. Res.* **41,** 201–217.

Keller, E. F. (1996). The biological gaze. In *FutureNatural. Nature, Science, Culture,* Robertson, G., Mash, M., Tickner, L., Bird, J., Curtis, B., and Putnam, T. (Eds.), pp. 108–121. Routledge, London.

Knorr-Cetina, K. (1981). *The Manufacture of Knowledge: An Essay on the Constructivist and Contextual Nature of Science.* Pergamon Press, New York.

Knorr-Cetina, K. (1999). *Epistemic Cultures: How the Sciences Make Knowledge.* Harvard University Press, Cambridge, MA.

Kuper, A. (1999). *Culture: The Anthropologists' Account.* Harvard University Press, Cambridge, MA.

Latour, B. (1993). *We Have Never Been Modern.* Harvester Wheatsheaf, New York.

Latour, B. (1999). *Pandora's Hope: Essays on the Reality of Science Studies.* Harvard University Press, Cambridge, MA.

Latour, B., and Woolgar, S. (1979). *Laboratory Life: The Social Construction of Scientific Facts.* Sage, Beverly Hills, CA.

McCrone, J. (1999). *Going Inside: Tour Round a Single Moment of Consciousness.* Faber and Faber, London.

Nader, L. (Ed.) (1996). *Naked Science. Anthropological Inquiry into Boundaries, Power and Knowledge.* Routledge, New York.

Nagel, T. (1986). *The View from Nowhere.* Oxford University Press, Oxford, UK.

Nakahara, K., Hayashi, T., Konishi, S., and Miyashita, Y. (2002). Functional MRI of macaque monkeys performing a cognitive set-shifting task. *Science* **295,** 1532–1536.

Nielsen, F. A. (2001). Author co-citation analysis of articles from *NeuroImage. NeuroImage* **13,** 210.

Otto, T., and Pedersen, P. (2000). Tradition between continuity and invention: An introduction. *FOLK, J. Danish Ethnographic Soc.* **42,** 3–17.

Pickering, A. (Ed.). (1992). *Science as Practice and Culture.* Chicago University Press, Chicago.

Popper, K. R. (1972). *Objective Knowledge: An Evolutionary Approach.* Oxford University Press, Oxford, UK.

Premack, D., and Premack, A. J. (1994). Why animals have neither culture nor history. In *Companion Encyclopaedia of Anthropology. Humanity, Culture and Social Life*, Ingold, T. (Ed.), pp. 350–365. Routledge, London.

Roepstorff, A. (2001a). Brains in scanners: an umwelt of cognitive neuroscience. *Semiotica* **134,** 747–765.

Roepstorff, A. (2001b). Facts, styles and traditions. Studies in the ethnography of knowledge. Ph.D. dissertation, Aarhus sity, Department of Social Anthropology.

Roepstorff, A. (2001c). Insiders and outsiders unite! Science and science studies in/of the 21st century. In *Science Under Pressure,* Vol. 2001/1, Siune, K. (Ed.), pp. 107–122, The Danish Institute for Studies in Research and Research Policy, Aarhus, Denmark.

Roepstorff, A. (2002). Transforming subjects into objectivity. An ethnography of knowledge in a brain imaging laboratory. *FOLK, J. Danish Ethnographic Soc.* **44,** 145–170.

Roepstorff, A. (2003). A double dissociation in twentieth century psychology? *J. Consciousness Studies* **10**(1), 62–67.

Roepstorff, A., and Frith, C. (2003). What's at the top in the top-down control of action?—Script-sharing and "top-top" control of action in cognitive experiments. *Psychol. Res.* (in press).

Shapin, S., and Shaffer, S. (1985). *Leviathan and the Air-Pump: Hobbes, Boyle and the Experimental Life.* Princeton University Press, Princeton, NJ.

Sokal, A. D. (1966). A physicist experiments with cultural studies. *Lingua Franca*, **6**(4), 62–64.

Steiner, F. (1956). *Taboo.* Cohen and West, London.

Varela, F. J. (1996). Neurophenomenology: a methodological remedy for the hard problem. *J. Consciousness Studies* **3,** 330–349.

Index

E

G

H

I

J

K

L

M

N

Q

R

S

T

W

X

Z